2
Ed
Tel: (780) 407-1843

ACUTE CARE SURGERY

Editors

L.D. Britt, MD, MPH, FACS, FCCM, FRCSEng (Hon), FRCSEd (Hon), FWACS (Hon), FRCSI (Hon)

Brickhouse Professor and Chairman
Department of Surgery
Eastern Virginia Medical School
Norfolk, Virginia

Andrew B. Peitzman, MD, FACS

Mark M. Ravitch Professor and Vice-Chair
Chief, Division of General Surgery
UPMC-Presbyterian
Pittsburgh, Pennsylvania

Philip S. Barie, MD, MBA, FIDSA, FCCM, FACS

Surgeon and Professor of Surgery
Department of Surgery
Weill Cornell Medical College
New York, New York

Gregory J. Jurkovich, MD, FACS

Chief of Surgery
Denver Health
Bruce M. Rockwell Distinguished Chair of Trauma
Professor and Vice-Chairman
University of Colorado School of Medicine
Denver, Colorado

New illustrations by BodyScientific International, LLC

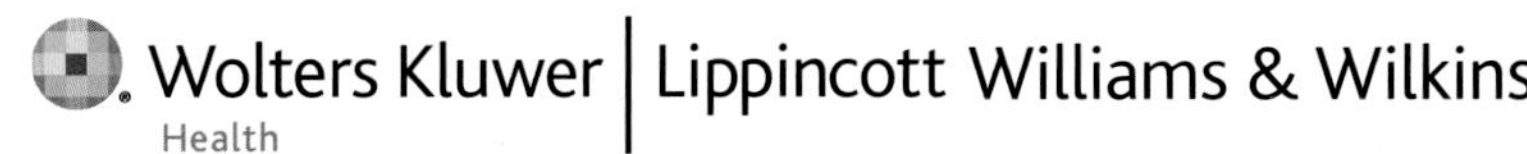

Philadelphia • Baltimore • New York • London
Buenos Aires • Hong Kong • Sydney • Tokyo

Acquisitions Editor: Brian Brown
Product Manager: Brendan Huffman
Production Manager: Alicia Jackson
Senior Manufacturing Manager: Benjamin Rivera
Marketing Manager: Lisa Lawrence
Design Coordinator: Holly McLaughlin
Production Service: SPi Global

Two Commerce Square
2001 Market Street
Philadelphia, PA 19103 USA
LWW.com

Printed in China

Library of Congress Cataloging-in-Publication Data
Acute care surgery / [edited by] L.D. Britt, Andrew B. Peitzman. — 1st ed.
p. ; cm.
Includes bibliographical references.
ISBN 978-1-60831-428-7 (hardback)
I. Britt, L. D. II. Peitzman, Andrew B.
[DNLM: 1. Emergency Treatment—methods. 2. Surgical Procedures, Operative—methods. 3. Wounds and Injuries—surgery. WO 700]
617.9—dc23

2011045998

To purchase additional copies of this book, call our customer service department at (800) 638-3030 or fax orders to (301) 223-2320. International customers should call (301) 223-2300.

Visit Lippincott Williams & Wilkins on the Internet: at LWW.com. Lippincott Williams & Wilkins customer service representatives are available from 8:30 am to 6 pm, EST.

10 9 8 7 6 5 4 3 2 1

RRS1203

CONTENTS

PREFACE

We are firmly committed to the tridisciplinary specialty—acute care surgery, which encompasses trauma, critical care, and emergency general surgery. This comprehensive textbook represents innumerable hours of dedication and sacrifice by us and the editors of this new edition along with the many accomplished contributors, who are recognized leaders in their respective areas of interest. The full spectrum of acute care surgery is expertly addressed in the 64 chapters included in this book, with each chapter highlighting cutting-edge advances in the field and underscoring state-of-the-art management paradigms.

In an effort to create the most definitive reference on acute care surgery, we have emphasized an evidence-based approach for all content included. Also, notable controversies are discussed in detail often accompanied by data-driven resolution.

Perhaps the most pivotal point in the process was the working retreat that we had in a makeshift conference room where we essentially had a marathon and critically reviewed each chapter for accuracy, relevance, and style. This process continued on an almost weekly basis until a consensus of high-level satisfaction was achieved for each chapter. Without hesitation or trepidation, we are dedicating this book to all the authors, whose tireless efforts contributed to the success of *Acute Care Surgery*. In addition, we graciously thank our family and friends for allowing us to spend some of our "free time" diligently working on this important project.

Khalid M. Abbed, MD
Chief
Yale Spine Institute
Director
Minimally Invasive Spine Surgery
Director
Oncologic Spine Surgery
New Haven, Connecticut

Herand Abcarian, MD
Professor
Department of Surgery
University of Illinois-Chicago
Chairman
Division of Colon and Rectal Surgery
Department of Surgery
John Stroger Hospital of Cook County
Chicago, Illinois

Sadaf S. Ahanchi, MD
Vascular Surgery Fellow
Department of Surgery
Eastern Virginia Medical School
Norfolk, Virginia

Babatunde H. Alamaroof, MD
Vascular Surgery Fellow
Department of Surgery
Eastern Virginia Medical School
Norfolk, Virginia

Louis H. Alarcon, MD
Associate Professor
Department of Surgery and Critical Care Medicine
Medical Director, Trauma Surgery
University of Pittsburgh School of Medicine
Pittsburgh, Pennsylvania

Juan Asensio, MD
Professor Surgery
Department of Surgery
University of Miami Miller School of Medicine
Director
Trauma Clinical Research, Training and Community Affairs
Department of Surgery
University of Miami Miller School of Medicine
Miami, Florida

Philip S. Barie, MD, MBA
Surgeon and Professor of Surgery
Department of Surgery
Weill Cornell Medical College
New York, New York

Graciela Bauza, MD
Assistant Professor
Department of Surgery
University of Pittsburgh Medical Center
Pittsburgh, Pennsylvania

Greg J. Beilman, MD
Professor and Vice Chair
Department of Surgery
University of Minnesota
Minneapolis, Minnesota

Timothy R. Billiar, MD
George Vance Foster Professor and Chair
Department of Surgery
University of Pittsburgh
Pittsburgh, Pennsylvania

Deanna Blisard, MD
Assistant Professor
Department of Critical Care Medicine
University of Pittsburgh Medical Center
Assistant Professor
Department of Surgery
University of Pittsburgh Medical Center
Pittsburgh, Pennsylvania

Karen J. Brasel, MD, MPH
Professor
Department of Surgery
Medical College of Wisconsin
Milwaukee, Wisconsin

L.D. Britt, MD, MPH
Brickhouse Professor and Chairman
Department of Surgery
Eastern Virginia Medical School
Norfolk, Virginia

D. Patrick Bryant, MD
Assistant Professor
Department of Surgery
Penn State University School of Medicine
Attending Physician
Division of Trauma and Critical Care
Milton S Hershey Medical Center
Hershey, Pennsylvania

Timothy G. Buchman, PhD, MD
Director, Emory Center for Critical Care
Professor of Surgery and Anesthesiology
Emory University School of Medicine
Atlanta, Georgia

Eileen Bulger, MD
Professor
Department of Surgery
University of Washington
Harborview Medical Center
Seattle, Washington

Matthew C. Byrnes, MD
Assistant Professor
Department of Surgery
University of Minnesota
Minneapolis, Minnesota
Trauma Surgeon
Department of Trauma
North Memorial Medical Center
Robbinsdale, Minnesota

Marc A. Camacho, MD, MS
Section Chief
Department of Emergency Radiology
Beth Israel Deaconess Medical Center
Instructor
Department of Radiology
Harvard Medical School
Boston, Maryland

Christopher J. Carlson, MD
Clinical Associate Professor
Division of Gastroenterology
University of Washington School of Medicine
Attending Physician
Harborview Medical Center
Seattle, Washington

Fitzgerald J. Casimir, MD
Instructor of Surgery
Division of Trauma and Surgical Critical Care
Vanderbilt University Medical Center
Nashville, Tennessee

Brian L. Chen, MD
Vascular Surgery Fellow
Department of Surgery
Eastern Virginia Medical School
Norfolk, Virginia

Walter K. Clair, MD, MPH
Assistant Professor
Department of Medicine
Vanderbilt University Medical Center
Medical Director
Department of Cardiac Electrophysiology
Vanderbilt Heart and Vascular Institute
Nashville, Tennessee

Raul Coimbra, MD, PhD
The Monroe E. Trout Professor of Surgery
Chief
Division of Trauma, Surgical Critical Care, and Burn
University of California San Diego
Executive Vice-Chairman
Department of Surgery
University of California San Diego
San Diego, California

Gustavo X. Cordero, MD
Orthopaedic Trauma Surgery Fellow
Department of Orthopaedic Surgery
University of Pittsburgh Medical Center
Pittsburgh, Pennsylvania

Edward E. Cornwell III, MD
LaSalle D. Leffall, Jr. Professor & Chairman of Surgery
Department of Surgery
Howard University College of Medicine
Washington, District of Columbia

Todd Costantini, MD
Clinical Fellow
Division of Trauma Surgical Critical Care, and Burns
University of California San Diego
San Diego, California

Francis L. Counselman, MD, CPE
Professor and Chairman
Department of Emergency Medicine
Eastern Virginia Medical School
Emergency Physicians of Tidewater
Norfolk, Virginia

Martin A. Croce, MD
Professor of Surgery
Chief, Trauma and Critical Care
Regional Medical Center at Memphis
University of Tennessee Health Science Center
Memphis, Tennessee

Giana Hystad Davidson, MD, MPH
Research Fellow
Department of Surgery
University of Washington
Harborview Medical Center
Seattle, Washington

Kimberly A. Davis, MD
Professor, Vice Chairman of Clinical Affairs
Department of Surgery
Yale University School of Medicine
Trauma Medical Director
Yale New Haven Hospital
New Haven, Connecticut

Jarrod D. Day, MD
Vascular Surgery Fellow
Department of Surgery
Eastern Virginia Medical School
Norfolk, Virginia

Michael E. de Vera, MD
Professor of Surgery
Chief of Transplant
Director, LLU Transplantation Institute
Loma Linda University
Loma Linda, California

Joseph DuBose, MD
Assistant Professor
Department of Surgery
University of Maryland Medical System, R Adams Cowley Shock Trauma Center
Director of Physician Education
Baltimore C-STARS
United States Air Force
Baltimore, Maryland

Soumitra R. Eachempati, MD
Professor of Surgery and Public Health
Departments of Surgery and Public Health
Weill Cornell Medical College
Director, Surgical ICU and Chief, Trauma Services
Department of Surgery
New York Weill Cornell Center
New York, New York

Bradley A. Erickson, MD
Assistant Professor
Department of Urology
University of Iowa College of Medicine
Iowa City, Iowa

Timothy C. Fabian, MD
Harwell Wilson Alumni Professor and Chairman
Department of Surgery
University of Tennessee Health Science Center
Memphis, Tennessee

David V. Feliciano, MD
Attending Surgeon
Atlanta Medical Center
Professor of Surgery
Mercer University School of Medicine
Atlanta, Georgia

Suzanne A. Fidler, MD, JD, CPHRM
Senior Director of Risk Management and Patient Safety
Department of Risk Management
Desert Regional Medical Center
Palm Springs, California

John Fildes, MD
Professor
Department of Surgery
University of Nevada School of Medicine
Medical Director & Chair
Department of Trauma
University Medical Center of Southern Nevada
Las Vegas, Nevada

Raquel Forsythe, MD
Assistant Professor
Department of Surgery and Critical Care Medicine
University of Pittsburgh Medical School
Pittsburgh, Pennsylvania

Heidi Frankel, MD
Professor of Surgery
Department of Surgery
University of Maryland Shock Trauma Center
Baltimore, Maryland

Richard L. Gamelli, MD
Robert J. Freeark Professor of Surgery
Loyola University Medical Center
Maywood, Illinois

Paul S. García, MD, PhD
Assistant Professor
Department of Anesthesiology
Emory University School of Medicine
Atlanta, Georgia
Staff Physician
Anesthesiology Department
Atlanta VA Medical Center
Decatur, Georgia

Mark Glazer, MD
Assistant Professor
Department of Medicine/Cardiovascular
Vanderbilt University Medical Center
Attending Physician
Division of Cardiology
Vanderbilt University Medical Center
Nashville, Tennessee

Amy J. Goldberg, MD
Professor of Surgery
Chief of Trauma/Surgical Critical care
Department of Surgery
Temple University School of Medicine
Philadelphia, Pennsylvania

Daniel Grabo, MD
Instuctor in Surgery
Division of Traumatology, Surgical Critical Care
and Emergency Surgery
Department of Surgery
University of Pennsylvania School of Medicine
Philadelphia, Pennsylvania

Gary S. Gruen MD
Professor
Department of Orthopaedic Surgery
University of Pittsburgh Scholl of Medicine
Attending Physician
University of Pittsburgh Medical Center
Pittsburgh, Pennsylvania

Carla Irene Haack, MD
Assistant Professor
Department of Surgery
Emory University School of Medicine
Atlanta, Georgia

Brian M. Hall, MD
Assistant Professor of Surgery
Department of Surgery
Stony Brook University School of Medicine
Stony Brook, New York

Elliott R. Haut, MD
Associate Professor
Departments of Surgery, Anesthesiology/Critical Care Medicine,
and Emergency Medicine
The Johns Hopkins University School of Medicine
Baltimore, Maryland

Sharon Henry MD
Anne Scalea
Professor of Trauma
University of Maryland School of Medicine
Baltimore, Maryland

F. Herrerias, MD
International Visiting Scholar/Research Fellow
Department of Surgery
Division of Trauma and Surgical Critical Care
University of Miami
Miami, Florida

Fernando Herrerías González, MD
Attending Physician
Department of General and Digestive Surgery
Hospital Universitari Arnau de Vilanova
Lleida, Spain

Amy N. Hildreth, MD
Assistant Professor
Department of Surgery
Wake Forest University School of Medicine
Winston-Salem, North Carolina

Vanessa P. Ho, MD, MH
Department of Surgery
Weill Cornell Medical College
New York, New York

Marcus K. Hoffman, MD
General Surgery Resident
Department of Surgery
University of Pittsburgh School of Medicine
Pittsburgh, Pennsylvania

W. Allen Hogge, MD, MA
Professor and Chair
Department of Obstetrics, Gynecology & Reproductive Science
University of Pittsburgh/Magee-Womens Hospital
Pittsburgh, Pennsylvania

David B. Hoyt, MD
Executive Director
American College of Surgeons
Chicago, Illinois

Jeremy M. Hsu, B.Pharm, MBBS
Clinical Lecturer
Department of Surgery
University of Sydney
Sydney, New South Wales, Australia
Consultant Surgeon
Department of Surgery
Westmead Hospital
Westmead, New South Wales, Australia

Steven Hughes, MD
Associate Professor and Chief
General Surgery, University of Florida
Gainesville, Florida

Maureen B. Huhmann, DCN, RD, CSO
Adjunct Assistant Professor
Department of Nutritional Sciences
University of Medicine and Dentistry of New Jersey
Newark, New Jersey

Rao R. Ivatury, MD
Professor
Department of Surgery
Virginia Commonwealth University
Chair
Division of Trauma, Critical Care and Emergency Surgery
Department of Surgery
VCU Medical Center
Richmond, Virginia

Uroghupatei P. Iyegha, MD
Surgery Resident
Department of Surgery
University of Minnesota
Minneapolis, Minnesota

Robert A. Izenberg, MD, CAPT MC USN
Assistant Professor of Surgery
Department of Surgery
F. Edward Hebert School of Medicine
Uniformed Services University of the Health Sciences
Bethesda, Maryland
Attending Surgeon
Department of Surgery
Naval Medical Center
San Diego, California

David G. Jacobs, MD
Professor
Department of Surgery
University of North Carolina School of Medicine
Chapel Hill, North Carolina
Associate Medical Director
F.H. "Sammy" Ross Trauma Institute
Carolinas Medical Center
Charlotte, North Carolina

Gregory J. Jurkovich, MD
Chief of Surgery
Denver Health
Bruce M. Rockwell Distinguished Chair of Trauma
Professor and Vice-Chairman
University of Colorado School of Medicine
Denver, Colorado

David M. Kashmer, MD, MBA
Section Chief
Trauma & Acute Care Surgery
Guthrie Health System
Center Valley, Pennsylvania

Leslie Kobayashi, MD
Assistant Clinical Professor of Surgery
Department of Surgery, Division of Trauma, Surgical Critical Care, and Burns
University of California San Diego
San Diego, California

Michael Krzyzaniak, MD
Research Fellow
Division of Trauma Surgical Critical Care, and Burns
University of California San Diego
San Diego, California

Daniel Lader, DDS
Attending Surgeon
Oral and Maxillofacial Surgery
St. Luke's Hospital and Health Network
Bethlehem, Pennsylvania

Anna M. Ledgerwood, MD
Professor
Department of Surgery
Wayne State University School of Medicine
Medical Director
Trauma Department
Detroit Receiving Hospital
Detroit, Michigan

Karen S. Lee, MD
Attending Radiologist
Department of Radiology
Beth Israel Deaconess Medical Center
Harvard Medical School
Boston, Massachusetts

Peter B. Letarte, MD
Chief of Neurological Surgery
Department of Surgery
Edward G. Hines Veterans Hospital
Hines, Illinois

Pamela A. Lipsett, MD, MHPE
Warfield M. Firor Professor of Surgery
Program Director, General Surgery and Surgical Critical Care
Co-Director of the Surgical Intensive Care Units
Johns Hopkins Hospital
Baltimore, Maryland

Frank Liu, MD
Assistant Professor
Department of Medicine
New York Presbyterian – Weill Cornell Center
Nephrologist
The Rogosin Institute
New York, New York

Lawrence Lottenberg, MD
Associate Professor of Surgery and Anesthesiology
Division of Acute Care Surgery
Department of Surgery
University of Florida College of Medicine
Gaiensville, Florida

Charles E. Lucas, MD
Professor
Department of Surgery
Wayne State University
Senior Attending
Department of Surgery
Detroit Receiving Hospital
Detroit, Michigan

Robert C. Mackersie, MD
Professor of Surgery
University of California, San Francisco
San Francisco General Hospital
San Francisco, California

Ronald V. Maier, MD
Jane and Donald D. Trunkey Professor and Vice-Chair
Surgery
University of Washington
Surgeon-in-Chief
Harborview Medical Center
Seattle, Washington

Kenneth L. Mattox, MD
Distinguished Service Professor
Department of Surgery
Baylor College of Medicine
Chief of Staff/Chief of Surgery
Ben Taub General Surgery
Houston, Texas

Addison K. May, MD
Professor
Department of Surgery and Anesthesiology
Vanderbilt University Medical Center
Nashville, Tennessee

F. Mazzini, MD
International Visiting Scholar/Research Fellow
Dewitt-Daughtry Family Department of Surgery
University of Miami
Miami, Florida
Attending Physician
Department of Surgery
Hospital Italiano de Buenos Aires
Buenos Aires, Argentina

Jack W. McAninch, MD
Professor
Department of Urology
University of California San Francisco
Chief of Urology
Department of Urology
San Francisco General Hospital
San Francisco, California

Shannon M. McCole, MD
Chairman and Residency Program Director
Assistant Professor
Department of Ophthalmology
Eastern Virginia Medical School
Norfolk, Virginia

Nathaniel McQuay Jr, MD
Assistant Professor of Surgery
Johns Hopkins University
Johns Hopkins Bayview Medical center
Baltimore, Maryland

Norman E. McSwain Jr, MD
Professor of Surgery, Tulane University
Medical Director, PreHosptial Trauma Life Support (PHTLS)
Trauma director, Spirit of Charity Trauma Center, ILH

J. Wayne Meredith, MD
Professor and Chair
Department of Surgery
Wake Forest University School of Medicine
Director
Division of Surgical Sciences
Wake Forest University School of Medicine
Winston-Salem, North Carolina

Frederick Moore, MD
Professor
Department of Surgery
Chief, Division of Acute Care Surgery
University of Florida
Gainesville, Florida

John A. Morris Jr, MD
Professor of Surgery and Biomedical Informatics
Department of Surgery
Vanderbilt University School of Medicine
Nashville, Tennessee

Michael L. Nance, MD
Professor
Department of Surgery
University of Pennsylvania School of Medicine
Director, Pediatric Trauma Program
Department of Surgery
The Children's Hospital of Philadelphia
Philadelphia, Pennsylvania

Lena M. Napolitano, MD
Professor of Surgery
Division Chief
Acute Care Surgery (Trauma, Burn, Critical Care, Emergency Surgery)
Director, Trauma and Surgical Critical Care
Associate Chair
Department of Surgery
University of Michigan
Ann Arbor, Michigan

Shawn Nessen, DO
Lieutenant Colonel, US Army Medical Corps
Deputy Commander Clinical Services
212th Combat Support Hospital
Miseau, Germany
Acute Care Surgeon
Division of Trauma and Critical Care
Landstuhl Regional Medical Center
Landstuhl, Germany

Jean Nickleach, MSIS, RD, CNSC
Inpatient Nutrition Coordinator
University of Pittsburgh Medical Center
Pittsburgh, Pennsylvania

Juan B. Ochoa, MD
Professor of Surgery and Critical Care
University of Pittsburgh
Pittsburgh, Philadelphia
Medical and Scientific Director
Nestle Health Care Nutrition
Nestle Health Science
North America

Grant E. O'Keefe, MD
Professor
Department of Surgery
University of Washington
Attending Surgeon
Department of Surgery
Harborview Medical Center
Seattle, Washington

Mickey M. Ott, MD
Assistant Professor of Surgery
Division of Trauma and Surgical Critical Care
Vanderbilt University Medical Center
Nashville, Tennessee

H. Leon Pachter, MD
The George David Stewart Professor & Chairman
Department of Surgery
New York University School of Medicine
New York, New York

Jean M. Panneton, MD
Professor of Surgery
Department of Surgery
Program Director and Chief
Division of Vascular Surgery
Eastern Virginia Medical School
Norfolk, Virginia

Michael D. Pasquale, MD
Chairman
Lehigh Valley Health Network
Professor of Surgery
University of South Florida College of Medicine
Allentown, Pennsylvania

Mayur B. Patel, MD
Instructor
Department of Surgery
Division of Trauma, Acute Care Surgery, & Surgical Critical Care
Vanderbilt University School of Medicine
Nashville, Tennessee

Abhijit S. Pathak, MD
Professor of Surgery
Department of Surgery
Temple University School of Medicine
Philadelphia, PA
Director, Surgical Intensive Care Unit
Temple University Hospital

Andrew B. Peitzman, MD
Mark M. Ravitch Professor and Vice-Chair
Chief, Division of General Surgery
UPMC-Presbyterian
Pittsburgh, Pennsylvania

Fredric M. Pieracci, MD, MPH
Staff Surgeon
Denver Health Medical Center
Assistant Professor of Surgery
Denver School of Medicine
University of Colorado
Denver, Colorado

Greta L. Piper, MD
Assistant Professor of Surgery
Yale School of Medicine
New Haven, Connecticut

Patricio Polanco, MD
General Surgery Resident
Department of Surgery
University of Pittsburgh
Pittsburgh, Pennsylvania

Basil A. Pruitt Jr, MD
Clinical Professor
Department of Surgery
University of Texas Health Science Center
San Antonio, Texas
Surgical Consultant
U. S. Army Institute of Surgical Research
Fort Sam Houston, Texas

Jennifer C. Roberts, MD
Resident
Department of Surgery
Medical College of Wisconsin
Milwaukee, Wisconsin

Aurelio Rodriguez, MD
Associate Director
Division of Trauma Surgery
Sinai Hospital
Baltimore, Maryland

Matthew R. Rosengart, MD, MPH
Associate Professor
Department of Surgery
University of Pittsburgh
Pittsburgh, Pennsylvania

Michael F. Rotondo, MD
Professor and Chairman
Department of Surgery
Brody School of Medicine
East Carolina University
Chief of Surgery
Vidant Medical Center
Greenville, North Carolina

Grace S. Rozycki, MD, MBA
Professor of Surgery
Emory University School of Medicine
Vice Chair for Academic Affairs
Director, Division of Trauma/SCC/Emergency General Surgery
Atlanta, Georgia

Edgardo S. Salcedo, MD
Instructor in Surgery
Division of Traumatology, Surgical Critical Care and Emergency Surgery
Department of Surgery
University of Pennsylvania School of Medicine
Philadelphia, Pennsylvania

Umut Sarpel, MD, MSc
Assistant Professor
Department of Surgery
New York University School of Medicine
New York, New York

Thomas M. Scalea, MD
Physician-in-Chief
R Adams Cowley Shock Trauma Center
Francis X Kelly Professor and Director
Program in Trauma
University of Maryland School of Medicine
Baltimore, Maryland

Matthew Schuchert, MD
Assistant Professor
Department of Cardiothoracic Surgery
University of Pittsburgh Medical Center
Pittsburgh, Pennsylvania

Vaishali Schuchert, MD
Assistant Professor
Department of Surgery
University of Pittsburgh School of Medicine
Assistant Professor
Department of Critical Care Medicine
University of Pittsburgh School of Medicine
Pittsburgh, Pennsylvania

C. William Schwab, MD
Professor of Surgery
Division of Traumatology, Surgical Critical Care & Emergency Surgery
Department of Surgery
University of Pennsylvania School of Medicine
Philadelphia, Pennsylvania

William R. Sexson, MD
Professor of Neonatology
Emory University School of Medicine
Professor, Emory Center for Ethics
Atlanta, Georgia

Marc J. Shapiro, MS, MD
Professor of Surgery and Anesthesiology
Department of Surgery
State University of New York-Stony Brook
Chief of General Surgery, Trauma, Critical Care Medicine and Burns
Department of Surgery
Stony Brook, New York

Peter A. Siska, MD
Assistant Professor
Department of Orthopaedic Surgery
University of Pittsburgh Medical Center
Pittsburgh, Pennsylvania

Ronald M. Stewart, MD
Jocelyn and Joe Straus Professor and Chairman
Department of Surgery
School of Medicine
University of Texas Health Science Center
San Antonio, Texas

David Streitman, MD
Assistant Professor
Department of Obstetrics, Gynecology & Reproductive Sciences
University of Pittsburgh School of Medicine/Magee-Womens Hospital
Pittsburgh, Pennsylvania

Ivan S. Tarkin, MD
Chief of Orthopaedic Trauma
Department of Orthopaedic Surgery
University of Pittsburgh Medical Center
Pittsburgh, Pennsylvania

Donald D. Trunkey, MD
Professor Emeritus
Department of Surgery
Oregon Health & Science University
Portland, Oregon

Leo L. Tsai, MD, PhD, MSc
Resident
Department of Radiology
Beth Israel Deaconess Medical Center
Boston, Massachusetts

Krista Turner, MD
Assistant Professor
Department of Surgery
The Methodist Hospital, Weill Cornell Medical College
Houston, Texas

Behroze A. Vachha, MD, PhD
Resident
Department of Radiology
Beth Israel Deaconess Medical Center, Harvard Medical School
Boston, Massachusetts

T. Vu, MD
Trauma Fellow
Department of Surgery
University of Miami School of Medicine
Miami, Florida

Brett H. Waibel, MD
Assistant Professor
Department of Surgery
Brody School of Medicine at East Carolina University
Greenville, North Carolina

Leonard J. Weireter Jr, MD
Arthur and Marie Kirk Family Professor of Surgery
Department of Surgery
Eastern Virginia Medical School
Norfolk, Virginia

Matthew Keith Whalin, MD, PhD
Resident Physician
Department of Anesthesiology
Emory University School of Medicine
Atlanta, Georgia

Robert D. Winfield, MD
Fellow, Trauma Surgery/Surgical Critical Care
Division of Trauma, Surgical Critical Care, and Burns
Department of Surgery
University of California—San Diego
San Diego, California

Brian Zuckerbraun, MD
Samuel P. Harbison Assistant Professor
Department of Surgery
University of Pittsburgh
Attending Physician
Department of Surgery
VA Pittsburgh Healthcare System
Pittsburgh, Pennsylvania

ACUTE CARE SURGERY: INTRODUCTION

Acute care surgery (ACS), an evolving tridisciplinary specialty, addresses the concern highlighted by Dr. William Steward Halsted when he stated that "...every important hospital should have on its resident staff of surgeons at least one who is well trained and able to deal with any emergency."[1] The evolution of ACS did not occur *de novo*. On the contrary, several forces created an optimal environment for its birth and development, including a precipitous decline in the surgical workforce that would be involved in the management of such emergencies, along with the well-documented short supply of specialty support in the acute care setting. A survey conducted by the American College of Emergency Physicians in 2005 showed that nearly three-quarters of emergency department medical directors believe they have inadequate on-call specialty coverage. In that same survey, orthopedic, plastic, and neurologic surgeons, as well as otolaryngologists and hand surgeons, were reported as being in short supply. A fact sheet entitled "The Future of Emergency Care," produced by the Institute of Medicine of the National Academies in 2006, corroborated these findings. Although some controversy still exists regarding scope of practice and the essential requirements for this specialty, ACS is a new and unique discipline. The label "acute care surgeon" has been erroneously applied to the "surgical hospitalists" and the "emergency general surgeons." However, the true definition of "acute care surgery" embodies three specialty components—trauma surgery, emergency general surgery, and surgical critical care (Figure 1).

As a result, the general principles of ACS are derived from these three specialties. The overarching principle, which transcends each of these three components, is early and expedient medical/surgical intervention. Whether managing a patient with perforated duodenal ulcer or enterotomies secondary to a gunshot wound to the abdomen, early diagnosis and expedient intervention make up the cornerstone of optimal management. There is no disharmony between the well-established tenets of trauma management and the general principles of ACS. While adhering to the basic priorities (airway, breathing, circulation, etc.) underscored in the primary survey is always prudent, such an emphasis needs to be tailored on a case-by-case basis in nontrauma surgical emergencies so that timely intervention is not delayed. For example, little attention has to be directed to the disability assessment, included in the primary survey, for a young patient who presents with a presumptive diagnosis of acute appendicitis and an obvious surgical abdomen. The same would be the case for many other nontrauma surgical emergencies. Because of the disparate disease entities and unique patient populations that can lead to surgical emergencies, it is unlikely and, perhaps, unnecessary that an all-encompassing management paradigm, such as Advanced Trauma Life Support (ATLS)[2], which is arguably the most accepted and successful practice guideline in American (and international) medicine—is actually needed. However, general principles of optimal management are, indeed, applicable even among special populations of patients with potential surgical emergencies. Such general principles are embedded in the thrust of surgical education that continually underscores the important role of surgical judgment and prioritization of patient management.

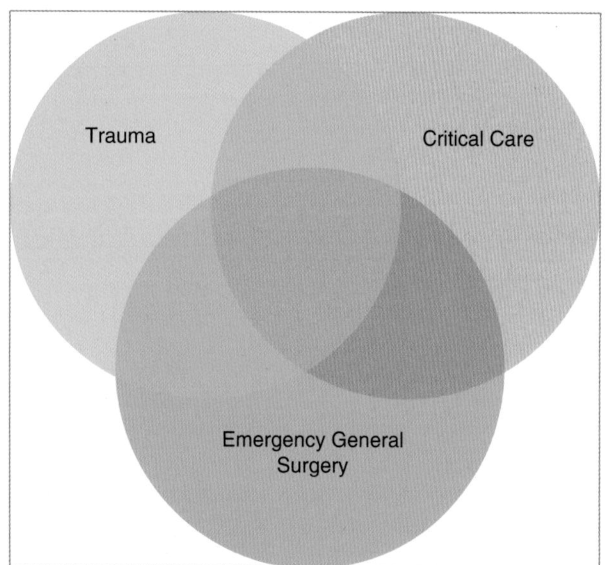

FIGURE 1. Acute care surgery: a tri-disciplinary specialty.

As articulated in a well-written commentary in a recent edition of the *New Yorker*, old age is the new demography.[3] The general principles of "acute care surgery" must adapt to this and other vulnerable populations. Between 2010 and 2050, there will be a substantial increase in the elderly population (Figure 2).[4] With the preexisting conditions, or comorbidities, increasing with age, the finding by Schloss[5] that the elderly require twice the time and effort of the general surgeon is even more relevant for the elderly patient in the acute care setting.

In addition, there are age-related physiologic changes that must be considered when managing the patients. Figure 3 represents a plausible treatment algorithm for this special population.

The accepted general principles of ACS management must be malleable enough that appropriate adjustments can be made for such age-related physiologic changes for this unique cohort of patients. Limited physiologic reserves should also be expected in the management of another vulnerable population—pediatric patients. For example, it is even more imperative to ensure environmental control (prevention of hypothermia) in management of the child in the acute care setting. Also, the health care provider team must be fully cognizant of the fact that hemodynamic instability is often a *late* finding in the pediatric patient population.

In addition to an aging population, each decade in the United States the population also increases by 25 million. With being an established trend toward specialization and a heavy emphasis on the elective practice, expert surgical management in the acute care setting needs to be both cultivated and fortified if optimal patient care is to be ensured for the injured and critically ill surgical patients. While a multifaceted approach will be needed to address this challenge, the establishment of the specialty, acute care surgery, is a major step in the right direction.

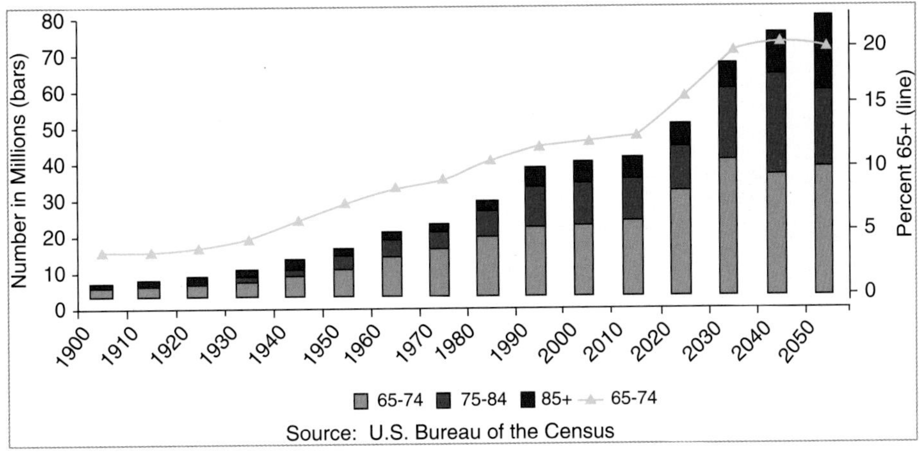

FIGURE 2. Growth of US population over age 65, 1900 to 2050, by age group.

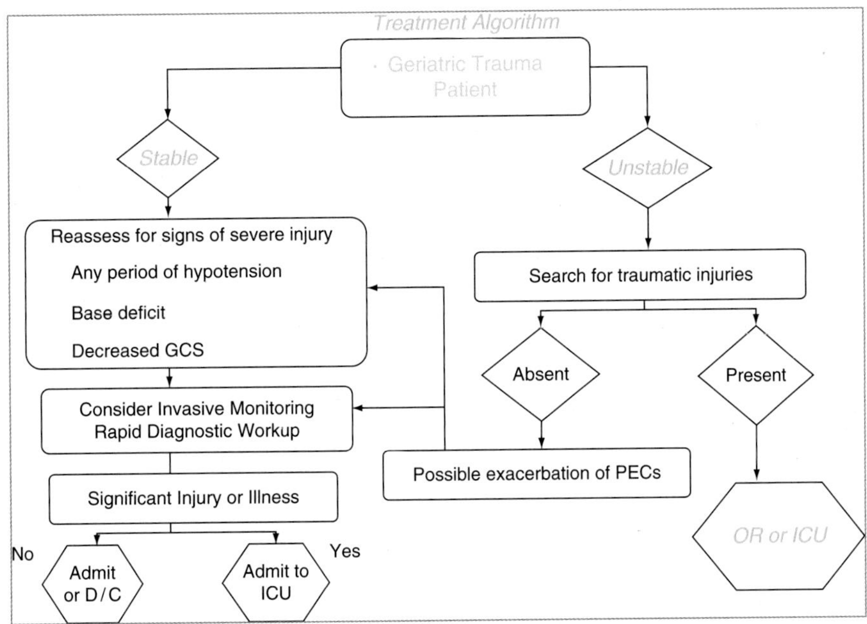

FIGURE 3. Geriatric trauma patient treatment algorithm.

References

1. Halsted WS. The training of the surgeon. *John Hopkins Hosp Bull.* 1904;15:267–275.
2. *American College of Surgeons Committee on Trauma: Advanced Trauma Life Support®*. 6th ed. Chicago, IL: American College of Surgeons; 1997.
3. Gawande A. (2007, April 30). The way we age now. Retrieved from http://www.newyorker.com/.
4. U.S. Bureau of Census, 2008.
5. Schloss EP. Beyond GMENAC—another physician shortage from 2010 to 2030? *N Engl J Med* 1988;318:920–922.

CHAPTER 1 ■ ACUTE CARE SURGERY: GENERAL PRINCIPLES

L.D. BRITT

ACUTE CARE SURGERY-GENERAL PRINCIPLES

Expedient assessment/intervention is the paramount axiom of acute care surgery management. This in no way undermines or devalues the merits of comprehensive assessments. On the contrary, prioritization of management—in an attempt to quickly address disease and injury that can rapidly result in severe morbidity and mortality—has always been the cornerstone of all aspects of medicine. Emergency operative intervention, precluding a comprehensive assessment and preoperative clearance, is indicated in some circumstances. In such case, the complete evaluation is done after stabilization of the patient. While the importance of preoperative clearance cannot be over emphasized, it often cannot (and should not) be implemented in the acute care setting for a risk benefit analysis of delaying surgical intervention would be unfavorable and detrimental to the health status of the patient. However, when appropriate, a systematic approach to preoperative clearance should be done.

The general principles of acute care surgery, in the nontrauma setting, must be applicable in the following areas of emergency general surgery and surgical critical care: (1) inflammation, (2) perforation, (3) obstruction, (4) bleeding, (5) ischemia, (6) necrosis, (7) hypoxia, and (8) infection.

CORE MANAGEMENT PRINCIPLES

In the nontrauma setting, the core management principles (the four Es) in acute care surgery are the following:

- Expeditious initial assessment
- End point–guided resuscitation
- Early intervention and definitive management (if possible)
- Essential physiologic monitoring

Expeditious Initial Assessment

Each of the presentations highlighted in Table 1.1 is time sensitive and, therefore, often necessitates a rapid, methodical, and accurate evaluation process. When applicable, this would entail obtaining a relevant history from the patient and possible family members or health providers caring for the patient. In addition, the patient should, initially, undergo a focused physical examination, which can be expanded to a full and complete exam, if emergency intervention does not preclude such an assessment. Integrated in the assessment and resuscitative phase should be the acquisition of the important laboratory values and any required imaging studies necessary to provide quality surgical care. Because of the broad spectrum of presentations in acute care surgery, there is some variability in the diagnostic/treatment paradigms although the core management principles remain the same. For example, the otherwise healthy young male patient who presents with relatively acute onset of right lower-quadrant pain (preceded by periumbilical pain), anorexia, and a fever is likely to have acute appendicitis. If physical exam confirms right lower-quadrant tenderness with localized peritoneal signs and no other remarkable abnormal findings, the patient should have ongoing resuscitation, antibiotics, and operative intervention for suspected acute appendicitis. While some physicians may advocate obtaining a CT scan, it is not essential in this setting. Also, if a patient presents toxic with diffuse peritonitis and has associated comorbidities suggestive of secondary peritonitis (e.g., perforated duodenal ulcer), he/she should be considered for surgery. Any patient with an acute surgical abdomen should not have intervention delayed by unnecessary imaging studies. However, the elderly patient, who has multiple comorbidities, presenting with an insidious onset of left lower-quadrant pain and tenderness elevated on abdominal palpation in this area will likely have diverticulitis. Radiologic imaging, specifically computed tomography (CT), would be essential in the diagnostic workup, disease classification, and management of this patient. A CT scan that demonstrates a contained pericolonic abscess secondary to a perforated inflamed diverticulum (Hinchey II classification) would dictate the need for CT scan–directed percutaneous drainage of the abscess and nonoperative management.

The importance of preoperative laboratory assessment cannot be overstated. Such an evaluation is needed to help determine if there are associated medical conditions that could adversely impact the postoperative course of a patient. However, in the acute care surgical setting, optimal preoperative evaluation, including imaging and laboratory studies, often cannot be accomplished (Algorithm. 1.1).

End Point–guided Resuscitation

Optimal resuscitation is imperative in the management of any patient in the acute care setting. It is a dynamic process that requires a continued assessment process to ensure that the targeted end points of resuscitation are achieved. The debate continues, however, over the optimal end points of resuscitation in trauma patients. Urine output, lactate levels, base deficit, gastric intramucosal pH, and direct determination of oxygen delivery and consumption are all proposed markers for end points of resuscitation. Irrespective of the end point chosen, the overarching goal in the resuscitation of patients is correction of inadequate organ perfusion and tissue oxygenation.

TABLE 1.1

BROAD SPECTRUM OF ACUTE CARE SURGERY (NONTRAUMA)—EMERGENCY GENERAL SURGERY AND SURGICAL CRITICAL CARE

INFLAMMATION	PERFORATION	OBSTRUCTION
e.g., appendicitis, diverticulitis, cholecystitis, cholangitis, pancreatitis, gastritis, gastric and duodenal ulcer disease	e.g., **hollow visceral rupture;** esophageal gastric duodenal small and large bowel appendiceal	e.g., **Airway** aspiration foreign body **Esophagus** stricture foreign body **Intestine** mechanical obstruction of small bowl or large bowel (adhesions, intussus-ception, volvolus) adynamic ileus **Biliary** bile duct obstruction (intra-and extra-luminal biliary pancreatitis
ACUTE BLEEDING	**ISCHEMIA**	**NECROSIS**
e.g., stress gastritis, esophageal and gastric variceal bleeding, gastric/duodenal ulcer disease, diverticulosis, hemorrhoidal bleeding, spontane-ous splenic/hepatic rupture, vascular aneurysmal rupture, iatrogenic	e.g., **mesenteric ischemia** non-occlussive embolic thrombotic **compartment syndrome** extremity abdominal thoracic	e.g., necrotizing fasciitis, gas gangrene, decubitus ulcers, and other open wounds
HYPOXEMIA	**INFECTION**	**MULTIPLE ORGAN FAILURE**
e.g., aspiration, pneumonia, acute lung injury, acute respiratory distress syndrome, pulmonary embolus	e.g., superficial and deep seated soft tissue abscesses, bacteremia, cath-eter sepsis, solid organ abscesses, suppurative cholangitis, septic shock	e.g., combined pulmonary, renal, and cardiovascular system failure (portends poor prognosis)

Inability to achieve adequate organ perfusion and tissue oxygenation can result in anaerobic metabolism with the development of acidosis and an associated oxygen debt. Scalea et al. reported that inadequate tissue perfusion can exist even when the conventional end points (e.g., blood pressure, heart rate, and urine output) of resuscitation are normal.[1]

Early Intervention and Definitive Management, If Possible

In the acute care setting, irrespective of the specific illness/injury encountered, early and often definitive intervention is the essential component of management. Specific treatment paradigms differ depending on the specific disease entity and its unique presentation (Algorithms. 1.2-1.6).

GENERAL PRINCIPLES—TRAUMA SETTING

Prior to focusing on the specific anatomical region where there is an obvious traumatic injury, an initial assessment of the entire patient is imperative.

The concept of initial assessment includes the following components: (1) rapid primary survey, (2) resuscitation, (3) detailed secondary survey (evaluation), and (4) reevaluation. Such an assessment is the cornerstone of the Advanced Trauma Life Support (ATLS) program. Integrated into primary and secondary surveys are specific adjuncts. Such adjuncts include the application of electrocardiographic monitoring and the utilization of other monitoring modalities such as arterial blood gas determination, pulse oximetry, the measurement of ventilatory rate and blood pressure, insertion of urinary or gastric catheters, and incorporation of necessary x-rays and other diagnostic studies, when applicable, such as focused abdominal sonography for trauma (FAST) exam, other diagnostic studies (plain radiography of the spine/chest/pelvis and CT), and diagnostic peritoneal lavage (DPL). Determination of the right diagnostic study depends on the mechanism of injury and the hemodynamic status of the patient.

The focus of the primary survey is to both identify and expeditiously address immediate life-threatening injuries. Only after the primary survey is completed (including the initiation of resuscitation) and hemodynamic stability is addressed should the secondary survey be conducted, which entails a head-to-toe (and back to front) physical examination, along with a more detailed history.

PRIMARY SURVEY

Only the emergency care disciplines of medicine have a two-tier approach to their initial assessment of the patient, with primary and secondary surveys as integral components. As highlighted above, the primary survey is designed to quickly detect life-threatening injuries. Therefore, a

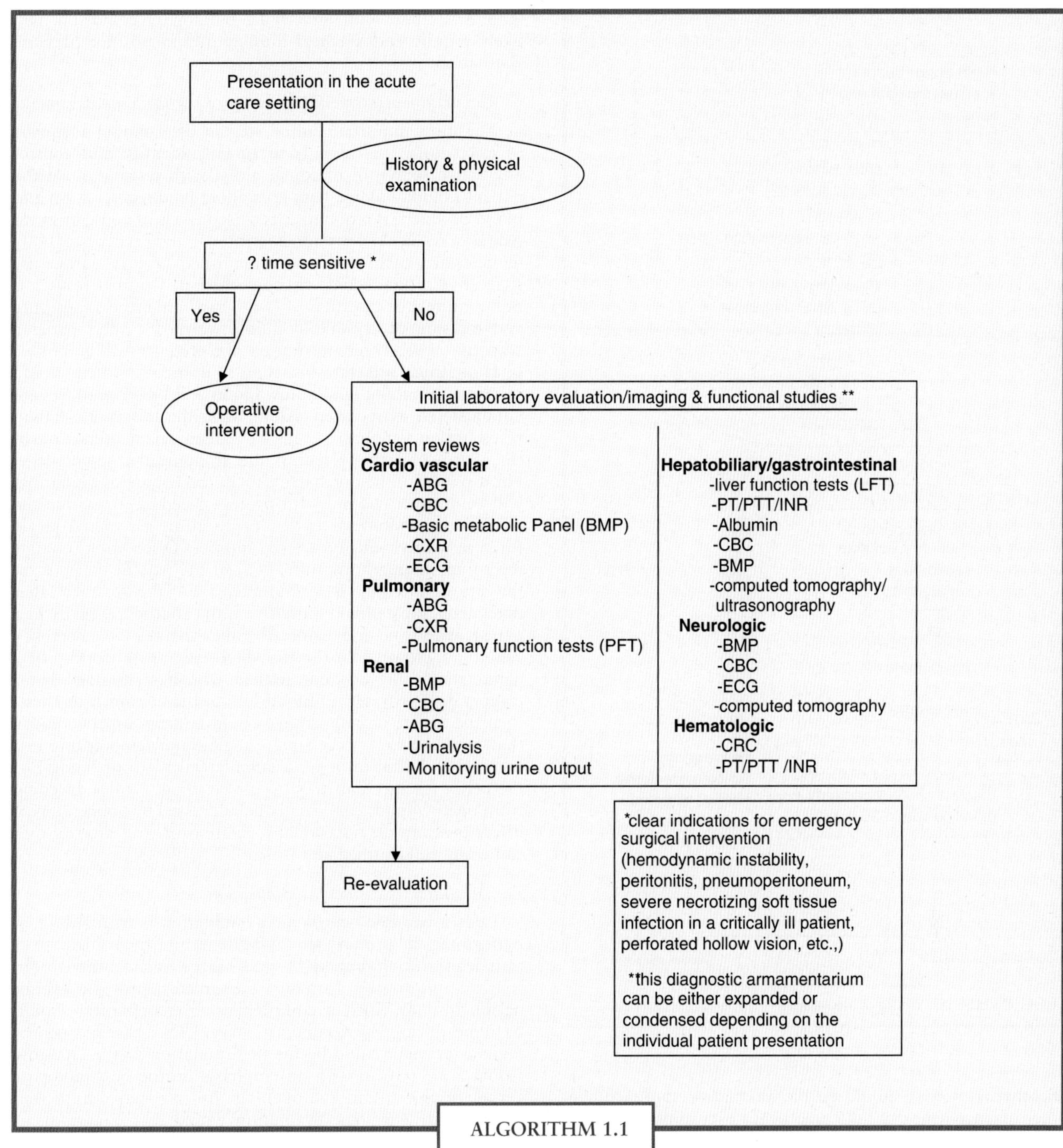

ALGORITHM 1.1 Preoperative assessment.

universal approach has been established with the following prioritization:

- Airway maintenance (with protection of the cervical spine)
- Breathing (ventilation)
- Circulation (including hemorrhage control)
- Disability (neurologic status)
- Exposure/environmental control

Such a systematic and methodical approach (better known as the ABCDEs of the initial assessment) greatly assists the surgical/medical team in the timely management of those injuries that could result in a poor outcome.

A. Airway assessment/management (along with cervical spine protection)

Because loss of a secure airway could be lethal within 4 minutes, airway assessment/management always has the highest priority during the primary survey of the initial assessment of any injured patient, irrespective of the mechanism of injury or the anatomical wound. The chin lift and jaw thrust maneuvers are occasionally helpful in attempting to secure a patient airway. However, in the trauma setting, the airway management of choice is often translaryngeal, endotracheal intubation. If this cannot be achieved due to an upper airway obstruction or some technical difficulty, a surgical airway (needle or surgical

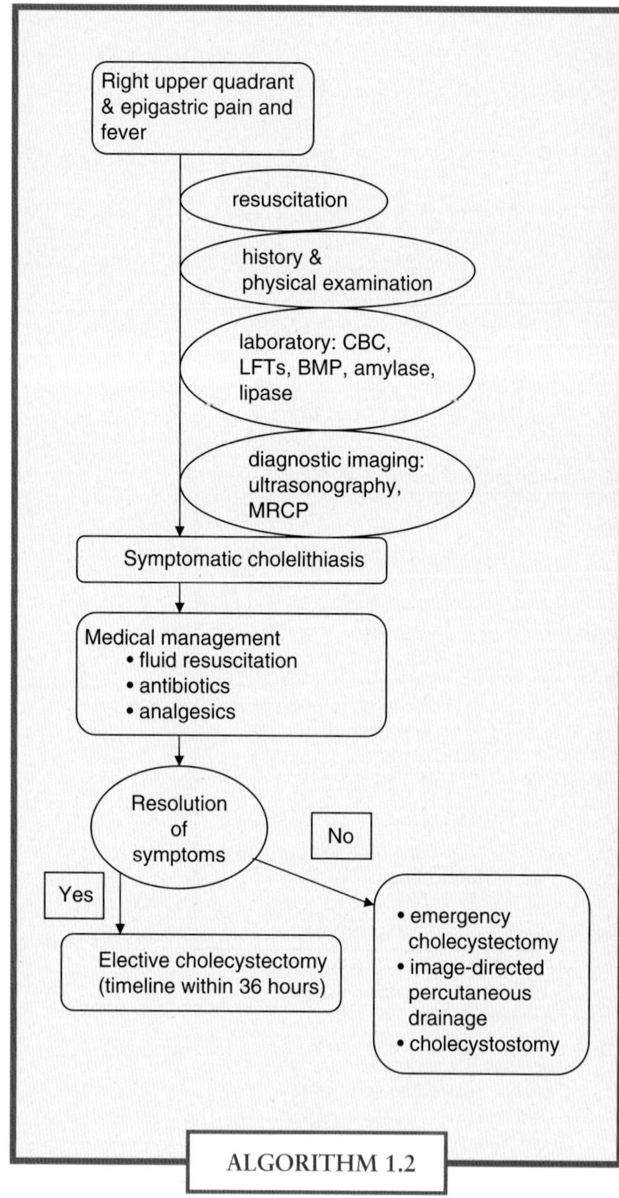

ALGORITHM 1.2 Acute cholecystitis.

cricothyroidotomy) should be the alternative approach. No other management can take precedence over appropriate airway control. Until adequate and sustained oxygenation can be documented, administration of 100% oxygen is required.

B. Breathing (ventilation assessment)

An airway can be adequately established and optimal ventilation still not be achieved. For example, such is the case with an associated tension pneumothorax (other examples include a tension hemothorax, open pneumothorax, or a large flail chest wall segment). Worsening oxygenation and an adverse outcome would ensue unless such problems are expeditiously addressed. Therefore, assessment of breathing is imperative, even when there is an established and secure airway. A patent airway but poor gas exchange will still result in a poor outcome. Tachypnea, absent breath sounds, percussion hyperresonance, distended neck veins, and tracheal deviation are all consistent with inadequate gas exchange. Decompression of the pleural space with a needle/chest tube insertion should be the initial intervention for a pneumo-/hemothorax. A large flail chest, with underlying pulmonary contusion, will likely require endotracheal intubation and positive pressure ventilation.

C. Circulation assessment (adequacy of perfusion management)

The most important initial step in determining adequacy of circulatory perfusion is to quickly identify and control any active source of bleeding, along with restoration of the patient's blood volume with crystalloid fluid resuscitation and blood products, if required. Decreased levels of consciousness, pale skin color, slow (or nonexistent) capillary refill, cool body temperature, tachycardia, or diminished urinary output are suggestive of inadequate tissue perfusion. Optimal resuscitation requires the insertion of two large-bore intravenous lines and infusion of crystalloid fluids (warmed). Adult patients who are severely compromised will require a fluid bolus (2 L of Ringer's lactate or saline solution). Children should receive a 20 mL/kg fluid bolus. Blood and blood products are administered as required. Along with the initiation of fluid resuscitation, emphasis needs to remain on identification of the source of active bleeding and stopping the hemorrhage. For a patient in hemorrhagic shock, the source of blood loss will be an open wound with profuse bleeding, or within the thoracic or abdominal cavity, or from an associated pelvic fracture with venous or arterial injuries. Disposition (operating room, angiography suite, etc.) of the patient depends on the site of bleeding. For example, a FAST assessment that documents substantial blood loss in the abdominal cavity in a patient who is hemodynamically labile dictates an emergency celiotomy. However, if the expedited diagnostic workup of a hemodynamically unstable patient who has sustained blunt trauma demonstrates no blood loss in the abdomen or chest, then the source of hemorrhage could be from a pelvic injury that would likely necessitate angiography/embolization if external stabilization (e.g., a commercial wrap or binder) of the pelvic fracture fails to stop the bleeding. Profuse bleeding from open wounds can usually be addressed by application of direct pressure or, occasionally, ligation of torn arteries that can easily be identified and isolated.

D. Disability assessment/management

Only a baseline neurologic examination is required when performing the primary survey to determine neurologic function deterioration that might necessitate surgical intervention. It is inappropriate to attempt a detailed neurologic examination initially. Such a comprehensive examination should be done during the secondary survey. This baseline neurologic assessment could be the determination of the Glasgow Coma Scale (GCS), with an emphasis on the best motor or verbal response, and eye opening. An alternative approach for a rapid neurologic evaluation would be the assessment of the pupillary size and reaction, along with establishing the patient's level of consciousness (alert, responds to visual stimuli, responds only to painful stimuli or unresponsive to all stimuli). The caveat that must be highlighted is that neurologic deterioration can occur rapidly and a patient with a devastating injury can have a lucid interval (e.g., epidural hematoma). Because the leading causes of secondary brain injury are hypoxia and hypotension, adequate cerebral oxygenation and perfusion are essential in the management of a patient with neurologic injury.

E. Exposure/environmental control

To perform a thorough examination, the patient must be completely undressed. This often requires cutting off the garments to safely expedite such exposure. However, care must be taken to keep the patient from becoming hypothermic. Adjusting the room temperature and infusing warmed intravenous fluids can help establish an optimal environment for the patient.

SECONDARY SURVEY

The secondary survey should not be started until the primary survey has been completed and resuscitation initiated, with some evidence of normalization of vital signs. It is imperative that this head-to-toe evaluation be performed in a detailed manner to detect less obvious or occult injuries. This is particularly important in the unevaluable (e.g., head injury or severely intoxicated) patient. The physical examination should include a detailed assessment of every anatomical region, including the following:

- Head
- Maxillofacial
- Neck (including cervical spine)
- Chest
- Abdomen
- Perineum (including the rectum and genital organs)
- Back (including the remaining spinal column)
- Extremities (musculoskeletal)

A full neurologic examination needs to be performed, along with an estimate of the GCS score if one was not done during the primary survey. The secondary survey and the utilization (when applicable) of the diagnostic adjuncts previously mentioned will allow detection of more occult or subtle injuries that could, if not found, produce significant morbidity and mortality. When possible, the secondary survey should include a history of the mechanism of injury, along with vital information regarding allergies, medications, past

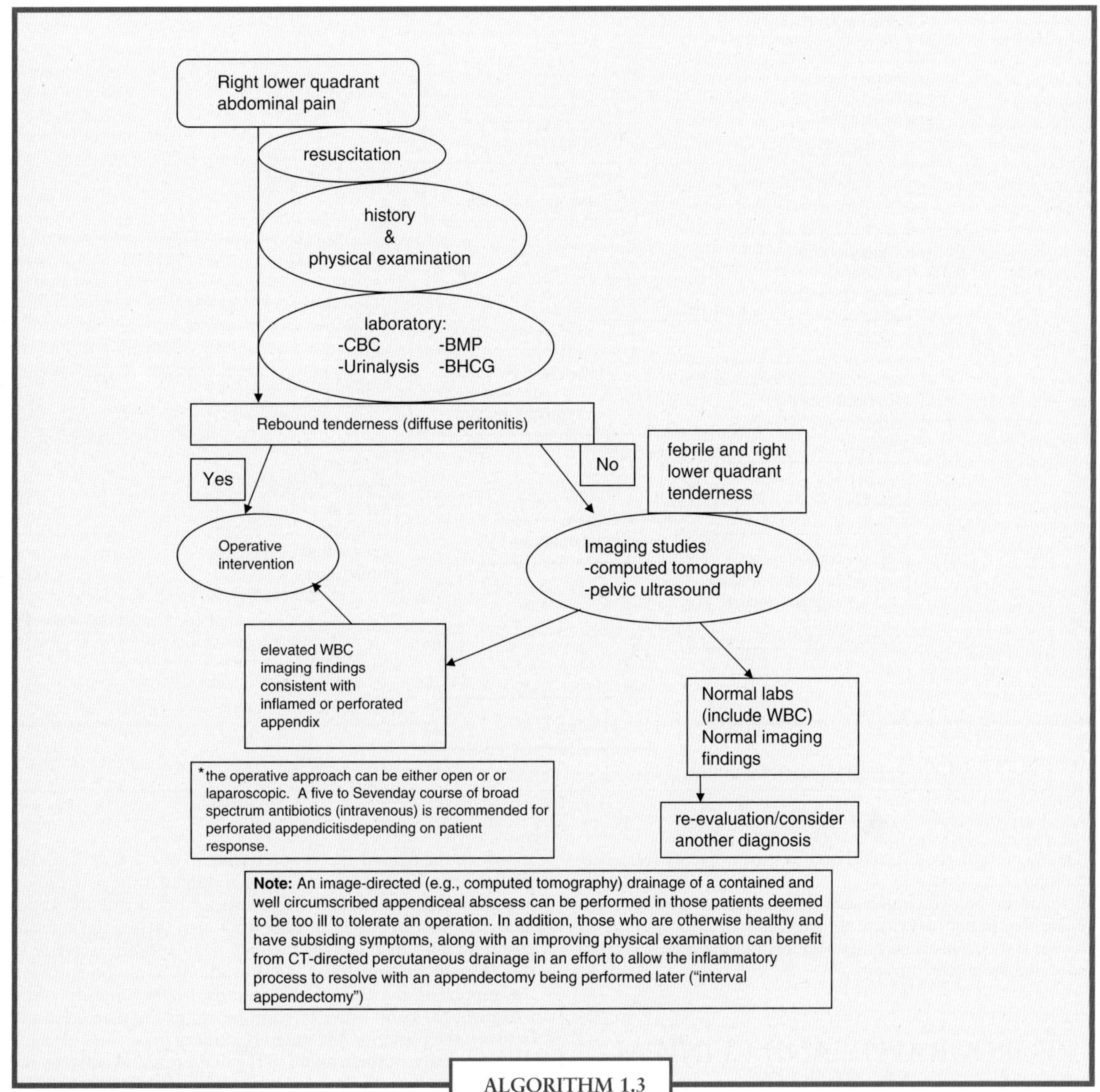

ALGORITHM 1.3 Appendicitis

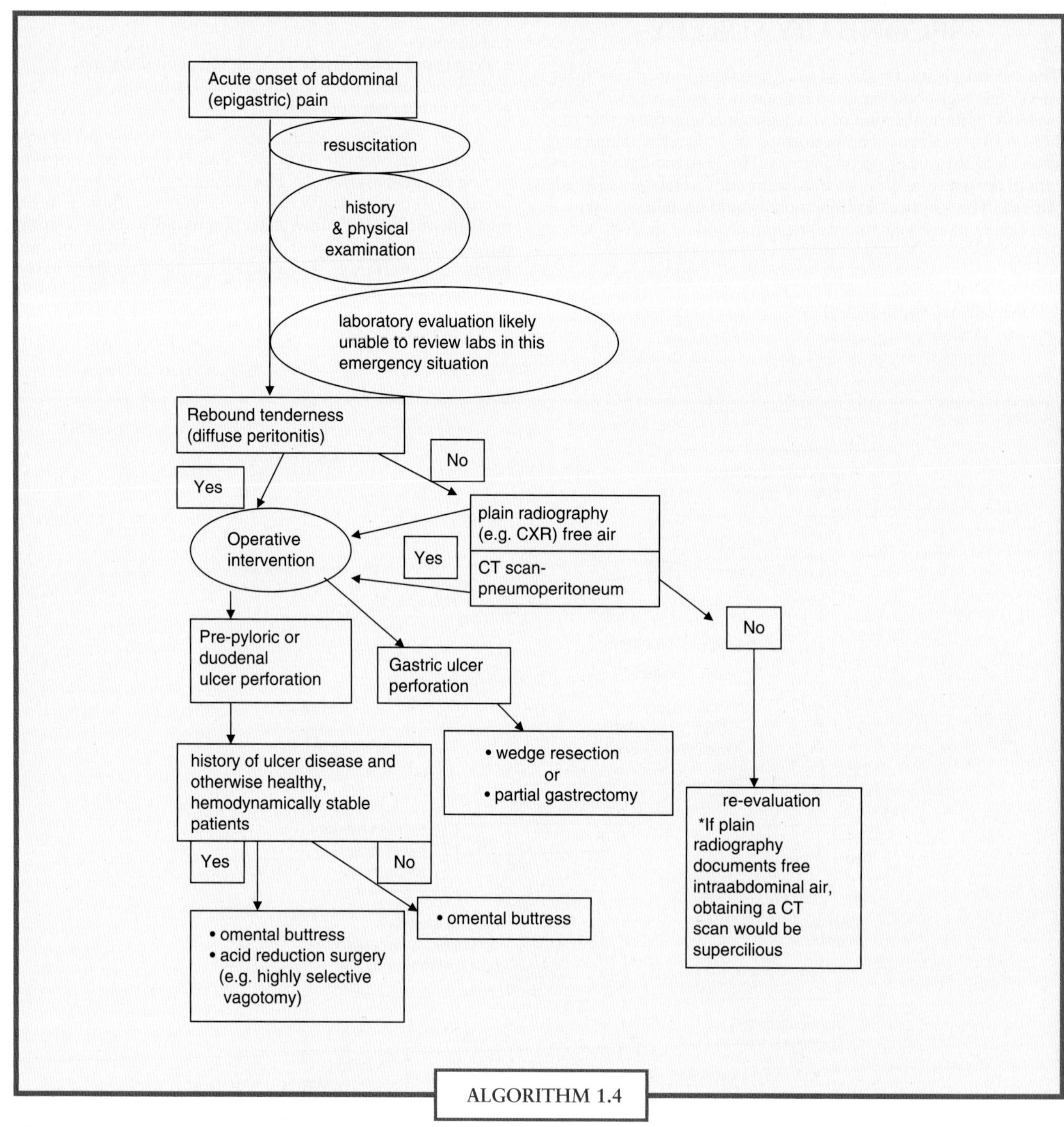

ALGORITHM 1.4 Perforated ulcer (duodenal and gastric).

illnesses, recent food intake, and pertinent events related to the injury.

It cannot be overemphasized that frequent reevaluation of the injured patient is critical to detect any deterioration in the patient status. This sometimes requires repeating both the primary and secondary surveys.

TOPOGRAPHY AND CLINICAL ANATOMY

The abdomen is often defined as a component of the torso that has as its superior boundary the left and right hemidiaphragm, which can ascend to the level of the nipples (4th intercostal space) on the frontal aspect and to the tip of the scapula in the back. The inferior boundary of the abdomen is the pelvic floor. For clinical purposes, it is helpful to further divide the abdomen into four areas: (1) anterior abdomen (below the anterior costal margins to above the inguinal ligaments and anterior to the anterior axillary lines), (2) intrathoracic abdomen (from the nipple or the tips of the scapula to the inferior costal margins), (3) flank (inferior scapular tip to the iliac crest and between the posterior and anterior axillary lines), and (4) back (below the tips of the scapula to the iliac crest and between the posterior axillary lines). The majority of the digestive system and urinary tract, along with a substantial network of vasculature and nerves, are contained with the abdominal cavity. A viscera-rich region, the abdomen can often be the harbinger for occult injuries as a result of penetrating wounds, particularly

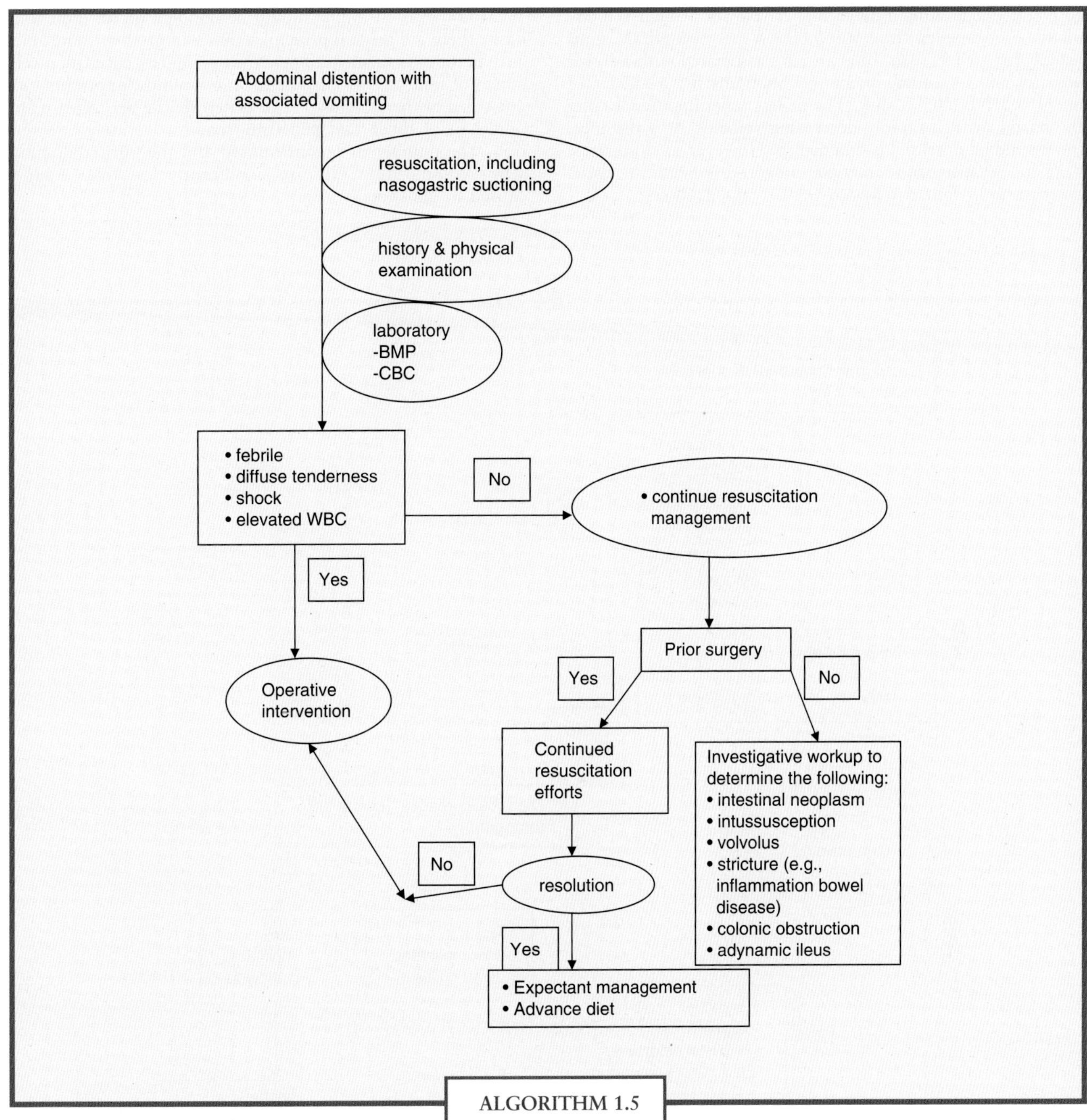

ALGORITHM 1.5 Small bowel obstruction.

in the unevaluable abdomen as the result of a patient's compromised sensorium.

Mechanism of Injury—Penetrating Trauma

In addition to the hemodynamic status of the patient, important variables in the decision making in the management of penetrating abdominal injuries are both the mechanism and location of injury (see "Physical Examination"). The kinetic energy generated by hand-driven weapons, such as knives and sharp objects, is substantially less than caused by firearms. Although not always evident, it is important to know the length and width of the wound along with the depth of penetration of the weapon or device that caused the stab injury. For example, a stab injury usually results in a long, more shallow wound that does not penetrate the peritoneum. Local wound management is the primary focus for these injuries with no concern for any potential intra-abdominal injury.[2] Although there are some stab wounds that do not penetrate the peritoneal cavity, such cannot just be assumed without some formal determination or serial abdominal examinations to assess for worsening abdominal tenderness or the development of peritoneal signs.

There is notable variability among the full spectrum of firearms in the civilian setting, with this arsenal including handguns, rifles, shotguns, and airguns. The kinetic energy, which correlates with the wounding potential, is dependant on mass and velocity (KE = $1/2\ mv^2$). Therefore, the higher the velocity (v), the greater the wounding potential.[3] Because the barrel is longer in a rifle than a handgun, the bullet has more time to accelerate, generating a much higher velocity. A high-velocity missile is propelled at 2,500-5,000 ft per second. Airguns usually fire pellets (e.g., BBs) and are associated with a lower velocity and wounding potential. Shotguns fire a cluster of metal pellets, called a shot. The pellets separate after leaving the barrel, with a rapidly decreasing velocity. At a distance, the wounding potential is diminished. However, at close range (<15 ft), because of the increase in aggregate mass, the tissue destruction is similar to a high-velocity missile injury.

Although each injury should be handled on an individual basis, there are general principles that will provide some guidance in the management of penetrating injuries based on mechanism of injury. With respect to stab wounds, approximately one-third of the wounds do not penetrate the peritoneum and only half of those that penetrate require operative intervention. The number of organs injured and the intra-abdominal sepsis complication rate are significantly less than wounds caused by gunshots.[4,5]

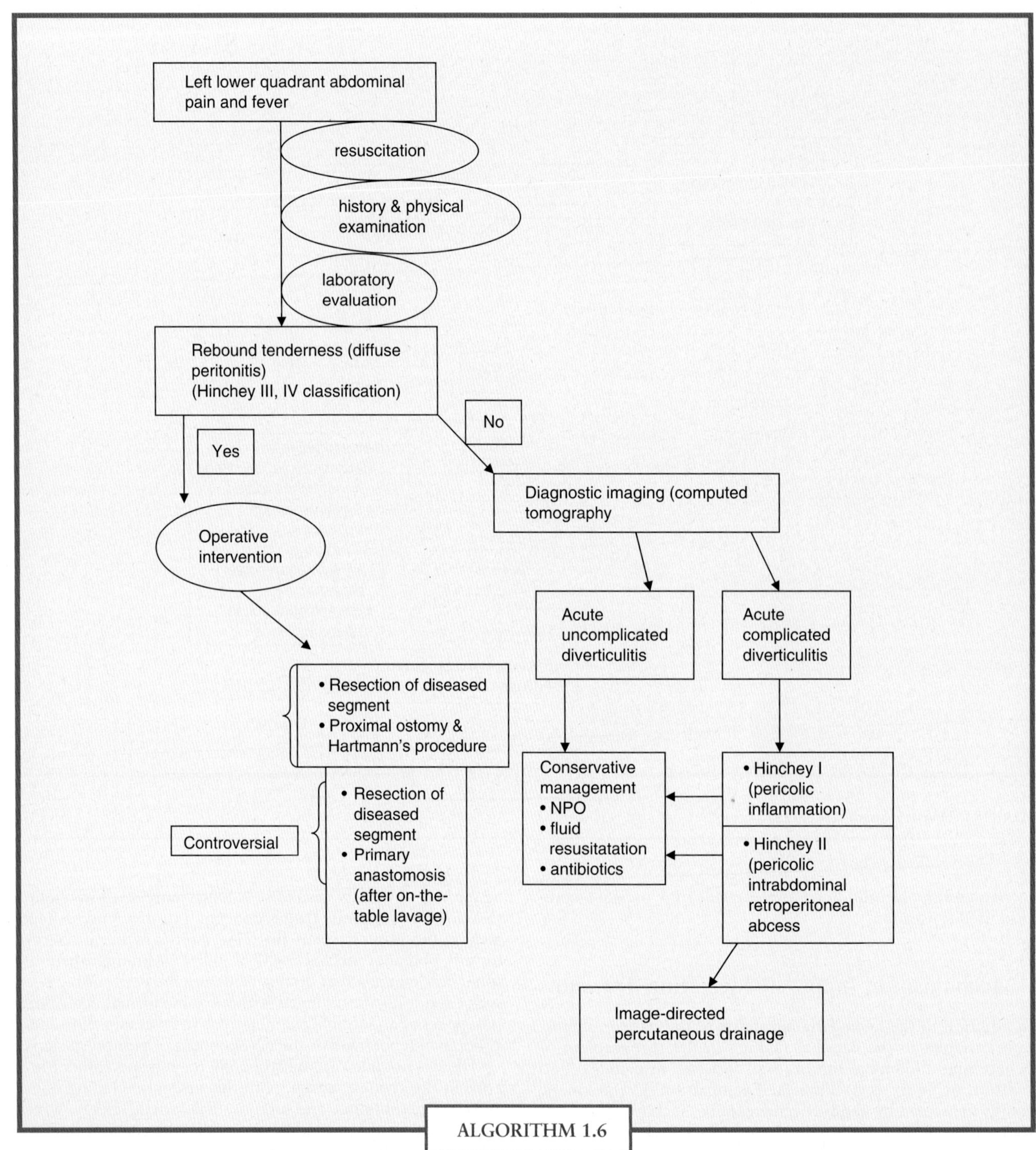

ALGORITHM 1.6 Diverticulitis

PHYSICAL EXAMINATION

A complete and thorough physical examination of the entire body is essential in the management of penetrating abdominal injury. There are some findings (Table 1.2) on physical examination that are absolute indications for operative intervention. The components of the physical exam should include careful inspection, palpation, and auscultation.

In addition to determination of the location, extent, and the number of wounds, inspection can sometimes determine the trajectory of the missile or other wounding agent and, consequently, guide management decisions. For example, a patient with a documented, superficial tangential gunshot wound (low-velocity), with no other remarkable physical findings, would likely be managed expectantly (observation). However, if a penetrating abdominal injury results in a patient presenting with an evisceration, exploratory laparotomy would be the management option of choice. Palpation will enable the examiner to elicit abdominal tenderness or frank peritoneal signs, along with detection of abdominal distention and rigidity. On occasion, missiles can be palpated lodged in the soft tissue. Unless in a controlled and sterile setting such as the operative theater, probing of a wound should be avoided. Auscultation is also an important component of the physical examination. It can detect diminished or absent bowel sounds that could be suggestive of evolving peritonitis. Also, auscultation could detect a trauma-induced bruit, suggestive of a vascular injury. The examiner must be keenly aware that there are situations in which the abdominal exam will be unreliable due to possible spinal cord injury or a patient's altered mental state.

DIAGNOSTIC STUDIES

Even with penetrating injuries, the abdomen is notorious for hiding its secrets—occult injuries. Access to an extensive diagnostic armamentarium is imperative in the optimal management of these injuries. Strongly advocated by some for abdominal stab wounds, local wound exploration has the advantage of allowing the patient to be discharged from the trauma bay or emergency department, if surgical exploration of the wound fails to demonstrate penetration of the posterior fascia and peritoneum. However, if the patient goes to the operating room for other injuries, the local wound exploration should be done in the surgical suite with better lighting and a more sterile environment. A positive finding during local wound exploration dictates a formal laparotomy or laparoscopy. However, even with local wound exploration as a guide, the nontherapeutic laparotomy rate can be high, given that only a third of the patients with stab wounds to the anterior abdomen require therapeutic laparotomy.[6,7] In the patient who has an evaluable abdomen, serial abdominal examinations would be an acceptable alterative to local wound exploration, to determine the need for operative intervention (selective management). Local would exploration should only be done for stab wounds to the anterior abdomen. Such an approach is potentially too hazardous for thoracoabdominal penetrating injuries and back/flank wounds. Plain radiography (abdomen/pelvis/chest) can be pivotal in documenting the presence of missiles and other foreign bodies and determining the trajectory of the injury tract, particularly for wounds from firearms. Also, the presence of free air might be confirmed by plain radiography. Unless there is concern about a retained broken blade, there is little utility for plain radiography for stab injuries.[8] The DPL developed by David Root, in 1965, was a major advance in the care of the hemodynamically labile patient who sustained blunt trauma.[9] With the advent of FAST and rapid CT, DPL has limited utility. DPL has never had a broad appeal in the diagnostic evaluation of penetrating abdominal wounds. Although some have advocated its use with tangential wounds of the abdominal wall, the technique has failed to receive widespread support.[10] Its reliability in detecting clinically important injuries sustained as a result of penetrating abdominal injuries has been a prevailing concern.[11-13] The reported sensitivity and specificity of DPL for abdominal stab wounds are 59%-96% and 78%-98%, respectively.[14] Also, DPL is a poor diagnostic modality for detection of diaphragmatic and retroperitoneal injuries.

Diagnostic imaging has had the greatest impact in changing the face of trauma management with CT taking the lead in this area. Its ubiquitous presence in the management of blunt abdominal trauma is well established. However, it is becoming an important diagnostic study in the evaluation of penetrating abdominal injuries. In addition to its excellent sensitivity in detection of pneumoperitoneum, free fluid, and abdominal wall/peritoneal penetration, CT is helpful in identifying the tract of the penetrating agent. Hauser et al. recommended the use of "triple contrast" CT in the assessment of penetrating back and flank injuries.[15] CT scan evaluation is an essential diagnostic tool in the increasing advocacy for selective management of abdominal gunshot wounds, obviating the need for mandatory surgical exploration.[16] However, there still remain two major limitations of CT: detection of intestinal perforation and diaphragmatic injury.

Unless the injury is confined to the solid organ of the abdomen, such as the liver or spleen, the matrix of intestinal gas patterns makes detection of penetrating injuries difficult. Kristensen et al.[17] were one of the first teams to introduce the role of ultrasonic scanning as part of the diagnostic armamentarium in trauma management. Kimura and Otsuka[18] endorsed using ultrasonography in the emergency room for evaluation of hemoperitoneum. FAST does not have the same broad application in the evaluation of penetrating trauma as it does in blunt trauma assessment. Rozycki et al.[19] reported on the expanded role of ultrasonography as the "primary adjuvant modality" for the injured patient assessment. Rozycki also reported that FAST examination was the most accurate for detecting fluid within the pericardial sac. Such a finding would be confirmatory for a cardiac injury and possible cardiac tamponade, given a mechanism of injury that could result in an injury to the heart.

As a diagnostic modality, laparoscopy is not a new innovation. Other specialists have been utilizing this operative intervention for several decades. However, it was formally introduced as a possible diagnostic procedure of choice for specific torso wounds when Ivatury et al.[20] critically evaluated laparoscopy in penetrating abdominal trauma. Fabian et al.[21] also reported on the efficacy of diagnostic laparoscopy in a prospective analysis.

With no conventional diagnostic tool that can conclusively rule out a diaphragmatic laceration or rent, diagnostic laparoscopy becomes the study of choice for penetrating thoracoabdominal injuries, particularly left thoracoabdominal wounds

TABLE 1.2

ABSOLUTE INDICATIONS FOR EXPLORATORY LAPAROTOMY IN PENETRATING ABDOMINAL INJURIES

A. Peritonitis
B. Evisceration
C. Impaled object
D. Hemodynamic instability
E. Associated bleeding from natural orifice
F. Documented pneumoperitoneum

(Algorithm. 1.7). Laparoscopy can also be used to determine peritoneal entry from a tangential penetrating injury.

Penetrating Abdominal Injuries and the Hemodynamically Stable and Unstable Patient

As highlighted above, the management principles in patients who sustain penetrating abdominal injuries and remain hemodynamically stable depend on the mechanism and location of injury, along with the hemodynamic status of the patient. Irrespective of the patient's hemodynamic parameter, the Adult Trauma Life Support (ATLS) protocol should be strictly followed upon arrival of the patient to the trauma bay (Algorithms. 1.8-1.11).

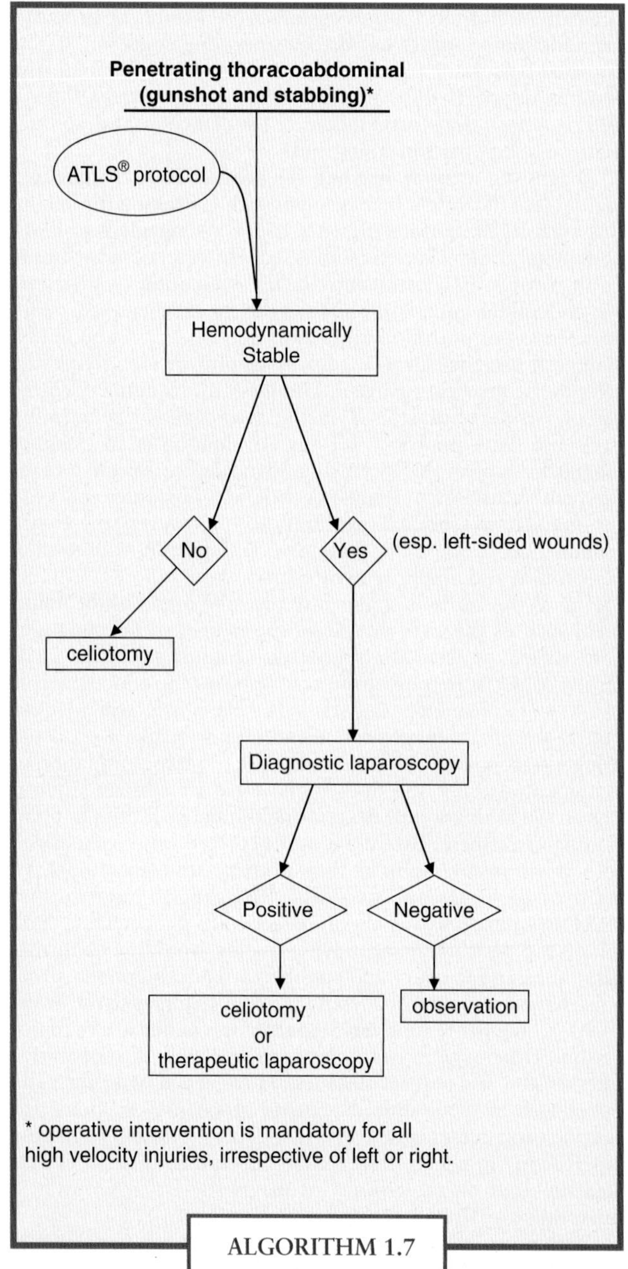

ALGORITHM 1.7 Management algorithm for penetrating thoracoabdominal injury.

Trauma Laparotomy The operative theater should be large enough to accommodate more than one surgical team, in the event the patient requires simultaneous procedures to be performed. In addition, the room should have the capability of maintaining room temperature as high as the lower 80's °F to avoid hypothermia. Also, a rapid transfusion device should be in the room to facilitate the delivery of large fluid volume and ensure that the fluid administration is appropriately warm.

Abdominal exploration for trauma has basically four imperatives: (1) hemorrhage control, (2) contamination control, (3) identification of the specific injury (ies), and (4) repair/reconstruction. The abdomen is prepared with a topical antimicrobial from sternal notch to bilateral midthighs and extending the prep laterally to the side of the operating room table followed by widely draping the patient. Such preparation allows expeditious entry into the thorax if needed and possible vascular access or harvesting. Exploration is initiated with a midline vertical incision that should extend from the xiphoid to the symphysis pubis to achieve optimal exposure.

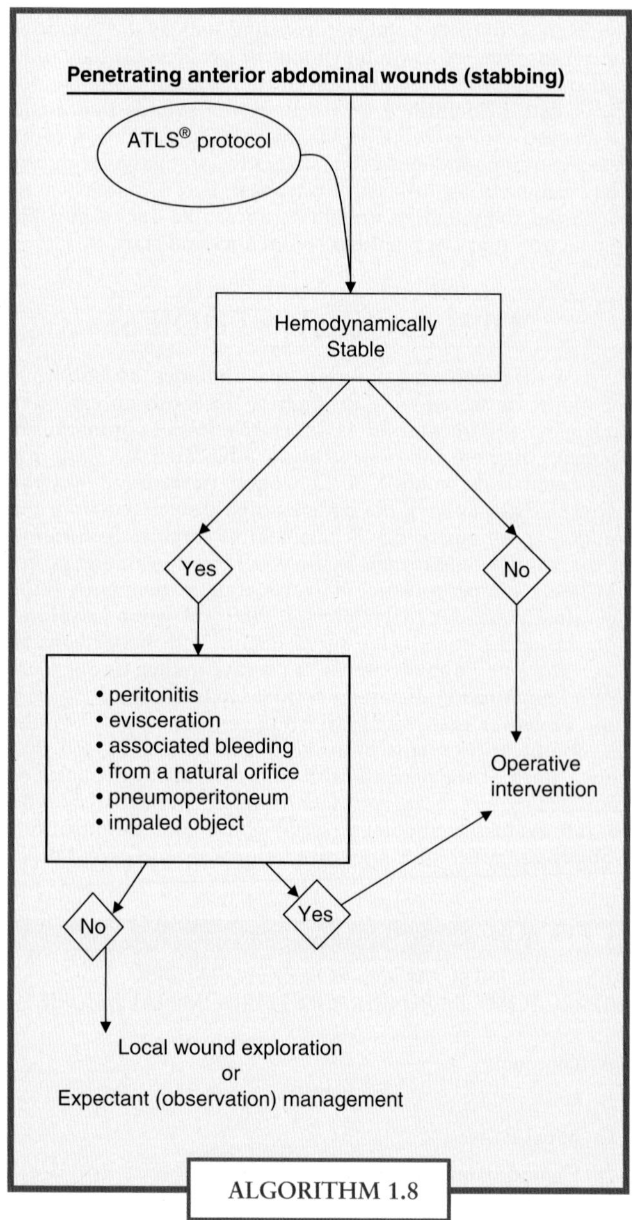

ALGORITHM 1.8 Management algorithm for penetrating anterior abdominal injuries.

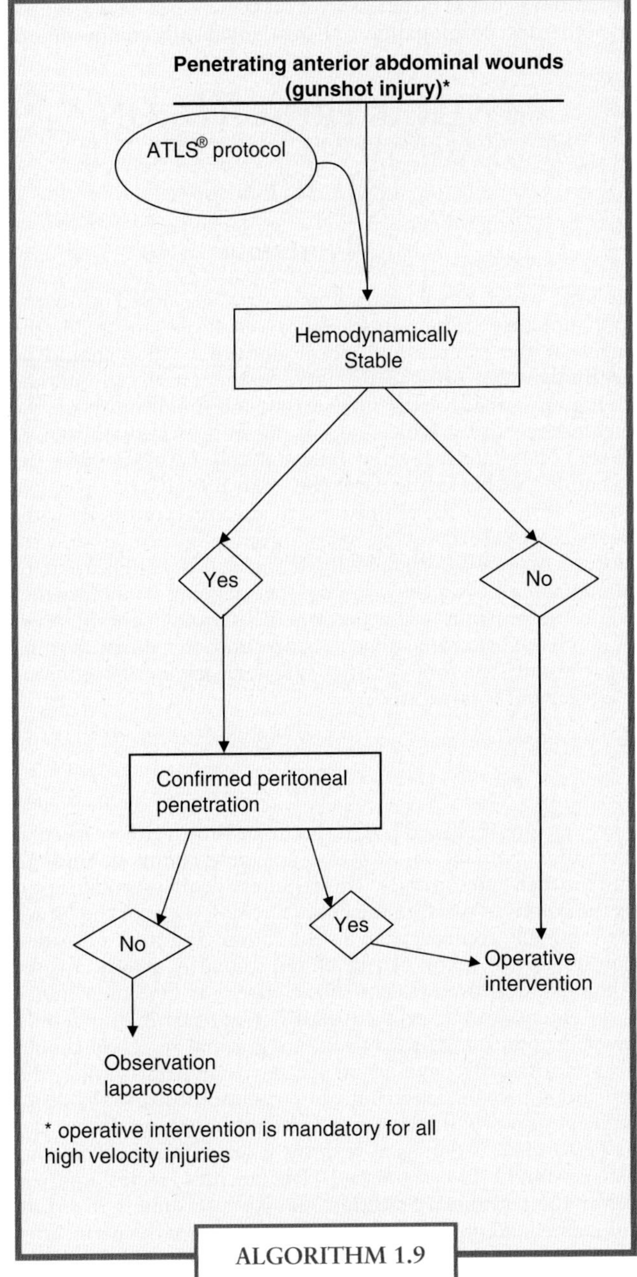

ALGORITHM 1.9 Management algorithm for penetrating abdominal injuries.

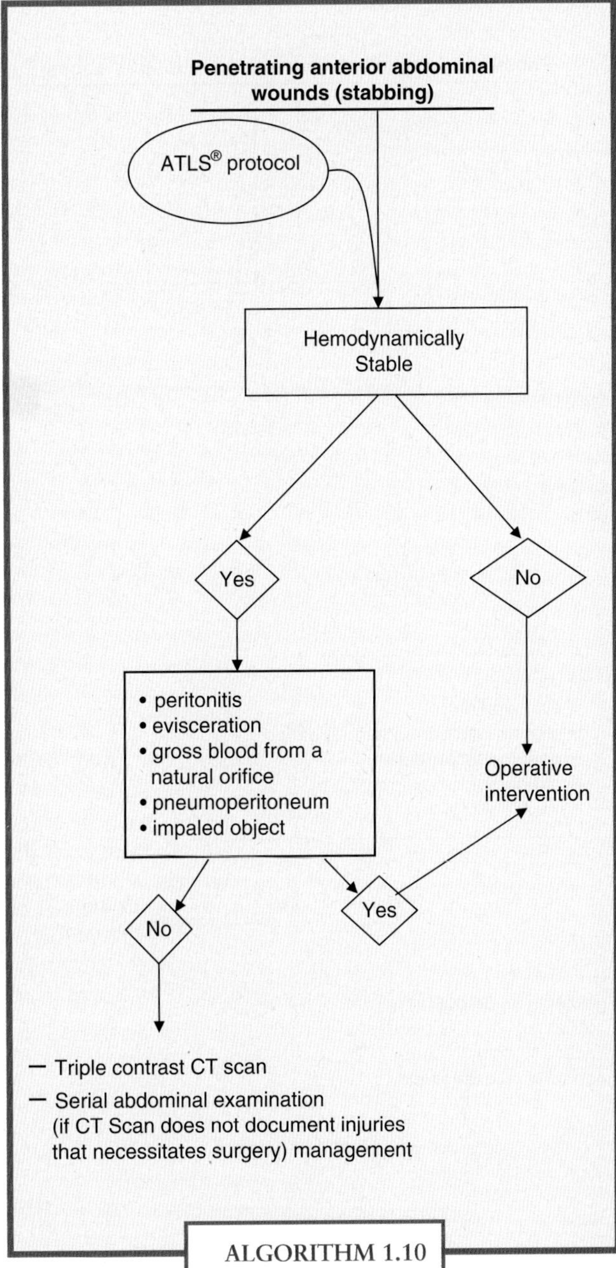

ALGORITHM 1.10 Management algorithm for penetrating abdominal injuries.

The first priority upon entering the abdomen is control of exsanguinating hemorrhage. Such control can usually be achieved by direct control of the lacerated site or obtaining proximal vascular control. After major hemorrhage is controlled, blood and blood clots are removed. Abdominal packs (radiologically labeled) are used to tamponade any bleeding and allow identification of any injury bleeding. The preferred approach to packing is to divide the falciform ligament and retract the anterior abdominal wall. This will allow manual placement of the packs above the liver. Abdominal packs should also be placed below the liver. This arrangement of the packs on the liver creates a compressive tamponade effect. After manually eviscerating the small bowel out of the cavity, packs should be placed on the remaining three quadrants, with care taken to avoid iatrogenic injury to the spleen. During the packing phase after ongoing hemorrhage has been controlled, the surgeon should communicate with the anesthesia team that major hemorrhage has been controlled and that this would be an optimal time to establish a resuscitative advantage with fluid/blood/blood product administration.

The next priority is control or containment of gross contamination. This begins with the removal of the packs from each quadrant—one quadrant at a time. Packs should be removed from the quadrants that you least suspect to be the source for blood loss, followed by removal of the packs from the final quadrant; the one that you believe is the area of concern.

After control of major hemorrhage has been achieved, any evidence of gross contamination must be addressed immediately. Obvious leakage from intestinal injury can be initially controlled with clamps (e.g., Babcock clamp), staples, or sutures. The entire abdominal gastrointestinal tract needs to be inspected, including the mesenteric and antimesenteric border of the small and large bowel, along with the entire

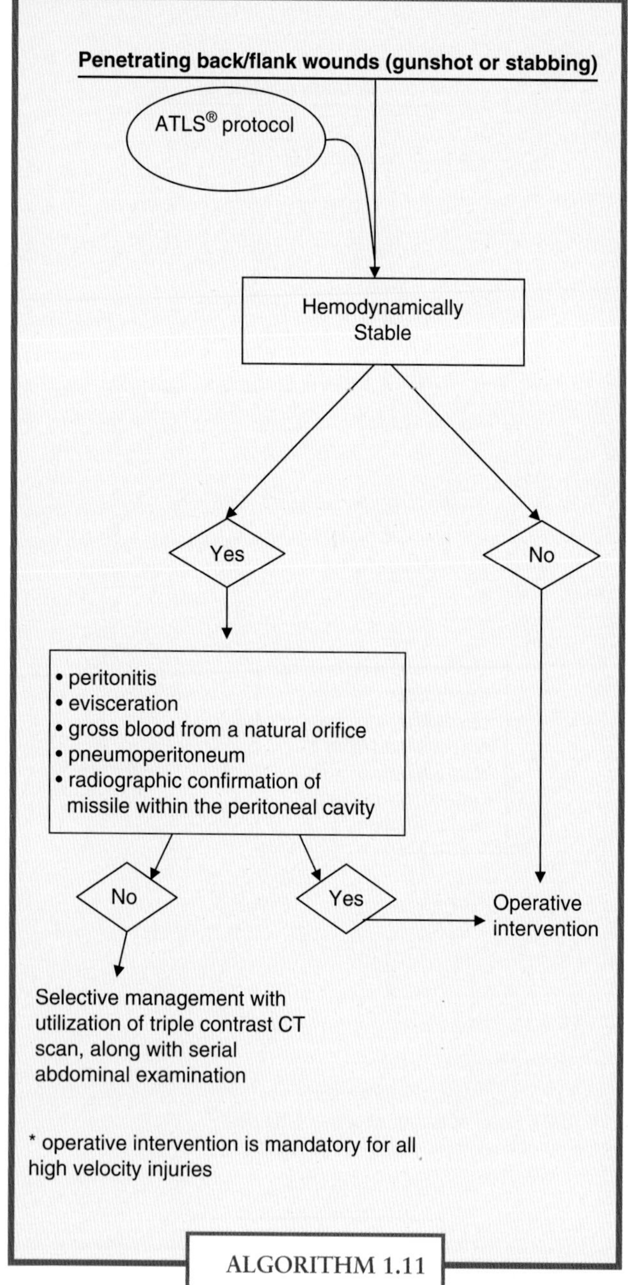

ALGORITHM 1.11 Management algorithm for penetrating back/flank injury.

mesentery. Rents in the diaphragm should also be closed to prevent contamination of the thoracic cavity.

Further identification of all intra-abdominal injuries should be initiated. Depending on the mechanism of injury and the estimated trajectory of wounding agent, a thorough and meticulous abdominal exploration should be performed, including exploring the lesser sac to inspect the pancreas and the associated vasculature. In addition, mobilization of the C-loop of the duodenum (Kocher maneuver) might be required, along with medical rotation of the left or right colon for exposure of vital retroperitoneal structures.

The final component of a trauma laparotomy is definitive repair, if possible, of specific injuries. As will be highlighted later in the chapter, the status of the patient dictates whether each of the components of a trauma laparotomy can be achieved at the index operation. A staged celiotomy ("damage control" laparotomy) might be necessary if the patient becomes acidotic, hypothermic, coagulopathic, or hemodynamically compromised.

GENERAL PRINCIPLES IN MANAGEMENT OF SPECIFIC INJURIES

Small Intestine

Isolated small bowel enterotomies can be closed primarily with nonabsorbable sutures for a one-layer closure. If the edges of the enterotomy appear nonviable, they should be gently debrided prior to primary closure. However, multiple contiguous small bowel holes or an intestinal injury on the mesenteric border with associate mesenteric hematoma will likely necessitate segmental resection and anastomosis of the remaining viable segments of the small bowel. The operative goal is always the reestablishment of intestinal continuity without substantial narrowing of the intestinal lumen, along with closure of any associated mesenteric defect. Application of noncrushing bowel claps can contain ongoing contamination while the repair is being performed. Although a hand-sewn or stapler-assisted anastomosis is operator dependant, trauma laparotomies are time-sensitive interventions and expeditious management is imperative.

Colon

The segment of injured bowel should be thoroughly inspected, particularly missile injuries that are most common, through and through enterotomies. This requires adequate mobilization of the colon to visualize the entire circumference of the bowel wall. Initially controversial, an enterotomy (right- or left-sided injuries) of the colon can be closed primarily, irrespective of contamination or transient shock state.[22] If the colon injury is so extensive that primary repair is not possible or would severely compromise the lumen, a segmental resection should be performed. Depending on the environmental setting, the remaining proximal segment can be anastomosed to the distal segment or a proximal ostomy and Hartmann's procedure can be performed. If the distal segment is long enough, a mucous fistula should be established. Documented rectal injuries, below the peritoneal reflection, should necessitate a diverting colostomy and presacral drainage (exiting from the perineum). Such drainage is, however, not universally endorsed.

Stomach/Duodenum

With respect to penetrating wounds of the stomach, the anterior and posterior aspects of the stomach need to be meticulously inspected for accompanying through-and-through injuries. Penetrating injuries of the stomach should be repaired primarily after debridement of nonviable edged. The primary repair can either be single layer with nonabsorbable suture or double layer closure with an absorbable suture (e.g., Vicryl) for the first layer and the second layer closed with nonabsorbable sutures (e.g., silk) Few penetrating injuries of the stomach or primary repairs of a through-and-through gastric injury would compromise the gastric lumen. Duodenal injuries can be repaired primarily in a one- or two-layered fashion if the penetration is less than half the circumference of the duodenum. However, for more complex duodenal injuries, an operative procedure is needed to divert gastric contents away from the injury site (where closure of the wound has been attempted). Pyloric exclusion with the establishment of a gastrojejunostomy is such a procedure.[23-25]

Pancreas

Superficial or tangential penetrating wounds of the pancreas, without injury to the main pancreatic duct, can be externally drained. However, a penetrating injury that transects the pancreas, including the main pancreatic duct, requires extirpation of the distal pancreas (distal pancreatectomy), particularly if the transection site is to the left of the superior mesenteric vessels. A more proximal penetrating pancreatic injury can generally be managed by wide drainage. If a proximal injury involves the main pancreatic duct, with associated complex duodenal injury (e.g., injury to the ampulla), pancreatoduodenectomy may be necessary. Thus, the indication for pancreatoduodenectomy is combined destructive injury to both the duodenum and pancreas; the operation in essence completes the procedure that the injury has functionally necessitated. Unfortunately, because of the rich vascular network surrounding the pancreas, penetrating pancreatic wounds can be lethal injuries.

Spleen

Most penetrating splenic injuries, particularly gunshot wounds, require splenectomy. To visualize the entire spleen, it should be mobilized to the midline by division of its ligamentous attachments. Superficial penetrating injuries of the spleen can sometimes be managed by either splenorrhaphy or application of a topical hemostatic agent. Splenorrhaphy can be by pledgeted repair or an omental buttress. However, complex repair of the spleen is not a prudent approach in the always time-sensitive trauma setting.

Gallbladder and Liver

Penetrating injuries to the gallbladder dictate the need for extirpation. There is no role for primary repair of a penetrating wound to the gallbladder.

Liver injuries are common in both blunt and penetrating trauma. The majority of injuries are superficial or minor and require no surgical repair. Simple application of pressure or a hemostatic agent or fibrin glue will constitute definitive management of the majority of these injuries. The argon beam coagulation, also a helpful adjunct, in superficial hepatic injuries with persistent oozing generates ionizing energy through an argon gas stream that causes rapid coagulation. The operative armamentarium for complex penetrating hepatic injuries is highlighted in Table 1.3.

Genitourinary System

Less than 10% of patients with penetrating abdominal wounds sustain genitourinary tract injury; the majority are renal. Penetrating injuries that result in a grade IV (cortical/calyceal injury and associated vascular injury with contained hemorrhage) or grade V (shattered kidney and vascular avulsion) invariably necessitate nephrectomy, particularly if there is a viable

TABLE 1.3

LIVER INJURY SCALE OF THE AAST

GRADE[a]	TYPE OF INJURY	INJURY DESCRIPTION	ICD-9[b]	AIS-90[c]
I	Hematoma	Subcapsular, <10% surface area	864.01 864.11	2
	Laceration	Capsular tear, <1 cm parenchymal depth	864.02 864.12	2
II	Hematoma	Subcapsular, 10%-50% surface area; intraparenchymal, <10 cm in diameter	864.01 864.11	2
	Laceration	1-3 cm parenchymal depth, <10 cm in length	864.03 864.13	2
III	Hematoma	Subcapsular, >50% surface area or expanding; ruptured subcapsular or parenchymal hematoma; intraparenchymal hematoma >10 cm or expanding	864.04	3
	Laceration	>3 cm parenchymal depth	864.14	3
IV	Laceration	Parenchymal disruption involving 25%-75% of hepatic lobe or 1-3 Couinaud's segments within a single lobe	864.04 864.14	4
V	Laceration	Parenchymal disruption involving >75% of hepatic lobe or >3 Couinaud's segments within a single lobe		5
	Vascular	Juxtahepatic venous injuries; i.e., retrohepatic vena cava/central major hepatic veins		5
VI	Vascular	Hepatic avulsion		6

[a]Advance one grade for multiple injuries, up to grade III.
[b]ICD, International Classification of Diseases, 9th Revision.
[c]AIS, Abbreviated Injury Score.

contralateral kidney. Lacerations or more superficial wounds of the kidney might require renorrhaphy, with approximation of the disrupted capsule with pledgeted sutures or a prosthetic (mesh) wrap. Absorbable interrupted suture should be used and all repairs should be drained. The injury pattern may dictate the need for a partial nephrectomy. Ureteral injuries can be difficult to identify in penetrating wounds with an accompanying retroperitoneal hematoma. When possible, the ureter should be repaired primarily with interrupted absorbable suture over a double J stent. A complete transection of the ureter requires debridement of the nonviable edges, spatulation of the ends, and primary repair over a stent. All repair sites should be adequately drained. If the anastomosis cannot be performed in a tension-free fashion, a bladder flap (Boari) could be surgically constructed, with implantation of the proximal segment of the transected ureter into the flap. A psoas "hitch" might be required if there is any tension on the flap and the tunneled ureter.

Penetrating injury to the intraperitoneal bladder requires surgical repair. After confirmation that there is no involvement of the trigone, the bladder should be closed with a two-layer closure with absorbable suture (the second layer incorporates Lembert sutures to imbricate the first layer). Suprapubic drainage should only be done selectively; however, a Foley's catheter should be left in place.

Retroperitoneal Hematoma

The retroperitoneum, an organ-rich region, has several vital structures that can be injured when its boundaries are penetrated. It can be a major potential site for hemorrhage in patients sustaining either penetrating or blunt trauma due to the substantial vascularity along with bleeding that can occur from an associated solid organ wound (e.g., kidney). In the central region (Zone 1) of the retroperitoneum resides the abdominal aorta, celiac axis, and the superior mesenteric artery, vena cava, and proximal renal vasculature. The lateral retroperitoneum (Zone 2) encompasses the proximal genitourinary system and its vasculature. The pelvic retroperitoneum (Zone 3) contains the iliac arteries, veins, and their tributaries. In addition to the vasculature and the kidneys (plus ureters) highlighted above, the retroperitoneum contains the second, third, and fourth portion of the duodenum, along with the pancreas, the adrenals, and the intrapelvic portion of the colon and rectum. Table 1.4 underscores the management principles of trauma-related retroperitoneal hematomas. Ideally, proximal (and when applicable, distal) control needs to be achieved prior to exploration of a retroperitoneal hematoma. For retroperitoneal hematomas in Zone 1, irrespective of a penetrating or blunt mechanism, mandatory exploration is required. Also, retroperitoneal hematoma in any of the three zones requires exploration for all penetrating injuries. For Zone 2 retroperitoneal hematomas resulting from blunt trauma, all pulsatile or expanding hematomas should undergo exploration. Gross extravasation of urine also necessitates exploration. Zone 3 (pelvic retroperitoneum) hematomas should be explored only for penetrating injuries to determine if there is a specific intrapelvic colorectal, ureteral, or vascular injury. However, such an approach should not be taken for blunt trauma, for the injury would likely be venous and application of an external compression device would be the preferred intervention. An arterial injury could be addressed by arteriography/embolization.

Intra-abdominal Packing and "Damage Control" Strategy

"Damage control" strategy, popularized by Rotondo et al., is a staged celiotomy strategy that was initially made operationally visible by Mattox and Feliciano. Although this approach was not actually developed by them, Mattox and Feliciano certainly popularized the technique and made it acceptable for

TABLE 1.4

KIDNEY INJURY SCALE OF THE AAST

GRADE[a]	TYPE OF INJURY	INJURY DESCRIPTION	ICD-9[b]	AIS-90[c]
I	Contusion	Microscopic or gross hematuria, urologic studies normal	866.00 866.02	2
	Hematoma	Subcapsular, nonexpanding without parenchymal laceration	866.11	2
II	Hematoma	Nonexpanding perirenal hematoma confined to renal retroperitoneum	866.01	2
	Laceration	Parenchymal depth of renal cortex (>1.0 cm) without urinary extravasation	866.11	2
III	Laceration	Parenchymal depth of renal cortex (>1.0 cm) without collecting system rupture or urinary extravasation	866.02 866.12	3
IV	Laceration	Parenchymal laceration extending through the renal cortex, medulla, and collecting system	866.02	4
	Vascular	Main renal artery or vein injury with contained hemorrhage	866.12	4
V	Laceration	Completely shattered kidney	866.03	5
	Vascular	Avulsion of renal hilum, which devascularizes kidney	866.13	5

[a]Advance one grade for biliateral injuries up to grade III.
[b]ICD, International Classification of Diseases, 9th Revision.
[c]AIS, Abbreviated Injury Score.

use in this country.[26-30] Irrespective of the name given to this strategy of surgically managing only immediate life-threatening injuries (along with intra-abdominal packing and rapid temporary closure of the abdominal cavity), the goal is the same—avoid the potential irreversibility of sustained acidosis, hypothermia, coagulopathy, and hemodynamic lability by delaying definitive operative management until the patient can be stabilized in the intensive care unit. Although "damage control" is most frequently used in association with severe hepatic wounds, other organ injuries, including vascular wounds, can necessitate this staged celiotomy approach with hepatic packing and a rapid, creative abdominal closure.

Mechanism of Injury—Blunt Trauma

The management paradigm of blunt abdominal has evolved over the last few decades. For example, the emphasis on the physical examination, plain x-radiography, laboratory findings, and DPL has shifted to greater reliance on CT and ultrasonography. Treatment for visceral injury has traditionally been operative but many forms of solid organ injury can now be managed nonoperatively or with minimally invasive and interventional radiology techniques. Management of the multiply injured trauma patient at level I trauma centers with state-of-the-art techniques has now conclusively shown significantly improved patient outcome and survival.[31]

CURRENT DIAGNOSTIC AND IMAGING TECHNIQUES

Focused Abdominal Sonography for Trauma

One of the most recent advances in the workup of the acutely injured patient is the use of bedside ultrasonography for detection of cardiac and intra-abdominal injury. Known as FAST, the technique's noninvasive nature allows the operator to perform an exam simultaneously during the initial resuscitation and stabilization of a multiply injured trauma patient. The technique may thereby provide evidence of significant hemorrhage early in the course of evaluation. An ultrasound probe is used to examine four key windows for fluid; the subxiphoid area permits visualization of the pericardium, the left subcostal area visualization of the splenorenal recess, right subcostal area visualization of Morison's pouch, and the suprapubic area visualization of the pelvic cul-de-sac (Fig. 1.1). The presence of fluid may indicate presence of cardiac tamponade, intra-abdominal hemorrhage, hollow viscus perforation, hemoperitoneum, or ascites. False-positive results secondary to preexisting ascites or false negatives due to operator error or body habitus are the main limitations. Scanning the suprapubic area with distension of the urinary bladder will enhance the sensitivity of the exam for the detection of pelvic fluid.

A threshold of at least 200 mL of fluid in the abdominal cavity is necessary for detection; intra-abdominal injuries must be associated with the presence of this much free fluid for a positive finding.[32] Reported sensitivities range between 73% and 88% and specificity between 98% and 100%.[33] Accuracy rates range from 96% to 98%. FAST is an inexpensive, rapid, portable, noninvasive technique that can be performed in serial fashion if patient stability changes.[34-36] Additionally, it obviates the risk of exposing pregnant females to radiation. Positive findings in stable patients can be further evaluated with CT or DPL while unstable patients with a positive finding may be taken to the operating room for emergent exploration. Workup of a patient with a reliable abdominal exam may be complete with a negative FAST in the absence of abdominal signs or symptoms. However, in the patient with significant mechanism of injury, we generally follow a negative FAST with CT of the chest and abdomen.

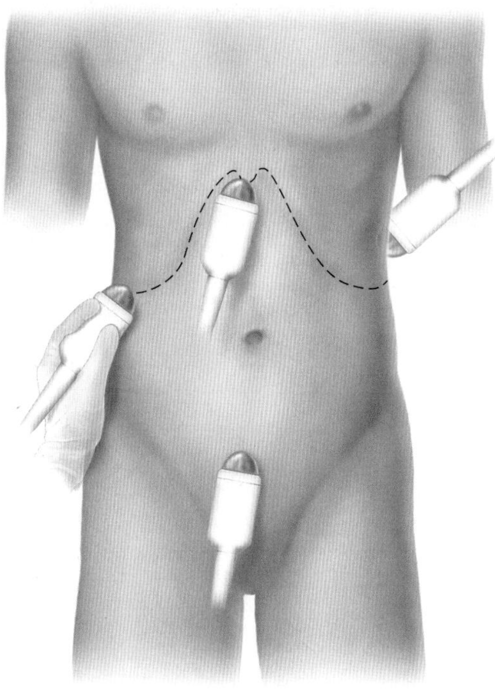

FIGURE 1.1. Schematic showing sonographic windows for (1) subxiphoid, (2) left subcostal, (3) right subcostal and suprapubic areas. Distension of the urinary bladder either prior to Foley's catheter placement or by installation of 150-200 mL normal saline will enhance sensitivity. (Redrawn from Rozycki GS, Ochsner MG, Schmidt JA, et al. A prospective study of surgeon-performed ultrasound as the primary adjuvant modality for injured patient assessment. *J Trauma.* 1995;39:492-498; discussion 498-500.)

Computed Tomography

Technologic advances in CT have revolutionized the initial management of trauma patients over the past two decades. Multidetector scanners have dramatically improved resolution and accuracy of these imaging studies. Negative predictive values as high as 99.63% have been reported for patients sustaining major mechanisms of blunt trauma, allowing the use of CT as a reliable and noninvasive screening tool for screening patients with blunt abdominal trauma. In light of modern-day CT capabilities, prospective data have demonstrated that patients with an important mechanism and a benign abdomen can be released from the emergency department if a CT scan of the abdomen shows no evidence of visceral injury provided that there are no other reasons for hospitalization.[37]

CT reliably identifies injuries in solid organs such as the spleen, liver, and kidney because of their vascular anatomy, demonstrating disruption of normal architecture, associated free fluid, and the so-called vascular blush. Similar grading scales have been developed to allow for accurate classification and determination of management plan (Tables 1.3-1.5).[38,39]

Detection of bowel injury via CT in patients who are intoxicated, intubated, or have associated closed head injury or other distracting injuries can present a diagnostic challenge in the absence of a reliable abdominal exam. The incidence of blunt bowel injury varies from series to series but is generally

TABLE 1.5

SPLEEN INJURY SCALE OF THE AAST

GRADE[a]	TYPE OF INJURY	INJURY DESCRIPTION	ICD-9[b]	AIS-90[c]
I	Hematoma	Subcapsular, <10% surface area	865.01 865.11	2
	Laceration	Capsular tear, <1 cm parenchymal depth	865.02 865.12	2
II	Hematoma	Subcapsular, 10%-50% surface area; intraparenchymal, <5 cm in diameter	865.01 865.11	2
	Laceration	1-3 cm parenchymal depth, which does not involve a trabecular vessel	865.02 865.12	2
III	Hematoma	Subcapsular, >50% surface area or expanding; ruptured subcapsular or parenchymal hematoma		3
	Laceration	Intraparenchymal hematoma >5 cm or expanding	865.03	3
		>3 cm parenchymal depth or involving trabecular vessels	865.13	
IV	Laceration	Laceration involving segmental or hilar vessels producing major devascularization (>25% of spleen)		4
V	Laceration	Completely shattered spleen	865.04	5
	Vascular	Hilar vascular injury, which devascularizes spleen	865.14	5

[a]Advance one grade for multiple injuries, up to grade III.
[b]ICD, International Classification of Diseases, 9th Revision.
[c]AIS, Abbreviated Injury Score.

reported in the 1%-5% range in all blunt trauma patients admitted to level 1 trauma centers.[40] A high index of suspicion is predicated on mechanism of injury and physical exam findings such as abdominal wall tattooing or seat belt sign. CT findings may be direct such as extravasation of oral contrast or pneumoperitoneum, or more commonly, indirect such as bowel wall thickening, stranding of the mesentery, or free fluid in the absence of solid organ injury. Indirect findings may be fairly nonspecific and secondary to bowel edema from resuscitation or preexisting ascites. Reproductive-age females may have a small amount of normal or "physiologic" pelvic fluid present, sometimes adding to the complexity of the evaluation. Patients on positive pressure ventilation or with substantial barotrauma may develop mediastinal or subcutaneous emphysema that can tract through the peritoneum or retroperitoneum and give the appearance of free air. Great care in the radiologic interpretation and close clinical correlation are necessary in such cases. The liberal use of DPL may prevent nontherapeutic laparotomy. Obviously, when significant doubt remains, abdominal exploration may be necessary to confirm an injury.

The role of oral contrast in the evaluation of the acutely injured patient has recently come under question. Little time is usually available in the emergent setting to permit adequate opacification of the small bowel. Patients are further at risk for aspiration of the contrast media and administration often requires placement of a nasogastric tube. Reports have shown that elimination of oral contrast media does not lead to an increased incident of missed bowel injury.[41,42] Many centers have now safely eliminated the use of oral contrast media from their routine trauma protocols, expediting management and ease of patient care. Resuscitation edema may cause a hazy appearance around the head of the pancreas and duodenal c-loop, raising the question of a pancreatic or duodenal injury. Further clarification in this situation can be obtained via repeat CT scan with the administration of oral contrast and the injection of 300-500-mL bolus of air down the nasogastric tube may make pneumoperitoneum obvious.

CT may also be of importance in identification in patients with arterial hemorrhage related to pelvic fracture. CT may demonstrate an arterial blush or large hematoma in the vicinity of a pelvic fracture, indicating the need for pelvic arteriography or pelvic external fixation. A "CT cystogram" may also be helpful and eliminate redundancy of x-ray evaluation. The Foley's catheter is clamped after placement in the trauma bay. Real-time interpretation as the CT is performed by the evaluating physician, which may dictate further delayed images or a formal three-view (anterior/posterior, lateral, and post void views) cystogram.

SPECIFIC ORGAN INJURY

The Spleen

The spleen is the most commonly injured intra-abdominal organ followed by the liver and small bowel in blunt trauma patients. The spleen's location in the left upper quadrant lends susceptibility to injury from broken ribs, deceleration, and blunt percussion forces. Clinically, patients with splenic injury may present with hypotension, left upper-quadrant pain or tenderness to palpation or diffuse peritonitis from extravasated blood. Referred pain to the left shoulder on deep inspiration, in face of splenic hematoma, is known as Kehr's sign.

NONOPERATIVE MANAGEMENT

Most series indicate that 60%-80% of patients presenting with blunt splenic injury can be managed nonoperatively at level I or II trauma centers.[43] Facilities without the resources and experience of a bonafide trauma team may not safely meet the demands of nonoperative management and should consider patient transfer.[44] Patients selected for nonoperative management must have stable vital signs, be free of peritoneal signs or other concern for hollow viscus injury, and have no evidence of free extravasation of IV contrast from the splenic parenchyma.

Considerable debate remains regarding risk factors for failure of nonoperative management. Higher American Association for the Surgery of Trauma (AAST) splenic injury grade, age >55 years, moderate to large hemoperitoneum, subcapsular hematoma, and portal hypertension have all been suggested to increase the risk of failure. Early reports in the evolution of nonoperative management regarding ASST grade did not demonstrate higher failure rates for higher grade injury. More recent reports using high-resolution multidetector CT scanners allow better assessment of injury grade. The data from these studies show that patients with injury grades III-V to be at increased risk for nonoperative failure.[45-47] Age continues to be controversial subject matter in the literature, with numerous reports claiming that age >55 years *is* or *is not* a risk factor for failure.[48,49] Documentation of a moderate or large hemoperitoneum is suggestive of a major injury and should be considered an important factor in individual patient assessment.

Patients with splenic subcapsular hematoma or history of portal hypertension are specific subgroups of patients who deserve special consideration. Patients with subcapsular hematoma in our experience tend to ooze from the raw parenchymal surface and further disrupt the capsule, leading to more raw surface area to bleed. These patients are at increased risk for delayed rupture 6-8 days following injury and may already be discharged from the hospital if they have isolated injury. Furthermore, splenic embolization is not an effective treatment of this condition because it usually necessitates coiling of the main splenic artery, which can lead to substantial pain and abscess formation. History of portal hypertension or cirrhosis, while not an absolute contraindication to nonoperative management, certainly should raise concerns. The general risks of laparotomy in a Childs B or C cirrhotic need to be carefully weighed against the risk of ensuing and worsening coagulopathy. This scenario may, indeed, call for main splenic artery embolization. None of these risk factors alone should dictate the decision to proceed immediately to operative intervention. Nonoperative management does reduce hospital length of stay and transfusion requirement; however, the morbidity of splenectomy should remain low in any surgeon's hands. Overall, the patient's condition including comorbidities, coagulopathy, and other problems (such as traumatic brain injury, aortic injury, and suspicion for concomitant hollow viscus injury) factor into the decision-making process. No one undergoing nonoperative management should ever succumb to splenic hemorrhage.

BLUNT SPLENIC INJURY—GENERAL PRINCIPLES OF MANAGEMENT

Approximately 20% of patients initially undergoing nonoperative management of blunt splenic injury require further intervention (Algorithm. 1.12). Failure has been associated with the presence of a contrast blush in up to two-thirds of these patients.[50] The presence of a contained contrast blush within the parenchyma of the spleen represents pseudoaneurysm formation of a branch of the splenic artery. Angioembolization is now commonly used to selectively occlude the arterial branches containing these injuries.[51] Implementation of this salvage technique at centers that routinely screen for the presence of pseudoaneurysm has increased the success of nonoperative management to 90% or greater. Pseudoaneurysm formation has been observed in even grade I and II injuries and may not be present on the initial imaging.[52] Therefore, follow-up CT scan is recommended on all patients with splenic trauma within 24-48 hours after injury. If these images show stable injuries without pseudoaneurysm formation, expectant management may ensue.

Long-term data are unavailable concerning the risk of outpatient or delayed rupture, but the incidence is low and has been reported to be about 1.4%.[53] The average date to readmission for delayed splenectomy after discharge was 8 days in this study. Lower grade (I and II) injuries tend to heal more quickly and most injuries are healed by 5-6 weeks.[54] However, approximately 20% of blunt splenic injuries will not show complete healing and may be at risk for pseudocyst formation. CT should be repeated in 6 weeks for grade I and II injuries and 10–12 weeks in grades III-V before reinstating patients to normal activity.

Splenectomy

Patients requiring urgent or emergent intervention for splenic hemorrhage may develop hypothermia, coagulopathy, and visceral edema. The most expeditious and safest course of action under these conditions is removal of the spleen. The general assumption of abdominal exploration for trauma is that there are known and, possibly, unknown injuries. The operative approach is via a midline vertical incision that allows the best exposure and facilitates temporary abdominal closure should visceral edema or damage control measures be necessary. Standard operating procedure is similar to that previously highlighted in the section, "Management of Penetrating Abdominal Trauma."

With respect to performing a splenectomy, a self-retaining (Buckwalter, Thompson, Rochard, etc.) retractor is used to expose the left upper quadrant. The spleen is retracted medially with some downward compression and the posterior attachments can be taken with the cautery. Once these attachments are freed, the spleen can be mobilized medially for optimal exposure. The assistant stands on the left side of the table and supports the spleen while the surgeon ligates short gastric and hilar vessels. Being careful to avoid the tail of the pancreas, a large clip, placed on the specimen side of the splenic hilum, will reduce back-bleeding and expedite the procedure. Once the spleen has been removed, the splenic fossa is inspected for further bleeding with a rolled laparotomy pad.

Splenorrhaphy

Hemodynamically stable patients found to have small to moderate amounts of parenchymal hemorrhage at laparotomy may be candidates for splenic preservation. The spleen is mobilized into the wound using the same technique as for splenectomy. The injury to the spleen is assessed and decision is made whether to resect a portion if the parenchymal injury extends into the hilum or if arterial bleeding is coming from within the splenic laceration itself. If the decision is made to resect the upper or lower pole, the parenchyma is divided with the cautery and the associated hilar vessels are taken with clamps and ties. Any arterial bleeding from the parenchyma is controlled with suture ligature and the cautery is used to control oozing from the parenchyma. A tongue of omentum is then sutured into the laceration or to the raw surface of the remaining spleen in the

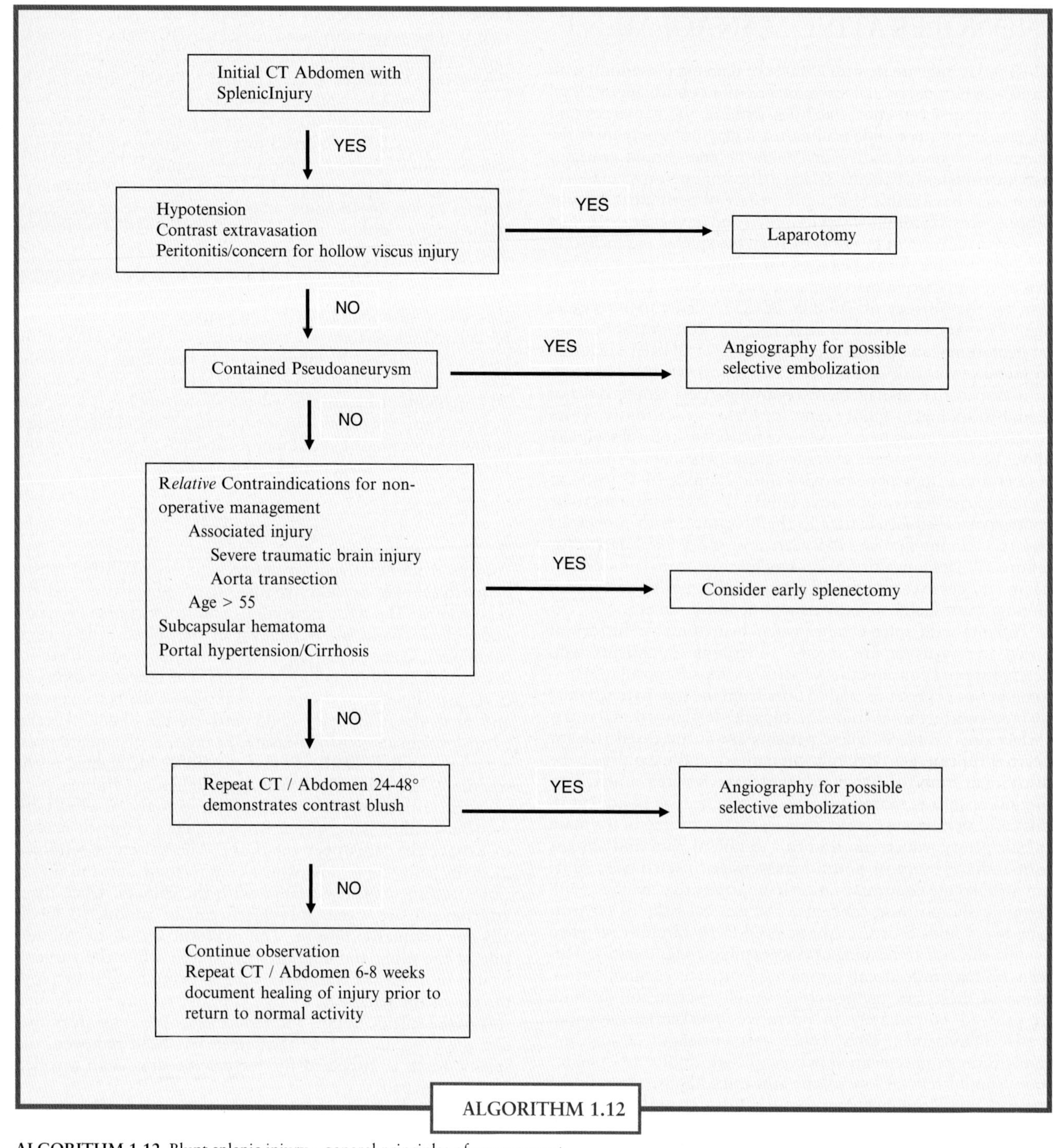

ALGORITHM 1.12 Blunt splenic injury—general principles of management.

case of resection. Approximately 50% of the spleen is required to preserve adequate phagocytic and immunologic function. If this cannot be achieved, a splenectomy is probably the best option, with appropriate postsplenectomy immunization.[55,56]

THE LIVER

The liver is susceptible to the same blunt force mechanisms as the spleen, making it the second most frequently injured intra-abdominal organ. Similar to the spleen, nonoperative management of blunt liver injury has reduced transfusion requirements, hospital length of stay, and mortality.[57-60] Angiographic embolization of arterial injury has also reduced the morbidity and mortality of liver trauma. Complications of nonoperative management such as biloma and liver abscess can usually be managed with minimally invasive techniques as well. What is imperative in the management scheme is to know when to take the patient immediately to the operating room for active hemorrhage versus attempting nonoperative management with angioembolization. The liver is obviously not as expendable an organ as the spleen, and there is no substitute for an in-depth knowledge and experience handling hepatic injuries.

Nonoperative Management

Similar to the experience with blunt splenic trauma, routine use of CT has revolutionized the management of blunt hepatic trauma. The most recent data show that 70%-85% of all patients presenting with blunt liver injury can be managed nonoperatively.[61,62] Patients must be hemodynamically stable, free of peritoneal signs or other evidence of bowel injury, and have absence of contrast extravasation. Worsening grade of injury makes nonoperative management less likely but injury grade alone should *not* dictate the decision to intervene.[63,64] Patients should have stable systolic blood pressure >90 mm Hg with a heart rate <100 bpm after controlling other possible sources of extraabdominal blood loss, such as orthopedic and soft tissue injuries. Failure from subsequent liver hemorrhage occurs in 0.4%-5% of patients and failure due to missed injury of other intra-abdominal organs, such as the kidney, spleen, pancreas and bowel, occurs in 0.5%-15% of patients.[65] The results of these data are summarized in Table 1.6. It is difficult to tell the specific cause of immediate surgery in the earlier reports because laparotomy for *all* causes, such as associated splenic hemorrhage, was included.

Angiographic embolization is a useful adjunct in the management of blunt hepatic trauma both in nonoperative patients and those who have undergone damage control laparotomy in a number of small series.[66-70] Intravenous contrast extravasation from the liver parenchyma into the peritoneal cavity and contrast contained within the parenchyma of the liver associated with a large amount of intraperitoneal blood on initial CT scan are emergent situations mandating angiographic embolization or surgery.[71] If bleeding appears to originate from the retrohepatic vena cava or hepatic veins and it is ongoing, emergent exploration is the only option because arterial embolization is ineffective in these scenarios. Patients with labile blood pressure and parenchymal injury may be better served with emergent exploration depending on the time necessary to assemble the angiography team. However, if angiography is readily available, favorable results have been obtained transporting patients to the angiography suite with ongoing resuscitation for arterial bleeding.[72] Patients requiring significant resuscitation during a successful embolization procedure may still be at risk for abdominal compartment syndrome and should have bladder pressures monitored.[73]

Patients with contrast extravasation contained within the liver parenchyma without significant associated hemoperitoneum are less worrisome but should probably undergo arteriogram for further assessment. A perceived contrast blush on CT scan is associated with bleeding identified at angiography in 60% of patients.

Operative Management

Bleeding from minor liver injuries (grades I and II) usually stops spontaneously and surgical intervention is rarely required.[74] Occasionally, patients may require exploration for other injuries after abdominal trauma in the presence of minor liver trauma. Nonbleeding liver injuries should be left alone. In the face of coagulopathy or hypothermia, minor hepatic injuries may present with persistent oozing. In such cases, topical hemostatic agents, with or without perihepatic packing, may be all that is necessary to stop the bleeding if the patient is being adequately resuscitated.

Major liver injuries (grades III-V) are more likely to bleed and require surgical intervention. Because grade IV and V liver injuries can present formidable technical challenges even in the hands of the most capable individuals, a variety of surgical techniques have been developed for their management.

Large liver wounds should be quickly inspected to get some idea about the degree of hemorrhage and packed initially. Anesthesia should be notified about anticipated blood loss and blood availability checked. Vital signs and resuscitation status should be reviewed. Bleeding should be contained with packing and direct pressure until anesthesia has had time to "catch up." Remaining focused and well organized, as well replenishing intravascular volume is invaluable in the management of any trauma patient.

The most direct approach at this point is to remove the packing and visually inspect for bleeding vessels, which can be individually ligated. Debridement of devitalized tissue using finger fracture technique will expose additional bleeding vessels, which may have retracted into the surrounding parenchyma. If bleeding prevents adequate visualization of the surgical field, the next step should be vascular control of the portal triad (e.g., Pringle's maneuver). This maneuver is easiest to perform for the person standing on the left of the patient. This individual places the fingers of the left hand into the foramen of Winslow and he/she uses the thumb to palpate for the cord of tissue running into the caudal surface of the liver. Once this structure is suspected, its identity can generally be confirmed by appreciating the pulse in the hepatic artery. A hole is then created in the hepatoduodenal ligament using blunt finger dissection. A noncrushing vascular clamp or a half-inch Penrose's drain or vessel loop can be double-looped around the porta and cinched down with a Kelly clamp. We prefer the latter technique because it seems to be less obtrusive to further manipulation of the liver and may be less traumatic to the structures of the porta hepatis.

TABLE 1.6

FAILURE RATES FOR NONOPERATIVE MANAGEMENT OF LIVER TRAUMA

STUDY (YEAR)	NUMBER OF PATIENTS	IMMEDIATE SURGERY (%)	OVERALL FAILURE RATE (%)	LIVER FAILURE RATE (%)	OTHER FAILURE RATE (%)
Meredith (1994)	116	48	3	3	0
Croce (1995)	136	18	11	5	6
Pacther (1996)	404	53	1.2	0.7	0.5
Malhotra (2000)	661	15	7	3	4
Velmahos (2003)	78	29[a]	15	0	15
Christmas (2005)	561	32[b]	1.8	0.4	1.4

Other Failure refers failure due to injuries from other intra-abdominal organs such as the spleen, kidney, pancreas, or bowel.
[a]15% for liver bleeding.
[b]13% for liver bleeding.

If a Pringle's maneuver does not adequately decrease liver bleeding, then concern for hepatic vein or retrohepatic caval injury should be entertained. Obtaining adequate exposure in deep liver wounds or in juxtahepatic caval injuries is of utmost importance. The falciform ligament is taken off the diaphragm posteriorly to the bare area. The right and left triangular ligaments are dissected with the cautery, along extension to the corresponding coronary ligaments. Further dissection of the coronary ligaments to the bare area will allow full mobilization of the liver into the surgical field. Careful dissection of the bare area will allow access to the suprahepatic inferior vena cava. If the plane in the bare area is difficult to develop, a transverse incision in the diaphragm here will gain access to the pericardium and intrapericardial control of the inferior vena cava can be achieved. Total hepatic isolation can be achieved with a Pringle's maneuver and vascular control of the infrahepatic, suprarenal inferior vena cava, and the suprahepatic intra-abdominal or intrapericardial inferior vena cava. The physiologic stress of this technique may not be well tolerated in patients with severe shock and clamp times <20-30 minutes should be maintained.

INTESTINE

A missed intestinal injury may have devastating consequences. Therefore, the basic principle in the management of hollow viscus injuries is operative intervention. In general, the surgical management is straightforward: debridement of any devitalized tissue and primary closure of a simple enterotomy. However, for more destructive injuries, segmental resection and primary anastomosis (or stomal formation) will likely be required.

Knowledge of the AAST organ injury grading scale is helpful in describing wounds of the bowel[75] (Tables 1.7 and 1.8). Grade I injury is contusion or partial thickness laceration of the bowel wall without perforation. Grade II injury is a full-thickness wound involving <50% of the bowel wall circumference. Grade III is a laceration comprising >50% of the bowel wall circumference without complete transection. Grades IV and V injuries represent complete transection of the bowel wall and transection with segmental tissue loss or devascularization of the mesentery, respectively. The terms destructive and nondestructive simplify the terminology; nondestructive wounds are those injuries that can be managed with debridement and primary suture enterorrhaphy and are comprised of grades I through III. Destructive wounds necessitate resection of an entire segment of the bowel due to loss of colonic integrity or devascularization of the mesentery and encompass grades IV and V.

The distinction between destructive and nondestructive wounds is important in terms of the prescribed management. Nondestructive wounds of the large or small bowel can generally be repaired without further consideration. Most small bowel and large destructive injuries should be resected and reconstituted unless "damage control" management is planned.[74,76-78]

LUNG AND CHEST WALL

The most common lung injury in blunt trauma is pulmonary contusion. These specific injuries are managed expectantly and supportively. Extensive injury will likely dictate the need for endotracheal intubation and the administration of positive pressure ventilation to optimize oxygenation. A thoracotomy will likely be required for left or right mainstem bronchial tears with associated major airleak. Other indications for early operative intervention include a massive hemothorax (1,500 mL or greater or blood initially evacuated from the pleural space upon insertion of a chest tube or >200 mL per hour of blood chest tube drainage for successive hours). Operative fixation or chest wall stabilization by plating fractured ribs has gained some popularity for multiple rib fractures or a flail chest.[79,80]

TABLE 1.7

AAST SMALL BOWEL INJURY SCALE

GRADE[a]	TYPE OF INJURY	DESCRIPTION OF INJURY	ICD-9[b]	AIS-90[c]
I	Hematoma	Contusion or hematoma without devascularization	863.20-863.31	2
	Laceration	Partial thickness, no perforation		2
II	Laceration	Laceration <50% of circumference	863.20-863.31	3
III	Laceration	Laceration ≥50% of circumference without transaction		3
IV	Laceration	Transection of the small bowel	863.20-863.31	4
V	Laceration	Transection of the small bowel with segmental tissue loss	863.20-863.31	4
	Vascular	Devascularized segment		4

[a]Advance one grade for multiple injuries, up to grade III.
[b]ICD, International Classification of Diseases, 9th Revision.
[c]AIS, Abbreviated Injury Score.

TABLE 1.8

AAST COLON INJURY SCALE

GRADE[A]	TYPE OF INJURY	DESCRIPTION OF INJURY	ICD-9[B]	AIS-90[C]
I	Hematoma	Contusion or hematoma without devascularization	863.40 863.44	2
	Laceration	Partial thickness, no perforation	863.40 863.44	2
II	Laceration	Laceration ≤50% of circumference	863.50 863.54	3
III	Laceration	Laceration >50% of circumference	863.50 863.54	
IV	Laceration	Transection of the colon	863.50 863.54	4
V	Laceration	Transection of the colon with segmental tissue loss	863.50 863.54	4

ICD-9:4, .51 = ascending; 42, .52 = transverse; 43, .53 = descending; .44, .54 = rectum.
[a]Advance one grade for multiple injuries, up to grade III.
[b]ICD, International Classification of Diseases.
[c]AIS, Abbreviated Injury Score.

ACUTE CARE SURGERY—GENERAL PRINCIPLES: SUMMARY

As highlighted above, the core principle of acute care surgery is expeditious and effective medical/surgical management, with early diagnosis an essential element. Many of the general principles of trauma management are applicable in the nontrauma setting. However, each specific disease entity has its own unique diagnostic/management paradigm that is covered throughout the textbook. Depending on the regional geography, the disease (nontrauma) entities that are most commonly encountered by the acute care surgeon are outlined in Table 1.9.

The severity of the disease and the stage of presentation, along with the status of the patient (e.g., hemodynamic stability) will often dictate the specific course of management (operative vs. nonoperative approach).

TABLE 1.9

COMMONLY ENCOUNTERED DISEASE ENTITIES

Appendicitis
Intestinal obstruction
Diverticulitis and deep (cartilage) of tissue, abscesses
Necrotizing soft tissue infection
Biliary diseases
Pancreatitis
Gastrointestinal bleeding
Mesentery ischemia
Inflammatory intestinal disease
Perforated hollow viscus

References

1. Abramson D, Scalea TM, Hitchcock R, et al. Lactate clearance and survival following injury. *J Trauma*. 1993;35:584.
2. Rouse DA. Patterns of stab wounds: a six year study. *Med Sch Law.* 1994;34:67-71.
3. Dimaio VJM. *Gunshot Wounds: Practical Aspects of Firearms, Ballistics, and Forensic Techniques*. Boca Raton, FL: CRC Press; 1985:163-226, 257-265.
4. Moore EE, Dunn EL, Moore JB, et al. Penetrating abdominal index. *J Trauma*. 1981;21:439-442.
5. Croce MA, et al. Correlation of abdominal trauma index and injury severity score with abdominal septic complications in penetrating and blunt trauma. *J Trauma*. 1992;32:380-392.
6. Demernada D, Rabinowitz B. Indications for operation in abdominal stab wounds. *Ann Surg*. 1987;205:129-132.
7. Shore, RM Gottlieb MM, Webb R, et al. Selective management of abdominal stab wounds. *Arch Surg*. 1988;123:1141-1145.
8. Kester DE, Andrassy RJ, Aust JB. The value and cost effectiveness of abdominal roentgenograms in the evaluation of stab wounds to the abdomen. *Surg Gynenol Obstet*. 1986;162:337.
9. Root HD, Hauser CW, McKinley CR, et al. Dianostic peritioneal lavage. *Surgery*. 1965;57:633.
10. Merlotti GJ, et al. Use of peritoneal lavage to evaluate abdominal penetration. *J Trauma*. 1985;25:228.
11. Thal ER. Peritoneal lavage: reliability of RBC count in patients with stab wounds to the chest. *Arch Surg*. 1984;119:579.
12. Oreskovich MR, Crrico CJ. Stab wounds of the anterior abdomen: analysis of management plan using local wound exploration and quantative peritoneal lavage. *Ann Surg*. 1983;198:411.
13. Alyono D, Morrwo CE, Perry JF Jr. RE-appraisal of diagnostic peritoneal lavage criteria for operation in penetrating and blunt trauma. *Surgery*. 1982;92:751.
14. Feliciano DV, et al. Five hundred open taps or lavages in patients with abdominal stab wounds. *Am J Surg*. 1984;148:772.
15. Hauser CJ, et al. Triple contrast computed tomography in the evaluation of penetrating posterior abdominal injuries. *Arch Surg*. 1987;122:1112.
16. Demetriades D, Cahralambides D, Lakhoo M, et al. Gunshot wounds of the abdomen: the role of selective conservative management. *Br J Surg*. 1996;78:220.
17. Kristensen JK, Bueman B, Kuhl E. Ultrasonic scanning in the diagnostic splenic hematoma. *Acta Chir Scand*. 1971;137:653-657.
18. Kimura A, Otsuka T. Emergency center ultrasonography in the evaluation of hemoperitoneum: a prospective study. *J Trauma*. 1991;31:20.
19. Rozycki GS, Ochsner MG, Schmidt JA, et al. A prospective study of surgeon-performed ultrasound as the primary adjuvant modality for injured patient assessment. *J Trauma*. 1995;39:492-498.
20. Ivatury RR, Simon RJ, Stahl WM. A critical evaluation of laparoscopy in penetrating abdominal trauma. *J Trauma*. 1993;34:822.

21. Fabian TC, Croce MA, Stewart RM, et al. A prospective analysis of diagnostic laparoscopy in trauma. *Ann Surg*. 1993;217:557.
22. George SM, Fabian TC, Voeller GR, et al. Primary repair of colon wounds. *Ann Surg*. 1989;209:728-734.
23. Vaughan G, Grazie O, Graham D, et al. The use of pylric exclusion in the management of severe duodenal injuies. *Am J Surg*. 1977;134:785.
24. Cogbill T, Moore EF, Feliciano DV, et al. Conservative management of duodenal traumas: a multi-center perspective. *J Trauma*. 1990;30:1461.
25. Asensio J, Feliciano DV, Britt LD, et al. Management of complex duodenal injuries. *Curr Probl Surg*. 1993;30:1023-1093.
26. Rotondo MF, Schwab CW, McGonigal MD, et al. "Damage control": an approach for improved survival in exsanguinating penetrating abdominal injury. *J Trauma*. 1993;35:375-381.
27. Shapiro MB, Jenkins DH, Schwab CW, et al. Damage control: collective review. *J Trauma*. 2000;49:969-978.
28. Feliciano DV, Mattox KL, Jordan GL. Intraabdominal packing for control of hepatic hemorrhage: a reappraisal. *J Trauma*. 1981;21:285-291.
29. Burch JM, Ortiz VB, Richardson RJ, et al. Abbreviated laparotomy and planned reoperation for critically injured patients. *Ann Surg*. 1992,215:476-483.
30. Hirschberg A, Mattox KL. Planned reoperation for severe trauma. *Ann Surg*. 1995;222:3-8.
31. MacKenzie EJ, et al. A national evaluation of the effect of trauma-center care on mortality. *N Engl J Med*. 2006;354(4):366-378.
32. Branney SW, et al. Quantitative sensitivity of ultrasound in detecting free intraperitoneal fluid. *J Trauma*. 1995;39(2):375-180.
33. Hoff WS, et al. Practice management guidelines for the evaluation of blunt abdominal trauma: the East practice management guidelines work group. *J Trauma*. 2002;53(3):602-615.
34. Rozycki GS, et al. A prospective study of surgeon-performed ultrasound as the primary adjuvant modality for injured patient assessment. *J Trauma*. 1995;39(3):492-498; discussion 498-500.
35. Boulanger BR, et al. Emergent abdominal sonography as a screening test in a new diagnostic algorithm for blunt trauma. *J Trauma*. 1996;40(6):867-874.
36. Branney SW, et al. Ultrasound based key clinical pathway reduces the use of hospital resources for the evaluation of blunt abdominal trauma. *J Trauma*. 1997;42(6):1086-1090.
37. Livingston DH, et al. Admission or observation is not necessary after a negative abdominal computed tomographic scan in patients with suspected blunt abdominal trauma: results of a prospective, multi-institutional trial. *J Trauma*. 1998;44(2):273-280; discussion 280-282.
38. Moore EE, et al. Organ injury scaling: spleen and liver (1994 revision). *J Trauma*. 1995;38(3): 323-324
39. Moore EE, et al. Organ injury scaling: spleen, liver, and kidney. *J Trauma*. 1989;29(12):1664-1666.
40. Holmes JF, et al. Performance of helical computed tomography without oral contrast for the detection of gastrointestinal injuries. *Ann Emerg Med*. 2004;43(1):120-128.
41. Stafford RE, et al. Oral contrast solution and computed tomography for blunt abdominal trauma: a randomized study. *Arch Surg*. 1999;134(6): 622-626; discussion 626-627.
42. Allen TL, et al. Computed tomographic scanning without oral contrast solution for blunt bowel and mesenteric injuries in abdominal trauma. *J Trauma*. 2004;56(2):314-322.
43. Bee TK, et al. *Failures of* splenic nonoperative management: is the glass half empty or half full? *J Trauma*. 2001;50(2):230-236.
44. Peitzman AB, et al. Blunt splenic injury in adults: Multi-institutional Study of the Eastern Association for the Surgery of Trauma. *J Trauma*. 2000;49(2):177-187; discussion 187-189.
45. Weinberg JA, et al. The utility of serial computed tomography imaging of blunt splenic injury; still worth a second look? *J Trauma*. 2007;62(5):1143-1147; discussion 1147-1148.
46. Gaarder C, et al. Nonoperative management of splenic injuries: improved results with angioembolization. *J Trauma*. 2006;61(1):192-198.
47. Haan JM, et al. Splenic embolization revisited: a multicenter review. *J Trauma*. 2004;56(3):542-547.
48. Meyers JG, et al. Blunt splenic injuries: dedicated trauma surgeons can achieve a high rate of nonoperative success in patients of all ages. *J Trauma*. 2000;48(5):801-805: discussion 805-806.
49. Cocanour CS, et al. Age should not be a consideration for nonoperative management of blunt splenic injury. *J Trauma*. 2000;48(4):606-610: discussion 610-612.
50. Schurr MJ, et al. Management of blunt splenic trauma: computed tomographic contrast blush predicts failure of nonoperative management. *J Trauma*. 1995;39(3):507-512; discussion 512-513.
51. Raikhlin A, et al. Imaging and transcatheter arterial embolization for traumatic splenic injuries: review of the literature. *Can J Surg*. 2008;51(6):464-472.
52. Davis KA, et al. Improved success in nonoperative management of blunt splenic injuries: embolization of splenic artery pseudoaneurysms. *J Trauma*. 1998;44(6):p. 1008-1013: discussion 1013-1015.
53. Zarzaur BL, et al. The real risk of splenectomy after discharge home following nonoperative management of blunt splenic injury. *J Trauma*. 2009;66(6):1531-1536; discussion 1536-1538.
54. Savage SA, et al. The evolution of blunt splenic injury: resolution and progression. *J Trauma*. 2008;64(4):1085-1091; discussion 1091-1092.
55. Holdsworth RJ, Irving AD, Cuschieri A. Postsplenectomy sepsis and its mortality rate: actual versus perceived risks. *Br J Surg*. 1991;78(9):1031-1038.
56. American Academy of Pediatrics. Committee on Infectious Diseases. Policy statement: recommendations for the prevention of pneumococcal infections, including the use of pneumococcal conjugate vaccine (Prevnar), pneumococcal polysaccharide vaccine, and antibiotic prophylaxis. *Pediatrics*. 2000;106(2 pt 1):362-366.
57. Croce MA, et al. Nonoperative management of blunt hepatic trauma is the treatment of choice for hemodynamically stable patients. Results of a prospective trial. *Ann Surg*. 1995;221(6):744-753; discussion 753-755.
58. Malhotra AK, et al. Blunt hepatic injury: a paradigm shift from operative to nonoperative management in the 1990s. *Ann Surg*. 2000;231(6):804-813.
59. Delius RE, Frankel W, Coran AG. A comparison between operative and nonoperative management of blunt injuries to the liver and spleen in adult and pediatric patients. *Surgery*, 1989;106(4):788-792; discussion 792-793.
60. Christmas AB, et al. Selective management of blunt hepatic injuries including nonoperative management is a safe and effective strategy. *Surgery*. 2005;138(4):606-610; discussion 610-611.
61. Velmahos GC, et al. High success with nonoperative management of blunt hepatic trauma: the liver is a sturdy organ. *Arch Surg*. 2003;138(5): 475-480; discussion 480-481.
62. David Richardson J, et al. Evolution in the management of hepatic trauma: a 25-year perspective. *Ann Surg*. 2000;232(3):324-330.
63. Meredith JW, et al. Nonoperative management of blunt hepatic trauma: the exception or the rule? *J Trauma*. 1994;36(4):529-534; discussion 534-535.
64. Pachter HL, et al. Status of nonoperative management of blunt hepatic injuries in 1995: a multicenter experience with 404 patients. *J Trauma*. 1996;40(1):31-38.
65. Wahl WL, et al. The need for early angiographic embolization in blunt liver injuries. *J Trauma*. 2002;52(6):1097-1101.
66. Johnson JW, et al. Hepatic angiography in patients undergoing damage control laparotomy. *J Trauma*. 2002;52(6):1102-1106.
67. Mohr AM, et al. Angiographic embolization for liver injuries: low mortality, high morbidity. *J Trauma*. 2003;55(6):1077-1081; discussion 1081-1082.
68. Hagiwara A, et al. The usefulness of transcatheter arterial embolization for patients with blunt polytrauma showing transient response to fluid resuscitation. *J Trauma*. 2004;57(2):271-276; discussion 276-277.
69. Misselbeck TS, et al. Hepatic angioembolization in trauma patients: indications and complications. *J Trauma*. 2009;67(4):769-773.
70. Asensio JA, et al. Approach to the management of complex hepatic injuries. *J Trauma*. 2000;48(1):66-69.
71. Fang JF, et al. Classification and treatment of pooling of contrast material on computed tomographic scan of blunt hepatic trauma. *J Trauma*. 2000;49(6):1083-1088.
72. Ciraulo DL, et al. Selective hepatic arterial embolization of grade IV and V blunt hepatic injuries: an extension of resuscitation in the nonoperative management of traumatic hepatic injuries. *J Trauma*. 1998;45(2):353-358; discussion 358-359.
73. Maxwell RA, et al. Secondary abdominal compartment syndrome: an underappreciated manifestation of severe hemorrhagic shock. *J Trauma*. 1999;47(6):995-999.
74. Moore EE, et al. Organ injury scaling, II: Pancreas, duodenum, small bowel, colon, and rectum. *J Trauma*. 1990;30(11):1427-1429.
75. Pachter HL, et al. Significant trends in the treatment of hepatic trauma. Experience with 411 injuries. *Ann Surg*. 1992;215(5):492-500; discussion 500-502.
76. Cayten CG, Fabian TC, Garcia VF, et al. Patient management guidelines for penetrating colon injury. *Eastern Association of the Surgery of Trauma*, 1998. Trauma Practice Guidelines(http://www.east.org).
77. Chavarria-Aguilar M, et al. Management of destructive bowel injury in the open abdomen. *J Trauma*. 2004;56(3):560-564.
78. Demetriades D, et al. Penetrating colon injuries requiring resection: diversion or primary anastomosis? An AAST prospective multicenter study. *J Trauma*. 2001;50(5):765-775.
79. Ahmed Z, Mohyuddin Z. Management of flail check injury: Internal fixation versus endotracheal intubation and ventilation. *J Thorac Cardiothorac Surg*. 1995;110:1676.
80. Voggenreiter G, Neudeck F, Aufmolk M, et al. Operative chest wall stabilization in flail chest—outcomes of patients with or without pulmonary contusion. *J Am Coll Surg*. 1998;187:130.

CHAPTER 2 ■ TRAINING IN ACUTE CARE SURGERY

GREGORY J. JURKOVICH

Training in acute care surgery has been formalized in an advanced surgical training fellowship that is currently endorsed and sponsored by the American Association for the Surgery of Trauma (AAST).[1,2] The AAST is a professional surgical society that was founded in 1938 and has been the academic home for trauma surgeons in North America. The curriculum for acute care surgery fellowships is outlined below (Table 2.1), as well as detailed on the AAST Web site (http://www.aast.org/Library/AcuteCareSurgery/Default.aspx).

Fundamental to this training is an emphasis on the three main components of acute care surgery: trauma, surgical critical care, and emergency general surgery. Key structural components of the curriculum are that it is 2 years in length and includes within its content an Accreditation Council on Graduate Medical Education (ACGME)-approved surgical critical care residency, as well as advanced surgical training in trauma care and emergency general surgical care. Applicants must have finished an ACGME-approved general surgery residency. Throughout this chapter, the term "residency" means a formal training program approved by the Surgery Residency Review Committee (RRC) of the Accreditation Council for Graduate Medical Education. The term "fellowship" means a formal training program that is similar to ACGME-accredited residencies, but is *not an* ACGME-accredited program. Current examples of such "fellowships" include minimally invasive surgery, acute care surgery, transplantation, breast surgery, and others. Some fellowships are generally in newer or developing fields and are considering seeking formal ACGME accreditation in the future. Other fellowships (including some established ones) are less inclined to seek ACGME overnight due to the reimbursement restrictions on resident care mandated by federal funding sources and the increasingly stringent additional requirements (e.g., duty hour limitations).

The curriculum includes a dedicated minimum of 9 months of surgical critical care, as mandated by the ACGME for accredited surgical critical care residencies. In the majority of the programs, this results in having a 1-year surgical critical care fellowship, along with an additional year of clinical operative experience in trauma and emergency general surgery. Only a program with an ACGME-accredited surgical critical care residency can be eligible for AAST approval for an acute care surgery training program.

The remaining 12-15 months are focused on operative rotations in emergency and elective surgery, with the expectation that there will be at least 12 months of acute care surgical on-call experience, or a minimum of 52 nights of trauma and emergency general surgery call. The 12-15 months of operative rotations have as a foundation time spent on an active acute care surgical service. This is ideally supplemented by three specific rotations in thoracic, vascular, and hepatobiliary–pancreatic surgery, with the expectation that these rotations will provide supplemental and advanced exposure to surgical skills and patient care challenges that often are inadequate in core general surgery training. It is felt that these three specific areas of advanced specialty training are needed to fully prepare a surgeon for the clinical challenges of emergency trauma and nontrauma surgery.

While there is considerable flexibility allowed in these new training fellowships, it is suggested that there is time spent on trauma orthopedics and neurosurgical services, with additional elective time to be allocated to meet the needs of the trainee. The expectation is that trainees will be competent in the management of a wide spectrum of acute care surgical needs and have specific operative competency in the procedures listed in Table 2.2.

In summary, the clinical component of these fellowships includes the following key areas:

1. The program should supply the necessary volume and variety of trauma, critical care, and emergency general surgery to ensure adequate training of fellows.
2. Each fellow must have ample opportunity and responsibility for the care of patients with acute surgical problems, and the operative experience must be consistent with developing competency in technical skills and procedures required to provide acute surgical care.
3. Elective general surgery is an essential component of the training of acute care surgeons.
4. Emergency surgical call and trauma call are mandatory components of the training curriculum. Fellows will take a minimum of 52 trauma and emergency surgery night calls during the 2-year fellowship.
5. Elective operative experience in thoracic, vascular, and complex hepatobiliary and pancreatic procedures are strongly encouraged as a means of developing competency in the management of acute surgical emergencies in these anatomic regions.
6. Working knowledge of the diagnosis, management, and operative treatment of neurosurgical and orthopedic injuries is expected.
7. Experience with the use of interventional radiology techniques is encouraged.
8. Experience and competency with diagnostic upper and lower gastrointestinal (GI) endoscopy and bronchoscopy are encouraged.

As of early 2011, there were seven formally approved training sites, one pending approval, with another estimated 10-20 programs in various stages of considering submitting applications for approved training sites.

The history of how the AAST became the sponsoring organization and pushed the development of acute care surgery fellowships is worthy of comment. Trauma surgery as a unique academic surgical specialty had its roots in the urban county hospitals of the United States, although it has always been the specialty of military surgeons. Those spheres of influence overlapped at the end of the Vietnam War, with the lessons learned in that massive trauma resuscitation experience being applied to the civilian trauma centers that had begun to develop in the late 1960s.[3] Primarily due to the charismatic and academically focused leadership in Chicago (Freeark), Dallas (Shires), and San Francisco (Blaisdell), followed by regional trauma systems in Illinois (Boyd) and Maryland (Cowley) in the early 1970s, the urban county hospitals had by necessity become hospitals for the most critically injured blunt and penetrating trauma patients.[4] The American College of Surgeons (ACS) recognized this trend, and its inherent value in patient care, and began to advocate for trauma centers and trauma surgeons via the Committee on Trauma (ACS/COT). The publication of the

TABLE 2.1

ACUTE CARE SURGERY CURRICULUM

REQUIRED CLINICAL ROTATION	LENGTH
Surgical critical care including:	
• Trauma/surgical critical care, including other relevant critical care rotations	9-12 mo
• This portion of the fellowship must comply with ACGME requirements for a surgical critical care residency	
Emergency and elective surgery:	12-15 mo
Total	**24 mo**
SUGGESTED EMERGENCY AND ELECTIVE SURGERY ROTATIONS	**LENGTH**
• Trauma/emergency surgery (required)	2-3 mo
• Thoracic	2-3 mo
• Transplant/hepatobiliary/pancreatic	2-3 mo
• Vascular/interventional radiology	2-3 mo
• Orthopaedic surgery	1 mo
• Neurological surgery	1 mo
• Electives	1-3 mo
• Recommended: burn surgery and pediatric surgery	
• Additional: endoscopy, imaging, plastic surgery, etc.	
Total	**12 mo**

Notes to Curriculum Outline

It is a requirement that over the 2-y fellowship, trainees participate in acute care surgery call for no less than 12 mo. Fellows are required to take 52 night calls in trauma and emergency surgery during the 2-y fellowship.

1. Flexibility in the timing of these rotations and the structure of the 24-mo training should be utilized to optimize the training of the fellow.
2. Rational for out-of-system rotations for key portions of the training must be based on educational value to the fellow.
3. Acute care surgery fellowship sites must have RRC approval for surgical critical care residency.
4. Experience in elective surgery is an essential component of fellowship training.
5. An academic environment is mandatory, and fellows should be trained to teach others and conduct research in acute care surgery.

sentinel document "Optimal Hospital Resources for Care of the Seriously Injured" first occurred in 1976 and has spurred over 30 years of formalized trauma center and trauma system development in the United States that is the template for how regionalization of care can occur.

Those who pursued a trauma career during this period fondly remember the golden age of trauma surgery from the mid-1970s to the late 1980s.[5] Mentorship was a decisive factor. The trauma surgeon was regarded as the master technician (Blaisdell, Carrico, Davis, Freeark, Lucas, Ledgerwood, Mattox, Shires, Moore, Feliciano) who operated confidently and effectively in the neck, chest, abdomen, and pelvis and repaired any injured blood vessel. After exposure to the "trauma service," residents initially bent on a career in cardiac surgery or transplant surgery often changed direction because of exposure to these individuals during surgical training. This was a time of novel operative techniques and frequent trauma operations. The annual program of the AAST was replete with presentations on innovative operative techniques (hepatic tractotomy, splenorrhaphy, pyloric exclusion; cervical, thoracic, abdominal, and peripheral vascular reconstruction). As poignantly stated by Tom Cogbill in the editorial entitled "Eraritjaritjaka," "I had no thought of choosing surgery as a career until the third year surgery rotation at the Denver General Hospital. In less than a day I felt as if I had been thrown into a busy field hospital on the edge of some unknown battlefield. The Knife and Gun Club lived up to its reputation night after night. Each day was more exciting than the day before... I looked with great admiration upon... attending surgeons for their excellent decision making and technical skills."[6] Eraritjaritjaka is an archaic poetic expression in Arunta, which means "full of desire for something that has been lost."

Indeed, by 1990, a number of critical events radically changed the scope of practice for trauma surgery, but perhaps none so subtly yet dramatically as the progressive reduction in operative procedures and marked increased responsibility for nonoperative care of the injured patient; these became synonymous with a disenfranchisement of the specialty as a viable surgical career. The advent of computed tomographic scanning ushered in nonoperative management of solid organ injuries that has become the rule rather than the exception. A successful national emphasis on injury prevention lessened the injuries from motor vehicle crashes, and the operative management for blunt torso trauma became infrequent. Penetrating trauma, at one time the most prevalent indication for thoracic, abdominal, and vascular operations in urban trauma centers, became much less common for reasons that are still debated in social science circles. The emergence of other surgical specialists (thoracic, vascular, otolaryngology) additionally diverted many injuries away from trauma surgery, and angioembolization and endovascular stenting further decreased operative intervention. A report by Richardson and Miller in 1992[6] verified this trend away from trauma surgery as a desirable field, noting that only 8% of graduating surgical residents were interested in trauma.

Concurrent with these events, surgical critical care emerged as a viable discipline with strong academic interests and challenging physiology, and trauma surgeons became absorbed in delivering comprehensive care for all injured patients, with some developing a primary interest and focus of practice in

TABLE 2.2

OPERATIVE MANAGEMENT PRINCIPLES AND TECHNICAL PROCEDURE REQUIREMENTS OF ACUTE CARE SURGERY FELLOWSHIP

AREA/PROCEDURE	ESSENTIAL	DESIRABLE
AIRWAY		
Cricothyroidotomy	×	
Nasal and oral endotracheal intubation including rapid sequence induction	×	
Tracheostomy, open and percutaneous	×	
HEAD/FACE		
Nasal packing (for complex facial fracture bleeding)	×	
ICP monitor		×
Lateral canthotomy		×
Ventriculostomy		×
NECK		
Exposure and definitive management of vascular and aerodigestive injuries	×	
Elective neck dissection		×
Parathyroidectomy		×
CHEST		
Advanced thoracoscopic techniques as they pertain to the described conditions	×	
Bronchoscopy: diagnostic and therapeutic for injury, infection, and foreign body removal	×	
Damage control techniques	×	
Definitive management of empyema: decortication (open and video-assisted thoracic surgery [VATS])	×	
Diaphragm injury, repair	×	
Exposure and definitive management of cardiac injury, pericardial tamponade	×	
Exposure and definitive management of esophageal injuries and perforations	×	
Exposure and definitive management of thoracic vascular injury	×	
Exposure and definitive management of tracheobronchial and lung injuries	×	
Pulmonary resections	×	
Spine exposure: thoracic and thoracoabdominal	×	
VATS for management of injury and infection	×	
Partial left heart bypass		×
Repair blunt thoracic aortic injury: open or endovascular		×
ABDOMEN AND PELVIS		
Abdominal wall reconstruction following resectional debridement for infection, ischemia	×	
Advanced laparoscopic techniques as they pertain to the described procedures	×	
Damage control techniques	×	
Exposure and definitive management of duodenal injury	×	
Exposure and definitive management of gastric, small intestine, and colon inflammation, bleeding, perforation, and obstructions.	×	
Exposure and definitive management of gastric, small intestine, and colon injuries	×	
Exposure and definitive management of major abdominal and pelvic vascular injury	×	
Gastrostomy (open and percutaneous) and jejunostomy	×	
Hepatic resections	×	
Management of abdominal compartment syndrome	×	
Management of all grades of liver injury	×	

(Continued)

TABLE 2.2

OPERATIVE MANAGEMENT PRINCIPLES AND TECHNICAL PROCEDURE REQUIREMENTS OF ACUTE CARE SURGERY FELLOWSHIP (*Continued*)

AREA/PROCEDURE	ESSENTIAL	DESIRABLE
Management of pancreatic injury, infection, and inflammation	×	
Management of rectal injury	×	
Management of renal, ureteral, and bladder injury	×	
Management of splenic injury, infection, inflammation, or disease	×	
Pancreatic resection and debridement	×	
Exposure and definitive management of major abdominal and pelvic vascular rupture or acute occlusion		×
Management of acute operative conditions in the pregnant patient		×
Management of injuries to the female reproductive tract		×
Place IVC filter		×
EXTREMITIES		
Amputations, lower extremity (hip disarticulation, above knee, below knee, trans-met.)	×	
Damage control techniques in the management of extremity vascular injuries, including temporary shunts	×	
Exposure and management of lower extremity vascular injuries	×	
Exposure and management of upper extremity vascular injuries	×	
Fasciotomy, lower extremity	×	
Radical soft issue debridement for necrotizing infection	×	
Acute thromboembolectomy		×
Applying femoral/tibial traction		×
Fasciotomy, upper extremity		×
Hemodialysis access, permanent		×
On-table arteriography		×
Reducing dislocations		×
Splinting fractures		×
OTHER PROCEDURES		
Skin grafting	×	
Treatment of hypothermia	×	
Lower GI endoscopy		×
Operative management of burn injuries		×
Thoracic and abdominal organ harvesting for transplantation		×
Upper GI endoscopy		×
PEDIATRIC SURGICAL PROCEUDRES		
Inguinal hernia repair		×
Trauma management		×
Treatment of bowel obstruction		×
Ventral hernia repair		×

this largely nonoperative specialty. The new specialty of emergency medicine further compounded these changes, as these physicians sought to be the primary hospital-based responders to trauma and directors of trauma resuscitation and evaluation. In response, the ACS/COT promulgated guidelines for the physical presence of the trauma surgeon in the Emergency Department for initial evaluation of the injured patient and the intensive care unit to provide nonoperative supportive care, all in an effort to provide a continuity of care and surgical presence that support surgeon primacy in caring for the injured patient. While clearly well intended, the guidelines became regulations in many states and translated into frequent nocturnal excursions to the ED to oversee initial care of head injuries and multiple fractures, forcing onerous mandatory in-house call, with decreasing operative experience.

A further destructive consequence was the practice of divorcing elective procedures from trauma surgery. While the stated rationale was that the trauma surgeon was preoccupied with ED and SICU responsibilities, it often was the case that the trauma surgeons were prohibited from having an elective practice by either hospital administrators or private practice community surgeons who not only did not want to do trauma care but also did not want the trauma surgeons, who were paid by the hospital, to compete for their referrals. The net result was that trauma surgery—once a predominantly operative service—became a largely nonoperative field with disproportionate demands on lifestyle. Esposito et al convincingly articulated that trauma surgery was in the midst of an identity crisis, a feeling that was not lost on competing emergency physicians, some of whom felt they should be assuming the lead in trauma care.[7,8]

These forces combined with other social, demographic, and economic pressures to develop a crisis in trauma care. New graduates in all medical specialties were congregating to "controllable lifestyle" specialty practices; there was increasing unavailability of surgeons committed to the injured patient; the high economic pressures on hospitals to pay "on-call" surgeons of every conceivable specialty of what some would consider to be outrageous or at least disproportionate pay for simply being available, while the trauma surgeons provided the bulk of clinical care. While a disruptive lifestyle, extended work hours, poor reimbursement, risk of blood-borne infections, and medicolegal risk are to a degree shared by all surgical disciplines, the unique challenge confronting trauma surgeons was the shrinking scope of operative practice. The unique challenge confronting societal health care was the increasing cost of medical care, the unavailability of surgeons willing to provide emergency call, and the decreased availability of general surgeons well versed and comfortable with the management of all types of surgical emergencies, including trauma.[9,10]

Recognizing these challenges and the changing face of general surgery, the trauma community developed an active response to patient and provider needs. Representative members of the AAST, Eastern Association for the Surgery of Trauma, Western Trauma Association, and American College of Surgeons Committee on Trauma (ACS/COT) met in August of 2002 to consider the future of trauma surgery in light of the changing demographics and economics of trauma care. That initial meeting was cochaired by David Hoyt, MD, president of the AAST, and Wayne Meredith, MD, chairman of the ACS Committee on Trauma. The AAST was assigned primary responsibility for developing a plan of action, and Dr. Hoyt appointed Gregory J. Jurkovich, MD, chairman of an ad hoc committee, to accomplish just that. This became a standing committee of the AAST in the fall of 2006 and has subsequently been chaired by Dr. Grace Rozycki (2008-2010) and John Fildes (2010-2014). Further details of the history behind the organization of this committee and its workings to develop the acute care surgery training fellowship are referenced.[1,2]

The primary recommendation of this committee was that the AAST should take a leadership role in defining, developing, and promoting a new postgraduate training fellowship. It was believed this fellowship should be built on a foundation of "general surgery," meaning it would follow core general surgery training, currently a 5-year ACGME residency in the United States. The primary purpose of this new training fellowship would be to define and train a surgeon with expertise in trauma, critical care, and emergency general surgery. It was expected that this broad training would allow for great flexibility in local practice patterns, including encouraging an elective practice in general surgery if desired. This training paradigm, and the fellowships and specialty practice patterns it has spawned, have come to be known as acute care surgery.

The details of this 2-year fellowship have been described already. Extensive exposure and direct care of the injured patient are the bedrock of this fellowship, combined with surgical critical care and emergency general surgery. Academic activities are expected of these trainees, and a core curriculum including operative experience has been mandated. Finally, a measurement of knowledge (multiple choice test) in trauma and general surgical emergencies has been developed.

It is clear this fellowship is in its infancy. However, in a recent survey of program directors of ACGME-approved surgical critical care programs, of which there are 95 programs offering 189 residency positions, 57% responded that they are considering incorporating an acute care surgery fellowship training paradigm.[11] In 2005, the American Board of Surgery initially established advisory councils for trauma, burns, and surgical critical care along with gastrointestinal surgery, surgical oncology, and transplant surgery. These advisory councils were in addition to component boards in pediatric surgery and vascular surgery.[12] In 2010, the Trauma, Burns, and Surgical Critical Care Advisory Council was made a component board, with ongoing discussions on the pathway to board-certification status for acute care surgery training. Programs are advertising acute care surgery positions, hospitals are recruiting to acute care surgery positions, other medical specialties are talking about acute care surgery, and importantly, medical students and residents are asking questions about a career in acute care surgery. Indeed, the dilemma of limited or restricted elective operative prerogative for trauma surgeons has been most conspicuous in university hospitals where general surgery has become maximally fragmented, compounded by the existence of financially powerful cardiothoracic, vascular, transplant, and interventional radiology services. Many of these academic centers have embraced at least part of the true acute care surgery practice concept, incorporating "emergency general surgery" into the trauma service with or without a critical care practice as a solution to the lack of availability of a "general surgeon."[13-17] And while many criticisms have been leveled at the concept and development of this training paradigm, it has gained traction because it is fulfilling a need.

This is the practice paradigm that most "trauma surgeons" identify with as we enter the 2nd decade of the 21st century. In reality, while the name is new, the practice paradigm of acute care surgery is not. Academic urban county hospitals, now often called "safety net hospitals," have always employed this model to ensure optimal care of the injured patient, convinced that emergent torso trauma surgery and elective general surgery are inseparable.[4,13] Moreover, this has always been the scope of practice for rural trauma surgeons.[18-20] Acute care surgery training is likely to become one of the pathways of specialization following core general surgery training and the one that best develops broadly trained general surgeons who will embrace the challenges of surgical emergencies and critical care.

References

1. Acute care surgery: trauma, critical care, and emergency surgery. *J Trauma*. 2005;58(3):614-616.
2. Committee on the Future of Trauma Surgery. The acute care surgery curriculum. *J Trauma*. 2007;62(3):553-556.
3. Blaisdell FW. Development of the city-county (public) hospital. *Arch Surg*. 1994;129(7):760-764.
4. Moore EE. Acute care surgery: the safety net hospital model. *Surgery*. 2007;141(3):297-298.
5. Moore EE, et al. Acute care surgery: Eraritjaritjaka. *J Am Coll Surg*. 2006;202(4):698-701.
6. Richardson J, Miller F. Will future surgeons be interested in trauma care? Results of a resident survey. *J Trauma*. 1992;32:229-235.
7. Esposito TJ, et al. Making the case for a paradigm shift in trauma surgery. *J Am Coll Surg*. 2006;202(4):655-667.
8. Green S. Trauma Surgery: discipline in crisis. *Ann Emerg Med*. 2008;53(1):199-206.
9. Esposito TJ, et al. Why surgeons prefer not to care for trauma patients. *Arch Surg*. 1991;126(3):292-297.
10. Dorsey E, Jarjoura D, Rutecki G. Influence of controllable lifestyle on recent trends in specialty choice by US medical students. *JAMA*. 2003;290(9):1173-1178.

11. Napolitano LM, et al. Challenging issues in surgical critical care, trauma, and acute care surgery: a report from the Critical Care Committee of the American Association for the Surgery of Trauma. *J Trauma.* 2010;69(6):1619-1633.
12. *ABS New Letter.* Winter 2005. http://home.absurgery.org/default.jsp?newsletter&ref=news. Accessed February 16, 2006.
13. Ciesla DJ, et al. The academic trauma center is a model for the future trauma and acute care surgeon. *J Trauma.* 2005;58(4):657-661; discussion 661-662.
14. Earley AS, et al. An acute care surgery model improves outcomes in patients with appendicitis. *Ann Surg.* 2006;244(4):498-504.
15. Diaz JJ Jr, et al. Acute care surgery: a functioning program and fellowship training. *Surgery.* 2007;141(3):310-316.
16. Hoyt DB, Kim HD, Barrios C. Acute care surgery: a new training and practice model in the United States. *World J Surg.* 2008;32(8):1630-1635.
17. Reilly PM, Schwab CW. Acute care surgery: the academic hospital's perspective. *Surgery.* 2007;141(3):299-301.
18. Finlayson SR. Surgery in rural America. *Surg Innov.* 2005;12(4):299-305.
19. Vangelisti G. Training in rural surgery: a resident's perspective. *Bull Am Coll Surg.* 2003;88(5):18-20.
20. Hunter J, Deveny K. Training the rural surgeon. *Bull Am Coll Surg.* 2003;88(5):13-17.

CHAPTER 3 ■ PATHOPHYSIOLOGY OF ACUTE ILLNESS AND INJURY

TIMOTHY R. BILLIAR AND MARCUS K. HOFFMAN

In the setting of an acute surgical illness, the patient's body responds to stresses resulting from tissues in distress and often from microbial invasion. This results in profound changes in the function of most organs and systems. Most of these changes are adaptive. The range and extent of the responses depend on not only the type of insult but also host factors (see Table 3.1). When excessive, the responses designed to allow the host to adapt can become dysregulated or excessive and hence maladaptive. Timely intervention can limit the untoward consequences. However, an appreciation of both the adaptive and maladaptive response can assist with care decisions that can impact patient outcomes.

Systemic responses are secondary to a combination of factors including neurohormonal responses, release of bioactive molecules from damaged or injured tissues, or infectious organisms or elaborated products. The extent to which tissue damage and invasive infection contribute to the host response can vary considerably by the type of insult. For example, in cholangitis, minimal tissue damage occurs but bacteremia can be substantial. Likewise with gastrointestinal ulceration, a small area of tissue necrosis can result in diffuse peritonitis and sepsis if there is free perforation.

As local disease processes become more extensive, a systemic response ensues. Patients may exhibit tachycardia, tachypnea or carbon dioxide retention, or temperature elevation above 38°C or below 36°C. Complete blood counts may reveal leukocytosis of 12K white blood cells/mm^3 (WBC) or higher, depression below 4K, or bandemia. Having at least two of the aforementioned physiologic changes or laboratory values defines a patient as having systemic inflammatory response syndrome (SIRS) and, in the setting of infection, defines a patient as having sepsis. However, in the clinical setting, a patient is usually referred to as being "septic" when he or she has sepsis and some form of organ dysfunction, such as altered mental status or oliguria. Patients have progressed to septic shock when they develop hypotension resistant to fluid boluses.

Along the spectrum of localized inflammation to septic shock, the surgeon must determine how well a patient is compensating and how much physiologic reserve the patient has remaining. A systematic approach to evaluating patients in acute care surgery allows for an appropriate global evaluation of the patient. Several scoring systems have been developed to estimate the physiologic status of the patient. Among the most predictive is the Acute Physiology and Chronic Health Evaluation II (APACHE II) classification system (see Fig. 3.1). Although not often calculated acutely, this classification system assesses parameters of organ and system function that should be part of the evaluation of acutely ill surgical patients.

CARDIOVASCULAR

Patients with coronary artery disease, congestive heart failure, or severe valvular problems will not tolerate drastic hemodynamic changes seen in severe systemic inflammation. With coronary artery disease, atherosclerosis prevents demand-driven vasodilation that can result in ischemia and myocardial damage in the setting of sustained tachycardia as seen with SIRS. Aside from a history of previous myocardial infarction, coronary artery bypass grafting or percutaneous coronary interventions, coronary disease should be suspected in any patient with diabetes mellitus, smoking history, hyperlipidemia, and peripheral vascular disease.

Congestive heart failure and valvular disease do not drastically change the management of patients presenting with acute surgical issues but may necessitate more invasive hemodynamic monitoring as ongoing resuscitation occurs. Resuscitation should not be limited due to these comorbidities as aggressive resuscitation will likely correct disturbances in low cardiac output. Consideration must be given to heart rate control as tachycardia can lead to inefficient cardiac contractility, pulmonary edema, and hypotension. The development of atrial fibrillation in a patient with or without a cardiac history should cue the surgeon into the fact that the heart is irritated in the current physiologic state.

In a compensated state, the cardiovascular system will maintain a sinus rhythm and an acceptable blood pressure. In states of intravascular depletion, vascular resistance will increase via increased vessel tone to maintain a mean arterial pressure for perfusion of vital organs. This attempt at compensation is seen as a narrowed pulse pressure, as the diastolic pressure is elevated from increased vascular tone and the systolic pressure drops from decreased preload. For maintenance of cardiac output with decreased preload and resultant decreased stroke volume, the heart rate will increase.

Decompensated states of the cardiovascular system can be either obvious or arbitrary. Obvious states are the development of new nonsinus rhythms (e.g., atrial fibrillation) and the occurrence of myocardial ischemia or acute coronary syndromes. Arbitrary decompsensated states lie along the same spectrum of compensated states, but occur further along, such as when a patient has a sinus tachycardia in the 160 bpm range or when mean arterial pressure drops below 55 mm Hg.

Therapeutic interventions begin with the insertion of an arterial line for continuous blood pressure monitoring, frequently followed by central venous catheterization if there is any doubt about the volume status of a patient. Pulmonary artery or Swan-Ganz catheters may be placed if large hemodynamic changes are expected in the setting of known severe aortic or mitral valve dysfunction or if the etiology of hypotension and cardiac dysfunction is unknown. Resuscitation begins with isotonic crystalloid fluids and may need to be supplemented with vasopressors depending on the degree of volume depletion (prolonged vomiting or lack of oral intake), presence of septic response (high cardiac output, peripheral vasodilation, high mixed venous oxygen saturations), and patient parameters such as high central venous pressure in the presence of low mean arterial pressure.

PULMONARY

Relevant respiratory history includes both previous and current smoking, known diagnosis of chronic obstructive pulmonary disease (COPD), pulmonary medications

TABLE 3.1

PATIENT FACTORS ASSOCIATED WITH INCREASED MORTALITY

DISEASE/INTERVENTION	
Necrotizing soft tissue Infectionsinfections	Age > 60, DM, acute renal failure,
Emergent colorectal surgery	Age
Perforated peptic ulcer	Age, number of comorbidities, NSAIDs or corticosteroid use
Upper GI bleed	Age, CHF, hepatic failure, malignancy, IBD, renal disease, DM, CAD, corticosteroid use
Appendectomy	Age, ASA Class IV or V, complete dependence functional status, insulin controlled DM, COPD, chronic corticosteroid use, current pneumonia, history of bleeding disorder
Cholecystectomy	Age > 60, ASA Class III–V

DM, diabetes mellitus; NSAIDs, nonsteroidal anti-inflammatory drugs; GI, gastrointestinal; CAD, coronary artery disease; COPD, chronic obstructive pulmonary disease; IBD, inflammatory bowel disease; CHF, congestive heart failure; ASA, American Society of Anesthesiologists.

including inhalers or prednisone, or shortness of breath with activity. Patients with COPD may decompensate and develop hypoxemia or hypercapnia and carbon dioxide narcosis. For patients with appreciable pulmonary comorbidities, patients and their families should be aware that mechanical ventilation could be required for days to weeks while the patient's respiratory status is optimized for extubation following surgery. Septic patients may develop acute respiratory distress syndrome and require low tidal volume ventilation and early tracheostomy.

THE APACHE II SEVERITY OF DISEASE CLASSIFICATION SYSTEM

PHYSIOLOGIC VARIABLE	HIGH ABNORMAL RANGE						LOW ABNORMAL RANGE		
	+4	+3	+2	+1	0	+1	+2	+3	+4
TEMPRATURE – rectal (°C)	$\geq 41^{+}$	39^{+} 40.9^{-}		$38.5^{+}\cdot 38.9^{-}$	$36^{+}\cdot 38.4^{-}$	$34^{+}\cdot 35.9^{-}$	$32^{+}\cdot 39.9^{-}$	$30^{+}\cdot 31.9^{-}$	$\leq 29.9^{+}$
MEAN ARTERIAL PRESSURE – mm Hg	≥160	130.159	110.129		70.109		50.69		≤49
HEART RATE (ventricular response)	≥180	140.139	110.139		70-109		55.69	40-54	≤39
RESPIRATORY RATE – (non-ventilated or ventilated)	≥50	35.49		25-34	12-24	10-11	6.9		≤5
OXYGENATION: $A\text{-}aDO_2$, or PaO_2 (mm Hg) a. FIO, ≥ 0.5 record $A\text{-}aDO_2$	≥500	150.499	200-349		<200				
b. FIO, < 0.5 record only PaO_2					$PO_1 > 70$	$PO_1 > 61.70$		$PO_1 > 55.60$	$PO_1 > 56$
ARTERIAL pH	≥7.7	76.759		7.5-7.59	7.33-7.49		7.25-7.32	7.15-7.24	≤7.15
SERUM SODIUM (mMol/Li)	≥160	160.179	155-159	150-154	130-149		120-129	151-119	≤110
SERUM POTASSIUM (mMol/Li)	≥7	66.9		5.5-5.3	3.5-5.4	3-3.4	2.5-2.9		≤2.5
SERUM CREATININE (mg/100 ml) (Double pone score 1 or acute renal failure)	≥35	23.4	1.5-1.9		0.6-1.4		<0.6		
HEMATOCRIT (%)	≥60		50-59.9	45-49.9	30-45.9		20-29.9		≤20
WHITE BLOOD COUNT (total/mm3) (in 1.000 %)	≥40		20-39.9	15-19.9	3-14.9		1-2.9		<1
GLASCOW COMA SCORE (GCS) Score = 15minus acutal GCS									
[A] Tcial ACUTE PHYSIOLOGY SCOPE (APS) Sumof the 12 individual variable points									
Setu HCo, (venous mMeol) (Not preferred, use if no ABGs)	≥52	41.51 g		32.40 g	22.31 g		18.21 g	15.17 g	<15

[B] **AGE POINTS:**
Assign points to age as follows:

AGE(yrs)	Points
≤44	0
45-54	2
55-64	3
65-74	5
≥75	6

[C] **CHRONIC HEALTH POINTS:**
If the patient has a history of severe organ system insufficiency or is immuno copromised assign points as follows:

a. for nonoperative or emergency poscoprative patien– 5 points
or
b. for efective postoperative patients – 2 points

DEFINITIONS

Organ Insuficiency or immune-compromised state must have been evident prior to this hospital admission and conform to the following critenis.

LIVER Biopsy prowen crihisic and documented portal hypertension, spidoses of past upper GI bleeding as Inbuted to portal hypertension, or prior episodes of hepatic failure/encephalopathy/coma

CAROIOVASCULAR : New York Heart Association Class IV
RESPIRATORY: Chronic restrictive, obstructive, or vascular disease resulting in severe exercise restriction, i.e. unable to climb stairs or perform household dulies; or documented chronic hypoxia, hypercapnia, secondary polycythemia, severe pulmonary hyperten sion (> 40 mm/Hg), or respirato dependency.

RENAL : Receiving crhonic cialysis.

IMMUND COMPROMISED : The patient has received theraphy that suppresses resistance to infection, e.g. immumnosuppression, chemotherapy, radiation, long term of recent high dose streoids, or has a disease that is sufficiently advanced to suppress resistance to infection, e.g., Iruhemia, lymphomia, AIDS.

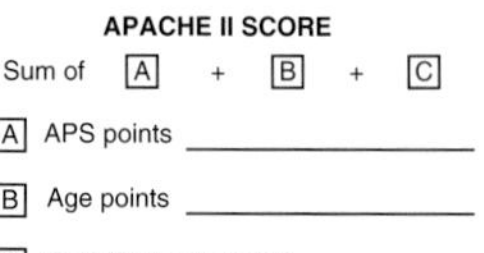

APACHE II SCORE
Sum of [A] + [B] + [C]
[A] APS points ________
[B] Age points ________
[C] Chronic Health points ________
Toeal APACHE II ________

FIGURE 3.1. The APACHE II severity of disease classification system. (From Knaus WA, Draper EA, Wagner DP, et al. APACHE II: a severity of disease classification system. *Crit Care Med*. 1985;13:818-829.)

In most situations in acute care surgery, the lungs do not sustain a direct insult with the exception of possible aspiration pneumonitis during episodes of emesis. Instead, pulmonary dysfunction occurs as the result of systemic response to infection or hemorrhagic shock. The lungs appear to be especially sensitive to the "mediator storm" that occurs in the setting of SIRS. In states of metabolic acidosis via lactate, diabetic ketoacidosis, etc., the patient will become tachypneic to develop a compensatory respiratory alkalosis.

Respiratory decompensation and failure becomes imminent when patients show signs of accessory muscle use, head bobbing, or nostril flaring. First-line interventions of supplemental oxygen via nasal cannula or face mask should occur immediately. Chest radiograph and auscultation should also be performed to look for other causes of respiratory difficulty that could be corrected, such as wheezing and bronchospasm responsive to bronchodilators or large pleural effusions causing respiratory compromise. The next step in the majority of cases is intubation and mechanical ventilation.

RENAL

Renal failure is frequently seen with other comorbidities, especially diabetes and coronary artery disease, and should prompt further medical history interrogation. Urinary catheter placement and monitoring of urine output should occur early in patients with systemic illness. Basic metabolic panels should be reviewed and compared with previous values. Elevation in blood urea nitrogen (BUN) or creatinine can be indicative of intravascular volume depletion, which can occur due to a number of factors including decreased oral intake, increased vascular permeability, and peripheral vasodilation depending on the level of systemic inflammation occurring. Hyponatremia is of significance as it is commonly seen in necrotizing soft tissue infections.

Determination of the function of the renal system is difficult to perform. Gold standards involve measurements of inulin clearance. Creatinine is used as a surrogate marker, and various formulas have been created based on studies of 24-hour creatinine clearance. As such, estimated glomerular filtration rate (eGFR) presumes that the serum level of creatinine is indicative of current renal function. However, if renal function is acutely declining and clearing less creatinine, eGFR would be an overestimate of the current function. This would only be revealed in subsequent serum creatinine level on the following day.

A more accurate indicator of current renal function may be urine output. A simplified method of conceptualizing urine output is classifying it as adequate, marginal, inadequate, and anuric. Urine output of approximately 0.5 mL/kg/h has been used as acceptable urine production for adults. New-onset anuria would indicate decompensation as metabolites would not be actively cleared from the blood.

Interventions for renal dysfunction should be directed toward resuscitation to a normovolemic state with appropriate mean arterial pressures. Disturbances in potassium, magnesium, and phosphorus should be corrected. Acute renal failure may necessitate continuous renal replacement therapy, but this commonly does not need to be performed within the first hours of presentation unless the patient meets criteria for emergent dialysis.

ENDOCRINE

Patients with long-standing diabetes mellitus are prone to have underlying coronary artery disease and chronic kidney disease, and, as such, their cardiac and renal statuses must be further investigated. Blood glucoses levels obtained at the time of presentation may be indicator of systemic inflammation. Insulin-dependent diabetics who normally have well-regimented control of their blood glucoses may present with elevated but not alarmingly high levels or may report requiring higher-than-average units of insulin in the previous 24 hours. Normal blood glucose levels indicate a compensated or normal state while slightly elevated glucose levels indicate a partially decompensated state.

Extremely elevated glucose levels are indicative of a decompensated state, as seen in diabetic ketoacidosis and nonketotic hyperosmolar hyperglycemia. Both states of decompensation must be treated with volume resuscitation and intravenous insulin drips. Concerning hyperkalemia will frequently lead to hypokalemia with the aforementioned interventions. While debate exists surrounding the exact range of blood glucose levels that are ideal, glycemic control should be implemented as hyperglycemia is associated with worse outcomes.

Patients with conditions requiring chronic oral steroids, that is, prednisone, are at risk of acute adrenocortical insufficiency. In patients who are already at risk for developing septic shock, it is extremely difficult to differentiate sepsis and adrenal insufficiency. Adrenocorticotropic hormone stimulation test with cosyntropin takes hours to perform correctly. If necessary, testing can be performed at a later time when it is certain that the patient is stabilized. Patients are presumably in a compensated adrenal state unless they have inexplicable hemodynamics that appear to be refractory to both intravenous fluids and vasoactive medications. Patients with this decompensated picture may have a history of chronic steroid use, but this is not a prerequisite for developing acute adrenocortical insufficiency. In this patient population, treatment with IV hydrocortisone 100 mg every 6-8 hours empirically should be given if there is concern for adrenocortical insufficiency.

NEUROLOGIC

Altered mental status or delirium may be a sign of systemic inflammation or bacteremia. Altered mental status can be the only presenting symptom in bacteremic elderly patients, as is frequently seen in urinary tract infections and urosepsis. In most cases, a family member or medical power of attorney will be able to describe the patient's neurologic baseline. Patients who are not alert and oriented to their baseline level are neurologically decompensated. Interventions may include keeping a family member or staff at bedside to reorient the patient, antipsychotic medications for agitated patients who will not reorient, and intubation for the obtunded patient not protecting his or her airway.

HEMATOLOGIC

Systemic inflammation usually results in leukocytosis and possibly the presence of bands on the peripheral smear but on occasion will result in a depressed WBC count. These changes might not be seen in a patient on chemotherapeutic agents or immunosuppressive medications (transplant patients or patients with autoimmune disorders such as rheumatoid arthritis). Questions to patients should focus on family or personal history of bleeding or clotting disorders and medications with anticoagulant or antiplatelet properties, specifically warfarin, clopidogrel, and aspirin. Unexpected elevation in international normalized ratio (INR) should prompt investigation into liver disease, especially if the platelet count is on the lower end of normal or frankly thrombocytopenic. Hemoglobin and hematocrit levels on the high end of normal may further suggest intravascular volume depletion.

Therapeutic intervention should be geared toward maintaining an acceptable hemoglobin and hematocrit, platelet count, and INR. Packed red blood cell transfusion may be indicated, understanding that volume resuscitation may also contribute to low hematocrit levels through dilution. Platelet counts should be kept above 50K in the perioperative setting and periprocedural settings for interventional radiology or endoscopy. Elevated INR can be corrected with fresh frozen plasma and/or intravenous phytonadione (vitamin K) depending on timing of interventions.

HEPATIC AND METABOLIC

In obtaining information from a patient, one must query recent weight loss or weight gain and alcohol history, both current and remote alcohol use. Recent unexpected weight loss may cue the surgeon into the duration of the disease process at hand or the presence of another medical problem. Correlating this to an albumin level will give the surgeon an indication to the nutritional status of the patient, which is useful in determining how well a patient will recover from an operation. Prealbumin level gives a better picture of the nutritional status as it is not affected by liver dysfunction, but this laboratory value is not always readily available in most institutions. Unexpected weight gain should prompt investigation into worsening cardiac, renal, or hepatic function.

A considerable alcohol history should focus attention on determining if the patient has cirrhosis. While there are numerous causes of cirrhosis and liver damage, alcohol intake is the most common cause within the United States. On physical exam, one may palpate an enlarged liver or spleen, note a fluid wave on abdominal exam, or find peripheral musculoskeletal wasting with abdominal protuberance. Jaundice may be present, but jaundice without other exam findings generally does not occur. Laboratory findings may include thromobocytopenia or a platelet count on the lower spectrum of normal, elevated prothrombin time (PT) and INR, elevated bilirubin, low albumin, and low sodium. Along a spectrum of acute hepatic dysfunction, patients may have elevated ammonia levels, elevated PTs, and in severe cases, elevated lactate levels. Aside from correcting laboratory abnormalities, cirrhosis is an important comorbidity in the management of acute care surgery patients as it portends to higher risks of morbidity and mortality regardless of surgical intervention.

When presented with a patient, the surgeon must perform a systematic evaluation to determine the level of insult the patient is experiencing (from localized inflammation to septic shock) and the comorbid conditions of the patient. This knowledge allows one to ascertain the degree to which the patient is compensating and the physiologic reserve for further compensation or insult. The surgeon can then take this information into consideration when determining how to manage the various problems that are presented in acute care surgery. Depending on the nature of the surgical emergency, it may be prudent to delay surgery while hematologic and volume abnormalities are corrected. However, for many surgical emergencies (e.g., life-threatening hemorrhage and ischemic bowel), this is not an option, and efforts to correct abnormalities should occur simultaneous to emergent surgical interventions.

MEDIATORS OF INJURY

Discussion of the pathophysiology of acute care surgery would not be complete without mention of mediators. The disease processes that present to the acute care surgeon are varied from the hemorrhage-reperfusion physiology seen with gastrointestinal bleeds to overt sepsis seen with necrotizing fasciitis.

Pattern recognition receptors allow for signaling through both pathogen-associated and danger-associated molecular patterns. The Toll-like receptors bind a variety of exogenous ligands including flagellin from bacterial flagella and lipoteichoic acid and lipopolysaccharide (LPS) of gram-positive and gram-negative bacteria cell walls, respectively. Toll-like receptor 4 (TLR4) recognizes LPS and mediates signalings seen in overt gram-negative sepsis. LPS-TLR4 signaling leads to degradation of inhibitor of κB. This releases NF-κB, allowing its transport into the nucleus and up-regulating the transcription of a multitude of genes involved in innate and adaptive immunity, including cytokine production. TLR4 recognizes endogenous molecules including high-mobility group box 1 (HMGB1), a nonhistone nuclear protein that peaks in the blood within minutes of sterile injury. Elevated levels of HMGB1 have been associated clinically with weight loss, food aversion, and shock.

At the level of microvasculature, multiple changes occur. With hemorrhage and reperfusion, endothelial cells undergo uncoupling of the mitochondrial electron transport chain. Cytochrome c generates reactive oxygen species. In the setting of low flow and relative hypoxic conditions, xanthine oxidoreductase that normally reduces nicotinamide adenine dinucleotide to nicotinamide adenine dinucleotide phosphate is posttranslationally modified to become xanthine oxidase. With reperfusion, superoxide and hydrogen peroxide are generated. Endothelium also generates nitric oxide (NO) through the enothothelial NO synthase in response to a variety of stimuli including hypoxia, cellular injury, or endotoxin. NO causes vascular dilation and reduction in platelet adhesion and aggregation. Up-regulation of the inducible NO synthase isoform in multiple cell types may contribute to the excessive vasodilation seen in septic shock and also contribute to end organ injury in hemorrhagic shock.

At the site of injury, platelets are activated, releasing a variety of factors including serotonin, platelet activating factor, prostaglandin E_2, and thromboxane. Platelet activation leads to clot formation and chemoattraction of neutrophils and macrophages. Endothelium undergoes up-regulation of intercellular adhesion molecule-1 (ICAM-1) when exposed to the cytokines tumor necrosis factor-α (TNFα) or interleukin 1 (IL1). The presence of ICAM-1 on endothelium allows for binding by beta-integrin on leukocytes that can then migrate into the surrounding tissue to the site of injury.

As cytokine production increases at the site of injury, they begin to act systemically. TNFα rises early in inflammation and induces glucocorticoid release, cachexia, and muscle catabolism. IL1 also peaks early in inflammation. One of its clinically distinguishable effects is the production of prostaglandins in the anterior hypothalamus resulting in fever. IL6 has longer half-life in circulation than TNFα or IL1 and induces the production of acute phase proteins (e.g., C-reactive protein) by the liver as well further inducing neutrophil activation. Simultaneous to proinflammatory response, some cytokines function to dampen and control inflammation. IL10 is known to attenuate the inflammatory response to TNFα.

While cytokine levels or profiles currently are not part of clinical practice, studies have been performed in recent years to investigate their utility. One investigation in adult appendicitis (85 patients) found elevated WBC, CRP, IL6, and IL10 when comparing patients who had appendicitis with those who had negative surgical explorations. In pediatrics, one study involved 105 patients admitted with presumed appendicitis and observed for 6 hours before undergoing appendectomy. The highest specificity was in patients who had both leukocytosis and elevated IL6. Multiple studies in the ensuing years will need to be performed before cytokine levels become part of accepted clinical practice.

References

1. Abraldes JG, Bosch J. The treatment of acute variceal bleeding. *J Clin Gastroenterol.* 2007;41:S312-S317.
2. Bongard FS, Sue DY, Vintch JRE. *Current Critical Care Diagnosis and Treatment.* New York, NY: McGraw-Hill Medical; 2008.
3. Cainzos M, Gonzalez-Rodriguez FJ. Necrotizing soft tissue infections. *Curr Opin Crit Care* 2007;13:433.
4. Chiu PWY, Ng EKW. Predicting poor outcome from acute upper gastrointestinal hemorrhage. *Gastroenterol Clin North Am.* 2009;38:215-230.
5. Cinel I, Opal SM. Molecular biology of inflammation and sepsis: a primer. *Crit Care Med.* 2009;37:291.
6. Hall JB, Schmidt GA, Wood LDH. *Principles of Critical Care.* New York, NY: McGraw-Hill Medical Pub. Division; 2005.
7. Harboe KM, Bardram L. The quality of cholecystectomy in Denmark: outcome and risk factors for 20,307 patients from the national database. *Surg Endosc.* 2011;25:1630-1641.
8. Hofer JE, Nunnally ME. Taking the septic patient to the operating room. *Anesthesiol Clin.* 2010;28:13.
9. Knaus WA, Draper EA, Wagner DP, et al. APACHE II: a severity of disease classification system. *Crit Care Med.* 1985;13:818.
10. Margenthaler JA, Longo WE, Virgo KS, et al. Risk factors for adverse outcomes after the surgical treatment of appendicitis in adults. *Ann Surg.* 2003;238:59.
11. McGillicuddy EA, Schuster KM, Davis KA, et al. Factors predicting morbidity and mortality in emergency colorectal procedures in elderly patients. *Arch Surg.* 2009;144:1157.
12. Møller MH, Adamsen S, Thomsen RW, et al. Preoperative prognostic factors for mortality in peptic ulcer perforation: a systematic review. *Scand J Gastroenterol.* 2010;45:785-805.
13. Oscarsson A, Fredrikson M, Sörliden M, et al. Predictors of cardiac events in high risk patients undergoing emergency surgery. *Acta Anaesthesiol Scand.* 2009;53:986-994.
14. Rushing GD, Britt LD. Reperfusion injury after hemorrhage: a collective review. *Ann Surg.* 2008;247:929.
15. Sarani B, Strong M, Pascual J, et al. Necrotizing fasciitis: current concepts and review of the literature. *J Am Coll Surg.* 2009;208:279-288.
16. Schwartz SI, Brunicardi FC, Andersen DK, et al. Schwartz's principles of surgery. New York, NY: McGraw-Hill, Medical Pub. Division; 2010.
17. Türkyilmaz Z, Sönmez K, Karabulut R, et al. Sequential cytokine levels in the diagnosis of appendicitis. *Scand J Clin Lab Invest.* 2006;66:723-732.
18. Yildirim O, Solak C, Kocer B, et al. The role of serum inflammatory markers in acute appendicitis and their success in preventing negative laparotomy. *J Invest Surg.* 2006;19:345-352.

CHAPTER 4 ■ SHOCK STATES IN ACUTE CARE SURGERY

JEREMY M. HSU AND RONALD V. MAIER

Shock is the clinical end result of inadequate tissue perfusion. The currently accepted concept was first described in 1918 by Walter B. Cannon.[1] There are multiple causes of shock; however, the common pathway is an imbalance in oxygen delivery and utilization, and ultimately cellular dysfunction. Cellular hypoxia induces the production of inflammatory mediators that may further compromise tissue perfusion through changes in the microvasculature. If this vicious cycle is not interrupted, multiorgan failure (MOF) and death result.[2] The clinical manifestations of shock are due to the autonomic neurohumoral responses to hypoperfusion and the resulting organ dysfunction.

This chapter describes the pathogenesis of shock and discusses the diagnostic and therapeutic options in current management.

PATHOGENESIS AND ORGAN RESPONSE TO SHOCK

At the cellular level, shock results in cellular hypoxia. Initially, the injury to cells is reversible; however, if it is not corrected, cell death ensues. The hallmarks of *reversible injury* are reduced oxidative phosphorylation with subsequent depletion of energy stores in the form of adenosine triphospate (ATP) and cellular swelling caused by failure of the sodium pump. In addition, massive influx of calcium occurs due to failure of the calcium pump, causing mitochondrial dysfunction. When injury becomes irreversible, the plasma membrane is disrupted; lysosomal enzymes enter the cytoplasm and digest the cell, resulting in *necrosis*.

Cellular hypoxia also predisposes to *reperfusion injury*, where new damaging processes are set in motion, causing the death of cells that might have recovered otherwise. Increased amounts of reactive oxygen and nitrogen species are generated from parenchymal and endothelial cells as well as infiltrating leucocytes.[3] These free radicals may be produced as a result of mitochondrial damage and incomplete reduction of oxygen. Endogenous cellular antioxidant mechanisms are compromised, favoring the accumulation of free radicals. Increased calcium may also enter the reperfused cells, damaging mitochondria and producing further free radicals. Hypoxic cells produce cytokines and increased expression of adhesion molecules, which recruit circulating neutrophils to reperfused tissue. The resulting inflammation generates additional tissue injury. Activation of the complement system also contributes to reperfusion injury. Select IgM antibodies are predisposed to deposit in hypoxic tissue, and when blood flow is resumed, complement proteins bind to the deposited antibodies, thus causing activation and subsequent inflammation and cell injury.

Cardiovascular Response

Decreased tissue perfusion results in the release of epinephrine and norepinephrine from the adrenal medulla due to decreased afferent impulses from the arterial baroreceptors. Systemic vascular resistance (SVR) rises to maintain adequate perfusion of the heart and brain, at the expense of perfusion to the skin, kidneys, and, primarily, the gastrointestinal tract via splanchnic vasoconstriction. This peripheral vasoconstriction occurs primarily in the arterioles, mediated by $\alpha 1$ receptors. However, vasoconstriction also occurs in the precapillary and postcapillary sphincters and the small veins and venules. This results in a reduced hydrostatic pressure distal to the precapillary sphincter that leads to reabsorption of interstitial fluid into the vascular space. This reabsorption functions to restore intravascular volume and is known as transcapillary refill.

Cardiac output (CO), the product of stroke volume and heart rate (HR), is a major determinant of tissue perfusion. Decreased intravascular volume leads to a reduction in ventricular preload, which in turn results in a diminished stroke volume. Compensation occurs to a degree with an increase in HR. However, shock also causes a reduction in myocardial compliance, resulting in a decreased ventricular end-diastolic volume and thus stroke volume at any given ventricular filling pressure.

Neurohumoral Response

Sustained compensatory mechanisms exist to restore intravascular volume, maintain central perfusion, and mobilize metabolic and osmotic substrates. Disinhibition of the vasomotor center results in increased adrenergic output and decreased vagal activity. Decreased renal blood flow leads to renin release. Renin induces the formation of angiotensin I, which is then converted to angiotensin II. This is a potent vasoconstrictor and stimulates aldosterone release by the adrenal cortex. Aldosterone contributes to restoration of the intravascular volume by enhancing sodium reabsorption in the cortical collecting duct, in exchange for potassium and hydrogen. Hypovolemia, as well as an increase in serum osmolarity, leads to the release of antidiuretic hormone. This has a direct vasoconstrictive effect on vascular smooth muscle and also increases reabsorption of water in the distal renal tubule. The peripheral vasoconstriction is countered by circulating vasodilators including prostacyclin and nitric oxide and, more importantly, the products of local metabolism such as adenosine. This balance between the various vasoconstrictor and vasodilator effects determines local perfusion in a deleterious, repeating hypoxia–reperfusion cycle. Additionally, shock causes release of stress hormones: ephinephrine, adrenocorticotrophic hormone (ACTH), cortisol, and glucagon. This results in glycogenolysis, lipolysis, gluconeogenesis, and insulin resistance causing a negative nitrogen balance and a high extracellular concentration of glucose. This increase in glucose acts as a major osmotic agent for intravascular restitution and anaerobic energy supply. Insulin-independent tissues such as the brain and heart have a substantial increase in glucose utilization.

Pulmonary Response

The pulmonary vascular bed responds to shock much in the same way as the systemic vascular bed. The relative increase in pulmonary vascular resistance (PVR), particularly in septic shock, may exceed that of the SVR, potentially resulting in acute right heart failure. Shock results in tachypnea that reduces tidal volume and increases both dead space and minute ventilation, producing an early respiratory alkalosis. Hypoxia occurs due to diffuse alveolar damage, resulting in acute lung injury and subsequent acute respiratory distress syndrome (ARDS). These disorders are characterized by noncardiogenic pulmonary edema secondary to widespread pulmonary capillary and alveolar injury. Hypoxemia results from a significant ventilation–perfusion mismatch, and lung compliance is reduced due to loss of surfactant and lung volume, particularly functional residual capacity, in conjunction with an increase in intra-alveolar and interstitial edema.[4,5]

Renal Response

The kidneys respond to hypoperfusion by conserving sodium and water, with subsequent decreased urine output. Acutely, oliguria in the face of hypovolemia represents renal success, not renal failure. Early aggressive volume replacement has reduced the frequency of acute renal failure. Acute tubular necrosis is mostly due to the multifactorial interaction of shock, sepsis, nephrotoxic agents, and rhabdomyolysis. These toxic insults cause necrosis of tubular epithelium and tubular obstruction by cellular debris with back-leak of filtrate. Prolonged renal hypoperfusion results in a depletion of renal ATP stores with subsequent impairment of renal function and ultimate failure.

Inflammatory Response

The progression of shock is influenced by activation of the innate immunoinflammatory system. There is also a simultaneous anti-inflammatory response and suppression of the adaptive immune system in those surviving the initial insult. Excesses of both proinflammatory and anti-inflammatory responses are detrimental. An uncontrolled proinflammatory response results in a systemic inflammatory response syndrome, which may lead to continuing shock and MOF.[6,7] Excessive anti-inflammatory responses and adaptive immune suppression increase the susceptibility to secondary nosocomial infections.

The complement cascade is activated by hypoxia and tissue injury, resulting in the generation of anaphylatoxins C3a and C5a. Direct complement fixation in injured tissues can progress to the C5-C9 attack complex, resulting in further cell damage. In addition, concomitant coagulation cascade activation causes microvascular thrombosis, with subsequent fibrinolysis and repeated episodes of ischemic/reperfusion injury. Thrombin is a potent inflammatory mediator that increases activation of neutrophils, leading to further microvascular injury.

The membrane Toll-like receptors are a major source of monocyte/macrophage activation. These receptors recognize damage-associated molecular patterns and pathogen-associated molecular patterns, which are released following tissue injury and pathogenic microbial organisms. Monocytes and macrophages are major regulators of the inflammatory response. Macrophages release proinflammatory cytokines such as interleukin 1 and 6 and tumor necrosis factor α (TNF-α). These produce many of the shock features including hypotension, lactic acidosis, and respiratory failure. Interleukin 8 is a potent neutrophil chemoattractant and up-regulates neutrophil adhesion molecules to enhance aggregation, adherence, and damage to the vascular endothelium.

Eicosanoids, such as prostaglandins, leukotrienes, and thromboxane A2, are vasoactive and immunomodulatory products that affect vascular resistance as well as capillary permeability. LTB4 attracts neutrophils and stimulates the formation of reactive oxygen species.

CLASSIFICATION OF SHOCK STATES

Although the cellular effects of shock are the common pathway regardless of the primary cause, a classification scheme is useful to delineate the underlying process. It is important to note that a combination of two or more causes of shock frequently occurs. The primary importance of classifying the type of shock lies in the recognition of the precipitating event, and initiating appropriate therapy to correct this original cause, while simultaneously carrying out resuscitation. There are five broad categories of shock as outlined in Table 4.1.

GENERAL APPROACH TO SHOCK

The main priorities when dealing with shock include appropriate monitoring in an intensive care setting, prompt correction of tissue perfusion, and perhaps most importantly, correction or treatment of the precipitating cause. Careful and continuous assessment of physiological status and response to therapy is essential.

Physiologic Monitoring

Physiologic monitoring of the patient in shock commences with the "vital signs," and progresses as needed, using increasing technology and invasiveness.

Heart rate is commonly elevated in response to intravascular volume loss, to maintain adequate CO. This tachycardia becomes pathologic when HR exceeds 120-130 beats per minute. Above this rate, there is insufficient diastolic time to adequately fill the ventricles, resulting in decreased stroke volume. A rapid decrease in HR after a volume challenge can be a useful indicator of hypovolemia. In contrast, bradycardia is associated with severe physiologic derangement, usually hypoxia and impending cardiovascular collapse. It is also seen in conjunction with neurogenic shock, as a result of disruption to the cardiac sympathetic fibers. Frequent use of beta-blockers to treat baseline cardiac disease also produces inappropriate HR responses.

Blood pressure (BP) is a crude measure of tissue perfusion. Hypotension results in inadequate tissue perfusion;

TABLE 4.1

CLASSIFICATION OF SHOCK STATES

CLASSIFICATION	SPECIFIC CLINICAL CAUSES
Hypovolemic	Hemorrhage, trauma, third-space loss (burns, pancreatitis, bowel obstruction)
Obstructive	Pericardial tamponade, tension pneumothorax, pulmonary embolus
Cardiogenic	Myocardial infarct, cardiac failure, arrhythmias, blunt cardiac injury
Distributive	sepsis, neurogenic, anaphylaxis
Endocrine	Adrenal insufficiency

however, the exact definition of hypotension is variable, depending on the individual patient. Elderly patients, in particular, are frequently hypertensive at baseline and may not be perfusing tissues adequately at a "normal" BP. Chronic use of antihypertensives also makes reliance on BP as a measurement of shock inaccurate. BP may be measured noninvasively or invasively. Both methods are subject to dynamic response artifacts that may result in inaccurate measurements. Obese patients frequently have unreliable BP measurements due to positioning and poor cuff compression. Mean arterial pressure (MAP) is usually consistent, regardless of measurement method and artifact, and is thus preferred.

Urine output is often decreased in shock in an attempt to preserve and restore intravascular volume. Oliguria is one of the earliest signs of inadequate tissue perfusion. Improvement of urine output is a key monitor for shock resuscitation.

Temperature may help define etiology of shock and provide prognostic value. Hypothermia results as an imbalance between heat loss and the body's ability to generate and maintain metabolic energy. Clinically important hypothermia occurs when the core temperature is <35°C. Hypothermia is associated with an increase in sympathetic drive with resulting peripheral vasoconstriction, end-organ hypoperfusion, and metabolic acidosis from anaerobic respiration. In addition, hypothermia may exacerbate coagulopathy by causing dysfunction of the intrinsic and extrinsic coagulation pathways, as well as platelet activity. There is a markedly increased mortality in shocked patients with hypothermia.[8,9]

Pulse oximetry is a useful method of continuously monitoring arterial oxygen saturation. It utilizes the differential light absorption characteristics of oxyhemoglobin and deoxyhemoglobin to calculate the percentage saturation of oxygenated hemoglobin in blood. Pulse oximetry provides an indication of the degree of hypoxia as well as the assessment of oxygen transport balance.[10]

Biochemical markers are used to identify shock in early stages. The biochemical analysis of shock is based on the shift from aerobic to anaerobic metabolism with a resulting increase in lactate production and decreased clearance due to impaired hepatic function.[11] Shock is also associated with a base deficit on arterial blood gas analysis. The base deficit is defined as the amount of fixed base or acid that must be added to an aliquot of blood to restore the pH to 7.40. Any patient with a lactate of ≥4 mmol/L or a base deficit of ≥6 mEq/L should be considered to be in shock until proven otherwise.[12]

Invasive Hemodynamic Monitoring

Most patients in the intensive care unit (ICU) may be managed safely without the use of a pulmonary artery catheter (PAC or Swan-Ganz catheter).[13] However, in those patients with major ongoing blood loss, fluid shifts and/or underlying cardiac dysfunction, a PAC may be helpful. The current generation of PACs has been improved from the original catheter allowing measurement of pulmonary artery pressures, and continuous hemodynamic and oxygen transport assessment. The PAC is inserted percutaneously via the subclavian or internal jugular vein, to lie in the pulmonary artery.

The circulatory system consists of the systemic and pulmonary vasculature circuits connected in series. Two pressures are generated by each circuit: an outgoing pressure (MAP or mean pulmonary arterial pressure) and an incoming pressure or preload (pulmonary artery occlusion pressure [PAOP] or central venous pressure [CVP]), respectively. These pressures can be used to calculate the afterload of each circuit (SVR or PVR). Therefore, three variables are measured by the PAC: pressure, volume, and flow. From these measured variables, a number of calculated variables may be obtained, which can be useful in guiding resuscitative therapy. Table 4.2 outlines the hemodynamic variables obtained with a PAC.

TABLE 4.2

HEMODYNAMIC VARIABLES

VARIABLE	UNIT	NORMAL RANGE
MEASURED VARIABLES		
Systolic blood pressure (SBP)	mm Hg	90-140
Diastolic blood pressure (DBP)	mm Hg	60-90
Systolic pulmonary artery pressure (PASP)	mm Hg	15-30
Diastolic pulmonary artery pressure (PADP)	mm Hg	4-12
Pulmonary artery occlusion pressure (PAOP) or pulmonary capillary wedge pressure (PCWP)	mm Hg	2-12
Central venous pressure (CVP)	mm Hg	0-8
Heart rate	beats/min	Variable
Cardiac output	L/min	4-8
Right ventricular ejection fraction (RVEF)	Fraction	0.4-0.6
CALCULATED VARIABLES		
Mean arterial pressure (MAP) (SBP + 2 × DBP)/3	mm Hg	70-105
Mean pulmonary artery pressure (MPAP) (PAS + 2 × PAD)/3	mm Hg	9-16
Cardiac index (CI) CO/Body Surface Area (BSA)	$L/min/m^2$	2.8-4.2

TABLE 4.2

HEMODYNAMIC VARIABLES (*Continued*)

VARIABLE	UNIT	NORMAL RANGE
Stroke volume CO/HR	mL/beat	50-100
Systemic vascular resistance (SVR) [(MAP – CVP)/CO] × 80	dyn·s·cm^{-5}	700-1,600
Pulmonary vascular resistance (PVR) [(MPAP – PAOP)/CO] × 80	dyn·s·cm^{-5}	20-130
Left ventricular stroke work (LVSW) SV(MAP – PAOP) × 0.0136	g·m	60-80
Right ventricular stroke work (RVSW) SV(MPAP – CVP) × 0.0136	g·m	10-15
Right ventricular end-diastolic volume index (RVEDVI) SVI/RVEF	mL/m^2	60-100

Preload optimization is essential in the initial resuscitation of all forms of shock. CVP and PAOP are commonly used to estimate preload. The Frank-Starling law defines preload in terms of myocardial fibril length at end diastole. As this is not measureable, several assumptions are made to utilize PAOP to assess the preload of the left ventricle. First, left ventricular end-diastolic volume is assumed to be proportional to myofibril length. Second, assuming that ventricular compliance is constant, end-diastolic volume is equal to end-diastolic pressure. Third, assuming that mitral valve function is normal, left ventricular end-diastolic pressure is equal to mean left atrial pressure (LAP). Fourth, properly transduced PAOP is equal to LAP. Similar assumptions are applicable to the use of CVP in estimating preload status of the right ventricle. While indirectly a surrogate for intravascular volume, overall these pressures correlate poorly with volumes.[14] In addition, many of these assumptions are invalid in the critically ill patient due to changes in ventricular compliance, contractility, and intrathoracic pressures. Therefore, the trend (rather than absolute values of PAOP and CVP measurements) in response to therapeutic interventions is more useful and valid.

With the improvement in technology, current-generation PACs also allow a volumetric, as opposed to pressure-based, estimate of intravascular volume status. The right ventricular end-diastolic volume index (RVEDVI) is an accurate indicator of the effect of right ventricular preload on ventricular volume and thus output. Use of RVEDVI is significantly more accurate than PAOP or CVP in estimating cardiac preload and has been associated with a decrease in mortality and MOF when used in part as an end point of resuscitation.[15-17]

There is ongoing debate as to the utility and safety of PACs. A multicenter study in a mixed ICU population suggested that the use of a PAC was associated with an increased mortality.[18] Also, several studies have suggested that there is no advantage to using a PAC versus a CVP monitor in the treatment of a mixed population of patients with adult respiratory distress syndrome.[19] As a result, additional methods of volumetric preload assessment have been developed. Lithium dilution cardiac output (LiDCO) is a noninvasive method for measuring CO. It requires only an arterial pressure catheter and a central venous catheter. Lithium dilution is used to calibrate a pulse pressure algorithm, which allows continuous CO assessment.[20] Although comparable with PACs, the LiDCO method does not allow continuous assessment of oxygen transport. The major problem is the loss of reliability in the acutely unstable patient.

In addition to measurements of CO, indicators of preload responsiveness including systolic and pulse pressure variation (SPV and PPV) can be obtained. These variations have been derived from observations in mechanically ventilated patients, where cyclical changes due to respiration are induced in the vena cava, pulmonary artery, and aortic blood flow. It is important to note that these arterial pressure variations are not an indicator of volume status, nor a direct marker of cardiac preload. Rather, SPV and PPV are indicators of the position on the Frank-Starling curve. Patients on the flat portion of the curve are insensitive to cyclical changes in preload induced by mechanical ventilation. Conversely, arterial pressure variations are increased in patients who are on the steep portion of the preload curve.[21-23] Thus, a PPV of >12% or SPV >5 mm Hg is indicative of preload responsiveness and need for increased intravascular volume.[20-23] The variables obtained by this method can be affected by aortic regurgitation, cardiac arrhythmia including tachycardia, irregular breathing, damped arterial line, or marked peripheral arterial vasoconstriction.

Esophageal Doppler ultrasound and transesophageal echocardiography have also been utilized in the hemodynamic assessment and monitoring of critically ill patients.[24] These modalities provide information about global and ventricular function of the heart. End-diastolic volume may be assessed and has been shown to be more accurate than PAOP in the estimate of optimal preload status. Again, while these methods are comparable to several measurements obtained with PAC use, they do not allow continuous assessment of cardiopulmonary function and provide only a "snapshot" view of a complex, potentially rapidly changing physiology. In addition, these methods suffer the common problem of noninvasive monitors in that the algorithms and validation studies have been performed in relatively healthy patients. Algorithms used to calculate CO and stroke volume may be flawed in critically ill patients with severe shock.

Invasive Oxygen Transport Monitoring

In addition to the hemodynamic variables obtained with the PAC, determination of oxygen content in arterial and venous blood, together with CO and hemoglobin concentration, allows calculation of oxygen delivery, oxygen consumption, and oxygen-extraction ratio. The shock state induces an imbalance between oxygen demand and oxygen supply, resulting in anaerobic metabolism, lactic acidosis, and cell death. Table 4.3 outlines the oxygenation variables that may be obtained.

The assessment of oxygen transport begins with the calculation of oxygen content in blood. The majority of oxygen is bound to hemoglobin (>98%). Less than 2% is dissolved in plasma due to oxygen's low solubility coefficient. Delivery of oxygen to the tissues is highly dependent upon the hemoglobin concentration as well as the ability of red blood cells to unload oxygen, which is dependent on the 2,3-diphosphoglycerate (2,3 DPG) content and its loss during blood banking storage. Oxygen delivery (DO_2) and consumption (VO_2) may be calculated by utilizing cardiac index (CI), arterial oxygen content (CaO_2), and mixed venous oxygen content (CvO_2).

The oxygen content in the pulmonary end capillary is at its highest, as none of the oxygen has been consumed by the tissues or diluted by unsaturated blood. As the blood leaves the heart, the oxygen content is reduced due to introduction of unsaturated blood from three sources. The first is bronchial blood, which empties into the pulmonary veins. The second is intrapulmonary shunt, which may be significantly higher in those patients with pulmonary dysfunction or in shock. The third is venous blood from the thebesian veins, which drain directly into the left ventricle after supplying the myocardium. Therefore the arterial O_2 concentration can be calculated as the amount of oxygen bound to arterial hemoglobin + oxygen dissolved in arterial plasma.

After extraction of oxygen by the tissues, the blood is returned to the heart. The partial pressure of mixed venous oxygen tension (PvO_2) can be measured by a venous blood gas or via the intra-atrial port of the PAC. The venous oxygen content of blood as it returns to the heart is calculated as the amount of oxygen bound to venous hemoglobin + oxygen dissolved in venous plasma.

The difference between arterial and venous oxygen content (CaO_2 - CvO_2) represents the amount of oxygen extracted by the tissues. It is often elevated in shock due to increased oxygen demands and decreased oxygen delivery. A CaO_2 - CvO_2 of >5.5 mL O_2/dL or >35% suggests that CO is inadequate to optimally meet cellular oxygen demands.[25] Ideally, adequate resuscitation should generate a mixed oxygen saturation of >0.70.

As seen in the calculation for oxygen delivery, an important factor is hemoglobin concentration. Previously, it was thought that a hemoglobin concentration of 10-13 g/dL was optimal for oxygen delivery; however, recent studies have suggested that transfusion to this level provides no benefit in critically ill patients and is associated with a decrease in survival. A hemoglobin concentration of <7-8 g/dL is recommended as the level required to trigger a blood transfusion, in the absence of recent acute myocardial infarct, unstable angina, or ongoing blood loss.[26] Blood transfusion to maximize oxygen delivery must be balanced against the potentially harmful effects and increased risks of infection, immunosuppression, and organ failure associated with transfusion of banked blood.

TABLE 4.3

OXYGEN TRANSPORT VARIABLES

VARIABLE	UNIT	NORMAL RANGE
MEASURED VARIABLES		
Arterial oxygen tension (PaO_2)	mm Hg	70-100
Arterial carbon dioxide tension ($PaCO_2$)	mm Hg	35-50
Arterial oxygen saturation (SaO_2)	fraction	0.93-0.98
Mixed venous oxygen saturation (SvO_2)	fraction	0.70-0.78
Mixed venous oxygen tension (PvO_2)	mm Hg	36-42
Hemoglobin (Hb)	g	13-17
CALCULATED VARIABLES		
Oxygen delivery (DO_2) $CaO_2 \times CO \times 10$	mL/min	800-1,600
Oxygen consumption (VO_2) $(CaO_2 - CvO_2) \times CO \times 10$	mL/min	150-400
Arterial oxygen content (CaO_2) $(1.34 \times Hb \times SaO_2) + (PaO_2 \times 0.0031)$	mLO_2/dL blood	16-22
Mixed venous oxygen content (CvO_2) $(1.34 \times Hb \times SvO_2) + (PvO_2 \times 0.0031)$	mLO_2/dL blood	12-17
Arteriovenous O_2 difference $CaO_2 - CvO_2$	mLO_2/dL blood	3.5-5.5
Oxygen extraction ratio (O_2ER) $[1 - (VO_2/DO_2)$	Fraction	0.22-0.32

GENERAL SHOCK TREATMENT PRINCIPLES

There are three priorities in the treatment of shock. First, the diagnosis and underlying cause of shock must be diagnosed and corrected. Second, resuscitation for shock must rapidly restore tissue perfusion and optimize oxygen delivery, hemodynamics, and cardiac function. Third, end-organ failure must be prevented or function supported. Often, resuscitation will be initiated prior to or simultaneously with identifying the underlying etiology.

For resuscitation, a reasonable goal of therapy is to achieve normal mixed venous oxygen saturation and arteriovenous oxygen-extraction ratio, while simultaneously, the elevated SVR should return to normal. Oxygen delivery may be enhanced by improving hemoglobin concentration, arterial oxygen saturation and CO, individually or simultaneously.[27] An algorithm for the resuscitation of the shocked patient is shown in Algorithm 4.1.

Fluid Therapy for Shock

A decreased CVP and oxygen delivery were key features noted in the early investigations of hemorrhagic shock, and a prolonged decrease in oxygen delivery led to a reduction in oxygen consumption. After successful fluid resuscitation, oxygen delivery and consumption increased above baseline for several hours. Failure of the patient to achieve this adequate response to resuscitation was almost universally fatal. Thus, restoration of hemodynamics and oxygen transport with fluid and inotropes became the primary paradigm of shock treatment. However, it is important to note that excessive use of either modality has been shown to be detrimental to patient outcomes and survival.

It was noted by Shires et al. that additional fluid replacement beyond the actual amount of blood loss, due to ongoing interstitial "third spacing" loss, was required to improve outcomes in hemorrhagic shock.[28,29] These data led to the appropriate practice of aggressive, early fluid resuscitation. However, over time, complications from excessive fluid therapy began

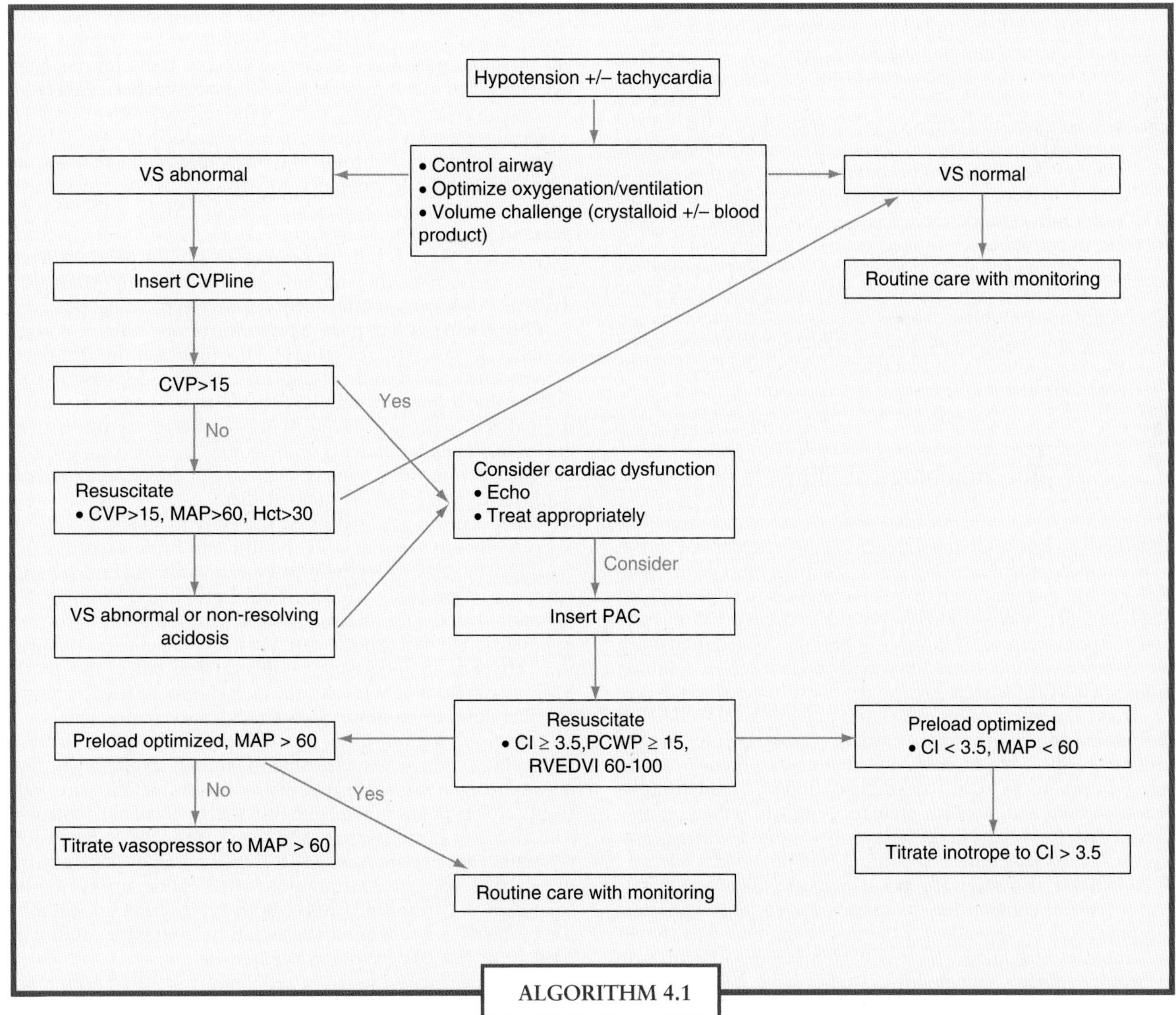

ALGORITHM 4.1 An algorithm for shock resuscitation. (VS, vital signs; CVP, central venous pressure; HCt, hematocrit; ECHO, echocardiogram; PAC, pulmonary artery catheter; CI, cardiac index in (L per minute) per m^2; PCWP, pulmonary capillary wedge pressure in mm Hg; RVEDVI, right ventricular end-diastolic volume index.)

to appear, such as ARDS, abdominal compartment syndrome, and detrimental elevations in intracranial pressures. Currently, resuscitation volumes have become more judicious, and earlier use of blood components is advocated.

Crystalloids are balanced salt solutions widely used as resuscitative fluids. They restore the extracellular volume, decreasing the transfusion requirement after hemorrhagic shock and restoring adequate volume in most cases. Crystalloids are inexpensive and readily available. Lactated Ringer's solution is isotonic and rapidly replaces the loss of interstitial fluid, without worsening any pre-existing electrolyte abnormality. However, recent investigations have identified the proinflammatory effects of lactated Ringer's solution containing the D(-) isomer of lactate found in some commercial forms of lactated Ringer's. D(-) lactate has been shown to increase neutrophil adhesion and increase production of reactive oxygen species.[30,31] These adverse effects of crystalloid resuscitation are not found with L(-) lactate isomer formulations. In addition, lactated Ringer's contains potassium and must be used cautiously if renal function is impaired or unknown.[32] Normal saline solution is also effective in the resuscitation of shocked patients. Large-volume administration of normal saline, though, is associated with a hypernatremic, hyperchloremic metabolic acidosis. This acidosis complicates the resuscitation of the critically ill patient.

Colloids theoretically remain in the intravascular space for a longer period compared with crystalloids, due to the increased molecular size. Commonly used colloids include albumin, modified fluid gelatin, dextran 70, dextran 40, and hydroxyethyl starch. Despite widespread use since the early 20th century, there has been no demonstrated benefit to colloid use.[33] In fact, colloid albumin infusion has been shown to increase mortality as well as prolong the resuscitation phase and delay postresuscitation diuresis. Albumin may also depress circulating immunoglobulin levels and reduce endogenous albumin synthesis. Given the lack of benefit and increased cost, colloids cannot be recommended in the current management of shock.[34]

Pharmacological Support

Pharmacological agents affecting preload, cardiac contractility, and afterload can be of major benefit in the treatment of shock. Importantly, optimal intravascular restoration must always precede cardiac augmentation. Inotropic support may be required when adequate preload fails to provide sufficient CO to meet tissue oxygen demands.[35] Pressor support may be required when the systemic vasculature is abnormally dilated with a resulting diminished SVR, as seen particularly with hyperdynamic septic shock. The effect of inotropes and pressors is dependent on the specific adrenergic receptor affinity (Table 4.4). In cases of primary cardiac dysfunction, vasodilators can reduce cardiac oxygen demand by reducing afterload and/or by dilating the venous system and reducing preload. Afterload reduction may preserve stroke volume in the failing myocardium, whereas preload reduction may relieve pressure-driven pulmonary edema.

Dopamine is a naturally occurring catecholamine that is a precursor of epinephrine. Its affinity for various adrenergic receptors is dose dependent. Low-dose dopamine was shown to augment renal blood flow and glomerular filtration rate in healthy subjects, but multiple studies have failed to demonstrate that low-dose dopamine prevents acute renal failure in critically ill patients.[36] At moderate doses, dopamine has mainly beta effects and primarily improves cardiac contractility, but at the expense of increased HR. Higher doses stimulate alpha receptors resulting in an increase in peripheral vascular resistance, BP, and oxygen consumption by the myocardium. Dopamine must be carefully titrated in each patient due to the variable dose-dependent affinity for adrenergic receptors.

Dobutamine is a synthetic catecholamine that predominantly affects beta receptors. When its chronotropic effects are minimal, the inotropic effects of dobutamine have little effect on myocardial oxygen demand because it also induces peripheral vasodilatation. However, this decrease in SVR limits its utility in patients with risk of hypotension. Dobutamine is an excellent agent if cardiac augmentation is required to optimize oxygen delivery once intravascular volume has been function supported.

Epinephrine is released physiologically in response to stress. Beta effects predominate at pharmacological doses, resulting in increased stroke volume, cardiac contractility, and noteworthy tachycardia, with peripheral vasodilatation. At higher doses, alpha-adrenergic receptors are stimulated with subsequent vasoconstriction and increased myocardial oxygen demand. In addition, cardiac arrhythmias and renal and splanchnic vasoconstriction all limit the prolonged use of high-dose epinephrine. It should be considered as a short-term agent in patients with refractory cardiac dysfunction not responsive to other agents.

Norepinephrine has both alpha and beta receptor effects; however, it is predominantly an alpha-adrenergic agonist. Combined alpha and beta stimulation typically results in an increase in afterload and glomerular perfusion pressure, with preservation of CO. It has been shown to be of most benefit in septic patients.[37] Adequate volume resuscitation must occur prior to use, due to the risk of tissue hypoperfusion from excessive vasoconstriction in the hypovolemic patient.

Isoproterenol is a synthetic catecholamine with major beta-adrenergic effects. Chronotropy may predominate over its inotropic effects. In conjunction with the peripheral vasodilatation, CO and pulse pressure increase. Myocardial oxygen demand is greatly increased, and the tachycardia limits coronary filling. As a result, isoproterenol should be considered only in those patients with hemodynamically important bradycardia, as a temporizing agent before electrical pacing.

Phenylephrine has pure alpha effects and thus increases peripheral vascular resistance. This increase in afterload increases cardiac workload and may cause a decrease in CO and stroke volume. It may be considered as a first-line agent for patients with neurogenic shock; however, its use is generally restricted to patients who require pressor support and cannot tolerate other agents such as dopamine and norepinephrine due to excessive tachycardia.

Vasopressin is released physiologically in shock. It acts on V1 receptors in vascular smooth muscle to cause vasoconstriction and increase receptivity to catecholamines. Endogenous vasopressin levels are decreased after prolonged hemorrhagic or septic shock. This relative deficiency may explain refractory hypotension in those shock states. In patients with septic shock, it is effective in increasing peripheral resistance and MAP. Vasopressin has no inotropic effects. It should be used at physiological doses to minimize associated pressor requirements.

Amrinone and milrinone are steroid-like phosphodiesterase antagonists, which increase smooth muscle cyclic adenosine monophosphate (cAMP) and alter calcium metabolism. Inotropic effects predominate with minimal positive chronotropy. The risk for vasodilatation and aggravation of hypotension is significant. The increase in CO with minimal demands on myocardial oxygen consumption offers some utility in the treatment of cardiogenic shock. Both agents have a long half-life of nearly 3 hours and thus should be used with caution in patients at risk of developing hypotension.

Nitroprusside is a potent arterial and venous smooth muscle vasodilator of very short duration. Afterload is reduced, leading to an increase in CO and stroke volume. Hypotension may limit its use, particularly in cases of inadequate preload. Nitroprusside use for more than 48 hours requires monitoring of serum thiocyanate levels and arterial pH to detect complications of cyanide toxicity.

TABLE 4.4

HEMODYNAMIC EFFECTS OF INOTROPES/PRESSORS

		SITE OF ACTION					HEMODYNAMIC RESPONSE				
		HEART		VESSELS							
DRUG	METABOLISM	β1	β2	α1	β2	V1	RENAL PERFUSION	CO	SVR	BP	HR
Isoproterenol 1-20 μg/min	Renal	+++	+++		+++		↑	↑↑	↔	↔/↑	↑↑
Dobutamine 2-40 μg/kg/min	Hepatic	+++	+		+		↔/↑	↑↑	↓	↔/↑	↑↑
Milrinone[a] 50 μg/min load 0.375-0.75 μg/kg/min	Hepatic						↔	↑↑	↓	↔/↓	↑
Epinephrine 2-10 μg/min	Renal	+++	+++	+++	++		↔	↑↑	↔/↑	↑↑	↑↑
Norepinephrine 2-12 μg/min	Renal	++	+	+++			↔	↑	↑↑	↑↑	↔/↑
Phenylephrine 40-100 μg/min	Renal			+++			↔/↓	↔	↑↑	↑	↔
Vasopressin 0.01-0.04 U/min	Renal/ Hepatic					+++	↔	↔	↑↑	↑	↔
Dopamine[b]	Hepatic										
2-5 μg/kg/min (low)		+	+	+	+		↔	↔/↑	↔/↓	↔/↑	↔/↑
5-15 μg/kg/min (med)		++	++	+	+		↔	↑↑	↔/↑	↑	↑
15-50 μg/kg/min (high)		+++	++	+++	++		↔/↓	↑↑	↑↑	↑↑	↑↑

α1, vasoconstriction peripheral arterioles; β1, myocardial inotropy, chronotropy, enhanced AV conduction; β2, chronotropy, vasodilation mesenteric/skeletal bed, bronchodilation; V1 vasoconstriction peripheral arterioles, CO, cardiac output; SVR, systemic vascular resistance; BP, blood pressure; HR, heart rate.

[a]Milrinone: inhibits phosphodiesterase 3 resulting in increase in cAMP.

[b]Dopamine: dopamine receptor stimulation at low dose vasodilates mesenteric/coronary/renal beds.

Nitroglycerin predominantly affects the venous capacitance system. It is an effective treatment for acute myocardial ischemia, as it reduces excessive preload and ventricular end-diastolic pressure, thereby reducing myocardial oxygen demand.

END POINTS OF SHOCK RESUSCITATION

Resuscitation is an ongoing process, which requires constant assessment and modification dependent on the patient's response to therapy. End points can be categorized as either global or regional indicators of perfusion.[38] While BP and HR are commonly used global measures, they are relatively poor determinants of tissue oxygenation. Patient age and pre-existing medical conditions are frequent confounding influences.

Mixed venous oxygen saturation (SvO_2) can be measured continuously with a PAC. The continuously measured SvO_2 correlates well with oxygen extraction ratios calculated by laboratory measurements of arterial and mixed venous oxygen saturation, hemoglobin concentration, and CO.[39] SvO_2 is a global indicator of oxygen supply–demand balance but does not indicate the adequacy of perfusion of any individual vascular bed. A low SvO_2 (<0.65) always indicates an unfavorable imbalance in the delivery and consumption of oxygen. A high SvO_2 (>0.78) may exist in conditions of inadequate utilization such as sepsis, pregnancy, cirrhosis, and inflammation and is difficult to interpret. It implies a maldistribution of peripheral blood flow. There may be vascular areas of oxygen delivery in excess of consumption, but may be in conjunction with other areas of inadequate oxygen delivery. Therapeutic interventions should be aimed toward achieving an SvO_2 of approximately 0.7.[40]

Arterial lactate concentrations increase in conditions of shock, but can be misleading. The shift from aerobic to anaerobic metabolism causes accumulation of hydrogen ions and lactate, resulting in acidosis and cellular death. However, an elevation in lactate may be due to several mechanisms. Ongoing anaerobic metabolism and decreased lactate metabolism due to hepatic and/or renal hypoperfusion increases lactate levels. Lactate may accumulate in tissues during periods of hypoperfusion and wash out into the central circulation when perfusion to these relatively hypoxic tissues is restored. Excessive lactate production may occur in tissues that depend on glycolysis for energy production despite adequate oxygen delivery. Elevated serum lactate levels are not specific in detecting abnormal regional perfusion, and may also reflect "washout" from anaerobic tissues caused by a period of hypoperfusion that has already resolved. Importantly, a positive response toward correction during resuscitation is associated with a better prognosis.[41,42] However, "normal clearance" of lactate is controversial. The half-life of lactate in patients with normal renal and hepatic function is estimated between 2 and 4 hours. In the presence of shock, the half-life may be significantly longer. Aggressive resuscitation may result in a slight increase in lactate due to peripheral washout. This should generally correct early, and the trend should be a steady decrease.[43]

Base deficit predicts fluid resuscitation requirements, similar to lactate, but normalizes rapidly with restoration of aerobic metabolism, making it a useful end point for guiding resuscitation.[44] The magnitude of base deficit is a predictor of mortality in trauma patients.[43] As with lactate, the base deficit trend toward normal should be the intended goal of resuscitation.

The splanchnic circulation is affected early and most importantly in shock. *Gastric tonometry* has been used to measure intramucosal pH, because of loss of buffering capacity provided by the extensive submucosal blood flow, and thus provides information about a single vascular bed.[45] Increasing intramucosal acidosis indicates inadequate oxygen delivery to the intestinal mucosa and thus may be used to guide resuscitation.[46] However, the logistic difficulty of the technology and interpretation of the data has restricted the widespread use of this method.[47]

FEATURES AND MANAGEMENT OF SPECIFIC FORMS OF SHOCK

Although, the end result of impaired tissue perfusion is common to all forms of shock, specific treatment options exist for specific shock states. The hemodynamic patterns seen with specific forms of shock are shown in Table 4.5. Early recognition of these patterns helps identify the underlying etiology.

TABLE 4.5

HEMODYNAMIC PATTERNS FOR SHOCK TYPES

TYPE	CO	SVR	PAOP	CVP	SVO_2
Hypovolemic	↓	↑	↓	↓	↓
Cardiogenic					
Left ventricular MI	↓	↑	↑	N, ↑	↓
Right ventricular MI	↓	↑	N, ↓	↑	↓
Obstructive					
Pericardial tamponade	↓	↑	↑	↑	↓
Pulmonary embolism	↓	↑	↑	↑	↓
Distributive					
Early	↑, N, ↓	↑, N, ↓	N	N,↑	N, ↑
Early after fluid administration	↑	↓	N,↑	N,↑	↑, N, ↓
Late	↓	↑	N	N	↓
Hypoadrenal	↓	N, ↓	↑, ↓	↑, ↓	↓

CO, cardiac output; SVR, systemic vascular resistance; PAOP, pulmonary artery occlusion pressure; CVP, central venous pressure; SvO_2, mixed venous oxygen saturation; MI, myocardial infarction; N, normal.

Hypovolemic Shock

The most common form of shock results from loss of red cell mass and plasma, or the loss of plasma volume alone. Physical findings stem from the cardiovascular and neurohumoral responses to shock. The signs include cold, clammy skin, tachycardia, hypotension, oliguria, and impaired mentation. Hypovolemic shock can be stratified into four classes depending on the degree of volume loss (Table 4.6).

The condition is readily diagnosed when there is hemodynamic instability and the source of volume loss is obvious. Remember, after acute hemorrhage, hemoglobin and hematocrit values do not change until compensatory fluid shifts occur or exogenous fluid is administered. Plasma loss alone results in hemoconcentration, and free water loss leads to hypernatremia. With more subtle or chronic volume losses, the etiology may be much more difficult to ascertain. A high degree of suspicion for hypovolemia should exist following all injuries or major gastrointestinal fluid losses.

In cases of hemorrhage, the focus must be on definitive hemorrhage control rather than merely aggressive replacement. Simultaneous judicious resuscitation should also occur; however, volume cannot be given rapidly enough to match massive hemorrhage.[48] In accordance with Starling's law, stroke volume and CO increase with an increase in preload. Therefore, resuscitation is initiated with a rapid infusion of isotonic saline or a balanced salt solution such as Ringer's lactate. There is no additional benefit to the initial use of colloid solutions, and in trauma patients, colloids are associated with an increased mortality.[34] Evidence of continuing or severe blood loss requires simultaneous replacement with cross-matched packed red blood cells, as well as other coagulation components including fresh frozen plasma, cryoprecipitate, and platelets. In the presence of severe or prolonged hypovolemia, inotropic support may be required to maintain adequate ventricular function, but only after blood volume has been restored.

Current concepts in the resuscitation of hemorrhagic shock include limited volume administration to restore or maintain low to normal BP and "damage control" or hemostatic resuscitation. In 1994, Bickell et al.[49] produced the landmark paper demonstrating improved mortality in those patients with penetrating torso trauma, who had a restrictive crystalloid resuscitation prior to surgical control of bleeding. The underlying premise is sound, in that aggressive restoration prior to definitive hemorrhage control may actually worsen bleeding. Interestingly, this is not a new concept. In 1918, Cannon wrote, "Injection of a fluid that will increase BP carries danger in itself. Hemorrhage in the case of shock may not have occurred to a large degree because the BP is too low, and the flow too scant to overcome the obstacle offered by a clot. If the pressure is raised before the surgeon is ready to check any bleeding that may take place, blood that is sorely needed may be lost." In addition, recent military conflicts in Iraq and Afghanistan have demonstrated benefit with a resuscitative strategy based on earlier replacement of blood and coagulation products in severely injured patients. There are military and emerging civilian data to suggest that early implementation in massive transfusion of a 1:1:1 ratio of packed red cells:fresh frozen plasma:platelets transfusion strategy results in improved mortality, ventilator-free days, and ICU length of stay.[50-54]

Hypovolemic shock may still exist despite normal or increased total body fluid volume, when such volume is not intravascular. An increase in interstitial fluid occurs in severe trauma, pancreatitis, intestinal obstruction, and burns. This is a result of both microcirculatory failure and the systemic inflammatory effect and resulting massive capillary leak. Thus, patients will require resuscitation in excess of their apparent intravascular loss. If this inadequate intravascular volume is not recognized, underresuscitation and continued tissue hypoperfusion will continue. Thus, multiple parameters should be followed to ensure adequate resuscitation and restoration of perfusion.

Obstructive Shock

Obstructive shock results from a mechanical barrier to normal CO. Reduced cardiac compliance leads to inadequate diastolic filling. Pericardial tamponade occurs due to acute or chronic collections of fluid in the pericardial space. This may be a result of trauma, myocardial rupture, and aortic dissection. Tension pneumothorax causes mediastinal shift with subsequent compression of the great venous structures, again impairing preload. Pulmonary embolus may occasionally cause profound circulatory collapse. Mechanical obstruction occurs as a result of massive clot (saddle embolus) or by pulmonary hypertension due to the release of proinflammatory mediators in response to the acute embolus.

TABLE 4.6

CLASSIFICATION OF HYPOVOLEMIC SHOCK

	CLASS I	CLASS II	CLASS III	CLASS IV
Blood loss (mL)	Up to 750	750-1,500	1,500-2,000	≥2,000
Blood loss (%)	Up to 15	15-30	30-40	≥40
Pulse rate	<100	>100	>120	≥140
Blood pressure	Normal	Normal	Decreased	Decreased
Pulse pressure	Normal/Increased	Decreased	Decreased	Decreased
Capillary refill	Normal	Decreased	Decreased	Decreased
Respiratory rate	14-20	20-30	30-40	>35
Urine output (mL/h)	>30	20-30	5-15	Negligible
Mental status	Slightly anxious	Anxious	Confused	Lethargic
Fluid replacement	Crystalloid	Crystalloid	Crystalloid + blood	Crystalloid + blood

Adapted from American College of Surgeons Committee on Trauma. Advanced Trauma Life Support for Doctors, 8th edition.

The diagnosis of obstructive shock is often based on a combination of clinical findings, chest radiograph, and echocardiography. Pulmonary embolus is most commonly diagnosed with CT–angiography. The classic clinical findings of pericardial tamponade include hypotension, jugular venous distension, and muffled heart sounds (Beck's triad). An echocardiogram will demonstrate the fluid in the pericardial sac. Immediate pericardiocentesis or surgical decompression is indicated. Tension pneumothorax is suspected clinically when hypotension, decreased ipsilateral breath sounds, ipsilateral hyperresonance, tracheal deviation away from the affected side, and jugular venous distension are present. Treatment consists of immediate needle or tube thoracostomy. Pulmonary embolus is treated with therapeutic heparinization, while associated hemodynamic collapse may require surgical or endovascular embolectomy and/or angiographic thrombolysis.

Cardiogenic Shock

Cardiogenic shock is a result of pump failure. This may be due to myocardial infarction (MI), cardiomyopathy, ventricular outflow obstruction, acute valvular failure, ventricular filling defects, or cardiac arrhythmias.[55] Most commonly, shock is a consequence of acute MI.[56] Clinical findings include peripheral vasoconstriction, oliguria, and pulmonary and peripheral edema. A pre-existing cardiac history and other physical findings including pulmonary crepitations, cardiac murmurs, an S3 gallop, and jugular venous distension are also suggestive of cardiogenic shock. Decreased CO, with an elevated PAOP, is diagnostic. Differentiation between right- and left-sided heart failure is essential, as the management is significantly different.[57] Shock from right-sided failure is treated with ongoing volume resuscitation to improve ventricular preload. Left-sided failure often requires inotropic support and limited resuscitation. Shock due to cardiac arrhythmias often requires chemical or electrical cardioversion.

Cardiogenic shock tends to be self-perpetuating. Myocardial perfusion is dependent on the duration of diastole and the pressure gradient between the coronary artery and the left ventricle. Overly aggressive fluid resuscitation is not well tolerated and is likely to be harmful to a patient with the compromised myocardial function resulting from cardiogenic shock.

Distributive Shock

Distributive shock is a result of widespread vasodilatation and pooling of blood in the periphery. There is often a preservation or increase in CO early in the course. Septic shock is the classic example of hyperdynamic shock; however, other conditions such as anaphylaxis and severe liver dysfunction also result in a similar presentation.

Septic shock is manifested early by a decrease in SVR, normal to low PAOP, and increased CO. Despite elevated CO, oxygen extraction is impaired, in part due to mitochondrial dysfunction. This is also due to excessive blood flow to areas of normal metabolic demand and hypoperfusion of areas with increased demand. In later stages of septic shock, myocardial depression occurs, and the hemodynamics mimic that of cardiogenic shock. Septic shock is a result of complex interplay between microbial constituents and the immunologic response. Bacterial endotoxin is a lipopolysaccharide cell wall constituent of gram-negative bacteria, which induces release of proinflammatory cytokines.[58] In addition, gram-positive organisms may secrete superantigens, which are polyclonal T-lymphocyte activators that induce release of high levels of proinflammatory cytokines with resulting severe systemic inflammatory response as seen with Group A streptococcal infections.

This massive release of cytokines results in three major sequelae: thrombosis, increased vascular permeability, and vasodilatation. Proinflammatory cytokines result in increased tissue factor production, while reducing fibrinolysis by increasing PAI-1 expression. Activated thrombin is itself a major activator of proinflammatory cytokines. Other anticoagulant factors such as thrombomodulin and protein C are also decreased. The procoagulant tendency is further exacerbated by decreased blood flow at the level of small vessels. Together, these effects promote the deposition of fibrin-rich thrombi in small vessels, often throughout the body, thus contributing to tissue hypoperfusion and consumptive depletion of coagulation factors. The increase in vascular permeability causes leakage of fluid into the interstitium, resulting in tissue edema that may impede blood flow and diffusion of oxygen into tissues. Systemic vasodilatation and resulting hypotension are aggravated by the production of NO and the increases in vasoactive inflammatory mediators.[59]

Sepsis causes insulin resistance and hyperglycemia. The release of stress hormones and catecholamines along with proinflammatory cytokines such as TNF-α and IL-1 all drive gluconeogenesis. Insulin resistance occurs due to the cytokine and glucagon impairment of GLUT-4 surface expression, a glucose transporter.

The goals of septic shock treatment are to maintain tissue perfusion and institute appropriate empiric antibiotic treatment prior to culture results, insulin therapy for hyperglycemia, and, if applicable, infection source control. Intravenous fluid requirements may be high, and often a pressor agent such as norepinephrine and/or vasopressin is required to counter the systemic vasodilatation. Early implementation of goal-directed therapy has been demonstrated to improve outcomes in septic shock.[60,61] Steroids have not been shown to be effective; however, activated protein C has been shown to improve mortality in selected cases of severe septic shock with more than one organ failure.[62,63]

Neurogenic shock is another form of distributive shock, which occurs as a result of a spinal cord injury above the upper thoracic level. Disruption of the sympathetic outflow leads to peripheral vasodilatation, bradycardia, and hypotension. There is a relative expansion of the intravascular space through vasodilatation, particularly of venous capacitance vessels, and this is initially treated with judicious fluid administration. Often a pressor agent is required, and the bradycardia may require atropine to counter the unopposed parasympathetic influence, or an inotrope/pressor such as dopamine or norepinephrine. In most cases, hypotension resolves within 24-48 hours. Overresuscitation with fluid must be avoided. The diagnosis of neurogenic shock must be a process of exclusion, as it is often associated with other traumatic injuries involving concomitant blood loss.

Neurogenic shock should not be confused with spinal shock, which is defined as a loss of sensation and motor paralysis with initial loss of reflexes that gradually return. No circulatory compromise is associated with this condition and thus should not be considered a shock state.

Anaphylaxis is a severe form of Type I hypersensitivity. Exposure to the offending agent results in massive histamine release, with subsequent dermatologic reaction, respiratory obstruction, and hypotension. Occasionally, the reaction is severe enough to produce shock through myocardial depression along with massive capillary leak and edema formation. Treatment consists of volume replacement, epinephrine, steroids, and histamine receptor antagonists.

Endocrine Shock

The normal host response to critical illness is an increase in cortisol secretion to maintain homeostasis. Hypoadrenal shock occurs when unrecognized adrenal insufficiency complicates the host response to the stress induced by critical illness or major surgery.[64] Adrenocortical insufficiency may occur as a result of chronic exogenous corticosteroid use. In addition, trauma and sepsis may also induce a relative hypoadrenal state. Hypovolemia with a decrease in SVR and CO occur in hypoadrenal shock. Administration of physiologic doses of steroids to correct the relative hypoadrenal state results in stabilization of hemodynamics and possible survival benefits.[65,66] The diagnosis is established by using an ACTH stimulation test. Empiric treatment is with dexamethasone, as this does not interfere with ACTH stimulation test. If the diagnosis is confirmed by low or no response to ACTH, treatment should consist of hydrocortisone, with tapering as the patient achieves hemodynamic stability.[67] Adjunctive volume resuscitation and pressor support should also continue.

SUMMARY

Shock is a common condition that is associated with a high mortality. Although the cellular pathways are largely similar, the etiology is varied and complex. Early recognition of inadequate tissue perfusion should trigger aggressive goal-directed therapy. Key data regarding hemodynamic and oxygenation transport variables should be obtained promptly. Correction of the underlying cause in conjunction with early resuscitation reduces the potentially fatal complication of end-organ dysfunction and failure.

References

1. Cannon W, Fraser J, Cowell E. The preventative treatment of wound shock. *JAMA*. 1918;70(9):618.
2. Matsuda N, Hattori Y. Systemic inflammatory response syndrome (SIRS): molecular pathophysiology and gene therapy. *J Pharmacol Sci*. 2006;101(3):189-198.
3. Rotstein OD. Modeling the two-hit hypothesis for evaluating strategies to prevent organ injury after shock/resuscitation. *J Trauma*. 2003;54(5 Suppl):S203-S206.
4. Ventilation with lower tidal volumes as compared with traditional tidal volumes for acute lung injury and the acute respiratory distress syndrome. The Acute Respiratory Distress Syndrome Network. *N Engl J Med*. 2000;342(18):1301-1308.
5. Goodman ER, et al. Role of interleukin 8 in the genesis of acute respiratory distress syndrome through an effect on neutrophil apoptosis. *Arch Surg*. 1998;133(11):1234-1239.
6. Baue AE. MOF, MODS, and SIRS: what is in a name or an acronym? *Shock*. 2006;26(5):438-449.
7. Darville T, Giroir B, Jacobs R. The systemic inflammatory response syndrome (SIRS): immunology and potential immunotherapy. *Infection*. 1993;21(5):279-290.
8. Gentilello LM, et al. Is hypothermia in the victim of major trauma protective or harmful? A randomized, prospective study. *Ann Surg*. 1997;226(4):439-447; discussion 447-449.
9. Jurkovich GJ, et al. Hypothermia in trauma victims: an ominous predictor of survival. *J Trauma*. 1987;27(9):1019-1024.
10. Neff TA. Routine oximetry. A fifth vital sign? *Chest*. 1988;94(2):227.
11. Kruse JA, et al. Lactate levels as predictors of the relationship between oxygen delivery and consumption in ARDS. *Chest*. 1990;98(4):959-962.
12. Davis JW, Shackford SR, Holbrook TL. Base deficit as a sensitive indicator of compensated shock and tissue oxygen utilization. *Surg Gynecol Obstet*. 1991;173(6):473-476.
13. Swan HJ, et al. Catheterization of the heart in man with use of a flow-directed balloon-tipped catheter. *N Engl J Med*. 1970;283(9):447-451.
14. Calvin JE, Driedger AA, Sibbald WJ. Does the pulmonary capillary wedge pressure predict left ventricular preload in critically ill patients? *Crit Care Med*. 1981;9(6):437-443.
15. Cheatham ML, et al. Right ventricular end-diastolic volume index as a predictor of preload status in patients on positive end-expiratory pressure. *Crit Care Med*. 1998;26(11):1801-1806.
16. Diebel L, et al. End-diastolic volume versus pulmonary artery wedge pressure in evaluating cardiac preload in trauma patients. *J Trauma*. 1994;37(6):950-955.
17. Durham R, et al. Right ventricular end-diastolic volume as a measure of preload. *J Trauma*. 1995;39(2):218-223; discussion 223-224.
18. Connors AF Jr, et al. The effectiveness of right heart catheterization in the initial care of critically ill patients. SUPPORT Investigators. *JAMA*. 1996;276(11):889-897.
19. Wheeler AP, et al. Pulmonary-artery versus central venous catheter to guide treatment of acute lung injury. *N Engl J Med*. 2006;354(21):2213-2224.
20. Sundar S, Panzica P. LiDCO systems. *Int Anesthesiol Clin*. 2010;48(1):87-100.
21. Cannesson M, Vallet B, Michard F. Pulse pressure variation and stroke volume variation: from flying blind to flying right? *Br J Anaesth*. 2009;03(6):896-897; author reply 897-899.
22. Michard F. Changes in arterial pressure during mechanical ventilation. *Anesthesiology*. 2005;103(2):419-428; quiz 449-445.
23. Michard F, et al. Relation between respiratory changes in arterial pulse pressure and fluid responsiveness in septic patients with acute circulatory failure. *Am J Respir Crit Care Med*. 2000;162(1):134-138.
24. Singer M, Bennett ED. Noninvasive optimization of left ventricular filling using esophageal Doppler. *Crit Care Med*. 1991;19(9):1132-1137.
25. Hayes MA, et al. Elevation of systemic oxygen delivery in the treatment of critically ill patients. *N Engl J Med*. 1994;330(24):1717-1722.
26. Hebert PC, et al. A multicenter, randomized, controlled clinical trial of transfusion requirements in critical care. Transfusion Requirements in Critical Care Investigators, Canadian Critical Care Trials Group. *N Engl J Med*. 1999;340(6):409-417.
27. Moore FA, et al. Inflammation and the Host Response to Injury, a large-scale collaborative project: patient-oriented research core—standard operating procedures for clinical care. III. Guidelines for shock resuscitation. *J Trauma*. 2006;61(1):82-89.
28. Shires GT. Pathophysiology and fluid replacement in hypovolemic shock. *Ann Clin Res*. 1977;9(3):144-150.
29. Shires GT, Carrico CJ, Coln D. The role of the extracellular fluid in shock. *Int Anesthesiol Clin*. 1964;2:435-454.
30. Alam HB, et al. Effect of different resuscitation strategies on neutrophil activation in a swine model of hemorrhagic shock. *Resuscitation*. 2004;60(1):91-99.
31. Rhee P, et al. Lactated Ringer's solution resuscitation causes neutrophil activation after hemorrhagic shock. *J Trauma*. 1998;44(2):313-319.
32. Canizaro PC, Prager MD, Shires GT. The infusion of Ringer's lactate solution during shock. Changes in lactate, excess lactate, and pH. *Am J Surg*. 1971;122(4):494-501.
33. Velanovich V. Crystalloid versus colloid fluid resuscitation: a meta-analysis of mortality. *Surgery*. 1989;105(1):65-71.
34. Finfer S, et al. A comparison of albumin and saline for fluid resuscitation in the intensive care unit. *N Engl J Med*. 2004;350(22):2247-2256.
35. Miller PR, Meredith JW, Chang MC. Randomized, prospective comparison of increased preload versus inotropes in the resuscitation of trauma patients: effects on cardiopulmonary function and visceral perfusion. *J Trauma*. 1998;44(1):107-113.
36. Bellomo R, et al. Low-dose dopamine in patients with early renal dysfunction: a placebo-controlled randomised trial. Australian and New Zealand Intensive Care Society (ANZICS) Clinical Trials Group. *Lancet*. 2000;356(9248):2139-2143.
37. Marin C, et al. Renal effects of norepinephrine used to treat septic shock patients. *Crit Care Med*. 1990;18(3):282-285.
38. Goodrich C. Endpoints of resuscitation: what should we be monitoring? *AACN Adv Crit Care*. 2006;17(3):306-316.
39. Burchell SA, et al. Evaluation of a continuous cardiac output and mixed venous oxygen saturation catheter in critically ill surgical patients. *Crit Care Med*. 1997;25(3):388-391.
40. Velmahos GC, et al. Endpoints of resuscitation of critically injured patients: normal or supranormal? A prospective randomized trial. *Ann Surg*. 2000;232(3):409-418.
41. Abramson D, et al. Lactate clearance and survival following injury. *J Trauma*. 1993;35(4):584-588; discussion 588-589.
42. Nguyen HB, et al. Early lactate clearance is associated with improved outcome in severe sepsis and septic shock. *Crit Care Med*. 2004;32(8):1637-1642.
43. Englehart MS, Schreiber MA. Measurement of acid-base resuscitation endpoints: lactate, base deficit, bicarbonate or what? *Curr Opin Crit Care*. 2006;12(6):569-574.
44. Davis JW, Kaups KL, Parks SN. Base deficit is superior to pH in evaluating clearance of acidosis after traumatic shock. *J Trauma*. 1998;44(1):114-118.
45. Chang MC, et al. Gastric tonometry supplements information provided by systemic indicators of oxygen transport. *J Trauma*. 1994;37(3):488-494.
46. Ivatury RR, et al. Gastric mucosal pH and oxygen delivery and oxygen consumption indices in the assessment of adequacy of resuscitation after trauma: a prospective, randomized study. *J Trauma*. 1995;39(1):128-134; discussion 134-136.
47. Taylor DE, et al. Measurement of gastric mucosal carbon dioxide tension by saline and air tonometry. *J Crit Care*. 1997;12(4):208-213.
48. Gann DS, et al. Impaired restitution of blood volume after large hemorrhage. *J Trauma*. 1981;21(8):598-603.
49. Bickell WH, et al. Immediate versus delayed fluid resuscitation for hypotensive patients with penetrating torso injuries. *N Engl J Med*. 1994;331(17):1105-1109.

50. Duchesne JC, Holcomb JB. Damage control resuscitation: addressing trauma-induced coagulopathy. *Br J Hosp Med (Lond).* 2009;70(1):22-25.
51. Duchesne JC, et al. Damage control resuscitation in combination with damage control laparotomy: a survival advantage. *J Trauma.* 69(1):46-52.
52. Duchesne JC, et al. Damage control resuscitation: the new face of damage control. *J Trauma.* 69(4):976-990.
53. Holcomb JB, et al. Increased plasma and platelet to red blood cell ratios improves outcome in 466 massively transfused civilian trauma patients. *Ann Surg.* 2008;248(3):447-458.
54. Gunter OL Jr, et al. Optimizing outcomes in damage control resuscitation: identifying blood product ratios associated with improved survival. *J Trauma.* 2008;65(3):527-534.
55. Alonso DR, et al. Pathophysiology of cardiogenic shock. Quantification of myocardial necrosis, clinical, pathologic and electrocardiographic correlations. *Circulation.* 1973;48(3):588-596.
56. Goldberg RJ, et al. Cardiogenic shock after acute myocardial infarction. Incidence and mortality from a community-wide perspective, 1975 to 1988. *N Engl J Med.* 1991;325(16):1117-1122.
57. Roberts N, et al. Right ventricular infarction with shock but without significant left ventricular infarction: a new clinical syndrome. *Am Heart J.* 1985;110(5):1047-1053.
58. Cuschieri J, et al. Modulation of endotoxin-induced endothelial function by calcium/calmodulin-dependent protein kinase. *Shock.* 2003;20(2):176-182.
59. Sharma S, Kumar A. Septic shock, multiple organ failure, and acute respiratory distress syndrome. *Curr Opin Pulm Med.* 2003;9(3):199-209.
60. Rivers E, et al. Early goal-directed therapy in the treatment of severe sepsis and septic shock. *N Engl J Med.* 2001;345(19):1368-1377.
61. Rivers EP, et al. The influence of early hemodynamic optimization on biomarker patterns of severe sepsis and septic shock. *Crit Care Med.* 2007;35(9):2016-2024.
62. Bernard GR. Drotrecogin alfa (activated) (recombinant human activated protein C) for the treatment of severe sepsis. *Crit Care Med.* 2003;31 (1 suppl):S85-S93.
63. Bernard GR, et al. Efficacy and safety of recombinant human activated protein C for severe sepsis. *N Engl J Med.* 2001;344(10):699-709.
64. Lipiner-Friedman D, et al. Adrenal function in sepsis: the retrospective Corticus cohort study. *Crit Care Med.* 2007;35(4):1012-1018.
65. Annane D, et al. Effect of treatment with low doses of hydrocortisone and fludrocortisone on mortality in patients with septic shock. *JAMA.* 2002;288(7):862-871.
66. Barquist E, Kirton O. Adrenal insufficiency in the surgical intensive care unit patient. *J Trauma.* 1997;42(1):27-31.
67. Sprung CL, et al. Hydrocortisone therapy for patients with septic shock. *N Engl J Med.* 2008;358(2):111-124.

CHAPTER 5 ■ BASIC OPERATIVE TECHNIQUES IN TRAUMA AND ACUTE CARE SURGERY

RAO R. IVATURY

Trauma and acute care surgery is an exciting field that offers a wide spectrum of operative experience, which ranges from elective to semielective to truly emergent, in body sites and cavities from head to toe and also from minimally invasive techniques to the "maximally" invasive procedures (e.g., "trap-door" approach to the left subclavian vessels). The basic principles of these divergent procedures are essentially the same: adequate exposure, control of bleeding and contamination, attention to patient physiology, and most importantly "do no harm." The scope of acute care surgery practice is so vast that a discussion of it can only be a sketch. This chapter, therefore, outlines the accepted techniques of exposure and treatment of various injuries and diseases in different anatomic sites. A brief introduction into minimally invasive approach follows, since that will surely be the state-of-the-art in the next decade. The reader is encouraged to supplement this chapter with atlas of operative and anatomic details.

OPERATIVE APPROACH TO NECK TRAUMA

In a landmark 1969 article, Monson et al. arbitrarily divided the neck into three clinical zones.[1] Zone I is defined as the area between the suprasternal notch and the cricoid cartilage, Zone II is the region between the cricoid and the angle of the mandible, and Zone III lies above the angle of the mandible. Zone II injuries are accessible via standard cervical approaches and do not present operative difficulty. Zone I injuries by definition involve the thoracic inlet with potential injuries to major vessels, and Zone III injuries are problematic because of the difficulty in obtaining distal control. Direct operative approach is therefore preferred for Zone II, while angiography may be helpful in the other zones.[2,3]

The patient should be placed in a prone position with both arms tucked, if possible. As long as there is no concurrent spine injury, a shoulder roll should be placed to extend the neck and the table placed in a semi-Fowler's position to aid in the operative exposure. The entire thorax and abdomen should be prepped in case of Zone I injury for accessing the chest and abdomen for potential multicavitary injuries. The groin and both thighs are prepped and draped for possible saphenous vein harvest.

Innominate and Subclavian Vessel Injury

Operative exposure of Zone I vascular injuries varies with the stability of the patient. If the patient is hemodynamically unstable with a large hemothorax or excessive bleeding from the chest tube, an anterolateral thoracotomy (high in the 3rd or 4th intercostal space) will allow apical packing to tamponade the bleeding from innominate or proximal subclavian vessels. This can be done in the trauma bay of the emergency department for the patient in extremis. In the stable patient, a median sternotomy in the O.R. is a good approach for the innominate and the right subclavian vessels. For the left subclavian artery, the incision may be extended along the sternocleidomastoid or the clavicle. This approach is superior to the morbid "trap-door" incision. The second and third portions of the subclavian are best approached by an incision along the clavicle with extension along the sternocleidomastoid, if necessary (Fig. 5.1). Subperiosteal resection of the mid or medial one-third of the clavicle will allow excellent exposure. The majority of these vascular injuries may be managed by simple lateral repair or end-to-end anastomosis. Occasionally, a saphenous vein graft may be necessary. In stable patients with a subclavian pseudoaneurysm or intimal injuries, endovascular stent grafts are an increasingly attractive option.

Carotid Artery Injury

Carotid exposure is obtained via a skin incision made along the anterior border of the sternocleidomastoid muscle (Figs. 5.1-5.3). The carotid sheath and its contents are readily identifiable. The venous and lymphatic structures are retracted in a lateral direction. Proximal and distal exposure of the carotid arteries is obtained after identifying the ansa cervicalis and 12th cranial nerve (Fig. 5.2). Digital pressure or a side-biting vascular clamp can be used to control hemorrhage while obtaining control. Proximal injury to the carotid at its aortic or subclavian origin requires more extensive exposure than the simple neck incision. Median sternotomy is the most commonly employed approach. A supraclavicular incision is useful for exposure in some cases, and dislocation or resection of the clavicle may improve the exposure (Fig. 5.1).

High Zone III injuries resulting in distal internal carotid laceration or disruption can be problematic in exposure and control. Anterior subluxation of the mandible can improve exposure, but only by about 2 cm. Osteotomy of the mandibular ramus may provide better exposure and mobility. Placement of a Fogarty balloon catheter to provide distal vascular control can be lifesaving during these maneuvers. Depending on the surgeon's experience in operating around the base of the skull, intraoperative assistance from either a maxillofacial surgeon or a neurosurgeon is advisable in difficult cases. Once proximal and distal control are secured, a Fogarty balloon catheter is carefully passed to remove any thrombus, and both proximal and distal ends are flushed with heparinized saline. A 5-O or 6-O monofilament polypropylene suture is used for the repair and handled with appropriate vascular technique. Except for tangential lacerations where primary repair is possible by lateral arteriorrhaphy, end-to-end anastomosis is often difficult, because the transected ends of the artery retract. Care must be taken to inspect for and repair any intimal flap at this time. This can often be done by incorporating the intimal defect into the laceration repair by utilizing a series of interrupted sutures. Also, the lumen of the artery must not be narrowed by this primary repair; if so, vein patch or interposition graft will be required. If there is a considerable destruction of the carotid artery, interposition grafting is warranted, preferably utilizing autologous tissue. Saphenous vein is generally the ideal conduit.

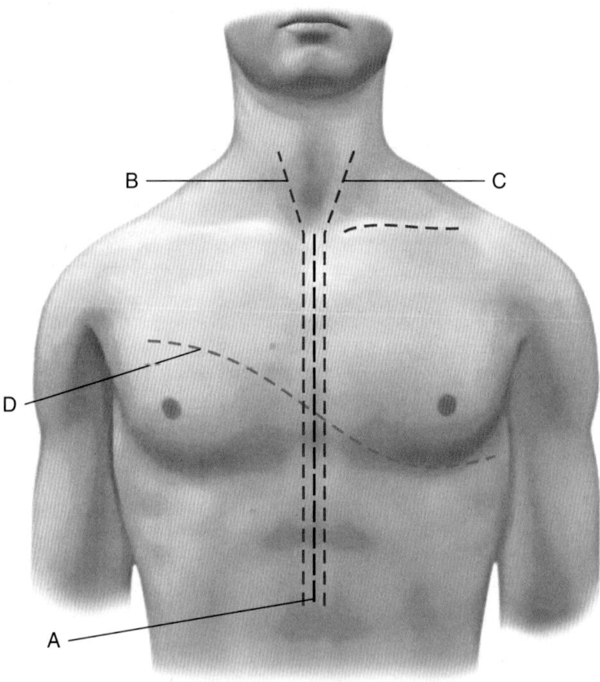

FIGURE 5.1. Operative approaches to neck and chest: **A:** standard median sternotomy for ascending aorta, innominate, cardiac injuries. **B:** Median sternotomy with extension to right neck for innominate, right subclavian, and common carotid artery injuries. Extension along the right clavicle will provide access to distal right subclavian vessels. **C:** Median sternotomy with left neck extension for left common carotid, aortic arch, and left subclavian vessel injuries. Extension along the left clavicle will provide access to distal left subclavian vessel injuries. **D:** Left anterolateral thoracotomy with extension to right chest as a clamshell incision providing access to all chest structures.

If adequate autologous conduit is not available, synthetic material may be used. The choice between woven Dacron and ePTFE is based on a surgeon's preference, as neither represents an ideal substitute for a vein graft.[3] If anatomy permits, the external carotid artery can be divided at a distal location, and transposed to the internal carotid artery. The use of a temporary shunt is not mandated by the available data. Increasingly, percutaneous transluminal placement of endovascular devices has become an alternative option to surgical repair.

Vertebral Artery Injury[4]

Vertebral artery injury,[4] fortunately, is not common. As warned by Matas "A glance at the surgical anatomy of this vessel as it lies deeply hidden in the skeleton of the neck, only escaping at short intervals from its osseous canal, to become immediately invested by the very important and vital cervical nerves as they issue from the spinal foramina, will at once remind us of the magnitude of the purely technical difficulties in the way of its atypical ligation, and of the errors of diagnosis that must be incurred."

If the identification and exposure of the vertebral artery injury is uncomplicated during neck exploration, proximal and distal surgical ligation of the injured vessel is performed. If encountered at neck exploration, the following steps are indicated: (1) Gauze packing at the site of bleeding and (2) exposure of the subclavian artery by dividing the origin of sternomastoid from the clavicle and proximal control of the origin of the subclavian artery. The neck incision is carried posterior to the ear with division of the attachment of sternomastoid and splenius capitis muscle. Distal ligation may be performed by dividing the splenius capitis and sternomastoid attachments to the mastoid, palpation of the transverse process of the atlas, and exposing the vertebral artery between the axis and atlas. Bone wax or other hemostatic agents can be used to pack and compress this area, or "blind" application of surgical clips deep into the wound may staunch the bleeding (Fig. 5.3A-C). The difficult dissection of the vertebral artery makes angiographic embolization an attractive option. Current data support the conclusion that most vertebral artery injuries can safely be managed without an operation or by angiographic embolization. Surgical intervention should be reserved for patients with severe bleeding or where embolization has failed.

Venous Injury

Injury to the innominate, subclavian, axillary, or internal jugular veins may be the source of severe hemorrhage. These veins can be ligated if the destruction is severe. In the case of severe bilateral jugular venous injury, ligation will carry significant clinical consequences. In this setting, reconstruction with an autologous conduit is advisable.[3]

Cervical Esophagus

Exposure is obtained by a left neck incision along the anterior border of the sternocleidomastoid muscle with medial retraction of the carotid vessels. Adequate mobilization behind the trachea and palpation of the nasogastric tube facilitate identification of the esophagus. The recurrent laryngeal nerve needs to be protected in the dissection and frequently may be palpated or visualized (Fig. 5.2). The esophageal perforation is identified either by direct visualization or with the help of intraluminal saline or dye. The perforation is repaired in either one or two layers. Neither the number of suture layers nor the type of suture material (absorbable or nonabsorbable) seem to influence the incidence of fistulization after the repair. If the operative exploration is delayed, repair may be difficult because of extensive inflammation in the area. In either instance (early or delayed operation), wide drainage is the key to success. Closed suction drains (Jackson- Pratt) usually are preferred.[5]
Laryngotracheal injury in the neck is uncommon but can be produced by blunt trauma, seat belt injury, or penetrating injuries. These injuries should be suspected with subcutaneous emphysema, soft tissue air in x-rays, or changes in phonation and blood in the aerodigestive tract. Primary repair with absorbable sutures without tracheostomy is the ideal approach. Tracheostomy through the injury, as once recommended, is not the preferred option. More complex injuries to the larynx are best handled with the help of ENT surgeons because of long-term complications and the need for corrective procedures.[6]

OPERATIVE APPROACHES TO CHEST TRAUMA

Emergency Department Thoracotomy

The usual incison is a left anterolateral thoracotomy (Fig. 5.1). For right-sided penetrating wounds and suspected injuries in the right chest, thoracotomy may be commenced as a right

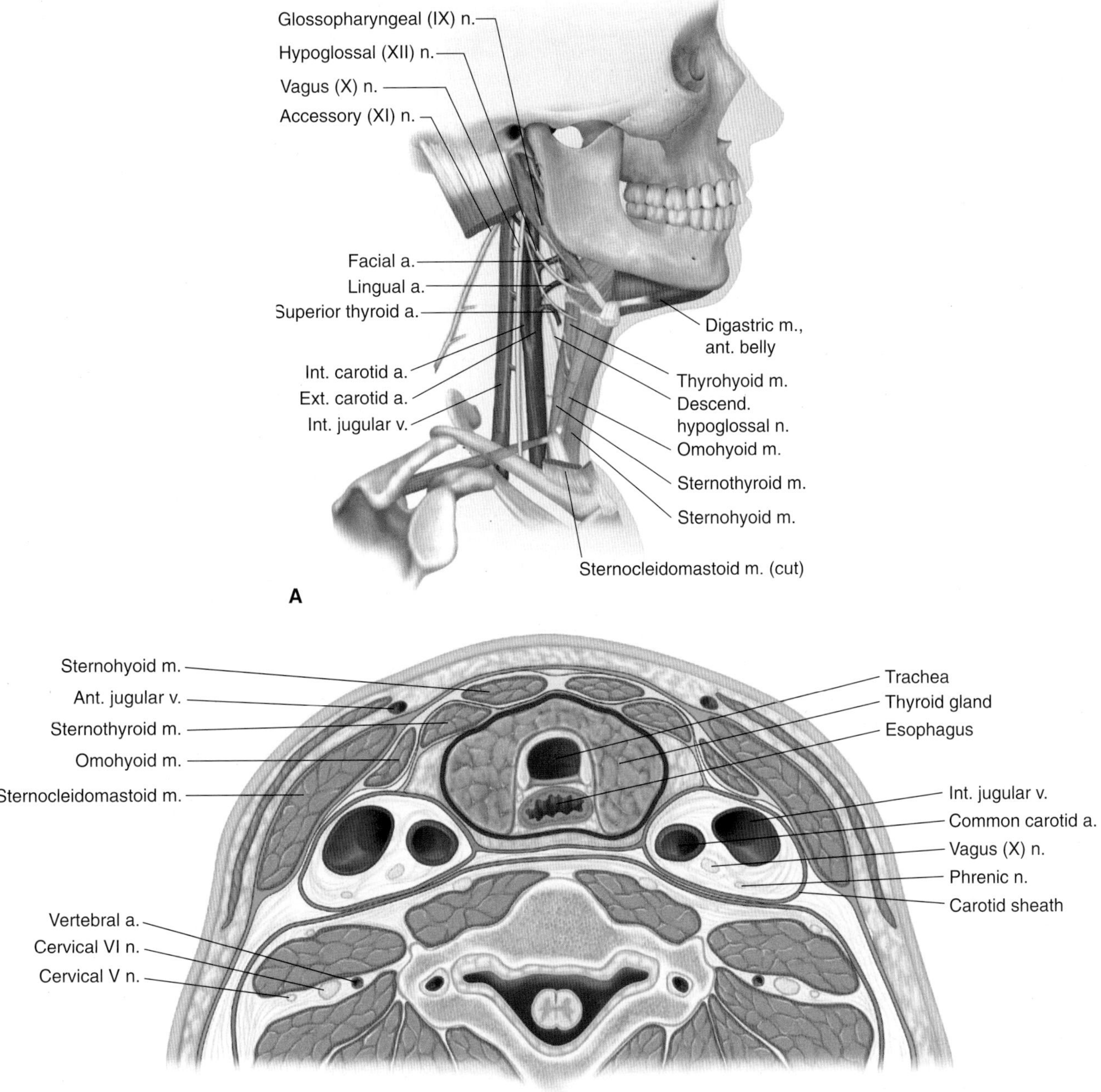

FIGURE 5.2. **A,B:** Anatomy of neck demonstrating the important structures in neck exploration. The cross section shows the carotid sheath and its contents and the anatomy of trachea and esophagus.

anterolateral thoracotomy and, if cardiac arrest has occurred and open cardiac massage is needed, a separate left anterolateral thoracotomy may be added. The usual incision is in the 4th or 5th intercostal space, extending as a sweeping curve into the axilla. If exposure is inadequate or for bilateral thoracic injuries, the incision may be extended across the sternum into the right chest as a "clam shell" thoracotomy. This provides outstanding exposure but one has to look for the transected internal mammary arteries and ligate them. When a patient is in extremis from a penetrating injury at the thoracic inlet and a massive hemothorax, a higher (3rd intercostal space) incision provides access to the thoracic vessels at the inlet that can be compressed manually while the patient is transported to the Operating Room.

Once inside the chest, a rapid assessment of the pericardium is made.[7] Tense, bluish pericardium suggests tamponade and is relieved by a knife anterior to the phrenic nerve. The pericardiotomy is then extended with a scissors parallel to the nerve. In the presence of a cardiac laceration, cardiorrhaphy may be achieved by staples, sutures, or gentle traction on a Foley catheter balloon inserted through the laceration (Figs. 5.4 and 5.5). Active hemorrhage from pulmonary lacerations is controlled by clamping the hilum of the lung manually with fingers or by placing a vascular clamp across. Some surgeons recommend "a lung twist" after the inferior pulmonary ligament is divided. These maneuvers also aid in the prevention of air embolism and aspiration of blood into the uninjured lung. Active hemorrhage from the apex of the pleural cavity suggests a subclavian vessel injury. Temporary tamponade of the vessels may be achieved by packing with large lap pads or pressure with a fist. The patient, if resuscitated, is then moved to the operating room. Cardiorrhaphy is completed by interrupted sutures with pledgets, taking care not to occlude the coronary vessels, if the wounds are adjacent to them. Most bleeding pulmonary injuries are best treated by resectional debridement.[8] In penetrating abdominal

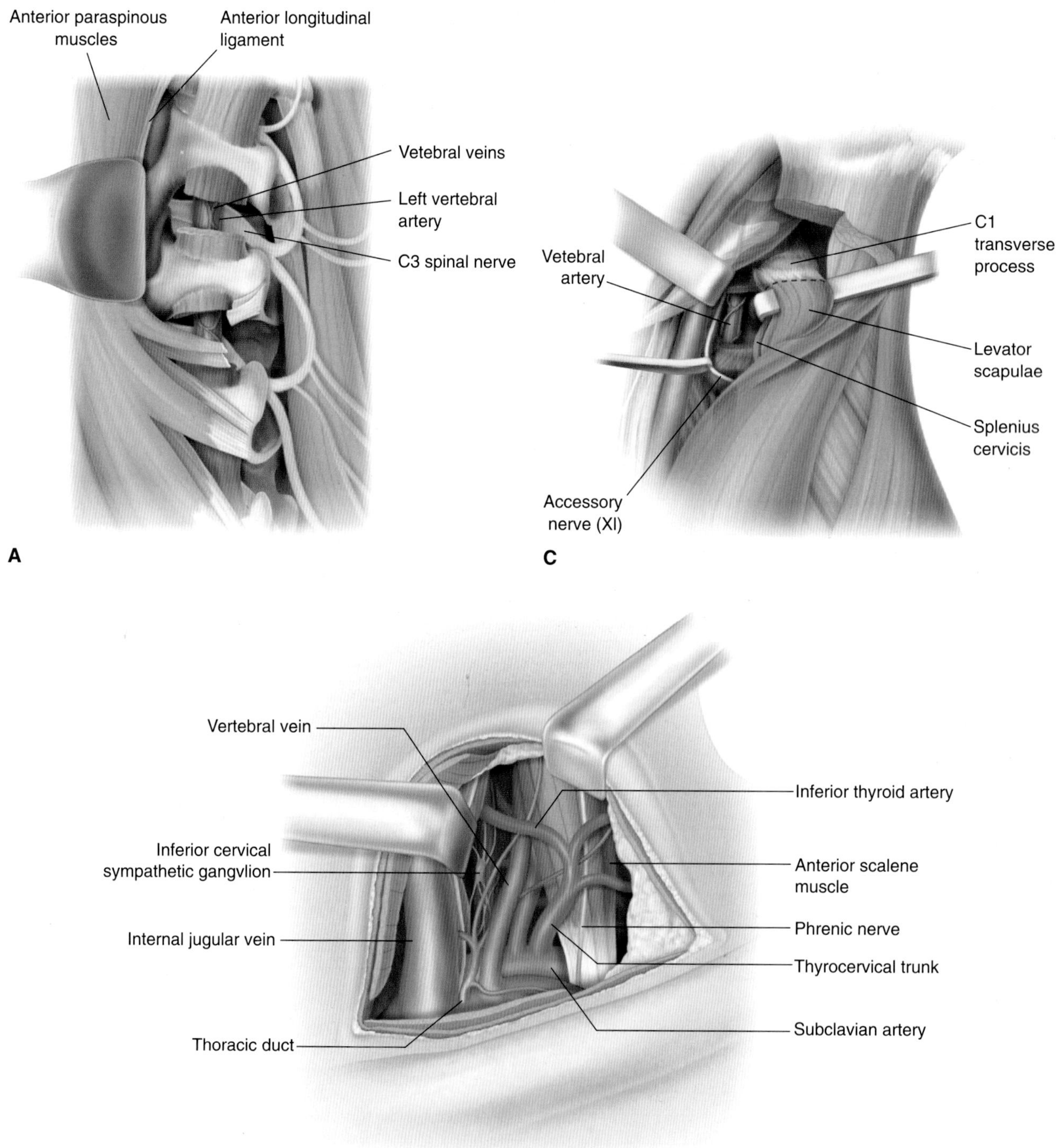

FIGURES 5.3. **A:** Anatomy of the vertebral artery, showing the course surrounded by cervical transverse processes. Exposure is facilitated by retraction of the anterior paraspinous muscles and anterior longitudinal ligament. **B:** Exposure of proximal vertebral artery by a supraclavicular incision, exposing the thyrocervical trunk from the subclavian artery. **C:** Exposure of the distal vertebral artery by sternocleidomastoid incision, dividing its origin from the mastoid process and dividing the levator scapulae and the splenius cervicis muscles.

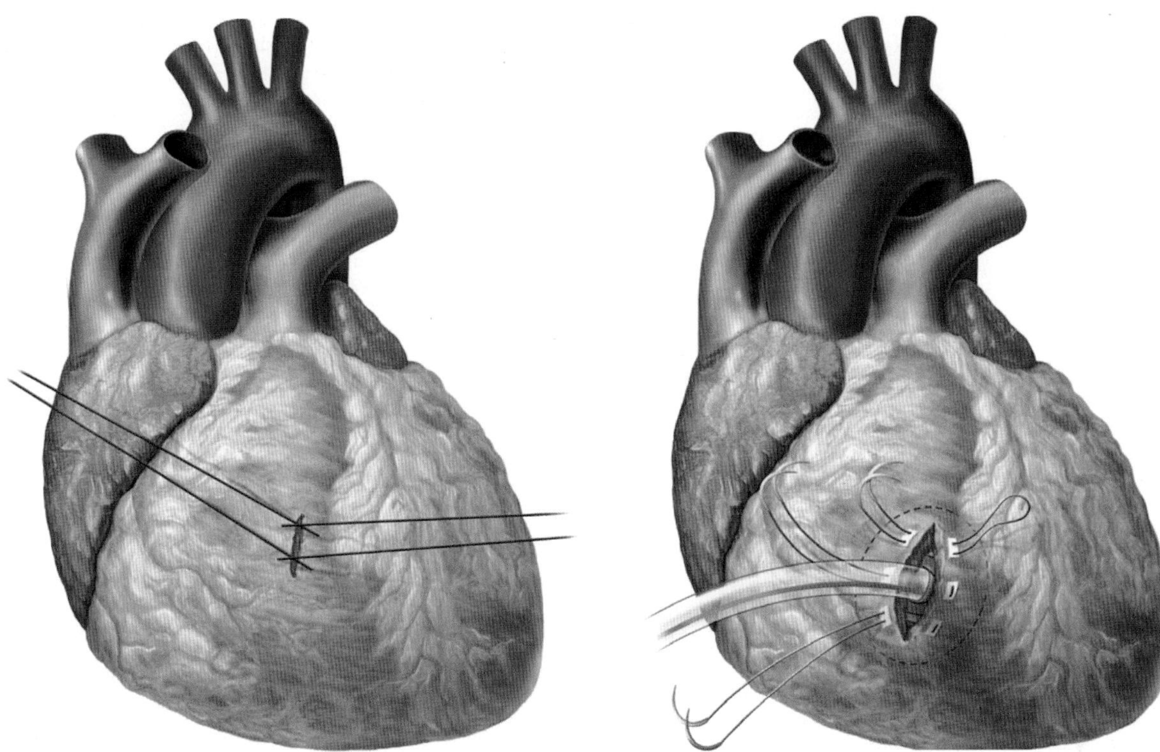

FIGURES 5.4 AND 5.5. Cardiac repair with sutures crisscrossed to close the laceration and control of hemorrhage with placement of a Foley catheter with the balloon inflated.

wounds with continuing hemorrhage, the descending thoracic aorta may be occluded initially by finger compression over the spine. Blunt finger dissection of the aorta must be performed for a proper application of a thoracic aortic clamp. A Penrose drain around the aorta applied as a tourniquet is a useful alternative technique. While doing these maneuvers, beware of injury to the esophagus or the intercostal vessels. Open cardiac massage, if needed, is best performed by a two-handed technique. Beware of the surgeon's fingers causing a rent in the soft, hypoxic ventricle.

Pitfalls of ERT: The potential problems of ERT include improperly placed incisions with severe limitation of exposure, incision through the female breast, iatrogenic injury to the lung, intercostal or internal mammary vessels, pericardium, lung, phrenic nerve, and coronary vessels. Hasty and inexperienced efforts at descending thoracic aortic occlusion may result in injury to the aorta, intercostal vessels, or the esophagus. The uncontrolled, desperate nature of Emergency Department Thoracotomy is a setup for injury to the operating team by sharp objects.

Injury to the Thoracic Esophagus

Operative repair is the treatment of choice for free thoracic perforations, for injuries diagnosed both early (<24 hours) or late (>24 hours). The presence of systemic sepsis, pneumothorax, pneumomediastinum or pneumoperitoneum is indication for early thoracotomy and repair.[5]

The operative approach consists of thoracotomy on the side of the leak (left thoracotomy for lower esophageal injury and right thoracotomy for upper esophageal injury), exposure of the esophagus, and thorough debridement of all necrotic tissue. The perforation is identified and closed. In penetrating trauma, multiple perforations are not uncommon and should be sought diligently. The choice of suture material for closure of the perforation is variable between surgeons, as is the necessity for a two-layered closure with inner absorbable and outer nonabsorbable sutures. While various tissues are recommended as buttress for the suture, Richardson[5] used buttress by either muscle or pleura. Sternocleidomastoid muscle is used to buttress or primarily close the defects in the neck, and a flap of diaphragm is often used for thoracic perforation. Patients with perforated cancer or severe underlying disease may need esophagectomy. Whichever method is used, it is critical to drain the area extensively, usually with large caliber chest tubes placed in the vicinity of the esophageal repair.

Treatment of delayed recognition of the perforation: The problems of delayed treatment involve extensive mediastinitis, necrosis of the esophageal wall, and the difficulty of effectively closing the perforation, even with various buttressing methods. Even when repair is technically feasible, subsequent breakdown of the repair is the rule rather than the exception. It is in such patients that "exclusion" procedures were practiced at one time, largely replaced in recent times by esophageal stenting. In selected patients with controlled sepsis, esophageal irrigation and wide drainage of the mediastinum and pleural cavity are viable options.[5]

Control of Intrathoracic Bleeding

Pulmonary lacerations are best approached by localized debridement–resection of the injured lung. Staplers are useful to accomplish this rapidly and effectively. Only rarely is formal lobectomy needed. Pneumonectomy is reserved for extensive injury to the hilum and is even more uncommon.

Intercostal vessel bleeding requiring operative control can easily be performed through a thoracotomy.

Damage-control Procedures in the Chest

These are not uncommon with success of early transport and emergency resuscitation in patients with severe injury.

As described by Wall and associates, "Damage control in the chest consists of different technical maneuvers to use quicker and technically less demanding operations to accomplish the same goal."[9] These include resuscitative thoracotomy, nonanatomically stapled lung resections, pulmonary tractotomy, en masse lobectomy/pneumonectomy, intravascular shunts and vascular ligation instead of repair. The chest incision is provisionally closed by prosthetic patches or towel clips.

Tracheobronchial Injury

Richardson[6] presented a personal series of laryngotracheal injuries recently and pointed out the infrequency of these injuries and the resultant limitation of experience. This report is mandatory reading to be prepared to deal with these injuries. The basic lessons are clear: tracheal injury in the neck from blunt trauma needs resection and reanastomosis of the trachea. The need for complete excision of damaged cartilage was emphasized. The repair may be performed through the neck with a sternal extension. For injury near the carina, a right thoracotomy is preferred. Mainstem bronchial injury represents a major problem, especially from penetrating trauma. Involvement of the pulmonary hilum with major vascular injuries forces a pneumonectomy, a highly lethal procedure, especially when performed on the patient in shock. For blunt bronchial injury, end-to-end anastomosis is feasible. Preservation of pulmonary tissue is clearly preferable. Richardson[6] emphasized the poor long-term prognosis of these patients. Fortunately, these injuries are relatively uncommon and the inexperienced surgeon is admonished to call senior thoracic surgeons for help.

OPERATIVE APPROACH TO ABDOMINAL TRAUMA

Solid Organ Injury

Exploratory celiotomy is clearly indicated in patients with suspected hollow viscus injury or hemodynamic instability with solid organ injury. Prep the patient from chin to midthighs and table-to-table laterally (be prepared for possible resuscitative thoracotomy, median sternotomy, or availability of the groins for vascular access or saphenous vein harvesting). The abdomen is explored by a long midline incision. After evacuation of the peritoneal cavity of all blood, the abdomen is packed in all the quadrants and serially explored. Control the most active bleeding first.

Liver. Perihepatic packs and manual compression of the liver by an assistant will reduce bleeding from the liver. Exploration of the abdominal cavity is rapidly completed. Intestinal perforation, if present, is swiftly closed to prevent continued contamination of the peritoneal cavity. The various options in the operative treatment of the injured liver can then be considered.

Approximately 50%-60% of the liver lacerations, especially after penetrating trauma, are minor capsular tears that have stopped bleeding at the time of laparotomy. These capsular tears and minor parenchymal lacerations may be left alone. Grade II injuries are deeper lacerations, especially central in location and may be actively bleeding at operation. Hemostasis can temporarily be achieved by pressure. If bleeding resumes after releasing the tamponade, liver sutures of an absorbable material may be applied in an interlocking mattress fashion. A better alternative is to explore the laceration by a hepatotomy and individually ligate the bleeding vessels. If a diffuse bleeding continues, absorbable mattress sutures buttressed by pledgets of gelfoam can be used to compress the parenchyma and achieve hemostasis. The majority of liver injuries, fortunately, can be controlled by these simple methods.

Burst injuries due to blunt trauma and large-caliber missile wounds cause greater destruction of the parenchyma of the liver, often involving both lobes and require more "complex repairs." Ancillary techniques as autotransfusion by a cell saver, blood warmers to combat hypothermia and massive transfusion protocols with emphasis on high Fresh Frozen Plasma (FFP) to packed cell ratios, and appropriate resuscitation are crucial for a successful outcome. Adequate mobilization of the liver by dividing its ligamentous attachments enables the organ to be delivered into the operative wound and facilitate manual compression of the liver.

Occlusion of the portal triad or Pringle's maneuver reduces vascular inflow to the liver and consequently may reduce bleeding from the liver laceration. It consists of sliding the operator's hand into the lesser sac and occluding the free edge of the lesser omentum and its contained portal and hepatic vessels between the fingers. If the procedure is effective in slowing the hemorrhage from the liver laceration, a vascular clamp may be applied across the free edge of the omentum. With reduction in the rate of bleeding by portal occlusion, the liver laceration can be evaluated to control bleeding vessels by direct visualization and ligation. Deeper lacerations may be explored by the finger-fracture technique popularized by Pachter et al.[10] The parenchyma of the liver is teased between the surgeon's fingers so that the hepatic vessels are exposed as threads traversing the teased liver substance (Fig. 5.6). These can then be individually ligated. The process is continued till the entire laceration is explored and hemostasis is achieved. The staplers are an invaluable adjunct in this setting.

In the patient with large stellate fractures or deep lacerations of the liver, the finger-fracture technique of hemostasis and debridement of nonviable liver tissue inevitably results in large defects in the hepatic lobes. Minor bleeding, usually of venous origin, may persist from the raw surfaces of the divided liver. A graft of viable omentum with an intact vascular supply can be used to fill in this dead space and control the venous bleeding (Fig. 5.7). This living tissue acts not only as a pack to control bleeding, but may serve also as a rich source of macrophages to help minimize the risk of subsequent sepsis.

HEPATIC RESECTION.

Anatomic lobectomy, or formal hepatic resection even though underemphasized in recent years, has its role. Polanco et al.[11] recently analyzed 216 patients with complex liver injury and noted 21 anatomic segmentectomies, 23 nonanatomic resections, 3 left lobectomies, 8 right lobectomies, and 1 hepatectomy with orthotopic liver transplant. The overall mortality was 17.8%, but only 9% from liver injury. Despite these impressive results, the consensus opinion in this country favors resectional debridement. Selective vascular ligation of hepatic artery, once popular, is now less commonly applied to hepatic trauma. If active bleeding persists after resectional debridement or packing, angiographic embolization is the preferred method. On the other hand, do not leave the operating room if control of surgical bleeding has not been achieved.

Despite these various techniques, in a small number of patients, approximately 2%-5%, profuse bleeding persists and may relate to the onset of coagulopathy. Massive red cell

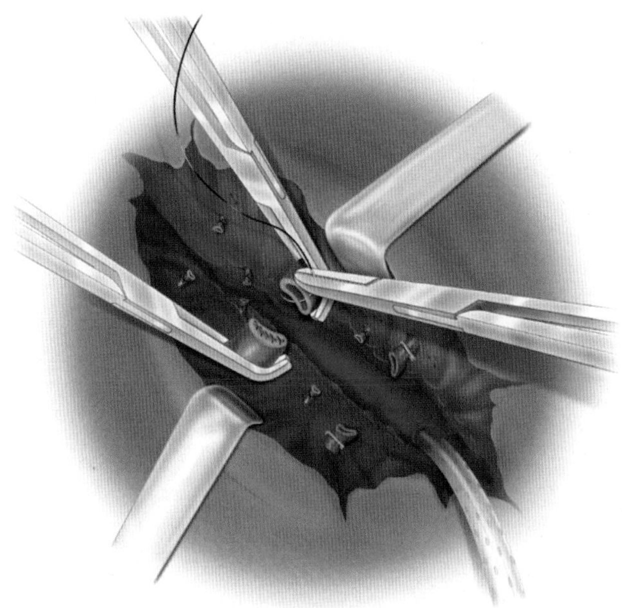

FIGURE 5.6. Hepatotomy with vascular ligation.

transfusion, hypothermia, and acidosis contribute to the development of coagulation defects. The liver injury, which may have stopped bleeding, may start to bleed diffusely without controllable points of hemorrhage. "Liver packing" has emerged as an important advance to control this "nonmechanical" bleeding.[12] In such patients, perihepatic packing, abbreviated laparotomy, damage control resuscitation with hepatic angiography as an adjunct have emerged as the treatment of choice. The technique of packing is by Kerlix rolls tightly in the crevices of the liver injury and over the raw areas of the resected liver. Additional packs are placed around the liver and between the organ and the diaphragm and the lateral abdominal wall. The laparotomy is abbreviated, and the patient is taken to the ICU for resuscitation. The packs are removed in 24-48 hours, when

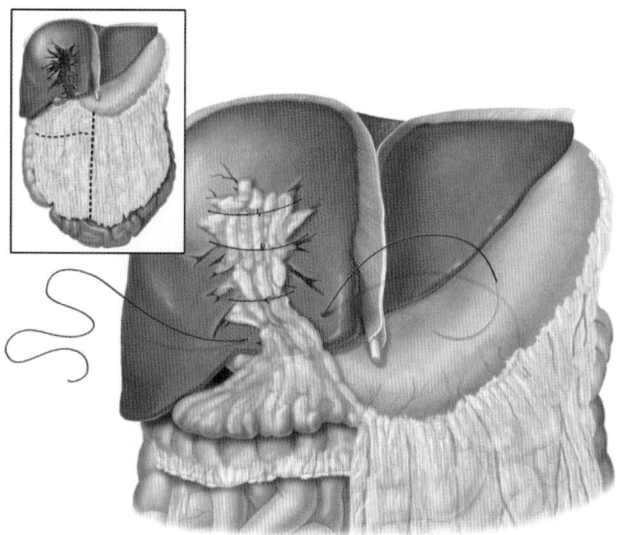

FIGURE 5.7. Omental packing after debridement–resection of liver.

the coagulation factors have been replaced and the coagulopathy corrected. Pack removal is accomplished by copious irrigation with normal saline. The raw areas of the liver are carefully inspected and nonviable tissue is debrided. The liver laceration is drained extensively with closed suction drains.

As opposed to external tamponade, internal tamponade is a valuable method in patients with missile wounds of the liver that traverse the entire thickness of the lobes, an injury too extensive to control without a major resection. In such patients, a method of internal tamponade by a "Penrose pack," made by passage of a red rubber catheter through the missile tract and pulling a wad of Penrose drains tied to the end of the catheter through the laceration. The Penrose pack acts as a tamponading plug and controls the bleeding. The drains, brought to the exterior through the flank, also serve to drain the laceration. A similar result may be achieved by using a sterilized Sengstaken-Blakemore tube. The management of retrohepatic venous injuries is discussed under the section on abdominal vascular trauma.

Spleen. Except for high-grade splenic injuries with hemodynamic instability, nonoperative management of splenic trauma is the rule. In patients with penetrating trauma with multiple injuries and in unstable patients, splenectomy is the preferred treatment. Complete mobilization of the spleen from its ligaments, control and division of the splenic vessels at hilum, attention to the short gastric vessels and the tail of the pancreas are some of the technical details that need emphasis. Splenorrhaphy is an option when circumstances are favorable for repair: hemodynamic stability and absence of major associated injuries. Techniques include sutures with buttress of omentum, strips of gelfoam or absorbable mesh; partial splenectomy or splenic wrap with absorbable mesh[13] (Figs. 5.8-5.10).

PANCREATODUODENAL COMPLEX.[14-16] At celiotomy, the important findings suggestive of injury to the duodeno-pancreatic complex[14,16] are bile staining of the retroperitoneum, small bubbles of entrapped air in the periduodenal tissues, small periduodenal hematoma, fat necrosis or saponification of tissues in the upper abdomen. Kocherization (mobilization of the C-loop of the duodenum from its retroperitoneal attachment) facilitates inspection of DI, DII, and a portion of DIII as well as allows evaluation of the pancreatic head, periampullary area, and distal common bile duct. The Cattell-Braasch maneuver consists of mobilization of the hepatic flexure of the colon, sharp dissection of the small bowel attachment from the ligament of Treitz to the right lower quadrant, and cephalad displacement of the small bowel. This brings D III into view along with the body of the pancreas. DIV may be evaluated by mobilization of the ligament of Treitz (Figs. 5.11 and 5.12).

The surgical management of these injuries depends on hemodynamic stability, severity of duodenal injury, and the presence and severity of associated pancreatic injury. In the hemodynamically unstable patient, the optimal treatment is an abbreviated laparotomy with rapid, provisional closure of the duodenum by simple methods such as suture, stapling, and rapid resection without establishing continuity. Control of bleeding supersedes duodenal repair. In hemodynamically stable patients with lower-grade lesions of the duodenum and pancreas from civilian penetrating wounds and without delay in diagnosis and treatment, the vast majority of duodenal injuries may be managed by simple procedures of primary repair, duodenoduodenostomy, or duodenojejunostomy. Segmental resection and primary end-to-end duodenoduodenostomy is usually feasible when dealing with injuries to DI, DIII, or DIV.

Complex repairs: Only a small number of duodenal injuries require more involved procedures; complex grades of injuries as defined above, delayed diagnosis, or forced delayed

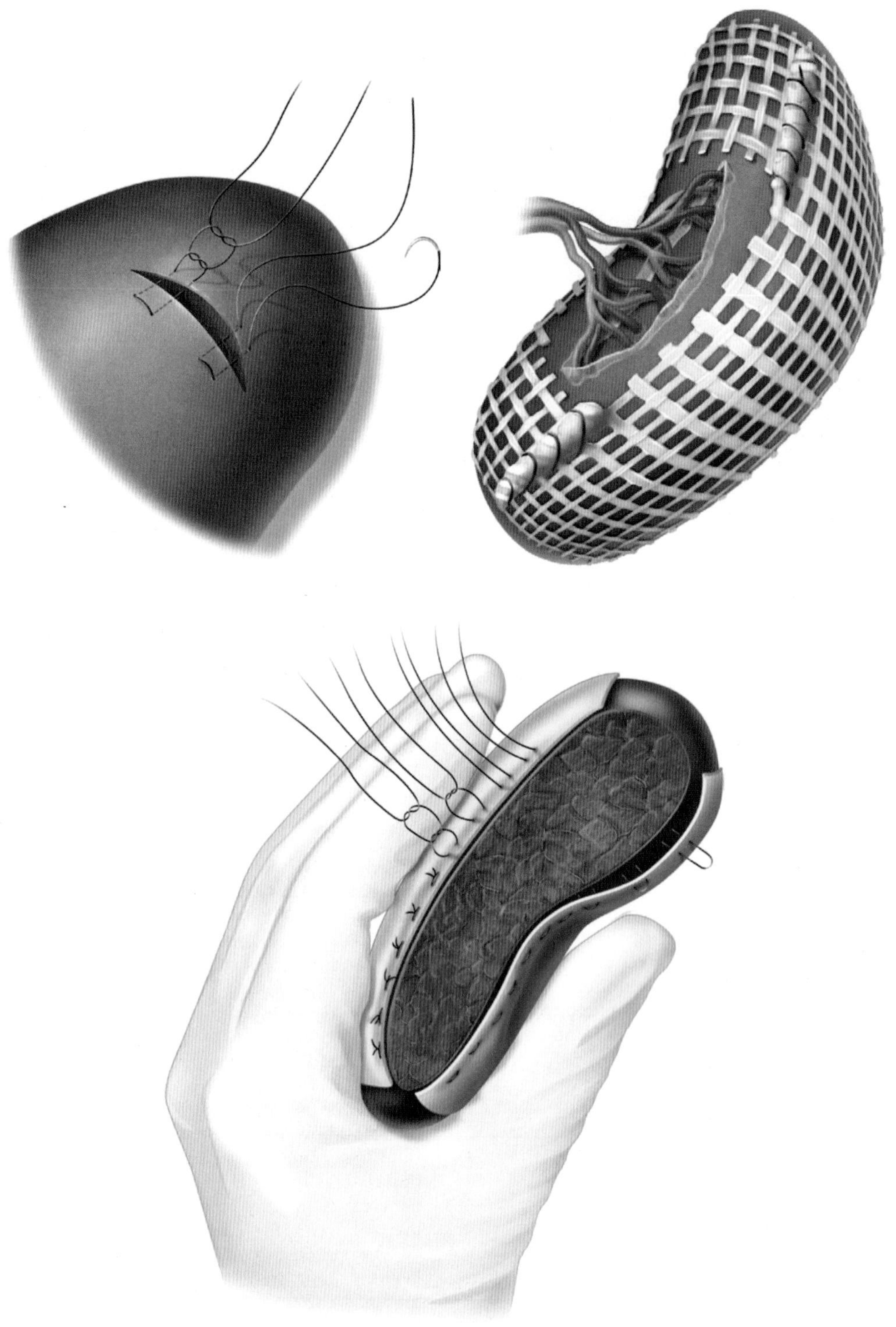

FIGURES 5.8-5.10. Technics of splenic salvage with sutures, mesh wrap, and partial splenectomy.

treatment by initial damage control procedure. Adjunctive operative procedures are often added to protect the duodenal suture line. Triple ostomy, particularly valuable when dealing with high-grade lesions in the difficult region of DII, consists of gastrostomy, duodenostomy, and jejunostomy. The duodenostomy may be antegrade, proximal to the injury site or retrograde, via a jejunostomy. Serosal patch and pedicled mucosal grafts are not often used currently. One preferred option when dealing with large duodenal defects is resection and end-to-end duodenoduodenostomy or, especially in DII: either side-to-end or end-to-end Roux-en-Y duodenojejunostomy or a side-to-side duodenojejunostomy. These complex procedures, however, are seldom used in large series of duodenal injuries.

Duodenal exclusion (Figs. 5.13 and 5.14): The principle of duodenal exclusion is to divert gastric secretions away from

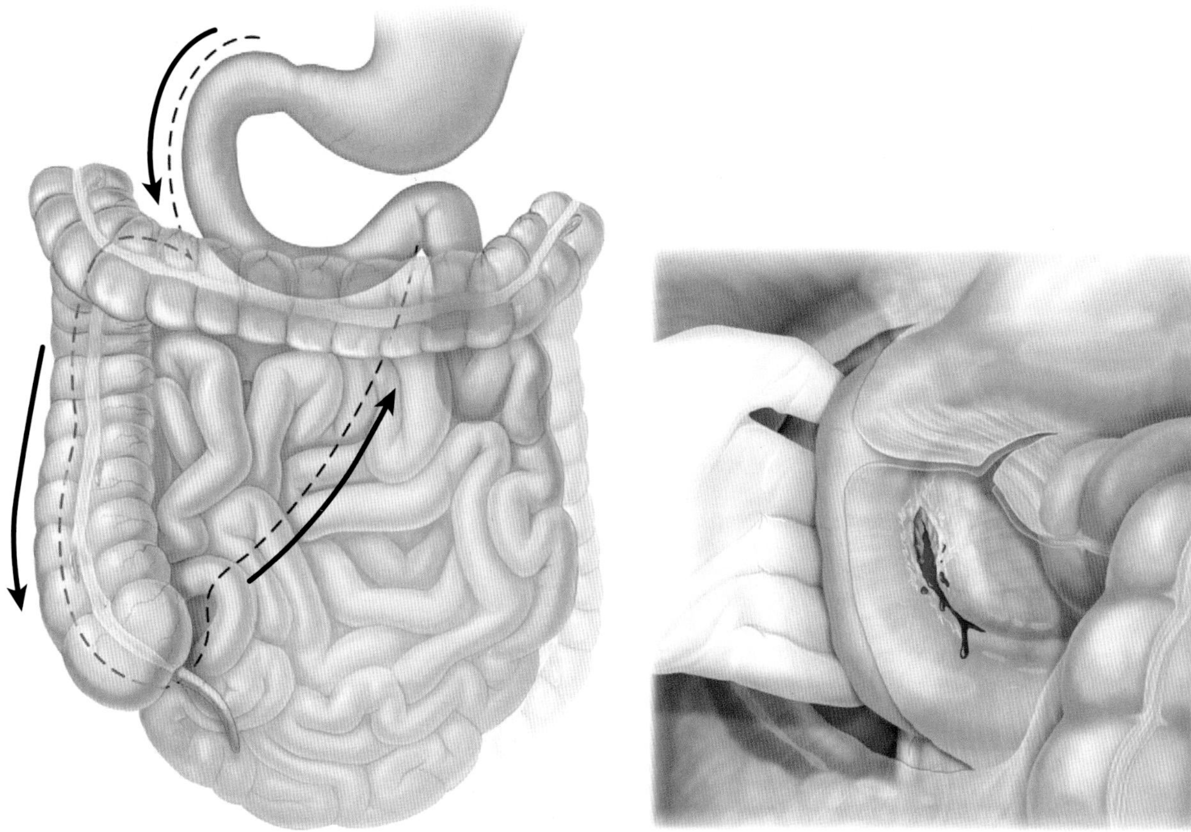

FIGURES 5.11 AND 5.12. The Cattell-Braasch and Kocher maneuvers for exposure of duodenum and pancreas.

the duodenal repair and allow time for adequate healing of repair and is currently performed as pyloric exclusion. This procedure consists of primary repair of the duodenal wound, closure of the pylorus with nonabsorbable sutures accomplished through a gastrotomy incision on the greater curvature of the antrum, or placement of a staple line across the pylorus. A gastrojejunostomy is then performed at the gastrotomy site. Injury to the extrahepatic biliary system may be present and should be sought. Total or near-total transection of the common duct should be treated by biliary-enteric anastomosis. Lateral repair will lead to stenosis.[15] Pancreaticoduodenectomy is the ultimate option for extensive injuries causing uncontrollable peripancreatic hemorrhage, distal bile duct and proximal pancreatic duct or ampullary injury with extensive

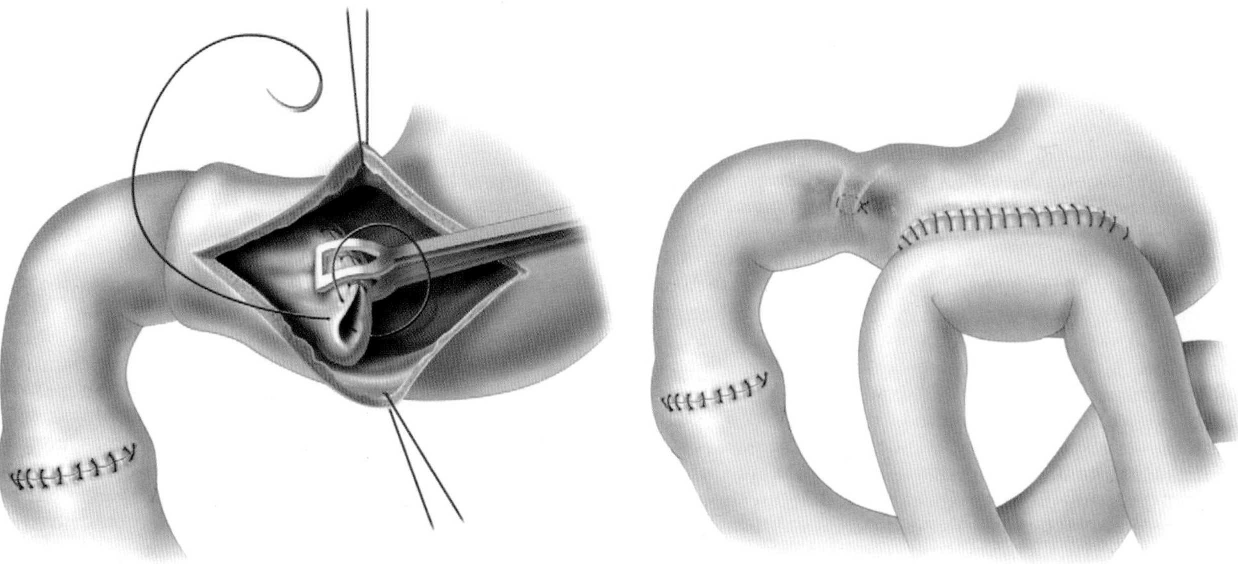

FIGURES 5.13 AND 5.14. Pyloric exclusion procedure with gastrojejunostomy.

tissue destruction, and combined devascularizing injury to the duodenum and head of the pancreas. Abbreviated laparotomy in unstable patients with staged reconstruction should make this a rare operation for trauma.

Pancreas[16]

The majority of pancreatic injuries require operative treatment.[16] In the case of penetrating abdominal injury, laparotomy is the rule rather than the exception. In addition to the pancreatic injury, major associated wounds of the vascular structures around the organ, namely, the superior mesenteric vessels, portal vein, splenic vessels, inferior vena cava (IVC), and the aorta are found. Pancreatic injury, under these circumstances, takes a lesser priority than the vascular injuries. Control of bleeding and appropriate resuscitation are the immediate goals. If the patient is unstable with hypothermia, acidosis, and coagulopathy, "damage control" or an abbreviated laparotomy is indicated. In such circumstances, addressing the pancreatic injury may be deferred until the second laparotomy.

In stable patients, thorough pancreatic exploration is vital to avoid missed injury. This mandates complete visualization and bimanual palpation of the pancreas. Exploration is indicated with peripancreatic hematoma or bile staining around the duodenum or when penetrating injury traverses the lesser sac. The duodenum may be kocherized for exposure of the head of the pancreas. The lesser sac is opened and division of peritoneum along the lower border of the pancreas allows complete mobilization of the gland. All hematomas and lacerations must be explored for hemostasis. Establishing major ductal integrity is the goal: often, this can be determined by the depth and site of the laceration. In the body and tail, large and deep lacerations may be treated as if the duct is injured. In the head of the organ, it is often difficult to investigate the duct. Intraoperative ERCP is often difficult. Intraoperative pancreatography is seldom used now. If there is a concomitant duodenal laceration, the ampulla may be cannulated and a small amount of methylene blue injected to verify the ductal intergrity.. Drainage is the most critical part of pancreatic injury management. For the minor grades of injuries (Grade I and II), it is the definitive treatment. For the major grades, it is an important component of treatment. Drainage must be adequate and, preferably, of the closed suction type as opposed to sump drainage. Drains must be left in place for at least 7-10 days to establish a pancreatic fistula, should a leak from the major duct occur. Minor leaks usually stop spontaneously, without any untoward sequelae.

Resection is the preferred method of treatment of major injuries to the left of the superior mesenteric vessels. Distal pancreatectomy may be rapidly accomplished by mobilizing the gland and stapling with 4.5 mm staples. If the major duct is readily identified in the stump of the gland, it may be ligated with a nonabsorbable suture. No special treatment for the resection line is necessary apart from control of bleeding. The area is drained widely. Often, the spleen is removed because of patient instability or concomitant injury to the spleen. In stable patients with favorable anatomy, splenic salvage may be accomplished by dissecting the splenic vessels from the pancreas and removing only the distal gland.

Injury in the head of the pancreas (to the right of superior mesenteric vessels) is difficult to treat. Subtotal resection is indicated for a totally disrupted gland but is avoided if the body and tail are uninjured, since 85%-90% resection will result in pancreatic exocrine or endocrine insufficiency. In such patients, the author prefers to establish wide drainage in the region of the injury, accepting the formation of a fistula. Pyloric exclusion may be added, especially in the presence of associated high-grade injuries to the duodenum.[14]

Pancreatoduodenectomy is the ultimate treatment for the most severe combined pancreatoduodenal injuries. Current opinion reserves this procedure for devascularizing lesions of both the duodenum and pancreas. The operation may be done as a single-stage or multiple-stage procedure, depending on the stability of the patient. The infrequency with which this operation is required is quite evident in all the series; <2%.

It is important to emphasize the current trend toward conservative approach to pancreatic injuries. Resection is only performed when the remnant can be handled effectively (e.g., distal pancreatectomy). In general, enteric anastomoses to the pancreas is best avoided since the normal gland, as is often found in these patients, handles sutures very poorly and the morbidity of pancreato-enteric leaks is enormous. For complex lacerations in the head, we prefer drainage, pyloric exclusion with gastrojejunostomy, and a feeding jejunostomy.

Enteric Injury

In abbreviated operations for hemodynamic instability: contamination control from enteric perforation is important. After packing all quadrants of abdomen to reduce bleeding, all the blood in the peritoneal cavity is evacuated. Rapid visualization of the appropriate part of GI tract will identify the perforations or lacerations. These can be closed by placing Allis or Babcock clamps on the edges of the lacerations. Marking the areas of injury with these clamps, the bowel is "run" from the stomach to the rectosigmoid junction. Next, exploration of the bleeding sites must be done to control bleeding: from the solid organs and the mesentery. If a "damage control" procedure is elected, rapid closure of the intestinal lesions is the goal to facilitate abbreviated laparotomy. Several techniques are available to accomplish this: a rapid running suture incorporating all the layers of the bowel and rapid stapling of the bowel wall to close the lacerations' rapid resection of the segment of bowel where multiple lacerations are present. The segment of bowel containing multiple lacerations may be resected quickly and the ends of the bowel ligated with umbilical tapes

Stable patient: After closure of enteric perforations, the peritoneal cavity should be thoroughly irrigated to clear contaminated fluid before embarking on definitive repairs.

Next, the GI tract is inspected again from the stomach to the rectosigmoid to find all perforations. The gastroesophageal junction, the fundus of the stomach, posterior lacerations of the stomach, and all retroperitoneal portions of bowel are difficult areas that need special attention (Figs. 5.15-5.19).

Stomach. All areas of the stomach must be visualized. The G-E junction and the fundus of the stomach may be brought into view by pulling the stomach down while holding the body of the organ by Babcock forceps. These areas may then be inspected and palpated. The lesser sac is entered by dividing the gastrocolic ligament and the posterior wall of the stomach is inspected and palpated in its entirety, proceeding from the right to the left, reaching the posterior aspect of the first portion of the duodenum. Beware of the posterior gastric wall high on the fundus near the G-E junction, where injury can be missed. Evaluation of the duodenum is described above.

Small Bowel. The entire small bowel, from the duodenal-jejunal junction to the ileocecal wall must be carefully "run" visualizing both walls of the bowel. Special attention must be given to injuries near the mesenteric border. Small perforations may be hidden in this area behind the mesenteric attachment. All major mesenteric avulsions and rents must be carefully exposed and hemostasis secured by ligation of individual vessels or running a suture in the free edge of the rent. This maneuver,

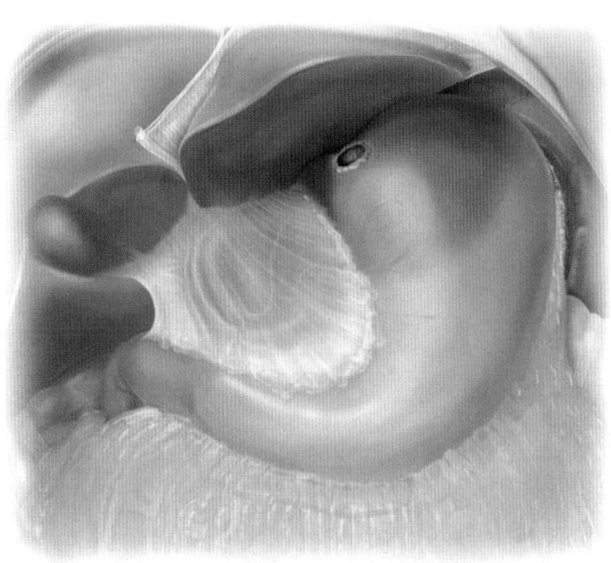

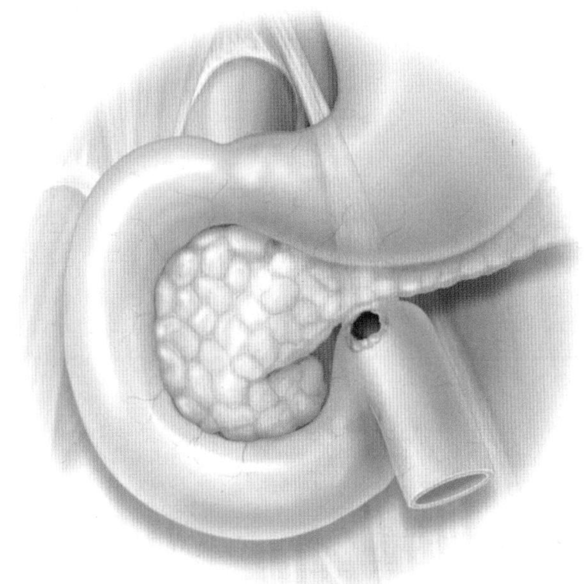

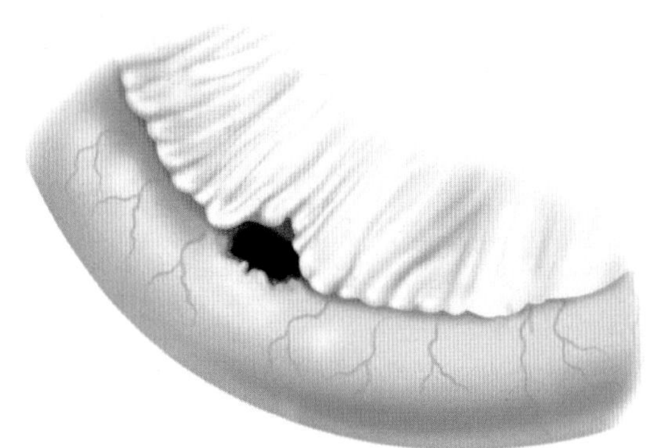

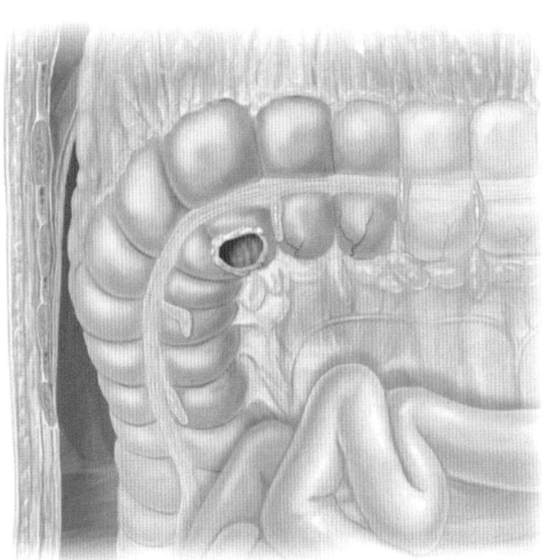

FIGURES 5.15-5.19. "Potential sites of missed injuries" that deserve careful appraisal: G-E junction, ligament of Treitz, mesenteric border of bowel, posterior wall of transverse colon, extraperitoneal rectum.

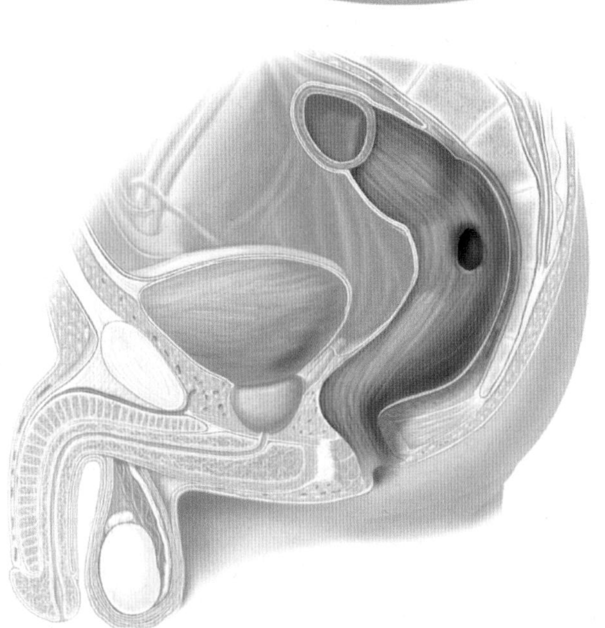

as well as major rents in the mesentery may lead to ischemia of the segment of the bowel and must be sought. If bowel viability is doubtful and there is no risk for short-gut syndrome, these segments of doubtful viability are best resected.

Colon. The entire colon must be visually inspected. In areas of suspected injury, the colon must be mobilized from its retroperitoneal attachments to inspect the posterior wall. In patients with excessive fat and thick omentum, colon perforations may be hidden near the omental attachment to the transverse colon. Hepatic and splenic flexures high under the liver and the spleen and the rectosigmoid at the peritoneal reflection are the other areas that need special attention. Hematomas adjacent to bowel wall must be completely unroofed to expose bowel wall in order not to miss a perforation. One must never accept an odd number of holes in bowel unless one of the perforations has been proven to be tangential beyond any doubt.

In general, injuries from stab wounds and low-velocity gun shot wounds are small perforations of the bowel that may be repaired after debridement of the edges and control of bleeding from the edges. Injuries from blunt trauma are large rents that may need more extensive repairs or resection and anastomosis. Lacerations in the bowel wall are repaired in the transverse axis so as not to narrow the lumen. Perforations in close proximity (e.g., GSW × 2) may be combined into one and repaired. Multiple perforations in a small segment of the small bowel are best treated by resection of the segment of the intestine back to healthy edges and anastomosis in an end-to-end fashion. The mesenteric defect of the bowel segment is then closed to prevent subsequent herniation of bowel loops. A GIA stapler can be effective in resection and anastomosis of the bowel. Repair or anastomosis may be performed by a variety of techniques and is one of personal preference. No definitive data support one technique over the other: single versus two layers, interrupted versus continuous sutures, and sutured versus stapled anastomoses. It is better to avoid, in the author's opinion, stapled anastomoses when dealing with edematous bowel such as in delayed diagnosis of bowel injuries. Gastric lacerations have a propensity to bleed after repair because of the generous vascularity of the stomach. Traditionally, therefore, a two-layered repair is preferred: inner hemostatic running suture of absorbable suture and outer nonabsorbable sutures. Lacerations near the pylorus may be treated by a pyloroplasty so that pyloric channel is not narrowed.

The majority of nondestructive colon injuries may be repaired primarily with excellent results. Current opinion supports repair of the colon wounds even at reexploration after "damage control" surgery; if the colon is not edematous, the lesion does not require resection, and other conditions, locally and systemically, are favorable. Majority of the trauma centers do not recommend a primary colocolic anastomosis at the first or reexploratory operations, unless the conditions are extremely favorable. Colostomy is the safest approach under these circumstances. Intraperitoneal rectal injuries may be treated by mobilization of the rectosigmoid and primary repair. Proximal colostomy is the preferred treatment for an extraperitoneal rectal injury. Presacral drainage, colorectal washout are recommended by some for high-velocity wounds of the rectum. Their benefit in the management of all rectal wounds is unproven. If the lesion is easily approachable by proctoscopy, repair may be performed. Otherwise, repair of the lesion is not a high priority as long as the feces are diverted by a proximal colostomy.

Abdominal Vascular Injury[17-22]

Injury to abdominal vessels accounts for 27%-33% of all vascular trauma treated in urban trauma centers.[17-22] Approximately 95% of these are from penetrating trauma and occur in 10% of admissions with stab wounds and 25% with gunshot wounds. These injuries are rarely isolated and multiple visceral injuries as well as multiple vascular injuries are common. About 10% of patients with penetrating abdominal vascular injuries will present to the ED in an agonal state, without vital signs and with a distended abdomen. In these patients, a rapid left anterolateral thoracotomy in the ED will facilitate occlusion of the descending thoracic aorta with the hope of reducing intra-abdominal bleeding. However, the results of this approach have been disappointing with a survival of only 2%-7%. Some patients also need ED thoracotomy because of cardiac arrest. Survival in these circumstances is even less.

Patients who are stable or can be stabilized by resuscitative thoracotomy are rapidly transported to the operating room. The entire torso as well as the upper thighs is rapidly prepped and draped into the operative field. In hypotensive patients, a preliminary anterolateral thoracotomy may be indicated in order to prevent extensive blood loss when the distended abdomen is decompressed. Laparotomy is performed through a long midline incision from the xiphoid to the pubis.

Suspecting vascular injury: Abdominal vascular injury may be suspected by the presence of a large amount of blood in the abdomen or the presence of hematoma. The vascular zones of the abdomen are the midline Zone I (supramesocolic and inframesocolic), Zone II on either side located in the perinephric gutters, and Zone III in the pelvis. All hematomas in these zones incorporate vascular structures and need to be explored. The presence of an expanding hematoma or brisk, bright red blood through penetrating wounds will suggest a major vascular injury.

The next step is to evacuate intraperitoneal blood rapidly and pack the abdomen with laparotomy pads. The point of hematoma or bleeding is compressed manually. Volume replacement and maintenance of physiologic stability are the next goals. Proximal and distal control is rapidly obtained by dissection, often facilitated by the hematoma. Exposure of individual blood vessels is described below. The laceration(s) are repaired by the usual vascular techniques, the abdomen is irrigated with warm saline, and minor points of bleeding are ligated or sutured. Bowel perforations are temporarily closed so that contamination of the peritoneal cavity will not continue. At this point, a decision is made whether to continue with the operation or to abbreviate the laparotomy for damage control, as discussed in other chapters.

Abdominal Aorta. In the patients with hematoma in the supramesocolic space, it is important to obtain proximal control of the aorta at the aortic hiatus in the diaphragm, if not obtained already in the left chest by thoracotomy and cross-clamping in the chest (Figs. 5.20-5.23).

Abdominal control is first accomplished by medial mobilization of all the left-sided intra-abdominal viscera including the kidney (the so-called Mattox's maneuver), Figure 5.24. This will allow exposure of the celiac axis, the SMA as well as the origin of the renal arteries. An alternative approach for the suprarenal, infra-SMA abdominal aorta is by an extensive Kocherization of the duodenum medially and by incision of the retroperitoneal tissue to the left of IVC. Once proximal control is achieved, the aorta is dissected distally, exposing the perforation(s). Bleeding may, at this time, be controlled by manual compression either by sponge sticks or hand. In the majority of patients, the injuries to the suprarenal aorta are small defects in the wall that can be closed with a continuous suture of 3 or 4 polypropylene after debridement. More extensive loss in the aortic wall needs resection of a part of the aorta and insertion of an interposition graft, usually of 12-14 mm, of Dacron or PTFE. Fortunately, these injuries are not common and the majority of the series have fewer than 20 patients each with a mean survival of about 30%.

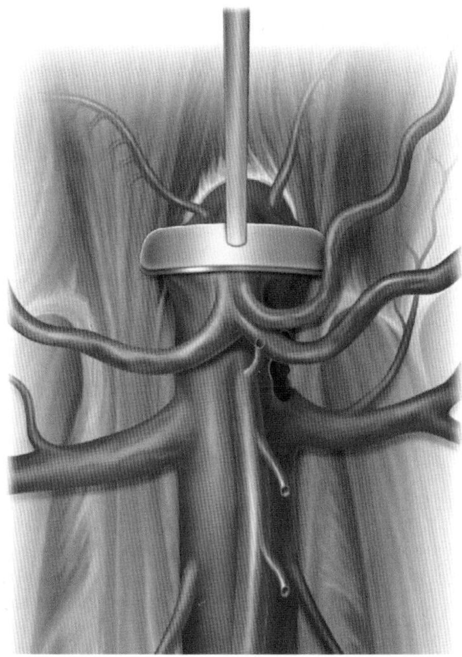

FIGURE 5.20. Aortic compression against the spine. The same effect may be obtained by two sponge forceps on either side of the aorta with a rolled gauge holding them.

Infrarenal aortic injury is easier to expose and manage by the same principles.

Celiac Axis Injury

Exposure of celiac axis is by medial rotation of viscera, as described above. Injury to the celiac axis is usually treated with ligation because of the lack of any short-term morbidity, if the SMA is patent.

Superior Mesenteric Vessels. Exposure of SM vessels is difficult and may be achieved as described for the aorta. Injury to the superior mesenteric vein also may require division of the neck of the pancreas to expose the confluence of splenic and portal veins. More distal injury may be exposed by dissection through an incision in the root of the mesentery. More proximal injury may be approached through the lesser sac and mobilization of the pancreas. Small lateral injuries are treated with 5.0 or 6.0 polypropylene suture while extensive injuries require a synthetic graft from the aorta. It is usual to plan a second-look operation after repair of SMA to detect bowel ischemia early. These injuries have a high mortality (45%-75%) because of the difficulty in exposure. Proximal injuries are best treated by ligation and a second-look operation. More distal injuries in the transverse mesocolon should always be repaired because of the high risk of bowel ischemia.

Infrahepatic Vena Cava. Injury to the IVC presents as a large hematoma next to the duodenum or with active bleeding from this site. This is best exposed by mobilization of the cecum, ascending colon, and hepatic flexure medially (Figs. 5.25 and 5.26). The C-loop of the duodenum is mobilized medially by Kocherization of the duodenum. Proximal and distal compression by sponge sticks may facilitate the exposure of the IVC rent. Usually, a large amount of bleeding will ensue, requiring manual compression of the bleeding IVC. One useful technique is to apply pressure with sponge to control the bleeding, slow withdrawal of the pack to expose small segments of the caval injury and controlling the perforation(s) with rapid application of a Satinsky clamp on the vessel. One useful technique is to approximate the edges of the laceration with Allis clamps progressively, as the pack is withdrawn. The laceration is then closed with polypropylene sutures.

A wound in the suprarenal IVC is best approached by obtaining proximal control above the renal veins by retracting the liver superiorly and applying compression on the IVC against the spine at this level. A rapid exposure of both renal veins and IVC will facilitate control of the entire IVC and exposure of the injury. Injuries to the inferior vena cava are repaired by a transverse suture of 5.0 polypropylene.

The posterior laceration IVC must be identified and repaired. The best approach for this is to repair the posterior laceration through the anterior laceration by direct visualization. The IVC may also be rotated to approach the posterior aspect. Ligation of the lumbar veins may facilitate this exposure and repair of the posterior perforation.

In the profoundly hypotensive patient who is coagulopathic, ligation of the IVC is an option. It is, of course, poorly tolerated by the patient in profound hypovolemia but occasional survival is possible

Portal Venous Injury, Hepatic Artery Injury, or Retrohepatic Vena Caval Injury

Massive bleeding from the hepatoduodenal ligament or from behind the liver is indicative of these injuries. Exposure of the first two is obtained by dissection in the free edge of the lesser sac and identification of the portal vein in its posterior plane. More proximal portal venous injuries at the confluence of splenic and superior mesenteric veins require transection of the neck of the pancreas. Lateral venorrhaphy is the preferred mode of repair of the portal vein. Occasionally, an end-to-end anastomosis may be necessary. More complex repairs are not needed since ligation of the portal vein is a viable option. Injured hepatic artery may be ligated and this is usually well tolerated as long as the portal vein is patent.

Bleeding from behind the liver, which is not easily controlled by a Pringle's maneuver, suggests a retrohepatic venous injury. If the bleeding can be controlled by packing, this may be all that is needed. Continuing bleeding demands exposure and repair of the bleeding veins.

Retrohepatic Venous Injury

Retrohepatic venous injury should be suspected in the presence of rapid bleeding or a large retroperitoneal hematoma behind the liver or when the bleeding is not controlled by portal triad occlusion. Once there is a suspicion of a retrohepatic venous injury, the area should be packed with laparotomy pads, portal triad occlusion completed, and preparation made for massive transfusions. Mobilization of the liver and gentle dissection may, on occasion, visualize the hepatic venous injury and repair may be carried out. More frequently, these maneuvers only accentuate the bleeding. If an atriocaval shunt and vascular isolation of the liver is decided upon, the midline celiotomy incision should be extended as a median sternotomy to gain control of the supradiaphragmatic vena cava. While a variety of tubes have been used for the shunt, a wide (no. 36) chest tube or an endotracheal tube are readily available and

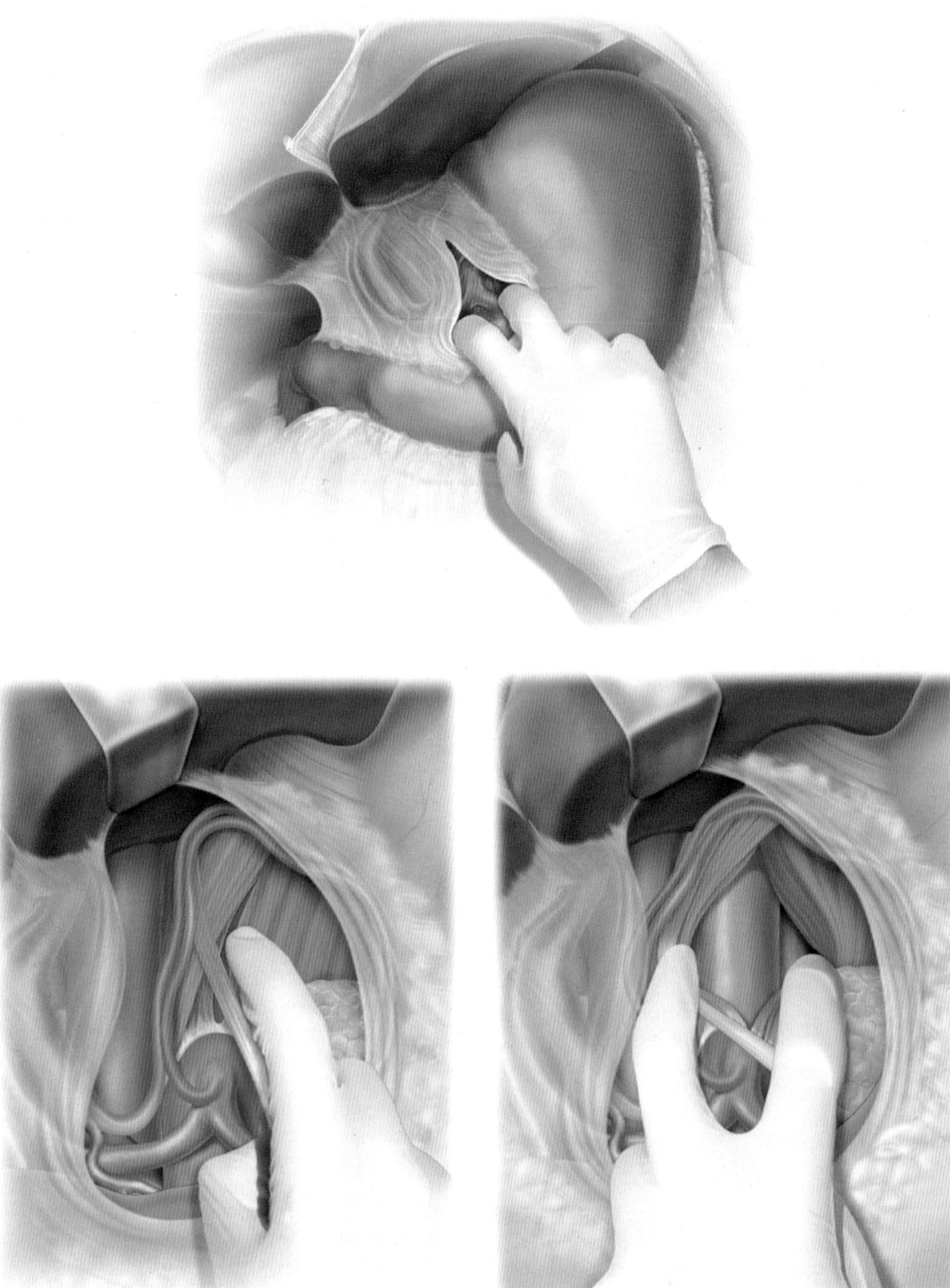

FIGURES 5.21-5.23. Control of supra-celiac abdominal aorta.

serve the purpose well. Vascular isolation is achieved by securing the tube at the intrapericardial vena cava and suprarenal vena cava with umbilical tapes. The open end of the shunt beyond the atrial appendage can be used for rapid transfusion. Once vascular isolation is completed, the area of the perihepatic veins can be explored and repaired. The use of an endotracheal tube and inflation of the balloon in the suprarenal cava obviates the need for isolating the suprarenal cava.

While these steps in achieving vascular isolation of the liver by an atriocaval shunt appear relatively simple, in practice, the method is fraught with pitfalls and dangers. Burch et al.[22] analyzed a 11-year experience with 35 patients with atriocaval shunts from Ben Taub hospital. This is the largest series of this technique yet published. They highlighted many of the pitfalls of this technique and noted that 7 patients had a total of 8 technical problems in the insertion of the shunt. These included late placement in 3 patients, tourniquets below the renal veins in 2 patients, and injury to suprarenal vena cava in 2 patients. Six of the 35 survived. All of the survivors had gunshot wounds of the retrohepatic vena cava. None of the patients who required either a resuscitative thoracotomy or concomitant hepatic resection survived.

Dissatisfied by the high mortality of atriocaval shunting for juxtahepatic venous injury, Pachter et al.[10] recommended (1)

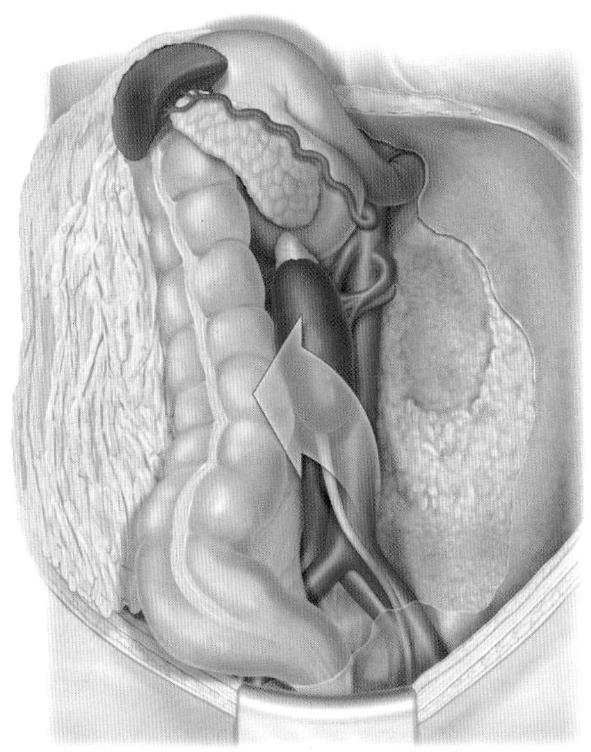

FIGURE 5.24. Modified left visceral rotation to expose the supra and infra renal aorta.

compression of the injury site while resuscitation is in progress; (2) early diagnosis of the injury by failure of Pringle's maneuver to staunch bleeding; (3) prolonged portal triad occlusion (up to 1 hour) using topical hypothermia and steroids; and (4) extensive finger fracture of the liver parenchyma up to the site of vascular injury and primary repair or ligation of the venous injury. It should be borne in mind that not all juxtahepatic venous injuries require atriocaval shunting. On occasion, the injury may be visible on lobar mobilization and be amenable to repair by the placement of a Babcock or Satinsky clamp. Ligation of the injured hepatic vein is a viable option in patients with a tenuous physiologic status. Finally, it needs to be reiterated that tight perihepatic packing can control bleeding from injured retrohepatic venous injury and may serve as the definitive treatment.

Renal Pedicle. Injury to the renal pedicle presents as a lateral hematoma. Renal artery injury is often associated with aortic tear and the fastest and safest approach is nephrectomy after making sure that there is a contralateral kidney. In more stable conditions, these lateral hematomas are best explored after preliminary control of the renal pedicle (Figs. 5.27 and 5.28). This can be achieved by dissection at the root of the mesocolon and opening the retroperitoneum. Injuries to the renal veins are exposed as described for inferior vena cava. Small lacerations can be repaired by lateral venorrhaphy with 5-0 or 6-0 prolene sutures. In more extensive injury or with venous ligation, nephrectomy is the most expeditious recourse. Lateral perirenal hematomas from blunt trauma are often left unexplored by the majority, especially if there is no injury to the calyceal system. Blunt renal artery lesions are rarely encountered. Renal salvage after penetrating

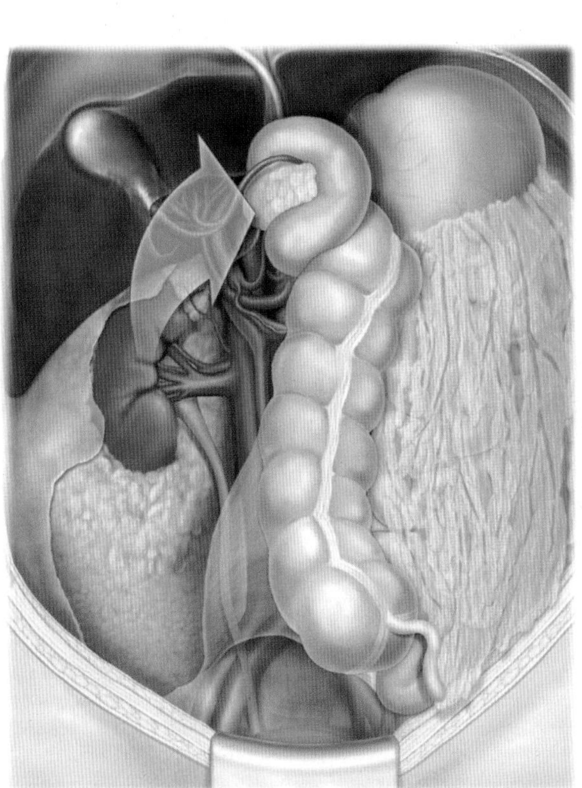

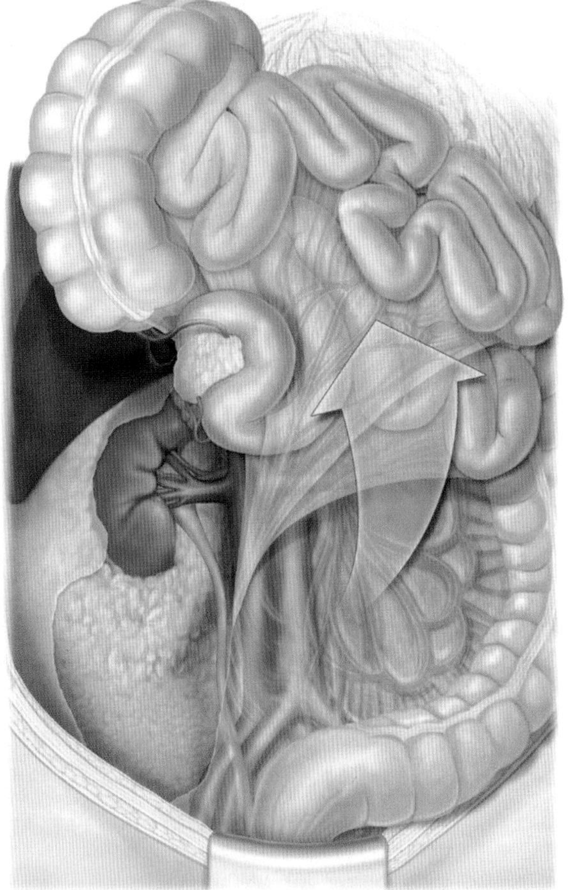

FIGURE 5.25 AND 5.26. Right-sided visceral rotation to expose the IVC, parts of the aorta, ureter, and the retroperitoneum.

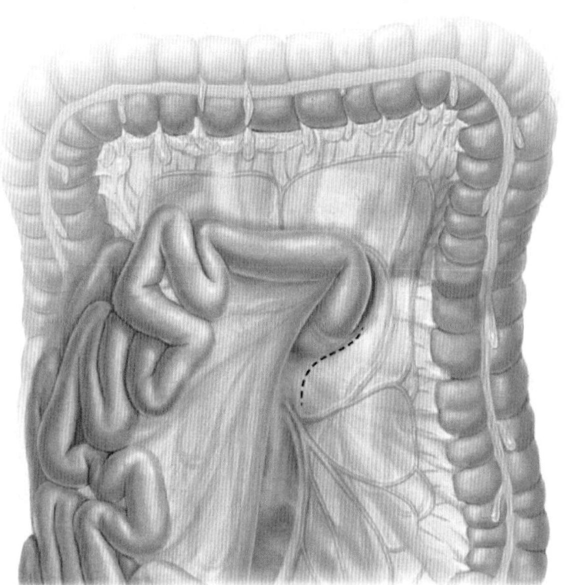

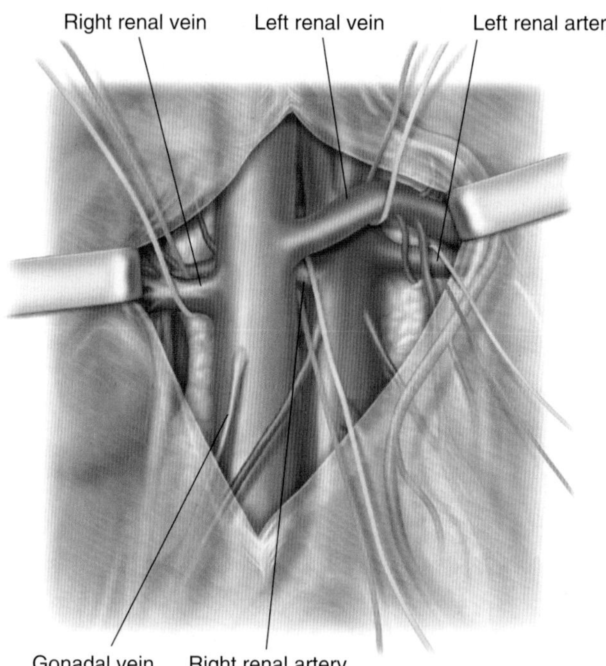

FIGURES 5.27 AND 5.28. Preliminary isolation of renal vessels before exploring a perinephric hematoma.

renovascular injuries is only 30%-40%. Renal preservation after injury to the renal parenchyma is possible by a variety of techniques outlined by Figures 5.29-5.31.

In the presence of a lateral pelvic hematoma, iliac vessel injury should be suspected. These are usually from penetrating trauma, but may be due to pelvic fractures from blunt trauma. Proximal and distal vascular control may be obtained at the aortic bifurcation and at the inguinal ligament. The internal iliac artery may need to be controlled to prevent back bleeding and may be ligated, if torn. Lateral repair or vein interposition graft is the optimal management approach for the external iliac artery. This is a critical artery and ligation has a high probability of resultant limb loss. Extra-anatomic bypass may be necessary when limb viability is threatened. Injury to the iliac veins is more difficult to control, especially at the confluence of veins. Ligation of the injured iliac vein is a better option than interposition grafts, if lateral venorrhaphy is not possible. This should be followed by a fasciotomy of the ipsilateral leg. The survival from these injuries will depend upon the presence of associated injuries. Isolated arterial injuries carry a survival rate of 87%, while it was about 94% for isolated iliac venous injuries.

In summary, the presence of major abdominal vascular injury is apparent early. In patients who are stable to reach the operating room, a reasonable survival may be expected. The exceptions are wounds of suprarenal aorta and the retrohepatic veins. With increasing appreciation of physiology and the application of principles of "damage control," as discussed below, survival is much improved in recent series.

Minimally Invasive Surgery in Trauma and Acute Care Surgery[23]

Laparoscopy can play a major role in the evaluation and management of the stable patient with penetrating trauma to the abdomen.[23,24] Laparoscopy is invaluable in the evaluation of thoracoabdominal wounds (the so-called intrathoracic abdomen). Laparoscopy also has a role in selected patients with missile wounds with doubtful trajectory through the peritoneal cavity. Selective management of abdominal gunshot wounds can be accomplished without morbidity. A significant number of patients with minor grades of hemoperitoneum, minor lacerations of liver and spleen, and nonexpanding mesenteric hematomas away from bowel wall can be managed without laparotomy successfully. It is noteworthy that recent experience is encouraging in the problematic issue of bowel injury—a high index of suspicion and a low threshold for laparotomy in the presence of hematomas near or around the bowel wall and a greater proficiency in running the small bowel and mobilizing the retroperitoneal colon.

Operative Technique. A 10-mm 30 degree forward-seeing laparoscope is inserted via a 10-mm trocar placed by cutdown into the peritoneal cavity with intra-abdominal pressures limited to 15 mm Hg. First, peritoneal violation is confirmed. A 10-mm camera port is created at the suprapubic region for alternative use and two 5-mm ports are placed at right and left paramedian sites. The surgeon inspects the stomach, omentum, transverse colon, and diaphragm on the patient's left side from the umbilical camera port with the patient in the reverse Trendelenburg's position. The pancreas and the posterior gastric wall are inspected after the scope is introduced into the lesser sac if a hematoma or fluid accumulation is found in the lesser sac. Next, the pelvic organs are inspected with the patient in Trendelenburg position. For complete evaluation of the ascending colon and the small bowel, the laparoscope is inserted into the suprapubic camera port, and with atraumatic grasping forceps through the umbilical port and the left paramedian port, the bowel is "run." By changing the position to the right, the surgeon runs the proximal one-third of the small bowel and the descending colon. Once all injuries are assessed, the surgeon can decide upon laparoscopic repair, open laparotomy or hand-assisted laparoscopic resection, and anastomosis of the bowel. Some of the therapeutic procedures now successfully performed in trauma include hemostasis of bleeding solid organs, splenectomy, cholecystectomy, distal pancreatectomy,

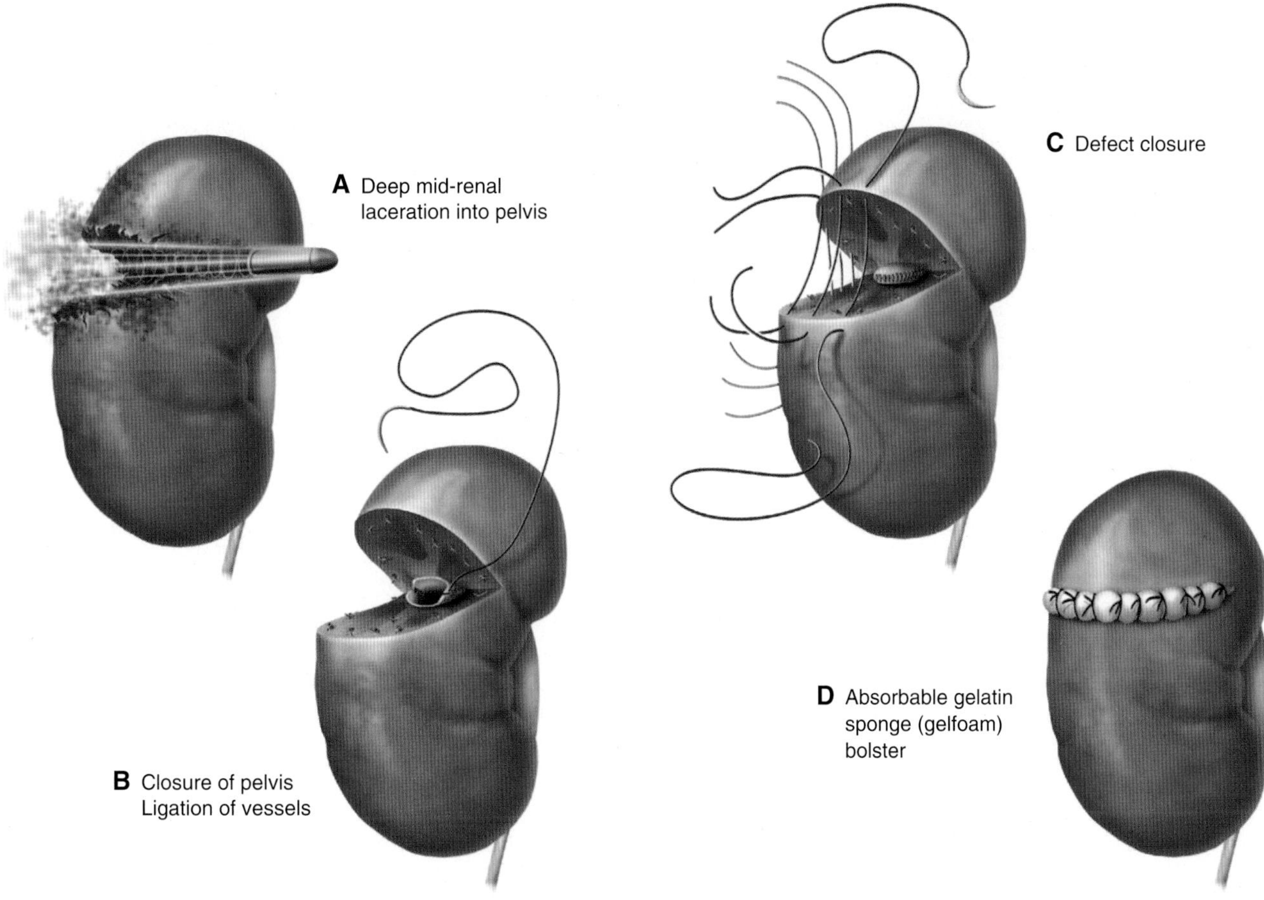

FIGURES 5.29 AND 5.30. Techniques of renorrhaphy.

repair of diaphragm lacerations with intracorporeal sutures or staples, and repair or resection and anastomosis of perforated hollow organs with laparoscopy-assisted procedures. A careful honest evaluation of his/her own surgical expertise, patient stability, adequacy of available in staff and tools are important prerequisites for the surgeon in the success of minimally invasive techniques in trauma.

Diagnostic and Therapeutic Laparoscopy in the Evaluation of Acute Abdomen

The principles of diagnostic laparoscopy are increasingly applied to acute care surgery.[26-28] A recent meta-analysis on the subject confirmed the excellent role in establishing the diagnosis of acute cholecystitis and intestinal ischemia in critically ill patients at level 2 and 3 evidence, as well as in cardiac surgery patients to exclude abdominal catastrophes. It is well tolerated if performed by trained acute care surgeons. The role of laparoscopy in the diagnosis of acute appendicitis in women has been confirmed as superior to CT scan. Therapeutic laparoscopy is increasingly applied in selected patients with small bowel obstruction, incarcerated hernias, perforated peptic ulcer, adnexal pathology, and acute diverticulitis. In some instances, randomized studies have proven the superiority of laparoscopic-assisted surgery over conventional open procedures (e.g., sigmoid resection for complicated acute diverticulitis).[28] The therapeutic arm of minimally invasive surgery is expanding rapidly.

The Role of Thoracoscopy in Trauma[25]

Both laparoscopy and thoracoscopy[25] are useful techniques for evaluating the diaphragm after penetrating trauma. Thoracoscopy provides excellent visualization of the posterior recesses of the thoracic cavity, areas often not well seen with the laparoscope. Consequently, it should be the preferred approach for posterior wounds from the posterior axillary line to the spine. For an anterior lower chest wound with potential injury to the dome of the diaphragm, thoracoscopy can confirm the injury, facilitate evacuation of residual blood and clots from the hemithorax, and also permit easy repair of the diaphragm. In the absence of a pneumothorax and if the wound is anterior and low in the interspaces, laparoscopy offers the following advantages: (1) An unnecessary thoracostomy tube may be avoided and (2) abdominal injuries can be assessed. Thoracoscopy may be performed by routinely available instruments such as sponge forceps, lung clamp, Yankauer suction. General endotracheal anesthesia with a double lumen tube is commonly used to allow collapse of the lung on the injured side. The full lateral decubitus position, as for a posterolateral thoracotomy, provides the best visualization of the diaphragm with the mediastinum shifting away. The modified lateral position with the patient's torso propped up with a "bean bag" and the arm suspended above the head with a screen works well, should an abdominal exploration become necessary. The optimal positioning of the camera and accessory ports is in the shape of a baseball diamond with the camera at the home plate, the area of interest at second base, and the additional

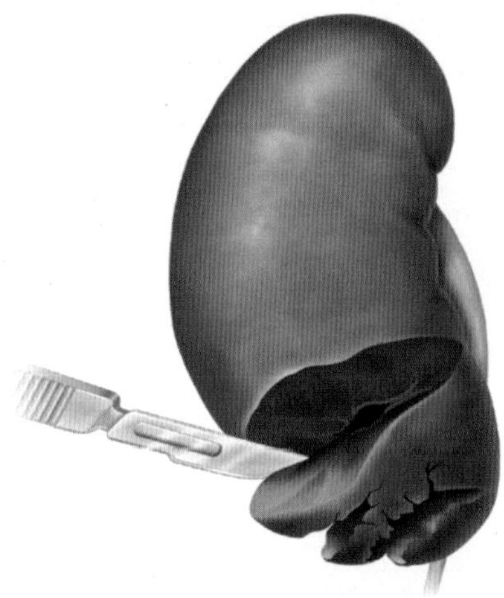
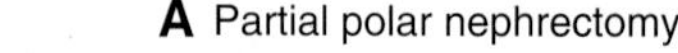
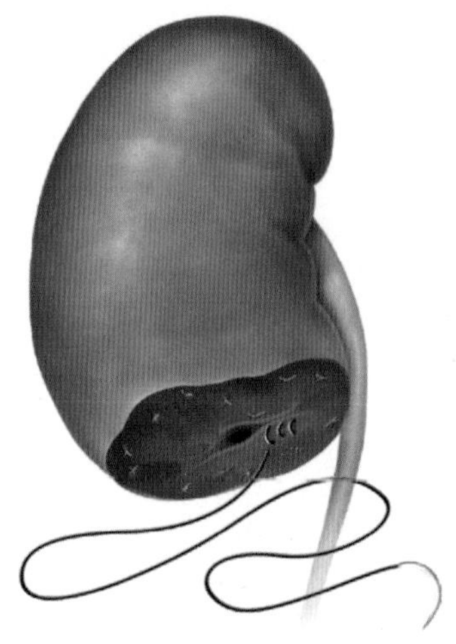
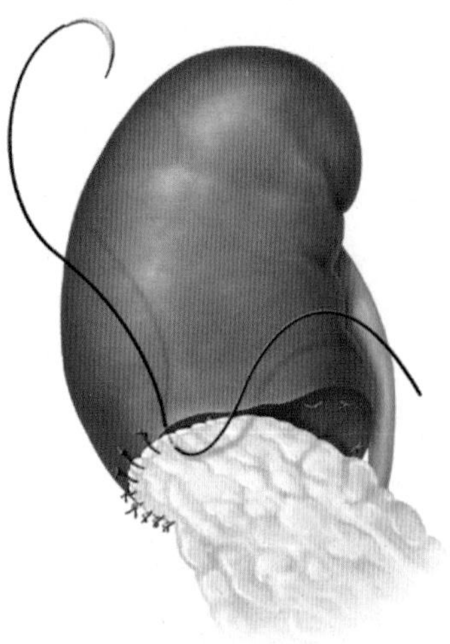

A Partial polar nephrectomy **B** Collecting system closure **C** Omental pedicle flap

FIGURE 5.31. Technique of partial nephrectomy.

ports at first and third bases. The initial incision for the camera placement is in the 6th or 7th space or at the site of the tube thoracostomy. The placement of additional ports may be determined after the initial inspection with the thoracoscope. Generally, three or four ports are needed and should be placed so that they may be incorporated into the thoracotomy incision, should one become necessary.

Ports placed in the 3rd interspace provide excellent exposure of the apical region. Posteriorly placed (in the scapular line) port in the 3rd or 4th space provides access to the carina on the right and peritracheal regions on both sides. For inspection of the diaphragm, the camera is placed in the 5th interspace, in the anterior axillary line for anterior wounds and posterior axillary line for posterior wounds. The thoracic cavity is suctioned of all blood and clots and rapidly inspected for active bleeding. The chest wound is probed with a blunt clamp to indicate the area of the diaphragm at greatest risk. The area of concern is easily inspected with suitable retraction of the lung and mediastinum. Occasionally, herniated omentum or abdominal structures mark the presence of a diaphragmatic wound and hernia. These may be reduced, the diaphragm repaired, and the abdomen investigated by laparoscopy. For clotted hemothorax, the thoracic cavity is emptied of all blood and clots and one or more chest tubes are inserted into the chest under thoracoscopic guidance. Irrigation of the chest and efficient emptying of the chest by the thoracoscope will help prevent subsequent residual hemothorax or empyema. The ideal timing is within the 1st week after thoracic injury.

With increasing technical expertise and advanced training in minimally invasive surgery, both laparoscopy and thoracoscopy have become applicable for both diagnostic and therapeutic indications in trauma and acute care surgery.

DAMAGE CONTROL (ABBREVIATED LAPAROTOMY)[29-31]

No discussion of surgical procedures for trauma and acute care surgery can be complete without a mention of "damage control" surgery[29-31] discussed in detail elsewhere in this text.

First discussed by Stone in 1983, the technique involved saving the day for another day in battle by truncation of laparotomy, intra-abdominal packing for tamponade of mechanical bleeding, and subsequent completion of definitive surgical repair when the patient is in better physiologic condition.

Damage control consists of three separate parts: rapid control of hemorrhage and contamination; intra-abdominal packing and temporary abdominal closure (Part I), correction of hypothermia by rewarming; correction of coagulopathy; fluid resuscitation and optimization of tissue perfusion (Part II) and reexploration for definitive management of injuries and abdominal closure (Part III). This concept of abbreviated laparotomy and non-closure of abdomen has lead to profound advantages in the management of severely unstable trauma patients. These principles are now being applied to various aspects of acute care surgery. Morgan et al.[30] demonstrated this in 8 patients with exsanguinating hemorrhage and severe sepsis related to pancreatic surgery. Similar application of damage control can be applied to all critically ill patients with acute abdominal conditions.

BASIC OPERATIVE APPROACHES IN EXTREMITY INJURIES[32]

While a complete discussion of extremity surgery is beyond the scope of this chapter, the principles that deserve emphasis are temporary prevention of hemorrhage by pressure dressings or tourniquet and prompt identification and definition of impaired perfusion.[32] Arterial inflow/venous outflow is quickly reestablished by insertion of temporary intraluminal shunts, external fixators to stabilize fractures, debridement of necrotic soft tissues, and completion of fasciotomy for suspected or confirmed compartment syndromes.: This is "damage control" extremity surgery. Following orthopedic stabilization at a second operative procedure, the shunts are removed and a reversed autogenous saphenous vein graft from an uninjured lower extremity is used to restore arterial continuity. Venous drainage is reestablished even temporarily, accepting the inevitable clotting of these repairs and grafts in the venous system. Coverage of vascular suture lines and conduits under healthy tissue is the next important principle. Finally, the importance of primary amputation of unsalvageable mangled extremity to save the patient's life, while a difficult decision, cannot be overemphasized.

SUMMARY AND CONCLUSION

The basic operative techniques in trauma and acute care surgery follow the time-honored principles of caring for the critically ill or injured patient: emergency priorities focusing on restoration of normal physiology as rapidly as possible before anatomic repairs. Proficiency in acute care surgery is synonymous with the ability to use all of the currently available techniques.

References

1. Monson DO, Saletta JD, et al. Carotid vertebral trauma. *J Trauma.* 1969;9:987-999.
2. Ivatury RR, Stoner MC. Penetrating cervical vascular injury. In: Rich NM, Mattox KL, Hirshberg A, eds. *Vascular Trauma.* 2nd ed. Philadelphia, PA: Elseiver Saunders; 2004.
3. Ledgerwood AM. Neck: vascular injuries. In: Ivatury RR, Cayten CG, eds. *The Textbook of Penetrating Trauma.* Philadelphia, PA: Williams & Wilkins; 1996.
4. Yee LF, Olcott EW, Knudson MM, Lim RC Jr. Extraluminal, transluminal, and observational treatment for vertebral artery injuries. *J Trauma.* 1995;39:480-486.
5. Richardson JD. Management of esophageal perforations: the value of aggressive surgical treatment. *Am J Surg.* 2005;190(2):161-165.
6. Richardson JD. Outcome of tracheo-bronchial injuries: a long-term perspective. *J Trauma.* 2004;56:30-36.
7. Ivatury RR. Resuscitative thoracotomy. In: Ivatury RR, Cayten CG, eds. *The Textbook of Penetrating Trauma.* Philadelphia, PA: Williams & Wilkins; 1996.
8. Cothren C, Noore EE, Biffl WL, et al. Lung-sparing techniques are associated with improved outcomes compared with anatomic resection for severe lung injuries. *J Trauma.* 2002;53:483-487.
9. Wall MJ Jr, Soltero E. Damage control for thoracic injuries. *Surg Clin North Am.* 1997;77(4):863-878.
10. Pachter HL, Spencer FC, Hofstetter SR, et al. The management of juxtahepatic venous injuries without an atriocaval shunt. *Surgery.* 1986;99:569-575.
11. Polanco P, Leon S, Pineda, et al. Hepatic resection in the management of complex injury to the liver. *J Trauma.* 2008;65(6):1264-1269.
12. Feliciano DV, Mattox KL, Burch JM, et al. Packing for control of hepatic hemorrhage. *J Trauma.* 1986;26:738-743.
13. Britt LD. Spleen. In: Britt LD, Trunkey DD, Feliciano DV, eds. *Acute Care Surgery Principles and Practice.* Springer; 2007.
14. Ivatury RR, Rohman M, Nallathambi M, et al. The morbidity from traumatic injuries of the extra-hepatic biliary system. *J Trauma.* 1985;10:967-973.
15. Feliciano DV, Martin TD, Cruse PA, et al. Management of combined pancreatoduodenal injuries. *Ann Surg.* 1987;205:673-680.
16. Stawicki SP, Schwab CW. Pancreatic trauma: demographics, diagnosis, and management. *Am Surg.* 2008;74(12):1133-1145.
17. Feliciano DV. Abdominal vessels. In: Ivatury RR, Cayten CG, eds. *The Textbook of Penetrating Trauma.* Baltimore, MD: William & Wilkins; 1996:702-715.
18. Carrillo EH, Spain DA, Wilson MA, Miller FB, et al. Alternatives in the management of penetrating injuries to the iliac vessels. *J Trauma.* 1998;44:1024-1029.
19. Porter JM, Ivatury RR, Islam SZ, et al. Inferior vena cava injuries: noninvasive follow_up of venorrhaphy. *J Trauma.* 1997;42:913-917.
20. Asensio JA, Demetriades D, Hoyt DB. Vascular injuries: complex and challenging injuries. *Part 1: Surg Clin of North Am.* 2001;81.
21. Hoyt DB, Coimbra R, Potenza BM. Anatomic exposures for vascular injuries. *Surg Clin North Am.* 2001;81:1299-1330.
22. Burch JM, Feliciano DV, Mattox KL. The atriocaval shunt. Facts and fiction. *Ann Surg.* 1988;207:555-568.
23. Zantut L, Ivatury R, Smith S, et al. Diagnostic & therapeutic laparoscopy for penetrating abdominal traima: a multicenter experience. *J Trauma.* 1997:42:825-831.
24. Lin HF, Wu JM, Tu CC, et al. Value of diagnostic and therapeutic laparoscopy for abdominal stab wounds. *World J Surg.* 2010;34:1653-1662.
25. Ivatury RR. Thoracoscopy for trauma. *Eur J Trauma Emerg Surg.* 2010;36:15-18.
26. Stefanidis D, Richardson WS, Chang L, et al. The role of diagnostic laparoscopy for acute abdominal conditions: an evidence-based review. *Surg Endosc.* 2009;23:16-23.
27. Sauerland S, Agresta F, Bergamaschi R, et al. Laparoscopy for abdominal emergencies: evidence-based guidelines of the European Association for Endoscopic Surgery. *Surg Endosc.* 2006;20(1):14-29.
28. Klarenbeek BR, Veenhof AA, Bergamaschi R, et al. Laparoscopic sigmoid resection for diverticulitis decreases major morbidity rates: a randomized control trial: short-term results of the Sigma Trial. *Ann Surg.* 2009;249:39-44.
29. Rotondo MF, Schwab CW, McGonigal MD, et al. "Damage control": an approach for improved survival in exsanguinating penetrating abdominal injury. *J Trauma.* 1993;35:375-383.
30. Morgan K, Mansker D, Adams DB. Not just for trauma patients: damage control laparotomy in pancreatic surgery. *J Gastrointest Surg.* 2010;14(5):768-772.
31. Subramanian A, Balentine C, Palacio CH, et al. Outcomes of damage-control celiotomy in elderly nontrauma patients with intra-abdominal catastrophes. *Am J Surg.* 2010;200(6):783-788.
32. Sise MJ, Shackford SR. Extremity vascular trauma. In: Rich NM, Mattox KL, Hirshberg A, eds. *Vascular Trauma.* 2nd ed. Philadelphia, PA: Elseiver Saunders; 2004.

CHAPTER 6 ■ DAMAGE CONTROL MANAGEMENT/OPEN ABDOMEN

BRETT H. WAIBEL AND MICHAEL F. ROTONDO

HISTORY AND EVOLUTION OF DAMAGE CONTROL

While historically the management of the injured patient was done by the general surgeon, treating these patients like an elective surgery patient, with attempts at definitive repair at onset, failed to obtain satisfactory results, mainly due to fundamental differences in physiology and anatomic issues. The multisystem trauma patient has the potential for severely destructive injuries across multiple organs and/or body spaces usually not seen with the elective surgery patient. In addition, a prolonged time from injury to definitive care allows for ongoing bleeding and visceral contamination, resulting in altered physiology on presentation. The elective surgery patient presents with stable physiology, and does not suffer from uncontrolled bleeding or visceral contamination generally. Finally, the initial evaluation between these patients is necessarily different. The multisystem trauma patient may not have the physiologic reserve to undergo extensive evaluation and imaging commonly utilized with elective surgical patients. Furthermore, the shock state common in emergent trauma patients often prevents the patient from being able to provide a basic medical history. It is these essential differences of altered physiology, delay of presentation, complications from ongoing bleeding and contamination, and limited or absent preoperative medical history and evaluation that make the traditional attempt of definitive repair at presentation often futile. Ongoing bleeding from coagulopathy, initial physiologic failure from unresuscitatable shock, and subsequent multiple organ system failure later in the patient's hospital course present specific challenges that defy conventional therapy.[1-3]

While this problem was known and discussed in the first half of the 20th century, it was not until the early 1980s that the foundations for a solution were placed. H. Harlan Stone presented work in aborting laparotomy for coagulopathic bleeding using abdominal packing and Burch with hepatic injuries demonstrated improvement in outcomes over traditional approaches.[4,5] However, the term "damage control" and its sequence was not defined and refined until the 1990s by Rotondo and Schwab.[6-9]

While initially developed for abdominal injury with uncontrolled hemorrhage, damage control concepts have expanded into other areas, including vascular surgery and orthopedics.[10,11] These concepts have even altered the way the military organizes its treatment of severely injured soldiers.[12-15] In emergent general surgery, damage control techniques have been applied to those patients who develop similar physiologic instability and intolerance of the shock state.[16-20] However, with the aggressive resuscitation employed along with damage control, the incidence of abdominal compartment syndrome (ACS) and open abdomens has increased.[21,22] The increased exposure to open abdomens has allowed surgeons to gain experience in their management with development of multiple methods of obtaining temporary abdominal closure. Additionally, recognition of ACS, both in trauma and with intra-abdominal catastrophe, and its treatment has probably been a huge source of the improved outcomes in both patient populations.[16,22,23]

New strategies have been devised to reduce the volume of resuscitation as well as deal with the metabolic alterations the shock state and the resuscitation itself creates. Permissive hypotension and "damage control resuscitation" using fresh frozen plasma in a 1:1 ratio with packed red blood cell have been recently debated in the literature.[24-28] Many novel strategies involving transfusion ratios, alternative fluids, and hemostatic dressings are currently being evaluated.[29] As resuscitative technique and our understanding of control of physiology prior to operative intervention improve, the need for damage control and its adjuncts may decrease.

DAMAGE CONTROL INDICATIONS

In the traditional approach by general surgeons, control of bleeding and contamination were achieved and followed immediately with definitive repair and closure of the abdomen at the first surgery. The core concepts of damage control surgery evolved out of the failure of traditional approaches to exsanguinating hemorrhage from traumatic injury. Damage control changed the traditional sequence via termination of the initial laparotomy after cessation of hemorrhage and control of contamination, preferably before the development of physiologic exhaustion as noted by the development of acidosis, coagulopathy, and hypothermia ("the bloody vicious cycle").[30] Instead, definitive repair is delayed until after reestablishment of the patient's physiology in the ICU. Abdominal closure may even be delayed further if the resuscitation required to treat the patient would lead to ACS (Table 6.1).

The decision to carry out a damage control procedure should be made early in the operation, before the development of hypothermia, acidosis, and coagulopathy. Waiting for the development of this triad to abbreviate the operation reduces the success of damage control surgery, as the components of this triad interact to worsen ongoing hemorrhage, ultimately leading to the patient's demise.[31] While temperature below 35°C, pH below 7.2 or base deficit exceeding 8, and evidence of coagulopathy clinically or via laboratory are often discussed as indications for abbreviating the operation in favor of damage control, no definitive values exist for consideration of a damage control procedure.[32-34]

In addition to physiology parameters, another indication for damage control is the presence of multiple injuries, both within and without the operative field, which would exceed the patient's physiologic reserve to definitively repair. Complex injuries, such as those combined to the pancreas and duodenum, may require exceedingly long operative times. Preferably, the damage control laparotomy should be <90 minutes in duration.[35]

TABLE 6.1

INDICATIONS FOR DAMAGE CONTROL

1. Hemodynamic instability
2. Coagulopathy on presentation or during operation (clinical or laboratory)
3. Severe metabolic acidosis (pH < 7.2 or base deficit > 8)
4. Hypothermia (< 35° C)
5. Prohibitive operative time required to repair injuries (>90 minutes)
6. High-energy blunt torso trauma
7. Multiple penetrating torso injuries
8. Multiple visceral injuries with major vascular trauma
9. Multiple injuries across body cavities
10. Massive transfusion requirements (> 10 units packed red blood cells)
11. Presence of injuries better treated with nonsurgical adjuncts

Injuries outside of the operative field are easily forgotten, especially those across multiple body cavities. Continuing or recurrent hemorrhage from these sites can hasten a patient's advance toward physiologic collapse and may not be immediately identifiable by the operative team. Hemorrhage control should be treated as a continuum across body cavities and regions, with the surgeon starting at the perceived most compelling source of hemorrhage and expeditiously moving to other sites as the situation develops, keeping in mind sites that are outside the operative field.

Injuries that may be better treated with adjuncts, such as angiographic embolization of hepatic or pelvic injuries, are another potential indication for damage control surgery.[36] When identified intraoperatively, such an injury can be temporized with packing followed by angioembolization. The variation in physiologic reserve across different patient populations must also be considered. The elderly, young, and those with multiple medical comorbidities have less tolerance for prolonged surgical procedures.

Thus, constant reevaluation of the patient is needed to identify those patients who would benefit from an abbreviated operative approach and subsequent aggressive secondary resuscitation. The evolving physiology, time for repair, concurrent injuries and their effects on the patient, and the patient themselves all factor into the decision to abbreviate the operation to prevent collapse of the patient's physiology.

DAMAGE CONTROL SEQUENCE

When first conceptualized for exsanguinating truncal trauma, damage control focused upon management of ongoing hemorrhage and visceral contamination from abdominal injuries (part 1). This was followed by reestablishment of the patient's physiology in the intensive care unit (part 2) before definitive repair in the operation room (part 3) and closure of the abdominal wall (part 4). With further process improvement, the significance of the prehospital setting (ground zero) and expansion of damage control to extra-abdominal injury began to be evaluated (Algorithm. 6.1). A description of the process in the exsanguinating abdominal trauma patient follows, though many parallels can be noted in other emergent surgery patients, such as those with abdominal sepsis.

GROUND ZERO: PREHOSPITAL CARE/INITIAL RESUSCITATION

The prehospital care received by the trauma patient can have profound implications on their outcomes. The need for rapid transport or transfer to definitive care cannot be overemphasized.[37,38] Theories on resuscitation have arisen recognizing the potential of traditional methods of focusing on increasing hydrostatic pressure to normal levels to restore tissue perfusion to destabilize clots and increase bleeding, which may have a deleterious effect upon the patient.[39] A moderate resuscitation goal to systolics of 80-90 mm Hg with concomitant signs of end-organ perfusion during transport may be more prudent for patients with prolonged transfer times.[24,40] Some militaries are resuscitating only to the presence of a radial pulse and cleared sensorium in austere environs.[41-43] Prehospital hypotension, despite resolution before arrival at the hospital, should be considered a warning sign for a more severely injured patient with the potential for a prolonged operation.[44] Communication between the transporting crew and hospital personnel before arrival allows for mobilization of resources to prevent delays in the care of the unstable trauma patient.

Advanced Trauma Life Support is the foundation for care at this stage.[45] Airway management and correction of breathing disorders using adjuncts like endotracheal intubation and tube thoracostomy are well described. Circulation assessment with point control of hemorrhage and alignment of fractures should be performed. Resuscitation is begun via large bore intravenous and occasionally intraosseous catheters using a combination of isotonic crystalloid and blood product. A rapid evaluation using adjuncts, such as focused abdominal sonography in trauma, diagnostic peritoneal lavage, tube thoracostomy, and radiographic imaging of the chest and pelvis, to identify sites of ongoing hemorrhage is performed. The rapidity and ease of the mentioned adjuncts makes them particularly useful, but are not absolute. Diaphragm injuries can allow for transmission of blood between cavities. The areas prone to unobserved bleeding in an unstable patient are intrathoracic, intraperitoneal, pelvic/retroperitoneal, or long bone fracture sites. One must not forget the potential for bleeding prior to arrival from external wounds, especially those associated with the scalp. Generally, fluid in the peritoneal cavity with hypotension will lead to a celiotomy, while large volume loss from tube thoracostomy (>1,500 mL) or ongoing drainage (>200 mL per hour over 3-4 hours) indicates the need for a thoracotomy. Localization of ongoing hemorrhage allows for better planning of operative intervention and can be performed in <20 minutes.

PART 1: CONTROL OF HEMORRHAGE AND CONTAMINATION (INITIAL LAPAROTOMY)

The initial operative intervention is the focus of the next phase. The goal is an abbreviated operation for control of mechanical hemorrhage and visceral contamination. The operation is abbreviated to prevent depletion of the patient's physiologic reserve and initiation of nonmechanical (coagulopathic) hemorrhage. After evacuation of the peritoneal cavity, hemorrhage control is established using abdominal packing, especially with hepatic, retroperitoneal, and pelvic injuries. Shed blood can be collected using a variety of techniques for return to the patient; however, they remove the clotting factors, leading to a coagulopathy without the concomitant use of plasma and cryoprecipitate replacement.

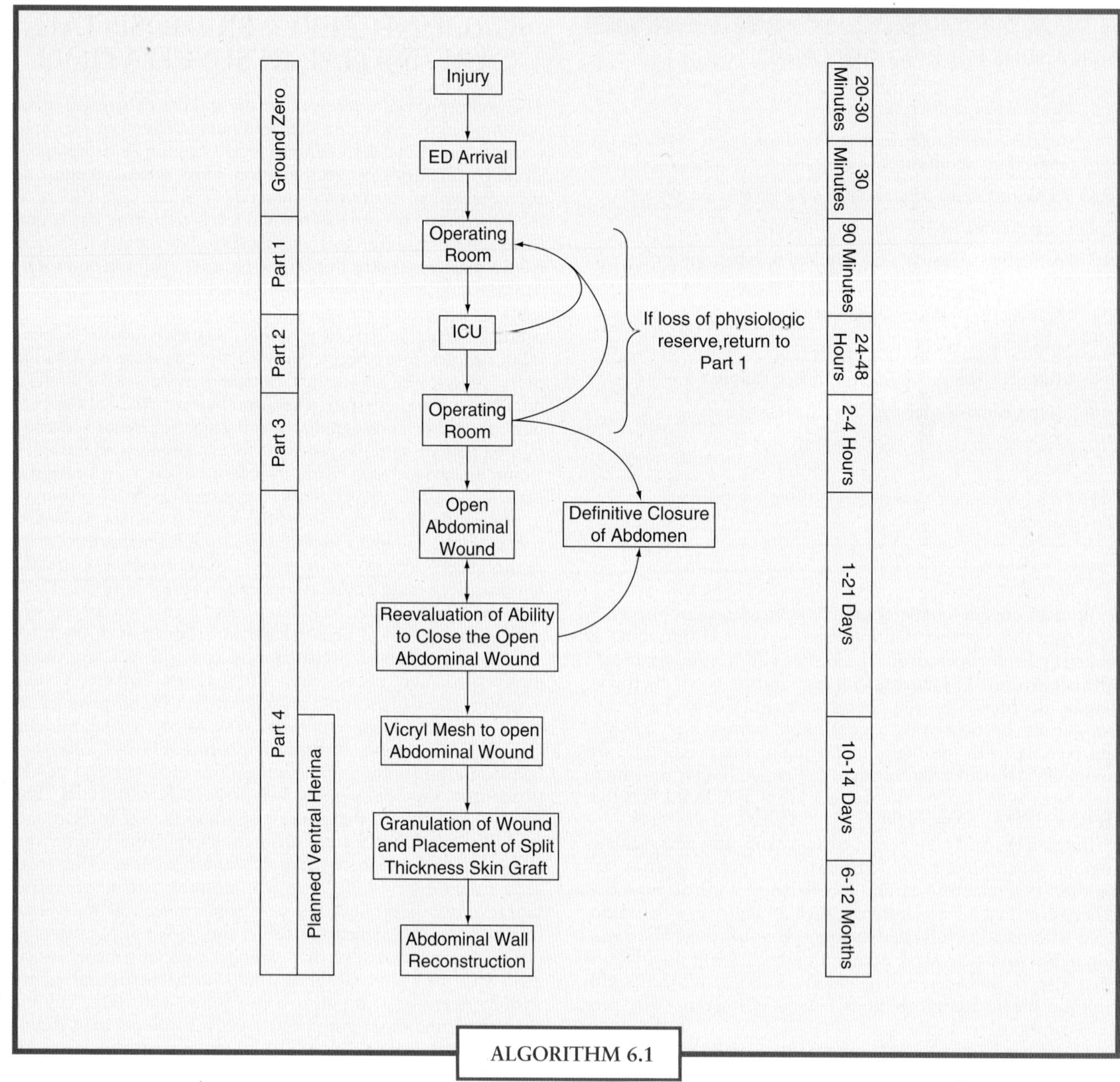

ALGORITHM 6.1 Damage control timeline.

While specifics of operative intervention are described elsewhere, some underlying themes can be established.[46,47] Central is full exposure of the injuries to identify ongoing bleeding and contamination. Numerous maneuvers, including Kocher, Mattox, Aird, and Cattell-Braasch, allow for exposure of the retroperitoneal structures as needed. Suture ligation and control of the vascular pedicle of solid organs is commonly used to gain rapid control of ongoing hemorrhage. Some solid organs, such as the spleen or isolated kidney with normal contralateral kidney, may be sacrificed if repair times are prohibitively prolonged. Those vessels that provide end-organ supply or outflow to vital organs/regions, such as the suprarenal vena cava and portal vein, however, require repair. Shunting techniques are available to allow temporary restoration of flow during the resuscitation (part 2) phase before definitive repair (part 3) while reducing ischemic injury.[48-53] A large variety of hemostatic agents have entered the market over the last few years.[54] While human data is limited to case series, animal data does exist showing improved outcomes in hemorrhage control. Some early generation agents released large amounts of thermal energy, leading to burns of uninjured tissues.[55,56] Adjuncts, such as angiography with embolization, may be needed to obtain hemorrhage control in inaccessible areas, such as the pelvis.

Control of intestinal injuries causing contamination of the peritoneal cavity is the second important objective. Closure of the visceral wound with suture or stapling techniques can easily and quickly control ongoing contamination. Formal repairs are avoided in the unstable patient with intestines left in discontinuity until definitive repair is performed in part 3 of damage control.

Positioning in the operating room is important, especially with multiple compartment injuries. The combined thoracic/abdominal compartment injuries are not suited by either a supine or decubitus position used in abdominal or thoracic trauma. The taxicab hailing position will often allow for practical exploration of both compartments (Fig. 6.1). The patient is placed in a supine position with the chest laterally rotated 30 degrees anterior to the coronal plane using folded blankets to one side based upon preoperative evaluation. The arm can be included into the operative field if manipulation is required. The position also allows for sternotomy if needed.

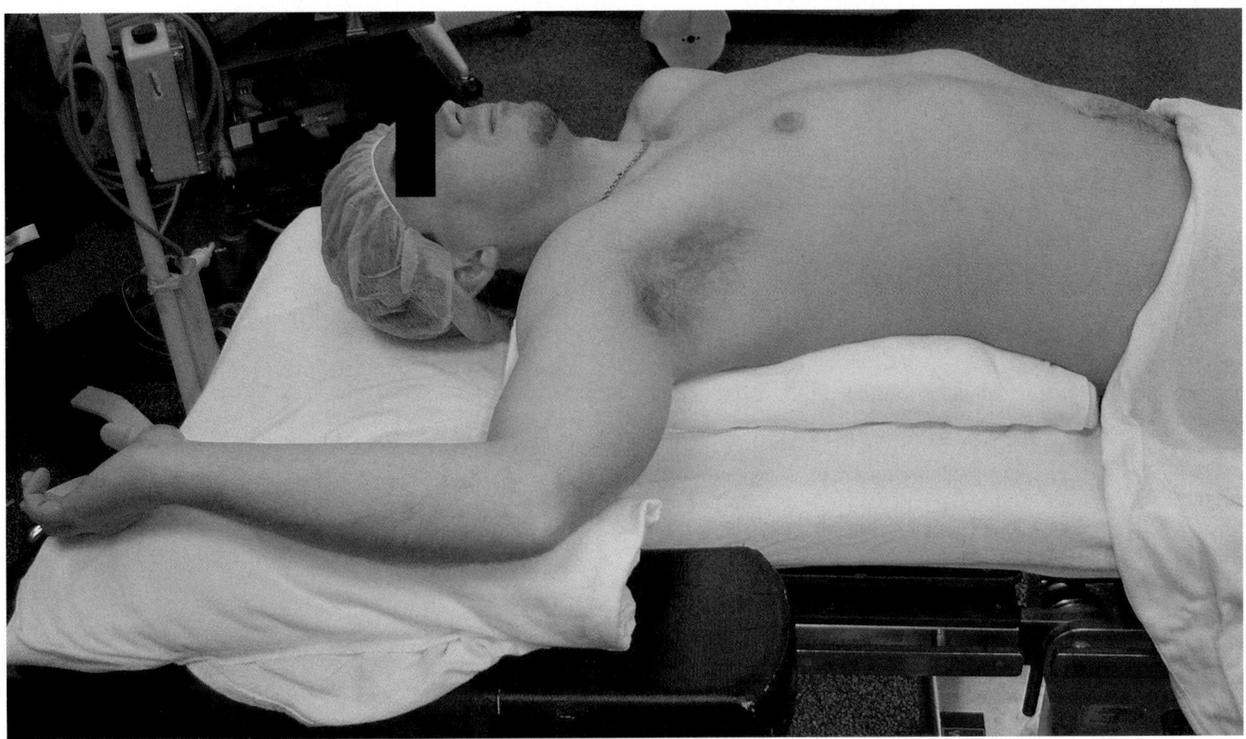

FIGURE 6.1. Taxi cab hailing position: note torso rotation to 30 degrees anterior to coronal plane with blankets. Arm abducted to 90 degrees for exposure of chest wall.

Temporary abdominal closures can further decrease the time in the operating room. Use of the abdominal pack or vacuum-assisted abdominal dressing allows for rapid reentry while preserving fascial integrity for latter closure.[57-61] In addition, effluent from the abdominal cavity can be managed and quantified to facilitate the ongoing resuscitation.

PART 2: RESUSCITATION IN INTENSIVE CARE UNIT

After the initial operation, the patient is transferred to the intensive care unit to reestablish the patient's physiology by aggressive resuscitation with intravenous fluids and blood products in conjunction with correction of hypothermia, acidosis, and coagulopathy. The fluid choice for resuscitation can have major effects. The use of normal saline in large volumes leads to a hyperchloremic (nongap) metabolic acidosis.[62] Animal models suggest the potential for proinflammatory mediator stimulation with lactated Ringer's solution.[63,64] Colloids have been suggested as an substitute resuscitative fluid; however, evidence of superiority to crystalloid does not exist, and maybe even increases mortality in trauma patients.[65-67] Hypertonic saline reduces inflammatory mediator activation in animal models, but has failed to show superior improvements in mortality or morbidity in clinical trials.[68-71] Isotonic crystalloids (normal saline/lactated Ringer's solution) are used for the majority of resuscitations.

A debate over transfusion policies in patients requiring massive transfusion protocols (>10 units packed red blood cell in first 24 hours) rages.[25-28,72-83] A host of articles on transfusion ratios have been published since 2007 with the military's report on improved survival with a 1:1:1 platelet:plasma:pRBC transfusion ratio compared to the traditional 1:4 to 1:5 plasma:pRBC ratio. While most of the civilian literature supports this aggressive transfusion policy in a small group of patients (1%-3% of civilian trauma patients), not all studies have shown survival benefits. In addition, the optimal ratio of plasma to red blood cells has yet to be fully determined. Massive transfusion is not without complications, including the potential for acute transfusion reactions, electrolyte disorders (hypocalcemia and hyperkalemia), acidosis, hypothermia, dilutional coagulopathy, and alteration of red blood cell morphology and oxygen-binding affinity.[54]

Recombinant factor VIIa has also been evaluated for its potential in hemorrhage control due to the acquired coagulopathy of trauma. Multiple case reports and one single randomized controlled trial have been done with variable results.[84-98] On the whole, it appears to reduce the transfusion requirements, especially if given early in the course of acquired coagulopathy, and correct the coagulation profile, but mortality does not appear to be improved. The recent multicenter CONTROL trial was discontinued for futility due to low mortality rates.[99] Also, the potential for thromboembolic events has been argued given its mechanism of action.[100] Other compounds, such as prothrombin complex concentrates (PCCs), are also now being evaluated. While having a history of clinical use in hemorrhage from vitamin K antagonist coagulopathy and hemophilia with inhibitors, animal models are being developed for trauma with PCCs.[101-109]

While induced hypothermia has shown benefit in some elective surgical interventions, hypothermia on arrival to definitive care (spontaneous hypothermia) has shown almost uniform negative consequences in trauma patients.[110-117] A depletion of energy levels in the hypothermic trauma patient compared to the elective surgical patient exists.[118-121] Some of this depletion may be due to metabolic exhaustion and inability to restore the adenosine triphosphate supply, while some may be due to uncontrolled shivering in the prehospital setting and the energy consumption associated with it.[122] Recent studies on hypothermia in trauma patients have used a temperature of 36°C to define hypothermia compared to the cooler 35°C in older studies, with identification that the effects of hypothermia occur at warmer temperatures than previously thought.[115-117,123,124] While hypothermia has some potential positive effects on cellular preservation, especially in the central nervous system, a multitude of negative effects are noted, including alterations in metabolism and drug clearance, altered renal function and diuresis, electrolyte disturbances due to ion shift and renal loss, and inhibition of the coagulation pathways and platelet dysfunction.[125] Given the increased risk of death associated with hypothermia in trauma, expedient rewarming of the patient is recommended. A multitude of noninvasive and invasive measures, including intravascular heat exchange catheters and body cavity lavage, exist.[126] However, whether prevention of hypothermia in the prehospital setting translates into improved outcomes has yet to be shown.

Metabolic issues must also be addressed during this phase. In addition to electrolyte disturbances that need to be expediently corrected, hyperglycemia is commonly present in these critically ill patients. Strict glycemic control with aggressive insulin therapy has become commonplace since Van den Berghe's 2001 study; yet, more recent studies have given variable results.[127-133] A recent meta-analysis found that intensive insulin therapy increased the risk of hypoglycemia without a survival benefit in critically ill patients; though a survival benefit was noted in the surgical population when stratified by patient type (mixed, medical, or surgical).[134] Given these recent studies, some have concluded that targeting age-normal glucose levels in units not equipped or accustomed to aggressive insulin therapy should be avoided and instead to target "to maintain blood glucose levels as close to normal as possible without evoking unacceptable fluctuations, hypoglycemia, and hypokalemia".[135]

While multiple resuscitation endpoints have been described, no single test is ideal.[136-138] Even once vital signs are normalized, the majority of patients exhibit evidence of inadequate tissue perfusion and oxygenation.[139] Given the poor response of traditional vital signs, such as heart rate and blood pressure, to detect shock, alternative measures are being developed, such as shock index and heart rate variability.[140-150] Resuscitation should continue until the shock state has resolved as determined by multiple methods of evaluation. While the medical critical care literature general shows a lack of efficacy of pulmonary artery catheter-based resuscitation, surgical literature tends to support its use, especially with right ventricular end-diastolic volume index (RVEDVI) pulmonary catheters.[151-153] This discrepancy probably exists due to the differences in the patients themselves and volumes used to resuscitate between medical and surgical disease processes. A RVEDVI pulmonary catheter can help guide the resuscitation volume and pressure use in the difficult resuscitation.

Generally, once hemorrhage is controlled, the patient can be resuscitated and prepared for return to the operating room in the following 24-48 hours. While normalization of vitals usually occurs rapidly, a short period of time to regain true physiologic reserve is needed. In hypothermic trauma patients, the energy stores lag behind normalization of vitals, even beyond 24 hours from injury.[119] Failure to regain a stable physiology in a short time is an indication that ongoing bleeding is present or the patient is developing an ACS. This should hasten the return to the operating room for reexploration before recovery of the patient's physiology.

Care should be taken to prevent iatrogenic injuries during this and subsequent phases. Inappropriate ventilator strategies can produce or extend injury. The ARDSNet studies demonstrate the ventilator as a major inducer of pulmonary injury and acute respiratory distress syndrome (ARDS).[154-157] A lung protective strategy of 4-6 mL/kg of lean body weight should be used. Sedation and analgesia are commonly needed to promote synchrony between the patient and ventilator with these strategies.[158] A small group of patients may even require neuromuscular blockade to achieve synchrony; however, their use has not shown improvement in either mortality or oxygen consumption in ARDS. Their use has been associated with higher prevalence of myopathy and neuropathy, especially with renal or hepatic dysfunction or asthma.[159-163]

ACS is a common complication seen in the severely injured patient. While normal intra-abdominal pressure is 5-7 mm Hg, pressures above 12 mm Hg are designated intra-abdominal hypertension.[164-166] In some patients, the increased visceral edema is noted at the initial surgery manifested by the inability to return the visceral block to the peritoneal cavity; while in others, a delayed presentation with development during the resuscitation takes place.[22] ACS, the clinical entity hallmarked by hypotension, increased ventilatory pressures, and oliguria in the presence of intra-abdominal hypertension, should be routinely monitored for by checking bladder pressure measurements.[167,168] Clinical examination and abdominal circumference measurements correlate poorly with intra-abdominal pressure as the elasticity of the abdominal wall is not a linear function of distention.[169-171] While intra-abdominal pressures exceeding 30 mm Hg are most associated with ACS, patients have been noted to develop this syndrome with pressures below this level.[172] In 2006, the World Society of Abdominal Compartment Syndrome (WSACS) defined ACS as sustained intra-abdominal pressures above 20 mm Hg associated with new organ dysfunction or failure.[166]

The physiologic effects of ACS are global. The cardiovascular system undergoes an increase in peripheral vascular resistance from compression of the vascular beds and increased sympathetic signaling while venous return to the heart via the inferior vena cava is decreased due to the increased abdominal and thoracic pressures.[173-175] Additionally, cardiac compression causes atrial natriuretic peptide secretion to decrease, resulting in further fluid sequestration. Eventually, the patient becomes unresponsive to volume loading.[176] Pressure measurements (central venous pressure, pulmonary capillary wedge pressure) from pulmonary artery catheters become uncoupled to volume status.[177] In this situation, RVEDVI, which does not depend upon pressure measurements, becomes the best measure of volume status.[136,152] Ultimately, a cycle of hypotension treated with volume resuscitation leads to further edema and increases in intra-abdominal pressures that worsen the clinical syndrome.

Increases in ventilatory pressures occur with ACS. While impediment of diaphragm movement from increased intra-abdominal pressure is present, resulting in 20%-80% of the intra-abdominal pressure being transmitted intrathoracic, other factors are involved.[178] Typically in these patients, aggressive volume resuscitation has led to increased chest wall edema and extravascular lung water, resulting in decreased pulmonary compliance.[179] Furthermore, increases in positive end-expiratory pressures (PEEP) are used to help in the recruitment of lung lost to a decline in negative pleural pressures that result in ventilation–perfusion mismatch, especially in the lower lung lobes. The combination of elevated PEEP along with transmission of intra-abdominal pressures results in increased intrathoracic pressures, which can further act to decrease cardiac return and output.[180] The increase in intrathoracic pressures coupled with a decline in pulmonary compliance leads to the increase in ventilatory pressures needed for lung expansion.

Renal function impairment, noted by oliguria or anuria, is the third clinical component of ACS and is independent of volume expansion and maintenance of cardiac output.[181,182] Outside of direct compression of the ureters from a pelvic hematoma, ureteral compression is not a cause of the renal failure as stenting fails to correct the oliguria. While mixed results have been seen in studies on direct renal parenchymal compression, compression of the renal vein creates ACS like failure, probably due to renal venous hypertension and decreased blood flow in the kidney.[183-185] Additionally, a decline in the filtration gradient probably occurs as the increase in intra-abdominal pressure exceeds proximal tubular pressures, leading to a decrease in glomerular filtration rate. Activation of the renin-angiotensin-aldosterone pathway further worsens oliguria with increases in antidiuretic hormone and aldosterone.[186,187] The combination of decreased cardiac output and renal venous compression along with parenchymal compression and endocrine alterations leads to the "dose-dependent" oliguria and anuria of ACS.

In addition to the aforementioned systems, ACS affects other body systems. Visceral blood flow is almost uniformly decreased and may be a component in intestinal anastomosis failure.[188-191] Additionally, bacterial translocation appears to increase with increased intra-abdominal pressures.[192,193] Transmission of intra-abdominal pressures is associated with increased intracranial pressures.[194-196] Some have advocated decompressive laparotomy for patients with head injury and intracranial hypertension.[197-199] Additionally, abdominal wall blood flow is altered with increasing intra-abdominal pressures.[200] Closure with increased tension and relative tissue ischemia may result in tissue necrosis and fascial dehiscence to further complicate management of the abdominal wound.

Risk factors include severe hemorrhagic shock, damage control surgery (especially with fascial closure), and elevated penetrating abdominal trauma index. Elevated pulmonary peak pressures and low gastric mucosal pH also correlate with its development.[201] Aggressive fluid resuscitation has been linked in several studies with volumes in excess of 10 L crystalloid, 10 units packed red blood cells (massive transfusion), 0.25 L/kg of crystalloid, or 6 L of crystalloid or units of packed cells in 6 hours associated with an incidence between 5% and 30%, depending on the patient population and definition used for ACS.[22,202,203] Tighter abdominal closures, including primary fascial closure, have the highest incidence of ACS, death, ARDS, and multiple organ failure; however, use of the temporary abdominal closures does not guarantee its prevention.[204-206] The development of ACS in patients with temporary abdominal closures has a higher mortality than in those patients with an open abdomen without development of ACS.[207] It is through delays in identification and commencing therapy that increases in morbidity and mortality occur.[208] Recognition and treatment with decompression of the abdominal cavity improves perfusion and organ function.[209,210] In one prospective study, the mortality of severity-adjusted patients with an open abdomen approached that of patients without an open abdomen with aggressive monitoring and treatment of ACS based upon the WSACS guidelines.[23,211]

PART 3: DEFINITIVE INJURY REPAIR (SUBSEQUENT LAPAROTOMY)

Once the patient's physiologic reserve has been restored, definitive repair can be undertaken (Table 6.2). Abdominal packing is removed and a complete examination with identification of all injuries and control of remaining errant bleeding points is performed. Uncontrolled hemorrhage, hemodynamic instability, or inability to undergo a prolonged operation would prompt an abbreviated laparotomy for control of hemorrhage and visceral contamination followed by return to the ICU for resuscitation.

The definitive repairs required will depend upon the injury and organ system concerned; however, one should consider limiting the use of prosthetic material in a contaminated wound and the need to return to the operating room for further washouts prior to definitive closure. Some repairs can be considered that would not have been undertaken in a traditional, single operative setting. For example, isolated colon injuries have traditionally been treated with an ostomy; however, in a resuscitated patient, one might consider a primary anastomosis, especially if the patient would poorly tolerate an ostomy.[212] The abdomen should be thoroughly irrigated upon completion of repairs. Closed suction drains should be used, when necessary. While definitive closure of the abdomen is preferred, a temporary abdominal closure may be required. One should attempt to ensure the intestines are located below the fascial level. The omentum is useful in providing coverage of the abdominal viscera to provide additional protection from injury.

TABLE 6.2

SEQUENCE OF DEFINITIVE REPAIR

1. Careful removal of packs
2. Inspection/identification of all injuries
3. Control of remaining errant bleeding points
4. Definitive gastrointestinal repair
5. Thorough abdominal washout
6. Avoid stomas and tube enterostomies, if possible
7. Nasoenteric feeding tube placement
8. Closed suction drainage, if needed
9. Temporary vs. definitive abdominal wound closure
10. Tracheostomy, if needed
11. Radiographic evaluation for retained packing before definitive abdominal closure

Stomas and tube enterostomies should be avoided if possible owing to potential complications, as considerable changes in abdominal wall geometry can occur in the critically ill patient.[213-215]. However, nutritional support is incredibly essential in this patient population.[216] Postpyloric nasoenteric feeding tubes provide continuous feeding, even during return trips to the operating room. Initiation of enteral feeds should be delayed in unstable patients because of the possibility for intestinal ischemia, but ought to be started after physiology is restored and proven stable. Even with an open abdomen, early enteral feeding is possible and associated with reduced septic complications.[217-220] Earlier primary fascial closure, lower fistula rates, and decreased cost compared to patients with later (>4 days) enteral feeding was noted in one study of open abdomens.[221]

Since acute lung injury and ARDS manifest themselves during the 2nd and 3rd hospital days and can prolong ventilator requirements for several weeks, consideration of a tracheostomy should be made early.[222-228] Ventilator circuit disruption after onset of pulmonary dysfunction can have devastating consequences; a tracheostomy provides for a more secure airway during this tenuous time. While early tracheostomy may decrease ventilator days and ICU stay, a high degree of misclassification may exist in this literature.[229]

PART 4: OPEN ABDOMINAL WOUNDS AND DEFINITIVE ABDOMINAL CLOSURE

Before definitive abdominal closure is obtained, a radiographic evaluation is made. Given the rapid nature of the initial operations and use of packing, closing counts cannot be trusted. Imaging allows for further evaluation that retained foreign bodies are not present and provides for a permanent record of complete pack removal.

Primarily due to the aggressive resuscitation used with damage control at present, approximately 40%-70% of patients cannot initially have primary fascial closure.[59,60,230] Temporary closures are desirable for patients undergoing repeated operations or have a distended visceral block preventing closure without ACS developing. While closing an abdomen, increases in airway pressure above 10 mm Hg from baseline indicate that fascial closure should be delayed.

Multiple temporary closure methods are available (Table 6.3).[57-59,61,230-236] Optimally, a temporary closure should control the viscera while preventing additional peritoneal cavity contamination or visceral injury. The abdomen should be sealed and effluent controlled to preserve skin/soft tissue integrity. The closure should avoid unnecessary tension to prevent subsequent ACS. Finally, fascial integrity should be preserved for latter use during definitive closure.

When closure of the abdomen is not initially possible, skin closure techniques, silo placement, or vacuum pack techniques are most commonly used. Skin closure techniques using suture or towel clips, while the easiest closures that maintain domain while avoiding fascial injury, are rarely watertight and create (towel clips) radiographic artifacts, complicating diagnostic and therapeutic adjuncts.[237] Silo placement (Bogota bag) has been replaced by vacuum-assisted abdominal closures due to their dynamic properties.[238-242] The vacuum pack dressing (Barker technique abdominal dressing) is formed from commonplace supplies and can be done outside the operating room.[57-59] An impervious dressing, created from a perforated plastic drape or surgical towel wrapped in Ioban (3M, St Paul, MN), is positioned between the visceral block and abdominal wall to prevent adhesions while allowing effluent to egress the peritoneal cavity. An interposition layer of Kerlex (Kendall, Mansfield, MA) rolls with embedded closed suction drains is placed next. A final layer of Ioban over the wound maintains a watertight system for skin preservation while suction is applied to the embedded drains for control of peritoneal fluids (Fig. 6.2). Commercial vacuum-assisted dressings, such as the KCI V.A.C. and ABThera (Kinetic Concepts, Inc., San Antonio, TX) and Renasys systems (Smith & Nephew, Inc., St. Petersburg, FL), exist. The internal portions of the dressing are replaced with a protected polyurethane sponge that facilitates fluid collection while providing continuous medial traction on the fascial edges to help prevent domain loss (Fig. 6.3).

If definitive closure is further delayed, other techniques are employed. Sequential abdominal wall closure with temporary abdominal dressings in the remaining defect is one option. Vacuum-assisted dressings can be used with interpositional meshes, and decreases in multiple organ system failure, ACS, necrotizing fasciitis, and fistula formation have been seen with interpositional mesh use.[243-246] No single mesh is entirely ideal. Some meshes, such as Vicryl (polyglactic acid, Ethicon, Somerville, NJ) and Dexon (polyglycolic acid, Davis and Geck, Danbury, CT), have low tensile strength and are prone to tearing. The polypropylene meshes (Marlex, Bard, Billerica, MA; Prolene, Ethicon, Somerville, NJ; Surgipro, US Surgical, Norwalk, CT) have higher tensile strength but are associated with higher fistula rates (15%-50%) due to an aggressive inflammatory reaction.[247] Gore-Tex (polytetrafluoroethylene, Gore and Associates, Flagstaff, AZ) mesh, while nonadherent and strong, has a high infection rate in this setting due to its design.

TABLE 6.3

CLOSURE OF OPEN ABDOMINAL WOUNDS

1. Immediate term
   a. Skin closure only (suture or towel clips)
   b. Vacuum-assisted abdominal dressing
2. Intermediate term
   a. Sequential fascial closure
   b. Sequential skin closure
   c. Interpositional mesh placement
   d. Vacuum-assisted abdominal dressing
3. Long term (planned ventral hernia)
   a. Interpositional Vicryl mesh placement followed by split thickness skin grafting and abdominal wall reconstruction

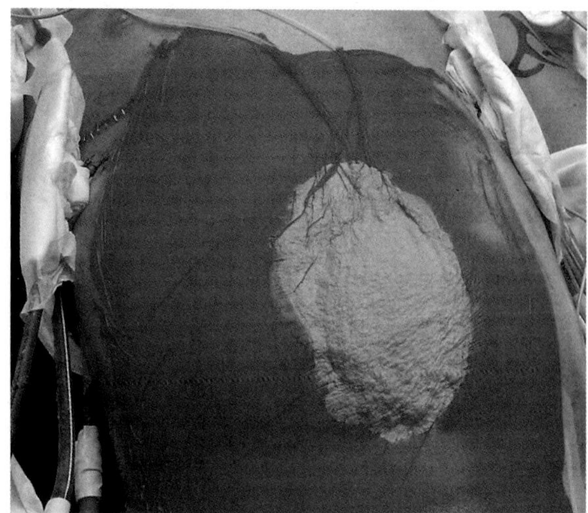

FIGURE 6.2. Barker technique vacuum pack abdominal dressing.

While closure rates vary greatly in the literature, fascial closure can be achieved in most patients.[248] Interpositional meshes have fascial closure rates from 22%-88%, with most of the literature in the lower part of that range.[232,244,247,249,250] Vacuum-assisted techniques range from 29%-100%, with most studies on the higher end without increase in morbidity or mortality.[59,60,248,251-258] Only one prospective study has directly compared interpositional mesh to vacuum-assisted abdominal dressings, with no difference in fascial closure rates between them (26% vs. 31%, respectively).[259] More complex closures with permanent synthetic meshes and fascial releases or extensive skin flaps are avoided at this stage, as they carry increased infection and wound complication rates. They also complicate or prevent abdominal wall reconstruction techniques, such as component separation, at later dates.[61]

For patients for whom definitive closure is not achievable, a planned ventral hernia with subsequent abdominal wall reconstruction is a viable option. An absorbable interpositional mesh (Vicryl) is placed and followed with a split thickness skin graft once granulation tissue appears (generally 10-14 days). After 6-12 months, the underlying viscera will fall away from the skin graft, indicating that the abdominal wall reconstruction can be done then. Waiting beyond 12 months will not improve the operative field, but loss of domain issues becomes more frequent. Tissue expanders or flaps may be needed if soft tissue coverage is insufficient.[247,260] If sufficient fascia is present for closure, then a fascial closure is performed, potentially with a mesh onlay. However, an underlay mesh (allograft or prosthetic) in a subfascial or retrorectus position and/or component separation are usually necessary for abdominal wall reconstruction.[261-265] Allograft meshes have begun to be used to bridge defects, but long-term outcomes are unknown.[252,266-269] The possibility for tissue regeneration and infection resistance compared to synthetics makes them potentially superior in the future. Survivors with a planned ventral hernia feel decreased levels of physical, social and emotional health, but with definitive abdominal reconstruction, return to the general population baseline.[270]

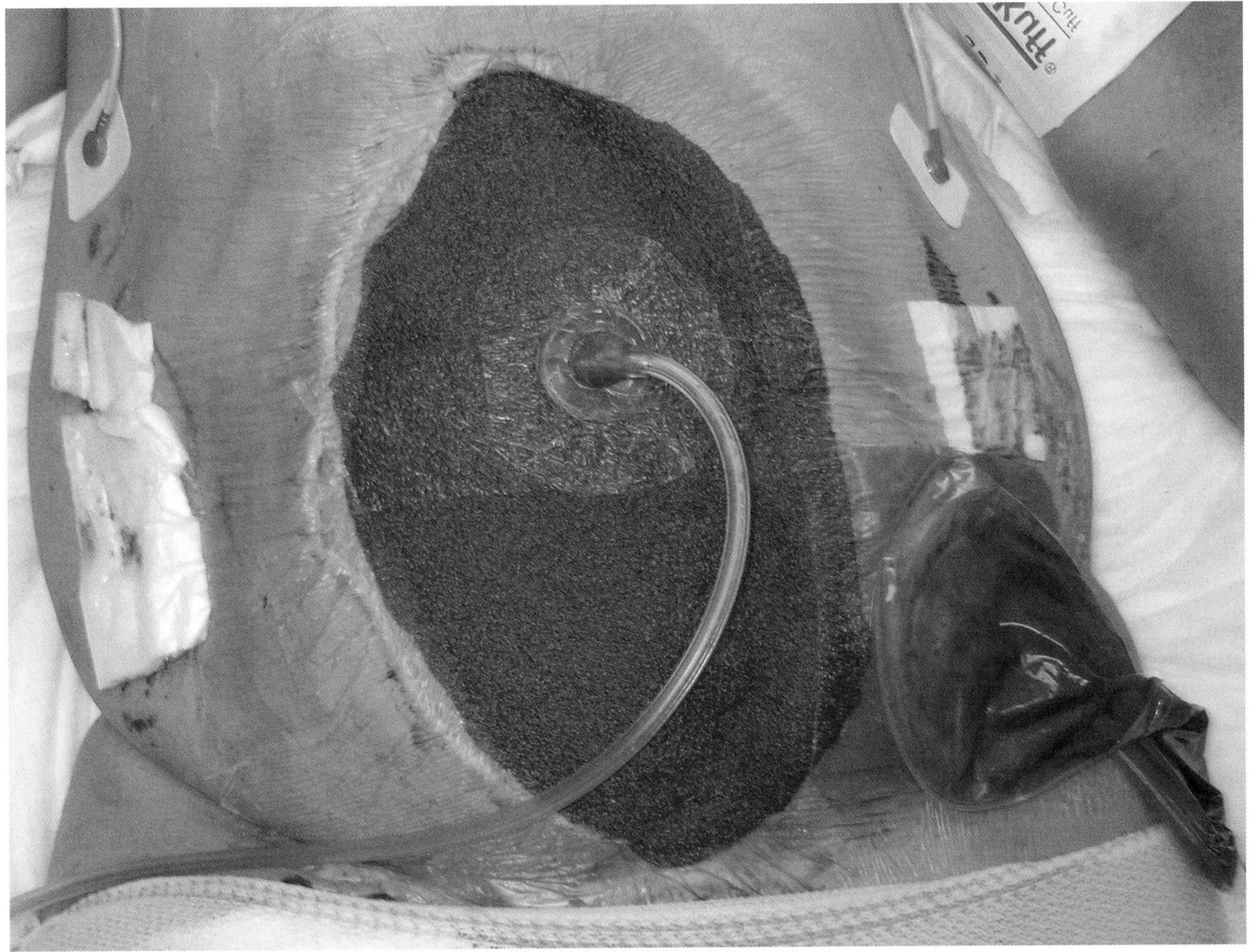

FIGURE 6.3. KCI V.A.C. system.

COMPLICATIONS AND DAMAGE CONTROL

Complications occur primarily in two time periods with damage control. The initial intervention and resuscitation phase has complications related to the sequelae of shock, injury, and resuscitation. These include ACS, missed injuries, and intra-abdominal infections. The later complications of enterocutaneous fistula are found during an open abdominal phase.

Given the ill nature of the patient at presentation, missed injuries have a higher potential to exist. Some injuries, such as those to the diaphragm, retroperitoneal structures (duodenum, ureters, bladder, and rectum), and difficult-to-expose structures (posterior wall of stomach, pancreas, GE junction, retroperitoneal colon, and mesenteric border of bowel), are more common due to anatomy. Repeated examinations can improve capture of these injuries, but damage control is not a substitute for complete injury identification and control.[271,272] The missed unusual or insufficiently controlled vascular injury invariably leads to the patient's death.

Intra-abdominal infection rates vary from 10% to 70% and appear linked to the duration abdominal packs are retained.[273-275] The interval between washouts, however, is highly variable depending on the clinical situation. More frequent washouts promote less abscess formation, but increase the risk of fistula formation with more bowel manipulation. While usual surveillance methods are used in damage control patients, weekly abdominal CT scans for abscess surveillance may be needed in those patients with persistent fever or leukocytosis. Ventilator-associated pneumonia and catheter-related infections are also common in the damage control patients.

Enterocutaneous fistula formation depends upon several factors, including the nature of the injuries, the degree of bowel manipulation, and care and closure technique of the open abdomen. While higher rates have been noted in the literature, fistula rates generally vary between 1% and 15%.[230,259,276,277] Unfortunately, they tend to be the more aggressive enteroatmospheric fistulae that occur within the granulating bed of the open abdominal wound with lower nonsurgical closure rates than typical fistula (around 25%).[232] When encountered, standard therapies of bowel rest and total parenteral nutrition are begun. While many techniques exist in the literature beyond use of frequent dressing changes and suction drains, all fall short of ideal in controlling the caustic effluent.[278-283] Thus, different strategies must be known as individual patients will have differing responses to a therapy. If effluent control can be obtained, a skin graft may be useful for placement of an enterostomal appliance, and the fistula managed as an ostomy. Fistula closure is normally deferred until abdominal wall reconstruction and is associated with increased complications.[284]

DAMAGE CONTROL AND ABDOMINAL SEPSIS

Emergency general surgery has adopted the techniques of damage control and the open abdomen. Many of the management concerns of the damage control trauma patient and the abdominal sepsis patient during the resuscitation and open abdomen phases overlap. The open abdomen allows for instant access to the peritoneal cavity and improved peritoneal toilet with control of effluent, when further debridement is needed or source control cannot be obtained due to patient hemodynamic instability.[16] The present studies have been small, often with mixed populations of abdominal sepsis, trauma, and ACS, and vary concerning mortality between the open and closed abdomen cohorts.[17-20,285,286] The prevention of ACS probably has most influence on outcomes after an operation for peritonitis.

However, alterations to the damage control sequence are needed for abdominal sepsis patients. An intra-abdominal catastrophe without hemorrhage needs initial stabilization of vitals, which with aggressive resuscitation can generally be done in a few hours, preceding operative intervention to prevent hemodynamic collapse on anesthesia induction. The operative goal is source control and wide drainage of the surgical process. A temporary abdominal closure is used when multiple operations are needed for debridement/source control, significant visceral edema prevents closure or further resuscitation has a high risk of creating an ACS, or the patient's hemodynamic instability precludes further operative intervention. Afterward, resuscitation is performed again. The development of a distributive shock, which is generally self-limiting to a few days, is common after operative intervention in an infected surgical field. The heretofore described open abdomen techniques can be used to manage the open abdominal wound, especially with control of effluent from the abdominal wound. They do not replace wide drainage of the surgical field, however. Compared to patients with traumatic injury, fascial closure rates may be lower.[287]

ACKNOWLEDGMENT

We would like to thank Dr Christopher Durham for help with the taxi cab hailing position figure.

References

1. Cinat ME, Wallace WC, Nastanski F, et al. Improved survival following massive transfusion in patients who have undergone trauma. *Arch Surg.* 1999;134:964-970.
2. Krishna G, Sleigh JW, Rahman H. Physiological predictors of death in exsanguinating trauma patients undergoing conventional trauma surgery. *Aust N Z J Surg.* 1998;68:826-829.
3. Ciesla DJ, Moore EE, Johnson JL, et al. A 12-year prospective study of post injury multiple organ failure: has anything changed? *Arch Surg.* 2005;140:432-440.
4. Stone HH, Strom PR, Mullins RJ. Management of the major coagulopathy with onset during laparotomy. *Ann Surg.* 1983;197:532-535.
5. Burch JM, Ortiz VB, Richardson RJ, et al. Abbreviated laparotomy and planned reoperation for critically injured patients. *Ann Surg.* 1992;215:476-484.
6. Rotondo MF, Schwab CW, McGonigal MD, et al. "Damage Control": an approach for improved survival in exsanguinating penetrating abdominal injury. *J Trauma.* 1993;35:375-382.
7. Johnson JW, Gracias VH, Schwab CW, et al. Evolution in damage control for exsanguinations penetrating abdominal trauma. *J Trauma.* 2001;51:261-269.
8. Rotondo MF, Zonies DH. The damage control sequence and underlying logic. *Surg Clin North Am.* 1997;77:761-777.
9. Hoey BA, Schwab CW. Damage control surgery. *Scand J Surg.* 2002;91:92-103.
10. Porter JM, Ivatury RR, Nassoura ZE. Extending the horizons of "Damage Control" in unstable trauma patients beyond the abdomen and gastrointestinal tract. *J Trauma.* 1997;42:559-561.
11. Pape HC, Giannoudis P, Krettek C. The timing of fracture treatment in polytrauma patients: relevance of damage control orthopedic surgery. *Am J Surg.* 2002;183:622-629.
12. Sebesta J. Special lessons learned from Iraq. *Surg Clin N Am.* 2006;86:711-726.
13. Holcomb JB, Helling TS, Hirschberg A. Military, civilian, and rural application of the damage control philosophy. *Mil Med.* 2001;166:490-493.
14. Eiseman B, Moore EE, Meldrum DR, et al. Feasibility of damage control surgery in the management of military combat casualties. *Arch Surg.* 2000;135:1323-1327.
15. Blackbourne LH. Combat damage control surgery. *Crit Care Med.* 2008;36:S304-S310.
16. Schecter WP, Ivatury RR, Rotondo MF, et al. Open abdomen after trauma and abdominal sepsis: a strategy for management. *J Am Coll Surg.* 2006;203:390-396.
17. Stawicki SP, Brooks A, Bilski T, et al. The concept of damage control: extending the paradigm to emergency general surgery. *Injury.* 2008;39:93-101.
18. Cipolla J, Stawicki SP, Hoff WS, et al. A proposed algorithm for managing the open abdomen. *Am Surg.* 2005;71:202-207.
19. Finlay IG, Edwards TJ, Lambert AW. Damage control laparotomy. *Br J Surg.* 2004;91:83-85.
20. Horwood J, Akbar F, Maw A. Initial experience of laparotomy with immediate vacuum therapy in patients with severe peritonitis. *Ann R Coll Surg Engl.* 2009;91:681-687.
21. Maxwell R, Fabian T, Croce M, et al. Secondary abdominal compartment syndrome: an underappreciated manifestation of severe hemorrhagic shock. *J Trauma.* 1999;47:995-999.
22. Balogh Z, McKinley BA, Cocanour CS, et al. Supranormal trauma resuscitation causes more cases of abdominal compartment syndrome. *Arch Surg.* 2003;138:637-643.
23. Cheatham ML, Safcsak K. Is the evolving management of intra-abdominal hypertension and abdominal compartment syndrome improving survival? *Crit Care Med.* 2010;38:402-407.
24. Holcomb JB. Damage control resuscitation. *J Trauma.* 2007;62:S36-S37.
25. Beekley AC. Damage control resuscitation: a sensible approach to the exsanguinating surgical patient. *Crit Care Med.* 2008;36:S267-S274.
26. Kashuk JL, Moore EE, Johnson JL, et al. Postinjury life threatening coagulopathy: is 1:1 fresh frozen plasma: packed red blood cells the answer? *J Trauma.* 2008;65:261-271.
27. Snyder CW, Weinberg JA, McGwin G, et al. The relationship of blood product ratio to mortality: survival benefit or survival bias? *J Trauma.* 2009;66:358-364.
28. Scalea TM, Bochicchio KM, Lumpkins K, et al. Early aggressive use of fresh frozen plasma does not improve outcome in critically injured trauma patients. *Ann Surg.* 2008;248:578-584.
29. Sambasivan CN, Schreiber MA. Emerging therapies in traumatic hemorrhage control. *Curr Opin Crit Care.* 2009;15:560-568.
30. Moore EE. Staged laparotomy for the hypothermia, acidosis, and coagulopathy syndrome. *Am J Surg.* 1996;172:405-410.
31. Aoki N, Wall MJ, Zupan B, et al. Predictive model for survival at the conclusion of a damage control laparotomy. *Am J Surg.* 2000;180: 540-545.
32. Asensio JA, Petrone P, Roldan G, et al. Has evolution in awareness of guidelines for institution of damage control improved outcome in the management of the posttraumatic open abdomen? *Arch Surg.* 2004;139:209-214.
33. Asensio JA, McDuffie L, Petrone P, et al. Reliable variables in the exsanguinated patient which indicate damage control and predict outcome. *Am J Surg.* 2001;182:743-751.
34. Moore EE, Burch JM, Franciose RJ, et al. Staged physiologic restoration and damage control surgery. *World J Surg.* 1998;22:1184-1191.
35. Hirshberg A, Sheffer N, Barnea O. Computer simulation of hypothermia during "damage control" laparotomy. *World J Surg.* 1999;23:960-965.
36. Carrillo EH, Spain DA, Wohltmann CD, et al. Interventional techniques are useful adjuncts in nonoperative management of hepatic injuries. *J Trauma.* 1999;46:619-624.
37. Young JS, Bassam D, Cephas GA, et al. Interhospital versus direct scene transfer of major trauma patients in a rural trauma system. *Am Surg.* 1998;64:88-92.
38. Esposito TJ, Sanddal ND, Hansen JD, et al. Analysis of preventable trauma deaths and inappropriate trauma care in a rural state. *J Trauma.* 1995;39:955-962.
39. Revell M, Greaves I, Porter K. Endpoints for fluid resuscitation in hemorrhagic shock. *J Trauma.* 2003; 54(suppl):S63-S67.
40. Soreide E, Deakin CD. Pre-hospital fluid therapy in the critically injured patient-a clinical update. *Injury.* 2005;36:1001-1010.
41. Rhee P, Koustova E, Alam HB. Searching for the optimal resuscitation method: recommendations for the initial fluid resuscitation of combat casualties. *J Trauma.* 2003;54(suppl):S52-S62.
42. Dawes R, Thomas GOR. Battlefield resuscitation. *Curr Opin Crit Care.* 2009;15:527-535.
43. McManus J, Yershov AL, Ludwig D, et al. Radial pulse character relationships to systolic blood pressure and trauma outcomes. *Prehosp Emerg Care.* 2005;9:423-428.

44. Schenarts PJ, Phade SV, Agle SC, et al. Field hypotension in patients who arrive at the hospital normotensive: a marker of severe injury or crying wolf? *NC Med J*. 2008;69:265-269.
45. American College of Surgeons Committee on Trauma. *Advanced Trauma Life Support for Doctors*. 2nd ed. Chicago, IL: American College of Surgeons; 2008.
46. Hirshberg A, Mattox KL. *Top Knife. The Art And Craft of Trauma Surgery*. Castle Hill Barns, UK: TFM Publishing Ltd; 2005.
47. Jacobs LM, Gross RI, Luk SS, eds. *Advanced Trauma Operative Management (ATOM)*. Woodbury, CT: Cine-Med, Inc; 2004.
48. Reilly PM, Rotondo MF, Carpenter JP, et al. Temporary vascular continuity during damage control: intraluminal shunting of proximal superior mesenteric artery injury. *J Trauma*. 1995;39:757-760.
49. Rasmussen TE, Clouse WD, Jenkins DH, et al. The use of temporary vascular shunts as a damage control adjunct in the management of wartime vascular injury. *J Trauma*. 2006;61:8-15.
50. Starnes BW, Beekley AC, Sebesta JA, et al. Extremity vascular injuries on the battlefield: tips for surgeons deploying to war. *J Trauma*. 2006;60:432-442.
51. Gifford SM, Eliason JL, Clouse D, et al. Early versus delayed restoration of flow with temporary vascular shunt reduces circulating markers of injury in a porcine model. *J Trauma*. 2009;67:259-265.
52. Glass GE, Pearse MF, Nanchahal J. Improving lower limb salvage following fractures with vascular injury: a systematic review and new management algorithm. *J Plast Reconstr Aesthet Surg* 2009;62:571-579.
53. Chambers LW, Green DJ, Sample K, et al. Tactical surgical intervention with temporary shunting of peripheral vascular trauma sustained during operation Iraqi freedom: one unit's experience. *J Trauma*. 2006;61:824-830.
54. Perkins JG, Cap AP, Weiss BM, et al. Massive transfusion and nonsurgical hemostatic agents. *Crit Care Med*. 2008;36(suppl):S325-339.
55. Rhee P, Brown C, Martin M, et al. QuikClot use in trauma for hemorrhage control: case series of 103 documented uses. *J Trauma*. 2008;64:1093-1099.
56. Cox ED, Schreiber MA, McManus J, et al. New hemostatic agents in the combat setting. *Transfusion*. 2009;49(suppl):248S-255S.
57. Schein M, Saadia R, Jamieson JR, et al. The 'sandwich technique' in the management of the open abdomen. *Br J Surg*. 1986;73:369-370.
58. Brock WB, Barker DE, Burns RP. Temporary closure of open abdominal wounds: the vacuum pack. *Am Surg*. 1995;61:30-35.
59. Barker DE, Kaufman HJ, Smith LA, et al. Vacuum pack technique of temporary abdominal closure: a 7 year experience with 112 patients. *J Trauma*. 2000;48:201-206.
60. Barker DE, Green JM, Maxwell RA, et al. Experience with vacuum-pack temporary abdominal wound closure in 258 trauma and general and vascular surgical patients. *J Am Coll Surg*. 2007;204:784-793.
61. Vargo D, Richardson JD, Campbell A, et al.; for the Open Abdomen Advisory Panel. Management of the open abdomen: from initial operation to definitive closure. *Am Surg*. 2009;75(suppl):S1-S22.
62. Ho AM, Karmakar MK, Contardi LH, et al. Excessive use of normal saline in managing traumatized patients in shock: a preventable contributor to acidosis. *J Trauma*. 2001;51:173-177.
63. Rhee P, Burris D, Kaufmann C, et al. Lactated Ringer's solution resuscitation causes neutrophil activation after hemorrhagic shock. *J Trauma*. 1998;44:313-319.
64. Watters JM, Tieu BH, Todd SR, et al. Fluid resuscitation increases inflammatory gene transcription after traumatic injury. *J Trauma*. 2006;61:300-309.
65. Rizoli SB. Crystalloids and colloids in trauma resuscitation: a brief overview of the current debate. *J Trauma*. 2003;54(suppl):S82-S88.
66. Choi P, Yip G, Quinonez LG, et al. Crystalloid vs. colloids in fluid resuscitation: a systematic review. *Crit Care Med*. 1999;27:200-210.
67. Perel P, Roberts I, Pearson M. Colloids versus crystalloids for fluid resuscitation in critically ill patients. *Cochrane Database Syst Rev*. 2007;(4):CD000567.
68. Bulger EM, Jurkovich GJ, Nathes AB, et al. Hypertonic resuscitation of hypovolemic shock after blunt trauma. A randomized controlled trial. *Arch Surg*. 2008;143:139-148.
69. Cooper DJ, Myles PS, McDermott FT, et al. Prehospital hypertonic saline resuscitation of patients with hypotension and severe traumatic brain injury. A randomized controlled trial. *JAMA*. 2004;291:1350-1357.
70. Bunn F, Roberts IG, Tasker R, et al. Hypertonic versus near isotonic crystalloid for fluid resuscitation in critically ill patients. *Cochrane Database Syst Rev* 2004;(3):CD002045.
71. Kramer GC. Hypertonic resuscitation: physiologic mechanisms and recommendations for trauma care. *J Trauma*. 2003;54(suppl):S89-S99.
72. Spinella PC, Holcomb JB. Resuscitation and transfusion principles for traumatic hemorrhagic shock. *Blood Rev*. 2009;23:231-240.
73. Stansbury LG, Dutton RP, Stein DM, et al. Controversy in trauma resuscitation: do ratios of plasma and red blood cells matter? *Transfus Med Rev*. 2009;23:255-265.
74. Duchesne JC, Hunt JP, Wahl G, et al. Review of current blood transfusions strategies is a mature level I trauma center: were we wrong for the last 60 years? *J Trauma*. 2008;65:272-278.
75. Zink KA, Sambasivan CN, Holcomb JB, et al. A high ratio of plasma and platelets to packed red blood cells in the first 6 hours of massive transfusion improves outcomes in a large multi-center study. *Am J Surg*. 2009;197:565-570.
76. Borgman MA, Spinella PC, Perkins JG, et al. The ratio of blood products transfused affects mortality in patients receiving massive transfusions at a combat support hospital. *J Trauma*. 2007;63:805-813.
77. Sperry JL, Ochoa JB, Gunn SR, et al. An FFP:PRBC transfusion ratio >/= 1:1.5 is associated with a lower risk of mortality after massive transfusion. *J Trauma*. 2008;65:986-993.
78. Gunter Jr OL, Au BK, Isbell JM, et al. Optimizing outcomes in damage control resuscitation: identifying blood product ratios associated with improved survival. *J Trauma*. 2008;65:527-534.
79. Teixeira PG, Inaba K, Shulman I, et al. Impact of plasma transfusion in massively transfused trauma patients. *J Trauma*. 2009;66:693-697.
80. Holcomb JB, Wade CE, Michalek JE. Increased plasma and platelet to RBC ratios improves outcome in 466 massively transfused civilian trauma patients. *Ann Surg*. 2008;248:447-458.
81. Maegele M, Lefering R, Paffrath T, et al. Red blood cell to plasma ratios transfused during massive transfusion are associated with mortality in severe multiple injury: a retrospective analysis from the Trauma Registry of the Deutsche Gesellschaft fur Unfallchirurgie. *Vox Sang*. 2008;95:112-119.
82. Perkins JG, Cap AP, Spinella PC, et al. An evaluation of the impact of platelets used in the setting of massively transfused trauma patients. *J Trauma*. 2009;66(suppl):S77-S84.
83. Cotton BA, Gunter OL, Isbell JM, et al. Damage control hematology: impact of a defined exsanguination protocol on mortality and blood utilization. *J Trauma*. 2008;64:1177-1183.
84. Kenet G, Walden R, Eldad A, et al. Treatment of traumatic bleeding with recombinant factor VIIa. *Lancet*. 1999;354:1879.
85. Martinowitz U, Kenet G, Segal E, et al. Recombinant activated factor VII for adjunctive hemorrhage control in trauma. *J Trauma*. 2001;51:431-439.
86. O'Neill P, Bluth M, Gloster E, et al. Successful use of recombinant activated factor VII for trauma-associated hemorrhage in a patient without pre-existing coagulopathy. *J Trauma*. 2002;52:400-405.
87. Dutton R, Hess J, Scalea T. Recombinant factor VIIa for control of hemorrhage: early experience in critically ill trauma patients. *J Clin Anaesth*. 2003;15:184-188.
88. Eikelboom J, Bird R, Blythe D, et al. Recombinant activated factor VII for the treatment of life-threatening haemorrhage. *Blood Coagul Fibrinolysis*. 2003;14:713-717.
89. Dutton R, McCunn M, Hyder M, et al. Factor VIIa for correction of traumatic coagulopathy. *J Trauma*. 2004;57:709-718.
90. Udy A, Vaghela M, Lawton G, et al. The use of recombinant activated factor VII in the control of hemorrhage following blunt pelvic trauma. *Anaesthesia*. 2005;60:613-616.
91. Harrison T, Laskosky J, Jazaeri O, et al. "Low dose" recombinant activated factor VII results in less blood and blood product use in traumatic hemorrhage. *J Trauma*. 2005;59:150-154.
92. Geeraedts L, Kamphuisen P, Kassjager H, et al. The role of recombinant factor VIIa in the treatment of life-threatening haemorrhage in blunt trauma. *Injury*. 2005;36:495-500.
93. Holcomb J, Hoots K, Moore F. Treatment of acquired coagulopathy with recombinant activated factor VII in a damage control patient. *Mil Med*. 2005;170:287-290.
94. Benharash P, Bongard F, Putnam B. Use of recombinant factor VIIa for adjunctive hemorrhage control in trauma and surgical patients. *Am Surg*. 2005;71:776-780.
95. McMullin NR, Kauvar DS, Currier HM, et al. The clinical and laboratory response to recombinant factor VIIa in trauma and surgical patients with acquired coagulopathy. *Curr Surg*. 2006;63:246-251.
96. Rizoli SB, Nascimento Jr B, Osman F, et al. Recombinant activated coagulation factor VII and bleeding trauma patients. *J Trauma*. 2006;61:1419-1425.
97. Perkins JG, Schreiber MA, Wade CE, et al. Early versus late recombinant factor VIIa in combat trauma patients requiring massive transfusion. *J Trauma*. 2007;62:1095-1101.
98. Boffard KD, Riou B, Warren B, et al. for the NovoSeven Trauma Study Group. Recombinant factor VIIa as adjunctive therapy for bleeding control in severely injured trauma patients: two parallel randomized, placebo-controlled, double-blind clinical trials. *J Trauma*. 2005;59:8-18.
99. Dutton R, Hauser C, Boffard K, et al. Scientific and logistical challenges in designing the CONTROL trial: recombinant factor VIIa in severe trauma patients with refractory bleeding. *Clin Trials*. 2009;6:467-479.
100. O'Connell KA, Wood JJ, Wise RP, et al. Thromboembolic adverse events after use of recombinant human coagulation factor VIIa. *JAMA*. 2006;295:293-298.
101. Dickneite G, Dörr B, Kaspereit F, et al. Prothrombin complex concentrate versus recombinant Factor VIIa for reversal of hemodilutional coagulopathy in a porcine trauma model. *J Trauma*. 2010;68:1151-1157.
102. Dickneite G, Pragst I. Prothrombin complex concentrate vs fresh frozen plasma for reversal of dilutional coagulopathy in a porcine trauma model. *Br J Anaesth*. 2009;102:345-354.
103. Kalina M, Tinkoff G, Gbadebo A, et al. A protocol for the rapid normalization of INR in trauma patients with intracranial hemorrhage on prescribed Warfarin therapy. *Am Surg*. 2008;74:858-861.
104. Schick KS, Fermann JM, Jauch KW, et al. Prothrombin complex concentrate in surgical patients: retrospective evaluation of vitamin K antagonist reversal and treatment of severe bleeding. *Crit Care*. 2009;13:R191.

105. Bruce D, Nokes TJC. Prothrombin complex concentrate (Beriplex P/N) in severe bleeding: experience in a large tertiary hospital. *Crit Care.* 2008;12:R105.
106. Tanaka KA, Szlam F, Dickneite G, et al. Effects of prothrombin complex concentrate and recombinant activated factor VII on vitamin K antagonist induced anticoagulation. *Thromb Res.* 2008;122:117-123.
107. Pabinger I, Brenner B, Kalina U, et al. Prothrombin complex concentrate (Beriplex P/N) for emergency anticoagulation reversal: a prospective multinational clinical trial. *J Thromb Haemost.* 2008;6:622-631.
108. Treur MJ, McCracken F, Heeg B, et al. Efficacy of recombinant activated factor VII vs. activated prothrombin complex concentrate for patients suffering from haemophilia complicated with inhibitors: a Bayesian meta-regression. *Haemophilia.* 2009;15:420-436.
109. Dickneite G. Prothrombin complex concentrate versus recombinant factor VIIa for reversal of coumarin anticoagulation. *Thromb Res.* 2007;119:643-651.
110. Luna GK, Vaier RV, Pavlin EG, et al. Incidence and effect of hypothermia in seriously injured patients. *J Trauma.* 1987;27:1014-1018.
111. Jurkovich GJ, Greiser WB, Luterman A, et al. Hypothermia in trauma victims: an ominous predictor of survival. *J Trauma.* 1987:27:1019-1024.
112. Martin RS, Kilgo PD, Miller PR, et al. Injury-associated hypothermia: an analysis of the 2004 National Trauma Data Bank. *Shock.* 2005;24:114-118.
113. Wang HE, Callaway CW, Peitzman AB, et al. Admission hypothermia and outcome after major trauma. *Crit Care Med.* 2005;33:1296-1301.
114. Shafi S, Elliott AC, Gentilello L. Is hypothermia simply a marker of shock and injury severity or an independent risk factor for mortality in trauma patients? Analysis of a large national trauma registry. *J Trauma.* 2005;59:1081-1085.
115. Arthurs Z, Cuadrado D, Beekley A, et al. The impact of hypothermia on trauma care at the 31st combat support hospital. *Am J Surg.* 2006;191:610-614.
116. Waibel BH, Schlitzkus LL, Newell MA, et al. Impact of hypothermia (below 36°C) in the rural trauma patient. *J Am Coll Surg.* 2009;209:580-588.
117. Waibel BH, Durham CA, Newell MA, et al. Impact of hypothermia in the rural, pediatric trauma patient. *Pediatr Crit Care Med.* 2010;11:199-204.
118. Johannigman JA, Johnson DJ, Roettger P. The effect of hypothermia on liver adenosine triphosphate (ATP) recovery following combined shock and ischemia. *J Trauma* 1992;32:190-195.
119. Seekamp A, van Griensven M, Hildebrand F, et al. Adenosine-triphosphate in trauma-related and elective hypothermia. *J Trauma.* 1999;47:673-683.
120. Eidelman Y, Glat PM, Pachter HL, et al. The effects of topical hypothermia and steroids on ATP levels in an in vivo liver ischemia model. *J Trauma.* 1994;37:677-681.
121. Hildebrand F, Giannoudis PV, van Griensven M, et al. Pathophysiologic changes and effects of hypothermia on outcome in elective surgery and trauma patients. *Am J Surg.* 2004;187:363-371.
122. Badjatia N, Strongilis E, Prescutti M, et al. Metabolic benefits of surface counter warming during therapeutic temperature modulation. *Crit Care Med.* 2009;37:1893-1897.
123. Eastridge BJ, Jenkins D, Flaherty S, et al. Trauma system development in a theater of war: experiences from Operation Iraqi Freedom and Operation Enduring Freedom. *J Trauma.* 2006;61:1366-1373.
124. Husum H, Olsen T, Murad M, et al. Preventing post-injury hypothermia during prolonged prehospital evacuation. *Prehospital Disaster Med.* 2002;17:23-26.
125. Polderman KH. Mechanisms of action, physiological effects, and complications of hypothermia. *Crit Care Med.* 2009;37(suppl):S186-S202.
126. Giesbrecht GC. Emergency treatment of hypothermia. *Emerg Med.* 2001;13:9-16.
127. Van den Berghe G, Wouters P, Weekers F, et al. Intensive insulin therapy in critically ill patients. *N Engl J Med.* 2001;345:1359-1367.
128. Van den Berghe G, Hermans G, Meersseman W, et al. Intensive insulin therapy in the medical ICU. *N Engl J Med.* 2006;354:449-461.
129. Vlasselaers D, Milants I, Desmet L, et al. Intensive insulin therapy for patients in paediatric intensive care: a prospective randomized controlled study. *Lancet.* 2009;373:547-556.
130. Brunkhorst FM, Engel C, Bloos F, et al. Intensive insulin therapy and pentastarch resuscitation in severe sepsis. *N Engl J Med.* 2008;358:125-139.
131. Arabi YM, Dabbagh OC, Tamim HM, et al. Intensive versus conventional insulin therapy; a randomized controlled trial in medical and surgical critically ill patients. *Crit Care Med.* 2008;36:3190-3197.
132. De La Rosa Gdel C, Donado JH, Restrepo AH, et al. Strict glycaemic control in patients hospitalized in a mixed medical and surgical intensive care unit: a randomized clinical trial. *Crit Care.* 2008;12:R120.
133. Finfer S, Chittock DR, Su SY, et al. Intensive versus conventional glucose control in critically ill patients. *N Engl J Med.* 2009;360:1283-1297.
134. Griesdale DEG, de Souza RJ, van Dam RM, et al. Intensive insulin therapy and mortality among critically ill patients: a meta-analysis including NICE-SUGAR study data. *CMAJ.* 2009;180:821-827.
135. Van den Berghe G, Schetz M, Vlasselaers D, et al. Intensive insulin therapy in critically ill patients: NICE-SUGAR or Leuven blood glucose target? *J Clin Endocrinol Metab.* 2009;94:3163-3170.
136. Cheatham ML, Safcsak K, Block EFJ, et al. Preload assessment in patients with an open abdomen. *J Trauma.* 1999;46:16-22.
137. Porter JM, Ivatury RR. In search of the optimal end points of resuscitation in trauma patients: a review. *J Trauma.* 1998;44:908-914.
138. Cocchi MN, Kimlin E, Walsh M, et al. Identification and resuscitation of the trauma patient in shock. *Emerg Med Clin N Am.* 2007;25:623-642.
139. Tisherman SA, Barie P, Bokhari R, et al. Clinical practice guideline: endpoints of resuscitation. *J Trauma.* 2004;57:898-912.
140. Rady MY, Nightingale P, Little RA, et al. Shock index: a reevaluation in acute circulatory failure. *Resuscitation.* 1992;23:227-234.
141. Rady MY, Smithline HA, Blake H, et al. A comparison of the shock index and conventional vital signs to identify acute, critical illness in the emergency department. *Ann Emerg Med.* 1994;24:685-690.
142. Rady MY, Rivers EP, Nowak RM. Resuscitation of the critically ill in the ED: responses of blood pressure, heart rate, shock index, central venous oxygen saturation, and lactate. *Am J Emerg Med.* 1996;14:218-225.
143. Birkhahn RH, Gaeta TJ, Terry D, et al. Shock index in diagnosing early acute hypovolemia. *Am J Emerg Med.* 2005;23:323-326.
144. Zarzaur BL, Croce MA, Fischer PE, et al. New vitals after injury: shock index for the young and age x shock index for the old. *J Surg Res.* 2008;147:229-236.
145. Zarzaur BL, Croce MA, Magnotti LJ, et al. Identifying life-threatening shock in the older injured patient: an analysis of the National Trauma Data Bank. *J Trauma.* 2010;68:1134-1138.
146. Grogan EL, Morris JA Jr, Norris PR, et al. Reduced heart rate volatility: an early predictor of death in trauma patients. *Ann Surg.* 2004;240:547-554.
147. Norris PR, Ozdas A, Cao H, et al. Cardiac uncoupling and heart rate variability stratify ICU patients by mortality: a study of 2088 trauma patients. *Ann Surg.* 2006;243:804-814.
148. Morris JA Jr, Norris PR, Ozdas A, et al. Reduced heart rate variability: an indicator of cardiac uncoupling and diminished physiologic reserve in 1,425 trauma patients. *J Trauma.* 2006;60:1165-1174.
149. Proctor KG, Atapattu SA, Duncan RC. Heart rate variability index in trauma patients. *J Trauma.* 2007;63:33-43.
150. King DR, Ogilvie MP, Pereira BM, et al. Heart rate variability as a triage tool in patients with trauma during prehospital helicopter transport. *J Trauma.* 2009;67(3):436-440.
151. The National Heart, Lung, and Blood Institute ARDS Clinical Trails Network. Comparison of two fluid-management strategies in Acute Lung Injury. *N Engl J Med.* 2006;354:1-12.
152. Chang MC, Miller PR, D'Agostino R, Meredith JW. Effects of abdominal decompression on cardiopulmonary function and visceral perfusion in patients with intra-abdominal hypertension. *J Trauma.* 1998;44:440-445.
153. Cheatham ML, Safcsak K, Zoha Z, et al. Right ventricular end-diastolic volume index as a predictor of preload status in abdominal compartment syndrome. *Crit Care Med.* 1998;26(suppl):A38.
154. The Acute Respiratory Distress Syndrome Network. Ventilation with lower tidal volumes as compared with traditional tidal volumes for acute lung injury and the acute respiratory distress syndrome. *N Engl J Med.* 2000;342:1301-1308.
155. Gajic O, Dara SI, Mendez JL, et al. Ventilator-associated lung injury in patients without acute lung injury at the onset of mechanical ventilation. *Crit Care Med.* 2004;32:1817-1824.
156. Lionetti V, Recchia FA, Ranieri VM. Overview of ventilator-induced lung injury mechanisms. *Curr Opin Crit Care.* 2005;11:82-86.
157. Schreiber TC, Boyle III WA. Lung injury caused by mechanical ventilation. *Contemp Crit Care.* 2005;3:1-11.
158. Klein Y, Blackbourne L, Barquist ES. Non-ventilatory-based strategies in the management of acute respiratory distress syndrome. *J Trauma.* 2004;57:915-924.
159. De Jonghe B, Lacherade JC, Sharshar T, et al. Intensive care unit-acquired weakness: risk factors and prevention. *Crit Care Med.* 2009. 37(suppl):S309-S315.
160. Hall JB, Schweickert W, Kress JP. Role of analgesics, sedatives, neuromuscular blockers, and delirium. *Crit Care Med.* 2009;37(suppl):S416-S421.
161. Behbehani NA, Al-Mane F, D'Yachkova Y, et al. Myopathy following mechanical ventilation for asthma: the role of muscle relaxants and corticosteroids. *Chest.* 1999;115:1627-1631.
162. Leatherman JW, Fluegel WL, David WS, et al. Muscle weakness in mechanically ventilated patients with severe asthma. *Am J Respir Crit Care Med.* 1996;153:1686-1690.
163. Murray M, Cowen J, DeBlock H, et al. Clinical practice guidelines for sustained neuromuscular blockade in the adult critically ill patient. *Crit Care Med.* 2002;30:142-156.
164. Sanchez NC, Tenofsky PL, Dort JM, et al. What is normal intra-abdominal pressure? *Am Surg.* 2001;67:243-247.
165. De Keulenaer BL, De Waele JJ, Powell B, et al. What is normal intra-abdominal pressure and how is it affected by positioning, body mass and positive end-expiratory pressure? *Intensive Care Med.* 2009;35:969-976.
166. Malbrain ML, Cheatham ML, Kirkpatrick A, et al. Results from the international conference of experts on intra-abdominal hypertension and abdominal compartment syndrome. I. Definitions. *Intensive Care Med.* 2006;32:1722-1732.
167. Burch JM, Moore EE, Morre FA, et al. The abdominal compartment syndrome. *Surg Clin North Am* 1996;76:833-842.
168. Iberti TJ, Kelly K, Gentili DR, et al. A simple technique to accurately determine intra-abdominal pressure. *Crit Care Med.* 1987;15:1140-1142.

169. Kirkpatrick AW, Brenneman FD, McLean RF, et al. Is clinical examination an accurate indicator of raised intra-abdominal pressure in critically injured patients? *Can J Surg*. 2000;43:207-211.
170. Barnes GE, Laine GA, Giam PY, et al. Cardiovascular responses to elevation of intra-abdominal hydrostatic pressure. *Am J Physiol*. 1985;248:R208-R213.
171. Obeid F, Saba A, Fath J, et al. Increases in intra-abdominal pressure affect pulmonary compliance. *Arch Surg*. 1995;130:544-548.
172. Cheatham ML. Abdominal compartment syndrome. *Curr Opin Crit Care*. 2009;15:154-162.
173. Ivankovich AD, Miletich DJ, Albrecht RF, et al. Cardiovascular effects of intraperitoneal insufflation with carbon dioxide and nitrous oxide in the dog. *Anesthesiology*. 1975;42:281-287.
174. Diamant M, Benumof JL, Saidman LJ. Hemodynamics of increased intra-abdominal pressure. *Anesthesiology*. 1978;48:23-27.
175. Robotham JL, Wise RA, Bromberger-Barnea B. Effects of changes in abdominal pressure on left ventricular performance and regional blood flow. *Crit Care Med*. 1985;13:803-909.
176. Balogh Z, McKinley BA, Cacanour CS, et al. Patients with impending abdominal compartment syndrome do not respond to early volume loading. *Am J Surg*. 2003;186:602-608.
177. Cullen DJ, Coyle JP, Teplick R, et al. Cardiovascular, pulmonary, and renal effects of massively increased intra-abdominal pressure in critically ill patients. *Crit Care Med*. 1989;17:118-121.
178. Murtoh T, Lamm WJE, Embree LJ, et al. Abdominal distension alters regional pleural pressure and chest wall mechanics in pigs in vivo. *J Appl Physiol*. 1991;70:2611-2618.
179. Schachtrupp A, Graf J, Tons C, et al. Intravascular volume depletion in a 24-hour porcine model of intra-abdominal hypertension. *J Trauma*. 2003;55:734-740.
180. Burchard KW, Ciombor DM, McLeod MK, et al. Positive end expiratory pressure with increased intra-abdominal pressure. *Surg Gynecol Obstet*. 1985;161:313-318.
181. Harman PK, Kron IL, McLachlan HD, et al. Elevated intra-abdominal pressure and renal function. *Ann Surg*. 1982;196:594-597.
182. Sugrue M, Jones F, Deane SA, et al. Intra-abdominal hypertension is an independent cause of postoperative renal impairment. *Arch Surg*. 1999;134:1082-1085.
183. Doty JM, Saggi BH, Sugerman HJ, et al. Effect of increased renal venous pressure on renal function. *J Trauma*. 1999;47:1000-1003.
184. Doty JM, Saggi GH, Blocher CR, et al. Effects of increased renal parenchymal pressure on renal function. *J Trauma*. 2000;48:874-877.
185. Stone HH, Fulenwider JT. Renal decapsulation in the prevention of post-ischemic oliguria. *Ann Surg*. 1977;186:343-355.
186. Le Roith D, Bark H, Nyska M, et al. The effect of abdominal pressure on plasma antidiuretic hormone levels in the dog. *J Surg Res*. 1982;32:65-69.
187. Bloomfield G, Blocher C, Fakhry I, et al. Elevated intra-abdominal pressure increases plasma renin activity and aldosterone levels. *J Trauma*. 1997;42:997-1005.
188. Cadwell CB, Ricotta JR. Changes in visceral blood flow with elevated intraabdominal pressure. *J Surg Res*. 1987;43:14-20.
189. Diebel LN, Dulchavsky SA, Wilson RF. Effect of increased intra-abdominal pressure on mesenteric arterial and intestinal mucosal blood flow. *J Trauma*. 1992;33:45-49.
190. Diebel LN, Wilson RF, Dulchavsky SA, et al. Effect of increased intra-abdominal pressure on hepatic arterial, portal venous, and hepatic microcirculatory blood flow. *J Trauma*. 1992;33:279-283.
191. Behrman SW, Bertken KA, Stefanacci HA, et al. Breakdown of intestinal repair after laparotomy for trauma: incidence, risk factors, and strategies for prevention. *J Trauma*. 1998;45:227-233.
192. Eleftheriadis E, Kotzampassi K, Papanotas K, et al. Gut ischemia, oxidative stress and bacterial translocation in elevated abdominal pressure in rats. *W J Surg*. 1996;20:11-16.
193. Diebel LN, Culchavsky SA, Brown WJ. Splanchnic ischemia and bacterial translocation in the abdominal compartment syndrome. *J Trauma*. 1997;43:852-855.
194. Bloomfield GL, Ridings PC, Blocher CR, et al. Effects of increased intra-abdominal pressure upon intracranial and cerebral perfusion pressure before and after volume expansion. *J Trauma*. 1996;40:936-943.
195. Bloomfield GL, Ridings PC, Blocher CL, et al. A proposed relationship between increased intra-abdominal, intrathoracic, and intracranial pressure. *Crit Care Med*. 1997;25:496-503.
196. Citerio G, Vascotto E, Villa F, et al. Induced abdominal compartment syndrome increases intracranial pressure in neurotrauma patients: a prospective study. *Crit Care Med*. 2001;29:1466-1471.
197. Bloomfield GL, Dalton JM, Sugerman HJ, et al. Treatment of increasing intracranial pressure secondary to the acute abdominal compartment syndrome in a patient with combined abdominal and head trauma. *J Trauma*. 1995;39:1168-1170.
198. Joseph DK, Dutton RP, Aarabi B, et al. Decompressive laparotomy to treat intractable intracranial hypertension after traumatic brain injury. *J Trauma*. 2004;57:687-695.
199. Scalea TM, Bochicchio GV, Habashi N, et al. Increased intra-abdominal, intrathoracic, and intracranial pressure after severe brain injury: multiple compartment syndrome. *J Trauma*. 2007;62:647-656.
200. Diebel L, Saxe J, Dulchavsky S. Effect of intra-abdominal pressure on the abdominal wall blood flow. *Am Surg* 1992;58:573-576.
201. McNelis J, Marini CP, Jurkiewecz A, et al. Predictive factors associated with the development of abdominal compartment syndrome in the surgical intensive care unit. *Arch Surg*. 2002;137:133-136.
202. Ertel W, Oberholzer A, Platz A, et al. Incidence and clinical pattern of the abdominal compartment syndrome after "damage control" laparotomy in 311 patients with severe abdominal and/or pelvic trauma. *Crit Care Med*. 2000;28:1747-1753.
203. Malbrain ML, Chiumello D, Pelosi P, et al. Prevalence of intra-abdominal hypertension in critically ill patients: a multicenter epidemiological study. *Intensive Care Med*. 2004;30:822-829.
204. Mayberry JC, Mullins RJ, Crass RA, et al. Prevention of abdominal compartment syndrome by absorbable mesh prosthesis closure. *Arch Surg*. 1997;132:957-962.
205. Ivatury RR, Porter JM, Simon RJ, et al. Intra-abdominal hypertension after life-threatening penetrating abdominal trauma; prophylaxis, incidence, and clinical relevance to gastric mucosal pH and abdominal compartment syndrome. *J Trauma*. 1998;44:1016-1023.
206. Offner PJ, de Souza AL, Moore EE, et al. Avoidance of abdominal compartment syndrome by absorbable mesh prosthesis closure. *Arch Surg*. 1997;132:957-962.
207. Gracias VH, Braslow B, Johnson J, et al. Abdominal compartment syndrome in the open abdomen. *Arch Surg*. 2002;137:1298-1300.
208. Biffl WL, Moore EE, Burch JM, et al. Secondary abdominal compartment syndrome is a highly lethal event. *Am J Surg*. 2001;182:645-648.
209. Meldrum DR, Moore FA, Moore EE, et al. Prospective characterization and selective management of the abdominal compartment syndrome. *Am J Surg*. 1997;174:667-673.
210. De laet IE, Ravyts M, Vidts W, et al. Current insights in intra-abdominal hypertension and abdominal compartment syndrome: open the abdomen and keep it open! *Langenbecks Arch Surg*. 2008;393:833-847.
211. Cheatham ML, Malbrain ML, Kirkpatrick A, et al. Results from the international conference of experts on intra-abdominal hypertension and abdominal compartment syndrome. II. Recommendations. *Intensive Care Med*. 2007;33:951-962.
212. Miller PR, Chang MC, Hoth JJ, et al. Colonic resection in the setting of damage control laparotomy: is delayed anastomosis safe? *Am Surg*. 2007;73:606-610.
213. Block EFJ, Cheatham ML, Bee TK. Percutaneous endoscopic gastrostomy in patients with an open abdomen. *Am Surg*. 2001;67:913-914.
214. Duchesne JC, Wang YZ, Weintraub SL, et al. Stoma complications: a multivariate analysis. *Am Surg*. 2002;68:961-966.
215. Shellito PC. Complications of abdominal stoma surgery. *Dis Col Rect*. 1998;41:1562-1572.
216. McKibbin B, Cresci G, Hawkins M. Nutrition support for the patient with an open abdomen after major abdominal trauma. *Nutrition*. 2003;19:563-566.
217. Moore EE, Jones TN. Benefits of immediate jejunostomy feeding after major abdominal trauma-a prospective, randomized study. *J Trauma*. 1986;26:874-881.
218. Kudsk KA, Croce MA, Fabian TC, et al. Enteral versus parenteral feeding. Effects on septic morbidity after blunt and penetrating abdominal trauma. *Ann Surg*. 1992;215:503-511.
219. Moore FA, Feliciano DV, Andrassy RJ, et al. Early enteral feeding, compared with parenteral, reduces postoperative septic complications. The results of a meta-analysis. *Ann Surg*. 1992;216:172-183.
220. Dissanaike S, Pham T, Shalhub S, et al. Effect of immediate enteral feeding on trauma patients with an open abdomen: protection from nosocomial infections. *J Am Coll Surg*. 2008;207:690-697.
221. Collier B, Guillamondegui O, Cotton B, et al. Feeding the open abdomen. *JPEN*. 2007;31:410-415.
222. Ahmed N, Kuo Y-H. Early versus late tracheostomy in patients with severe traumatic head injury. *Surg Infect*. 2007;8:343-347.
223. Agle SC, Kao LS, Moore FA, et al. Early predictors of prolonged mechanical ventilation in major torso trauma patients who require resuscitation. *Am J Surg*. 2006;192:822-827.
224. Shirawi N, Arabi Y. Bench-to-bedside review: early tracheostomy in critically ill trauma patients. *Crit Care* 2006;10:201. http://ccforum.com/content/10/1/201
225. Goettler CE, Fugo JR, Bard MR, et al. Predicting the need for early tracheostomy: a multifactorial analysis of 992 intubated trauma patients. *J Trauma*. 2006;60:991-996.
226. Dunham CM, Ransom KJ. Assessment of early tracheostomy in trauma patients: a systematic review and meta-analysis. *Am Surg*. 2006;72:276-281.
227. Arabi Y, Haddad S, Shirawi N, et al. Early tracheostomy in intensive care trauma patients improves resource utilization: a cohort study and literature review. *Crit Care*. 2004;8:R347-R352.
228. Bouderka MA, Fakhir B, Bouaggad A, et al. Early tracheostomy versus prolonged endotracheal intubation in severe head injury. *J Trauma*. 2004;57:251-254.
229. Goettler CE, Waibel BH, Watkins F, et al. Predicting tracheostomy in traumatized ICU patients. *Crit Care Med*. 2009;37(suppl):A356.
230. Mayberry JC. Bedside open abdominal surgery: utility and wound management. *Crit Care Clin*. 2000;16:151-172.

231. Garner GB, Ware DN, Cocanour CS, et al. Vacuum-assisted wound closure provides early fascial reapproximation in trauma patients with open abdomens. *Am J Surg*. 2001;182:630-638.
232. Tremblay LN, Feliciano DV, Schmidt J, et al. Skin only or silo closure in the critically ill patient with an open abdomen. *Am J Surg*. 2001;182:670-675.
233. Markley MA, Mantor PC, Letton RW, et al. Pediatric vacuum packing wound closure for damage control laparotomy. *J Pediatr Surg*. 2002;37:512-514.
234. Sherck J, Seiver A, Shatney C, et al. Covering the "open abdomen": a better technique. *Am Surg*. 1998;64:854-857.
235. Smith LA, Barker DE, Chase CW, et al. Vacuum pack technique of temporary abdominal closure: a four year experience. *Am Surg*. 1997;63:1102-1107.
236. Losanoff JE, Richman BW, Jones JW. Temporary abdominal coverage and reclosure of the open abdomen: frequently asked questions. *J Am Coll Surg*. 2002;195:105-115.
237. Feliciano DV, Burch JM. Towel clips, silos and heroic forms of wound closure. In: Maull KI, Cleveland HC, Feliciano DV, et al. eds. *Advances in Trauma and Critical Care*. Vol. 6. St. Louis, MO: Mosby-Year Book; 1991:231-250.
238. Fox VJ, Miller J, Nix AM. Temporary abdominal closure using an i.v. bag silo for severe trauma. *AORN J*. 1999;6:530-535, 537, 539-541.
239. Argenta LC, Morykwas MJ. Vacuum-assisted closure: a new method for wound closure and treatment: clinical experience. *Ann Plast Surg*. 1997;38:563-576.
240. Morykwas MJ, Argenta LC, Shelton-Brown EI, et al. Vacuum-assisted closure: a new method for wound control and treatment: animal studies and basic foundation. *Ann Plast Surg*. 1997;38:553-562.
241. MullnerT, Mrkonjic L, Kwasny O, et al. The use of negative pressure to promote the healing of tissue defects: a clinical trial using the vacuum sealing technique. *Br J Plast Surg*. 1997;50:194-199.
242. Garner GB, Ware DN, Cocanour CS, et al. Vacuum-assisted wound closure provides early fascial reapproximation in trauma patients with open abdomens. *Am J Surg*. 2001;182:630-638.
243. Vertrees A, Greer L, Pickett C, et al. Modern management of complex open abdominal wounds of war: a 5-year experience. *J Am Coll Surg*. 2008;207:801-809.
244. Mayberry JC, Mullins RJ, Crass RA, et al. Prevention of abdominal compartment syndrome by absorbable mesh prosthesis closure. *Arch Surg*. 1997;132:957-962.
245. Oelschlager BK, Boyle EM, Johansen K, et al. Delayed abdominal closure in the management of ruptured abdominal aortic aneurysms. *Am J Surg*. 1997;173:411-415.
246. Rasmussen TE, Hallet JW, Noel AA, et al. Early abdominal closure with mesh reduces multiple organ failure after ruptured abdominal aortic aneurysm repair: guidelines from a 10 year case control study. *J Vasc Surg*. 2002;35:246-253.
247. Jernigan TW, Fabian TC, Croce MA, et al. Staged management of giant abdominal wall defects. *Ann Surg*. 2003;238:349-357.
248. Miller PR, Thompson JT, Faler BJ, et al. Late fascial closure in lieu of ventral hernia: the next step in open abdomen management. *J Trauma*. 2002;53:843-849.
249. Ciresi DL, Cali RF, Senagore AJ. Abdominal closure using non-absorbable mesh after massive resuscitation prevents abdominal compartment syndrome and gastrointestinal fistula. *Am Surg*. 1999;65:720-724.
250. Miller RS, Morris Jr JA, Diaz Jr JJ, et al. Complications after 344 damage control open celiotomies. *J Trauma*. 2005;59:1365-1374.
251. Miller PR, Meredith JW, Johnson JC, et al. Prospective evaluation of vacuum-assisted fascial closure after open abdomen: planned ventral hernia rate is substantially reduced. *Ann Surg*. 2004;239:608-614.
252. Teixeira PG, Salim A, Inaba K, et al. A prospective look at the current state of open abdomens. *Am Surg*. 2008;74:891-897.
253. Garner GB, Ware DN, Cocanour CS, et al. Vacuum-assisted wound closure provides early fascial reapproximation in trauma patients with open abdomens. *Am J Surg*. 2001;182:630-638.
254. Stone PA, Hass SM, Flaherty SK, et al. Vacuum-assisted fascial closure for patients with abdominal trauma. *J Trauma*. 2004;57:1082-1086.
255. Perez D, Wildi S, Demartines N, et al. Prospective evaluation of vacuum-assisted closure in abdominal compartment syndrome and severe abdominal sepsis. *J Am Coll Surg*. 2007;205:586-592.
256. Suliburk JW, Ware DN, Balogh Z, et al. Vacuum-assisted wound closure achieves early fascial closure of open abdomens after severe trauma. *J Trauma*. 2003;55:1155-1160.
257. Wondberg D, Larusson HJ, Metzger U, et al. Treatment of the open abdomen with the commercially available vacuum-assisted closure system in patients with abdominal sepsis: low primary closure rate. *World J Surg*. 2008;32:2724-2729.
258. Cothren CC, Moore EE, Johnson JL, et al. One hundred percent fascial approximation with sequential abdominal closure of the open abdomen. *Am J Surg*. 2006;192:238-242.
259. Bee TK, Croce MA, Magnotti LJ, et al. Temporary abdominal closure techniques: a prospective randomized trial comparing polyglactin 910 mesh and vacuum-assisted closure. *J Trauma*. 2008;65:337-342.
260. Rodriguez ED, Bluebond-Langner R, Silverman RP, et al. Abdominal wall reconstruction following severe loss of domain: The R Adams Cowley Shock Trauma Center algorithm. *Plast Reconstr Surg*. 2007;120: 669-680.
261. Fabian TC, Croce MA, Pritchard FE, et al. Planned ventral hernia: staged management for acute abdominal wall defects. *Ann Surg*. 1994;219:651-653.
262. Ramirex OM, Raus E, Dellen AL. "Components separation" method for closure of abdominal-wall defects: an anatomic and clinical study. *Plast Reconstr Surg*. 1990;86:519-526.
263. Ennis LS, Young JS, Gampper TJ, et al. The 'openbook' variation of component separation for repair of massive midline abdominal wall hernia. *Am Surg*. 2003;69:733-742.
264. Vargo D. Component separation in the management of the difficult abdominal wall. *Am J Surg*. 2004;188:633-637.
265. de Vries Reilingh TS, van Goor H, Rosman C, et al. 'Components separation technique' for the repair of large abdominal wall hernias. *J Am Coll Surg* 2003;196:32-37.
266. Scott BG, Welsh FJ, Pham HQ, et al. Early aggressive closure of the open abdomen. *J Trauma*. 2006;60:17-22.
267. Patton JH Jr, Berry S, Kralovich KA. Use of human acellular dermal matrix in complex and contaminated abdominal wall reconstructions. *Am J Surg*. 2007;193:360-363.
268. Singh MK, Rocca JP, Rochon C, et al. Open abdomen management with human acellular dermal matrix in liver transplant recipients. *Transplant Proc*. 2008; 40: 3541-354.
269. Diaz JJ Jr, Conquest AM, Ferzoco SJ, et al. Multiinstitutional experience using human acellular dermal matrix for ventral hernia repair in a compromised surgical field. *Arch Surg*. 2009;144:209-215.
270. Cheatham ML, Safcsak K, Llerena LE, et al. Long term physical, mental and functional consequences of abdominal decompression. *J Trauma*. 2003;56:237-242.
271. Enderson BL, Reath DB, Meadors J, et al. The tertiary trauma survey: a prospective study of missed injury. *J Trauma*. 1990;30:666-670.
272. Hirshberg A, Wall MJ, Mattox KL. Planned reoperation for trauma: a two year experience with 124 consecutive patients. *J Trauma*. 1994;37:365-369.
273. Morris JA Jr, Eddy VA, Blinman TA, et al. The staged celiotomy for trauma. Issues in unpacking and reconstruction. *Ann Surg*. 1993;217:576-586.
274. Shapiro MB, Jenkins DH, Schwab CW, et al. Damage control: collective review. *J Trauma*. 2000;49:969-978.
275. Martin RR, Byrne M. Postoperative care and complications of damage control surgery. *Surg Clin North Am*. 1997;77:929-942.
276. Nagy KK, Filder JJ, Mahr C, et al. Experience with 3 prosthetic materials in temporary abdominal wall closure. *Am Surg*. 1996;62:331-338.
277. Fischer PE, Fabian TC, Magnotti LJ, et al. A ten-year review of enterocutaneous fistulas after laparotomy for trauma. *J Trauma*. 2009;67:924-928.
278. Erdmann D, Drye C, Heller L, et al. Abdominal wall defect and enterocutaneous fistula treatment with vacuum-assisted closure (V.A.C.) system. *Plast Reconstr Surg*. 2001;108:2066-2068.
279. Subramaniam MH, Liscum KR, Hirshberg A. The floating stoma: a new technique for controlling exposed fistulae in abdominal trauma. *J Trauma*. 2002;53:386-388.
280. Cro C, George KJ, Donnelly J, et al. Vacuum assisted closure system in the management of enterocutaneous fistulae. *Postgrad Med J*. 2002;78:364-365.
281. Goverman J, Yelon JA, Platz JJ, et al. The 'Fistula VAC,' a technique for management of enterocutaneous fistulae arising within the open abdomen: report of 5 cases. *J Trauma*. 2006;60:428-431.
282. Jamshidi R, Schecter WP. Biological dressings for the management of enteric fistulas in the open abdomen. *Arch Surg*. 2007;142:793-796.
283. Al-Khoury G, Kaufman D, Hirshberg A. Improved control of exposed fistula in the open abdomen. *J Am Coll Surg*. 2008;206:397-398.
284. Connolly PT, Teubner A, Lees NP, et al. Outcome of reconstructive surgery for intestinal fistula in the open abdomen. *Ann Surg*. 2008;247:440-444.
285. Christou NV, Barie PS, Dellinger EP, et al. Surgical Infection Society intra-abdominal infection study. Prospective evaluation of management techniques and outcome. *Arch Surg*. 1993;128:193-198.
286. Adkins AL, Robbins J, Villalba M, et al. Open abdomen management of intra-abdominal sepsis. *Am Surg*. 2004;70:137-140.
287. Tsuei BJ, Skinner JC, Bernard AC. The open peritoneal cavity: etiology correlates with the likelihood of fascial closure. *Am Surg*. 2004;70:652-656.

CHAPTER 7 ■ AIRWAY MANAGEMENT

MATTHEW KEITH WHALIN, CARLA IRENE HAACK, TIMOTHY G. BUCHMAN, AND PAUL S. GARCIA

HISTORY, DEFINITIONS, AND BASICS

"There is nothing living that does not breathe, and nothing breathing that does not live."

—*Lectures on the Whole of Anatomy* (Harvey, 1653)

William Harvey's recognition of the importance of ventilation marked a turning point in medical history. Prior generations of practitioners followed the teachings of Galen who opined that the lungs existed to cool the heart. Following Harvey, 18th Century European communities organized "Rescue Societies" to save drowning victims.

As airway structures were increasingly recognized for their specific roles as conduits of gases destined for the alveoli; oral and nasal devices were developed for the specific purpose of resuscitation. These were naturally adapted to stabilize airways for use with first-generation inhalational anesthetics such as chloroform. Periodically, airway emergencies would occur. Tracheostomy, which had fallen into disrepute during the middle ages, reappeared as an essential tool for anesthesiologists when performed by John Snow (who famously delivered chloroform as an obstetrical anesthetic to Queen Victoria) to save a patient's life. As anesthesia itself disseminated through surgical practice, so did the need for surgical airway skills.

Fortunately, technology has made the need for emergent surgical airways rare. Airway management progressed from natural airways and "blind" techniques, through direct visualization, and is now facilitated by video tools including videolaryngoscopy and fiberoptic laryngobronchoscopy. As emergent surgical airways are performed less frequently, some of those skills have been lost, yet operative teams (surgeons and anesthesiologists) must find common strategies to ensure that the procedure can be performed safely when needed. The need is invariably urgent or emergent. Thus, consideration of alternative airway strategies (Plan A, Plan B..., surgical airway) is an essential part of every airway plan.

IS AN ARTIFICIAL AIRWAY NECESSARY?

Before selecting a strategy for securing an artificial airway in an acute care situation, practitioners must first ask themselves whether airway manipulation is necessary. Adequate surgical anesthesia can often be accomplished by either peripheral nerve blockade or neuraxial (spinal/epidural) techniques, especially where limb or pelvic surgery is required. While these skills require advanced training and in some cases specialized equipment not immediately available in all situations, infiltrative local anesthesia should also always be considered as an option for the procedurally trained acute care physician, as it has been used successfully in several trauma situations including cesarean section,[1] craniotomy for epidural hematoma,[2] and facial injury after motor vehicle accidents that include zygomatic arch fractures and multiple lacerations.[3] Irrespective of the situation, training in airway management is crucial for every acute care physician, because unexpected events are frequent occurrences[4] and preparedness is a high priority.

Herein, we define a "secured airway device" to be a patent conduit for gas exchange that is unlikely to fail through conventional manipulation of a patient's body position encountered during a perioperative period (including transport to/from stretchers, ICU beds, and operating room tables). A "definitive airway device" is defined as a patent conduit for gas exchange that involves the trachea and a specialized plastic connection, which universally fits most ventilators and manual ventilation equipment. Current advanced cardiac life support (ACLS) guidelines use a slightly broader term (the "advanced airway device") to describe tubular conduits that facilitate ventilation.[5] By this definition, some advanced airway devices require advanced skill and training (endotracheal tubes), while others require minimal skill and training (such as the supraglottic airways [see laryngeal mask airways (LMAs) and Combi-tubes below]). In most acute care situations, a definitive airway such as an oral endotracheal tube is preferred over the supraglottic advanced airway devices. However, certain scenarios necessitate the use of an LMA or Combi-tube (or even mask) on a temporary basis.

After placement, the position and patency of all airway devices must be confirmed as soon as possible by either direct means (visualization of conduit in trachea) or indirect means (e.g., end-tidal CO_2, blood gas results, or chest x-ray). The "gold standard" for accepting any airway device as functional is end-tidal CO_2 monitoring as it provides nearly instant physiologic confirmation of cardiac output and successful gas exchange. Because a secured airway device known to exist in the trachea is a definitive airway device and a definitive airway device becomes secured with either strong adhesive tape or through the use of a mechanical strap holder, these two terms will often be used interchangeably in clinical settings. Moreover, in clinical practice of acute care surgery, the word "device" is often omitted, as in "the patient's airway was secured."

To avoid confusion with specific anatomical structures, also referred to as airways, this shortening will be avoided. For this chapter, we will assume all secured airway devices are confirmed and all definitive airway devices are confirmed and subsequently secured unless explicitly noted.

COMMON DEVICES AND TIMING OF PLACEMENT

The three most common definitive airway devices in acute surgical care patients are the oral endotracheal tube (oral ETT), the nasal ETT, and the tracheostomy tube.[6] Besides specialized semipermanent tracheostomy tubes, these devices all contain an inflatable bulb designed as a barrier to prevent the entry of stomach contents or copious oral secretions into the conducting airways (see aspiration below). The choice of device will depend on several factors such as procedure site, ease of placement, and hemodynamic stability of the patient. In most patients, the oral ETT is the most efficient way to establish a definitive airway (see below for difficult airway considerations and intubation techniques). Because placement of an oral ETT is facilitated with neck extension (and in some instances flexion), precautions must be taken in patients with known or suspected cervical instability. Basal skull fractures are an absolute contraindication to nasal ETTs. Tracheostomy or needle cricothyrotomy as a bridge to tracheostomy (see end of Chapter) constitutes the default backup plan for any acutely ill patient in whom a definitive airway device cannot be established by other means. Although the oral ETTs are the most common airways in these patients, a tracheostomy is an acceptable (and sometimes desirable) plan "A" in patients with a suspected or known difficult airway who are likely to require mechanical ventilation for extended periods of time.

Protection of the airway is often used as a justification of the establishment of a definitive airway. Common wisdom holds that as a patient progresses through depressed levels of consciousness, the airway reflexes attenuate and the inability to cough and swallow secretions may lead to an increased risk of aspiration of stomach contents. It is prudent to consider the use of a definitive airway device in a patient whose Glasgow Coma Scale (GCS) is deteriorating. Many clinicians regard descent through a GCS of 9 as an indication to establish a definitive airway device, although the patient's history and baseline mental status must also be considered. While generally accepted as an indication for endotracheal intubation, a GCS of <9 is not necessarily a contraindication to extubation.

Aspiration has traditionally been associated with poor outcomes in trauma patients.[7,8] High morbidity and mortality is associated with the development of chemical pneumonitis or aspiration pneumonia. Prevention of aspiration is therefore a goal of airway protection. It is prudent to delay elective surgery until a patient has fasted for 8 hours or more, to allow time for gastric emptying. Some controversy surrounds the specific time interval. In 2011, the American Society of Anesthesiologists (ASA) revised their published guidelines to include special considerations for otherwise healthy patients not at increased risk for delayed gastric emptying. For these patients, the recommended minimum fasting period for clear liquids is 2 hours, and 6 hours for nonhuman milk and for light meals not containing fried or fatty food.[9] Regardless, major trauma can slow gastric emptying (as can diabetes and hiatal hernias) and, if possible, prophylactic treatment with antacids, H2-blockers, and agents that speed gastric motility are recommended as long as their administration does not impede more urgent treatments.

Other risks and complications associated with intubation are both less common and less severe than the failure either to mask ventilate or to establish a secure airway. Tooth, gum, and lip damage can occur with any oral manipulation. Nasal ETTs are traumatic to the nasal mucosa. Bleeding can be minimized with a topical vasoconstrictor, such as phenylephrine. The posterior pharynx can be inadvertently penetrated.[10] Such penetration is a major concern in patient who had previously received radiation treatment to the head, neck, or face.

MASK VENTILATION

Mask ventilation is the most fundamental and essential skill of airway management, yet it is undervalued from educational and clinical perspectives. Whether a patient requires sedation for a minor procedure or is facing pending respiratory failure, evaluation for potentially difficult mask ventilation should occur in tandem with evaluation for potential difficult intubation (see Tables 7.1 and 7.2). It is easy for mask ventilation to become an afterthought in the acute care setting since most patients in trauma surgery are generally intubated without masking to minimize aspiration risk (see section on Rapid Sequence Induction). When intubation fails in a patient who is easy to mask ventilate, there is time to call for help, retrieve additional equipment, or prepare for a surgical airway. In contrast, failed intubation of a patient who is difficult or impossible to mask ventilate can rapidly become a fatal situation. Thus, even in the setting of emergency surgery where time is of the essence, identification of the patient who is a potentially difficult to mask ventilate should prompt a discussion between the surgeons and anesthesiologists about contingency plans for failed intubation.

It is critical to rapidly assess the adequacy of mask ventilation and make adjustments (or abandon attempts at masking) in a timely fashion. As discussed in a recent review,[11] adequacy can be difficult to define. What is considered safe in the operating room may be of questionable security in the trauma helicopter or hospital elevator. The modern anesthesia machine in most operating rooms not only provides inhaled anesthesia but is well-equipped with several monitors capable of assessing adequacy of ventilation. The flexible bag connected to the anesthesia machine will deflate and inflate with the spontaneous ventilation of a patient as long as the mask is well-placed

TABLE 7.1

SUMMARY OF POOLED SENSITIVITY AND SPECIFICITY OF COMMONLY USED METHODS OF AIRWAY EVALUATION

EXAMINATION	SENSITIVITY (%)	SPECIFICITY (%)
Mallampati classification	49	86
Thyromental distance	20	94
Sternomental distance	62	82
Mouth opening	46	89

Data derived from Wilson ME, Spiegelhalter D, Robertson J, et al. Predicting difficult intubation. *Br J Anaesth*. 1988;61:211.

TABLE 7.2

ASSESSMENT AND PREDICTABILITY OF DIFFICULT MASK VENTILATION

CRITERIA FOR DIFFICULT MASK VENTILATION	
Inability for one anesthesiologist to maintain oxygen saturation >92%	
Irreparable gas leak around face mask	
Need for ≥4 L/min gas flow (or use of fresh gas flow button more than twice)	
No chest movement	
Two-handed mask ventilation needed	
Change of operator required	
INDEPENDENT RISK FACTORS FOR DIFFICULT MASK VENTILLATION	
PATIENT FEATURE	**ODDS RATIO**
Presence of a beard	3.18
Body mass index >26 ng/m^2	2.75
Lack of teeth	2.28
Age > 55 y	2.26
History of snoring	1.84

From Langeron O, Masso E, Huraux C, et al. Prediction of difficult mask ventilation. *Anesthesiology*. 2000;92:1229.

("sealed") to the face. It is important to recognize that the bag for manual ventilation in the operating room performs differently from the more familiar self-inflating (Ambu TM) bag. During manual ventilation in the apneic patient, the bag in the operating room will fail to reinflate with leakage of air, and often this is a clue that the mask may need to be readjusted (see C-E technique below). The digital readout of the exhaled tidal volume can also be used to confirm delivery of manually or machine-delivered ventilated breaths. Most importantly, a persistent end-tidal CO_2 ($etCO_2$) waveform on the capnograph signals gas exchange. With most sampling systems, $etCO_2$ will only appear after several breaths. Importantly, the appearance of $etCO_2$ verifies both ventilation and perfusion. This makes $etCO_2$ monitoring an especially important tool.

Outside of the operating room, it can be challenging to assess the adequacy of mask ventilation. Bag movement is unreliable as most emergency carts are stocked with self-inflating bags. Physical examination should reveal chest rise and breath sounds with spontaneous or manual ventilation. Although less reliable than $etCO_2$, the observation of condensation in the mask is a good sign that gas exchange is taking place. Similarly, maintenance or improvement in oxygen saturation (as measured by arterial blood gas or pulse oximetry) is another indirect method that provides confidence in one's ventilation technique. However, $etCO_2$ is quickly being recognized as the gold standard monitor of ventilation. The ASA's 2010 monitoring guidelines recommend $etCO_2$ monitoring for deep sedation and the 2010 ACLS guidelines encourage its use in CPR.[5] These guidelines may translate to increased availability of these monitors outside the operating room. Local administrators and their clinical leaders should include $etCO_2$ monitoring capability as they evaluate purchasing of new equipment.

Problems with mask ventilation can generally be classified into one of two categories: (1) difficulty creating an adequate seal or (2) obstruction to airflow. Examples of the former include patients with thick beards, edentulous patients, and patients with severe facial trauma. Obstruction to airflow may occur anywhere along the airway, from bronchoconstriction or masses within the lungs to larygnospasm to collapse of the upper airway in a patient with obstructive sleep apnea. Even in the absence of sleep apnea, morbid obesity can lead to enough extrathoracic pressure to impede mask ventilation. Chest compressions performed as part of cardiopulmonary resuscitation can divert mask ventilation breaths from the lungs to the stomach, and for this reason, current (as of 2010) ACLS guidelines mandate that cycles of 30 compressions followed by two quick breaths be continued until an advanced airway is in place.[5] Subtle improvements in the technique of mask ventilation as well as airway adjuncts can alleviate many cases of difficult mask ventilation.

In traditional one-handed masking, the practitioner's left hand is responsible not only for creating an adequate seal, but also for minimizing upper airway obstruction by providing jaw thrust. The left thumb and index finger form a "C" and apply the mask to the face, taking care not to compress the bridge of the nose or interfere with the eyes. The remaining three fingers are spread along the mandible to form an "E," with the fifth digit behind the angle of the jaw to maximize vertical thrust. Novices and trainees need to be constantly reminded to "lift the face to the mask" rather than pressing the mask on the face. It is also important to remember that the jaw thrust is very uncomfortable and should not be performed on conscious patients whose airway muscular tone is adequate to prevent their tongue from obstructing their airway.

At the first sign of difficulty with one-handed masking, two adjustment techniques are available to the lone practitioner. One is to use both hands to readjust the mask seal and provide maximal jaw thrust, as sometimes it is easier to maintain a strong jaw thrust with one hand than it is to create one with a single hand. Having optimized the seal and jaw thrust, the right hand goes back to squeezing the bag. The second technique is placement of airway adjuncts (orally or nasally), often followed by the two-handed readjustment described above.

Airway Adjuncts

Placement of an oral airway is often facilitated by using a wooden tongue depressor. Without a depressor, the oral airway should initially be inserted with the curve pointing away from the tongue, and then rotated to follow the curve of the tongue as the tip reaches the posterior pharynx. Either way, care must be taken to bring the tongue forward to open the airway, but not so far that it rests between the lower teeth and the oral airway (which could lead to laceration). It is important to select a size appropriate to the patient, though a size 10 (100 mm) oral airway is adequate for most adults. A properly placed oral airway is typically very effective at facilitating mask ventilation, but this adjunct should only be placed in patients with depressed levels of consciousness, as it sits at the base of the tongue and can be uncomfortable and stimulate a gag reflex.

Nasopharyngeal airways ("nasal trumpets") are better tolerated in awake patients, though they should be avoided in patients with known or suspected skull base fractures. The nasal airway should be long enough to extend past soft tissue obstruction but not so long as it contacts the base of the tongue as the trumpet could be occluded by a large tongue or stimulate a gag reflex. Usually, size 30-34 is appropriate for adults, but it is prudent to check the fit by holding it against the side of the face to see if it extends from the nare to the angle of the mandible using its natural curve.

When repositioning and airway adjuncts do not allow adequate one-handed masking, you should progress to two-handed masking or alternative approaches to airway management. Even experienced anesthesia providers using oral airways in routine cases deliver larger tidal volumes with two-handed masking, and a two-handed technique should be used as soon as practicable.[12] Most acute care situations involve either a self-inflating mask bag or an anesthesia machine, which necessitates the aid of a second provider to squeeze the bag. There are several approaches to two-handed masking, but one common method is to apply a seal with both thumbs and use the remaining fingers to maximize jaw thrust. In some situations, a third person is needed to depress the mask at an area of leak.

It is important to remember that the total volume of most adult-sized bags is 2 L and adverse effects of delivering the entire volume in some situations can occur. In patients with a full stomach, every attempt should be made to avoid delivering high volumes and pressures to prevent emesis from stomach distention. It is estimated that delivering pressures of over 20 cm H_2O can open the lower esophageal sphincter in patients with normal esophageal anatomy. Normal tidal volumes vary between 4 and 8 mL per kg of ideal body weight. Positive-end expiratory pressure (PEEP), most commonly accomplished through the use of a specialized valve, is a preferred method for maintaining recruitment of end alveoli during manual ventilation as opposed to delivering large tidal volumes. The respiratory rate must allow for an appropriate time of exhalation, especially in patients with chronic obstructive pulmonary disease who may be more prone to "breath-stacking" or auto-PEEP.

In an emergency situation, it is time-consuming and dangerous to progress through each of these modifications in a stepwise fashion. For these cases, it is prudent to immediately place a nasal or oral airway adjunct. Outside of the operating room where patient positioning may be suboptimal and monitors of the adequacy of ventilation are less accessible, it is appropriate to begin with two-handed masking if enough help is available. In situations of cardiac arrest, the acute care surgeon is often supervising resuscitation efforts and should be sure that ventilation is being optimized with oral airways and two-handed masking. As part of the quality improvement program at our level 1 trauma hospital, we found that these techniques were being used in only 25% of cardiac arrests in a 6-month sample set (manuscript in progress). Finally, it is important to remember that adequate mask ventilation should not be considered a long-term solution for most acute care situations as blood in the airway, facial edema and fluid shifts, or provider fatigue can quickly turn adequate mask ventilation into an airway emergency.

ENDOTRACHEAL INTUBATION

Direct Laryngoscopy: Evaluation and Performance

Should a patient require an advanced airway, whether for elective surgery or respiratory failure, an endotracheal tube is often the first choice. As with all aspects of airway management, planning and preparation are paramount even in critical situations. After taking the patient history and clinical situation into account, the next step in the process is evaluation of the airway.

Despite ongoing attempts to apply evidence-based medicine to the prediction of difficult intubations, existing tests suffer from low specificity.[13] We favor an airway evaluation that can be completed quickly and without complicated anatomical measurements or calculations. Bedside measurements in finger breadths are common. Every practitioner should be aware of exactly how many centimeters are spanned with two and with three finger breadths of his/her hand. Potentially difficult intubations are suggested by limited mouth opening, limited neck extension, limited ability to prognath the jaw, immobility of anterior neck tissues (e.g., radiation changes), and a short thyromental distance (<5 cm). The Mallampati classification (Fig. 7.1) refers to the view obtained by asking a patient sitting upright to open his mouth maximally and protrude his tongue. A view of the tonsillar pillars constitutes class I, view of part but not the entire uvula is class II, soft palate only is class III, and hard palate only is class IV. Identification of a class III or IV view raises concern for potentially difficult intubation. The test is properly performed without the patient phonating, but if a poor view does not improve with phonation, it is particularly worrisome. Practitioners must be aware that serial attempts at laryngoscopy lead to trauma, bleeding, and edema, all of which conspire to make the next attempt more difficult: every effort should be made to optimize conditions for the first attempt.

Preoxygenation is one of the cornerstones of preparation for intubation. It prolongs the time between apnea and desaturation not only by maximizing oxygen saturation of

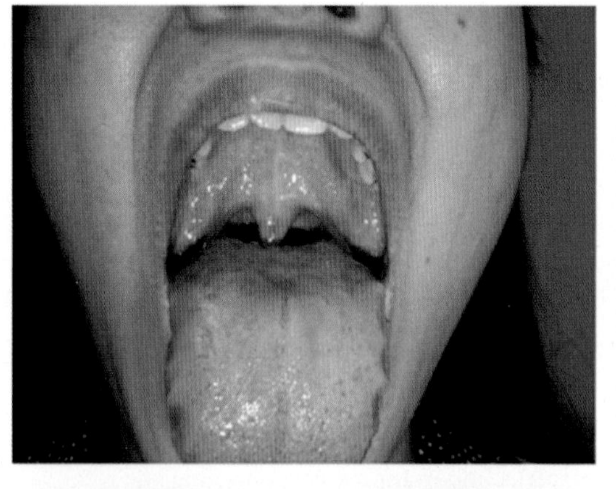

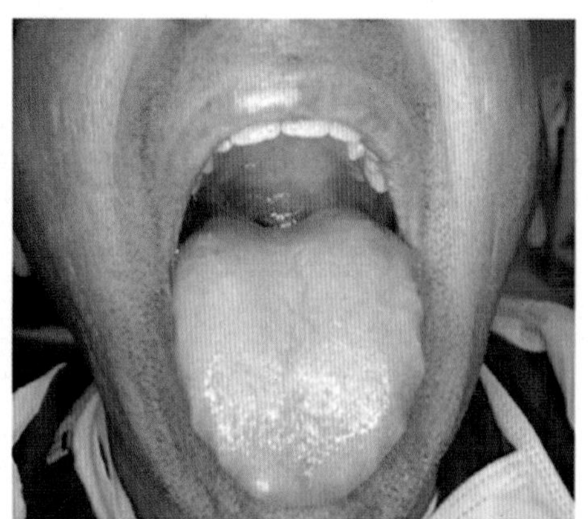

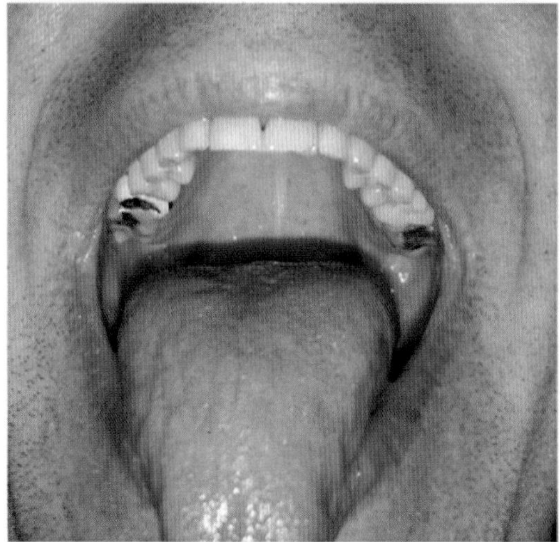

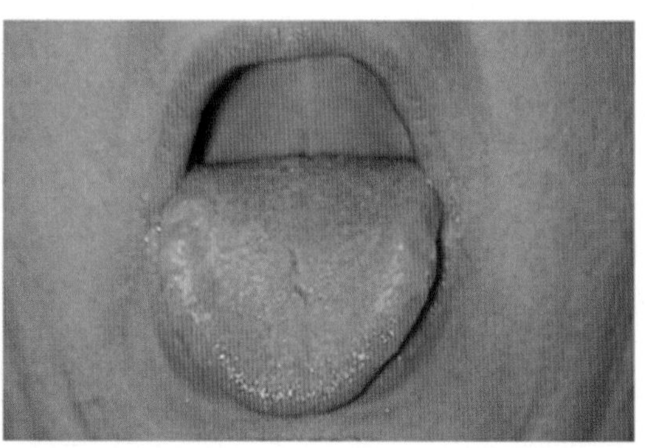

FIGURE 7.1. Photographic examples of Mallampati class. **A-D:** Mallampati I-IV. (From Barash PG, Cullen BF, Stoelting RK, et al. *Clinical Anesthesia*. 6th ed. Philadelphia, PA: Lippincott Williams & Wilkins, 2009.)

hemoglobin, but also by replacing the nitrogen in the patient's functional residual capacity with oxygen. One convenient endpoint to preoxygenation is delivery of oxygen to the spontaneously breathing patient until the measured expired oxygen concentration equals or exceeds 90%. Many critically ill patients will never reach this goal and outside of the operating room there is rarely access to a gas analyzer, so one must remain flexible in this regard. Even after a prolonged period of preoxygenation, patients who are obese or who have limited physiologic reserve can desaturate within seconds of becoming apneic. It is therefore essential to have all necessary equipment assembled, organized, and within easy reach. No matter what the setting, patient positioning often sets the stage for success or failure.

One aspect of positioning involves ergonomics. To facilitate visualization of the airway structures without leaning or bending, the patient should be moved up to the end of the bed and the height set so that his or her head comes to the level of the xiphoid process of the laryngoscopist. In emergent situations, it is sometimes necessary to intubate patients on the ground or in a lateral or prone position, but this increases the difficulty significantly. Another aspect of positioning involves the creation of a direct line of sight from the patient's mouth to his vocal cords. For patients with a normal body habitus, slight elevation of the head on a folded sheet and extension of the neck into a "sniffing position" can facilitate direct laryngoscopy. An obese patient should have her upper body on an incline sufficient to keep the angle of her jaw higher than her sternal notch (Fig. 7.2). When viewed from the side, the patient's upper body appears to be on a "ramp".

With the patient optimally positioned and preoxygenated, equipment should be arranged within easy reach. This equipment should include a rigid suction device, endotracheal tubes of the appropriate sizes, and working laryngoscopes. The suction device (typically a curved plastic "Yankauer" suction tip) is essential to clear debris or secretions obstructing view of the cords and to quickly remove emesis should it occur. The laryngoscope light source should be bright enough to create a spotlight on an object 5 or more centimeters from the tip. Laryngoscopes are designed to be held in the left hand. Laryngoscope blades come in two basic styles: straight and curved.

The most common straight blade is the Miller blade, first introduced in 1941. The tip of the blade is used to lift the epiglottis to develop a straight line of sight to the vocal cords. Its use requires great control since small movements can cause the epiglottis to slide off the end of the blade. It is also challenging to maintain a view while inserting the tube and it is sometimes useful to have an assistant pull on the right corner of the patient's mouth to create more space. Although straight blades are extremely effective in experienced hands, curved blades might be considered easier to master.

Robert Macintosh introduced a laryngoscope with a curved blade in 1943 and it remains widely used today. The flange facilitates displacement of the tongue to the left side of the mouth. The tip of the blade is placed in the vallecula and the laryngoscopist applies caudad and ventral force to develop a view of the vocal cords. With both the straight and curved blades, any rocking motion of the wrist will result in dental trauma. Such rocking motion is to be avoided, but a number of other techniques can often improve a poor view.

To create a direct line of vision to the vocal cords, it is sometimes necessary to lift the patients head off the bed and further extend the neck. The right hand can lift the head to develop the view and that position is maintained by the left hand while grasping the endotracheal tube in your right hand. Another useful technique is bimanual laryngoscopy, in which the laryngoscopist's right hand applies pressure at the cricoid cartilage dorsally, laterally, and longitudinally to bring the cords into view. An assistant can then be instructed to substitute his hand in order to keep the larynx in the identical position while the laryngoscopist places the endotracheal tube.

Even with these maneuvers, it is sometimes only possible to see the arytenoid cartilage. An experienced laryngoscopist will often use an endotracheal tube that has a stylet, which maintains the tube configured with an anterior curve in order to intubate the trachea semiblind. In these situations, or when only the epiglottis is visible, an endotracheal tube introducer (e.g., bougie or Eschmann catheter) may be helpful. Introducers are plastic tubes with some shape memory and a bend

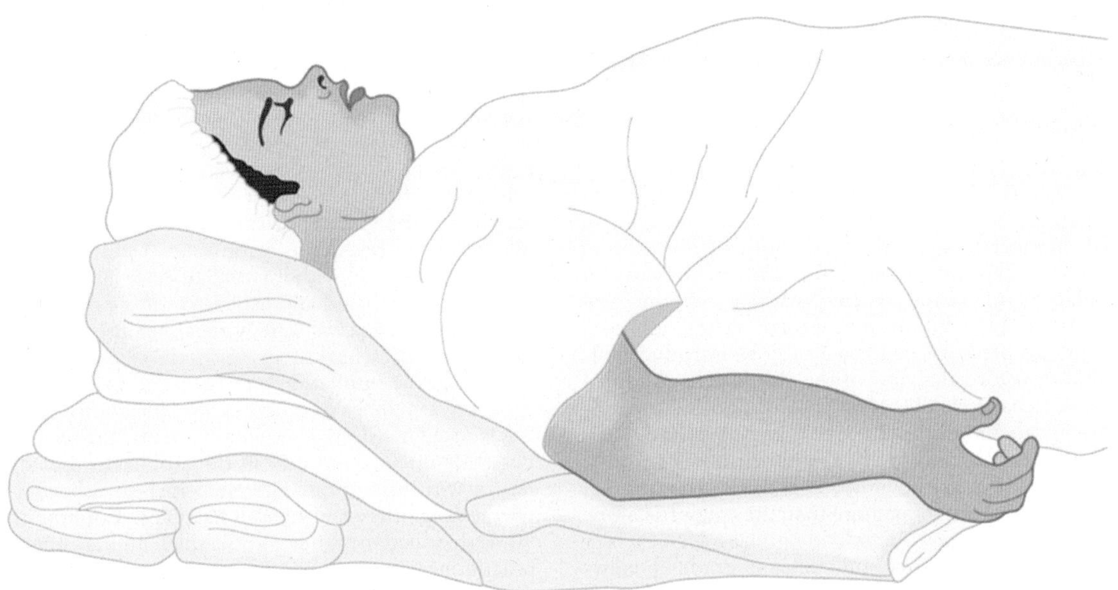

FIGURE 7.2. Achieving proper positioning of the obese patient for airway manipulation. (From Barash PG, Cullen BF, Stoelting RK, et al. *Clinical Anesthesia*, 6th ed. Philadelphia, PA: Lippincott Williams & Wilkins, 2009.)

2-3 cm from the tip. The tip is directed under the epiglottis and advanced gently until tactile resistance from the tracheal rings is felt. An endotracheal tube is then advanced over the introducer akin to the Seldinger technique for vascular cannulation. This technique is less straightforward than it seems; the endotracheal tube may be unable to move past the curve of the posterior pharynx or at the level of the epiglottis and may require additional manipulation (i.e., twisting) to move the tube into the trachea.

Following placement of an endotracheal tube, the operator is responsible for immediately seeking verification of proper placement. While condensation in the tube and chest movements with manual ventilation are reassuring signs of endotracheal placement, one must also auscultate the axillae for bilateral and symmetric breath sounds as well as verifying the absence of sounds over the stomach. Most importantly, there should be persistent exhaled CO_2 as assayed by a capnograph or a disposable color change device (but again recall that in a cardiac arrest there may be insufficient blood flow to carry CO_2 to the lungs). Advancement of the endotracheal tube too deep will result in an endobronchial intubation (typically in the right main stem). Some of the signs of endobronchial intubation are mimicked by many other conditions in the acutely ill: asymmetric breath sounds and low pulse oximetry. Hemodynamic instability can also be a sign of endobronchial intubation if the delivered tidal volume results in large enough intrathoracic pressures to periodically impede venous return through compression of the vena cava and right atrium. Endobronchial intubation should be suspected when increased peak airway pressures are noted (either quantitatively by digital monitor or qualitatively by difficult manual ventilation by bag).

Whenever the endotracheal tube location is in doubt, either immediate visualization with a fiberoptic broncoscope or else a chest x-ray should be used to confirm proper position. Besides the possibility of pneumothorax from high intrathoracic pressures, the consequences of an endobronchial intubation might be mild in comparison to the patient's overall acute health status and as long as ventilation is possible (even if suboptimal), the diagnosis of endobronchial intubation should not delay surgical intervention in the most acutely ill patient. However, we recommend confirmation of proper airway placement of endotracheal tubes (through end-tidal CO_2 monitoring) in most cases before proceeding with invasive procedures or surgery. It is also important to secure the endotracheal tube with tape or a specialized device to avoid airway disasters after a procedure has begun.

The Importance of Documentation

After intubation, it is important to document the type of blade used, number of attempts, and depth of the tube in an airway note. The note should comment on the ease of mask ventilation (one hand vs. two, with or without oral airway) and should mention any special techniques used (ramping, cricoid pressure, endotracheal tube introducer). It is also useful to record the view of the glottis. The modified Cormack and Lehane classification categorizes views as follows: entire vocal cords is grade 1, partial view of the cords is grade 2a, arytenoids only is 2b, epiglottis only is grade 3, and neither the glottis nor epiglottis is grade 4. The original system called grade 2 anything more than the epiglottis alone but less than the full cords. Subdividing class 2 gives very useful information since in one study 65% of grade 2b views were deemed difficult intubations versus only 13% of grade 2a views.[14]

If there is time, locating prior airway notes should be part of the airway evaluation. A history of difficult intubation should prompt special preparation for alternative techniques. Even a patient who was easy to intubate last year or last week may now be difficult due to weight gain, surgery, radiation treatment, or the development of edema, bleeding, or masses in the airway. If the overall evaluation of the airway suggests a potentially difficult mask or intubation, a clear plan with alternative strategies should be formulated in advance (see ASA Difficult Airway Algorithm, Algorithm 7.1, from American Society of Anesthesiologists).[15]

Alternatives to Direct Laryngoscopy

Endotracheal intubation can be achieved by a number of methods other than direct laryngoscopy. One such method is the use of a video laryngoscope such as the Glidescope or Pentax AWS. These systems have a miniature camera incorporated into the laryngoscope blade and connected to a viewing monitor. This allows the operator (and other team members) to "see around the corner" and can produce excellent views of the glottis when immobility of the neck, a large tongue, or a short thyromental distance would make a direct view nearly impossible. Nevertheless, this excellent view does not always translate into an easy intubation. Just as a direct line of sight allows a direct path for the endotracheal tube, so an indirect view implies a circuitous path for the tube to travel. A stylet is almost mandatory, and some systems come with specialized stylets to match the curve of the blade.

Another technique for indirect visualization of the glottis is fiberoptic bronchoscopy. Fiberoptic intubation was pioneered in the 1970s by Dr Andranik Ovassapian and remains the gold standard approach for a difficult airway. There are numerous variations on the technique, which are beyond the scope of this chapter. It allows placement of either nasal or oral endotracheal tubes in patients who are either apneic or spontaneously ventilating.

While fiberoptic intubation may be the gold standard in predicted difficult airways in elective surgery, only the most experienced providers should attempt this in the acute situation, and if unsuccessful, in an agreed upon time by the leaders of the surgical and anesthesia team, a surgical airway should be considered. In situations where visualization is not possible or emergencies in which specialized airway devices are not readily available, a retrograde wire technique may be used to facilitate endotracheal intubation. The method requires an 18-gauge angiocatheter connected to a syringe half-full with saline or lidocaine as well as a wire at least 70 cm long. With the angle of the angiocatheter directed cephalad, the cricothyroid membrane is entered slowly while continuously aspirating on the syringe. Entrance to the trachea is signaled by aspiration of air bubbles, at which point the syringe is held steady and the catheter advanced to its hub. After withdrawing the needle, position is reconfirmed by attaching the syringe to the catheter and withdrawing air once again. Then the wire is advanced cephalad and fished out of the mouth (or perhaps the nose) with forceps. The wire is then used to guide an oral or nasal endotracheal tube.

Retrograde intubation can be useful in an emergency but there are a number of potential complications. If the catheter is advanced too deep, it can inadvertently proceed through the posterior trachea and into in the esophagus and still give air return with aspiration. The endotracheal tube can get stuck on the epiglottis or arytenoid cartilage. Rotating the tube in 90-degree increments can sometimes address this, but some practitioners use a second wire to elevate the epiglottis.

The initial steps of placing an 18-gauge angiocatheter into the tracheal lumen are the same for needle cricothyrotomy as they are for retrograde intubation. By administering short bursts of high-flow oxygen through the angiocatheter

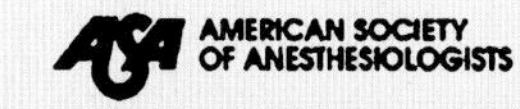

DIFFICULT AIRWAY ALGORITHM

1. Assess the likelihood and clinical impact of basic management problems:
   A. Difficult Ventilation
   B. Difficult Intubation
   C. Difficulty with Patient Cooperation or Consent
   D. Difficult Tracheostomy
2. Actively pursue opportunities to deliver supplemental oxygen throughout the process of difficult airway management
3. Consider the relative merits and feasibility of basic management choices:

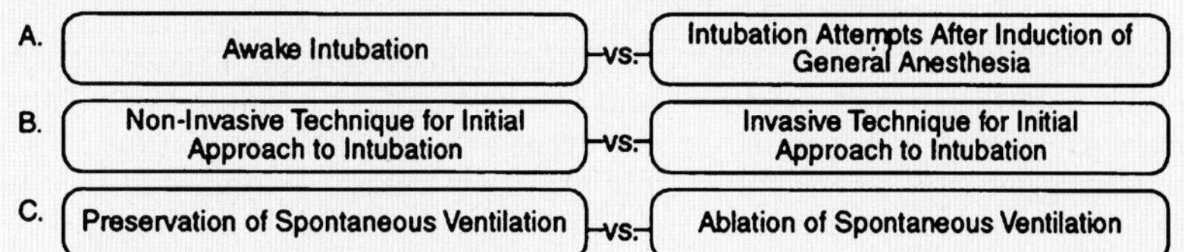

4. Develop primary and alternative strategies:

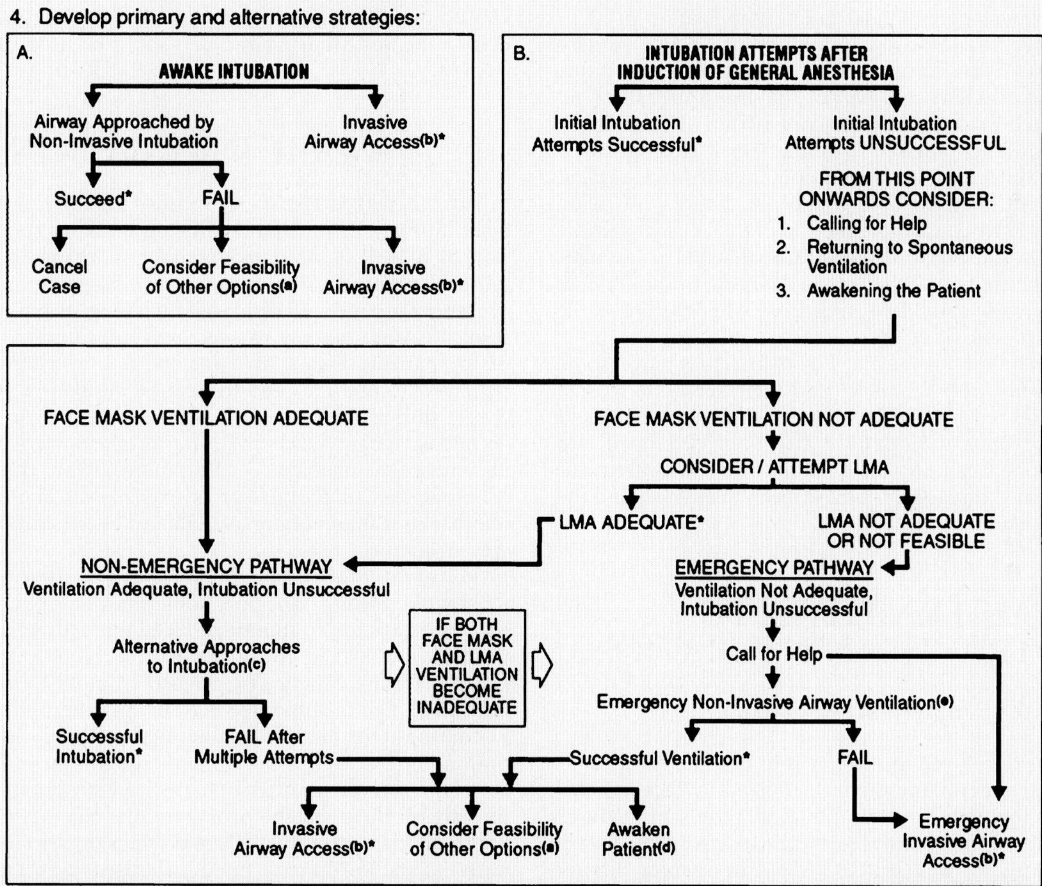

*** Confirm ventilation, tracheal intubation, or LMA placement with exhaled CO_2**

a. Other options include (but are not limited to): surgery utilizing face mask or LMA anesthesia, local anesthesia infiltration or regional nerve blockade. Pursuit of these options usually implies that mask ventilation will not be problematic. Therefore, these options may be of limited value if this step in the algorithm has been reached via the Emergency Pathway.

b. Invasive airway access includes surgical or percutaneous tracheostomy or cricothyrotomy.

c. Alternative non-invasive approaches to difficult intubation include (but are not limited to): use of different laryngoscope blades, LMA as an intubation conduit (with or without fiberoptic guidance), fiberoptic intubation, intubating stylet or tube changer, light wand, retrograde intubation, and blind oral or nasal intubation.

d. Consider re-preparation of the patient for awake intubation or canceling surgery.

e. Options for emergency non-invasive airway ventilation include (but are not limited to): rigid bronchoscope, esophageal-tracheal combitube ventilation, or transtracheal jet ventilation.

ALGORITHM 7.1

ALGORITHM 7.1 ASA difficult airway algorithm. (Adapted from practice guidelines for management of the difficult airway: an updated report by the american society of anesthesiologists task force on management of the difficult airway. *Anesthesiology*. 2003;98(5):1269-1277.)

into the conducting airways, oxygenation of the patient can be accomplished on an emergency basis. This procedure should only be viewed as a temporary measure until someone with experience in either retrograde intubation or more invasive techniques (see below) can provide definitive airway management. During delivery of high-flow oxygen via catheter, appropriate time must be given to allow for the egress of air from the lungs, or barotrauma will occur. For most surgeons, a cricothyroidotomy would be just as fast as and more reliable than retrograde intubation or needle cricothyrotomy.

CERVICAL SPINE PRECAUTIONS

Victims of blunt force or penetrating trauma may have acute surgical issues that take priority over known or suspected injury to the cervical spine. The management of airways in patients with possible neck injury that involves the cervical spine deserves special consideration. It is customary to have a second provider apply manual in-line stabilization prior to and throughout laryngoscopy. In a study of elective surgery patients, 55% of the in-line stabilization group had grade 3 or 4 vocal cord views and half of the group overall could not be intubated by direct laryngoscopy within 30 seconds by experienced anesthesiologists.[16] Another small study showed that in-line stabilization leads to a doubling of force applied by a Macintosh laryngoscope, which the authors postulate could paradoxically cause more motion of the cervical spine.[17] A number of studies have demonstrated that video laryngoscopes allow intubation with decreased motion of the cervical spine, and their use should be considered whenever available (reviewed in Dupanovic et al.[18]).

A blind technique called the Lightwand may have some utility in patients who cannot extend their neck due to suspected or confirmed cervical neck fractures. Custom semirigid camera or fiberoptic devices have also been developed and many practitioners can become quite proficient with frequent use, but a detailed discussion of these techniques is beyond the scope of this chapter.

ALTERNATIVES TO ENDOTRACHEAL INTUBATION

Laryngeal Mask Airway

The LMA was developed in the 1980s to provide an alternative to inhaled general anesthetics delivered by face mask.[19] In patients at low risk for aspiration undergoing procedures which do not require paralysis, the LMA provides a very effective airway. A well-seated LMA can sustain airway pressures up to 20 cm of water without an air leak. Many practitioners feel that they are best suited for cases in which the patient is spontaneously breathing, but LMAs have been successfully used with neuromuscular blockade.[20] The latest generation of devices (e.g., LMA ProSeal) claims a 30 cm of water seal and integrated channels for gastric venting and drainage. Although there are a few limited reports of this new device being used in nonacute laparotomies,[21] there is not enough evidence to support its routine use in acute trauma situations, and we recommend any supraglottic airway device only as a temporizing measure toward definitive airway management.

Although acute settings predispose to aspiration, the LMA has an important role in emergency airway management. As described in the ASA difficult airway practice guideline,[15] if initial intubation attempts fail and mask ventilation is not adequate, then successful placement of a LMA allows the luxury of time and pursuit of "nonemergency" strategies. For example, the LMA can act as a conduit for fiberoptic intubation via an exchange catheter. According to the 2010 ACLS guidelines,[5] an LMA constitutes as an advanced airway and therefore allows continuous chest compressions instead of cycles of CPR interrupted by ventilation.

Esophageal–Tracheal Combination Tubes

Although seldom placed in the hospital, airways such as the Combi-tube TM and laryngeal tube are mainstays of prehospital airway management. These devices are inserted blindly and have two cuffs: one supraglottic cuff and one tracheal. In the event of esophageal intubation with a Combi-tube TM, the breathing circuit is connected to a second lumen going to a sideport proximal to the tracheal cuff. After arrival to the hospital, leaders of the surgical and anesthesia teams should discuss when this should be changed to an endotracheal tube and what technique should be used to make this exchange.

AWAKE INTUBATION

In patients with marginal respiratory function, history of difficult intubation, anticipated difficult mask, or some combination thereof, it is safest to maintain spontaneous ventilation until an endotracheal tube is placed and its position confirmed. Whether the tube is to be placed by laryngoscope or fiberoptic bronchoscope, the key to success is appropriate preparation of the patient. This should include a conversation with the patient outlining the need for awake intubation and what to expect during the process. It is also important to administer an antisialagogue (such as 0.4 mg of glycopyrrolate given by intramuscular injection) 20-30 minutes before the procedure. Manipulation of the airway is extremely stimulating and a number of techniques are available to anesthetize various airway structures.

For nasal intubations, the nares can be topically anesthetized with viscous lidocaine, sometimes in conjunction with a vasoconstrictor to minimize bleeding. This can be accomplished with soaked cotton swabs (placed deep to block the sphenopalatine ganglia) or a nasal trumpet lubricated with lidocaine. The oropharynx may be anesthetized with either viscous or aerosolized lidocaine. Benzocaine spray is another option but carries the risk of methemoglobinemia. The vocal cords themselves are often anesthetized by spraying lidocaine directly on them via the bronchoscope channel (after warning the patient that this will make him or her cough). Alternatively, the cords may be anesthetized by a transtracheal block.

In patients with good landmarks, puncture of the cricothyroid membrane and injection of 4% lidocaine (1-3 mL) directly into the lumen can provide topical anesthesia of the trachea and larynx. This block is also referred to as a recurrent laryngeal nerve block since it locally anesthetizes the structures below the cords. Injection is performed at end expiration so that the solution is inhaled and then coughed cephalad. Vigorous coughing in and of itself may be deleterious in patients with unstable necks so use of this block should be considered with regard to clinical context. To minimize the risk of injury, either the needle should be withdrawn immediately after injection or an angiocatheter should be used for puncture with removal of the needle prior to injection of the lidocaine.

Anesthesia of the territory served by the superior laryngeal nerve may occur with transtracheal block as the local anesthetic is coughed onto the structures superior to the vocal cords. For more reliable anesthesia of the superior laryngeal nerve territory, however, blockade of the nerve itself is sometimes used. The nondominant hand is used to laterally displace the hyoid bone toward the side to be blocked. A 25-gauge needle is inserted at the level of the greater cornu of the hyoid bone and walked off the bone inferiorly until it pierces the thyrohyoid membrane. After negative aspiration of air or blood, 2 mL of 2% lidocaine is injected and the block is repeated on the contralateral side.

Since these techniques are often used in combination, it is important to be mindful of the total amount of local anesthetic delivered. The maximum dose of lidocaine varies between 4.5 mg/kg (lidocaine not mixed with epinephrine) and 7 mg/kg (lidocaine mixed with 1:200,000 epinephrine). Symptoms of lidocaine toxicity include perioral tingling, auditory or visual disturbance, and depressed consciousness. Once the endotracheal tube is placed, whether by laryngoscopy or fiberoptic bronchoscope, it is connected to the circuit and the cuff is gently inflated. After final confirmation of correct placement (either end-tidal CO_2 or collapse of the bag on inspiration), additional anesthetic, anxiolytic, sedative, and paralytic agents (as appropriate) are administered.

INVASIVE APPROACHES TO AIRWAY MANAGEMENT

Cricothyrotomy

Cricothyroidotomy is an ancient procedure (dating back to the 1500s) that remains a popular choice for rapid control of a difficult airway owing to its simplicity. It may be performed after initial endotracheal intubation attempts have failed or as the first attempt in the setting of craniofacial trauma. Properly trained individuals can even perform cricothyroidotomy in the field with good success.[22] One relative contraindication is young age as the risk for subglottic stenosis is higher than conventional tracheostomy.

Thus, emergent cricothyroidotomy should always be in the emergency airway algorithm and the necessary equipment kept at hand. Aseptic skin preparation, a scalpel and the tube destined to become the airway are all that is needed. Additional instruments may include forceps, a hemostat, some form of retractor, and suture. Frequently, a scalpel (No. 10 or No. 15 blade) is the only instrument used. The type of tube used can include cuffed endotracheal tubes with internal diameters of 5.0-7.0 mm or a tracheostomy tube (typically No. 6 or smaller). A rigid stylet can be useful in directing an endotracheal tube caudally, as it can occasionally direct itself retrograde toward the vocal cords upon insertion. While practitioners who are not surgically trained may favor the use of kits that employ "percutaneous" methods for the insertion of cricothyroidotomy tubes, familiarity and practice are important: these kits may contain advanced tools such as breakaway needles and should be mastered prior to their emergent need.

The surface anatomy of the neck should be assessed at the time initial airway attempts are being made or discussed. Skin should be cleansed quickly with antiseptic preparation solution and the anatomic landmarks clearly identified. Universal precautions should be maintained. Hyoid and cricoid cartilages are palpated, as the cricothyroid membrane lies between them. Landmark identification of anatomical structures is complicated by obesity, edema, the presence of facial/neck hair, and cervical spine immobilization devices. The right-handed surgeon is ideally positioned at the right side of the patient, and vice-versa. This facilitates the stabilization of the trachea and larynx by using the first three fingers of the nondominant hand on the superior cornu of the larynx, allowing the dominant hand the best access to the area of interest. Laryngeal stabilization is crucial as it will allow for palpation of critical structures in the event that visualization is lost. It should be maintained until the airway is secure. Once this has been accomplished, the dominant hand makes a generous (typically, 1.5-2 cm) longitudinal incision in the midline of the neck overlying the membrane. This incision is oriented vertically to decrease the chance of lacerating the anterior jugular veins. The pretracheal tissue and fascia are divided in this manner as well. The membrane is incised transversely. This step is frequently performed blindly, as bleeding or body habitus can make visualization difficult. Care is taken to not injure the posterior tracheal wall. The incision in the membrane is then dilated digitally (the fifth finger is often perfect) or with an instrument such as forceps or a hemostat. In older descriptions of the procedure, the handle of the scalpel is used to dilate the opening in the membrane, but this has been shown to increase the incidence of iatrogenic injury, and, thus, many practitioners are now abandoning this practice. The index finger of the nondominant hand should be used to maintain control of the cricothyroidotomy and guide insertion of the tube distally into the airway. The tube should be placed with the dominant hand, using a gentle, caudally curving motion. Care should be taken to position the tube above the carina, as there is a tendency toward endobronchial intubation due to the length of the tube. Endotracheal tubes should be exchanged for tracheostomy tubes, in a controlled setting, whenever possible. Verification of tube position is essential (as discussed above) and a high index of suspicion should be maintained for endobronchial intubation. If present, the cuff should be gently inflated as to prevent air leak; high cuff pressures (>25 cm H_2O) can damage the tracheal mucosa. Depending on the setting and available equipment, the tube should be secured to the neck with tape or suture. When using a tracheostomy tube, the obturator needs to be in the cannula to facilitate device placement. Once in position, the obturator is quickly removed before connecting to the circuit or reinflating manual ventilation bag (please see the section on "tracheostomy" for additional details on placement of tracheostomy tubes). The flange on the neck plate of the tracheostomy tube is then used to secure the tube in place using suture, tracheostomy ties, or both.

Tracheostomy

Tracheostomy is indicated for patients with prolonged requirements for mechanical ventilation, inability to clear airway secretions, and with difficulty weaning from the ventilator. Advantages include decreased dead space, improved pulmonary toilet and ease of suctioning, and ease of ventilator weaning. Elective tracheostomies can be performed open or percutaneously, with similar complication profile (mortality <1%) regardless of the operative approach. Emergent tracheostomies in the hands of an experienced surgeon are typically faster with an open technique. The tracheostomy tube is built with a neck plate and flange that is secured to the patient with a collar that encircles the neck. The neck plate is frequently sutured to the patient's skin using a permanent monofilament suture that remains in place until the tracheal stoma has matured.

The neck is extended to open the tracheal interspaces. The skin from the mandible to below the sternal notch should be cleansed with sterile prep. The skin incision is made over the tracheal rings below the cricoid cartilage in a transversely oriented fashion, approximately 2 cm in length. Care should be taken at this point to quickly identify and protect (or ligate) the anterior jugular veins as bleeding will obscure the view.

Open Tracheostomy

Once the subcutaneous fat and platysma have been divided, the anterior cervical fascia is encountered and divided along the midline—the strap muscles of the neck should then be separated along their midline raphe, taking care to control bleeding. The isthmus of the thyroid is frequently encountered at this point and requires division, either between clamps followed by suture ligation or with high-powered electrocautery. Care must be taken to avoid use of cautery in the trachea, since the combination of cautery and high oxygen concentration can lead to explosion and fire. Typically, we abandon the use of the cautery as soon as the thyroid isthmus is divided. The tracheal fascia is encountered next and opened to allow for exposure of the second and third tracheal rings. Once again, care must be taken upon opening of the trachea to assess the percent of inspired oxygen that is being used in ventilating the patient. History reveals that opening the trachea might be considered the most important part of the entire operation.[23]

Frequently used methods include inferiorly based flap (Björk method), or the linear tracheotomy. In the Björk method, the trachea is opened using a scalpel to create an inverted u-shaped flap that is one-half to two-thirds of the tracheal width, as viewed anteriorly. The transverse portion is created in the intercartilaginous region between the first and second rings, and then extended inferiorly to cut through the second tracheal ring, and possibly the third. The blood supply to the trachea enters laterally and thus, cautery can prove useful in providing hemostasis in the corners of the inferiorly based flap. A permanent suture on a taper is used to secure the tracheal flap to the skin, ensuring the patency of the tracheal stoma. This facilitates the replacement of the airway should it become dislodged. The endotracheal tube can then be withdrawn under direct visualization. Once the tip of the endotracheal tube is visualized at the top of the tracheal opening, the tracheostomy tube can be advanced into the airway with the obturator in place, with a gentle, posterior, and caudally curving motion. When a linear tracheotomy is used to open the trachea, the use of a tracheal spreader can allow visualization and placement of the tracheostomy tube. Once the tube is in the airway, the obturator is removed. If a dual-cannula tracheostomy tube is employed, the inner cannula must be in place before connecting to the breathing circuit. The position of the tube is verified by chest movement and the detection of end-tidal CO_2. The time between opening the trachea and connecting the circuit should be minimized to prevent collapse of alveoli.

Percutaneous Tracheostomy

A percutaneous approach using specialized kits provides a convenient alternative and with some practice can be used electively. The skin is anesthetized prior to prepping and draping. The initial incision is the same. The pretracheal soft tissues are dissected bluntly and the trachea is exposed. The endotracheal tube is then withdrawn to just below the vocal cords. The trachea is then punctured 1-2 rings caudad to the cricoid cartilage and a guidewire is advanced into the trachea. The tracheal puncture is then dilated to allow placement of the tracheal cannula.

PEDIATRIC CONSIDERATIONS

In general, the approach to pediatric airway management is similar to adults. However, there are important anatomical and physiologic differences between pediatric patients and adults. The infantile larynx is smaller, funnel-shaped (narrowest below the vocal cords), and more anterior when compared with adults (Fig. 7.3). For these reasons, most practitioners favor a straight blade for intubation. Although it is possible to estimate the appropriate size blade, tube, and depth of tube placement from a pediatric patient's age and weight, it is necessary to have a wide variety of sizes readily available (Table 7.3). A convenient rule of "thumb" is to choose an ETT, which is approximately the size (outer diameter) of the patient's little finger. Uncuffed tubes with a larger inner diameter to decrease airway resistance are at times favored for pediatric patients <6 years old. The ETT should not be forced into the trachea of young patients. In general, an air leak around the uncuffed tubes at pressures of 15-20 cm H_2O is considered appropriate.

Because the pediatric patient has a reduced FRC and higher oxygen consumption, desaturation occurs quicker and more dramatically than in adults. In spontaneously breathing neonates, desaturation due to apneic breathing is common and can be associated with drastic bradycardia (especially in the prematurely born). Premature children are also prone to retrolental fibroplasia, which is related to prolonged exposure to high FIO_2. The target for pulse oximetry should be 93%-95% with maintenance of PaO_2 between 60 and 80 mm Hg. Although, several rare congenital disorders are associated with craniofacial abnormalities and difficult intubation (Hurler's syndrome, Goldenhar's syndrome), Down's syndrome (Trisomy 21) is also frequently associated with specific challenges in airway management because of the phenotype, which includes short neck, small mouth, large tongue, and atlantooccipital instability.

Epiglottitis is a life-threatening pediatric infection that involves the upper airway. This acute infection is typically bacterial in origin, occurring most frequently in children 3-7 years old and is accompanied by dysphagia, stridor, salivation, and fever. A common mimic easily ruled out by plain x-ray films is croup (laryngotracheobronchitis). It can also present with stridor but is typically associated with a viral prodrome, gradual onset, and characteristic "barking" cough. It is generally recommended that pediatric patients with epiglottitis go directly to the operating room for airway management.

PHARMACOLOGY AND RAPID SEQUENCE INDUCTION

It is common for experienced practitioners to administer a variety of anesthetic drugs to both render the patient unconscious and block neuromuscular activity to optimize conditions for airway management prior to intubation. It is important to remember in acute care that these drugs may not be prudent in every situation. Many anesthetic drugs can cause hypotension in acutely ill patients, especially those who are hypovolemic from bleeding. In the pulseless patient, drugs are rarely necessary, but it may be necessary to temporarily halt chest compressions during the intubation.

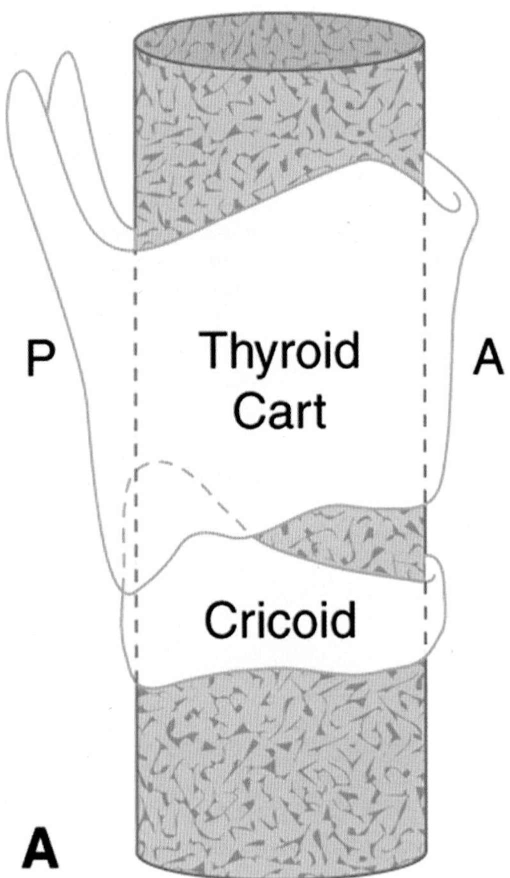

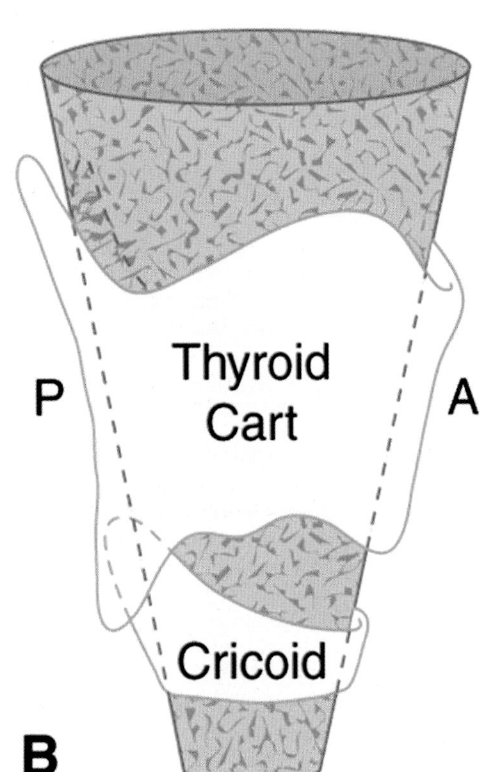

FIGURE 7.3. Comparison of the adult (**A**) versus pediatric (**B**) airway anatomy. (From Barash PG, Cullen BF, Stoelting RK, et al. *Clinical Anesthesia*. 6th ed. Philadelphia, PA: Lippincott Williams & Wilkins; 2009.)

Traditionally, etomidate has been considered a good choice for hemodynamic stability. However, hypotension can still occur after administration of this drug, especially if the patient is maintaining normotension from sympathetic overactivation by fear, pain, or drug intoxication (e.g., cocaine). Because the hypotensive patient undergoing trauma surgery is at high risk for awareness under anesthesia,[24,25] benzodiazepines are frequently administered during or shortly after induction, but their use has not been proven to decrease awareness.[26] Benzodiazepines, much like etomidate, may decrease blood pressure in certain situations. Scopolamine has been used in an attempt to facilitate amnesia in trauma patients with low blood pressure but its vagolytic effects on heart rate preclude routine administration. In general, one should avoid large doses of anesthetics and pain medicines known to depress cardiac activity and therefore opioids, propofol, and inhaled anesthetics should be titrated judiciously in patients suspected to be hypovolemic. Depending on the urgency of needed treatment, cautious dosing regimens of these drugs may delay valuable time to treatment.

The NMDA antagonist, ketamine, which has dissociative and pain-relieving qualities, is an interesting choice for induction and maintenance of anesthesia in acute care situations. In normovolemic subjects, it has some symapthomimetic activity. It is generally associated with an increase in heart rate and blood pressure; however, hypotension can occur similar to etomidate if the patient's hemodynamics are dependent on high sympathetic tone. Ketamine can complicate airway management by

TABLE 7.3

GUIDELINES FOR SIZE AND LENGTH OF TRACHEAL TUBES IN CHILDREN

AGE	INTERNAL DIAMETER (MM)	DISTANCE FROM LIPS TO MIDTRACHEA[a] (CM)
Premature	2.5	8
Full term	3.0	10
1–6 mo	3.5	11
6–12 mo	4.0	12
2 y	4.5	13
4 y	5.0	14
6 y	5.5	15
8 y	6.5	16[b]
10 y	7.0	17-18[c]
12 y	7.5	18-20
14 y	8.0-9.0	20-22

[a]Add 2-3 cm for nasal tubes.
[b]Females.
[c]Males.

increasing oral secretions and can complicate neurologic exams as it is associated with unpleasant dreams and nystagmus.

While neuromuscular blockade using succinylcholine and other neuromuscular blocking drugs have been viewed as mainstays of rapid airway management for decades, they may not be appropriate in all management situations. They should never be administered without sufficient anesthesia to decrease consciousness (including the obtunded patient). The administrators of these drugs should be highly trained and confident in their airway management skills as neuromuscular blocking drugs eliminate the patient's ability to generate diaphragmatic movements on a temporary basis and ventilation becomes the responsibility of the clinical team. The depolarizing neuromuscular blocker, succinylcholine, has many beneficial qualities for acute situations (e.g., rapid onset and short duration). However, it is essential to recall that after an adequate dose for intubation (1.0 mg per kg), there is no assurance that the drug's effects will disappear before detrimental or possibly fatal consequences of hypoxemia arise in situations where ventilation by mask or airway device is unsuccessful or impossible. This danger is magnified with the use of nondepolarizing neuromuscular blockers (e.g., rocuronium, vecuronium, cisatracurium) as their duration of action is enhanced. Although a novel cyclodextran molecule, sugammadex, is currently available in Europe for rapid reversal of aminosteroid based, nondepolarizing neuromuscular blocking agents (e.g., rocuronium and vecuronium). Should sugammadex be approved for use in the United States, the preference of neuromuscular blocking drugs in the acute setting may change.

Succinylcholine acts by first depolarizing the nicotinic acetylcholine receptors at the motor end plate before inactivating them. For this reason, muscle fasciculation and a transient increase in potassium is expected upon administration. In the acute trauma situation, succinylcholine is generally considered safe with the exception of patients suspected or known to have potassium levels high enough to cause EKG changes. Caution is also recommended for the use of succinylcholine in patients rehabilitating from extensive burns or large stroke as a large proportion of their regenerating muscle may have extrasynaptic acetylcholine receptors, which are more sensitive to the effects of succinylcholine. Use of succinylcholine in the acute burn or stroke patient is typically not a problem.

Rapid sequence induction (RSI) is a technique favored by many trained in airway management in situations where regurgitation and possible pulmonary aspiration of stomach contents is a major concern. No standard RSI technique exists,[27] but administration of an IV induction agent immediately followed by administration of fast-acting neuromuscular blockade (1.2-2.0 mg per kg succinylcholine, or 0.8-1.2 mg per kg rocuronium) without any mask ventilation are the major steps involved. In RSI, mask ventilation is avoided to prevent filling the stomach with air. Cricoid pressure, originally described by Sellick in the 1950s, is applied to hopefully occlude the esophagus with pressure from the trachea. The necessity and validity of this technique has been debated.[28,29] After the administered drugs have an appropriate time to circulate, an oral endotracheal tube is placed via direct laryngoscopy in an efficient and time-sensitive manner.

SUMMARY

Through medical knowledge and practical training, the physician who tends to the most acutely ill patient should be prepared to maintain ventilation and oxygenation in critical clinical situations. Despite the existence of a large set of clinical options and technical devices available to practitioners, extensive training in a subset of airway management options is sufficient as long as definitive and invasive techniques are part of their clinical repertoire. Each individual should approach the airway in the acutely ill patient with an honest evaluation of his or her skill set.

It is time-consuming and in some situations dangerous to exhaust all noninvasive techniques before proceeding to invasive techniques in acutely ill patients. Yet an appreciation for basic airway management principles such as preoxygenation, preprocedural airway evaluation, mask ventilation skills, and temporary use of an LMA is essential. Employment of these techniques can often turn a critical situation into one that is perhaps less acute and can prevent an urgent situation from becoming an emergent situation. A formal but flexible plan for airway management with good communication among the medical personnel involved is essential to favorable patient outcomes.

References

1. Fyneface-Ogan S, Uzoigwe SA. Caesarean section outcome in eclamptic patients: a comparison of infiltration and general anaesthesia. *West Afr J Med.* 2008;27(4):250-254.
2. Liu JT, et al. Emergency management of epidural haematoma through burr hole evacuation and drainage. A preliminary report. *Acta Neurochir (Wien).* 2006;148(3):313-317; discussion 317.
3. Mezitis M, Stathopoulos P, Rallis G. Use of a curved mosquito for reducing isolated zygomatic arch fractures. *J Craniofac Surg.* 2010;21(4):1281-1283.
4. Musawi AA, Andersson L. Use of topical as only anesthetic for suturing a traumatic facial laceration. *Dent Traumatol.* 2010;26(3):292-293.
5. Neumar RW, et al. Part 8. Adult advanced cardiovascular life support: 2010 American Heart Association guidelines for cardiopulmonary resuscitation and emergency cardiovascular care. *Circulation.* 2010;122(18 suppl 3): S729-S767.
6. Lee TS, Jordan JS. Pyriform sinus perforation secondary to traumatic intubation in a difficult airway patient. *J Clin Anesth.* 1994;6(2):152-155.
7. Wu J, et al. The analysis of risk factors of impacting mortality rate in severe multiple trauma patients with posttraumatic acute respiratory distress syndrome. *Am J Emerg Med.* 2008;26(4):419-424.
8. Raghavendran K, et al. Lung contusion: inflammatory mechanisms and interaction with other injuries. *Shock.* 2009;32(2):122-130.
9. Apfelbaum JL, Caplan RA, Connis RT, et al. Practice guidelines for preoperative fasting and the use of pharmacologic agents to reduce the risk of pulmonary aspiration: application to healthy patients undergoing elective procedures: an updated report by the American Society of Anesthesiologists Committee on Standards and Practice Parameters. *Anesthesiology.* 2011;114(3):495-511.
10. Ghaffari S. Forceful insertion of nasal tube may pierce the posterior nasopharyngeal mucosa. *Paediatr Anaesth.* 2006;16(9):997.
11. El-Orbany M, Woehlck HJ. Difficult mask ventilation. *Anesth Analg.* 2009;109(6):1870-1880.
12. Joffe AM, Hetzel S, Liew EC. A two-handed jaw-thrust technique is superior to the one-handed "EC-clamp" technique for mask ventilation in the apneic unconscious person. *Anesthesiology.* 2010;113(4):873-879.
13. Ghatge S, Hagberg CA. Does the airway examination predict difficult intubation? In: Fleisher LA, ed. *Evidence-Based Practice of Anesthesiology.* Philadelphia, PA: Saunders/Elsevier; 2009: 101-115.
14. Koh LK, Kong CE, Ip-Yam PC. The modified Cormack-Lehane score for the grading of direct laryngoscopy: evaluation in the Asian population. *Anaesth Intensive Care.* 2002;30(1):48-51.
15. Caplan RA, Benumof JL, Berry FA, Blitt CD, Bode RH, Cheney FW, Connis RT, Guidry OF, Nickinovich DG, Ovassapian A. Practice guidelines for management of the difficult airway: an updated report by the American Society of Anesthesiologists Task Force on Management of the Difficult Airway. *Anesthesiology.* 2003;98(5):1269-1277.
16. Thiboutot F, et al. Effect of manual in-line stabilization of the cervical spine in adults on the rate of difficult orotracheal intubation by direct laryngoscopy: a randomized controlled trial. *Can J Anaesth.* 2009;56(6):412-418.
17. Santoni BG, et al. Manual in-line stabilization increases pressures applied by the laryngoscope blade during direct laryngoscopy and orotracheal intubation. *Anesthesiology.* 2009;110(1): 24-31.
18. Dupanovic M, Fox H, Kovac A. Management of the airway in multitrauma. *Curr Opin Anaesthesiol.* 2010;23(2):276-282.
19. Brain AI. The laryngeal mask—a new concept in airway management. *Br J Anaesth.* 1983;55(8):801-805.
20. Maltby JR, et al. LMA-Classic and LMA-ProSeal are effective alternatives to endotracheal intubation for gynecologic laparoscopy. *Can J Anaesth.* 2003;50(1):71-77.
21. Borkowski A, et al. The applicability of the ProSeal laryngeal mask airway for laparotomies. *Anasthesiol Intensivmed Notfallmed Schmerzther.* 2005;40(8):477-486.

22. Gerich TG, et al. Prehospital airway management in the acutely injured patient: the role of surgical cricothyrotomy revisited. *J Trauma.* 1998;45(2):312-314.
23. Kinley CE. A technique of tracheostomy. *Can Med Assoc J.* 1965;92:79-81.
24. Bogetz MS, Katz JA. Recall of surgery for major trauma. *Anesthesiology.* 1984;61(1):6-9.
25. ErrandoCL, et al. Awareness with recall during general anaesthesia: a prospective observational evaluation of 4001 patients. *Br J Anaesth.* 2008;101(2):178-185.
26. Sandin RH, et al. Awareness during anaesthesia: a prospective case study. *Lancet.* 2000;355(9205):707-711.
27. El-Orbany M, Connolly LA. Rapid sequence induction and intubation: current controversy. *Anesth Analg.* 2010;110(5):1318-1325.
28. Ovassapian A, Salem MR. Sellick's maneuver: to do or not do. *Anesth Analg.* 2009;109(5):1360-1362.
29. Lerman J. On cricoid pressure: "may the force be with you". *Anesth Analg.* 2009;109(5):1363-1366.

CHAPTER 8 ■ PREOPERATIVE PREPARATION OF THE EMERGENCY GENERAL SURGERY PATIENT

KRISTA TURNER AND FREDERICK MOORE

Skillful perioperative care of acutely ill patients is a defining characteristic of the specialty of acute care surgery. Appropriate resuscitation and planning permit a safe operation and establish the patient's clinical trajectory. Prevailing literature on preoperative assessment emphasizes risk modification primarily for the elective patient. In an emergency situation, this luxury disappears, and the surgeon must attempt to reverse existing damage and prevent further loss quickly and based on limited information. The acute care surgeon encounters a wide spectrum of patients, with varying severity of chronic and acute illness. Although each patient will provide a unique challenge, the same concepts can be applied universally. It is helpful to follow an approach to the emergency general surgery patient similar to that to a trauma patient—initial evaluation and treatment based on urgency, followed by careful system evaluation prior to surgery.

PRIMARY SURVEY

Identification and Assessment

There is little doubt that the floridly ill 80-year-old woman with free air requires more attention prior to surgery than the healthy 18-year-old male with classic signs of early appendicitis. In between the two extremes are patients who may appear well on preliminary exam only to decompensate in the operating room later. Early identification of patients with subtle signs of shock can greatly affect their outcome when appropriately treated prior to surgery. Clinical assessment of these patients can often be limited, given the time constraints in some emergency situations.

The approach to the emergency surgery patient should include an initial brief history and physical to guide further decision making. Once a surgical emergency is established, the initial medical history can follow that of the "AMPLE" format used for obtaining a history in trauma patients. The "A" and "M" represent allergies and medications, for which particular attention should be paid to prescribed anticoagulants, insulin, and cardiovascular medications. The "P" prompts for listing of previous surgery or prominent medical problems. The "L" indicates the last meal and signifies a higher aspiration risk. The "E" refers to events that surrounded the inciting event. In the case of the emergency general surgery patient, this should focus on components of the acute illness that may attest to its severity.

Physical examination should have two components: one that focuses on the specific disease process and one that focuses on signs of systemic sequelae. The first identifies the need for surgery; the second quantifies the degree of illness. Establishing the diagnosis by physical exam is fundamental to general surgery practice. Examining the patient for systemic illness is of equal importance to the acute care surgeon. Criteria for systemic inflammatory response syndrome (SIRS) are nonspecific[1] but highly sensitive for any type of systemic duress experienced by the patient (i.e., bleeding or tachyarrhythmia) and should prompt further investigation (Table 8.1). Modifications to SIRS scoring can be used to increase specificity for particular systemic illness. To facilitate early identification and treatment of surgical sepsis, for example, we devised a validated screening tool that combined SIRS criteria with a second-level screen to extrapolate possible infectious processes.[1,2] Signs of shock can be obvious with tachycardia and hypotension, but cellular hypoperfusion may be ongoing without such outward signs. Signs of pending organ dysfunction and failure should be sought (Table 8.2).

Basic laboratory studies and x-rays can be valuable adjuncts to identifying the patient with systemic illness. Values on the general chemistry panel, such as low serum bicarbonate and elevated anion gap, can indicate tissue hypoxia. A concentrated hematocrit may also attest to hypovolemia. More specific indicators such as a base deficit, elevated lactate, or decreased oxygen saturation on a venous blood gas can confirm shock and guide resuscitation. A preoperative chest x-ray in the patient with cardiac or pulmonary disease can guide perioperative modalities.

Resuscitation

Similar to the trauma evaluation, the first encounter the surgeon has with the patient in need of emergency surgery may require immediate life-saving measures. Often the patient with presumed surgical pathology will be triaged as such by the emergency department and given less-than-astute attention once the surgeon has been contacted. The surgeon may then arrive to find the patient metabolically deranged to the point of extremis. Simple basic life support skills are then necessary.

Airway and Breathing This is not such an anatomical issue as it is with trauma patients, but the patency of the airway should still be evaluated. These patients may suffer from altered mentation secondary to shock and require airway protection. Tachypnea is often present to compensate for metabolic acidosis and is not well tolerated in the older patient. The use of accessory muscles of breathing, paradoxical respiratory effort, and apnea should all be signs to intubate and ventilate. Pulse oximetry can be used to assess adequacy of oxygenation; however, this can lag behind actual alveolar oxygenation, and a low-normal value should always be interpreted with caution. Anecdotally speaking, if it occurs to you that maybe you should intubate the patient, then you should.

The key to successful intubation is preparation. Always ensure that the appropriate personnel and equipment are available while providing oxygen by mask. Rapid sequence intubation may be achieved with an inducing agent and short-acting paralytic. Etomidate is often favored due to rapidity of action and relative lack of hemodynamic effect. The transient

TABLE 8.1

SYSTEMIC INFLAMMATORY RESPONSE SYNDROME (SIRS) CRITERIA

1	Heart rate > 90 beats/min
2	Respiratory rate > 20 breaths/min, or $Paco_2$ < 32 mm Hg
3	Temperature > 38°C or < 36°C
4	Leukocytes > 12,000/mm^3 or < 4,000/mm^3 or ≥ 10% juvenile neutrophil granulocytes

NOTE: Two out of four criteria establish the diagnosis for SIRS.

adrenal suppression induced by etomidate has raised concern, and studies are mixed regarding its safety for single use.[3,4] Chest x-ray should always be obtained to visualize the tip of the endotracheal tube and avoid right mainstem bronchus intubation for the duration of the ensuing operation.

Circulation Again, trauma resuscitation basics should be followed but are often neglected. Intravenous access upon evaluation of these patients is typically poor—a single 22-gauge peripheral in the hand is simply not adequate. If the classic "two large-bore peripheral IVs" cannot be obtained, then central venous access is necessary, preferably of large diameter, and placed in the chest or neck with ultrasound guidance.

Despite the type of shock, volume loading is the first step of resuscitation. Options include isotonic crystalloids, hypertonic saline, colloids, and blood products. Crystalloids are inexpensive and readily available. Initial bolus of 20 mL per kg of either normal saline or lactated Ringer's solution should be followed by reassessment and ongoing hydration. Hypertonic saline is promising for emergency use in that it may cause less edema and has a favorable immunologic profile. This has been particularly studied in patients with traumatic brain injury.[5] While relatively safe compared to colloid infusion, the administration of large amounts of saline for volume resuscitation carries the concern for hypernatremia, hyperosmolarity, and hyperchloremic metabolic acidosis.

Colloids may provide a greater volume expansion per amount infused, although the presence of leaky capillaries may negate this advantage. Given that it offers no advantage to crystalloid use and is of limited availability, albumin should be limited to specific patient populations.[6] Hydroxyethyl starch (HES) has likewise been proposed as a resuscitative colloid. Large volumes of HES should be used with caution, as doses exceeding 20 mL/kg/d can incite platelet dysfunction and renal failure in certain patient populations.[7,8]

Provision of blood products as a resuscitation fluid should be considered carefully. The risk of infection, immunosuppression, and transfusion reaction are well known.[9] Fresh frozen plasma (FFP), cryoprecipitate, and platelets also have utility as colloids based on the coagulation profile. Each has the same adverse transfusion profile as administering packed red blood cells (pRBCs) and should only be used in combination for hemorrhagic shock or for coagulopathy. The patient with ongoing bleeding should be treated with a hemostatic resuscitation strategy that involves transfusion of plasma, platelets, and pRBCs in a ratio that mimics that of whole blood and avoids large volumes of crystalloid infusion.[10] Monitoring ongoing transfusion with platelet count, hematocrit, thromboelastrography (TEG), and venous oxygen saturation will help guide further therapy. Hypotensive resuscitation in the hemorrhagic

TABLE 8.2

SIGNS AND SYMPTOMS OF ORGAN DYSFUNCTION

ORGAN SYSTEM	SYMPTOMS OR SIGNS	CAUSES
CNS	Mental status changes	↓ Cerebral perfusion
Circulatory	Tachycardia	Adrenergic stimulation, depressed contractility
Cardiac	Hypotension	Coronary ischemia
Systemic	New murmurs Hypotension ↓ JVP ↑ JVP	Depressed contractility secondary to ischemia or MDFs, right ventricular failure Valvular dysfunction, VSD ↓ SVR, ↓ venous return Hypovolemia, ↓ venous return Right heart failure
Respiratory	Tachypnea Cyanosis	Pulmonary edema, respiratory muscle fatigue, sepsis, acidosis Hypoxemia
Renal	Oliguria	↓ Perfusion, afferent arteriolar vasoconstriction
Skin	Cool, clammy	Vasoconstriction, sympathetic stimulation
Other	Lactic acidosis Fever	Anaerobic metabolism, hepatic dysfunction Infection

CNS, central nervous system; MDFs, myocardial depressant factors; VSD, ventricular septal defect; SVR, systemic vascular resistance patient is an additional emerging concept.[11] Measures to raise blood pressure (BP) with fluid administration may be counterproductive until bleeding is controlled. This approach should be used with caution as efforts to maintain vital organ perfusion (particularly the brain) should be the top priority.

Ongoing signs of shock despite adequate volume resuscitation will require the addition of vasopressors or inotropes. Sympathomimetics are the standard for raising the mean arterial pressure (MAP). Each vasopressor has advantages and disadvantages, although norepinephrine has emerged as one of the first-line agents for septic and cardiogenic shock.[12] Inotropes such as dobutamine or milrinone can be added if cardiac output remains low despite adequate volume loading and vasopressor provision. More advanced monitoring should be applied to help titrate inotrope effect.

Adjunctive measures to assist with hemorrhagic or septic source control may be considered as part of the resuscitation strategy. If interventional radiology is available and capable, a well placed drain or coil can stabilize the patient who is otherwise too acutely ill for the operating room. Shock resuscitation should be ongoing throughout this process with the intent of proceeding to the operating room for definitive control when it is safe to do so.

Endpoints of Resuscitation Deciding where surgical intervention fits into shock resuscitation may be difficult. For the less ill patient, providing a liter of crystalloid may be sufficient to restore signs of tissue perfusion prior to operating. For sicker patients, the surgical intervention is an integral part of the resuscitation and must be undertaken before any further improvement can be seen. More difficult yet, particularly in the elderly population, is the nonresponder for whom a surgical intervention will have no bearing on outcome and may put simply put the patient and family through undue duress. Luckily, most patients will fall short of this extreme.

The surgeon should have in mind what end points are to be met before operating. It is prudent that once resuscitation is initiated, the progress of the patient is closely monitored. All too often, an initial assessment and plan will be established, only to find several hours later that nothing has been accomplished. Likewise, "resuscitation" does not equal "extra few hours of sleep" for the surgeon whose patient presents in the middle of the night. While consideration should be given to availability of appropriate operating room staff based on time of day, physiologic optimization of the patient should take precedence.

For the patient in shock, various hemodynamic end points and modes of monitoring progress can be used both pre- and postoperatively. Basic monitoring in patients with shock includes heart rate and urinary output. Noninvasive BP measurements tend to give falsely elevated readings in patients who are hypotensive. An arterial catheter should therefore be placed when there is a concern for hypoperfusion. Central venous pressure (CVP) is often one of the first invasive measures employed. Although this has numerous confounders, resuscitation protocols often aim for a CVP of 12–15 mm Hg.[13] With the addition of pulmonary artery catheters, numerous additional hemodynamic parameters become available, although it is not clear that the appropriate end point is the normalization of these values, nor is it clear how these end points should be achieved. Arterial pressure waveform analysis is a promising modality. Utilizing an existing arterial catheter, it can provide reliable measures of cardiac output and volume status that can outperform pulmonary artery and central venous catheters for resuscitation.[14]

End points of tissue oxygenation may also be used for resuscitation. Mixed-venous oxygen saturation (SvO_2) has classically been employed as an estimate of global tissue perfusion, but requires a pulmonary artery catheter for measurement. Values <65% are associated with reduction in oxygen delivery, indicating reduced cardiac output or oxygen content of blood. Central venous oxygen saturation ($ScvO_2$) generates similar information from a standard central venous catheter, with values <70% significant.[15] Laboratory values such as lactate and base deficit can also help guide resuscitative efforts, with prognostic significance.[16,17] Near-infrared spectroscopy offers a method of monitoring tissue hemoglobin oxygen saturation (StO_2) in the skeletal muscle. Changes in skeletal muscle StO_2 correlate well with changes in oxygen delivery, base deficit, and lactate levels during active resuscitation.[18]

SECONDARY SURVEY: SYSTEM-BASED CONSIDERATIONS

A surgical emergency can often be the patient's first exposure to the health care system, leaving the surgeon to uncover previously undiagnosed medical problems. Special attention in the history should be given to previous problems with anesthesia, clotting disorders, as well as medications and substance use. Baseline functioning including mental status, activity level, and vital signs should also be established from family if the patient is unable to communicate. Careful physical examination can reveal other pertinent comorbidities. These include signs of pulmonary disease, vascular disease, cirrhosis, previous unmentioned surgery, and malnutrition, to name a few. The following describes components of the preoperative evaluation by system, with more pertinent topics discussed in detail.

Neurologic

Baseline function should be established through either the patient or family, particularly for elderly patients who may have dementia. Superimposed delirium from acute illness complicates this exam. Chronic neurologic disease should be ascertained, as numerous diseases such as muscular dystrophy, myasthenia gravis, multiple sclerosis, epilepsy, Parkinson's disease, and Alzheimer's disease may influence the type of anesthetic and paralytic agents used.

Substance Abuse and Dependency Patients undergoing emergency surgery often present with substance use disorders. Alcohol dependency poses the most dangerous risk to the patient in the perioperative period. Acute illness may impact the usual amount of alcohol ingested, initiating withdrawal sooner than expected. Administration of benzodiazepines prior to surgery reduces the dose of inhaled anesthetics required and prevents seizures. Preoperative morphine can help mediate the exaggerated stress response that is chronically suppressed by alcohol.[19] For the malnourished alcoholic, thiamine should be given prior to glucose administration to prevent Wernicke's encephalopathy. Nicotine and narcotic dependence should also be anticipated and treatment begun in the preoperative period. When initiated early, nicotine replacement therapy can reduce opioid requirement.[20] Narcotic dependence can be treated with short- as well as long-acting opioids, with clonidine added to help temper withdrawal symptoms.[21]

Analgesia Pain control prior to surgical evaluation is an area of debate. Concern for "masking the examination" hinders administration of appropriate analgesia and unnecessarily leaves the patient in pain. Meta-analysis of adult and pediatric patients treated with opiates shows a trend toward increased risk of altered physical exam, but no difference in subsequent management thereof.[22] Patients with chronic pain syndromes should be treated appropriately with their baseline dosing plus additional narcotics as needed for acute pain.

Pulmonary

Chronic Pulmonary Disease Patients with preexisting chronic pulmonary disease present an additional challenge for the surgeon. Emergency patients do not have the luxury of undergoing optimization or risk stratification before surgery, and therefore may present with ongoing atelectasis, respiratory infection, or bronchospasm. Smoking history and chronic obstructive pulmonary disease are clear risk factors for postoperative pulmonary complications such as pneumonia, pleural effusion, and respiratory failure.[23] Additional preoperative risks are low oxygen saturation, respiratory infection within the past month, age >80 years, and preoperative hemoglobin <10 mg per dL.[24] Avoiding these complications can be difficult in the immediate preoperative period, but a few strategies for risk reduction can be applied (Table 8.3).

Acute Lung Injury Acute lung injury (ALI) and Acute Respiratory Distress Syndrome (ARDS) are particularly devastating for the emergency patient. The combination of aggressive resuscitation strategies, profound inflammatory processes, and blood transfusions adds to this risk. Strategies to limit further barotrauma with restrictive tidal volumes (6 mL/kg), judicious use of positive end-expiratory pressure, and permissive hypercapnia have been described once the patient is diagnosed with ALI/ARDS.[25] Studies have also demonstrated that application of a low tidal volume protocol from the outset can prevent subsequent ALI/ARDS by limiting pulmonary cytokine production and inflammation.[26,27] While the initial tendency will be to increase s ventilation in these patients to help compensate for metabolic acidosis, these measures may lead to subsequent barotrauma, and use of lower tidal volumes should be encouraged.

Cardiovascular

Guidelines for preoperative cardiac assessment are abundant and revised frequently. These algorithms uniformly divert the patient directly to surgery for true emergency situations. Patients with acute coronary syndrome complicating their surgical disease should be treated according to American Heart Association/American College of Cardiology (AHA/ACC) guidelines for coronary revascularization.[28] Any attempt to temporize the acute surgical problem should be made in the face of ongoing cardiac ischemia. Coordinating care in a multidisciplinary manner for these patients is paramount. For the more common patient with stable cardiac disease, preparation for surgery is much less dramatic. The limited workup for these patients derived from the history, physical exam, and EKG can provide information regarding functional status. Preoperative optimization options are limited in a short time frame, but a few basic principles can be applied (Table 8.4).

Hypertension Although preoperative hypertension is an important predictor of postoperative morbidity, no data have established that this is remedied by preoperative treatment. This applies principally to those with long-standing moderate hypertension for which any attempt at acute reduction may result in relative hypoperfusion once general anesthesia is induced. Stage III hypertension (>180/110 mm Hg), however, requires control prior to surgery. Continuous intravenous esmolol, labetalol, nitroprusside, or nitroglycerin may be used, as may some of the newer calcium channel blockers such as nicardipine or clevidipine.[29] Invasive arterial BP monitoring for these patients is essential.

Beta-blockade Beta-blockers mitigate cardiovascular stress from surgery by suppressing catecholamine production and increasing stability of atherosclerotic plaques. Initial data regarding perioperative beta-blocker use in cardiovascular surgery demonstrated a decrease in myocardial ischemia, ventricular arrhythmias, and blunting of the hypertensive response in high-risk patients.[30,31] This led to a class I recommendation by the AHA for perioperative beta-blockade with a goal heart rate of 60 bpm for those patients with coronary ischemia undergoing vascular surgery. A class IIa recommendation was also made for patients with untreated hypertension, coronary artery disease, or other risk factors.[32]

With this evidence, perioperative beta-blockade was enthusiastically and liberally applied. Emerging data began to demonstrate unacceptable risks of bradycardia, hypotension, and stroke in certain patient populations.[33–36] When stratified per cardiac risk index, the relationship between perioperative beta-blockade and risk of death varied directly with cardiac risk: those with high risk (cerebrovascular or coronary artery disease, insulin-depending diabetes, creatinine >3 mg/dL,) showed a benefit, but those with low risk showed a trend toward harm.[37] Subsequent revisions to the ACC/AHA

TABLE 8.3

PREOPERATIVE INTERVENTIONS TO REDUCE THE RISK OF POSTOPERATIVE PULMONARY COMPLICATIONS

Incentive spirometry
Continue bronchodilators, inhaled steroids
Intravenous pulse steroids if active reactive airway disease
Restrictive fluid strategy
Antibiotics for active infection
Transfusion for critical hypoxemia
Maintain head of bed >30 degrees
Avoid noninvasive ventilation
Early intubation
Restrictive tidal volumes (6 mL/kg) on positive pressure ventilation
Short-acting neuromuscular blockade intra-op
Laparoscopy if able
Supplemental oxygen

TABLE 8.4

PREOPERATIVE INTERVENTIONS TO REDUCE THE RISK OF POSTOPERATIVE CARDIAC COMPLICATIONS

Aggressively correct electrolytes
Arterial catheter placement for BP measurement
Pulmonary artery catheter or transesophageal echo monitoring for high risk
Correct hemoglobin to 9 g/dL for those with coronary artery disease
Continue beta-blocker if on previously or if cardiac ischemia
Volume restriction in CHF patients
Adequate pain control to reduce stress
Supplemental oxygen

guidelines restrict class I indication for perioperative beta-blockade to those already on beta-blockers and to patients with known coronary ischemia undergoing high-risk surgery.[38]

Congestive Heart Failure Patients with congestive heart failure (CHF) should be cautiously managed prior to emergency surgery. Therapy is aimed at reducing ventricular filling pressures in addition to improving cardiac output. This may be a difficult balance in the face of ongoing disease processes such as vasodilatory shock or bleeding. Chronic disease may be complicated by acute ischemia or metabolic myocardial depression. Inotropes such as dobutamine or milrinone may be needed for those with systolic dysfunction. More invasive monitoring devices such as pulmonary artery catheters or continuous transesophageal echocardiography should be available intraoperatively for this patient population.

Preoperative administration of chronic medications used to treat CHF should be considered carefully. Beta-blockade has already been discussed and should be continued for those already on therapy but without ongoing hypotension.[39] Diuretics should be administered only if clinically indicated on physical exam. Ongoing angiotensin-converting enzyme (ACE) inhibitor administration should be avoided in those patients with hypotension or acute renal insufficiency, but otherwise may have a protective effect.[40] Digoxin should be held in the preoperative period, as therapy with the drug is associated with an increased cardiac risk in urgent surgical patients.[41]

Arrhythmias Perioperative atrial arrhythmias can contribute substantially to morbidity in the emergency surgical patient. Electrolytes should be aggressively corrected and home medications used for rate or rhythm control continued. Acute-onset atrial fibrillation with rapid ventricular response should be stabilized according to advanced cardiac life support protocol prior to proceeding to the operating room.[42] New arrhythmias should prompt investigation for ischemia, for which reperfusion may take precedence of acute surgical pathology. Patients with permanent pacemakers or implantable defibrillators should be identified preoperatively. If time permits, the device should be interrogated by the electrophysiology service. Otherwise, a magnet should be taped over the device en route to surgery. Magnets will reprogram pacing devices to asynchronous mode and will disable defibrillators, making them immune to electromagnetic interference that may be experienced in the operating room.

Renal

Acute kidney injury (AKI) is unfortunately commonplace in the emergency surgery patient and portends a bad outcome. The surgeon should correct issues such as hypovolemia, electrolyte disturbances, and acid/base prior to operating. Metabolic acidosis should be initially treated with volume resuscitation and correction of the underlying problem. If acidosis persists and is hemodynamically limiting, then temporizing measures with sodium bicarbonate, tromethamine (THAM), or immediate continuous renal replacement therapy should be considered.[43] Additional indications for emergent dialysis in the preoperative period (volume overload, intractable hyperkalemia, azotemia, pericarditis), whether for acute or chronic renal failure, should be considered and pursued if time permits.[44] For the patient with chronic renal failure, the surgeon should also be cognizant of appropriate positioning on the table to avoid compression of existing arteriovenous fistulas, as well as avoiding the subclavian vein for central venous catheter placement.

Acute Renal Dysfunction Most cases of renal impairment share the underlying pathology of hypoperfusion.[45] Pre-existing renal function and patient comorbidities such as hypertension, diabetes, and vascular disease play a critical role. Inflammatory and nephrotoxic factors, in combination with type of surgery, can exacerbate these baseline factors. Renal perfusion may be preserved by adequate volume resuscitation and goal-directed therapy.[46]

Contrast-induced Nephropathy Special consideration is given to the acutely ill patient facing exposure to contrast agents for either diagnosis or therapeutic purposes. Current guidelines for prevention of contrast-induced nephropathy (CIN) emphasize provision of isotonic fluid. Normal saline should be administered at 1 mL/kg/h for 24 hours, beginning 2–12 hours before contrast administration. The lowest dose and osmolality contrast should be used. *N*-acetylcysteine (Mucomyst) is often employed with a standard dose of 600 mg every 12 hours for four doses beginning before contrast is given. Although this drug is promising as a free-radical scavenger, the data show no improvement in renal function, despite a decrease in creatinine.[47] Meta-analysis of sodium bicarbonate for prevention of CIN likewise shows no benefit over isotonic saline administration.[48] Other nephrotoxic agents should likewise be avoided. These include ACE inhibitors, angiotensin II receptor blockers, and metformin.

Gastrointestinal

The emergency general surgery patient very often has some component of ileus and is therefore always considered at high aspiration risk. A nasogastric tube should be placed prior to induction of anesthesia to help empty the stomach and prevent voluminous aspiration. Premedication with H_2-receptor blockers is typically given in this patient population prior to induction as well. If the need for future enteral feeding access is anticipated, appropriate tubes can be made available in the operating room. Signs and symptoms of liver disease should be carefully elucidated. Further management of the cirrhotic is discussed below.

Abdominal Compartment Syndrome Intra-abdominal hypertension and abdominal compartment syndrome (ACS) should be considered in certain patients presenting with emergency abdominal pathology. The triad of oliguria, elevated peak airway pressures, and elevated intra-abdominal pressure (as obtained from bladder pressure readings) defines ACS, which can be from either a primary or secondary process.[49] When suspected or diagnosed preoperatively, the surgeon should proceed expeditiously to the operating room to avoid bowel ischemia and further kidney injury. Plans for leaving the fascia open should be made prior to starting the operation so that appropriate supplies are available.

Hematology

Transfusion The concept of liberally transfusing the patient prior to proceeding to the OR with the intention of "loading them up" should be abandoned. While certain patient populations are critically dependent on optimization of oxygen content of blood, most patients needlessly risk the adverse effects associated with transfusion. Patients with active bleeding are the exception, and strategies for transfusion in this population have been described above.

Tolerance for a lower hematocrit in critically ill patients has been supported by the Transfusion Requirements in Critical Care (TRICC) trial. This demonstrated that a restrictive transfusion strategy (hemoglobin trigger of 7 g/dL) is as at least as effective and may be superior to a liberal transfusion threshold of 10 g per dL.[50] This finding persisted for patients with coronary disease, with the exception of those with an acute ischemic event or unstable angina.[51] This was a select group of ICU patients who were considered to be euvolemic, and thus patients with active hemorrhage were excluded in this study and were not specifically identified.

A recent study using the National Surgical Quality Improvement Program (NSQIP) database examined patients undergoing noncardiac surgery.[52] An increase in mortality was shown for those older than 65 years when preoperative hematocrit levels deviated from normal. This was an observational study, however, and patients undergoing emergency surgery did not experience the same effect. A recent large prospective study likewise examined a restrictive versus liberal (hematocrit 24% vs. 30%) transfusion policy prior to cardiac surgery.[53] Thirty-day all-cause morbidity and mortality were the same for both groups; however, the number of units transfused was an independent risk factor for subsequent complications.

Anticoagulation Reversal When performing emergency surgery on anticoagulated patients, the surgeon must balance the risk of operative bleeding versus thromboembolism. For the patient with minimal clinical consequence of operative site bleeding and high risk of thromboembolism, a higher threshold should be given to acceptable INR levels or continuing anticoagulant therapy. High-risk patients with prosthetic valves in the mitral position, atrial fibrillation associated with mitral valve disease, and a history of thromboembolism should be placed on intravenous heparin therapy while warfarin is held. In this patient population, FFP may be administered to acutely reverse anticoagulation, with care taken to avoid volume overload. Vitamin K therapy should be avoided as the delayed effect will serve no purpose in the short term and complicate subsequent anticoagulation in the postoperative period.

Similarly, patients taking antiplatelet therapy should be treated with a risk/benefit approach. Prevalence of patients taking dual antiplatelet therapy with aspirin plus clopidogrel is increasing with expanding criteria for use in cardiovascular patients. Patients with bare metal coronary stents placed within the last 6 weeks or drug-eluting stents placed within the last 12 months should be considered at high risk of a fatal perioperative myocardial infarction.[54] As such, if bleeding risk is acceptable, the patient should be left on antiplatelet therapy without attempt to reverse the effects of platelet inhibition. For the patient on antiplatelet therapy without high risk of cardiac or cerebrovascular complications, a strategy to temporarily reverse platelet inhibition is desired. Ideally, platelet reactivity could be assessed by light transmittance aggregometry, but this test may be of limited availability, particularly in an emergency setting. If the bleeding risk is high, two to three pools of platelet concentrate should be administered to temporarily assist with clot formation. This strategy has been demonstrated to normalize platelet response in those treated with typical doses of clopidogrel plus aspirin.[55]

Thromboembolism Prophylaxis The risk for venous stasis and subsequent thromboembolic disease increases in the operative period due to vasodilation, inflammation, and immobilization. Most hospitals include the placement of mechanical antithrombotic devices (e.g., sequential compression devices) in the operating room checklist and emphasize placement prior to induction of anesthesia. Pharmacologic methods for deep venous thrombosis (DVT) prophylaxis are often not emphasized preoperatively; however, trials demonstrating heparin efficacy were performed with dosing started 1–2 hours before surgery.[56] Enoxaparin and subcutaneous heparin are therapeutically equivalent for preventing DVT, although renal clearance of enoxaparin makes dosing less predictable in those patients with compromised kidney function.[57] Patients at high risk of bleeding should at least have mechanical methods employed in the operating room.[58]

Endocrine

Hyperglycemia Observational evidence shows that patients with acutely elevated glucose preoperatively fare worse than those who are normoglycemic; however, no trials investigate whether acute correction demonstrates any benefit.[59] In 2001, Van den Berghe et al. published a large randomized controlled trial of surgical intensive care unit patients in which intensive insulin therapy (IIT) (target blood glucose [BG], 80–110 mg/dL) reduced in-hospital mortality by 34% when compared to standard therapy (target BG, 180–200 mg/dL).[60] This finding has been broadly applied and included in perioperative care guidelines, as well as included as a Surgical Care Improvement Project (SCIP) measure. Particular attention has been given to achieving normoglycemia intraoperatively, although results are mixed. Higher incidence of clinically manifest hypoglycemia, in addition to the findings from the NICE-SUGAR trial, has generally called into question the safety of IIT.[61] Guidelines from major societies now advocate a "reasonable, achievable, and safe" approach to tight glucose control acutely.[62]

Diabetic Ketoacidosis Diabetic ketoacidosis (DKA) is a serious diabetic emergency and should be aggressively treated preoperatively. The American Diabetic Association (ADA) defines DKA as glucose > 250 mg per dL, pH < 7.3, serum bicarbonate < 18 mmol per L, anion gap > 10, and presence of ketosis.[63] Typically, an infectious process initiates the process, so the emergency surgery patient with diabetes is at high risk. Treatment consists of aggressive hydration and provision of intravenous insulin. Electrolytes should be monitored every 2 hours, and hypokalemia corrected. When the serum glucose falls below 250 mg per dL, the IV fluid should be changed to 5% dextrose with 0.45% sodium chloride with subsequent glucose goal of 150–200 mg per dL. In the emergency setting, this process should be pursued at least with the goal of providing generous hydration and correction of hypokalemia prior to proceeding to the operating room.

Stress Dose Steroids Patients treated in the long term with exogenous steroids have a blunted hypothalamic–pituitary–adrenal axis response to surgical stress when compared to normal controls. Complete cessation of steroids in the perioperative period for those on long-term treatment can result in a 1%-2% incidence of hypotensive crisis with significant risk of death.[64] Based on these findings, the concept of "stress dose steroids" has been widely applied and is now dogma. There is no evidence that supraphysiologic doses of corticosteroids are necessary to prevent hemodynamic instability however. Numerous studies have failed to demonstrate any difference in perioperative BP when comparing normal steroid dosing with supraphysiologic levels.[65,66] Given the risks of corticosteroids (wound healing, immunosuppression, interaction with anesthetic agents, psychiatric disturbances), the concept of "stress dosing" above the baseline should be reexamined. Current guidelines recommend providing the patient with an intravenous dose equivalent to their baseline until oral medications can be resumed.[67] An important exception to this recommendation is the critically ill patient. Steroid-dependent patients requiring vasopressors should be tested for adrenal insufficiency and started on supraphysiologic doses of 100–150 mg intravenous hydrocortisone daily until hypotension resolves.[68]

Infectious Disease

Sepsis A large percentage of patients undergoing emergency surgery by the general surgeon will have an infectious etiology. For those patients without systemic signs of disease, management is straightforward: source control (surgery) and/or antibiotics. For those patients with sepsis (SIRS plus infection), management requires more skillful resuscitation. Treatment is based on primary source control, with resuscitative efforts to limit systemic inflammatory sequelae. The specifics of sepsis management are discussed later in the chapter as it pertains to intra-abdominal catastrophe.

Surgical Prophylaxis Surgical prophylaxis refers to the administration of antibiotics in the patient with no signs of infection in an effort to reduce the risk of postoperative wound infections. Clean cases in which the gastrointestinal tract, genitourinary tract, or respiratory tract are not entered do not routinely require antibiotic prophylaxis. This is rarely the case for emergency general surgery. Antibiotics should be chosen based on operative site and predominant bacterial flora to that area. Skin flora such as *staphylococci* and *streptococci* should be covered for most cases, with additional coverage of gram-negative flora and anaerobes for cases involving the gastrointestinal tract. Antibiotics should be redosed intraoperatively based on clearance profiles for that drug, as well as for cases in which blood loss is estimated over 1.5 L.

Guidelines from the Joint Commission on Accreditation of Healthcare Organizations (JCAHO) and SCIP provide common recommendations to further limit surgical site infection.[69] Antibiotics should be administered within 1 hour before surgical incision, but should be completed prior to skin incision to achieve maximal tissue penetration. True antibiotic prophylaxis should be completed within 24 hours of the case. Hair at the operative site should be clipped (not shaved). Additionally, hypothermia and hyperglycemia should be avoided. Specific antibiotics for use in general surgery are outlined in Table 8.5.

TABLE 8.5

SURGICAL ANTIMICROBIAL PROPHYLAXIS. COVERAGE FOR GENERAL SURGERY CASES—GASTROINTESTINAL

ANTIBIOTIC	INTRAOPERATIVE REDOSING INTERVAL
Cefotetan 2 g IV	none
Cefoxitin 1 g IV	every 4 h
Cefazolin 2 g IV[a]+	every 4 h
Flagyl 500 mg IV	every 8 h
Ampicillin/Sulbactam 3 g IV	every 6 h
Ertapenem 1 g IV	None
If penicillin allergy:	
Clindamycin 600 mg IV+	every 8 h
Gentamicin 5 mg/kg IV	none

[a]Substitute vancomycin for cefazolin in hospital with high MRSA rate

SPECIAL PATIENT POPULATIONS

Pregnant Patient

This is often one of the more feared patient populations undergoing emergency surgery. While now caring for two patients, the health of the mother takes precedence. Assessment of the pregnant patient with a surgical abdomen should proceed as in any patient, with a few additional concerns. A complete obstetric history should be obtained including issues with the current or prior pregnancies, last menstrual history, and gestational age. Most common causes of abdominal pain are similar to those in the general population and include appendicitis, cholecystitis, and bowel obstruction. Additional consideration should be given to those diagnoses more specific to pregnancy including ruptured ectopic pregnancy, abruptio placentae, rupture of uterus, preeclampsia, as well as pyelonephritis and rupture of visceral aneurysms.

Evaluation must be performed with an understanding of the physiologic changes that occur at varying points during pregnancy (Table 8.6).[70] Adjuncts to the physical exam include fetal heart tone monitoring and inclusion of a sterile speculum exam. Fetal heart tones should be continuously monitored pre- and postoperatively starting at 24 weeks of gestation. Mental status changes or seizures should prompt consideration for a diagnosis of eclampsia.

Expeditious and accurate diagnosis should take precedence over concerns for ionizing radiation when further workup is needed. Ultrasound is safe with a relatively high sensitivity and specificity for many intra-abdominal processes. This is also the test of choice for most gynecologic causes of abdominal pain. Use of ionizing radiation should be based on further need for diagnosis, and cumulative dosage should be limited to 5–10 rads during the first 25 weeks' gestation with no single dose exceeding 5 rads.[71] An abdominal/pelvis CT scan provides 5–10 rads of exposure; however, risk versus benefit of the scan should be considered. MRI without gadolinium is also considered safe in pregnancy, but time necessary to obtain such a scan should be considered in the workup and resuscitation.

Once in the operating room, additional considerations are necessary for the pregnant patient. Diminished maternal oxygen reserve and high risk for aspiration make early intubation essential. Aggressive fluid management should dominate the resuscitation, with use of vasopressors limited to phenylephrine due to its limited effects on uteroplacental perfusion. To assist with venous return, the patient should be positioned in left lateral position to move the fetus off of the vena cava. The coordination of care with an obstetrician is imperative. An obstetrician can assess fetal status, provide consultation for medication provision, assist if gynecologic or obstetric-related disease is found, and decide when emergent Caesarean section is required.

Morbidly Obese Patient

The preoperative evaluation and management of the morbidly obese (MB) patient requiring emergency surgery is challenging.[72] The first issue is making the correct diagnosis. Physical examination, plain radiography, and ultrasonography are notoriously inaccurate, and many of the super obese are too big to fit into the CT scanner. Once the decision to operate has been made, there are a variety of issues unique to this population. BP measurement by sphygmomanometry frequently overestimates BP, and an MB patient who has a normal BP may have occult hypoperfusion. Arterial lines are therefore recommended but difficult to place. Additionally, central venous catheters are frequently needed, but placement is cumbersome and risky. Airway management is especially problematic, and early consultation with an anesthesiologist is recommended.

TABLE 8.6

PHYSIOLOGIC CHANGES IN PREGNANCY

CARDIAC	PULMONARY	HEMATOLOGY
↑ cardiac output by 50%	↑ oxygen consumption by 20%	↑ blood volume by 50%
↓ blood pressure 5–15 mm Hg	↑ tidal volume	↑RBC volume by 30%
↑ heart rate by 15 bpm	↓functional reserve capacity	↓ hematocrit to 32%-34%
↓ systemic vascular resistance	↑ respiratory rate	
↓ central venous pressure	↑ PaO_2 to 104–108 mm hg	

Dosing of drugs is problematic because of the high volume of distribution and increased percentage of adipose tissue. Surgical site infections are much more common in the MB, but little is known about optimal dosing of antibiotics in emergency surgery.[73] In general, antibiotic dosing should be based on a 40% correction factor.[74] Adjusted body weight is calculated by the following formula: adjusted body weight = ideal body weight + 0.4 × (actual body weight – ideal body weight). It is also felt that more frequent dosing is required for prophylaxis against gram-negative organisms.[75] Consultation with a pharmacist or an infectious disease specialist, close drug level monitoring (when available), and dosing interval determination based on creatinine clearance are recommended.

MB patients experience appreciably higher rates of postoperative complications. They have a notably high risk for cardiac complications and should be managed as outlined in Table 8.4. It is important to remember that many MB patients have significant pulmonary hypertension that puts them at risk for right heart failure. MB patients are also at high risk to develop pulmonary complication and should be managed as outlined in Table 8.3. DVT and pulmonary embolism are major concerns with most data extrapolated from elective bariatric surgery patients.[76] There is no consensus on optimal dosing of heparin or whether to use unfractionated or low molecular weight heparin. A recent study recommended 7,500 units of unfractionated heparin three times daily for patients with a BMI > 50 and 5,000 units of unfractionated heparin three times daily for patients with a BMI < 50.[77] Finally, MB patients require unique equipment for their operation including bigger OR tables, lifts, and longer instruments.

Septic Shock Patients Requiring Emergency Laparotomy

The mortality of these patients has traditionally exceeded 40%, but more recently with the broader application of "damage control" laparotomy, the mortality has been reduced substantially.[78] The rationale for utilizing damage control in septic shock is different from traumatic shock. In traumatic shock, damage control is used when there is severe bleeding and the patient is at risk of entering the "bloody viscous cycle" (i.e., hypothermia, acidosis, and hypothermia), which leads to exsanguination and death. This type of bleeding is generally not a problem when operating on septic shock patients. As depicted in Algorithm 8.1, the problem in septic shock is that the patient presents in a persistent septic shock cycle that can progress to fulminant multiple organ failure (MOF) if nothing is done. They are too ill to tolerate a general anesthetic and need preoperative optimization prior to proceeding to the OR. Optimal timing of OR source control is not known; expert opinion guideline recommendations are that it should be completed by 6 hours.[79] The goal is to quickly optimize the patient, perform a rapid operative intervention for source control to break the cycle, and then return to the ICU for completion of resuscitation.

Preoperative optimization of septic shock can be protocolized based on recommendations by the Surviving Sepsis Campaign.[78] Intravenous volume resuscitation is initiated as measured by urine output and CVP. A fluid bolus of 20 mL per kg of lactated Ringer's should be given initially, with CVP pushed to >8 mm Hg. Norepinephrine is administered to maintain MAP > 65 mmHg. Further fluid boluses (up to a CVP of 12 mm Hg) are given to insure adequate urine output (>0.05 mL/kg), and weaning of the norepinephrine is attempted. Low-dose vasopressin is started in patients requiring persistent high doses of norepinephrine. Broad-spectrum antimicrobial agents (Table 8.7) should be infused within 1 hour.[80] Adrenal function is tested, and steroids are administered if relative adrenal insufficiency is proven. It usually takes 2–3 hours to optimize the patient prior to proceeding to the OR. As the operation begins, the decision is made on whether damage control is going to be utilized. Indications are persistent septic shock (most frequent), myocardial ischemia or serious arrhythmia, and critical hypoxia.

The goals of damage control are to (1) resect dead bowel, (2) limit ongoing contamination, (3) control bleeding (pack as necessary), and (4) have limited irrigation followed by temporary abdominal closure with a vacuum-assisted devise. The patient is returned to the ICU for continued resuscitation, optimization ventilation, rewarming, correction of

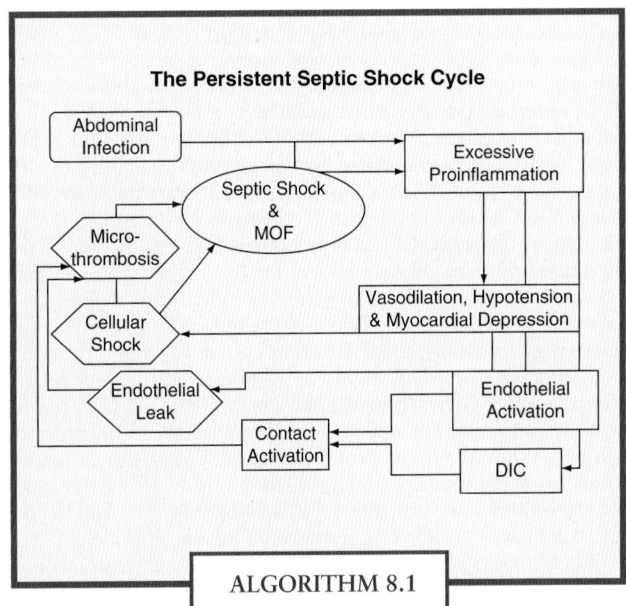

ALGORITHM 8.1 The persistent septic shock cycle.

TABLE 8.7

ANTIBIOTIC RECOMMENDATIONS BASED ON SUSPECTED SITE OF INFECTION

SUSPECTED SITE OF INFECTION	FIRST-LINE DRUG REGIMEN	SECOND-LINE DRUG REGIMEN
CAP	Ceftriaxone 1 g IV every 24 h ± azithromycin 500 mg IV/PO every 24 h	Levofloxacin 750 mg IV every 24 h
Suspected aspiration	CAP regimen + clindamycin 600 mg IV every 8 h or change ceftriaxone to piperacillin/tazobactam 4.5 g IV every 6 h	
Early VAP (<5 d)	Cefepime 2 g IV every 24 h	
Late VAP (pseudomonal risk)	Cefepime 2 g IV every 24 h + Vancomycin 15 mg/kg IV every 12 h + tobramycin 7 mg/kg IV	Ciprofloxacin 400 mg IV every 12 h + vancomycin 15 mg/kg IV every 12 h + tobramycin 7 mg/kg IV
UTI/urosepsis	Piperacillin/tazobactam 4.5 g IV every 6 h	Ciprofloxacin 400 mg IV every 12 h
Line infection	Remove line + vancomycin 1 g IV every 12 h + fluconazole 800 mg IV every 24 h (if risk for candidemia)	
Necrotizing fasciitis	Piperacillin/tazobactam 4.5 g IV every 6 h + vancomycin 15 mg/kg IV every 12 h + clindamycin 900 mg IV every 8 h	Ciprofloxacin 400 mg IV every 12 h + vancomycin 15 mg/kg IV every 12 h + clindamycin 900 mg IV every 8 h
Surgical site infections	Piperacillin/tazobactam 4.5 g IV every 6 h + vancomycin 15 mg/kg IV every 12 h	Ciprofloxacin 400 mg IV every 12 h + vancomycin 15 mg/kg IV every 12 h
Intra-abdominal	Imipenem/cilastatin 500 mg IV every 6 h + vancomycin 15 mg/kg IV every 12 h ± fluconazole 800 mg IV every 24 h	Ciprofloxacin 400 mg IV every 12 h + metronidazole 500 mg IV every 8 h + vancomycin 15 mg/kg IV every 12 h + fluconazole 800 mg IV every 24 h

NOTE: All doses are based on normal renal/hepatic function.
IV, intravenous; PO, per mouth.

coagulopathy, monitoring of bladder pressures, and implementation of routine ICU care (e.g., stress gastritis prophylaxis, DVT prophylaxis, tight glucose control, lung protective ventilation). After stabilization (usually within 24 hours), the patient is returned to the OR for definitive surgery and abdominal wall closure.

Cirrhotic Patient

The mortality rate for emergency surgery in a cirrhotic patient is prohibitive. Consequently, the first question is to determine whether operative intervention is really needed. Individual patient risk can be estimated by calculating the Child-Turcott-Pugh Score (Table 8.8).[81] Estimated mortality rate for emergency surgery in Class A (5 or 6 points) patients is 10%, in class B (7–9 points) is 30%, and in Class C (> 9 points) exceeds 80%.[82] Given that bleeding is major risk of operating on cirrhotic patients, correction of coagulopathy is imperative.[83] Vitamin K deficiency is common in cirrhotic patients due to malnutrition, and single dose of 10 mg is recommended. This is not going to help in the short run, and therefore, FFP should be administered to lower INR < 1.6 if feasible. Given the short half-life of factor VII (3–5 hours) in FFP, additional FFP will need to be administered just prior to surgery. Point-of-care measures such as TEG analysis can guide transfusion of plasma product, reducing considerably the amount of FFP required for hemostasis.[84] If fibrinogen levels < 100 mg per dL, administer 10 units of cryoprecipitate, and if platelet count < 20,000/mm^3, administer 6 units of platelets. 1-Deamino-8-D-arginine vasopressin (DDAVP) can improve platelet function by releasing large amounts of von Willebrand factor and should be considered in cases of refractory coagulopathy.

Hypovolemia contributes to hypoperfusion with worsening hepatic function and AKI setting the stage for MOF and death. On the other hand, hypervolemia will contribute to worsening of postoperative pulmonary dysfunction (due to increased pulmonary edema and effusion) and ascites. Therefore, a central venous catheter in the internal jugular vein should be placed under ultrasound guidance. Recognizing the limitations of a single CVP measurement in assessing volume status, it is important to follow the trends in the CVP with volume loading. Additionally, because high-risk cirrhotic patients have lower BP due to vasodilation, placement of a radial arterial

TABLE 8.8

CHILD-TURCOTTE-PUGH (CTP) SCORE TO ASSESS SEVERITY OF CIRRHOSIS

	POINTS		
PARAMETER	1	2	3
Total bilirubin (mg/dL)	<2	2–3	>3
Serum albumin (g/dL)	>3.5	2.8–3.5	<2.8
INR	<1.7	1.71–2.20	>2.20
Ascites	None	Medication control	Refractory
Encephalopathy	None	Grade I-II	Grade III-IV

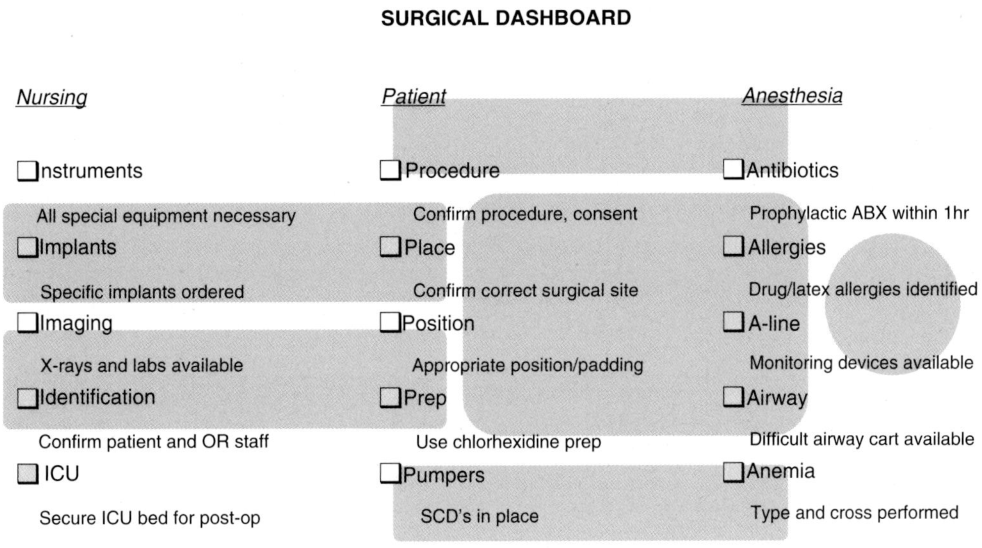

SURGICAL DASHBOARD

Nursing	*Patient*	*Anesthesia*
☐ Instruments	☐ Procedure	☐ Antibiotics
All special equipment necessary	Confirm procedure, consent	Prophylactic ABX within 1hr
☐ Implants	☐ Place	☐ Allergies
Specific implants ordered	Confirm correct surgical site	Drug/latex allergies identified
☐ Imaging	☐ Position	☐ A-line
X-rays and labs available	Appropriate position/padding	Monitoring devices available
☐ Identification	☐ Prep	☐ Airway
Confirm patient and OR staff	Use chlorhexidine prep	Difficult airway cart available
☐ ICU	☐ Pumpers	☐ Anemia
Secure ICU bed for post-op	SCD's in place	Type and cross performed

FIGURE 8.1. Operating room dashboard

line for more accurate BP measurement is prudent, and norepinephrine should be used to maintain a MAP > 60 mm Hg. In the mechanically ventilated patient, a minimally invasive monitor can be used to assess stroke volume variation and cardiac output.[85]

In regard to volume loading, crystalloid with high sodium content should be avoided to minimize postoperative ascites. However, cirrhotic patients who are hyponatremic and have a metabolic alkalosis may benefit from some normal saline during the preoperative period. Of note, FFP and pRBCs transfusions are good volume expanders and should be administered if indicated. Albumin is another option for volume expansion for the cirrhotic with hypoproteinemia. The last consideration is appropriate antibiotics. The cirrhotic patient should be considered an immunocompromised host and should receive extended prophylaxis for fungal infection. Given the high risk of AKI, aminoglycosides should be avoided.

THE OPERATING ROOM

Smooth transition from preoperative resuscitation to operating room to recovery requires thorough communication with the surgical team and anticipation of a myriad of problems. When possible, the surgeon should make a preemptive trip to the operating room to check the physical properties of the room and discuss the patient with the nursing and anesthesia staff. Careful attention should be paid to the temperature of the room, availability of special equipment (hemostatic agents, retractors, wound management systems, stapling devices, etc.), and positioning of the table. This is particularly important for off-hours cases in which available staff may not be familiar with equipment typical to general cases. If at all possible, involve the help of consulting surgeons or other physicians earlier rather than later. This includes specialty services such as gynecology, urology, orthopedics, vascular surgery, or interventional radiology. The operating room is a high-risk area for communication failure. The team must function at a high level to avoid undue harm to the patient, particularly in an emergency situation. Checklists have been devised to verify clinical information and confirm that specific preventative measures have been taken. The use of checklists before surgery can improve patient outcomes, operating room efficiency, and patient safety indicators.[86,87] We have devised a surgical dashboard that contains essential elements of emergency general surgery (Fig. 8.1).

CONCLUSION

Caring for the emergency surgical patient can be a challenging but rewarding experience. Good resuscitation principles are essential, but so too is the ability to obtain details thorough secondary examination. Basic components of preparation include shock resuscitation, early interventions with appropriate medication, coagulopathy reversal, and appreciation for cardiopulmonary disease, which may require a more nuanced approach. Adequate preparation can help avoid common pitfalls in the operating room. More importantly, attention to these early interventions can improve the ultimate outcome for patients.

References

1. Bone RC, Balk RA, Cerra FB, et al. Definitions for sepsis and organ failure and guidelines for the use of innovative therapies in sepsis. The ACCP/SCCM Consensus Conference Committee. American College of Chest Physicians/Society of Critical Care Medicine. *Chest*. 1992;101(6):1644–1655.
2. Moore LJ, Jones SL, Kreiner LA, et al. Validation of a screening tool for the early identification of sepsis. *J Trauma*. 2009;66(6):1539–1546; discussion 1546–1547.
3. Tekwani KL, Watts HF, Sweis RT, et al. A comparison of the effects of etomidate and midazolam on hospital length of stay in patients with suspected sepsis: a prospective, randomized study. *Ann Emerg Med*. 2010;56(5):481–489.
4. Warner KJ, Cuschieri J, Jurkovich GJ, et al. Single-dose etomidate for rapid sequence intubation may impact outcome after severe injury. *J Trauma*. 2009;67(1):45–50.
5. Pascual JL, Maloney-Wilensky E, Reilly PM, et al. Resuscitation of hypotensive head-injured patients: is hypertonic saline the answer? *Am Surg*. 2008;74(3):253–259.
6. Finfer S, Bellomo R, Boyce N, et al. A comparison of albumin and saline for fluid resuscitation in the intensive care unit. *N Engl J Med*. 2004;350(22):2247–2256.
7. Schortgen F, Lacherade JC, Bruneel F, et al. Effects of hydroxyethylstarch and gelatin on renal function in severe sepsis: a multicentre randomised study. *Lancet*. 2001;357(9260):911–916.
8. Franz A, Bräunlich P, Gamsjäger T, et al. The effects of hydroxyethyl starches of varying molecular weights on platelet function. *Anesth Analg*. 2001;92(6):1402–1407.
9. van de Watering LM, Hermans J, Houbiers JG, et al. Beneficial effects of leukocyte depletion of transfused blood on postoperative complications in

patients undergoing cardiac surgery: a randomized clinical trial. *Circulation.* 1998;97(6):562–568.

10. Plotkin AJ, Wade CE, Jenkins DH, et al. A reduction in clot formation rate and strength assessed by thrombelastography is indicative of transfusion requirements in patients with penetrating injuries. *J Trauma.* 2008;64 (2 suppl):S64–S68.
11. Bickell WH, Wall MJ, Pepe PE, et al. Immediate versus delayed fluid resuscitation for hypotensive patients with penetrating torso injuries. *N Engl J Med.* 1994;331(17):1105–1109.
12. Müllner M, Urbanek B, Havel C, et al. Vasopressors for shock. *Cochrane Database Syst Rev.* 2004;(3):CD003709.
13. Bendjelid K, Romand J. Fluid responsiveness in mechanically ventilated patients: a review of indices used in intensive care. *Intensive Care Med.* 2003;29(3):352–360.
14. Hata JS, Stotts C, Shelsky C, et al. Reduced mortality with noninvasive hemodynamic monitoring of shock. *J Crit Care.* 2011;26(2):224.e1–e8.
15. Reinhart K, Kuhn H, Hartog C, et al. Continuous central venous and pulmonary artery oxygen saturation monitoring in the critically ill. *Intensive Care Med.* 2004;30(8):1572–1578.
16. Nguyen HB, Rivers EP, Knoblich BP, et al. Early lactate clearance is associated with improved outcome in severe sepsis and septic shock. *Crit Care Med.* 2004;32(8):1637–1642.
17. Rixen D, Raum M, Bouillon B, et al. Base deficit development and its prognostic significance in posttrauma critical illness: an analysis by the trauma registry of the Deutsche Gesellschaft für unfallchirurgie. *Shock.* 2001;15(2):83–89.
18. Santora RJ, Moore FA. Monitoring trauma and intensive care unit resuscitation with tissue hemoglobin oxygen saturation. *Crit Care.* 2009;13(suppl 5):S10.
19. Spies C, Eggers V, Szabo G, et al. Intervention at the level of the neuroendocrine-immune axis and postoperative pneumonia rate in long-term alcoholics. *Am J Respir Crit Care Med.* 2006;174(4):408–414.
20. Møller AM, Villebro N, Pedersen T, et al. Effect of preoperative smoking intervention on postoperative complications: a randomised clinical trial. *Lancet.* 2002;359(9301):114–117.
21. Gowing L, Farrell M, Ali R, et al. Alpha2-adrenergic agonists for the management of opioid withdrawal. *Cochrane Database Syst Rev.* 2009;(2):CD002024.
22. Ranji SR, Goldman LE, Simel DL, et al. Do opiates affect the clinical evaluation of patients with acute abdominal pain? *JAMA.* 2006;296(14):1764–1774.
23. Smetana GW, Lawrence VA, Cornell JE. Preoperative pulmonary risk stratification for noncardiothoracic surgery: systematic review for the American College of Physicians. *Ann Intern Med.* 2006;144(8):581–595.
24. Canet J, Gallart L, Gomar C, et al. Prediction of postoperative pulmonary complications in a population-based surgical cohort. *Anesthesiology.* 2010;113(6):1338–1350.
25. Ventilation with lower tidal volumes as compared with traditional tidal volumes for acute lung injury and the acute respiratory distress syndrome. The Acute Respiratory Distress Syndrome Network. *N Engl J Med.* 2000;342(18):1301–1308.
26. Gajic O, Dara SI, Mendez JL, et al. Ventilator-associated lung injury in patients without acute lung injury at the onset of mechanical ventilation. *Crit Care Med.* 2004;32(9):1817–1824.
27. Pinheiro de Oliveira R, Hetzel MP, dos Anjos Silva M, et al. Mechanical ventilation with high tidal volume induces inflammation in patients without lung disease. *Crit Care.* 2010;14(2):R39.
28. Antman EM, Hand M, Armstrong PW, et al. 2007 focused update of the ACC/AHA 2004 guidelines for the management of patients with ST-elevation myocardial infarction: a report of the American College of Cardiology/American Heart Association Task Force on Practice Guidelines. *J Am Coll Cardiol.* 2008 15;51(2):210–247.
29. Marik PE, Varon J. Perioperative hypertension: a review of current and emerging therapeutic agents. *J Clin Anesth.* 2009;21(3):220–229.
30. Mangano DT, Layug EL, Wallace A, et al. Effect of atenolol on mortality and cardiovascular morbidity after noncardiac surgery. Multicenter Study of Perioperative Ischemia Research Group. *N Engl J Med.* 1996;335(23):1713–1720.
31. Poldermans D, Boersma E, Bax JJ, et al. The effect of bisoprolol on perioperative mortality and myocardial infarction in high-risk patients undergoing vascular surgery. Dutch Echocardiographic Cardiac Risk Evaluation Applying Stress Echocardiography Study Group. *N Engl J Med.* 1999;341(24):1789–1794.
32. Eagle KA, Berger PB, Calkins H, et al. ACC/AHA guideline update for perioperative cardiovascular evaluation for noncardiac surgery—executive summary a report of the American College of Cardiology/American Heart Association Task Force on Practice Guidelines (Committee to Update the 1996 Guidelines on Perioperative Cardiovascular Evaluation for Noncardiac Surgery). *Circulation.* 2002;105(10):1257–1267.
33. Yang H, Raymer K, Butler R, et al. The effects of perioperative beta-blockade: results of the Metoprolol after Vascular Surgery (MaVS) study, a randomized controlled trial. *Am Heart J.* 2006;152(5):983–990.
34. Juul AB, Wetterslev J, Gluud C, et al. Effect of perioperative beta blockade in patients with diabetes undergoing major non-cardiac surgery: randomised placebo controlled, blinded multicentre trial. *BMJ.* 2006;332(7556):1482.
35. Brady AR, Gibbs JSR, Greenhalgh RM, et al. Perioperative beta-blockade (POBBLE) for patients undergoing infrarenal vascular surgery: results of a randomized double-blind controlled trial. *J Vasc Surg.* 2005;41(4): 602–609.
36. Devereaux PJ, Yang H, Yusuf S, et al. Effects of extended-release metoprolol succinate in patients undergoing non-cardiac surgery (POISE trial): a randomised controlled trial. *Lancet.* 2008;371(9627):1839–1847.
37. Lindenauer PK, Pekow P, Wang K, et al. Perioperative beta-blocker therapy and mortality after major noncardiac surgery. *N Engl J Med.* 2005;353(4):349–361.
38. Fleisher LA, Beckman JA, Brown KA, et al. ACC/AHA 2007 guidelines on perioperative cardiovascular evaluation and care for noncardiac surgery: a report of the American College of Cardiology/American Heart Association Task Force on Practice Guidelines (Writing Committee to Revise the 2002 Guidelines on Perioperative Cardiovascular Evaluation for Noncardiac Surgery): developed in collaboration with the American Society of Echocardiography, American Society of Nuclear Cardiology, Heart Rhythm Society, Society of Cardiovascular Anesthesiologists, Society for Cardiovascular Angiography and Interventions, Society for Vascular Medicine and Biology, and Society for Vascular Surgery. *Circulation.* 2007;116(17):e418–e499.
39. Fonarow GC, Abraham WT, Albert NM, et al. Influence of beta-blocker continuation or withdrawal on outcomes in patients hospitalized with heart failure: findings from the OPTIMIZE-HF program. *J Am Coll Cardiol.* 2008;52(3):190–199.
40. Groban L, Butterworth J. Perioperative management of chronic heart failure. *Anesth Analg.* 2006;103(3):557–575.
41. Sear JW, Howell SJ, Sear YM, et al. Intercurrent drug therapy and perioperative cardiovascular mortality in elective and urgent/emergency surgical patientst. *Br J Anaesth.* 2001;86(4):506–512.
42. Neumar RW, Otto CW, Link MS, et al. Part 8: adult advanced cardiovascular life support: 2010 American Heart Association Guidelines for Cardiopulmonary Resuscitation and Emergency Cardiovascular Care. *Circulation.* 2010;122(18 suppl 3):S729–S767.
43. Kallet RH, Liu K, Tang J. Management of acidosis during lung-protective ventilation in acute respiratory distress syndrome. *Respir Care Clin N Am.* 2003;9(4):437–456.
44. Sykes E, Cosgrove JF. Acute renal failure and the critically ill surgical patient. *Ann R Coll Surg Engl.* 2007;89(1):22–29.
45. Mangano CM, Diamondstone LS, Ramsay JG, et al. Renal dysfunction after myocardial revascularization: risk factors, adverse outcomes, and hospital resource utilization. The Multicenter Study of Perioperative Ischemia Research Group. *Ann Intern Med.* 1998;128(3):194–203.
46. Brienza N, Giglio MT, Marucci M, et al. Does perioperative hemodynamic optimization protect renal function in surgical patients? A meta-analytic study. *Crit Care Med.* 2009;37(6):2079–2090.
47. Barrett BJ, Parfrey PS. Clinical practice. Preventing nephropathy induced by contrast medium. *N Engl J Med.* 2006;354(4):379–386.
48. Zoungas S, Ninomiya T, Huxley R, et al. Systematic review: sodium bicarbonate treatment regimens for the prevention of contrast-induced nephropathy. *Ann Intern Med.* 2009;151(9):631–638.
49. Ivatury RR, Porter JM, Simon RJ, et al. Intra-abdominal hypertension after life-threatening penetrating abdominal trauma: prophylaxis, incidence, and clinical relevance to gastric mucosal pH and abdominal compartment syndrome. *J Trauma.* 1998;44(6):1016–1021; discussion 1021–1023.
50. Hébert PC, Wells G, Blajchman MA, et al. A multicenter, randomized, controlled clinical trial of transfusion requirements in critical care. Transfusion Requirements in Critical Care Investigators, Canadian Critical Care Trials Group. *N Engl J Med.* 1999;340(6):409–417.
51. Hébert PC, Yetisir E, Martin C, et al. Is a low transfusion threshold safe in critically ill patients with cardiovascular diseases? *Crit Care Med.* 2001;29(2):227–234.
52. Wu W, Schifftner TL, Henderson WG, et al. Preoperative hematocrit levels and postoperative outcomes in older patients undergoing noncardiac surgery. *JAMA.* 2007;297(22):2481–2488.
53. Hajjar LA, Vincent J, Galas FRBG, et al. Transfusion requirements after cardiac surgery: the TRACS randomized controlled trial. *JAMA.* 2010;304(14):1559–1567.
54. Thachil J, Gatt A, Martlew V. Management of surgical patients receiving anticoagulation and antiplatelet agents. *Br J Surg.* 2008;95(12):1437–1448.
55. Vilahur G, Choi BG, Zafar MU, et al. Normalization of platelet reactivity in clopidogrel-treated subjects. *J Thromb Haemost.* 2007;5(1):82–90.
56. Collins R, Scrimgeour A, Yusuf S, et al. Reduction in fatal pulmonary embolism and venous thrombosis by perioperative administration of subcutaneous heparin. Overview of results of randomized trials in general, orthopedic, and urologic surgery. *N Engl J Med.* 1988;318(18):1162–1173.
57. Geerts WH, Bergqvist D, Pineo GF, et al. Prevention of venous thromboembolism: American College of Chest Physicians Evidence-Based Clinical Practice Guidelines (8th Edition). *Chest.* 2008;133(6 suppl):381S–453S.
58. Geerts WH, Bergqvist D, Pineo GF, et al. Prevention of venous thromboembolism: American College of Chest Physicians Evidence-Based Clinical Practice Guidelines (8th Edition). *Chest.* 2008;133(6 suppl):381S–453S.
59. Noordzij PG, Boersma E, Schreiner F, et al. Increased preoperative glucose levels are associated with perioperative mortality in patients undergoing noncardiac, nonvascular surgery. *Eur J Endocrinol.* 2007;156(1):137–142.
60. van den Berghe G, Wouters P, Weekers F, et al. Intensive insulin therapy in the critically ill patients. *N Engl J Med.* 2001;345(19):1359–1367.

61. Finfer S, Chittock DR, Su SY, et al. Intensive versus conventional glucose control in critically ill patients. *N Engl J Med*. 2009;360(13):1283–1297.
62. Moghissi ES, Korytkowski MT, DiNardo M, et al. American Association of Clinical Endocrinologists and American Diabetes Association consensus statement on inpatient glycemic control. *Endocr Pract*. 2009;15(4):353–369.
63. Kitabchi AE, Umpierrez GE, Murphy MB, et al. Hyperglycemic crises in diabetes. *Diabetes Care*. 2004;27(suppl 1):S94–S102.
64. Knudsen L, Christiansen LA, Lorentzen JE. Hypotension during and after operation in glucocorticoid-treated patients. *Br J Anaesth*. 1981;53(3):295–301.
65. Glowniak JV, Loriaux DL. A double-blind study of perioperative steroid requirements in secondary adrenal insufficiency. *Surgery*. 1997;121(2):123–129.
66. Bromberg JS, Baliga P, Cofer JB, et al. Stress steroids are not required for patients receiving a renal allograft and undergoing operation. *J Am Coll Surg*. 1995;180(5):532–536.
67. Brown CJ, Buie WD. Perioperative stress dose steroids: do they make a difference? *J Am Coll Surg*. 2001;193(6):678–686.
68. Lamberts SW, Bruining HA, de Jong FH. Corticosteroid therapy in severe illness. *N Engl J Med*. 1997;337(18):1285–1292.
69. Gagliardi AR, Fenech D, Eskicioglu C, et al. Factors influencing antibiotic prophylaxis for surgical site infection prevention in general surgery: a review of the literature. *Can J Surg*. 2009;52(6):481–489.
70. Hill CC, Pickinpaugh J. Trauma and surgical emergencies in the obstetric patient. *Surg Clin North Am*. 2008;88(2):421–440, viii.
71. Karam PA. Determining and reporting fetal radiation exposure from diagnostic radiation. Health Phys. 2000;79(5 suppl):S85–90.
72. King DR, Velmahos GC. Difficulties in managing the surgical patient who is morbidly obese. *Crit Care Med*. 2010;38(9 suppl):S478–S482.
73. Forse RA, Karam B, MacLean LD, et al. Antibiotic prophylaxis for surgery in morbidly obese patients. *Surgery*. 1989;106(4):750–756; discussion 756–757.
74. Pai MP, Bearden DT. Antimicrobial dosing considerations in obese adult patients. *Pharmacotherapy*. 2007;27(8):1081–1091.
75. Barbour A, Schmidt S, Rout WR, et al. Soft tissue penetration of cefuroxime determined by clinical microdialysis in morbidly obese patients undergoing abdominal surgery. *Int J Antimicrob Agents*. 2009;34(3):231–235.
76. Prystowsky JB, Morasch MD, Eskandari MK, et al. Prospective analysis of the incidence of deep venous thrombosis in bariatric surgery patients. *Surgery*. 2005;138(4):759–763; discussion 763–765.
77. Miller MT, Rovito PF. An approach to venous thromboembolism prophylaxis in laparoscopic Roux-en-Y gastric bypass surgery. *Obes Surg*. 2004;14(6):731–737.
78. Dellinger RP, Levy MM, Carlet JM, et al. Surviving Sepsis Campaign: international guidelines for management of severe sepsis and septic shock: 2008. *Crit Care Med*. 2008;36(1):296–327.
79. Moore LJ, Turner KL, Todd SR, et al. Computerized clinical decision support improves mortality in intra abdominal surgical sepsis. *Am J Surg*. 2010;200(6):839–843; discussion 843–844.
80. Fitousis K, Moore LJ, Hall J, et al. Evaluation of empiric antibiotic use in surgical sepsis. *Am J Surg*. 2010;200(6):776–782; discussion 782.
81. Farnsworth N, Fagan SP, Berger DH, et al. Child-Turcotte-Pugh versus MELD score as a predictor of outcome after elective and emergent surgery in cirrhotic patients. *Am J Surg*. 2004;188(5):580–583.
82. Mansour A, Watson W, Shayani V, et al. Abdominal operations in patients with cirrhosis: still a major surgical challenge. *Surgery*. 1997;122(4): 730–735; discussion 735–736.
83. Wu CC, Yeh DC, Lin MC, et al. Improving operative safety for cirrhotic liver resection. *Br J Surg*. 2001;88(2):210–215.
84. Wang S, Shieh J, Chang K, et al. Thromboelastography-guided transfusion decreases intraoperative blood transfusion during orthotopic liver transplantation: randomized clinical trial. *Transplant Proc*. 2010;42(7): 2590–2593.
85. Hofer CK, Senn A, Weibel L, et al. Assessment of stroke volume variation for prediction of fluid responsiveness using the modified FloTrac and PiCCOplus system. *Crit Care*. 2008;12(3):R82.
86. Haynes AB, Weiser TG, Berry WR, et al A surgical safety checklist to reduce morbidity and mortality in a global population. *N Engl J Med*. 2009;360(5):491–499.
87. Paull DE, Mazzia LM, Wood SD, et al. Briefing guide study: preoperative briefing and postoperative debriefing checklists in the Veterans Health Administration medical team training program. *Am J Surg*. 2010;200(5):620–623.

CHAPTER 9 ■ DIAGNOSTIC IMAGING IN ACUTE CARE SURGERY

BEHROZE A. VACHHA, LEO L. TSAI, KAREN S. LEE, AND MARC A. CAMACHO

The management of acute care surgical patients, as that of all patients, has largely benefited by advances in radiology. Current imaging techniques and modalities have vastly improved the ability to noninvasively diagnose and characterize disease and injury, which has largely supplanted the need for invasive exploratory surgery. Almost equally important, imaging can reliably exclude severe illness or injury in the acute presentation. This has resulted, for example, in a major shift in the management of trauma patients, in particular, with a greater emphasis on conservative management and reduction in the attendant morbidity and mortality introduced by surgical intervention and perisurgical (e.g. ICU) care.

There is a vast array of imaging modalities in the diagnostic armamentarium currently. While radiography, angiography, and nuclear medicine have undergone advances in their own right, the advances in magnetic resonance imaging (MRI), ultrasound (US), and, in particular, computed tomography (CT) have resulted in a major expansion in applications and extraordinary increases in utilization. This has led to justified concerns regarding health care costs, the need for outcomes research, and potential deleterious effects introduced by the imaging modalities themselves (e.g. radiation dose and CT). However, these imaging modalities each exhibit unique advantages that can be exploited for specific indications to help increase accuracy of, and decrease delays in, diagnosis. Additionally, these modalities also may have associated relative and absolute contraindications, which should be considered when considering utilization for a particular patient and clinical scenario.

In this chapter, we present these three imaging modalities in detail, introduce basic background concepts, and detail advantages and disadvantages as well as optimal target patient populations, clinical scenarios, and indications. Each subsection concludes with a gallery of images representing commonly encountered acute care surgical pathology, with detailed captions.

ULTRASOUND

Ultrasound is one of the most utilized and widespread diagnostic imaging modalities in medicine. Ultrasound images are generated by transmitting an ultrasonic pulse and detecting the amplitudes and delay times from returning acoustical echoes reflecting off of tissue interfaces. Typical operating frequencies range from 2 to 12 MHz. The major advantages of this modality include the ability to perform real-time noninvasive imaging without the use of ionizing radiation, its high degree of portability, its relatively low cost, and the capability to acquire images in an infinite number of planes. Additionally, by evaluating Doppler frequency shifts from moving blood, ultrasound can provide blood flow information by producing arterial or venous waveforms and quantitatively measuring blood flow velocities.

Ultrasound is particularly well suited to evaluate the abdomen and pelvis, owing to excellent acoustical windows provided by the liver, spleen, and bladder. The liver window provides a view of the gallbladder, pancreas, right kidney, heart, and right pleural space. The spleen is used to image the left kidney and left pleural space. A full bladder can allow a thorough assessment of the uterus and adnexa. Transvaginal, transrectal, transesophageal, and endoscopic probes are also available for more detailed imaging of the pelvis, prostate, rectum, heart, upper gastrointestinal tract, and pancreas. Ultrasound is also the primary imaging method used for assessment of the fetus, as no ionizing radiation or contrast materials are required, and the transmitted acoustic energy in typical obstetric examinations is accepted as safe.[1] Furthermore, thoracentesis,[2] paracentesis, superficial abscess drainage, percutaneous cholecystostomy, and other minimally invasive bedside procedures are commonly performed under real-time ultrasound guidance.

Common uses of ultrasound in the acute surgical setting include evaluation for acute cholecystitis (Fig. 9.1),[4–6] renal obstruction or calculi (Fig. 9.2), vascular occlusion,[7] ovarian or testicular torsion (Fig. 9.3),[9,10] and appendicitis (Fig. 9.4).[11] Because of its portability and real-time imaging capability, ultrasound is also often employed in the trauma setting to assess patients who may be too unstable for a CT examination. Ultrasound can readily evaluate for solid organ injury within the liver, spleen, and kidneys. Additionally, the Focused Assessment with Sonography for Trauma (FAST) exam is a common bedside ultrasound study used to detect free fluid within the peritoneal, pericardial, and pleural spaces as a first-step measure to identify an internal hemorrhage (Fig. 9.5).[13–15]

Drawbacks of ultrasound include its limited ability to assess the brain, thorax, and bowel due to the presence of tissue–air and tissue–bone interfaces that are nearly completely acoustically reflective and therefore prevent the penetration of ultrasound waves. Ultrasound imaging of obese patients is also challenging, often resulting in low-quality images due to poor penetration of the ultrasound beam. Additionally, ultrasound can be subject to imaging artifacts from oblique scattering and multiple reflections.[16] Most importantly, quality ultrasound imaging is highly dependent on operator skill and experience.

Table 9.1 summarizes the advantages and disadvantages of ultrasound.

Figures 9.1 through 9.5 demonstrate common acute care surgical pathology optimally diagnosed via ultrasound.

MAGNETIC RESONANCE IMAGING

Magnetic resonance imaging (MRI) is performed through manipulation of the magnetic moment of water hydrogen protons within a static magnetic field. The behavior of these

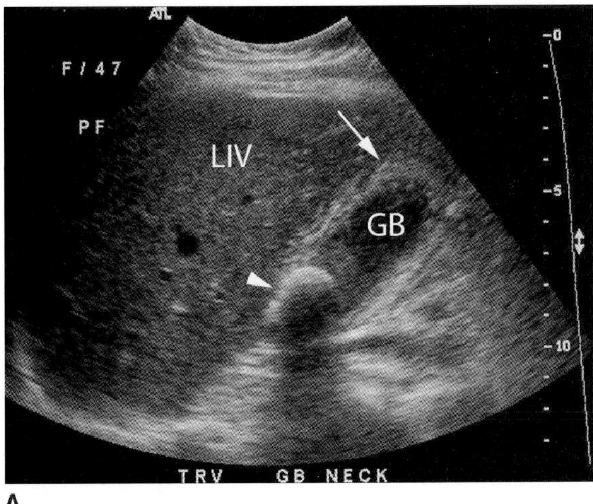

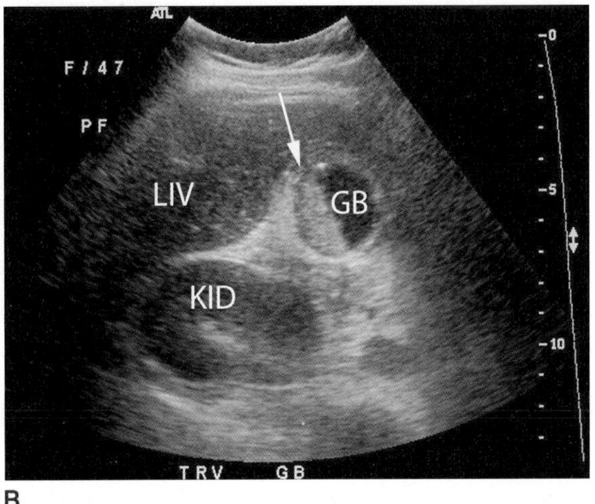

FIGURE 9.1. Acute cholecystitis. **A:** A sagittal view shows a dilated gallbladder with a thickened wall (*arrow*) and a large shadowing stone (*arrowhead*). **B:** A transverse view demonstrates the presence of layering hyperechoic sludge (*arrow*). Sonographic signs that favor acute cholecystitis include wall thickening > 3 mm, gallbladder dilation, impacted stone, the presence of a sonographic Murphy's sign, and pericholecystic fluid.[3] Acute cholecystitis was confirmed at surgery. GB, gallbladder; LIV, liver; KID, kidney.

moments, or spins, is directly related to the environment surrounding the water molecule through local effects such as magnetic fields from neighboring spins and energy exchange with nearby nuclei. Images are created after applying pulsed radiofrequency (RF) waves and magnetic field gradients at calculated times, then extracting spatial and temporal data from the subsequent signal patterns. Each programmed set of RF and gradient settings is referred to as a pulse sequence. The signal from protons within fat, protein, or free water can be isolated and highlighted through different pulse sequences, allowing for excellent soft tissue contrast that is superior to other cross-sectional imaging methods.[17] Isometric 3D MRI is now commonly used for multiplanar and curved reconstructions of vascular and ductal structures. Multiple types of contrast agents can be used to highlight the gastrointestinal tract, vascular structures, or bile ducts.[18,19] Interventional MRI continues to be an active area of research, particularly in oncology.[20]

A particular advantage of MRI is that this modality does not employ ionizing radiation, and, therefore, is favored whenever there is a particular desire to limit or avoid radiation exposure, such as in the evaluation of pregnant patients (Figs. 9.6-9.8).[22,23] MRI is also increasingly considered as a primary imaging modality in the evaluation of chronic diseases where the cumulative radiation dose from frequent follow-up CT examinations would be quite substantial. Inflammatory bowel disease is one such entity, where rapid pulse sequences

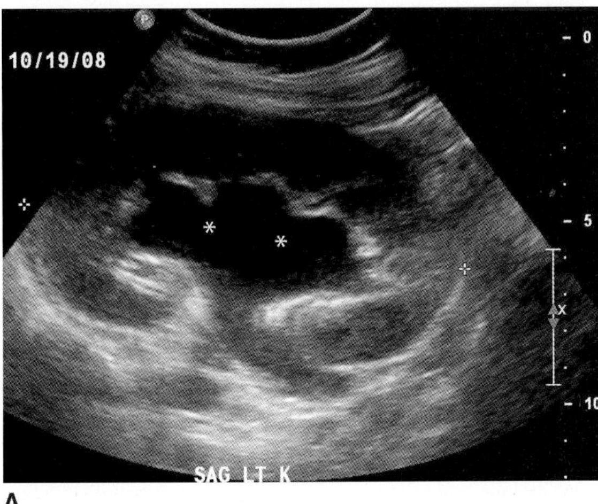

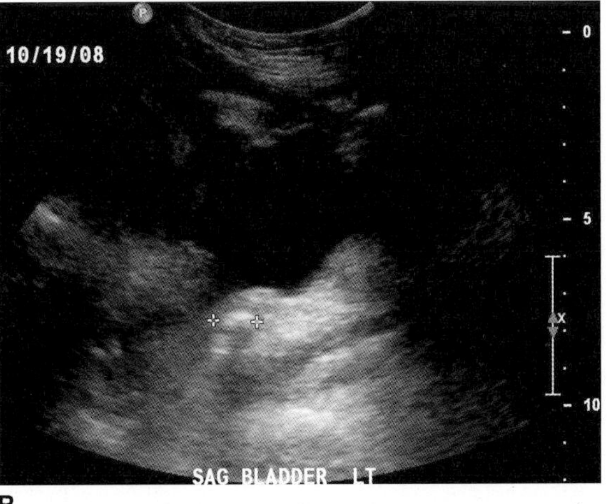

FIGURE 9.2. Hydronephrosis secondary to obstructing ureteral calculus. **A:** Moderate pelvic and calyceal dilation is present within the left kidney (*asterisk*). Urine and other simple fluids appear anechoic on ultrasound. The kidney is outlined by the caliper markers (+), and the cortex is appropriately homogeneous in echotexture. **B:** A 1-cm shadowing obstructive ureteral calculus, outlined by caliper markers (+), was found at the left ureterovesical junction.

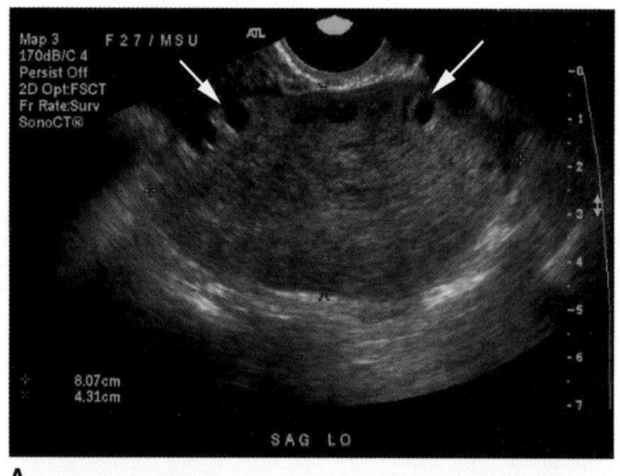

A

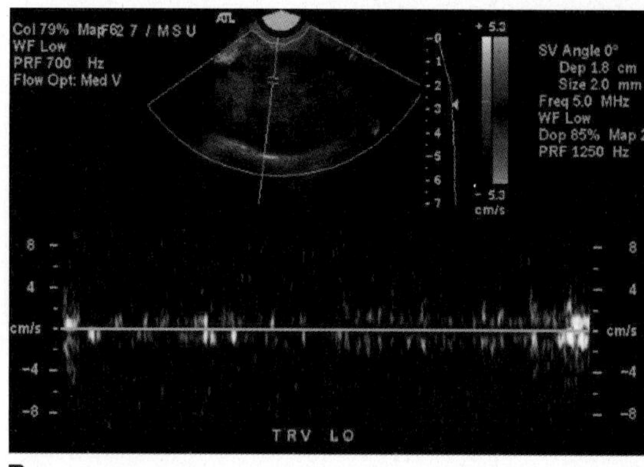

B

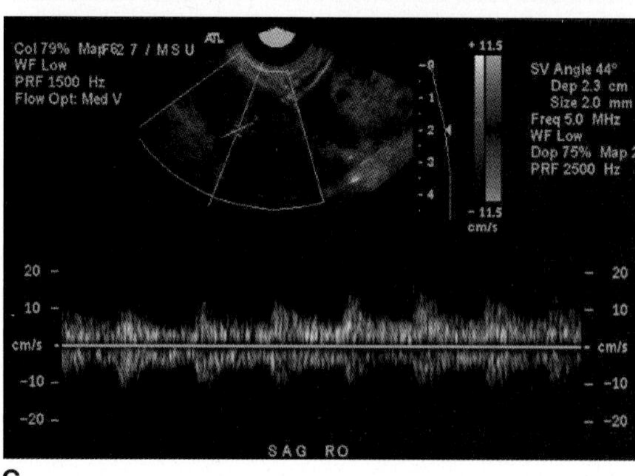

C

FIGURE 9.3. Ovarian torsion. **A:** Transvaginal sagittal grey-scale ultrasound image of the left ovary demonstrates an enlarged left ovary measuring up to 8 cm with small, peripherally located follicles (*arrows*) and slightly heterogeneous stroma. **B:** Duplex ultrasound image of the left ovary demonstrates absence of normal arterial or venous spectral Doppler waveforms. **C:** In contrast, the normal right ovary demonstrates normal arterial waveforms. Upon surgery, the left ovary was twisted 720 degrees. Ultrasound features of ovarian torsion include unilateral enlarged ovary >4 cm, peripherally located small follicles, coexistent mass within the torsed ovary, presence of free pelvic fluid, and visualization of a twisted vascular pedicle. On color Doppler imaging, absence of arterial flow is a classic feature of ovarian torsion, although preserved normal flow may also be seen.[8]

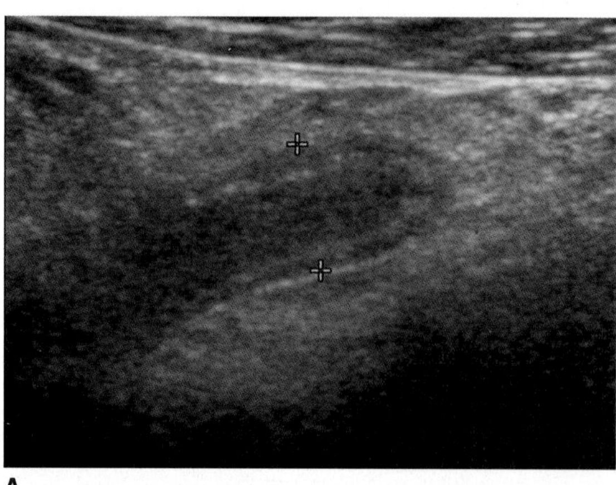

A

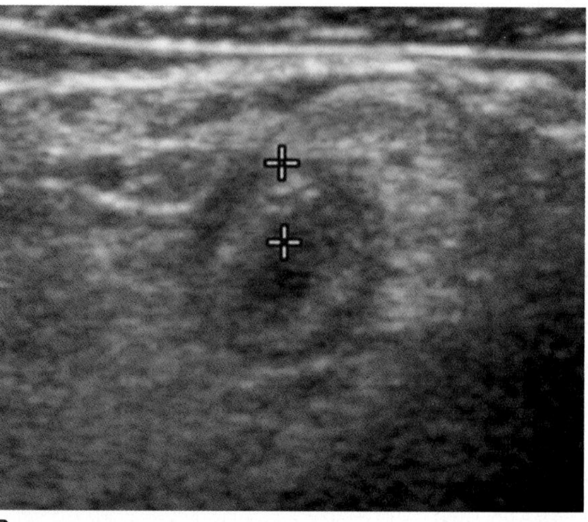

B

FIGURE 9.4. Acute appendicitis. **A:** Graded compression ultrasound imaging at the area of tenderness in the right lower quadrant demonstrates a tubular, blind-ending structure measuring 8 mm in diameter, as marked by the calipers (+), compatible with a dilated appendix, which was noncompressible. **B:** A transverse view demonstrates the appendix to have an abnormally thickened wall, as outlined by the calipers (+). Sonographic signs for appendicitis include a diameter >6 mm, lack of compressibility, echogenic periappendiceal fat, hyperemia on color Doppler imaging, the presence of an appendicolith, and the presence of adjacent fluid collections that would raise concern for rupture.[3] Acute appendicitis was confirmed upon surgery.

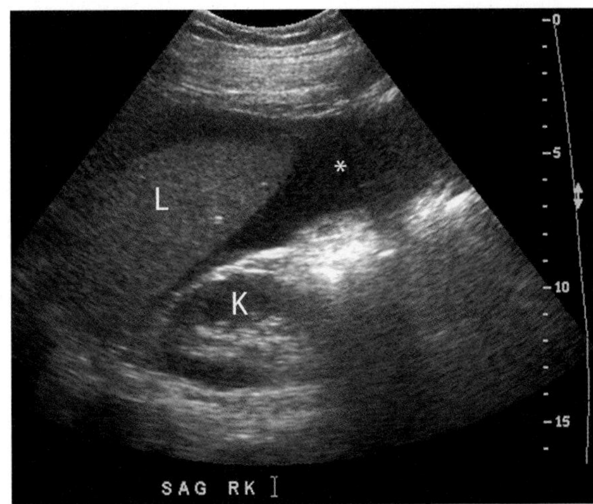

FIGURE 9.5. Hemoperitoneum in Morrison's pouch. A hypoechoic collection (*) is seen between the inferior edge of the right hepatic lobe (*L*) and the right kidney (*K*) in this patient with hemoperitoneum. Fresh blood appears hypoechoic on ultrasound. Acute clots are initially hyperechoic; the echogenicity diminishes with time.[12]

are now able to compensate for peristaltic motion, and T2-weighted, fluid-sensitive sequences are particularly useful for detecting fistulas or abscesses (Figs. 9.9 and 9.10).[25–27] While magnetic resonance cholangiopancreatography (MRCP) is commonly used for assessment of the biliary tree, liver, and pancreas for oncologic staging, surgical planning, or radiotherapy targeting,[28–31] in acute settings, MRCP is well suited for diagnosing emergent gallbladder and biliary tract conditions, including acute cholecystitis, choledocholithiasis, and acute cholangitis (Figs. 9.11 and 9.12).[32] Furthermore, magnetic resonance angiography provides an excellent alternative to CT for the imaging of vascular abnormalities (Fig. 9.13), particularly when iodinated contrast agents cannot be used due to contrast allergies or poor renal function.

Drawbacks of MRI include the need for a large static magnetic field to achieve an adequate signal-to-noise ratio, requiring large superconducting coils that are relatively expensive to maintain. An MRI suite must also be specially shielded to avoid signal interference from electromagnetic noise.

TABLE 9.1

ADVANTAGES AND DISADVANTAGES OF ULTRASOUND

ADVANTAGES	DISADVANTAGES
• No ionizing radiation	• Poor penetration through bone or air
• Real-time imaging	• Limited penetration in obese patients
• Safe for pregnant patients	• Highly dependent on operator skill
• Highly portable	
• Relatively low cost	
• Can provide quantitative measurements of vascular flow	

Furthermore, typical magnets have a narrow cylindrical bore that can induce claustrophobia and may not be able to accommodate obese patients or patients who require large support devices.

Another primary disadvantage of MRI is the inability to image patients with MRI-incompatible devices. The high magnetic field strengths of MRI are not compatible with ferromagnetic materials, such as many intracranial aneurysm clips. Additionally, RF pulses used to acquire MR images may interfere with electronic implants, including many current and older generations of cardiac pacemakers. MRI centers, therefore, require prescreening of all patients with a detailed checklist to ensure that the patient is safe for imaging and that all support equipment are MRI compatible.[34] Even the suspected presence of embedded metal within the orbits warrants further evaluation, typically with a radiograph, as fluctuations in magnetic fields can cause current-induced heating and particle movement. Furthermore, metallic implants that are deemed safe for MRI still cause local magnetic field artifacts that distort and obscure adjacent structures, thereby degrading image quality.

Contrast reactions with gadolinium-based agents can occur, as they do with CT agents; however, particular care must be paid to patients with severely impaired renal function, who have an increased risk of developing nephrogenic systemic fibrosis, or NSF. Typical symptoms include swelling and tightening of the skin within the extremities, but can progress to involve the internal organs, including skeletal muscle, myocardium, lungs, kidneys, and dura mater, with potentially fatal outcomes and no effective treatments.[34–36] The proposed pathogenesis is attributed to an abnormal activation of circulating fibrocytes as a response to residual gadolinium in tissues that has remained long after initial administration. Since the first description of NSF in 1997, there have been approximately 335 biopsy-confirmed cases worldwide, but virtually no new cases since 2008 due to widespread restrictions on gadolinium-based contrast use in patients with severe renal failure.[37] The use of intravenous gadolinium-based contrast agents is also not considered safe in pregnancy.[38] With the recent development of robust noncontrast MRI sequencing techniques, these issues related to contrast administration, fortunately, can be circumvented in many cases.

Motion-related artifacts are a common occurrence in MRI. Many sequences require the patient to lie still for a substantially longer amount of time than that needed for a CT or ultrasound, with some sequences lasting several minutes. Additionally, the total duration of an MRI examination can be lengthy compared to other modalities, typically lasting 40 minutes. As a result, sedation is often required in the pediatric population in order to obtain images free of motion artifact. Breath-hold imaging acquisitions can reduce the total imaging time and are frequently used to eliminate respiratory-related motion artifacts. Acutely ill patients who are unable to suspend their respiration, however, pose a challenge for MRI. The use of non–breath-hold, rapid imaging strategies can allow interpretable MR images to be acquired in these sicker patients.

Finally, MRI has a limited capability to image structures that have low water proton density. As a result, the detection of calcifications on MRI can be difficult. Furthermore, imaging of the lungs with MRI is particularly challenging as these structures contain mostly air and, therefore, generate little signal. The multiple air–tissue interfaces within the lung parenchyma also increase the rate of signal decay, further limiting the imaging of the pulmonary parenchyma.

Table 9.2 summarizes the advantages and disadvantages of MRI.

Figures 9.6 through 9.13 demonstrate common acute care surgical pathology optimally diagnosed via MRI.

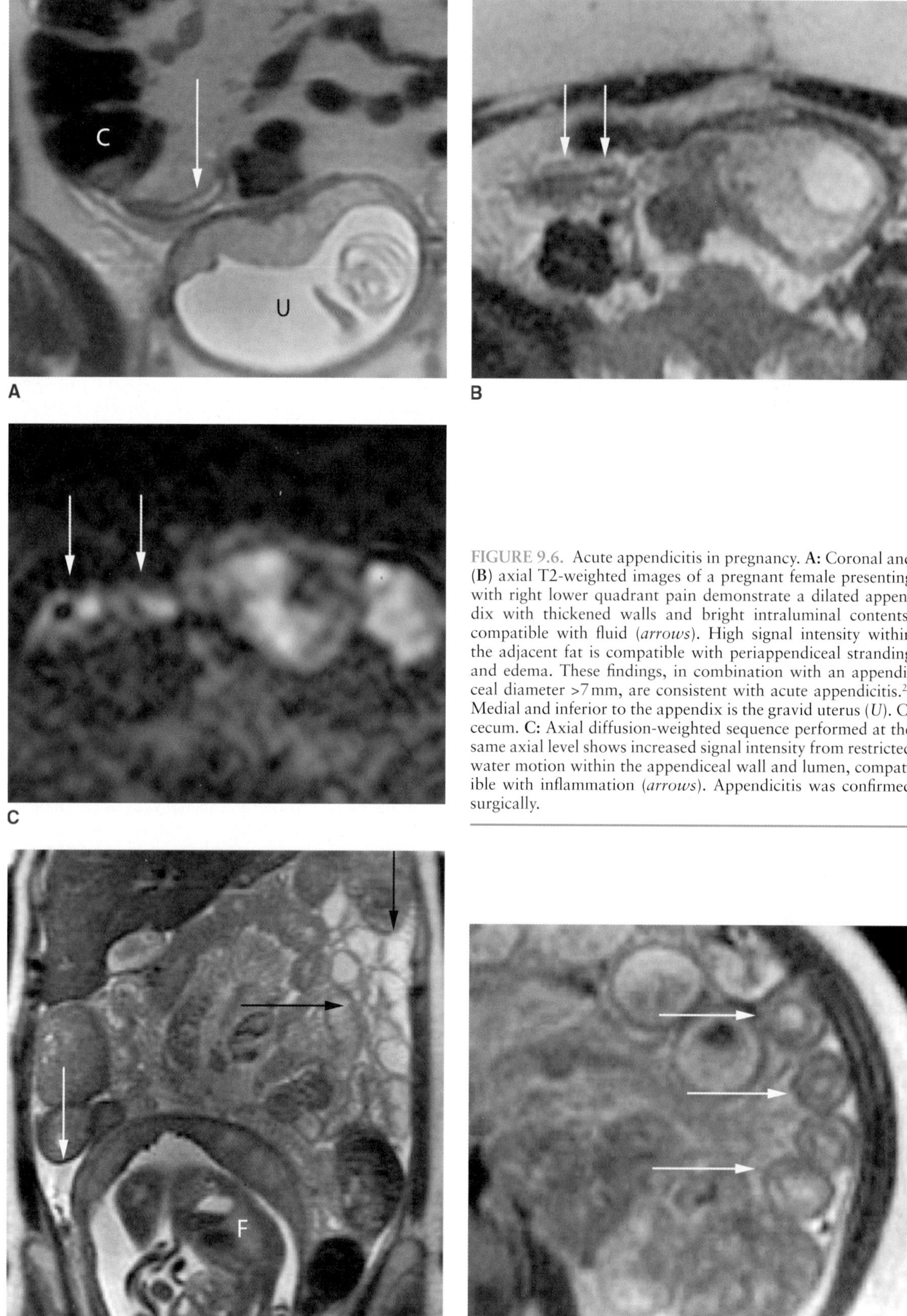

FIGURE 9.6. Acute appendicitis in pregnancy. **A:** Coronal and (**B**) axial T2-weighted images of a pregnant female presenting with right lower quadrant pain demonstrate a dilated appendix with thickened walls and bright intraluminal contents, compatible with fluid (*arrows*). High signal intensity within the adjacent fat is compatible with periappendiceal stranding and edema. These findings, in combination with an appendiceal diameter >7 mm, are consistent with acute appendicitis.[21] Medial and inferior to the appendix is the gravid uterus (*U*). C, cecum. **C:** Axial diffusion-weighted sequence performed at the same axial level shows increased signal intensity from restricted water motion within the appendiceal wall and lumen, compatible with inflammation (*arrows*). Appendicitis was confirmed surgically.

FIGURE 9.7. Ischemic bowel in pregnancy. **A:** Coronal T2-weighted image in a pregnant woman at 25 weeks' gestational age demonstrates fluid-filled loops of small bowel (*black arrows*) in the left abdomen with free intraperitoneal fluid (*white arrow*). F, fetus. **B:** Axial T2-weighted image demonstrates thickening of the proximal loops of small bowel with a target appearance compatible with mural edema. At surgery, the patient was discovered to have a small bowel volvulus secondary to an adhesion resulting in extensive small bowel ischemia. Ischemic bowel on MRI may demonstrate wall thickening and mural stratification or a target appearance, with high signal within the wall on T2-weighted imaging indicative of mural edema.[32,63]

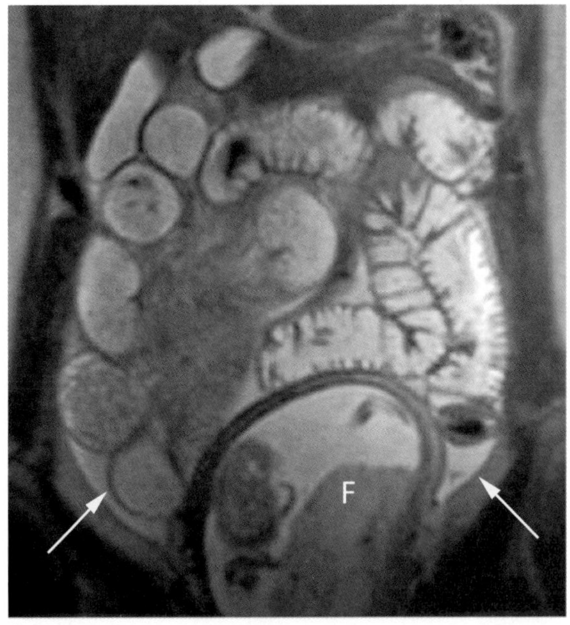

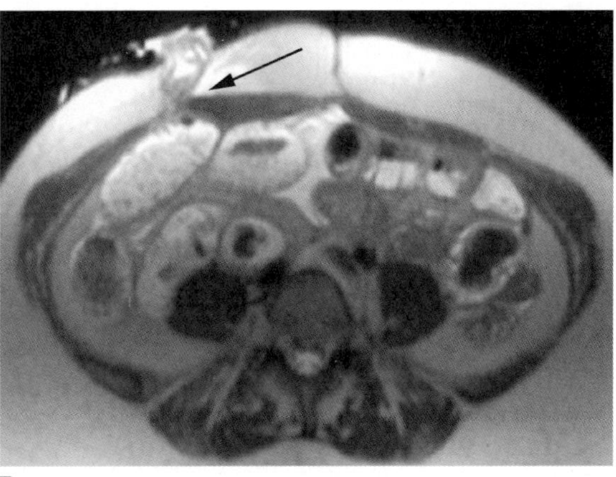

FIGURE 9.8. Small bowel obstruction in pregnancy. **A:** Coronal T2-weighted image in a pregnant female with a history of total colectomy for ulcerative colitis demonstrates diffusely dilated loops of small bowel and free fluid within the abdomen (*arrows*). F, fetus. **B:** Axial T2-weighted image shows dilated loops of small bowel with abrupt tapering within the end ileal loop and a transition point noted at the level of the ostomy due to a stricture (*arrow*).

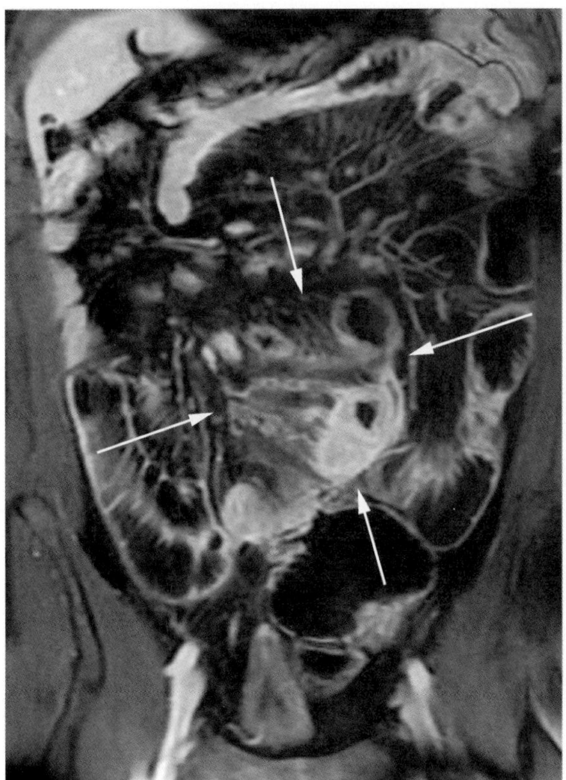

FIGURE 9.9. Active Crohn's disease. Coronal, fat-suppressed, T1-weighted image of the abdomen obtained after the administration of intravenous contrast demonstrates a matted, abnormal appearance to the loops of small bowel within the midline abdomen. These bowel loops show intense bowel wall enhancement, mural thickening, luminal narrowing, and adjacent mesenteric stranding and enhancement compatible with active inflammation (*arrows*).[24]

COMPUTED TOMOGRAPHY

Computed tomography (CT) is a method of acquiring and reconstructing the image of a thin cross section of an object on the basis of measurements of attenuation.[39] CT images eliminate the problem of superimposing tissues seen with conventional radiographs and provide higher contrast due to the absence of scatter.

Technical developments since the 1990s improved upon earlier conventional CT scanners by advancing helical or spiral technology, increasing speed of gantry rotation, increasing tube outputs to maintain adequate signal-to-noise ratios, and increasing the number of x-ray detector rows. The resultant significant improvements in image quality, acquisition speed, and hence patient throughput have led to a dramatic increase in the use of CT scanners as an essential diagnostic tool for multiple clinical applications.

Spiral CT scanners are of two types: single detector (SDCT) scanners and multi-detector (MDCT) scanners. SDCT scanners have a single row of detectors that are used to record data as the gantry rotates around the patient with the simultaneous translation of the patient through the gantry opening.[39,40] MDCT scanners have multiple parallel rows of x-ray detectors with each of the rows recording data independently as the gantry rotates. Compared to SDCT scanners, MDCT scanners allow for the simultaneous acquisition of multiple slices at higher tube rotation speeds, allowing significant reduction of acquisition times without compromising image quality, particularly along the z-axis (patient–table) direction. The benefit of faster scanning times with MDCT scanners is seen in the examination of uncooperative or critically ill patients who cannot reliably suspend breathing. Additionally, MDCT scanners allow images to be reconstructed with different thicknesses after image acquisition is completed. For these reasons, MDCT scanners have largely replaced SDCT in clinical practice.

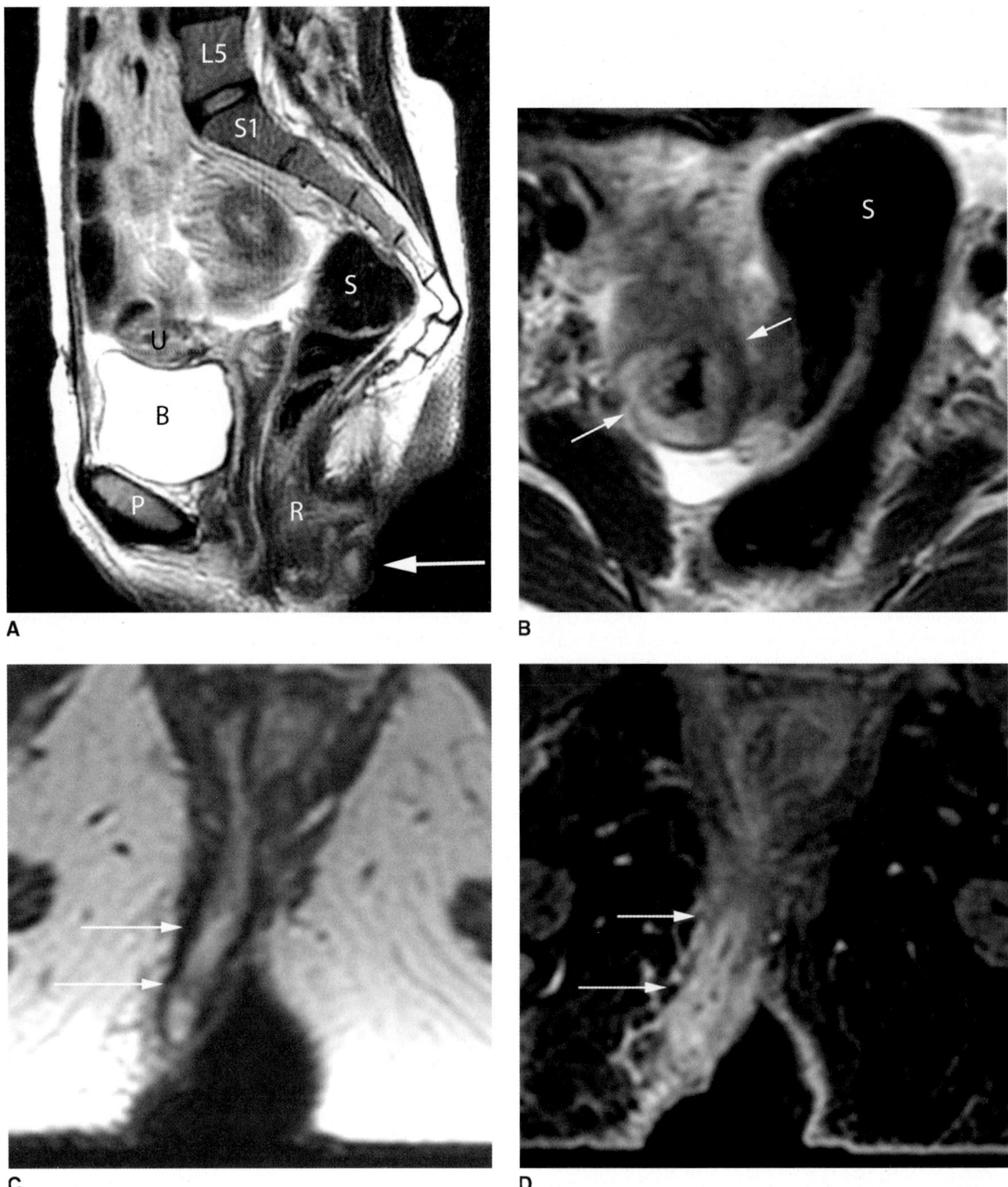

FIGURE 9.10. Complex Crohn's disease. **A:** Sagittal T2-weighted image of the pelvis demonstrates an abnormally thickened rectum (*R*) and distal sigmoid colon, in contrast to the proximal sigmoid colon (*S*), which appears normal. A superficial tract compatible with a perianal fistula is present (*arrow*). P, pubic symphysis; B, bladder; U, uterus, L5/S1: vertebral bodies. **B:** Axial T2-weighted image of the lower pelvis demonstrates abnormally thickened distal sigmoid colon (*arrows*). The adjacent proximal sigmoid is normal with smooth, thin walls. I: iliac bones. Axial (**C**) T2-weighted and (**D**) postcontrast T1-weighted fat-suppressed images of the perineum demonstrate a perianal fistula tracking along the right gluteal fold (*arrows*) with marked inflammatory enhancement within the fistula and surrounding soft tissues.

Contraindications/Limitations

Given the acuity and severity of illness or injury often encountered in acute care surgical services, the benefit of rapid and reliable diagnosis often exceeds risks that traditionally accompany CT. For the purpose of completeness, we present a discussion on relative contraindications with the caveat that utilization of CT (with or without intravenous contrast) often requires a careful evaluation of the risk–benefit ratio on a case-by-case basis, ideally via discussions between emergency medicine physicians and/or intensivists, surgeons, and radiologists.

Renal insufficiency and IV contrast: Contrast medium–induced acute renal failure or contrast-induced nephropathy (CIN) is defined as an absolute increase in the serum creatinine

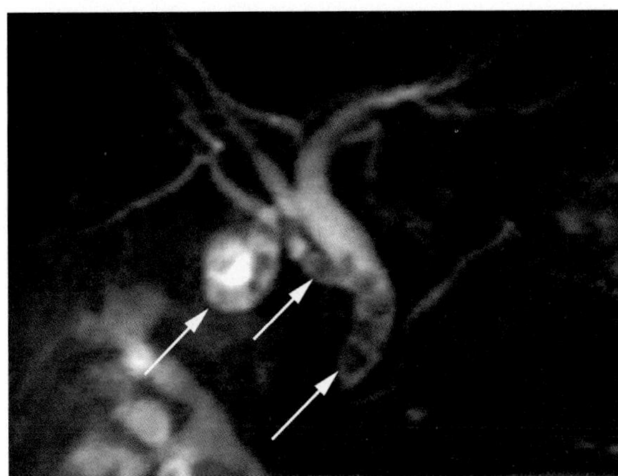

FIGURE 9.11. Choledocholithiasis. Coronal thick-slab heavily T2-weighted MRCP image of the biliary tree demonstrates multiple round filling defects within the gallbladder, cystic duct, and common bile duct (*arrows*) with mild intrahepatic and extrahepatic biliary dilatation.

concentration of at least 0.5 mg/dL or a relative increase of at least 25% from the baseline value.[41–43] The incidence of CIN ranges from less than 5% in the general population[43,44] to 12%-50% in those patients with associated risk factors including preexisting renal impairment and diabetes.[44] Fewer than 5% of patients who develop CIN require dialysis; the majority of patients develop mild renal failure.[43] The main goal is prevention of CIN, and most radiology practices routinely require determination of serum creatinine levels in patients prior to administration of IV contrast. Iso-osmolar nonionic contrast agents, lower doses of contrast agents (aided by increases in acquisition speed and improved resolution), preadministration hydration regimens, and an increased role for noncontrast studies, wherever possible, can help minimize the risk of CIN.[25,45] Additionally, the American College of Radiology has published guidelines regarding the use of contrast media in patients with renal impairment.[45]

Acute care surgical patients frequently present with predisposing risk factors for acute renal failure, namely hypovolemia, decreased renal perfusion, rhabdomyolysis, nephrotoxicity from polypharmacy, and multiorgan failure. The nephrotoxic effects of intravenous contrast are often, at least in part, mitigated by vigorous fluid resuscitation often undertaken in the usual course of care. Studies have proposed various pre-CT strategies, including oral acetylcysteine and intravenous sodium bicarbonate solution among others; however, benefits have inconsistently been demonstrated.[46–50] The time course of most acute surgical conditions usually precludes undertaking time-consuming pre-CT nephroprotective regimens for moderate impairment (estimated glomerular filtration rate [eGFR] between 45 and 60 mL per second). As previously stated, a case-by-case assessment of the risk–benefit ratio should be made with respect to precipitating risk factors, potential nephrotoxicity from IV contrast (including safety profile of type of contrast used and dose) and urgent time course of administration.

Contrast reactions and IV contrast: Adverse reactions with contrast agents are infrequent, ranging from 5%-12% for the ionic high-osmolality contrast media (HOCM) to 1%-3% for the nonionic low-osmolality contrast media (LOCM).[45,51] Immediate allergic reactions occur within an hour after injection of the contrast media and can be mild (nausea, vomiting, mild urticaria, pallor), moderate (severe vomiting, symptomatic urticaria, vasovagal reaction, mild bronchospasm, tachycardia secondary to transient mild hypotension) or severe (pulmonary edema, cardiac arrhythmias or arrest, circulatory collapse).[25,52] Delayed reactions occur hours to weeks after

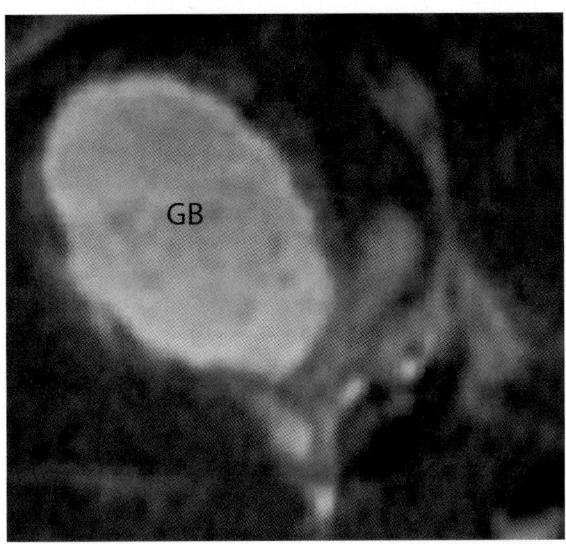

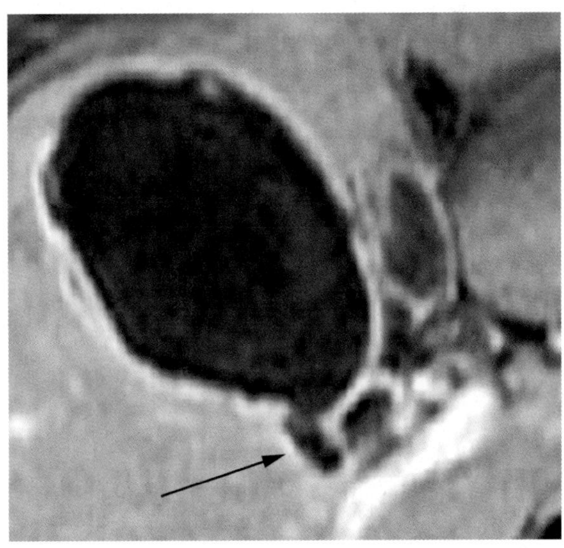

FIGURE 9.12. Gangrenous cholecystitis with perforation. **A:** Axial T2-weighted image of the abdomen demonstrates a distended gallbladder (GB) with a thickened and edematous wall. **B:** Postcontrast T1-weighted fat-suppressed axial image shows inhomogeneous enhancement of the gallbladder wall and disruption of mucosal enhancement with a contained perforation (*arrow*). Characteristic features of gangrenous cholecystitis on MRI include a patchy pattern of gallbladder wall enhancement with an interrupted rim of mucosal enhancement.[32,33]

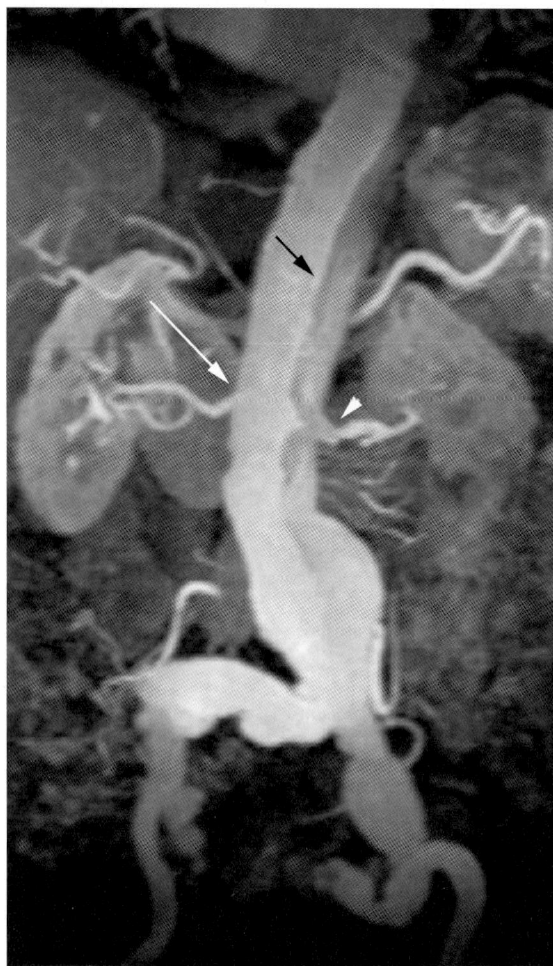

FIGURE 9.13. Abdominal aortic aneurysm with dissection. Coronal, contrast-enhanced, maximal-intensity projection image of the abdominal aorta demonstrates fusiform aneurysmal dilatation of the entire abdominal aorta with an extensive intimal flap (*black arrow*), compatible with dissection. The right renal artery is supplied by the true lumen (*white arrow*), while the left renal artery is supplied by the false lumen (*arrowhead*). Bilateral common iliac artery aneurysms are also present, with a more saccular, irregular appearance of the aneurysm on the right.

injection of the contrast medium and are usually self-limited and cutaneous (rash, erythema, urticaria and angioedema). Underlying medical conditions (asthma, heart disease, dehydration, renal disease, diabetes), medications (NSAIDS, IL-2, beta-blockers, biguanides), and prior reactions to contrast agents can predispose patients to contrast reactions. Allergy or sensitivity to seafood is not associated with an increased risk of allergic-type contrast reactions.[52] However, the history of anaphylactoid reaction to any allergen should raise concern of a potential such reaction to IV contrast. Premedication regimens with prednisone and histamine blocking agents (e.g. diphenhydramine and cimetidine) may be helpful in patients with previous allergic-type reactions to contrast media; however, such regimens are lengthy (typically at least 6 hours or more), again precluding utility in most acute care surgical settings.

Radiation: The technologic sophistication and improved clinical efficacy of CT imaging in the recent past have resulted in a dramatic increase in its use as a diagnostic and screening tool in a variety of clinical contexts. However, this widespread use has resulted in a significant increase in the population's cumulative exposure to ionizing radiation.[53,54]

Deleterious effects of ionizing radiation are divided into deterministic effects (skin erythema/necrosis, epilation, cataracts, sterility) and stochastic effects (carcinogenic and genetic effects). Deterministic effects assume a threshold (set at 2 Gy) below which no direct radiation-induced damage to tissues or organs occurs.[55] A recent study by Huda[56] demonstrated that representative organ-absorbed doses in CT were substantially lower than the threshold doses for the induction of deterministic effects. Patient cancer risk with CT imaging depends upon the dose and radiosensitivity of all exposed organs and tissues and is best quantified by the effective dose parameter, measured in milliSievert (mSv). At present, the dominant notion for stochastic effects is that no threshold dose exists. Instead, the "linear no-threshold" model accepted by many authors for stochastic effects posits a direct dose–response relationship between exposure to even low doses of radiation and the development of solid cancers.[54,57] Data most cited to provide support for this model have been extrapolated from survivors of the Hiroshima bombing, which were primarily obtained for high acute doses delivered at a high dose rate.[56] No other studies to date have verified the linear, no-threshold assumption about cancer associated with the low doses used in diagnostic imaging.[58]

Radiation doses associated with common diagnostic CT scans used in the acute care setting (Table 9.3) do not

TABLE 9.2

ADVANTAGES AND DISADVANTAGES OF MRI

ADVANTAGES	DISADVANTAGES
• No ionizing radiation	• Relatively long imaging times
• Safe for pregnant patients	• Relatively high cost
• Excellent soft tissue contrast	• Narrow magnet bore can exclude obese or claustrophobic patients
• Pulse sequences can be adjusted to highlight or suppress certain tissues	• Susceptibility and motion artifacts
• Multiplanar capability	• Many MRI-incompatible devices
• Angiography can be performed without IV contrast	• Limited imaging of low–proton density substances (e.g., lung, calcifications)

TABLE 9.3

ADVANTAGES AND DISADVANTAGES OF CT

ADVANTAGES	DISADVANTAGES
• High spatial resolution	• Significant ionizing radiation
• Excellent soft tissue contrast	• Risks from contrast-induced nephropathy (CIN) and adverse reaction (in cases with IV contrast administration)
• High-speed acquisition	• Relative high cost
• Wide array of applications, including noninvasive diagnostic angiography	• Remains prone to motion and other artifacts
• Multiplanar capabilities	

individually contribute to stochastic or deterministic risk when used appropriately.[59] However, there is growing concern about the radiation risk to patients due to the overuse of CT studies in lieu of non- or low-radiation dose alternatives, or due to multiple repeated exposures (NEJM). The American College of Radiology (ACR) supports the "as low as reasonably achievable" (ALARA) concept that encourages healthcare professionals to use the least amount of radiation needed in imaging exams to achieve the necessary results. Additionally, multiple technical options (x-ray beam filtration and collimation, manual tube current modulation tailored to patient size and indication, peak kilovoltage optimization, improved detector efficiency, noise-reduction algorithms) are now included in newer CT scanners in an effort to reduce the dose from CT exams.[60]

Overall, the deterministic and stochastic risk from urgent CT exams in the acute setting is overwhelmingly small relative to the diagnostic benefit for most acute care surgical indications. However, it is prudent to be aware of radiation dose particularly with regard to age of patient, imaging through radiosensitive organs, and repeated imaging. Consultation with radiologists to determine strategies that reduce radiation doses without compromising diagnostic accuracy or to determine applicability of nonionizing radiation alternative exams (e.g. MRI, US) will promote imaging that is both justified and optimally performed.

Table 9.3 summarizes the advantages and disadvantages of CT.

Figures 9.14 through 9.31 demonstrate common acute care surgical pathology optimally diagnosed via CT. Figures 9.14 through 9.23 depict common traumatic injuries and sequelae on CT. Figures 9.24 through 9.31 depict nontraumatic conditions.

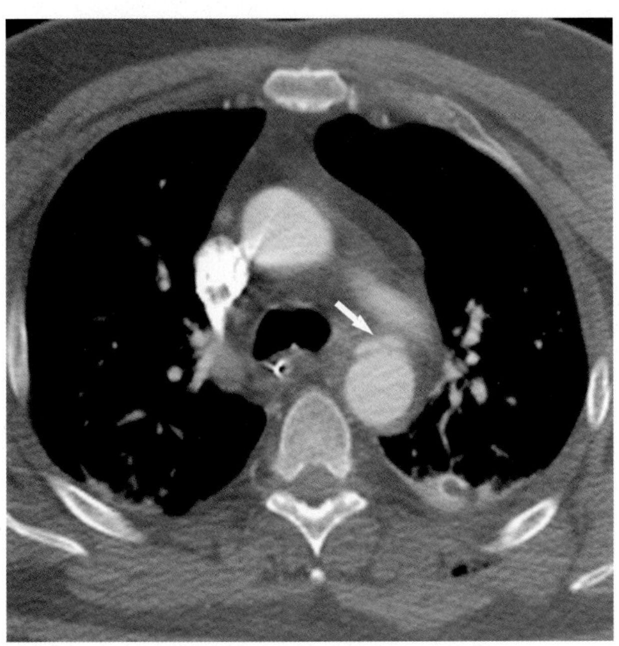
A

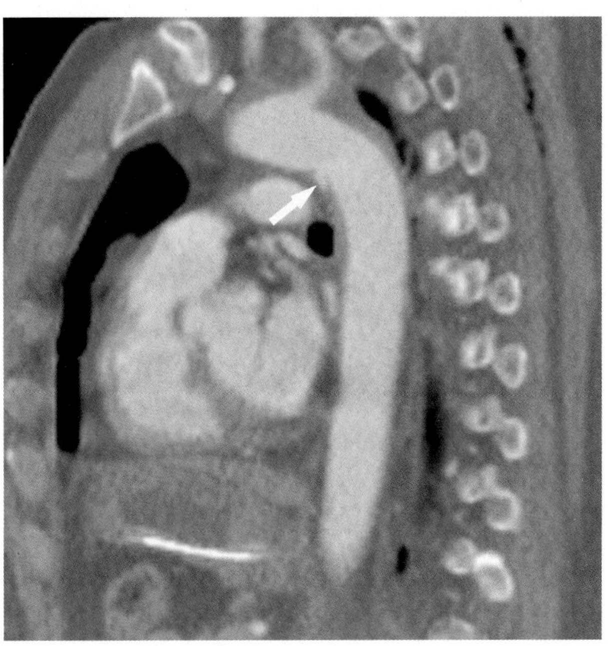
B

FIGURE 9.14. Acute traumatic aortic injury (ATAI). Coned views of (**A**) contrast-enhanced transverse (axial) slice and (**B**) sagittal reconstruction from chest CT. Contour irregularity at the proximal descending aorta (*white arrow*) represents pseudoaneurysm at the ligamentum arteriosum in the aortic isthmus. ATAI is due to abrupt deceleration resulting in injury at fixation sites: namely the aortic root, the isthmus at the ligamentum arteriosum, and the aortic hiatus. The injury at the isthmus represents the most common site of injury overall, and the most common presenting to the hospital. CT angiography has replaced the need for diagnostic thoracic angiography in the evaluation of trauma patients.[61,62]

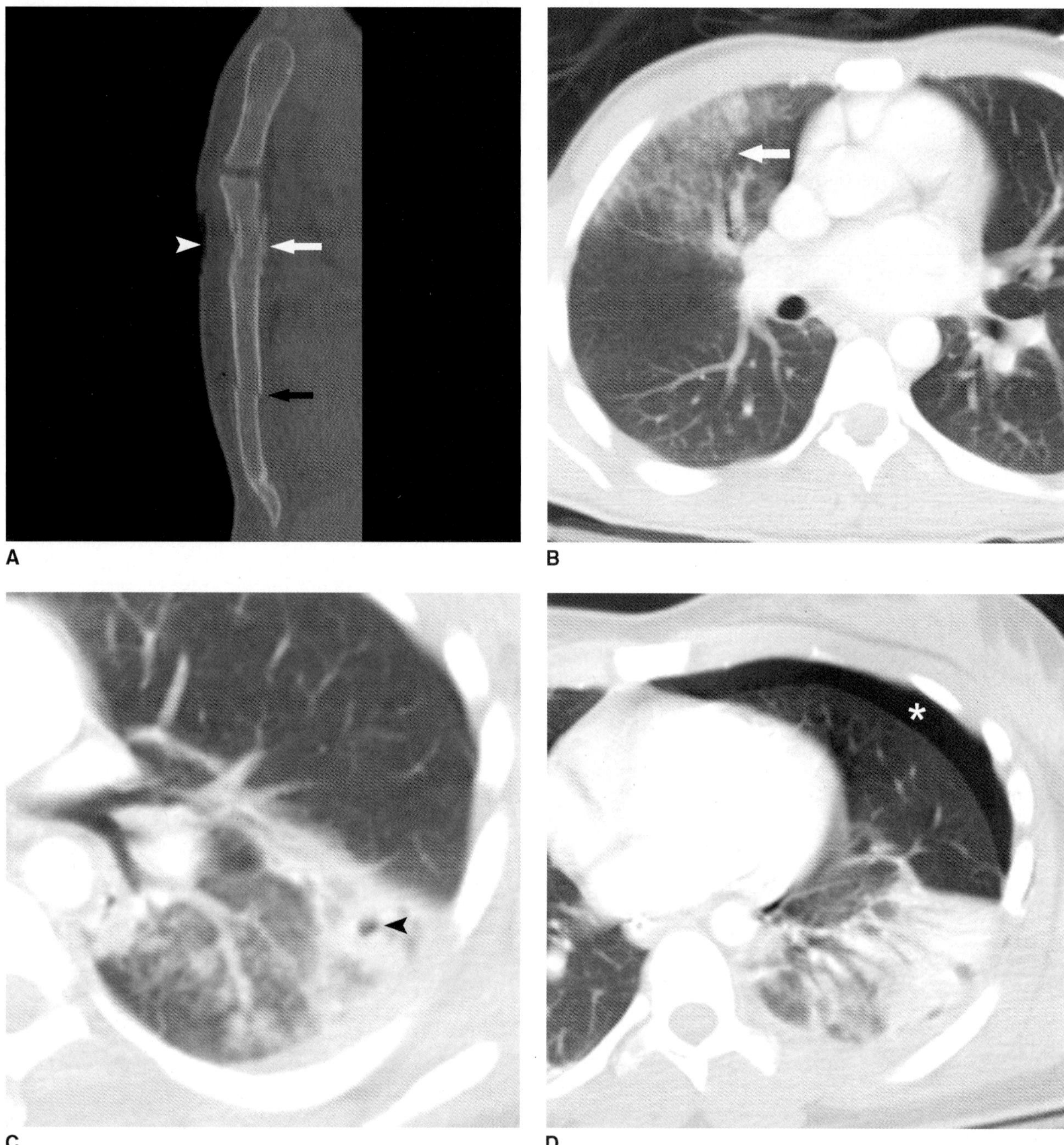

FIGURE 9.15. Chest trauma. **A:** Coned view from sagittal reconstruction of chest CT in bone windows demonstrating a minimally displaced fracture of the sternal body (*black arrow*), a commonly missed fracture prior to the routine use of such reconstructions from submillimeter thin slice multidetector CT. Note the pseudofractures (*arrow*) more cephalad due to respiratory motion, a common pitfall, which are invariably accompanied by corresponding irregularities of the skin surface (*arrowhead*). **B:** Coned view of anterior right lung from transverse (axial) slice demonstrating typical appearance of pulmonary contusions, geographic pattern of peripheral patchy opacities. **C:** Coned view of posterior left lung from transverse (axial) slice demonstrating a cystic lucency (*black arrowhead*) within an area of contusion representing a laceration. Lacerations are characterized by the surrounding lung injury and the clinical context of trauma. Completely air-filled lacerations are termed pneumatoceles, those filled with blood are termed hematomas.[64,65] **D:** Coned view of the left hemithorax from transverse (axial) slice demonstrating an anterior pneumothorax (*asterisk*), which was radiographically occult. Multiple studies have shown approximately 5%-15% of pneumothoraces are missed on initial conventional supine chest radiographs and subsequently seen at CT.[66–68]

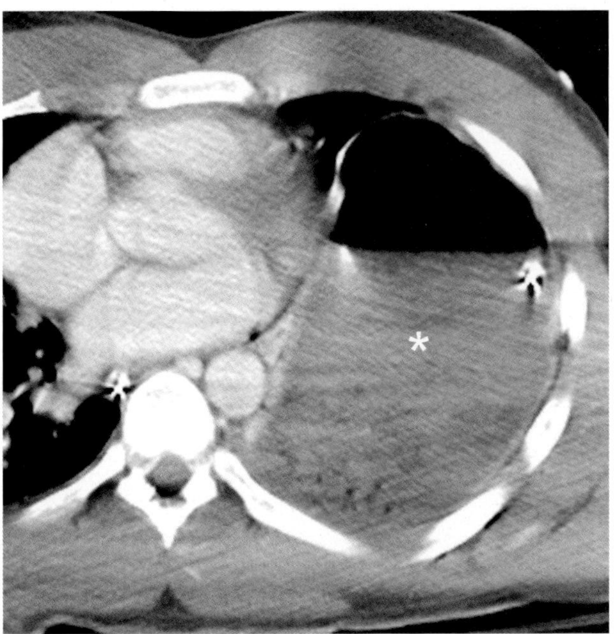

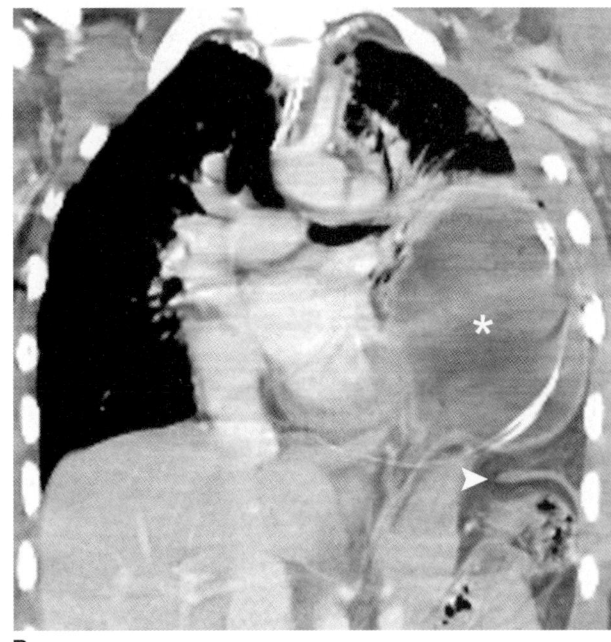

FIGURE 9.16. Traumatic diaphragmatic injury. **A:** Transverse (axial) and (**B**) coronal slices from contrast-enhanced chest CT. Note the stomach (*asterisk*) herniating into the left hemithrorax. The defect in the diaphragm [*arrowhead* in (**B**)] is typically best demonstrated on nonaxial reconstructions, coronal and/or sagittal.

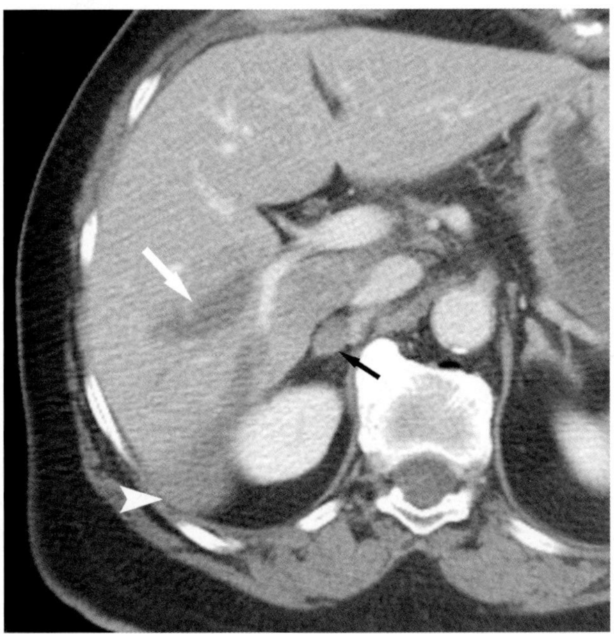

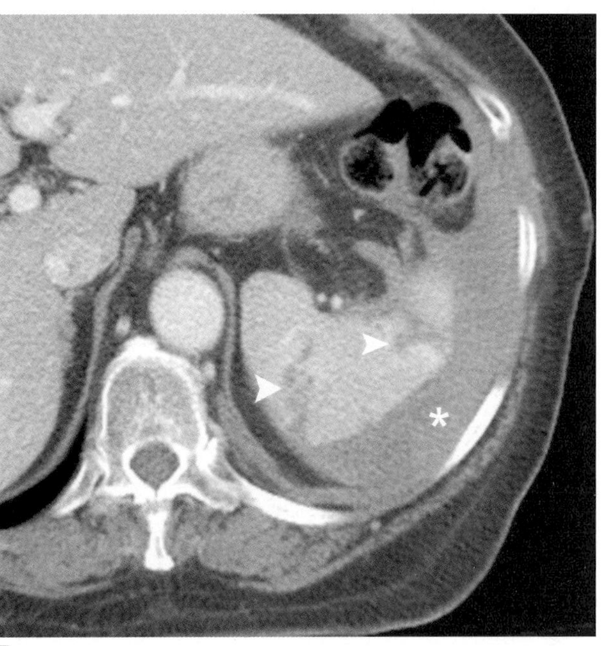

FIGURE 9.17. Abdominal trauma. **A:** Coned view of liver on transverse (axial) slice from abdominal CT demonstrating jagged linear hypoattenuated foci in the right hepatic lobe (*arrow*) typical of traumatic lacerations, with associated hepatorenal recess hemorrhage (*arrowhead*). Coincident right adrenal hematoma is also noted (*black arrow*, see **D**). **B:** (Different patient Coned view of the spleen on transverse (axial) slice from abdominal CT demonstrating lacerations of the spleen (*arrowheads*) with extensive perisplenic hemorrhage (*asterisk*).

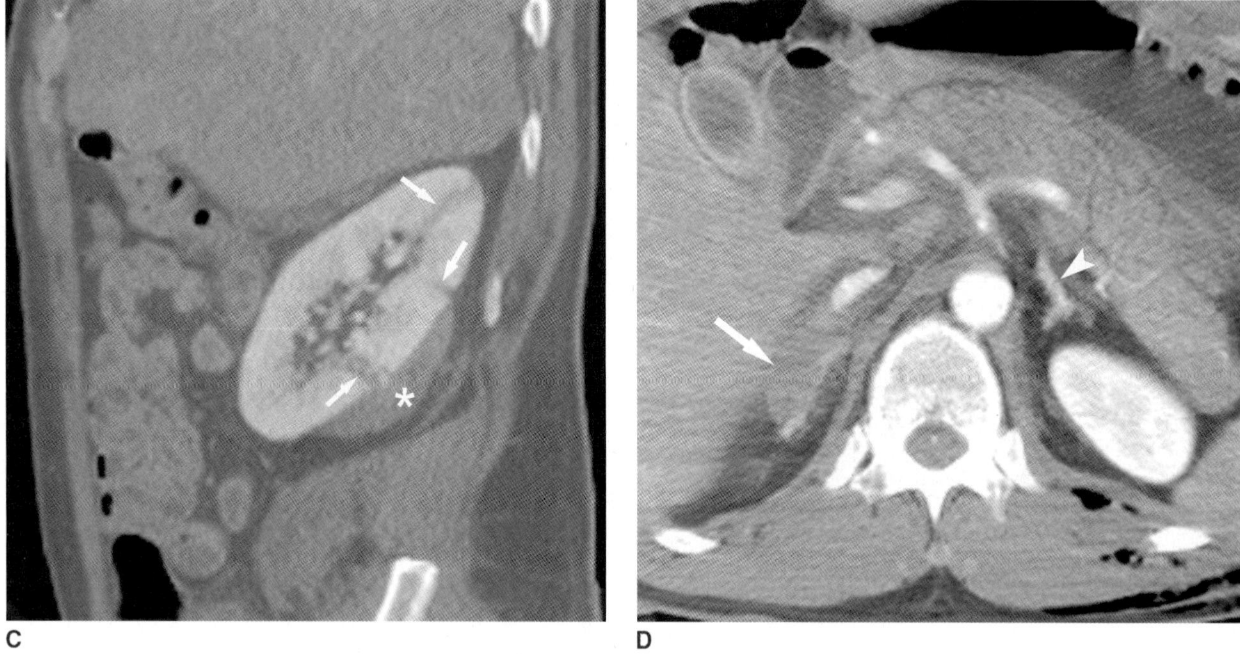

FIGURE 9.17. (*Continued*) **C:** (Different patient) Coned view of the right kidney on sagittal reconstruction from abdominal CT demonstrating multiple lacerations (*arrows*) with an adjacent perirenal hematoma (*asterisk*). **D:** (Different patient) Coned view of adrenal glands and other retroperitoneal structures on transverse (axial) slice from abdominal CT. The slightly hyperattenuated (hyperdense) left adrenal gland (*arrowhead*) is normal in shape. There is a right adrenal hematoma (*arrow*) with periadrenal hemorrhage. Adrenal hematoma can also manifest as an ovoid or round hyperdensity with surrounding stranding (*black arrow* in **A**).

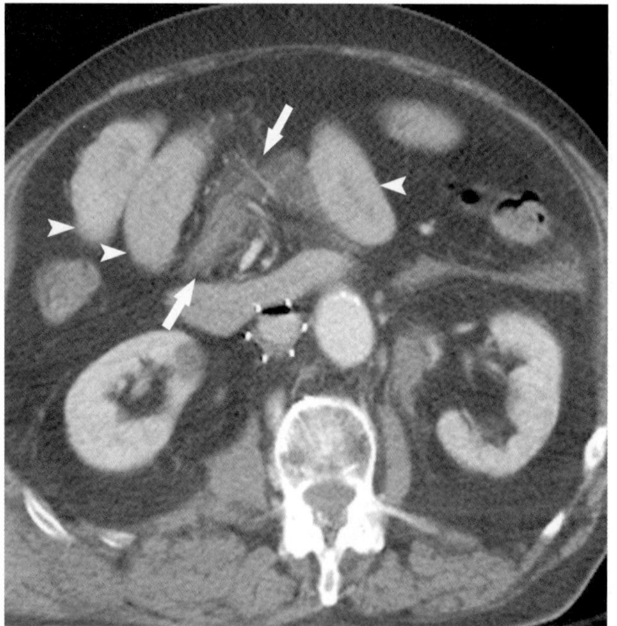

FIGURE 9.18. Bowel and mesenteric injury (BMI). Coned view from contrast-enhanced abdominal CT at level of midabdomen. Hazy ill-defined opacity in mesentery (between *white arrows*) supplying small bowel loops with circumferential wall thickening (*arrowheads*) representing BMI. Highly specific CT signs of BMI include bowel wall discontinuity, extraluminal air otherwise not explained, extraluminal contrast, mesenteric vascular extravasation, mesenteric vascular beading, or the termination of mesenteric vessels. Less specific CT signs include bowel wall thickening, abnormal bowel wall enhancement, mesenteric infiltration, or mesenteric hematoma. Surgical BMI is essentially present when one highly specific finding or two or more less specific findings are present.[69]

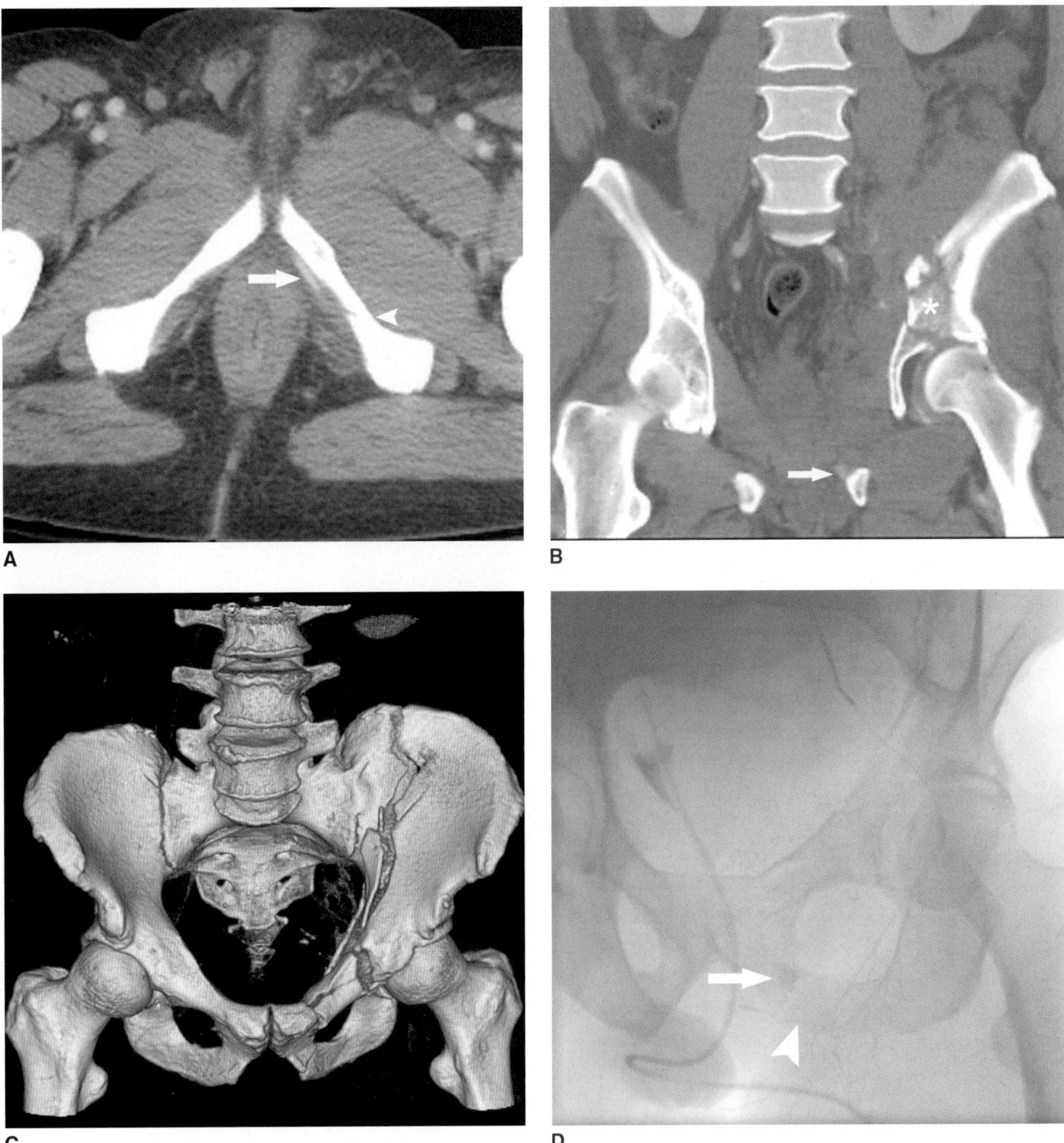

FIGURE 9.19. Pelvic trauma. **A:** Transverse (axial) and (**B**) coronal reconstructed slices from a pelvic CT with contrast. The linear focus of hyperattenuation along the course of the internal pudendal artery (*arrow*) is seen adjacent to a left inferior pubic ramus fracture (*arrowhead*) indicates active extravasation. Iliac/acetabular fractures are depicted in B (*asterisk*). **C:** Volume rendered reconstruction of the pelvis filtered for bone and contrast-enhanced vessels from the same data set as in A and B demonstrating extensive left pelvic fractures. Such reconstructions are useful for complex fracture patterns and to assist in preoperative planning as they can be rotated on an axis on the workstation. **D:** Coned view from conventional angiogram with a microcatheter (*arrowhead*) in the left internal pudendal artery and a faint contrast blush distally (*arrow*) indicating extravasation, corresponding to the abnormality on CT. This lesion was successfully embolized.

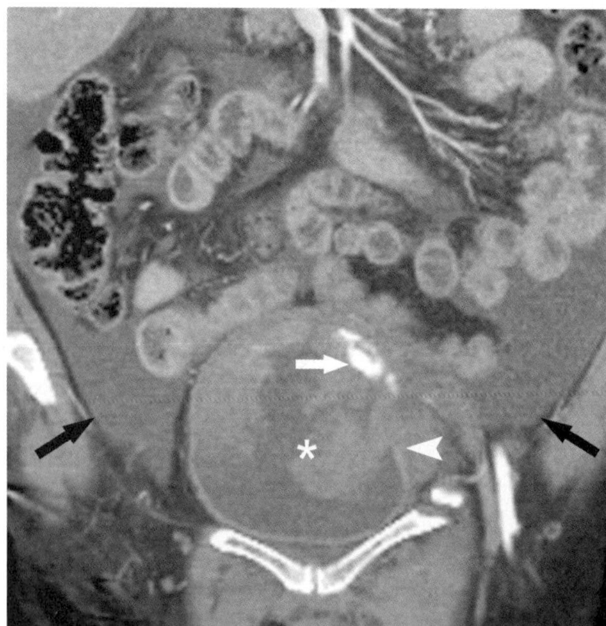

FIGURE 9.20. Bladder injury. Coned view of the bladder and pelvic structures from coronal reconstructed CT scan of the pelvis. There is mixed attenuation within the bladder lumen (*asterisk*) representing urine mixing with clot with a focus of very hyperattenuated material (*arrow*) representing active hemorrhage from an injured bladder wall artery. Note the discontinuity in the bladder wall representing intraperitoneal bladder injury (*arrowhead*) with intermediate attenuation fluid tracking in the pericolic gutters representing hemoperitoneum (*black arrows*).

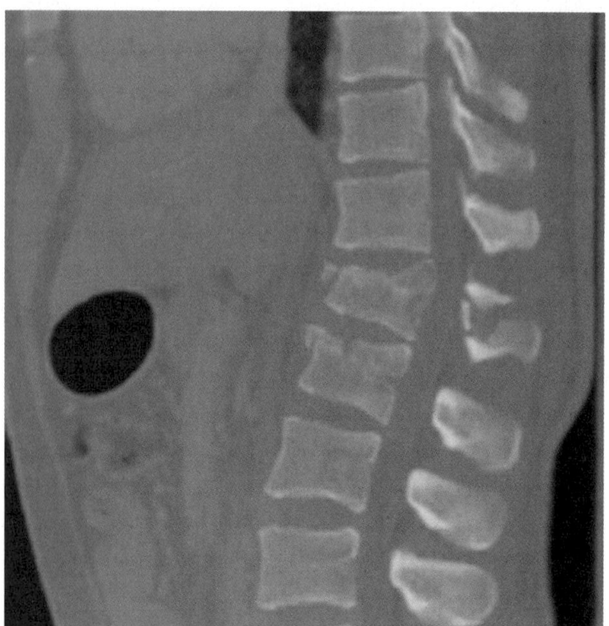

FIGURE 9.21. Thoracolumbar trauma. Sagittal reconstructed image in bone windows demonstrating a Chance fracture of T12 (*arrow*) and a superior endplate compression fracture of L1 (*arrowhead*). Multidetector CT of the torso allows high-resolution reconstructions of the spine and obviates the need for conventional radiography of thoracic and/or lumbar spines reducing costs, delay in diagnosis, and radiation dose.[70,71]

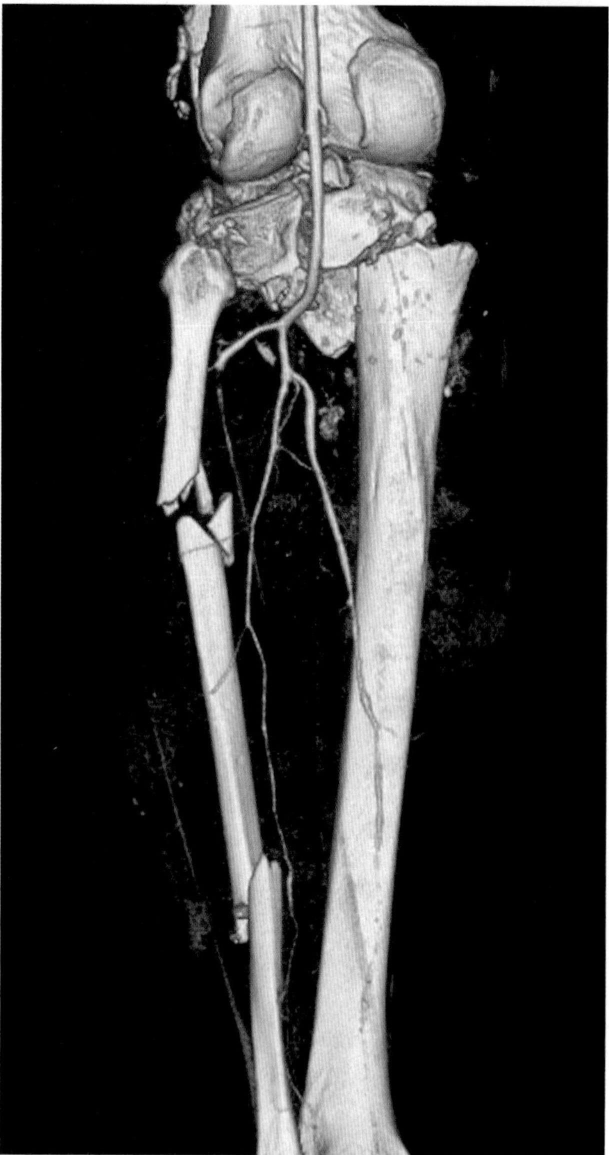

FIGURE 9.22. Extremity trauma. Volume-rendered reconstruction from a CT angiogram of the lower extremity filtered for high attenuation structures (bone and contrast-enhanced vasculature). CT angiography can be integrated into the initial CT examination to investigate possible or known extremity vascular injury supplanting diagnostic conventional angiography in select patients.[72]

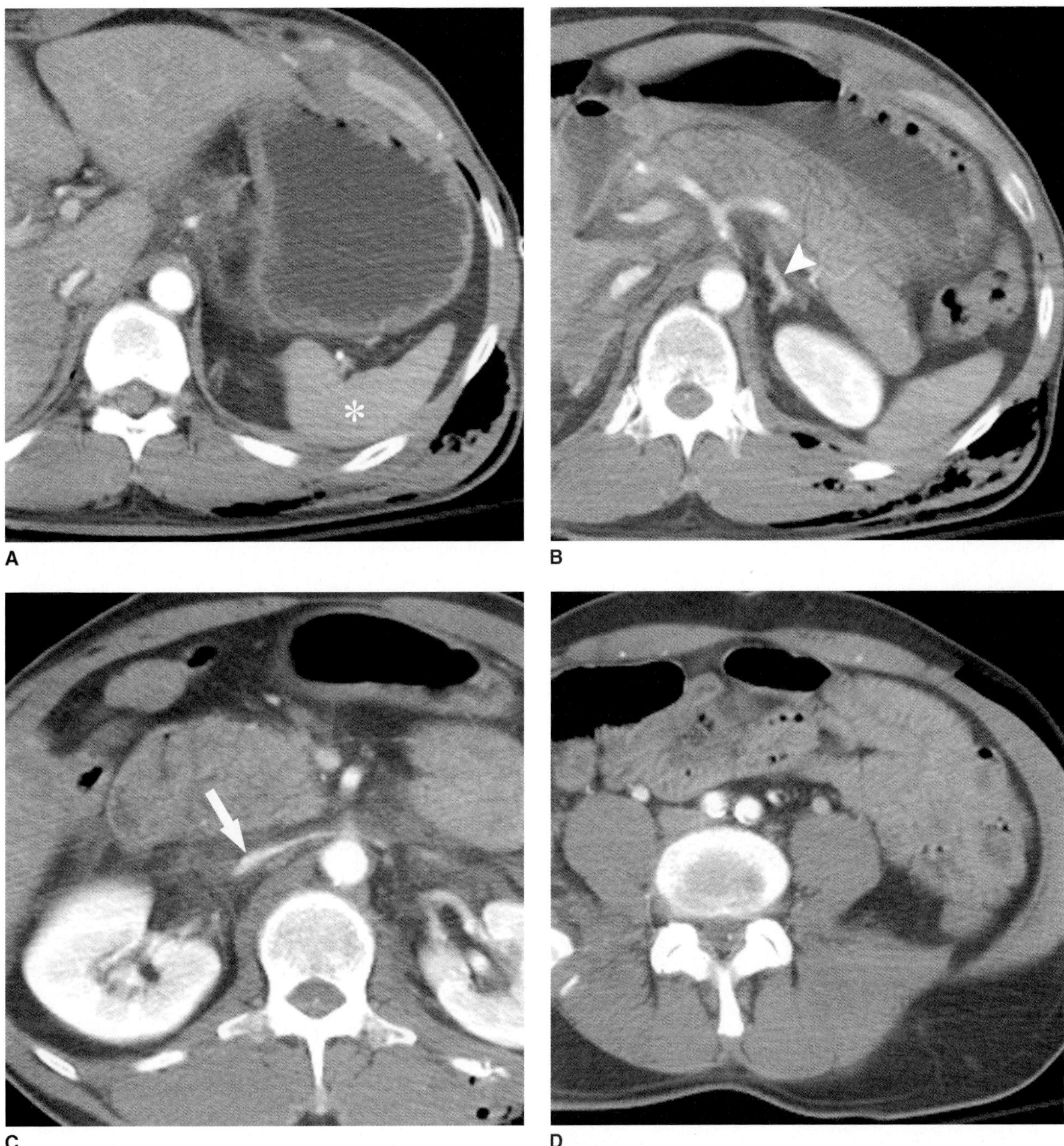

FIGURE 9.23. Hypovolemic shock. Coned views from transverse (axial) slices from contrast-enhanced abdominal CT demonstrating a small spleen (*asterisk* in **A**), a hyperattenuated left adrenal gland (*arrowhead* in **B**), a flat inferior vena cava (*arrow* in **C**), and hyperattenuated bowel mucosa (**D**) consistent with hypovolemic shock. The so-called hypoperfusion complex was first described in the pediatric radiology literature but now is largely accepted as indicative of shock in the adult patient population as well.

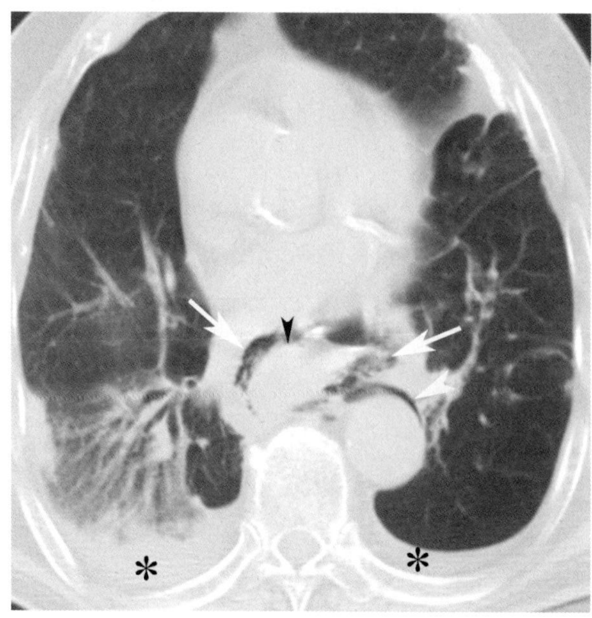

FIGURE 9.24. Esophageal perforation. Perforation of the distal esophagus following attempted dilation of an esophageal stricture is evidenced by extensive air in the mediastinum (*arrows*) and around the aorta (*white arrowhead*) on axial slice from noncontrast chest CT in lung windows. The esophagus (*black arrowhead*) is collapsed with thickened wall. Pleural effusions (*asterisk*) are common. Extraluminal mediastinal air and periesophageal contrast are the most specific findings.

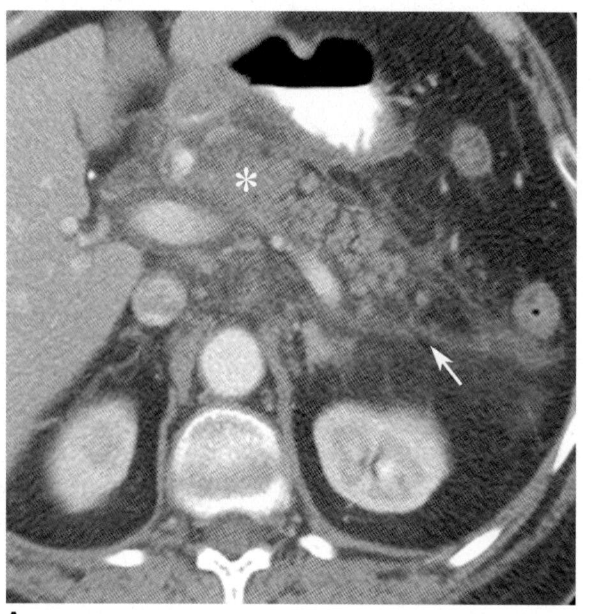

A

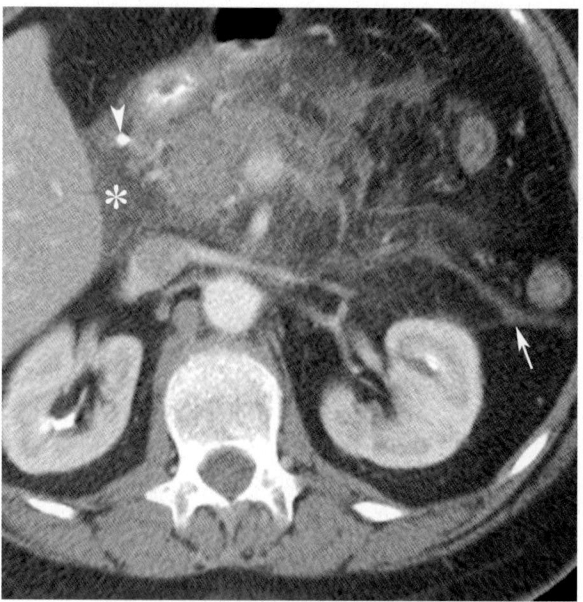

B

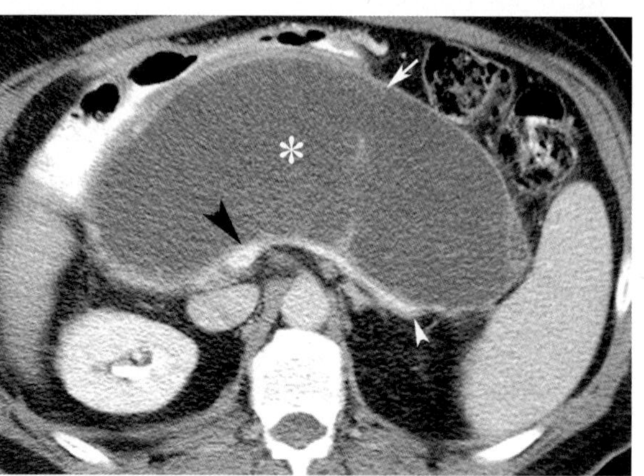

C

FIGURE 9.25. Acute pancreatitis. **A:** Coned view of the pancreas on transverse (axial) slice from abdominal CT demonstrating pancreatic edema at the junction of the pancreatic head and body (*asterisk*) with extensive surrounding peripancreatic stranding indicating acute pancreatitis. Inflammatory stranding is noted tracking along the Gerota's fascia (*arrow*). Uniform enhancement excludes pancreatic necrosis. **B:** Coned view of the pancreas on axial slice from abdominal CT from the same patient demonstrates tracking of the inflammation into the pericholecystic space (*asterisk*) and along Gerota's fascia (*arrow*). The patient is status postcholecystectomy (*arrowhead*). **C:** Coned view of the pancreatic region in a different patient demonstrates a well-defined oval fluid collection (*asterisk*) with a clearly defined capsule (*arrow*) occupying most of the pancreatic bed consistent with a pseudocyst. There is mass effect on the superior mesenteric (*black arrowhead*) and splenic (*white arrowhead*) veins; however, these opacify well with contrast.

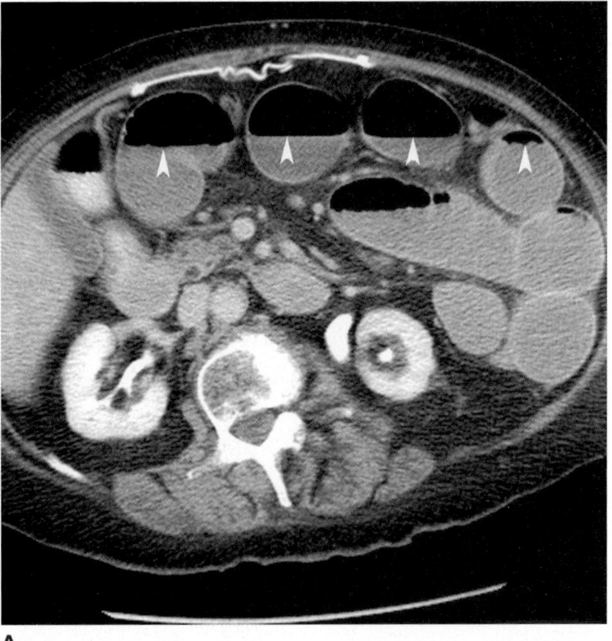

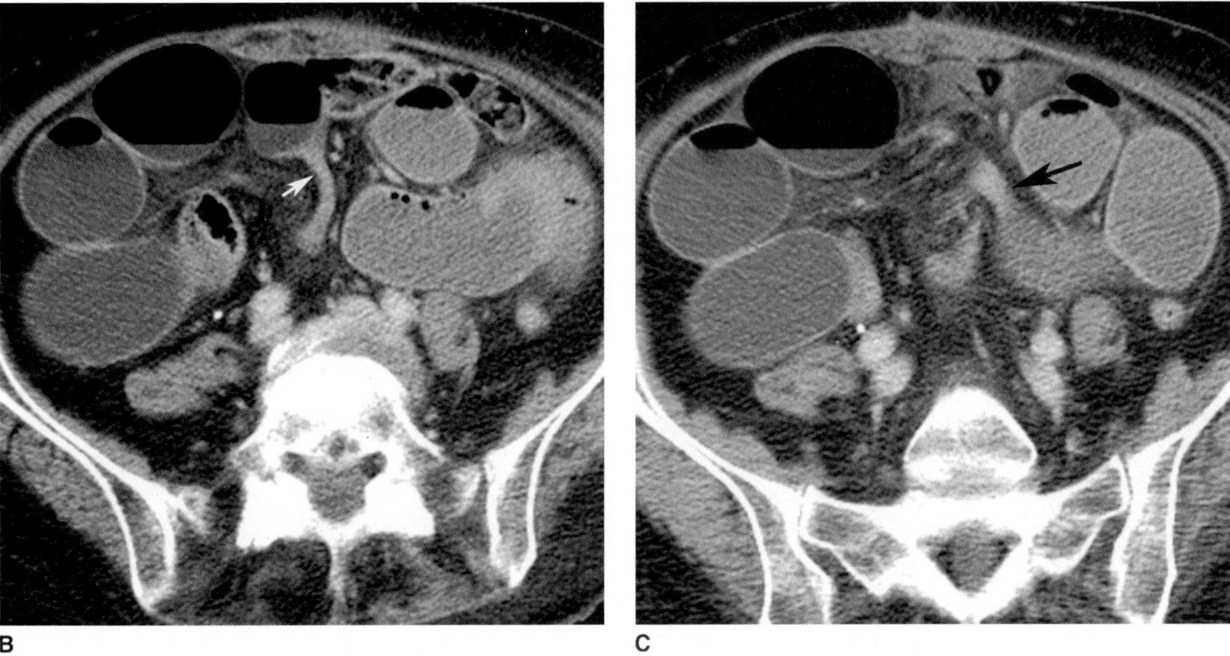

FIGURE 9.26. Small bowel obstruction. **A, B, C:** Coned views of the small bowel on transverse (axial) slices from abdominal CT demonstrate distended loops of small bowel with air fluid levels (*white arrowheads* in **A**) with abrupt transition point in the mid lower abdomen (*white arrow* in **B**). No ascites or bowel wall thickening noted to suggest ischemia. Surgery revealed adhesions, the most common etiology. Please note: It is very rare to see an actual adhesion on CT.[73]

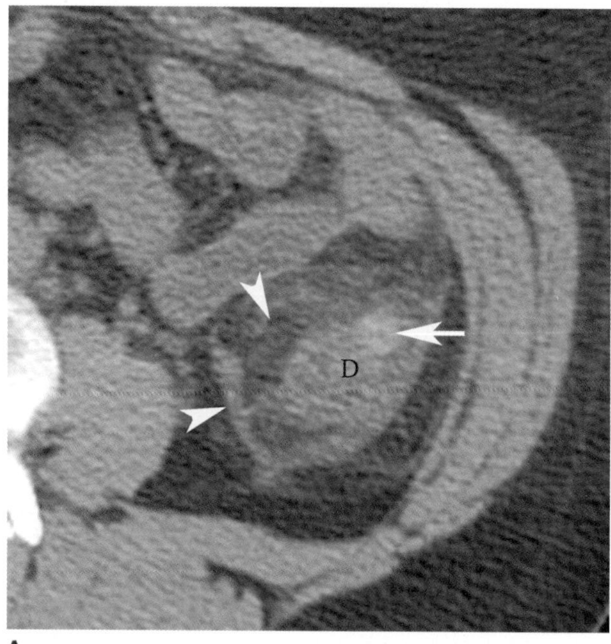

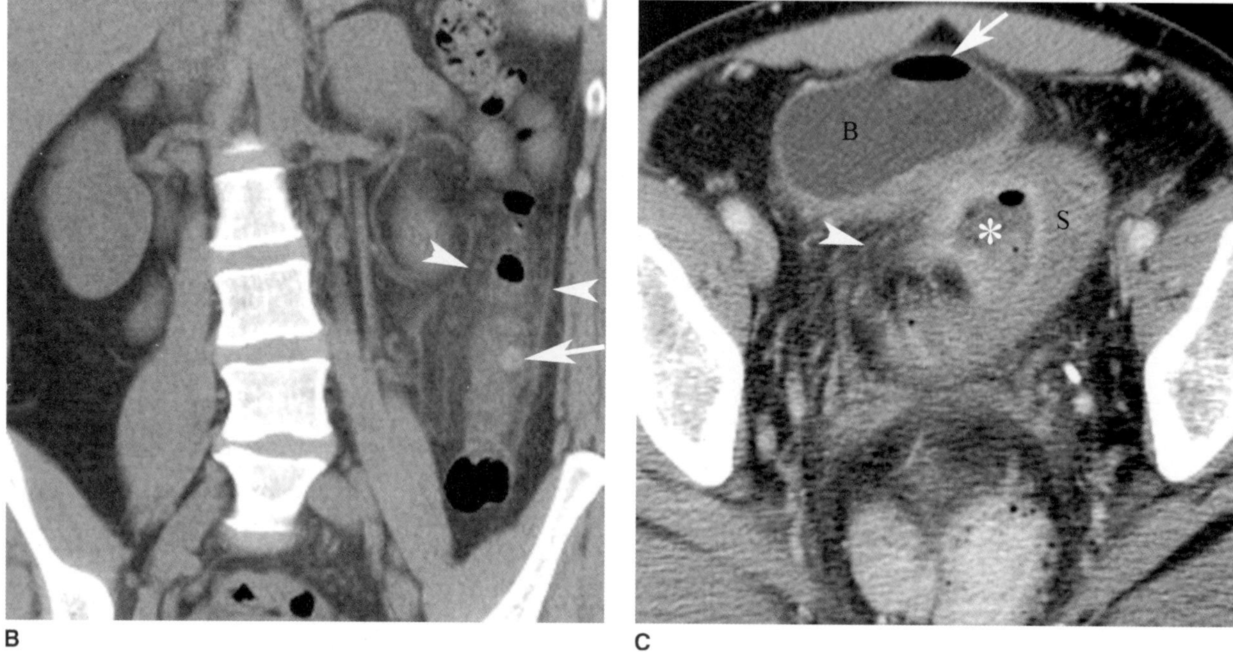

FIGURE 9.27. Acute diverticulitis. Coned views of the descending colon on axial (**A**) and coronal (**B**) slice from abdominal CT demonstrates wall thickening of the descending colon with pericolonic inflammation manifested by fascial thickening and stranding in the pericolic fat (*arrowheads*). A single diverticulum is noted in the inflamed portion of the descending colon (*arrow*). Findings represent uncomplicated acute diverticulitis. **C:** Coned views of the sigmoid colon on axial slice from abdominal CT in a different patient demonstrate thickened sigmoid colon with adjacent fat stranding (*arrowhead*) and rim enhancing collection along the medial aspect of the sigmoid colon consistent with abscess formation (*asterisk*). The abscess abuts the posterolateral aspect of the bladder with focus of air within the bladder (*arrowhead*) concerning for fistula formation. Abscess, sinus, or fistula may complicate diverticulitis. D, Descending colon; S, Sigmoid colon; B, Bladder.

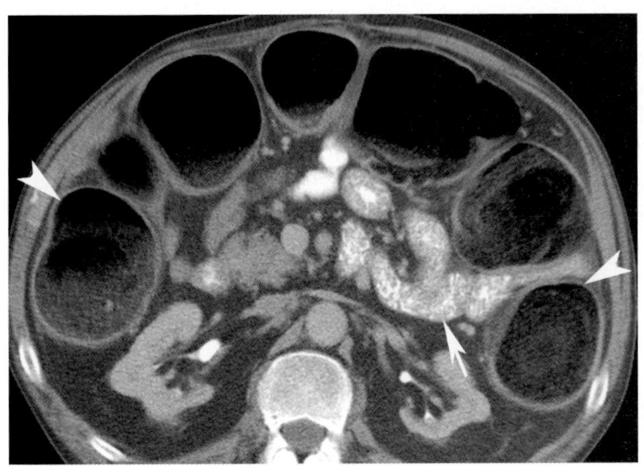

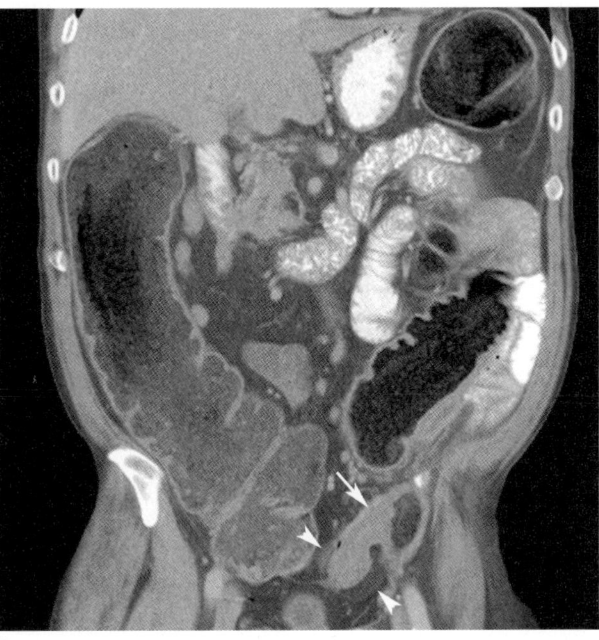

FIGURE 9.28. Large bowel obstruction. **A:** Coned view of the large bowel on axial slice from abdominal CT demonstrates dilation of the large bowel (*arrowheads*) from the cecum to the descending colon. The proximal small bowel is of normal caliber (*arrow*). **B:** Coned views of the large bowel on coronal slice from abdominal CT in the same patient demonstrate a transition point in the left lower quadrant at the junction of the descending colon and sigmoid colon (*arrow*). The bowel distal to the transition point demonstrates marked luminal narrowing, wall thickening, and pericolonic fat stranding consistent with inflammatory stricture (due to prior diverticulitis in this patient). The main causes of mechanical large bowel obstruction include colon cancer, diverticulitis, sigmoid volvulus, and cecal volvulus.[74]

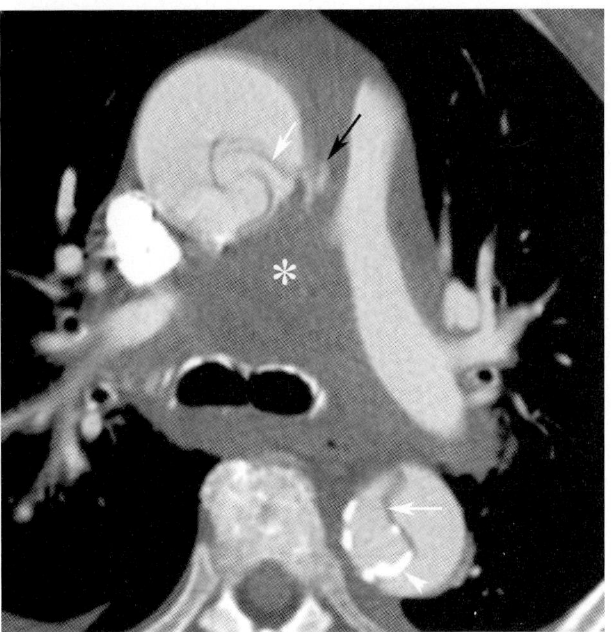

FIGURE 9.29. Acute aortic dissection. Coned views of the chest on axial slice from contrast-enhanced chest CT demonstrate a Stanford A aortic dissection involving the ascending and descending thoracic aorta. The intimal flap (*white arrows*) is lower in attenuation than the contrast opacified blood. Circumferential calcification (*arrowhead*) within the intima helps outline the true lumen. There is extraluminal contrast (*black arrow*) in the anterior mediastinum along the medial aspect of the ascending aorta concerning for rupture. There is also a large mediastinal hematoma (*asterisk*). CT is highly sensitive and specific (>95%) in the diagnosis of aortic dissection and helps determine the aortic branches involved.[40] Specificity for involvement of the ascending aorta can be increased with cardiac gating, which requires specialized protocols and radiologic consultation.

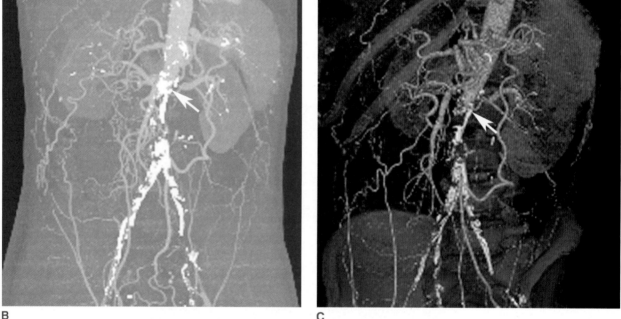

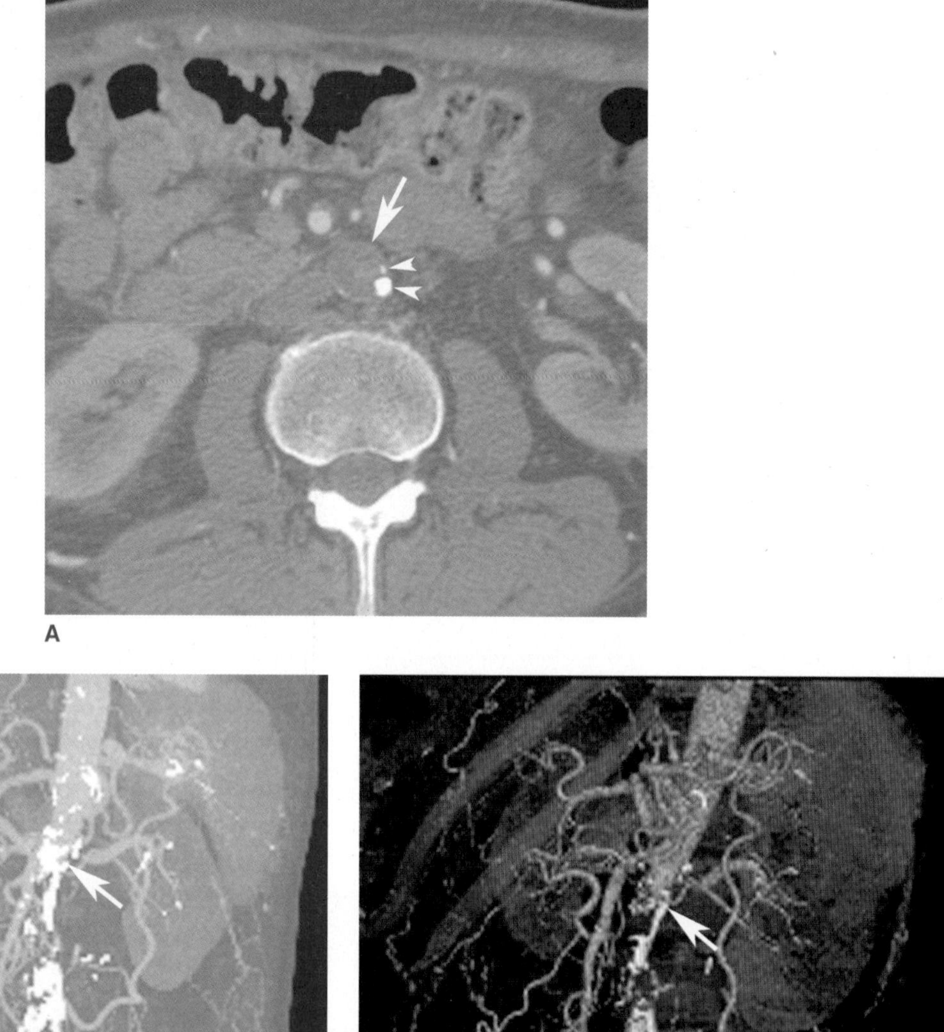

FIGURE 9.30. Aortic occlusion. **A:** Coned view of the abdominal aorta at the level of the kidneys on axial slice from abdominal CT demonstrates complete occlusion of the infrarenal abdominal aorta (*arrow*). Foci of atherosclerotic calcification are noted (*arrowheads*). **B:** Maximal intensity projection (MIP) and (**C**) volume-rendered (VR) images of the distal abdominal aorta in the same patient as (**A**) demonstrate occlusion of the infrarenal abdominal aorta (*arrow*), extensive atherosclerotic calcifications, and extensive collateral vessels.

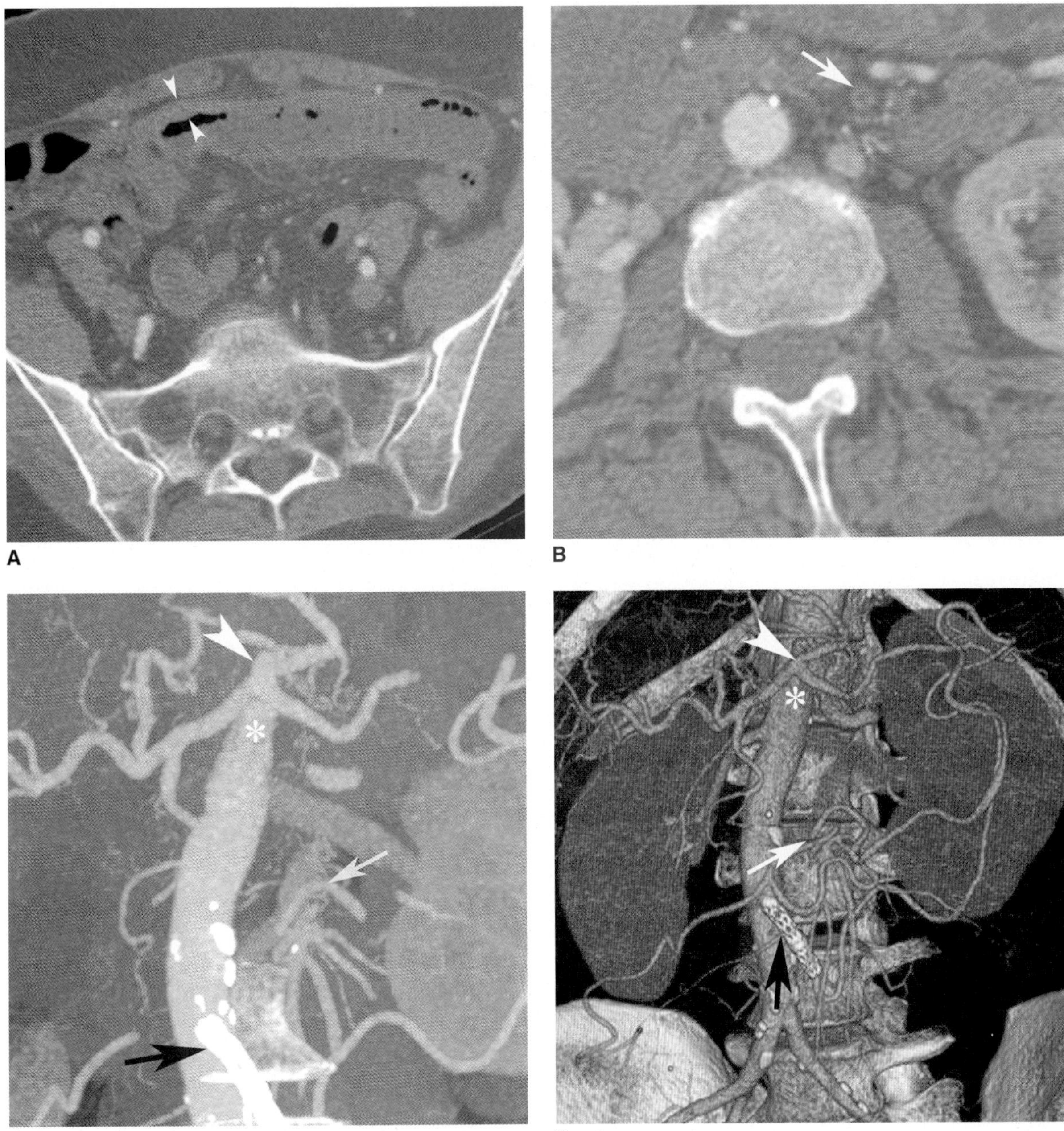

FIGURE 9.31. Mesenteric ischemia. **A:** Coned views of the small bowel in the mid lower abdomen on axial slice from abdominal contrast-enhanced CT in a patient with mesenteric ischemia demonstrates hypoenhancement of the bowel mucosa and mild bowel wall thickening (*arrowheads*) concerning for bowel ischemia. **B:** Coned views of the abdominal aorta abdomen on axial slice from abdominal contrast-enhanced CT in the same patient demonstrates thrombosed superior mesenteric artery (*arrow*). Findings of acute mesenteric ischemia included mesenteric arterial or venous thrombus, mesenteric venous gas, pneumatosis intestinalis, bowel-wall thickening, increased or decreased enhancement of the bowel wall. **C:** Maximal intensity projection (MIP) and (**D**) volume-rendered (VR) images of the abdominal aorta in the same patient as (A) and (B) demonstrate complete occlusion of the proximal portion of the superior mesenteric artery which is therefore not visualized (site of origin of the superior mesenteric artery is marked by *asterisk*). There is reconstitution of the distal portion of the superior mesenteric artery (*white arrow*). Celiac axis (*arrowhead*) is patent. Note the stent within the inferior mesenteric artery (*black arrow*).

References

1. Houston LE, Odibo AO, Macones GA. The safety of obstetrical ultrasound: a review. *Prenat Diagn*. 2009;29:1204-1212.
2. Feller-Kopman D. Ultrasound-guided thoracentesis. *Chest*. 2006;129:1709-1714.
3. Kurtz AB, Middleton WD. *Ultrasound*. St. Louis, MO: Mosby; 1996.
4. Kalimi R, Gecelter GR, Caplin D, et al. Diagnosis of acute cholecystitis: sensitivity of sonography, cholescintigraphy, and combined sonography-cholescintigraphy. *J Am Coll Surg*. 2001;193:609-613.
5. Rosen CL, Brown DF, Chang Y, et al. Ultrasonography by emergency physicians in patients with suspected cholecystitis. *Am J Emerg Med*. 2001;19:32-36.
6. Spence SC, Teichgraeber D, Chandrasekhar C. Emergent right upper quadrant sonography. *J Ultrasound Med*, 2009;28:479-496.
7. Somarouthu B, Abbara S, Kalva SP. Diagnosing deep vein thrombosis. *Postgrad Med*. 2010;122:66-73.
8. Chang HC, Bhatt S, Dogra VS. Pearls and pitfalls in diagnosis of ovarian torsion. *Radiographics*. 2008;28:1355-1368.
9. Bhatt S, Dogra VS. Role of US in testicular and scrotal trauma. *Radiographics*. 2008;28:1617-1629.

10. Kamaya A, Shin L, Chen B, et al. Emergency gynecologic imaging. *Semin Ultrasound CT MR*. 2008;29:353-368.
11. Rybkin AV, Thoeni RF. Current concepts in imaging of appendicitis. *Radiol Clin North Am*. 2007;45:411-422, vii.
12. Coelho JC, Sigel B, Ryva JC, et al. B-mode sonography of blood clots. *J Clin Ultrasound*. 1982;10:323-327.
13. Lee BC, Ormsby EL, McGahan JP, et al. The utility of sonography for the triage of blunt abdominal trauma patients to exploratory laparotomy. *AJR Am J Roentgenol*. 2007;188:415-421.
14. Tourtier JP, Ramsang S, Sauvageon X, et al. The utility of focused assessment with sonography in trauma as a triage tool. *J Trauma*. 2010;68:507-508; author reply 508.
15. Valentino M, Serra C, Zironi G, et al. Blunt abdominal trauma: emergency contrast-enhanced sonography for detection of solid organ injuries. *AJR Am J Roentgenol*. 2006;186:1361-1367.
16. Feldman MK, Katyal S, Blackwood MS. US artifacts. *Radiographics*. 2009;29:1179-1189.
17. Hashemi RH, Bradley WG, Lisanti CJ. *MRI: The Basics*. Philadelphia, PA: Lippincott Williams & Wilkins; 2010.
18. Morana G, Salviato E, Guarise A. Contrast agents for hepatic MRI. *Cancer Imaging*. 2007;7 Spec No A:S24-S27.
19. Waters EA, Wickline SA. Contrast agents for MRI. *Basic Res Cardiol*. 2008;103:114-121.
20. Tatli S, Morrison PR, Tuncali K, et al. Interventional MRI for oncologic applications. *Tech Vasc Interv Radiol*. 2007;10:159-170.
21. Pedrosa I, Zeikus EA, Levine D, et al. MR imaging of acute right lower quadrant pain in pregnant and nonpregnant patients. *Radiographics*. 2007;27:721-743; discussion 743-753.
22. Cobben LP, Groot I, Haans L, et al. MRI for clinically suspected appendicitis during pregnancy. *AJR Am J Roentgenol*. 2004;183:671-675.
23. Israel GM, Malguria N, McCarthy S, et al. MRI vs. ultrasound for suspected appendicitis during pregnancy. *J Magn Reson Imaging*. 2008;28:428-433.
24. Siddiki H, Fidler J. MR imaging of the small bowel in Crohn's disease. *Eur J Radiol*. 2009;69:409-417.
25. Benko A, Fraser-Hill M, Magner P, et al. Canadian Association of Radiologists: consensus guidelines for the prevention of contrast-induced nephropathy. *Can Assoc Radiol J*. 2007;58:79-87.
26. Handl-Zeller L, Hubsch P, Hohenberg G, et al. B-mode and color-coded Doppler sonography in irradiation planning in klippel-Trenaunay syndrome with Kasabach-Merritt symptoms. *Ultraschall Med*. 1989;10:41-43.
27. Lichtenstein GR, Schnall M, Herlinger H. MRI evaluation of Crohn disease activity. *Abdom Imaging*. 2000;25:229.
28. Al Samaraee A, Khan U, Almashta Z, et al. Preoperative diagnosis of choledocholithiasis: the role of MRCP. *Br J Hosp Med (Lond)*. 2009;70:339-343.
29. Darge K, Anupindi S. Pancreatitis and the role of US, MRCP and ERCP. *Pediatr Radiol*. 2009;39(suppl 2):S153-157.
30. Macdonald GA, Peduto AJ. Magnetic resonance imaging (MRI) and diseases of the liver and biliary tract. Part 1. Basic principles, MRI in the assessment of diffuse and focal hepatic disease. *J Gastroenterol Hepatol*. 2000;15:980-991.
31. Sandrasegaran K, Lin C, Akisik FM, et al. State-of-the-art pancreatic MRI. *AJR Am J Roentgenol*. 2010;195:42-53.
32. Pedrosa I, Guarise A, Goldsmith J, et al. The interrupted rim sign in acute cholecystitis: a method to identify the gangrenous form with MRI. *J Magn Reson Imaging*. 2003;18:360-363.
33. Watanabe Y, Nagayama M, Okumura A, et al. MR imaging of acute biliary disorders. *Radiographics*. 2007;27:477-495.
34. Shellock FG, Spinazzi A. MRI safety update 2008: part 2, screening patients for MRI. *AJR Am J Roentgenol*. 2008;191:1140-1149.
35. Abujudeh HH, Rolls H, Kaewlai R, et al. Retrospective assessment of prevalence of nephrogenic systemic fibrosis (NSF) after implementation of a new guideline for the use of gadobenate dimeglumine as a sole contrast agent for magnetic resonance examination in renally impaired patients. *J Magn Reson Imaging*. 2009;30:1335-1340.
36. Juluru K, Vogel-Claussen J, Macura KJ, et al. MR imaging in patients at risk for developing nephrogenic systemic fibrosis: protocols, practices, and imaging techniques to maximize patient safety. *Radiographics*. 2009;29:9-22.
37. Morris MF, Zhang Y, Zhang H, et al. Features of nephrogenic systemic fibrosis on radiology examinations. *AJR Am J Roentgenol*. 2009;193:61-69.
38. Shellock FG, Crues JV. MR procedures: biologic effects, safety, and patient care. *Radiology*. 2004;232:635-652.
39. Mahesh M. AAPM/RSNA physics tutorial for residents: Search for isotropic resolution in CT from conventional to multiple-row detector. *Radiographics*. 2002;22:949-962.
40. Webb WR, Brant WE, Major NM. *Fundamentals of Body CT*. Philadelphia, PA: Elsevier/Saunders; 2006.
41. Barrett BJ, Katzberg RW, Thomsen HS, et al. Contrast-induced nephropathy in patients with chronic kidney disease undergoing computed tomography: a double-blind comparison of iodixanol and iopamidol. *Invest Radiol*. 2006;41:815-821.
42. Gleeson TG, Bulugahapitiya S. Contrast-induced nephropathy. *AJR Am J Roentgenol*. 2004;183:1673-1689.
43. Herrada B, Agarwal J, Abcar AC. How can we reduce the incidence of contrast-induced acute renal failure? *Permanente J*. 2005;9.
44. Nguyen SA, Suranyi P, Ravenel JG, et al. Iso-osmolality versus low-osmolality iodinated contrast medium at intravenous contrast-enhanced CT: effect on kidney function. *Radiology*. 2008;248:97-105.
45. ACR. *Manual on Contrast Media Version* 7. 2010. Available at: http://www.acr.org/SecondaryMainMenuCategories/quality_safety/contrast_manual.aspx
46. Ellis JH, Cohan RH. Prevention of contrast-induced nephropathy: an overview. *Radiol Clin North Am*. 2009;47:801-811, v.
47. Goldfarb S, McCullough PA, McDermott J, et al. Contrast-induced acute kidney injury: specialty-specific protocols for interventional radiology, diagnostic computed tomography radiology, and interventional cardiology. *Mayo Clin Proc*. 2009;84:170-179.
48. Hogan SE, L'Allier P, Chetcuti S, et al. Current role of sodium bicarbonate-based preprocedural hydration for the prevention of contrast induced acute kidney injury: a meta-analysis. *Am Heart J*. 2008;156:414-421.
49. McCullough PA, Bertrand ME, Brinker JA, et al. A meta-analysis of the renal safety of isosmolar iodixanol compared with low-osmolar contrast media. *J Am Coll Cardiol*. 2006;48:692-699.
50. Zoungas S, Ninomiya T, Huxley R, et al. Systematic review: sodium bicarbonate treatment regimens for the prevention of contrast-induced nephropathy. *Ann Intern Med*. 2009;151:631-638.
51. Singh J, Daftary A. Iodinated contrast media and their adverse reactions. *J Nucl Med Technol*. 2008;36:69-74; quiz 76-67.
52. Baerlocher MO, Asch M, Myers A. Allergic-type reactions to radiographic contrast media. *CMAJ*, 2010;182:1328.
53. Amis ES, Jr., Butler PF, Applegate KE, et al. American College of Radiology white paper on radiation dose in medicine. *J Am Coll Radiol*. 2007;4:272-284.
54. Lauer MS. Elements of danger–the case of medical imaging. *N Engl J Med*. 2009;361:841-843.
55. Huda W. *Review of Radiologic Physics*. Philadelphia, PA: Lippincott Williams & Wilkins; 2010.
56. Huda W, Vance A. Patient radiation doses from adult and pediatric CT. *AJR Am J Roentgenol*. 2007;188:540-546.
57. Brenner DJ, Hall EJ. Computed tomography—an increasing source of radiation exposure. *N Engl J Med*. 2007;357:2277-2284.
58. Mezrich RS. Radiation exposure from medical imaging procedures. *N Engl J Med*. 2009;361:2290; author reply 2291-2292.
59. Bettman MA. Selecting the right test and relative radiation dose as they relate to appropriateness criteria. *Image Wisely*. 2010:1-3.
60. Mayo-Smith WW. Protocol design. *Image Wisely*. 2010:1-3.
61. Mirvis SE, Shanmuganathan K. Diagnosis of blunt traumatic aortic injury 2007: still a nemesis. *Eur J Radiol*. 2007;64:27-40.
62. Steenburg SD, Ravenel JG. Acute traumatic thoracic aortic injuries: experience with 64-MDCT. *AJR Am J Roentgenol*. 2008;191:1564-1569.
63. Rha SE, Ha HK, Lee SH, et al. CT and MR imaging findings of bowel ischemia from various primary causes. *Radiographics*. 2000;20:29-42.
64. Miller LA. Chest wall, lung, and pleural space trauma. *Radiol Clin North Am*. 2006;44:213-224, viii.
65. Sangster GP, Gonzalez-Beicos A, Carbo AI, et al. Blunt traumatic injuries of the lung parenchyma, pleura, thoracic wall, and intrathoracic airways: multidetector computer tomography imaging findings. *Emerg Radiol*. 2007;14:297-310.
66. Ball CG, Kirkpatrick AW, Feliciano DV. The occult pneumothorax: what have we learned? *Can J Surg*. 2009;52:E173-179.
67. de Moya MA, Seaver C, Spaniolas K, et al. Occult pneumothorax in trauma patients: development of an objective scoring system. *J Trauma*. 2007;63:13-17.
68. Wall SD, Federle MP, Jeffrey RB, et al. CT diagnosis of unsuspected pneumothorax after blunt abdominal trauma. *AJR Am J Roentgenol*. 1983;141:919-921.
69. Brofman N, Atri M, Hanson JM, et al. Evaluation of bowel and mesenteric blunt trauma with multidetector CT. *Radiographics*. 2006;26:1119-1131.
70. Hauser CJ, Visvikis G, Hinrichs C, et al. Prospective validation of computed tomographic screening of the thoracolumbar spine in trauma. *J Trauma*. 2003;55:228-234; discussion 234-225.
71. Wintermark M, Mouhsine E, Theumann N, et al. Thoracolumbar spine fractures in patients who have sustained severe trauma: depiction with multi-detector row CT. *Radiology*. 2003;227:681-689.
72. Shah N, Anderson SW, Vu M, et al. Extremity CT angiography: application to trauma using 64-MDCT. *Emerg Radiol*. 2009;16:425-432.
73. Boudiaf M, Soyer P, Terem C, et al. Ct evaluation of small bowel obstruction. *Radiographics*. 2001;21:613-624.
74. Flasar MH, Goldberg E. Acute abdominal pain. *Med Clin North Am*. 2006;90:481-503.

CHAPTER 10 ■ HEMATOLOGIC ABNORMALITIES, COAGULOPATHY, AND TRANSFUSION THERAPY

LENA M. NAPOLITANO

HEMATOLOGIC ABNORMALITIES

Red Blood Cell Disorders

Anemia Anemia is common in critically ill and injured patients admitted to the intensive care unit (ICU), with >90% of patients anemic on ICU day 3.[1] Anemia in the ICU is associated with appreciable red blood cell (RBC) transfusion use (Table 10.1).[2–9] Furthermore, anemia persists after ICU discharge, with >50% of patients still anemic 6 months after ICU discharge.[10–12]

The World Health Organization defines anemia as Hb concentration <12 g/dL in women and <13 g/dL in men. Etiologies of anemia in the ICU include blood loss related to daily phlebotomy, hemodilution due to crystalloid fluid resuscitation, renal replacement therapies, renal disease, hemorrhage, occult blood loss from the gastrointestinal tract, bone marrow suppression due to diseases, drug-induced anemia, and nutritional deficiencies such as iron, folate, and vitamin B12 deficiency. In ICU patients with anemia and chronic kidney disease, treatment with erythropoietin-stimulating agents (ESAs) is indicated, with target hemoglobin concentrations no higher than 9 g/dL. Adjunctive iron treatment should be strongly considered, as optimal response to ESAs requires supplemental iron.

In most ICU patients, the etiology of anemia is "anemia of inflammation" or "anemia of chronic disease." Anemia of inflammation develops via three mechanisms: (1) impaired iron regulation, (2) shortened RBC life span, and (3) reduced rate of erythropoiesis related to inappropriate erythropoietin response. Hepcidin is the main iron regulatory hormone, made primarily in hepatocytes, and causes functional iron deficiency, hypoferremia, and iron-restricted erythropoiesis despite normal iron stores by blocking enteral iron absorption and shuttling iron into macrophages where it is unavailable for erythropoiesis (Fig. 10.1). Hepcidin concentrations are high in anemia of inflammation and anemia of chronic disease (ACD).[13]

ANEMIA: CLINICAL APPROACH TO DIAGNOSTIC EVALUATION

All ICU patients with anemia should undergo a diagnostic evaluation (Algorithm. 10.1) as for any patient with anemia. Determination of the causative factors for anemia will allow appropriate anemia management, which will aid in avoiding RBC transfusion solely for the treatment of anemia.

ANEMIA AND DIAGNOSIS OF IRON DEFICIENCY IN THE INTENSIVE CARE UNIT

Iron deficiency is difficult to diagnose in intensive care unit (ICU) patients, since most will have high ferritin levels related to inflammation. In these patients, one should check blood zinc protoporphyrin concentration, which will be high in iron deficiency. In the presence of inflammation, true iron deficiency is defined by a ferritin < 100 ng/mL and a TSAT < 20%, whereas functional iron deficiency is defined by ferritin > 100 ng/mL and a TSAT < 20% (Algorithm 10.2).

Total iron deficit (TID) can be calculated using the Ganzoni formula: TID (mg) = weight (kg) × (ideal Hb − actual Hb) (g/dL) × 0.24 + depot iron (500 mg). According to this formula, a person weighing 70 kg with a Hb concentration of 9 g/dL would have a body iron deficit of about 1,400 mg. Following the administration of oral iron, it takes 2–2.5 weeks for the Hb to start rising, 2 months for it to return to normal levels, and 6 months for iron stores to be replete. In anemia of inflammation or ACD, enteral iron absorption is problematic due to high hepcidin concentrations, which block enteral iron absorption, and intravenous (IV) iron should be considered. A number of safe IV iron formulations are now available for use (Table 10.2).

Polycythemia Polycythemia is not common in critical care and is defined as Hgb > 18.5 g/dL (men) > 16.5 g/dL (women) or Hgb > 17 g/dL (men) > 15 g/dL (women) if associated with a sustained increase of >2 g/dL from baseline that cannot be attributed to correction of iron deficiency. The most common cause of polycythemia is hypoxia secondary to pulmonary disease. A low-serum erythropoietin concentration in the polycythemic patient suggests the diagnosis of polycythemia vera. Management of polycythemia is control of the underlying cause (i.e., removal of an erythropoietin-secreting tumor) and limited phlebotomy as indicated if symptoms are present.

Platelet Disorders

Platelet disorders are common in the ICU. Thromboctyopenia occurs often in critical illness, perhaps in up to 41% of patients.[14] Thrombocytosis and functional platelet disorders are less common and are found in up to 25% of ICU patients. Systematic evaluation of platelet disorders in critical care is essential to accurate identification and management of the cause. Importantly, thrombocytopenia has been associated with adverse outcomes. In contrast, thrombocytosis has been associated with improved outcomes in the ICU.

Thrombocytopenia Thrombocytopenia is defined as a platelet count of <150,000/mm³ or <150 × 10⁹/L. The normal range for platelet count in adult humans is 150–450 × 10⁹/L. Thrombocytopenia may result from decreased production or increased destruction of platelets. A patient is at risk for spontaneous bleeding when the platelet count fall below 20,000 and may warrant platelet transfusion.

The reported incidence of thrombocytopenia in the critical care setting varies from 23% to 41% and is associated with mortality rates between 38% and 54% in retrospective studies.[15–22] Although the incidence of severe thrombocytopenia (platelet counts lower than 50 × 10⁹/L) is lower (10%–17%), the association with adverse outcomes is even stronger. Sepsis

TABLE 10.1

RESULTS OF EPIDEMIOLOGIC STUDIES ON ANEMIA AND BLOOD TRANSFUSION IN CRITICAL CARE

	n	MEAN ADMISSION HEMOGLOBIN (g/dL)	PERCENTAGE OF PATIENTS TRANSFUSED IN ICU (%)	MEAN TRANSFUSIONS PER PATIENT (U)	MEAN PRE-TRANSFUSION HEMOGLOBIN (g/dL)	MEAN ICU LENGTH OF STAY (D)	ICU MORTALITY (%)	HOSPITAL MORTALITY	ADMISSION APACHE II (MEAN)
ABC Trial[a] (Western Europe)	3534	11.3 ± 2.3	37.00	4.8 ± 5.2	8.4 ± 1.3	4.5	13.50	20.20%	14.8 ± 7.9
Crit Study[b] (USA)	4892	11.0 ± 2.4	44.10	4.6 ± 4.9	8.6 ± 1.7	7.4 ± 7.3	13.00	17.60%	19.7 ± 8.2
TRICC Investigators[c] (Canada)	5298	9.9 ± 2.2	25	4.6 ± 6.7	8.6 ± 1.3	4.8 ± 12.6	22	–	18 ± 11
North Thames Blood Interest Group[d] (UK)	1247	–	53.40	5.7 ± 5.2	8.5 ± 1.4	–	21.50	–	18.1 ± 9.1

[a]Vincent JL, Baron J-F, Reinhart K, et al. Anemia and blood transfusion in critically ill patients. *JAMA*. 2002;288:1499–1507.
[b]Corwin HL, Gettinger A, Pearl RG, et al. The CRIT study. Anemia and blood transfusion in the critically ill: current clinical practice in the United States. *Crit Care Med*. 2004;32:39–52.
[c]Hebert PC, Wells G, Martin C, et al. A Canadian survey of transfusion practices in critically ill patients. *Crit Care Med*. 1998;26:482–487.
[d]Rao MP, Boralessa H, Morgan C, Soni N, Goldhill DR, Brett SJ, Boralessa H, Contreras M: Blood component use in critically ill patients. *Anaesthesia*. 2002, 57:530–534
Data are expressed as mean ± standard deviation. ABC, Anemia and Blood Transfusion in Critical Care; APACHE, Acute Physiology and Chronic Health Evaluation; ICU, intensive care unit; TRICC, Transfusion Requirements in Critical Care.
From: Napolitano LM. Scope of the problem: epidemiology of anemia and use of blood transfusions in critical care. *Critical Care*. 2004;8(suppl 2):S1-S8.

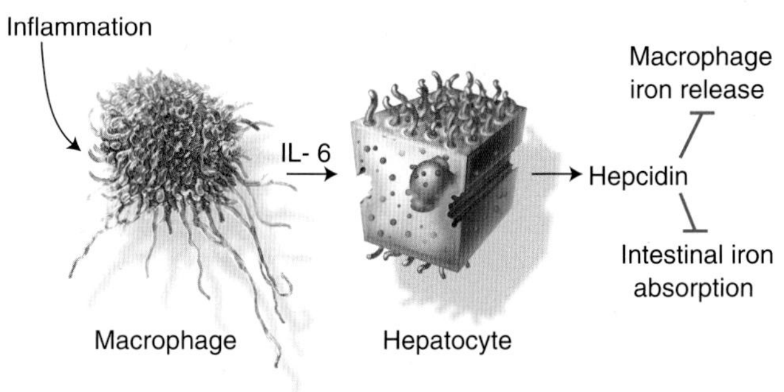

FIGURE 10.1. Hepcidin and the anemia of critical illness. Regulation of hepcidin production in inflammation. Inflammation leads to macrophage elaboration of IL–6, which acts on hepatocytes to induce hepcidin production. Hepcidin inhibits macrophage iron release and intestinal iron absorption, leading to hypoferremia.

and hemodilution are common etiologies of thrombocytopenia in critical illness, but heparin-induced thrombocytopenia (HIT) is one potential etiology that warrants serious consideration in all patients.

DIAGNOSTIC EVALUATION OF THROMBOCYTOPENIA IN THE INTENSIVE CARE UNIT

Systematic evaluation of the numerous potential etiologies of thrombocytopenia in critical care is essential to accurate identification and management of the cause (Table 10.3). Sepsis is the most common etiology of thrombocytopenia in critical illness, accounting for 48% of cases of thrombocytopenia.[23] However, >25% of intensive care unit (ICU) patients have more than one cause of thrombocytopenia.[8] Drug-induced thrombocytopenias present diagnostic challenges, because many of the multiple medications administered to ICU patients may be the cause.[24] One such commonly administered drug is heparin—the most common cause of drug-induced thrombocytopenia due to immune mechanisms.

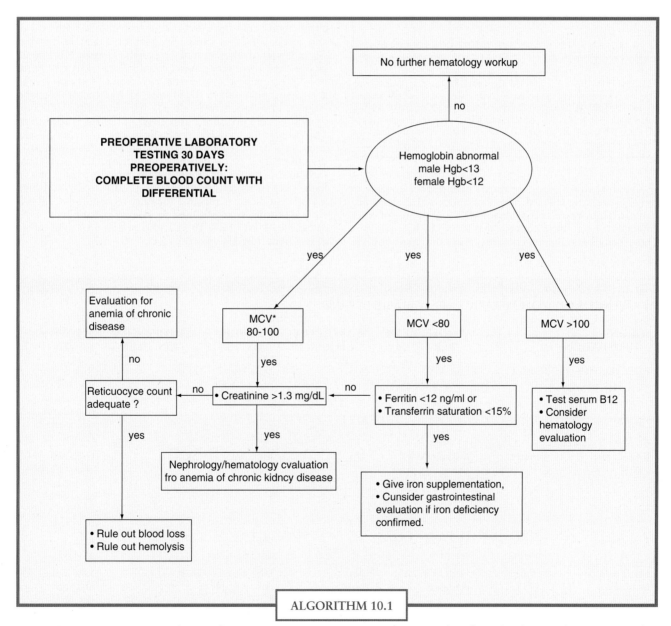

PREOPERATIVE LABORATORY TESTING 30 DAYS PREOPERATIVELY: COMPLETE BLOOD COUNT WITH DIFFERENTIAL

→ Hemoglobin abnormal
male Hgb<13
female Hgb<12

- no → No further hematology workup
- yes → MCV* 80-100
  - yes → • Creatinine >1.3 mg/dL
    - yes → Nephrology/hematology cvaluation fro anemia of chronic kidncy disease
    - no → Reticuocyce count adequate ?
      - no → Evaluation for anemia of chronic disease
      - yes → • Rule out blood loss • Rule out hemolysis
- yes → MCV <80
  - yes → • Ferritin <12 ng/ml or • Transferrin saturation <15%
    - yes → • Give iron supplementation, • Cunsider gastrointestinal evaluation if iron deficiency confirmed.
    - no → • Creatinine >1.3 mg/dL
- yes → MCV >100
  - yes → • Test serum B12 • Consider hematology evaluation

ALGORITHM 10.1

ALGORITHM 10.1 Diagnostic evaluation of anemia in acute care surgery patients. From: Goodnough LT, Shander A, et al. "Detection, evaluation, and management of anemia in the elective surgical patient." *Anesth Analg.* 2005;101(6):1858–1861.

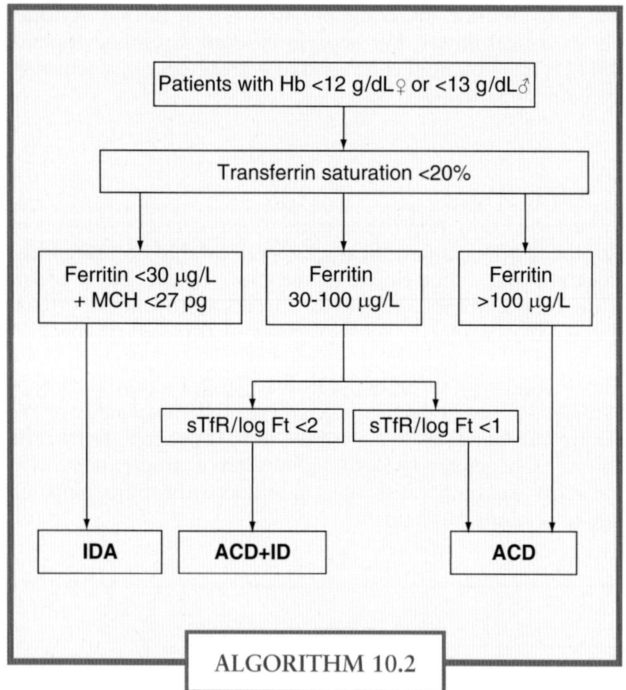

ALGORITHM 10.2 A simplified algorithm for the diagnosis of iron deficiency anemia. ACD, anemia of chronic disease; Hb, hemoglobin; ID, iron deficiency; IDA, iron deficiency anemia; MCH, mean corpuscular hemoglobin; sTfR, serum transferring receptor. From: Muñoz M, García-Erce JA, Remacha AF. Disorders of iron metabolism, part II: iron deficiency and iron overload. *J Clin Pathol.* 2011;64:287–296.

The three most important causes of thrombocytopenia in the ICU are drug-induced thrombocytopenia, HIT, and disseminated intravascular coagulation (DIC). A number of other etiologies of thrombocytopenia may occur in ICU patients. These include autoimmune or alloimmune thrombocytopenia (ITP), posttransfusion purpura, the thrombotic microangiopathies [thrombotic thrombocytopenic purpura (TTP) and hemolytic uremic syndrome (HUS)], and the HELLP (hemolysis, elevated liver enzymes, and low platelets) syndrome. TTP most commonly presents with a pentad of thrombocytopenia (with purpura), RBC fragmentation, renal failure, neurologic dysfunction, and fever.

Drugs can induce thrombocytopenia by a number of mechanisms. In addition to those that are directly cytotoxic, thiazide diuretics, interferon, and alcohol can cause thrombocytopenia by inhibiting platelet production in the bone marrow. More commonly, drug-induced thrombocytopenia results from the immunologic destruction of platelets. Drugs can induce antibodies to platelets either by acting as a hapten or by functioning as an innocent bystander. Drugs such as gold salts and interferon can induce an ITP-like disorder. Some common ICU drugs that are associated with thrombocytopenia are detailed in Table 10.4.

HEPARIN-INDUCED THROMBOCYTOPENIA

Heparin-induced thrombocytopenia (HIT) is an anticoagulant-induced *prothrombotic* disorder. HIT is an immune-mediated adverse drug effect characterized by platelet activation, hypercoagulability, and increased risk of thrombosis, both venous and arterial. HIT is caused by platelet-activating heparin-dependent antibodies of immunoglobulin G class. HIT should be considered when the platelet count falls to $<150 \times 10^9$/L (or by >50% from baseline) between days 5 and 14 of exposure to any heparinoid product. Rapid-onset HIT can occur if heparin is given to a patient who already has circulating HIT antibiotics, usually due to heparin given in the last 5–100 days. Thrombocytopenia in HIT is usually moderate – mean platelet count 60×10^9/L – and recovers within a few days of heparin discontinuation. Some patients will develop HITT—HIT and thrombosis (venous or arterial) with associated high rates of limb loss and mortality, ranging from 10% to 20%. A high index of suspicion is required for early recognition of HIT. A clinical scoring system is used to identify patients with HIT, called the "4 Ts" (Table 10.5), with a pretest probability score of 6–8 indicating high risk for HIT.

TABLE 10.2

INTRAVENOUS (IV) IRON PREPARATIONS AVAILABLE FOR USE

IRON PREPARATION		MOLECULAR WEIGHT (MW)	TEST DOSE REQUIRED?	DOSING ISSUES	ADMINISTRATION TIMING	ADVERSE EVENTS
Ferric gluconate	Ferrlicit	Low MW, unstable complex	No	Dose limitation 62.5 mg	Slow	Risk of labile iron toxicity, oversaturation of iron transport system
Iron sucrose	Venofer	Medium MW, semistable	No	Max single dose 200 mg	Slow	High pH of solution, lowest rate of adverse events reported
Iron dextran	Dexferrum, Imferon	High MW, stable complex	Yes	High single dose possible	Slow	Risk of anaphylaxis
Ferric carboxymaltose	Ferinject	High MW, stable complex	No	High single dose possible	Fast	Low immunogenic potential
Ferumoxytol	Feraheme, iron oxide nanoparticles	High MW, stable complex	No	High single dose possible	Fast	Minimal

TABLE 10.3

POTENTIAL ETIOLOGIES OF THROMBOCYTOPENIA

Common causes
- Hemodilutional (postresuscitation and perioperative)
- Sepsis and healthcare-associated infections
- Drug-induced thrombocytopenias, including HIT
- Peripheral platelet consumption or destruction
- DIC
- MT
- Lab error-clumping secondary to EDTA in test tube need smear to examine

Less common causes
- Liver disease
- Hypersplenism
- Primary marrow disorder, bone marrow failure
- Antiphospholipid antibody syndrome/lupus anticoagulant
- Immune thrombocytopenias (ITP, TTP, PTP)
- Intravascular devices (IABP, LVAD, ECMO, pulmonary artery catheter)

HIT, heparin-induced thrombocytopenia; DIC, disseminated intravascular coagulation; ITP, idiopathic thrombocytopenic purpura; PTP, posttransfusion purpura; TTP, thrombotic thrombocytopenic purpura;
IABP, intra-aortic balloon pump; LVAD, left ventricular assist devices; ECMO, extracorporeal membrane oxygenation.

TABLE 10.4

COMMON DRUGS THAT CAN INDUCE THROMBOCYTOPENIA

Quinidine
Amiodarone
Captopril
Thiazide diuretics
Ibuprofen
Phenytoin
Carbamazepine
Glibenclamide
Gold
Tamoxifen
Cimetidine
Ranitidine
Sulfonamides
Vancomycin
Piperacillin

Once HIT is strongly suspected in a critically ill patient, prompt discontinuation of all heparin and administration of an alternative nonheparin anticoagulant (commonly a direct thrombin inhibitor, DTI, Table 10.6) should be initiated. The principles of treatment for suspected or confirmed HIT include the "Six A's" (Table 10.7).[25] Do not wait for the laboratory confirmation of HIT prior to initiation of a DTI—this is associated with increased risk for thrombosis and adverse outcome. When evaluating a patient for HIT, one must also consider a number of other potential etiologies of thrombocytopenia (Table 10.8).[26]

HIT diagnosis is confirmed with either a positive anti-PF4/polyanion-IgG enzyme immunoassay or a positive platelet activation assay (i.e., serotonin-release assay). Once platelet count has normalized, warfarin should be initiated with a low maintenance dose (specifically, no loading dose) and overlapped with the nonheparin anticoagulant until the target international normalized ratio has been reached and for a minimum of 5 days. The duration of warfarin therapy should be standard for venous thromboembolism (VTE), for a minimum of 6 months with consideration for a more extended course depending on clinical circumstances related to the thromboembolic event.

TABLE 10.5

A CLINICAL SCORING SYSTEM USED TO DIAGNOSE HIT: THE "FOUR T'S"

CLINICAL SCORING SYSTEM USED TO DIAGNOSE HIT: THE "FOUR T'S"			
	POINTS (0, 1, OR 2 FOR EACH OF THE FOUR CATEGORIES): MAXIMUM SCORE = 8		
	2	1	0
Thrombocytopenia	>50% platelet decrease to nadir ≥20	30%–50% platelet decrease, or nadir 10–19, or >50% decrease secondary to surgery	<30% platelet decrease, or nadir < 10
Timing[a] of onset of platelet decrease (or other sequelae of HIT)	Days 5–10 or ≤ day 1 with recent heparin (past 30 days)	>Day 10 or timing unclear; or < day 1 with recent heparin (past 31–100 days)	<Day 4 (no recent heparin)
Thrombosis or other sequelae	Proven new thrombosis, skin necrosis, or acute systemic reaction after IV unfractionated heparin bolus	Progressive or recurrent thrombosis, erythematous skin lesions, suspected thrombosis (not proven)	None
Other cause of platelet decrease	None evident	Possible	Definite

[a]First day of immunizing heparin exposure considered day 0. Pretest probability score: 6–8 indicates high; 4–5, intermediate; and 0–3, low.
Adapted from Warkentin TE. Heparin-induced thrombocytopenia: diagnosis and management. *Circulation*. 2004;110:e454-e458.

TABLE 10.6

NONHEPARIN ANTICOAGULANTS FOR HIT TREATMENT

DRUG	MECHANISM	APPROVED FOR HIT	HALF-LIFE	MONITORING	DOSING	CLEARANCE
Fondaparinux	Long-acting AT3-dependent inhibition of factor Xa	Not approved for HIT treatment in the United States	Long (24 h); avoids potential for rebound hypercoagulable state	Direct (anti-Xa levels): accurate drug levels obtained	Not established for HIT, but consider 7.5 mg once daily (prophylaxis dose is 2.5 mg daily)	Renal
Danaparoid	Long-acting AT3-dependent inhibition of factor Xa	Not approved for HIT, not available in the United States, Approved for HIT in Canada, Europe, Australia, New Zealand and Japan.	Long (17–20 h) avoids potential for rebound hypercoagulable state	Direct (anti-Xa levels): accurate drug levels obtained	Bolus: 2250 U IV only in life-or limb-threatening thrombosis;infusion, 400 U/h × 4 h, then 300 U/h × 4 h, then 200 U/h IV, subsequently adjusted by anti-Xa levels (target, 0.5–0.8 anti-Xa U/mL)	Renal
Argatroban	Direct thrombin inhibitor (DTI)	Approved for HIT treatment in the United States	Short (40–50 min); potential for rebound hypercoagulable state	Indirect (APTT): risk for DTI underdosing due to APTT elevation for non-DTI factors	No bolus; initial rate, 0.5–2 μg/kg/min (adjust to APTT); reduce in liver disease	Hepatobiliary
Lepirudin	Direct thrombin inhibitor (DTI)	Approved for HIT treatment in the United States	Short (80 min); potential for rebound hypercoagulable state	Indirect (APTT): risk for DTI underdosing due to APTT elevation for non-DTI factors	No bolus; initial rate, 0.10 mg/kg/h (adjust to APTT); reduce dose for renal dysfunction	Renal
Bivalirudin	Direct thrombin inhibitor (DTI)	Not approved for HIT treatment in the United States	Short (25 min); potential for rebound hypercoagulable state	Indirect (APTT): risk for DTI underdosing due to APTT elevation for non-DTI factors	Not established; no bolus; initial dose, 0.15–0.20 mg/kg/h has been suggested	Enzymic metabolism

APTT, activated partial thromboplastin time.
Adapted from: Warkentin TE, Greinacher A, Koster A, et al. Treatment and prevention of heparin-induced thrombocytopenia. American College of Chest Physicians evidence-based clinical practice guidelines. 8th ed. *Chest.* 2008;133(suppl 6):340S–380S.

TABLE 10.7

THE PRINCIPLES OF TREATMENT FOR SUSPECTED OR CONFIRMED HIT: THE "SIX A'S"

Two "Do's"	1. Avoid and discontinue all heparin (including low molecular weight heparin) 2. Administer an alternative nonheparin anticoagulant with a DTI
Two "Don'ts"	3. Await platelet recovery before initiation of warfarin anticoagulation 4. Avoid platelet transfusions
Two diagnostics	5. Anti-PF4/heparin antibody test for confirmation 6. Assess for lower extremity deep venous thrombosis

Adapted from: Napolitano LM, Warkentin TE, AlMahameed A, Nasrawy SA. Heparin-induced thrombocytopenia in the critical care setting: diagnosis and management. *Crit Care Med.* 2006;34:2898–2911.

Thrombocytopenia Treatment In the bleeding patient, platelet transfusion is most commonly required. HIT is treated with heparin discontinuation and substitution of an alternative anticoagulant (DTI). Plasma exchange with fresh frozen plasma is the most effective treatment for TTP. HUS is best treated with supportive therapy including dialysis. Corticosteroids and splenectomy are the mainstays of therapy for ITP.

Thrombocytosis Thrombocytosis is defined as a platelet count above the normal value, in general, > 400–600,000/mm^3 or > 400–600 × 10^9/L (normal in adults—150–450 × 10^9/L). Thrombocytosis is classified into primary and secondary forms. *Primary (Clonal) thrombocytosis* is due to clonal thrombopoiesis and most often occurs in chronic myeloproliferative or in some myelodysplastic disorders. *Secondary (Reactive) thrombocytosis* is the most common form of thrombocytosis and is due to a variety of underlying conditions involving an acute phase reaction. These include trauma, surgery, bleeding, malignancy, infection, and inflammatory diseases.[27–29] (Table 10.9) Thrombocytosis is common (up to 25% of ICU patients) in the critically ill and is associated with improved outcome.

TABLE 10.8

COMPARISON OF SELECTED THROMBOCYTOPENIC DISORDERS THAT SHOULD BE CONSIDERED WHEN EVALUATING A PATIENT FOR HEPARIN-INDUCED THROMBOCYTOPENIA (HIT)

DISORDER	COMMON CLINICAL MANIFESTATIONS	USEFUL CLINICAL LABORATORY ANALYSES	COMMENTS
Heparin-induced thrombocytopenia (HIT)	>50% present with thrombosis; venous thrombosis > arterial.	Anti-heparin/PF4 antibody testing (ELISA, functional assays).	Temporal relationship with heparin or LMWH therapy.
Antiphospholipid syndrome (APS)	Recurrent venous and/or arterial thromboembolic complications; recurrent fetal loss.	Anticardiolipin antibody and anti-β_2-glycoprotein I antibody testing (ELISA); lupus anticoagulant testing.	Autoimmune disorder, either primary or associated with other rheumatologic conditions (e.g., lupus); in some cases, may be drug-induced (e.g., procainamide).
Dissesminated intravascular coagulation (DIC)	Hemorrhagic or thromboembolic events predominate, depending on underlying cause and clinical course.	PT, PTT, thrombin time, fibrinogen, D-dimer.	May be acute (e.g., associated with sepsis, obstetric complications, severe trauma) or chronic (e.g., associated with cancer, aortic aneurysm). DIC can complicate severe HIT.
Thrombotic thrombocytopenic purpura (TTP)	Neurologic manifestations may include stroke, TIA, altered mental status, seizures; other symptoms include fever, renal insufficiency.	Microangiopathic hemolytic changes on blood film, elevated LDH, decreased ADAMTS13 levels.	Associated with severe ADAMTS13 deficiency due to inhibitors in most patients; may be seen in patients taking ticlopidine or clopidogrel, or with other drugs, (e.g., cyclosporine, tacrolimus, mitomycin). Microangiopathy can also be seen in severe HIT with associated DIC.
Drug-induced thrombocytopenia (non-heparin)	Petechiae, purpura, and other hemorrhagic symptoms with severe thrombocytopenia.	Isolated thrombocytopenia, may be severe.	Associated with multiple drugs (e.g., abciximab, quinine, multiple antibiotics).
Post-transfusion purpura (PTP)	Hematoma, ecchymoses, purpura.	Severe thrombocytopenia that begins approximately 5 days after blood product use.	Temporal relationship to transfusion therapy; most common in multiparous females. The timing of PTP approximately one week after surgery can mimic HIT.

LMWH indicates low molecular weight heparin; DIC, disseminated intravascular coagulation; ELISA, enzyme-linked immunosorbent assay; TIA, transient ischemic attack; PT, prothrombin time; PTT, partial thromboplastin time; LDH, lactate dehydrogenase; ADAMTS13, a disintegrin and metalloproteinase with thrombospondin components–13.

Common clinical manifestations focus on thrombotic versus hemorrhagic symptoms. Comments include relationships to other disorders and/or drugs that need to be considered. HIT has also been reported to occur concomitantly in patients with antiphospholipid syndrome or DIC

From: Ortel TL. Heparin-induced thrombocytopenia: when a low platelet count is a mandate for anticoagulation. *Hematology Am Soc Hematol Educ Program.* 2009:225–232.

TABLE 10.9

MAJOR CAUSES OF THROMBOCYTOSIS

1. Primary (clonal) thrombocytosis (chronic myeloproliferative diseases)
   Essential (primary) thrombocythemia
   Other myeloproliferative disorders (chronic myelogenous leukemia, polycythemia vera, myeloid metaplasia, and myelofibrosis)
2. Familial thrombocytosis
3. Secondary (reactive) thrombocytosis
   Acute hemorrhage
   Trauma
   Major surgery
   Iron deficiency anemia, hemolytic anemia
   Postsplenectomy
   Recovery ("rebound") from thrombocytopenia
   Malignancies
   Chronic inflammatory and infectious diseases (inflammatory bowel disease, connective tissue disorders, temporal arteritis, tuberculosis, and chronic pneumonitis)
   Acute inflammatory and infectious diseases
   Response to intense exercise
   Reaction to drugs (vincristine, epinephrine, all-*trans*-retinoic acid, cytokines, and growth factors)

Thrombocytosis Treatment The greatest challenge in formulating a treatment plan for ICU patients is to correctly diagnose the cause of thrombocytosis. Treatment for patients with reactive thrombocytosis should be directed at the underlying disease. The abnormal platelet count itself does not increase the risk for thrombotic complications. Therefore, antiplatelet or platelet-lowering therapy is not indicated. In contrast, clonal thrombocytosis often needs treatment to reduce platelet counts, especially for high risk patients.[30] This group includes those with a history of bleeding or thrombotic complications, age > 60 years, other cardiovascular risk factors or extremely high platelet counts (>1,500 × 10^9/L).[31] Some of the agents employed to decrease platelet counts include hyroxyurea, interferon-α, and anagrelide. Low-dose aspirin (40–325 mg) has been used to reduce the risk of thrombosis in patients with platelet counts < 1,500 × 10^9/L.[32] Platelet apheresis and phlebotomy have been used to decrease platelet counts rapidly in patients with life-threatening complications from thrombocytosis. An algorithmic approach to the management of thrombocytosis is depicted in Algorithm 10.3.[33]

COAGULOPATHY

Hypercoagulable States

Hypercoagulable States (Thrombophilia) Hypercoagulable states should be considered in ICU patients who develop venous or arterial thrombosis. Hypercoagulable states are classified as inherited or acquired. Acquired thrombophilia is related to risk factors or predisposing conditions for thrombosis, including surgery, trauma, malignancy, central venous catheter, use of oral contraceptives, and others. Inherited thrombophilia is a genetic tendency to VTE. Factor V Leiden is the most common cause of inherited thrombophilia, accounting for 40%–50% of cases. The prothrombin 20210A gene mutation and deficiencies in protein S, protein C, or antithrombin account for most of the remaining cases of inherited thrombophilia. Patients with possible hypercoagulable states should undergo diagnostic testing for thrombophilia with a comprehensive panel of diagnostic tests (Table 10.10). Prior to the initiation of diagnostic testing for hypercoagulable states, it is important to assess whether the patient is on medication or has preexisting clinical conditions that may confound interpretation of laboratory tests for evaluation of thrombophilia (Table 10.11).[34]

Treatment of Hypercoagulable States Initial treatment of venous or arterial thrombosis in an ICU patient is systemic anticoagulation. Antithrombin, protein C, or protein S deficiency carry VTE recurrence rates of 5%–15% per year, a relative increase of 2.5 compared with rates in the absence of thrombophilia. Patients heterozygous for factor V Leiden or the prothrombin G20210A mutation are much less prone to VTE recurrence with a relative risk of 1.3–1.4; VTE recurrence rates are fivefold greater with homozygosity or double heterozygosity. A mild/moderate increase in homocysteine level is associated with a 2.5 increased risk for recurrent VTE. Long-term anticoagulant therapy is recommended in selected high-risk hypercoagulable states after a first spontaneous VTE episode in antithrombin, protein C or protein S deficiency, and for patients homozygous or doubly heterozygous for factor V Leiden and/or the prothrombin mutation. For patients with lower risk for recurrence, they are treated with anticoagulation for 6 months, and then imaging for residual thrombosis or D-dimer testing is performed at the end of anticoagulant therapy, and the results are used to determine likelihood of VTE recurrence.

Coagulopathies ICU patients with coagulation defects have a four- to fivefold increased risk for bleeding compared to patients with a normal coagulation status. Diagnostic testing for coagulopathy in critically ill patients requires a panel of comprehensive tests including prothrombin time (PT), activated partial thromboplastin time, thrombin time (TT), fibrinogen, fibrin degradation products, platelet count, and bleeding time (Table 10.12).[35]

DIC is a syndrome caused by systemic intravascular activation of coagulation with formation of microvascular thrombi with clotting factor consumption and occurs in patients with infection, malignancy, trauma, amniotic fluid embolism, and others. DIC manifests as prolonged plasma clotting times, thrombocytopenia, reduced plasma fibrinogen concentration, raised plasma fibrin-degradation products, and sometimes microangiopathic hemolysis (Algorithm. 10.4). The most frequent cause of DIC is sepsis, with reduced protein C concentrations resulting in decreased endogenous fibrinolysis. ICU patients with severe sepsis or septic shock may manifest abnormalities in coagulation testing, but plasma should not be transfused unless the patient has evidence of clinical bleeding (Surviving Sepsis Guidelines, 2008).[36] In cases of DIC, where thrombosis predominates, such as arterial or VTE severe purpura fulminans associated with acral ischemia or vascular skin infarction, therapeutic doses of heparin should be considered. Patients with sepsis-induced DIC may progress to purpura fulminans, a rapidly progressive thrombotic disorder with hemorrhagic infarction of the skin and dermal vascular thrombosis. Protein C concentrations should be measured in patients with purpura fulminans. In patients with severe limb-threatening purpura fulminans and low-protein C levels, replacement with exogenous protein C should be considered. Meningococcal and pneumococcal sepses are common causes of purpura fulminans and DIC. Treatment of DIC is supportive with aggressive treatment of the underlying cause of the DIC. Treatment of bleeding in DIC requires blood component replacement therapy with plasma, platelets, and cryoprecipitate.[37]

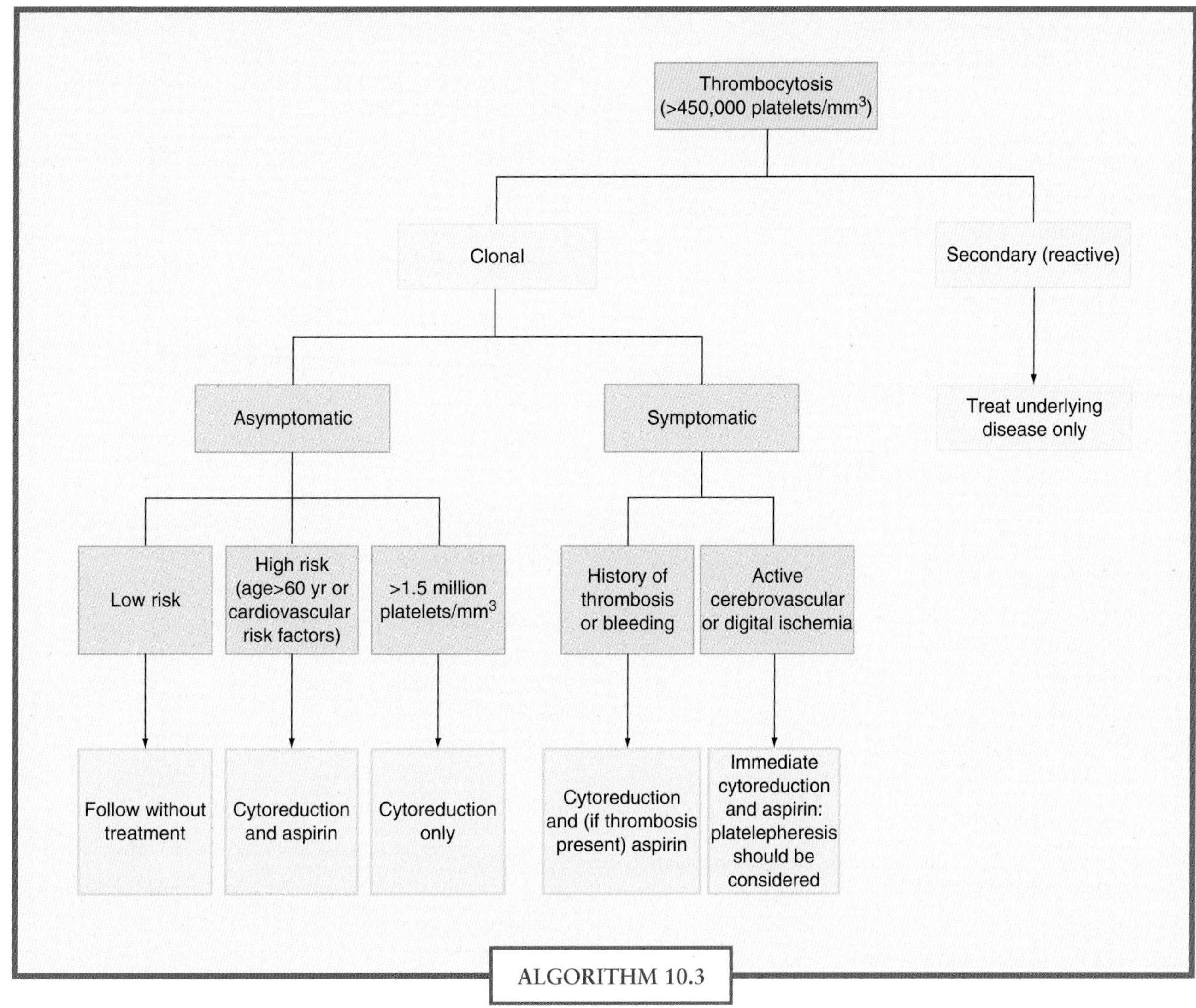

ALGORITHM 10.3 Approach to the management of thrombocytosis. From: Schafer AI. Thrombocytosis: Current Concepts [Review]. *N Engl J Med.* 2004;350:1211–1219.

Acute Traumatic Coagulopathy and Hemostatic Resuscitation

Hemorrhage is a major cause of trauma deaths and coagulopathy exacerbates hemorrhage. Trauma patients with severe hemorrhage have early hyperfibrinolysis in addition to coagulopathy (dilutional and consumptive).[38–40] Uncontrolled hemorrhage in trauma leads to the lethal triad of acidosis, hypothermia, and coagulopathy. Most severely injured patients are coagulopathic at hospital admission, before resuscitation interventions (Algorithm. 10.5).

Prompt reversal of coagulopathy using "hemostatic resuscitation" with early use of blood component therapy is advocated as the optimal practice for patients requiring massive transfusion (MT). It is recognized that increased early use of plasma is associated with increased risk for acute lung injury (ALI) and acute respiratory distress syndrome (ARDS), but is associated with decreased mortality. An emerging consensus for hemostatic resuscitation in patients requiring MT is as follows:

- Expedite the control of hemorrhage to prevent consumptive coagulopathy and thrombocytopenia and reduce the need for blood products.
- Limit isotonic crystalloid infusion to prevent dilutional coagulopathy and thrombocytopenia.
- Hypotensive resuscitation (SBP, 80–100 mm Hg) until definitive hemorrhage control is established
- Transfuse blood products in a 1:1:1 ratio of RBCs/FFP/platelets (one five-pack of pooled platelets counted as 5 U).
- Frequent laboratory monitoring (arterial lactate to assess adequacy of resuscitation, ionized calcium, and electrolytes)

TRANSFUSION THERAPY

Indications for Transfusion of Blood Components in the Intensive Care Unit

Red Blood Cell Transfusion RBC transfusion is common in intensive care unit (ICU) patients, with 40%–50% receiving RBC transfusion during the ICU stay. The Transfusion Requirements in Critical Care (TRICC) trial confirmed that ICU patient 30-day mortality was not different in patients randomized to a restrictive (transfuse if hemoglobin < 7 g/dL) or liberal (transfuse if hemoglobin < 10 g/dL) transfusion strategy.[41] Guidelines for RBC transfusion in ICU patients recommend transfusion when hemoglobin < 7 g/dL in most ICU patients (see Guideline Executive Summary, Table 10.13). In

TABLE 10.10

DIAGNOSTIC TESTING FOR HYPERCOAGULABLE STATES

A panel of diagnostic tests is used to evaluate patients with possible hypercoagulable states:
Complete blood count
Activated Protein C (APC) resistance test
Prothrombin 20210A mutation
Antithrombin III activity
Protein C activity
Protein S activity
ELISA anti-PF4 antibody (for HIT diagnosis)
Cardiolipin antibody (IgG and IgM)
B2-glycoprotein–1 antibody (IgG and IgM)
Lupus anticoagulant
Homocysteine levels
Factor VIII activity
Fibrinogen (clottable)
Fibrinogen antigen
Plasminogen activity
Hexagonal phospholipid neut
Dilute Russel's viper venom
Aspirin and/or plavix resistance (VerifyNow rapid assay)

ICU patients with acute cardiac ischemia, the recommendation is to transfuse RBCs if hemoglobin < 8 g/dL.[42]

INDICATIONS:
These evidence-based guidelines for RBC transfusion in adult trauma and critical care[43,44] recommended the following:

1. RBC transfusion is indicated for patients with evidence of hemorrhagic shock.
2. RBC transfusion may be indicated for patients with evidence of acute hemorrhage and hemodynamic instability or inadequate oxygen delivery.
3. A "restrictive" strategy of RBC transfusion (transfuse when Hb < 7 g/dL) is as effective as a "liberal" transfusion strategy (transfusion when Hb < 10 g/dL) in critically ill patients with hemodynamically stable anemia, except possibly in patients with acute myocardial ischemia.
4. The use of only Hb concentration as a "trigger" for transfusion should be avoided. Decision for RBC transfusion should be based on individual patient's intravascular volume status, evidence of shock, duration and extent of anemia, and cardiopulmonary physiologic parameters.
5. In the absence of acute hemorrhage, RBC transfusion should be given as single units.
6. RBC transfusion should not be considered as an absolute method to improve tissue oxygen consumption in critically ill patients.

Technical Aspects RBC serology requires transfusion from patient with compatible ABO and Rhesus (Rh) groups. In patient with multiple transfusion subgroup (A1, A2) and other groups (MN, K, D, L), compatibility becomes necessary. Crossmatched blood should be used unless unavailable or in emergent situations. Rewarming blood products is a necessity as they are cold in storage.

TABLE 10.11

MEDICATIONS AND CLINICAL CONDITIONS THAT CONFOUND INTERPRETATION OF THROMBOPHILIA LABORATORY TESTING

CLINICAL CIRCUMSTANCE	AFFECTED FACTOR
Estrogens	Low Proteins S Elevated AT III
Oral contraceptives and pregnancy	APC resistance + Elevated proteins S
Inflammation/sepsis/burn injury/ polytrauma	Elevated factor VIII Low AT III Low protein S
Heparin	Low AT III
Warfarin	Low protein C and S Elevated AT III
Liver disease, disseminated intravascular coagulation	Low AT III Low protein C and S
Asparaginase chemotherapy	Low AT III
Vitamin K deficiency	Low protein C and S
Acute thrombosis	Low protein C and S
Increased factor VIII or factor II, and circulating lupus anticoagulant	APC resistance
Nephrotic syndrome	Low AT III Low protein S

Abbreviations: APC, activated protein C; AT III, antithrombin III.
Prior to diagnostic testing for hypercoagulable states, it is important to assess whether the patient is on medications that may confound interpretation of these laboratory tests.
From: Houbballah R, LaMuraglia GM. Clotting problems: diagnosis and management of underlying coagulopathies. *Semin Vasc Surg.* 2010;23(4):221–227.

Room temperature is acceptable for slow and low volume transfusions but for substantial and MTs using a blood warmer is necessary to prevent hypothermia. Blood tubing with a filter should be used for transfusions, but the use of microfilters (30–40 μm pores) has not been associated with reduced complications. All patients must be monitored during RBC transfusions, with patient vital signs including temperature monitored during and after completion of RBC transfusions.

In Patients with Bleeding or Hemorrhagic Shock

Uncrossmatched blood (Type O) is used if the patient has hemodynamic instability due to hemorrhagic shock and crossmatched blood is not yet available. Type-specific blood is used as soon as possible for hemorrhagic shock to minimize exposure to anti-A and anti-B antibodies in type O blood. In patients requiring RBC transfusion in hemorrhagic shock, transfusion rate depends on bleeding rate, and we should not rely on hemoglobin as an assessment of adequacy of blood resuscitation.

COMPLICATIONS.
Citrate toxicity: metabolic alkalosis and hypocalcemia with low levels of ionized calcium in patients with impaired liver function or with MTs

Electrolytes: low ionized calcium, hyperkalemia, and hypokalemia

Hypothermia with MT, transfusion-related febrile reactions

TABLE 10.12

COMPARISON OF HEMOSTATIC TESTING FOUND WITH COMMON MEDICATIONS AND DISEASE STATES IN CRITICALLY ILL PATIENTS

CONDITION	PT	APTT	FIBRINOGEN	FDP	PLATELETS	BT	TT
UFH	Normal or prolonged[a]	Prolonged	Normal	Normal	Normal	Normal	Prolonged
LMWHs	Normal or prolonged[a]	Normal or minimally prolonged	Normal	Normal	Normal	Normal	Normal or minimally prolonged
Direct factor Xa inhibitors	Normal or prolonged[a]	Normal or minimally prolonged	Normal	Normal	Normal	Normal	Normal
Direct thrombin inhibitors	Prolonged	Prolonged	Normal	Normal	Normal	Normal	Prolonged
Coumadin	Prolonged	Normal or prolonged[b]	Normal	Normal	Normal	Normal	Normal
Vitamin K deficiency	Prolonged	Prolonged	Normal	Normal	Normal	Normal	Normal
Hepatic Insufficiency	Prolonged	Normal or prolonged	Low or normal	Normal or elevated	Low	Normal or prolonged	Prolonged
DIC	Normal or prolonged	Normal or prolonged	Normal or low	Elevated	Low	Prolonged	Prolonged
Dilution	Prolonged	Prolonged	Low or normal	Normal	Low	Normal or prolonged	Normal or prolonged
von Willebrand Disease	Normal	Prolonged	Normal	Normal	Normal	Prolonged	Normal
Lupus anticoagulant	Normal or prolonged	Prolonged	Normal	Normal	Normal	Normal	Normal
Thrombocytopenia	Normal	Normal	Normal	Normal	Low	Normal or prolonged	Normal

BT, bleeding time; DIC, disseminated intravascular coagulation; FDP, fibrin degradation product; LMWH, low-molecular-weight heparin; TT, thrombin time; UFH, unfractionated heparin. See Table 10.2 for expansion of other abbreviations.

[a]At supratherapeutic dosages.

[b]Early in coumadin treatment. From: Wheeler AP, Rice TW. Coagulopathy in critically ill patients, part 2: soluble clotting factors and hemostatic testing. *Chest.* 2010;137(1):185–194.

Anaphylactoid reactions; hemolytic reactions

Transfusion-associated immunomodulation: increased risk for infections

Graft versus host disease

Transfusion related acute lung injury (TRALI)

Transfusion-associated circulatory overload (TACO)

Infection: by contamination from donor (decreasing incidence) or contamination from manipulation

Fresh Frozen Plasma Transfusion

Indications. Fresh frozen plasma (FFP) should be transfused to patients requiring MT. The optimal amount of FFP required in MT patients is controversial. The guidelines[45] recommend plasma:RBC ratio of 1:3 or more during MT with the use of coagulation studies and clinical evidence of bleeding as a guide. The guidelines did not recommend for or against plasma transfusion to patients undergoing surgery in the absence of MT. FFP should be transfused in patients with warfarin therapy–related intracranial hemorrhage but could not recommend for or against transfusion of plasma to reverse warfarin anticoagulation in patients without intracranial hemorrhage. The guidelines suggested against plasma transfusion for other selected groups of patients, including those with liver disease, hemophilia (A&B), other factor deficiency, and antithrombin deficiency in a situation requiring anticoagulation with heparin.

Technical Aspects. FFP transfusion has the same technical aspects as RBC transfusion including using crossmatched plasma for transfusions avoiding a reaction between patient RBCs and donor antibodies. ABO compatibility is required, but Rh compatibility is not required.

Complications. Identical to RBC transfusion keeping in mind that citrate content is higher in FFP and potassium transfer is not an issue. TRALI has a higher incidence with plasma transfusions.

Platelet Transfusion

Indications Prophylactic platelet transfusions are indicated in patients at risk of bleeding, for platelet count < 10×10^9/L. Therapeutic platelet transfusions are required in hemorrhage

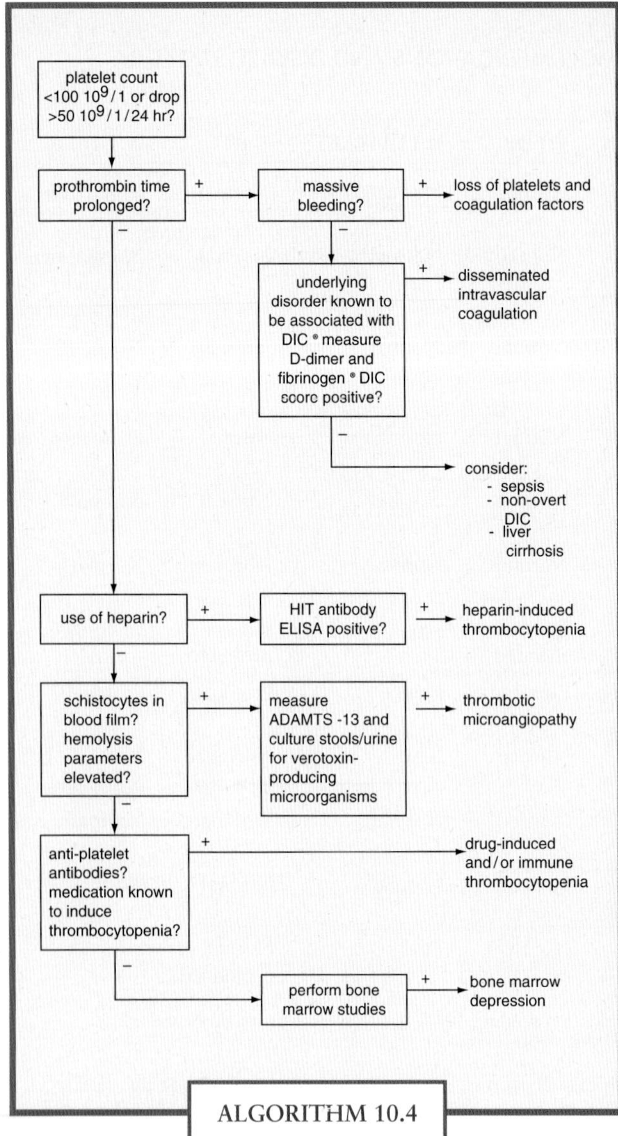

ALGORITHM 10.4 Differential diagnostic algorithm for coagulation abnormalities in the ICU. DIC, disseminated intravascular coagulation; ELISA, enzyme-linked immunosorbent assay; HIT, heparin-induced thrombocytopenia. From: Levi M, Opam SM. Coagulation abnormalities in critically ill patients. *Crit Care.* 2006;10(4):222.

to maintain platelet count > 100 × 10^9/L, which is required to create stable clot and minimize rebleeding risk. In elective surgery, platelet transfusions may or may not be required, dependent on the procedure being performed, and, in general, platelet counts > 50 × 10^9/L are adequate.[46,47]

Transfusion of one platelet pool and 1 U of apheresis platelets will typically increase the platelet count of an adult by 20,000–40,000/μL. A posttransfusion platelet count should be obtained 10 minutes to 1 hour after transfusion for best assessment of transfusion effectiveness. Platelet counts obtained later may not allow for differentiation between immune and nonimmune causes of platelet transfusion refractoriness. The corrected count increment (CCI) is usually the best assessment of transfusion effectiveness. A 1-hour CCI greater than 5,000 is typically considered a satisfactory response.[48] Causes of an inadequate response to platelet transfusion include the following:

- Insufficient dosage
- Incomplete transfusion

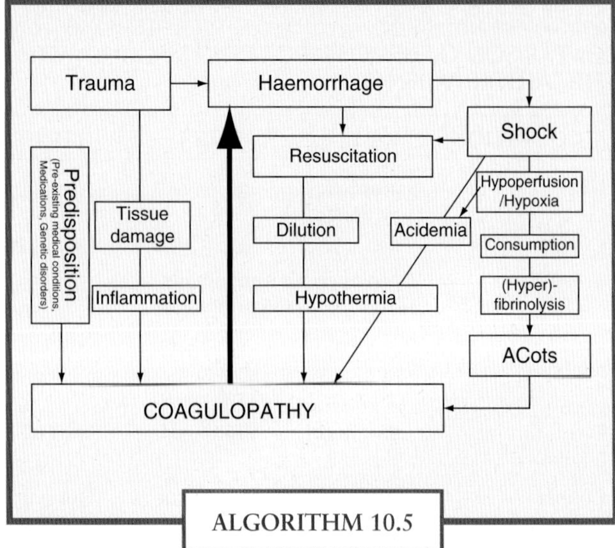

ALGORITHM 10.5 Acute coagulopathy of trauma. The main contributing factors and potential mechanisms implicated in the acute coagulopathy of trauma. Hemorrhage in the severely injured patient may lead to shock that causes acidemia and hypothermia further triggering coagulopathy, typically termed the "lethal triad." Injudicious fluid resuscitation is closely linked to dilutional coagulopathy and hypothermia. Trauma in combination with shock causing hypoperfusion and hypoxia can also cause the "Acute Coagulopathy of Trauma-Shock" (ACoTS) associated with anticoagulation and hyperfibrinolysis. The clinical significance of inflammation for the development of acute traumatic coagulopathy still has to be fully elucidated. From Wafaisade A, Wutzler S, Lefering R, et al. Trauma Registry of DGU. Drivers of acute coagulopathy after severe trauma: a multivariate analysis of 1987 patients. *Emerg Med J.* doi:10.1136/emj.2009.088484 and Hess JR, Brohi K, Dutton RP, et al. The coagulopathy of trauma: a review of mechanisms. *J Trauma.* 2008;65:748–54.

- Transfusion of platelet concentrates near date of expiration
- Immune refractoriness. ABO antigens are weakly expressed on platelets and usually are not an important consideration in platelet transfusions. However, some patient may benefit from ABO-matched platelet transfusions. Antibodies to platelet-specific antigens are rare causes of transfusion refractoriness. HLA antibodies may cause platelet transfusion refractoriness. HLA antigens are expressed on platelets, and HLA antibodies are common in multiply transfused patients and parous women. Patients with immune refractoriness may benefit from crossmatched or HLA-matched platelets.
- Splenomegaly
- Consumption
- Bleeding, intravascular coagulation, intravascular platelet activation, graft versus host disease (GVHD), or sepsis may decrease platelet survival

Contraindications to platelet transfusions include TTP and heparin-HIT.

Technical Aspects Platelet transfusions require ABO compatibility, and RhD-negative platelet concentrates should be given, when possible, to RhD-negative patients and women in particular. A randomized controlled international multicenter trial (SToP) comparing two dosing strategies for platelet transfusion [standard-dose (300–600 × 10^9 platelets/product, equivalent to pooled five-pack of whole blood-derived platelets) or low-dose (150–<300 × 10^9 platelets/product) platelets] in patients with chemotherapy-HIT was stopped early due to a higher rate of bleeding in patients receiving the low-dose prophylactic platelet transfusions.[49]

TABLE 10.13

EXECUTIVE SUMMARY FROM CLINICAL PRACTICE GUIDELINE: RBC TRANSFUSION IN ADULT TRAUMA AND CRITICAL CARE

A. Recommendations Regarding Indications for RBC Transfusion in the General Critically Ill Patient

1. RBC transfusion is indicated for patients with evidence of hemorrhagic shock. (Level 1)
2. RBC transfusion may be indicated for patients with evidence of acute hemorrhage and hemodynamic instability or inadequate oxygen delivery. (Level 1)
3. A "restrictive" strategy of RBC transfusion (transfuse when Hb <7 g/dL) is as effective as a "liberal" transfusion strategy (transfusion when Hb <10 g/dL) in critically ill patients with hemodynamically stable anemia, except possibly in patients with acute myocardial ischemia. (Level 1)
4. The use of only Hb level as a "trigger" for transfusion should be avoided. Decision for RBC transfusion should be based on an individual patient's intravascular volume status, evidence of shock, duration and extent of anemia, and cardiopulmonary physiologic parameters. (Level 2)
5. In the absence of acute hemorrhage RBC, transfusion should be given as single units. (Level 2)
6. Consider transfusion if Hb <7 g/dL in critically ill patients requiring mechanical ventilation (MV). There is no benefit of a "liberal" transfusion strategy (transfusion when Hb <10 g/dL) in critically ill patients requiring MV. (Level 2)
7. Consider transfusion if Hb <7 g/dL in resuscitated critically ill trauma patients. There is no benefit of a "liberal" transfusion strategy (transfusion when Hb <10 g/dL) in resuscitated critically ill trauma patients. (Level 2)
8. Consider transfusion if Hb <7 g/dL in critically ill patients with stable cardiac disease. There is no benefit of a "liberal" transfusion strategy (transfusion when Hb <10 g/dL) in critically ill patients with stable cardiac disease. (Level 2)
9. RBC transfusion should not be considered as an absolute method to improve tissue oxygen consumption in critically ill patients. (Level 2)
10. RBC transfusion may be beneficial in patients with acute coronary syndromes (ACS) who are anemic (Hb ≤8 g/dL) on hospital admission. (Level 3)

B. Recommendations Regarding RBC Transfusion in Sepsis

1. There are insufficient data to support Level 1 recommendations on this topic.
2. The transfusion needs for each septic patient must be assessed individually since optimal transfusion triggers in sepsis patients are not known and there is no clear evidence that blood transfusion increases tissue oxygenation. (Level 2)

C. Recommendations Regarding RBC Transfusion in Patients at Risk for or With Acute Lung Injury (ALI) and ARDS

ALI and ARDS are common clinical sequelae of massive transfusion. Prior studies have suggested that RBC transfusion is associated with respiratory complications, including ALI and ARDS that remains even after adjusting for potential confounders.

1. There are insufficient data to support Level 1 recommendations on this topic.
2. All efforts should be initiated to avoid RBC transfusion in patients at risk for ALI and ARDS after completion of resuscitation. (Level 2)
3. All efforts should be made to diagnose and report transfusion-related ALI (TRALI) to the local blood bank because it has emerged as a leading cause of transfusion-associated morbidity and mortality, despite underdiagnosis and underreporting. (Level 2)
4. RBC transfusion should not be considered as a method to facilitate weaning from MV. (Level 2)

D. Recommendations Regarding RBC Transfusion in Patients With Neurologic Injury and Diseases

1. There are insufficient data to support Level 1 Recommendations on this topic.
2. There is no benefit of a "liberal" transfusion strategy (transfusion when Hb <10 g/dL) in patients with moderate-to-severe traumatic brain injury. (Level 2)
3. Decisions regarding blood transfusion in patients with subarachnoid hemorrhage (SAH) must be assessed individually since optimal transfusion triggers are not known and there is no clear evidence that blood transfusion is associated with improved outcome. (Level 3)

E. Recommendations Regarding RBC Transfusion Risks

1. There are insufficient data to support Level 1 Recommendations on this topic.
2. RBC transfusion is associated with increased nosocomial infection (wound infection, pneumonia, sepsis) rates independent of other factors. (Level 2)
3. RBC transfusion is an independent risk factor for MOF and SIRS. (Level 2)
4. There is no definitive evidence that prestorage leukocyte depletion of RBC transfusion reduces complication rates, but some studies have shown a reduction in infectious complications.(Level 2)
5. RBC transfusions are independently associated with longer ICU and hospital length of stay, increased complications, and increased mortality. (Level 2)
6. There is a relationship between transfusion and ALI and ARDS. (Level 2)

F. Recommendations Regarding Alternatives to RBC Transfusion

1. There are insufficient data to support Level 1 recommendations on this topic.
2. Recombinant human erythropoietin (rHuEpo) administration improves reticulocytosis and hematocrit and may decrease overall transfusion requirements. (Level 2)
3. Hemoglobin-based oxygen carriers (HBOCs) are undergoing investigation for use in critically ill and injured patients but are not yet approved for use in the United States. (Level 2)

TABLE 10.13

EXECUTIVE SUMMARY FROM CLINICAL PRACTICE GUIDELINE: RBC TRANSFUSION IN ADULT TRAUMA AND CRITICAL CARE (*Continued*)

G. Recommendations Regarding Strategies to Reduce RBC Transfusion

1. There are insufficient data to support Level 1 recommendations on this topic.
2. The use of low-volume adult or pediatric blood sampling tubes is associated with a reduction in phlebotomy volumes and a reduction in blood transfusion. (Level 2)
3. The use of blood conservation devices for reinfusion of waste blood with diagnostic sampling is associated with a reduction in phlebotomy volume. (Level 2)
4. Intraoperative and postoperative blood salvage and alternative methods for decreasing transfusion may lead to a significant reduction in allogeneic blood usage. (Level 2)
5. Reduction in diagnostic laboratory testing is associated with a reduction in phlebotomy volumes and a reduction in blood transfusion. (Level 2)

From: Napolitano LM, Kurek S, Luchette FA, et al; American College of Critical Care Medicine of the Society of Critical Care Medicine; Eastern Association for the Surgery of Trauma Practice Management Workgroup. Clinical practice guideline: red blood cell transfusion in adult trauma and critical care. *Crit Care Med.* 2009;37(12):3124–3157.

Complications Technical issues (related to platelet unit contamination and infection risk), platelet's function (deep venous thrombosis), and immune effects (alloimmunization and hemolysis from residual ABO antibodies). Some patients will be refractory to platelet transfusions, defined as failure to achieve an appropriate increment after receiving two consecutive transfusions with fresh ABO-compatible platelets (Algorithm. 10.6). Measurement of platelet count 30 and 60 minutes following platelet transfusion will determine adequacy of platelet transfusion host response.

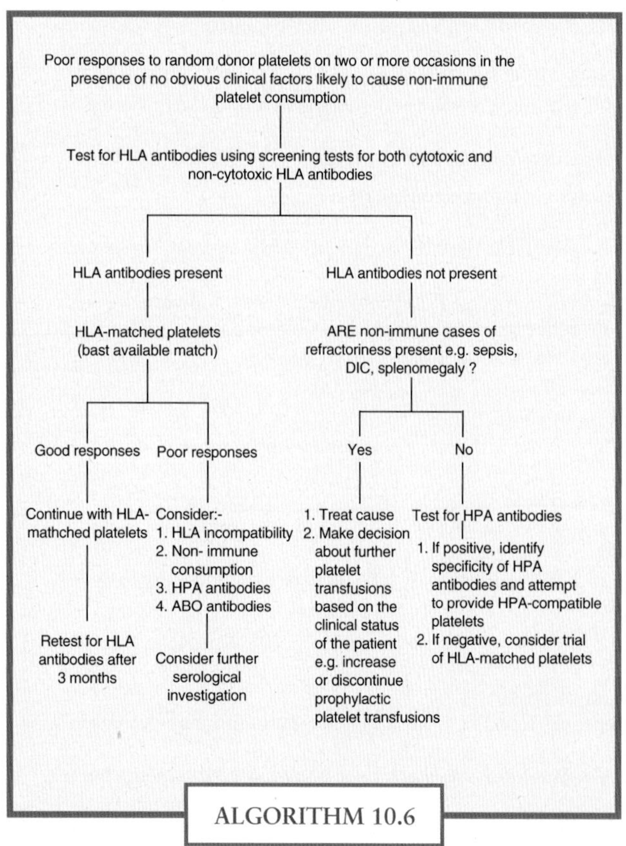

ALGORITHM 10.6 Diagnostic evaluation in patient refractory to platelet transfusions.

Cryoprecipitate Transfusion

Indications Cryoprecipitate is a diverse product containing factor VIII, von Willebrand factor, fibrinogen, fibronectin, factor XIII, and platelet microparticles. The most common current indication for the use of cryoprecipitate is in patients with hypofibrinogenemia in the setting of massive hemorrhage. It is also indicated for von Willebrand disease and hemophilia A (factor VIII deficiency).[50]

Technical Aspects Same as all blood products but ABO compatibility is not necessary.

Complications Similar to all blood products and in case of large volume of ABO-incompatible cryoprecipitate is used, the recipient may develop a positive DAT and, very rarely, mild hemolysis.

BLOOD TRANSFUSION IN TRAUMA

Traumatic injuries are common and account for almost 15% of all allogeneic RBC transfusion use in the United States. Control and treatment of hemorrhage is a critical aspect of trauma care, particularly in patients with hemorrhagic shock.[51] Despite major advances in the treatment of hemorrhagic shock, hemorrhage remains a leading cause of early death in both civilian and military trauma. Failure to control and treat hemorrhage promptly in such patients resulted in a "Bloody Vicious Cycle" (Algorithm. 10.7) of hemorrhage, resuscitation, hemodilution, and coagulopathy, leading to more hemorrhage.[52–54]

At present, the only oxygen-carrying resuscitation fluid available for use in patients with traumatic injuries is allogeneic RBC transfusion. The aim of treatment of hemorrhagic shock with RBC transfusion is the rapid and effective restoration of an adequate blood volume to maximize tissue oxygen delivery. Furthermore, the goal of transfusion of blood and blood products is to maintain the patient's blood composition within safe limits with regard to hemostasis, oxygen-carrying capacity, oncotic pressure, and biochemistry. Therefore, the additional administration of other blood components (in addition to RBCs) is necessary for the prevention of dilutional coagulopathy and dilutional thrombocytopenia.

The Advanced Trauma Life Support course of the American College of Surgeons recommends starting two large-bore IVs

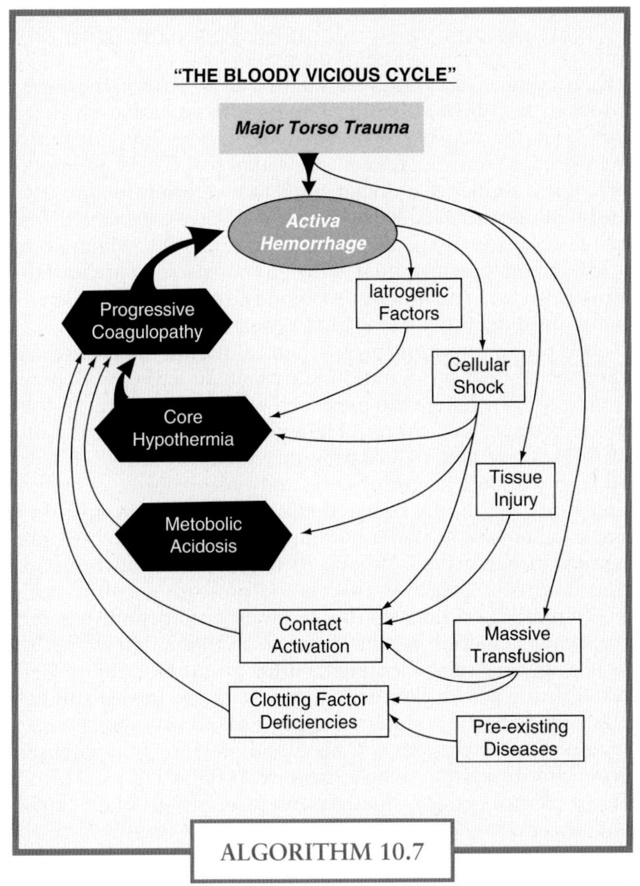

ALGORITHM 10.7 The pathogenesis of the "bloody vicious cycle" following major torso trauma is multifactorial, but usually manifests as a triad of refractory coagulopathy, progressive hypothermia, and persistent metabolic acidosis. From: Moore EE. Thomas G. Orr Memorial Lecture. Staged laparotomy for the hypothermia, acidosis, and coagulopathy syndrome. *Am J Surg* 1996;172(5):405–410.

in patients who are seriously injured and, if they are hypotensive, giving 2 L of isotonic crystalloid solution.[55] If the patient remains hypotensive in shock, then RBCs should be transfused. These guidelines were based on the recognition that prolonged shock frequently led to organ failure that could be prevented by fluid resuscitation. Most frequently, uncrossmatched RBC units are administered to trauma patients requiring emergent RBC transfusion, and the increasing use of uncrossmatched RBC transfusion has been identified as an independent predictor of mortality and the need for MT.[56] The use of fresh whole blood has also been required in the combat casualty setting due to a lack of sufficient stored blood products, and therefore these combat casualty reports also document administration of fresh whole blood.[57]

Massive Transfusion

Massive transfusion (MT) is required as a treatment for uncontrolled hemorrhage, and trauma is the most common etiology.[58–60] Massive blood transfusion is commonly defined as administration of ≥10 U of allogeneic RBCs to an individual patient or transfusion of more than one blood volume in 24 hours. Other "dynamic" definitions of MT have been used, particularly in order to initiate MT institutional protocols.[61–67] Risk factors for MT in trauma include tachycardia, hypotension, acidosis, penetrating mechanism, hemoperitoneum by sonography, and anemia.[68] Several predictive models for MT have been developed, with all variables necessary to calculate the score easily available within upon emergency room arrival.[69–71]

Trauma patients requiring MT have high mortality rates, ranging from 19% to 84%. Data from more recent studies document a significant reduction in mortality in trauma patients requiring MT, with most recent series reporting a mortality rate of approximately 30%–58% (Table 10.14).[72] Mortality is directly related to the severity of the hemorrhagic shock and the total number of PRBC units transfused.[73] Interestingly, in a single-center retrospective study of trauma patients requiring MT of more than 50 U of blood products in the first 24 hours,

TABLE 10.14

MORTALITY RATES ASSOCIATED WITH MT IN PUBLISHED STUDIES

STUDY	YEAR	PATIENTS	MEAN # RBC UNITS	MORTALITY RATE (%)
Phillips	1987	56	33	61
Wudel	1991	92	33	48
Cosgriff	1997	–	24	43
Velmahos	1998	141	32	69.5
Cinat	1999	45	63	71
Vaslef	2002	44	33	57
Como	2004	147	25	39
Huber-Wagner	2007	1062	19.5	35–60
Mitra	2007	119	8 in 4 h	27.7
Gonzalez	2007	97	–	30
Borgman	2007	246	–	19–65
Holcomb	2008	467	–	26–59
Duchesne	2008	135	–	55.5
Maegele	2008	713	–	24.3–45.5
Sperry	2008	415	14	33.5
Knudson	2010	380	28	54.5 (30)

the overall mortality was 57%, but there was no significant difference in mortality rate between patients who received >75 U of blood products in the 1st day versus those who received 51–75 U.[74]

Strategies to Reduce Complications Associated with Massive Transfusion

Massive transfusion (MT) protocols should be established with standardized policies to reduce complications related to transfusion therapy. Adverse effects of MT and strategies to reduce these adverse effects are shown in Table 10.15.

Massive Transfusion and Coagulopathy

The standard goal of massive transfusion (MT) in past years was to supply isotonic crystalloids and plasma-poor RBC concentrates to maintain normovolemia and tissue oxygen supply. This, however, frequently led to dilutional coagulopathy, which was frequently aggravated and accelerated by hypothermia, acidosis, shock-induced impairment of hepatic function, DIC due to tissue injury, and increased consumption of clotting factors and platelets at extensive wound sites in injured patients.

We now recognize that patients who have sustained severe hemorrhage and require MT commonly have an early and profound coagulopathy that is present on admission and worsens with PRBC transfusion due to dilutional and consumptive coagulopathy.[75–78] Traditional resuscitation techniques using large amounts of crystalloid and PRBCs without other blood products can exacerbate this coagulopathy.[79] Therefore, another key aim of modern MT protocols is the timely administration of plasma and platelet concentrates as required to halt microvascular bleeding induced by impaired hemostasis.[80,81]

Hypotensive or Delayed Resuscitation

The concept of delaying resuscitation or only resuscitating to a low to low-normal blood pressure ("hypotensive resuscitation") in the actively hemorrhaging patient until definitive hemorrhage control has been advocated based on a number of preclinical studies that documented that vigorous fluid resuscitation in uncontrolled hemorrhagic shock was associated with increased hemorrhage and decreased survival.[82] Maintaining a low-blood pressure goal with "hypotensive resuscitation" aims to reduce the amount of blood lost through the site of injury until definitive hemorrhage control is achieved.

In a randomized prospective clinical trial of immediate versus delayed fluid resuscitation in patients (n = 598) with penetrating torso trauma who presented with a prehospital systolic blood pressure of ≤ 90 mm Hg with an overall mortality rate of 34%, there was significantly increased mortality (38% vs. 30%, p = 0.04), length of stay, and postoperative complication rates in the immediate versus the delayed group.[83] In a single-center study that randomized patients (n = 110) presenting in hemorrhagic shock to one of two fluid resuscitation protocols (target systolic blood pressure > 100 mm Hg vs. 70 mm Hg) titrated to this endpoint until definitive hemostasis was achieved, no difference in overall survival (92.7% in both groups) was identified. Although no mortality benefit was identified with hypotensive resuscitation in this study, it was noted that a number of study limitations were present: failure to achieve target systolic blood pressure in hypotensive group (mean systolic blood pressure 100mm Hg vs. 114mm Hg in control group); small sample size; mix of blunt (49%) and penetrating (51%) trauma patients and lengthy time for duration of active hemorrhage (2.97 ± 1.75 hours vs. 2.57 ± 1.46 hours, p = 0.20). Despite the limitations of these clinical studies, "hypotensive" resuscitation has become increasingly accepted in the prehospital resuscitation phase of trauma, prior to definitive hemorrhage control, since aggressive fluid resuscitation may increase bleeding.[84]

TABLE 10.15

STRATEGIES TO REDUCE COMPLICATIONS WITH MASSIVE TRANSFUSION

COMPLICATION	STRATEGIES TO REDUCE COMPLICATION
Hypothermia	Warm the room Surface warm the patient with heating blankets and heating lamps Heat and humidity inspired gases for ventilators Warm all IV fluids and blood products administered
Coagulopathy	Transfuse RBC: FFP in 1:1 ratio Check coagulation testing, including fibrinogen Transfuse cryoprecipitate if fibrinogen concentration low
Thrombocytopenia	Transfuse platelets to keep platelet count >100,000 to form stable clot
Electrolyte abnormalities	Calcium depletion occurs secondary to citrate chelation, correct with calcium IV Measure blood potassium, calcium (ionized), and magnesium concentrations Replete electrolytes to normal values as indicated
Acid-base disorders	Sodium bicarbonate or tromethamine for severe metabolic acidosis with hemodynamic instability or renal failure
TRALI	Use restrictive transfusion strategy once hemorrhage controlled Use FFP from men or nulliparous women
TACO	Discontinue crystalloid fluid resuscitation Consider IV diuretic use

Hemostatic Resuscitation

Acidosis, hypothermia, and coagulopathy were identified more than 20 years ago as a deadly triad for patients presenting with exsanguinating hemorrhage. This led to fundamental changes in initial management of severely injured patients. Despite these major advances, hemorrhage remains a leading cause of early death in trauma patients. Recent studies report most severely injured patients to be coagulopathic at admission, before resuscitation interventions, and that traditional MT practices grossly underestimate what is needed to correct the coagulopathy.

Since hemorrhage is a major cause of trauma deaths and coagulopathy exacerbates hemorrhage and is commonly seen during major trauma, prompt reversal of coagulopathy using "hemostatic resuscitation" has been advocated as the optimal practice for MT in trauma.[85,86] Reversal of coagulopathy involves normalization of body temperature, elimination of the causes of DIC, and transfusion with FFP, platelets, and cryoprecipitate as needed. Some have advocated that coagulopathy can best be avoided or reversed when severe trauma victims are transfused with at least the equivalent of whole blood.[87,88]

A study in combat casualty care identified that the ratio of blood products transfused affected mortality in patients receiving MTs at a combat support hospital.[26] They performed a retrospective chart review of 246 patients at a US Army combat support hospital, each of who received a MT (≥10 U of PRBCs in 24 hours). They identified that a high 1:1.4 plasma to PRBC ratio was independently associated with improved survival to hospital discharge, primarily by decreasing death from hemorrhage. The authors concluded that MT protocols should utilize a 1:1 ratio of plasma to PRBCs for all patients who are hypocoagulable with traumatic injuries.[89,90]

The practice of hemostatic resuscitation was initiated in military combat casualty care,[91] but has also been examined in civilian trauma, and the concept is now being applied to other patient populations requiring massive blood transfusion for severe hemorrhage. Multiple clinical studies in civilian trauma patient populations have addressed the topic of hemostatic resuscitation as well.[92–97] A recent systematic review of 37 studies, most of which were observational in nature, documented that in patients undergoing MT, plasma infusion at high plasma:RBC ratios was associated with a significant reduction in the risk of death (OR, 0.38, 95% CI: 0.24–0.60) and multiple organ failure (OR 0.40, 95% CI: 0.26–0.60; Fig. 10.2). However, the quality of this evidence was very low due to substantial unexplained heterogeneity and several other biases. In patients undergoing surgery without MT, plasma infusion was associated with a trend toward increased mortality (OR, 1.22; 95% CI: 0.73–2.03). Plasma transfusion was associated with increased risk of developing ALI (OR, 2.92; 95% CI: 1.99–4.29).[98] Evidence-based practice guidelines for plasma transfusion by the American Society of Hematology recommended that plasma be transfused to patients requiring MT, however could not recommend a specific plasma:RBC ratio.[99]

Although hemostatic resuscitation has been associated with reduced mortality in these retrospective studies, we must recognize that there are potential adverse effects associated with transfusion of blood component therapy, including fresh frozen plasma and platelets. A number of studies have documented increased risk for ALI and ARDS with both blood and plasma transfusions.[100–102] TRALI is now the leading cause of transfusion-associated mortality, even though it is probably underdiagnosed and underreported.[103–105]

Massive Transfusion Protocols

Massive transfusion (MT) protocols have long been in place at major trauma centers for the treatment of patients with severe hemorrhagic shock.[106] In the past, MT protocols provided PRBCs, but still required the clinician to issue specific requests for other blood component therapy, including FFP and platelets. Furthermore, it was recommended that transfusion of these additional blood components wait until laboratory evidence of dilutional and consumptive coagulopathy and thrombocytopenia were present. In the current era, MT protocols now focus on the *prevention* of coagulopathy and thrombocytopenia.

As we have noted above, a 1:1:1 ratio (i.e., equal parts PRBCs, FFP, and platelets) for blood component therapy is now recommended for MT based on a more physiologic regimen similar to whole blood transfusion. This approach has been named "Hemostatic Resuscitation" and focuses on the early correction of coagulopathy, which is thought to be associated with improved survival. MT protocols have now been revised to include other blood component therapy in addition to RBC units and have been associated with improved outcomes in trauma.[107–110]

A multicenter prospective observational study of severely injured trauma patients who require blood transfusions is underway (PROMMTT, Prospective Observational Multicenter Massive Transfusion study[111]) and aims to further investigate MT protocols that are associated with improved outcome. The results of this observational study will inform the development of a future randomized clinical trial that will test these protocols.

MORTALITY

	OR	Lower limit	Upper limit	Events/Total Plasma	Events/Total Control
Borgman, 2007	0.29	0.61	0.51	31/162	38/84
Cotton, 2009	0.46	0.28	0.75	54/125	88/141
Holcomb, 2008	0.58	0.40	0.84	87/252	102/214
Kashuk, 2008	0.44	0.22	0.88	23/59	44/74
Maegele, 2008	0.59	0.42	0.81	76/229	222/484
Teixeira, 2008	0.18	0.12	0.28	58/226	103/157
Scalea, 2008	1.49	0.63	3.53		
Snyder, 2009	0.84	0.47	1.50		
Duchesne, 2008	0.05	0.02	0.13	19/71	56/64
Dente, 2009	0.12	0.02	0.67	7/50	4/7
	0.38	0.24	0.60		

OR and 95% CI: 0.01 0.1 0.25 1 1.5 3.5 — Favors higher plesma ratio / Favors lower plesma ratio

Heterogeneity : p = 0.01 : I^2 = 85%
Quality of evidence : Very low⊕ OOO

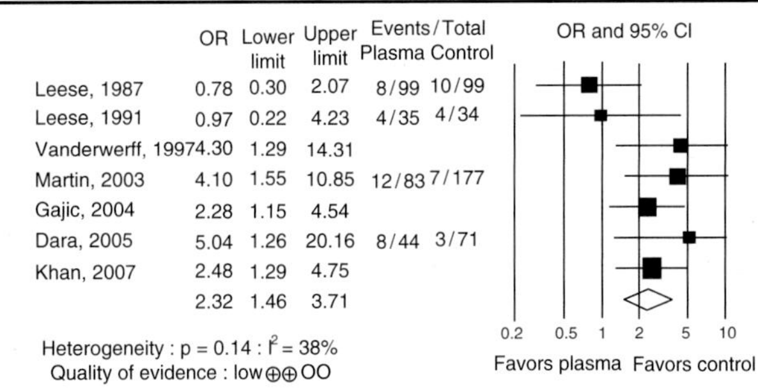

FIGURE 10.2. In patients undergoing MT, plasma infusion at high plasma:RBC ratios was associated with a significant reduction in the risk of death (OR 0.38, 95% CI: 0.24–0.60) and increased risk for ALI. From: Murad MH, Stubbs JR, Gandhi MJ, et al. The effect of plasma transfusion on morbidity and mortality: A systematic review and meta-anaylsis. *Transfusion.* 2010;50:1370–1383.

Transfusion After Hemorrhage Control

Once the definitive hemorrhage control has been established, a restrictive approach to blood transfusion should be implemented. Guidelines for transfusion in the trauma patient have been established as a standard operating procedure to guide RBC transfusion therapy for critically ill patients after the immediate resuscitation phase and to minimize the adverse consequences of potentially unnecessary transfusions. This protocol considers that the acute hemorrhage has been controlled, the initial resuscitation has been completed, and the patient is stable in the ICU with no evidence of ongoing bleeding (Algorithm. 10.8). This guideline advocates a trigger for PRBC transfusion of hemoglobin < 7 g/dL (or a hematocrit < 21%), even in patients with a history of cardiovascular disease.[112]

The recent report of the findings of the FOCUS trial confirms the use of a lower transfusion trigger in patients with stable anemia. The Transfusion Trigger Trial for functional outcomes in cardiovascular patients undergoing surgical hip fracture repair (FOCUS, sponsored by the National Heart, Lung and Blood Institute)[113] randomized 2,016 patients with asymptomatic anemia to a transfusion Hb trigger < 8 versus < 10 g/dL in 47 medical centers in the United States and Canada (8/2004–2/2009). No difference in cardiovascular outcomes (4.3 vs. 5.2%) or in-hospital mortality (2 vs. 1.4%) was identified.[114]

Efficacy of Red Blood Cell Transfusion in Trauma and Associated Risks

Adverse effects may occur with the transfusion of stored human red blood cells (RBCs). It has been documented that as human blood is stored, hemolysis occurs and increased concentrations of free hemoglobin are present in these units of blood.[115] Abnormal hemolysis in an individual RBC unit may be caused by several factors including inappropriate handling during processing of blood, inappropriate or extended duration of storage, bacterial hemolysins, antibodies that cause complement lysis, defects in the RBC membrane, or an abnormality in the blood donor. The acceptable level of hemolysis has not been established in North America, but the value of 1% is currently used to assess biocompatibility of blood storage materials.[116]

Increasing free plasma hemoglobin in aged stored RBC units, in addition to generating reactive oxygen species such as the hydroxyl and superoxide radicals, is also a potent scavenger of nitric oxide. Nitric oxide, which is normally produced by the endothelium, regulates basal vasodilator tone, inhibits platelet and hemostatic activation, and reduces superoxide concentration through radical–radical scavenging. The vasodilator activity of nitric oxide is possible only because most hemoglobin is normally compartmentalized within erythrocytes. As free hemoglobin concentration increased in aged stored allogeneic RBCs, a vasoconstrictive effect is evident (Fig. 10.3). It has been documented that RBC transfusion was

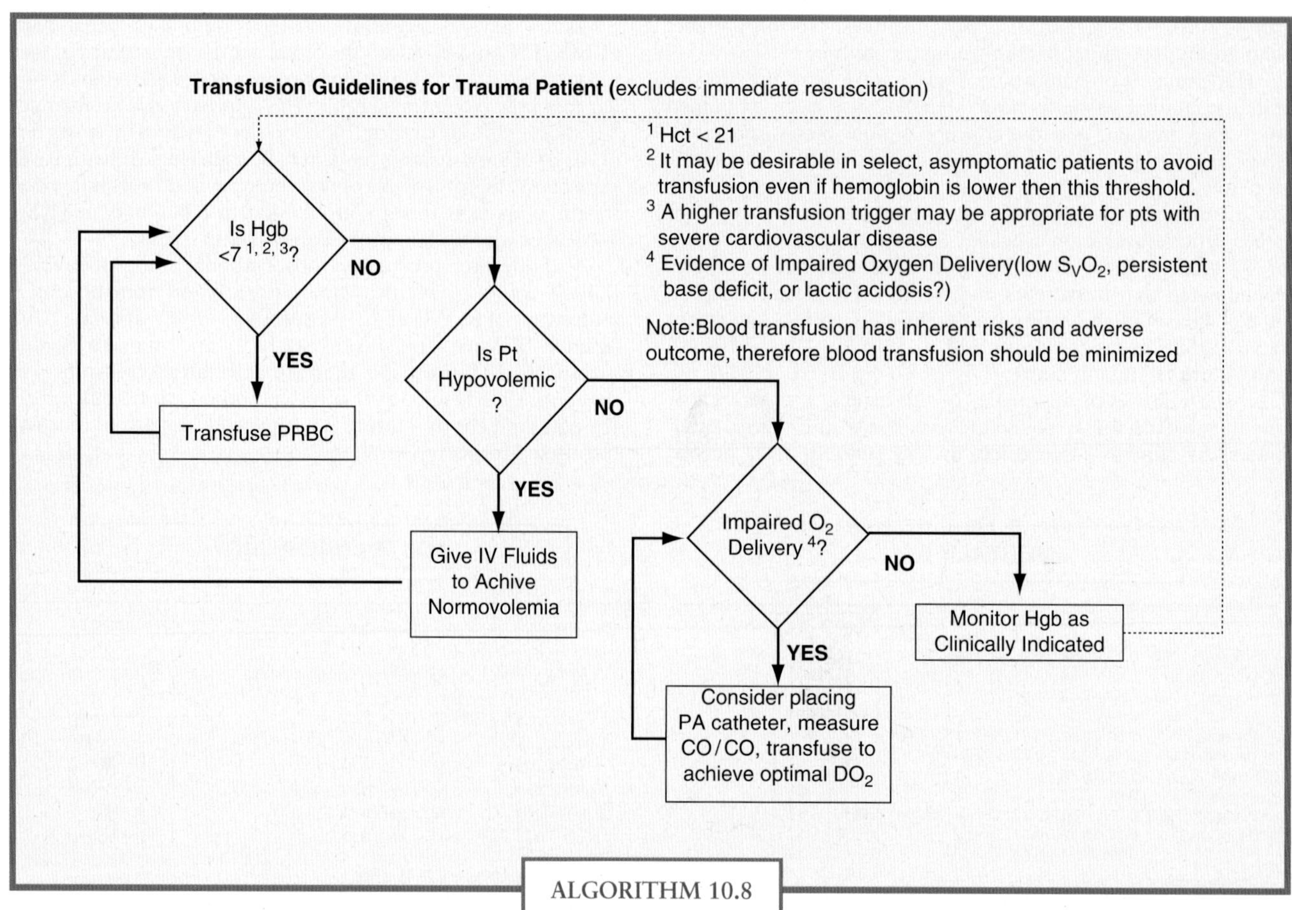

ALGORITHM 10.8 Guidelines for transfusion in the trauma patient have been established as a standard operating procedure to guide PRBC transfusion therapy for critically ill patients after the immediate resuscitation phase and to minimize the adverse consequences of potentially unnecessary transfusions. From: West MA, Shapiro MB, Nathens AB, et al. Guidelines for transfusion in the trauma patient. Inflammation and host response to injury, a large-scale collaborative project: patient-oriented research core—standard operating procedures for clinical care. *J Trauma.* 2006;61:436–439.

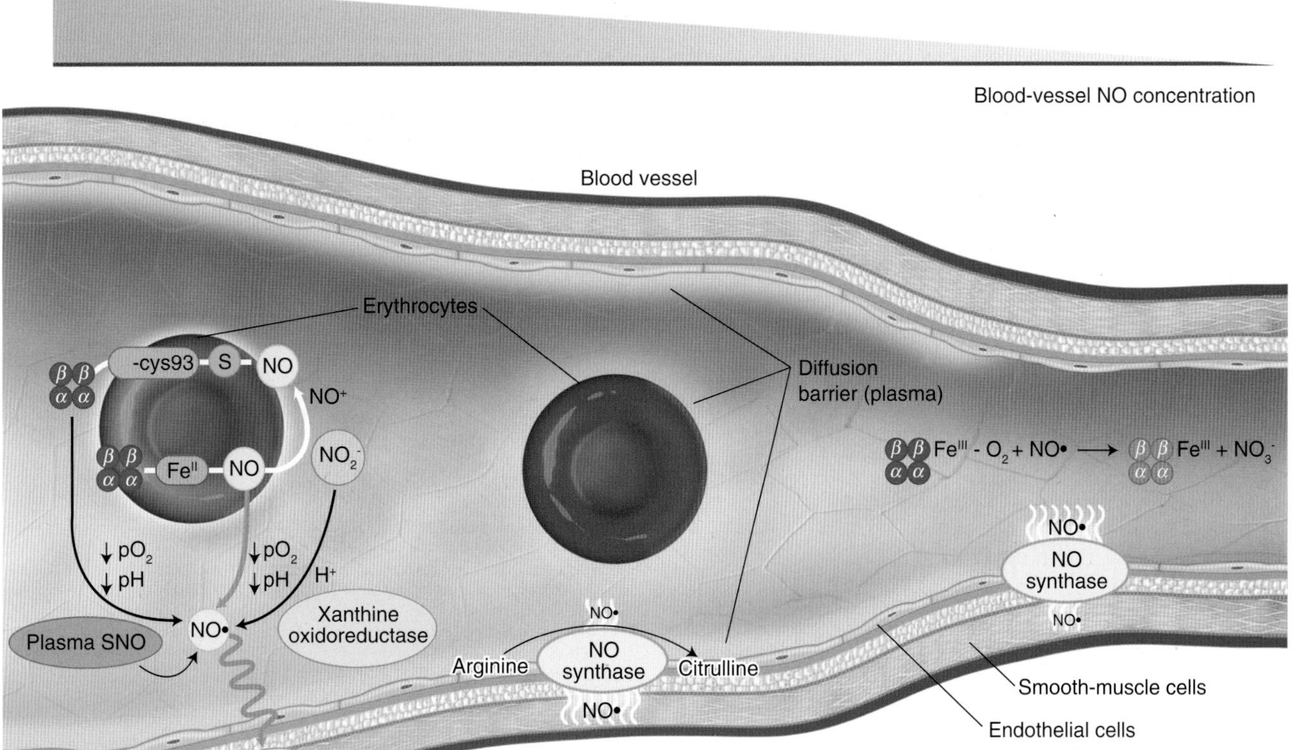

FIGURE 10.3. A model of the interactions of nitric oxide (NO) with erythrocytes and cell-free Hb in an arterial blood vessel. The diagram illustrates the major processes regulating NO concentration in blood vessels during pharmacologic nitric oxide delivery (**left**), under normal conditions (**center**), and under pathologic conditions, such as acute or chronic hemolysis (**right**). The overall blood-vessel NO concentration is depicted by the width of the blue band above the vessel. Within the vessel, smooth-muscle cells and a layer of endothelial cells are shown. Free Hb binds NO resulting in vascular constriction on the right side of the figure. Aged stored RBC units with increased hemolysis and early generation HBOCs may both have increased free hemoglobin concentrations and induce vasoconstriction in blood vessels.

associated with a significant increase in pulmonary vascular resistance index, which was not evident in the control cohort that received 5% albumin instead.[117]

The clinical consequences of red cell storage in trauma and the critically ill are particularly concerning (Fig. 10.4).[118] Duration of red cell storage has been associated with adverse outcomes including increased mortality.[119] In patients undergoing cardiac surgery, transfusion of red cells that had been stored for more than 2 weeks was associated with a significantly increased risk of postoperative complications as well as reduced short-term and long-term survival.[120] The multicenter Age of Blood Evaluation (ABLE) trial in the resuscitation of critically ill patients is ongoing, randomizing patients to the transfusion of fresh leuko-reduced RBCs (stored less than 8 days) versus transfusion of standard issue RBCs stored 2 to 42 days.[121]

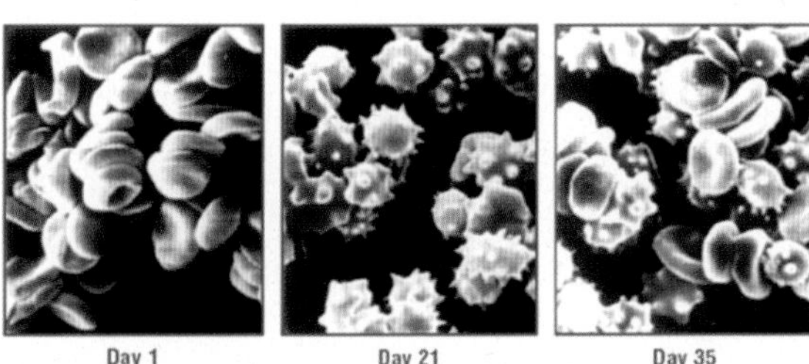

FIGURE 10.4. Changes in RBCs during storage. Scanning electron micrographs of RBCs isolated from stored blood on days 1, 21, and 35. During storage, the shape of RBCs changes gradually from normal discoid to echinocytes (dented or shriveled). Reproduced with permission from Hovav et al. *Transfusion.* 1999;39:277–281.

Additional studies have documented significant risks associated with RBC transfusion[122–124] and lack of efficacy.[125,126] Recent evidence suggests that in adult trauma patients, when used for treatment of anemia, RBC transfusion is associated with increased morbidity and mortality, and, therefore, current RBC transfusion practices may require reevaluation, and alternative oxygen-carrying resuscitation fluids warrant investigation.

Conclusion

Hematologic abnormalities, particularly anemia, are common in ICU patients. A careful diagnostic evaluation should be performed in all patients with anemia to determine if treatable etiologies are present. Blood transfusion is commonly used in surgical and ICU patients. Blood and blood products are scarce resources and should be reserved for treatment of patients with acute hemorrhage. Surgical and critically ill patients with anemia who are hemodynamically stable can tolerate hemoglobin concentrations of 7 g/dL. Transfusion of the bleeding patient with RBCs and other blood products requires careful vigilance during the acute resuscitative and recovery phases. At present, RBC transfusion is the only oxygen-carrying resuscitation fluid for treatment of severe hemorrhagic shock. Newer protocols using "hemostatic resuscitation" advocate concomitant early use of plasma, and some studies report improved survival. This strategy has resulted in more liberal use of RBCs and blood products in the acute resuscitation for massive hemorrhage. Additional multicenter studies are warranted to confirm this survival benefit with hemostatic resuscitation. However, following definitive cessation of hemorrhage, all efforts to minimize the use of RBC transfusion is warranted. Efforts to reduce blood transfusion in acute care surgery require a multidisciplinary effort including the use of institutional and unit-based transfusion protocols, educational efforts, and preventive strategies to reduce blood loss.

References

1. Sihler KC, Napolitano LM. Anemia of inflammation in critically ill patients. *Intensive Care Med.* 2008;23(5):295-302.
2. Napolitano LM. Scope of the problem: epidemiology of anemia and use of blood transfusions in critical care. *Crit Care.* 2004;8(Suppl 2):S1-S9.
3. Vincent JL, Baron JF, Reinhart K, et al. ABC (anemia and blood transfusion in critical care) investigators. Anemia and blood transfusion in critically ill patients. *JAMA.* 2002;288:1499-1507.
4. Vincent JL, Sakr Y, Sprung C, et al. Are blood transfusion associated with greater mortality rates? Results of the Sepsis Occurrence in Acutely Ill Patients (SOAP) Study. *Anesthesiology.* 2008;108:31-39.
5. Corwin HL, Gettinger A, Pearl RG, et al. The CRIT Study: anemia and blood transfusion in the critically ill—current clinical practice in the United States. *Crit Care Med.* 2004;32:39-52.
6. Hebert PC, Wells G, Blajchman MA, et al. A multicenter, randomized, controlled clinical trial of transfusion requirements in critical care. Transfusion requirements in critical care investigators, Canadian Critical Care Trials Group. *N Engl J Med.* 1999;340:409-417.
7. Rao MP, Boralessa H, Morgan C, et al. Blood component use in critically ill patients. *Anesthesia.* 2002;57:530-534.
8. Walsh TS, Garrioch M, Maciver C, et al. Audit of Transfusion in Intensive Care in Scotland Study Group. Red cell requirements for intensive ca re units adhering to evidence-based transfusion guidelines. *Transfusion.* 2004;44:1405-1411.
9. Walsh TS, McClelland DB, Lee RJ, et al. Prevalence of ischemic heart disease at admission to intensive care and its influence on red cell transfusion thresholds: Multicenter Scottish Study. *Br J Anaesth.* 2005;94:445-452.
10. Bateman AP, McArdle F, Walsh TS. Time course of anemia during six months follow up following intensive care discharge and factors associated with impaired recovery of erythropoiesis. *Crit Care Med.* 2009;37(6):1906-1912.
11. Napolitano LM. Review: scope of the problem: epidemiology of anemia and use of blood transfusions in critical care. *Crit Care.* 2004;8(Suppl 2):S1-S8.
12. Napolitano LM, Corwin HL, Fink MP. Anemia in critical care: etiology, treatment and prevention (In Editorial). *Critl Care.* 2004;8(suppl 2):S1-S64.
13. Sihler KC, Raghavendran K, Westerman M, et al. Hepcidin in trauma: linking injury, inflammation, and anemia. *J Trauma.* 2010;69(4):831-837.
14. Levi M, Lowenberg EC. Thrombocytopenia in critically ill patients. *Semin Thromb Hemost.* 2008;34(5):417-424.
15. Baughman RP, Lower EE, Flessa HC, et al. Thrombocytopenia in the intensive care unit. *Chest.* 1993;104:1243-1247.
16. Hanes SD, Quarles DA, Boucher BA. Incidence and risk factors of thrombocytopenia in critically ill trauma patients. *Ann Pharmacother.* 1997;31:285-289.
17. Stéphan F, Hollande J, Richard O, et al. Thrombocytopenia in a surgical intensive care unit: incidence, risk factors and outcome. *Chest.* 1999;115:1363-1370.
18. Marshall JC, Cook DJ, Christou NV, et al. Multiple organ dysfunction score: a reliable descriptor of a complex clinical outcome. *Crit Care Med.* 1995;23:1638-1652.
19. Strauss R, Wehler M, Mehler K, et al. Thrombocytopenia in patients in the medical intensive care unit: bleeding prevalence, transfusion requirements, and outcome. *Crit Care Med.* 2002;30:1765-1771.
20. Cawley MJ, Wittbrodt ET, Boyce EG, et al. Potential risk factors associated with thrombocytopenia in a surgical intensive care unit. *Pharmacotherapy.* 1999;19:108-113.
21. Akca S, Haji-Michael P, de Mendonca A, et al. Time course of platelet counts in critically ill patients. *Crit Care Med.* 2002;30:753-756.
22. Vanderschueren S, De Weerdt A, Malbrain M, et al. Thrombocytopenia and prognosis in intensive care. *Crit Care Med.* 2000;28:1871-1876.
23. Levi M. Platelets in sepsis. *Hematology* 2005;10(suppl 1):129-131.
24. Drews RE. Critical issues in hematology: anemia, thrombocytopenia, coagulopathy and blood product transfusions in critically ill patients. *Clin Chest Med.* 2003;24:607-622.
25. Napolitano LM, Warkentin TE, AlMahameed A, et al. Heparin-induced thrombocytopenia in the critical care setting: Diagnosis and management. *Crit Care Med.* 2006;34:2898-2911.
26. Ortel TL. Heparin-induced thrombocytopenia: when a low platelet count is a mandate for anticoagulation. *Hematology Am Soc Hematol Educ Program.* 2009;225-232.
27. Schafer AI. Thrombocytosis and thrombocythemia. *Blood Rev.* 2001;15(4):159-166.
28. Schafer AI. Thrombocytosis. *N Engl J Med.* 2004;350(12):1211-1219.
29. Powner DJ, Hoots WK. Thrombocytosis in the NICU. *Neurocrit Care.* 2008;8(3):471-475.
30. Finazzi G, Harrison C. Essential thrombocythemia. *Semin Hematol.* 2005;42(4):230-238.
31. Harrison CN. Essential thrombocythaemia: challenges and evidence-based management. *Br J Haematol.* 2005;130(2):153-165.
32. Solberg LA Jr. Therapeutic options for essential thrombocythemia and polycythemia vera. *Semin Oncol.* 2002;29(3, suppl 10):10-15.
33. Schafer AI. Thrombocytosis: current concepts. Review article. *N Engl J Med.* 2004;350:1211-1219.
34. Houbballah R, LaMuraglia GM. Clotting problems: diagnosis and management of underlying coagulopathies. *Semin Vasc Surg.* 2010;23(4):221-227.
35. Wheeler AP, Rice TW. Coagulopathy in critically ill patients. Part 2-soluble clotting factors and hemostatic testing. *Chest.* 2010;137(1):185-194.
36. Dellinger RP, Levy MM, Carlet JM, et al. Surviving Sepsis Campaign: international guidelines for management of severe sepsis and septic shock: 2008. *Crit Care Med.* 2008;36(1):296-327. Erratum in: *Crit Care Med.* 2008;36(4):1394-1396.
37. Levi M, Toh CH, Thachil J, Watson HG. Guidelines for the diagnosis and management of disseminated intravascular coagulation. British Committee for Standards in Haematology. *Br J Haematol.* 2009;145(1):24-33.
38. Brohi K, Cohen MJ, Ganter MT, et al. Acute coagulopathy of trauma: hypoperfusion induces systemic anticoagulation and hyperfibrinolysis. *J Trauma.* 2008;64(5):1211-1217; discussion 1217.
39. Frith D, Goslings JC, Gaarder C, et al. Definition and drivers of acute traumatic coagulopathy: clinical and experimental investigations. *J Thromb Haemost.* 2010;8(9):1919-1925.
40. Hess JR, Brohi K, Dutton RP, et al. The coagulopathy of trauma: a review of mechanisms. *J Trauma.* 2008;65:748-754.
41. Hébert PC, et al. A multicenter, randomized, controlled clinical trial of transfusion requirements in critical care. Transfusion Requirements in Critical Care Investigators, Canadian Critical Care Trials Group. *N Engl J Med.* 1999;340(6):409-417. Erratum in: *N Engl J Med.* 1999;340(13):1056.
42. Napolitano LM, et al. Clinical practice guideline: red blood cell transfusion in adult trauma and critical care. *Crit Care Med.* 2009;37(12):3124-3157.
43. Napolitano LM, Kurek S, Luchette FA, et al. American College of Critical Care Medicine of the Society of Critical Care Medicine; Eastern Association for the Surgery of Trauma Practice Management Workgroup. Clinical practice guideline: red blood cell transfusion in adult trauma and critical care. *Crit Care Med.* 2009;37(12):3124-3157. Erratum in: *Crit Care Med.* 2010;38(7):1621.
44. Napolitano LM, Kurek S, Luchette FA, et al. EAST Practice Management Workgroup; American College of Critical Care Medicine (ACCM) Taskforce of the Society of Critical Care Medicine (SCCM). Clinical practice guideline: red blood cell transfusion in adult trauma and critical care. *J Trauma.* 2009;67(6):1439-1442.
45. Roback, J. D., S. Caldwell, et al. Evidence-based practice guidelines for plasma transfusion. *Transfusion.* 2010;50(6):1227-1239.
46. British Committee for Standards in Haematology, Blood Transfusion Task Force. Guidelines for the use of platelet transfusion. *Br J Haematol.* 2003;122(1):10-23.
47. Contreras, M. Consensus conference on platelet transfusion. Final statement. *Blood Rev.* 1998;12(4):239-240.
48. Butch SH, Davenport RD, Cooling L. Blood Transfusion Policies and Standard Practices of the University of Michigan, July 2010. http://www.pathology.med.umich.edu/bloodbank/manual/
49. Heddle NM, Cook RJ, Tinmouth A, et al.; SToP Study Investigators of the BEST Collaborative. A randomized controlled trial comparing standard- and low-dose strategies for transfusion of platelets (SToP) to patients with thrombocytopenia. *Blood.* 2009;113(7):1564-1573.
50. Callum JL, Karkouti K, Lin Y. Cryoprecipitate: the current state of knowledge. *Transfus Med Rev.* 2009;23(3):177-188.
51. Holcomb JB. Methods for improved hemorrhage control. *Crit Care.* 2004;8:S57-S60.
52. Cosgriff N, Moore EE, Sauaia A, et al. Predicting life-threatening coagulopathy in the massively transfused trauma patient: hypothermia and acidoses revisited. *J Trauma.* 1997;42:857-861.
53. Moore EE. Thomas G. Orr memorial lecture. Staged laparotomy for the hypothermia, acidosis, and coagulopathy syndrome. *Am J Surg.* 1996;172:405-410.

54. McKinley BA, Gonzalez EA, Balldin BC, et al. Revisiting the "Bloody Vicious Cycle". *Shock*. 2004;21(suppl 2):47.
55. ATLS® for Doctors Student Manual with DVD, 8th ed. American College of Surgeons. http://www.facs.org/trauma/atls/index.html.
56. Inaba K, Teixeira PG, Shulman I, et al. The impact of uncross-matched blood transfusion on the need for massive transfusion and mortality: analysis of 5,166 uncross-matched units. *J Trauma*. 2008;65(6):1222-1226.
57. Repine TB, Perkins JG, Kauvar DS, et al. The use of fresh whole blood in MT. *J Trauma*. 2006;60:S59-S69.
58. Sihler KC, Napolitano LM. Massive transfusion: New insights. *Chest*. 2009;136(6):1654-1667.
59. Sihler KC, Napolitano LM. Complications of massive transfusion. *Chest*. 2010;137(1):209-220.
60. Harvey MP, Greenfield, TP, Sugrue ME, et al. Massive blood transfusion in a tertiary referral hospital. Clinical outcomes and haemostatic complications. *Med J Aust*. 1995;163:356-359.
61. Mollison PL, Engelfreit CP, Contreras M. Transfusion in oligaemia. In: *Blood Transfusion in Clinical Medicine*. Oxford: Blackwell Science, 1997; p. 47.
62. Levy, JH. MT coagulopathy. *Semin Hematol*. 2006;43:S59-S63.
63. Lim RC, Olcott C, Robinson AJ. Platelet response and coagulation changes following massive blood replacement. *J Trauma*. 1973;13:577-558.
64. *Advanced Trauma Life Support for Doctors: Student Course Manual*. 8th ed. Chicago, IL: American College of Surgeons; 2008.
65. Wudel JH, Morris JA, Yates K. MT: outcome in blunt trauma patients. *J Trauma*. 1991;31:1-7.
66. Moltzan CJ, DA Anderson, J Callum, et al. The evidence for use of recombinant factor VIIa in massive bleeding: development of a transfusion policy framework. *Transfus Med*. 2008;18:112-120.
67. Fakhry SM, Sheldon GF. MT in the surgical patient. In: Jeffries LC, Brecher ME, ed. *MT*. Bethesda, MD: American Association of Blood Banks; 1994
68. Schreiber MA, Perkins J, Kiraly L, et al. Early predictors of MT in combat casualties. *J Am Coll Surg*. 2007;205:541-545.
69. Cotton BA, Dossett LA, Haut ER, et al. Multicenter validation of a simplified score to predict massive transfusion in trauma. *J Trauma*. 2010;69(suppl 1):S33-S39.
70. Maegele M, Lefering R, Wafaisade A, et al.; Trauma Registry of the Deutsche Gesellschaft fur Unfallchirurgie (TR-DGU). Revalidation and update of the TASH score: a scoring system to predict the probability for massive transfusion as a surrogate for life-threatening haemorrhage after severe injury. *Vox sang*. 2011;100(2):231-238.
71. Nunez TC, Voskresensky IV, Dossett LA, et al. Early prediction of massive transfusion in trauma: simple as ABC (assessment of blood consumption)? *J Trauma*. 2009;66(2):346-352.
72. Mahambrey TD, Fowler RA, Pinto R, et al. Early massive transfusion in trauma patients: Canadian single-centre retrospective cohort study. *Can J Anaesth*. 2009;56(10):740-750.
73. Como JJ, Dutton RP, Scalea TM, et al. Blood transfusion rates in the care of acute trauma. *Transfusion*. 2004;44:809-813.
74. Vaslef SN, Knudsen NW, Neligan PJ, et al. MT exceeding 50 units of blood products in trauma patients. *J Trauma*. 2002;53:291-296.
75. Brohi K, Cohen MJ, Ganter MT, et al. Acute coagulopathy of trauma: hypoperfusion induces systemic anticoagulation and hyperfibrinolysis. *J Trauma*. 2008;64(5):1211-1217.
76. Cohen MJ, Brohi K, Ganter MT, et al. Early coagulopathy after traumatic brain injury: the role of hypoperfusion and the protein C pathway. *J Trauma*. 2007;63(6):1254-1261; discussion 1261-1262.
77. Frith D, Goslings JC, Gaarder C, et al. Definition and drivers of acute traumatic coagulopathy: clinical and experimental investigations. *J Thromb Haemost*. 2010;8(9):1919-1925.
78. MacLeod JB, Lynn M, McKenney MG, et al. Early coagulopathy predicts mortality in trauma. *J Trauma*. 2003;55:39-44.
79. Hardy JF, DeMoerloose P, Samama CM. The coagulopathy of MT. *Vox Sang*. 2005;89:123-127.
80. Hellstern P, Haubelt H. Indications for plasma in MT. *Thromb Res*. 2002;107(suppl 1):S19-S22.
81. Erbert WN, Perry DJ. Plasma and plasma products in the treatment of massive hemorrhage. *Best Pract Res Clin Haematol*. 2006;19:97-112.
82. Stern SA. Low-volume fluid resuscitation for presumed hemorrhagic shock: helpful or harmful? *Curr Opin Crit Care*. 2001;7:422-430.
83. Bickell WH, Wall MJ, Pepe PE, et al. Immediate versus delayed fluid resuscitation for hypotensive patients with penetrating torso injuries. *N Engl J Med*. 1994;331:1105-1109.
84. Napolitano LM. Resuscitation endpoints in trauma. *Transfus Altern Transfus Med*. 2005;6(4):6-14.
85. Holcomb JB, Hoyt D, Hess JR. Damage control resuscitation: the need for specific blood products to treat the coagulopathy of trauma. *Transfusion*. 2006;46:685-686.
86. Johansson PI, Stensballe J. Hemostatic resuscitation for massive bleeding: the paradigm of plasma and platelets—a review of the current literature. *Transfusion*. 2010;50(3):701-710.
87. Ho AM, Karmakar MK, Dion PW. Are we giving enough coagulation factors during major trauma resuscitation? *Am J Surg*. 2005;190: 479-484.
88. Ho AM, Dion PW, Cheng CA, et al. A mathematical model for fresh frozen plasma transfusion strategies during major trauma resuscitation with ongoing hemorrhage. *Can J. Surg*. 2005;48:470-478.
89. Holcomb JB, Hess JR (eds.). Early MT: state of the art—Conference Proceedings. US Army Institute of Surgical Research, Ft. Sam, Houston. TX. May 26-27, 2005 J Trauma 2006;60:S1-S2.
90. Fox CJ, Gillespie DL, Cox D, et al. Damage control resuscitation for vascular surgery in a combat support hospital. *J Trauma*. 2008;65:1-9.
91. Simmons JW, White CE, Eastridge BJ, Mace JE, Wade CE, Blackbourne LH. Impact of policy change on US Army combat transfusion practices. *J Trauma*. 2010;69(suppl 1):S75-S80.
92. Gonzalez EA, Moore FA, Holcomb JB, et al. Fresh frozen plasma should be given earlier to patients requiring MT. *J Trauma*. 2007;62:112-119.
93. Holcomb JB, Wade CE, Michalek JE, et al and The Trauma Outcomes Group. Increased plasma and platelet to RBC ratios improves outcome in 466 massively transfused civilian trauma patients. *Ann Surg*. 2008;248(3):447-458.
94. Scalea T, Bochicchio G, Lumpkins K, et al. Early aggressive use of fresh frozen plasma (FFP) does not improve outcome in critically injured trauma patients. *Ann Surg*. 2008;248(4):578-584.
95. Duchesne JC, Hunt JP, Wahl G, et al. Review of current blood transfusion strategies in a mature level 1 trauma center: were we wrong for the last 60 years? *J Trauma*. 2008;65(2):272-276.
96. Maegele M, Lefering R, Paffrath T, et al; Working Group on polytrauma of the German Society of Trauma Surgery (DGU). Red blood cell to plasma ratios transfused during MT are associated with mortality in severe multiple injury: a retrospective analysis from the Trauma Registry of the Deutsche Gesellschaft fur Unfallchirurgie. *Vox Sanguinis*. 2008;95:112-119.
97. Sperry JL, Ochoa JB, Gunn SR, et al.; Inflammation the Host Response to Injury Investigators. An FFP:PRBC transfusion ratio >/= 1:1.5 is associated with lower risk of mortality after MT. *J Trauma* 2008;65(5):986-993.
98. Murad MH, Stubbs JR, Gandhi MJ, et al. The effect of plasma transfusion on morbidity and mortality: a systematic review and meta-analysis. *Transfusion*. 2010;50(6):1370-1383.
99. Roback JD, Caldwell S, Carson J, et al.; American Association for the Study of Liver; American Academy of Pediatrics; United States Army; American Society of Anesthesiology; American Society of Hematology. Evidence-based practice guidelines for plasma transfusion. *Transfusion*. 2010;50(6):1227-1239.
100. Khan H, Belsher J, Yilmaz M, et al. Fresh-frozen plasma and platelet transfusions are associated with development of acute lung injury in critically ill medical patients. *Chest*. 2007;131:1308-1314.
101. Gajic O, Yilmaz M, Iscimen R, et al. Transfusion from male-only versus female donors in critically ill recipients of high plasma volume components. *Crit Care Med*. 2007;35:1645-1648.
102. Netzer G, Shas CV, Iwashyna TJ, et al. Association of RBC transfusion with mortality in patients with acute lung injury. *Chest*. 2007;132:1116-1123.
103. Toy P, Popovsky MA, Abraham E, et al.; National Heart, Lung and Blood Institute Working Group on TRALI. Transfusion-related acute lung injury: definition and review. *Crit Care Med*. 2005;33:721-726.
104. Gajic E. Rana R, Winters JL, et al. Transfusion-related acute lung injury in the critically ill: prospective nested case-control study. *Am J Respir Crit Care Med*. 2007;176:886-891.
105. Rubenfeld GD, Caldwell E, Peabody E, et al. Incidence and outcomes of acute lung injury. *N Engl J Med*. 2005;353:1685-1693.
106. Malone DL, Hess JR, Fingerhut A. MT practices around the globe and a suggestion for a common MT protocol. *J Trauma*. 2006;60:S91-S96.
107. Cotton BA, Gunter OL, Isbell J, et al. Damage control hematology: the impact of a trauma exsanguination protocol on survival and blood product utilization. *J Trauma*. 2008;64:1177-1182.
108. Johansson PI, Stensballe J, Rosenberg I, et al. Proactive administration of platelets and plasma for patients with a ruptured abdominal aortic aneurysm: evaluating a change in transfusion practice. *Transfusion*. 2007;47:593-598.
109. Johansson PI. The blood bank: from provider to partner in treatment of massively bleeding patients. *Transfusion*. 2007;47:176S-181S
110. Johansson PI, Bochsen L, Stensballe J, et al. Transfusion packages for massively bleeding patients: the effect on clot formation and stability as evaluated by TEG. *Transfus Apher Sci*. 2008;39:3-8.
111. http://www.uth.tmc.edu/cetir/PROMMTT/index.html.
112. West MA, Shapiro MB, Nathens AB, et al. Guidelines for transfusion in the trauma patient. Inflammation and host response to injury, a large-scale collaborative project: patient-oriented research core—Standard operating procedures for clinical care. *J Trauma*. 2006;61:436-439.
113. Carson JL, Terrin ML, Magaziner J, et al.; FOCUS Investigators. Transfusion trigger trial for functional outcomes in cardiovascular patients undergoing surgical hip fracture repair (FOCUS). *Transfusion*. 2006;46(12):2192-2206.
114. Carson JL et al. Transfusion Trigger Trial for Functional Outcomes in Cardiovascular Patients Undergoing Surgical Hip Fracture Repair (FOCUS) trial results. Orlando, FL: Late-breaker presented at the American Heart Association Scientific Session; 2009.
115. Gammon RR, Strayer SA, Avery NL, et al. Hemolysis during leukocyte-reducction of stored red blood cells. *Ann Clin Lab Sci*. 2000;30(2):195-199.
116. Sowemimo-Coker SO. Red blood cell hemolysis during processing. *Transfus Med Rev* 2002;16(1):46-60.
117. Fernandes CJ Jr, Akamine N, De Marco FV, et al. Red blood cell transfusion does not increase oxygen consumption in critically ill septic patients. *Crit Care*. 2001;5(6):362-367.

118. Tinmouth A, Fergusson D, Yee IC, et al.; ABLE Investigators; Canadian Critical Care Trials Group. Clinical consequences of red cell storage in the critically ill. *Transfusion.* 2006;46(11):2014-2027.
119. Spinella PC, Carroll CL, Staff I, et al. Duration of red blood cell storage is associated with increased incidence of deep vein thrombosis and in-hospital mortality in patients with traumatic injuries. *Crit Care.* 2009;13(5);R151.
120. Koch CG, Li L, Sessler DI, et al. Duration of red cell storage and complications after cardiac surgery. *N Engl J Med.* 2008;358(12):1229-1239.
121. Age of Blood Evaluation (ABLE) trial. http://www.controlled-trials.com/ISRCTN44878718/.
122. Napolitano LM. Cumulative risks of early red blood cell transfusion. *J Trauma.* 2006;60(6 suppl):S26-S34.
123. Malone DL, Dunne J, Tracy JK et al. Blood transfusion, independent of shock severity, is associated with worse outcome in trauma. *J Trauma.* 2003;54(5):898-905.
124. Dunne JR, Malone DL, Tracy JK, et al. Allogeneic blood transfusion in the first 24 hours after trauma is associated with increased SIRS and death. *Surg Infect (Larchmt).* 2004;5(4):395-404.
125. Napolitano LM, Corwin HL. Efficacy of blood transfusion in the critically ill [Review]. *Crit Care Clin.* 2004;20(2):255-568.
126. Marik PE, Corwin HL. Efficacy of red blood cell transfusion in the critically ill: a systematic review of the literature. *Crit Care Med.* 2008;36(9):2667-2674.

CHAPTER 11 ■ NUTRITION IN ACUTE CARE SURGERY

JUAN B. OCHOA AND JEAN NICKLEACH

Modern care of the acutely ill surgical patient cannot be conceived without the provision of adequate nutrition. Nutrition has evolved far beyond that of being solely "supportive." Nutrition intervention therapy, in addition to providing the necessary nutrients to maintain normal metabolic processes, plays other essential roles including maintenance of mucosal integrity, modulation of immune responses, and protection against oxidative stress, among others. Nutrition intervention therapy is a powerful tool for the acute care surgeon that, when used adequately, beneficially affects patient outcomes; conversely, when poorly applied, it can cause increased morbidity and mortality and increase cost.[1] This chapter reviews the basic principles to assist the clinician with successful utilization of nutrition intervention.

Humans need food, water, and electrolytes. When digested and absorbed by the gastrointestinal tract, nutrients provide the basic elements to meet the energetic and metabolic needs for normal activity, growth and repair of cells and tissues. Under normal circumstances, a human adult is capable, through the process of eating and drinking, of ingesting a balanced amount of nutrients to meet his/her daily needs. This process occurs naturally and is regulated by physiologic processes such as hunger, thirst, and craving. Notwithstanding the epidemic of obesity, most humans achieve an equilibrium maintaining adequate hydration and electrolyte balance while satisfying the needs of macro- and micronutrients.

Eating and drinking are dramatically disrupted in the acutely ill surgical patient, obligating the clinician to replace the natural process of food intake. Balanced intravenous electrolyte solutions resolve most needs for water and electrolyte replacement and thus permit moderate periods of starvation. Ideally, resumption of oral intake is possible within a short amount of time after injury or operation; being the "golden standard," spontaneous normal eating should be allowed whenever possible.

Until 1968, a patient without a functional gastrointestinal tract was condemned to die of starvation. Evidence that total parenteral nutrition (TPN) could maintain normal growth and activity of growing pups ushered in the modern era of nutrition.[2] TPN coupled with the continued growth and sophistication of enteral diets now permits the provision of adequate nutrition intervention therapy so that normal cellular activities and tissue growth and repair can proceed. Despite its progress, any form of nutrition intervention, other than promotion of spontaneous oral intake, is artificial and does *not* replace the physiologic process of eating. Also, the nutrients provided by either TPN or total enteral nutrition (TEN) cannot be mistaken for normal food intake. As such, nutrition intervention therapy is comparable to other form of medical therapy and is associated with benefits when adequately ordered and delivered; side effects, some of which can be unexpected; and risks including severe complications and even death.

NUTRIENT UTILIZATION DURING NORMAL STATES OF HEALTH

The purpose of the creation of nutritional requirement guidelines has been the optimization of the human diet. Recommended dietary allowances (RDA) were developed by the government to sufficiently cover the nutritional requirements of most individuals (97% of the population). The Dietary Reference Intakes (DRIs) recommendations were introduced in 1997 to broaden the RDA. The DRIs include the RDA as well as adequate intakes (AIs) to provide guidance for those nutrients for which there is no RDA (i.e., vitamin D, vitamin K, fiber) or acceptable macronutrient distribution range to describe the range of intake for a particular energy source that is associated with reduced risk of chronic disease while providing intakes of essential nutrients (i.e., fat).[3] Human nutrition requirements vary widely from individual to individual depending upon multiple variables including age, gender, activity, and presence of illness. Despite their limitations, published RDA and DRI for normal states of health have provided the basis for comparisons of what is needed in the acutely ill surgical patient (Table 11.1).[3]

Protein balance (also called nitrogen balance) is a result of equal intake versus protein loss. Average healthy male adult intake necessary to maintain nitrogen balance is 0.75 g/kg/d.[3] Proteins (and amino acids) are the sole source of nitrogen, which can be measured in different nutrients, in tissues, and in urine. The average nitrogen conversion factor for mixed foods is 6.25 and is utilized universally to determine protein content. Protein losses include shed skin, losses in stool, and losses in urinary nitrogen that occur as a result of normal protein turnover.

Protein turnover is governed by anabolism and catabolism, two independent and carefully regulated processes, and balance is achieved when the same amount of protein is deposited as is broken down. Within the catabolic process, protein is broken down into amino acids. Approximately 80% of the amino acids are utilized back for the formation of new protein with loss of the remaining 20%. Illness alters both protein catabolism and anabolism in different ways. Generally, illness leads to a negative nitrogen balance, meaning that protein catabolism predominates over that of anabolic processes.

Investigators have identified several protein compartments in the body including skeletal, visceral, and circulatory compartments. Skeletal muscle constitutes a primary source of protein during stress, and its destruction is prioritized to protect visceral protein (defined as the protein compartment contained in vital organs). Plasma circulating proteins including albumin and prealbumin, although small as a compartment, are important in that they have been used as biomarkers of nutritional status. However, synthesis of albumin and prealbumin is profoundly affected by inflammatory

TABLE 11.1

RECOMMENDED INTAKES FOR MACRONUTRIENTS

MACRONUTRIENT	DIETARY REFERENCE INTAKES
Total fat	20%-33% energy[a]
Saturated fat	As low as possible
Cholesterol	As low as possible
Linoleic acid	11–17 g/d[b]
α-linolenic acid	1.1–1.6 g/d
Carbohydrates	130 g/d
Added sugars	No more than 25% energy
Total fiber	21–38 g/d[b]
Protein	46–56 g/d

NOTE: Amounts above are recommended for men and women from ages 19 to 70.
[a]Acceptable macronutrient distribution range.
[b]Adequate intake.
Source: Insitute of Medicine. *Food and Nutrition Board. Dietary Reference Intakes for Energy, Carbohydrate, Fiber, Fat, Fatty Acids, Cholesterol, Protein, and Amino Acids (Macronutrients).* Washington, DC: National Academy of Sciences; 2005.

states, and changes in their plasma concentrations are not specific to the nutritional status of the patient during acute illness, thereby limiting their value as reliable biomarkers of nutrition status.[4]

Protein can be used as an energy source roughly providing a similar amount of calories per gram as that of carbohydrates. In the absence of carbohydrate intake, certain amino acids contained in protein (e.g., alanine) become obligate sources of glucose (gluconeogenesis), an essential process during prolonged fasting.

Lipids perform multiple essential functions; they are essential for the cell membrane architecture, serve as the substrate for the formation of signaling molecules and hormones, and are the most important source of energy storage. Healthy myocardium primarily uses fatty acids as its energy source.[5,6] Lipids often become the primary source of energy during acute surgical illness.

Glucose is an essential compound for cell function providing energy for anaerobic and aerobic metabolism. Several tissues including erythrocytes, the brain, and parts of the renal parenchyma are obligate users of glucose. Small amounts of glucose can be stored in the muscle as glycogen, although these stores are exhausted within the first 48 hours of fasting. Dietary carbohydrates, which include monosaccharides, disaccharides, and polysaccharides, vary considerably in their presentation with more complex carbohydrates, such as starch, forming chains of monosaccharides. Glucose, a monosaccharide, is readily absorbed into the circulation while complex carbohydrates require enzymatic breakdown (e.g., amylase) before absorption. The impact of a dietary carbohydrate on circulating glucose (and therefore insulin release) is called the glycemic index (GI) and is inversely proportional to its complexity. The GI value is derived from the area under the curve for the increase in blood glucose after the ingestion of a set amount of carbohydrate in a food during the 2-hour postprandial period.[7] Complex carbohydrates require a functional gastrointestinal tract for their absorption and digestion while glucose can be delivered directly into the circulation as in TPN. The rate of breakdown and absorption is proportional to the rise in circulating blood sugar and subsequent insulin response. For this reason, GI is often used to calculate the glycemic load, an indicator of glucose response or insulin demand that is induced by total carbohydrate intake. It is calculated by multiplying the weighted mean of the dietary GI by the percentage of total energy from carbohydrate. The utilization of GI in combination with glycemic load is important in patients with insulin resistance or underlying diabetes mellitus.[8]

Micronutrients are also essential for survival. Micronutrients include vitamins, co-vitamins, and minerals. All micronutrients are contained in a balanced diet, although specific deficiencies may be observed with relative frequency. In addition, disease imposes the need for supraphysiologic supplementation of specific micronutrients (Table 11.2). The importance of micronutrients in management of the acutely ill surgical patient cannot be overstated, although an exhaustive discussion of this topic goes beyond the scope of the chapter. We provide a partial list of most frequently mentioned micronutrients to raise awareness of their importance.[3,8–11]

NUTRIENT UTILIZATION DURING ACUTE SURGICAL ILLNESS

Survival in the acutely ill surgical patient is influenced by neuroendocrine and immune activation including the release of inflammatory signals. As a result, noticeable metabolic

TABLE 11.2

SELECTED MICRONUTRIENT REQUIREMENTS

MICRONUTRIENT	NORMAL SERUM LEVELS	DRI—MALES (19–70 Y)	DRI—FEMALES (19–70 Y)
Vitamin C[9]	0.2–2.0 mg/dL (serum ascorbic acid)	90 mg	75 mg
Vitamin D[10]	30.0–74.0 ng/mL (25-hydroxy-vitamin D)	600 IU	600 IU
Vitamin E[9]	5–20 μg/mL (serum tocopherol)	15 mg alpha tocopherol	15 mg alpha tocopherol
Iron[12]	Male: 12–300 ng/mL; female: 12–150 ng/mL (serum ferritin) 30% (transferrin saturation)	8 mg	8–18 mg
Magnesium[11]	1.7–2.2 mg/dL (serum magnesium)	400–420 mg	320 mg
Selenium[9]	46–143 μg/dL (serum selenium)	55 μg	55 μg
Zinc[12]	11–19 mmol/L (serum zinc)	11 mg	8 mg

changes include an increased catabolic response, hyperglycemia, appreciable alteration in lipid utilization as an energy source, changes in synthesis and breakdown of visceral proteins, and alterations in the availability of certain micronutrients, such as amino acids and iron.

Increased protein catabolism that exceeds anabolic responses is a hallmark of the catabolic response of physical injury, be it trauma or surgery.[12] Protein losses (negative nitrogen balance) are higher than those observed with a simple starvation response. Following surgery, muscle is used as an essential source of amino acids necessary for the generation of glucose and for tissue repair and healing. Skeletal muscle serves the purpose of being the "protein store" of the body; during prolonged illness, protein becomes the "limiting" macronutrient often long before exhaustion of lipid stores ensues. As a result, protein depletion following acute care surgery leads to severe malnutrition and muscle deconditioning.[13] Thus, the major focus of nutrition intervention therapy is achieving a positive nitrogen balance as a means to prevent protein malnutrition and improve outcome.

There have been many attempts at restoring protein anabolism in the acutely ill through the provision of increased amounts of calories and protein above that of the daily normal requirements. These therapeutic strategies have been called by different names including hyperalimentation or the correction for "stress factors" that are artificially used to calculate increased metabolic requirements. The use of TPN has been a preferred treatment strategy, as it is easy to provide large amounts of calories through this route. These well-intentioned strategies have, however, failed to show benefit and in some cases are known to produce harm.[14] Failure to achieve positive nitrogen balance through dietary means alone has forced nutrition investigators and surgeons alike to focus on control of inflammation as a means to reverse the catabolic response.

The immune (inflammatory) response to acute surgical illness plays a key role in the catabolic responses observed in acute care surgery. Tumor necrosis factor, initially known as cachectin, increases muscle breakdown. Interleukin-1 increases metabolic rate and generates a febrile response. The rate of protein catabolism and negative nitrogen balance is proportional to the severity of the inflammatory response. As a result, progression towards protein malnutrition is accelerated in critically ill patients. Resolution of the inflammatory response leads to restoration between anabolic and catabolic processes and gives opportunity to an effective nutrition intervention therapy.

Insulin resistance often follows acute surgery and is frequently associated with hyperglycemia and poor utilization of glucose as an energy source. In addition, glycogen stores as a source of glucose are exhausted within the first 48 hours, making lipids a preferred fuel following surgery. The exhaustion of glucose along with insulin resistance obligates cells to utilize amino acids (particularly alanine and glutamine) as a mechanism for gluconeogenesis. Ketogenesis (from lipid oxidation) is also increased. Lipid mobilization is therefore observed, and it is common detect moderate amounts of hyperlipidemia in the acutely ill surgical patient. A depletion of circulating lipids and cholesterol is considered a marker of ensuing malnutrition and portends a poor prognosis.[15]

Little is known about the utilization of many micronutrients following acute care surgery. The use of supraphysiologic quantities of antioxidants and other micronutrients including selenium, zinc, and vitamin C have been suggested as an important adjunct to therapy in acute surgical illness. For example, vitamin C is now used routinely in high quantities during the resuscitation of burn patients. The results of ongoing studies are still not in, however, and therefore, prescription of high levels of these micronutrients should be reserved for the instances where they have found to be deficient.

The provision of the necessary substrate for cellular proliferation and repair and for the satisfaction of the energy needs in a given individual is an essential aspect of nutrition intervention therapy. As, such the acute care surgeon is obligated to provide a careful design and delivery of a well-balanced nutrition intervention.

THE PHYSIOLOGIC RESPONSE TO STARVATION AS A STARTING POINT IN THE DESIGN OF NUTRITION INTERVENTION THERAPY

Acutely ill surgical patients are often unable to maintain spontaneous food intake. As a result, many patients undergo periods of starvation, which can be prolonged at times. Starvation response has been used as a starting point to design nutritional intervention therapies. Starvation is a physiologic process. During times of famine, a series of carefully orchestrated genetic/metabolic responses occur aimed at preserving macro- and micronutrients to sustain normal organ function. The starvation response "buys time" for the individual. Several remarkable features are observed during starvation including that of decreased protein turnover (catabolism) and careful preservation of energy stores.

Obligatory protein loss in the normal individual is balanced through protein intake. As protein intake decreases, negative nitrogen balance ensues. However, in the starved individual protection of protein stores is achieved through a decrease in protein turnover.[16] Thus, in the normal individual up to 15 g of nitrogen are lost per day and need to be replaced. An otherwise healthy human subjected to starvation will decrease nitrogen loss to approximately 5 g per day. This essential adaptive process protects muscle mass and prolongs the time to the development of malnutrition.[17]

Obligatory protein loss during starvation (5 g per day) is necessary for the generation of glucose and is essential for survival. Obligatory protein loss in starved individuals can be abrogated through the provision of small amounts of glucose (700 calories a day). This process is known as the *protein-sparing effect of glucose* and decreases muscle loss considearbly.

Preservation of energy during starvation is also remarkable.[18] Starved individuals will spontaneously reduce their daily activities to meet the limited amount of energy intake. In addition, starved individuals will decrease their resting metabolic rate and thermal responses.[17] This is probably secondary to decreased catecholamine turnover and action; and decreased peripheral conversion of thyroxine (T4) to the active triiodothyronine (T3).[16] Clinical manifestations of decreased energy consumption are characteristic and include reduced interaction with the environment (apathy), hypothermia, and bradycardia.

Prolonged starvation inevitably leads to depletion of nutrients and the onset of malnutrition, a pathologic process characterized by organ dysfunction. Malnutrition negatively affects all disease processes and is associated with dramatic increases in morbidity and mortality. Malnutrition is surprisingly frequent in surgical and institutionalized patients, affecting up to one-third of patients. Attempts at its early identification and correction should be promptly instituted.

In contrast to the normal individual, acutely ill patients appear unable to mount a protective starvation response. As a result, progression towards malnutrition occurs more rapidly. In fact, patients with late multiple organ failure in the ICU will exhibit characteristics of severe malnutrition. Nutrition intervention therapy attempts to prevent the progression towards malnutrition observed in the critically ill.

STARVATION: A PHYSIOLOGIC PROCESS IN THE ACUTELY ILL?

Some short periods of starvation are almost inevitable in the acutely ill surgical patient. For example, care of hemodynamically unstable patients requires all attention toward stabilization. In this environment, nutrition intervention becomes secondary and is frequently forgotten. It is progressively clear, however, that acutely ill (particularly critically ill) surgical patients tolerate even modest starvation poorly. In fact, better outcomes including possibly decreased mortality are observed when nutrition intervention is started early—ideally within the first 24 hours of arrival to the intensive care unit.

NUTRITIONAL INTERVENTION THERAPY

The provision of nutrients necessary to support metabolic processes is essential for the acutely ill surgical patient. However, in addition to playing a "supportive role," nutrition intervention plays essential therapeutic roles in prevention of muscle loss and increasing nitrogen retention, modulation of immune responses, and preservation of gastrointestinal function (Table 11.3).

NUTRITION INTERVENTION TEAM; MORE THAN JUST THE DOCTOR

The continued process of specialization in the care of the acutely ill surgical patient requires specialized teams that, working together, result in improved outcomes for these complex patients. The push for specialization is a result of increased knowledge and technology along with complex social and economic reasons that encourage consultative processes rather than care by only one individual. Such is the case for the formation of acute pain support teams, the emergence of the infection preventionists, and the appearance of specialized nutrition support teams. It is essential to learn how to interact with these multiple teams to produce coordinated, seamless care. Traditional nutrition support, similar to other specialties, has evolved into complex nutrition intervention teams that deliver specialized nutrition intervention (Table 11.4).

Nutrition education for medical students appears to be a logical and essential component of training. However, several studies have shown that there have been major deficiencies for decades.[19,20] For example, only 25% of medical schools provide at least 25 hours or more of nutrition education to medical students during their entire 4 years of training.[21] Formal nutrition education does not appear to improve during residency training either. Major deficiencies in physician knowledge on the topic of nutrition is by no means a problem limited to the United States as it has been also reported in other countries.

Nutrition support teams first evolved to provide technical and logistical support for the provision of TPN. Typically, these teams comprise a group of people with multiple disciplines including physicians, dietitians, pharmacists, nurses, and sometimes social workers. Nutrition support teams improve the quality of nutrition intervention therapy and prove cost-effective.[22] Today, nutrition support teams focus their function on consulting services for optimization of enteral nutrition and prevention of the misuse of TPN.

TABLE 11.3

GOALS OF FEEDING

Primary goals	Decrease protein loss Increasing nitrogen retention Promotion of healing
Secondary goals	Modification of the Inflammatory response Preservation of gastrointestinal function Protection of gastrointestinal mucosa Preservation of gut-associated lymphoid tissues

TABLE 11.4

HOW TO USE SPECIALIZED NUTRITION INTERVENTION TEAMS

Consult early, particularly in complex patients.
Develop a comprehensive nutrition intervention strategy (plan) Plan both short- and long-term goals
Act on the plan with careful targeted interventions
Start nutrition intervention therapy as early as possible
Monitor for side effects
Use specialized nutrition intervention following clear indications and guidelines

HOW TO CALCULATE NUTRITIONAL GOALS

A considerable amount of research currently focuses on determination of the number and type of calories that should be provided to the acutely ill patient. It is interesting that such a basic question (i.e., how many calories should we order?) remains unanswered. Several observations demonstrate that the accumulation of a caloric debt (10,000 cal during the first week) is associated with increased morbidity and mortality.[23] Most scientific societies and clinical guidelines advocate 20–25 kcal/kg/d, regardless of the patients' metabolic state.[1] These goals attempt to achieve a middle road between overfeeding and starvation. Ongoing prospective trials currently are underway and promise to better determine the ideal amounts of calories to be provided.

To accurately assess the nutritional needs of a patient, the nutrition clinician must obtain a thorough history from the patient, family members, and medical records. Parameters that need to be identified include relevant anthropometrics such as height, current weight, weight changes over time, and a dietary history to identify any potential nutritional imbalances prior to current hospitalization. Once a valid weight history is obtained, various methods are employed to calculate estimated energy and protein goals for the patient. The Harris-Benedict Equation, Mifflin-St Jeor Equation, and the Ireton-Jones Energy Expenditure equation are among current methods available for energy estimation[3,24–27] (Table 11.5). However, a common equation utilized for daily practice due to brevity and convenience is the "kcal/kg" formulation. There

TABLE 11.5

SELECT ADULT NUTRITIONAL ASSESSMENT EQUATIONS

NUTRITIONAL ASSESSMENT METHOD	FORMULA	HISTORY
Calorie per kilogram	25–35 cal/kg[25,26]	Extrapolated from the WHO calculations. Estimated based on nonobese population.[26] ASPEN recommends that predictive energy requirements should fall within the range of 20–35 cal/kg.[25]
World Health Organization	Women: 18–30 y = 15.3(weight in kg) + 679 30–60 y = 11.6(weight in kg) + 879 >60 y = 8.8(weight in kg) + 1,128(height in m) − 1,071 Men: 18–30 y = 14.7(weight in kg) + 496 30–60 y = 8.7(weight in kg) + 829 >60 y = 9.2(weight in kg) + 637(height in m) − 302	Developed by FAO/WHO in 1974 for a healthy population.[27]
Harris Benedict	Women: REE = [655 + 9.6(weight in kg) + 1.7(height in cm)] ÷ 4.7(age in years) Men: REE = [66 + 1.37(weight in kg) + 5(height in cm)] ÷ 6.8(age in years)	Developed in 1919 from studies of indirect calorimetry of 239 men and women. Random error calculations female equation ($r^2 = 0.53$), male calculation ($r^2 = 0.75$).[26,28]
Ireton-Jones equations	Ventilator dependent: EEE = 1,784 − 11(a) + 5(w) + 244(s) + 239(t) + 804(b) Spontaneous breathing: EEE = 629 − 11(a) + 25(w) − 609(o) a = age (years) w = body weight (kg) s = sex (male = 1, female = 0) t = trauma (present = 1, absent = 0) b = burn (present = 1, absent = 0) o = obesity [BMI > 27] (present = 1, absent = 0)	Developed for critically ill and hospitalized patients using indirect calorimetry.[26,28]
Mifflin-St. Jeor	Women: REE = −161 + 10(weight in kg) + 6.25(height in cm) − 5(age) Men: REE = 5 + 10 (weight in kg) + 6.25(height in cm) − 5(age)	Developed in 1990 from studies of 247 women and 251 men. ($r^2 = 0.71$)[28]
DRIs for energy	Women: EEE = 354 − 6.91(age) + PA[9.36(weight in kg) + 726(height in m)] Men: EEE = 662 − 9.53(age) + PA[9.36(weight in kg) + 539.6(height in m)] PA (physical activity coefficient) Sedentary = 1.00 Low active = 1.11 Active = 1.25 Very active = 1.48	Developed in 2002 by the Institute of Medicine from studies of doubly labeled water for use in a healthy population.[29]

REE, resting energy expenditure; EEE, estimated energy expenditure.

is limited evidence in the literature supporting what weight to use to calculate these formulas, especially in the obese patient. Guidelines published in 2009 by ASPEN and SCCM have summarized an approach based on body mass index (BMI) to estimate kcal and protein requirements[1] (Table 11.6).

Estimations may lead to over- or underassessment of caloric needs based on patient scenarios, including obesity; thus, indirect calorimetry via a metabolic cart may be used in the ICU to ascertain a more concrete estimate of the Measured Resting Energy Expenditure. Also, indirect calorimetry calculates a respiratory quotient (CO_2 produced/O_2 consumed), which may validate the results of the study and also may lead to identification of over- or underfeeding. Despite limited evidence of benefit and inconvenience, indirect calorimetry remains the "golden standard" tool to assess caloric goals in the ICU.

MACRO- AND MICRONUTRIENTS GOALS

The proportion of carbohydrates, lipids, and protein to be provided to a patient can vary depending on the metabolic needs of the patient, the disease process, and the route of delivery of nutrients. Nutrition intervention (i.e., oral diet, enteral nutrition, or parenteral nutrition) should be adjusted to correct issues related to carbohydrate (i.e., hyperglycemia), protein (i.e., azotemia), or fat (i.e., severe hypertriglyceridemia) ingestion. Micronutrient imbalances should be adjusted with separate intravenous or oral supplementation; nutrition intervention should provide the minimum recommended amounts of micronutrients.

NUTRITION INTERVENTION THERAPY

All patients who come under the care of the acute care surgeon require nutrition intervention. As such, an early decision to proactively evaluate and determine a nutrition intervention plan (strategy) is strongly recommended; otherwise, nutrition intervention therapy can be delayed; delay in initiation of nutrition intervention therapy negatively affects clinical outcomes. In the acute care setting, an initial nutrition assessment should be performed on first encounter with the patient as soon as other basic priorities (such as the presence of shock) are managed.

Nutrition intervention therapy strategies fall into five categories including controlled starvation, spontaneous oral intake, provision of oral nutritional supplements, use of enteral nutrition (TEN), and use of TPN. The risks, benefits, and alternatives to these interventions are described below.

An order to stop volitional oral intake *Nil Per Os* (NPO) is frequently written on admission for the acutely ill surgical patient and may be necessary for several reasons. First, the disease process suffered by an acutely ill surgical patient may prevent adequate oral intake. Such is the case of patients with intestinal obstruction, protracted nausea, or vomiting from acute pancreatitis or in the case of poor splanchnic perfusion observed in intestinal ischemia or in shock. In addition, the clinician may determine that oral intake increases the risk of complications (such as aspiration) during procedures or surgical interventions. Control of oral intake thus serves an important role in the care of the acutely ill surgical patient. *Nil per Os* is predicated under the assumption that moderate periods of starvation are well tolerated by the patient without metabolic or clinically identifiable consequences. In fact, it is frequently suggested (and practiced) that patients can be safely maintained NPO for a week or more. This assumption easily leads to complacency in the plan and execution of an adequate nutrition intervention strategy.

Increasing evidence, however, suggests that even moderate periods of starvation may be detrimental in the acutely ill patient. For example, Lewis has provided two meta-analyses that compare early oral/enteral nutrition demonstrating an appreciable decrease in infections and postoperative mortality.[28] Similar observations have been made in critically ill patient populations in whom the provision of early enteral nutrition is associated with decreased mortality when compared to patients who are kept NPO.[1] This information suggests that in the acutely ill patient, even short periods of starvation are poorly tolerated and that every effort should be made to provide comprehensive nutrition intervention.

Two mechanisms that lead to poor outcomes with only moderate periods of starvation have been studied. The first includes the accumulation of a caloric deficit.[24] The second is the fact that profound pathologic changes occur in the gastrointestinal tract upon starvation. These changes can lead to decreased digestive capacity, increased bacterial growth, poor wound healing (particularly of gastrointestinal anastomosis) and impaired immune responses. Evidence that the prophylactic provision of TPN early after surgery fails to decrease postoperative complications (in patients who are otherwise NPO), suggests that negative outcomes in the surgical patient are a consequence of failing to maintain adequate gastrointestinal function through the provision of enteral intake while reaching delivery of caloric goals early on may not be as important.

Every effort has to be made, therefore, to provide early nutrition intervention, ideally in the form of oral or enteral nutrition. To do this, the surgeon (and her/his team), need to minimize the amount of time a patient is maintained NPO, through daily assessment and discussion. Enteral nutrition is the best alternative to normal oral intake when the patient's capacity to eat or swallow is impaired.

There have been some traditional barriers that prevent physicians from considering the use of the gastrointestinal

TABLE 11.6

GUIDELINES FOR THE PROVISION AND ASSESSMENT OF NUTRITION SUPPORT THERAPY IN THE ADULT CRITICALLY ILL PATIENT

BMI	ASSESSMENT (WT)	CALORIC GOALS (KCAL/KG)	PROTEIN GOALS (G/KG)
<30	Actual	25	1.5
30–34.9	Ideal	22	2.0
35–39.9	Ideal	22	2.0
≥40	Ideal	22	2.5

tract and achieving successful nutrition intervention and, as a result, unnecessarily prolong starvation. These include

- The use of nasogastric tubes. Nasogastric tube utilization varies considerably among surgeons denoting the lack of data to support routine utilization. Nasogastric tubes output is used as a measure to assess resolution of ileus, despite the lack of evidence that this is the case. Routinely, patients with nasogastric tubes are maintained NPO. There is a significant lack of data on the indications and utilization of nasogastric tubes. A meta-analysis performed on patients undergoing elective colon surgery suggests that even though nasogastric tubes decrease the incidence of vomiting, there is an increase in respiratory tract infections, probably as a result of increased aspiration.[29] There is also no evidence that nasogastric tubes protect gastrointestinal anastomoses. Other data demonstrate that nasogastric tubes offer no benefit for patients with acute pancreatitis. Thus, routine use of nasogastric tubes cannot be advocated. When the clinician finds it necessary to use a nasogastric tube, it should be removed as soon as possible.
- Waiting for bowel sounds and passing of flatus. The assumption that ileus is routinely observed postoperatively and this prevents successful oral intake prompts clinicians to keep the patient NPO. The presence of bowel sounds and the passage of flatus are used as evidence of recovery and are frequently awaited to start oral intake. Both assumptions may prevent early nutrition intervention. In fact, early oral intake may provide a substantial stimulus for resolution of ileus. Furthermore, there is no evidence that the lack of bowel sounds predicts success or failure of oral/enteral feeding.
- The use of a "clear fluid diet." A transition clear fluid diet is frequently utilized to "test" tolerance and used as a transition phase between being NPO and receiving a regular diet. No clear benefit has been observed with these diets, and they are of no physiologic or therapeutic value. Clear diets delay adequate oral intake and may cause substantial electrolyte imbalance. Clear diets should be avoided if possible.
- "Protecting the anastomosis" by keeping the patient NPO. A frequent reason to avoid oral or enteral intake is the idea that luminal food may harm a fresh anastomosis. Growing evidence demonstrates that oral/enteral intake is not associated with increased anastomotic leaks and in fact may even be protective. For example, Lewis, in a meta-analysis of early oral/enteral intake in elective surgery patients demonstrated a trend toward decreased anastomotic breakdown, although this did not achieve statistical significance.[28,30] Rodent studies demonstrate that allowing oral intake is associated with increased burst strength and collagen deposition at the anastomotic site.

In addition to the above, other interventions may help in achieving a successful early oral/enteral intake including

- Multimodality pain control with the use of combinations of opioids and nonsteroidal anti-inflammatory agents (NSAIDS). Nausea and vomiting are frequent side effects observed with the use of opioids. In addition, opioid utilization decreases gastrointestinal motility and may prolong postoperative ileus. Combination of opioids with NSAIDS objectively achieves better pain control than single-modality therapy and may decrease the side effects associated with opioid utilization. Objectively, the utilization of NSAIDS improves tolerance to an oral diet and decreases hospital length of stay.[31]
- Regulation of the amount of IV fluids and avoidance of major electrolyte disturbances. Judicious use of intravenous fluids is an important issue in the care of the acutely ill surgical patient. Avoidance of excess intravenous fluids has been associated in some critically ill patient populations with better outcome, without an increase in the incidence of acute renal failure. Similarly, large fluid shifts associated with major electrolyte imbalances such as hypokalemia and hypomagnesemia may be associated with poor gastrointestinal motility and ileus. These should be avoided through early and daily correction.
- Understanding that meeting 100% caloric goals through oral or enteral intake may not be necessary at least early on. Perhaps one of the most important areas of current controversy revolves around the amount of caloric intake a patient should receive during acute illness.[23] Studies performed in critically ill patients and in patients after surgery demonstrate that patients receiving enteral nutrition will only receive 50%-70% of estimated caloric goals and they receive fewer calories when compared to patients receiving TPN. Despite evidence of decreased caloric intake, better outcomes are observed with the use of early oral intake/enteral nutrition when compared to TPN.[1] In addition, the use of higher caloric intake may be associated with risk of overfeeding and increased side effects including nausea, vomiting, bloating, or diarrhea. This has led to the creation of guidelines suggesting that during the first week in the intensive care unit, meeting only 50%-65% of caloric goals may be sufficient.[1]
- The issue of optimal caloric intake remains controversial. A recent analysis of outcomes in intensive care units in Canada demonstrated that while outcomes in the patients with normal BMI and in overweight patients was independent of caloric intakes, an increased mortality was associated with poor caloric intakes in the patients with lower-than-normal BMI and in the severely obese patients.[32] In addition, others have demonstrated that an accumulated caloric deficit is associated with poorer outcome in the critically ill. To solve this controversy, ongoing trials comparing the use of enteral nutrition alone or in combination with TPN (to meet caloric goals not met with enteral nutrition) are under way. We await the results of these trials as they may result in considerable paradigmatic changes in practice.
- Nutritional (biological) value of oral intake. Education as to the biological value of food intake is essential for all clinicians involved. All too often, early oral intake is confused with allowing the patients oral intake without supervision or guidance and result in the consumption of products with poor nutritional value. Oral intake in patients should be carefully guided to provide higher protein intake. The utilization of high-lipid diets (i.e., typical American diet) is associated with delayed gastric emptying and potential bloating and poor tolerance.

The utilization of oral nutritional supplements may facilitate the delivery of a balanced nutrition intake with the provision of a balanced amount of macro- and micronutrients in the early postoperative period. Oral nutritional supplements may help avoid the misuse of "clear diets" or inappropriately balanced diets and allow simplified postoperative transition to a regular diet. In contrast to the elective surgery, there is, however, little evidence in acute care surgery that oral nutritional supplements are associated with benefits in outcome. Nevertheless, the use of high-protein oral supplements has been associated with improved outcomes including a decrease in mortality in elderly and malnourished patients with hip fractures. In addition, perioperative utilization of oral nutrition supplements containing arginine, omega 3 fatty acids, and nucleotides are associated with a dramatic decrease in infections and other complications (including anastomotic breakdown) in patients undergoing elective surgery.[33] Thus, careful use of oral nutritional supplements may prove to be of benefit in the acute care surgery setting.

Enteral nutrition is delivered via a feeding tube using liquid diets, bypassing the processes of mastication and swallowing. As with oral intake, enteral nutrition should be started as soon as possible. There are different forms of access to the gastrointestinal tract. Deciding whether a patient needs enteral access should be part of the nutrition intervention strategy and determined early. It is particularly important to determine the type of enteral access to use in a patient with planned surgery, as the trip to the operating room provides an optimal opportunity for the placement of an enteral access device. All too often, patients leave the operating room without a plan or decision as to the type of placement of enteral access, unnecessarily delaying or complicating nutrition intervention.

Types of enteral access:

- Nasoenteric feeding tubes. These tubes are placed through the nose and advanced either to the stomach (nasogastric), duodenum, or proximal jejunum (nasoenteric). These tubes tend to be of small caliber (10–12 French) and made of flexible materials. Feeding tubes are used for short-term enteral access and can remain for 6 weeks or even longer. Feeding tubes are technically easier to place than other forms of enteral access. However, complications during their placement can arise, and thus, placement should be performed only by personnel with adequate experience. For example, misplacement of the feeding tube into the airway can lead to severe complications, including the inadvertent infusion of formula into the lung, perforation of the lung, pneumothorax, or even death. The reported incidence of airway misplacement of feeding tubes is 2%, which suggests that this complication may be observed several thousand times a year in the United States alone.[34]

Protocols and technology are available to avoid or detect feeding tube misplacement and are strongly recommended as part of quality improvement in any given institution. For example, at the University of Pittsburgh, the routine use of a trained Enteral Access Team and x-rays when the feeding tube is advanced to 35 cm effectively detects airway misplacement, prior to tube advancement into the more distal airway or lung. In addition, other devices including CO_2 detectors are used. With these strategies, complications from feeding tube misplacement can be effectively eliminated.

Controversy exists as to whether the tip of the feeding tube should lie in the stomach or more distally. Advocates suggest that more distal feeding facilitates meeting caloric goals and decreases the rate of pneumonia. In contrast, others suggest that attempts to place feeding tubes through the pylorus unnecessarily delay starting enteral nutrition.

- Gastrostomy tubes are inserted into the stomach and exit the abdomen generally in the left upper quadrant. Gastrostomy tube insertion can be performed percutaneously in the radiology or endoscopy suite (percutaneous endoscopic gastrostomy—PEG) or through open surgery. Gastrostomy tubes allow easy access to the stomach and can be kept indefinitely. Tube extensions of gastrostomy tubes that extend through the pylorus into the duodenum or jejunum are commercially available and may facilitate early enteral feeding.
- Jejunostomy tubes are placed directly into the jejunum. Similar to gastrostomy tubes, they can be placed percutaneously or in open or laparoscopic surgery. Jejunostomy tubes are associated with considearble complication rates and should be used with caution and by clinicians who have sufficient expertise in placement and care.

TPN was successfully developed in 1968.[2] Its utilization ushered the modern era of nutrition and was first tested in animal models and then in patients with severe malnutrition and a nonfunctional gastrointestinal tract. When carefully used, TPN provides an invaluable resource: a therapy that has undoubtedly saved countless numbers of lives since its inception.

Learning how to use TPN however, is not easy, requiring dedication, careful monitoring of the patient for complications, and a thorough understanding of its limitations and side effects. The most obvious barrier to the successful utilization of TPN is the false idea that it provides an interchangeable substitute to oral intake or to enteral nutrition. This misconception leads to overutilization of TPN in patients with otherwise functional gastrointestinal tracts. For example, a prospective randomized trial performed by Moore and colleagues in trauma patients demonstrated a significant increase in complications in the group receiving TPN when compared to those receiving enteral nutrition. Like any other form of medical therapy, misuse and overuse of TPN leads to increased complications including infections, hyperglycemia and other metabolic disorders, and, in some cases, increased mortality.

The use of TPN in the acute care surgery setting is indicated when it is clear that enteral nutrition will fail or has failed. As such, there is controversy as to how soon TPN should be started. The use of "prophylactic" TPN "just in case" EN fails has so far proved to be of no benefit and is not advocated. Guidelines suggest that TPN should be started within 7 days and can be started earlier in the patient who has underlying severe malnutrition.

It is important to avoid the complications associated with TPN. First, it is essential to avoid overfeeding and thus careful attention to meeting but not exceeding caloric goals is important. Use of indirect calorimetry as a means of carefully determining caloric goals is suggested, particularly in the obese and morbidly obese patient in whom calculations based on weight may be erroneous. In some instances, clinicians withhold the use of lipid formulations during the first week, particularly in the United States, where only omega-6 lipid formulas are available. Excess amounts of glucose are also avoided. In contrast, protein delivery in the form of amino acids is more liberally delivered at rates of 1.5–2.0 g/kg/d.

SIDE EFFECTS OF NUTRITION INTERVENTION THERAPY

Overfeeding

Strategies aimed at "hyperalimentation" advocated providing 30 kcal/kg/d or more. Measures to proportionately give even more calories using so called "stress factors" were also suggested. Far from achieving the therapeutic goals intended, hyperalimentation led to overfeeding with unintended severe deleterious consequences, increased morbidity, and mortality (Table 11.7). Hyperalimentation should NOT be used in modern acute care surgery. Although acute care surgery has been associated with a catabolic stress state, attempts to correct negative energy balance through the use of hypercaloric diets have not improved clinical outcome. Rather, overfeeding of the critically ill patient has led to metabolic morbidity, longer ICU and hospital length of stay,[35,36] *greater mortality* rates,[37] *longer duration* on mechanical ventilators,[38–41] and higher rates of infectious complications.[46,47]

A study done by Reid[47] identified patient populations within the ICU who were more prone to receive overfeeding. Most commonly, patients who received nutrition through multiple routes, especially nutrient-dense EN and PN in combination, were overfed. Patients with ICU stays >16 days and those with tracheostomies were also at risk for overfeeding.

Refeeding syndrome was first described as a severe metabolic disturbance leading to death in famine (severely malnourished) victims who were offered aggressive nutrition intervention.

TABLE 11.7

COMPLICATIONS AND METABOLIC CONSEQUENCES AND OF OVERFEEDING IN THE ACUTE CARE SURGICAL PATIENT

COMPLICATION	SOURCES	NOTES[40]
Azotemia	40–42	
Fat-overload syndrome	40	
Glucosuria	43	
Hepatic steatosis	39–41, 44	
Hyperammonemia	42	
Hypercapnia	38–41,46	
Hyperglycemia	38, 40, 41, 44, 45, 47	Exacerbates underlying hyperglycemia associated with critically ill state
Hypertonic dehydration	40, 42	Indicated by azotemia and hypernatremia
Hypertriglyceridemia	39, 41	
Metabolic acidosis	40, 41	

Refeeding is commonly observed as a fluid and electrolyte disorder, and can include hypophosphatemia, hypomagnesemia, and hypokalemia. In addition, organ dysfunction including neurologic, pulmonary, cardiac, neuromuscular, and hematologic complications is observed. *Refeeding syndrome* occurs within a few days of initiation of nutrition intervention. The mechanisms that lead to the development of major electrolyte imbalances suggest that increased insulin release due to a change in the primary metabolic fuel source from fat to carbohydrate is the result of increased cellular uptake of electrolytes. Severe electrolyte imbalance such as hypokalemia can lead to cardiac irritability; depletion of phosphates can lead to muscle dysfunction and rhabdomyolysis. Refeeding syndrome can be observed in hospitals and may not follow the classic clinical patterns previously described, but should be suspected after initiation of nutrition intervention. Patients need to be monitored closely for abnormalities in phosphate, potassium, magnesium, glucose, and thiamine. Deficiencies should be promptly corrected.

Hyperglycemia and Glucose Control

Hyperglycemia can occur as a result of many potential issues present in the acute care surgery patient. Hyperglycemia associated with insulin resistance occurs in acutely ill patients due to adaptive activation of endocrine responses, including increased release of catecholamines, cortisol, and glucagon and a reduced capacity for glucose uptake. Meaningful debates as to the degree of glucose control with the use of insulin have ensued for the last 10 years and have caused a fair amount of confusion. Limitations in the accuracy of glucose metering technology along with significant differences in glucose intake (mostly through the use of TPN) have produced wide variations in practice. The results of the NICE-SUGAR trial demonstrate that tight glucose control (70–110 mg per dL) is impractical and may result in considearble side effects. Conversely, blood sugar levels above 200 mg per dL are consistently associated with poor outcomes. Management of hyperglycemia with pharmacological interventions (i.e., insulin) and reasonable carbohydrate intake improves morbidity and mortality in the surgical ICU.[48,49]

Remember that an important cause of hyperglycemia in acute care surgical patients is overfeeding—a major problem associated with the TPN where glucose intake may be excessive. As mentioned earlier in this chapter, overfeeding is associated with negative outcome; avoid overfeeding. Use of indirect calorimetry can assist with a more exact determination of caloric needs.

Hypertriglyceridemia

Hypertriglyceridemia is a potential complication of parenteral lipids. Parenteral lipids are cleared from the serum by the enzyme lipoprotein lipase. Hypertriglyceridemia occurs if the rate or duration of the lipid provision exceeds the enzyme's clearance capacity. Patients with hyperglycemia, renal failure, pancreatitis, or sepsis may be at higher risk for hypertriglyceridemia[50] Dosage of the lipids should not exceed 2.5 g/kg/d. Patients receiving parenteral lipids should be regularly monitored for hypertriglyceridemia. If elevated triglycerides occur, lipids in TPN should be reduced or provided on a cyclical schedule three or four times a week.

Azotemia

Azotemia can result from acute or chronic renal failure, gastrointestinal bleed, overfeeding, or administration of excessive amounts of protein in TPN. If azotemia results from renal failure and the patient is receiving dialysis, there is no need to restrict protein intake as dialysis will correct the azotemia. The presence of azotemia in the absence of renal failure may indicate GI bleed or overfeeding protein. For patients with a GI bleed, EN is typically contraindicated, and TPN should be initiated.

Gastrointestinal Intolerance

Gastrointestinal intolerance can occur following the initiation of enteral nutrition. This can manifest as vomiting, bloating, and diarrhea. Many of these symptoms are temporary and will resolve with a brief decrease in feeding rate. Additionally, medications can be helpful in symptom management. Prokinetic agents can assist with the management of nausea and vomiting. The addition of antidiarrheals, soluble fiber, or change to a peptide-based formula can assist with bloating and diarrhea. It may appear that patients experiencing gastrointestinal intolerance should discontinue EN and initiate TPN; it is important to remember that EN is associated with improvement in intestinal permeability in comparison to TPN.[51] For this reason, it is more desirable to pursue aggressive symptom management and maintain EN.

SPECIALIZED NUTRITION INTERVENTION

Specialized nutrition formulas have evolved to provide nutrition interventions for optimized care of specific patient populations. Some of these formulas may be difficult to use and may be associated with serious side effects. Thus, the clinician is encouraged to, in conjunction with specialized nutrition teams, develop protocols for their use.

Immunonutrition

One of the most controversial and confusing areas of nutrition intervention is the use of immunonutrition. As the name implies, immunonutrients are food components that alter the inflammatory response to illness. An increasing list of immunonutrients is seen in Table 11.8. Due to the complexity and incomplete understanding of the role of these nutrients in the care of the acutely ill surgical patient, the acute care surgeon is encouraged to consult specialized nutrition intervention teams.

Arginine supplementation has been utilized in many different patient populations including the acutely ill medical patient, trauma, elective surgery patient. It has also been studied in chronic illnesses such as peripheral vascular disease and coronary artery disease. To date, Level 1 evidence of benefit (with over 28 randomized studies performed) is observed only in patients undergoing elective surgery when used in combination with omega 3 fatty acids and nucleotides. In elective surgery patients, the use of immunonutrients as an oral supplement (ideally started preoperatively and continued postoperatively) is associated with a 38%-61% reduction in postoperative infections and other complications such as anastomotic dehiscence. Improved outcomes are translated into decreased length of stay and an appreciable cost benefit. All surgical patient populations studied so far appear to benefit, including patients with head and neck cancer, patients undergoing cardiac surgery, and patients undergoing gastrointestinal surgery.

TABLE 11.8

A PARTIAL LIST OF IMMUNONUTRIENTS

Amino acids
Arginine. Improves T-lymphocyte function, may increase the production of nitric oxide
Glutamine. Induces heat shock protein 70 along with multiple other metabolic effects
Lipids
Omega 3 fatty acids. Modulate inflammatory response
Micronutrients
Zinc. Supplemented in patients with open wounds
Vitamin C is used as an antioxidant. May have important clinical roles in burn patients

Immunonutrition with the use of arginine, omega 3 fatty acids, and nucleotides in trauma patients also holds promise, with some studies suggesting appreciable benefit. In trauma patients, however, there are limitations in the amount of volume that can be delivered enterally, preventing adequate dosing of the immunonutrients. A large controversy for the use of arginine in the septic patient still exists.

Glutamine is another intensely studied immunonutrient. The metabolism of glutamine when given enterally is noticeably different than when given intravenously due to enteric metabolism. Glutamine, when placed in solution, has a short half-life. To overcome this problem, parenteral presentations of glutamine as a dipeptide have been developed. These are currently not commercially available in the United States. The use of intravenous glutamine is associated with decreased mortality in sepsis.

Omega 3 fatty acid supplementation is also used extensively. Omega 3 fatty acids modify prostaglandin production and may alter lipid composition of the cell membrane. The modern American diet is particularly low in omega 3 fatty acids. Omega 3 fatty acids are used primarily to modulate the inflammatory response.

Nutrition for the Obese Patient

It is estimated that 25% of the patients in the intensive care units in the United States are obese with a BMI > 30. The combined prevalence of overweight (BMI > 25) and obesity in the general population is above 50%. Significant variations in obesity exist among the different States and is more frequently observed among patients with lower socioeconomic status. The incidence of obesity-related complications increases considerably in the hospital, as this patient population has an increased incidence of multiple chronic illnesses including diabetes, hypertension, coronary artery disease, and others.

The management of the obese, acutely ill surgical patient is particularly challenging. Evidence in Canada of clinical practices in intensive care units demonstrates that obese patients are grossly underfed, possibly increasing morbidity and mortality. The traditional methods of calculating caloric intake are grossly inaccurate in this patient population. Thus, the utilization of indirect calorimetry is encouraged in these patients. Controversy as to the number of calories and protein provided exists; current guidelines are therefore a compromise and attempt to provide a rational approach to the care of the obese patient and suggest that these patients should receive higher protein loads with a moderate restriction in calories.

THE FUTURE

Considerable advances in knowledge and technology suggest that nutrition intervention will evolve appreciably in the years to come. Recently, for example, specialized immune cells (myeloid-derived suppressor cells) that tightly regulate the availability of certain amino acids have been described in different patient populations, including after surgery and trauma, in certain cancers, and in chronic infections such as tuberculosis. Myeloid-derived suppressor cells express enzymes such as arginase and create states of arginine deficiency, which ultimately result in profound T-cell suppression and the incapacity to produce nitric oxide. It is thought, currently, that myeloid-derived suppressor cells worsen prognosis in these illnesses, particularly contributing to increased infections in the surgical and in the trauma patient. The development of carefully tailored diets aimed at overcoming the effects of myeloid-derived suppressor cells promises to become an integral part of the care of the acutely ill surgical patient.

References

1. McClave SA, Martindale RG, Vanek VW, et al. Guidelines for the Provision and Assessment of Nutrition Support Therapy in the Adult Critically Ill Patient: Society of Critical Care Medicine (SCCM) and American Society for Parenteral and Enteral Nutrition (A.S.P.E.N.). *J Parenter Enteral Nutr.* 2009;33(3):277-316.
2. Dudrick SJ. History of parenteral nutrition. *J Am Coll Nutr* 2009;28(3):243-251.
3. Institute of Medicine. *Food and Nutrition Board. Dietary Reference Intakes for Energy, Carbohydrate, Fiber, Fat, Fatty Acids, Cholesterol, Protein, and Amino Acids (Macronutrients).* Washington, DC: National Academy of Sciences; 2005.
4. Fuhrman MP, Charney P, Mueller CM. Hepatic proteins and nutrition assessment. *J Am Diet Assoc.* 2004;104(8):1258-1264.
5. Ballard FB, Danforth WH, Naegle S, et al. Myocardial metabolism of fatty acids. *J Clin Invest.* 1960;39:717-723.
6. Nelson RH, Prasad A, Lerman A, et al. Myocardial uptake of circulating triglycerides in nondiabetic patients with heart disease. *Diabetes.* 2007;56(2):527-530.
7. Barclay AW, Petocz P, McMillan-Price J, et al. Glycemic index, glycemic load, and chronic disease risk—a meta-analysis of observational studies. *Am J Clin Nutr.* 2008;87(3):627-637.
8. Institute of Medicine. *Food and Nutrition Board. Dietary Reference Intakes for Vitamin A, Vitamin K, Arsenic, Boron, Chromium, Copper, Iodine, Iron, Manganese, Molybdenum, Nickel, Silicon, Vanadium, and Zinc.* Washington, DC: National Academy of Sciences; 2001.
9. Institute of Medicine. *Food and Nutrition Board. Dietary Reference Intakes for Calcium, Phosphorus, Magnesium, Vitamin D, and Fluoride.* Washington, DC: National Academy of Sciences, 1997.
10. Institute of Medicine. *Food and Nutrition Board. Dietary Reference Intakes for Vitamin C, Vitamin E, Selenium, and Carotenoids.* Washington, DC: National Academy of Sciences; 2000.
11. Institute of Medicine. *Food and Nutrition Board. Dietary Reference Intakes for Calcium and Vitamin D.* Washington, DC: National Academy of Sciences; 2010.
12. Russell AP. Molecular regulation of skeletal muscle mass. *Clin Exp Pharmacol Physiol.* 2010;37(3):378-384.
13. Thornton FJ, Schaffer MR, Barbul A. Wound healing in sepsis and trauma. *Shock.* 1997;8(6):391-401.
14. Martindale RG, McClave SA, Vanek VW, et al. Guidelines for the provision and assessment of nutrition support therapy in the adult critically ill patient: Society of Critical Care Medicine and American Society for Parenteral and Enteral Nutrition: Executive Summary. *Crit Care Med.* 2009;37(5):1757-1761.
15. Kaysen GA. Biochemistry and biomarkers of inflamed patients: why look, what to assess. *Clin J Am Soc Nephrol.* 2009;4(suppl 1):S56-S63.
16. Vellai T, Takacs-Vellai K. Regulation of protein turnover by longevity pathways. *Adv Exp Med Biol.* 2010;694:69-80.
17. Finn PF, Dice JF. Proteolytic and lipolytic responses to starvation. *Nutrition.* 2006;22(7-8):830-844.
18. Rabinowitz JD, White E. Autophagy and metabolism. *Science.* 2010;330(6009):1344-1348.
19. Committee on Nutrition in Medical Education Food and Nutrition Board CoLSNRC. *Nutrition Education in U.S. Medical Schools.* Washington, DC: National Academies Press; 1985.
20. Winick M. Nutrition education in medical schools. *Am J Clin Nutr.* 1993;58(6):825-827.
21. Adams KM, Lindell KC, Kohlmeier M, et al. Status of nutrition education in medical schools. *Am J Clin Nutr.* 2006;83(4):941S-944S.
22. Schneider PJ. Nutrition support teams: an evidence-based practice. *Nutr Clin Pract.* 2006;21(1):62-67.
23. Stapleton RD, Jones N, Heyland DK. Feeding critically ill patients: what is the optimal amount of energy? *Crit Care Med.* 2007;35(9 suppl):S535-S540.
24. American Society for Parenteral and Enteral Nutrition (ASPEN) Board of Directors. Guidelines for the use of parenteral and enteral nutrition in adult and pediatric patients. *Jof Parenter Enteral Nutr.* 2002;26(1SA):138SA.
25. Edel J, Murray M, Schurer W, et al. Nutriton assessment of adults. In: Rychlec G, ed. *Manual of Clinical Dietetics.* 6th ed. Chicago, IL: American Dietetic Association; 2000:3-38.
26. Frankenfield D. Energy and macrosubstrate requirements. In: Gottschlich M, ed. *The Science and Practice of Nutrition Support.* Dubuque: Kendall-Hunt; 2001:31-52.
27. World Health Organization. Energy and protein requirements. Report of a joint FAO/WHO/UN Expert Consultation. Geneva: World Health Organization; 1985.
28. Lewis SJ, Andersen HK, Thomas S. Early enteral nutrition within 24 h of intestinal surgery versus later commencement of feeding: a systematic review and meta-analysis. *J Gastrointest Surg.* 2009;13(3):569-575.
29. Wolkewitz M, Vonberg RP, Grundmann H, et al. Risk factors for the development of nosocomial pneumonia and mortality on intensive care units: application of competing risks models. *Crit Care.* 2008;12(2):R44.
30. Lewis SJ, Egger M, Sylvester PA, et al. Early enteral feeding versus "nil by mouth" after gastrointestinal surgery: systematic review and meta-analysis of controlled trials. *BMJ.* 2001;323(7316):773-776.
31. Holte K, Kehlet H. Postoperative ileus: progress towards effective management. *Drugs.* 2002;62(18):2603-2615.
32. Alberda C, Gramlich L, Jones N, et al. The relationship between nutritional intake and clinical outcomes in critically ill patients: results of an international multicenter observational study. *Intensive Care Med.* 2009;35(10):1728-1737.
33. Marik PE, Zaloga GP. Immunonutrition in high-risk surgical patients: a systematic review and analysis of the literature. *J Parenter Enteral Nutr.* 2010;34(4):378-386.
34. de Aguilar-Nascimento JE, Kudsk KA. Clinical costs of feeding tube placement. *J Parenter Enteral Nutr.* 2007;31(4):269-273.
35. Hise ME, Halterman K, Gajewski BJ, et al. Feeding practices of severely ill intensive care unit patients: an evaluation of energy sources and clinical outcomes. *J Am Diet Assoc.* 2007;107(3):458-465.
36. Bryk J, Zenati M, Forsythe R, et al. Effect of calorically dense enteral nutrition formulas on outcome in critically ill trauma and surgical patients. *J Parenter Enteral Nutr.* 2008;32(1):6-11.
37. Krishnan JA, Parce PB, Martinez A, et al. Caloric intake in medical ICU patients: consistency of care with guidelines and relationship to clinical outcomes. *Chest.* 2003;124(1):297-305.
38. Baudouin SV, Evans TW. Nutritional support in critical care. *Clin Chest Med.* 2003;24(4):633-644.
39. Kitchen P, Forbes A. Intravenous nutrition in critical illness. *Curr Opin Gastroenterol.* 2001;17(2):150-153.
40. Klein CJ, Stanek GS, Wiles CE III. Overfeeding macronutrients to critically ill adults: metabolic complications. *J Am Diet Assoc.* 1998;98(7):795-806.
41. Plank LD, Hill GL. Energy balance in critical illness. *Proc Nutr Soc.* 2003;62(2):545-552.
42. Mechanick JI, Brett EM. Nutrition and the chronically critically ill patient. *Curr Opin Clin Nutr Metab Care.* 2005;8(1):33-39.
43. Sandström R, Drott C, Hyltander A, et al. The effect of postoperative intravenous feeding (TPN) on outcome following major surgery evaluated in a randomized study. *Ann Surg.* 1993;217(2):185-195.
44. Grau T, Bonet A. Caloric intake and liver dysfunction in critically ill patients. *Curr Opin Clin Nutr Metab Care.* 2009;12(2):175-179.
45. Reeds D. Near-normal glycemia for critically ill patients receiving nutrition support: fact or folly. *Curr Opin Gastroenterol.* 2010;26(2):152-155.
46. Jeejeebhoy KN. Enteral and parenteral nutrition: evidence-based approach. *Proc Nutr Soc.* 2001;60(3):399-402.
47. Reid C. Frequency of under- and overfeeding in mechanically ventilated ICU patients: causes and possible consequences. *J Hum Nutr Diet.* 2006;19(1):13-22.
48. Fahy BG, Sheehy AM, Coursin DB. Glucose control in the intensive care unit. *Crit Care Med.* 2009;37(5):1769-1776.
49. Griesdale DE, de Souza RJ, van Dam RM, et al. Intensive insulin therapy and mortality among critically ill patients: a meta-analysis including NICE-SUGAR study data. *CMAJ.* 2009;180(8):821-827.
50. Llop J, Sabin P, Garau M, et al. The importance of clinical factors in parenteral nutrition-associated hypertriglyceridemia. *Clin Nutr.* 2003;22(6):577-583.
51. Heys SD, Ogston KN. Peri-operative nutritional support: controversies and debates. *Int J Surg Investig.* 2000;2(2):107-115.

CHAPTER 12 ■ SEPSIS

TODD W. COSTANTINI, MIKE KRZYZANIAK, AND RAUL COIMBRA

DEFINITION

Sepsis is a common cause of morbidity and mortality in the surgical intensive care unit (SICU) accounting for an estimated 700,000 cases per year in the United States.[1] Sepsis is defined by the presence of infection in addition to a systemic inflammatory response syndrome (SIRS). Clinically, SIRS can manifest as fever, leukocytosis, tachycardia, and/or tachypnea. Severe sepsis is defined as sepsis with concomitant organ dysfunction. Septic shock is characterized by sepsis with persistent hypotension (systolic blood pressure < 90 mm Hg or mean arterial pressure [MAP] < 60) despite volume resuscitation.[2] Sepsis is currently the 10th most common cause of death in the United States, accounting for over 34,000 deaths per year.[3] Mortality rates for patients admitted with sepsis approach 20%-30%, with increased mortality seen in the nonwhite population and the elderly.[1]

PATHOPHYSIOLOGY

Sepsis occurs as a result of a complex set of interactions, incited by an invading pathogen, which result in a substantial host inflammatory response and activation of both the complement and coagulation cascades. While these responses are essential to control and eradicate the infecting microorganism, they are also capable of causing major damage to host tissues.

MICROBIAL FACTORS

Gram-positive bacteria, gram-negative bacteria, fungi, and parasites are capable of causing sepsis. Gram-negative bacteria have a cell wall that contains lipopolysaccharide (LPS) on its outer layer. The pathogenicity of gram-negative bacteria is due to LPS, which elicits an innate immune response. Extensive studies using animal models have characterized the ability of LPS to cause a significant host inflammatory response, with pathophysiologic responses similar to those seen in humans with sepsis.[4] Studies in human volunteers have further confirmed the toxicity of endotoxin itself, showing that injection of small concentrations of LPS causes fever, activation of inflammatory cells, and increased cytokine production.[5]

Until recently, gram-negative bacteria were the most common cause of sepsis in the ICU. There has been an increase in the incidence of gram-positive bacteria causing severe sepsis, now identified as the causative bacteria in up to 50% of the cases.[6] Gram-positive bacteria exert their pathogenic effects through the release of exotoxins and contain an outer polysaccharide capsule that protects against phagocytosis. Gram-positive bacteria contain a thick peptidoglycan layer that forms the cell wall. It is the peptidoglycan layer of gram-positive bacteria that is recognized by inflammatory cells of the innate immune system. Fungi remain a rare cause of severe sepsis, causing approximately 5% of cases.

INFLAMMATORY RESPONSE

The innate immune system is responsible for recognizing an invading microorganism. The innate immune system consists of peripheral blood mononuclear cells and polymorphonuclear leukocytes (PMNs). These cells recognize pathogen-associated molecular patterns (PAMPs), which are displayed by gram-positive bacteria, gram-negative bacteria, fungi, parasites, and viruses. Sepsis also results in the release of damage-associated molecular patterns (DAMPs), which are released by damaged or dying host tissues. The innate immune system initiates an inflammatory response when these PAMPs and DAMPs bind to pattern recognition receptors on host inflammatory cells.[7] In sepsis, there are high levels of DAMPs and PAMPs released, which can cause an exaggerated response from inflammatory cells, resulting in damage to host tissues.[8]

The toll-like receptor (TLR) family is an example of pattern recognition receptors that are key mediators of this inflammatory response. TLR expression is up-regulated, and TLR receptor reactivity is enhanced in patients with sepsis.[9] TLR-4 has been shown to be the receptor that binds to LPS, triggering the activation of multiple inflammatory signaling cascades.[10,11] The importance of the TLR-4 receptor in sepsis has been well documented in animal models using TLR-4 knockout and mutant mice.[12] These studies have shown that mice with mutations in their TLR4 gene exhibit endotoxin tolerance and are unable to mount an inflammatory response upon exposure to LPS.[13]

Binding of a PAMP to the TLR receptor activates numerous intracellular signaling pathways that up-regulate the production of transcriptional factors. These transcriptional factors, including nuclear factor-kappa B (NF-KB), activator protein-1 (AP-1), and phosphoinositide 3-kinase (PI3K)/Akt, activate the inflammatory response resulting in the production of cytokines, acute phase proteins, and inducible nitric oxide synthase (iNOS). Proinflammatory cytokines such as tumor necrosis factor-alpha (TNF-α) and interleukin (IL)-1β exert several downstream effects that propagate the inflammatory response. Studies in animal models of sepsis have shown that there is a relationship between increased TNF-α production and the development of organ failure and septic shock.[14] TNF-α exerts these effects through the production of other proinflammatory mediators such as leukotrienes and prostaglandins, which together mediate the inflammatory response in sepsis by increasing capillary leak, causing damage to epithelial and endothelial barriers and increasing adhesion molecules on both inflammatory cells and vascular endothelial cells. The PMN is the primary effector cell that mediates the acute inflammatory response to invading microorganisms. Activated PMNs bind to adhesion molecules expressed on endothelial cells allowing for diapedesis into the tissues. There, PMNs respond to the pathogen through phagocytosis, degranulation, and oxidative burst. Oxidative burst results in the release of reactive oxygen species (ROS), which leads to bacterial killing. While PMN activation and degranulation is essential in neutralizing the invading pathogen, the release of ROS can also be deleterious to the host tissues, resulting in organ injury.

COMPLEMENT ACTIVATION

The complement cascade is a part of the innate immune system that responds to invading pathogens. The complement system is composed of circulating plasma proteins that are normally in their inactive state. This system is highly regulated, as activation of the complement cascade can be damaging to host tissues. Once activated by a stimulus such as the presence of microorganisms, proteins of the complement system become activated. These activated complement proteins are responsible for lysis of bacteria and viruses, and for opsonization of bacteria resulting in phagocytosis by other inflammatory cells.

The complement cascade can be activated through three different pathways.[15] In the classic pathway, complement proteins are activated by immunoglobulin-G (IgG) or IgM bound to an antigen. The classic pathway is also activated by acute phase proteins that are produced in response to invading pathogens. The alternate pathway of complement activation occurs when complement binds directly to the PAMPs displayed by bacteria, viruses, and fungi and does not rely on antibodies binding to the pathogen. The mannose-binding lectin pathway is similar to the classic pathway of complement activation. Mannose-binding lectin is produced by the liver in response to infection and binds to the surface of invading pathogens, initiating the complement cascade. Activation of the complement system also alters the coagulation cascade, linking these two pathways in the response to sepsis.

COAGULATION

Sepsis increases the procoagulant balance in the host resulting in increased risk of small vessel thrombosis, decreased microcirculatory blood flow, and possible tissue ischemia. Inflammation is a potent activator of tissue factor that can initiate the coagulation cascade.[16] Activated tissue factor complexes with factor VIIa ultimately resulting in the conversion of prothrombin to thrombin. Thrombin then converts fibrinogen into fibrin leading to the formation of thrombus. The importance of sepsis-induced tissue factor activation was demonstrated in a study by de Jonge et al.[17] in which a tissue factor pathway inhibitor decreased coagulation activation after exposure to endotoxin. Sepsis also decreased the presence of anticoagulant factors in the blood, further shifting the procoagulant balance. The effects of activated protein C, antithrombin III, and the tissue factor pathway inhibitor are diminished in response to inflammation.

Disseminated intravascular coagulation (DIC) is a frequent complication in septic patients. DIC is characterized by the activation of the coagulation cascade resulting in fibrin activation and microvascular thrombosis, which is accompanied by consumption of coagulation factors and platelets.[18] Decreased microcirculatory blood flow caused by microvascular thrombosis can result in tissue ischemia and organ failure. Consumption of coagulation factors and platelets puts patients at risk for serious bleeding complications and may require transfusion of blood products. In a bleeding patient with DIC, platelets should be maintained at >20-30 × 10,[9] cryoprecipitate given to maintain fibrinogen concentration > 100 mg per dL, and fresh frozen plasma given to correct the PT and PTT.[19] Replacement therapy may be needed repeatedly until the underlying cause of DIC is treated as consumption of blood products will continue. Treatment of DIC is focused on treating the source of sepsis, as DIC typically resolves upon treatment of the underlying cause of infection.

MULTIPLE ORGAN FAILURE

The exaggerated host response to the septic insult can lead to major tissue injury, end organ dysfunction, and ultimately multiple organ failure (MOF). In fact, mortality rates in critically ill septic patients have been shown to be related to the magnitude of the host inflammatory response, rather than to the type of bacteria responsible for the infection or the extent of the infectious insult.[20] MOF is an important cause of mortality in critically ill patients, with mortality rates directly related to the number of organ systems that have failed. ICU patients who develop MOF have a 20-fold increased mortality compared to ICU patients who do not develop MOF, as well as a significantly increased ICU and hospital length of stay.[21] Therefore, the timely diagnosis and prompt treatment of the septic patient is essential for improved outcomes in this population.

DIAGNOSIS OF SEPSIS

Patients suspected to have sepsis should be monitored closely for signs of the SIRS response and evidence of end organ dysfunction. Prompt identification of the source of infection is a cornerstone in the treatment of sepsis. It is critically important to obtain specimens for culture including blood, urine, sputum, peritoneal fluid, abscess drainage, and catheter tips. It is vital that these cultures be obtained prior to beginning broad-spectrum antibiotic therapy. Culture specimens obtained following administration of antibiotics may prevent the identification of the organism responsible for the septic insult and later limit the ability of the clinician to properly tailor antimicrobial therapy. It is important to note that a clear microbiologic source of sepsis is not identified through cultures in at least one-third of cases.[22] Prompt imaging is also important in the diagnosis of the septic source, including plain radiographs and CT scans. Imaging studies should be chosen based on the clinical presentation and the presumed source of infection.

Identification of laboratory markers of sepsis or surrogates to measure the response of the septic patient is the topic of considerable research efforts. Biomarkers may play several roles in the clinical setting, including identification of patients at risk for an adverse outcome related to sepsis, to diagnose sepsis and inform treatment decisions, to rule out sepsis, for risk stratification, to monitor the response to treatment, and for use as a surrogate end point to monitor the effect of various treatment strategies.[23] The diverse host response to microbial infection and sepsis make identification of clinically reliable markers quite difficult.

Currently biomarkers are not widely used in the clinical setting to diagnose or guide the treatment of the septic patient. While hundreds of unique biomarkers have been proposed as possible markers of sepsis, a few potentially promising candidates have been studied. C-reactive protein (CRP) has been used for several years in an attempt to guide the management of septic patients. CRP has long been used as a marker of generalized inflammation. CRP levels increase within 6 hours of the onset of infection, with CRP levels doubling every 8 hours as the infection persists. CRP levels have been shown to peak near 36 hours after the onset of infection, with levels 1,000 times higher than normal physiologic levels.[24] CRP levels that remain persistently elevated in patients with sepsis are associated with worse outcomes.[25] CRP levels may help guide the effectiveness of antibiotic therapy in the septic patient, with decreasing CRP levels of the first 48 hours indicating effective antimicrobial therapy.[26]

Procalcitonin (PCT) is a precursor molecule of calcitonin, which has been shown to be released in response to inflammation and infection. Recent studies suggest that PCT may be a superior marker of inflammation compared to CRP.[27] Increases in circulating PCT are related to the severity of sepsis, with PCT levels decreasing after institution of appropriate antibiotic therapy.[28,29] In a study of healthy volunteers injected with endotoxin, PCT levels peaked within 6 hours and maintained a plateau between 8 and 24 hours after injection.[30] Decreased PCT levels between days 2 and 3 are associated with improved survival and may represent a way to monitor the effectiveness of antibiotic therapy.[31] Measurement of PCT may allow for the rapid identification of patients at risk for developing sepsis; however, further randomized control trials are needed to further define its clinical utility.

MANAGEMENT OF SEPSIS AND SEPTIC SHOCK

In the setting of acute organ dysfunction with or without hypotension, the speed and appropriateness of therapy are crucial to achieving treatment goals. In 2008, phase II of the Surviving Sepsis Campaign was published with clear guidelines for the treatment of sepsis and septic shock.[32] Since publication of those guidelines, sepsis bundles have emerged to eliminate piecemeal application of the guidelines and to make it easier for clinicians to bring the guidelines into practice.[33] In the surgical setting, life-threatening oxygenation, ventilation, and circulation deficits must be addressed quickly with complete interrogation of the patient for source of infection. Swift action with appropriate decision making is key in reducing mortality.

Specific treatment guidelines, protocols, and bundles have been shown to reduce morbidity and mortality of severe sepsis and septic shock in addition to reducing health care costs.[34-37] Although no study has been designed to give evidence of a clear causal relationship between adherence to SSC guidelines and reduction in mortality, these observational studies do provide a strong association between reduced mortality and use of the guidelines, whether in bundle format or not. Levy et al.[34] reported on the >15,000 patients registered in the SSC database and found a reduction in mortality from 37% to 30.8% over 2 years with use of SSC guidelines. Two additional studies demonstrate that compliance with a 6-hour bundle is significantly associated with an up to 50% reduction in mortality.[35,37]

Despite the attractive evidence supporting a benefit of the SSC, the guidelines that were produced have had their shortcomings. The initial goals of the campaign were to reduce the mortality related to sepsis by 25% over 5 years and provide a backbone for quality improvement in the treatment of severe sepsis and septic shock. Over the 5-year course, only a 20% reduction in mortality was achieved.[38] Although commendable, this is still regarded as failure. The majority of studies report <50% compliance with all or a major portion of the guidelines. This illustrates the difficulty in producing a large global shift in management strategies. The education, implementation, mentoring, and compliance to new policies and procedures have countless obstacles, be it resources, funding, or agreement to change practice patterns. Finally, a causal relationship between the implementation of the guidelines and an establishment of the reduction in mortality must be made through firm research, likely prospective in nature.[39]

EARLY PHASE OF MANAGEMENT

Vital signs, central venous pressure, urinary output, and physical findings do not adequately assess tissue hypoxia in severe disease. Early goal-directed therapy gives specific resuscitation end points that give a more accurate picture of adequate tissue perfusion and oxygenation (Algorithm. 12.1). Resuscitation end points include not only global indicators of perfusion (i.e., heart rate, blood pressure, urine output) but also mixed venous oxygen saturation, arterial lactate concentration, based deficit, and pH.[40] Specifically, within the first 6 hours of onset of severe sepsis or septic shock, intravascular volume should be increased to achieve CVP 8-12 mm Hg and vasopressors should be initiated for MAP < 65 mm Hg, vasodilators for MAP > 90 mm Hg. If central venous oxygen saturation measured within the superior vena cava or right atria is <70%, transfusion of packed red blood cells could be considered to achieve a hematocrit of ≥ 30%, especially in cases of active cardiac ischemia. If all these parameters are met and $ScvO_2$ remains <70%, initiation of inotropic support was recommended. Identification of the source of infection and initiation of antibiotic therapy are also of utmost importance. Initiation of broad-spectrum antibiotics, preferably after multiple blood cultures have been obtained, is absolutely necessary as early as possible. Ideally, the source of infection is also identified and addressed within the first 6 hours of presentation. Use of and compliance with early goal-directed therapy produced a statistically significant increased achievement of resuscitation end points and significant reduction of in-hospital, 28-, and 60-day mortality.[40]

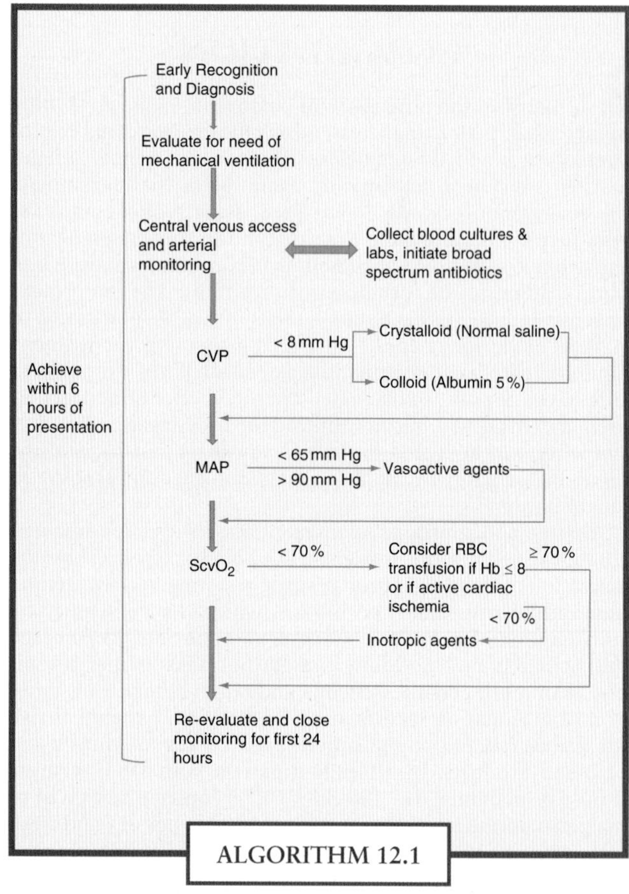

ALGORITHM 12.1 This chart represents the specific goals and indicators as an example of how to manage the septic patient upon presentation.

FLUID RESUSCITATION

There has been much debate over the use of crystalloid or colloid to expand intravascular volume in hypotensive, septic patients. Two large meta-analyses produced differing results in choice of crystalloid versus colloid. Choi et al.[41] found no difference with respect to mortality and pulmonary edema. However, subgroup analysis in trauma patients did seem to favor crystalloid over colloid. Schierhout and Roberts[42] concluded a 4% increased risk of mortality when using colloid over crystalloid for initial resuscitation. One study attempted to measure the distribution of 5% albumin versus normal saline in the treatment of critically ill patients. Ultimately, through specific scientific measurements, the change in extracellular fluid volume to include both the plasma volume (intravascular) and the interstitial volume (edema) was expanded relatively equally per given MAP.[43] Although nearly three times more normal saline was needed to achieve that of 5% albumin, the cost benefit greatly favored normal saline. The SAFE trial demonstrates equivalent outcomes of either 4% albumin or normal saline in the resuscitation of critically ill patients in the ICU.[44]

The 2008 Surviving Sepsis Campaign recommends using fluid challenges to achieve an adequate cardiac filling pressure while still affecting change in overall hemodynamics. Once hemodynamic improvement is lost, fluid administration should be slowed. Overall, there is no clear consensus whether colloid or crystalloid is superior over the other. Clinicians must use good judgement in making individual assessments based on patient needs and severity of disease.

OXYGEN DELIVERY

The state of sepsis on a systemic level is a mismatch of oxygen delivery with oxygen extraction. The combination of the two leads to an oxygen debt within tissues. Oxygen delivery can be manipulated in several ways, ultimately leaving the disorder of tissue oxygen extraction in inflammatory states as the root of organ dysfunction. As the inflammatory cascade progresses leading to vascular permeability and tissue edema, oxygen extraction only becomes more difficult. Early goal-directed therapy has a clear algorithm for increasing oxygen delivery. Initially, volume resuscitation is stressed, followed by vasoactive agents with or without blood transfusion to achieve the desired $ScvO_2$ of ≥ 70%, and finally adding inotropic agents. The Surviving Sepsis Campaign advocates either blood transfusion to Hct ≥ 30% or adding inotropic agents to achieve goal $ScvO_2$ ≥ 70%. Hébert et al.[45] demonstrated that a restrictive transfusion strategy to maintain hemoglobin concentration between 7 and 9 g per dL was associated with significantly reduced in-hospital, 30-day, and 60-day mortality compared to liberal strategy between 10 and 12 g per dL. With the exception of a subset population of patients with active ongoing cardiac ischemia, these recommendations applied to critically ill patients once euvolemia was obtained with initial resuscitation. With respect to transfusion of other human blood products, transfusion of fresh frozen plasma to correct coagulopathy should be based on circumstances in which the patient is actively bleeding or in anticipation of surgery or procedure. Platelet transfusion is indicated when counts are <5,000 per mm^3 regardless of lack of ongoing bleeding, considered when counts are between 5,000 and 30,000 per mm^3, and to achieve goal of ≥ 50,000 for invasive procedure.[32]

In conjunction with raising the oxygen content of blood via transfusion, the second component of increasing oxygen delivery is affecting cardiac output after achieving a target MAP of ≥65 mm Hg. The SSC recommends either dopamine or norepinephrine as first-line vasopressor support for septic patients with hypotension. However, dopamine is favored as the vasopressor of choice if there is no contraindication.[32] Physiologic dosage of vasopressin (0.03 U per minute) may be added as an adjunct with expectation that vasopressin will have the same effect as norepinephrine alone. In the setting of low $ScvO_2$ after adequate fluid resuscitation, MAP ≥ 65 mm Hg, and if adequate hematocrit has been achieved, the use of an inotropic agent is recommended.[40,46] There has been debate that increasing cardiac index to levels above the normal maximal average, the "supranormal" range, may have benefit by restoring hemostasis sooner and repaying the oxygen debt. Two randomized, controlled trials, however, failed to show a benefit in mortality with supranormal cardiac indices.[46,47] In fact, a study Hayes et al. was terminated prematurely due to an increase in mortality in patients achieving supranormal physiologic conditions.

SOURCE CONTROL AND ANTIBIOTICS

Admissions to the SICU with the diagnosis of sepsis often result from specific infection. In the United States, the most common sites of infection are the respiratory tract (56.8%), the bloodstream (26.9%), the renal/urinary tract (22.2%), and the abdomen (16.6%).[48] Many of these infections require surgical or invasive intervention to control the source of infection quickly. Pathologies such as necrotizing fasciitis, ascending cholangitis, closed-loop bowel obstruction, or intestinal perforation can be treated quickly and not necessarily definitively and still have a major impact on morbidity and mortality. Often, a lower physiologic insult is the more appropriate choice. SSC guidelines recommend that source control be achieved within 6 hours of admission to the hospital/ICU.[32] For example, if available, percutaneous transhepatic cholangiography with drain placement by an interventional radiologist may be more appropriate and less stressful on a patient than operative choledochotomy for the treatment of cholangitis.

Line sepsis is a not uncommon consequence of prolonged ICU stay and can often be difficult to diagnose. Lines are frequently empirically removed or exchanged over guidewire to eliminate them as the source of infection. Older methods of blood culture often did not yield an expeditious answer and would frequently take days to determine if the indwelling catheter was truly the source of infection. New developments in laboratory technology can now provide automatic detection of microbial growth in blood cultures and measure the time elapsed between bottle inoculation and time to positivity. These technologies can provide answers within hours as opposed to days. One retrospective study found that a faster time to positivity between blood drawn centrally versus peripherally could effectively determine if the septic source was the indwelling catheter or another source.[49] Special attention should be given to the patient who presents with severe diarrhea and a history of even a single dose of antibiotics, especially clindamycin or cefoxitin, with a white blood cell count > 30 × 10^9 per mL. These patients should be empirically treated for *C. diff* colitis with either oral vancomycin or combination of oral vancomycin and intravenous metronidazole.[50]

In addition to source control, the initialization of antimicrobial therapy is of utmost importance (Table 12.1). SSC guidelines recommend the start of broad-spectrum antimicrobials happen as soon as possible and within the first hour.[32] If difficulty arises in obtaining blood cultures, this should not hinder the start of appropriate antimicrobial coverage. A study by Kumar et al. demonstrated that the duration a

TABLE 12.1

ANTIMICROBIAL THERAPY IN THE TREATMENT OF SEPSIS AND SEPTIC SHOCK

SUSPECTED SOURCE	COMMUNITY ACQUIRED			HIGH RISK/HEALTH CARE ASSOCIATED		
	1ST LINE	2ND LINE	3RD LINE	1ST LINE	2ND LINE	3RD LINE
Pulmonary Abdominal Urinary	Ceftriaxone	Ampicillin/ sulbactam	Carbepenem	4th generation cephalosporin (Cefepime or Ceftazidine)	Carbepenem (Meropenem/ Imipenem)	Pipericillin/ tazobactam
	Add fluoroquinolone or macrolide if needed			Add aminoglycoside or MRSA agent if needed		
Soft tissue	Cefazolin in MRSA low concern	Vancomyin if MRSA high concern	Daptomycin	Vancomycin	Linezolid Daptomycin Tigecycline	
Immunocompromised	Consider adding empiric antifungal or antiparasitic agent			Consider adding empiric antifungal or antiparasitic agent		

De-escalation of therapy according to organism sensitivities must occur as they become available and should occur within 4–5 d.

patient spends hypotensive prior to initiating broad-spectrum, antimicrobials has a direct effect on mortality. Time is truly of the essence. In their study, starting appropriate antimicrobials within the first hour was associated with a survival rate of 79.9%; the average rate of decline in survival was 7.6% per hour; by the sixth hour, if effective antimicrobials were not initiated, mortality rate was an abysmal 58%.[51] Therefore, empiric broad-spectrum antimicrobials (potentially providing double coverage) to cover all possible organisms based on the suspected source of infection must be initiated as soon as possible.

GLUCOSE MANAGEMENT

In critical illness, diabetics and nondiabetics often experience differences in glucose management from baseline. Infection, physiologic stress, and sepsis cause hyperglycemia. In 2001, Van den Berghe et al.[52] conducted a prospective, randomized, controlled trial comparing intensive insulin therapy via continuous insulin infusion versus conventional methods. With goal blood glucose maintained between 80 and 110 mg per dL, they demonstrated a marked reduction in overall in-hospital mortality. They also found that the greatest reduction in mortality occurred within the subgroup of patients with MOF from a septic focus. In another study, hyperglycemia was associated with increased mortality independent of severity of illness.[53] Additionally, unstable angina, acute myocardial infarction, congestive heart failure, arrhythmia, ischemic and hemorrhagic stroke, GI bleeding, acute renal failure, pneumonia, and pulmonary embolism were significantly associated with hyperglycemia and adjusted mortality. Since that time, several studies have evaluated the hypoglycemic events related to an intensive insulin regimen with concerns of ill effects related to hypoglycemia.

Two recent meta-analyses concluded that there was no benefit in mortality with intensive insulin regimens versus conventional therapy.[54,55] Most notably and recently, the NICE-SUGAR study compared an intensive insulin group with target glucose of 80-110 mg per dL to a more conventional group with goal blood glucose of <180 mg per dL. That study demonstrated not only a lower mortality rate in the conventional group but also a significantly lower number of hypoglycemic events (6.8% in the intensive group vs. 0.5% in the conventional group).[56] The deleterious effects of hypoglycemia are not completely categorized and to date, no causal relationship between increased mortality and hypoglycemia has been established. The current data are retrospective in nature but do provide compelling conclusions that warrant further study. For example, one retrospective study in trauma patients found that both mild and moderate levels of hypoglycemia were associated with mortality.[57] Corneille et al. further suggest that hyperglycemia should be minimized and any hypoglycemia excursions should be avoided. Another convincing study suggests the danger of hypoglycemic events during tight glucose-control strategies in severely brain-injured patients. Oddo et al.[58] demonstrated via cerebral microdialysis that tight glucose control (80-120 mg per dL) was associated with decreased cerebral glucose availability and increased mortality.

Although subgroup analysis of one study does demonstrate a significant reduction in septicemia/bacteremia of surgical ICU patients with intensive insulin therapy,[55] further investigation must be done to determine ideal blood glucose ranges for different subsets of patient disease and possibly demographics. At this time, both the American Association of Clinical Endocrinologists and the American Diabetes Association have published consensus recommendations for target blood glucose concentrations in both critically ill and noncritically ill patients.[59] The most appropriate approach to glycemic control appears to be intravenous insulin administration to maintain a blood glucose targeted between 140 and 180 mg per dL in critically ill patients, irrespective of cause of critical illness. The one exception may be the patient with evidence of bacteremia in the surgical ICU.

CORTICOSTEROIDS

Controversy still exists over when and if to give the septic patient exogenous corticosteroids. The diagnosis of adrenal insufficiency also remains a controversial topic. Previously, the diagnosis could be made with a baseline random cortisol level <15 μg per dL or with failure of an increase of ≥9 mg per dL after ACTH stimulation. The retrospective CORTICUS study concluded that the change in cortisol level after corticotropin stimulation test was associated with improved clinical outcome. It was not, however, associated with improvement in mortality or with baseline cortisol level.[60] These findings are further supported in a study by Briegel et al.,[61] which concluded that only patients who have been adequately fluid resuscitated and continue to require high-dose vasopressors for longer than 1 hour should receive hydrocortisone.

An article that appeared in *Chest* in 2009 defined the critical illness–related corticosteroid insufficiency as a complex physiologic state of relative adrenal insufficiency given the severity of an individual's illness.[62,63] This definition further clouds the picture and makes for an absolute recommendation over the subject nearly unobtainable. Further evidence exists for a component of corticosteroid resistance, similar to insulin resistance, in an inflammatory state but will not be elaborated upon here. A recent Cochrane Review published in 2009 analyzed available prospective data and found that prolonged, low-dose corticosteroid treatment (200-300 mg hydrocortisone or equivalent per day) for severe sepsis and septic shock may have a lowering effect on all-cause mortality.[64] In contrast, the PROGRESS worldwide registry suggests that low-dose corticosteroid therapy is associated with higher mortality rates.[65] However, given the retrospective nature of the study, it is important to acknowledge that this relationship is truly an association and not a causal relationship. This study attempted to characterize the global use of steroids in the treatment of severe sepsis and septic shock. Given the most recent guidelines to treatment, one interesting finding in the study was that 14.2% of patients globally received corticosteroids without any evidence of shock.

Current recommendations for the usage of corticosteroids in critical illness are in situations of hypotension refractory to high-dose vasopressors in the volume-resuscitated patient. Dosing of hydrocortisone or equivalent should be between 200 and 300 mg per day divided over two to three doses with the optional addition of mineralocorticoid, fludrocortisone, 50 mg daily for patients with vasopressor-dependent septic shock for a period of 5 days.[32,63,64] Special attention should be given to any patient that has received etomidate, even single dose, for induction of anesthesia as this may suppress adrenal function for up to 48 hours.[66] The use of etomidate is therefore not recommended for use in critical illness.[32]

RECOMBINANT HUMAN ACTIVATED PROTEIN C

The use of recombinant human activated protein C is based on the results of two large randomized, controlled trials. The PROWESS study demonstrated a reduction of in-hospital mortality at 28 days compared to placebo, especially in high-risk groups defined as APACHE II score of ≥ 25 or sepsis with MOF.[67] This led to FDA approval of the use of recombinant activated protein C and the appearance of Xigris (Eli Lilly). The ADDRESS trial sought the benefit of recombinant human activated protein C in the low-risk population defined as APACHE II score < 25 or sepsis with single organ failure. This study determined that low-risk populations received no mortality benefit from the administration of recombinant human activated protein C. Another interesting finding in subgroup analysis within ADDRESS was that a significant number of surgical patients suffered more bleeding events during the drug infusion compared to placebo.[68] In October 2011, Xigris was withdrawn from the market and should no longer be considered for the treatment of patients with sepsis.[32]

SUPPORTIVE ICU CARE

The supportive management strategy must be tailored to the individual patient. However, there are some adjunctive treatments with benefit regardless of the condition of the patient. Stress gastric ulceration is a well-characterized consequence of critical illness that can lead to significant upper GI bleeding. Although no specific study has looked at the septic patient, it is reasonable to extrapolate data looking at general ICU populations. Current SSC guidelines recommend the use of either a proton pump inhibitor (1B evidence) or H2-blocker (1A evidence).[32] Research, however, questions the effectiveness of H2-blockers at maintaining the gastric pH high enough for a long enough duration to be effective.[69] Without respect to cost, proton pump inhibitors do appear to be a better choice for stress ulcer prophylaxis based on duration of gastric pH above goal of 3.5.

DVT prophylaxis in the critically ill patient has also been extensively studied. There is no question that critically ill patients need to be on DVT prophylaxis unless there is a specific contraindication such as ongoing bleeding or low platelet count at risk for spontaneous bleeding. In 1996, a randomized, double-blinded trial in critically ill trauma patients concluded that low molecular weight heparin was superior to unfractionated heparin in prevention of both distal and proximal DVT.[70] There is, however, a paucity of data in the critically ill surgical patient to effectively recommend one treatment strategy. Although, based on available literature, low-dose–molecular-weight heparin, either 40 mg per day or 30 mg twice daily, would appear to be the best option for the critically ill patient at high risk for DVT or VTE.

The nutritional supplementation of the septic patient is of utmost importance. Since the disease state is characterized by an increase in energy expenditure and catabolism, the septic patient absolutely needs nutritional support. Early nutritional support improves wound healing and immune function and has been shown to prevent intestinal mucosal breakdown. Parenteral nutrition carries with it an increased risk of line infection and may predispose to concurrent fungal infection. Thus, enteral nutrition is preferred even in the setting of decreased enteric motility associated with sepsis. Not only has research demonstrated that enteral nutrition is safe and effective in sepsis,[71] but the addition of glutamine to the enteral diet may have positive effects on host immune response.[72] In general, the septic patient should receive enteral nutrition as early as possible unless contraindicated by major GI hemorrhage, bowel obstruction, or uncorrected hemodynamic instability.[73]

The decision to initiate mechanical ventilation on a patient can be a complex issue. Frequently, however, the effect of MOF associated with septic shock requires mechanical ventilation to improve oxygenation. The reduction in oxygen saturation, increased work of breathing, increased respiratory rate, reduction of PaO_2, or any two in combination are sufficient justification to initiate mechanical ventilation. When choosing a ventilation strategy, there is clear evidence produced by the ARDSNet trial supporting lower tidal volume ventilation.[74] Current recommendations from the ARDSNet trial and supported by the most recent SSC guidelines include tidal volume of ≥6-8 mL per kg as long as plateau pressure can be maintained ≤ 30 cm H_2O.[32,74] SSC goes on to suggest that permissive hypercapnia (allowing $PaCO_2$ to rise above premorbid baseline) be allowed in ALI/ARDS if the strategy minimizes plateau pressures to acceptable levels while maintaining adequate oxygenation.[32]

When addressing the need for renal replacement therapy, guidelines are mixed as to whether continuous or intermittent therapy is more efficacious. Renal replacement needs arise when a patient becomes uremic, hyperkalemic, or acidotic, or reaches toxic drug levels. Volume overload is categorized as a relative indication. Professional opinion typically leans toward continuous renal replacement as a gentler means of both fluid management and control of blood ions and toxins. However, within the literature, there is no clear advantage of intermittent dialysis versus continuous renal replacement. As far as administration of exogenous bicarbonate is concerned, current guidelines recommend only administering exogenous bicarbonate solution to a goal of pH of ≥7.15.[32] The best course of action is to work closely with a nephrologist in an interdisciplinary approach to meet the individual patient's needs.

ABDOMINAL SEPSIS FOR THE ACUTE CARE SURGEONS: KEY CONCEPTS

Abdominal sepsis is defined when sepsis or septic shock are secondary to intra-abdominal infection (IAI). Mortality of abdominal sepsis varies from 25% to 70%.[75-79]

The basic principles in the management of abdominal sepsis include early diagnosis, immediate and adequate drainage or removal of the source of infection, which can be accomplished by formal operative intervention (laparotomy with or without laparostomy) or less invasive techniques such as percutaneous drainage, appropriate antimicrobial therapy, and supportive critical care measures to prevent or immediately treat organ dysfunction.[80]

According to the International Sepsis Forum Consensus Conference, an IAI is an infection of any intra-abdominal organ with or without peritoneal involvement (peritonitis).[81,82] A complicated IAI implies diffuse peritoneal involvement (peritonitis) usually due to a perforated viscus. Only rarely, these cases may present as a contained abscess or minimal peritonitis.[83] Peritonitis is a complex disease process and has been traditionally divided into primary, secondary, and tertiary depending on its cause and extent. In general, the clinical course of peritonitis depends on the microbiology, the anatomical location, the degree of localization, and the presence of correctable anatomical derangements involving abdominal viscera.[81]

Primary peritonitis, also known as primary peritoneal infection or spontaneous bacterial peritonitis, is characterized by the absence of an identifiable anatomical derangement in the intra-abdominal viscera. The source of infection cannot be attributed to a gastrointestinal problem.

Secondary peritonitis, also known as secondary peritoneal infection, occurs in the presence of a clearly defined anatomical derangement of an intra-abdominal organ such as perforated viscus. The most common organisms are part of the indigenous flora of the gastrointestinal tract. Gastroduodenal perforations may be accompanied by *Candida* infections. Polymicrobial isolates remain the hallmark of IAIs.[84] Escherichia coli is the most common aerobe isolate, whereas *Bacteroides* is the most common anaerobe.[85-87] Enterococci are more commonly isolated in high-risk patients who failed antimicrobial treatment for IAI. When enterococci are isolated, *Enterococcus faecalis* and *Enterococcus faecium* account for 90% and 10% of episodes, respectively.[88-91]

Other enteric gram-negative bacteria such as *Pseudomonas aeruginosa* and *Acinetobacter* species have become an important problem more recently because of the increasing resistance to many antimicrobials. They occur more commonly in high-risk, debilitated individuals, in those who have received antimicrobials previously, in postoperative patients, and in those receiving immunosuppressant therapy.[86] *Staphylococcus aureus* is also a potential pathogen with inherent antibiotic resistance issues.[92] Table 12.2 presents the most common bacteria found in the biliary and GI tract.

In secondary peritonitis, antimicrobial therapy against gram-negative enteric pathogens and gram-positive and gram-negative anaerobic bacteria is indicated. Enterococci, yeast, or fungi are not routinely treated, unless the patient has developed IAI after prior operation or is considered high risk for infection caused by one of these pathogens.[93]

TABLE 12.2

COMMON BACTERIA FOUND IN DIFFERENT INTRA-ABDOMINAL ORGANS

INTRA-ABDOMINAL ORGAN	COMMON BACTERIA
Stomach	Streptococci *Lactobacillus* spp.
Bilary tract	*E. coli* *Klebsiella* spp. Enterococci
Proximal small bowel	*E. coli* *Lactobacillus* spp. Streptococci Diphtheroids Enterococci
Distal small bowel	*Bacteroides fragilis* *Clostridium* spp. *E. coli* *Enterobacter* spp. *Klebsiella* spp. Peptostreptococci Enterococci
Large bowel	*Bacteroides* spp. *Clostridium* spp. *E. coli* *Enterobacter* spp. *Klebsiella* spp. Peptostreptococci Enterococci

The antimicrobial options, currently used in IAIs and secondary peritonitis can be found in two recent publications.[86,94] The duration of treatment is dependent on the type of infection, the immunologic status of the host, and the response to the initial treatment. In general, a course of 7-10 days of antimicrobial therapy is adequate for the treatment of patients with a normal immune system who have localized peritonitis or an intra-abdominal abscess. Patients with generalized peritonitis usually receive a longer course (10-14 days) of antimicrobial therapy. Treatment with antibiotics should continue until the infection has subsided. Culture results are important to adjust antimicrobial therapy and to detect resistance to treatment, a common cause of treatment failure and increased mortality.

Tertiary peritonitis can be defined as peritonitis that persists or recurs 48 hours following apparently successful management of primary or secondary bacterial peritonitis (source control procedure). Cultures usually show growth of nosocomial flora including coagulase-negative staphylococci, *Candida*, *Enterococci*, *Pseudomonas*, and Enterobacter.[79,93,95] The management of tertiary peritonitis is challenging due to the increased likelihood of infection with multidrug-resistant organisms.

SOURCE CONTROL

Source control is a critical element in the management of IAI and sepsis.

It is defined as "all physical measures undertaken to eliminate a source of infection, to control ongoing contamination, and to restore premorbid anatomy and function."[96] Management success is determined by the elimination of the source and control of ongoing contamination. Restoration of anatomy and function may be performed in a delayed fashion to avoid prolongation of the initial surgical intervention in patients already physiologically and metabolically challenged (damage control strategy). Source control includes four basic principles of care: drainage, debridement plus device removal, decompression, and restoration of anatomy and function. Surgical or less invasive techniques such as image-guided percutaneous drainage of abscess may be used.

Patients with diffuse peritonitis are advised to undergo an emergency surgical procedure as soon as possible, even if ongoing measures to restore physiologic stability need to be continued during the procedure; for hemodynamically stable patients without evidence of acute organ failure, an urgent approach should be taken, intervention may be delayed for as long as 24 hours if appropriate antimicrobial therapy is given, and careful clinical monitoring is provided. Source control measures should be implemented as soon as possible following successful initial resuscitation.

Delay in diagnosis and prompt resuscitation of the patient with abdominal sepsis usually leads to delays in source control. The overuse of diagnostic tests, particularly imaging, as well as extensive evaluation in the emergency department, without focusing on quick resuscitation, correction of coagulation and electrolyte disturbances, early antibiotic administration, and early intervention has a negative impact on outcome.[93,97]

Preoperative optimization of the septic patient with a severe IAI should happen quickly, last no more than 2-3 hours, and it should not delay operative intervention.

References

1. Martin GS, Mannino DM, Eaton S, et al. The epidemiology of sepsis in the United States from 1979-2000. *N Engl J Med.* 2003;348:1546-1554.
2. Levy MM, Fink MP, Marshall JC. 2001 SCCM/ESICM/ACCP/ATS/SIS International Sepsis Definitions Conference. *Crit Care Med.* 2003;31:1250-1256.
3. Heron M, Hoyert DL, Murphy SL, et al. Deaths: Final data for 2006. National vital statistics report. Volume 57, No. 14. National Center for Health Statistics, 2009.
4. Rittirsch D, Hoesel LM, Ward PA. The disconnect between animal models of sepsis and human sepsis. *J Leukoc Biol.* 2007;81:137-43.
5. Abraham E. Alterations in cell signaling in sepsis. *Clin Infect Dis.* 2005;41:S459-S464.
6. Bone RC. Gram positive organisms and sepsis. *Arch Int Med.* 1994;154:26-34.
7. Cinel I, Opal SM. Molecular biology of inflammation and sepsis: A primer. *Crit Care Med.* 2009;37:291-304.
8. Rittirsch D, Flierl MA, Ward PA. Harmful molecular mechanisms in sepsis. *Nat Rev Immunol.* 2008;8:776-787.
9. Williams DL, Ha T, Li C, et al. Modulation of tissue toll-like receptor 2 and 4 during the early phases of polymicrobial sepsis correlates with mortality. *Crit Care Med.* 2003;31:1808-1818.
10. Ozinsky A, Underhill DM, Fontenot JD, et al. The repertoire for pattern recognition of pathogens by the innate immune system is defined by cooperation between Toll-like receptors. *PNAS.* 2000;97:13766-13771.
11. Salamao R, Martins PS, Brunialti KC, et al. TLR signaling in patients with sepsis. *Shock,* 2008;30:73-76.
12. Poltorak A, He X, Smirnova I, et al. Defective LPS signaling in C3H/HeJ and C57BL/10ScCr mice: mutations in Tlr4 gene. *Science.* 1998;282:2085-2088.
13. Qureshi ST, Larivière L, Leveque G, et al. Endotoxin-tolerant mice have mutations in Toll-like receptor 4. *J Exp Med.* 1999;189:615-625.
14. Tracey KJ, Fong Y, Hesse DG, et al. Anti-cachectin/TNF monoclonal antibodies prevent septic shock during lethal bacteremia. *Nature.* 1987;330:662-664.
15. Goldfarb RD, Parrillo JE. Complement. *Crit Care Med.* 2005;33:S482-S484.
16. Schouten M, Wiersinga WJ, Levi M, et al. Inflammation, endothelium, and coagulation in sepsis. *J Leukol Biol,* 2008;83:536-545.
17. de Jonge E, Dekkers PE, Creasey AA, et al. Tissue factor pathway inhibitor dose-dependently inhibits coagulation activation without influencing the fibrinolytic and cytokine response during human endotoxemia. *Blood.* 2000;95:1124-1129.
18. Zeerleder S, Hack CE, Wuillemin WA. Disseminated intravascular coagulation in sepsis. *Chest.* 2005;128:2864-2875.
19. Lieberman HA and Weitz IC. Disseminated intravascular coagulation. In: Hoffman R, Benz EJ, Shattil SJ, et al., eds. *Hematology: Basic Principles and Practice.* Philadelphia, PA: Elsevier; 2009, 1999-2009.
20. Marshall JC, Sweeney D. Microbial infection and the septic response in critical surgical illness: Sepsis, not infection, determines outcome. *Arch Surg.* 1990;125:17-23.
21. Barie PS, Hydo LJ. Epidemiology of multiple organ dysfunction syndrome in critical surgical illness. *Surg Infect.* 2000;1:173-183.
22. Sands KE, Bates DW, Lanken PN, et al. Epidemiology of sepsis syndrome in 8 academic medical centers. *JAMA.* 1997;278:234-224.
23. Marshall JC, Reinhart K, et al. Biomarkers of sepsis. *Crit Care Med.* 2009;37:2290-2298.
24. Vigushin DM, Pepys MB, Hawkins PM. Metabolic and scintigraphic studies studies of radioiodinated human C-reactive protein in health and disease. *J Clin Invest.* 1993;91:1351-1357.
25. Lobo SM, Lobo FR, Bota DP, et al. C-reactive protein levels correlate with mortality and organ failure in critically ill patients. *Chest.* 2003;123:2043-2049.
26. Schmidt X, Vincent JL. The time course of blood C-reactive protein levels in relation to the response to initial antimicrobial therapy in patients with sepsis. *Infection.* 2008;36:213-219.
27. Becker KL, Snider R, Nylen ES. Procalcitonin assay in systemic inflammation, infection, and sepsis: Clinical utility and limitations. *Crit Care Med.* 2008;36:941-952.
28. Assicot M, Gendrel D, Carsin H, et al. High serum procalcitonin concentrations in patients with sepsis and infection. *Lancet.* 1993;341:515-518.
29. Uzzan B, Cohen R, Nicolas P, et al. Procalcitonin as a diagnostic test for sepsis in adults after surgery or trauma: a systematic review and meta-analysis. *Crit Care Med.* 2006;34:1996-2003.
30. Dandona P, Nix, P, Wilson MF, et al. Procalcitonin increases after endotoxin injection in normal subjects. *J Clin Endocrinol Metab.* 1994;79:1705-1708.
31. Charles PE, Tinel C, Barbar S, et al. Procalcitonin kinetics within the first days of sepsis: relationship with the appropriateness of antibiotic therapy and the outcome. *Crit Care.* 2009;13:R38.
32. Dellinger RP, et al. Surviving Sepsis Campaign: international guidelines for management of severe sepsis and septic shock: 2008. *Crit Care Med.* 2008;36:296-327.
33. Levy MM, Pronovost PJ, Dellinger RP, et al. Sepsis change bundles: Converting guidelines into meaningful change in behavior and clinical outcome. *Crit Care Med.* 2004;32:S595-S597.
34. Levy MM, Dellinger RP, Townsend SR, et al. The surviving sepsis campaign: Results of an international guideline-based performance improvement program targeting severe sepsis. *Crit Care Med.* 2010;38:367-374.
35. Gao F, Melody T, Daniels DF, et al. The impact of compliance with 6-hour and 24-hour sepsis bundles on hospital mortality in patients with severe sepsis: a prospective observational study. *Crit Care.* 2005;9:R764-R770.
36. Ferrer R, Artigas A, Suarez, D, et al. Effectiveness of treatments for severe sepsis: A prospective, multicenter, observational study. *Am J Respir Crit Care Med.* 2009;180;861-866.
37. Castellanos-Ortega A, Suberviola B, Garcia-Astudillo LA, et al. Impact of the surviving sepsis campaign protocols on hospital length of stay and mortality in septic shock patients: results of a three-year follow-up quasi-experimental study. *Crit Care Med.* 2010;38:1036-1043.
38. Marshall JC, Dellinger RP, Levy M. The surviving sepsis campaign: a history and perspective. *Surg Infect.* 2010;11(3):275-281.
39. Finfer S. The surviving sepsis campaign: Robust evaluation and high-quality research is still needed. *Crit Care Med.* 2010;28(2):367-374.
40. Rivers E, et al. Early goal-directed therapy in the treatment of severe sepsis and septic shock. *N Engl J Med.* 2001;345:1368-1377.
41. Choi PT, et al. Crystalloids vs. colloids in fluid resuscitation: a systematic review. *Crit Care Med.* 1999;27:200-210.
42. Schierhout G, Roberts, I. Fluid resuscitation with colloid or crystalloid solutions in critically ill patients: a systematic review of randomised trials. *BMJ.* 1998;316:961-964.
43. Ernest D, Belzberg AS, Dodek PM. Distribution of normal saline and 5% albumin infusions in septic patients. *Crit Care Med.* 1999;27:46-50.
44. Finfer S, et al. A comparison of albumin and saline for fluid resuscitation in the intensive care unit. *N Engl J Med.* 2004;350:2247-2256.
45. Hébert PC, et al. A multicenter, randomized, controlled clinical trial of transfusion requirements in critical care. Transfusion Requirements in Critical Care Investigators, Canadian Critical Care Trials Group. *N Engl J Med.* 1999;340:409-417.
46. Hayes MA, et al. Elevation of systemic oxygen delivery in the treatment of critically ill patients. *N Engl J Med,* 1994;330:1717-1722.
47. Gattinoni L, et al. A trial of goal-oriented hemodynamic therapy in critically ill patients. SvO2 Collaborative Group. *N Engl J Med.* 1995;333:1025-1032.
48. Vincent JL, et al. International study of the prevalence and outcomes of infection in intensive care units. *JAMA.* 2009;302:2323-2329.
49. Blot F, et al. Earlier positivity of central-venous- versus peripheral-blood cultures is highly predictive of catheter-related sepsis. *J Clin Microbiol.* 1998;36:105-109.
50. Leclair MA, et al. Clostridium difficile infection in the intensive care unit. *J Intensive Care Med.* 2010;25:23-30.
51. Kumar A, et al. Duration of hypotension before initiation of effective antimicrobial therapy is the critical determinant of survival in human septic shock. *Crit Care Med.* 2006;34:1589-1596.

52. van den Berghe G, et al. Intensive insulin therapy in the critically ill patients. *N Engl J Med.* 2001;345:1359-1367.
53. Falciglia M, Freyberg RW, Almenoff PL. Hyperglycemia-related mortality in critically ill patients varies with admission diagnosis. *Crit Care Med.* 2009;37:3001-3009.
54. Preiser JC, Devos P. Clinical experience with tight glucose control by intensive insulin therapy. *Crit Care Med.* 2007;35(suppl):S503-S507.
55. Wiener RS, Wiener DC, Larson RJ. Benefits and risks of tight glucose control in critically ill adults: a meta-analysis. *JAMA.* 2008;300:933-944.
56. Finfer S, et al. Intensive versus conventional glucose control in critically ill patients. *N Engl J Med.* 2009;360:1283-1297.
57. Corneille MG, Villa C, Wolf S, et al. Time and degree of glycemic derangement are associated with increased mortality in trauma patients in the setting of tight glycemic control. *Am J Surg.* 2010;200:832-838.
58. Oddo M, Schmidt JM, Carrera E, et al. Impact of tight glycemic control on cerebral glucose metabolism after severe brain injury: A microdialysis study. *Crit Care Med.* 2008;36:3233-3238.
59. Moghissi ES. Reexamining the evidence for inpatient glucose control: New recommendations for glycemic targets. *Am J Health Syst Pharm.* 2010;67:S3-S8.
60. Lipiner-Friedman D, et al. Adrenal function in sepsis: the retrospective Corticus cohort study. *Crit Care Med.* 2007;35(4):1012-1018.
61. Briegel J, Kilger E, Schelling G. Indications and practical use of replacement dose of corticosteroids in critical illness. *Curr Opin Crit Care.* 2007;13:370-375.
62. Marik PE, et al. Recommendations for the diagnosis and management of corticosteroid insufficiency in critically ill adult patients: consensus statements from an international task force by the American College of Critical Care Medicine. *Crit Care Med.* 2008;36:1937-1949.
63. Marik PE. Critical illness-related corticosteroid insufficiency. *Chest.* 2009;135:181-193.
64. Annane D, Bellissant E, Bollaert PE, et al. Corticosteroids in the treatment of severe sepsis and septic shock in adults. *JAMA.* 2009;301(22):2362-2375.
65. Beale R, Janes JM, Brunkhorst FM, et al. Global utilization of low-dose corticosteroids in severe sepsis and septic shock: a report from the PROGRESS registry. *Crit Care.* 2010;14:R102.
66. Vinclair M, et al. Duration of adrenal inhibition following a single dose of etomidate in critically ill patients. *Intensive Care Med.* 2008;34:714-719.
67. Bernard GR, et al. Efficacy and safety of recombinant human activated protein C for severe sepsis. *N Engl J Med.* 2001;344:699-709.
68. Abraham E, et al. Drotrecogin alfa (activated) for adults with severe sepsis and a low risk of death. *N Engl J Med.* 2005;353:1332-1341.
69. Terzi Coelho CB, et al.,Ranitidine is unable to maintain gastric pH levels above 4 in septic patients. *J Crit Care.* 2009;24:627.e7-627.e13.
70. Geerts WH, et al. A comparison of low-dose heparin with low-molecular-weight heparin as prophylaxis against venous thromboembolism after major trauma. *N Engl J Med.* 1996;335:701-707.
71. Moore FA, Moore EE. The evolving rationale for early enteral nutrition based on paradigms of multiple organ failure: a personal journey. *Nutr Clin Pract.* 2009;24:297-304.
72. McQuiggan M, et al. Enteral glutamine during active shock resuscitation is safe and enhances tolerance of enteral feeding. *J Parenter Enteral Nutr.* 2008;32:28-35.
73. Morrell MR, Micek ST, Kollef MH. The management of severe sepsis and septic shock. *Infect Dis Clin North Am.* 2009;23:485-501.
74. ARDS Network. Ventilation with lower tidal volumes as compared with traditional tidal volumes for acute lung injury and the acute respiratory distress syndrome. *N Engl J Med.* 2000;342:1301-1308.
75. Barie PS, Vogel SB, Dellinger EP, et al. A randomized, doubleblind clinical trial comparing cefepime plus metronidazole with imipenem-cilastatin in the treatment of complicated intra-abdominal infections. Cefepime Intra-abdominal Infection Study Group. *Arch Surg.* 1997;132:1294-1302.
76. De Waele J, Blot S. Critical Issues in the Clinical Management of Complicated Intra-Abdominal Infections. *Drugs.* 2005;65:1611-1620.
77. Farthmann EH, Schoffel U. Principles and limitations of operative management of intraabdominal infections. *World J Surg.* 1990;14:210-217.
78. Garcia-Sabrido Jl, Tallado JM, Christou NV, et al. Treatment of severe intra-abdominal sepsis and/or necrotic foci by an 'open-abdomen' approach. Zipper and zipper-mesh techniques. *Arch Surg.* 1988;123:152-156.
79. Pieracci FM, Barie FS. Management of severe sepsis of abdominal origin. *Scand J Surg.* 2007;96:184-196.
80. Marshall JC, Maier RV, Jimenez M, et al. Source control in the management of severe sepsis and septic shock: an evidence-based review. *Crit Care Med.* 2004;32:S513-S526.
81. Calandra T, Cohen J. The international sepsis forum consensus conference on definitions of infection in the intensive care unit. *Crit Care Med.* 2005;33:1538-1548.
82. Solomkin JS, Hemsell DL, Sweet R, et al. Evaluation of new anti-infective drugs for the treatment of intraabdominal infections. Infectious Diseases Society of America and the food and Drug Administration. *Clin Infect Dis.* 1992;15(suppl 1): S33-S42.
83. Nathens AB, Rotstein OD, Marshall JC. Tertiary peritonitis: clinical features of a complex nosocomial infection. *World J Surg.* 1998;22:158-163.
84. Weigelt J. Empiric treatment options in the management of complicated intra-abdominal infections. *Cleve Clin J Med.* 2007;74(suppl 4):S29-S37.
85. Marshall JC. Intra-abdominal infections. *Microbes Infect.* 2004;6:1015-1025.
86. Mazuski JE, Sawyer RG, Nathens AB, et al. The Surgical Infection Society guidelines on antimicrobial therapy for intra-abdominal infections: Evidence for the recommendations. *Surg Infect.* 2002;3:175-233.
87. Solomkin JS, Mazuski JE, Baron EJ, et al. Guidelines for the selection of anti-infective agents for complicated intra-abdominal infections. *Clin Infect Dis.* 2003;37:997-1005.
88. Burnett RJ, Haverstock DC, Dellinger EP, et al. Definition of the role of enterococcus in intraabdominal infection: analysis of a prospective randomized trial. *Surgery.* 1995;118:716-723.
89. de Vera ME, Simmons RL. Antibiotic-resistant enterococci and the changing face of surgical infections. *Arch Surg.* 1996;131:338-342.
90. Dougherty SH. Role of enterococcus in intraabdominal sepsis. *Am J Surg.* 1984;148:308-312.
91. Hopkins JA, Lee JCH, Wilson SE. Susceptibility of intra-abdominal isolates at operation: a predictor of postoperative infection. *Am Surg.* 1993;59:791-796.
92. Smith TL, Pearson ML, Wilcox KR, et al. Emergence of vancomycin resistance in *Staphylococcus aureus*. *N Engl J Med.* 1999;340:493-501.
93. Malangoni MA. Contributions to the management of intra-abdominal infections. *Am J Surg.* 2005;190:255-259.
94. Solomkin JS, Mazuski JE, Bradley JS, et al. Diagnosis and management of complicated intra-abdominal infection in adults and children: guidelines by the surgical infection society and the infectious diseases society of America. *Clin Infect Dis.* 2010;50:133-164.
95. Malangoni MA. Evaluation and management of tertiary peritonitis. *Am Surg.* 2000;66:157-161.
96. Schein M, Marshall J. *Source Control: A Guide to the Management of Surgical Infections.* Berlin, Germany: Springer-Verlag; 2002.
97. De Waele JJ. Early source control in sepsis. *Langenbecks Arch Surg.* 2010;395:489-494.

CHAPTER 13 ■ ANTIBIOTIC USE AND MISUSE

PHILIP S. BARIE AND VANESSA P. HO

Traditionally, surgeons were only involved with infections that required invasive measures for treatment (e.g., complicated intra-abdominal infections and skin/soft tissue infections [cSSTIs]). However, surgical patients are particularly vulnerable to nosocomial infections; therefore, the acute care surgeon must be concerned with the prevention and treatment of all infections that affect surgical patients, including surgical site infections (SSIs), central line–associated bloodstream infections (CLABSIs), urinary tract infections (UTIs), and hospital- or ventilator-associated pneumonia (HAP/VAP). Trauma patients are particularly vulnerable to infections of injured tissue as well as nosocomial infections related to environmental factors (e.g., hypothermia), host immunosuppression (e.g., inadequate glycemic control), and therapeutic interventions (e.g., multiple incisions and catheters, blood transfusion).[1,2] The overall incidence of infection following trauma is estimated to be 25%[3–6]; trauma patients may be twice as likely to become infected as critically ill general surgery patients.[7] These disease states are discussed elsewhere in this volume; this chapter discusses the use and misuse of antibiotics for prophylaxis and therapy.

Considering that the development of a postoperative infection has a negative impact on surgical outcomes, recognizing and minimizing risk and an aggressive approach to the diagnosis and treatment of such infections go hand in hand. Infection is preventable to some degree, and every acute care surgeon must do his or her utmost to prevent infection. An ensemble of tactics is required, because no single method, including antibiotic prophylaxis, is universally effective. Infection control is paramount. It must always be remembered that surgical illness and injury are immunosuppressive, as are many critical care therapeutics. Surgical incisions and traumatic wounds must be handled gently, inspected daily, and dressed if necessary using strict asepsis. Drains and catheters must be avoided if possible and removed as soon as practicable. Prophylactic and therapeutic antibiotics, whether empiric or directed against a known infection, must be used optimally so as to minimize antibiotic selection pressure on the development of multidrug-resistant (MDR) pathogens.

INFECTION CONTROL

General principles of surgical care, critical care, and infection control must be adhered to at all times. As but a few examples, resuscitation must be rapid, yet precise; both over- and under-resuscitation increase the risk of infection. Pathology must be identified and treated as soon as possible. Central venous catheters inserted under suboptimal barrier precautions (i.e., lack of cap, mask, sterile gown, and sterile gloves for the operator and a full-bed drape for the patient) must be removed and replaced (if necessary) by a new puncture at a new site as soon as the patient's condition permits. Drains should be avoided and removed as soon as possible if required.[8] Detailed evidence-based guidelines for the general prevention of SSI,[9] CLABSI,[10,11] and VAP have been published.[12,13] Hand hygiene is the most effective means to reduce the spread of infection, yet compliance is a continual challenge.[14]

Endogenous flora are the source of most human pathogens. Skin surfaces, artificial airways, gut lumen, wounds, catheters, and inanimate surfaces (e.g., bed rails, computer terminals) may become colonized.[15] Any break in natural epithelial barriers (e.g., incisions, percutaneous catheters, airway or urinary catheters) creates a portal of entry for invasion of pathogens. The fecal–oral route is the most common manner by which pathogens reach the portal, but health care workers facilitate the transmission of pathogens on their hands.[15] In this context, antibiotics should be considered an essential component, but not a panacea, and certainly not as a substitute for best practices in all aspects of patient care.

Unfortunately, selection pressure from long-term overuse of antibiotics is a major factor in the emergence of MDR pathogens such as methicillin-resistant *Staphylococcus aureus* (MRSA), vancomycin-resistant enterococci (VRE), and gram-negative bacilli (e.g., *Klebsiella* spp., *Acinetobacter* spp., *Stenotrophomonas* spp., *and Pseudomonas aeruginosa*)[16–19] (Table 13.1) that have developed numerous mechanisms to express resistance to antibiotics. Fortunately, adherence to optimal prescribing practices, sometimes known as *antimicrobial stewardship*,[20] can improve the microbial ecology of the facility or unit and preserve the efficacy of the few extant antibiotics for MDR pathogens. Reduction of usage of antibiotics that exert substantial selection pressure (e.g., vancomycin, fluoroquinolones, third-generation cephalosporins) can be used to manage outbreaks and restore susceptibility.[19,21–24]

PHARMACOKINETICS AND PHARMACODYNAMICS

Pharmacokinetics (PK) describes the principles of drug absorption, distribution, and metabolism.[25] Dose–response relationships are influenced by dose, dosing interval, and route of administration. Plasma and tissue drug concentrations are influenced by absorption, distribution, and elimination, which in turn depend on drug metabolism and excretion. Serum drug concentrations may or may not correlate, depending on tissue penetration, but to the extent that they do, relationships between local drug concentration and effect are described by pharmacodynamic (PD) principles (see below).[25]

Bioavailability describes the percentage of drug dose that reaches the systemic circulation. Bioavailability is 100% after intravenous administration, but after oral administration is affected by absorption, intestinal transit time, and hepatic metabolism, if any. *Half-life* ($T_{1/2}$), the time required for the serum drug concentration to reduce by one-half, reflects both *clearance* and *volume of distribution* (V_D).[25] The V_D is independent of a drug's clearance or $T_{1/2}$ and is used to estimate the plasma drug concentration achievable from a given dose. Volume of distribution varies substantially due to pathophysiology; reduced V_D may cause a higher plasma drug concentration for a given dose, whereas fluid overload and hypoalbuminemia (which decrease drug binding) increase V_D, making dosing more complex. For example, dosing of hydrophilic drugs such as beta-lactams may need to be increased in the early phases of sepsis owing to the expansion of the extracellular space due to fluid resuscitation and alterations in microvascular permeability.[26]

TABLE 13.1

CAUSES AND CONSEQUENCES OF BACTERIAL RESISTANCE AS RELATED TO ANTIBIOTIC SELECTION PRESSURE

INITIAL THERAPEUTIC AGENT	EMERGENT RESISTANT BACTERIA	TREATMENT OF RESISTANT BACTERIA
Fluoroquinolones	MRSA	Vancomycin, others (Table 13.18)
	MDR gram-negative bacilli	Carbapenem or polymyxin or tigecycline (not for *Pseudomonas*)
	C. difficile infection	Vancomycin or metronidazole or fidaxomicin
Vancomycin	VRE	Tigecycline, linezolid, daptomycin
	VISA	Ceftaroline, tigecycline, linezolid, daptomycin
Cephalosporins	VRE	Tigecycline, linezolid, daptomycin
	MDR gram-negative bacilli	Carbapenem or polymyxin or tigecycline (not for *Pseudomonas*)
	C. difficile infection	Vancomycin or metronidazole or fidaxomicin
Carbapenems	MDR gram-negative bacilli	Carbapenem or polymyxin or tigecycline (not for *Pseudomonas*)
	S. maltophilia	Trimethoprim/sulfamethoxazole
	C. difficile infection	Vancomycin or metronidazole or fidaxomicin

MDR, multidrug resistant; MDR gram-negative bacilli include producers of extended-spectrum beta-lactamases, metallo-beta-lactamases, and carbapenemases; MRSA, methicillin-resistant *Staphylococcus aureus*; VISA, vancomycin-intermediate *Staphylococcus aureus*; VRE, vancomycin-resistant *Enterococcus*.

Clearance refers to the volume of fluid from which drug is eliminated completely per unit of time, regardless of the mode of elimination (e.g., metabolism, excretion, or dialysis); knowledge of drug clearance is important to determine the dose of drug necessary to maintain a steady-state concentration. Most drugs are metabolized by the liver to polar compounds for eventual renal excretion, which may occur by filtration or either active or passive transport. The degree of filtration is determined by molecular size and charge and by the number of functional nephrons. In general, if ≥40% of active drug (including active metabolites) is eliminated unchanged in the urine, a dosage adjustment is required if renal function is decreased.

PDs are unique for antibiotic therapy, because drug–patient, drug–microbe, and microbe–patient interactions must be accounted for.[25] The key drug interaction is with the microbe rather than the host. Microbial physiology, inoculum characteristics (i.e., size, quorum sensing, presence of a device-related biofilm),[27,28] microbial growth phase, mechanisms of resistance, the microenvironment (e.g., local pH), and the host's response are important factors to consider. Because of microbial resistance, mere administration of the "correct" drug may not be microbicidal if an adequate dose/concentration is not achieved.[29,30] *In vitro* results may be irrelevant if bacteria are inhibited only by drug concentrations that cannot be achieved clinically.

Antibiotic PD parameters determined by laboratory analysis include *the minimal inhibitory concentration* (MIC), the lowest serum drug concentration that inhibits bacterial growth (MIC_{90} refers to 90% inhibition) (Fig. 13.1). However, some antibiotics may suppress bacterial growth at subinhibitory concentrations (*postantibiotic effect*, PAE).[26,31] Appreciable PAE can be observed with aminoglycosides and fluoroquinolones for gram-negative bacteria, and with some β-lactam drugs (notably carbapenems) against *S. aureus*. However, MIC testing may not detect resistant bacterial subpopulations within the inoculum (e.g., "heteroresistance" of *S. aureus*),[32] which may be selected for by therapy, overgrow in the ecologic vacuum caused by treatment, and cause clinical failure.

Sophisticated analytic strategies utilize both PK and PD, for example, by determination of the peak serum concentration: MIC ratio, the duration of time that plasma concentration remains above the MIC (fT>MIC), and the area of the plasma concentration-time curve above the MIC (the *area under the curve* or AUC). Accordingly, aminoglycosides exhibit concentration-dependent killing,[31,33] whereas beta-lactam agents exhibit efficacy determined by time above the MIC.[34] For beta-lactam antibiotics with short $T_{1/2}$, it may be efficacious to administer by continuous infusion,[25,35,36] although prolonged intermittent infusion may accomplish the same while freeing up vascular access for other medications

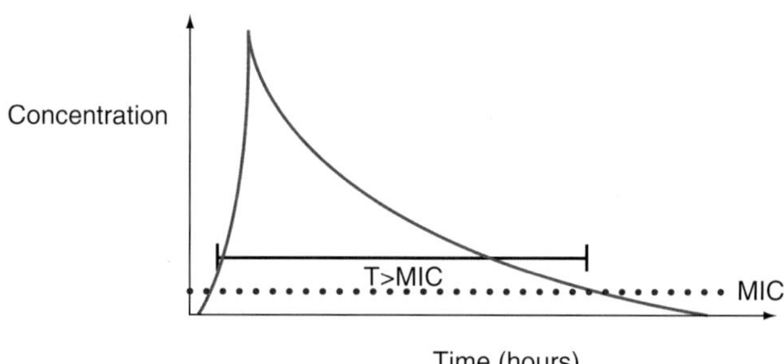

FIGURE 13.1. A stylized elimination curve is shown for a single bolus dose of a parenteral antibiotic. Some drugs (e.g., aminoglycosides) exhibit concentration-dependent bactericidal activity; a peak concentration/minimum inhibitory concentration (MIC) ratio >10 is optimal for bacterial killing. Beta-lactam agents exhibit time-dependent bactericidal activity; the proportion (fT) of time above the MIC should be at least 40% for optimal killing. Efficacy of still other drugs (e.g., vancomycin, fluoroquinolones) is reflected by the AUC, a method of measurement of the bioavailability of a drug based on a plot of blood concentrations sampled at frequent intervals. The AUC is directly proportional to the total amount of unaltered drug in the patient's blood. A ratio of AUC: MIC > 400 is associated with optimal antibacterial effect and minimization of the development of resistance.

for a period of time each dosing interval. Some agents (e.g., fluoroquinolones, vancomycin) exhibit both properties; bacterial killing increases as drug concentration increases up to a saturation point, after which the effect becomes concentration-independent. An $AUC:MIC_{24h} > 125$ is associated with optimal effect and reduced risk of developing resistance, whereas some authors recommend an $AUC:MIC_{24h} > 400$ if treating a MDR pathogen. A framework for considering the dosing of individual antibiotics according to PK/PD principles is presented in Table 13.2.

Antibiotic Prophylaxis

Prophylactic antibiotics are used most often to prevent SSIs, for which the benefit has been proved in many circumstances. However, only the incision itself is protected, and only while it is open and thus vulnerable to inoculation. If not administered properly, antibiotic prophylaxis is ineffective and may be harmful. Antibiotic prophylaxis of surgery does not prevent postoperative nosocomial infections, which actually occur at an increased rate after prolonged prophylaxis,[37,38] selecting for more resistant pathogens when infection does develop.[8,38]

Four principles guide the administration of antimicrobial agent for prophylaxis of a surgical incision: safety; an appropriate narrow spectrum of coverage of relevant pathogens; little or no reliance upon the agent for therapy of infection (owing to the possible induction of resistance with heavy usage); and administration within 1 hour before surgery and for a defined, brief period of time thereafter (no more than 24 hours [48 hours for cardiac surgery]; ideally, a single dose).[39] According to these principles, quinolones or carbapenems are undesirable agents for surgical prophylaxis, although ertapenem and quinolone prophylaxis have been endorsed by the Surgical Care Improvement Project (SCIP) for prophylaxis of elective colon surgery (the latter with metronidazole for penicillin-allergic patients) (Table 13.3). The SCIP recommendations do not consider emergency surgery.

The spectrum of bacterial contamination of surgical sites is well described.[40] Clean surgical procedures affect only skin structures and other soft tissues. Clean-contaminated procedures are characterized by controlled opening of a hollow viscus (e.g., elective aerodigestive or genitourinary tract surgery). Contaminated procedures introduce a large inoculum of bacteria into a normally sterile body cavity, but too briefly for infection to become established during surgery (e.g., penetrating abdominal trauma, enterotomy during adhesiolysis for mechanical bowel obstruction). Dirty procedures are those performed to control established infection (e.g., colon resection for perforated diverticulitis).

Most SSIs are caused by gram-positive cocci; therefore, prophylaxis should be directed primarily against staphylococci for clean cases and high-risk clean-contaminated upper abdominal surgery. A first-generation cephalosporin is preferred in almost all circumstances (Table 13.4), with clindamycin used for penicillin-allergic patients.[39] If gram-negative or anaerobic coverage is required, a second-generation cephalosporin, or the combination of a first-generation agent plus metronidazole, is the regimen of first choice. Vancomycin prophylaxis is generally not recommended, except in institutions where the incidence of MRSA infection is high (>20% of all SSIs caused by MRSA).

The optimal time to administer parenteral antibiotic prophylaxis is within 1 hour prior to incision.[41] Antibiotics given sooner are ineffective, as are agents given after the incision is closed. A 2001 audit of prescribing practices in the United States indicated that only 56% of patients who received prophylactic antibiotics did so within 1 hour prior to the skin incision[42]; timeliness was documented in only 76% of cases in a 2005 audit in US Department of Veterans Affairs hospitals.[42]

TABLE 13.2

PHARMACOKINETICS OF BACTERIAL KILLING: IMPLICATIONS FOR ANTIBIOTIC DOSING

CHARACTERISTIC	DRUGS	THERAPEUTIC GOAL	TACTIC
Time-dependent (no or minimal PAE); fT > MIC > 70% ideal	Carbapenems Cephalosporins Linezolid Penicillins	Maintain drug concentration	Maximize duration of exposure with prolonged or continuous infusion[a]
Time-dependent, concentration-enhanced (with PAE) $AUC:MIC_{24h} > 125$; $AUC:MIC_{24h} > 400$ for MDR pathogens?	Clindamycin Glycylcyclines Macrolides Streptogramins Tetracyclines Vancomycin	Maximize effectiveness of bacteriostatic/weak bactericidal antibiotics with prolonged PAEs. PAE is concentration-dependent	Maximize drug dosage[b] consistent with avoidance of toxicity
Concentration-dependent (with PAE)	Aminoglycosides Daptomycin Fluoroquinolones Ketolides Metronidazole Polymyxins	PAE is concentration-dependent. Achieve C_{max} ([peak]) MIC >10	Maximize peak concentration[c]

[a]Continuous or prolonged infusion of linezolid is not recommended, as efficacy has not been established.
[b]Examples of maximized drug dosages include clindamycin 900 mg q8h rather than 600 mg q6h, and vancomycin 15 mg/kg/d for patients with normal renal function. Larger doses of tigecycline (a glyclcyline) and streptogramins (e.g., quinupristin/dalfopristin) may be limited by increased toxicity.
[c]Examples of dosing to achieve maximized peak drug concentrations include single daily-dose aminoglycoside therapy and metronidazole 1 g q12h rather than 500 mg q8h. Prolonging the dosing interval is not recommended for polymyxins, owing to a negligible PAE.
See text for additional explanations.
AUC, area under the concentration–time curve; Cmax, maximum drug concentration (peak concentration); fT, proportion of time; MIC, minimum inhibitory concentration; MDR, multidrug-resistant; PAE, postantibiotic effect.

TABLE 13.3

SURGICAL CARE IMPROVEMENT PROGRAM: APPROVED ANTIBIOTIC PROPHYLACTIC REGIMENS FOR ELECTIVE SURGERY

TYPE OF OPERATION	ANTIBIOTIC(S)
Cardiac (including CABG)[a], vascular[b]	Cefazolin or cefuroxime or vancomycin[c]
Hip/knee arthroplasty[b]	Cefazolin or cefuroxime or vancomycin[c]
Colon[d,e,f]	Oral: neomycin sulfate plus either erythromycin base or metronidazole, administered for 18 h before surgery Parenteral: cefoxitin or cefotetan or ertapenem or cefazolin plus metronidazole or ampicillin–sulbactam
Hysterectomy[e]	Cefazolin or cefoxitin or cefotetan or cefuroxime or ampicillin–sulbactam

[a]Prophylaxis may be administered for up to 48 h for cardiac surgery; for all other cases, the limit is 24 h.
[b]For beta-lactam allergy, clindamycin or vancomycin is an acceptable substitute for cardiac, vascular, and orthopedic surgery.
[c]Vancomycin is acceptable with a physician-documented justification for use in the medical record.
[d]For beta-lactam allergy, clindamycin plus gentamicin, a fluoroquinolone, or aztreonam; or metronidazole plus gentamicin or a fluoroquinolone are acceptable choices.
[e]For colon surgery, either oral or parenteral prophylaxis alone, or both combined, are acceptable.
[f]For beta-lactam allergy, either clindamycin plus gentamicin, a fluoroquinolone, or aztreonam; or metronidazole plus gentamicin or a fluoroquinolone or clindamycin monotherapy, is an acceptable choice.
CABG, coronary artery bypass grafting.

Most inappropriately timed first doses of prophylactic antibiotic occur too early.[41,42] Antibiotics with short half-lives (<2 hours, e.g., cefazolin or cefoxitin) should be redosed every 3–4 hours during surgery if the operation is prolonged or bloody.[43] Even though SCIP specifies a 24-hour limit for prophylaxis, single-dose prophylaxis (with intraoperative redosing, if indicated) is equivalent to multiple doses for the prevention of SSI.[44] Prolonged prophylaxis increases the risk of nosocomial infections unrelated to the surgical site, and the emergence of MDR pathogens. Both pneumonia and vascular catheter–related infections have been associated with prolonged prophylaxis,[37,38,45,46] as has the emergence of SSI caused by MRSA.[8]

Recent US data show that only 40% of patients who receive antibiotic prophylaxis do so for <24 hours.[47] As a result of ischemia caused by surgical hemostasis, antibiotic penetration into the incision immediately after surgery is questionable until neovascularization occurs (24–48 hours). Antibiotics should not be given to "cover" indwelling drains or catheters, in lavage or irrigation fluid,[48] or as a substitute for poor surgical technique.

Antibiotic prophylaxis is indicated for most clean-contaminated and contaminated (or potentially contaminated) operations. Antibiotic prophylaxis is indicated for high-risk biliary surgery; high risk is conferred by age >70 years, diabetes mellitus, or a recently instrumented biliary tract (e.g., biliary stent). By contrast, antibiotic prophylaxis is usually not indicated for elective laparoscopic cholecystectomy[49]; meta-analysis of 12 trials revealed no benefit compared with placebo for prevention of SSI (odds ratio [OR] 1.07, 95% confidence interval [CI], 0.59–1.94; $p = 0.99$), or "overall infection," "major infection," or "distant infection." Emergency cholecystectomy (regardless of technique) is performed most commonly for acute cholecystitis, for which antibiotic administration would be therapeutic, not prophylactic.

Antibiotic prophylaxis of clean surgery is controversial. Where bone is incised (e.g. craniotomy, sternotomy) or a prosthesis is inserted, antibiotic prophylaxis is generally indicated. Meta-analysis of randomized controlled trials shows a decrease of SSI rate for groin hernia surgery,[50] especially when nonabsorbable mesh is implanted. Twelve randomized clinical trials (6,705 patients) were identified, six of which used prosthetic material (hernioplasty). Infection rates were 2.9% and 3.9% in the prophylaxis and control groups, respectively (OR 0.64, 95% CI 0.48-0.85). Patients with herniorrhaphy had infection rates of 3.5% and 4.9% in the prophylaxis and control groups, respectively (OR 0.71, 95% CI 0.51–1.00). Patients with hernioplasty had infection rates of 1.4% and 2.9% in the prophylaxis and control groups, respectively (OR 0.48, 95% CI 0.27-0.85).

The incidence of SSI is higher for abdominal wall incisional hernia repair than for groin hernioplasty, especially for open surgery as compared with laparoscopic repair,[51,52] and is increased dramatically if an enterotomy occurs during adhesiolysis.[53] Because of the known risk of SSI, antibiotic prophylaxis is warranted, but has not been examined with rigor.

Arterial reconstruction with a prosthetic graft, especially infrainguinal, is an example of clean surgery where the risk of infection is substantial. Meta-analysis[54] of 23 randomized, controlled trials of prophylactic antibiotics for peripheral arterial reconstruction demonstrated that prophylaxis reduced the risk of SSI by approximately 75%, and early graft infection by about 69%. There was no benefit to prophylaxis for more than 24 hours, of antibiotic bonding to the graft material itself, or preoperative bathing with an antiseptic agent compared with unmedicated bathing.

Skin closure of a contaminated or dirty incision increases the risk of SSI, but few good studies evaluate the multiplicity of wound closure techniques used by surgeons. "Open abdomen" techniques of temporary abdominal closure for management of trauma or severe peritonitis are utilized increasingly. Antibiotic prophylaxis of the open abdomen is probably not indicated[55] (Table 13.5), although an inability to achieve primary abdominal closure is associated with several nosocomial infections (pneumonia, bloodstream infection, and SSI) and substantially increased cost from prolonged length of stay, but not mortality.[56]

Drains placed in incisions may cause more infections than they prevent. Epithelialization of the wound is prevented,

TABLE 13.4

APPROPRIATE CEPHALOSPORIN PROPHYLAXIS FOR SELECTED OPERATIONS

OPERATION	ALTERNATIVE PROPHYLAXIS IN SERIOUS PENICILLIN ALLERGY
First-Generation Cephalosporin (i.e., Cefazolin, Cefuroxime)	
Cardiovascular and thoracic	
Median sternotomy	Clindamycin (for all cardiovascular and thoracic cases except amputation)
Pacemaker insertion	
Vascular reconstruction involving the abdominal aorta, insertion of a prosthesis, or a groin incision (except carotid endarterectomy, which requires no prophylaxis)	
Implantable defibrillator	
Pulmonary resection	
Lower limb amputation	Gentamicin and metronidazole
General	
Cholecystectomy (high risk only)	Gentamicin
Gastrectomy (high risk only: not uncomplicated chronic duodenal ulcer)	Gentamicin and metronidazole
Hepatobiliary	Gentamicin and metronidazole
Major debridement of traumatic wound	Gentamicin
Genitourinary (ampicillin plus gentamicin is a reasonable alternative)	Ciprofloxacin
Gynecologic	
Cesarean section (STAT)	Metronidazole or doxycycline, after cord clamping
Hysterectomy (cefoxitin is a reasonable alternative)	Doxycycline
Head and neck/oral cavity	
Major procedures entering oral cavity or pharynx	Gentamicin and clindamycin or metronidazole
Neurosurgery	
Craniotomy	Clindamycin, vancomycin
Orthopedics	
Major joint arthroplasty	Vancomycin[b]
Open reduction of closed fracture	Vancomycin[b]
Second-generation (i.e., cefoxitin)[c]	
Appendectomy	Metronidazole plus gentamicin
Colon surgery[d]	
Surgery for penetrating abdominal trauma	

[a]Should be given as a single intravenous dose just before the operation. Consider an additional dose if the operation is prolonged longer than 3–4 h.
[b]Primary prophylaxis with vancomycin (i.e., for the non–penicillin-allergic patient) may be appropriate for cardiac valve replacement, placement of a non-tissue peripheral vascular prosthesis, or total joint replacement in institutions where a high rate of infections with methicillin-resistant *S. aureus* or *S. epidermidis* has occurred. The precise definition of "high rate" is debated. A single dose administered immediately before surgery is sufficient unless operation lasts for more than 6 h, in which case the dose should be repeated. Prophylaxis should be discontinued after a maximum of two doses but may be continued for up to 48 h.
[c]An intraoperative dose should be given if cefoxitin is used and the duration of surgery exceeds 3–4 h, because of the short half-life of the drug. A postoperative dose is not necessary but is permissible for up to 24 h.
[d]Benefit beyond that provided by bowel preparation with mechanical cleansing and oral neomycin and erythromycin base is debatable.

TABLE 13.5

ANTIBIOTIC PROPHYLAXIS OF TRAUMA-SUMMARY OF EVIDENCE AND PUBLISHED GUIDELINES

CLINICAL SITUATION	AGENT (IF ANY)	DOSE/DURATION	EVIDENCE CLASS
Bites (mammalian)[65,66]			
"High-risk" <12–24 h postinjury	Amoxicillin/clavulanic acid (bites of the hand; deep puncture crushed or devitalized tissue, overt contamination)	875 mg BID × 3 d	II
Burn debridement[67]	Cefazolin or piperacillin/tazobactam	Higher doses or prolonged infusion	III
Craniotomy[68,69]			
Elective Emergency	Cefazolin	≤24 h perioperative Insufficient data	I
Cutaneous wounds (acute)[70–72]	Topical	Systemic oral	Not recommended
Closed long bone fractures[73,74]	Cefazolin	Single-dose	I
Facial fractures[75–79]			
(Midface, including open, with or without sinus involvement)	Cefazolin	≤24 h perioperative only	III
Mandible Orbital floor	Cefazolin	≤24 h perioperative only Insufficient	III
Open abdomen[55]	Not indicated		III
Open extremity fractures[80]			
Grade I extremity	Cefazolin	24–48 h	I
Grade II extremity	Cefazolin	48 h	II
Grade III extremity	*Single* broad-spectrum agent (aminoglycoside second agent not recommended)	48 h	III
Gunshot fractures-no ORIF	Not indicated		I
Multiple "washouts"	Prolongation not indicated	Insufficient	
Penetrating abdominal trauma[81]			
No hollow viscus injury	Second-generation cephalosporin	Single dose	I
Hollow viscus injury (including colon injury)	Second-generation cephalosporin	≤24 h	I
Placement of intracranial pressure monitor (including ventriculostomy)[82–84]	Not indicated		III
Skull fracture[85–87]		Not recommended	I
Basilar skull fracture with/without cerebrospinal fluid leak, adult or pediatric	Open, depressed	Insufficient	
Thoracotomy			
Emergency		Insufficient	
Traumatic brain injury[88]			
Tube thoracostomy[89]		Insufficient	
Emergency	First-generation cephalosporin	≤24 h	III

ORIF: Open reduction.internal fixation.

and the drain becomes a conduit, holding open a portal for invasion by pathogens colonizing the skin. Several studies of drains placed into clean or clean-contaminated incisions show that the rate of SSI is not reduced[57,58]; in fact, the rate is increased.[59–62] Considering that drains pose this risk, they should be used as little as possible and removed as soon as possible.[63] Under no circumstances should prolonged antibiotic prophylaxis be administered to "cover" indwelling drains.

For trauma, antibiotic prophylaxis may be required for operative management, but may also be indicated to prevent traumatic wounds from becoming infected. Obviously, the principle of administration within 1 hour before surgical incision does not apply in the latter case. Moreover, many surgical procedures performed for trauma are likely to be in a contaminated field (e.g., penetrating trauma, open reduction/internal fixation of open fractures). Likewise, as many as three-quarters of traumatic wounds are likely to be contaminated to some degree, the likelihood of infection is increased when the degree of contamination is higher.[64] The evidence for antibiotic prophylaxis of traumatic injury is presented in Table 13.5.[55,65–89] The evidence is most robust for penetrating abdominal trauma, for which no more than 24 hours of prophylaxis with a second-generation cephalosporin (or equivalent) is recommended, even for colon injury. Weaker data sets that have been subjected to robust analysis include the evidence for prophylaxis of open extremity fractures.

PRINCIPLES OF ANTIBIOTIC THERAPY

Antimicrobial therapy is a mainstay of the treatment of infections, but widespread overuse and misuse of antibiotics have led to an alarming increase in MDR pathogens (Table 13.1). New agents and innovative ways to administer existing antibiotics may allow shorter courses of therapy, which is desirable for cost savings and control of microbial ecology. Effective therapy with no toxicity requires a careful but expeditious search for the source of infection and an understanding of the principles of PK (see above).

Evaluation of Possible Infection

Absent a fever, any of hypotension, tachycardia, tachypnea, confusion, rigors, skin lesions, respiratory manifestations, oliguria, lactic acidosis, leukocytosis, leukopenia, immature neutrophils (i.e., bands >10%), or thrombocytopenia may indicate a workup for infection and immediate empiric therapy. A new temperature elevation is usually the trigger for an evaluation for the presence of infection (hence, "fever workup"). However, some infected patients do not manifest fever, and may be even be hypothermic. Such patients include elderly patients; those with open abdominal wounds, end-stage liver disease, or chronic kidney disease; and patients taking anti-inflammatory or anti-pyretic drugs. Moreover, fever in the early postoperative period often has a non-infectious cause, hence fever does not equate with infection (Table 13.6).[90,91] The acute care surgeon must also bear in mind that non-infectious and infectious causes of fever may coexist, and that an infected patient may harbor more than one discrete focus of infection.

Antibiotics should not be given until evaluation has occurred, including the collection of specimens for culture. Therefore, evaluation must be expeditious, as delay in antibiotic administration is associated with an increased risk of death.[92–95] It is mandatory to remove the surgical dressing to inspect the incision as part of any fever evaluation. However, if an incision is opened and cultured, a deep culture specimen should be collected; swabbing an open wound superficially or collecting fluid from drains (if present) for culture is un-helpful because the likelihood of colonization is high. A chest x-ray is optional for evaluation of early postoperative fever unless mechanical ventilation, physical examination, abnormal blood gases, or pulmonary secretions suggest a high yield. Urinalysis or culture is not mandatory in the early postoperative period unless there is reason by history or examination to suspect a UTI. After trauma, UTI is common only after injury to the urinary tract.[96]

Traditional diagnostic criteria have low specificity for the diagnosis of HAP/VAP; therefore, culture of a lower respiratory tract sample is mandatory for nosocomial pneumonia prior to administration of antibiotics. There is controversy regarding methods of sputum specimen collection (invasive vs. noninvasive) and specimen analysis (semiquantitative vs. quantitative). The crucial issue in diagnosis of HAP/VAP is whether a sputum isolate reflects colonization rather than infection. Endotracheal suction aspirates have lower specificity than deep specimens collected by bronchoalveolar lavage or protected-specimen brush, due to an increased likelihood of contamination of the former by oropharyngeal flora,[97] although it is unclear if this makes a difference clinically. A meta-analysis of randomized trials that compared outcomes of patients with VAP managed with invasive versus noninvasive sampling showed no difference in mortality,[98] although patients in the invasive group were more likely to undergo narrowing of the antimicrobial regimen or cessation of therapy.

Blood cultures should be obtained from febrile patients when clinical evaluation does not suggest a non-infectious cause. The venipuncture site should be cleaned with either 2% chlorhexidine gluconate in 70% isopropyl alcohol or 1–2% tincture of iodine. Povidone–iodine (10%) is acceptable but not bactericidal until dry; false-positive blood cultures may result from premature specimen collection.[99] For adults, a minimum 20–30 mL sample of blood is drawn at a single time from a single site; additional guidelines apply for blood cultures taken from new or existing central venous catheters.[91] The minimum inoculum for an adult blood culture should be 10 mL/bottle. The cumulative yield of pathogens is optimized when three blood cultures (i.e., six bottles inoculated) with adequate volume (20–30 mL each) are drawn.[100] The sensitivity of blood culturing for detection of true bacteremia or fungemia is related to many factors, most importantly the volume of blood drawn and obtaining the cultures before initiation of anti-infective therapy.[100]

TABLE 13.6

MISCELLANEOUS CAUSES OF FEVER RELATED TO NON-INFECTIOUS STATES

Acalculous cholecystitis
Acute myocardial infarction
Acute respiratory distress syndrome (fibroproliferative phase)
Adrenal insufficiency
Cytokine release syndrome
Fat embolism
Gout
Hematoma
Heterotopic ossification
Immune reconstitution inflammatory syndrome (IRIS)
Infarction of any tissue
Intracranial hemorrhage (trauma or vascular etiology)
Myocardial infarction
Pancreatitis
Pericarditis
Pulmonary infarction
Stroke
Thyroid storm
Transfusion of blood or blood products
Transplant rejection
Tumor lysis syndrome
Venous thromboembolic disease
Withdrawal syndromes (e.g., drug, alcohol)

Empiric Antibiotic Therapy

Empiric antibiotic therapy must be administered judiciously, but expeditiously. Injudicious therapy could result in undertreatment of established infection, or unnecessary therapy in the setting of sterile inflammation or bacterial colonization; either may be deleterious. Inappropriate therapy (e.g., delay,[92,101] therapy misdirected against usual pathogens, failure to treat MDR pathogens) leads unequivocally to increased mortality.[93–95] There is urgency because delay in initiation of empiric antibiotic therapy of as little as 30–60 minutes can result in increased mortality.[101,102] Current guidelines for the diagnosis and management of severe sepsis recommend that empiric antibiotic therapy be instituted with 1 hour of presentation.[103]

Antibiotic choice is based on several interrelated factors (Tables 13.7–13.9). Paramount is activity against identified or likely (for empiric therapy) pathogens, presuming infecting and colonizing organisms can be distinguished, and that narrow-spectrum coverage is always desired. Estimation of likely pathogens depends on the disease process believed responsible; whether the infection is community-, health care–, or hospital-acquired; and whether MDR organisms are present, or likely to be. Local knowledge of antimicrobial resistance patterns is essential, even at the unit-specific level. Patient-specific factors of importance include age, debility, immunosuppression, intrinsic organ function, prior allergy or other adverse reaction, and recent antibiotic therapy. Institutional factors of importance include guidelines that may specify a particular therapy, formulary availability of specific agents, outbreaks of infections caused by MDR pathogens, and antibiotic control programs.

Antibiotic stewardship programs[20] support optimal antibiotic administration, including physician prescribing patterns, computerized decision support, administration by protocol, and formulary restriction programs. Owing to the increasing prevalence of MDR pathogens, it is crucial for initial empiric antibiotic therapy to be targeted appropriately, administered according to PK/PD principles, given in sufficient dosage to assure bacterial killing, narrowed in spectrum (*de-escalation*)[104] as soon as possible based on microbiology data and clinical response, and continued only as long as necessary.[105] Appropriate antibiotic prescribing not only optimizes patient care but supports infection control practice and preserves microbial ecology.[20,104]

TABLE 13.7

FACTORS INFLUENCING ANTIBIOTIC CHOICE

Activity against known/suspected pathogens
Disease/pathogen believed responsible (see Table 13.8)
Distinguish infection from colonization
Narrow-spectrum coverage most desirable
Antimicrobial resistance patterns

Patient-specific factors
  Location prior to presentation—home versus health care facility
  Recent prior antibiotic therapy?
  Severity of illness?
  Age?
  Immunosuppression
  Organ dysfunction
  Allergy

Institutional guidelines/restrictions
  Institutional approval required?
  Agent available immediately?

Logistics
  Onset, dose, and dosing interval
  Single or multiple agents?
  Duration of infusion and course of therapy

Choice of Antibiotic Numerous agents are available for therapy (Table 13.10).[106,107] Agents may be chosen based on spectrum, whether broad or targeted (e.g., antipseudomonal, antianaerobic), in addition to the above factors. If a nosocomial gram-positive pathogen is suspected (e.g., wound or SSI, CLABSI, HAP/VAP) or MRSA is endemic, empiric vancomycin (or linezolid) is appropriate. Some authorities recommend dual-agent therapy for serious *Pseudomonas* infections (i.e., an antipseudomonal beta-lactam drug plus an aminoglycoside), but evidence of efficacy is mixed.[108–111] Combination therapy of a specific pathogen (e.g., "double coverage" of *Pseudomonas*) may actually worsen outcomes. Meta-analysis of β-lactam monotherapy versus β-lactam/aminoglycoside combination therapy for immunocompetent patients with sepsis (64 trials, 7,586 patients) found no difference in either mortality (RR 0.90, 95% CI 0.77–1.06) or the development of resistance.[109] Clinical failure was more common with combination therapy, as was the incidence of acute kidney injury. Regardless of the specifics of the choice that is made, initial empiric therapy of any infection caused potentially by either a gram-positive or gram-negative bacterium (e.g., HAP/VAP, hospital-acquired intra-abdominal infection) must include activity against all likely pathogens.[106,112–114]

Optimization of Therapy Conventional antibiotic dosing may not apply to the critically ill or injured patient.[26] Higher doses may be required for MDR isolates,[26,115–117] increased extracellular volume,[26,118] decreased serum albumin concentration,[119] or increased glomerular filtration rate (e.g., morbid obesity,[120] burns, traumatic brain injury,[121] multiple trauma). Underdosing of antibiotics is a major factor for the development of resistance during therapy and failure thereof.[116] By contrast, lower doses may be required with multiple organ dysfunction syndrome,[122] acute kidney injury, and chronic kidney disease (see below and Chapter 52). Dosing of vancomycin and aminoglycosides may be monitored via measurement of drug concentrations in serum,[123–125] and may be useful to limit toxicity.[126] Therapeutic drug concentration monitoring is possible for a host of other antibiotics, although not widely available.

The practical and financial challenges of performing PK studies in critically ill patients have made valuable mathematical modeling such as Monte Carlo simulation (MCS) to perform virtual clinical trials.[127] In order to utilize MCS, four conditions must be present: (1) A robust population PK model must be available for the patient population of interest; (2) descriptors of the effect of covariates that influence PK are needed; (3) the susceptibility of bacteria to the modeled antibiotic must be known; and (4) a PK/PD target must be associated with efficacy. Probability of target attainment outputs describe the proportion of patients who will achieve a prespecified PD target for any given MIC. Such analyses can then inform dosing decisions to achieve a high likelihood of achieving PK/PD targets for organisms with different MICs.

Zelenitsky et al. provided a useful example of MCS for interpreting the optimal methods for dosing meropenem, piperacillin/tazobactam, cefepime, and ceftobiprole in

TABLE 13.8

RANK ORDER OF KEY BACTERIAL PATHOGENS IN ICU INFECTIONS (BY INCIDENCE)

	BLOOD STREAM INFECTION[a]	URINARY TRACT INFECTION[a]	PNEUMONIA[b]
Gram-positive	1: Coag-neg staphylococci 2: *Enterococcus* 3: *S. aureus*	1: *Enterococcus* 2: Coag-neg staphylococci 3: *S. aureus*	1: *S. aureus*
Gram-negative	1: *Enterobacter* 2: *P. aeruginosa* 3: *K. pneumoniae* 4: *E. coli*	1: *E. coli* 2: *P. aeruginosa* 3: *K. pneumoniae* 4: *Enterobacter*	1: *P. aeruginosa* 2: *Enterobacter* 3: *K. pneumoniae* 4: *Acinetobacter* 5: *E. coli*

[a]Yeast are also important pathogens in blood stream and UTIs.
[b]Yeast are seldom pathogens in nosocomial infection, except for solid-organ transplant recipients and patients undergoing antineoplastic chemotherapy.
Coag-neg, coagulase-negative.

critically ill patients.[128] For meropenem, at MICs up to 8 mcg/mL, the probability of achieving 40% fT > MIC was 96%, 90%, and 61% for 3-hour infusions of 2 g q8h, 1 g q8h, and 1 g q12h, respectively, in patients with creatinine clearances ≥50, 30–49, and 10–29 mL/min, respectively. Target attainment was 75%, 65%, and 44% for these same dosing regimens as 0.5 hour infusions.

Continuous or prolonged infusion of beta-lactam agents may be the optimal way to administer these drugs[129–132] (Figs. 13.2 and 13.3). Lengthened fT > MIC is achieved, increasing the likelihood of therapeutic success, especially against organisms with higher MICs, while minimizing the possibility of the development of resistance. Prolonged infusions may accomplish the same without monopolizing an intravenous line. Clinical reports support the use of prolonged infusions of beta-lactam antibiotics,[133–135] sometimes at lower total dose when highly susceptible organisms are being treated. However, adoption into clinical practice is not widespread.[136] Continuous-infusion vancomycin has been described,[137] but is not recommended currently (Table 13.11).

Vancomycin has been a mainstay of therapy of infections of critically ill patients, but MICs for vancomycin against MRSA have been increasing, even within the susceptible range. As a result, MIC cutpoints for resistance of *S. aureus* have been revised downward to minimize the chance of ineffective therapy (Table 13.12),[138] and higher doses of vancomycin are recommended (Table 13.11),[124,125] although at a greater risk of nephrotoxicity. Mortality in patients with MRSA HAP, VAP, and HCAP increases as a function of the vancomycin MIC, even for strains with MIC values within the susceptible range (Table 13.13).[139,140] The use of vancomycin therapy in patients with MRSA infections caused by isolates with MICs between 1 and –2 mg/mL should be undertaken with caution. Adequate therapeutic concentrations may not be achievable for *S. aureus* isolates with MICs >2 mcg/mL,[141] so alternative therapy should be considered. Linezolid retains generally excellent activity,[142] but resistance to daptomycin is being reported.[143]

Aminoglycoside therapy is resurgent owing to limited options for treatment of MDR pathogens that have resulted

TABLE 13.9

BACTERIAL RESISTANCE: PROBLEM INFECTIONS AND PATHOGENS

INFECTION	ORGANISMS			
	MRSA	VRE	ESBL	CARBAPENEMASES
CAP	+ (CA-MRSA)			
VAP	++++		++	++
UTI		+	++	
Soft tissue	++++ (CA-MRSA)	+	++	+
CLABSI	++++	+	+	+

CA-MRSA, community-acquired methicillin-resistant *S. aureus*; CAP, community-acquired pneumonia; CLABSI, central line–associated blood stream infection; ESBL, extended-spectrum beta lactamase; VAP, ventilator-associated pneumonia; VRE, vancomycin-resistant *Enterococcus*.
The number of (+) indicators reflects relative prevalence.

TABLE 13.10

ANTIBACTERIAL AGENTS FOR EMPIRIC USE

Antipseudomonal
Piperacillin–tazobactam
Cefepime, ceftazidime
Imipenem-cilastatin, meropenem, doripenem
? Ciprofloxacin, levofloxacin (depending on local susceptibility patterns)
Aminoglycoside
Polymyxins (polymyxin B, colistin [polymyxin E])
Targeted-Spectrum
Gram-positive
Glycopeptide (e.g., vancomycin, telavancin)
Lipopeptide (e.g., daptomycin; not for known/suspected pneumonia)
Oxazolidinone (e.g., linezolid)
Gram-negative
Third-generation cephalosporin (not ceftriaxone)
Monobactam
Polymyxins (polymyxin B, colistin [polymyxin E])
Anti-anaerobic
Metronidazole
Broad-Spectrum
Piperacillin–tazobactam
Carbapenems
Fluoroquinolones (depending on local susceptibility patterns)
Tigecycline (plus an anti-pseudoomonal agent)
Trimethoprim–sulfamethoxazole (used primarily for CA-MRSA, *Stenotrophomonas*)
Anti-anaerobic
Metronidazole
Carbapenems
Beta-lactam/beta-lactamase combination agents
Tigecycline
Anti-MRSA
Ceftaroline
Daptomycin (not for use against pneumonia)
Minocycline
Linezolid
Telavancin
Tigecycline (not in pregnancy or for children under age 8 y)
Vancomycin

from the increasing prevalence of extended-spectrum beta-lactamase (ESBL)-producing strains and the emergence of carbapenemases, although use as part of an empiric therapy regimen remains debated.[108,109,123] Single daily-dose aminoglycoside therapy ensures that a peak:MIC concentration ratio >10 will be achieved to optimize therapy. A dose of gentamicin or tobramycin (7 mg/kg) or amikacin (20 mg/kg) is administered and a trough concentration is determined at 23-hour postdose (some protocols call for an intermediate determination as well, at approximately 16-hour post-dose, so that the elimination curve can be determined with greater precision). A trough concentration of 0.5–2 mcg/mL is sought for gentamicin or tobramycin, whereas a trough concentration of 5–10 mcg/mL is ideal for amikacin. Outcomes are comparable or better compared with conventional dosing, with decreased toxicity. Single-daily-dose aminoglycoside therapy has not been validated for children, pregnant patients, patients with burns, patients aged >70 years, or treatment of bacterial endocarditis.

Infections caused by highly resistant or pan-resistant gram-negative bacilli pose a major problem. Carbapenems, tigecycline, and polymyxins (see below) retain useful activity

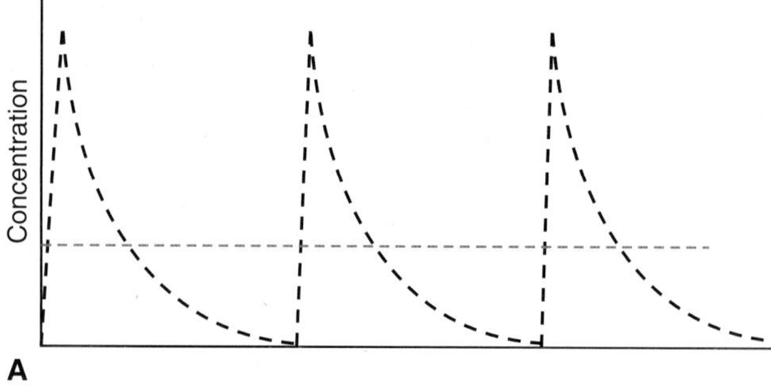

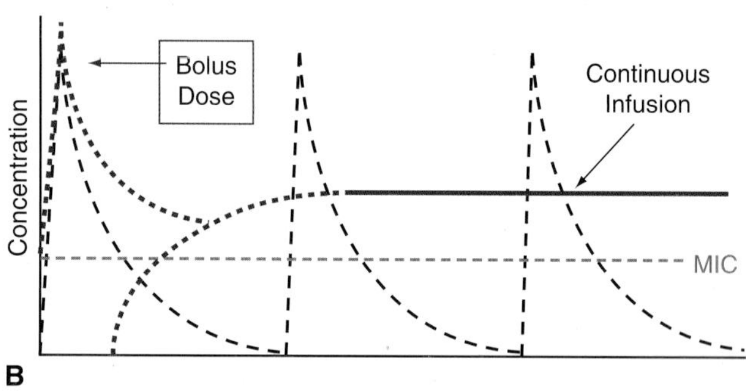

FIGURE 13.2. **A:** Stylized curves of bolus 30-min infusions of antibiotic at 6-h intervals. The proportion of time (fT) above the minimum inhibitory concentration (MIC) must be at least 40% for bactericidal activity in most cases. If the MIC is low, this can be achieved with conventional dosing, but not for organisms with higher MICs. **B:** Continuous infusion of antibiotic after an initial loading dose (*dotted lines*) is depicted. Not only is fT:MIC higher, but the antibiotic becomes effective against organisms with higher MICs, depending on the rate of continuous infusion. Lower total daily doses of antibiotic may be used against bacteria with low MICs. For drugs that exhibit time-dependent bactericidal activity (e.g., beta-lactams), this is the ideal mode of administration, provided vascular access is sufficient.

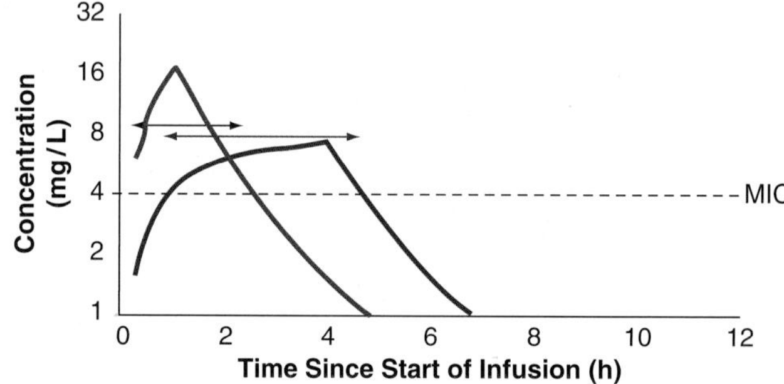

FIGURE 13.3. A conventional bolus dose of antibiotic with a 30-min infusion and a 6-h dosing interval is compared with the same drug given as a 4-h infusion over the same dosing interval. fT:MIC is doubled (compare the lengths of the *short* and *long double arrows*), while organisms with higher MICs can still be treated. The interruption allows the intravenous line to be used for fluid or other medication during the hiatus, without compromising bactericidal action.

TABLE 13.11

VANCOMYCIN MIC INTERPRETIVE CRITERIA FOR *S. AUREUS*

OLD BREAKPOINTS		NEW BREAKPOINTS	
Susceptible	≤4 mg/L	Susceptible	≤2 mg/L
Intermediate	8–16 mg/L	Intermediate	4–8 mg/L
Resistant	≥32 mg/L	Resistant	≥16 mg/L

From FDA Lowers Vancomycin Breakpoints for Staph Infections. May 1, 2008. Available at: http://news.idsociety.org/idsa/issues/2008-05-01/. Accessed July 5, 2011.
MIC: minimal inhibitory conccentration.

against ESBL-producing organisms. MDR non-fermenting gram-negative bacilli (e.g., *P. aeruginosa*, *Acinetobacter* spp., *Stenotrophomonas* spp., and carbapenemase-producing Enterobacteriaceae) may require therapy with a polymyxin, high-dose carbapenem by prolonged infusion, or unusual combinations of agents that have demonstrated synergy *in vitro*, but remain of uncertain clinical utility.[106,107,143,144]

Duration of Therapy

The end point of antibiotic therapy is largely undefined, because quality data are few. If cultures are negative, empiric antibiotic therapy should be stopped in most cases after no more than 48–72 hours. Unnecessary antibiotic therapy increases the risk of MDR infection; therefore, prolonged therapy with negative cultures is usually unjustifiable. The morbidity of antibiotic therapy also includes allergic reactions, development of nosocomial superinfections, (e.g., fungal, enterococcal, and *Clostridium difficile*–related infections), organ toxicity, reduced yield from subsequent cultures, and vitamin K deficiency with coagulopathy or accentuation of warfarin effect.

If infection is evident, treatment is continued as indicated clinically, but the microbiology data should be examined to see if the antibiotic regime can be de-escalated to a narrower regimen (e.g., choosing a narrower-spectrum agent, changing multi-drug therapy to monotherapy). If empiric therapy has been appropriate, the need to escalate therapy at this point (e.g., choosing a more broad-spectrum agent, changing monotherapy to multi-drug therapy, adding antifungal therapy [see below]) should be a rare event.

Some infections can be treated with therapy lasting 4 days or less[105] (Table 13.14). Every decision to start antibiotics must be accompanied by an *a priori* decision regarding duration of therapy. A reason to continue therapy beyond the predetermined end point must be compelling. Bacterial killing is rapid in response to effective agents, but the host response may not subside immediately. Therefore, the clinical response of the patient should not be the sole determinant. There is increasing belief that shorter courses of antibiotic therapy that were used previously are equally effective with fewer side effects, and that therapy should continue to a predetermined end point, after which it should be stopped.

TABLE 13.12

SUMMARY OF VANCOMYCIN DOSING GUIDELINES

THERAPEUTIC VANCOMYCIN DOSE ADJUSTMENT AND DRUG MONITORING

Dosage

- Initial vancomycin dosages should be calculated on the basis of actual body weight, including for obese patients. IV vancomycin 15–20 mg/kg/dose (actual body weight) every 8–12 h, not to exceed 2 g per dose, is recommended for most patients with normal renal function
- For seriously ill patients (e.g., those with sepsis, meningitis, pneumonia, or infective endocarditis) with suspected MRSA infection, a loading dose of 25–30 mg/kg (actual body weight) may be considered
- Subsequent dosage adjustments should be based on actual trough serum concentrations, obtained just before the fourth dose, to achieve targeted therapeutic concentrations. Trough vancomycin monitoring is recommended for serious infections and patients who are morbidly obese, have renal dysfunction (including those receiving renal replacement therapy), or have fluctuating volumes of distribution
- For serious infections, such as bacteremia, infective endocarditis, osteomyelitis, meningitis, pneumonia, and severe SSTI (e.g., necrotizing fasciitis) due to MRSA, vancomycin trough concentrations of 15–20 mcg/mL are recommended
- Monitoring of peak vancomycin concentrations is not recommended
- Doses of 1 g should be infused over 1 h. Doses of more than 1 g should be infused over 1.5- 2 h. Continuous infusion of vancomycin is not recommended[60,61]

Adapted from 124, 125
MRSA: methicillin-resistant S. aureus; SSTI: skin and soft tissue infection.

TABLE 13.13

CAUSES OF VANCOMYCIN FAILURE IN A SINGLE-CENTER COHORT OF 320 PATIENTS WITH DOCUMENTED MRSA BACTEREMIA. LOGISTIC REGRESSION ANALYSIS

PARAMETER PREDICTING FAILURE	ADJUSTED ODDS RATIO	95% CONFIDENCE INTERVAL OF VANCOMYCIN THERAPY
Infective endocarditis	4.55	2.26–9.15
Nosocomial acquisition of infection	2.19	1.21–3.97
Initial vancomycin trough concentration < 15 mcg/mL	2.00	1.25–3.22
Vancomycin MIC > 1 mcg/mL	1.52	1.09–2.49

MIC, minimum inhibitory concentration; MRSA, methicillin-resistant S. aureus.
From Patel N, Pai MP, Rodvold KA, et al. Vancomycin: We can't get there from here. *Clin Infect Dis.* 2011;52:969–974.

Procalcitonin has been evaluated extensively (11 randomized prospective trials) as a biomarker to guide duration of therapy.[105] Procalcitonin has been used to guide initiation of therapy in three trials, to end therapy in four trials, and as a guide to both in four trials. Without exception, clinical outcomes were unchanged (nine trials) or length of stay was reduced (two trials). Also without exception, procalcitonin monitoring was antibiotic sparing, reducing prescriptions of antibiotics by 32–72% in three trials and duration of therapy by 1.7–7.1 days in eight trials.

There are few data and no guidelines to inform the clinical approach to the patient who has failed a course of antibacterial therapy. There is not even a clear definition of what constitutes failure. Has the patient failed if the SIRS response persists after three days, or five or seven? When should antibiotics be changed? Is the antibiotic therapy well-chosen, but the patient has inadequate source control and requires operation (or reoperation)?[145] If a patient still has SIRS at the predetermined end point, it is more useful to stop therapy and reevaluate for persistent or new infection, MDR pathogens, and noninfectious causes of SIRS than to continue therapy uninformed or to add or change antibiotics without additional data.

MANAGING MICROBIAL ECOLOGY (INCLUDING OUTBREAKS)

Prescribing the same antibiotic regimen repeatedly is believed to lead to resistance by increasing antibiotic selection pressure on a unit. Intensive care units are frequently the epicenter of

TABLE 13.14

CURRENT RECOMMENDATIONS FOR DURATION OF THERAPY FOR SELECTED SERIOUS INFECTIONS

Bacterial Meningitis	
Gram-negative bacilli (e.g., postoperative)	21 d
Central Line-Associated Blood Stream Infection	
Coagulase-negative *Staphylococcus*	5–7 d
S. aureus	14 d[a]
Enterococcus spp.	7–14 d
Gram-negative bacilli	7–14 d
Candida spp.	14 d after the last positive blood culture
Complicated intra-abdominal infection	4–7 d
Pneumonia	
CAP[b]	≤5 d
VAP[b]	
Bacteria other than NFGNB	7 d
NFGNB	14 d

[a]If the patient is not immunosuppressed or neutropenic, the catheter has been removed, there is no recent placement of a prosthetic intravascular device, and there is neither evidence of endocarditis (by echocardiography) or suppurative thrombophlebitis (by ultrasound). Fever and bacteremia must resolve within 72 h, and there must be no evidence of metastatic infection by physical examination. If these conditions are not met, six weeks of therapy is recommended.
[b]Supported by one or more randomized, prospective trials, rather than expert opinion.
CAP, community-acquired pneumonia; NFGNB, nonfermenting gram-negative bacilli; VAP, ventilator-associated pneumonia
From Hayashi DL, Paterson DL. Strategies for reduction in duration of antibiotic use in hospitalized patients. *Clin Infect Dis.* 2011;52:1232–1240.

nosocomial infections caused by MDR bacteria. Prevention of bacterial resistance is paramount to achieving good outcomes of critical care, but outbreaks do occur invariably, and must be managed. The microbiology laboratory supports the provision of appropriate antibiotic therapy by providing clinicians with "antibiograms" to aid empiric antibiotic choice and by providing MICs of key antibiotics so that antibiotic dosing is optimized to PD targets. Laboratories also play a crucial role in the prevention of antibiotic resistance. Molecular epidemiologic evidence of an oligoclonal outbreak of infections orients prevention measures toward investigation of common environmental sources of infection and prevention of patient-to-patient transmission. The US Centers for Disease Control and Prevention (CDC) has published several guidelines for management of outbreaks cause by MDR organisms, including hand hygiene, isolation precautions, and environmental controls.[146–149]

By contrast, evidence of polyclonality shifts the emphasis for prevention of antibiotic resistance to antibiotic management strategies. Specific antibiotics are discussed below; selection strategies for individual patients have been outlined above. Restoration of microbial ecology at the unit-specific or institutional level requires a coordinated effort. It has been demonstrated that the selective withdrawal of antibiotics that exert high selection pressure (e.g., ceftazidime, vancomycin, fluoroquinolones) is restorative of antibiotic susceptibility.[22–24,150] Whether the ecology can be maintained is still hypothetical. The underlying hypothesis states that if homogeneity of prescribing leads to increased antibiotic selection pressure, then diversity of prescribing will prevent the development of resistance.[151] Truly random prescribing cannot occur; each clinician will have his or her favored regimens, and bias is inevitable. The so-called heterogeneity of prescribing can be enforced through tactics referred to as "mixing" or "cycling." These constructs are not identical, in that in the former one antibiotic is withdrawn from use at a time, whereas cycling utilizes only a single agent for a defined period. Neither approach is clearly superior,[152] but cycling has been tested more extensively and found to be an effective tactic for both interdiction and maintenance in surgical ICUs,[102,153–156] but it is not a panacea.[157] Questions still to be answered about antibiotic cycling include which agents comprise an optimal cycle, and at what interval to cycle them.

SPECTRA OF ANTIBIOTIC ACTIVITY

Susceptibility testing of specific organisms is necessary for management of serious infections (including all nosocomial infections). Recommendations focus on agents useful for the treatment of serious/nosocomial infections; not every agent within the class will receive mention. Recommended agents for specific organisms are guidelines only, because *in vitro* susceptibilities may not correlate with clinical efficacy. Exposure to certain agents has been associated with the emergence of specific MDR bacteria, which require a different empiric antibiotic choice or modification of a regimen if identified or suspected (Table 13.1).

Cell Wall–Active Agents: Beta-lactam Antibiotics

The beta-lactam antibiotic group consists of penicillins, cephalosporins, monobactams, and carbapenems. Within this group, several agents have been combined with beta-lactamase inhibitors to broaden the spectrum of activity. Several subgroups of antibiotics are recognized within the group, notably penicillinase-resistant penicillins and several "generations" of cephalosporins.

Penicillins Penicillinase-resistant semisynthetic penicillins include methicillin, nafcillin, and oxacillin. These agents are useful as therapy for sensitive strains of staphylococci, but not as empiric agents, because of high rates of MRSA. Virtually all enterococcal species are resistant. However, if the *S. aureus* isolate is susceptible, any of these drugs is the treatment of choice (TOC).

Except for carboxypenicillins and ureidopenicillins, penicillins retain little or no activity against gram-negative bacilli. Carboxypenicillins (ticarcillin and carbenicillin) and ureidopenicillins (azlocillin, mezlocillin, and piperacillin; sometimes referred to as acylampicillins) are no longer used without a beta-lactamase inhibitor in combination (BLIC), such as sulbactam, tazobactam, clavulanic acid, which enhance the effectiveness of the parent beta-lactam agent (piperacillin > ticarcillin > ampicillin), and to a lesser extent the inhibitor (tazobactam > sulbactam ~ clavulanic acid). Piperacillin–tazobactam has the widest spectrum of activity against gram-negative bacteria and reasonable potency against *P. aeruginosa*. Ampicillin–sulbactam is unreliable against *Escherichia coli* and *Klebsiella* (resistance rate ~ 50%), but it has useful activity against *Acinetobacter* spp. owing to the sulbactam moiety. All of the BLIC agents have excellent anti-anaerobic activity.

Cephalosporins More than twenty agents comprise the class; their characteristics vary widely. The heterogeneity of spectrum requires broad familiarity with all of these drugs. First- and second-generation agents are useful only for prophylaxis, uncomplicated infections, or for de-escalation when results of susceptibility testing are known. "Third-generation" agents have enhanced activity against gram-negative bacilli (some have specific antipseudomonal activity), but only ceftriaxone is active against gram-positive cocci (but not MRSA), and none against anaerobes. Cefepime, a "fourth-generation" cephalosporin, has antipseudomonal activity and activity against most gram-positive cocci, but not MRSA. Ceftaroline (usual dose, 600 mg intravenously every 12 hours) has not been classified, but has anti-MRSA activity unique among the cephalosporins while retaining modest activity comparable to first-generation agents against gram-negative bacilli.[158] None of the cephalosporins are useful against enterococci.

Third-generation cephalosporins, particularly ceftazidime, have been associated with the induction of ESBL production among many of the Enterobacteriaceae (Table 13.1). Activity is reliable only against non-ESBL–producing species of Enterobacteriaceae including *Enterobacter*, *Citrobacter*, *Providencia*, and *Morganella*, but not for empiric monotherapy against nonfermenting gram-negative bacilli (e.g., *Acinetobacter* spp., *P. aeruginosa*, *Stenotrophomonas maltophilia*).

The potential of cefepime for induction of ESBL production is less than that of ceftazidime, but it, too, has no activity against either enterococci or enteric anaerobes. Similar to the carbapenems, cefepime is intrinsically more resistant to hydrolysis by beta-lactamases, but not enough to be reliable against ESBL-producing bacteria.

Monobactams

Aztreonam, the single agent of this class, has activity against gram-negative bacilli comparable to the third-generation cephalosporins, but no activity against gram-positive organisms or anaerobes. Aztreonam is not a potent inducer of beta-lactamases. Resistance to aztreonam is widespread, but the drug remains useful for directed therapy against known susceptible strains, and may be used safely for penicillin-allergic patients because the incidence of cross-reactivity is low.

Carbapenems

Imipenem–cilastatin, meropenem, doripenem, and ertapenem are available in the United States. Imipenem–cilastatin, meropenem, and doripenem have the widest (and generally comparable) antibacterial spectrum of any antibiotics, with excellent activity against aerobic and anaerobic streptococci, methicillin-sensitive staphylococci, and virtually all gram-negative bacilli except *Acinetobacter* spp., *Legionella* spp., *Pseudomonas cepacia*, and *S. maltophilia*.[159] All carbapenems are superlative anti-anaerobic agents; thus, there is no reason to combine a carbapenem with metronidazole except, for example, to treat concurrent mild *C. difficile* colitis in a patient with a coexistent life-threatening infection that mandates carbapenem therapy.

Meropenem and doripenem have less potential for neurotoxicity than imipenem–cilastatin, which is contraindicated in patients with active central nervous system disease or injury (excepting the spinal cord), because of the rare (~0.5%) appearance of myoclonus or generalized seizures in patients who have received high doses (with normal renal function) or inadequate dosage reductions with renal insufficiency. Ertapenem is not useful against *Pseudomonas* spp., *Acinetobacter* spp., *Enterobacter* spp., or MRSA, but its long half-life permits once-daily dosing.[160] Ertapenem is highly active against ESBL-producing Enterobacteriaceae and also has less potential for neurotoxicity. With all carbapenems, disruption of host microbial flora may lead to superinfections (e.g., fungi, *C. difficile*, *Stenotrophomonas*, resistant enterococci).

CELL WALL–ACTIVE AGENTS: LIPOGLYCOPEPTIDES

Vancomycin, a soluble lipoglycopeptide, is bactericidal, but tissue penetration is universally poor, which limits its effectiveness. Both *S. aureus* and *S. epidermidis* are usually susceptible to vancomycin, although MICs for *S. aureus* are increasing, requiring higher doses for effect,[124,125] and leading to rates of clinical failure that exceed 50% in some reports[140] (Table 13.13). *Streptococcus pyogenes*, group B streptococci, *S. pneumoniae* (including penicillin-resistant *S. pneumoniae*-PRSP), and *C. difficile* are susceptible. Most strains of *E. faecalis* are inhibited (but not killed) by attainable concentrations, but *E. faecium* is increasingly VRE.

Telavancin, a synthetic derivative of vancomycin, has been approved for treatment of cSSTI.[161] There appears to be a dual mechanism of action, including cell membrane disruption and inhibition of cell wall synthesis. The drug is active against MRSA, pneumococci including PRSP, and vancomycin-susceptible enterococci with MICs <1 mcg/mL. The most common side effects are taste disturbance, nausea, vomiting, and headache. There may be a small increased risk of acute kidney injury. The usual dose is 10 mg/kg, infused intravenously over 60 minutes, every 24 hours for 7–14 days; dosage reductions are necessary in renal insufficiency. No information is available regarding dosing during renal replacement therapy.

Cell Wall–Active Agents: Cyclic Lipopeptides

Daptomycin has potent, rapid bactericidal activity against most gram-positive organisms. The mechanism of action is via rapid membrane depolarization; potassium efflux; arrest of DNA, RNA, and protein synthesis; and cell death. Daptomycin exhibits concentration-dependent killing (Table 13.2), and has a long half-life (8 hours). A dose of 4 mg/kg once daily is recommended for cSSTI, versus 6 mg/kg/d for bacteremia. Daptomycin is excreted in the urine; therefore, the dosing interval should be increased to 48 hours when creatinine clearance <30 mL/min. No antagonistic drug interactions have been observed. Daptomycin is active against most aerobic and anaerobic gram-positive bacteria, including MDR strains such as MRSA, MRSE, VRE, *Peptostreptococcus* spp., *C. perfringens*, and *C. difficile*. Resistance to daptomycin has been reported for both MRSA and VRE.[143] Importantly, daptomycin must not be used for the treatment of pneumonia or empiric therapy when pneumonia is in the differential diagnosis, even when caused by a susceptible organism, because daptomycin penetrates lung tissue poorly and is also inactivated by pulmonary surfactant.[162]

Cell Wall–Active Agents: Polymyxins

Polymyxins are cyclic, cationic peptide antibiotics that have fatty acid residues[163]; two (polymyxins B and E, or colistin) have been used clinically. Polymyxins bind to the anionic bacterial outer membrane, leading to a detergent effect that disrupts membrane integrity. High affinity binding to the lipid A moiety of lipopolysaccharide may have a endotoxin-neutralizing effect. Commercial preparations of polymyxin B are standardized, but those of colistimethate (the less-toxic prodrug of colistin that is administered clinically) are not, so dosing depends on which preparation is being supplied. Most recent reports describe colistimethate use, but the drugs are therapeutically equivalent.

Dosing of polymyxin B is 1.5–2.5 mg/kg (15,000–25,000 U/kg) daily in divided doses, whereas dosing of colistimethate ranges from 2.5–6 mg/kg/d, also in divided doses. The diluent is voluminous, adding substantially to daily fluid intake. Data on PK are scant, but the drugs exhibit rapid concentration-dependent bacterial killing against a wide variety of gram-negative bacilli, including most isolates of *E. coli*, *Klebsiella* spp., *Enterobacter* spp., *P. aeruginosa*, *S. maltophilia*, and *Acinetobacter* spp. Excellent activity persists despite the widespread emergence of MDR pathogens. Combinations of polymyxin B or colistimethate and rifampin exhibit synergistic activity *in vitro*.[107] Tissue uptake is poor, but both intrathecal and inhalational administration have been described. Clinical response rates for respiratory tract infections appear to be lower than for other sites of infection.

Polymyxins fell out of favor due to nephro- and neurotoxicity, but the emergence of MDR pathogens has returned them to clinical use. Up to 40% of colistimethate-treated patients (5–15% for polymyxin B) will have an increase of serum creatinine concentration, but seldom is renal replacement therapy required. Neurotoxicity (5–7% for both) usually becomes manifest as muscle weakness or polyneuropathy.

PROTEIN SYNTHESIS INHIBITORS

Several classes of antibiotics, although dissimilar structurally and having divergent spectra of activity, exert their effects via binding to bacterial ribosomes and inhibiting protein synthesis. This classification is valuable mechanistically, linking several classes of antibiotics conceptually that have few clinically useful members.

Aminoglycosides

Although aminoglycosides were once disdained for their toxicity, a resurgence of aminoglycoside use has occurred as resistance to newer antibiotics (especially third-generation cephalosporins and fluoroquinolones) has developed. Gentamicin, tobramycin, and amikacin are still used frequently. Aminoglycosides bind to the bacterial 30S ribosomal subunit, inhibiting protein synthesis. Gentamicin has modest activity against gram-positive cocci; otherwise, the spectrum of activity of the several agents is nearly identical. Prescribing decisions should be based upon toxicity and local resistance patterns. Nevertheless, the potential for toxicity is real, and aminoglycosides are now seldom first-line therapy, except in a synergistic combination to treat a serious *Pseudomonas* infection, enterococcal endocarditis, or an infection caused by an MDR gram-negative bacillus. As second-line therapy, these drugs are highly efficacious against the Enterobacteriaceae but less active against *Acinetobacter* and have limited activity against *P. cepacia*, *Aeromonas* spp., and *S. maltophilia*.

Aminoglycosides kill bacteria most effectively with a concentration peak:MIC > 10; therefore, a loading dose is necessary, and serum drug concentration monitoring is performed.[123] Marked dosage reductions are necessary in renal insufficiency, but the drugs are dialyzed, and a maintenance dose should be given after each hemodialysis treatment.

Tetracyclines

Tetracyclines bind irreversibly to the 30S ribosomal subunit, but they are bacteriostatic only. Widespread resistance limits their utility in the hospital setting (with the exceptions of doxycycline, minocycline, and tigecycline [IV only]). Tetracyclines are active against anaerobes; *Actinomyces* can be treated successfully. Doxycycline is active against *Bacteroides fragilis*, but used seldom for the purpose. All tetracyclines are contraindicated in pregnancy and for children under the age of 8 years, owing to dental toxicity.

Tigecycline is a novel glycylcycline derived from minocycline (both are now available parenterally).[164] With the major exceptions of *Pseudomonas* spp. and *Proteus mirabilis*, the spectrum of activity is broad, including many MDR gram-positive and -negative bacteria, including MRSA, VRE, and *Acinetobacter* spp. Tigecycline overcomes typical bacterial resistance to tetracyclines because a modification at position 9 of its core structure enables high-affinity binding to the 30S ribosomal unit. Tigecycline is active against aerobic and anaerobic streptococci, staphylococci, MRSA, MRSE, and enterococci, including VRE. Activity against gram-negative bacilli is directed against Enterobacteriaceae including ESBL-producing strains, *Pasteurella multocida*, *Aeromonas hydrophila*, *S. maltophilia*, *Enterobacter aerogenes*, and *Acinetobacter* spp. Anti-anaerobic activity is excellent.

Concern has been raised recently by a post-hoc analysis that the mortality of tigecycline-treated patients is higher in pooled Phase 3–4 clinical trials, including unpublished registration trials.[165] The adjusted risk difference for all-cause mortality based on a random effects model stratified by trial weight was 0.6% (95% CI 0.1–1.2) between tigecycline and comparator agents. However, an independent meta-analysis found no such survival disadvantage in an analysis of eight published randomized controlled trials (4,651 patients).[166] Overall, no difference was identified for the pooled clinically- (OR 0.92, 95% CI 0.76–1.12) or microbiologically evaluable populations (OR 0.86, 95% CI 0.69–1.07) from the trials.

Oxazolidinones

Oxazolidinones bind to the ribosomal 50S subunit, preventing complexing with the 30S subunit. Assembly of a functional initiation complex for protein synthesis is blocked, preventing translation of mRNA. This mode of action is novel, in that other protein synthesis inhibitors permit mRNA translation but then inhibit peptide elongation. Linezolid is bacteriostatic against most susceptible organisms. The ribosomes of *E. coli* are as susceptible to linezolid as those of gram-positive cocci, but, with minor exceptions, gram-negative bacteria are oxazolidinone-resistant, because oxazolidinones are excreted from bacterial cells by efflux pumps.

Linezolid is equally active against MSSA and MRSA, vancomycin-susceptible enterococci and VRE, and against susceptible and PRSP pneumococci. Most gram-negative bacteria are resistant, but *Bacteroides* spp. are susceptible. Linezolid requires no dosage reduction in renal insufficiency, and exhibits excellent tissue penetration, but it is uncertain whether that provides clinical benefit in treatment of cSSTI or HAP/VAP.[167] Meta-analysis suggests that linezolid is equivalent to vancomycin for HAP/VAP,[168] but some clinicians believe that linezolid should supplant vancomycin as first-line therapy for serious infections caused by gram-positive cocci.

The Macrolide–Lincosamide–Streptogramin Family

Clindamycin The only lincosamide in active clinical use in surgical practice is clindamycin, which also binds to the 50S ribosome. Clindamycin has good antianaerobic activity (although *B. fragilis* resistance is increasing) and reasonably good activity against susceptible gram-positive cocci (not MRSA or VRE). Clindamycin is used occasionally for anaerobic infections and is preferred over vancomycin for prophylaxis of clean surgical cases in penicillin-allergic patients[115] (Table 13.8). Because clindamycin inhibits exotoxin production *in vitro*, it has been advocated in preference to penicillin as first-line therapy of invasive *S. pyogenes* infections.

DRUGS THAT DISRUPT NUCLEIC ACIDS

Fluoroquinolones

Fluoroquinolones inhibit bacterial DNA synthesis by inhibiting DNA gyrase, which folds DNA into a superhelix in preparation for replication. The fluoroquinolones exhibit a diminishing spectrum of activity, excellent oral absorption and bioavailability, and numerous toxicities (e.g., photosensitivity, cartilage [especially in children] and tendon damage, prolongation of the QTc interval). These agents have a marked propensity to develop (and induce, see Table 13.1) resistance. Ciprofloxacin, levofloxacin, and moxifloxacin (which has some anti-anaerobic activity) are available parenterally and orally. Several others have been withdrawn from the market or were never approved owing to toxicity.

Fluoroquinolones are most active against enteric gram-negative bacteria, particularly the Enterobacteriaceae and *Haemophilus* spp. There is some activity against *P. aeruginosa*, *S. maltophilia*, and gram-negative cocci. Activity against gram-positive cocci is variable, being least for ciprofloxacin and best for moxifloxacin. Ciprofloxacin is most active against *P. aeruginosa*. However, rampant overuse of fluoroquinolones is rapidly causing resistance that may limit severely the future usefulness of these agents.[169] Fluoroquinolone use has been associated with the emergence of resistant *E. coli*, *Klebsiella* spp., *P. aeruginosa* and MRSA.[170,171] Fluoroquinolones prolong the QTc interval and may precipitate the ventricular dysrhythmia *torsade de pointes*, so electrocardiographic measurement of the QTc interval before and during fluoroquinolone therapy is important. Also, fluoroquinolones interact with warfarin to cause a rapid, marked prolongation of the international normalized ratio, so warfarin anticoagulation must be monitored closely during therapy.

CYTOTOXIC ANTIBIOTICS

Metronidazole

Metronidazole is active against nearly all anaerobes, and many protozoa that parasitize human beings. Metronidazole has potent bactericidal activity, including activity against *B. fragilis*, *Prevotella* spp., *Clostridium* spp. (including *C. difficile*), and anaerobic cocci, although it is ineffective in actinomycosis. Resistance remains rare and of negligible clinical importance.

Metronidazole causes DNA damage after intracellular reduction of the nitro group of the drug. Acting as a preferential electron acceptor, it is reduced by low-redox potential electron transport proteins, decreasing the intracellular concentration of the unchanged drug and maintaining a transmembrane gradient that favors uptake of additional drug. The drug thus penetrates well nearly all tissues, including neural tissue, making it effective for deep-seated infections and bacteria that are not multiplying rapidly. Absorption after oral or rectal administration is rapid and nearly complete. The $T_{1/2}$ of metronidazole is 8 hours, owing to an active hydroxy metabolite. Intravenous metronidazole is usually administered every 8–12 hours in recognition of the active metabolite, but once-daily dosing is possible.[172] No dosage reduction is required for renal insufficiency, but the drug is dialyzed effectively, and administration should be timed to follow dialysis if twice-daily dosing is used. PK in patients with hepatic insufficiency suggest a dosage reduction of 50% with marked impairment.

Trimethoprim–Sulfamethoxazole (TMP–SMX)

Sulfonamides exert bacteriostatic activity by interfering with bacterial folic acid synthesis, a necessary step in DNA synthesis. Resistance is widespread, limiting use. The addition of sulfamethoxazole to trimethoprim, which prevents the conversion of dihydrofolic acid to tetrahydrofolic acid by the action of dihydrofolate reductase (downstream from the action of sulfonamides), accentuates the bactericidal activity of trimethoprim.

The combination of TMP–SMX is active against *S. aureus*, *S. pyogenes*, *S. pneumoniae*, *E. coli*, *P. mirabilis*, *Salmonella* and *Shigella* spp., *Yersinia enterocolitica*, *S. maltophilia*, *L. monocytogenes*, and *Pneumocystis jirovici*. Used for UTIs, acute exacerbations of chronic bronchitis, and *Pneumocystis* infections, TMP–SMX is a TOC for infections caused by *S. maltophilia* and outpatient (and sometimes inpatient) treatment of infections caused by CA-MRSA.

A fixed-dose combination of TMP–SMX of 1:5 is available for parenteral administration. The standard oral formulation is 80:400 mg, but lesser and greater strength tablets are available. Oral absorption is rapid and bioavailability is nearly 100%. Tissue penetration is excellent. Ten mL of the parenteral formulation contains 160:800 mg drug. Full doses (150–300 mg TMP in 3–4 divided doses) may be given if creatinine clearance is >30 mL/min, but the drug is not recommended when the creatinine clearance is <15 mL/min.

ANTIBIOTIC TOXICITIES

Beta-lactam Allergy

Allergic reaction is the most common toxicity of beta-lactam antibiotics. The incidence is approximately 7–40/1,000 treatment courses of penicillin,[173] and is more likely to be provoked by parenteral therapy. A history of penicillin allergy is sought commonly, and reported by 5–20% of patients (far in excess of the true incidence), therefore most serious reactions occur in patients with no history. Patients with a prior reaction have a four- to sixfold increased risk of another reaction compared to the general population, but the risk decreases with time, from 80–90% skin test reactivity at 2 months, to 20% reactivity at 10 years. The risk of cross-reactivity between penicillins and other beta-lactams (carbapenems and cephalosporins) is ~5%, being highest for first-generation cephalosporins.[173] There is negligible cross-reactivity to monobactams.

"Red Man" Syndrome

Tingling and flushing of the face, neck, or thorax may occur with parenteral vancomycin therapy but are less common than fever, rigors, or local phlebitis. The cause is believed to be histamine release due to local hyperosmolality. Although a hypersensitivity reaction, "red man" syndrome is not a true allergy owing to the clear association with too-rapid infusion of the drug (<1 hour for a 1 g dose, or <1.5–2 hours for a larger dose). Too-rapid infusion can also cause hypotension. A maculopapular rash due to hypersensitivity occurs in about 5% of patients.

Nephrotoxicity

All aminoglycosides are nephrotoxic, with little to distinguish among them. Aminoglycosides do not provoke inflammation, thus there is no allergic component to any manifestation of aminoglycoside toxicity. Mechanisms of toxicity include ischemia and toxicity to the renal proximal tubular cell (PTC).[174] Ultimately, injury manifests as necrosis of the PTC, reduction of the glomerular filtration rate, and decreased creatinine clearance but is usually reversible, and the need for renal replacement therapy is rare. Aminoglycoside nephrotoxicity is accentuated by frequent dosing, older age, sodium and volume depletion, acidemia, hypokalemia, hypomagnesemia, and coexistent liver disease. The risk of injury is ameliorated by single-daily-dose therapy.[123] If renal function deteriorates, it is advisable to discontinue therapy unless treatment is for a life-threatening infection.

Vancomycin nephrotoxicity is on the increase, owing to higher dosing and concurrent administration of other nephrotoxins.[124–126] Nephrotoxicity of polymyxins may be unavoidable; the need to use an agent with known nephrotoxic potential to treat serious infections caused by MDR gram-negative bacilli exists when alternatives are few or none.

Ototoxicity

Aminoglycosides cause cochlear or vestibular toxicity that is usually irreversible, and may develop after the cessation of therapy.[175] Repeated exposures create cumulative risk. Most patients develop either cochlear toxicity or a vestibular lesion, but rarely both. Cochlear toxicity can be subtle, because few patients have baseline audiograms, and formal screening is undertaken seldom. Few patients complain of hearing loss, yet when sought, the incidence of cochlear toxicity may be more than 60%. Clinical hearing loss may occur in 5–15%

of patients. Ototoxicity caused directly by vancomycin is documented poorly in the literature and may not occur unless vancomycin is coadministered with another ototoxin (e.g., aminoglycoside, furosemide). Hearing loss attributed to vancomycin is really neurotoxicity, manifesting as auditory nerve damage, tinnitus, and high-frequency hearing loss of acuity. There is no correlation between ototoxicity and nephrotoxicity for drugs that cause both (e.g., aminoglycosides, vancomycin).

AVOIDING TOXICITY: ADJUSTMENT OF ANTIBIOTIC DOSAGE

Hepatic Insufficiency

The liver metabolizes and eliminates drugs that are too lipophilic for renal excretion. The cytochromes P_{450} (a gene superfamily consisting of more than 300 different enzymes) oxidize lipophilic compounds to water-soluble products. Oxidation in particular is disrupted when liver function is impaired. Other enzymes metabolize drugs by conjugating them with sugars, amino acids, sulfate, or acetate to facilitate biliary or renal excretion.

Drug dosing in hepatic insufficiency is complicated by insensitive clinical assessments of liver function, and changing metabolism as the degree of impairment fluctuates (e.g., resolving cholestasis). Changes in renal function with progressive hepatic impairment add considerable complexity. Renal blood flow is decreased in cirrhosis, and glomerular filtration is decreased in cirrhosis with ascites. Adverse drug reactions are more frequent with cirrhosis than other forms of liver disease. The effect of liver disease on drug disposition is thus difficult to predict for individual patients.[176] Generally, a dosage reduction of up to 25% of the usual dose is considered if hepatic metabolism is 40% or less and renal function is normal (Table 13.15). Greater dosage reductions (up to 50%) are advisable if the drug is administered chronically, there is a narrow therapeutic index, protein binding is reduced considerably, or the drug is excreted renally and renal function is severely impaired.

Renal Insufficiency

Renal drug elimination depends on glomerular filtration, tubular secretion, and reabsorption, any of which may be altered with renal dysfunction. Kidney disease or acute kidney injury may affect hepatic as well as renal drug metabolic pathways. Drugs whose hepatic metabolism is likely to be disrupted in renal insufficiency include aztreonam, penicillins, several cephalosporins, macrolides, and carbapenems.

Accurate estimates of renal function are important in patients with mild-to-moderate renal dysfunction, because the clearance of many drugs by renal replacement therapy actually makes management easier. Factors influencing drug clearance by hemofiltration include molecular size, aqueous solubility, plasma protein binding, equilibration kinetics between plasma and tissue, and the apparent V_D. New high-flux polysulfone dialysis membranes can clear molecules up to 5 kDa efficiently (the molecular weight of vancomycin is 1.486 kDa). The need to dose patients during or after a renal replacement therapy treatment must be borne in mind; during continuous renal replacement therapy, the estimated creatinine clearance is approximately 15–25 mL/min in addition to the patient's intrinsic clearance.[177] For sustained low-efficiency dialysis, clearance rates of 60–100 mL/min may be achieved.[178] Cefaclor, cefoperazone, ceftriaxone, chloramphenicol, clindamycin, cloxacillin and dicloxacillin, doxycycline, erythromycin, linezolid, methicillin/nafcillin/oxacillin, metronidazole, rifampin, and tigecycline do not require dosage reductions in renal failure (Table 13.15). Conditions vary substantially from patient to patient, so dosing must be individualized and supported by therapeutic drug level monitoring when available.[179] Prolonged infusion of beta-lactam agents is not precluded.[180]

TABLE 13.15

ANTIBIOTICS THAT REQUIRE DOSAGE REDUCTION FOR HEPATIC AND RENAL INSUFFICIENCY

Hepatic
- Aztreonam
- Cefoperazone
- Chloramphenicol
- Clindamycin
- Erythromycin
- Isoniazid
- Linezolid
- Metronidazole
- Nafcillin
- Quinupristin/dalfopristin
- Rifampin
- Tigecycline

Renal
- Aminoglycosides
- Aztreonam
- Carbapenems
- Cephalosporins (most)
- Chloramphenicol
- Fluoroquinolones
- Macrolides (except erythromycin and fidoxamycin)
- Penicillins
- Polymyxins
- Sulfonamides
- Trimethoprim/sulfamethoxazole
- Vancomycin

PROPHYLAXIS AND THERAPY OF FUNGAL INFECTIONS

Fungi are ubiquitous heterotrophic eukaryotes, resilient to environmental stress and adaptable to diverse environments. The most important human pathogens are the yeasts and the molds. Invasive mycoses have emerged as a major cause of morbidity and mortality in hospitalized surgical patients. The incidence of nosocomial candidemia in the United States is approximately 8/100,000 population, at a cost of approximately $1 billion/year. Fungemia is the fourth most common type of blood stream infection in the United States, but many surgical patients develop invasive infections without positive blood cultures. Host or therapeutic immunosuppression, organ transplantation, implantable devices, and human immunodeficiency virus infection have all changed the landscape of fungal pathogenicity. The surgical ICU population is an extremely high-risk group.[181] Several conditions (both patient dependent and disease specific) are independent predictors for invasive fungal infection, including ICU length of stay, extent of medical comorbidity, host immune suppression, and the number of medical devices present. Neutropenia, diabetes mellitus, new-onset renal replacement therapy, central venous catheterization, total parenteral nutrition, broad-spectrum antibiotic administration, bladder catheterization, azotemia, diarrhea, corticosteroid therapy, and mechanical ventilation have also been associated with candidemia.[182,183]

Central Venous Catheters

Many episodes of candidemia represent a CLABSI. In non-neutropenic subjects, the most common portals of entry for catheter contamination (and subsequent infection) are from skin during catheter placement, manipulation of an indwelling catheter, and cross-infection among ICU patients attributed to health care workers. Other possible sources for primary catheter colonization include contaminated parenteral nutrition solution, multiple medication administration with repetitive violation of the sterile fluid path, and the presence of other medical devices. The secondary route of contamination for devices in direct contact with the blood stream (e.g., pacemakers, cardiac valves, joint prostheses) is candidemia originating from the gastrointestinal tract. Endogenous flora are also the most common source in neutropenic and other immunosuppressed patients. Once the catheter is contaminated, a stereotypical series of events occurs: Yeast adhere to the catheter surface and develop hyphae that integrate into a biofilm that increases in size and tridimensional complexity. Biofilms are the main reservoirs for candidemia secondary to contaminated medical devices, as they induce stasis and sequester the fungi from antimycotic medication and the immune response. In general, catheter removal is indicated following the diagnosis of systemic fungal infections and fungemia. Antifungal agents are usually continued for a defined period after blood cultures become negative after the catheter is removed (Table 13.14),[105] and *Candida* endophthalmitis should be ruled out (see below).

Prediction of Invasive Candida *Infection*

Overgrowth and recovery of *Candida* spp. from multiple sites (even from asymptomatic patients) carry a high likelihood of invasive candidiasis. Risk factors for the development of *Candida* colonization include female gender, antibiotic therapy prior to an ICU admission, a prolonged stay in the ICU, and multiple gastrointestinal operations.[184] The source of the pathogen in the surgical context is most frequently the gastrointestinal tract. Because colonization with *Candida* spp. presages invasive disease, it is desirable to identify and characterize patients further in terms of risk. Surveillance cultures may be used to screen ICU patients. Several scoring systems have been proposed to quantify the risk of invasive fungal infection (Table 13.16).[185–189] Comparisons between the *Candida* colonization index and the *Candida* score are few, but the *Candida* score may perform better.[190,191] The other scoring systems are less well validated.

The use of broad-spectrum antibiotics is a well-documented risk factor for fungal colonization and subsequent infection. Interrelations between bacteria and fungi in human disease are complex. *Candida* may enhance the pathogenicity of certain bacteria, but not others, and this interaction remains to be elucidated.[192] Antibiotics that have some antianaerobic therapy are associated with substantial increases in colony counts of yeast flora of the gut, whereas antibiotics with poor anaerobic activity are less likely to produce this effect.

PROPHYLAXIS OF FUNGAL INFECTION

The substantial morbidity and mortality of invasive fungal infections has led to the practice of administering prophylactic antifungal agents (usually fluconazole) to critically ill patients. Early on, concern was raised that increasing use of azole antifungals would lead to increased resistance to the agents.[193,194] A randomized, placebo-controlled trial of enteral fluconazole 400 mg/d was conducted among 260 critically ill surgical patients with an ICU length of stay of ≥3 days in a tertiary-care surgical ICU.[195] After adjusting for potentially confounding effects of the Acute Physiology and Chronic Health Evaluation (APACHE) III score, days to first dose, and fungal colonization at enrollment, the risk of fungal infection was reduced by 55% in the fluconazole group, but no difference in mortality was observed.

Four randomized studies comparing fluconazole to placebo for prevention of fungal infections in the surgical ICU were subjected to meta-analysis.[196] The studies enrolled 626 patients but used differing dosing regimens of fluconazole. All trials were double-blind; two were multicenter studies. Fluconazole prophylaxis reduced the incidence of fungal infections considerably (pooled OR 0.44; 95% CI 0.27-0.72; $p < 0.001$) but was not associated with a survival advantage (pooled OR for mortality 0.87; 95% CI 0.59–1.28). The absence of a survival advantage may reflect the paucity of data and a need for further study. Current guidelines recommend fluconazole prophylaxis for "high-risk" patients[197] (Table 13.17).

Antifungal Prophylaxis of Solid Organ Transplant Recipients

Solid organ transplantation is life-saving for end-stage organ failure, but invasive fungal infections remain a major cause of morbidity and mortality. Various tactics of prevention have been tested, including both systemic and topical antifungal prophylaxis. Currently, data support the use of antifungal prophylaxis with fluconazole in liver, lung, small bowel, and pancreas transplant recipients[197] (Table 13.17).

In a meta-analysis of randomized, placebo-controlled trials with fluconazole prophylaxis, the incidence of fungal infections was appreciably reduced; however, there was no survival advantage, similar to antifungal prophylaxis of critically ill general surgical patients.[198] A systematic review and meta-analysis of antifungal prophylaxis in liver transplant recipients evaluated ten randomized trials (1,106 patients) of any prophylactic antifungal regimen versus either no antifungal agent or another antifungal regimen.[199] Fluconazole prophylaxis did not reduce mortality (RR 0.84, 95% CI 0.54–1.30) but did reduce invasive fungal infections (RR 0.28, 95% CI: 0.13-0.57), while not increasing colonization or infection with azole-resistant fungi.

PRINCIPLES OF ANTIFUNGAL THERAPY

Candidemia is defined as (1) one blood culture that grows *Candida* spp. and either histologically documented invasive candidiasis, or ophthalmic examination consistent with candidal endophthalmitis; (2) at least two blood cultures obtained at different times from a peripheral vein that grow the same *Candida* spp.; or (3) one blood culture obtained peripherally and one blood culture obtained through an indwelling central

TABLE 13.16

SCORING SYSTEMS FOR RISK STRATIFICATION FOR INVASIVE CANDIDIASIS

***Candida* Colonization Index**[185]	
Number of cultures sites positive for the identical yeast isolate, divided by the number of sites cultured. At least three sites should be cultured (oral mucosa, axillae, rectum, gastric contents, and urine). A score ≥0.5 points is considered high risk for subsequent infection. Discrimination statistics were not reported	
***Candida* Score**[186]	
Five dichotomous variables are awarded points. A summed total score of ≥2.5 points is strongly predictive of invasive fungal infection (sensitivity 81%, specificity 75%, c statistic = 0.847)	
Total parenteral nutrition	1 point
Surgery on ICU admission	1 point
Multifocal *Candida* species colonization	1 point
Severe sepsis	2 points
Ostrosky-Zeichner Score (2007)[187]	
Prediction rule that provides a dichotomous risk assessment based on the presence of at least three risk factors. Relative risk 5, sensitivity 0.27, specificity 0.93, positive predictive value 0.13, negative predictive value 0.97, accuracy 0.90	
Any systemic antibiotic (days 1–3 of the ICU stay) *or*	
Central venous catheter (days 1–3) *and*	
At least two of the following: • Total parenteral nutrition (days 1–3) • Any renal replacement therapy (days 1–3) • Any major surgery (days 7 to 0) • Pancreatitis (days 7 to 0) • Any steroid use (days 7 to 3) • Any other immunosuppression (days –7 to 0)	
Ostrosky-Zeichner Modified Score (2011)[188]	
Prediction rule that provides a dichotomous risk assessment based on the presence of at least three risk factors. Relative risk 4, sensitivity 0.50, specificity 0.83, positive predictive value 0.10, negative predictive value 0.97, accuracy 0.81	
Mechanical ventilation > 48 h (days 1–4) *and*	
Any systemic antibiotic (days 1–3 of the ICU stay) *and*	
Central venous catheter (days 1–3) *and*	
At least one of the following: • Total parenteral nutrition (days 1–3) • Any renal replacement therapy (days 1–3) • Any major surgery (days –7 to 0) • Pancreatitis (days –7 to 0) • Any steroid or other immunosuppression (days –7 to 0)	
Shorr Candidemia Score[189]	
A simple, equal-weight score (one point each) differentiated reasonably well among patients admitted with a blood stream infection, with a c statistic of 0.70	
Age < 65 y	
Temperature ≤ 98°F or severe altered mental status	
Cachexia	
Hospitalization within the previous 30 d	
Admission from another health care facility	
Need for mechanical ventilation	

venous catheter, both of which grow identical *Candida* spp.. Patients with one positive blood culture drawn through an intravenous line and a positive semiquantitative catheter tip culture (>15 colony-forming units [cfu]) are not considered infected unless they satisfy one of the above criteria.

Severe nonbloodstream candidal infections are defined as *Candida* spp. isolated from a normally sterile body site, and the presence of at least one of the following: fever (>38.5°C) or hypothermia (<36°C), unexplained prolonged hypotension (systolic blood pressure <80 mm Hg > 2 hours, unresponsive to volume challenge), or absence of response to adequate antibiotic treatment for a suspected bacterial infection. *Candida* spp. pneumonia (which some authorities believe does not exist in immunocompetent hosts) requires the recovery of >10^5 cfu/mL of *Candida* spp, in bronchoalveolar lavage fluid, in addition to the appearance of a new infiltrate on CXR. Invasive

TABLE 13.17

SYNOPSIS OF CLINICAL PRACTICE GUIDELINES FOR THE MANAGEMENT OF CANDIDIASIS: INFECTIOUS DISEASES SOCIETY OF AMERICA-2009

Antifungal Prophylaxis for Solid-Organ Transplant Recipients, and Patients Hospitalized in Intensive Care Units

- Solid-organ transplant recipients:

Postoperative antifungal prophylaxis for liver (A-I), pancreas (B-II), and small bowel (B-III) transplant recipients at high risk of candidiasis, daily for 7–14 d

Fluconazole (200–400 mg [3–6 mg/kg]
Liposomal amphotericin B (L-AmB) (1–2 mg/kg)

- Patients hospitalized in the ICU:

Fluconazole (400 mg [6 mg/kg] daily) is recommended for high-risk patients in adult units that have a high incidence of invasive candidiasis (B-I)

Treatment of Identified Candidemia in Non-neutropenic Patients

- Initial therapy for most adult patients (A-I):

Fluconazole (loading dose of 800 mg [12 mg/kg] and then 400 mg [6 mg/kg] daily) or echinocandin
Caspofungin: loading dose of 70 mg and then 50 mg daily, or
Micafungin: 100 mg daily, or
Anidulafungin: loading dose of 200 mg and then 100 mg daily is recommended

- An echinocandin for is favored for patients with moderate-to-severe illness or for patients who have had recent azole exposure (A-III). Fluconazole is recommended for patients who are less critically ill and who have had no recent azole exposure (A-III). The same therapeutic approach is advised for children, with attention to differences in dosing
- Transition from an echinocandin to fluconazole is recommended for patients who have isolates that are likely to be susceptible to fluconazole (e.g., *Candida albicans*) and who are clinically stable (A-II)
- For infection due to *C. glabrata*, an echinocandin is preferred (B-III). Transition to fluconazole or voriconazole therapy is not recommended without confirmation of isolate susceptibility (B-III). For patients who received fluconazole or voriconazole initially, who have improved clinically, and who have negative follow-up cultures, continuation of the azole to completion of therapy is reasonable (B-III)
- For infection due to *C. parapsilosis*, treatment with fluconazole is recommended (B-III). Patients who have received an echinocandin initially, who have improved clinically, and who have negative follow-up cultures, continuation of the echinocandin to completion of therapy is reasonable (B-III)
- Amphotericin B deoxycholate (AmB-d) 0.5–1.0 mg/kg daily, or a lipid formulation of AmB (LFAmB) 3–5 mg/kg daily, are alternatives if there is intolerance to or limited availability of other antifungal agents (A-I). Transition from AmB-d or LFAmB to fluconazole is recommended if isolates are likely to be susceptible to fluconazole (e.g., *C. albicans*) and the patient is stable clinically (A-I)
- Voriconazole 400 mg (6 mg/kg) twice daily for two doses and then 200 mg (3 mg/kg) twice daily thereafter is effective for candidemia (A-I), but there is little advantage over fluconazole, and is recommended as step-down oral therapy for selected cases of candidiasis due to *C. krusei* or voriconazole-susceptible *C. glabrata* (B-III)
- The recommended duration of therapy for candidemia without obvious metastatic complications is for 2 weeks after documented clearance of *Candida* from the bloodstream and resolution of symptoms attributable to candidemia (A-III)
- Intravenous catheter removal is strongly recommended (A-II)

Empirical Treatment for Suspected Invasive Candidiasis in Non-neutropenic Patients

- Empirical therapy for suspected candidiasis in nonneutropenic patients is similar to that for proven candidiasis (B-III)

Fluconazole (loading dose of 800 mg [12 mg/kg] and then 400 mg [6 mg/kg] daily)
Caspofungin (loading dose of 70 mg and then 50 mg daily)
Anidulafungin (loading dose of 200 mg and then 100 mg daily)
Micafungin (100 mg daily)

- AmB-d (0.5–1.0 mg/kg daily) or LFAmB (3–5 mg/kg daily) are alternatives if there is intolerance to or limited availability of other antifungals (B-III)
- Empirical antifungal therapy should be considered for critically ill patients with risk factors for invasive candidiasis and no other known cause of fever, based on clinical assessment of risk, serologic markers for invasive candidiasis, or culture data from nonsterile sites (B-III)

NOTE: Strength of evidence-based recommendations is shown in parentheses.
Adapted from 197.

TABLE 13.17

ANTIFUNGAL AGENTS

ANTIFUNGAL AGENT	INDICATIONS	ROUTES/DOSAGE
Amphotericin B	*Candida albicans* (>95%) *C. glabrata* (95%), *C. parapsilosis* (>95%) *C. krusei* (>95%), *C. tropicalis* (99%) *C. guilliermondii*; *C. lusitaniae* Variable activity: *Aspergillus* spp., ferrous *Trichosporon beigelii* *Fusarium* spp., *Blastomyces dermatitidis*	IV: 0.5–1.0 mg/kg/d over 2–4 h Oral: 1 mL oral suspension, swish and swallow 4× daily, times 2 weeks
Amphotericin B liposomal (less nephrotoxicity)	*C. albicans* (>95%), *C. glabrata* (>95%) *C. parapsilosis* (>95%), *C. krusei* (>95%) *C. tropicalis* (99%), *C. guilliermondii*, *C. lusitaniae* Variable activity: *Aspergillus* spp.	IV: 3–5 mg/kg/d
Amphotericin B colloidal dispersion (less nephrotoxicity)	*C. albicans* (>95%), *C. glabrata* (>95%) *C. parapsilosis* (>95%), *C. krusei* (>95%) *C. tropicalis* (99%), *C. guilliermondii*; *C. lusitaniae* Variable activity: *Aspergillus* spp.	IV: 3–5 mg/kg/d
Amphotericin B lipid complex (less nephrotoxicity)	*C. albicans* (>95%), *C. glabrata* (>95%) *C. parapsilosis* (>95%), *C. krusei* (>95%) *C. tropicalis* (99%), *C. guilliermondii*, *C. lusitaniae* Variable activity: *Aspergillus* spp.	IV: 5 mg/kg/d
Ketoconazole	*C. albicans*	
Voriconazole	*Aspergillus* spp., *Fusarium* spp., *C. albicans* (99%) *C. glabrata* (99%), *C. parapsilosis* (99%) *C. tropicalis* (99%), *C. krusei* (99%), *C. guilliermondii* (>95%) *C. lusitaniae* (95%)	PO: 200–400 mg/daily IV: 6 mg/kg Q12 ×2 and then 4 mg/kg IV every 12 h PO: >40 kg, 200 mg every 12 h; <40 kg, 100 mg every 12 h
Fluconazole	*C. albicans* (97%) *C. glabrata* (85–90% resistant/intermediate) *C. parapsilosis* (99%) *C. tropicalis* (98%) *C. krusei* (5%) Fungistatic against *Aspergillus* spp.	Candidiasis: Prophylaxis (IV or oral): 100–400 mg/d Invasive: 400–800 mg/d Oropharyngeal: 200 mg day 1 and then 100 daily for 2 weeks
Itraconazole	Fungicidal to *Aspergillus* spp., *C. albicans* (93%) *C. glabrata* (50%), *C. parapsilosis* (45%) *C. tropicalis* (58%), *C. krusei* (69%) *C. guilliermondii*, *C. lusitaniae* Blastomycosis, histoplasmosis, chromomycosis	IV: Load 200 mg IV 2× daily × 4 doses and then 200 mg 4× daily maximum 14 d Oral: 200 mg every daily or 2× daily Life-threatening: load 600–800/d × 3–5/d and then 400–600 mg/d
Caspofungin	*C. albicans*, *C. glabrata*, *C. parapsilosis*, *C. tropicalis*, *C. krusei*, *C. guilliermondi*, *C. lusitaniae*	IV: 70 mg IV and then 50 mg IV every day
Micafungin	*C. albicans*, *C. glabrata*, *C. parapsilosis*, *C. tropicalis*, *C. krusei*, *C. guilliermondii*, *C. lusitaniae*	IV: 100–200 mg IV daily
Anidulafungin	*C. albicans*, *C. glabrata*, *C. parapsilosis*, *C. tropicalis*, *C. krusei*, *C. guilliermondii*, *C. lusitaniae*	Esophageal candidiasis: IV: 100 mg IV day 1, 50 mg/d thereafter Candidemia: IV: 200 mg IV day 1, 100 mg/d thereafter
Flucytosine	Not effective for *C. krusei* Effective for *C. albicans*, *C. tropicalis*, *C. parapsilosis*, *C. lusitaniae*	PO: 50–150 mg/kg/d divided QID
Nystatin	*C. albicans*	100,000 U swish and swallow QID
Clotrimazole	"Thrush" (usually not cultured)	Oral troches daily for 14 d

fungal infections in non-neutropenic ICU patients are treated if histology or cytopathology shows yeast cells or pseudohyphae from a needle aspiration or biopsy (excluding mucous membranes), a positive culture obtained aseptically from a normally sterile and clinically or radiologically abnormal site consistent with infection (excluding urine, sinuses, and mucous membranes), or positive percutaneous blood culture in patients with temporally related clinical signs and symptoms compatible with the relevant organism. Survival is more likely from candidemia than other forms of invasive candidiasis, and is strongly influenced negatively by critical illness.[200]

Antifungal Agents in the Practice of Acute Care Surgery

The repertoire of antifungal agents has expanded with the introduction of less-toxic formulations of amphotericin B, improved triazoles, echinocandins, and other agents that target the fungal cell wall.[201] Table 13.18 presents a list of available antifungal agents. Amphotericin B is a natural polyene macrolide that binds primarily to ergosterol, the principal sterol in the fungal cell membrane, leading to disruption of ion channels, production of oxygen free radicals, and apoptosis. It is active against most fungi and penetrates into cerebrospinal fluid. Tissue concentrations are not usually affected by hemodialysis. Infusion-related reactions can occur in up to 73% of patients with the first dose and often diminish during continued therapy. Amphotericin B–associated nephrotoxicity can lead to azotemia and hypokalemia, although acute potassium release with rapid infusion can occur and lead to cardiac arrest. Amphotericin B lipid formulations allow for higher dose administration with lessened nephrotoxicity, but whether outcomes are enhanced is unproved.

Nystatin is a polyene similar in structure to amphotericin B, and is currently used topically for *C. albicans*. Flucytosine, a fluorinated pyrimidine analog that is converted to 5-fluorouracil, causes RNA miscoding and inhibits DNA synthesis. It is available in the United States in oral form only, and has been used with amphotericin B for synergism against *Candida* spp., but in general there is scant evidence that any dual-agent therapy regimen for fungal infections is beneficial.[202]

The azoles inhibit the cytochrome P_{450}–dependent enzyme, 14-alpha reductase, altering fungal cell membranes through accumulation of abnormal 14-alphamethyl sterols. Fluconazole and itraconazole are available in oral and parenteral formulations and are active against *Candida* spp. except *C. krusei*, and *Fusarium* spp. Itraconazole is active against *Aspergillus* spp. As mentioned previously, *C. glabrata* and *C. krusei* resistance has been observed with fluconazole. The tissue concentrations of both fluconazole and itraconazole are influenced by many agents, such as antacids, H_2-antagonists, isoniazid, phenytoin, and phenobarbital. Biofilms produced by *Candida* spp. are penetrated by fluconazole and most other antifungal agents.[203,204]

Second-generation anti-fungal triazoles include posaconazole, ravuconazole, and voriconazole. They are active against *Candida* spp., including fluconazole-resistant strains, and *Aspergillus* spp. For the latter, voriconazole is emerging as the TOC.[205,206]

The echinocandins include caspofungin, micafungin, and anidulafungin, each of which is approved therapy for candidiasis and candidemia, but third-line treatment for invasive aspergillosis.[207] Due to their distinct mechanism of action, disrupting the fungal cell wall by inhibiting (1->3)-β-D-glucan synthesis, the echinocandins can theoretically be used in combination with other standard antifungal agents.[202] The echinocandins have activity against *Candida* spp. and *Aspergillus* spp. but are not reliably active against other fungi. Echinocandin activity is excellent against most *Candida* spp. but moderate against *C. parapsilosis*, *C. guilliermondii*, and *C. lusitaniae*. Echinocandins exhibit no cross-resistance with azoles or polyenes.[208] Prospective randomized trials have demonstrated that micafungin is non-inferior to caspofungin for therapy of invasive candidiasis,[209] and as effective as liposomal amphotericin B.[210]

With the proliferation of non-*albicans Candida* infections owing to widespread use of fluconazole, empiric therapy regimens recommend either an echinocandin or a lipid formulation of amphotericin B as the first-line agent for therapy of seriously or critically ill patients[199,211] (Tables 13.16 and 13.17). Once the pathogen has been identified as *Candida*, therapy may be de-escalated to fluconazole except for *C. glabrata* and *C. krusei*, for which continuation therapy with an echinocandin may be indicated (Table 13.18).

TABLE 13.18

USUAL SUSCEPTIBILITIES OF *CANDIDA* SPECIES TO SELECTED ANTIFUNGAL AGENTS

CANDIDA SPP.	FLUCONAZOLE	ITRACONAZOLE	VORICONAZOLE (NOT STANDARDIZED)	AMPHOTERICIN B	CASPOFUNGIN (NOT STANDARDIZED)
C. albicans	S	S	S	S	S
C. tropicalis	S	S	S	S	S
C. parapsilosis	S	S	S	S	S to I (?R)
C. glabrata	S-DD to R	S-DD to R	S to I	S to I	S
C. krusei	R	S-DD to R	S to I	S to I	S
C. lusitaniae	S	S	S	S to R	S

I, Intermediate; R, resistant; S, susceptible; S-DD, susceptible-dose dependent (increased MIC may be overcome by higher dosing, such as 12 mg/kg/d fluconazole).

References

1. Bochicchio GV, Joshi M, Bochicchio KV, et al. Early hyperglycemic control is important in critically injured trauma patients. *J Trauma.* 2007;63:1353-1358.
2. Claridge JA, Sawyer RG, Schulman AM, et al. Blood transfusions correlate with infections in trauma patients in a dose-dependent manner. *Am Surg.* 2002;68:566-572.
3. Barie PS. Eachempati SR, Pieracci FM. Infection. In: Feliciano DV, Mattox KL, Moore EE, eds. *Trauma.* 6th ed. New York, NY: McGraw-Hill; 2008:363-393.
4. Stillwell M, Caplan ES. The septic multiple trauma patient. *Infect Dis Clin North Am.* 1989;3:155-183.
5. Dente CJ, Tyburski JG, Wilson RF, et al. Ostomy as a risk factor for posttraumatic infection in penetrating colon injuries: univariate and multivariate analyses. *J Trauma.* 2000;49:628-634.
6. Papia G, McLellan BA, el-Helou P, et al. Infection in hospitalized trauma patients: incidence, risk factors, and complications. *J Trauma.* 1999;47:923-927.
7. Wallace WC, Cinat M, Gornick WB, et al. Nosocomial infections in the surgical intensive care unit: a difference between trauma and surgical patients. *Am Surg.* 1999;65:987-990.
8. Manian FA, Meyer PL, Setzer J, Senkel D. Surgical site infections associated with methicillin-resistant *Staphylococcus aureus*: do postoperative factors play a role? *Clin Infect Dis.* 2003;36:863-868.
9. Mangram AJ, Horan TC, Pearson ML, et al. Guideline for prevention of surgical site infection, 1999. Hospital Infection Control Practices Advisory Committee. *Infect Control Hosp Epidemiol.* 1999;20:250-278.
10. O'Grady NP, Alexander M, Burns MA, et al., and the Healthcare Infection Control Practices Advisory Committee (HICPAC). Guidelines for the prevention of intravascular catheter-related infections. *Clin Infect Dis.* 2011;52:e1-e32.
11. Mermel LA, Mermel MA, Bouza E, et al. Clinical practice guidelines for the diagnosis and management of intravascular catheter-related infection: 2009 update by the Infectious Diseases Society of America. *Clin Infect Dis.* 2009:49:1-45.
12. Minei JP, Nathens AB, West M, et al. Inflammation and the host response to injury large scale collaborative research program investigators. Inflammation and the host response to injury, a large-scale collaborative project: patient-oriented research core-standard operating procedures for clinical care. II. Guidelines for prevention, diagnosis and treatment of ventilator-associated pneumonia (VAP) in the trauma patient. *J Trauma.* 2006;60:1106-1113.
13. Guidelines for the management of adults with hospital-acquired, ventilator-associated, and healthcare-associated pneumonia. *Am J Respir Crit Care Med.* 2005;171:388-416.
14. Erasmus V, Daha TJ, Brug H, et al. Systematic review of studies on compliance with hand hygiene guidelines in hospital care. *Infect Control Hosp Epidemiol.* 2010;31:283-294.
15. Dancer SJ. The role of environmental cleaning in the control of hospital-acquired infection. *J Hosp Infect.* 2009;73:378-385.
16. zur Wiesch PA, Kouyos R, Engelstadter J, et al. Population biological principles of drug-resistance evolution in infections diseases. *Lancet Infect Dis.* 2011;11:236-247.
17. Hawkey PM, Jones AM. The changing epidemiology of resistance. *J Antimicrob Chemother.* 2009;64(suppl 1):i3-i10.
18. Wilcox MH. The tide of antimicrobial resistance and selection. *Int J Antimicrob Agents.* 2009;34(suppl 3):S6-S10.
19. Tacconelli E. Antimicrobial use: risk driver of multidrug resistant organisms in healthcare settings. *Curr Opin Infect Dis.* 2009;22:352-358.
20. Dellit TH, Owens RC, McGowan JE Jr, et al., Infectious Diseases Society of America and Society of Healthcare Epidemiology. Infectious Diseases Society of America and Society of Healthcare Epidemiology of America guidelines for developing an institutional program to enhance antimicrobial stewardship. *Clin Infect Dis.* 2007;44:159-177.
21. May AK, Melton SM, McGwin G, et al. Reduction of vancomycin-resistant enterococcal infections by limitation of broad-spectrum cephalosporin use in a trauma and nurn intensive care unit. *Shock.* 2000;14:259-264.
22. Rice LB, Eckstein EC, DeVente J, et al. Ceftazidime-resistant *Klebsiella pneumoniae* isolates recovered at the Cleveland Department of Veterans Affairs Medical Center. *Clin Infect Dis.* 1996;23:118-124.
23. Patterson JE, Hardin TC, Kelly CA, et al. Association of antibiotic utilization measures and control of multiple-drug resistance in *Klebsiella pneumoniae. Infect Control Hosp Epidemiol.* 2000;21:455-458.
24. Rahal JJ, Urban C, Segal-Maurer S. Nosocomial gram-negative resistance in multiple gram-negative species: experience at one hospital with squeezing the resistance balloon at multiple sites. *Clin Infect Dis.* 2002;34: 499-503.
25. DiPiro JT, Edmiston CE, Bohnen JMA. Pharmacodynamics of antimicrobial therapy in surgery. *Am J Surg.* 1996;171:615-622.
26. McKenzie C. Antibiotic dosing in critical illness. *J Antimicrobial Chemother.* 2011;66(suppl 2):ii25-ii31.
27. Lazar V, Chifiriuc MC. Architecture and physiology of microbial biofilms. *Roum Arch Microbiol Immunol.* 2010;69:95-107.
28. Wright JS III, Jin R, Novick RP. Transient interference with staphylococcal quorum sensing blocks abscess formation. *Proc Natl Acad Sci U S A.* 2005;102:169-1696.
29. Kiffer CR, Mendes C, Kuti JL, Nicolau DP. Pharmacodynamic comparisons of antimicrobials against nosocomial isolates of *Escherichia coli, Klebsiella pneumoniae, Acinetobacter baumannii*, and *Pseudomonas aeruginosa* from the MYSTIC surveillance program: the OPTAMA program, South America 2002. *Diagn Microbiol Infect Dis.* 2004;49:109-116.
30. Lipman J, Boots R. A new paradigm for treating infections: "Go hard and go home." *Crit Care Resusc.* 2009;11:276-281.
31. Mueller EW, Bouchard BA. The use of extended-interval aminoglycoside dosing strategies for the treatment of moderate-to-severe infections encountered in critically ill surgical patients. *Surg Infect (Larchmt).* 2009;10:563-570.
32. Anstead GM, Owens AD. Recent advances in the treatment of infections due to resistant *Staphylococcus aureus. Curr Opin Infect Dis.* 2004;17:549-555.
33. Kashuba AD, Bertino JS Jr, Nafziger AN. Dosing of aminoglycosides to rapidly attain pharmacodynamic goals and hasten therapeutic response by using individualized pharmacokinetic monitoring of patients with pneumonia caused by gram-negative organisms. *Antimicrob Agents Chemother.* 1998;42:1842-1844.
34. Thomas JK, Forrest A, Bhavnani SM, et al. Pharmacodynamic evaluation of factors associated with the development of bacterial resistance in acutely ill patients during therapy. *Antimicrob Agents Chemother.* 1998;42:521-527.
35. Benko AS, Cappelletty DM, Kruse JA, et al. Continuous infusion versus intermittent administration of ceftazidime in critically ill patients with suspected Gram-negative infections. *Antimicrob Agents Chemother.* 1996;40:691-695.
36. Lau WK, Mercer D, Itani KM, et al. Randomized, open-label, comparative study of piperacillin-tazobactam administered by continuous infusion versus intermittent infusion for treatment of hospitalized patients with complicated intra-abdominal infection. *Antimicrob Agents Chemother.* 2006;50:3556-3561.
37. Hoth JJ, Franklin GA, Stassen NA, et al. Prophylactic antibiotics adversely affect nosocomial pneumonia in trauma patients. *J Trauma.* 2003;55:249-254.
38. Velmahos GC, Toutouzas KG, Sarkisyan G, et al. Severe trauma is not an excuse for prolonged antibiotic prophylaxis. *Arch Surg.* 2002;137:537-541.
39. Bratzler DW, Houck PM, Surgical Infection Prevention Guideline Writers Workgroup: an advisory statement from the National Surgical Infection Prevention Project. *Am J Surg.* 2005;189:395-404.
40. Barie PS. Surgical site infections: epidemiology and prevention. *Surg Infect* 2002;3(suppl 1):S9-S21.
41. Classen DC, Evans RS, Pestotnik SL, et al. The timing of prophylactic administration of antibiotics and the risk of surgical-wound infection. *N Engl J Med.* 1992;326:281-286.
42. Hawn MT, Gray SH, Vick CC, et al. Timely administration of prophylactic antibiotics for major surgical procedures. *J Am Coll Surg.* 2006;203:803-811.
43. Zaneti G, Giardina R, Platt R. Intraoperative redosing of cefazolin and risk for surgical site infection in cardiac surgery. *Emerg Infect Dis.* 2001;7:828-831.
44. McDonald M, Grabsch E, Marshall C, Forbes A. Single- versus multiple-dose antimicrobial prophylaxis for major surgery: a systematic review. *Aust N Z J Surg.* 1998;68:388-396.
45. Namias N, Harvill S, Ball S, et al. Cost and morbidity associated with antibiotic prophylaxis in the ICU. *J Am Coll Surg.* 1999;188:225-230.
46. Fukatsu K, Saito H, Matsuda T, et al. Influences of type and duration of antimicrobial prophylaxis on an outbreak of methicillin-resistant *Staphylococcus aureus* and on the incidence of wound infection. *Arch Surg* 1997;132:1320-1325.
47. Bratzler DW, Houck PM, Richards C, et al. Use of antimicrobial prophylaxis for major surgery: baseline results from the National Surgical Infection Prevention Project. *Arch Surg.* 2005;140:175-182.
48. Platell C, Papadimitriou JM, Hall JC. The influence of lavage on peritonitis. *J Am Coll Surg.* 2000;191:672-680.
49. Yan RC, Shen SQ, Chen ZB, et al. The role of prophylactic antibiotics in laparoscopic cholecystectomy in preventing postoperative infection: a meta-analysis. *J Laparoendosc Adv Surg Tech A.* 2011;21:301-306.
50. Sanchez-Manuel FJ, Lozano-García J, Seco-Gil JL. Antibiotic prophylaxis for hernia repair. *Cochrane Database Syst Rev.* 2007;3:CD003769.
51. Kaafarani HM, Kaufman D, Reda D, Itani KM. Predictors of surgical site infection in laparoscopic and open ventral incisional herniorrhaphy. *J Surg Res.* 2010;163:229-234.
52. Swenson BR, Camp TR, Mulloy DP, Sawyer RG. Antimicrobial-impregnated surgical incise drapes in the prevention of mesh infection after ventral hernia repair. *Surg Infect (Larchmt).* 2008;9:23-32.
53. LeBlanc KA, Elieson MJ, Corder JM 3rd. Enterotomy and mortality rates of laparoscopic incisional and ventral hernia repair: a review of the literature. *JSLS.* 2007;11:408-414.

54. Stewart A, Evers PS, Earnshaw JJ. Prevention of infection in arterial reconstruction. *Cochrane Database Syst Rev.* 2006;3:CD003073.
55. Miller RS, Morris JA Jr, Diaz JJ Jr, et al. Complications after 344 damage-control open celiotomies. *J Trauma.* 2005;59:1365-1370
56. Vogel TR, Diaz JJ, Miller RS, May AK, et al. The open abdomen in trauma: do infectious complications affect primary abdominal closure? *Surg Infect.* 2006;7:433-441.
57. Al-Inany H, Youssef G, Abd ELMaguid A, et al. Value of subcutaneous drainage system in obese females undergoing cesarean section using Pfannenstiel incision. *Gynecol Obstet Invest.* 2002;53:75-78.
58. Magann EF, Chauhan SP, Rodts-Palenik D, et al. Subcutaneous stitch closure versus subcutaneous drain to prevent wound disruption after cesarean delivery: a randomized clinical trial. *Am J Obstet Gynecol.* 2002;186:1119-1123.
59. Siegman-Igra Y, Rozin R, Simchen E. Determinants of wound infection in gastrointestinal operations. The Israeli study of surgical infections. *J Clin Epidemiol.* 1993;46:133-140.
60. Noyes LD, Doyle DJ, McSwain NE. Septic complications associated with the use of peritoneal drains in liver trauma. *J Trauma.* 1998;28:337-346.
61. Magee C, Rodeheaver GT, Golden GT, et al. Potentiation of wound infection by surgical drains. *Am J Surg.* 1976;131;28:14-20.
62. Vilar-Compote D, Mohar A, Sandoval S, et al. Surgical site infections at the National Cancer Institute in Mexico: a case-control study. *Am J Infect Control.* 2002;28:14-20.
63. Barie PS. Are we draining the life from our patients? *Surg Infect.* 2002;3:159-160.
64. Weigelt JA. Risk of wound infections in trauma patients. *Am J Surg.* 1985;150:782-784.
65. Bites (mammalian). *Clin Evid.* (Online) 2010 Jul 27:pli 0914. Accessed at http://clinicalevidence.bmj.com/ceweb/conditions/wnd/0914/0914.jsp.
66. Quinn JV, McDermott D, Rossi J, et al. Randomized controlled trial of prophylactic antibiotics for dog bites with refined cost model. *West J Emerg Med.* 2010;11:435-441.
67. Dailey AJ, Lipman J, Venkatesh B, et al. Inadequate antimicrobial prophylaxis during surgery: a study of beta-lactam levels during burn debridement. *J Antimicrobial Chemother.* 2007;60:166-169.
68. Korinek AM, Baugnon T, Goimard JL, et al. Risk factors for adult nosocomial meningitis after craniotomy: role of antibiotic prophylaxis. *Neurosurgery.* 2008;62(suppl 2):532-539.
69. Barker FG 2nd. Efficacy of prophylactic antibiotics against meningitis after craniotomy: a meta-analysis. *Neurosurgery.* 2007;60:887-894.
70. Singer AJ, Dagum AB. Current concepts: current management of cutaneous wounds. *N Engl J Med.* 2008;359:1037-1042.
71. Dire DJ, Coppola M, Dwyer DA. A prospective evaluation of topical antibiotics for preventing infections in uncomplicated soft-tissue wounds repaired in the ED. *Acad Emerg Med.* 1995;2:4-10.
72. Cummings P, Del Beccaro MA. Antibiotics to prevent infection of simple wounds: a meta-analysis of randomized trials. *Am J Emerg Med.* 1995;13:396-400.
73. Gillespie WJ, Walenkamp GH. Antibiotic prophylaxis for surgery of proximal femoral and other closed long bone fractures. *Cochrane Database Syst Rev.* 2010;3:CD000244.
74. Slobogean GP, Kennedy SA, Davidson D, O'Brien PJ. Single- versus multiple-dose prophylaxis in the surgical treatment of closed fractures: a meta-analysis. *J Orthop Trauma.* 2008;22:284-289.
75. Lauder A, Jalisi S, Spiegel A, et al. Antibiotic prophylaxis in the management of complex midface and frontal sinus trauma. *Laryngoscope.* 2010;10:1940-1945.
76. Lovato C, Wagner JD. Infection rates following perioperative prophylactic antibiotics versus postoperative extended regimen prophylactic antibiotics in surgical management of mandibular fractures. *J Oral Maxillfac Surg.* 2008;67:827-832.
77. Kyzas PA. Use of antibiotics in the treatment of mandible fractures: a systematic review. *J Oral Maxillofac Surg.* 2011;69:1129-1145.
78. Andreasen JO, Jensen SS, Schwartz O, Hilerup Y. A systematic review of prophylactic antibiotics in the surgical treatment of maxillofacial fractures. *J Oral Maxillofac Surg.* 2006;64:1664-1668.
79. Martin B, Ghosh A, mackway-Jones K. Antibiotics in orbital floor fractures. *Emerg Med J.* 2003;20:66.
80. Hauser CJ, Adams CA Jr, Eachempati SR, Council of the Surgical Infection Society. Prophylactic antibiotic use in open fractures: an evidence-based guideline. *Surg Infect. (Larchmt)* 2006;6:379-405.
81. Luchette FA, Borzotta AP, Croce MA, et al. Practice management guidelines for prophylactic antibiotic use in penetrating abdominal trauma: the EAST Practice Management Guidelines Work Group. *J Trauma.* 2000;48:508-518.
82. Bratton SL, Chestnut RM, Ghajar J, et al. Guidelines for the management of severe traumatic brain injury. IV. Infection prophylaxis. *J Neurotrauma.* 2007;24(suppl 1):S26-S31.
83. May AK, Fleming SB, Carpenter RO, et al. Influence of broad-spectrum antibiotic prophylaxis on intracranial pressure monitor infections and subsequent infectious complications in head-injured patients. *Surg Infect.* 2006;7:409-417.
84. Stoikes NF, Magniotti LJ, Hodges TM, et al. Impact of intracranial pressure monitor prophylaxis on central nervous system infections and bacterial multi-drug resistance. *Surg Infect. (Larchmt)* 2008;503-508.
85. Villalobos T, Arango C, Kubills P, Rathore M. Antibiotic prophylaxis after basilar skull fractures: a meta-analysis. *Clin Infect Dis.* 1998;27: 364-369.
86. Ali B, Ghosh A, Mackway-Jones K. Antibiotics in compound depressed skull fractures. *Emerg Med J.* 2002;19:552-553.
87. Ratilal B, Costa J, Sampaio C, Looke D, Dendle C. Antibiotic prophylaxis for preventing meningitis in patients with basilar skull fractures. *Cochrane Database Syst Rev.* 2006;(1):CD004884.
88. Dunn LT, Foy PM. Anticonvulsant and antibiotic prophylaxis in head injury. *Ann R Coll Surg Engl.* 1994;76:147-149.
89. Luchette FA, Barrie PS, Oswanski MF, et al. Practice management guidelines for prophylactic antibiotic use in tube thoracostomy for traumatic hemopneumothorax: the EAST Practice Management Guidelines Work Group. Eastern Association for Trauma. *J Trauma.* 2000;48:753-757.
90. Barie PS, Hydo LJ, Eachempati SR. Causes and consequences of fever complicating critical surgical illness. *Surg Infect.* 2004;5:145-159.
91. O'Grady NP, Barie PS, Bartlett JG, et al. Guidelines for evaluation of new fever in critically ill adult patients: 2008 update from the American College of Critical Care Medicine and the Infectious Diseases Society of America. *Crit Care Med.* 2008;36:1330-1349. Erratum in *Crit Care Med* 2008;36:1992.
92. Barie PS, Hydo LJ, Shou J, et al. Influence of antibiotic therapy on mortality of critical surgical illness caused or complicated by infection. *Surg Infect.* (Larchmt) 2005;6:41-54.
93. Kollef MH, Ward S, Sherman G, et al. Inadequate treatment of nosocomial infections is associated with certain empiric antibiotic choices. *Crit Care Med.* 2000;28:3456-3464.
94. Alvarez-Lerma F. Modification of empiric antibiotic treatment in patients with pneumonia acquired in the intensive care unit: ICU-Acquired Pneumonia Study Group. *Intensive Care Med.* 1996; 22:387-394.
95. Garnacho-Montero J, Garcia-Garmendia JL, Barrero-Almodovar A, et al. Impact of adequate empirical antibiotic therapy on the outcome of patients admitted to the intensive care unit with sepsis. *Crit Care Med.* 2003; 31:2742-2751.
96. Golob JF Jr, Claridge JA, Sando MJ, et al. Fever and leukocytosis in critically ill trauma patients: it's not the urine. *Surg Infect.* (Larchmt) 2008;9:49-56.
97. Pieracci FM, Barie PS. Strategies in the prevention and management of ventilator-associated pneumonia. *Am Surg.* 2007;73:419-432.
98. Shorr AF, Sherner JH, Jackson WL, Kollef MH. Invasive approaches to the diagnosis of ventilator-associated pneumonia: a meta-analysis. *Crit Care Med.* 2005;33:46-53.
99. Trautner BW, Claridge JE, Darouiche RO. Skin antisepsis kits containing alcohol and chlorhexidine gluconate or tincture of iodine are associated with low rates of blood culture contamination. *Infect Control Hosp Epidemiol.* 2002;23:397-401.
100. Cockerill FR 3rd, Wilson JW, Vetter EA, et al. Optimal testing parameters for blood cultures. *Clin Infect Dis.* 2004;38:1724-1730.
101. Kumar A, Roberts D, Wood KE, et al. Duration of hypotension before initiation of effective antimicrobial therapy is the critical determinant of survival in human septic shock. *Crit Care Med.* 2006;34:1589-1596.
102. Barie PS, Hydo LJ, Shou J, et al. Influence of antibiotic therapy on mortality of critical surgical illness caused or complicated by infection. *Surg Infect. (Larchmt)* 2005;6:41-54.
103. Dellinger RP, Levy MM, Carlet JM, et al., International Surviving Sepsis Campaign Guidelines Committee; American Association of Critical-Care Nurses; American College of Chest Physicians; American College of Emergency Physicians; Canadian Critical Care Society; European Society of Clinical Microbiology and Infectious Diseases; European Society of Intensive Care Medicine; European Respiratory Society; International Sepsis Forum; Japanese Association for Acute Medicine; Japanese Society of Intensive Care Medicine; Society of Critical Care Medicine; Society of Hospital Medicine; Surgical Infection Society; World Federation of Societies of Intensive and Critical Care Medicine. Surviving Sepsis Campaign: international guidelines for management of severe sepsis and septic shock: 2008. *Crit Care Med.* 2008;36:296-327. Erratum in: *Crit Care Med.* 2008;36:1394-1396.
104. Kollef MH, Micek ST. Strategies to prevent antimicrobial resistance in the intensive care unit. *Crit Care Med.* 2005;33:1845-1853.
105. Hayashi DL, Paterson DL. Strategies for reduction in duration of antibiotic use in hospitalized patients. *Clin Infect Dis.* 2011;52:1232-1240.
106. Giamarellou H. Treatment options for multidrug-resistant bacteria. *Expert Rev Antiinfect Ther.* 2006;4:601-618.
107. Rahal JJ. Novel antibiotic combinations against infections with almost completely resistant *Pseudomonas aeruginosa* and *Acinetobacter* species. *Clin Infect Dis.* 2006;43:S95-S99.
108. Aarts MA, Hancock JN, Heyland D, et al. Empiric antibiotic therapy for suspected ventilator-associated pneumonia: a systematic review and meta-analysis of randomized trials. *Crit Care Med.* 2008;36:108-117.
109. Paul M, Benuri-Silbiger I, Soares-Weiser K, et al. Beta-lactam monotherapy versus beta-lactam-aminoglycoside combination therapy for sepsis in immunocompetent patients: systematic review and meta-analysis of randomized trials. *BMJ.* 2004;328:668-672.
110. Kumar A, Zarychanski R, Light B, et al. Early combination antibiotic therapy yields improved survival compared with monotherapy in septic shock: a propensity-matched analysis. *Crit Care Med.* 2010;38:1773-1785.

111. Ost DE, Hall CS, Joseph G, et al. Decision analysis of antibiotic and diagnostic strategies in ventilator-associated pneumonia. *Am J Respir Crit Care Med*. 2003;168:1060-1067.
112. American Thoracic Society. Guidelines for the management of adults with hospital-acquired, ventilator-associated, and healthcare-associated pneumonia. *Am J Respir Crit Care Med*. 2005;171:388-410.
113. Solomkin JS, Mazuski JE, Bradley JS, et al. Diagnosis and management of complicated intra-abdominal infection in adults and children: guidelines by the Surgical Infection Society and the Infectious Diseases Society of America. *Surg Infect. (Larchmt)* 2010;11:79-109.
114. Kollef MH, Kollef KE. Antibiotic utilization and outcomes for patients with clinically suspected VAP and negative quantitative BAL cultures results. *Chest*. 2005;128:2706-2713.
115. Hosein S, Udy AA, Lipman J. Physiological changes in the critically ill patient with sepsis. *Curr Pharm Biotechnol*. 2011 May 10 [Epub ahead of print].
116. Thomas JK, Forrest A, Bhavnani SM, et al. Pharmacodynamic evaluation of factors associated with the development of bacterial resistance in acutely ill patients during therapy. *Antimicrob Agents Chemother*. 1998;42:521-527.
117. Zelenitsky SA, Ariano RE, Zhanel GG. Pharmacodynamics of empirical antibiotic monotherapies for an intensive care unit (ICU) population based on Canadian surveillance data. *J Antimicrob Chemother*. 2011;66:343-349.
118. Koomanachai P, Bulik CC, Kuti JL, Nicolau DP. Pharmacodynamic modeling of intravenous antibiotics against gram-negative bacteria collected in the United States. *Clin Ther*. 2010;32:766-779.
119. Ulldemolins M, Roberts JA, Rello J, et al. The effects of hypoalbuminaemia on optimizing antibacterial dosing in critically ill patients. *Clin Pharmacokinet*. 2010;50:99-110.
120. Pieracci FM, Barie PS, Pomp A. Critical care of the bariatric patient. *Crit Care Med*. 2006;34:1796-1804.
121. Udy A, Boots R, Senthuran S, et al. Augmented creatinine clearance in traumatic brain injury. *Anesth Analg*. 2010;111:1505-1510.
122. Ulldemolins M, Roberts JA, Lipman J, Rello J. Antibiotic dosing in multiple organ dysfunction syndrome. *Chest* 2011;139:1210-1020.
123. Kashuba AD, Bertino JS Jr, Nafziger AN. Dosing of aminoglycosides to rapidly attain pharmacodynamic goals and hasten therapeutic response by using individualized pharmacokinetic monitoring of patients with pneumonia caused by gram-negative organisms. *Antimicrob Agents Chemother*. 1998;42:1842-1844.
124. Rybak MJ, Lomaestro BM, Rotschaefer JC, et al. Vancomycin therapeutic guidelines: a summary of consensus recommendations from the Infectious Diseases Society of America, the American Society of Health-System Pharmacists, and the Society of Infectious Diseases Pharmacists. *Clin Infect Dis*. 2009;49:325-327.
125. Liu C, Bayer A, Cosgrove SE, et al. Clinical practice guidelines by the Infectious Diseases Society of America for the treatment of methicillin-resistant *Staphylococcus aureus* infections in adults and children. *Clin Infect Dis*. 2011;52:e18-e55.
126. Lodise TP, Patel N, Lomaestro BM, et al. Relationship between initial vancomycin concentration-time profile and nephrotoxicity among hospitalized patients. *Clin Infect Dis*. 2009;49:507-514.
127. Roberts JA, Kirkpatrick CM, Lipman J. Monte Carlo simulations: maximizing antibiotic pharmacokinetic data to optimize clinical practice for critically ill patients. *J Antimicrob Chemother*. 2011;66:227-231.
128. Crandon JL, Ariano RE, Zelenitsky SA, et al. Optimization of meropenem dosage in the critically ill population based on renal function. *Intensive Care Med*. 2011;37:632-638.
129. Nicasio AM, Ariano RE, Zelenitsky SA, et al. Population pharmacokinetics of high-dose, prolonged-infusion cefepime in adult critically ill patients with ventilator-associated pneumonia. *Antimicrob Agents Chemother*. 2009;53:1476-1481.
130. Kim A, Kuti JL, Nicolau DP. Probability of pharmacodynamic target attainment with standard and prolonged-infusion antibiotic regimens for empiric therapy in adults with hospital-acquired pneumonia. *Clin Ther*. 2009;31:2765-2678.
131. Ong CT, Kuti JL, Nicolau DP; OPTAMA Program. Pharmacodynamic modeling of imipenem-cilastatin, meropenem, and piperacillin-tazobactam for empiric therapy of skin and soft tissue infections: a report from the OPTAMA Program. *Surg Infect. (Larchmt)* 2005;6:419-426.
132. Kotapati S, Kuti JL, Nicolau DP. Pharmacodynamic modeling of beta-lactam antibiotics for the empiric treatment of secondary peritonitis: a report from the OPTAMA program. *Surg Infect. (Larchmt)* 2005;6:297-304.
133. Benko AS, Cappelletty DM, Kruse JA, et al. Continuous infusion versus intermittent administration of ceftazidime in critically ill patients with suspected Gram-negative infections. *Antimicrob Agents Chemother*. 1996;40:691-695.
134. Lau WK, Mercer D, Itani KM, et al. Randomized, open-label, comparative study of piperacillin-tazobactam administered by continuous infusion versus intermittent infusion for treatment of hospitalized patients with complicated intra-abdominal infection. *Antimicrob Agents Chemother*. 2006;50:3556-3561.
135. Lodise TP Jr, Lomaestro B, Drusano GL. Piperacillin-tazobactam for *Pseudomonas aeruginosa* infection: clinical implications of an extended-infusion dosing strategy. *Clin Infect Dis*. 2007;44:357-363.
136. Dulhunty JM, Paterson D, Webb SA, Lipman J. Antimicrobial utilisation in 37 Australian and New Zealand intensive care units. *Anaesth Intensive Care*. 2011;39:231-237.
137. Roberts JA, Taccone FS, Udy AA, et al. Vancomycin dosing in critically ill patients: robust methods for improved continuous-infusion regimens. *Antimicrob Agents Chemother*. 2011;55:2704-2709.
138. FDA lowers breakpoints for staph infections. http://news.idsociety.org/idsa/issues/2008-05-01. Accessed June 20, 2011.
139. Haque NZ, Zuniga LC, Peyrani P. Relationship of vancomycin minimum inhibitory concentration to mortality in patients with methicillin-resistant *Staphylococcus aureus* hospital-acquired, ventilator-associated, or health-care-associated pneumonia. Improving Medicine through Pathway Assessment of Critical Therapy of Hospital-Acquired Pneumonia (IMPACT-HAP) Investigators. *Chest* 2010;138:1356-1362.
140. Kullar R, Davis SL, Levine DP, Rybak MJ. Impact of vancomycin exposure on outcomes in patients with methicillin-resistant *Staphylococcus aureus* bacteremia: support for consensus guideline suggested targets. *Clin Infect Dis*. 2011;52:975-981.
141. Patel N, Pai MP, Rodvold KA, et al. Vancomycin: we can't get there from here. *Clin Infect Dis*. 2011;52:969-974.
142. Farrell DJ, Mendes RE, Ross JE, et al. LEADER program results for 2009: an activity and spectrum analysis of linezolid using 6,414 clinical isolates from the United States (56 medical centers). *Antimicrob Agents Chemother*. 2011 Jun 13 [Epub ahead of print].
143. Kelley PG, Gao W, Ward PB, Howden BP. Daptomycin non-susceptibility in vancomycin-intermediate *Staphylococcus aureus* (VISA) and heterogeneous-VISA (hVISA): implications for therapy after vancomycin treatment failure. *J Antimicrob Chemother*. 2011;66:1057-1060.
144. Bulik CC, Nicolau DP. Double-carbapenem therapy for carbapenemase-producing *Klebsiella pneumoniae*. *Antimicrob Agents Chemother*. 2011;55:3002-3004.
145. Marshall JC, Maier RV, Jimenez M, Dellinger EP. Source control in the management of severe sepsis and septic shock: an evidence-based review. *Crit Care Med*. 2004;32:S513-S526.
146. Siegel JD, Rhinehart E, Jackson M, Chiarello L; the Healthcare Infection Control Practices Advisory Committee. Management of multidrug-resistant organisms in healthcare settings, 2006. http://www.cdc.gov/hicpac/mdro/mdro_2.html. Accessed June 8, 2011.
147. Siegel JD, Rhinehart E, Jackson M, Chiarello L, the Healthcare Infection Control Practices Advisory Committee. 2007 Guideline for isolation precautions: preventing transmission of infectious agents in healthcare settings. http://www.cdc.gov/ncidod/dhqp/pdf/isolation2007.pdf. Accessed June 8, 2011.
148. Sehulster LM, Chinn RYW, Arduino MJ, et al. Guidelines for environmental infection control in health-care facilities. Recommendations from CDC and the Healthcare Infection Control Practices Advisory Committee (HICPAC). Chicago, IL: American Society for Healthcare Engineering/American Hospital Association; 2004. Accessed June 8, 2011.
149. Boyce JM, Pittet D. Guideline for hand hygiene in health-care settings recommendations of the healthcare infection control practices advisory committee and the HICPAC/SHEA/APIC/IDSA hand hygiene task force. http://www.cdc.gov/mmwr/preview/mmwrhtml/rr5116a1.htm. Accessed June 8, 2011.
150. Kollef MH, Vlasnik J, Sharpless L, et al. Scheduled change of antibiotic classes: a strategy to decrease the incidence of ventilator-associated pneumonia. *Am J Respir Crit Care Med*. 1997;156(4 Pt 1):1040-1048.
151. Sandiumenge A, Diaz E, Rodriguez A, et al. Impact of diversity of antibiotic use on development of antimicrobial resistance. *J Antimicrob Chemother*. 2006;57:1197-1204.
152. Bal AM, Kumar A, Gould IM. Antibiotic heterogeneity: from concept to practice. *Ann N Y Acad Sci*. 2010;1213:81-91.
153. Raymond DP, Pelletier SJ, Crabtree TD, et al. Impact of a rotating empiric antibiotic schedule on infectious mortality in an intensive care unit. *Crit Care Med*. 2001;29:1101-1108.
154. Smith RL, Evans HL, Chong TW, et al. Reduction in rates of methicillin-resistant *Staphylococcus aureus* infection after introduction of quarterly linezolid-vancomycin cycling in a surgical intensive care unit. *Surg Infect. (Larchmt)* 2008;9:423-431.
155. Evans HL, Sawyer RG. Preventing bacterial resistance in surgical patients. *Surg Clin North Am*. 2009;89:501-519.
156. Dortch MJ, Fleming SB, Kauffmann RM, et al. Infection reduction strategies including antibiotic stewardship protocols in surgical and trauma intensive care units are associated with reduced resistant gram-negative healthcare-associated infections. *Surg Infect. (Larchmt)* 2011;12:15-25.
157. Curtis L. Need for both antibiotic cycling and stringent environmental controls to prevent *Pseudomonas* infections. *Surg Infect. (Larchmt)* 2009;10:163-173.
158. Kaushik D, Rathi S, Jain A. Ceftaroline: a comprehensive update. *Int J Antimicrob Agents*. 2011;37:387-395.
159. Rodloff AC, Goldstein EJ, Torres A. Two decades of imipenem therapy. *J Antimicrob Chemother*. 2006;58:916-929.
160. Zhanel GG, Johanson C, Embil JM, et al. Ertapenem: review of a new carbapenem. *Expert Rev Anti Infect Ther*. 2005;31:23-39.
161. Chang MH, Kish TD, Fung HB. Telavancin: a lipoglycopeptide antibiotic for the treatment of complicated skin and skin structure infections caused by gram-positive bacteria in adults. *Clin Ther*. 2010;32:2160-2185.

162. Silverman JA, Mortin LI, Vanpraagh AD, et al. Inhibition of daptomycin by pulmonary surfactant: in vitro modeling and clinical impact. *J Infect Dis*. 2005;191:2149-2152.
163. Landman D, Georgescu C, Martin DA, Quale J. Polymyxins revisited. *Clin Microbiol Rev*. 2008;21:449-465.
164. Stein GE, Craig WA. Tigecycline: a critical analysis. *Clin Infect Dis*. 2006;43:518-524.
165. http://www.fda.gov/Drugs/DrugSafety/ucm224370.htm. Accessed June 8, 2011.
166. Cai Y, Wang R, Liang B, et al. Systematic review and meta-analysis of the effectiveness and safety of tigecycline for treatment of infectious disease. *Antimicrob Agents Chemother*. 2011;55:1162-1172.
167. Eckmann C, Dryden M. Treatment of complicated skin and soft-tissue infections caused by resistant bacteria: value of linezolid, tigecycline, daptomycin and vancomycin. *Eur J Med Res*. 2010;15:554-563.
168. Walkey AJ, O'Donnell MR, Weiner RS. Linezolid vs. glycopeptide antibiotics for the treatment of suspected methicillin-resistant *Staphylococcus aureus* nosocomial pneumonia. *Chest*. 2011;139:1148-1155.
169. Nseir S, Di Pompeo C, Soubrier S, et al. First-generation fluoroquinolone use and subsequent emergence of multiple drug-resistant bacteria in the intensive care unit. *Crit Care Med*. 2005;33:283-289.
170. Livermore DM, Woodford N. The beta-lactamase threat in Enterobacteriaceae, Pseudomonas and Acinetobacter. *Trends Microbiol*. 2006;14:413-420.
171. Charbonneau P, Parienti JJ, Thibon P, et al. Fluoroquinolone use and methicillin-resistant *Staphylococcus aureus* isolation rates in hospitalized patients: a quasi experimental study. *Clin Infect Dis*. 2006;42:778-784.
172. Sprandel KA, Drusano GL, Hecht DW, et al. Population pharmacokinetic modeling and Monte Carlo simulation of varying doses of intravenous metronidazole. *Diagn Microbiol Infect Dis*. 2006;55:303-309.
173. Demoly P, Romano A. Update on beta-lactam allergy diagnosis. *Curr Allergy Asthma Rep*. 2005;5:9-14.
174. De Broe ME, Giuliano RA, Verpooten GA. Aminoglycoside nephrotoxicity: mechanism and prevention. *Adv Exp Med Biol*. 1989;252:233-245.
175. Bates DE. Aminoglycoside ototoxicity. *Drugs Today*. 2003;39:277-278.
176. Roberts JA, Lipman J. Antibacterial dosing in intensive care: pharmacokinetics, degree of disease and pharmacodynamics of sepsis. *Clin Pharmacokinet*. 2006;45:755-773.
177. Trotman RL, Williamson JC, Shoemaker DM, et al. Antibiotic dosing in critically ill adult patients receiving continuous renal replacement therapy. *Clin Infect Dis*. 2005;41:1159-1166.
178. Bogard KN, Peterson NT, Plumb TJ, et al. Antibiotic dosing during sustained low-efficiency dialysis; Special considerations in adult critically ill patients. *Crit Care Med*. 2011;39:560-570.
179. Choi G, Gomersall CD, Tian Q, et al. Principles of antibacterial dosing in continuous renal replacement therapy. *Blood Purif*. 2010;30:195-212.
180. Patel N, Scheetz MH, Drusano GL, Lodise TP. Determination of antibiotic dosage adjustments in patients with renal impairment: elements for success. *J Antimicrob Chemother*. 2010;65:2285-2290.
181. Vincent JL, Anaissie E, Bruining H et al. Epidemiology, diagnosis and treatment of systemic *Candida* infections in surgical patients under intensive care. *Intensive Care Med*. 1998;24:206-216.
182. Blumberg HM, Jarvis WR, Soucie JM, et al. Risk factors for candidal bloodstream infections in surgical intensive care unit patients: the NEMIS prospective multicenter study. *Clin Infect Dis*. 2001;33:177-186.
183. Paphitou NI, Ostrosky-Zeichner L, Rex JH. Rules for identifying patients at increased risk for candidal infections in the surgical intensive care unit: approach to developing practical criteria for systematic use in antifungal prophylaxis trials. *Med Mycol*. 2005;43:235-243.
184. Chow JK, Golan Y, Ruthazer R, et al. Risk factors for albicans and non-albicans candidemia in the intensive care unit. *Crit Care Med*. 2008;36:1993-1998.
185. Pittet D, Monod M, Suter PM, et al. *Candida* colonization and subsequent infection in critically ill surgical patients. *Ann Surg*. 1994;220:751-758.
186. Leon C, Ruiz-Santana S, Saavedra P, et al. A bedside scoring system ("Candida score") for early fungal treatment in non-neutropenic critically ill patients with *Candida* colonization. *Crit Care Med*. 2006;34:730-737.
187. Ostrosky-Zeichner L, Sable C, Sobel J, et al. Multicenter retrospective development and validation of a clinical prediction rule for nosocomial invasive candidiasis in the intensive care setting. *Eur J Clin Microbiol Infect Dis*. 2007;26:271-276.
188. Ostrosky-Zeichner L, Pappas PG, Shoham S, et al. Improvement of a clinical prediction rule for clinical trials on prophylaxis for invasive candidiasis in the intensive care unit. *Mycoses*. 2011;54:46-51.
189. Shorr AF, Tabak YP, Johannes RS, et al. Candidemia on presentation to the hospital: development and validation of a risk score. *Crit Care*. 2009;13:R156.
190. Kratzer C, Graninger W, Lassnigg A, Presterl E. Design and use of *Candida* scores at the intensive care unit. *Mycoses*. 2011 May 3 [Epub ahead of print].
191. Leon C, Ruiz-Santana S, Saavedra P, et al., Cava Study Group. Usefulness of the "*Candida* score" for discriminating between *Candida* colonization and invasive candidiasis in non-neutropenic critically ill patients: a prospective multicenter study. *Crit Care Med*. 2009;37:1624-1633.
192. Sawyer RG, Adams RB, May AK, et al. Development of *Candida albicans* and *C. albicans/Escherichia coli/Bacteroides fragilis* intraperitoneal abscess models with demonstration of fungus-induced bacterial translocation. *J Med Vet Mycol*. 1995;33:49-52.
193. Rocco TR, Reinert SE, Simms HH. Effects of fluconazole administration in critically ill patients: analysis of bacterial and fungal resistance. *Arch Surg*. 2000;135:160-165.
194. Gleason TG, May AK, Caparelli D, et al. Emerging evidence of selection of fluconazole-tolerant fungi in surgical intensive care units. *Arch Surg*. 1997;132:1197-1201.
195. Pelz RK, Hendrix CW, Swoboda SM, et al. Double-blind placebo-controlled trial of fluconazole to prevent candidal infections in critically ill surgical patients. *Ann Surg*. 2001;233:542-548.
196. Shorr AF, Chung K, Jackson WL, et al. Fluconazole prophylaxis in critically ill surgical patients: a meta-analysis. *Crit Care Med*. 2005;33:1928-1935.
197. Pappas PG, Kauffman CA, Andes D, et al., Infectious Diseases Society of America. Clinical practice guidelines for the management of candidiasis: 2009 update by the Infectious Diseases Society of America. *Clin Infect Dis*. 2009;48:503-535.
198. Brizendine KD, Vishin S, Baddley JW. Antifungal prophylaxis in solid organ transplant recipients. *Expert Rev Anti Infect Ther*. 2011;9:571-581.
199. Playford EG, Webster AC, Sorrell TC, Craig JC. Systematic review and meta-analysis of antifungal agents for preventing fungal infections in liver transplant recipients. *Eur J Clin Microbiol Infect Dis*. 2006;25:549-561.
200. Horn DL, Ostrosky-Zeichner L, Morris MI, et al. factors related to survival and treatment success in invasive candidiasis or candidemia: a pooled analysis of two large, prospective, micafungin trials. *Eur J Clin Microbiol Infect Dis*. 2010;29:223-229.
201. Chen SC, Playford EG, Sorrell TC. Antifungal therapy in invasive fungal infections. *Curr Opin Pharmacol*. 2010;10:522-530.
202. Ostrosky-Zeichner L. Combination antifungal therapy: a critical review of the evidence. *Clin Microbiol Infect*. 2008;14(suppl 4):65-709.
203. Mukherjee OK, Zhou G, Munyon R, Ghannoum MR. *Candida* biofilm: a well-designed protected environment. *Med Mycol*. 2005;43:191-208.
204. Al-Fattani MA, Douglas LJ. Penetration of *Candida* biofilms by antifungal agents. *Antimicrob Agents Chemother*. 2004;48:3291-3297.
205. Herbrecht R, Denning DW, Patterson TF, et al. Voriconazole versus amphotericin B for primary therapy of invasive aspergillosis. *N Engl J Med*. 2002;347:408-415.
206. Kullberg BJ, Sobel JD, Ruhnke M, et al. Voriconazole versus a regimen of amphotericin B followed by fluconazole for candidaemia in non-neutropenic patients: a randomised non-inferiority trial. *Lancet*. 2005;366:1435-1442.
207. Glöckner A. Antifungal therapy in invasive fungal infections. Treatment and prophylaxis of invasive candidiasis with anidulafungin, caspofungin and micafungin: review of the literature. *Eur J Med Res*. 2011;16:167-179.
208. Anidulafungin. *Med Lett Drugs Ther*. 2006;48:43-44.
209. Pappas PG, Rotstein CM, Betts RF. Micafungin versus caspofungin for treatment of candidemia and other forms of invasive candidiasis. *Clin Infect Dis*. 2007;45:883-893.
210. Kuse ER, Chetchoyisakd P, da Cunha CA, et al. Micafungin versus liposomal amphotericin B for treatment of candidaemia and invasive candidosis: a phase III randomized trial. *Lancet*. 2007;369:1519-1527.
211. Bassetti M, Mikulska M, Viscoli C. Bench-to-bedside review: therapeutic management of invasive candidiasis in the intensive care unit. *Crit Care*. 2010;14:244.

CHAPTER 14 ■ PAIN MANAGEMENT

SHARON HENRY

Pain is a normal response to tissue injury or stimuli that can result in injury if sustained. This response results in neurochemical reactions that produce the perception of pain. In addition, there are humoral, sympathetic, and metabolic sequelae to pain. When pain is not controlled or poorly controlled, these humoral, sympathetic, and metabolic sequelae may be pathologic and produce serious side effects. In addition, without the development of adequate and powerful pain relievers, performing any major surgical procedure would be impossible, as successful surgical treatment requires that the pain produced by the procedure be adequately controlled.

Fredrich Wilhein Adam Sertürner isolated the active component of opium in 1806. He named this new constituent morphine after Morpheus, the Greek god of dreams. This discovery, among others, has allowed complex surgery to be developed. In 1884, cocaine was recognized as an effective local anesthetic. This allowed surgeons to perform surgery without producing substantial pain and obviated the need for systematic analgesics. As surgical complexity increased, the management of the resultant pain has continued to be a difficult problem to adequately resolve. In addition, postoperative pain is not the only form of acute pain that needs to be relieved. Pain from trauma, burns, and medical conditions like pancreatitis must also be managed.

From the 1950s until the late 1980s, pain management consisted of intramuscularly administered opioids on a fixed or *pro re nata* (prn) schedule.[1] This approach was used for its familiarity and safety and did not require specialized training or personnel. Additionally, the gradual onset of action of intramuscularly administered medication allowed time to monitor for side effects. Although arguably fairly safe, we now recognize that this approach is not efficacious. Intramuscular analgesia results in wide variability in medication levels and therefore fluctuations in pain levels (Fig. 14.1). Advances in perioperative care have transformed many procedures from mandating prolonged hospital care to requiring only abbreviated hospitalization or allowing for discharge on the day of the procedure. The management of postoperative pain under these circumstances can be even more challenging. Thus, it is important that the acute care surgeon is knowledgeable about the modalities and medications available to help control acute pain.

EPIDEMIOLOGY AND SCOPE

More than 73 million operative procedures are performed annually in the United States. Perhaps not surprisingly, 75% of patients report experiencing pain postoperatively, with 80% of those rating it as moderate or severe.[2] Pain management has become the rallying cry of insurers and governmental regulatory organizations. The American Pain Society urges health professionals to consider pain the fifth vital sign. The Joint Commission on Accreditation of Healthcare Organizations in 2000 declared pain management a patient right, as well as an education and training issue. They emphasized quantitative aspects of pain and encouraged systematic assessment and safe management[3] (Table 14.1). The United States Congress even declared 2001–2010 the "Decade of Pain Control and Research." Despite this, a 2003 survey of postoperative patients found that 70% of patients reported having experienced moderate or severe to extreme pain at some time during their postoperative period.[4]

Increased attention is now being focused on assessing and controlling perioperative pain. An analysis of reasons for readmission from same day surgery demonstrated that pain was the most frequent cause (36%).[5] There are a myriad of factors that lead to inadequate pain control[6] (Table 14.2). One of the most important factors in the difficulty of managing pain is related to our ability to quantify it. Pain is highly subjective. Individual variation regarding tolerance to noxious stimuli is substantial. At the same time, if we are to be successful in managing pain, it is important to have a mechanism to quantify pain and to assess the efficacy of treatment of pain.

Many physicians and nurses who care for patients in pain on a daily basis misjudge the intensity of their patients' pain and the efficacy of medications given for treatment of that pain. Use of autonomic and behavioral responses by the clinician to determine pain intensity and to judge response to medication is error prone.[7] For instance, tachycardia and hyperventilation may reflect anxiety or even the anticipation of pain. There are cultural and individual differences in the expression of pain. Some people remain impassive during even the most excruciatingly painful experiences, while others are loudly vocal and demonstrative of relatively minor pain. A nonrandomized study of patients in the emergency department of a tertiary care teaching hospital demonstrated the inconsistency between patient and caregiver perception of acute pain. In this study, caregivers consistently rated patients' pain lower than the patients' own rating.[8]

For this reason, the best estimation of a patient's pain and its response to treatment is the patient's perception. Several pain scales have been developed to standardize pain measurement. Visual analog scales are useful assessment tools.[9] They are simple, sensitive, and reproducible instruments that allow the patient to give a numerical score to the severity of the pain they are experiencing (Fig. 14.2A). Use of such scales allows the nurse and/or physician to assess the efficacy of intervention by comparison of scores before and after intervention. If such scales are to be used, it is imperative that the patient be conscious and have the cognitive ability to express themselves. Behavioral scales are appropriately used when patients are unable to communicate verbally (Fig. 14.2D). Many factors affect the perceived intensity of postoperative pain and these include the following:

1. Preexisting pain
2. Anxiety
3. Age
4. Type of operative procedure performed

Anxiety is often an emotional reaction in anticipation of pain. Anxiety can produce autonomic stimulation such as an increased heart rate. It can also cause any stimulation to be perceived as painful.[10] Although the mechanism is not fully elucidated, there is support for the notion that there is age-related decrease in pain perception and report.[11]

The site of surgery may also be the most important determinant of postoperative pain.[12] Operative procedures associated with the highest analgesic consumption are emergency, major,

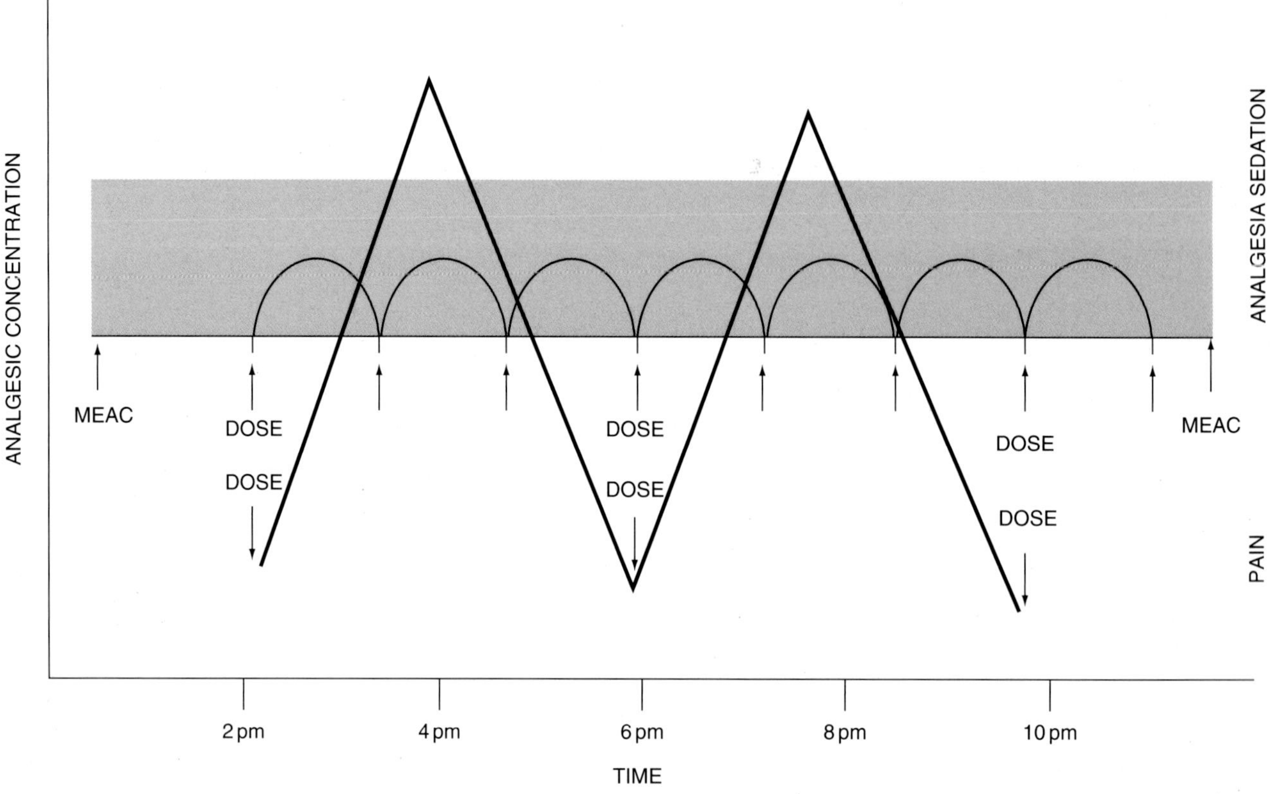

FIGURE 14.1. PCA paradigm. The relationship between plasma opioid concentration (ordinate), dosing interval (abscissa), and analgesic effect (*Z* axis), defining therapeutic effectiveness.

and abdominal surgeries. The most painful operative procedures are as follows:

1. Orthopedic procedures with major joints surgery
2. Thoracic procedures
3. Open abdominal procedures

TABLE 14.1

JCAHO PAIN MANAGEMENT STANDARDS

- *Rights and Ethics*. Recognize the right of individuals to appropriate assessment and management of pain
- *Assessment of Persons with Pain*. Assess the existence and, if so, the nature and intensity of pain in all patients, residents, or client
- As part of this standard, the organization also determines and ensures staff competency in pain assessment and management, and incorporates training on pain assessment and management in the orientation of new clinical staff
- *Care of Persons with Pain*. Establish policies and procedures that support the appropriate prescribing or ordering of effective pain medications
- *Education of Persons with Pain*. Educate patients, residents, and clients and families about effective pain management
- *Continuum of Care*. Address the individual's needs for symptom management in the discharge planning process
- *Improvement of Organization Performance*. Incorporate pain management into the organization's performance measurement and improvement program

Analgesic requirements can be estimated based on an assessment of the likely intensity of postoperative pain.[13]

Sequelae of uncontrolled or poorly controlled pain following surgery are well documented. Many of these are listed in Table 14.3.

PHYSIOLOGY OF PAIN

Pain can be defined as "an unpleasant sensory and emotional experience associated with actual or potential tissue damage, or described in terms of such damage."[14] Pain is an individual and subjective experience. It is influenced by a multitude of factors that include culture, previous pain events, mood, beliefs, and an ability to cope. Pain that is of recent onset with

TABLE 14.2

FACTORS CONTRIBUTING TO INADEQUATE PAIN MANAGEMENT

Fear of addiction (patient and healthcare provider)
Fear of respiratory depression
Difficulty adjusting dosage
Difficulty measuring pain
Relegation to staff with insufficient experience or training
Over or under dosing resulting from variable requirements
Fluctuating blood levels
Lag between request and administration
Reliance on routine orders to save time

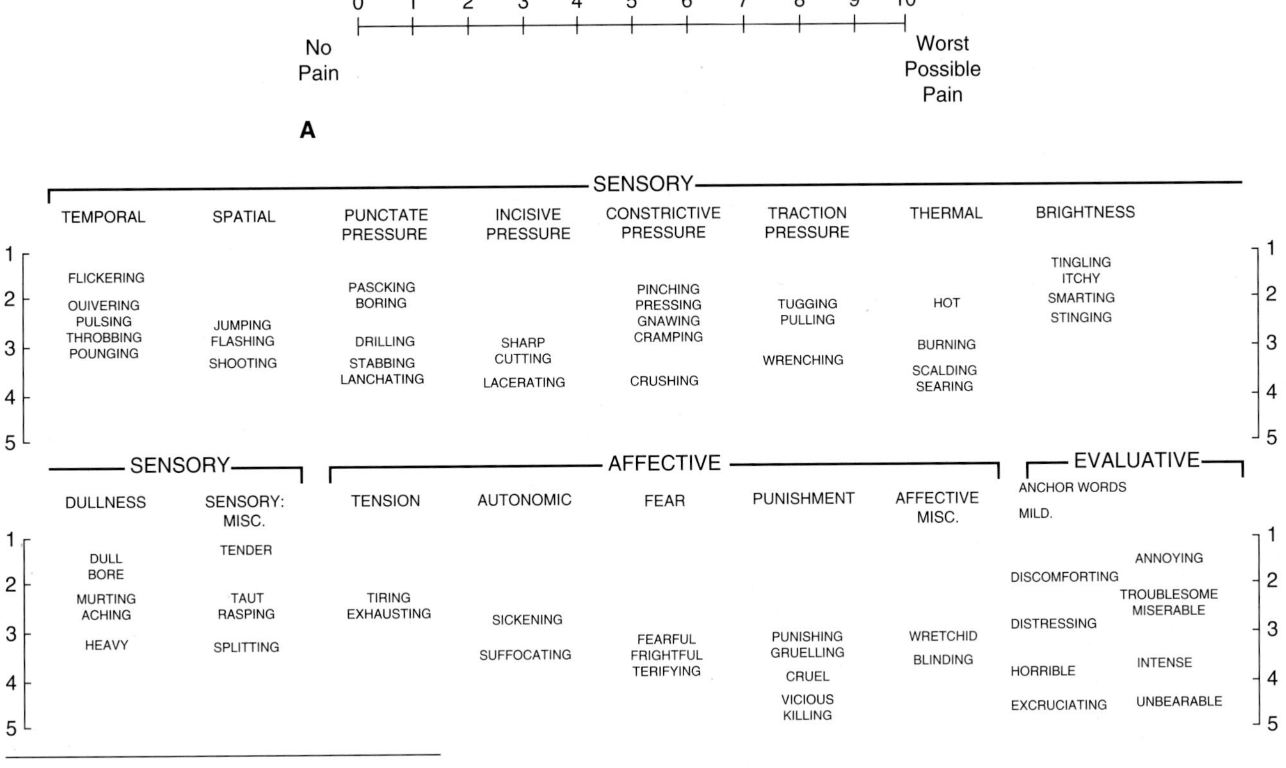

0 No Hurt | 2 Hurts Little Bit | 4 Hurts Little More | 6 Hurts Even More | 8 Hurts Whole Lot | 10 Hurts Worst

Wong-Baker FACES Pain Rating Scale

C

Behavioral/Observational Pain Assessment Tools

Observation	0	1	2	Score
Breathing	Normal	Occasional labored, short periods of hyperventilation	Noisy Labored, long periods of hyperventilation, Cheyne-Stokes respirations	
Negative vocalization	None	Occasional moan or groan, Low level speech with negative disapproving quality	Repeated troubled calling out Loud moaning or groaning, crying	
Facial expressions	Smiling or inexpressive	Sad, Frightened, Frown	Facial grimacing	
Body Language	Relaxed	Tense, distressed pacing or fidgeting	Rigid, fist clenched, knees pulled up or pushing away, striking out	
Consolability	No need to console	Distracted or reassured by voice or touch	Unable to console, distract or reassure	

D

FIGURE 14.2. Pain assessment tools. **A.** Visual analog scale. **B.** Verbal pain scales Classification of words used to describe pain. (Redrawn from Burchiel K, ed. *Surgical Management of Pain*. Thieme, 2002.) **C.** Faces pain scale for pediatrics. (Redrawn from Wong DL, Hockenberry-Eaton M, Wilson D, et al. *Whaley and Wong's Nursing Care of Infants and Children*, 6th ed. St. Louis, MO: Mosby; 1999:1153.) **D.** Behavioral pain scale recommended for use in demented patients. (Redrawn from Sinatra RS, de Leon-Cassasola OA, Viscusi ER, et al., eds. *Acute Pain Management*. New York, NY: Cambridge University Press; 2009:157.)

TABLE 14.3

SEQUELAE OF UNCONTROLLED OR POORLY CONTROLLED PAIN FOLLOWING SURGERY

- Slow recovery
- Increased postoperative morbidity
- Decreased mobility leading to thromboembolic complications
- Prolonged abnormal pulmonary function
- Nausea and vomiting
- Renin–angiotensin aldosterone activation
- Increased catecholamines
- Increased systemic vascular resistance, cardiac work, myocardial oxygen consumption
- Increased secretion of catabolic hormones (cortisol, glucagon, growth hormone)
- Inhibition of anabolic hormones (insulin and growth hormone)
- Muscle wasting
- Fatigue
- Immunoincompetence
- Impaired phagocytosis
- Impaired wound healing
- Enhanced sensitization of nociceptors
- Increased muscle spasm
- Visceral somatic ischemia and acidosis
- Renal hypoperfusion

a presumed short duration and can be related to a distinct process is termed acute pain. In general, the injured site and its periphery are the sites of ongoing pain, and as healing progresses, pain is diminished and finally disappears. Pain that persists for more than 3–6 months beyond the time required for healing or has no identifiable cause is termed chronic pain.

Pain perception requires the integration of peripheral and central processes. Nociception links the site of tissue damage and the electrochemical events that lead to the perception of pain. At the site of injury, peripheral sensory fibers that are widely distributed throughout the body in the skin, muscle, joints, viscera, and meninges are activated by mechanical, thermal, and chemical stimulus. This stimulus is transduced into an electrical signal.

Pain is perceived when there is nociceptive afferent transmission to the spinal cord and through the dorsal horn to higher centers. The A-δ myelinated fibers transmit the location and quality of the stimulus to the neothalamus and the higher cortex.[15] This prompts rapid withdrawal from the stimulus. Peripheral unmyelinated C fibers establish multiple synaptic connections within the brainstem, the midbrain nuclei, and the limbic system. When peripheral nerve injury occurs, several endogenous chemicals are released. These include bradykinin, histamine, serotonin, eicosanoids, and substance P. These substances, which are also involved in inflammation, activate receptors on sensory afferents beginning nociceptive transmission. This electrical stimulus is then transmitted to the spinal cord.

Prostaglandins, leukotrienes, and bradykinin act together to enhance the activation of the primary afferent terminal. Neurotransmitters including substance P, neurokinin A, and calcitonin gene-related peptide are released and cause increased permeability of blood vessels. Edema is produced and more vasoactive substances are released amplifying the response and spreading the pain outward from the initial locus. Thus infection, inflammation, and ischemia can lead to stimulation of an array of chemical mediators such as prostaglandins and histamines that can sensitize receptors to increase the perception of pain (peripheral sensitization).[16]

Peripheral sensitization can lead to central sensitization. Inhibitory modulation is also possible. The dorsal horn of the spinal cord contains μ, δ, and κ opioid receptors both pre- and postsynaptically. Inhibitory neuropeptides are also released after nociceptive stimulation. Alpha-adrenergic receptors also modulate nociceptive information. These receptors are found in high concentration in the substantia gelatinosa, and α_2 adrenergic receptors are found in the dorsal horn. Centrally, multiple areas of the brain are involved in pain perception. These areas (limbic system, areas in the cortex and the thalamus) interact with the psychological and environmental factors to produce the pain experience[17].

Classification

Pain is classified as nociceptive, neuropathic, or psychogenic. Nociceptive pain can be further characterized as somatic or visceral. Somatic pain results from activation of receptors in the cutaneous and deep tissues. It is usually well localized and described as throbbing, aching, or gnawing. Visceral pain occurs when organs that are innervated by the sympathetic nervous system are injured. It is often difficult to localize and described as aching, squeezing, dragging, or pressure like. It is produced by distension, mucosal irritation, traction, or torsion on mesenteric attachments or ischemia and necrosis. Pain in tissues distant from the pathologic condition (referred pain) is sometimes produced. This is thought to occur as a result of dual innervation of multiple structures or central convergence of impulses.

Neuropathic pain results from aberrant somatosensory pathways. This includes phantom limb pain associated with amputation as well as reflex sympathetic dystrophy, which is typically accompanied by vasomotor changes. Neuropathic pain is often described as dysesthetic. The pain is often a sensation that is not the usual recognizable discomfort. It may be itching, stinging, burning, squeezing, or numbness. It is decidedly uncomfortable, even intolerable. There is often a continuous component onto which is added an intermittent element. This is often described as an electric shock or jolt or lancing pain. Many patients have an abnormal sensory threshold and may have dysesthesia, hyperalgesia, allodynia, hyperesthesia, or hyperpathia.[18] Psychological stress, anxiety, and depression can influence the perception of pain in ways that make it difficult to determine if they are the cause or the effect. Anxious patients have increased perceived pain and may even have more complications from surgery.[19,20]

Assessment

Pain can be classified in a variety of ways. It can be described by the mechanism such as nociceptive versus neuropathic. The time relative to injury as in acute or chronic may also be used to describe pain. The etiology of the pain, such as cancer or postoperative pain, may be used to classify pain. Pain reactions are individual. Strong emotions are often associated with pain. Depression, anxiety and fear may alter pain perception. Objective physiologic responses to pain do occur. These include hypertension, tachycardia, sweating, and tachypnea. Grimacing, restlessness, and immobility are other typical physical signs of pain.

The use of behavioral cues or physiologic responses, though seemly objective, is inaccurate and suffused with the biases of the observer. This method is best reserved for those who are cognitively limited or nonverbal. Observer pain scores are notoriously unreliable.

Patient self-reporting is the best tool available for assessing pain. Several tools have been developed for use in clinical practice and are valid and reliable measures of pain intensity. They are the Numeric Rating scale, the Verbal Descriptor scale, the Visual analog scale, and the Faces Pain scale (Fig. 14.2A-D). These are one-dimensional scales and are most appropriate for assessing acute pain following trauma or operation. Multidimensional tools abstract information regarding the characteristics of the pain and its effect on the patient's life. These tools allow the emotional and physiological responses of patients to be accounted for and are more appropriate for accessing chronic pain. The McGill pain questionnaire is an example. It is a lengthy tool that incorporates categories encompassing the three major dimensions of pain: sensory, affective, and evaluative. This makes it an excellent tool to evaluate different modes of therapies and different analgesics. Its length and complexity make it a less useful clinical tool.[21]

Pathophysiology

Poorly controlled acute pain has the potential to produce deleterious effects that can lead to a host of complications, increased length of hospitalization, and even death. Several alterations in physiology are known to occur. Peripheral sensitization occurs at the site of injury and areas adjacent to it. This response is produced by the release of a combination of local mediators like bradykinin, serotonin and histamine, and cytokines like interleukin-1 beta (IL-1β) and IL-6. Additionally, sympathetic and sensory nerve endings release substance P and norepinephrine that further enhance pain sensitivity. Secondary hyperalgesia is the delayed alteration in noxious sensitivity seen in nontraumatized areas around the site of injury. Changes in spinal cord, brainstem, and limbic cortex pathways result in altered pain perception. Excitatory amino acids, aspartate, and glutamate act on *N*-methyl-D-aspartate (NMDA) and α-amino-3-hydroxy-5-methyl-4-isoxazole propionic acid receptors. Activation of these receptors increases the responsiveness of dorsal horn neurons to noxious input. Initially there is increased firing which is short lived followed by second longer lived period of enhanced sensitivity that does not require further noxious stimulation. This second phase of pain is much more difficult to control. This is the neurochemical basis for splinting. Pain is perceived at dermatomes above and below the site of injury and exacerbated by movement.[22]

Increased secretion of catabolic hormones occurs after extensive tissue injury. Cortisol, glucagon, growth hormone, and catecholamines are increasingly secreted, while insulin and testosterone are diminished. These hormones have the ability to negatively impact recovery through increased glucose, protein, and fat turnover producing hyperglycemia and negative nitrogen balance. Muscle wasting and fatigue can lead to prolonged convalescence. Immunoglobulin synthesis may be diminished leading to increase infection risk (Fig. 14.3).

Nociceptive transmissions stimulate preganglionic sympathetic neurons on the lateral horns. This produces adaptive responses designed to maintain blood pressure and cardiac output. Prolonged pathologic alterations in blood flow may occur and produce regional hypoperfusion and end organ dysfunction. The Renin–angiotensin system is activated and there is increased platelet activation. A variety of negative sequela results from uncontrolled pain. Tachycardia and increased afterload are a consequence of adrenergic stimulation. Renin–angiotensin stimulation produces hypervolemia that can be compounded with hypoventilation from splinting and congestive heart failure, and hypoxia can follow. Increased platelet aggregation produced by the activation of arachidonic acid cascade can lead to coronary artery occlusion and myocardial infarction. Appreciable pulmonary changes can accompany poorly managed pain in the abdomen and chest. Splinting leads to hypoventilation with loss of functional residual capacity and inability to clear secretions. This predisposes to the development of pneumonia. Preexisting pulmonary disease magnifies this effect. Platelet aggregation in combination with immobility leads to an increased risk of thromboembolic phenomenon[23] (Table 14.3).

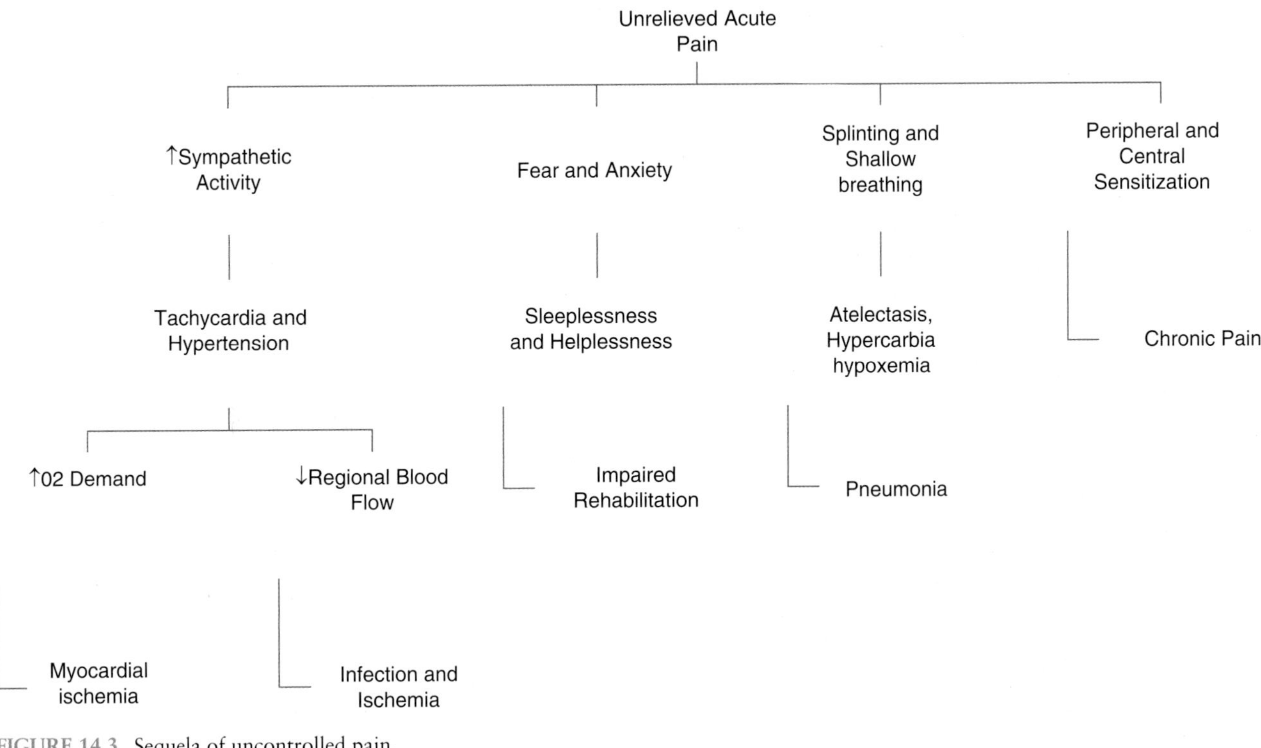

FIGURE 14.3. Sequela of uncontrolled pain.

THERAPY

Education

Before discussing potential medications for the management of pain, it is appropriate to remember the multidimensionality of pain perception. Pain is influenced by a variety of factors that include anxiety and psychosocial issues; the pain response can be affected by appropriate preparation of the patient. In the case of planned elective surgery, anxiety related to the unknown has the potential to create a circumstance where pain is magnified. Therefore, one of the most important aspects of preoperative preparation is providing information with regard to postoperative expectations.

The cognitive and emotional response to pain should not be minimized. Attempts at addressing these can lead to improved success in pain management. Psychoeducational care or information provided in preparation for surgery is beneficial at alleviating stress associated with surgery, recovery, and postoperative pain. Such measures as providing information on timing of procedures, functions of healthcare providers, pain and discomfort information skills teaching, like coughing and deep breathing, relaxation techniques, alleviating concerns, encouraging question, and problem solving are beneficial and without adverse effect though frequently omitted.[24] This approach is most applicable to patients undergoing elective procedures. Patients being treated for injury and illness can benefit from a similar philosophy of disclosure and teaching.

Medication

The World Health Organization recognized that millions of people worldwide suffer from acute and chronic pain because of a lack of standardized approach to pain management. In an effort to facilitate the adequate treatment of pain, the analgesic ladder was devised. This ladder provides for a stepwise increase in strength of the medication provided for pain relief. It was devised 20 years ago for the treatment of pain related to cancer, but the principles apply to the treatment of acute pain as well[25] (Fig. 14.4).

The first rung begins with nonopioids such as nonsteroidal anti-inflammatory drugs (NSAID), aspirin, and acetaminophen. These medications are appropriate for control of mild to moderate pain like headaches and musculoskeletal pain. Table 14.4 lists the commonly used drugs and their half-life and dosage. Aspirin was isolated from the bark of the willow tree in the 18th Century and found to have analgesic properties. Salicylic acid was subsequently synthesized in 1860 and used for its analgesic, antipyretic, and anti-inflammatory effects. Its gastrointestinal side effects were quickly recognized.[26]

Acetominophen is equal to aspirin in its analgesic effects but has no anti-inflammatory properties. The mechanism and exact site of action are not fully known. It seems to work by increasing the pain threshold. The pathway may involve inhibition of the nitric oxide pathway mediated by a variety of neurotransmitter receptors including NMDA and substance P. Acetominophen is metabolized by the liver through conjugation with glucuronide and sulfate and oxidation via the cytochrome P450 oxidative pathway. An intermediate metabolite conjugates with glutathione and is then further metabolized.[27] Acetominophen daily dosing must be monitored to assure that overdosing does not occur. Hepatotoxicity with doses in excess of 4 g/d is often irreversible and can be compounded by alcohol use.[28] Both acetaminophen and NSAIDs can be combined with narcotic analgesics to decrease the required dose of narcotic.

Ibuprofen is the most highly prescribed of the NSAIDs representing one-third of NSAID use. The drug has antipyretic and anti-inflammatory effects, is rapidly absorbed, and has high bioavailability. Ibuprofen is secreted in high concentration in synovial fluid. It is metabolized by the liver and excreted as a glucuronide conjugate in the urine. Ketorolac was the first injectable NSAID available in the United States. Ketorlac has longer time to onset of analgesic action, that is, 30–60 minutes. It is often given prior to the end of surgery to

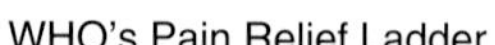

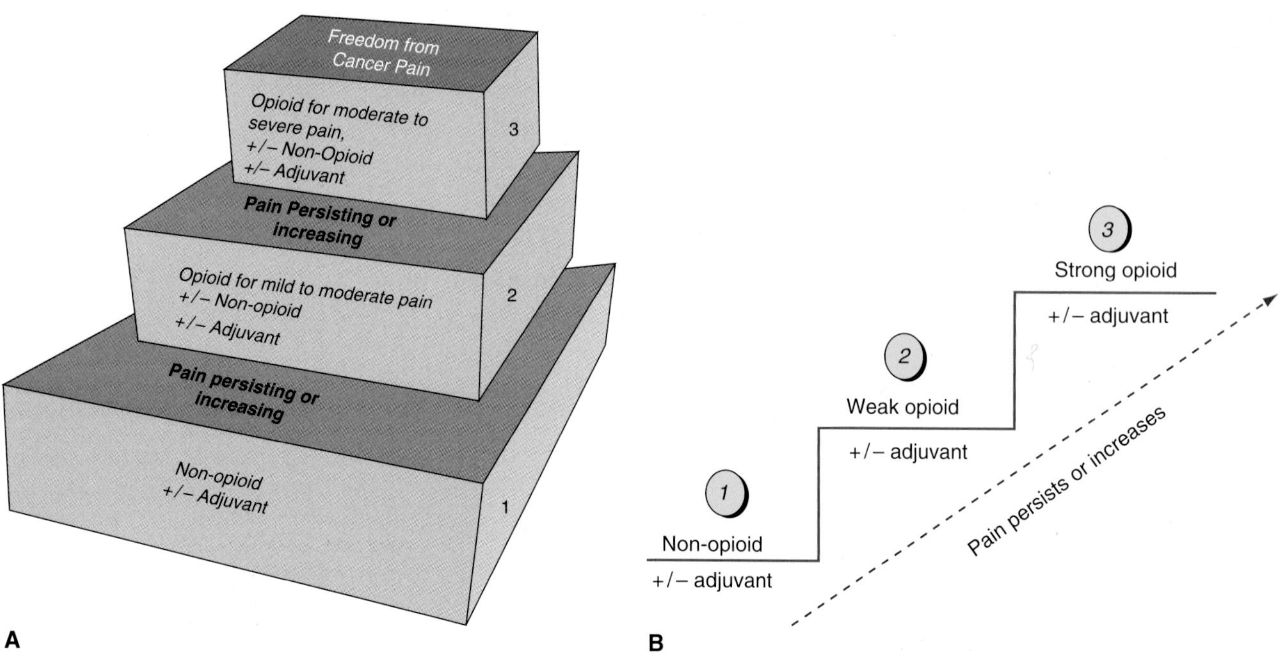

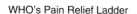

FIGURE 14.4. World Health Association "Pain Ladder." (Modified from http://www.who.int/cancer/palliative/painladder/en/)

TABLE 14.4

NONSTEROIDAL ANTI-INFLAMMATORY DRUGS

GENRIC NAME	HALF-LIFE (H)	DOSE SCHEDULE	STARTING DOSE (MG/D)	MAXIMUM DOSE (MG/D)	COMMENTS
Acetominophen	2–4	Q 4–6 h	1,400	4,000	Overdose produces hepatic toxicity not anti-inflammatory
Aspirin[a]	3–12	Q 4–6 h	1,400	6,000	Dose related GI toxicity
Choline magnesium trisalicylate	8–12	Q 12 h	1,500 × 1 then 1,000 Q 12		Less GI toxicity and no platelet dysfunction
Ibuprofen[a]	3–4	Q 4–8 h	1,200	4,200	Can delay fracture healing and has antiplatelet activity
Naproxen sodium[a]	13	Q 12 h	550	1,100	Can delay fracture healing and has antiplatelet activity
Ketorolac[a]	4–7	Q 4–6 h	30	120	Parental formulation. Higher doses associated with renal toxicity
Celecoxib[a]	11	Q 12 h	400	400	Lower GI toxicity, less platelet activity, increased adverse myocardial events

[a]Reduce dose in elderly and renal insufficiency.

reduce postoperative pain. It is not used alone for severe pain but may have narcotic sparing effect.

The side effects of NSAIDs can be considerable. NSAIDS are less sedating and do not cause ileus or constipation like narcotics. However, they do have several dose-dependent side effects that may limit their usefulness in specific patient populations. The cardiovascular side effects are the most concerning and have been highlighted recently in the lay press. By inhibition of the cyclooxygenase pathway leading to prostacyclin inhibition without concomitant thromboxane A_2 inhibition, NSAIDs can predispose to hypertension and thrombosis resulting in myocardial infarction and stroke. Gastrointestinal side effects are also well recognized. Symptomatic ulcers developed in 1%-4% of users annually. NSAIDs have also been implicated in the development of colitis and enteropathy. The intestinal wall becomes more permeable and bacterial translocation may occur.[29] Both aspirin and NSAIDs affect platelet function. Platelet aggregation is affected resulting in a 30% increase in bleeding time. Unlike aspirin, the impact that NSAIDs have on the platelet is reversible. Renal dysfunction caused by NSAIDs usually follows prolonged use. Through their effects on prostaglandins, rennin, and aldosterone release, NSAIDs may result in reduced renal blood flow and impaired excretion of water and electrolytes. Patients with preexisting dysfunction, advanced age, cirrhosis, cardiac disease, or hypovolemia are at high risk for renal complications from these medications.

When nonopioids fail to control pain, the WHO recommends stepping up to a "weak opioid." These include codeine, dihydrocodeine, and tramadol. Tramadol is an opioid agonist that weakly inhibits serotonin and norepinephrine reuptake. Codeine and hydrocodone must be converted to morphine by the enzyme CYP 2D6, a member of the cytochrome P450 mixed oxidase system. Some 20% of the populations is deficient in this enzyme and would, therefore, not get an analgesic response. Medications like amiodarone, fluoxetine, haloperidol, paroxetine, propafenone, propoxyphene, quinidine, ritonavir, terbinafine, and thioridazine inhibit this enzyme.[30] Many believe that these medications provide poor pain relief and should not be used.

The final rung in the WHO "pain ladder" is the strong opioid. Strong opioid medications should be considered if pain relief is not adequate. As important as the medication is the timing and route of administration. When medication dosage is inappropriately timed or administered via a route in which the absorption is erratic, poor pain control can result. In addition, respiratory depression, constipation, ileus, pruritus, over sedation, dysphoria, and physical dependence can occur. Opioids bind to the opiate receptors in the dorsal horn, central gray matter, medial thalamus, amygdala, and limbic cortex. In the periphery, they act on injured tissue to reduce inflammation. In the dorsal horn, they prevent the transmission of the nociceptive impulse and supraspinally they activate inhibitory pathways that then descend to the spinal level. Synthetic and naturally occurring opiates are structurally similar and bind to receptors in a dose-dependent manner. Table 14.5 contains a representative list with their relative strengths.

Opioids have no specific maximum dose. However, at high doses the side effects become troublesome and apnea, sedation, and confusion become more common. Morphine metabolites, morphine-3- and morphine-6-glucuronide, may build up. Morphine-3-glucuronide may cause myoclonus and hyperalgesia. Morphine-6-glucuronide is a more potent analgesic. Some side effects may be mistaken for inadequately treated pain, leading to the provision of higher doses of medication leading to further toxicity (Fig. 14.5). Patients with impaired renal function are at increased risk as the metabolites are excreted in the urine.[31]

While analgesia must be individualized for each patient, a number of principles exist that allow the practitioner to approach pain management wisely. The goal of analgesia should be to prevent pain if at all possible. "Breaking the pain cycle" and trying to prevent the pain from being severe will result in a patient who is far more comfortable and one who will use fewer total milligrams of analgesics.

Early on, it may be difficult to estimate how much analgesic will be required. This is a dynamic process that requires a certain amount of trial and error. During this phase, the ideal medication should have rapid onset and a relatively short half-life. This will allow the practitioner to titrate the dose to get the patient comfortable. Thus, during this phase, short acting intravenous medication is ideal. When one is able to estimate

TABLE 14.5

OPIOID ANALGESICS

DRUG	STRENGTH	ROUTE OF ADMINISTRATION	RECEPTOR	EFFECT
Morphine (gold standard)	Strong for severe pain	PO/IV/IM/SC/epidural	Mu	Analgesia, decreased respiration, constipation, nausea/vomiting, euphoria, dependence, tolerance
Hydromorphone	Strong for severe pain	PO/IV	Mu	Analgesia, decreased respiration, constipation, nausea/vomiting, euphoria, dependence, tolerance
Methadone	Strong for severe pain	PO/IV	Mu	Analgesia, decreased respiration, constipation, nausea/vomiting, euphoria, dependence, tolerance
Fentanyl	Strong for severe pain	PO/IV/epidural/transcutaneous	Mu	Analgesia, decreased respiration, constipation, nausea/vomiting, euphoria, dependence, tolerance
Oxycodone/ Oxycodone XR	Mild to moderate pain	PO	Mu	Analgesia, decreased respiration, constipation, nausea/vomiting, euphoria, dependence, tolerance
Codeine	Mild to moderate pain	PO	Mu	Analgesia, decreased respiration, constipation, nausea/vomiting, euphoria, dependence, tolerance
Propoxyphene	Mild to moderate pain	PO	Mu	Analgesia, decreased respiration, constipation, nausea/vomiting, euphoria, dependence, tolerance
Tramadol	Mild to moderate pain	PO/IV	Central acting	Minimal sedative and respiratory effects
Butorphanol	Strong for severe pain	PO/IV/transnasal	Delta, Kappa	Analgesia, sedation, no dependence, no respiratory depression, psychomimetic, paranoia
Buprenophine	Strong for severe pain	PO/IV	sigma	Psychomimetic, paranoia

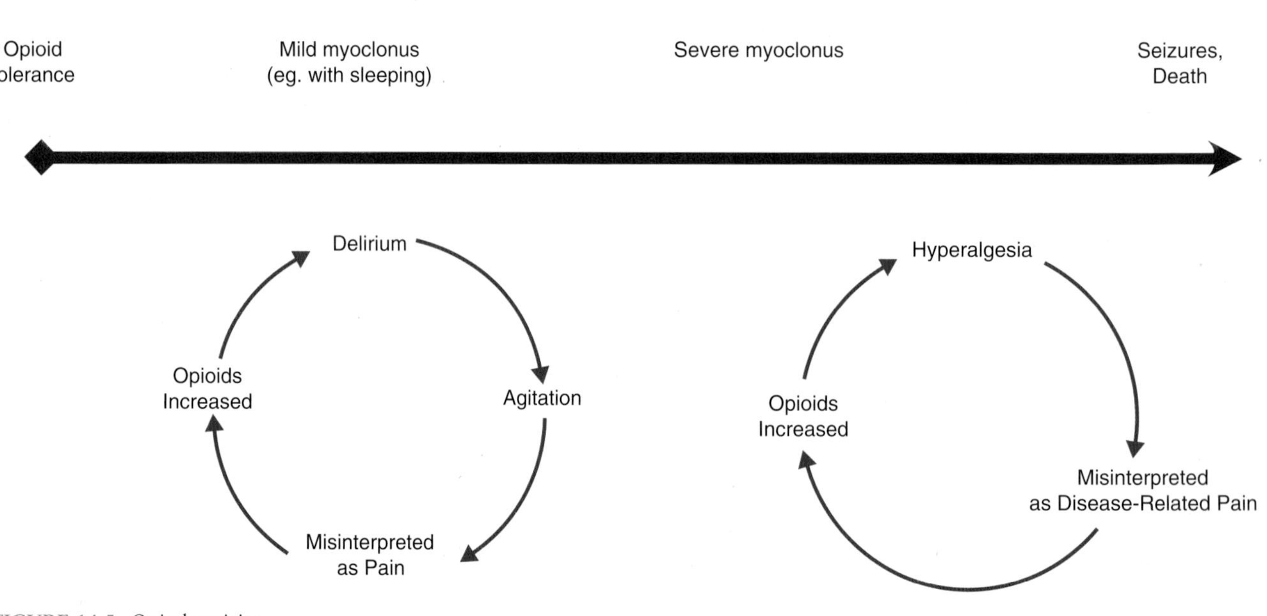

FIGURE 14.5. Opiod toxicity.

the severity of pain, and how much medication will be necessary, longer acting agents can be titrated into the regimen.[32]

After injury or operation, the gastrointestinal tract may not be the wisest way to deliver analgesics. However, as GI motility recovers, oral analgesics become extremely attractive. Their longer duration means that dosing need only occurs a few times a day. It is wise to still supplement longer acting analgesics with shorter acting drugs to treat any breakthrough pain that may occur in between doses of the longer acting medication.[33] For patients who have prolonged GI dysmotility or have other reasons why oral analgesics are not possible, cutaneous narcotics or sublingual agents can also be quite effective.

Early on, medications can be administered either by the nursing staff or via a patient-controlled analgesic (PCA) pump. PCA is attractive, as it gives the patient control over their own pain regimen. PCA pumps can be designed with or without a basal rate. The patient can then press the button for additional pain medicine as needed. A Cochrane review demonstrated that PCA provided slightly better pain control and increased patient satisfaction when compared with conventional methods. Patients tended to use higher doses of medication with PCA and suffered a higher occurrence of itching, but otherwise adverse effects were similar between groups. This allows for a smoother, more constant analgesia.[34] Studies demonstrate that IV PCA are safe and provide efficient analgesia.[35]

Medications can also be delivered via an epidural catheter. Medications can be administered directly into the epidural space and/or can be controlled by the patient using a PCA pump.

As patients may have several components to their pain, multiple drug regimens often make sense. Addition of an anxiolytic and/or an antispasmotic may potentiate the effect of a pure analgesic. An anti-inflammatory agent may also be quite helpful, particularly after bony or soft-tissue injury where edema is quite common.

Multiple routes of administration are available for opiates including oral, transbuccal, transnasal, transcutaneous, subcutaneous, intravenous, intramuscular, and rectal. Intravenous and/or PCA routes are best used when titration is necessary. However, meta-analysis has failed to demonstrate significant clinical advantage of IV PCA over prn. VAS scores were decreased in a statistically though not clinically significant way. The side effects were equivalent.[36] Less rigorous data do show 67% of patients having moderate-to-severe pain when treated with IM analgesia versus 35% treated with IV PCA and 20% with epidural PCA.[37] Sustained analgesia can be accomplished using long acting opioids or controlled release morphine; these drugs are not useful for rapid titration because of their extended half-life. Intrathecal, epidural, and even intra-articular administration has been advocated. They are most often combined with a local anesthetic.[38]

In a meta-analysis, epidural PCA has been shown to provide superior analgesia to systemic intravenous opioids. This effect was most apparent with activity on the first postoperative day. There was additionally a decreased incidence of nausea and sedation but an increased incidence of urinary retention and pruritis.[36] A meta-analysis of epidural analgesia in patients undergoing abdominal or thoracic surgery demonstrated a decreased risk of postoperative pneumonia, but that the degree of efficacy has decreased over the last decade. This is likely due to provision of improved analgesia for those who did not receive an epidural catheter.[39]

The epidural administration of analgesia is associated with a low but potentially catastrophic incidence of adverse effects. These include epidural hematoma, epidural or spinal abscess, and catheter dislodgement. The incidence of epidural abscess may be as high as 1 in 2000 in diabetics with a mortality of 18% in patients who develop spinal abscess. Other less common complications include intracranial subdural hematoma, transverse myelitis, local anesthetic toxicity and hypotension, and cardiac arrest.[40] The side effects of opiate medications often require the addition of medications to combat these symptoms. These medications may include cathartics, stool softeners, antiemetic, antipruritics, and stimulants.

Local anesthetics provide excellent analgesia. They can be injected locally at the site of surgery, used to block specific nerves, or be administered intrathecally or by epidural. Catheters can be left in place to provide ongoing delivery of medication by continuous infusion or a filled reservoir (Table 14.6). There has been suggestion that infiltration of the surgical site prior to incision prevents the nociceptive input from changing the excitability of the central nervous system. The theory is that NMDA-induced stimulation is blocked and release of inflammatory mediators prevented. Although this seems logical, there is no meaningful globally supportive literature. There is support for infiltration of ilioinguinal and iliohypogastric nerves prior to herniorrhapy.[41] When general anesthesia is administered and prn analgesia is provided, higher concentration of stress hormones, more intense pain, more substantial catabolism, and greater immune impairment are seen than when regional local anesthetic blockade is used.[42] Local anesthetics can be used to supplement narcotics and decrease the intensity of incisional pain in the early postoperative period.

TABLE 14.6

COMMONLY USED TECHNIQUES FOR ADMINISTERING LOCAL ANESTHESIA

Peripheral blocks

- Ilioinguinal/hypogastric (e.g., herniorrhaphy)
- Paracervical (e.g., dilation/curettage, cone biopsy)
- Penile (e.g., circumcision)
- Peroneal/femoral/saphenous/tibial/sural (e.g., podiatric)
- Femoral/obturator/lateral femoral cutaneous/sciatic (e.g., leg)
- Brachial plexus/axillary/ulnar/median/radial (e.g., arm or hand)
- Peribulbar/retrobulbar (e.g., ophthalmologic procedures)
- Mandibular/maxillary (e.g., oral surgery)
- IV regional (Bier block) (e.g., arms, legs)

Tissue infiltration and wound instillation

- Cosmetic and wound procedures (e.g., blepharoplasty, nasal, septum, endosinus)
- Excision of masses and biopsies (e.g., breast, axilla, lipomas)
- Field blocks or "splash" technique (e.g., hernia repair, vasovasotomy)
- Laparoscopic procedures (e.g., cholecystectomy, tubal ligation)
- Arthroscopic procedures (e.g., knees, shoulders)

Topical analgesia

- Eutectic mixture of local anesthetics (e.g., skin lesions)
- Lidocaine spray (e.g., bronchoscopy, endoscopy, hernia repair)
- Lidocaine gel or cream (e.g., circumcision or urologic or oral surgery)
- Cocaine paste (e.g., nasal or endosinus surgery, hernia repair)
- Lidocaine gel or cream (e.g., circumcision or urologic or oral surgery), cocaine paste (e.g., nasal or endosinus surgery)

Source: Reprinted from White PL. The role of non-opioid analgesic techniques in the management of pain after ambulatory surgery. *Anesth Analg*. 2002;94:577–585, with permission.

TABLE 14.7

ADJUVANT ANALGESICS

CLASS	INDICATION	EXAMPLES	DOSING	STARTING DOSE (mg/d)	DAILY DOSE (mg/d)
Tricyclic antidepressants	Continuous neuropathic pain	Amitriptyline, imipramine	Nightly dose	10–25	50–100
Anticonvulsants	Lancinating neuropathic pain	Carbamazepine, valproate, clonazcpam	Q 8 h Q 8 h Q 12 h	200 500 0.5	400–1,600 730–2,000 2–5
Second-generation anti-convulsants	Antihyperalgesia	Gabapentin, pregabalin	5–7 h 6 h	100 150	3,600 300
Muscle relaxants	Acute musculoskeletal Pain	Cyclobenzaprine (recommended only for short-term use), baclofen, carisoprodol methocarbamol	18 h 2–4 h 2 h 2 h	15 10 750 6,000	30 30 1,050 3,000

Ketamine blocks calcium channels within the NMDA receptor complex thereby decreasing neuron responsiveness to noxious stimuli in the dorsal horn. Ketamine is administered with benzodiazepams to counteract the psychotomimetic effects. It may also produce excess salivation and cardiac stimulation. Ketamine may also prevent opiate-related activation of pronociceptive systems and opiate tolerance through complex incompletely elucidated mechanisms.[43]

The addition of antiseizure or antidepressant medications may benefit patients who have evidence of neuropathic pain. Amitriptyline, carbamazepine, gabapentin, and tramadol have all been shown to be effective in treating neuropathic pain. The most common side effects are anticholinergic, sexual dysfunction, cognitive impairment, sedation, and orthostatic hypotension. Gabapentin, a second-generation antiepileptic drug, is also effective in treating neuropathic pain. Adverse effects include somnolence, dizziness, ataxia, fatigue, nystagmus, and weight gain. Pregabalin has a similar efficacy and adverse event profile.[44] Table 14.7 contains a list of adjunctive medications.

OTHER TREATMENT

Paravertebral nerve blocks result in excellent pain control evidenced by VAS score measurement and fewer side effects versus thoracic epidural in patients undergoing thoracotomy. Sciatic nerve block with continuous infusion and femoral nerve block with continuous infusion are shown to provide excellent analgesia and decrease in phantom limb pain.[45]

Meditation, massage, and acupuncture are other therapies that may have a role in pain management. As yet insufficient standardization of studies precludes unqualified support.[46]

References

1. Ferrante FM, VadeBancouer TP. *Postoperative Pain Management.* New York, NY: Churchill Livingstone, Inc; 1993:1–15.
2. Warfield CA, Kahn CH. Acute pain management: programs in U.S. hospitals and experiences and attitudes among U.S. adults. *Anesthesiology.* 1995;83:1090–1094.
3. Phillips DM. JCAHO pain management standards are unveiled. *JAMA.* 2000;284:428–429.
4. Apfelbaum JL, Chen C, Mehta S, et al. Postoperative pain experience: results from a national survey suggest postoperative pain continues to be undermanaged. *Anesth Analg.* 2003;97:534–540.
5. Polmano RC, Dunwoody CF, Krenzischek DA, et al. Perspective on pain management in the 21st century. *J Perianesth Nurs.* 2008;23:s4–s14.
6. Brennan F, Carr D, Cousins M. Pain management: a fundamental human right. *Anesth Anag.* 2007;105:205–221.
7. Thorn BE, Rich MA, Boothby JL. Pain beliefs and coping attempts: conceptual model building. *J Pain.* 1999;8:167–171.
8. Guru V, Dubinsky I. The patient vs. caregiver perception of acute pain in the emergency department. *J Emerg Med.* 2000;18(1):7–12.
9. Farrar JT, Young JP, LaMoreaux L, et al. Clinical importance of changes in chronic pain intensity measured on an 11-point numerical rating scale. *Pain.* 2001;94:149–158.
10. Caceres C, Burns CW. Cardiovascular reactivity to psychological stress may enhance subsequent pain sensitivity. *Pain.* 1997;69(3):237–244.
11. Gibson SJ, Helme RD. Age related difference in pain perception and report. *Clin Geriatr Med.* 2001;17(3):433–456, v–vi.
12. Parkerhouse J, Lambrechts W, Simpson BRJ. The incidence of postoperative pain. *Br J Anaesth.* 1961;33:345.
13. Kehlet H, Wilkinson RC, Fischer BJ, et al. PROSPECT: evidence-based, procedure-specific postoperative pain management. *Best Pract Res Clin Anaesthesiol.* 2007;21(1):149–159.
14. Mersky H. Classification of chronic pain: description of chronic pain syndromes and definition of pain terms. *Pain.* 1986;3(suppl):S1.
15. Carr DB, Goudas LC. Acute pain. *Lancet.* 1999;353:2051–2058.
16. Vadivelu N, Whitney CJ, Sinatra RS. Pain pathways and acute pain processing. In: Sinatra RS, deLeon-Casasola OA, Ginsberg B, et al., eds. *Acute Pain Management.* New York, NY: Cambridge University Press; 2009:3–17.
17. Raj PP. Characteristics, classification, and assessment of acute postoperative pain. In: Raj PP, ed. *Current Review of Pain.* Philadelphia, PA: Current Medicine; 1994:17–36.
18. Gracely RH, Lynch SA, Bennett GJ. Painful neuropathy: altered central processing maintained dynamically by peripheral input. *Pain.* 1992; 51:175–194.
19. Jamison RN, Parris WCV, Maxon WS. Psychological factors influencing recovery from outpatient surgery. *Behav Res Ther.* 1987;25:31–37.
20. Gil KM, Ginsburg B, Muir M, et al. Patient controlled analgesia in postoperative pain: the relation of psychological factors to pain and analgesic use. *Clin J Pain.* 1990;6:1370–1420.
21. Dunwoody CJ, Krenzischek DA, Pasero C, et al. Assessment, physiological monitoring, and consequences of inadequately treated acute pain. *J Perianesth Nurs.* 2008;23:S15–S27.
22. Brennan TJ, Zahn PK, Pogatzki-Zahn EM. Mechanisms of incisional pain. *Anesthesiol Clin N Am.* 2005;23:1–20.
23. Desborough JP. The stress response to trauma and surgery. *Br J Anaesth.* 2000;85:109–117.
24. Power I. Recent advances in postoperative pain therapy. *Br J Anaesth.* 2005;95:43–51.
25. World Health Organization. Pain relief and palliative care. In: Clinical Management if HIV and AIDS at District and PHC Levels. 1998.
26. Jones R. Nonsteroidal anti-inflammatory drug prescribing: past, present and future. *Am J Med.* 2001;110:4S–7S.
27. McNeil-PPC, Inc. www.tylenoprofessional.com/pharmacology. 2010.
28. Scanzello DR, Moskowit NK, Gibrofsky A. The post NSAID era: what to use now for pharmacologic treatment of pain and inflammation in osteoarthritis. *Curr Rheumatol Rep.* 2008;10:49–56.
29. Buttgereit F. Gastrointestinal toxic side effects of nonsteroidal anti-inflammatory drugs and cyclooxygenase-2–specific inhibitors. *Am J Med.* 2001;3:13–19.
30. Berger J. In: Silverstein J, Rooke GA, Rees JG, et al., eds. *Pain Management in Geriatric Anesthesiology.* New York, NY: Springer; 2008.

31. Burton AW. Acute, chronic and cancer pain. *Meth Mol Med.* 2003;84:267–283.
32. Etches R. Patient controlled analgesia. *Surg Clin North Am.* 1999;79:297–312.
33. Portenoy RK, Hagen NA. Breakthrough pain: definition, prevalence and characteristics. *Pain.* 1990;41:273–281.
34. Hudcova J, McNicol E, Quah C, et al. Patient controlled opioid analgesia versus conventional opioid analgesia for postoperative pain. *Cochrane Database Syst Rev.* 2006;(4):CD003348.
35. Popping DM, Zahn PK, Van Aken HK, et al. Effectiveness and safety of postoperative pain management: a survey of 18 925 consecutive patients between 1998 and 2006 (2nd revision): a database analysis of prospectively raised data. *Br J Anaesth.* 2008;101(6):832–840.
36. Liu SS, Wu CL. The effect of analgesic technique on postoperative patient-reported outcomes including analgesia: a systematic review. *Anesth Analg.* 2007;105:789–808.
37. Dolin SJ, Cushman JN, Bland JM. Effectiveness of acute postoperative pain management: I. Evidence from published data. *Br J Anaesth.* 2002;89:409–423.
38. Heitz JW, Witkowski TA, Viscusi ER. New and emerging analgesics and analgesic technologies for acute pain management. *Curr Opin Anaesthesiol.* 2009;22:608–617.
39. Popping DM, Elia N, Marret E, et al. Protective effects of epidural anesthesia on pulmonary complications after abdominal and thoracic surgery. *Arch Surg.* 2008;143:990–999.
40. Ballantyne JC, Kupelnick B, McPeek B, et al. Does the evidence support the use of spinal and epidural anesthesia for surgery? *J Clin Anesthes.* 2005;17:382–391.
41. White PF. The role of non-opioid analgesic technique in the management of pain after ambulatory surgery. *Anesth Analg.* 2002;94:577–585.
42. Kehlet J, Holte K. Effect of postoperative analgesia on surgical outcome. *Br J Anaesth.* 2001;87:62–72.
43. Himmelseher S, Durieux ME. Ketamine for perioperative pain management. *Anesthesiology.* 2005;102(1):211–220.
44. Shipton D. Post-surgical neuropathic pain. *ANZ J Surg.* 2008;78:548–555.
45. Evans H, Stelle S, Nielsen KC, et al. Peripheral nerve blocks and continuous catheter techniques. *Anesthesiol Clin N Am.* 2005;23:141–162.
46. Sun Y, Gan J, Dubose W, et al. Acupuncture and related techniques for postoperative pain: a systematic review of randomized controlled trials. *Br J Anaesth.* 2008;101:151–160.

CHAPTER 15 ■ ACUTE CARE SURGERY IN SPECIAL POPULATIONS

C. WILLIAM SCHWAB, DANIEL J. GRABO, EDGARGO S. SALCEDO, AND MICHAEL L. NANCE

ACUTE CARE SURGERY IN THE ELDERLY

Introduction

Surgical emergencies are diverse and challenging for the acute care surgeon. In patients over 60 years, age-related anatomic and physiologic changes as well as preexisting medical conditions can alter clinical presentation and management and have considerable impact on outcomes. As the population of elderly increases globally, it is important for all surgeons to understand how "aging" affects the presentation and progression of acute surgical disease.

In 1900, only 40% of the population lived to age 65; a century later, over 80% live past 65 years.[1] Two population trends will impact the age characteristics of elder patients in the near future. Significant increases in the population over 65 years will occur with the aging of the "baby boomers," the post World War II generation born between 1946 and 1964. This large cluster of seniors will accelerate the percentage of elderly.[2] The number of persons over age 65 years is expected to increase by 70 million persons by 2030.[3,4] Concomitantly, improvements in life expectancy suggest that the younger cohorts of elderly will live longer and enjoy a more active lifestyle and better health.[5] Improvements in longevity have already led to a steady increase in the numbers of the "oldest old," those over 85 years; by 2030, the number of seniors over age 80 will increase to 19.5 million persons.[3] As these two cohorts (boomers and the "oldest old") age, they will experience the common age-related chronic health conditions, consequences of senility, and the disabilities of "wearing out." They will require increasing prescription and over-the-counter drug use, physician office visits, and trips to the emergency department (ED).[6,7]

Injuries will be the most common surgical emergency among elders. While older Americans are injured at lower rates than those under the age of 65 (7,980/100,000 vs. 10,230/100,000 in 2005), they have higher injury mortality rates (118/100,000 vs. 50/100,000).[8] The percentage of emergency hospital admissions for injury increases with patient age, as well as hospitalization for injury.[4] The same types of injury are experienced in younger people; however, injury pattern, effect, postinjury course, and outcomes differ substantially.[9] Seniors aged 65–74 are usually more active and have injury patterns more similar to younger adults (motor vehicle crashes (MVSs) and falls from heights), and as they pass age 80, activity decreases, and the age-related changes, decreased vision, osteoarthritis, balance problems, low-level falls are dominant.

The presence and severity of preexisting disease, American Society of Anesthesiologist (ASA) physical status classification grade, delays in diagnosis, and time to surgery have substantial effects on morbidity and mortality.[10] Some have suggested that increasing age is an independent risk factor for operative mortality, while others report conflicting results.[10,11]

Physiologic Changes Associated with Aging

The combination of normal age-related changes that affect each organ system and the presence of chronic disease states result in a declining physiologic reserve and an enhanced susceptibility to disease.[12] The result is a diminished ability to handle the "stress" of surgery, trauma, and infection.

Cardiovascular System Cardiovascular disease is common, seen in 80% of patients over 80 years of age.[13] As the heart ages, a progressive loss of myocytes occurs with subsequent enlargement of the remaining myocytes, leading to reduced compensatory capacity and myocardial dysfunction.[14] Cardiac function is often affected by depressed myocardial contractility, decreased compliance in response to preload, and poor response to endogenous and exogenous catecholamines. Fibrosis of autonomic tissue causes conduction abnormalities, arrhythmias, and heart block.[15] Maintenance of cardiac output is difficult in elderly patients as the aged heart responds poorly to endogenous and exogenous catecholamines and is often preload dependent.[14] Cardiac medications, such as beta-blockers, calcium channel blockers, or digitalis, can blunt reflexive- or catecholamine-induced tachycardia. Arteriosclerotic vascular disease, common as we age, predisposes to impaired blood flow to organs.

Pulmonary System Respiratory function declines as the chest wall stiffens, respiratory muscles weaken, and lung elasticity decreases.[13] Arterial oxygenation decreases due to alveolar collapse and resultant diminished surface area for gas exchange.[16,17] Diminished pulmonary compliance, an inability to mount an effective cough, and impaired gas exchange often result in respiratory insufficiency and failure, especially in the setting of acute illness or injury. The elderly patient developing respiratory distress may appear comfortable as changes in chemoreceptor and respiratory drive are altered.[14] Inadequately treated postoperative or injury-related pain results in poor inspiratory effort, atelectasis, and pneumonia.[18] Epidural analgesia/anesthesia is an adjunct or alternative to commonly used enteral and parenteral opioids and nonsteroidal anti-inflammatory drugs (NSAIDs).

Renal System Structural and functional changes occur in the kidney as we age. Structural changes include decrease in effective renal cortex, resulting in 20%–25% cortical loss, hyalinization of blood vessel walls, and decrease in the number of glomeruli.[19] Functionally, decreased glomerular filtration rate (GFR) and impaired renal tubule reabsorption and secretion result in problems with solute clearance, acid–base balance, and fluid homeostasis. Hormonal responses of the renin-angiotensin-aldosterone axis and antidiuretic hormone are blunted. Despite decreased renal function, serum creatinine concentrations can remain within the normal range due to a decrease in lean body mass (BM) and creatinine production.[14] For this reason, serum creatinine concentration alone is an inadequate measure of renal function; creatinine clearance measurement or calculation based on age and BM should be used.

Gastrointestinal System Gastrointestinal function is relatively preserved; however, the catabolic state induced by critical illness or injury leads to rapid muscle breakdown. Protein-deficient malnutrition develops more rapidly in the elderly, and 17%–65% of acutely hospitalized patients become malnourished.[14] Impaired nutrition is related to an increased mortality in older patients requiring mechanical ventilation and is an independent risk factor for infection, impaired wound healing, and longer ICU stays. Early and sufficient nutritional support reduces hospital length of stay, mechanical ventilation days, and results in improved outcomes.[20,21]

Neurologic System Many neurologic and cognitive changes occur in the elderly.[12] Cortical atrophy becomes more rapid after age 60 based on several studies of postmortem human brains.[22] Pathologic changes such as amyloid deposition and arteriosclerotic cerebrovascular disease affect most past 80 years.[13] Decreases in cerebral blood flow and brain oxygen consumption can manifest as blunted sensation (visual, auditory, and tactile), altered cognition, and blunted pain perception. Anxiety, agitation, and delirium are more common in the postoperative and posttrauma period and more difficult to manage. Alterations in cerebellar function, gait, balance, and vision increase the risk of injury, especially falls.

Pharmacology There is an altered response to many drugs in the elderly.[23] Older patients often have an exaggerated response to central nervous system (CNS) active drugs due to underlying decline in CNS function and increased sensitivity to benzodiazapines, anesthetics, and opioids. A decreased effect of beta-adrenergic agents exacerbates the changes in autonomic function, leading to decreased baroreceptor reflex and orthostasis. Lastly, caution is advised with all nephrotoxic agents, such as iodinated contrast solutions, antibiotics, diuretics, and vasoactive medications.[12]

Clinical Presentation

The elderly can present with atypical symptoms or nonspecific complaints for surgical conditions.[24] Moreover, the history of the present illness may be difficult, and even impossible to elucidate secondary to dementia or previous neurologic insult (stroke). The medical history is often complex and unless supplemented by a family member or caregiver may be incomplete. Systemic response and findings on physical examination are often benign, especially with abdominal problems and soft tissue infections.

Abdominal pain is the main complaint in 15% of ED visits for older patients. Many physicians report greater difficulty with diagnosis and management of abdominal pain in older patients. In addition, abdominal and pelvis computerized tomography (CT) frequently adds critical information, with change in the diagnosis of acute abdominal pain in elderly patients.[25] Thus, early surgical consultation, directed computed tomography, and inpatient monitoring and observation are required for the elderly with a suspected surgical illness.

Perioperative Management of the Elderly

Increasing age in and of itself is not indicative of increased mortality, and many scoring systems have been developed to predict mortality for the elderly patient undergoing emergency surgery.[26] Nearly all scoring systems have clinical limitations because of time and amount of data required to calculate the score. The Acute Physiology and Chronic Health Evaluation II score (APACHE II) has been studied for its preoperative predictive value as well as its intended purpose of predicting ICU mortality. The Reiss Index compiles age, urgency of surgery, ASA score, presence of malignancy, and diagnosis in predicting mortality in patients undergoing laparotomy. Although the ASAs classification of fitness for surgery was not devised as a risk assessment tool, it has been used for many years in most emergent surgical cases (Table 15.1: ASA Score).[27] In six studies observing mortality after emergency surgery in the elderly, increasing ASA grade was associated with increased mortality irrespective of age. This subjective and simple-to-calculate score has been shown to be a good estimate of mortality risk even in octogenarians.[28]

As stated, the prevalence of chronic disease is quite high in the elderly. The National Center for Health Statistics reported that 80% of Americans over age 65 live with one chronic medical condition and 50% have at least two.[29] Chronic hypertension, arthritis, coronary heart disease, and diabetes are common. The management of these diseases requires medications (both prescription and over the counter), which further alter physiology and can affect a nontargeted organ. For example, NSAIDs can have deleterious effects on gastric mucosa, and beta-blockers can blunt a normal tachycardic response to hypovolemia. Thus, evaluation of the older patient with a surgical emergency is complex, and in many emergent cases complete preoperative assessment and risk stratification is impossible.

The current American College of Cardiology/American Heart Association (ACC/AHA) guidelines for cardiac risk stratification for patients undergoing noncardiac surgery can be used for preoperative assessment.[30] While the guidelines are primarily focused on patients undergoing elective noncardiac surgery, the guidelines list a Class I recommendation for patients in need of emergency surgery. These patients should proceed to the operating room without extensive preoperative cardiac assessment, followed by subsequent perioperative surveillance and postoperative risk assessment and risk factor management. The basic clinical evaluation should include a careful history and physical examination, pertinent laboratory tests (complete blood count to assess for anemia, which can impose stress on the cardiovascular system), and ECG to aid in determining the presence of active cardiac conditions. In elective surgery patients, the presence of unstable coronary artery disease, severe hypertension, uncompensated heart failure, valvular disease, or severe arrhythmia would lead to delay in surgery. However, in the emergent setting, where the risk of

TABLE 15.1

ASA GRADE

ASA GRADE	DESCRIPTION
ASA 1	Normal healthy patient
ASA 2	Patient with mild systemic disease
ASA 3	Patient with severe systemic disease
ASA 4	Patient with severe systemic disease that is a constant threat to life
ASA 5	Moribund patient who is not expected to survive

ASA, American Society of Anesthesiologists.
Modified from Owens WD, Felts JA, Spitznagel EL. ASA physical status classifications: a study of consistency ratings. *Anesthesiology.* 1978;49:239–243.

delaying the surgery would affect mortality, maximal medical therapy is instituted, and the procedure is performed. Most emergent general surgery procedures include the abdomen and fall into the intermediate cardiac risk category (1%–5%), including cardiac death and nonfatal myocardial infarction (MI).

The most frequent cause of morbidity and mortality in the elderly surgical patient is underlying cardiovascular disease.[14] Atrial fibrillation (AF) is the most common arrhythmia (1% of the general population over 60 years) and occurs in 5% of noncardiac surgical intensive care patients.[31] Advanced age (over 60), higher Injury Severity Score in trauma and increased Simplified Acute Physiology Score II, as well as catecholamine use and fluid and transfusion therapy are major risk factors for AF.[32] Patients who develop AF have considerably longer ICU length of stay, hospital length of stay, and higher mortality. Asymptomatic, hemodynamically stable patients can be treated pharmacologically with calcium channel blockers, beta-blockers, amiodarone, or digitalis to achieve either rate control or chemical cardioversion. Side effects of these medications are common. Electrical cardioversion is used for hemodynamically unstable patients or electively, often with cardiology consultation for patients with refractory AF.[33]

MI is the leading cause of postoperative death in patients over 80 years.[14] Preexisting cardiovascular disease and postoperative stressors including emergence from anesthesia and major fluid shifts contribute to myocardial ischemia and infarction in the elderly. Most postoperative MIs occur in the first 72 hours after surgery, and many are "silent." Thus, a high index of suspicion for cardiac ischemia must be present when an older patient presents with tachycardia, hemodynamic abnormalities, or chest pain. Initial management includes hemodynamic stabilization and support while addressing the underlying acute disease process, in addition to aspirin and heparin (where appropriate), beta-blockers, oxygen, and pain relief. Early cardiology consultation should be sought, particularly when coronary revascularization is beneficial.

The ACC/AHA guidelines of 2009 gave a class I recommendation that patients who were receiving beta-blockers on an outpatient basis be continued in the perioperative period.[34] Initiation and titration of beta-blockers in the perioperative setting for patient undergoing noncardiac emergency general surgery (intermediate risk) is controversial and requires cardiac risk stratification and recommendations usually made by a cardiologist. Many elderly patients have undergone percutaneous coronary intervention (PCI) with or without stent(s) (bare-metal or drug-eluting). Most are on antiplatelet therapy in the periprocedure time frame or long term to prevent stent thrombosis and subsequent MI. The ACC/AHA guidelines recommend maintenance of patients on antiplatelet therapy in the perioperative period, especially if drug-eluting stents were used. If drug-eluting stents were placed within 1 year of presentation for emergent surgery, then dual antiplatelet therapy should be considered. Obviously, the bleeding risks versus antiplatelet and coronary protective benefits must be evaluated on a case-by-case basis.

Other situations arise in which treatment of chronic medical conditions with antiplatelets or anticoagulants is necessary, such as peripheral arterial disease, deep venous thrombosis (DVT), and AF. Aspirin irreversibly inhibits platelet activity for the lifetime of the platelet (~7–10 days). Clopidogrel, however, has a long half-life and will affect newly transfused platelets. Platelet transfusion is the classic modality of treatment for platelet-associated coagulopathy. Desmopressin or DDAVP has been described in treating uremic platelet–associated coagulopathy and aspirin-induced platelet dysfunction.[35] Fresh plasma or fresh frozen plasma (FFP) has traditionally been used to reverse warfarin-induced coagulopathy. 10 mL/kg–15 mL/kg of FFP transfusion is often needed, which can result in as many as 4–6 units of plasma transfused (800–1200 mL).[36] In elderly patients with limited cardiopulmonary reserve, pulmonary edema can result. Alternatives to FFP do exist. Vitamin K is usually administered via the intravenous route (5mg or 10 mg) in the bleeding patient with warfarin-induced coagulopathy. Intravenous Vitamin K produces a more rapid response but has been associated with anaphylaxis.[37] Recombinant activated factor VIIa (rFVIIa) was initially described in the treatment of hemophilia and more recently has been used to treat moderate coagulopathy in traumatic brain injury.[38,39] rFVIIa enhances the thrombin-generating potential of activated platelets and aids in the activation of thrombin-activated fibrinolytic inhibitor, which results in a stable hemostatic plug that is resistant to premature lysis. A single dose of rFVIIa has been shown to be safe and effective in this cohort. Prothrombin complex concentrates are derived from human plasma, undergo viral inactivation, and contain vitamin K-dependent coagulation factors (II, VII, IX, and X). In the acute setting, such as traumatic brain injury, prothrombin complex concentrates have been shown to be effective in elderly patients in decreasing time to reversal of international normalized ratio.[40]

Perioperative respiratory insufficiency and failure are common and the need for mechanical ventilation is common in the elderly.[41] In addition, acute lung injury occurs more frequently with a higher mortality (60%) when compared to younger age groups.[42] Recognition and aggressive management of chronic pulmonary disease, such as chronic obstructive pulmonary disease and asthma, can minimize postoperative respiratory complications. Attention to postoperative and postinjury pain control with patient-controlled analgesia and epidural anesthesia is beneficial to the elderly patient.[43,44] Epidural or regional anesthesia promotes ambulation and provides excellent pain control while minimizing systemic opioids. In particular, patients over 65 years are susceptible to major complications after blunt thoracic trauma with even a few isolated rib fractures; mortality increases with increasing numbers of rib fractures in the elderly. Early use of mechanical ventilation that promotes spontaneous breathing and minimal barotrauma are the mainstays in management.

Specific Considerations

The common surgical emergencies in the older patient are injury and trauma, especially musculoskeletal, and diseases related to the abdomen, vascular insufficiency, and soft tissue infections.

Trauma The leading causes of nonfatal injury in older Americans are (1) falls, (2) pedestrian struck by automobiles, (3) MVC, and (4) violence.[8] Falls have become the main cause of hospitalizations for the elderly.[24] While younger adults tend to fall from heights (ladders), older adults fall from standing or sitting positions.[45] Up to 6% of falls result in fractures, with 1%–2% of these being hip fractures.[24] Pelvic fractures in the elderly have a higher risk of bleeding and of requiring interventional control.[46] Age-related changes in vision, hearing, cognition, and reflexes contribute to the higher rate of MVC in the elderly, but different driving patterns lead to more MVCs during the day. Elders account for more than 20% of automobile-pedestrian fatalities.[9] Violence is an unfortunate reality in the elderly, as older patients are more susceptible to unintentional injury and abuse.

The initial trauma evaluation and workup follow the principles of the Advanced Trauma Life Support (ATLS™) course with special attention to recognize preexisting medical conditions, chronic medications, and altered physiologic responses.[47] In addition, while resuscitation is ongoing, contacting family, caregivers, or physicians for medical information, health status, medications, and advanced directives is important. A heightened suspicion for occult injury, blunted cardiovascular response, and potential for early deterioration is required. Early use of ultrasound, placement of invasive monitoring or echocardiography to determine volume status and cardiac performance is helpful. Pain control is essential but should be given in smaller interval doses. Establishment of baseline mental status is important and early brain CT is critical in all cases. An age-related approach to patient care is presented in Table 15.2: Age-Related Approach to Patient Care.

Abdomen While the incidence of peptic ulcer disease in decreasing in the general population, the incidence of hospitalization and mortality due to gastric and duodenal ulcer in the elderly remains high.[48] This phenomenon can be attributed to the high prevalence of *Helicobacter pylori* infection and the increasing use of ulcerogenic medications, such as aspirin and NSAIDs. The treatment option for the management of perforated gastric ulcer begins with nonoperative measures, which include nasogastric decompression, analgesics, proton pump inhibitors, and appropriate antibiotics.[49] Mortality approaches 5% for nonoperative management of perforated peptic ulcer; therefore, this approach is advocated with caution in those over age 70. Patient history and overall stability will determine if nonresectional surgery with omental patching is more appropriate than definitive acid-reducing operation.[50,51] Recent studies have advocated the use of laparoscopic exploration, peritoneal lavage, and gastric or duodenal omental patching with excellent outcomes.[52]

Patients over age 80 with gallstone disease are more likely to present with obstructive jaundice or biliary colic.[53] Nonoperative management has a high failure rate and mortality (17%). Laparoscopic and open cholecystectomy in patients over 80 years for complicated choledocholithiasis requiring endoscopic sphincterotomy is associated with increased morbidity and mortality.[54] Failure to perform early cholecystectomy often leads to readmission with an increased percentage of those patients requiring open procedures. Thus, early laparoscopic cholecystectomy is the standard of care even in the face of a multitude of comorbidities.[55] Percutaneous cholecystostomy with interval cholecystectomy remains an option in the acutely ill and septic patient.[56]

Small bowel obstruction is a common reason for emergency surgical admission. Postoperative adhesions are by far the most common etiology of small bowel obstruction, with hernia (internal and external), malignancy, and inflammatory bowel disease accounting for the rest.[57,58] A high index of suspicion for necrotic bowel is necessary in the evaluation of the elderly patient with vague complaints and misleading signs and symptoms of abdominal pain, distention, and emesis. Delay in operation can result in loss of viable bowel and possible loss of life. The principles for fluid resuscitation with correction of electrolyte abnormalities, radiographic evaluation, and management are similar for younger patients with the caveat of performing laparotomy in cases without prompt improvement.

Colorectal emergencies are common in the elderly. In cases of bleeding, perforation, and obstruction, resection with creation of an ostomy is often the safest procedure. Emergency resection and primary anastomosis can be performed with an acceptable leak (6%) and mortality (9%) rates in the elderly who present with left-sided obstructing colorectal cancer, minimal soilage, and favorable physiology.[59] Acute appendicitis presents late in the course and is more complicated and lethal.[60,61] While abdominal CT is useful in the diagnosis of appendicitis and laparoscopic appendectomy has been shown to be beneficial in terms of improved postoperative pain, neither has affected outcome with respect to mortality in the elderly population.[62–64] Early appendectomy remains the mainstay of treatment and the most effective means to avoid

TABLE 15.2

AGE-RELATED APPROACH TO PATIENT CARE

Treatment Axioms, 55 through 69 Years

1. Assume some mild decrease in physiologic reserve.
2. Suspect the presence of some common disease of middle age (diabetes, hypertension).
3. Suspect use of prescription or over-the-counter medication.
4. Assume the patient is competent to provide an accurate medical history.
5. Look for subtle signs of organ dysfunction (ABG, EKG).
6. Assume TBI with history of LOC or cognitive abnormalities and obtain head CT.
7. Proceed with standard diagnostic and management schemes.

Treatment Axioms, 70 through 80 Years

1. Accept the presence of age related and acquired physiologic alterations.
2. Accept the presence of medications to control acquired diseases. Assume higher incidence of previous surgery and transfusion.
3. Determine competency for medical history; involve relatives and personal physician.
4. Aggressively monitor patient and control physiologic parameters to optimize cardiac performance.
5. Brain imaging is mandatory for any alterations in cognition.
6. Proceed with standard diagnostic and management schemes, including early, aggressive operative management.
7. Be aware of poor outcomes, especially with severe injury to the CNS; check for advanced directives.

Treatment Axioms, 80 Years or Older

1. Proceed as in items 1 through 5 for patients 70 through 80 years of age.
2. Assume a poor outcome with moderately severe injury, especially in the CNS or any injury causing physiologic disturbance.
3. After aggressive initial resuscitation and diagnostic maneuvers, examine item 2 and discuss appropriateness of care with patient and/or family members.
4. Attempt to be humane; recognize the legal and ethical controversies involved; consider early ethics consultation and social services.

Modified from Schwab CW, Kauder DR. Trauma in the geriatric patient. *Archives of Surgery*, 1992;127:701–706.

perforation, abscess formation, and sepsis. Interval appendectomy performed after a period of conservative management with antibiotics and percutaneous drainage for perforated appendicitis and periappendiceal abscess can be beneficial in adults.[65] The prevalence of diverticular disease increases to 50%–70% in those over the age of 65.[66] Chronic health conditions have been associated with poor outcomes in acute diverticulitis. Conservative management of acute noncomplicated diverticulitis with bowel rest, analgesia, and antibiotics are the initial treatment. Recurrent episodes are less well tolerated, and early resectional therapy should be considered. Surgery is reserved for abscess, perforation, or peritonitis.[67]

Hernias Elective repair of abdominal wall and groin hernias is one of the most common general surgical operations.[68] Emergencies, including obstruction, incarceration, and strangulation are frequent. External hernia repair has a 5% overall mortality, and this is largely associated with bowel resection for necrosis.[69–71] Other risk factors for unfavorable outcomes are advanced age, ASA class, coexistent disease, late presentation, and misdiagnosis. Older, stable patients who present with incarcerated body wall hernias should undergo attempts at manual reduction with appropriate sedation and analgesia as long as there are no signs of peritonitis or local cellulitis over the hernia. If reduction is successful, the patient should be observed in the hospital. If the patient develops abdominal pain, fever, tachycardia, or leukocytosis, emergent abdominal exploration to inspect the viscera and hernia repair should be completed. If attempted reduction fails or if the patient has signs or symptoms of strangulation or bowel necrosis, urgent operative intervention is necessary. If the peritoneal fluid is abnormal or the bowel is compromised, inadequately visualized, or reduces into the abdomen prior to inspection, full abdominal exploration is recommended for visceral inspection.

Vascular emergencies Mesenteric ischemia is uncommon but has a high mortality approaching 90%.[72] The three primary etiologies are acute mesenteric ischemia (arterial embolism or thrombus), mesenteric vein thrombosis, and nonobstructive mesenteric ischemia (low flow state). It is essential to maintain a high index of suspicion in the elderly patient who presents with abdominal pain out of proportion to physical exam findings and a history of comorbidities consistent with vascular disease or cardiac dysrhythmia. While angiography remains the gold standard as a diagnostic and therapeutic tool in acute mesenteric ischemia, CT angiography (CTA) is more readily available and commonly used. CTA also gives information about mesenteric vein thrombosis, bowel wall thickening, and pneumatosis. Management focuses on volume resuscitation and broad-spectrum antibiotics followed by operative exploration to determine bowel viability, resection, second-look procedures, and occasionally damage control procedures.

Acute lower extremity ischemia is a common surgical emergency, and the early recognition of symptoms can lead to limb salvage. Patients commonly present within a few hours of the ischemic event with the 6 "Ps": pain, pallor, paresthesias, paralysis, poikilothermia, and pulselessness (a late finding). A complete history and physical exam (with a detailed vascular pulse exam) will help elucidate the preexisting cardiovascular comorbidities that may have predisposed to the event, as well as the findings that identify the etiology of the event, that is, AF and embolus. The Rutherford Criteria have been used to grade the clinical severity of acute limb ischemia and are indicative of whether emergent surgical intervention is indicated and whether the limb is salvageable.[73] Category II (sensory loss, possible muscle weakness, and inaudible arterial doppler signals) represents a threatened limb that is salvageable with immediate therapy, and in category III (profound sensory loss and muscle weakness and inaudible arterial and venous doppler signals), the patient has substantive disease with an unsalvageable limb that will require amputation. Imaging should examine both inflow and outflow anatomy. Arteriography is the gold standard with magnetic resonance angiography and CTA becoming more common. Initial therapy includes systemic heparinization followed by thrombolysis, mechanical thrombectomy, or open revascularization. Endovascular advances and interventional percutaneous techniques are now common, and early consultation with a vascular surgeon is recommended. In the elderly patient, especially with substantial comorbidity and limited activity level, amputation may be a better option than surgical revascularization.

Skin and Soft Tissue The presence of underlying skin conditions and chronic disease states, such as diabetes, place the elderly at high risk for skin and soft tissue infections.[74] Necrotizing soft tissue infections (NSTI) are caused by microbial invasion of the subcutaneous tissues (SC) that occurs either through external trauma or direct spread from perforated viscus or urogenital organ.[75] Most NSTIs are polymicrobial in nature and occur in the perineal and trunk area, often in immunocompromised patients, diabetics, and patients with peripheral vascular disease. Because of nonspecific findings and a variable time course to fulminant disease, a high index of suspicion must exist to diagnose NSTI expeditiously. Erythema, pain beyond the margins of erythema, woody induration of the soft tissues, and swelling are common findings. CT of the involved body region often demonstrates inflammatory changes, abscesses, and fascial edema. Laboratory findings are nonspecific and include elevated white blood cell count and hyponatremia. The gold standard in diagnosis is operative exploration with the findings of "dishwater" or foul-smelling discharge, necrosis, and loss of normal resistance of the fascia to finger dissection. The mainstay of therapy for NSTI is wide surgical debridement well beyond the rim of cellulitis.[75] Prompt operation and adequacy of initial debridement are the most important determinants of survival. Broad-spectrum antibiotics are initiated and should include coverage for gram-positive, gram-negative, and anaerobic organisms. Antibiotic coverage for methicillin-resistant *Staphylococcus aureus* (MRSA) is also recommended. IV immune globulin and hyperbaric oxygen are additional therapies that have been described. Patients who survive NSTI have high morbidity, often necessitate multiple operations, and require prolonged ICU care. V.A.C. Therapy, nutritional support, and physical therapy are the additional mainstays of the long-term therapy. Outcomes in those over 70 years are poor.

Ethical and End-of-Life Issues

The primary objective of ICU care is to survive the acute threat to life. Success is achieved 75%–90% of the time, yet 20% of all deaths occur in the ICU.[76] Most of these are older patients in their 8th, 9th, and 10th decades. The Society for Critical Care Medicine (SCCM) guidelines call for shared decision making between the health care team, the patient, and the patient's family. Furthermore, even in cases of withdrawal or withholding of support, continued care and symptom management for dying patients is beneficial to both patient and family. Nearly 80% of the deaths that occur in the ICU occur after a decision has been made to limit life support measures (do not resuscitate or DNR).[77] Most DNR decisions are made within the first week of ICU admission, and decisions to withdraw or withhold treatments are usually made around day 7. Older age, more severe illness or injury are associated with earlier end-of-life decisions. Advances in critical care medicine and technology have complicated decisions regarding futility and withholding or withdrawing of care. Critically ill patients who have decision-making capacity have the right to determine their level of care and treatment.[78] When elderly patients are unable to participate in decision making, advanced directive and communication with family (next-of-kin, and power of attorney) must guide the health care team.

ACUTE CARE SURGERY AND PREGNANCY

Introduction

Caring for the pregnant woman presents a unique challenge to the acute care surgeon as there are two patients to manage: the mother and the fetus. The guiding management principle is that optimal care delivered to mother is the best initial treatment to the fetus. Often, managing the pregnant patient with a surgical emergency or critical injury is a multidisciplinary effort with input from the surgeon, obstetrician, anesthesiologist, and neonatologist.

Approximately 6%–7% of pregnancies are complicated by trauma, which is the leading nonobstetric cause of maternal death. The mechanisms of trauma for pregnant patients are most commonly motor vehicle collision (49%), fall (25%), and assault (18%). Penetrating trauma and burns comprise the minority of patients.[79]

General surgical procedures will be required in approximately 1 in 500 pregnant patients.[80] The incidence of surgical diseases in the pregnant population is similar to the nonpregnant population. Presenting clinical patterns for these conditions are commonly the same for pregnant patients as for nonpregnant patients. However, expected anatomic and physiologic changes during pregnancy and the normal spectrum of symptoms associated with the pregnancy itself can make prompt diagnosis and management challenging.[81] The section to follow will review the expected changes in pregnancy and the management approaches for the most commonly encountered acute care surgical scenarios.

Normal Physiologic Changes Associated with Pregnancy

Women undergo substantial physiologic changes as they progress through the trimesters of pregnancy. These changes involve virtually every organ system. It is essential for the acute care surgeon to be familiar with the nature of these normal changes to interpret a given patient's physiologic status, diagnostic maneuvers, and clinical trajectory appropriately.

Intravascular Volume Volume expansion in pregnancy is profound and progresses throughout pregnancy until it plateaus at 32–34 weeks of gestation. The volume expansion occurs to maintain perfusion to organs and the growing uteroplacental interface. The larger plasma volume also prepares the mother for blood loss associated with giving birth. Total body water (TBW) increases by 4–5 L and is regulated by changes in the renin-angiotensin-aldosterone system, which results in increased sodium reabsorption and water retention. Most of the increased TBW is found in the fetus, placenta, and amniotic fluid. Maternal blood volume augmentation is comprised of increased plasma volume (1,200–1,300 mL) and increased red blood cell volume (300–400 mL). The much larger increase in plasma volume when compared to red blood cell volume explains why the normal hematocrit in late pregnancy is lower, 31%–35% (physiologic anemia of pregnancy). These changes allow an otherwise healthy pregnant patient to sustain blood loss volumes up to 1,500 mL before manifesting signs and symptoms of hypovolemia.[82]

Cardiovascular System Consistent with the increase in intravascular volume to maintain organ and fetal perfusion, the cardiovascular system undergoes changes to achieve the same goals. Cardiac output increases by 50% to 6 L/min in the first two trimesters of pregnancy, primarily due to an increase in stroke volume. An increase in heart rate also occurs gradually throughout pregnancy, contributing to augmented cardiac output, reaching 10–20 beats per minute faster by the third trimester.[82,83]

As pregnancy progresses, uterine blood flow increases to approximately 25% of the total maternal cardiac output at term. Because uteroplacental perfusion lacks autoregulatory mechanisms, fetal perfusion relies primarily on maternal mean arterial blood pressure (MAP). Accordingly, maneuvers that result in decreasing maternal MAP or cardiac output may compromise fetal perfusion. A patient in the supine position during the second half of pregnancy will have compression of the vena cava and impaired venous return causing a decrease in cardiac output to as much as 30%.[82,83] Therefore, as a rule, all females in the second and third trimesters are positioned with the right side of the torso bumped up, shifting the weight of the uterus and fetus to the left. In addition, care should be taken when administering anesthesia of medications that can alter hemodynamics.

The hormone, progesterone, causes blood vessels to vasodilate. Coupled with the low resistance of the placental perfusion bed, systemic vascular resistance in pregnancy decreases by 15%. Resultant decreases in systolic and diastolic blood pressures by 5–15 mm Hg are observed by the end of the second trimester with a return to the prepregnancy range by term. Vasodilation also results in greater venous distensibility and higher venous pressures, particularly in the lower extremities.[82]

Physical findings associated with these cardiovascular changes of pregnancy include increased peripheral edema, mild tachycardia, jugular venous distension, and mild hypotension (depending on trimester). These expected changes in cardiovascular physiology warrant careful interpretation when evaluating a pregnant patient for emergency surgery.[82]

Pulmonary System Anatomical changes in the abdomen and chest wall account for a variety of changes in pulmonary mechanics during pregnancy. Resting lung volume decreases by 5% as the diaphragm elevates with displacement of the abdominal viscera by the enlarging uterus. Minute ventilation, the product of tidal volume and respiratory rate, increases in pregnancy by 30%–50%. The increase is primarily due to an increase in tidal volume as the respiratory rate in pregnancy is largely unchanged. This increase in minute ventilation results in a decrease in $PaCO_2$ levels (40 mm Hg down to 32 mm Hg) and is believed to be due to the increased levels of progesterone, a respiratory stimulant. The lower baseline $PaCO_2$ in pregnancy provides the necessary gradient to facilitate the transfer of carbon dioxide across the placenta from the fetal circulation to the maternal circulation for elimination.[82,83]

Oxygen demand increases during pregnancy because of the increased oxygen consumption of the maternal systems and the presence of the placenta and fetus. In total, these factors diminish maternal oxygen reserve. Difficult endotracheal intubation is a leading cause of morbidity and mortality in the pregnant patients. Airway edema and the generalized increase in BM of pregnancy contribute to airway obstruction and reduced glottis opening, and as such, smaller endotracheal tubes may be required.[82]

Renal System GFR increases as a result of the decreased vascular resistance and increased cardiac output. Alterations in sodium reabsorption result in water retention and plasma expansion. The higher GFR translates into decreased serum creatinine concentrations. It is important to consider the increased GFR during pregnancy to make appropriate adjustments to doses of medications cleared by the renal system. Glycosuria is a common finding during pregnancy.[82,83]

Anatomically, the collecting system dilates during pregnancy. This is mediated partially by the smooth muscle relaxing effect of progesterone. Also, the enlarging uterus compresses the distal ureters (right greater than left) in the pelvis, which also contributes to collecting system dilation. These expected findings should be noted and carefully interpreted on radiographic evaluation in the context of the patient's clinical symptoms. The ensuing urine stasis predisposes pregnant women to urinary tract and renal infections as well as renal stones.[82]

Gastrointestinal System The main alterations in the gastrointestinal system are due to the enlarging uterus in the abdomen causing cephalad displacement of the abdominal and pelvic viscera and general relaxation of smooth muscle. Intraperitoneal structures shift in position, resulting in unusual presentations of common surgical conditions. Similarly, the operative approach for managing common surgical conditions may require adjustment in incision selection to account for the gravid uterus.[82] Overall gastrointestinal motility and especially gastric emptying slow during pregnancy. The larger stomach volume and slower motility predispose pregnant women to aspiration when sedation is required during evaluation or management.[82]

Hematologic System As previously stated, the physiologic anemia of pregnancy is due to the proportionately larger increase in plasma volume compared to red blood cell volume. In addition to this dilutional anemia, iron stores are transferred to the fetus, a contributing factor to the anemia of pregnancy. Leukocytosis is observed during pregnancy and marked during labor that is endocrinologically mediated. This finding should not be mistaken for a marker of infection. Platelet counts remain relatively unchanged in pregnancy.[82,83]

The most noteworthy changes in the hematologic system during pregnancy involve the coagulation system. Essentially all procoagulant factors increase in pregnancy. Coupling this with a concomitant decrease in fibrinolysis puts the pregnant patient in a hypercoagulable state.[82,83] The incidence of venous thromboembolic events including DVT and pulmonary embolism (PE) has been shown to be five times higher in pregnant patients.[84] Following emergency surgery and trauma when additional factors of immobility, endothelial injury, and inflammatory mediators are exaggerated, the risk of DVT is even higher. As such, careful attention must be paid to DVT prophylaxis when managing pregnant patients, who often require pharmacologic prophylaxis.

Specific Considerations

Trauma The leading presenting mechanism of injury for the pregnant patient is blunt trauma after motor vehicle collision or fall.[85] As with all trauma patients, the evaluation of the pregnant trauma patient follows ATLS™ protocol beginning with a primary survey to identify and address any life-threatening injuries. The expected changes of pregnancy must be carefully interpreted and managed in the context of the patient's stage of pregnancy, mechanism of injury, signs, and symptoms. Foremost is the potential for a difficult airway, decreased oxygen reserves, and a full stomach. Substantial blood loss can occur before any changes in maternal hemodynamics are evident, manifesting first as fetal distress. Positioning the gravid patient in some degree of left lateral decubitus or manually displacing the uterus to the left side improves venous return by relieving pressure on the inferior vena cava.[86] Early fetal assessment is essential as even if the mother's vital signs are normal, the fetus may be inadequately perfused. Tocodynamometry and electronic fetal monitoring aids the diagnosis and treatment. Continuous monitoring is preferred and should be performed when the fetus is beyond 20–24 weeks.[79] Approximate gestational age can be estimated by examination of fundal height with a fundus palpable at the umbilicus, corresponding to 20 weeks.[87] Fetal viability is likely beyond 26 weeks gestation, and birth weight may have more impact than actual gestation age, with fetuses born <500 g less likely to survive.[88]

The following points are added in the care of the pregnant patient: palpation of the uterus for tenderness or contractions and pelvic examination to evaluate for fluid, bleeding, membrane integrity, and cervical status. Vaginal bleeding is concerning for abruptio placentae, which is the leading cause of fetal demise after maternal shock and death. Uterine rupture, though rare, is possible with considerable blunt trauma. Physical examination of the abdomen will reveal pain, palpable fetal anatomy and/or inability to palpate the uterus, or abnormal uterine shape or position.[86]

The secondary survey and appropriate adjunct diagnostic tests are employed to identify other injuries. The risk for potential harm to the fetus under 8 weeks gestation (during organogenesis) should not overshadow the necessity for radiographic imaging of the injured pregnant patient when there is need for accurate diagnosis. Radiation exposure of <0.1 Gy is considered safe; refer to Table 15.3: Absorbed Radiation Dose for radiation doses of specific imaging studies.[87] Again, the best initial management of the fetus is the optimal resuscitation, diagnosis, and care of the mother linked to early fetal assessment.[79],[86]

In addition to the standard battery of blood tests, a Kleihauer-Betke test is sent for Rh-negative patients. If the test demonstrates fetal blood in the maternal circulation, an appropriate dose of Rh immune globulin should be administered within 72 hours of injury. Alternatively, one can forego Kleihauer-Betke test and administer the Rh immune globulin to all known Rh-negative women.[79]

TABLE 15.3

ABSORBED RADIATION DOSE

RADIOGRAPHIC STUDY	ABSORBED DOSE (RADS)
Cervical Spine Series	0.0005
Anteroposterior Chest	0.0025
Thoracic Spine Series	0.01
Anteroposterior Pelvis	0.2
Lumbosacral Spine Series	0.75–1.0
Head CT Scan	0.05
Chest CT Scan	<1.0
Abdomen–Pelvic CT Scan	3.0–9.0
Limited Upper Abdomen CT Scan	<1.0

Modified from Tinkhoff G. Care of the Pregnant Trauma Patient. In Peitzman A, Rhodes M, Schwab CW, et al. eds. The Trauma Manual. 2008, 3rd ed. Philadelphia, PA: Lippincott, Williams & Wilkins Publishers.

Surgical Emergencies Most acute abdominal emergencies present with the typical signs and symptoms described for surgical disease. Prompt surgical intervention minimizes both maternal and fetal risks. Diagnosis, however, may be delayed and difficult due to the normal biologic alterations in anatomy and physiology of pregnancy or the mother's misinterpretation of symptoms. Consultation with an obstetrician should assure appropriate perioperative monitoring of the mother and fetus.[81]

The most common nonobstetric surgical condition affecting pregnant patients is acute appendicitis. This comprises 25% of nonobstetric operative interventions in pregnancy. The rate of perforated appendicitis in pregnant women is higher than in the nonobstetric population and correlates with maternal and fetal morbidity and mortality. The rates of preterm contractions are appreciable secondary to uterine irritation from peritonitis, and preterm labor and delivery can reach 50% in the third trimester.[81]

The anatomic position of the appendix changes as the uterus enlarges and in most women relocates to the right upper quadrant by late pregnancy.[89] The progressive displacement of the appendix fosters missed and delayed diagnosis and higher rates of perforation. Also, the enlarging uterus may impair the ability of the omentum and surrounding bowel to wall off an inflamed appendix. Rebound tenderness and guarding is less common due to the increased laxity of the abdominal musculature and the position of the uterus between the appendix and the anterior abdominal wall.[81]

However, diagnosis of acute appendicitis can be challenging, particularly late in gestation. Ultrasound is the most common initial imaging approach as it is noninvasive, sensitive, widely available, and low risk. The specificity and sensitivity of ultrasound is operator-dependent. CT scan and MRI are both highly sensitive and specific for the diagnosis and used whenever there is high clinical suspicion and ultrasound exam is normal or inadequate. CT scan exposes the fetus to considerable ionizing radiation. Although MRI avoids radiation, its long-term effects have not been proven in long-term follow-up studies. Any use of radiation or magnetic imaging should be discussed with the mother.

The risks and benefits associated with operation must always be evaluated. Appendectomy appears to be well tolerated by the mother and fetus. The laparoscopic approach versus open approach is based on surgeon preference, uterine size, and position of the appendix. After the second trimester, laparoscopy becomes increasingly challenging. The open technique for trocar placement should be used for any laparoscopic approach to avoid injury to the uterus. The only indication for delay in surgery is active labor in which appendectomy should be performed immediately after delivery. Cesarean delivery is indicated if there is evidence of appendiceal rupture, sepsis, or septic shock. With both the open or laparoscopic approach, initial incision or trocar configuration may be altered due to the variable position of the appendix throughout pregnancy. The false-positive rate of appendicitis on pathology is higher, but acceptably so, in pregnant women as the risks to mother and fetus are significant with the complications from a delay in diagnosis.[81]

Biliary tract disease is the second most common nonobstetric surgical condition. Signs and symptoms are typical, but Murphy's sign may not be elicited as frequently. Ultrasound examination is warranted in any pregnant woman with a complaint of right upper-quadrant abdominal pain. The clinical presentation of acute cholecystitis in pregnant patients is similar to that of age-matched nonpregnant women.[81] Symptomatic cholelithiasis is commonly managed conservatively at first. Bowel rest, intravenous fluids, and pain control with or without antibiotics are the mainstays of treatment. If successful and with no recurrent episodes or escalation of clinical signs or symptoms, patients are scheduled to have an elective cholecystectomy after delivery. Obviously, the risks of delayed cholecystectomy are those of progression of biliary disease or failure of conservative management.[81] Some advocate early surgical intervention to avoid the increased morbidity of complications from delayed management. The laparoscopic approach has been shown to be uniformly safe for mother and fetus. The ideal time to operate is in the second trimester because organogenesis is complete in the fetus, but the anatomic changes are not as marked in the mother.[90] Again, the open technique for initial trocar placement is safest and minimal uterine manipulation is recommended. Patients with acute cholecystitis or symptomatic choledocholithiasis are at higher risk for complication such as cholangitis or gallstone pancreatitis. If these conditions develop, maternal mortality rates and fetal loss rates increase dramatically. Intervention should not be delayed in such cases. Open or laparoscopic cholecystectomy with choledochotomy and drainage is one surgical approach. Operation with postoperative endoscopic retrograde cholangiopancreatography and sphincterotomy with or without stent placement is another acceptable option.[81]

While bowel obstruction is uncommon in pregnancy, it is the third most common reason for nonobstetric laparotomy. Nearly 60% of bowel obstruction in pregnant women is caused by adhesions from prior surgery, including previous cesarean section. Volvulus is more common in the pregnant patient and occurs more frequently during times of rapid changes in uterine size, such as during the second trimester and postpartum period.[81] Treatment of bowel obstruction during pregnancy is the same as for the nonpregnant patient. While umbilical hernia is very common in pregnancy due to abdominal wall alterations, incarceration and strangulation are uncommon.[91] Consideration should be given to repair reducible hernias electively in the postpartum period. Attempts at reduction of incarcerated hernias should be made with appropriate sedation and analgesia when no signs of cellulitis around the hernia or peritoneal signs are present. If reduction is successful, a period of observation in the hospital is warranted to monitor for signs of bowel necrosis. Operative repair is urgently undertaken for the irreducible hernia or in the case of the patient who develops peritoneal signs or fetal distress after reduction.

Anal lesions including thrombosed external hemorrhoids and anal fissures are common during pregnancy and the postpartum period.[92] Risk factors include maternal dyschezia, postdate delivery, larger babies, and perineal lacerations.[81] Treatment of hemorrhoids and anal fissures during pregnancy initially is conservative. Symptoms can be improved with topical anesthetics and steroid creams. Rubber band ligation can provide considerable improvement for patients with second- and third-degree internal hemorrhoids.[93] Intractable disease can be treated with surgical hemorrhoidectomy when fetal viability is achieved or in the postpartum period. Hemorrhoidectomy is reserved for third- and fourth-degree internal hemorrhoids, acute thrombosis, and strangulated hemorrhoids.[81]

Venous thromboembolism (VTE) is a leading cause of morbidity and mortality in the pregnant patient. DVT occurs with equal frequency in each trimester and postpartum period and is more common in the left leg.[94] PE, however, is more common during the postpartum period than during pregnancy. Diagnosis of DVT is difficult during pregnancy as the typical signs of leg swelling and pain are common. Unilateral pain and increase in leg size require evaluation for DVT. Venous compression ultrasonography is the diagnostic test of choice as it is noninvasive, safe, and inexpensive. Treatment of DVT requires anticoagulation. Low-molecular-weight heparins (LMWH) are replacing unfractionated heparin as the treatment of choice, and warfarin is only used in the postpartum period due to its teratogenic effects. Current recommendations are for anticoagulation for 3–6 months including 6 weeks postpartum. Longer courses of treatment (12 months) are required for patients with recurrent VTE and history of hypercoagulable state.

PEDIATRIC SURGERY FOR THE ACUTE CARE SURGEON

Introduction

The acute care surgeon should be familiar with the basic principles of pediatric physiology and the common presentation, diagnosis, and treatment of surgical diseases that affect young children and adolescents. In general, the acute care surgeon will be commonly asked to evaluate children and adolescents for injuries and multisystem trauma.[95] In addition, a number of common emergencies related to the abdomen, body wall, and groin make up an appreciable part of the work of the emergency surgeon. This section will address only a few surgical emergencies. The emergency surgeon should work closely with a pediatrician and pediatric surgeon if available. General surgeons who practice in a more remote location or in an environment where pediatric consultation is unavailable must be familiar with stabilization of the common surgical conditions of the very young child including pyloric stenosis, as well as emergency management of abdominal wall defects (gastroschisis and omphalocele).

Pediatric Anatomy and Physiology

Anatomy The unique anatomic and physiologic characteristics of the child will impact the patterns of injury and response when compared to adults. Children have a smaller BM, making them more susceptible to equivalent energy transfers and also at risk for hypothermia. The child's bony skeleton is more compliant due to incomplete calcification. As a result, energy is transmitted more readily to internal organs leading to injury, often in the absence of external signs or fractures.

Fluid Management The surgical care of the pediatric patient demands an understanding of the unique physiology that is manifested with each phase of development. A newborn infant's TBW is approximately 75% of BM.[96] This high percentage of TBW decreases rapidly in the first year of life and then trends down to 60% of BM by adolescence, approaching that of an adult. Maintenance fluid replacements must consider obligate fluid losses such as urine production, gastrointestinal losses, skin and respiratory losses, and basal metabolic requirements.[97] A weight-based algorithm (4-2-1 rule) is used to calculate fluid needs. One-quarter normal saline is usually appropriate in newborns. One-half normal saline can be used in children over 2 years old as their renal function approaches that of adults. The addition of dextrose is necessary in young children as hepatic glycogen stores are limited and must be supplemented.

Hypovolemia and Hemorrhage In children and adolescents, severe illness can result in hypovolemia, and injury can result in considerable blood loss.[98] The evaluation and management of circulation in the pediatric patient includes recognition of circulatory compromise and the principles of resuscitation with crystalloid and blood products. In children and adolescents, the primary response to hypovolemia, whether from severe illness or hemorrhage, is tachycardia (Table 15.4): Systemic Responses to Blood Loss in Pediatric Patients. Normal vital functions by age group are listed in Table 15.5: Vital Functions. Compensatory mechanisms, that is, vasoconstriction, are robust in the child and can mask the hypoperfusion and decreases in blood pressure typically seen in the adult with hypovolemia and hemorrhage. This compensation may result in a false sense of stability until much later in the clinical course. Hypotension in the pediatric patient should be treated aggressively. When shock is suspected, fluid resuscitation with boluses of 20 mL/kg of a balanced crystalloid solution is titrated to clinical response of heart rate, urine output, capillary refill, and level of consciousness as monitors of cardiac output. There is no data to support colloid over crystalloid infusion based on mortality difference. Failure to improve hemodynamic abnormalities following initial crystalloid resuscitation, particularly in the setting of trauma, raises the suspicion of hemorrhage and prompts the need to consider administration of warmed packed red blood cells (type specific or O negative in 10 mL/kg aliquots).[98] Normalization of heart rate, capillary refill <2 seconds, normal pulses and warm extremities, urine output (>2 mL/kg/h for infants, >1.5 mL/kg/h for younger children and >1 mL/kg/h for older children),

TABLE 15.4

SYSTEMIC RESPONSES TO BLOOD LOSS IN PEDIATRIC PATIENTS

SYSTEM	MILD BLOOD VOLUME LOSS (<30%)	MODERATE BLOOD VOLUME LOSS (30%–45%)	SEVERE BLOOD VOLUME LOSS (>45%)
Cardiovascular	Increased heart rate; weak, thready peripheral pulses; normal systolic blood pressure (80–90 + 2 × age in years); normal pulse pressure	Markedly increased heart rate; weak, thready central pulses; absent peripheral pulses; low normal systolic blood pressure (70–80 + 2 × age in years); narrowed pulse pressure	Tachycardia followed by bradycardia; very weak or absent central pulses; absent peripheral pulses; hypotension (<70 + 2 × age in years); widened pulse pressure (or undetectable diastolic blood pressure)
Central Nervous System	Anxious; irritable; confused	Lethargic; dulled response to pain[a]	Comatose
Skin	Cool, mottled; prolonged capillary refill	Cyanotic; markedly prolonged capillary refill	Pale and cold
Urine Output[b]	Low to very low	Minimal	None

[a]The child's dulled response to pain with this degree of blood loss (30%–45%) may be indicate by a decreased response to IV catheter insertion.
[b]After initial decompression by urinary catheter. Low normal is 2 mL/kg/h (infant), 1.5 mL/kg/h (younger child), 1 mL/kg/h (older child), and 0.5 mL/kg/h (adolescent). IV contract can falsely elevate urinary output.
Reproduced with permission from American College of Surgeons Committee on Trauma. *Advanced Trauma Life Support for Doctors ATLS Student Course Manual.* 8th ed. Chicago, IL: American College of Surgeons; 2008.

TABLE 15.5

VITAL FUNCTIONS

AGE GROUP	WEIGHT RANGE (IN KG)	HEART RATE (BEATS/MIN)	BLOOD PRESSURE (MM HG)	RESPIRATORY RATE (BREATHS/MIN)	URINARY OUTPUT (ML/KG/H)
Infant 0–12 mo	0–10	<160	>60	<60	2.0
Toddler 1–2 y	10–14	<150	>70	<40	1.5
Preschool 3–5 y	14–18	<140	>75	<35	1.0
School age 6–12 y	18–36	<120	>80	<30	1.0
Adolescent 13 y	36–70	<100	>90	<30	0.5

Reproduced with permission from American College of Surgeons Committee on Trauma. *Advanced Trauma Life Support for Doctors ATLS Student Course Manual.* 8th ed. Chicago, IL: American College of Surgeons; 2008.

and normal mental status are the endpoints of resuscitation for the pediatric patient with hypovolemia or hemorrhage.[98] Due to the high ratio of body surface area to BM in children, limited subcutaneous fat and thinner skin, the resultant increase in heat exchange with the environment leads to hypothermia. External warming efforts, such as warm resuscitation room, heat lamps, and warm blankets in addition to internal warming fluids should be employed. In the setting of severe hypovolemic shock, venous access is paramount and is preferably established peripherally. If unobtainable, intraosseous infusion via a bone marrow needle (18 gauge in infants, 15 gauge in young children) or femoral venous line is appropriate.

Specific Considerations

Trauma Injury is the most common reason for an ED visit for a child. Motor vehicle-associated injuries, whether the child is occupant, pedestrian, or cyclist, are the most common causes of injury death in children of all ages. Drowning, fire, abuse, and falls are all important causes of injury in pediatric patients. The principles of trauma management follow the standard put forth in the ATLS™ and PALS courses.[98,99] Head injuries are the most common cause of death and long-term disability in the pediatric trauma population. Hypotension and hypoxia from associated injuries will have an adverse effect on outcome associated with intracranial injury. Thoracic injuries in children are uncommon (only 8% of all injuries) but should serve as a marker for other organ system injury. Rarely do injuries in the chest require operative intervention. In abdominal trauma, single and even multiple solid organ injury can be managed nonoperatively if the child is hemodynamically stable without signs of peritonitis. Spinal cord injury is fortunately uncommon in children with only 5% of all spinal cord injuries occurring in the pediatric age group. The management of skeletal trauma in the child is similar to that for the adult. However, due to the potential for injury of the growth plate, management will often require consultation with an orthopedic surgeon familiar with these injuries. Special attention must be given to the possibility of nonaccidental trauma (i.e., child abuse) in the evaluation of all children suffering injury, trauma, and burns.

Triage is essential to effective functioning of regional trauma systems and to the proper care of the injured patient. The Pediatric Trauma Score (PTS) is an adaptation of the Revised Trauma Score (RTS) and used often to triage pediatric trauma patients to the appropriate trauma center.[100] The RTS is based on physiologic measurements on initial evaluation including blood pressure, respiratory rate, and Glasgow Coma Scale. The PTS is the sum of the severity grade of each category (weight, airway, blood pressure, level of consciousness, fracture, and wounds). The PTS reliably predicts the potential for death and severe disability. In general, injured children with a PTS less than 8 should be triaged to an appropriate pediatric trauma center, because of high potential for mortality and morbidity.

Surgical Emergencies Both congenital and acquired conditions can result in emergency surgical disease. Many neonatal surgical emergencies, such as (congenital diaphragmatic hernia and abdominal wall defects, etc.) are diagnosed *in utero* allowing planned postnatal care. Other newborns may present with surgical emergencies such as necrotizing enterocolitis or intestinal atresia, and the oncall emergency surgeon may be consulted to evaluate these infants. Malrotation causing midgut volvulus is perhaps the most feared abdominal emergency presenting in the newborn period. Malrotation occurs in 1:100 to 1:500 live births with most patients (90%) presenting within the first year of life.[101] Bilious emesis is the most common presenting symptom (93%) and should prompt expeditious evaluation and surgical consultation.[102] Bilious emesis and other signs of obstruction in infants warrant immediate investigation and consultation as delays in diagnosis and treatment threaten intestinal viability. Plain films of the abdomen may give information on the bowel gas pattern but cannot exclude the possibility of malrotation or volvulus. A contrast study to confirm normal positioning of the ligament of Treitz and retroperitoneal course of the duodenum is the gold standard for assessment. If symptomatic malrotation is present, after expeditious resuscitation, the child is taken to the operating room for a Ladd's procedure. A Ladd's procedure involves reduction (counterclockwise detorsion) of the volvulus (if present), division of abnormal peritoneal attachments or Ladd's bands, broadening of the mesentery, and appendectomy. Frankly necrotic bowel should be resected with anastomosis or diversion based on the stability of the child. If the viability of the bowel is uncertain, temporary closure and planned second look at 24 hours is recommended. The bowel is returned to abdomen with the cecum and colon in the left hemiabdomen and the small bowel in the right.

Acute appendicitis remains the most common surgical emergency in children. Obstruction of the appendiceal lumen by fecalith or lymphoid hyperplasia is thought to lead to appendiceal distention, venous congestion, edema, and finally ischemia. Delay in treatment can lead to perforation, peritonitis, and abscess. The diagnosis of appendicitis in the pediatric patient can be particularly challenging due to the inability of the child to accurately express the classic signs or symptoms associated with appendicitis. As such, appendiceal perforation at the time of presentation is not uncommon in young children. Clinical symptoms of pain, malaise, nausea, and vomiting are matched with findings of fever, leukocytosis (white blood cells >12,000/mm^3), and C-reactive protein > 3 mg/dL in distinguishing appendicitis from other diagnoses in pediatric patients who present to the ED with abdominal pain.[103] In addition, right lower-quadrant abdominal ultrasound is a useful screening tool with a negative predictive value of 95%, and in the case of an indeterminate ultrasound or diagnostic uncertainty, abdominal CT should be employed.[104] Alternatively, for patients with an unclear clinical picture, hospital admission and reexamination is recommended. The treatment of acute appendicitis is appendectomy. Guidelines for antibiotics in pediatric patients with acute appendicitis recommend a single dose of preoperative broad-spectrum antibiotics for nonperforated appendicitis that is to be treated by appendectomy.[105] The intraoperative findings will help determine the choice of antibiotics, route of administration (intravenous or oral), and duration of therapy postoperatively. Initial nonoperative management of perforated appendicitis with IV antibiotics, percutaneous drainage of abscess where appropriate, and interval appendectomy (at 6 weeks) showed no improvement in outcomes with regard to total hospitalization, recurrent abscess rates, or overall charges when compared to initial laparoscopic appendectomy.[106] However, interval appendectomy may prove beneficial in selected cases of complicated appendicitis. Antibiotics are continued as clinical parameters such as fever, pain, leukocytosis, and bowel function are followed. Laparoscopic appendectomy is becoming the preferred procedure in children despite a slight risk of postoperative abscess requiring drainage.[107] Open technique remains the approach in complicated appendicitis or if the surgeon cannot safely complete the laparoscopic operation.

Inguinal hernias are present in 1%–3% of newborn males, in females less so. Problems related to inguinal hernias are a common reason for ED evaluation. Incarceration and strangulation are uncommon but may have severe consequences. Longer wait times for elective repair of inguinal hernia in infants and young children are associated with an increased risk of incarceration.[108] Additional risk factors for incarceration are age <1 year, female sex, and ED visit. In cases of incarceration, attempts at reduction are indicated for those infants and young children who do not manifest signs or symptoms of peritonitis or scrotal erythema.[109] To reduce a hernia, steady, gentle manual pressure is directed along the canal for several minutes to reduce the contents back through the external and internal inguinal rings and into the abdominal cavity. Judicious use of sedation can be useful in reduction efforts. There is limited literature on the clinical practice of sedation and analgesic medication use for nonoperative reduction of incarcerated inguinal hernia.[110] For children <1 year of age, or in cases that are particularly difficult to reduce, hospital admission and nonemergent hernia repair during the same hospitalization are recommended. If reduction is unsuccessful, emergency operation to reduce the hernia contents and close the sac is undertaken. In cases with suspected bowel ischemia or necrosis, a thorough assessment of the bowel is necessary. Gangrenous bowel should be resected with primary anastomosis possible in most cases. If the hernia contents reduce without inspection and there is concern regarding the viability of the intestine, further assessment should be performed either by abdominal exploration or laparoscopy. Umbilical hernias are very common in young children. Unlike inguinal hernias, however, most spontaneously close before 4 years of age. As such, surgery prior to this time is generally limited to those patients with incarceration or strangulation. Such complications are rare but mandate urgent exploration and repair.[111]

Intussusception is a common cause of intestinal obstruction occurring in young children. There is a slight male predominance (3:2 male to female ratio), and most occur between 3 months and 3 years of age. Often an episode of gastroenteritis or viral syndrome will precede the presentation of episodic ("colicky") abdominal pain. The prodromal illness is postulated to cause intestinal lymphoid hyperplasia that, in turn, acts as a lead point with the invagination of a proximal portion of the intestine (intussusceptum) into the distal portion (intussuscipiens). Initial management is directed at fluid resuscitation. Abdominal radiograph suggestive of free air or evaluation consistent with peritonitis warrants abdominal exploration. The majority of intussusceptions are ileocolic and can be diagnosed and managed with air or contrast enema. Ultrasound has also been advocated for diagnosis of intussusception. The classic "target" sign is diagnostic. Radiologic reduction can then be attempted and ultrasound used to confirm a satisfactory result. Radiologic reduction is successful in the vast majority of cases. When radiologic attempts at reduction are unsuccessful, abdominal exploration is warranted. Depending on the level of comfort of the surgeon, such cases can be performed laparoscopically or open.[112] Necrotic segments of bowel or bowel that cannot be reduced in the operating room should be resected. The choice of anastomosis or diversion should be based on the clinical status of the patient. Much less commonly, the intussusceptions involves just the small bowel. Symptomatic small-bowel intussusceptions are often seen in the postoperative setting and typically require operative reduction. Asymptomatic small-bowel intussusception may be observed as an incidental finding and does not mandate intervention.

Ovarian torsion is an infrequent cause of abdominal pain in girls, and may be confused with other conditions.[113] Among females age 1–20 years, there is an estimated 4.9/100,000 incidence of ovarian torsion, and more than 50% of the patients will require oophorectomy.[114] Nonspecific abdominal pain, nausea, and vomiting occur most frequently, and up to 10% of patients may have a palpable abdominal mass. WBC and CRP values are lower in ovarian torsion than in appendicitis. Ultrasound is beneficial in diagnosis and for determining the adequacy of blood flow to the torsed ovary. CT scan can also help when presentation and ultrasound findings are not definitive. Laparoscopy is the surgical procedure of choice as it aids in the diagnosis of abdominal pain of unclear etiology and can effectively accomplish detorsion of the ovary.[115] In cases of uncertain viability of the ovary, detorsion and planned second-look laparoscopy is of value. Preservation of any ovarian tissue is desirable.

Testicular torsion is most common in adolescent males and requires urgent diagnosis and management.[116] Acute onset and short duration of pain (<6 hours), high-riding testicle, and loss of cremasteric reflex are all associated with testicular torsion. Ultrasound is frequently used to confirm diagnosis; however, if doppler sonography and clinical exam are unreliable, all children presenting with acute scrotal pain in whom testicular torsion is suspected should undergo scrotal exploration.[117] Salvage rates approach 95% if operative detorsion and orchiopexy is performed within 6 hours. Neonates are best served with inguinal incisions as an associated hernia or tumor might be present. A transscrotal incision along the midline raphe is appropriate in older children unless preoperative assessment raises suspicion for testicular malignancy or incarcerated hernia. If the testicle is not viable, an orchidectomy should be performed. The detorsion technique follows the rule that the torsed testicle is twisted toward the midline along the axis of the spermatic cord. As such, detorsion reverses this process. If the testicle is successfully detorsed and regains viability, it should be appended to the wall of the scrotum. Likewise, through the same midline incision, the contralateral testicle should be sutured to the wall of the respective hemi-srotum to prevent torsion.

References

1. Gorina Y, Hoyert D, Lentaner H, et al. *Trends in Causes of Death Among Older Persons in the United States*. Aging Trends, No. 6. Hyattsville, MD: National Center for Health Statistics; 2006.
2. Vincent G, Velkoff V. The next four decades, the older population in the United States: 2010 to 2050/current population reports, 2010, the U.S. Census Bureau, Washington DC.
3. Goulding M, Rogers M, Smith S. Public health and aging: trends in aging—United States and Worldwide. *Mort Morb Wkly Rev.* 2003;52:101-106.
4. Bernstein A, Hing E, Moss A, et al. *Health Care in America: Trends in Utilization*. Hyattsville, MD: National Center for Health Statistics; 2003.
5. Manton K, Gu X, Lowrimore G. Cohort changes in active life expectancy in the U.S. elderly population: experience from the 1982–2004 National Long-Term Care Survey. *J Gerontol B Psychol Sci Soc Sci.* 2008;63:S269-S281.
6. Cherry D, Lucas C, Decker S. *Population Aging and the Use of Office-Based Physician Services*. NCHS Data Brief No. 41. Hyattsville, MD: National Center for Health Statistics; 2010.
7. National Center for Health Statistics. *Health, United States, 2009: With Special Feature on Medical Technology*. Hyattsville, MD; 2010.
8. Centers for Disease Control and Prevention, National Center for Injury Prevention and Control. Web Based Injury Statistics Query and Reporting System (WISQARS). Accessed online December 8, 2010. http://www.cdc.gov/injury/wisqars/index.html
9. Schwab CW, Kauder DR. Trauma in the geriatric patient. *Arch Surg.* 1992;127:701-706.
10. Arenal JJ, Bengoenchea-Beeby M. Mortality associated with emergency abdominal surgery in the elderly. *Can J Surg.* 2003;46:111-116.
11. Turrentine FE, Wang H, Simpson VB, et al. Surgical risk factors, morbidity, and mortality in elderly patients. *J Am Coll Surg.* 2006;203:865-877.
12. Aalami OO, Fang TD, Song HM, et al. Physiologic features of aging persons. *Arch Surg.* 2003;138:1068-1076.
13. Colloca G, Santoro M, Gambassi G. Age-related changes and perioperative management of elderly patients. *Surg Oncol.* 2010;19:124-130.
14. Menaker J, Scalea TM. Geriatric care in the surgical intensive care unit. *Crit Care Med.* 2010;38:S452-S459.
15. Marik PE. Management of the critically ill geriatric patient. *Crit Care Med.* 2006;34:S176-S182.
16. Brandstetter RD, Kazemi H. Aging and the respiratory system. *Med Clin North Am.* 1983;67:419-431.
17. El Solh AA, Ramadan FH. Overview of respiratory failure in older adults. *J Intensive Care Med.* 2006;21;345-351.
18. Rosenthal RA, Kavic SM. Assessment and management of the geriatric patient. *Crit Care Med.* 2004;4:S92-S105.
19. Luckey AE, Parsa CJ. Fluids and electrolytes in the aged. *Arch Surg.* 2003;138:1055-1060.
20. Barr J, Hecht M, Flavin KE, et al. Outcomes in critically ill patients before and after the implementation of an evidence-based nutrition management protocol. *Chest.* 2004;125:1446-1457.
21. Neumayer LA, Smout RJ, Horn HG, et al. Early and sufficient feeding reduces length of stay and charges in surgical patients. *J Surg Res.* 2001;95:73-77.
22. Ho KC, Roessman U, Straumfjord JV, et al. Analysis of brain weight. I. Adult brain weight in relation to sex, race, and age. *Arch Pathol Lab Med.* 1980;104:635-639.
23. Bowie MW, Slattum PW. Pharmacodynamics in older adults: a review. *Am J Geriatr Pharmacother.* 2007;5:263-303.
24. Samaras N, Chevalley T, Samaras D, et al. Older patients in the emergency department: a review. *Ann Emerg Med.* 2010;56:261-269.
25. Esses D, Birnbaum A, Bijur P, et al. Ability of CT to alter decision making in elderly patients with acute abdominal pain. *Am J Emerg Med.* 2004;22:270-272.
26. Rix TE, Bates T. Pre-operative risk scores for prediction of outcome in elderly people who require emergency surgery. *World J Emerg Surg.* 2007;2:16.
27. Owens WD, Felts JA, Spitznagel EL. ASA physical status classifications: a study of consistency ratings. *Anesthesiology.* 1978;49:239-243.
28. Rubinfeld I, Thomas C, Berry S, et al. Octogenarian abdominal surgical emergencies: not so grim a problem with the acute care surgery model? *J Trauma.* 2009;67:983-987.
29. Centers for Disease Control and Prevention. *The State of Aging and Health in America 2007*. Atlanta, GA: CDC; 2007.
30. Fleisher LA, Beckman JA, Brown KA, et al. ACC/AHA 2007 Guidelines on perioperative cardiovascular evaluation and care for noncardiac surgery. *Circulation.* 2007;116:1970-1996.
31. Seguin P, Signouret T, Laviolle B, et al. Incidence and risk factors of atrial fibrillation in a surgical intensive care unit. *Crit Care Med.* 2004;32:722-726.
32. Seguin P, Laviolle B, Maurice A, et al. Atrial fibrillation in trauma patients requiring intensive care. *Intensive Care Med.* 2006;32:398-404.
33. Fuster V, Ryden L, Cannom D, et al. ACC/AHA/ESC 2006 Guidelines for the management of patients with atrial fibrillation. *Circulation.* 2006;114:701-752.
34. Fleisher LA, Beckman JA, Brown KA, et al. 2009 ACCF/AHA Focused update on perioperative beta blockade incorporated into the ACC/AHA 2007 guidelines on perioperative cardiovascular evaluation and care for noncardiac surgery. *Circulation.* 2009;120:e169-e276.
35. Peter FW, Benkovic C, Muehlberger T, et al. Effects of desmopressin on thrombogenesis in aspirin-induced platelet dysfunction. *Br J Haemotol.* 2002;117:658-663.
36. Baker RI, Coughlin PB, Gallus AS, et al. Warfarin reversal: consensus guidelines, on behalf of the Australasian Society of Thrombosis and Haemostasis. *Med J Aust.* 2004;181:492-497.
37. Hirsh J, Fuster V, Ansell J, et al. American Heart Association/American College of Cardiology Foundation guide to warfarin therapy. *Circulation.* 2003;107:1692-1711.
38. McQuay N, Cipolla J, Franges EZ, et al. The use of recombinant activated factor VIIa in coagulopathic traumatic brain injury requiring emergent craniotomy. Is it beneficial? *J Neurosurg.* 2009;111:666-671.
39. Ng HJ, Lee LH. Recombinant activated clotting factor VII (rFVIIa) in the treatment of surgical and spontaneous bleeding episodes in hemophilic patients. *Vasc Health Risk Manag.* 2006;2:433-440.
40. Kalina M, Tinkoff G, Ghadebo A, et al. A protocol for the rapid normalization of INR in trauma patients with intracranial hemorrhage on prescribed warfarin therapy. *Am Surg.* 2008;74:858-861.
41. Behrendt CE. Acute respiratory failure in the United States: incidence and 31-day survival. *Chest.* 2000;118:1100-1105.
42. Rubenfeld GD, Caldwell E, Peabody E, et al. Incidence and outcome of acute lung injury. *N Engl J Med.* 2005;353:1685-1693.
43. Schulz-Stubner S. The critically ill patient and regional anesthesia. *Curr Opin Anesthesiol.* 2006;19:538-544.
44. Simon BJ, Cushman J, Barraco R, et al. Pain management guidelines for blunt thoracic trauma. *J Trauma.* 2005;59:1256-1267
45. Sarani B, Temple-Lykens B, Kim P, et al. Factors associated with mortality and brain injury after falls from the standing position. *J Trauma.* 2009;67:954-958.
46. Henry SM, Pollak AN, Jones AL, et al. Pelvic fracture in geriatric patients: a distinct clinical entity. *J Trauma.* 2002;53:15-20.
47. American College of Surgeons Committee on Trauma. *Advanced Trauma Life Support for Doctors ATLS Student Course Manual.* 8th ed. Chicago, IL: American College of Surgeons; 2008: Chapter 11.
48. Pilotto A, Franceschi, M, Maggi S, et al. Optimal management of peptic ulcer disease in the elderly. *Drugs Aging.* 2010;27:545-558.
49. Crofts TJ, Kenneth GM, Park MB, et al. A randomized trial of nonoperative treatment for perforated peptic ulcer. *N Engl J Med.* 1989;320:970-973.
50. DiCarlo I, Toro A, Sparatore F, et al. Emergency gastric ulcer complications in elderly. Factors affecting the morbidity and mortality in relation to therapeutic approaches. *Minerva Chir.* 2006;61:325-332.
51. Millat B, Fingerhut A, Borie F. Surgical treatment of complicated duodenal ulcers: controlled trials. *World J Surg.* 2000;24:299-306.
52. Bertleff MJ, Lange JF. Laparoscopic correction of perforated peptic ulcer: first choice? A review of literature. *Surg Endosc.* 2010;24:1231-1239.
53. Arthur JD, Edwards PR, Chagla LS. Management of gallstone disease in the elderly. *Ann R Coll Surg Engl.* 2003;85:91-97.
54. Leardi S, DeVita F, Pietroletti R, et al. Cholecystectomy for gallbladder disease in elderly aged 80 years and over. *Hepatogastroenterology.* 2009;56:303-306.
55. Riall TS, Zhang D, Townsed C, et al. Failure to perform cholecystectomy for acute cholecystitis in elderly patients is associated with increased morbidity, mortality, and cost. *J Am Coll Surg.* 2009;210:668-677.
56. Morse BC, Smith JB, Lawdahl RB, et al. Management of acute cholecystitis in critically ill patients: contemporary role for cholecystostomy and subsequent cholecystectomy. *Am Surg.* 2010;73:708-712.
57. Sufian S, Matsumoto T. Intestinal obstruction. *Am J Surg.* 1975;130:9-14.
58. Tekin A, Kucukkartallar T, Aksoy F, et al. Intestinal herniation as a major cause of intestinal obstruction. *Med Principles Pract.* 2008;17:400-403.
59. Poon RT, Law WL, Chu KW, et al. Emergency resection and primary anastomosis for left-sided obstructing colorectal carcinoma in the elderly. *Br J Surg.* 1998;85:1539-1542.
60. Eldar S, Nash E, Sabo E, et al. Delay of surgery in acute appendicitis. *Am J Surg.* 1997;173:194-198.
61. Gurleyik G, Gurleyik E. Age-related clinical features in older patients with acute appendicitis. *Eur J Emerg Med.* 2003;10:200-203.
62. Harrell AG, Lincourt AE, Novitsky YW, et al. Advantages of laparoscopic appendectomy in the elderly. *Am Surg.* 2006;72:474-480.

63. Hui TT, Major KM, Avita I, et al. Outcome of elderly patients with appendicitis: effect of computed tomography and laparoscopy. *Arch Surg.* 2002;137:995-998.
64. Wang YC, Yang HR, Chung LB, et al. Laparoscopic appendectomy in the elderly. *Surg Endosc.* 2006;20:887-889.
65. Lugo JZ, Avgerinos DV, Lefkowitz AJ, et al. Can interval appendectomy be justified following conservative treatment of perforated appendicitis? *J Surg Res.* 2010;164:91-94.
66. Liu CK, Hsu HH, Cheng SM. Colonic diverticulitis in the elderly. *Int J Gerontol.* 2009;3:9-15.
67. Comparato G, Pilotto A, Franze A, et al. Diverticular disease in the elderly. *Dig Dis.* 2007;25:151-159.
68. Nilsson H, Stylianidis G, Haapamaki M, et al. Mortality after groin hernia surgery. *Ann Surg.* 2007;245:656-660.
69. Arenal JJ, Rodriguez-Vielba P, Gallo E, et al. Hernias of the abdominal wall in patients over the age of 70 years. *Eur J Surg.* 2002;168:460-463.
70. Derici H, Unalp HR, Bozdag AD, et al. Factors affecting morbidity and mortality in incarcerated abdominal wall hernias. *Hernia.* 200711:341-346.
71. Kulah B, Duzkan AP, Moran M, et al. Emergency hernia repair in elderly patients. *Am J Surg.* 2001;182:455-459.
72. Cangemi JR, Picco MF. Intestinal ischemia in the elderly. *Gastroenterol Clin North Am.* 2009;38:527-540.
73. Rutherford RB, Baer JD, Ernst C, et al. Recommended standards for reports dealing with lower extremity ischemia: revised version. *J Vasc Surg.* 1997;26:517-538.
74. Anderson DJ, Kaye KS. Skin and soft tissue infection in older adults. *Clin Geriatr Med.* 2007;23:595-613.
75. Sarani B, Strong M, Pascual J, et al. Necrotizing fasciitis: current concepts and review of the literature. *J Am Coll Surg.* 2009;208:279-288.
76. Truog RD, Campbell ML, Curtis JR, et al. Recommendations for end-of-life care in the intensive care unit: a consensus statement by the American College of Critical Care Medicine. *Crit Care Med.* 2008;36:953-963.
77. Meisser A, Genga KR, Studart FS, et al. Epidemiology of and factors associated with end-of-life decisions in a surgical intensive care unit. *Crit Care Med.* 2010;38:1060-1068.
78. Pawlik TM, Curley SA. Ethical issues in surgical palliative care: am I killing the patient by "letting him go"? *Surg Clin North Am.* 2005;85:273-286.
79. Chames MC, Pearlman MD. Trauma during pregnancy: outcomes and clinical management. *Clin Obstet Gynecol.* 2008;51:398-408.
80. Parangi S, Levine D, Henry A, et al. Surgical gastrointestinal disorders during pregnancy. *Am J Surg.* 2007;193:223-232.
81. Dietrich CS III, Hill CC, Hueman M. Surgical diseases presenting in pregnancy. *Surg Clin North Am.* 2008;88:403-419.
82. Hill CC, Pickinpaugh J. Physiologic changes in pregnancy. *Surg Clin North Am.* 2008;88:391-401.
83. Yeomans ER, Gilstrap LC III. Physiologic changes in pregnancy and their impact on critical care. *Crit Care Med.* 2005;33:S256-S258.
84. Toglia MR, Weg JG. Venous thromboembolism during pregnancy. *N Engl J Med.* 1996;335:108-114.
85. Shah AJ, Kilcline BA. Trauma in pregnancy. *Emerg Med Clin North Am.* 2003;21:615-629.
86. American College of Surgeons Committee on Trauma. *Advanced Trauma Life Support for Doctors ATLS Student Course Manual.* 8th ed. Chicago, IL: American College of Surgeons; 2008: Chapter 12.
87. Tinkhoff G. Care of the pregnant trauma patient. In: Peitzman A, Rhodes M, Schwab CW, et al. eds. *The Trauma Manual.* 3rd ed. Philadelphia: Lippincott, Williams & Wilkins Publishers; 2008;515-523.
88. Moore, Keith, Persaud, T. eds. *The Developing Human: Clinically Oriented Embryology.* 8th ed. Philadelphia, PA: Saunders Publishers; 2003.
89. Nathan L, Huddleston JF. Acute abdominal pain in pregnancy. *Obstet Gynecol Clin North Am.* 1995;22:55-67.
90. Dhupar R, Smaldone GM, Hamad GG. Is there a benefit to delaying cholecystectomy for symptomatic gallbladder disease during pregnancy? *Surg Endosc.* 2010; 24:108-112.
91. Gbolade BA, Daw EG. Strangulated umbilical hernia in pregnancy. *J Obstet Gynecol.* 1993;13:353-354.
92. Abramowitz L, Sobhani I, Benifla JL, et al. Anal fissure and thrombosed external hemorrhoids before and after delivery. *Dis Colon Rectum.* 2002;45:650-655.
93. Nisar PJ, Scholefield JH. Managing haemorrhoids. *BMJ.* 2003;327: 847-851.
94. Dresang LT, Fontaine P, Leeman L, et al. Venous thromboembolism during pregnancy. *Am Fam Physician.* 2008;77:1709-1716.
95. Stanton B, Behrman RE. Overview of pediatrics. In: Kliegman RM, Behrman RE, Jenson HB, Stanton BF, eds. *Nelson Textbook of Pediatrics.* 18th ed. Philadelphia, PA: Saunders Elsevier; 2007: Chapter 1.
96. Greenbaum LA. Electrolyte and acid-base disorders. In: Kliegman RM, Behrman RE, Jenson HB, Stanton BF, eds. *Nelson Textbook of Pediatrics.* 18th ed. Philadelphia, PA: Saunders Elsevier; 2007: Chapter 52.
97. Greenbaum LA. Maintenance and replacement therapy. In: Kliegman RM, Behrman RE, Jenson HB, Stanton BF, eds. *Nelson Textbook of Pediatrics.* 18th ed. Philadelphia, PA: Saunders Elsevier; 2007: Chapter 53.
98. American College of Surgeons Committee on Trauma. *Advanced Trauma Life Support for Doctors ATLS Student Course Manual.* 8th ed. Chicago, IL: American College of Surgeons; 2008: Chapter 10.
99. American Academy of Pediatrics. American Heart Association. *Pediatric Advanced Life Support.* Provider Manual, Chapter 1. 2006.
100. American College of Surgeons Committee on Trauma. *Advanced Trauma Life Support for Doctors ATLS Student Course Manual.* 8th ed. Chicago, IL: American College of Surgeons; 2008: Appendix C.
101. Applegate KE, Anderson JM, Klatte EC. Intestinal malrotation in children: a problem-solving approach to the upper gastrointestinal series. *Radiographics.* 2006;5:1485-1500.
102. Nehra D, Goldstein AM. Intestinal malrotation: varied clinical presentation from infancy through adulthood. *Surgery.* 2011;149:386-393.
103. Kwan KY, Nager AL. Diagnosing pediatric appendicitis: usefulness of laboratory markers. *Am J Emerg Med.* 2010;28:1009-1015.
104. Neufeld D, Vainrib M, Buklan G, et al. Management of acute appendicitis: an imaging strategy in children. *Pediatr Surg Int.* 2010;29:167-171.
105. Lee SL, Islam S, Cassidy LD. Antibiotics and appendicitis in the pediatric population: an American Pediatric Surgery Association outcomes and clinical trials committee systematic review. *J Pediatr Surg.* 2010:45;2181-2185.
106. St. Peter SD, Aguayo P, Fraser JD, et al. Initial laparoscopic appendectomy versus initial nonoperative management and interval appendectomy for perforated appendicitis with abscess: a prospective, randomized trial. *J Pediatr Surg.* 2010;45:236-240.
107. Jen HC, Shew SB. Laparoscopic versus open appendectomy in children: outcomes comparison based on statistical analysis. *J Surg Res.* 2010;16:113-117.
108. Zamakhshary M, To T, Guan J, et al. Risk of incarceration of inguinal hernia among infants and young children awaiting elective surgery. *Can Med Assoc J.* 2008;170:1001-1005.
109. Ruddy RM. Procedures. In: Ludwig S, Fleisher GR, Henreting FM, eds. *Textbook of Paediatric Emergency Medicine.* 5th ed. Baltimore, MD: Williams & Wilkins, 2006;1917-1918.
110. Al-Ansari K, Sulowski C, Ratnapalan S. Analgesia and sedation practices for incarcerated inguinal hernia in children. *Clin Pediatr.* 2008;47: 766-769
111. Papgrigoriadis S, Browse DJ, Howard ER. Incarceration of umbilical hernias in children: a rare but important complication. *Pediatr Surg Int.* 1998;14:231-232.
112. Zitsman JL. Pediatric minimal-access surgery: update 2006. *Pediatrics.* 2006;118:304-308.
113. Chang YJ, Yan DC, Kong MS, et al. Adnexal torsion in children. *Pediatr Emerg Care.* 2008;24:534-537.
114. Guthrie BD, Adler MD, Powell EC. Incidence and trends of pediatric ovarian torsion hospitalizations in the United States, 2000–2006. *Pediatrics.* 2010;125:532-538.
115. Oltmann SC, Fischer A, Barber R. et al. Cannot exclude torsion—a 15 year review. *J Pediatr Surg.* 2009;44:1212-1217.
116. Beni-Israel T, Goldman M, Bar Chaim S, et al. Clinical predictor for testicular torsion as seen in the pediatric ED. *Am J Emerg Med.* 2010;28: 786-789.
117. Murphy FL, Fletcher L, Pease P. Early scrotal exploration in all cases is the investigation and intervention of choice in the acute paediatric scrotum. *Pediatr Surg Int*, 2006;22:413-416.

CHAPTER 16 ■ PREHOSPITAL TRAUMA CARE

NORMAN E. MCSWAIN JR

This chapter is divided into two parts: the first is what the acute care surgeon (ACS) needs to know about the care provided to the patient before the patient arrives in the hospital and the second is a kinematics discussion for understanding the mechanism of injury (MOI). In the best of Emergency Medical Services (EMS) systems, the prehospital providers manage the injured patient for at least the first half of the proverbial "Golden Hour." It is the responsibility of the ACS to make sure that these providers understand the care of the trauma patient during this critical time period. This care may ultimately determine the outcome for the injured patient. The ACS must teach these principles to the person caring for his or her patient in the field.

Patient care begins when the first person reaches the patient. It does not start when the patient arrives in the hospital. From his experiences in the Spanish American War, Dr. Nicholas Senn, the 49th president of the American Medical Association, surgeon general of the Wisconsin National Guard, and founder of the Association of Military Surgeons stated *"The fate of the wounded rests in the hands of one who applies the first dressing."* He was probably quoting the German physician, Johann Nepomuk von Nussbaum from the early 1800s.[1]

If physicians believe that the care in their particular community in the prehospital period is not good, then they have the duty to teach the prehospital providers the correct methods.

The American College of Surgeons endorsed PreHosptial Life support (PHTLS) training, which is an excellent example of a physician–prehospital provider educational collaboration.[2] Involvement with this educational program will go a long way to achieving these educational goals by the ACS.

The philosophy of the continuum of care, which begins in the field and continues to rehab, is an important part of the ACS's career. The ACS must ensure that the prehospital provider provides this management for trauma patients before they get to the emergency department (ED). Mismanagement in the first 30–90 minutes of care and when the patient is with the prehospital provider is critical to the outcome. It is perhaps more critical than the care provided in the ED. "The die is cast" if the prehospital care is not good.

This chapter addresses the important points of the prehospital provider's training and education. Although there are several providers who care for the patient in many locations, the goals of patient care should be the same, but the steps are different. *There is one patient with the same disease in the same condition who requires the same care by different providers using different skills at different locations* (Tables 16.1 and 16.2).

Each of these providers has different skills, different resources, and different short-term goals. They each provide *definitive care* in the situation that they encounter the patient (Table 16.3).

The aim is to provide definitive/appropriate care for the patient as quickly as possible in each individual area and then move to the next area; for example, for the patient who is acidotic in the ED with uncontrolled hemorrhage, the *definitive emergency department is for hemorrhage control.* This patient needs to be in the Operating room (OR) for hemorrhage control with clamps and ligatures (factor XIV). Keeping the patient in the ED to give crystalloids, factor VII, factor IX, prothrombin clotting complex, or to get additional images such as the CT, is inappropriate. The patient needs to be either in the OR or in the interventional radiology suite with 10 minutes in the ED for the beginning resuscitation. The patient now needs to move on.

The same concept applies to the prehospital environment. For the patient with uncontrolled hemorrhage or potential uncontrolled hemorrhage, *definitive field care* is rapid movement of the patient to the hospital after control of all visible hemorrhage. The steps are appropriate airway and ventilation management, control of external hemorrhage, packaging for transport, and rapid movement to the trauma center. The patient does not need detailed secondary survey in the field. This can be done during transport if time allows or can be deferred if the transport time is short. Correct *definitive field care* is getting the patient to a setting where hemorrhage control (damage control surgery) and restoration of energy production are aerobic with metabolism (damage control resuscitation), and can be done as quickly as possible. In the urban areas, this means bypassing a nearby community hospital to go to a trauma center.

It does not mean overloading the patient with crystalloid. Hypotensive resuscitation is the correct management in the field and in the hospital until hemorrhage control can be obtained.

The term "scoop and run" is an incorrect process and should never be the correct method of patient care either in the ED or in the field. This term implies that no care is provided for the patient when transport to the next level of care is imminent. For the prehospital provider, "scoop and run" means placing the patient on the stretcher and racing at high speed to the closest hospital. This method of patient care began to disappear when Dr. J.D. "Deke" Farington wrote his paper entitled "Death in a Ditch," which was published in the Bulletin of the American College of Surgeons in 1967[3] (Box 16.1). Fortunately for the trauma patient, such an approach to patient care no longer exists in most of the United States. Unfortunately, this process continues to exist in many third world countries, usually due to a lack of proper trauma education for prehospital providers and lack of funding to provide this education. Just as "scoop and run" is the worst possible approach of addressing the patient's needs, equally poor is attempting to address all of the patient's needs in the prehospital arena either in the field or in the back of the ambulance.[4] The judgment of the provider based on an understanding of the patient's needs will define the extent of the field care.

The question for the Emergency Medical Technician (EMT) to answer is "what is best for the patient" and "where can this care best be provided." In the management of any patient, one has to consider the needs of the patient and the ability of the provider to address those needs at a given time and a specific place where the patient currently is located. The provider should assess the patient and provide care according to the situation, the condition of the patient, the abilities of the provider, and the resources available at the scene. This is addressed by understanding principles and preferences. A principle is the specific medical needs of the patient. The preference is how the provider can best address such needs.[5] (Table 16.4)

The foundation of patient care is based on certain principles of identification and management of the patient's condition.

TABLE 16.1

CONTINUUM OF CARE

- Begins in the field
- Location of care
  - Field
  - Transportation
  - Emergency Department
  - OR
  - ICU
  - Floor
  - Rehabilitation
- Ends when return to full activity

The preferences of how these principles are accomplished are based on the following four separate concepts: (1) the *situation* the patient and the provider are in at the time of their interaction, (2) the *condition* of the patient, (2) the *skill and knowledge* of the provider, and (4) the *equipment, resources, and supplies* that the provider has to work with at the time.

As an example, the principle is that the airway must be opened. The preference is how it is to be opened. Multiple options are available to the EMT: jaw lift, jaw thrust, nasal airway, oral airway, endotracheal tube, and cricothyrotomy. Scene conditions, situation, and patient condition will dictate which airway option is utilized. An unruly crowd on scene or hazardous weather conditions outside may dictate a rapid, basic-level airway, such as an oral airway or bag valve mask (BVM). This may change in the ambulance with more protection for the patient and the providers. The situation may change more in the ED with different equipment and skills for the provider.

The EMTs in the prehospital arena must be trained with the skills to manage the patient appropriately in a field setting.

The principles are the same, but there are different preferences depending on where the patient is located (Tables 16.3 and 16.4).

Besides principles and preferences, the other concept that requires understanding is definitive care of the patient in the field for the specific patient. Definitive field care will vary depending on the etiology. A patient with *cardiac arrest* needs definitive care of restoring the rhythm and cardiac output. This can be done in the field at the paramedic level.[6] A diabetic patient can be managed definitively in the field using glucose or insulin. A severe trauma patient most likely is suffering from hemorrhage. The hemorrhage cannot be managed in the field definitively. The patient must be transported as quickly as possible to an appropriate facility that can provide such care. The care that might be required is an expedient celiotomy to control the hemorrhage. In the urban setting, the arena for this definitive management is the trauma center that has the availability of trauma surgeons, emergency physicians, operating rooms, and a blood bank. These are the essential components. Just as it is incorrect for the EMS provider to spend more than 10 minutes in the field with a critical hemorrhaging patient, so is it incorrect for this same patient to stay more than 10 minutes in the resuscitation room.

In the rural setting, there is usually no hospital with an immediately available surgeon, operating room, and blood bank. The hemodynamically compromised patient should go to a trauma center in the urban area, but in the rural area, to the closest appropriate facility for stabilization of definitive management. EMS is a critical component of the health care network. Triage is an essential feature of prehospital care. Approximately 5% of the patients that are injured require the facilities of a trauma center. A well-trained provider has the knowledge to understand the patient's specific condition and understand where the patient can best get the most optimal care.

TABLE 16.2

STEPS OF CARE (BASED ON LOCATION)

- Primary
  - Field
  - Transport
- Secondary
  - Emergency Department
- Tertiary
  - OR
  - ICU
  - Floor
- Quaternary
  - Rehab
  - Home

TABLE 16.3

DEFINITIVE CARE

- Definitive FIELD care
- Definitive Emergency Department care
- Definitive OPERATING ROOM care
- Definitive ICU care
- Definitive FLOOR care
- Definitive REHAB care

RURAL TRAUMA ORGANIZATION SYSTEM

Trauma care in the rural communities has been less than that available in the urban area for two major reasons: (1) lack of money to equip staff and train the hospital and EMS personnel and (2) skill deterioration in both groups with lack of severe trauma care experience in the smaller hospitals.

BOX 16.1

DEATH IN THE DITCH[3]

"Come on fellow, we'll take you and your wife to the hospital."

He was pulled from the car, placed on a stretcher, and carried to the ambulance.

Ruth soon was placed on a similar rig. The door was slammed closed and the driver and his helper got into the front seat. The ambulance leaped forward with a screech from the tires and a shriek from the siren.

"Death in the ditch"

JD, 'Deke' Farrington MD 1967

TABLE 16.4

PRINCIPLES AND PREFERENCES

- Principles - Standard of Care
- Preferences -How can YOU as the provider achieve the standard
- *Situation of the encounter*
- Condition *of the patient*
- Ability of the provider
  - *Knowledge*
  - *Skill*
  - *Experience*
- Resources available

TABLE 16.5

TRAUMA DESIGNATION PROTOCOLS

- Directly to the trauma center from the field
  - ACS anatomic or physiologic injuries
  - CDC Revised level 1, 2 or 3[8] Bypass all hospitals unless
    - Time of transport >50 min
    - Airway problem that EMS cannot handle in the unit
    - Severe shock and needs blood or plasma during transport
    - DOA
- MOI alone to closest appropriate facility
- Patient choice does not count for bypass to trauma center
- Any patient short stopped is immediately accepted by trauma center when problem is solved
- Trauma center does not go on diversion unless;
  - Mechanical or electrical difficulties

Three trauma patients require simultaneous OR

Staff and equipment availability will always be difficult in the rural communities but the training is available to improve competence when the patient does present for care.

The first step in proper management is appropriate *field triage* and transport of the patient to the appropriate hospital. This must be coupled with an assessment of the strengths of all the hospitals in an area with appropriate bypass or delivery of the patient to the correct facility. Part of the well-developed regional trauma system is an agreement among the hospitals involved to accept the patients when presented and to either treat or stabilize those patients and quickly move them to the appropriate facility.

Such a rural trauma system could be modeled after the Joint Theater Trauma System (JTTS) Military Echelon Casualty management system.[7] Patients are taken to facilities dedicated to a specific level of care. When that care has been achieved, the patient is moved on to the next level. An example of this system in action is military personnel seen by medics (Echelon 1) and taken to an Echelon 2 facility where damage control surgery (DCS) is done (hemorrhage control only) and damage control resuscitation is initiated. The patient is sent directly from the OR to an Echelon 3 facility where definitive care is provided (or the second step of DCS). Within 24 hours when the patient is still in the ICU, he or she is moved to an Echelon 4 facility for additional definitive care if needed. Finally within 4–6 days of the injury, the patient is moved to the United States for follow-up care and rehab.

Approximately 10% of civilian injured patients will need assessment in a trauma center. The other 90% should be assessed and treated in the rural community hospital. About 80% of the patients with MOI alone will be discharged within 6 hours of admission into the ED. Of the remaining 20%, almost all will have orthopedic injures that also do not require the expertise of the trauma surgeon and can be better served by providing treatment close to the patient's family and home. Stated differently, MOI alone is not adequate reason for transporting a patient to a trauma center. These patients should be treated in the appropriate rural or regional hospital. This will also ensure financial support to the local community and community hospitals. The patients, who may require the expertise and resources of the trauma center, can be assessed in the community hospital and then transferred to the trauma center, if necessary. The additional benefit of this type of triage will prevent an overload in the trauma center with patients, who can easily be treated elsewhere (Table 16.5). It is the responsibility of the rural area to understand the resources in the various hospitals and to triage and transport patients to the appropriate hospital.

CONTINUUM OF PATIENT CARE

Patient care should be a continuum from the time the first person sees the patient until the patient is discharged to home. There should be interlinking of the various locations and individuals who provide the care, with prehospital care being an important component of this continuum. The prehospital assessment and care will vary depending on the condition of the patient. A 4 minute ride to the hospital, a 40 minute ride to the hospital, and a 4 hour ride to the hospital are vastly different rides and will require different judgments based on the knowledge[2] of the prehospital providers.

Priorities include initial airway management and ensuring adequate ventilation, and if possible, control of hemorrhage. External extremity hemorrhage is controlled with direct pressure and if that fails, then by tourniquet application. Torso hemorrhage control process in the field is only superficial pressure ; therefore, the optimal management is to get the patient to surgical care as quickly as possible. Fracture stabilization is next in priority and intravenous access/resuscitation can often be initiated en route to the hospital.

Patient care is provided based on principles, and these principles must meet the needs of the specific patient involved and the medical conditions present. Situation and available resources impact this decision. The prehospital provider makes a *judgment based on this knowledge*.[2]

Although the situation and location of patient care varies, the same basic process and the same attention to quality care exist throughout. There are unique steps, procedures, and techniques that are required to appropriately manage the patient in the prehospital arena—just as there are in the ED, the operating room, or other areas of patient care. This is the continuum of care through the time from injury to discharge. The basic concepts originate from the Advanced Trauma Life Support (ATLS) guidelines: primary assessment, resuscitation, secondary assessment, and definitive care. The degree of detail, the specific procedures, and the training of the providers will vary in each step according to the needs of the patient and the situation in which care is provided. The *ACSs* understand this concept and how they mesh in each situation to provide the best care for their patients.

HISTORY

The history of prehospital care, as the history of trauma, has chronicled major advances during active times of war. Those steps have been enhanced in times of peace (Tables 16.6 and 16.7).

The origin of prehospital care is credited to Baron Larrey, Napoleon's surgeon. He first recognized that leaving a patient for 3–30 days in the field with his or her injury was not in the best interest of the patient nor of their General (Napoleon). Therefore, he devised a system of rapid response in the field, with the rapid transport of the patient to a close medical facility to provide care. Care was provided both in the field and en route to the hospital with well-trained individuals. This remains the fundamental hallmark of prehospital care in the 21st Century: (1) rapid response to the field, (2) well-trained personnel who provide care in the field and en route to the hospital, (3) rapid transport of the patient to an appropriate hospital, (4) hospital near the site of injury, and (5) well-trained personnel in the hospital to provide care. With increasing emphasis on prioritization of management and with the advancement of patient transport systems, prehospital care continued to evolve.

TABLE 16.6

CHANGES IN MEDICAL CARE BROUGHT ABOUT BY WARS

- Napoleon Wars—Larrey
  - Foundation elements of prehospital care
  - Rapid response
  - Trained attendants
  - Close hospitals
- War Between the States (1861–1864)
  - Reinstitution of Larrey Principles
  - Development of Medical Corps
  - Rapid response vehicles
  - Trained and equipped ambulance personnel
- WWI
  - Thomas Splint
  - Ground evacuation
- WWII
  - Training of corpsmen in early management of injured soldiers
  - Plasma
- Korea
  - Use of helicopter for rapid transportation
  - Front-line hospitals (MASH)
- Vietnam
  - Advanced scene care by corpsmen
  - IV
  - Airway
  - Bypass CAS for MASH
  - Large volumes of crystalloid resuscitation
- Iraq/Afghanistan
  - Advanced care en route to the next medical care
  - Damage control surgery
  - Damage control resuscitation
  - Military Echelon of Casualty Management
  - Tourniquets/hemostatic agents
  - Interosseous vascular access
  - Permissive hypotension

TABLE 16.7

CHANGES INITIATED FROM THE CURRENT CONFLICTS

Committee on Tactical Combat Casualty Care (CoTCCC)
Tactical Combat Casualty Care Educational Course (TCCC)
Joint Theater Trauma System (JTTS)
Joint Theater Trauma Registry (JTTR)
Military Echelon Casualty Management (MECM)
Medical Evacuation (CCAT)
Hemorrhage control
Tourniquets
Hemostatic agents
Resuscitation
Surgical management
Interosseous Access
Field Assessment
Field trauma management
Permissive hypotension

These principles were lost in the early years of the War Between the States (1861–1865). In the first battle of Manassas (Battle of Bull Run), July 1861, injured patients were left in the field for up to 7 days before being transported. In addition, the transferring personnel were poorly trained. Medicinal alcohol was used liberally, and overall patient care was generally poor. This defect was addressed and changed by Jonathan Letterman (1824–1872) when he was made the commandant of the medical teams and they moved from the Quartermaster Corps to the Medical Corps.

PREHOSPTIAL TIME

R Adams Cowley, MD, the founder of Maryland Institute of EMS (MIEMS), developed the slogan "the golden hour" to emphasize the importance of getting a patient to definitive hospital care as soon as possible. While the 60 minute timeline should not be interpreted literally, emphasis should be placed on expeditious and effective care in order to adequately address severe injuries and critical illness. The need to move quickly for patients needing torso, extremity, and neck hemorrhage control is critical.[9]

Prior to the mid 1980s, when Dr. Crowley demonstrated the importance of a trauma center for providing timely management, the concept of limited time in the field was not well understood based on the "Golden Hour." The prehospital scene care and transport can be as little as 10–12 minutes in a well-run metropolitan EMS system or 25–30 minutes in a well-run suburban system. In the rural setting, the transport times can be hours after the initial traumatic event occurred. Prehospital time can be even longer in a wilderness setting. During this period of time, significant pathophysiologic changes can occur, resulting in deterioration of the patient's physiologic state, which can negatively affect survival, or create complications or long-term disability.

Similarly, delay should not occur in the ED for unneeded assessment or in opening the abdomen in the ED. Directing this process is the responsibility of the ACS.

PREHOSPITAL EDUCATION AND SURGICAL CONTROL OF PREHOSPITAL CARE

Once in the surgeon's hands and in the hospital, the outcome for the patient can be substantially affected by the care, or lack thereof, that occurred in the field. For this reason, *the complete trauma care of the patient, both before and after arrival in the hospital, must be* ***under the control of the surgeon***. This is from the instant the injury occurs until the patient is discharged from the hospital. This is the important continuum of trauma care. Fragmentation of patient care by a committee of providers is not in the best interest of the patient. Each may have a different perspective. Someone must be in charge.

For the surgeon to be involved in the prehospital care does not mean that the surgeon must be physically present in the field physically on every run. However, the surgeon must be present philosophically in the field by being involved in the education of the prehospital provider, understanding what happens in the field, engaging in quality assurance, and having confidence in the EMTs' ability and skill. The EMTs must appreciate this presence. This is achieved by (1) spending time with them, providing education both in the ED and in their classroom experiences, and (2) riding with them on the street and understanding the conditions under which they carry out their responsibilities in the field, working with the EMS committee of the medical society or the trauma center. This does not negate the responsibility of the emergency medicine physicians' involvement in EMS.

PREHOSPITAL CARE SYSTEM

Prehospital care is divided into two distinct components: (1) the EMS system and (2) the physiology, pathophysiology, and management of the trauma patient in the field. The same components are used in the hospital but in a different environment, that is, prevention of anaerobic metabolism by assuring oxygen of the RBC in the lung with delivery of those RBCs to the tissue. A major part of this process is hemorrhage control in the hospital environment. After all, "trauma is a surgical disease from beginning to end."[10] The ACS must understand and appreciate both components of care in the field, just as s/he must understand the hospital system and the physiology, pathophysiology and management of patient care in order to function effectively.

From the beginning of a surgeon's education in medical school, the day-to-day system in which the ACS functions in the hospital becomes apparent in the form of surgical schedules, patient admission, QA processes, peer review, morbidity and mortality conferences, and management of patient records including discharge summaries and operative notes. Such system information and much of the clinical/scientific information in the realm of prehospital care are often not taught to the surgeon in training. In order to ensure optimal patient care, it is imperative for the ACS to understand all of the key elements of the prehospital network and be involved in their teaching.

EMS SYSTEM AND PERSONNEL

An EMS system is to EMS and the EMT as the hospital is to medicine and the individual physician. It is the EMS system that provides a "home" for the EMTs, supervision of their function, quality assurance of their practice, delineation of their privileges, definition of their scope of practice, and financial support of the organization to provide patient care. But it does even more. The EMS system allows the hospital to get the critical and debilitated patients into the ED. Greater than 40% of the hospital admissions come through the ED. Patients would somehow get to the ED without EMS but not with the appropriate care en route and not to the correct hospital that is prepared to handle their specific problem.
The key to running an effective EMS system is strong physician oversight and quality control with attention to the details of patient outcome, skill utilization, skill success, proper judgment, and of the run report analysis.

Initially, there was only the EMT-A (Ambulance) certification available. In the early 1970s, the U. S. Department of Transportation codified the EMT into three levels, which with some small exceptions and modifications are the national standard of the 21st century. These are the EMT-Basic, EMT-Intermediate, and EMT-Paramedic. These have been abbreviated into EMT-B, EMT-I, and EMT-P. Many discussants further abbreviate this to use the term "EMT" meaning the basic EMT and "paramedic" meaning the EMT paramedic. Further references will utilize the terms EMT-B, EMT-I, and EMT-P and for the individual levels, EMT as a generic term indicating all three levels.

EMT-B

The EMT-Basic has completed a minimum of 110 contact hours of training following the objectives as outlined in the U. S. Department of Transportation's (DOT) National Standard Curriculum and tested either by the National Registry for EMTs or the individual state license exams or both. Depending on the state, reregistration is required every 2–4 years to maintain that license. Each state has varying criteria for this reregistration. EMS runs are approximately 1/3 trauma, 1/3 medical, and 1/3 cardiac. The EMT-B training program is divided essentially along these lines with emphasis on life- or limb-threatening injuries such as cardiac arrest, airway problems, childbirth, hemorrhage control, fracture immobilization, and seizures.

Additional training includes defensive driving, utilization of communication systems, ethics, legal issues, and run report writing.

EMT-I

The EMT-Intermediate has been trained to the level of an EMT-B, frequently has 1 or 2 years experience on the streets functioning as an EMT-B and takes approximately 200 hours of additional education, which includes IV fluid administration, advanced airway management, automatic defibrillation and in some states, limited use of drugs.

EMT-P

The EMT-Paramedic is trained with an increased emphasis on the utilization of cardiac drugs, medication for pain control, airway assistance (RSI in some systems), and seizure management. The drugs on the EMS unit usually consist of advanced blood pressure cardiac medications, glucose and insulin for the management of diabetic patients, pain and seizure medication, which would include morphine, a sedative, rapid sequence intubation (RSI) drugs and, perhaps, fentanyl or ketamine. The training program to reach the EMT-P level varies from state to state, but it is traditionally in the range of 1,000 to 1,200 hours in addition to the EMT-I. This includes not only didactic lectures, but time in various patient care areas, in the hospital such as the operating room, ER, ICU, and a supervised field internship. At the completion of the training program, the student takes the state examination, the examination of the National Registry of EMTs, or both to obtain a license to function at the ALS level. Reregistration to maintain this license is required every 2–4 years depending on the state. The reregistration depends on sustainment education in trauma, cardiac, and medical conditions, as well as skill demonstration and practice such as IVs and endotracheal intubation and a backup airway.

A growing number of EMS services throughout the United States are utilizing RSI with drug control, for airway management. Research results of the use of RSI in the field have been mixed, with respect to effectiveness; it is believed to be less effective with shorter transport time.

EMT-PARAMEDICS WITH A PHYSICIAN

There is a fourth level of care that is used by some systems in the United States and Canada, which is with a physician as part of the medical response system. Much literature in North America has indicated that the use of a physician prolongs the EMS run, delays transports, and has a negative impact on outcome. However, in Central and South America, many services rely on physicians to provide field care. In Europe, many services use only nurses for prehospital care.

Many systems in the United States in the early 21st century have begun to have a physician riding the streets with a supervisor. This physician provides radio medical control, medical supervision, and education on the scene, and adds to the quality assurance process. This type of arrangement has been thought to be effective especially in the urban areas for immediate and retrospective medical control (see below) as medical director (this is usually an emergency medicine resident), and responds to scenes on an ad lib basis, and some systems, usually not in the United States, have a full-time physician assigned to the ambulance.

COMMUNICATIONS

Prehospital communication systems are divided into two major categories:

1. Dispatch/administrative communications with the EMS system control
2. Medical communications with the hospital or physician

In the United States, most of the EMS dispatch is done by an emergency citizen access arrangement, using the 9-1-1 patient access phone number. The communication arrangement may be separated into police, fire, and EMS, but some communities combine fire and EMS. Other communities combine law enforcement and EMS. There are some communities, especially in rural areas, in which all three components are combined into one unit. Other countries have a similar communication system, but a different phone number.
Regardless of the system used, the function is

Notification: to receive a phone call from a patient, a family member, or a bystander and identify the type of call

Dispatch: to send the appropriate vehicle and personnel and provide assistance by the telephone to the caller while the ambulance is en route

Scene: to survey the scene (see scene survey below), identify additional resources or backup that are required, notify the dispatch of such needs, begin to address patient care, and get the patient ready for transport to the hospital

Transport: to ensure movement of the patient to the correct hospital for care of the condition(s) found

Urban EMS response times are highlighted in Table 16.8. It is clear from the table that even the best of systems use half of the "Golden Hour" in the field. The assessment and transport times will change based on the density of the population and the difficulty of the terrain.

AeroEMS (AEMS) has been used with questionable results to address the needs of rural America. Unfortunately in the United States, the AEMS has been frequently overused. Both patients and the AEMS personnel have suffered death. It is possible to set up a good aeromedical triage process[11], but most medical directors and AEMS systems refuse to accept that responsibility.

A medical communication system can be set up utilizing a cell phone or radio communicating to a hospital and the medical control physician. Both systems are used by some services. Medical communication has three components:

1. Notification to the hospital of the patient's condition and the expected time of arrival
2. Transmission of electronic data, which may be beneficial to the hospital either to prepare for the arrival of the patient or to enhance the care of the patient while en route (Electrocardiogram are commonly used, but photos have their supporters)
3. Medical control physician or a trained nurse to alter care from the usual guidelines that have been developed for the EMS system and provide specific care for a specific patient

The transmission of electronic data, such as EKGs, has been found to be of limited use. Training of the EMT to read the EKGs and to provide care on previously developed protocols by the EMS system have been found to be much more effective. This is another example of providing an EMT with knowledge and allowing appropriate decisions to be made in the field.

Most systems now have fairly in-depth guidelines that direct EMT care without the need to contact the hospital for initial orders. Further orders and advanced medical directions can be utilized and are especially helpful with long transport times such as in rural areas or with the use of arrow medical transportation systems.

A statewide system, rather than a local one, has many advantages and improves survival. (13)

PROTOCOLS VERSUS STANDING ORDERS

The terms "protocols" and "standing orders" have produced much misunderstanding and confusion since the early days of EMS, when these terms were not properly defined. The definitions in current use are as follows:

- *Standing orders* describe the initial care (and occasionally follow-up care) *prior to* communicating with medical control.

TABLE 16.8

URBAN EMS RESPONSE TIMES

Notification	2–3 min
Assessment	3–8 min
Scene time	5–10 min
Transport	3–8 min
Ideal total prehospital time = ≤30 min	

- *Protocols* are strict orders developed by medical control as to how to provide patient care. The EMS personnel are not allowed to modify them based on the situation, conditions, or other variables on the scene or during transport unless dictated by direct medical control.
- *Guidelines* are plans for medical care that have been approved by the medical or the community EMS committee. The latter allows the EMS personnel to think and to respond to patient needs based on what is found and the situations at the time of the call.

MEDICAL CONTROL

EMTs at all levels work as surrogates of physicians. In most states, they work on the license of the medical director of the EMS service. They are not independent practitioners. The various state licenses do not allow independent nonphysician practitioners to exist within the EMS. Some fire-based systems such as in Louisiana and other states are trying to enact legislation to make fire services exempt from statewide or even local standards and allow the fire chief (who is not a physician and may have no medical training) to provide medical control, critique the medical care given in the field, and circumvent any state standards of patient care. These types of attempts to blunt the improvement of patient care should be defeated. Patient care should always be top priority.

The critical factors in quality care of the patient and the function of EMS[12] in the medical care system have three phases of medical control:

- *Prospective*
  - Initial development of the EMS system and development of needed modifications as the system matures and medical knowledge improves
  - Prior to dispatch of the unit
- *Immediate*
  - While the EMTs are in the field caring for the patients
  - Real time
  - Direct (online) medical control
- *Retrospective*
  - After the unit returns based on discussions or run report review
  - Quality assurance, discipline, education
  - Indirect (off-line) medical control

Direct Medical Control (Online)

Direct medical control is a function of a physician or designee answering the radio and talking directly to the EMTs in the field. The EMTs explain the situation, the scene, the condition of the patient, scene care provided, specify the care to be provided en route and ask for further direction in the management of the patient if required. Further direction can range from bringing the patient to the hospital as quickly as possible to providing specific drugs or undertaking procedures for the health of the patient either prior to transport or while the patient is being transported.

Several studies have shown that well-trained EMTs with effective guidelines who are allowed to make judgments based on knowledge and experience produce better outcomes in shorter scene times than those forced to use communications for all decisions.

Indirect Medical Control (Off-line)

Indirect medical control is the retrospective analysis of the run reports, analysis of statistics gained from compiling various data points from the field such as scene times, response times, time on the scene, skills, attempted versus successful procedure, knowledge and skills, and the most difficult of all, assessment of the judgment used by the EMTs in the management of the patient. Such data can be used to change protocols, add or subtract personnel or vehicles, change the ambulance placement strategy, protocol redesign, sustainment education, redesign, and skills practiced. Such quality assessment can improve the outcome of patient care.

ASSESSMENT AND MANAGEMENT IN THE FIELD

Assessment in the field is composed of two separate steps: Assessment of the scene (safety and situation) and assessment of the patient. Safety comes first.

Situation

Patient: What is the situation of the injured patients? What happened? What is the MOI? Number of patients? Overview of the condition of the patients.

Resources: Does the number of patients or the conditions exceed the resources available? How many patients are present? Is there anyone on the scene who can provide information about the situation, about any of the patients, or about additional patients who are not visible?

Safety

An injured rescuer provides no benefit to the patient if he or she gets injured. In fact, this complicates the state of affairs by adding to the number of people needing care and reducing the number of caregivers at the scene. Therefore, the safety of the rescuers is paramount.

The next component of safety is that of the patients. Chemicals, weather, perpetrators of the incident, unruly bystanders, fire, etc. are all potential hazards in an area. Questions that should always be asked by the EMS team of themselves, other professionals on the scene, and bystanders are: Are there any biological or chemical hazards in the area? Is there an unknown liquid on the ground? Is there an unusual cloud or smell in the air? Is there gasoline on the ground? Is there a fire risk? Is the patient's car in a precarious situation? Is the scene secure from the perpetrators of the incident? Is law enforcement needed?

Initial Assessment

The patient care starts when the first provider touches the patient and continues until the patient does not need further care. There are many similarities in the initial assessment on the scene and the initial assessment in the ED as both are a continuum of the same process of care for the same patient. In fact, the ATLS pattern of the initial assessment was based on a similar system used by EMS. The basic goal of the initial assessment on the scene is also similar to the basic goal of the initial assessment in the ED, in the OR, in the ICU, and on the floor. What is wrong with the patient and what steps are necessary to be able to transport the patient to the next level of care? In the field, the next level of care is the ED. In the ED, the next level of patient care is generally the operating room, the ICU, or advanced diagnostic techniques.

Just as wasting time in the ED delays moving the patient to the next level, so it is on the scene, except perhaps more so. Almost never is the field the best place to assess or to care for the trauma patient. The patient should be moved into the ambulance as quickly and as safely as possible, and the ambulance should be en route to the ED quickly, while following the dictum of "*do no further harm*".

Do no further harm means sins of *omission*, as well as sins of *commission*. Scoop and Run or to move the patient quickly without assuring that the airway is open, that the patient is breathing, that the patient has cardiac output, or without stabilizing the fractures, are sins of *omission*. Starting unnecessary IVs, doing the secondary survey in the field when the patient is crashing, doing unnecessary diagnostic tests in the field such as otoscopic evaluations, auscultation of the abdomen, cervical spine clearance, and ultrasound of anything are examples of sins of *commission*. Both of these do further harm to the patient and should not be a part of field care. Another major sin of commission is the delay in critical patient care by taking up something not critical for survival. This occurs in the field, in the ED, and in getting the patient's abdomen opened in the OR. The components of the initial assessment (primary survey, resuscitation, secondary survey, definitive care) are present in the field just as they are in the ED (PHTLS). The methods and the extent to which they are used are different. There are two major differences:

1. For the severely injured patient with hemodynamic instability, the secondary survey may never be completed in the field or in the ED. The intent of the prehospital provider should be devoted to managing life- and limb-threatening conditions while transporting the patient to the hospital. Other less severe conditions are of lesser priority.
2. The equipment used, the skills, the process of patient care is extremely different when carried on outside in the rain, snow, with a large crowd of people around, when a patient is trapped in the vehicle, or when the perpetrator of the crime may still be in the area than in the warm, dry, controlled environment of the ER or the operating room.

In addition, in the hospital, there are frequently nurses, house staff, and other personnel to provide assistance to the physician providing this care. In the field, there are only the two EMTs and, occasionally, personnel from the fire department or law enforcement department who may or may not understand completely the job of the EMT. Nor does the occasional participant in field care know where all of the supplies in the "truck" are.

In most EMS services, only two EMTs ride on a unit. One may be at an advanced level or one may be at a basic level. Occasionally, in some services, there is a trained first responder available for additional help either from the fire department, law enforcement, or a volunteer first responder in some rural areas. Manpower limitation in the field is a major factor, which can slow prehospital care. For example, the care that must be provided by two providers for a trauma patient who requires intubation includes the following:

Immobilize the patient's spine
Place the backboard in position
Apply the cervical collar
Secure the patient to the backboard
Start airway management such as oral airway or intubation
Assess proper management of the airway
Secure the endotracheal tube into position
Load the patient in the unit
Notify the hospital of impending arrival and the patient's condition
Drive the ambulance
Recheck Endotracheal tube (ET) position after movement
Check vital signs
Start an IV if appropriate
Assess for other injuries
etc.

In the hospital, there are several individuals who participate in resuscitation. Such luxury does not exist in the field. Field care is different from the ED, OR, of ICU care. In each area, the basics of care are the same and have the same goals; however, the providers are trained to operate in different situations and the resources are developed for the specific situations encountered. Therefore, their specific goals will be different.

Primary Survey

As part of the scene assessment and the primary survey, a general impression of the patient's condition is obtained immediately upon seeing the patient. In the first few seconds, the patient is assessed for the MOI, for example, when the EMT finds the patient lying in a ditch, or lying in the street with a motorcycle 30 feet away, or leaning over the steering wheel without the deployed air bag, or lying in the street with blood coming from the chest and clothes soaked with blood. Each of these provides a general impression of what is going on and prepares the prehospital care provider with a general direction toward what needs to be quickly accomplished prior to initiation of transport.

Efficiency in the field is critically important if the patient is to be moved to the hospital safely and rapidly. The initial review must identify what is wrong with the patients; what has to be done to stabilize their condition prior to getting them into the ambulance; what care would need to be provided en route to the hospital; and which hospital is best equipped with the proper resources and is immediately ready to handle the patient's specific condition. Also important is triage: the assessment of which patients are the most severely injured, and who will require attention first.

The objective of the field primary survey is to identify the severity of the patients' injuries so that they can be taken to the right hospital so that the injuries will cause no further harm.

A: Airway The airway can be managed in the field as in the hospital by manual, mechanical, or transtracheal methods.

Techniques available to verify the correct placement of an airway device (oral, nasal, supraglottic or endotracheal intubation) are divided into two groups: clinical assessment and adjunctive devices depending on the device. Depending on the device, various methods will be helpful.

Clinical assessment includes the following:

1. Identification of bilateral breath sounds and absence of air sounds over the epigastrium
2. Observation of chest rising or falling during ventilation
3. Direct observation of the tube passing through the cords
4. Observation of fogging (vapor condensation in the endotracheal tube).

Adjunctive devices include:

1. Esophageal detector
2. Carbon dioxide monitor
3. Colorimetric carbon dioxide detector
4. Endotracheal carbon dioxide monitor (capnography)
5. Pulse oximeter.[13]

None of these methods are 100% accurate. Therefore, all of the clinical assessment should be used unless impractical. In addition, at least one (preferably two) of the adjunctive techniques should be added.

Airway Backup. As with any technique, there should always be a backup technique/plan available should the primary technique fail. The ultimate device and the first step in most cases is the BVM. A study by Stockinger showed similar survival rates with both BVM and ET placement.[1]

B: Breathing and ventilation. The first step for the prehospital provider in assuring that red cells are adequately oxygenated to deliver the oxygen to the tissue cells is an open airway. The second step is to assure adequate volume expansion of the lungs (Ficke principle). Traumatic conditions that interfere with lung expansion include the physical limitation of expansion (pneumothorax), reduced expansion of the chest cavity (rib pain), and reduced neurological drive (high spinal fracture, brain injury, or alcohol or drug excess).

BVM ventilation is the initial mechanical approach to getting air into the lungs and the continuing approach if the patient cannot be intubated (no RS1 protocols, training, skills, or proximity to hospital). As stated above, some studies have shown that the outcome using BVM ventilation and endotracheal intubation is the same. Unfortunately, in the United States, randomized trials are prohibited. Most are retrospective or prospective with historical controls.

If thoracic decompression is needed for the management of a pneumothorax, the needle should be long enough to reach the thoracic cavity. Military studies have shown this to be >3.25 inch. Some experts have suggested bilateral needle insertion on all prehospital cardiac arrest patients.

C: Cardiac. The American College of Surgeons/Committee on Trauma (ACS/COT) and the National Association of EMS Physicians (NAEMSP) have developed a position paper outlining when to and when not to initiate Cardiopulmonary resuscitation (CPR) in the field on a trauma patient. This has been verified recently at the COT resident paper competition.[14]

The most important component of "C" is hemorrhage control (discussed below under resuscitation).

D: Disability. The major goal is the assessment of the brain as an end organ for perfusion and oxygenation. A mental status examination at this point is for gross assessment or a head injury such as unequal pupils and appropriate stating with the Glascow Coma Score.

Resuscitation

The resuscitation phase of prehospital care is also different from the resuscitation in the ED. Intravenous fluid administration, as an example, is carried out en route to the hospital and not in the field as this would delay transportation. It is more difficult to start an IV in a crowded, moving ambulance than in an ER with the stable platform on which the patient is lying. However, IV access is possible with >95% success rate in a moving ambulance if necessary for good patient care. In 2012, the accepted approach to fluid replacement will be in the ratio 1:1:1 for RBC, plasma, and platelet. The prehospital step is fluid resuscitation with the goal of 80–90 mm Hg systolic pressure and rapid movement to facility where RBC and plasma are immediately available.

Secondary Survey

Another difference between patient care in the back of an ambulance versus the ED is the removal of all of the patient's clothes in the ED to do an adequate secondary survey. Environment, bystanders, and other conditions dictate that the patient's clothes usually should not be removed prior to the putting the patient in the ambulance. While en route, the patient must remain stable against the backboard and the stretcher; therefore, removing the straps to cut the clothes free is difficult and usually not productive to the long-term outcome of the patient (unless severe hemorrhage is present). However, the assessment can be incomplete if the clothes are not removed as major injuries such as a hemorrhage from the thigh can be missed. Spinal immobilization often complicates a complete secondary assessment. The EMT's assessment is limited to those parts of the body that are freely visible while immobilized.

In most situations, therefore, the secondary survey is not completed prior to arrival at the hospital. The general principle of immobilization, as a unit on the long backboard, is frequently the best method of transporting the patient and stabilizing all the fractures or potential fractures.

However, life-threatening injuries such as external hemorrhage, airway problems, pneumothorax, and flail chest should be addressed while providing rapid transport to the trauma center or local hospital. The backboard is a useful device for moving a patient to the stretcher in the field and off the stretcher in the ED. However, cervical collar use with the backboard is contraindicated in penetrating trauma without a neurological deficit, as (1) there is no benefit, (2) it delays transportation, and (3) it restricts assessment and management such as BVM ventilation.

Definitive Field Care

Like other steps in the assessment and management of the patient, definitive care in the field is different from definitive care in the ED. The definitive prehospital care is appropriate packaging and delivery of the patient safely and quickly to the ED.

SHOCK AND FLUID RESUSCITATION

The primary emphasis for the prehospital provider's knowledge base should be the following:

- Reestablishment of energy production at the cellular level when anaerobic metabolism has replaced aerobic metabolism
- Improved oxygenation of the tissue cells can be hampered by either (1) lack of oxygenation of the red cells in the lungs, (2) lack of delivery of the red cells to the tissue cells (Fick Principle), or (3) over resuscitation with crystalloid producing increased interstitial fluid, restricting oxygen transfer.
- Understanding of the physiology of fluid replacement
- Bernoulli theorem of fluid loss from an injured vessel
- Resuscitation of controlled versus uncontrolled hemorrhage

Energy Production

Metabolism produces injury utilizing oxygen and glucose as fuel with by-products of carbon dioxide and water. There are two pathways to achieve energy production: one with and one without oxygen. Aerobic metabolism is the most efficient and produces a large amount of adenosine triphosphate versus anaerobic metabolism, 38:2 per cycle.

Additionally, anaerobic metabolism increases the production of lactic and anaerobic acids with resultant total body acidosis. The increased acid will result in an increased ventilatory rate, which may be the first sign of early shock. Tachypnea frequently precedes tachycardia and certainly precedes hypotension. Reduced energy product produces hypothermia. This change provides assessment techniques. The so-called triangle of death (hypotension, acidosis, and coagulopathy) is the outcome of decreased energy production and *symptom* of shock *not the cause*.

The outcome of a prolonged hypoperfusion will result in impairment of organ function up to and including organ death. Many of the complications that occur result from hypoperfusion and hypo oxygenation in the first hour of patient care when EMS is with the patient. These may not manifest themselves for several hours or days.

Physiology of Fluid Replacement

The determination of how and what fluids to use for resuscitation depends on the type of shock and the presence of *controlled or uncontrolled* hemorrhage.

With controlled hemorrhage, the patient can be resuscitated back to normal hemodynamics without concern. Conversely with uncontrolled hemorrhage, increasing the blood pressure and flow back to normal can significantly increase the blood loss. With controlled hemorrhage, low-volume resuscitation is preferred.

Resuscitation of the blood volume, using fluids alone (such as Ringer's Lactate), has three potential negative outcomes:

- Large volumes of Ringer's lactate without replacing red cells dilutes the red cell mass. This reduces the delivery of oxygen to the tissue cells.
- The return of blood pressure to the normal range may dislodge a clot and initiate active bleeding. It also produces a higher transmural pressure (intravascular vs. extraocular pressure), which increases the rate of flow of blood from the injured vessel (Bernoulli's Principle).
- High-volume crystalloid resuscitation, which remains in vascular system only a very short period of time, produces significant edema and decreases the function of the lung, kidneys, and other organs.
- High-volume crystalloid resuscitation creates a dilutional coagulopathy.

In face of *uncontrolled* hemorrhage, volume resuscitation in the field should be intravenous, with no attempts to increase blood pressure > 90 mm Hg to maintain oxygen delivery. In a short-term transport situation, <20 minutes from the hospital and without traumatic brain injury, IV access only with less that 500 mL of fluid is the accepted management approach. For longer transportation, the recommendation of the Committee on Tactical Combat Casualty Care (CoTCCC) for military care is an acceptable option, which advocates pulse as the main assessment tool. Rate and character abnormality in the pulse (weak and thready) indicates resuscitation fluid should be given every 30 minutes if necessary. Crystalloid should not routinely be administered in this situation. Short-term use of volume-restricted resuscitation method in one study demonstrated that there was increased mortality rate associated with hemorrhage from the thoracic cavity, but no clinically significant changes in hemorrhage from other parts of the body.

However, it is logical to believe that based on the Bernoulli Theorem, increasing intraluminal blood pressure without increasing the external tissue pressure will cause greater blood loss and therefore increased mortality rate (Table 16.9).

A decrease in the intramural pressure will decrease the transmural pressure and therefore reduce the rate of leakage out of the hole in the vessel. Conversely, an increase in the intramural pressure will increase the transmural pressure and thereby increase the rate of blood flow out of the hole. This is the theory behind the restricted fluid resuscitation technique.

TABLE 16.9

MODIFIED BERNOULLI THEOREM

Rate of leakage ~ Size of the hole × transmural pressure
Transmural pressure = intraluminal pressure/extramural pressure

Therefore, the appropriate resuscitation in uncontrolled hemorrhage is as follows:

- Reduction of intravascular pressure (hypotensive resuscitation and/or tourniquet)
- Increased extra luminal pressure (direct wound pressure and pressure bandages)
- The addition of external hemostatic agents or nontourniquetable wounds (torso) must be accompanied with 3–5 minutes of direct pressure on the wound site after application of agent.
- Movement of patient as quickly as possible to factor XIV (hemostats and ligation of bleeding vessels)

Assessment

There are a variety of maneuvers that have been successfully used to quickly assess the level of shock in a trauma patient. Pulse. Three components of the pulse need to be evaluated on initial arrival of EMS personnel.

- Rate—slow or fast tachycardia indicates, at the very least, compensated shock. A very slow pulse (<50) could indicate the early onset of bradycardia associated with myocardial ischemia.
- Strength—strong versus thready
- Location. A radial pulse indicates adequate perfusion with the systolic pressure somewhere above 80 to 90 mm Hg. The absence of a similar pulse indicates that the pressure is probably below 70 systolic and absence of carotid pulse indicates that systolic blood pressure is 50 to 60 mm Hg or less.
- Ventilation rate, increased rate, indicates increased acid production at the cellular level (anaerobic metabolism) and generalized acidosis

Skin color: Pink versus cyanotic versus pale.
Skin temperature: Cool and clammy versus warm and dry.
Capillary refilling time: Greater than 2 seconds

All of these signs are in themselves not a test of shock, but a test of perfusion of that portion of the body wherein they are detected. Perfusion can be a function of cardiac dysfunction, reduced blood volume, a function of interruption of the blood supply proximal to the point of assessment. Hypothermia, vascular trauma, dehydration, or a variety of conditions can reduce the perfusion to the point of all of the above changes.

Blood Pressure: An important sign of shock, however, hypotension is frequently not noted until 30 to 40% of the blood volume has been lost. Therefore, it is a late sign. The afore-mentioned parameters (pulse rate, skin color, temperature, etc.) are earlier indicators of possible shock.

Transtracheal airway

Although there are three methods of transtracheal airway management, the **tracheostomy** is not an emergency procedure, either in the hospital or outside of the hospital. Therefore, EMTs are not taught this technique. Percutaneous transtracheal ventilation and surgical cricothyroidotomy are the transtracheal airway management options emphasized.

Percutaneous transtracheal placement of a large 14 or 12 gauze needle directly into the trachea is a quick and effective technique. It requires less train and sustainment training than a cricothyroidotomy.

Ventilation can be accomplished by connecting an oxygenation administration catheter to a 15 liter per minute oxygen source. Continuous flow, without pressure bags, is effective as long as the patient has spontaneous ventilation. Oxygenation without compromising CO2 build-up has been accomplished for 45 minutes without difficulty.

Surgical cricothyrotomy can be effective but requires extensive training and retraining to maintain proficiency.

Spinal Immobilization

Backboard Immobilization The critically injured patient should be immobilized to the backboard providing a stable transfer platform. The transportation of the patient to an appropriate facility to address these issues takes precedence over neurological assessment.

Without a neurological defect, there is no indication for immobilizing the cervical spine in penetrating neck trauma. The patient should be rapidly transported to the hospital without immobilization. The long backboard can be used as a device for moving the patient, if necessary; however, the cervical collar does not need to be added.

Cervical collar application Even the best of cervical collars, including the "hard" cervical collar, provide only about 50%–60% restriction in motion in the three standard positions of anterior/posterior, lateral flexion, and rotation. The soft cervical collar is ineffective in immobilizing the neck and is not indicated in acutely injured patients.

Field Helmet Removal

Removal of motorcycle, bicycle, and football helmets is taught and practiced by every EMT in training. Physicians are generally not taught how to remove a helmet and almost none have practiced it on a consistent basis. Therefore, it is appropriate for EMS personnel to remove helmets in the field to better immobilize the patient for transport.

Traction splints: For a fractured or suspected fractured femur, the traction splint is an excellent device. Early literature from World War I reports that the use of the Thomas Whole Ring or the Thomas Half Ring Splint on soldiers receiving femur injuries reduce the mortality rate by 80%. More recent analysis of these reports indicates that the reduction of mortality may well have been closer to the range of 40%, but nonetheless, this is a significant change by the use of such a device.

KINEMATICS (MECHANISM OF INJURY)

Critical to understanding the potential of injury in a patient is the MOI. Upwards of 95% of injuries can be anticipated before even examining the patient by understanding the energy exchange on the human body at the time of impact. These are based on some very simple laws of energy and motion.

1. Body at rest or body in motion will remain in that state until acted upon by some outside force.
2. Energy can be neither created nor destroyed, but it can be changed in form.
3. Mass × acceleration = force = mass × deceleration
4. Kinetic energy = mass/2 × velocity^2

Laws of Energy and Motion

Newton's first law of motion states that a body at rest will remain at rest and a body in motion will remain in motion unless acted on by an outside force.

The *law of conservation of energy combined with Newton's second law of motion describes* that energy cannot be created or destroyed but can be changed in form. The motion of the vehicle is a form of energy. When the vehicle is started, the gasoline burns inside the cylinder, producing motion of the piston, which turns the crankshaft and then the wheels. To stop the vehicle, the motion (energy) must be changed to another form, for instance, the bending of the frame in a crash or the heat of the brake drums or disk and the tires when the breaks are applied for control.

Mass × acceleration = force = mass × deceleration

Force (energy) is required to put a structure into motion. This force (energy) is required to create a specific speed. The speed imparted is dependent on the weight (mass) of the structure. Once this energy is passed on to the structure and it is placed in motion, the motion will remain until the energy is given up. (Newton's first law of motion).

An example of this process is the gun and the patient. In the chamber of a gun is a cartridge that contains gunpowder. When the gunpowder is ignited, it burns rapidly creating energy that pushes the bullet out of the barrel at a great speed. This speed is equivalent to the weight of the bullet and the amount of energy produced by the burning of the gunpowder or force. To slow down (Newton's first law of motion), the bullet must give up its energy into the structure that it hits. This will produce an explosion in the tissue that is equal to the explosion that occurred in the chamber of the gun when the initial speed was given to the bullet.

Kinetic energy is a function of an object's weight and speed. The relationship between weight and speed as it affects kinetic energy is as follows:

Kinetic energy = One-half the mass times the velocity squared

$$KE = \frac{1}{2}mv^2$$

The velocity is exponential and the mass is linear. In a collision between a small car and a semitrailer truck or between a car and a pedestrian, the advantage goes to the vehicle with the most energy (mass and speed).

This loss of energy will be exchanged into the tissue particles and put them into motion.

The same phenomenon occurs in the moving automobile, the falling patient from a building, or the explosion of an improvised explosive device (IED)

The inverse relationship between stopping distance and injury also applies to falls. A person has a better chance of surviving a fall if he or she lands on a compressible surface, such as deep powder snow versus terminating on to a hard surface, such as concrete. The compressible material (i.e., the snow) increases the stopping distance and absorbs at least some of the energy rather than allowing all the energy to be absorbed by the body. The result is decreased injury and damage to the body. This principle applies with a restraining belt or an airbag. An unrestrained driver will be more severely injured than a restrained driver. The restraint system, rather than the body, will absorb a significant portion of the damage energy.

Once an object is in motion and has energy in the form of motion, for the object to come to a complete rest, the object must lose all its energy by converting the energy to another form or transferring it to another object. For example, if a vehicle strikes a pedestrian, the pedestrian is knocked away from it. Although the vehicle is somewhat slowed by the impact, the greater force of the vehicle imparts much more acceleration to the lighter-weight pedestrian.

The energy in terms of acceleration imparted to the pedestrian is much more than the energy lost by the vehicle as it slows down. The softer body parts of the pedestrian versus the harder body parts of the vehicle also means more damage to the pedestrian than to the vehicle.

Energy Exchange between a Solid Object and the Human Body As the human body collides with a solid object, or vice versa, the number of body tissue particles that are impacted by the solid object determines the amount of energy exchange that takes place. This transfer of energy produces the damage (injury) that occurs to the patient. The greater the energy exchange, the greater the damage.

The energy exchange produces similar response in the patient. The number of tissue particles affected is determined by (1) the density (particles per volume) of the tissue and (2) the size of the contact area of the impact.

The outcome of the energy exchange is determined by the organs involved.

Cavitation Many games are based on the physics principle of energy exchange from one object to a cluster of other objects. The cluster is broken apart. The game of bowling is a classic example. The bowling ball is rolled down the hardwood floor aimed at a rack of pins in the middle of the lane. The energy given to the ball by the bowler breaks the rack apart. Pool is a similar game. The force of muscle motion of the arm is applied to the cue ball through the cue stick. The ball goes down the table to the rack of balls at the other end and exchanges the energy of motion and mass of the cue ball, into the rack of balls, which are broken apart.

A similar force on the human body occurs when the energy of the moving bullet transmits the energy into the tissues of the body and "blows them apart." This creates a cavity. The initial cavity is temporary and is produced by the rapid displacement of the tissue particle. This cavity cannot be seen a few seconds after the penetrating object has passed. The elastic tissue such as in muscle, lung, or even the liver must be mentally reconstructed as the patient is assessed. The permanent cavity can be seen or partially seen when the injured patient is assessed.

An analogy is to visualize the side of steel barrel hit with a baseball bat. Examine the dent made in the steel barrel by the baseball bat. Take the same baseball bat and swing it with the same force into a roll of foam rubber and examine the foam rubber. The cavity is directly away from the movement of the baseball bat. After the initial impact, there is no visible cavitation or dent although the hitter knows that such a cavitation was produced at the time of impact.

Such are the changes that occur within the human body, particularly when the force is spread out over an area too wide to penetrate the skin (blunt trauma). The elastic tissue of the body reforms the cavity quickly but not the damage created by the energy exchange.

For simplicity sake and ease of understanding, the forces are divided into blunt and penetrating trauma. However, the only difference in these two forces is the penetration of the object into the tissue and the direction of the cavitation.

BLUNT TRAUMA

The energy exchange in blunt trauma has four components: shear, compression (crush), overpressure (paper bag effect), and cavitation. Each, to a greater or lesser extent, is involved in every crash. These are the results of deceleration if the body suddenly stops or acceleration if the body is suddenly put into motion away from the point of impact.

To better understand the forces of blunt trauma, these are divided into motor vehicle crashes (automobiles, motorcycles, and pedestrians), falls, and blasts.

Vehicular Collisions

Vehicular impacts are further subdivided according to the direction of the forces and the vehicle in which the patient was riding. There are five separate types of collision each of which has its own individual patterns: frontal, rear, side impact, rotational impact, and rollover. As a general rule, the patient is injured on the same side as the vehicle.

Frontal: The occupant riding in the vehicle is traveling at a speed produced by the energy created in the engine from the burning of gasoline. When this vehicle strikes an immovable object directly in the front, the vehicle rapidly slows as the bending metal absorbs the energy of the momentum of this speed. If the car stops and the occupant inside the vehicle stops, then all of the energy of the momentum was absorbed by the vehicle or the patient. There are two types of energy absorption. The first shows energy absorbed locally on the front of the vehicle as energy is absorbed onto the frame.

In most modern cars, the energy of the motion of the occupant is absorbed as the energy is dissipated into the stretching of the seat belt, and the impact into the air bag in the best scenario. However, if neither safety device is available, such energy is dissipated into the tissues of the body as the passenger impacts the dash board, steering column, windscreen, or supporting pillars.

Generally, the unstrained occupant will follow two pathways, forward into the dash board or into the steering column as the energy of the vehicle is absorbed and stops (or a combination of the two): one, with the head as the lead point of the human missile, the "up and over" pathway and the second, where the knee is the lead point of the human missile into the dash or the floor. "Down and Under."

Down and Under: The vehicle stops its forward motion against some immovable object. The frame or front is bent as it absorbs the energy. The continued forward motion of the occupant's lower torso impacts the knees into the dash. The dash stops the forward motion of the knees, but the continued energy of the torso pushes into the upper portion of the lower extremity. This energy is absorbed by dislocation of the knee, fracture along the shaft of the femur, or if the femur remains intact, the pelvis continues to travel forward with the acetabulum overriding the head of the femur. The result is a posterior dislocation at the hip. As the lower half of the torso comes to rest, the upper half of the torso continues forward, bending at the hips and impacts the dash or the steering column with the patient's head or chest.

Up and Over: The chest is the lead point of the human missile. The sternum stops its forward motion against the steering column, but the continued motion of the posterior thoracic wall from behind bends and eventually fractures the ribs. The lungs are compressed between the forward motion of the posterior thoracic wall and the anterior components of the ribs and/or sternum. The heart is compressed between the vertebral column and the sternum.

If the energy forces are such that the head becomes the lead point of the human missile which impacts into the "A" pillow, the wind screen, or the roof of the car, the anterior part of the skull stops its forward motion, but the continued motion of the posterior skull pushed by the momentum of the torso fractures the area of the impact. The continued energy momentum of the brain produces compression, crush, or lacerations of the brain matter itself.

The brain is not attached to the inside of the skull, but floats in the cerebral spinal fluid. Once the skull stops, the brain continues to move forward until the energy of the momentum is absorbed by compression against the skull. This can result in contusion and laceration of the brain. Parts of the fractured skull may stick into the brain tissue itself.

The separation of the trailing edge of the brain from the back of the skull can tear the vessels loose, producing hemorrhage. This is the cause of the so-called contra coups injury. If the top of the skull is the impact point then base of the brain travels away from the base of the skull and the stretch is through the foramen magnum and the cerebrum can be pulled away from the spinal cord at the brain stem.

Once the head has stopped its forward motion, the continued momentum of the torso from behind distributes energy onto the unprotected cervical vertebrae, producing compression, hyperextension, or hyperflexion injuries. Such injuries to the cervical spine can lead to spinal cord damage at the time of impact or are unstable, leading to further injury to the patient en route to the hospital or in the hospital. Therefore, the entire spine must be appropriately protected on a backboard and a cervical collar.

Concomitant energy exchange can occur in the chest and abdomen. The anterior chest stops abruptly against the steering column. The posterior chest wall only stops when its energy of forward motion has been absorbed. This energy absorption is onto the ribs, resulting in lateral fractures, compression of the lung (pulmonary contusion) or compression of the heart. Rapid reduction of the intrathoracic volume and increase in intrathoracic pressure (overpressure) [Boyles law] can rupture the lung (like a paper bag hit with the hand), tearing the parenchyma and producing a pneumothorax. Although a sharp edge of the fractured rib can lacerate the lung, the paper bag effect is more common.

The descending aorta is firmly attached to the posterior chest wall and vertebrae, while the heart and the aortic arch are relatively mobile. The heart and the arch can decelerate at a different rate from the descending aorta. This produces shear forces at the junction of the arch and the descending aorta. The shear results in a tear of the aorta at that point. If the rupture extends into the thoracic cavity, immediate exsanguination results. In 20% or so of the situations, the blood is contained within the adventitia surrounding the aorta as a pseudoaneurysm. Such a pseudoaneurysm remains intact for several hours to several days.

The abdomen is also a closed container. The abdominal organs can be compressed between the posterior and anterior abdominal wall (crush of the liver, spleen, pancreas, or kidney) causing, for example, shear of the vascular attachments of the solid organs during differential change in motion such as deceleration (spleen and kidney); shear of the liver around the ligamentum teres (especially in down and under pathway); and overpressure to the abdominal cavity (diaphragmatic rupture into either the left or right pleural cavity).

As a starting point to estimate the energy potential and direction of the crash, a description of the damage to the vehicle by the EMTs to the trauma team, gives the ACS a visual picture of the initial energy exchange. The same type of damage occurs to the patient as happened to the vehicle.

Lateral: Lateral impact collisions are frequently the result of an intersection (T-bone) crash. This actually results in two types of collision patterns. One vehicle is involved in a lateral impact collision, the other in a frontal collision. A careful description of the crash will allow the ACS to assess the potential injuries to the individual patients.

At the time of the collision, the occupants in the target vehicle are usually traveling in a forward direction. The bullet vehicle impacts the target vehicle from the side. This energy exchange accelerates the target vehicle in the direction of the impact and away from the bullet vehicle. The unrestrained occupants remain in the forward motion until impacted by the interior of their own vehicle. This (1) crushes the side of the patient at the impact point, (2) rapidly accelerates the patient away from the point of the impact. The occupant on the near side receives more energy exchange than the far side as the door and "B" pillows come into direct contact with the occupant. This contact and acceleration to lateral motion initially affects in four motions:

1. Impact on the femur tends to push the femoral head into and through the acetabulum. As the force continues, the door contacts the pelvis proper.
2. Impact to the lateral chest wall, the shoulder, or both. This compression fractures ribs (flail chest), contuses the lung in the chest and crushes the liver or spleen (depending on the site of the impact), and produces pulmonary contusions or pneumothorax. The acceleration, in the lateral direction, produces shear of the aorta and vascular attachment of abdominal organs. The descending aorta is attached to the torso or the spine and moves with it. The arch of aorta and the heart are not attached and move only when pulled. Approximately 25% of aortic shear injuries occur in lateral impact collisions. Approximately 75% occur as a result of frontal collisions.
3. The arm and shoulder, if positioned inside the door below the window, are impacted by the door. This compresses the upper arm and produces a fracture of the humerus, compression fractures of the ribs, and possible pulmonary contusion or intrathoracic overpressure injures. A clavicle fracture is also possible.
4. The lateral acceleration of the torso pulls the head into motion by the attachments of the neck as a secondary effect. The center of gravity of the head is anterior and superior to the attachment of the skull to cervical spine at the foramen magnum. This action causes rotation of the head toward the impact and lateral flexion of the neck in the same direction. This opens the facets on the contralateral side of the spine and rotation of the upper vertebra as the head turns. Dislocations, lateral compressing fractures, and jumped facets result.

Rear: The target vehicle is stopped or moving at a significant slower rate than the bullet vehicle as the contact between the two vehicles transpires. The bullet vehicle imparts a significant amount of its energy to accelerate the target vehicle and all components inside the car, which are attached to the car. Those components not tied to the car (which includes the occupants) start to move forward only as the parts of the vehicle such as the seats add force to them. Some of the energy is absorbed in the springs of the seat. Those portions of the occupant that touch the seat are accelerated almost simultaneously with the vehicle.

Those body parts not touching the seat (e.g., when the head is above the head rest), are accelerated by their attachments to the body. Only if the acceleration force reaches or exceeds 15*g* is the energy exchange at a high enough level to cause significant damage to the occupant. When the energy exchange is below 15*g*, the acceleration of the thorax out from under the head produces only ligaments or muscle strain.

Since the acceleration forces are in line with the body posterior to anterior, except as noted above with spinal injuries, the injuries to the occupant at the initial impact are minimal. Much force is absorbed by the springs. Additional injuries can occur if there is a second collision with the target vehicle being pushed forward into another target vehicle and the collision suddenly becomes frontal.

Rotational: If the initial impact is off-center, that part of the vehicle stops the forward motion while the rest of the vehicle continues in forward motion. This puts the current rotation

around this pivot point, and therefore the occupants can receive collisions of either frontal or lateral or both.
Rollover: In a rollover collision, the unbelted occupant flies freely throughout the passenger compartment and impacts all aspects of the vehicle. The patterns associated with these injuries are extremely difficult to predict.

Falls

The 'g'-force on earth is 32 feet per second per second (feet/s^2). The potential patient's speed significantly increases over time and distance. The greater the distance of the fall, the more energy the potential patient has when the bottom of his or her fall is reached and the energy of the falling patient suddenly stops. The initial impact is on that part of the body that makes contact first, but there is continued energy/motion of those other components that have not stopped their fall. Even though the impacting point has stopped, the continued energy of the torso, head, brain, intra-abdominal and thoracic organs must absorb the energy exchange. This includes all of the bones as well. The old adage of "in a fall one breaks his S" is very true. The energy compresses the concavity of the S and stretches the convexity. The neck of the femur, posterior lumbar spine, anterior thoracic spine, and posterior cervical spines are all aligned to encounter this energy exchange. Compression fractures such as the talus into the tibia, the calcaneus itself, the shaft of the femur and tibia are vulnerable. Deceleration/sheer injuries will occur to the kidneys, spleen, liver, and arch of the aorta.

The multiple other directions and the energy exchange in them can be figured out with just a little imagination on the part of the provider.

Motorcycle Collisions

Three different types of collisions are associated with motor cycle crashes: (1) ejection or partial ejection of the biker and impact with another object with the body parts pinned between the motorcycle tank/engine and the impacted object; (2) the unprotected (unhelmeted) head and skull hitting the object or the roadway; (3) "laying the bike down" to prevent impact with another object but sliding on the road and losing skin and other tissue during the slide.

Blast Force

Blast injuries are a result of four separate mechanisms. The primary zone, in which overpressure injuries cause damage to air-filled organs; the secondary zone, where injury is caused by flying particles and debris; the tertiary zone, where the victim becomes a missile and is thrown a distance, often into another object; and the quaternary zone where injuries are from radiation or bacterial contamination.

Penetrating Trauma

Energy Penetrating trauma is a result of the energy exchange onto the human body, impacting only a limited surface area with enough energy at the penetration site to penetrate the skin.

In blunt trauma, the energy exchange to the body produces compression forces from the initial impact, and the differential motion of the body and the organs produces shear at the point of organ attachment from the acceleration or deceleration of the tissue.

In penetrating trauma, the compression forces and stretch forces are involved. The compression forces are from the direct impact of the missile as it goes through the organs and stretch from the cavitation that surrounds the bullet pathway. The amount of energy exchange occurring on the human body to produce injury is a result of the direct impact of the penetrating object onto the human tissue. The amount of energy varies proportional to the number of tissue particles hit. The *size of the frontal area* of the penetrating object and the *density* of the tissue impacted determines the number of tissue particles hit and therefore the amount of energy exchange that occurs.

Density of body tissue is a continuum, but can be simplistically put into three categories: air density, soft (water) tissue density, and bone density. The least amount of energy exchange would occur when the bullet impacts an object containing significant amounts of air, such as the lung. The greatest amount of energy exchange would occur when the bullet impacts a very dense tissue like bone. Soft tissue density (water density) is intermediate between the two and includes solid organs and muscle.

The size of the frontal area of impact depends on the characteristics of the bullet itself. Important variables include the spin imparted to the bullet as it comes out of the barrel and the shape of the bullet (which are constructed in such a manner so that the bullet flies aerodynamically as straight as possible passing through the air).
The frontal surface area of the bullet is increased by three variables:

1. *Profile modification* such as a hollow point bullet that expands and spreads (mushrooms) on impact.
2. *Tumbling* of the bullet to present a broad side. At the 90° angle point of the rotation, the greatest exchange of energy occurs.
3. *Fragmentation* can either occur as the missile is leaving the muzzle such as a shotgun or can fragment after impact. A third level of fragmentation is explosion of the bullet after entering the body.

The two factors that influence the severity of the injury from a penetrating object are the amount of energy exchange that occurs and the organs that are involved.

The amount of energy exchange can be grossly estimated prior to examining the patient in the operating room by dividing penetrating objects into three groups based on energy.

- Low energy: a knife that creates no temporary cavity and only lacerates tissue.
- Medium energy: generally a handgun with a muzzle velocity of <1,000 feet per second and creates a temporary cavity some five to seven times the diameter of the missile.
- High-energy weapon: high velocity greater than 2,000 feet per second and can create a temporary cavity as much as 20 times the diameter of the missile. A lower velocity but a higher mass such as a shotgun or even IED produces such injuries.

SUMMARY

Patient care begins at the site of the incident and when rehabilitation is complete. Patient care is a continuum of care from beginning to end. The care of the injured is not disparate. Patient care does not start when the patient reaches the ED nor does it stop when the ED elevator doors close as the patient goes to the OR. The first step in this care is field management and transportation. Prehospital care is not a separate happening, but a component of the whole. The assessment, (primary care, resuscitation, secondary survey, and definitive care) is the same throughout, albeit each different stage (emergency department, OR, ICU, etc.) has different levels of care and the skills of the providers are different, nonetheless it is one team from beginning to end with different providers and different locations, but there is one patient with one disease.

The ACS should have knowledge of the entire process. If the ACS ignores the prehospital component, patients may be treated in such a manner that is not compatible with the in-hospital component. The ACS has obligation to assess what the EMS personnel are providing and to educate both in the classroom and to critique at the end of each run.

Newer techniques in the management of patient in the last few years have included damage control, hypotensive resuscitation, reduced use of crystalloids, and more appropriate patient triage, particularly in the rural areas.

Appropriate prehospital management is essential in achieving optimal patient care.

References

1. Smith DC. Senn Nicholas: The Origins of the Association of Military Surgeons of the United States. *Military Medicine*, 1999;164(4):243-246.
2. Salomone J, Pons P, eds. *NAEMT: PHTLS Basic and Advanced Prehospital Trauma Life Support*. 7th ed. St. Louis, MO: Elsevier; 2011.
3. Farrington JD. Death in Ditch. *Am Coll Surg Bull*. 1967;52(3):121-132.
4. Stiell IG, Nesbitt LP, Pickett W, et al. The OPALS Major Trauma Study: impact of advanced life-support on survival and morbidity. *Can Med Assoc J*. 2008;178(9):1141-1152.
5. McSwain NE Jr. The Science and Art of Prehospital Care: Principles, Preferences and Critical Thinking. In: Salomone J, Pons P, eds. *PHTLS: Basic and Advanced Prehospital Trauma Life Support, Chapter 3*. 7th ed. St. Louis, MO: Elsevier; 2011:34-41.
6. Nichol G, Aufderheide TP, Eigel B, et al. Regional systems of care for out-of-hospital cardiac arrest: A policy statement from the American Heart Association. *Circulation*. 2010;121(5):709-729.
7. Erich J. The new Salvation Army. How the U. S. military is keeping soldiers alive and what it means for EMS. *Emerg Med Serv*. 2005;34(5): 53-57, 104.
8. Field Triage Decision Scheme: The National Trauma Triage Protocol. Atlanta, GA: Centers for Disease Control and Prevention; 2010.
9. Newgard CD, Schmicker RH, Hedges JR, et al. Emergency Medical Services Intervals and Survival in Trauma: assessment of the "Golden Hour" in a North American Prospective. *Ann Emerg Med*. 2010;55(3):235. e4-246.e4.
10. McSwain NE. Prehospital care from napoleon to mars: the Surgeon's Role. *J Am Coll Surg*. 2005;200(4):487-504.
11. Lubin JS, Delbridge TR, Cole JS, et al. EMS and Emergency Department Physician Triage: injury severity in Trauma Patients Transported by Helicopter. *Prehosp Emerg Care*. 2005;9(2):198-202.
12. McSwain NE Jr. Medical control—what is it? *JACEP*. 1978;7(3):114-116.
13. Sagraves SG, Newell MA, Bard MR, et al. Tissue oxygenation monitoring in the field: a new EMS vital sign. *J Trauma*. 2009;67(3):441-443; discussion 443-444.
14. McSwain NE. 2003 Clinical Congress, American College of Surgeons, "Scudder Oration on Trauma: Prehospital Care from Napoleon to Mars: The Surgeon's Role". Chicago, IL, October 21, 2003.

CHAPTER 17 DISASTER PREPAREDNESS AND MASS CASUALTY MANAGEMENT

LEONARD J. WEIRETER JR

Police find car bomb in Times Square

A crude car bomb of propane, gasoline and fireworks was discovered in a smoking Nissan Pathfinder in the heart of Times Square on Saturday evening, prompting evacuation of thousands of tourists and theatergoers.......... "We were very lucky" said Mayor Michael Bloomberg. "We avoided what could have been a very deadly event"
New York Times May 1, 2010

Storms Cut through Midwest, killing 5

Hundreds of homes and businesses were damaged or destroyed Friday in Kansas, Kentucky, Illinois, Missouri and West Virginia prompting several state of emergency declarations.
New York Times May 9, 2009

Imagine for a moment being on duty in a hospital adjacent to either scene above. The destruction of the second versus the absolute luck involved in avoiding the tragedy of the first is mind boggling. How would you, as an individual, your hospital and its staff, or your community at large have responded to either event? Who would be in charge? Where would injured patients go? How would they get there? How did they get here so fast? How would we, or could we, treat them? Where are the necessary supplies? What about the worried family members flocking to the hospital to find family members? Where do they go? How do I find out who goes with whom? What do we do with the ordinary patient traffic of the day in light of either of these events?

The easy answer is that "they" will take care of it. Unfortunately, the "they," usually thought of as a governmental agency, is not able to respond fast enough in the first hours to substantially impact the situation. The "they" realistically is "us." Disaster and mass casualty situations have distinct defining characteristics that need to be understood to appreciate the mindset change needed to deal with the problems.[1] Command and control is paramount but its mechanisms are not obvious to the individuals who spend most of their professional time in hospitals engaged in routines of care. How we view patient care needs to fundamentally change in such situations. Finally, unless we are committed to understanding these differences and practicing the responses demanded, we will be doomed to fail. At that point, we will be tasked with answering why we weren't better prepared only to realize that there is no good reason. The ultimate goal of such a response is to make ours a resilient community, that is, to build a community that can withstand the insult and return to normal structure and function with minimal deformation. To this end, the objective of this chapter is to begin to lay a foundation to support "us" as we develop a methodology to accomplish this goal.

DEFINITIONS

A disaster or mass casualty event in some ways depends on where you are at the time. A two-car, five-victim crash on the interstate may be routine to the urban level 1 trauma center but devastating to the much smaller critical access hospital in a rural county. The crux of the definition lies not in numbers or severity of injuries but in relation to the capability and resources of the responding community, be that EMS or hospital. Once the demands of the response outstrip the available resources, the situation warrants the label disaster or mass casualty. Frequently, the outstripped resources represent more than just local capabilities but expand to regional if not national capabilities. The occurrence of such events is thought sufficiently rare that two things occur. First, we believe we will never be called upon to deal with such catastrophe; thus, we have little need to be prepared. Second, the event is attributed to a random, fate-driven, unpredictable occurrence over which we have no control at any level. Unfortunately, the student of history soon discovers the fallacy underlying both of these assumptions. Recent history, well documented in the lay press, is replete with examples of both natural and man-made events that fulfill the definition of needs exceeding resources at several levels. Further study of this history will reveal patterns that are common to all such events. This knowledge can form the core around which response methodologies can be developed. Rather than try to develop unique solutions for every imaginable occurrence, we can build on the common themes present in the disaster situation and the needed response. A template can be developed, trained, critiqued, and refined until there is a cogent understanding and response methodology in place.

Disasters can be natural, such as hurricane, tornado, earthquake, or flooding. They can be man-made, intentional or unintentional, such as the bombing of a building, fire through carelessness or an industrial accident in a commercial district of a city or rural area. They can be finite such as a building collapse that is confined in a particular time and place or ongoing, such as an open forest wildfire that will spread through hundreds of acres over weeks or flooding subsequent to a hurricane, the effects of which persist months if not longer. Despite the seemingly endless possibilities, there are lessons to learn if we are attentive enough. Specific injury patterns are associated with different mechanisms. Common to all these disasters is environmental exposure, either as heat or hypothermia. Burns are common. Blast effects are common as explosions frequently accompany many of these events. Inhalation of substances dispersed into the air is very common. Exposure to chemicals or radiation is common. Very important and frequently overlooked is the psychological effects of the event on both the victim population and the responding caregivers.

The importance to us as surgeons is that we are looked to as an important cog in the wheel of first responders. The infrastructure our trauma systems are built on will become paramount in mounting this response. Our background in rapid situational analysis and decision making makes us well versed in the skills now needed to overcome the event at hand. Unfortunately, we have backed away from engaging this challenge. Unfortunately, or fortunately, we are a key component of the response system the public will look to in the face of such events. This response is not empiric though. It is very different from everyday practice, even in the busiest of trauma centers. It is not even accorded any part of routine medical training at any level.

PHASES OF THE DISASTER

Important to recognize here is that the disaster has a life cycle as does any other organism. Appreciation of the phases of this cycle is a key starting point as we begin to develop our response methodology. The initial phase of the response is characterized by utter chaos. Normalcy is gone, leadership is nonexistent, and hysteria and fear prevail. How long this phase lasts is difficult to determine. Urban areas with rapid response times of organized police, fire, and rescue units may do a better job of curtailing the chaos than more rural communities just by nature of time and distance. What is true though is that until trained staff can superimpose a command and control structure, the chaos will continue. While the chaos is unabated, the population remains at risk and the situation will continue to escalate (Table 17.1).

The initial response and reorganization phase is characterized by the imposition of crisis management. This begins with the arrival of the first responders. A command structure is set up and a situational assessment made. A security methodology to minimize further injury is established. Search and rescue operations begin and patients are moved to appropriate locations. One caveat here is that good training, planning, and rehearsal will shorten the time required to set up this phase of the response. In the absence of such preparation, this may never get off the ground until far too late in the evolution of the disaster.

The initial response phase gives way to the site clearing phase. The transition can be thought of as the transition from crisis management to consequence management. Search and rescue may move to search and recovery as victims are rarely found alive beyond 48 hours after the event. Debris is cleared. Causalities are moved to hospitals for definitive care.

Finally, the event enters the phase of late recovery. Definitive medical care is rendered. Infrastructure is rebuilt. A rigorous critique of the situation and the response is carried out. The psychological health of the victims and responders is assessed and treatment plans developed. The community determines what it needs to return to normal.[2] None of this happens a priori. How we begin to accomplish this follows next.

TABLE 17.1

PHASES OF A DISASTER RESPONSE

1. Chaos
2. Initial response/reorganization {Crisis management} • Establish command post • Needs assessment • Security and safety procedures • Casualty evacuation to casualty collection areas (CCAs)
3. Site clearing • Search and rescue/recovery • Casualty distribution from CCAs to hospitals • Initial hospital medical care {Consequence management}
4. Late recovery • Rebuilding infrastructure • Definitive hospital medical care/secondary casualty distribution • Provider and casualty mental health follow-up • Postevent critique and analysis of disaster response • Community recovery

(From Stein M. Hirshberg A. Medical consequences of terrorism: the conventional weapons threat. *Surg Clin North Am.* 1999;1537–1552.)

PLANNING

Military history can teach us much about planning. Dwight Eisenhower emphasized the planning process, not the plan per se, as the important component. George Patton espoused that plans need to be as simple and flexible as possible and made by those who will actually carry them out. All hospitals are required by the Joint Commission to have and rehearse a disaster plan on a regular basis. Thinking back to the last disaster plan discussion, much less drill, you may have participated in may give you some insight into the magnitude of the planning and preparation efforts of your institution. The disaster management cycle is illustrated in the accompanying diagram (Fig. 17.1). Ideally, we would like to begin by realizing what we need to prepare for, prepare for it, and then respond when tasked to do so. Historically, we frequently attempt to respond to the situation and make up a plan as we go. Hardly optimal. Plans are only as good as the assumptions they are based on. There are several elements deemed essential to a realistic plan (Table 17.2). There need to be valid assumptions about the threats faced; there needs to be some dependence on past performance critique; a systems approach that pulls together all components of the organization is important; everyone expected to participate in the execution of the plan needs to be part of the planning process; everyone needs to know and accept the plan; the expected participants need to be educated in the plan, both in a didactic and practical sense. Finally, the plan needs to be field tested, revised accordingly, and then retested.[3,4]

The first essential component of planning is to carry out a Hazard Vulnerability Analysis (HVA). This is a realistic assessment of the likelihood of particular events in your community. Both natural and man-made events need to be considered. For instance, living along the southeast coast of the United States, hurricane and flooding would need to be considered high on that list. Several such templates are available on the Internet, but without a realistic assessment of one's own location, the exercise is futile and the planning assumptions flawed.

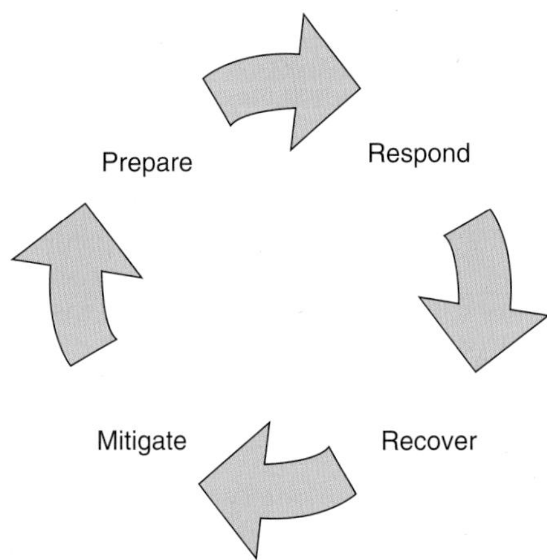

FIGURE 17.1. The disaster response cycle. We usually begin by responding to an incident rather than preparing to mitigate the consequences of the event. (From *Disaster Management and Emergency Preparedness Course Manual.* Chicago, IL: American College of Surgeons Committee on Trauma; 2010 with permission.)

TABLE 17.2

ESSENTIAL ELEMENTS OF DISASTER PLANNING

- Valid assumptions of injury patterns, threats, human behavior, and needs
- A basis in the results of past disasters and established disaster response principles
- An interorganizational or "systems" approach of many elements working together
- Inclusion of the participants in a disaster response in the planning process
- Knowledge and acceptance of the plan by the participants in the disaster response
- Training and education of the participants
- Regular drills and exercises to test a plan's workability and revise as necessary

From *Disaster Management and Emergency Preparedness Course Manual*. Chicago, IL: American College of Surgeons Committee on Trauma; 2010.

TABLE 17.3

KEY QUESTIONS TO BE ADDRESSED IN A HOSPITAL DISASTER PLAN

1. Will the hospital automatically activate the plan, or will there be a situational assessment validation?
2. What command structure will be used, and how will the hospital leaders be educated?
3. How will triage be coordinated with the other facilities and EMS agencies?
4. When and how will the medical decontamination team be implemented?
5. How will the hospital sustain its operation?
6. What are the primary sources of communication available, and how will these sources assist in interacting with the community and regional activities?
7. How will an alternate care site be established? Who makes decisions?
8. What are the expectations and requirements for documentation during a response? How will an official business summary be completed?
9. How will the evacuation plan be executed? What equipment items are needed? How will this plan be communicated?
10. How will the facility and surrounding area be secured?
11. What long-range psycho-emotional plans are needed?
12. Will the hospital's emergency response impact surrounding businesses? How will this impact be communicated?

From *Disaster Management and Emergency Preparedness Course Manual*. Chicago, IL: American College of Surgeons Committee on Trauma; 2010.

Once the HVA has been completed, comes the difficult task of assessing readiness to deal with any of the events listed (Table 17.3). Who to bring to this discussion is an important decision. All the constituents of the community will own part of the response; thus, all need to be part of this analysis and discussion. This moves beyond the hospital quickly and encompasses governmental and private sector entities. The EMS community, police, fire, the media, religious organizations, local industry, and employers who will be affected all need to come to the table, be educated in and contribute to the planning process. History is also an important contributor to this discussion.

To illustrate the point, consider for a moment a situation where water pressure and electricity to an entire region were lost, generators were inaccessible, supply chains destroyed, roads impassable, and the health care infrastructure gone. Hurricane Katrina in New Orleans certainly entailed all these problems. But Hurricane Hugo in South Carolina in 1989 did all the same. What lessons were transferable and learned from one to the other should be clear to the critical reader.

A few generalizations can be made as well as some methods of deluding ourselves noted. Klein and Weigelt[5] comment on four areas of failure in disaster response. A communication system that completely collapses; no clear lines of authority; inadequate scene and hospital security and a disorganized health care system that tries to deliver care to all patients without appropriate triage. These become key considerations in the planning process. Delusion is a grand frame of mind and we fall into it regularly when we engage in disaster planning. We stage disaster drills with sufficient warning to all involved parties, we hold them during daylight hours and plan them not to inconvenience daily operations. We are not realistic in our assumptions about the consumption of supplies and minimize the need for resupply.

Finally, we will never be able to engage the disaster response adequately if we are not prepared in our own lives. The distraction of the safety of our own families is powerful yet can be tempered by attention to detail and arranging a methodology to have sufficient materials on hand at home. There are a variety of resources to guide us here, and the CDC and FEMA Web sites are excellent sources for this level of preparation.

INCIDENT COMMAND

Probably the most critical initial function of a disaster response is the establishment of an effective command and control methodology. This becomes obvious when one considers that large-scale events require multiple agencies to respond, each with their own command structure. Even within a small hospital, the issues with who is in charge or who is tasked with what responsibility in a given circumstance can be confusing. The necessity of establishing a functioning structure to control all the moving pieces is clear. The Incident Command Structure (ICS) used today grew out of the California wildfire experiences of the 1970s. The difficulty with coordination of activities among multiple responding agencies forced a better mechanism. After several iterations, the National Incident Management System was put forth by the Department of Homeland Security. The ICS was determined to be a best practice and is now the operational standard for all emergency response systems in the United States. While the ICS has its origins as a field operations tool, the inhospital equivalent parallels the field tool in descriptions and functionality. The Hospital Emergency Incident Command System is the same modular system with the same titles and responsibilities. It is intended to facilitate the coordinated response in the hospital and smooth the field-to-hospital transition.

The principles of the ICS are simple and straightforward. The goal is the rapid imposition of a command and control system recognized by and agreed to by all response participants. Realizing that it can take up to 30 minutes to recoup every 5 minutes of chaos, such disaster situations induce a potent driver for such command and control systems. The ability to coordinate and escalate the response as needed is a key functionality of the ICS.

Structurally, the ICS allows expansion and contraction around several key positions (Algorithm. 17.1). The Incident Commander (IC) is the only position absolutely required in the construct. The concepts of unity of command and span of control are key factors that contribute to the functional success of this construct. Unity of command allows multiple agencies to coordinate activities under one overarching IC. The span of control is a recognition that everyone needs to report to only one clearly designated individual and that responders in leadership positions can only control a limited number of responders effectively, typically five to seven people. By keeping these lines of control well delineated and designated by job description rather than person, orderly progression and transfer of authority can occur.

Surrounding the IC are several key positions, all with clearly delineated responsibilities. Utilization of the same vocabulary for job titles and positions helps to ensure clear understanding of expectations and responsibilities. The IC has ultimate responsibility for all aspects of the response. The IC can delegate as seen appropriate by utilizing the staff surrounding and directly reporting to the IC. For instance, the safety officer is responsible for a safety assessment of the situation so that first responders do not unnecessarily endanger themselves. The Public Information Officer is the communication link, via the media, to the public to keep them informed of the situation. The liaison officer is tasked with coordination with other agencies as appropriate. These positions constitute the command staff.

There are four primary functionalities required to mount an effective response. All four report directly to the IC. Likewise, all four can expand or contract the response system beneath them as needed. These four are termed the general staff. They are the planning section, the operations section, the logistics section, and the finance and administration section.

The planning section is tasked with being the brains of the operation. Situational awareness is critical and keeping the IC informed of developments the key function. Likewise, the planning chief will direct the other sections as to the plan to be executed. Keeping ahead of developments and seeing where a preexisting response plan works well or needs modification are essential components of this position. The recorded lessons learned will be important in the after-action critique.

The operations section is the doer responsible for all aspects of the response. Arguably, all the other positions exist to support operations. Anything that requires something being done, from field search and rescue to evacuation to care, is the responsibility of operations.

The logistics section is responsible for all the material and manpower assets associated with the response effort. If it is needed to meet the demands of the disaster, logistics is responsible to get it or have it.

The finance and administration section is the record keeper for all activities associated with the response effort. Response personnel need time records maintained. Cost of materials needs to be tracked. Claims compensation needs to be determined. The overall cost of the response needs to be evaluated, in both human and fiscal terms, and mechanisms looked for that may bring cost savings in the future.

The interdependence of the four functionalities is very clear. The IC tasks operations with accomplishing a specific goal. The planning section informs the IC of the situation and how it compares to the predesigned response plan. Logistics supplies the people and supplies to accomplish the goal, and finance tracks the costs associated. What is also very clear is that this does not occur spontaneously. The great fallacy of Incident Command is that by assigning titles I have accomplished this goal. Individuals do not deserve one title or another based on seniority or everyday position. Without the proper education and opportunity to rehearse these positions in realistic drills, the system will fail. In similar fashion, multiple individuals need to be prepared to fulfill any role. There should be no key individual whose absence stymies the operation. Likewise, there needs to be provision for the smooth transition of individuals in a given position should the disaster continue for a prolonged time.

DEFINITIVE MEDICAL CARE

Up to this point, nothing has been said about the actual care of any injured patient or patients. That is because without the imposed structure of a disaster response plan that can function,

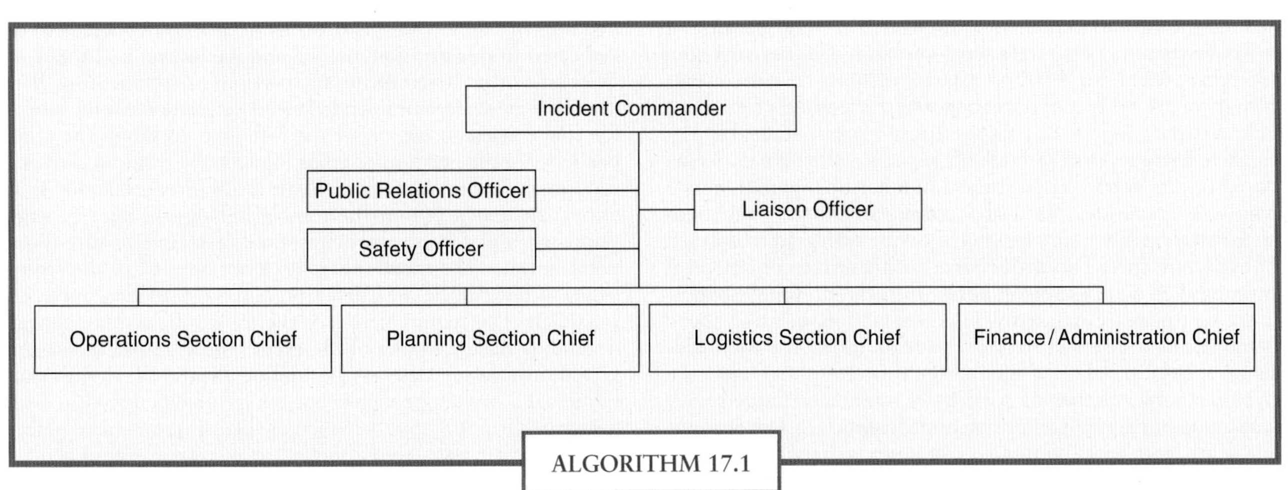

ALGORITHM 17.1 The incident command structure. (From *Disaster Management and Emergency Preparedness Course Manual*. Chicago, IL: American College of Surgeons Committee on Trauma; 2010 with permission.)

there is no definitive medical care. How to deliver care, where to do it, and who do we treat in what time frame are important questions that the response effort needs to answer. The mythology of disaster response needs to be appreciated as it will help guide our response.[4]

Popular mythology will contend that trained field personnel carry out initial field search and rescue operations. In reality, the survivors, or those less injured, perform this task. Similarly, the thought that the initial triage and treatment is done by trained providers is mythology. Survivors provide what they can and those injured who can move will self-transport to the closest health care facility. This uncovers another great myth, that patients are transported in an orderly fashion to appropriate hospitals. Victims of such events do not discriminate one type of hospital from another. All hospitals are equal and all are viewed as a safe haven for the injured. The hospital closest to the event will in all likelihood be flooded and overwhelmed by an influx of self-transported victims. By the very fact that these people were able to self-transport is indicative of their injury severity. The challenge for an individual hospital, and the larger response effort, is how to sort out those in need of immediate care from those with minimal or no injuries. Once identified, where do I send them and how do I do it? Can I provide the care I do everyday? Can I operate emergency services as I do every day when faced with such a circumstance?

TRIAGE

Modern American medical practice allows tremendous resource allocation toward any one patient regardless of the likelihood of survival. The resources that can be brought to bear usually so overwhelm the needs of the situation that the concept of rationing resources is virtually never considered. The modern trauma system is willing to accept tremendous overtriage in order to avoid undertriage at almost no consideration for the expenditure for that care. Quite the opposite when faced with a situation where, by definition, the resources needed to deal with a situation are outstripped by the demands of that situation. The triage process is arguably the most critical determinant of the success or failure of the response effort. Understanding the switch in mindset from an individual-based to a population-based health care ethic is crucial. The mechanics are straightforward but distinctly uncomfortable for the novice.

Triage is not a new or novel concept. The process of sorting based on severity of injury is used daily in emergency rooms around the nation. In reality, we do little real triage because of the overwhelming resources we command. The key first step to realize, when faced with a disaster or mass casualty event, is that we are no longer operating where the good of the individual is paramount. Rather, the distinctly public health perspective becomes operational and we now will make decisions based on the good of the greatest number or population as a whole. By definition, this means certain patients we would treat aggressively a few hours ago may now be relegated to delayed or expectant care. This is of course antithetical to our medical training, but without this mindset shift, the preventable mortality will increase markedly. Frykberg and associates[6–8] have demonstrated the effect of poor triage on mortality. An analysis of a large number of international events shows that the overwhelming number of patients is minimally injured with soft tissue or relatively minor orthopedic injuries. The percentage of patients with life-threatening injuries that are amenable to treatment under the constraints of treatment imposed by the event is approximately 20%. The challenge then becomes finding those 20%, initiating care in the field, and moving them expeditiously to definitive care. The concept of critical mortality, the death rate among that 20%, has become a marker of the success or failure of the response.

Categorization of the injured for triage purposes allows for rapid initial sorting to identify who needs the most immediate care.[9] While there are a number of methods available, there are common attributes that warrant discussion. The first pass at triage, done at or adjacent to the scene of the event, will sort victims into immediate or delayed categories. The immediate victim has a life-threatening injury or injuries and requires rapid treatment (Table 17.4). The qualifier here is that the treatment rendered needs to be simple to apply. Opening an airway, compressing hemorrhage, decompression of a tension pneumothorax, providing a rescue breath may fall into this category. Anything that ties up a rescuer beyond brief moments is not applicable. The delayed category victim is hemodynamically stable and can tolerate a period of no or minimal treatment without impacting mortality. Fractures, open or closed, soft tissue injuries, some penetrating wounds, and some burns will fall into this category.

Within the delayed care category, further subdivision is possible. Those with minimal injury, the colloquial walking wounded, need little more than simple first aid and are relegated to such care when available. More difficult is the concept of expectant care and those dead. Victims without signs of life are dead. This is not the time or place for heroics that may occur in the emergency department or trauma bay under more usual circumstances. No resuscitative effort should be expended. Expectant care is care rendered to victims critically injured but who are not amenable to treatment given the constraints of the situation. If the probability of survival is so low, if the resources consumed in treating this victim would detract from the care of other more salvageable victims thus jeopardizing them, then expectant care is rendered. That is not the same as no care, as analgesia and comfort are important. Equally important is that medical personnel need to be assigned to monitor this group of victims. They may show signs of improvement that justifies moving to a higher level of care. The situation may change, resources become available that were not available before, fewer critically injured present that anticipated and now the expectant victim may qualify for treatment.[10]

The mechanics of triage are as important as the philosophy. The role of the triage officer, the error tolerance of the system, and the movement of victims from one place to another to unclog or decongest the scene or nearest hospital need consideration.

The triage officer is the individual charged with the decision making regarding who gets treatment. The position needs to be dedicated to this decision making and the individual cannot be tasked to other assignments or locations simultaneously. The decisions made are not intended to be negotiations at the site of the triage decision but rather the definitive decision. The independence of the position is critical. Practically speaking, anyone can function as a triage officer. Realistically, they need good situational awareness of both the number and types of injuries being presented and the treatment resources available at any given point in time. The triage officer does not have to be the senior clinician but can be a qualified prehospital provider, nurse, or physician. The requirements for the triage officer may change depending on the nature of the event. For example, a surgeon versed in blast injuries may be well qualified to deal with causalities of a building collapse but poorly qualified to deal with a specific chemical spill or pandemic-like situation. The ability to work in a stressful environment, make rapid, sound clinical assessments, and maintain an awareness of the entire scope of the event and response are the critical job requirements.

In such a rapid-fire decision-making atmosphere, where large numbers of victims present simultaneously, errors will

TABLE 17.4

PRIMARY TRIAGE CATEGORIES

ACUTE	NONACUTE
(Immediate, Priority 1)	(Delayed, Minimal, Expectant, Dead)
Nonambulatory Patients with Physiologic Criteria • Airway: unstable • Breathing: present • Circulation: active bleeding, lack of pulse • 2 s capillary refill • Disability: not following simple command Low GCS ≤14 Motor GCS ≤5	**Walking Wounded** • Minimal soft tissue injuries • Superficial burns **Urgent, Non–Life-Threatening Injuries** • No airway compromise • No respiratory compromise • Extensive burns (deep, >30% TBSA) • Multiple orthopedic injuries
Exposure (Anatomic Criteria) • -4 body regions injured • Penetrating head wounds • Penetrating torso wounds	**Unsalvageable Injuries** • Unresponsive, not breathing • Traumatic amputation • Open head and chest wounds
Clinical Judgment and Expertise	

From *Disaster Management and Emergency Preparedness Course Manual.* Chicago, IL: American College of Surgeons Committee on Trauma; 2010.

happen. The system needs to develop error tolerance and the triage officer cannot be frozen by the possibility of error. As victims move through the system, they need to be re-triaged at subsequent stations. This reiterative methodology will minimize errors and allow rapid decompression of the incident zone and transport of victims to other areas for staging or care. If done correctly, the victims who reach the hospital, or point of definitive care, will be the critically injured most likely to benefit from aggressive care. The mandate of identifying the 20% critically injured and minimizing that mortality can now be tackled. In the absence of any of these, the system will become overrun with victims who do not need, or will not benefit from, immediate care and a key characteristic of effective triage missed. The point is that the process is dynamic and the rules change as the situation and response changes. For instance, the sudden, unexpected availability of personnel or material resources increases the number of victims that may be attended to, whereas the sudden loss of electrical power or depletion of supplies may well have the opposite effect. A lull in the influx of new injured victims may present an opportunity to address victims previously assigned to the expectant group. Unless the triage officer is aware of these nuances, opportunities will be lost.

There are two additional methods used to help the triage system that deserve consideration. Both entail movement of victims from the scene. The concept noted above moves victims to any of a number of casualty collection points. These points are removed from the incident scene but are not the hospital. Re-triage occurs and the victim can be "leap-frogged" from the field to any of the available hospitals in an attempt to minimize overloading any one hospital and rendering that hospital inoperable. The most critically injured victims would be transported to the closest hospital for definitive care while those less injured would be transported to hospitals at a greater distance from the scene. Secondary hospital distribution is a method of redistributing victims to other hospitals with capacity and capability to deal with them. This functionally off loads one hospital and minimizes the treatment delays that may be experienced. Both of these require a well-functioning regional incident command system with the knowledge of system-wide capabilities and the ability to move victims through the region.

The flip side of this process is undertriage. We accept tremendous overtriage every day to minimize undertriage. The process of mass casualty triage risks undertriage by its very nature. For this reason, the triage officer needs to be versed in the types of injuries presented. Different individuals with different qualifications may need to fill that role as the situation dictates. Additionally, the areas where less critically injured victims are assembled need to be staffed by medical personnel who can monitor for deterioration in clinical status, initiate appropriate treatment, and escalate care by moving the victim to a more urgent care area.

THE HOSPITAL RESPONSE

Up to this point, most of the emphasis in the discussion has been on the system-wide response to a disaster or mass casualty event. The specific role of the hospital now warrants consideration. Unless prepared, the hospital risks being overrun and rendered inoperable, not just for the disaster situation but for daily operations as well. When mobilized, the hospital incident command system will direct activities in the hospital and coordinate with other regional assets as required. Internally, there are two important concepts for the hospital to be aware of and be able to manipulate. One is the surge capacity and the other surge capability.[11] Surge capacity is the number or percentage of beds over and above maximum capacity the institution can mobilize. This is frequently up to 20% over and above the number of usually staffed beds in the hospital. Surge capability is the ability to staff those additional beds with appropriate nursing, paraprofessional, and other staff to make them usable. The effect of overtriage on surge capacity is clear. As overtriage exceeds 25%, the surge capacity is reduced dramatically. Hirshberg and associates demonstrated that with appropriate utilization of resources, the number of critically injured victims who can be treated can be increased without the concomitant decrease in the global level of care.[12–14]

The hospital will need to have in place plans for security, staff recall, resupply, and how to deal with other non–disaster-related aspects of daily care that will continue to go on simultaneously. Record keeping is a critical issue for the hospital. Accurate patient tracking and documentation of assessment and care rendered is required. The record keeping needs to be as simple as possible, using flowsheets that are well known to the staff and that do not require learning new systems. Communications can be expected to fail and the media will arrive looking for information. How well the hospital deals with these issues is a function of how well they planned for them.

SPECIFIC INJURY PATTERNS

A number of specific injury patterns require understanding if one is to effectively triage and treat these injuries. Blast injuries accompany explosions and are arguably one of the most common presenting injury patterns known. The common occurrence of bombings internationally makes knowledge of this particular pathophysiology germane to those who will respond to and treat these victims.[15]

The typical high energy explosive is capable of creating a blast wave that can exceed 4,000 m/s velocity. The incredibly rapid rise above ambient air pressure is responsible for the shatter ability of the blast. As the marked pressure head diminishes, there is a negative pressure phenomenon that sucks debris back toward the epicenter of the event. This blast wind, or to and fro air motion, gives the characteristic explosion followed by implosion.

The mechanics of the blast determines magnitude of injury. The initial force, distance from the center, interior versus exterior location, and open air or underwater are usually considered the mechanical factors at work determining magnitude of injury. Since the blast wave dissipates as the cube of the distance away from the center, mitigation of blast effect is straightforward if one is a modest distance away. Interior blasts allow reflection of energy with resultant magnification of effect. Water allows a greater distance for energy propagation due to the density of water compared to air.[16]

Blast injuries are categorized into one of four types (Table 17.5). Primary blast injury refers to the direct effect of the blast wave as it passes through the body. Air–water interfaces are especially prone to disruption as turbulence is most severe here. The lung is vulnerable in air blasts while the gastrointestinal tract is at risk underwater. Unfortunately, most victims of primary blast lung injury die as a result of cerebral or coronary air embolus. Those who do survive to hospitalization require treatment for severe pulmonary contusion or ARDS like pathophysiology.

Secondary blast injury arises from objects set in motion crashing into a victim. A special circumstance to be aware of is the ability to pack bombs with materials that act as shrapnel, causing a multitude of penetrating wounds scattered throughout the victim's body. These victims may look surprisingly well initially except for being pockmarked all over. A high degree of suspicion will evaluate these aggressively and determine the real extent of injury.

Tertiary blast injury occurs when a victim is picked up or thrown into other more stationary objects. By and large, secondary and tertiary injuries induce typical blunt injury patterns. Quaternary injuries refer to the indirect effects of the blast such as noxious inhaled materials, burns, crush injuries, and the like.

TABLE 17.5

MECHANISMS OF BLAST INJURY

CATEGORY	CHARACTERISTICS	BODY PART AFFECTED	TYPES OF INJURIES
Primary	Unique to HE, results from the impact of the over pressurization wave with body surfaces	Gas-filled structures are most susceptible lungs, GI tract, and middle ear	• Blast lung (pulmonary barotrauma • TM rupture and middle ear damage • Abdominal hemorrhage and perforation Globe (eye) rupture Compression (TBI without physical signs of head injury) • Traumatic amputations
Secondary	Results from flying debris and bomb fragments	Any body part may be affected	• Penetrating ballistic (fragmentation) or blunt injuries • Eye penetration (can be occult)
Tertiary	Results from individuals being thrown by the blast wind	Any body part may be affected	• Fractures • Closed and open brain injury
Quaternary	All explosion-related injuries, illnesses, or diseases not due to primary, secondary, or tertiary mechanisms Includes exacerbation or complications of existing conditions.	Any body part may be affected	• Burns (flash, partial, and full thickness) • Crush injuries • Closed and open brain injury • Asthma, COPD, or other breathing problems from dust, smoke, or toxic fumes • Angina • Hyperglycemia, hypertension

From *Disaster Management and Emergency Preparedness Course Manual.* Chicago, IL: American College of Surgeons Committee on Trauma; 2010.

The literature regarding the patterns of blast wounds is replete with descriptions of predictable patterns. Interestingly, most survivors are not critically injured. The severely injured are dead. Regardless, a victim with evidence of primary blast injury, head and/or torso injury, or amputation needs aggressive evaluation to preclude serious injury. A major issue with blast injury is that the naïve triage officer will be distracted by the visual appearance and not appreciate that many of these are soft tissue wounds that can be delayed several hours. The tendency for overtriage here needs to be mitigated.

A discussion of blast injury needs to mention the second hit phenomenon at least to make the triage and treatment teams aware of the concept. Secondary delayed explosions, either intentional or otherwise, have the potential to injure the responders and markedly complicate the response. A building explosion and collapse that 30 minutes later has an explosion of a fractured gas line, when the first responders are just on scene doing search and rescue, is a devastating event that needs to have mitigation before allowing first responders in the building. In a more nefarious construct, the intentional detonation of a secondary delayed device intended to injure the response teams is well described in this literature. This serves to reiterate the primary role of scene safety for the response providers. As much as possible, the scene needs to be secured before allowing rescue personnel access to the scene.[17]

The other common mechanisms of mass casualty include chemical exposure, radiologic exposure, and biologic agents. A detailed discussion of these agents is beyond the scope of this chapter. A few brief considerations are in order though.

Chemical agents have been used as weapons since antiquity and in recent history. Their detection can be very difficult and only by the recognition of specific clinical syndromes. Industrial incidents at least have requirements for posting potential toxins and the information is frequently forthcoming from the safety officers tasked to the job site. In either case, the responders need to protect themselves and provide decontamination of the victims prior to allowing entry to the hospital. The spectrum of personal protective gear and its use should be trained and drilled by all institutions that may need to respond to such events. Triage and decontamination needs to occur outside the hospital. Frequently, simply undressing the victim and washing with soap and water accomplishes the overwhelming majority of the decontamination. More specific decontamination may be dictated by special circumstances or exposure to specific agents. Any disaster plan needs to consider decontamination. Where it will occur, when it will occur, who will be responsible for operation of and maintaining the equipment and how will the victims be trafficked through the system are all integral questions the plan needs to address.

Nuclear or radiologic exposure induces panic quickly. The reality is that nuclear exposure is far easier to contend with than chemical exposure. The nuclear-exposed victim may be very ill but is a minimal threat to the health care team. Good decontamination is essential but, as with chemical exposure, undressing and showering or washing with soap and water is usually sufficient. Electromagnetic radiation, x-rays, and gamma rays have a high degree of penetration and induce the most damage. The victim though is not "radioactive" and not a real threat to the treatment team. Particle radiation, alpha and beta particles, penetrate minimally, need to be ingested for significant injury, and can be treated easily. Local effects are burn-like symptoms that require local treatment. Decontamination proceeds as noted above. If the treatment team exercises universal precautions, they will be well protected. Clothing taken from victims needs to be contained as does runoff water.

Medical care of nuclear and radiologic contamination is generally supportive. The psychologic effects of being irradiated may be more devastating than the physical consequences, and this will need to be addressed in the treatment algorithm for these victims. From the perspective of triage decision making, the time from irradiation to first emesis is critical. If emesis occurs within an hour of exposure, then the victim likely has had a lethal exposure and warrants supportive but expectant care. In such events, specific information can be obtained from the radiation safety officer on the IC's staff.

Biologic disasters are driven by microorganisms. While anthrax has been the agent of concern in the recent past, the experience with H1N1 may actually serve as a better example of how such a situation might unfold. Unlike a blast or chemical exposure event with its dramatic occurrence, the infectious disease and public health communities, through a process of syndromic surveillance, would piece together the clues from patterns of illness presenting to emergency departments, clinics, and private physician offices to come to the realization that an event was occurring. From the perspective of the disaster response plan, very little may need to change. If correctly developed, the flexibility and fluidity in the plan will direct response actions. H1N1 raised the specter of a pandemic and many organizations rehearsed scenarios to deal with the consequences.

RECOVERY

The goal of planning is to build resiliency in our community. That means we return to normal as soon as possible. It carries the additional mandate to mitigate future risk as much as possible. The issue now is that people are tired and want to get back to life as they knew it. Unfortunately, there is still a formidable task ahead. Two issues need to be clarified. One, the response personnel will have an emotional reaction to the events that need to be acknowledged and dealt with. Failure to so do will result in downstream psychological effects for some of the providers that may be crippling. A critical incident stress debriefing methodology should be offered to all members of the response system. These are small, unit-specific, not recorded meetings that allow people to process the emotional turmoil associated with the event. Resources should be available for individuals to help deal with the aftermath of the crisis. Additionally, we all need to be on the look out for personality changes exhibited by team members over the coming months, which provide clues that someone is not dealing with the aftermath well. New destructive habits, withdrawal and isolation, social disengagement, and decrement in job performance all point in this direction.

The second issue that is critically important is the after-action assessment of the event. This is a detailed critique of the response effort. This is the time to discuss triage decisions. This is the time to compare the plan going into the event with how well it is actually performed. The notes taken by participants become an important source of information at this juncture. Every aspect of the operation needs discussion, and all participants get a voice in the discussion. The lessons learned in this critique will form the template upon which the current disaster plan will be revised. That revision will set up the training and drilling agenda in the near future. The questions raised here pose the hypothetical situations, the what-if's that need to be accounted for going forward. This is not a simple or short meeting. This can be a very ego-threatening meeting at a time when ego strength is not especially strong. The importance of not losing these lessons is so high that we need to be aware, as much as possible, of the fragile nature of the discussants.

A common critique that arises from these sessions is that the disaster plan was completely inadequate. This is an indictment of a planning process carried out in a void, without appropriate clinical input and with no acknowledgement of the history of such events. Now is the time to correct that and develop an appropriate response methodology (Table 17.6).

This "predictable surprise" has been described by Bazerman and Watkins.[18] Their thesis is that most disasters are predictable but there are operational characteristics that actively interfere with adequate preparation. First of these is that the leadership knows a problem exists that will not fix itself. Additionally, everyone acknowledges that the problem is getting worse over time. Fixing the problem will be expensive in terms of material resource, human resource, and money. While there are great benefits to fixing the problem, uncertainty, delay and cost stand in the way. They further argue that we actually favor the status quo and a small group actually benefits from inaction. Lastly, the leadership gets little if any credit for prevention, so the incentive to move forward is minimal.

How to circumvent this blockade? Returning to the HVA discussed earlier is a good starting point. A realistic appraisal of the risk stratification, especially in light of the most recent experience, can begin to set the tone for revision of the disaster plan. Incorporating lessons from the disaster literature and then using imagination to think "out of the box" and engendering a discussion of possibilities begin to sharpen the revision discussions. Unfortunately, all the planning and imaging in the world will not compensate for a lack of education and rehearsal. The modified disaster plan now needs to be vetted and communicated to the participants who will execute it. The drills need to be realistic, inconvenient, and conducted at all times of the day so as to best mimic an actual occurrence.

SURGICAL VOLUNTEERISM

In the aftermath of the Haiti earthquake in January 2010, physicians came forward in large numbers to volunteer to help. Locally, these types of "mass volunteer" events contribute to confusion and interfere with the response. Frequently, the well-intentioned volunteer has no training, background, or experience in working in such circumstances. Austere environment medicine is dramatically different from our usual everyday work condition. While the intention is not to discourage volunteers, there does need to be an element of reality injected into the discussion.

There is no substitute for education and training to prepare one to work in such conditions. There are a variety of opportunities to gain this experience. The DMAT (Disaster Medical Assistance Teams) of FEMA are a common method. International Medical Surgical Response Teams (IMSuRT) are another. A number of national organizations, both governmental and private, can provide volunteer opportunities in a variety of venues around the world. Operation Giving Back of the American College of Surgeons offers a wide range of volunteer opportunities that can accomplish the same goals. The point is that preparation counts. Joining a credible organization that has experience in austere environments and that will provide a modicum of training prior to working in those environments will prepare one well to function in disaster situations. Locally, the situation is not very different. Well-trained and prepared providers will contribute to the success of a response effort. Not everyone needs to deploy overseas to understand how this medicine is different. The appropriate education to facilitate participation in disaster response can be obtained in a variety of ways. We all should obtain a minimum of training in disaster planning and response as part of our regular ongoing education. The American College of Surgeons offers a program designed to do this through the Disaster Management and Emergency Preparedness© course. Alternatively, the National Disaster Life Support curriculum offers an excellent introduction to disaster response planning and management. Regardless of how it is obtained, this knowledge base needs to be mastered before one can realistically contribute to such a response effort.

TABLE 17.6

COMMON RECOVERY PITFALLS

1. No postevent analysis and critique.
2. Planning based on the last disaster.
3. Excluding mental health in planning.
4. Forgetting local hazard vulnerability analysis.
5. While events may not be preventable, consequences may be lessened.
6. Not learning from prior disasters reported in the literature.
7. Mistaking the role of nonlocal assets in acute disaster response.

From *Disaster Management and Emergency Preparedness Course Manual*. Chicago, IL: American College of Surgeons Committee on Trauma; 2010.

SUMMARY

There is really very little surprise in the occurrence of a disaster or mass casualty event. History has a plethora of lessons to guide our response if we are willing to study and learn. Our reluctance to fully engage the planning, training, and drilling process probably reflects our belief that this will never happen here or to me. Unfortunately, as surgeons, we will be looked to as leaders, especially in events where trauma predominates. We need to be personally prepared, we need to push the senior administrative structures to support the planning and training effort, and we must continually advocate for integration of the disaster response plan across the entire community, encompassing the prehospital and hospital components. Once we have mastered these steps, we will have done all we can to build resiliency into our community. We may not be able to avoid a disaster or mass casualty situation, but we can be as well prepared as we possibly can to cope with it and minimize the subsequent damage.

Suggested Resources

Briggs SM, Brinsfield KH. Advanced Disaster Medical Response Manual for Providers. Harvard: International Trauma and Disaster Institute; 2003.

Disaster Management and Emergency Preparedness Course© developed by the ad hoc Committee on Disaster and Mass Casualty Management, Committee on Trauma American College of Surgeons 2006 *These are two excellent resources for a fairly rapid, in depth introduction to this topic.*

www.fema.gov *A wealth of information about US government resources and on-line educational offerings. The site also contains information about self-preparation at home.*

Hazard Vulnerability Analysis www.utmb.edu/emergency_plan/pdfs/HAZAARD%20VULNERABILITY%20ANALYSUIS%202009.pdf *A good demonstration of a tool and how to use it for risk assessment.*

Radiation Emergency Assistance Center/Training Site (REAC/TS) US Dept. of Energy orise.orau.gov/reacts.

US Army Medical Research Institute of Chemical Defense chemdef.apgea.army.mil *These last two are excellent resources for in-depth information about radiation and chemical contamination.*

References

1. Auf Der Heide E. *Disaster Response: Principles of Preparation and Coordination.* St. Louis, MO: CV Mosby; 1989.
2. Stein M, Hirshberg A. Medical consequences of terrorism: the conventional weapons threat. *Surg Clin North Am.* 1999;79:1537-1552.
3. Auf de Heide E. Principles of hospital disaster planning. In: Hogan DE, Burstein JL, eds. *Disaster Medicine.* Philadelphia, PA: Lippincott, Williams & Wilkins; 2002.
4. Auf de Heide E. The importance of evidence based planning. *Ann Energ Med.* 2006;47(1):34-49.
5. Klein JS, Weigelt JA. Disaster management: lessons learned. *Surg Clin North Am.* 1991;71:257-266.
6. Frykberg ER. Principles of mass casualty management following terrorist disasters. *Ann Surg.* 2004;239:319-321.
7. Frykberg ER. Triage: principles and practice. *Scan J Surg.* 2005;94:272-278.
8. Frykberg E, Weireter L, Flint L. 10 questions and answers about disasters and disaster response. *Bull Am Coll Surg.* 2010;95(3):6-13.
9. Cook CH, Muscarella P, Praba AC. Reducing over-triage without compromising outcomes in trauma patients. *Arch Surg.* 2001;136:752-756.
10. Hogan DE, Lariet J. Triage. In: Hogan DE, Burnstein JL, eds. *Disaster Medicine.* Philadelphia, PA: Lippincott Williams & Wilkins; 2002:10-15.
11. National Center for Injury Prevention and Control. *Updated in a Moment's Notice: Surge Capacity for Terrorists Bombings.* Atlanta, GA: Centers for Disease Control and Prevention; 2010.
12. Hirshberg A, Stein M, Walden R. Surgical resource utilization in urban terrorist bombing: a computer simulation. *J Trauma.* 1999;47:545-550.
13. Hirschberg A, Holcomb JB, Mattox KL. Hospital trauma care in multiple casualty incidents: a critical review. *Ann Emerg Med.* 2001;37:647-652.
14. Hirshberg A, Scott BG, Granchi T. How does bomb casualty load affect trauma care in urban bombing incidents? A quantitative analysis. *J Trauma.* 2004;57:446.
15. National Center for Injury Prevention and Control. *Interim planning guidance for preparedness and response to a mass casualty event resulting from terrorist use of explosives.* Atlanta, GA: Centers for Disease Control and Prevention; 2010.
16. Peleg K, Aharonson DL, Stein M. Terror related injuries: gunshots and explosions-characteristics, outcomes and implications for care. *Ann Surg.* 2004;293:311-318.
17. Jacobs LM, Burns KJ, Gross RI. Terrorism: a public health threat with a trauma system response. *J Trauma.* 2003;55:1014-1021.
18. Bazerman MH, Watkins DM. *Predictable Surprises: The Disasters You Should have Seen Coming and How to Prevent Them.* Cambridge: Harvard Business School Press; 2004.

CHAPTER 18 ■ INJURY PREVENTION

JENNIFER C. ROBERTS AND KAREN J. BRASEL

SCOPE OF THE PROBLEM

Webster defines the term accident as "an unforeseen and unplanned event or circumstance" and specifically when related to an injury as "an unexpected happening causing loss or injury which is not due to any fault or misconduct on the part of the person injured."[1] While this term is commonly used when talking about unintentional injury in both the medical community and lay press, it is a misnomer. "Accidents" are actually injuries that occur under predictable and preventable circumstances. Injuries result from physical damage sustained following exposure to harmful agents, such as heat, electricity, mechanical energy, radiation, and poisons. In the United States, 59 million or 1 in 4 Americans suffer an injury annually. This results in 36 million emergency department visits and nearly 2.9 million admissions each year.[2] Injuries are also a significant cause of mortality. Unintentional injury is the fourth leading cause of death overall, accounting for over 140,000 deaths (6.5% of all deaths) annually. In children, adolescents, and adults in the 1–44 age group, it is the leading cause of death.[3] When considering other leading causes of death such as cancer, heart disease, congenital abnormalities and HIV, unintentional injury accounts for more death and years of potential life lost before the age of 75 than the other leading causes of death combined.[3]

Death following trauma occurs in a predictable, trimodal distribution (Fig. 18.1). As depicted in the graph, more than half of the deaths occur within the first hour following injury. Particularly in individuals sustaining a head injury, those that do survive to definitive care often die from their injuries despite adequate care. As a result, it is clear that trauma prevention efforts are the only mode of injury prevention that can impact this population of victims.

The following chapter describes the early development of injury prevention, key thinkers in early prevention efforts, and the contribution the field of epidemiology has made to injury prevention. Attention is then focused on key principles that should be considered when developing injury prevention programs with special consideration given to the assessment of injury prevention effectiveness. Finally, the chapter provides specific examples where these principles have been successfully applied to both unintentional and intentional injury prevention.

FOUNDATIONS OF INJURY PREVENTION

An appropriate starting point for any discussion on injury prevention is John Gordon. In the 1940s, John Gordon first described injuries from an epidemiological perspective. He noted that, like other disease processes, unintentional injury occurs in predictable patterns. Specifically, he hypothesized that injuries were a result of an interaction between the host, the agent, and the environment.[4] This "epidemiological triad" forms the basis of modern epidemiological studies. While it is true that injuries affect specific individuals, studying patterns of injury across different social groups is crucial to prevent injury at a population level.

Whereas John Gordon laid the foundations for the beginning of injury prevention research, the first true leader in the field was William Haddon Jr. Realizing that injuries result from a transfer of energy from the vehicle to the host (human body), he expanded Gordon's epidemiological triad and formulated Haddon's Matrix. Haddon's matrix is best described as a grid with three rows and four columns. Each row represents different phases of an injury: pre-event, event, and post-event. The four columns represent different factors that influence the severity of the injury: host, vector, physical environment, and social environment. In the pre-event phase, each of the four factors influences the likelihood that an event will occur. In the event phase, the factors interact to influence the severity of the event. Lastly, in the post-event phase, each factor determines the overall outcome.[5] Consider an example where an intoxicated driver strikes an elderly pedestrian at night in a rural community (Table 18.1).

As a conceptual model, Haddon's Matrix has been an invaluable tool used in injury prevention. In addition, Haddon later went on to develop 10 different approaches specifically targeted to prevent or control human injury. Like the matrix, they can be broken down into three phases: pre-event, event, and post-event. In brief, the 10 general strategies with examples are[5]: (Table 18.2).

1. Prevent the creation of the hazard. Example: Laws to prevent the manufacture of certain poisons, drugs, weapons.
2. Reduce the amount of the hazard. Example: Speed limits, boating regulations, firework laws.
3. Prevent the release of the hazard. Example: Trigger locks for guns, nuclear waste management programs.
4. Modify the rate or spatial distribution of the hazard: Example: Antilock brakes, airbags, seat belts.
5. Separate, in time or space, the hazard from persons to be protected. Example: Isolation units in hospitals, pedestrian walkways.
6. Separate the hazard from persons to be protected by means of a mechanical barrier. Example: Exam gloves, helmets, hazardous material containers.
7. Modify the hazard to reduce the potential for injury. Example: Medications with fewer side effects, guardrails, guards on hand saws.
8. Make what is to be protected more resistant to damage from the hazard. Example: Immunizations, fire resistant clothing for children, earthquake resistant buildings.
9. Counter the damage that has already been done by the hazard. Example: Trauma systems, disaster response teams.
10. Stabilize, repair, and rehabilitate the damaged objects. Example: Critical care medicine, reconstructive surgery, physical therapy.

In the 1960s, Haddon noted that "It has been the consistent experience of public health agencies concerned with the reduction of other causes of morbidity and mortality that measures, which do not require the continued, active cooperation of the public, are much more efficacious than those that do."[5] The term "active intervention" now serves to describe injury prevention efforts that require people to perform an act or change in behavior such as putting on a seat belt or wearing a bicycle helmet. A "passive intervention" then is one in which

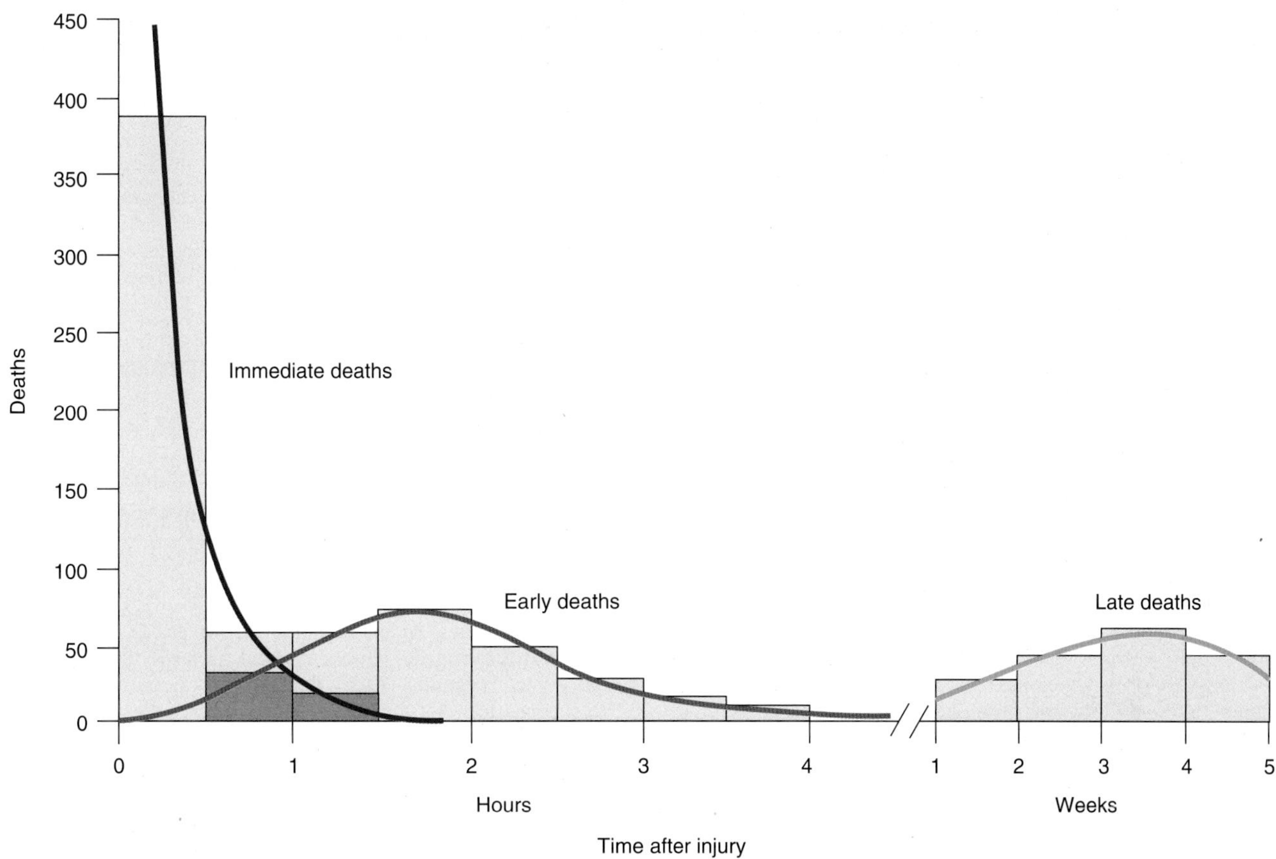

FIGURE 18.1. The trimodal distribution of trauma deaths as described in Trunkey DD. Trauma. *Sci Am.* 1983;249;28. (Reprinted from Feliciano D, Mattox K, Moore E. *Trauma.* 6th ed. New York: McGraw-Hill; 2008, with permission).

no action on the part of those being protected is required. Airbags are an example of a passive intervention. Intuitively, it makes sense that passive interventions are more efficacious in terms of preventing morbidity and mortality as the prevention is automatically built into the design of the intervention.

TABLE 18.1

HADDON'S 10 STRATEGIES TO PREVENT AND CONTROL INJURY

Pre-event phase
1. Prevent the creation of the hazard
2. Reduce the amount of the hazard
3. Prevent the release of the hazard.
Event phase
4. Modify the rate or spatial distribution of the hazard
5. Separate in time or space the hazard from persons to be protected
6. Separate the hazard from persons to be protected by means of a mechanical barrier
7. Modify the hazard to reduce the potential for injury
8. Make what is to be protected more resistant to damage from the hazard
Post-event phase
9. Counter the damage that has already been done by the hazard
10. Stabilize, repair, and rehabilitate the damaged objects

However, it is important to note that passive interventions usually require action on the part of society as a whole. As an example, in the late 1960s, to protect the public from unreasonable risk of injury following motor vehicle crashes (MVCs), the Federal Motor Vehicle Safety Standards (FMVSS) were put in place. The FMVSS are a set of regulations that describe the minimum safety performance requirement for motor vehicles, which must be met by all car manufactures.[6] Under the supervision of the National Highway Traffic Safety Administration, it has been estimated that approximately 10,000 to 30,000 lives per year have been saved since its implementation.[7,8]

CLASSIFICATION OF INJURY PREVENTION

It is clear that William Haddon has made notable contributions to the field of injury prevention. Through the interactions between phases and factors, Haddon's matrix is the foundation for newer concepts: primary, secondary, and tertiary prevention.[9] Primary prevention is described as the complete elimination of the hazardous event. Consider scald burns in children as an example. Young age is associated with an increased risk of scald injury.[10,11] Several studies have demonstrated that there is a clear relationship between water temperature and scald injury severity. Full-thickness burns can occur between 2 and 5 seconds at 60°C, and between 10 and 30 seconds at 55°C. At 52°C, 3 minutes of exposure is required to produce burns.[12,13] Logically, most scald burns due to tap water can be prevented by keeping the temperature in hot water heaters to

TABLE 18.2

EXAMPLE OF INTERACTIONS IN HADDON'S MATRIX

PHASE	HOST	VECTOR	PHYSICAL ENVIRONMENT	SOCIAL ENVIRONMENT
Pre-event	Impaired driver	Condition of vehicle headlights and breaks	Poor visibility	Traffic regulations
	Pedestrian crossing road	Vehicle speed	Road conditions Street signs	Law enforcement Local attitudes toward drunk driving
Event	Safety belt use	Airbags	Breakaway poles	Presence of local first responders and volunteers
	Hearing impaired pedestrian	Impact protection devices		
Post-event	Severity of injury	Severity of emotional distress of driver	Access to trauma center	Access to rehabilitation facilities
	Coping mechanisms of the injured			Community attitudes toward legal consequences

52°C or less. In 1983, Washington State passed a legislation requiring new water heaters to be set at 49°C. It also called for warning labels on water heaters, and annual notices for customers, homeowners, and landlords describing energy savings associated with lower water temperatures.[14] This legislation was extremely effective, as admissions for tap water scalds declined by 56% in two teaching hospitals in Washington state. More states adopted this legislation and since then scald-related death has decreased by half for all age groups and by 75% for children.[15]

While primary prevention efforts serve to eliminate the potential for injury before it occurs, this is not always possible. Secondary prevention minimizes the amount of injury that occurs when the event cannot be prevented. In a MVC, the most significant causes of injury occur during ejection, or collisions within the interior of the vehicle. Devices to dissipate kinetic energy in a more controlled fashion are designed to prevent this type of injury. There is little doubt that one such device, the seat belt, has saved thousands of lives (see following section on seat belts). A somewhat more controversial secondary prevention device is the airbag. Initially developed in the 1950s, first-generation airbags were made of nylon and were designed to deploy following a specific change in velocity. In 1989, the National Highway Traffic Safety Association (NHTSA) mandated the use of either driver airbags or automatic seat belts and by 1998 the NHTSA expanded this to include the installation of both driver and passenger airbags in all new cars. As a result, new patterns of injury associated with airbag deployment emerged. Particularly in children, there was an increase in facial fractures, cervical spine injuries, odontoid fractures, and extremity fractures in crashes with airbag deployment.[16–18] There was also an increase in both mild and moderate head injury when airbags are deployed.[19] As a result, second-generation airbags or "depowered" airbags are now mandated in new vehicles. Williams et al. has since reevaluated injuries associated with second-generation airbags and found that, when compared to no restraint device, airbags were associated with decreased odds of having a brain injury, or abdominal injury and had a decrease in infectious morbidity, hospital resource use, and mortality.[20]

Restraint devices have saved thousands of lives and are an excellent example of secondary prevention. Tertiary prevention can be thought of as efforts that will optimize the outcome after an injury has occurred. An example is the development of trauma centers and the trauma triage system. In the early 1970s, trauma patients were transported to the nearest hospital regardless of institutional resources. As the concept of specialized trauma centers evolved, in 1976 the American College of Surgeons (ACS) developed a document entitled "Resources for Optimal Care of the Injured Patient."[20] This resource outlined mechanistic, physiologic, and anatomic criteria that warranted transport to a trauma center following an injury. After its implementation, the first reports of improved morbidity and mortality associated with the use of specialized trauma centers emerged.[22] The American College of Surgeons Field Triage System is an extension of the "Resources" guidelines. This scheme has four steps[23]:

1. Assessment of vital signs, and level of consciousness.
2. Assessment of anatomic injury.
3. Assessment of the mechanism of injury with specific search for evidence of high-risk collisions (e.g., auto vs. pedestrian, motorcycle crash >20 mph).
4. Assessment of special patient or system considerations (e.g., age, burns, pregnancy).

The beneficial result of improved trauma systems is also considerable.[24] As an example, when controlling for other factors, in a study comparing mortality in Level I trauma centers versus non-trauma centers across 14 different states, MacKenzie et al.[25] found that the risk of death was considerably lower when patients were cared for at a trauma center.

TYPES OF PREVENTION EFFORTS

Whether primary, secondary, or tertiary prevention is the intent, the implementation of injury prevention strategies can be thought of according to the four "E's:" (1) Education, (2) Enforcement and legislation, (3) Engineering, (4) Economics. Education and efforts to promote behavioral change in high-risk groups have classically been the cornerstones of injury prevention design. This is based on the principle that knowledge will lead to behavioral changes. An example of a successful educational program is the "Just say no" campaign. As a part of the advertising strategy for the US "War on Drugs" in the late 1980s and 1990s, the slogan "Just Say No" was championed by the then first lady Nancy Reagan. When approached by an elementary school student who asked what the first lady would do if she was offered an illegal drug, Mrs. Reagan replied "Just say no." The phrase caught on immediately and led to the formation of thousands of "Just say no" groups across the United States. Mrs. Reagan visited drug rehabilitation and prevention institutions, and enlisted the help of several community groups, including the Girl Scouts of America and the Kiwanis Club to get the message out that drugs are harmful. "Just say no" also became a part of pop culture, appearing on popular television programs, in music videos, and on billboards across the United States.[26] While it is difficult to infer a causal relationship, the National Institute on Drug Abuse reported a significant decrease in marijuana, cocaine, and heroin use amongst high school students in the 1980s.[27]

Enforcement and legislation are also important in injury prevention. Despite adequate educational attempts, there are always individuals who will resist change, even when they may benefit from the improved outcome. As an example, despite considerable evidence to support the fact that restraint belts save lives and prevent serious injury, seat belt usage in the United States is not 100%. Currently, 30 states and the District of Columbia have primary enforcement laws where police may stop vehicles solely for occupants not wearing seat belts.[28] However, in states where primary enforcement laws are in place, 86% of occupants wear seat belts versus 78% of occupants in states where seat belt use is not enforced.[29]

Engineering and technology encompass a wide variety of topics, and may have the largest impact on injury when considering long-term benefits. Examples where engineering has been useful include the development of trigger locks on firearms, earthquake resistant buildings, and built-in protective devices on manufacturing equipment. Following the 1994 earthquake that struck Northridge California, a population-based cohort study was conducted to determine factors associated with increased physical injury. This study was unique in that it sought to examine how seismic risk factors, patient demographics, and building characteristics simultaneously interacted to produce injury compared to an exposure matched cohort. When controlling for other factors, building and seismic factors were identified, which independently increased risk of injury.[30] This information was useful to give back to engineers to target points of intervention.

Funding for injury prevention programs is generally inadequate. Within the community, there is a finite supply of volunteer services, not-for-profit organizations, and donations. Economic incentives (or penalties) can serve to reinforce legislative efforts when patient participation is required for successful prevention. Insurance companies, for example, have data on risk-taking behavioral patterns. Discounted premiums can then be offered to groups with lower risks (i.e., High school drivers who meet a minimum GPA). In a different example, consider the use of child car seats. It is well recognized that, particularly in the 0–4 age group, infants and young children do not fit into adult-sized seat belts and can suffer devastating injury if unrestrained in a MVC. All 50 states currently require child car seats. The success of this legislation is seen in the reduction in childhood deaths related to motor vehicles. When compared to 1994, where primary enforcement of child car seats was not mandatory, there were 682 deaths in the United States from MVCs compared with 471 deaths in 2006.[3,31]

EVALUATION OF INJURY PREVENTION STRATEGIES

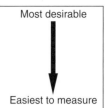

Whether the prevention strategy is education, legislation and enforcement, engineering or economic, critical evaluation of the effectiveness of a program is essential. Outcome assessment is vital to continue to fund strategies with proven benefit and is likewise useful to identify those that do not work. Many educational efforts consume a considerable amount of community resources and have excellent face validity, yet there may be little or no effect on outcomes. Alternatively, the outcomes affected may be only short-term or secondary endpoints. Educational programs teaching young children pedestrian safety illustrate this point. In a large meta-analysis that included 15 randomized controlled trials, which looked at the effectiveness of pedestrian safety education programs in preventing pedestrian versus motor vehicle collisions, education resulted in improved children's knowledge of road dangers and some changes in road crossing behaviors. However, the authors also concluded that the targeted "safe" behaviors in these trials were not necessarily related to decreased pedestrian injury risk.[32]

In an ideal situation, the outcomes an investigator wishes to prevent are those injuries that lead to death or major disability. In many situations, this is not possible. Injury outcomes can be described in a hierarchy. At the top are the serious outcomes that are desirable to prevent, yet difficult to access for change. Traveling downward are those that are more easy to assess for change, but of lesser importance in the prevention of serious outcomes.[33] (Fig. 18.2):

1. Death
2. Inpatient admissions following trauma
3. Injuries treated in the outpatient setting
4. All injuries
5. Behavioral change
6. Self-reported behavior
7. Measures of knowledge, attitudes, or intensions

1. Death	Most desirable
2. Injuries requiring inpatient treatment	↓
3. Injuries requiring outpatient treatment	
4. All injuries	
5. Behavioral changes	
6. Self-reported changes	
7. Measures of knowledge or beliefs	Easiest to measure

FIGURE 18.2. Hierarchy of outcomes associated with injury prevention techniques as described by Maier R, Mock C. Chapter 3. Injury prevention (Chapter). In: Feliciano D, Mattox K, Moore E, eds. *Trauma*. 6th ed.

The type of outcome measure selected for assessment depends on the population characteristics, type of intervention planned, and resources (particularly monetary) provided to the team. Clearly, all interventions should seek to impact those outcomes with the biggest impact (i.e., trauma resource utilization or mortality). This is not always possible for smaller projects. In those cases, the appropriate selection of a surrogate outcome measure with proven validity in similar situations may be beneficial. Regardless of the measure chosen, outcome assessment is crucial when developing an intervention.

THE PREVENTION OF UNINTENTIONAL INJURIES

MVC-related injures remain the leading cause of death for people between the ages of 1 and 34. In 2006, the total number of people killed in an MVC was 43,664, with vehicle-related deaths contributing 35.9% of the total unintentional mortality overall.[3] However, there have been many recent advances in automotive safety that have contributed to declining mortality over the last several years. The following section outlines some for individual discussion.

SAFETY BELTS, AIRBAGS, AND CHILD CAR SEAT RESTRAINTS

Saving an estimated 15,000 lives per year, seat belts are extremely effective in preventing injuries sustained in MVCs.[34] In 2001, as a part of the CDC's Motor Vehicle Injury Prevention program, the Task Force on Community Preventive Service concluded that seat belt laws and primary enforcement were effective and strongly recommended. The task force went on to recommend a goal of 92% overall seat belt use by 2010. In 2006, the overall prevalence in the United States was 82.4% with only four states achieving seat belt use rates >90% in self-reported surveys.[35] Interestingly, the 15 states with the highest levels of seat belt use also had primary enforcement laws. This is in contrast to 14 of the 15 states with the lowest levels of seat belt use that only had secondary enforcement or no enforcement at all.[35] So, while primary enforcement laws improve compliance with seat belt laws, there is still room for improvement nationwide.

As a form of active prevention, persuading occupants to wear seat belts remains a problem. The advent of airbags is intended to bypass the human element and as previously mentioned may contribute to decreased mortality.[30] However, combined use with a seat belt is required for enhanced safety.[36] Further, the use of a seat belt is also required to minimize airbag-related injuries.

Children represent a unique problem for injury prevention in that children and infants do not fit properly into adult-sized restraints. Also, there is evidence to suggest that restraint use among children depends upon the use of a restraint by their caregivers. Nearly 40% of children who are unrestrained travel in vehicles where the drivers are unrestrained themselves.[37] There is also an issue with the proper placement of a child in a car seat. In 2001, the National Highway Traffic Safety Administration (NHTSA) conducted a study to identify "critical misuses" of child seat restraints (CSRs). It found that 72.6% of observed caregivers had at least one critical misuse of CSRs. The commonly cited reasons were loose vehicle safety belt attachment, loose harness straps, misrouting of harness straps, parental customization of child safety seats, and CRSs being used beyond the manufacturer's expiration dates.[38]

Like CSRs, child booster seats reduce the risk of injury when compared to seat belts alone.[39] Currently, the NHTSA recommends booster seats for children until they are at least 8 years old or are >4′9″ tall. This recommendation stems from the fact that adult restraints still do not fit children in this age group. A properly placed booster seat elevates the child such that the shoulder restraint fits properly over the thorax and lap restraint over the pelvis. Currently, 38 states have adopted booster state requirements in addition to car and seat belt laws.[40]

In addition to restraint devices, children <12 years old should ride in the backseat. This eliminates the risk of injury from a front or passenger side airbag. In children and adolescents <16 years old, this is associated with a 40% reduction in the risk of serious injury.[41]

TRAFFIC REGULATIONS

The relationship between vehicle speed and injury is straightforward. The faster a vehicle is traveling, the more amount of energy that is transmitted and must be absorbed by the human body in a collision. One of the most successful traffic regulations resulting in the reduction of both morbidity and mortality was the adoption of a 55-MPH speed limit on major highways. Initially undertaken as an energy conservation measure, in 1973 congress passed legislation imposing a national maximum speed limit of 55 MPH. This resulted in the reduction of highway traffic fatalities from 54,000 in 1973 to 45,000 in 1974.[42] Eventually, the law was softened allowing for rural states to increase the speed limit to 65–75 MPH in selected areas. In 1995, citing personal freedom demands, this law was rescinded completely allowing states to control their own speed limits. This resulted in an estimated increase of fatalities by 9% and nonfatal injuries by 4%[42] Another study concluded that an estimated 2,985 lives may be saved a year if a nationwide speed limit of 65 MPH is adopted.[43] Restrictions on speed limits are not the only way to influence traffic patterns on a population level. Speed enforcement devices were developed based on the premise that enforcement requires speeding drivers to actually believe they will be caught. These pieces of equipment range from cameras over roadways to covert radar detection devices. A recent meta-analysis of 21 studies that measured the effect of SEDs on MVCs found that all reported a lower number of overall crashes (range 14%–72%), crashes causing injury (range 8%–46%), and crashes resulting in fatality (range 40%–45%).[44] Further, those trends were maintained over time. While the authors note that some of the methodologic quality was weak, speed enforcement devices remain a promising area for future research and intervention.

ALCOHOL

In addition to vehicle speed, drug- and alcohol-impaired driving is another important risk factor for motor vehicle-related morbidity and mortality. Estimates of alcohol-related injury use blood alcohol concentration (BAC) values reported to the Fatality Analysis Reporting System for analysis. In 2008, 11,773 people were killed in alcohol-related crashes. This amounts to one death every 45 minutes, and accounts for nearly one-third of all traffic-related deaths. It also poses a significant financial burden on the health care system.[45] The annual cost of alcohol-related injuries is estimated at more than $51 billion.[46] This problem does not just impact the adult population. More than two-thirds of childhood vehicular fatalities took place while riding with an impaired driver.[47]

There are common patterns in alcohol-related trauma. First, the rate of alcohol impairment in driver fatalities is four times higher at night than during the day (36% vs. 9%). Also, only 15% of alcohol-related fatalities occur during the week versus 32% on weekends. When breaking down the driver age and gender in fatal crashes where the driver had a BAC level of 80 mg/dL or higher, men are more commonly involved in a fatality and adults aged 21–24 (34%) have the greatest number of deaths. Motorcycle drivers account for the highest percentage of deaths by vehicle type (29%), followed by passenger cars, light trucks, and large trucks, respectively (23%, 23%, 2%).[48]

Given the magnitude of this problem, there are considerable resources and multiple modalities of intervention dedicated to reducing alcohol-related injuries. In terms of legislation, all 50 states, the District of Columbia, and Puerto Rico have adopted a BAC of 80 mg/dL as the legal limit for impaired driving. In 2008, this led to the arrest of over 1.4 million drivers.[49] This is only 1% of the 159 million self-reported episodes of adults driving under the influence of drink in the United States each year.[50] To increase the chance that impaired drivers will be stopped, many police agencies have increased the number of police patrols or the time officers spend patrolling. The effects of these efforts are promising. Despite some methodologic limitations, in a review performed on 32 studies testing the effects of increased police presence on traffic deaths, injuries, and crashes, a statistically significant reduction in total crashes and fatalities was identified.[51]

Enforcement efforts are clearly a large part of reducing alcohol-related injuries. However, there are a considerable amount of education programs directed at the same target population. Perhaps one of the most recognizable is Mothers Against Drunk Driving (MADD). MADD is a nonprofit organization that was formed by a Texas mother in 1980 following the death of her 13-year-old daughter from an intoxicated driver. The group now comprises over three million members, has nearly 600 community action teams with a chapter in every state.[52] Another group dedicated to education is Alcoholics Anonymous (AA). AA is an international organization that offers support via self-help groups using a 12-step approach.

Screening identifies up to 46% of the trauma population as having alcohol-use disorders.[53] Once a patient is identified as high risk for alcohol abuse, brief interventions designed to assist patients with reducing or eliminating their alcohol consumption are extremely successful. These interventions typically involve one or more short (<1 hour) sessions given as an inpatient.[54,55] Gentilello et al. reported a decrease in alcohol consumption by 21.8 drinks per week at 12 months in the intervention group versus a decrease of only 3.7 drinks per week in the control group. Importantly, this also correlated with a 48% reduction in injuries requiring hospital admission at 3 years follow-up.[56] Brief intervention programs are also cost effective. In the same study, trauma patients were randomized to a brief intervention versus control. The net benefit in reduced injury-related health care costs was $3.81 US dollars for every $1.00 spent on screening.[56] From this study and those documenting the feasibility of brief intervention programs in an acute care setting, the American College of Surgeons Committee on Trauma now requires all Level I and Level II trauma centers to have screening (for Level I and II centers) and brief intervention (for Level I centers) programs in place for trauma center verification.

HELMETS

Each year, approximately 900 people die from bicycle crashes.[57] Head injuries account for up to 75% of deaths among these patients despite the fact that this type of injury is largely preventable. For instance, between 1994 and 2005, 92% of deaths from bicyclists involved persons who were not wearing helmets.[58] Helmets protect cyclists from head and facial injuries, with an overall risk reduction in head and severe brain injuries of 63% to 88% across all age groups.[59] When mandatory helmet laws are enforced, there is an increase in helmet use from between 45% and 84% without any evidence to support any adverse effects of legislation.[59]

Like the use of bicycle helmets, motorcycle helmets considerably reduce mortality associated with crashes. Helmet use is associated with a 16% reduction in the odds for death. In addition to lives saved, one estimate of dollars saved due to ICU care related to head-injured motorcyclists is over $32 million.[60] Currently, 21 states have universal laws mandating the use of the helmet.[61] This has not always been the case. Historically, all but three states had mandatory helmet laws due to the requirement of such a law to receive federal highway funding. However, congress abolished the requirement and many states removed the helmet law requirement in the 1980s.

INJURY PREVENTION IN THE ELDERLY

As the population continues to age, geriatric trauma is increasing. Unintentional death is the ninth leading cause of death overall in those >65 years old, yet this accounts for 25% of injury-related deaths. The rate per 100,000 individuals is 113.2, which is double that of all other age groups.[3] It is also well established that geriatric trauma patients have worse outcomes compared to their younger counterparts. They have increased hospital length of stay, morbidity and case-fatality rates, particularly with less severe injuries.[62–64] The mechanism for this increased risk is thought to be due to preexisting medical conditions (PECs). PECs make it difficult for the elderly patients to rely on their own physiologic reserve in response to the stress of trauma. In a prevalence study, authors found that by age 60, 40% of the population has at least one chronic medical condition, with this percentage increasing to 69% of the population by age 75.[65]

Falls represent the most significant cause of morbidity and mortality in the elderly. In 2006, falls accounted for 45.4% of all geriatric unintentional trauma resulting in close to 16,650 deaths.[3] It is estimated that over one-third of community dwelling and half of institutionalized residents over the age of 65 will suffer at least one fall each year.[66,67] In 2005, falls accounted for 1.8 million trips to the emergency department, resulting in 430,000 admissions.[3] Between 20% and 30% of those falls resulted in moderate to severe injury, with the most common injuries reported as soft tissue injury, traumatic brain injury, and orthopedic fractures.[68,69] Unfortunately, patients with fall-related hip fractures often do not recover to their pre-fracture level of function.[70] This presents a significant burden to the health care system. In 2000, the direct costs were 19 billion in nonfatal falls and an additional $179 million in fatal falls.[69]

The prevention of falls in the elderly is multifactorial. The CDC recommends exercise programs designed to improve cardiovascular health as well as strength and coordination. Also, having a medical professional review both over-the-counter and prescription medications to avoid drug interactions and side effects, and performing yearly vision examinations is helpful. Additionally, reducing in home hazards by modifying home environment such as removing throw rugs, securing electrical cords, installing grab rails in bathrooms, and improving interior and exterior lighting is beneficial.[71] Fall prevention can also be instituted through population-based interventional programs. One example in Sweden is based on the World Health Organization Safe Communities model. In a multidisciplinary approach, members of the Red Cross, county authorities, sporting teams, and the Safety Council for the Elderly teamed up to promote safety initiatives. Some measures employed included home visits, distribution of brochures via mass media, community walking programs, and employing unskilled laborers to improve lighting in public places. Mortality rates and hospital admissions for fall injuries and unintentional injuries in geriatric patients were recorded for 1 year pre- and post-intervention in a population of 42,000 adults and in a control population from a nearby municipality. Results demonstrated a notable reduction in falls and unintentional injury in the intervention community while injuries remained the same in the control population.[72] The positive effect of population-based interventions was further supported in a recent Cochrane review where authors found that relative risk reduction in falls for well-designed interventional programs was between 6% and 33%.[73]

PREVENTION OF INTENTIONAL INJURY

According to the World Health Organization, intentional violent injury can be defined as one resulting from the "intentional use of physical force or power against oneself, another person, or group or community." Worldwide, more than 1.6 million people lose their lives to violence annually.[74]

In the United States, each year nearly 50,000 deaths and 2.2 million injuries are the result of violent crimes.[75] In 2000, the total costs due to injuries and deaths from violence in the United States totaled more than $70 billion. The majority, $64.4 billion or 92%, was due to lost productivity while $5.6 billion was spent on direct medical costs.[76] Traditionally thought to be an inevitable part of human life, fewer resources have been dedicated to the study and prevention of intentional, when compared with unintentional, injury. It wasn't until 1993 that the CDC created the division of violence prevention. Soon after, to provide researchers and communities with a better understanding of violent death, the National Violent Death Reporting System (NVDRS) was created. The NVDRS is a 17 state-based surveillance system that combines data from medical examiners, law enforcement, and vital statistics, which is designed to help design violent injury prevention efforts.[75]

With the help of increased interest in intentional injury prevention and the NVDRS, critical analysis of the root causes of intentional injury reveal that, like unintentional injury, the same factors, agent, host, and environment interact to produce injury in a predictable and preventable manner. As such, strategies using the "four E's" previously mentioned also apply to the prevention of intentional injury. The following sections describe the scope of several common types of intentional injury accompanied by prevention strategies.

HOMICIDE AND SUICIDE

Between the ages of 1 and 34, homicide is a leading cause of death. In 2006, over 18,000 people were victims of homicide representing over 600,000 potential years of life lost. Homicide affects specific populations at disproportionate rates. At nearly 5,700 deaths annually, homicide is the second leading cause of death in the 15–24 age group, with nearly 75% of the total victims being male. Minority populations are also unequally represented. Amongst African Americans between 10 and 24 years old, homicide is the leading cause of death. In the same age group, it is the second leading cause of death amongst Hispanics.[3]

Firearms are the most common method employed to commit homicide, used between 72% and 85% of the time between the ages of 15–34. Firearm availability is directly related to mortality; the correlation between the presence of a gun and suicide has been found to be 0.94, and homicide to be 0.75.[77] Also, guns are more likely to kill than any other weapon used in an assault.[78] Because of this, it is appealing to focus on prevention strategies that decrease the availability of firearms to the public. Although the law has now been repealed, the Firearms Control Regulations Act in the District of Columbia banned residents from owning handguns, automatic weapons, and unregistered firearms. It also called for guns at home to be "unloaded, disassembled, or bound by a trigger lock." This law resulted in a decline in homicides by 23% over a 10-year span. No such decline was noted in neighboring states where the ban did not apply.[79] In 2008, the US Supreme Court struck down the DC gun law on the basis that it violated the Second Amendment. Further attempts to limit the availability of firearms continue to meet resistance. Currently, the CDC recommends gun control laws that restrict ownership of handguns to those with a "clearly demonstrated need." They also call for greater enforcement of preexisting gun legislation such as waiting periods and background checks for those individuals purchasing firearms. (NCIP)

Like homicide, suicide is an important cause of morbidity and mortality in the United States. As the 11th leading cause of death overall, self-inflicted injury results in over 33,000 deaths and 359,000 visits to the emergency department each year. It represents the second leading cause of death in individuals aged 25–34.[76]. Risk factors for suicide include adolescent age, previous attempts at suicide, history of depression or mental illness, alcohol use, living alone, and having a recent adverse event. Gender and ethnicity also contribute, with men and American Indians affected disproportionately.[75]

Suicide prevention should involve strategies directed at high-risk groups. In particular, reducing the availability of means of suicide is beneficial. Safety barriers over bridges, catalytic converters that result in less toxic vehicle exhaust, changing home gas supply from toxic coal gas, and restriction of access to unsafe pesticides have effectively reduced rates of suicide.[80] Eliminating an easily accessible means of suicide ultimately does not lead to the choice of another method, but may lead to a decision to avoid committing suicide altogether.[81] The National Strategy for Suicide Prevention (NSSP) is a national program developed from the Department of Health and Human Services. The NSSP describes a public health approach to meet specific aims: prevent premature deaths due to suicide across the life span, reduce rates of suicidal behaviors, reduce harmful aftereffects associated with suicidal behaviors and their impact on family and friends, and promote opportunities to improve resiliency, resourcefulness, and respect for individuals, families, and communities affected by suicide. To achieve this, 11 specific goals complete with objectives and activities have been outlined.[82]:

1. Promote awareness that suicide is a public health problem that is preventable
2. Develop broad-based support for suicide prevention.
3. Develop and implement strategies to reduce the stigma associated with being a consumer of mental health, substance abuse, and suicide prevention services.
4. Develop and implement community-based suicide prevention programs.
5. Promote efforts to reduce access to lethal means and methods to self-harm.
6. Implement training for recognition of at-risk behavior and delivery of effective treatment.
7. Develop and promote effective clinical and professional practices.
8. Improve access to and community linkages with mental health and substance abuse services.
9. Improve reporting and portrayals of suicidal behavior, mental illness, and substance abuse in the entertainment and news media.
10. Promote and support research on suicide and suicide prevention.
11. Improve and expand surveillance systems.

In its current form, the NSSP is one of the first times a coordinated approach to suicide prevention by public and private sectors has been attempted in the United States.

DOMESTIC VIOLENCE

Domestic violence or intimate partner violence (IPV) can be defined as abusive behavior, physical or emotional, between two people in a close relationship. This includes single episodes, ongoing violence with current or former partners. There are four specific types of IPV.[83]

1. Physical violence causing physical injury such as hitting, kicking, or assault with a weapon
2. Threats ranging from words, gestures, and other messages of intent to cause either emotional or physical harm
3. Sexual violence including the use of physical or emotional force to compel a person to perform a sexual act, completed or not, and any sexual act involving a person unable to consent
4. Emotional violence such as threatening, harassing, intimidating, or controlling behaviors including the prevention of the victim to seek help from family or friends

Domestic violence affects 4.8 million women and 2.9 million men annually. This results in nearly 1,510 deaths, of which 78% are female.[75,84] In terms of financial burden, the medical, mental health, and costs due to lost productivity amount to more than $8.3 billion dollars.[85] It is important to note that these numbers are likely an underestimation of the scope of the problem as many victims do not report IPV to the proper authorities or friends and family.[84]

The majority of IPV involves men injuring their female partners. There are several risk factors, both individual and societal, for committing acts of IPV: alcohol and drug abuse, personal history of abuse, emotional disorders, low socioeconomic status, depression, marital instability, traditional gender norms, weak sanctions against domestic violence, and social norms supportive of violence.[86,88]

Domestic violence has a significant impact on overall health. In addition to acute physical injuries, victims of IPV are more likely to have prolonged health problems. In particular, victims adopt risky behaviors including smoking, drug, and alcohol abuse, and physical inactivity.[87,88,89] They are also at an increased risk of depression, chronic pain syndromes, psychosomatic and reproductive health consequences.[87] The longer the abuse persists and more severe the incident, the greater the impact on health.[87,88]

In the past, the majority of prevention efforts have focused on limiting abuse once it occurs. Focus has been on legislation and the criminal justice system. An example is a restraining order that prohibits an abuser from contacting his or her partner. Restraining orders are civil protective documents that attempt to prohibit contact between victims and their partners. Violating an order is then a criminal offense. Currently, all 50 states have some bit of legislation authorizing the use of general civil protective orders. There is some evidence to show that these orders are useful in deterring violence if they are in place for an entire year.[90] However, multiple studies have shown that these orders are violated between 23% and 70% of the time and do not necessarily result in arrests.[91,92] Furthermore, while women may feel safer and emotionally stronger after obtaining a protective order, it may serve to anger the recipient to the point of violence.[92]

Many efforts are led by women's outreach organizations and hotlines such as the National Domestic Violence Hotline, and shelters for abused persons. There is also a movement to target adolescents. The Safe Dates Program is a school-based intervention that focuses on educational efforts specifically directed at reducing dating violence. A treatment group of eighth and ninth graders in Johnston County North Carolina underwent a ten session curriculum developed to change norms associated with partner violence. At 4 years follow-up, compared with controls, those receiving the curriculum reported 56% to 92% less physical and sexual dating violence.[93] The results of this study are promising; however, continued research and outcome assessment is needed to identify those strategies that best impact interpersonal violence.

SUMMARY

Franklin D Roosevelt once said "Nothing happens by accident, if it happens, you can bet it was planned that way." While he was originally referring to politics, his statement also applies to both intentional and unintentional injury. Haddon first formalized the concept that injuries occur under specific and reproducible circumstances. As such, his matrix and basic prevention strategies should form the foundation of modern prevention efforts, whether primary, secondary, or tertiary prevention. Equally important is the critical evaluation of prevention programs. From small community programs to large-scale nationwide efforts, prevention efforts consume a substantial amount of resources in the United States. Well-designed outcome assessment tools are important to document the success of programs and justify further funds as well as identify those strategies that need modifying.

Unintentional injury has been the focus of the majority of prevention efforts. There is no question that the invention of seat belts combined with primary enforcement laws, mandatory airbag requirements in vehicles, and highway safety regulation like reduction in speed limits saves thousands of lives each year. Efforts in the prevention of intentional injury are less common, and have been less successful. It is likely that the social, political, and behavioral factors, such as alcoholism, mentioned previously are responsible for some of the gap between unintentional and intentional injury prevention successes. What is certain is that injury prevention is best attempted with a multidisciplinary, scientific approach at both a community and national level. It is in this way researchers and clinicians can have the largest impact on injury-related morbidity and mortality.

References

1. http://www.merriam-webter.com/dictionary/accident. Accessed March 28th, 2010.
2. CDC National center for injury prevention and control: ten leading causes of death, 2006. Atlanta Centers for Disease control 2006. Available online at www.cdc.gov/injury/wisqars/LeadingCauses.html. Accessed March 28th, 2010.
3. WISQARS fatal injuries: mortality reports. http://webappa.cdc.gov.proxy.lib.mcw.edu/sasweb/ncipc/mortrate.html. Accessed March 28th, 2010.
4. Gordon JE. The epidemiology of accidents. *Am J Pub Health*. 1949;39:504.
5. Haddon W Jr. Advances in the epidemiology of injuries as a basis for public policy. *Public Health Rep*. 1980;95(5):411–421.
6. Federal Motor Vehicle Safety Standards and Regulations. Brochure, HS 805 674. http://www.nhtsa.gov/cars/rules/import/fmvss/index.html. Accessed March 2010.
7. Robertson LS. Automobile safety regulations and death reductions in the United States. *Am J Public Health*. 1981;71(8):818–822.
8. Robertson LS. Automobile safety regulation: rebuttal and new data. *Am J Public Health*. 1984;74(12):1390–1394.
9. Runyan C. Using the Haddon matrix: introducing the third dimension. *Inj Prev*. 1998;4:302–307.
10. Baker SP, O'Neil B, Ginsburg M, et al. *The Injury Fact Book*. New York: Oxford University Press; 1992.
11. Katcher ML Scald burns from hot tap water. *JAMA*. 1981;246(11):1219–1222.
12. Moritz AR, Henriques FC. Studies of thermal injury: the relative importance of time and surface temperature in the causation of cutaneous burns. *Am J Pathol*. 1947;23:695–720.
13. The National Committee for Injury Prevention and Control: Injury Prevention: Meeting the Challenge. New York: Oxford University Press; 1989.
14. Washington State Substitute House Bill 177 (adding to RCW 19.27.130) 1983.
15. Erdmann T, Feldman K, Rivara F, et al. Tap water burn prevention: the effect of legislation. *Pediatrics*. 1991;88:572–577.
16. Blackskin MF. Patterns of fracture after air bag deployment. *J Trauma*. 1993;35:840–843.
17. Brooks CN. Maxillofacial and ocular injuries in motor vehicle crashes. *Ann R Coll Surg Engl*. 2004;86:149–155.
18. McGwin G Jr, Metzer J, Alonso JE, Rue LW. The association between occupant restraint systems and risk of injury in frontal motor vehicle collisions. *J Trauma*. 2003;54:1182–1187.
19. Huber CD, Lee JB, Yang KH, King AI. Head injuries in airbag equipped motor vehicles with special emphasis on AIS 1 and 2 facial and loss of consciousness injuries. *Traffic Inj Prev*. 2004;6:170–174.
20. Williams RF, Fabian TC, Fischer PE, et al. Impact of airbags on a Level I trauma center: injury patterns, infectious morbidity, and hospital costs. *J Am Coll Surg*. 2008;206(5):962–968; discussion 968–969. Epub 2008 Mar 4.
21. American College of Surgeons' Committee on Trauma: optimal hospital resources for care of the seriously injured. *Bull Am Coll Surg*, Sep 1976.
22. Campbell S, Watkins G, Kreis D. Preventable deaths in a self-designated trauma system. *Am Surg*. 1989;55:478–480.
23. Sasser SM, Hunt RC, Sullivent EE, et al. Guidelines for field triage of injured patients. Recommendations of the National Expert Panel on Field Triage. *MMWR Recomm Rep*. 2009; 58:1–35.
24. West J, Cales R, Gazzaniga A. Impact of regionalization: The Orange County experience. *Arch Surg*. 1983;118:740.
25. MacKenzie E, Rivara F, Jurkovich G, et al. A National Evaluation of the Effect of Trauma-Center Care on Mortality. *N Engl J Med*. 2006;354:366–378.
26. Benze JG Jr. *Nancy Reagan: On the White House Stage*. Lawrence, KA: University Press of Kansas; 2005.
27. NIDA InfoFacts: High School and Youth Trends. National Institute on Drug Abuse, NIH. http://www.nida.nih.gov/Infofacts/HSYouthtrends.html. Retrieved 2010-03-29.

28. National institute of highway safety. http://www.iihs.org/laws/ChildRestraint.aspx Accessed march 29, 2010.
29. National Highway Traffic Safety Administration: Traffic Safety Facts 2004. Washington, DC: National Center for Statistics and Analysis, US DOT, 2005.
30. Peek-Asa C, Ramirez M, Seligson H, et al. Seismic, structural, and individual factors associated with earthquake related injury. *Inj Prev.* 2003;9:62–66.
31. National Highway Traffic Safety Administration: www.nhtsa.dot.gov/people/NCSA, 2010. Accessed Mar 29, 2010
32. Duperrex O, Roberts I, Bunn F. Safety education of pedestrians for injury prevention. *Cohrane Database Syst Rev* 2002;(2). Art. No.: CD001531. DOI: 10.1002/14651858.CD001531
33. Maier R, Mock C. Chapter 3. Injury prevention (Chapter). In: Feliciano D, Mattox K, Moore E, eds. *Trauma.* 6th ed. New York: McGraw-Hill; 2008
34. http://www.cdc.gov/motorvehiclesafety/index.html Accessed Mar 29, 2010.
35. Beck, LF, Shults, RA. Seat belt use in states and territories with primary and secondary laws—United States, 2006. *J Safety Res.* 2009;40:469–472.
36. Crandall C, Olson L, Sklar D. Mortality reduction with air bag and seat belt use in head-on passenger car collisions. *Am J Epidemiol.* 2001;153:219–224.
37. Cody BE, Mickalide AD, Paul HP, et al. *Child Passengers at Risk in America: A National Study of Restraint Use.* Washington, DC: National SAFE KIDS Campaign; 2002.
38. Department of Transportation (US), National Highway Traffic Safety Administration (NHTSA), Traffic Safety Facts Research Note 2005: Misuse of Child Restraints: Results of a Workshop to Review Field Data Results. Washington, DC: NHTSA; 2006. http://www.nhtsa.dot.gov/people/injury/research/TSF_MisuseChildRetraints/images/809851.pdf. Accessed March 30th 2010.
39. Durbin DR, Elliott MR, Winston FK. Belt-positioning booster seats and reduction in risk of injury among children in vehicle crashes. *JAMA.* 2003;289(14):2835–2840.
40. http://www.nhtsa.dot.gov/people/injury/childps/BoosterSeatLaws_OverviewMaps07.pdf. Accessed Mar 30, 2010.
41. Durbin DR, Chen I, Smith R, et al. Effects of seating position and appropriate restraint use on the risk of injury to children in motor vehicle crashes. *Pediatrics.* 2005;115:305–309
42. NHTSA-FHWA, 1998. NHTSA-FHWA Report to Congress: The Effect of Increased Speed Limit in the Post-NMSL Era. National Highway Traffic Safety Administration and Federal Highway Administration DOT HS 808 637 NRD-31.
43. Shafi S, Gentilello L. A nationwide speed limit < or = 65 miles per hour will save thousands of lives. *Am J Surg.* 2007;193(6):719–722.
44. Wilson C, Willis C, Hendrikz JK, et al. Speed enforcement detection devices for preventing road traffic injuries. *Cochrane Database Syst Rev.* 2006(2). Art. No.: CD004607. DOI: 10.1002/14651858.CD004607.pub4.
45. Dept of Transportation (US), National Highway Traffic Safety Administration (NHTSA). *Traffic Safety Facts 2008: Alcohol-Impaired Driving.* Washington, DC: NHTSA; 2009. http://www-nrd.nhtsa.dot.gov/Pubs/811155.PDF accessed March 30 2010.
46. Blincoe L, Seay A, Zaloshnja E, et al. *The Economic Impact of Motor Vehicle Crashes, 2000.* Washington, DC: Dept of Transportation (US), National Highway Traffic Safety Administration (NHTSA); 2002.
47. Shults RA. Child passenger deaths involving drinking drivers—United States, 1997–2002. *MMWR* 2004;53(4):77–79.
48. http://www.nhtsa.dot.gov/staticfiles/DOT/NHTSA/Communication & Consumer Information/Articles/Associated Files/EconomicImpact2000.pdf. Accessed Mar 31st 2010.
49. Department of Justice (US), Federal Bureau of Investigation (FBI). *Crime in the United States 2008: Uniform Crime Reports.* Washington, DC: FBI; 2009. http://www.fbi.gov/ucr/cius2008/data/table_29.html Accessed Mar 30 2010.
50. Jones RK, Shinar D, Walsh JM. State of knowledge of drug-impaired driving. Dept of Transportation (US), National Highway Traffic Safety Administration (NHTSA); 2003.
51. Goss CW, Van Bramer LD, Gliner JA, et al. Increased police patrols for preventing alcohol-impaired driving. *Cochrane Database Syst Rev.* 2008(4). Art. No.: CD005242. DOI: 10.1002/14651858.CD005242.pub2.
52. Hamilton WJ. Mothers against drunk driving—MADD in the USA. *Inj Prev.* 2000;6(2):90–91.
53. Gentilello LM, Rivara FP, Donovan DM, et al. Alcohol interventions in a trauma center as a means of reducing the risk of injury recurrence. *Ann Surg.* 1999;230:473–483.
54. World Health Organization Brief Intervention Study Group. A crossnational trial of brief intervention with heavy drinkers. *Am J Public Health.* 1996; 86:948–955.
55. Dunn C, Donovan D, Gentilello L. Practical guidelines for performing alcohol interventions in trauma centers. *J Trauma* 1997;42:299.
56. Gentilello LM, Ebel BE, Wickizer TM, et al. Alcohol interventions for trauma patients treated in emergency departments and hospitals: a cost benefit analysis. *Ann Surg.* 2005;241:541–550.
57. Baker SP, Li G, Fowler C, et al. 1993 *Injuries to bicyclists: A national perspective.* Johns Hopkins University Injury Prevention Center, sponsored by the Snell Memorial Foundation; 1993
58. Insurance Institute for Highway Safety. *2005 Fatality Facts: Bicycles.* Arlington, VA: Insurance Institute for Highway Safety; 2005.http://www.iihs.org/research/fatality_facts/bicycles.html. Accessed Mar 30 2010.
59. Macpherson A, Spinks A. Bicycle helmet legislation for the uptake of helmet use and prevention of head injuries. *Cochrane Database Syst Rev.* 2008(3). Art. No.: CD005401. DOI: 10.1002/14651858.CD005401.pub3.
60. Croce MA, Zarzaur BL, Magnotti LJ, et al. Impact of motorcycle helmets and state laws on society's burden: a national study. *Ann Surg.* 2009;250(3):390–394.
61. Current US motorcycle and bicycle helmet laws. Available at: http://www.iihs.org/laws/HelmetUseCurrent.aspx. Accessed April 2, 2009.
62. Morris JA Jr, MacKenzie EJ, Damiano AM, et al.: Mortality in trauma patients: The interaction between host factors and severity. *J Trauma.* 1990;30:1476.
63. Hollis S, Lecky F, Yates DW, et al. The effect of pre-existing medical conditions and age on mortality after injury. *J Trauma.* 2006;61(5):1255–1260.
64. McGwin G Jr, MacLennan PA, Fife JB, et al. Preexisting conditions and mortality in older trauma patients. *J Trauma.* 2004;56(6):1291–1296.
65. Milzman DP, Boulanger BR, Rodriguez A, et al.: Pre-existing disease in trauma patients: A predictor of fate independent of age and injury severity score. *J Trauma.* 1992;32:236; discussion 243.
66. Hausdorff JM, Rios DA, Edelber HK. Gait variability and fall risk in community-living older adults: a 1-year prospective study. *Arch Phys Med Rehabil.* 2001;82(8):1050–1056.
67. Rubenstein LZ, Josephson KR, Robbins AS: Falls in the nursing home. *Ann Intern Med.* 1994;121:442.
68. Bell AJ, Talbot-Stern JK, Hennessy A. Characteristics and outcomes of older patients presenting to the emergency department after a fall: a retrospective analysis. *Med J Aust.* 2000;173(4):176–177.
69. Stevens JA, Corso PS, Finkelstein EA, et al. The costs of fatal and nonfatal falls among older adults. *Inj Prev.* 2006;12:290–295.
70. Magaziner J, Simonsick EM, Kashner TM, et al. Predictors of functional recovery one year following hospital discharge for hip fracture: a prospective study. *J Gerentology.* 1990;45:101–107.
71. http://www.cdc.gov/HomeandRecreationalSafety/Falls/adultfalls.html. Accessed 3-29-10.
72. Lindqvist K, Timpka T, Schelp L. Evaluation of an interorganizational prevention program against injuries among the elderly in a WHO Safe Community. *Public Health.* 2001;115:308–316.
73. McClure RJ, Turner C, Peel N, et al. Population-based interventions for the prevention of fall-related injuries in older people. *Cochrane Database Syst Rev.* 2005(1). CD004441. DOI: 10.1002/14651858.CD004441.pub2.
74. WHO Global Consultation on Violence and Health. *Violence: A Public Health Priority.* Geneva: World Health Organization; 1996.
75. http://www.cdc.gov/injury/wisqars/nvdrs.html Accessed 3-29-10.
76. Corso P, Mercy J, Simon T, et al. Medical costs and productivity losses due to interpersonal and self-directed violence in the United States. *Am J Prev Med.* 2007;32(6):474–482.
77. Wintemute GJ: Handgun availability and firearm mortality. *Lancet.* 1988;2:1136–1137.
78. Zimring FE: Firearms, violence and pubgc policy. *So/Am.* 1991;265:48–54.
79. Loftin C, McDowall D, Wiersema B, et al. Effects of restrictive licensing of handguns on homicide and suicide in the District of Columbia. *N Engl J Med.* 325:1615, 1991.
80. Hawton K, van Heeringen K. Suicide. *Lancet.* 2009;373(9672):1372–1381.
81. O'Carroll P, Rosenberg M, Mercy J. Suicide. In: Rosenberg M, Fenley M, et al., eds *Violence in America.* New York: Oxford University Press; 1991.
82. http://www.cdc.gov/ViolencePrevention/suicide.index.html. Accessed April 2, 2009.
83. http://www.cdc.gov/ViolencePrevention/intimatepartnerviolence/definitions.html Accessed April 1, 2009.
84. Tjaden P, Thoennes N. *Extent, Nature, and Consequences of Intimate Partner Violence: Findings from the National Violence Against Women Survey.* Washington, DC: Department of Justice (US); 2000.
85. Max W, Rice DP, Finkelstein E, et al. The economic toll of intimate partner violence against women in the United States. *Violence Vict.* 2004;19(3):259–272.
86. Garcia L, Soria C, Hurwitz EL. Homicides and intimate partner violence: a literature review. *Trauma Violence Abuse.* 2007;8(4):370–383.
87. http://www.cdc.gov/ViolencePrevention/intimatepartnerviolence/index.html
88. Koss MP, Koss PG, Woodruff WJ. Deleterious effects of criminal victimization on women's health and medical utilization. *Arch Int Med.* 1991;151:342–347.
89. Dickinson LM, et al. Health-related quality of life and symptom profiles of female survivors of sexual abuse. *Arch Family Med.* 1999;8:35–43.
90. Buzawa E, Hotaling G, Klein A. The response to domestic violence in a model court: Some initial findings and implications. *Behav Sci Law.* 1998;16:185–206.
91. Logan TK, Shannon L, Walker R, et al. Protective orders: questions and conundrums. *Trauma Violence Abuse.* 2006;7(3):175–205.
92. Harrell A, Smith B, Newmark L. *Court Processing and the Effects of Restraining Orders for Domestic Violence Victims.* Washington, DC: Urban Institute; 1993.
93. Foshee VA, Bauman KE, Ennett ST, et al. Assessing the long-term effects of the Safe Dates program and a booster in preventing and reducing adolescent dating violence victimization and perpetration. *Am J Public Health.* 2004;94(4):619–624.

CHAPTER 19 ■ RECOVERY AND REHABILITATION

ROBERT D. WINFIELD AND LAWRENCE LOTTENBERG

In trauma and emergency general surgery, a great deal of attention is often paid to the acute management of the injured or critically ill patient. While this focus reflects the initial and most time-sensitive aspects of patient care, it is important to remember that the traditional metrics of quality of care in this setting, namely, morbidity and mortality, tell us little about what is probably the most important outcome: the ability of the injured or ill individual to ultimately return to society as a functioning, productive citizen. This is reflected poignantly in the financial burden attributed to trauma by the CDC with 2000 data suggesting that injuries led to lifetime costs of $406 billion, with lost productivity costs totaling approximately $326 billion of this amount, or greater than four times the cost of medical care.[1] This chapter provides information on the complex multidisciplinary care essential to the recovery and rehabilitation of the injured or critically ill surgical patient. While the chapter places emphasis on post-trauma rehabilitation due to the data that exists in this field, the principles contained within are applicable to all of acute care surgery, and may be utilized as such.

ADMISSION OF THE PATIENT TO THE HOSPITAL

Whether it is a trauma patient or an emergency general surgery patient, recovery and rehabilitation should start on admission to the hospital, or upon first encounter with the acute care surgeon. The interview and history should include where the patient lives, as many acute surgical patients are from surrounding local areas, or conversely from out of the surrounding area (vacation, work, visiting relatives, etc.). Who the patient lives with is equally important, as the patient living alone has vastly different needs from one who has the support of a spouse, siblings, parents, or children. Living conditions, such as single family home, multilevel home, apartment, or as has been seen in most recent times, whether the patient is homeless, also clearly have a role in disposition planning. Frank, open discussions with the patient's family and friends will allow the clinician to gain valuable insight into the disposition planning that will need to be done once the primary surgical issues are resolved.

The physical examination of the acute surgical patient should also lead the physician to make certain early decisions about disposition. The multiple trauma patient with complex pelvic fractures and lower extremity fractures should lead one to conclude that ambulation may not be possible for weeks to months and a skilled nursing facility (SNF) may be a destination prior to a rehabilitation facility. A traumatic brain injury (TBI) will trigger a different set of potential destinations. An emergency general surgery patient who is going to receive a diverting or a permanent stoma will also present a different set of circumstances, and once again, open discussion with family members will yield important information regarding whether they will be comfortable caring for such a patient or whether a SNF may be needed.

MULTIDISCIPLINARY INPATIENT CONFERENCE FOR THE ACUTE CARE SURGERY PATIENT

Once the patient is admitted to the acute care hospital and once the surgical procedures have been performed, it is crucial to assemble a team of all the specialists involved in the patient's care to plan immediately for the acute and chronic care of the patient. Many acute care services have daily "sit-down" rounds with team members; however, it is the opinion of the authors that at a minimum, twice-weekly "multidisciplinary rounds" be held with a team of surgical attendings, surgical residents if in a teaching environment, staff nurses from the patient floor and the intensive care unit, physical therapist, occupational therapist, social workers, speech pathologists, dietician, rehabilitation intake specialist, quality assurance staff (trauma service coordinators), and on occasion clergy and ethics panel members. The optimal days for these twice-weekly conferences would be on Monday, after the weekend to discuss all the new admissions and on Friday, before the weekend to make destination disposition plans prior to the weekend. Such conferences should become part of standard policy and procedures on the acute care surgery service. Further, the use of frequently updated, electronically generated lists should comprise every element of the patient's status to reflect involvement of all the aforementioned disciplines. Trauma patients at designated or verified trauma centers may be bound by rules to have certain consultations from rehabilitation intake personnel and physicians within a certain time period varying from within 24 hours to 7 days of admission.

MULTIDISCIPLINARY REHABILITATION OF THE TRAUMA PATIENT

The multiply injured trauma patients must deal with the healing of both visible and invisible wounds following their traumatic insult. In order to provide optimal care, a team approach should be undertaken, and will necessarily incorporate specialists in a variety of fields to achieve the best possible outcome. As is true in the field of trauma as a whole, much has been learned about interdisciplinary rehabilitation as a result of military conflict. The recent campaigns in Iraq and Afghanistan have generated a new series of challenges that have led to innovative responses that may be employed by providers taking on the responsibility of recuperating and rehabilitating the multiply injured patient.

The Veterans Health Administration has outlined its system for interdisciplinary care, the Polytrauma System of Care (PSC), which grew out of the recognition of the complex care needs of the significant numbers of multiply injured soldiers returning from Iraq.[2,3] The PSC is a VHA-wide, regionalized, tiered system of care delivery (Algorithm. 19.1). At the core of each region is the Polytrauma Rehabilitation Center (PRC),

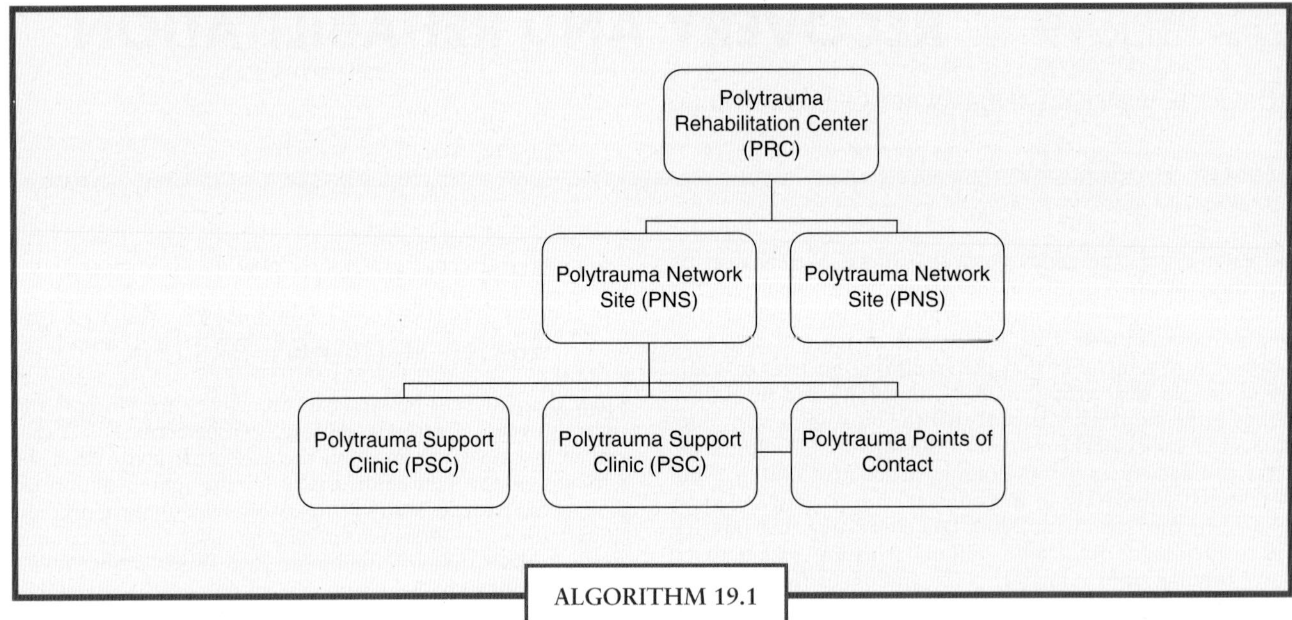

ALGORITHM 19.1 The Veterans Health Administration Polytrauma System of Care. (Adapted from Sigford BJ. To care for him who shall have borne the battle and for his widow and his orphan (Abraham Lincoln): the Department of Veterans Affairs polytrauma system of care *Arch Phys Med Rehabil.* 2008;89:160–162.)

which delivers comprehensive medical, surgical, and rehabilitative care within the setting of a tertiary medical center. The PRC offers all potential services needed by the multiply injured as well as their families, and doubles as a consultation and education center for practitioners employed in other components in the region of that PRC. The next tier is the Polytrauma Network Site (PNS), which is geared toward the delivery of postacute inpatient rehabilitative care and has the responsibility of ongoing coordination of rehabilitation services for veterans and their families within their local area. The final tier is delivered at the local level in the form of Polytrauma Support Clinic Teams that accept and refer veterans and provide rehabilitative care to those with stable needs, and Polytrauma Points of Contact, comprised of individuals (primarily social workers) at various VA sites who provide no direct rehabilitative services, but assist veterans in receiving needed care on a local level.

The PSC is guided by four tenets that govern care (Table 19.1). Proactive case management is carried out by nurses for clinical issues and social workers for psychosocial ones. Tasks include regular contact with patients to ensure appropriate execution of the plan of care, identifying changes in the social situation of the patient, coordinating resources, providing support and education, and helping patients make the transition from active duty to veteran status. As substantial, major multiple traumas often lead to long-term issues, the system is designed to deliver lifelong care via the PSC closest to the veteran. All centers within the system are linked by the Polytrauma Telehealth Network, which is a system of videoconferencing utilized in the coordinated care between practitioners, and in providing education and support to veterans and their families. Finally, severely injured veterans may require long-term care and assistance within facilities or within their homes, and the PSC is committed to providing this for injured veterans.

TABLE 19.1

KEY COMPONENTS OF THE VETERANS HEALTH ADMINISTRATION POLYTRAUMA SYSTEM OF CARE

Proactive case management
Delivery of lifelong care
Telehealth networking between care sites
Provision of long-term inpatient, outpatient, and home-based care for chronic illness and injury

Adapted from Sigford BJ. To care for him who shall have borne the battle and for his widow and his orphan (Abraham Lincoln): the Department of Veterans Affairs polytrauma system of care *Arch Phys Med Rehabil.* 2008;89:160–162.

While the PSC provides what is perhaps in theory a model system for the delivery of interdisciplinary care for the multiply injured, it is unlikely that such a system could be implemented in the current civilian health care environment in the United States. A complex system with multiple, sometimes divergent interests, in which centers compete against one another for business, in which payor concerns often dictate the location and level of care afforded, and in which long-term follow-up and care is a luxury rather than the standard, the delivery of optimal multidisciplinary care is a challenging process. That said, the components are in place, and the key aspects and providers will be reviewed individually.

Social Work

The social worker is at the core of post-injury care planning and coordination. According to the National Association of Social Workers, "professional social workers assist individuals and groups to restore or enhance their capacity for social functioning, while creating societal conditions favorable to their goals. The practice of social work requires knowledge of human development and behavior, of social, economic and cultural institutions, and of the interaction of all these factors."[4] One crucial example of an area in which social workers are widely utilized in U.S. Level I Trauma Centers is in the performance of screening and brief interventions for alcohol use.[5] The understanding possessed by the social workers of the interplay between psychiatric disorders, substance abuse, and the association of these factors with traumatic injury makes them ideally suited for this task, and for many of the other multidimensional challenges faced by the recovering injured.

Often times, it is the social worker who can really identify the impediments and challenges to a successful discharge from acute care to chronic care. The social worker is able to relate to the patient's home situation, source of income, viability of the family unit, and needs for the patient to transition to skilled nursing care, rehabilitation, or other areas prior to the patient returning to a functional life at home. It cannot be overemphasized how important a close, congenial relationship between the physician and the social worker is in implementing the recovery and rehabilitation of the acute care surgical patient.

Physical Therapy

Utilizing multimodality therapy methods to improve strength and flexibility, the goal of the physical therapist for the injured patient is to restore physical function and reduce the morbidity and discomfort resulting from injuries sustained. In the literature, the greatest amount of attention has been paid to the benefits of physical therapy following TBI, although there is a paucity of quality data regarding improvement in outcomes. In a recent review of 14 studies of efficacy in patients suffering TBI, Hellweg and Johannes[6] found support for high-intensity rehabilitation, serial casting and splinting, aerobic training, and aspects of functional training.

The physical therapist is often the first provider who will give physicians involved in acute care disposition for the patient; however, it is essential that the physicians, especially the orthopedic surgeons, write appropriate and accurate ambulation orders on each and every patient needing physical therapy consultation. The best time to write ambulation orders for orthopedic injuries is on admission if nonoperative management is to be done or immediately postoperatively in the post-op orders. Even patients in the intensive care unit should have range of motion, out of bed, or ambulation orders written early in the hospital stay. The therapist will then be able to indicate on subsequent visits with patients whether they will be able to go home with or without outpatient therapy, home with therapy, go to a SNF (usually for patients who are on required non-ambulation for more than a week), or on to a rehabilitation facility for intensive rehabilitation. At that point, consultation with the physiatrist and the rehabilitation intake specialist can be appropriately made and the social worker can begin planning.

Occupational Therapy

The occupational therapist works with post-injury patients to restore their ability to participate in the usual activities of daily living. While for many people, the term "occupation" is synonymous with one's employment, in this setting, it refers to "the breadth and meaning of everyday activity" for the recovering trauma patient, whether that be work-related, or simply the ability to perform usual functions in the home setting.[7] This should be seen as a parallel, but distinctly different, function to that served by the physical therapist, whose focus is more on redeveloping the strength and coordination necessary to do the function, rather than the performance of the function itself.

Speech–Language Pathology

The speech–language pathologist evaluates and treats disorders of speech, language, swallowing, and cognitive communication. This can be important for a variety of reasons, as the ability to speak, swallow, communicate, and understand may be adversely affected by TBI, intubation and tracheostomy, blast injuries to the eyes and ears, blunt or penetrating trauma to the structures key to these processes, or blunting of function due to ongoing emotional distress or medical therapies for pain or spasticity. As a result of the unique training and function of the speech–language pathologist, the Communication Sciences and Disorders Clinical Trials Research Group have recommended that injured veterans returning from Iraq and Afghanistan have access to these valuable providers as part of their multidisciplinary team.[8] Speech–language pathologists develop individualized plans of care tailored to the patients' needs. They may recommend alternative nutrition based upon aspiration risk when swallowing. This becomes particularly important in those patients who have had tracheostomies during their acute hospital phase and are either being decannulated or weaned from their tracheostomy. Finally, speech–language pathologists provide important education to patients, their family members and caregivers regarding impairments, disease processes, and compensatory strategies. This allows the recovering patient to identify strenghts and weaknesses to maintain swallowing, speech and language skills.

Neurocognitive Rehabilitation Services

Eighty-five thousand people suffer TBI leading to long-term disability each year in the United States, and twelve thousand people sustain spinal cord injuries over the same time frame.[1,9] Injuries to the central and peripheral nervous systems may result in a variety of forms of dysfunction, with communicative disorders, impairment of mobility, pain, and psychiatric disorders all being manifest. The rehabilitation of these patients can be particularly challenging, as it often involves relearning basic activities, developing compensation methods for loss of function, and employing nonstandard pain control regimens.[10] The neurocognitive rehabilitation specialist is familiar with the patterns of injury present in this population, and can play an integral role in developing patient-specific management plans.

Clinical Dietitian

The role of optimal nutrition in healing after injury and illness is well-established, and is an area of intense research.[11] A clinical dietitian utilizes his or her training to guide nutritional support, whether it be via the enteral or parenteral route, and can ensure that the nutritional needs of the patient with complex injuries and illnesses are met. There is data to suggest that use of the recommendations of registered dietitians enhances the quality of nutrition received, and that this has the potential to improve outcomes in long-term acute care (LTAC) patients.[12] The clinical dietitian should be consulted early to provide initial nutritional support, and his or her recommendations following reevaluation should be a part of each multidisciplinary patient care rounds.

Pain Management

The management of short- and long-term pain following injury is an expected component of post-injury recovery and rehabilitation. While most practitioners are accepting of the need for short-term pain control strategies, in an assessment of 50 soldiers receiving inpatient rehabilitation services at the Tampa PRC, 96% were found to have pain during their stay, and this led to impairments in physical, emotional, and social functioning.[13] There is some suggestion that the pain experienced both in the acute and rehabilitative phases can influence the ultimate development of chronic pain syndromes and eventual long-term disability.[13] Pain management specialists work alongside other practitioners to prescribe and provide multimodality therapy including medications, psychiatric and psychological therapy, regional nerve blockades, nerve stimulation, and other novel forms of pain management to improve both short- and long-term function following major injury.

Psychiatric Care

Depression and posttraumatic stress disorder are the two most commonly encountered psychiatric disorders following injury; however, several types of these disorders are seen, carrying with them implications for short- and long-term management.[14–16] Comorbid TBI as well as pain issues make post-injury psychiatric care multilayered and challenging. Studies from the University of Washington suggest that early intervention in patients screening positively for PTSD can improve outcomes through a collaborative approach that includes psychopharmacology, case management, and cognitive–behavioral therapy.[17] The inclusion of the psychiatric care provider is critical to this tactic and to similar efforts to treat depression and more rare post-injury psychiatric disorders, and represents an opportunity to improve long-term mental well-being.

Physiatry

As the patient transitions from the acute care setting to a rehabilitation center, it is vital to have a team leader familiar with the needs of patients requiring rehabilitation from illness and injury. Physiatrists are physicians who complete specific residency training in physical medicine and rehabilitation and are skilled at designing coordinated treatment plans in concert with the aforementioned specialists to deliver comprehensive care to alleviate discomfort and rehabilitate the sick and injured. There are about 8,300 board-certified physiatrists in the United States. Physiatrists also treat neurologic illness including stroke, brain injury, and spinal cord injury. Also, their scope of practice includes musculoskeletal injuries, pain syndromes, and sports injuries. Physiatrists treat patients of all ages in the three major areas of the diagnosis and treatment of musculoskeletal injuries and pain syndromes, electrodiagnostic medicine (electromyography), and of course the rehabilitation of patients with severe impairments.

Care for the Caregiver

The majority of the focus in post-injury care is on the recovery and rehabilitation of the injured individual; however, the recovery of the individual places incredible stress on the family and friends who provide support and direct care with the added stress of long-term emotional investment. Loved ones who serve in the role of caregiver face the difficult tasks of assisting with medical care, helping to coordinate the various components of the multidisciplinary care process on behalf of the recovering patient, and often times are responsible for bearing the financial burdens associated with recovery. In the VA PSC, the complicated nature of caregiver involvement is acknowledged, and efforts to incorporate family into the recovery and rehabilitation process and to provide them with therapy are ongoing.[18] This includes provision of housing, meeting basic needs, assisting financially, and providing therapy to anxious and grieving family members struggling with the reintegration of their loved one following injury. This method provides the opportunity to treat the whole patient, by recognizing that the depth and breadth of one's social support is the key to recovery, and that, at times, the family or friend requires own form of assistance to adjust to life after injury.

RECOVERY AND REHABILITATION ENVIRONMENTS

Much of the recovery following injury occurs outside of the hospital. The level and amount of supportive, professional care needed are dictated by the extent of the injuries, post-injury complications, and preexisting comorbidities. Different types of recovery sites provide these different levels of care, and these are reviewed here.

Long-Term Acute Care Facilities

Although critical illness is thought of as an issue primarily dealt with in the period surrounding and immediately following acute injury, approximately 3%-6% of patients fall under the category of being chronically critically ill.[19] For patients with ongoing critical illness unlikely to resolve in the short term, and due to the tremendous financial strain generated by the care of these individuals, LTAC facilities have been established and have the benefit of being exempt from the Medicare prospective payment system.[19] LTACs vary in the completeness of services offered, but provide the personnel and facilities to manage patients needing prolonged mechanical ventilation as well as other complex care including provision of parenteral nutrition, wound management, and on-site hemodialysis.

Skilled Nursing Facilities

SNFs exist in order to treat, manage, observe, and evaluate patients with subacute needs. This includes services requiring the services of skilled professionals, such as provision of injectable medications by nursing, physical and occupational therapy, and ongoing speech and language therapy.[20]. As with LTACs, SNFs vary with regard to the services offered, but generally provide a site of convalescence and rehabilitation for patients with lower acuity and fewer care needs.

Rehabilitation Centers

For patients whose long-term needs are primarily related to their ability to regain physical function, a rehabilitation center provides an environment in which providers of these services (physical and occupational therapy, speech–language pathologists, etc.) work together in an interdisciplinary fashion to meet patient needs. Nursing care can be provided in this environment, and physician care is provided by physiatrists; the medical needs of patients tend to be at a higher level than that seen in a SNF, and intensive rehabilitation efforts can be undertaken. The brain-injured patient must be of sufficient functioning level so as to follow commands to participate in rehabilitation.

Any rehabilitation center should be surveyed and approved by the Commission on Accredication of Rehabilitation Facilities (CARF), which is designed to provide standards for excellence for care of injured and ill patients.

Outpatient and Home-Based Recovery and Rehabilitation

For patients not requiring 24-hour nursing supervision or intensive rehabilitation, outpatient and/or home-based care may be arranged to allow the recovering patient to convalesce in a familiar and comfortable environment. Patients may receive a wide variety of services in this way, to include physical and occupational therapy, wound care, and injectable medications courtesy of visiting nurses, or the patient may visit an infusion center to receive intermittently dosed intravenous medications.

SUMMARY

The recovery and rehabilitation of the multiply injured or critically ill patient can be a challenge for patients, their caregivers, and their loved ones; however, this is clearly an important component of care as it focuses on the transition from being a patient to being a functioning member of society. This may require the assistance of a host of professionals, each with specialized training that can be employed to facilitate the process. Through the conflicts in Iraq and Afghanistan, the U.S. Armed Forces has recognized the value of a coordinated, multidisciplinary approach to this process, and through the PSC has created a model for delivery of care that is comprehensive in nature. Although the current civilian health care system in the United States possesses the manpower and features necessary to deliver this type of care, coordination of the various pieces needs to progress to the levels of the military and the Veterans Administration systems; however, with new legislation addressing the financing and delivery of health care and a developing interest in regionalization of services, opportunities may be emerging for the creation of a streamlined system of rehabilitative care, and a chance to maximize our ability to return the injured and sick to optimum levels of functioning and productivity.

References

1. Corso P, Finkelstein E, Miller T, et al. Incidence and lifetime costs of injuries in the United States. *Inj Prev*. 2006;**12**(4):212-218.
2. Sigford BJ. To care for him who shall have borne the battle and for his widow and his orphan (Abraham Lincoln): the Department of Veterans Affairs polytrauma system of care. *Arch Phys Med Rehabil*. 2008;89(1):160-162.
3. Strasser DC, Uomoto JM, Smits SJ. The interdisciplinary team and polytrauma rehabilitation: prescription for partnership. *Arch Phys Med Rehabil*. 2008;89(1):179-181.
4. General Fact Sheets. Social Work Profession. [cited 2011 February 2]; Available from: http://www.naswdc.org/pressroom/features/general/profession.asp.
5. Terrell F, Zatzick DF, Jurkovich GJ, et al. Nationwide survey of alcohol screening and brief intervention practices at US Level I trauma centers. *J Am Coll Surg*. 2008;207(5):630-638.
6. Hellweg S, Johannes S. Physiotherapy after traumatic brain injury: a systematic review of the literature. *Brain Inj*. 2008;22(5):365-373.
7. Occupational Therapy in Acute Care. American Occupational Therapy Association Fact Sheet 2009 [cited 2011 February 2]; Available from: http://www.aota.org/Consumers/Professionals/WhatIsOT/RDP/Facts/43243.aspx.
8. Cherney LR, Gardner P, Logemann JA, et al. The role of speech-language pathology and audiology in the optimal management of the service member returning from Iraq or Afghanistan with a blast-related head injury: position of the Communication Sciences and Disorders Clinical Trials Research Group. *J Head Trauma Rehabil*. 2010;25(3):219-224.
9. Sekhon LH, Fehlings MG. Epidemiology, demographics, and pathophysiology of acute spinal cord injury. *Spine (Phila Pa 1976)*. 2001;26 (24, suppl):S2-S12.
10. Gironda RJ, Clark ME, Ruff RL, et al. Traumatic brain injury, polytrauma, and pain: challenges and treatment strategies for the polytrauma rehabilitation. *Rehabil Psychol*. 2009;54(3):247-258.
11. Heyland DK, Heyland J, Dhaliwal R, et al. Randomized trials in critical care nutrition: look how far we've come! (and where do we go from here?). *JPEN J Parenter Enteral Nutr*. 2010;34(6):697-706.
12. Braga JM, Hunt A, Pope J, et al. Implementation of dietitian recommendations for enteral nutrition results in improved outcomes. *J Am Diet Assoc*. 2006;106(2):281-284.
13. Clark ME, Bair MJ, Buckenmaier CC III, et al. Pain and combat injuries in soldiers returning from Operations Enduring Freedom and Iraqi Freedom: implications for research and practice. *J Rehabil Res Dev*. 2007;44(2):179-194.
14. O'Donnell ML, Bryant RA, Creamer M, et al. Mental health following traumatic injury: toward a health system model of early psychological intervention. *Clin Psychol Rev*. 2008;28(3):387-406.
15. O'Donnell ML, Creamer MC, Parslow R, et al. A predictive screening index for posttraumatic stress disorder and depression following traumatic injury. *J Consult Clin Psychol*. 2008;76(6):923-932.
16. Steel J, Youssef M, Pfeifer R, et al. Health-related quality of life in patients with multiple injuries and traumatic brain injury 10+ years postinjury. *J Trauma*. 2010;69(3):523–530; discussion 530-531.
17. Zatzick DF, Roy-Byrne P, Russo JE, et al. Collaborative interventions for physically injured trauma survivors: a pilot randomized effectiveness trial. *Gen Hosp Psychiatry*. 2001;23(3):114-123.
18. Collins RC, Kennedy MC. Serving families who have served: providing family therapy and support in interdisciplinary polytrauma rehabilitation. *J Clin Psychol*. 2008;64(8):993-1003.
19. Carson SS, Bach PB, Brzozowski L, et al. Outcomes after long-term acute care. An analysis of 133 mechanically ventilated patients. *Am J Respir Crit Care Med*. 1999;**159**(5, pt 1):1568-1573.
20. *Medicare Coverage of Skilled Nursing Facility Care*. CMS, ed. U.S. Department of Health and Human Services; 2007.

CHAPTER 20 ■ THE EVOLUTION OF TRAUMA CARE IN THE UNITED STATES

DONALD D. TRUNKEY

PAST

The history of trauma care is inextricably linked to wars and wounds. Trauma antedates recorded history, and there are examples of anthropological findings showing trepanation of the skull dated to 10,000 BC. These skulls have been found in the Tigress-Euphrates Valley, along the shores of the Mediterranean, and in Meso-America. It is most likely these operations were done for depressed skull fractures, and possibly epidural hematomas. The surgery was most likely performed by priests or shamans within the various cultures. Some of these skulls show that the operation was done more than once; and there is ample evidence that there was success since there was healing of the man-made hole. There is also evidence that they were able to treat fractures and dislocations with successful knitting of the bones.

The first solid evidence for war wounds came from a mass grave found in Egypt and dated to approximately 2000 BC.[1] The bodies of 60 soldiers were found in a sufficiently well-preserved state to show mace wounds, gaping wounds, and arrows still in the bodies. The Smith Papyrus records the clinical treatment of 48 cases of war wounds and is primarily a textbook on how to treat wounds, most of which were penetrating. According to Majno, there were 147 recorded wounds in Homer's Iliad, with an overall mortality of 77.6%. Thirty-one soldiers sustained wounds to the head, all of which were lethal. The surgical care for a wounded Greek was crude at best. However, the Greeks did recognize the need for a system of trauma care, and theirs is one of the first examples of a trauma system. The wounded were given care in special barracks (*klisiai*) or in nearby ships. Drugs, usually derived from plants, were applied to wounds.

Further east, there was evidence of another trauma system that had been established by the Indian army. This was a system that rivaled that of the Greeks and Romans. India was divided into several kingdoms, and the Far East kingdom was Magadha. It was ruled by Ashoka, the third of the Maurya Dynasty. Ashoka was responsible for developing three sets of documents describing governance, the third of which described some of the care provided to his soldiers when he invaded the kingdom of Kalinga. The *Artasastra* documented that the Indian army had an ambulance service well-equipped with surgeons and women to prepare food and beverages and to bandage wounds. Indian medicine was specialized and it was the "shalyarara" (surgeon) who would be called upon to treat wounds. Shalyarara literally means "arrow remover," as the bow and arrow was the traditional weapon for Indians.

The Romans perfected the delivery of combat care and set up a system of trauma centers in all parts of the Roman Empire. These trauma centers were called "valetudinaria" and were built during the first and second centuries AD. The remains of 25 such centers have been found, but importantly, none were found in Rome or other large cities. It is noteworthy that there were 11 found in Roman Britannica, more than currently exist. Some of the valetudinaria were designed to handle a combat casualty rate of up to 10%. There was a regular medical corps within the Roman legions, and at least 85 army physicians are found in the records, mainly because they earned an epitaph.

The concept of shock was not appreciated during this period of time. In fact, it was not until the late 19th and early 20th centuries that shock was finally described.[2] The Greeks understood that hemorrhage could lead to death, and they also empirically treated this with herbs, specifically ephedra nebrodensis, which came from Sardinia. The same treatment was used in China, where it was called Ma-Hung, and it was also ephedra. It is most likely that these two distant cultures shared the discovery of ephedra via the "Silk Road." Hippocrates and Galen did not use the tourniquet. This was partially based on the evidence of Largus, who stated that if you took a pig stomach, filled it with liquid, and then wrapped a rope around it, tightening the rope would increase expulsion of the fluid out of the bag orifice.

Over the first millennium, military trauma care did not make any major advances until midway in the second millennium, just before the Renaissance. Arabic surgery did thrive for two to three centuries, but it was up to French military surgeons, who lived 250 years later, to bring trauma care into the Age of Enlightenment. Ambrose Paré (1510–1590) served four French kings during the time of the French and Spanish civil and religious wars.[3] His major contribution to treating penetrating trauma included the treatment of gunshot wounds, the use of ligature instead of cautery, and the use of nutrition during the post-injury period. Paré was much interested in prosthetic devices and designed a number of them for amputees.

It was Dominique Larrey, Napoleon's surgeon, who addressed trauma from a systematic and organizational standpoint.[4] Larrey introduced the concept of the "flying ambulance," the sole purpose of which was to provide rapid removal of the wounded from the battlefield. Larrey also introduced the concept of placing the hospital as close to the front lines as feasible to undertake wound surgery as soon as possible. His primary intent was to operate during the period of "wound shock" when there was an element of analgesia, most likely due to endorphins, but also to reduce infection in the postamputation period.

Larrey had an understanding of problems that were unique to military surgery and system development. Some of his contributions can best be appreciated by his efforts before Napoleon's Russian campaign. Larrey did not know which country

Napoleon was planning to attack, and there was even conjecture of an invasion of England. He left Paris on February 24, 1812, and was ordered to Mentz, Germany. Shortly thereafter, he went to Magdeberg and then on to Berlin, where he began preparation for the campaign, still not knowing precisely where the French army was headed. In his own words, "Previous to my departure from this capital, I organized six divisions of flying ambulances, each one consisting of eight surgeons. The surgeon-majors exercised their divisions daily according to my instructions, in the performance of operations and the application of bandages. The greatest degree of emulation and the strictest discipline were prevalent among all thc surgeons."

The 19th and 20th centuries were notable in the improvement of surgical care in combat. Antisepsis was introduced during our Civil War, and there was a gradual decline in patients who died from their wounds (Table 20.1) The surgical mortality for head, chest, and abdominal wounds also decreased after the First World War (Table 20.2). Between WWI and WWII, the first civilian trauma system was created in Austria by Böhler. Although initially designed for industrial accidents, by the time of WWII, it also included motor traffic accidents.

The most remarkable development of a statewide trauma system occurred early in the 1970s in Germany.[5] At that time, road traffic accidents accounted for 18,000 deaths annually. Since 1975, this has been reduced to approximately 7,000. In 1966, two trauma centers were started in the United States: one in Chicago at Cook County (Robert Freeark) and one in San Francisco (F. William Blaisdell). The first statewide trauma system was initiated in 1969 by R.A. Cowley in the state of Maryland. It was at approximately the same time that the American College of Surgeons Committee on Trauma (ACSCOT) started to develop criteria for trauma systems. In 1976, the first Optimal Criteria document was published, followed shortly thereafter by the ATLS course, which was designed for emergency physicians and surgeons, and defined criteria for resuscitation during the first hour following injury. Subsequently, there were two other significant developments by the ACSCOT, including the Multiple Trauma Outcome Study, which has now gone on to be the National Trauma Data Bank, and a verification program for existing trauma centers. The College recognized early on that the designation of trauma centers was a political and legal process, and the verification program simply examined patient medical records and program improvement documents to verify whether or not the hospital met the designation criteria. By 1995, a report in the *Journal of the American Medical Association* showed that five states had statewide trauma systems.[6] This was followed by another study in 1998 published in the *Journal of Trauma* documenting that the five states continued to meet all eight previously described criteria for trauma systems[7] and 28 states met at least six or seven criteria, whereas an additional four states met at least four criteria. Finally in 2006, another study evaluating the efficacy of trauma center care on mortality showed that the mortality from trauma was 7.6% in designated trauma centers compared to 9.5% in hospitals that were not designated.[8] One year after discharge, the significance continued with a mortality of 10.4% versus 13.8%. Another study published in 2006 from Florida showed that in counties with a trauma center, the mean fatality rate was 50% less than in counties without a trauma center.[9] It can be seen from this data that the effectiveness of a trauma center is irrefutable as shown by these two recent studies and the data from Germany. Finally, a more recent study shows that trauma centers are more cost effective than hospitals that are not trauma centers.[10]

TABLE 20.1

CIVIL WAR DEATHS

Union	
In Battle	110,070
Disease	224,586
Accidents, suicide	24,872
Total	**359,528**
Confederacy	
In Battle	94,000
Disease	164,000
Total	**258,000**
Total Union and Confederacy	**617,528**

Data from *The Medical and Surgical History of the War of the Rebellion*. Vol. 6, 2nd Issue. Washington, DC: Government Printing Office; 1875.

PRESENT

I think it is fair to state that the training of a general surgeon over the last 40 years has changed fairly dramatically. To illustrate this, I will compare my own training with the current resident training.

TABLE 20.2

SURGICAL MORTALITY FOR HEAD, CHEST AND ABDOMINAL WOUNDS (U.S. ARMY)

	HEAD		THORAX		ABDOMEN	
WAR	CASES	% MORTALITY	CASES	% MORTALITY	CASES	% MORTALITY
First World War	189	40	104	37	1,816	67
Second World War	2,051	14	1,364	10	2,315	23
Korean Conflict	673	10	158	8	384	9
Vietnam Conflict	1,171	10	1,176	7	1,209	9

Data from Trunkey D. History and development of trauma care in the United States. *Clin Orthop Relat Res*. 2000;374:36–46.

I spent 4 years in medical school between 1959 and 1963 at the University of Washington. During my senior year, I decided that I would go into internal medicine, and did a 3-month sub-internship on the medical wards at Harborview Hospital. At the end of 3 months, I was confused and disheartened because I had not enjoyed internal medicine that much. Unfortunately, there was a paucity of role models in surgery and I applied and got accepted to the University of Oregon in Portland to do a rotating internship. My first rotation was on general surgery with Dr. Dunphy. Within 3 weeks, I had made the decision to pursue surgery as a career. After my internship, I did 2 years in the military and then joined Dr. Dunphy at the University of California San Francisco for my residency between 1966 and 1971. This residency was a true general surgery training program. During that period of time, I did vascular surgery, thoracic surgery, general surgery, and I had 3 months of orthopedic surgery, 3 months of anesthesia, 3 months of pathology, and 2 months of neurosurgery. Following this training, I did an NIH trauma fellowship at Southwestern Medical Center in Dallas with Dr. Tom Shires. This was the same year that I first contacted the American Board of Surgery. I had sent in my cases, which were a little over 1,300. This was again reflective of a general surgery training program at that time. During a 4-month period with Dr. Jack Wiley, I did 137 major vascular cases and this did not include the vascular cases that I did at San Francisco General Hospital or in some of the community hospitals. I turned in almost 80 thoracic cases, of which approximately one-half were due to trauma and half were due to cancer and tuberculosis. I had also done a number of orthopedic procedures, including hip nailings, ORIF of femurs and tibias, and reduction of dislocations. I also had an equally good experience in neurosurgery. After submitting these cases, I did the written exam in November, and after passing this was immediately offered the oral exam in December. Every general surgeon remembers their board examiners, and I am no exception. Fortunately, I passed, and out of the 1,100 candidates that year, the failure rate was 18%. However, two-thirds of these individuals then went on to get specialty training, and the remaining one-third (300 diplomats) stayed in general surgery. How many went into rural practice or urban practice is not a number that I can determine.

Moving forward in time, I would now like to contrast my surgical training and my experiences with the American Board of Surgery. In 1975, I became a guest examiner and received an appointment to the Board in 1980. Interestingly, the same number of total residents was being examined and then this decreased slightly. However, the number that now goes into general surgery is approximately 200. This may be misleading, since a number of people who get specialty training also do general surgery. The year that I came on the American Board of Surgery, the Vascular Board had been just voted in the previous January and for reasons that I cannot explain, they made me chairman of the new certification committee for vascular surgery. This became a very contentious issue. One of the issues that impacted negatively on general surgery training was the decrease in the number of vascular cases residents were allowed to do. This has been compounded recently by the shift of vascular management to endovascular stents and interventional procedures. This has also been exacerbated by the creation of a subspecialty board in surgical oncology, and the separation of cardiothoracic into subspecialty boards of cardiac, thoracic, and pediatric cardiac surgery. Another issue in the 1980s was whether or not to have a certificate for trauma and acute care. Trauma was eventually eliminated from the process due to two surgeons on the board who were vehement that trauma was part of general surgery. Alex Walt argued persuasively that we should still proceed with critical care as a counter to anesthesiology and pulmonary medicine, who he thought would be the only ones who could do critical care if the American Board of Surgery did not provide for this. This eventually came to pass and although we tried to have a common certificate with anesthesiology, pulmonary medicine, and cardiology, this failed. Eventually, the critical care training in surgery became synonymous with trauma. Only time will tell what impact emergency general surgery will have on general surgery training.

Since my initial experiences with the Board, there have been many additional pressures and distractions placed on general surgery, not the least of which is subspecialization within general surgery, including hepatobiliary surgery and pancreatic surgery. Much of this subspecialization is ostensibly done because "experience" leads to better results. However, there is a caveat. In a wonderful article in the *British Medical Journal*, Sir David Carter made the following comments: "There is now abundant evidence that hospitals with higher volumes of activity tend to have better outcomes and emerging evidence that surgeons' volume of work is also a determinant of outcome. Certain cancers, cardiac surgery, liver transplantation, and vascular surgery show technical skill is vital, but it is by no means the only essential ingredient for success. Thorough training, compassion, sound judgment, good communication skills, and knowledge are all critically important. However, words of caution are needed. The relation is not linear; some low-volume units achieve good results, whereas higher levels of activity do not necessarily guarantee good outcome."[11] I would ask the question: why can we not teach general surgeons to achieve good results even if they have low volumes?

I articulated in the first portion of this introduction the evolution of trauma centers and trauma systems in the United States. The multiple distractions and pressures against general surgeons are felt keenly by the trauma community. It has been well-documented that many general surgeons, neurosurgeons, and orthopedic surgeons do not want to take trauma call.[12] The reasons articulated are busy elective practices that can be negatively impacted following the day after trauma call. Many of the patients do not have insurance and there is a fear of increased malpractice risk when one takes care of trauma patients.[13] This has led hospital administrators to initiate on-call pay for general surgeons and some specialty surgeons. This on-call pay varies from $1,000 a shift (general surgeons) up to $7,000 a shift for some of the specialties (neurosurgery). Some of these on-call pay schedules could be interpreted as greed versus need. I recently reviewed the American College of Surgeons data on Level I and II hospitals on the number of emergency procedures done by neurosurgery and orthopedic surgeons within the first 24 hours of admission. In 2008, there was a range of seven craniotomies to 137 craniotomies; the average was 43 per year. In 2009, it ranged from six craniotomies to 137 craniotomies per year, for an average of 62, which is a 50% increase over 2008. For orthopedic cases in 2008, the average was 494 cases with a range of 20 to 1,604. In 2009, it was 558 cases, with a range of 106–1,890. It does not take a mathematical genius to determine that the neurosurgeons average one craniotomy every seven to eight nights, and yet may be paid up to $7,000 a night just to take call. It is highly unlikely that Congress and/or the public will understand or be sympathetic to such payments, particularly with the increasing annual costs in health care and the median total compensation for surgeons. The public might be more sympathetic if hospitals reimburse the surgeons for uncompensated patient care services or assisted specialty groups in recruitment to fulfill trauma care need and obligations.

The Division of Advocacy and Health Policy of the American College of Surgeons has recently come out with a very timely white paper that highlights other issues impacting general surgery.[12] In the introduction of the article, it was pointed out that:

- "A majority of surgeons take ED call 5–10 days a month; some surgical specialists take call far more often."
- "Many surgeons provide on-call services simultaneously at two or more hospitals, and a notable number say they have difficulty negotiating their on-call schedules."
- "Hospital bylaws typically require surgeons to participate in on-call panels, although older individuals are often allowed to 'opt out,' and they are more frequently taking advantage of this option."
- "A notable number of surgeons have been sued by patients first seen in the ED, and some physicians are offered discounts on their liability coverage if they limit or eliminate ED call."

The Advocacy and Health Policy Division goes on to point out the importance of emergency rooms as a safety net for patients and their role in trauma care. A study by the Lewin group in 2002 showed that neurosurgeons, orthopedic surgeons, general surgeons, and plastic surgeons were among the specialists in short supply for emergency department (ED) call panels.[14] The Lewin study was confirmed by the Schumacher Group in 2003, reporting that one-third of EDs lacked surgeon specialty coverage, causing 76% of those responding to go on divert status.[15] More recently, similar surveys were conducted by the American College of Emergency Physicians in 2006, and they showed that nearly three-quarters of ED medical directors think that they have inadequate on-call specialist coverage, compared with two-thirds in 2004.[16] In the most recent survey, orthopedic, plastic, and neurologic surgeons, as well as otolaryngologists and hand surgeons, were reported as most often being in short supply. The American College of Surgeons Bulletin white paper also points out that surgeons are older, with a noteworthy number taking emergency call at 55 years or older. Furthermore, there is a decrease in surgeons providing charity care. The Emergency Medical Treatment and Active Labor Act (EMTALA), which was originally designed as an "antidumping" federal measure, has created a "dumping" problem: an unintended consequence. Finally, malpractice continues to be a problem to any surgeon who provides emergency care.

The crisis in general surgery is further compounded by two studies published by R. A. Cooper, who states, "The physician shortage is here now and will become worse by 2020, when the deficit may be as great as 200,000 physicians.[17,18] Many of these will be surgeons, gastroenterologists, and cardiologists." As noted above, there is a particular crisis in general surgery. Of the approximately 1,000 surgeons who successfully pass their boards, only 200–250 remain in general surgery. Most are getting subspecialty training, and very few of these want to take trauma call. There is also a decline in interest in general surgery because of lifestyle issues, gender, and mentorship. A particularly poignant study by Bland and Isaacs showed a trend toward lifestyle medical specialties rather than surgical specialties.[19] There is a fairly dramatic fall from 1978 to 2001 in the interest of fourth-year medical students in general surgery. Orthopedics may have slightly increased, but neurosurgery, otolaryngology, and urology have stayed relatively flat. There is a particular issue as it relates to gender. Graduating medical students are at least 50% female, and very few apply to general surgery (7% or a little more than 500 applicants). Part of this disinterest in general surgery is the hours of work during the surgical residency, part of it is lifestyle, part of it is a desire to combine a professional career with a traditional role as a mother, and part of it because the programs have not provided protective time so that they can do both. However, there seems to be some recent positive changes in application to surgical programs since the institution of the 80-hour work week.

Recently, the American Association for the Surgery of Trauma, working in concert with the American Board of Surgery, has proposed a solution to attracting medical students into trauma and critical care surgery and retaining them once they pass their boards. The proposed solution essentially expands trauma and surgical critical care to also include emergency general surgery. To accomplish this, it is most likely that surgeons would have to rotate in shifts to cover the hospital 24 hours a day. This might be particularly attractive to women and single parents who would have more control of their time, since they could do 12- to 13-hour shifts a month, leaving the rest of the time for parenting.

Another major problem by 2020 will be the 30% increase in the elderly population in hospitals. It used to be that the peak in death rate from injury was in the 16- to 24-year age group. We are now seeing a bimodal distribution, with an increased death rate in the elderly. The elderly are more active, and unfortunately, the mortality rate for Injury Severity Score >15 is 3.5 times more than those of their younger counterparts.[20] These patients spend more time in the intensive care unit, and unfortunately, do not always have a good return to independent living status or quality of life after their trauma episode.

The lack of general surgeons also impacts negatively on the Department of Defense (DOD) and its need for surgeons.[21–25] Approximately 20% of DOD surgeons are active-duty surgeons; 80% must come from the reserve. Studies after Desert Storm by the General Accounting Office showed that surgeons were not being trained properly for trauma, particularly the active-duty surgeons; however, the DOD has improved this during the past 4 years.

Another negative impact on trauma care is that many trauma centers are closing or downgrading their level of care. Since 2003, "dumping" has become an increasing problem for Level 1 and II trauma centers. This phenomenon is characterized by community hospitals calling the trauma centers and speaking to an emergency physician or surgeon, telling them they have a trauma case that they cannot provide care for, either because of a lack of personnel or because the patient's case is too complex. Many of these patients, once they reach the trauma center, are observed and then discharged the following morning.

Another issue for concern in trauma care is that rehabilitation beds are not available after a severe injury. The General Accounting Office performed a study showing that only one in eight patients with a traumatic brain injury receives appropriate rehabilitation after acute care.[10] Rehabilitation is particularly a problem for patients who have no insurance. I had a patient approximately 6 years ago who was 36 years old, married, and had four children—all boys. He started his own construction company, but unfortunately, he did not have enough money to buy health insurance, which would have cost $6,000 per year for a family of six. He fell while constructing a building and became paralyzed. As a result of the accident, his acute care was provided by my hospital free of charge, but we could not find a rehabilitation facility that would take him. We taught his wife the bare necessities of care for a paraplegic, but, obviously, he is at high risk for complications, and home care with his wife performing most of the care will not allow her to work and provide for the family.

There are other issues as well. Of some concern to acute care hospitals is the recent growth in free-standing ambulatory surgery centers. In many instances, these centers are owned by specialty surgeons, and one of the advantages to them is that they do not have to take night call. In addition, they often will not accept patients with Medicaid or Medicare insurance, thus increasing the burden on the "safety net" hospitals

Finally, we must address the issue of specialty surgical coverage to EDs, and specifically those that are designated trauma centers. The lack of consistent coverage, obviously, adversely affects outcomes, and when a hospital diverts, it puts more stress on other parts of the trauma system. Optimally, the solutions would come from professional societies that represent the surgical subspecialties. Not only does this problem apply to trauma centers in this country, but it also has an impact on our ability to deliver trauma care to the military.

FUTURE

This last section is to ponder on the future of emergency general surgery and trauma surgery. To do so, we have to ask the question: is there a future for trauma in general surgery, and is it good for the community we serve? I think the answer is an unequivocal "yes." In order for this to happen, however, we have to train a general surgeon who is comfortable working with the neck, chest, abdomen, and is comfortable dealing with vascular injuries and compartment syndromes (Table 20.3) This would include the mangled extremity, and in some instances, emergency neurosurgical and orthopedic procedures.

As stated in the previous section, there have been a number of negative impacts on training the general surgeon in the last 40 years. To summarize, these include:

- Establishment of vascular surgery boards and changes in the management of vascular disease and injury,
- The subspecialty of general surgical oncology,
- Changes in the boards within cardiothoracic surgery, which has now been fragmented into pediatric cardiac surgery, thoracic surgery, and cardiac surgery,
- Other surgery fellowships within the house of general surgery, including hepatobiliary and pancreatic fellowships.

The creation of these specialists and subspecialists has had a profound effect on the number of cases the general surgery resident has access to for training. An obvious solution to this problem is to establish opportunities for general surgeons to train in suburban and even rural hospitals where these cases are still being done by general surgeons. This would have tremendous advantage to the university program in establishing goodwill within these hospitals. Obviously, the "farming out" of these residents would have to be done in a very calculated and careful process. An associate program director would have to be appointed; legal requirements would have to be met; and a clear definition of what the surgical resident can do, the amount of proctorship, and the amount of supervision needed would have to be carefully defined. This might very well solve the issue of training somebody who is truly general surgery trained, and it would certainly help solve the demand for general surgeons who would go into rural surgical practice. The resident could then rotate back to the university hospital for experiences in pediatric surgery, trauma, and emergency general surgery. It would also be an opportunity to avoid having general surgery residents doing scut work on subspecialty surgical services.

The second issue regarding the future of emergency general surgery and trauma surgery relates to the overall shortage of general surgeons that has been predicted by Cooper and the number of medical students who even apply to general surgery. The link to this is the number of general surgeons, upon completion of their American Board of Surgery, who choose to go into subspecialties, leaving only 20%–25% who make general surgery their life endeavor. I personally think this is linked to issue number one discussed above. If we can make general surgery attractive by reestablishing the general surgeon as a true generalist from a surgical standpoint, in addition to making it intellectually challenging, this problem could be solved. Related to this is the issue of hours of work during training and later in the professional life. This would solve the gender issue as well. By doing shift work and having reasonable hours, such as the 80-hour work week for residency and 12-hour shifts as an attending, it would mean that in a 1-month period, almost half would be devoted to family and outside interests. It is of interest that the National Health Service in Great Britain has recently announced that their experiment with the 56-hour work week has been an abysmal failure.

The third issue is touched upon above, but I would like to expand on the rural general surgery issue. Many rural surgeons do trauma care, and staff Level III and Level IV hospitals. Many of these hospitals are so-called "critical access hospitals," of which there are 1,307 in the United States. These are critical to rural areas, and not only provide trauma care, but also emergency general surgery care. For example, in Oregon we have 22 of these critical access hospitals, 18 of which have a general surgeon on staff. Four of the hospitals have no general surgeon. These critical access hospitals get a marginal increase (5%) in Medicare payments. These hospitals are vital to the community they serve. They provide jobs and a service to the community. In order to encourage surgeons to go to rural areas to practice, we have established a 1-year training program in a community of 30,000 people in southwestern Oregon. During this 1-year period, the resident or residents who go there would do a wholly different type of general surgery and trauma care than in the parent university hospital (Table 20.4). These residents are usually on 24-hour call, and will assist three general surgeons who provide the care for this community. This 24-hour call can be very onerous if you're the only general surgeon in some of the smaller communities. One solution is to transfer emergency general surgery cases to a higher level of care. In at least one instance, the university hospital in Oregon has contracted to a hospital 30 miles away in a smaller community to take four out of seven night calls. If a patient comes into the hospital emergency room on the night the university is on-call, the patient is quickly transported to the university emergency room. This relieves the general surgeon from having to take call 24/7/365.

This does not solve all of the problems in the rural areas. Many of these surgeons have to get locums to come in and do 2 weeks of call so that they can go on vacation, and if they want to go to medical meetings, then they must work out some type of alternative call. This could possibly be solved by having general surgeons in these communities rotate to the university, where a faculty would go out and take a call for a week at a rural hospital. Another solution is to have at least one mid-level provider, such as a physician's assistant or a nurse practitioner, to take care of minor surgical problems like lacerations and reduction of closed fractures so that the surgeons can at least get a good night's rest.

TABLE 20.3

COMPARTMENT SYNDROMES

Cranial	Retro-orbital
Chest	Pericardium
Abdomen	Kidneys
Pelvis	Extremities
Spinal canal	

TABLE 20.4

EXPERIENCE IN RURAL SURGERY TRAINING PROGRAM[a]

GENERAL SURGERY		OTOLARYNGOLOGIC SURGERY	
Hernia	19	Tonsillar abscess	5
Breast	12	Tonsillectomy/adenoidectomy	6
Vascular[a]	14	Parotidectomy	3
Major Abdominal	57	Radical neck dissection	5
Thoracic[b]	6	Laryngectomy	2
Skin/soft tissue	11	Neck abscess	2
Appendectomies[c]	28	ORIF facial fracture	3
Cholecystectomies[d]	31	Thyroglossal duct cyst excision	3
Endoscopy	5	Facial plastics	7
Total	183	Other	4
		Total	40
ORTHOPEDIC SURGERY		**GYNECOLOGIC SURGERY**	
Hand	32	Cesarean section	9
Closed reduction of fracture	8	TAH/BSO[e]	14
ORIF of fracture (other)	18	Lap ovarian surgery	5
ORIF of hip fracture	14	Ectopic cases	3
Other	16	Other	12
Total	88	Total	43
UROLOGICAL SURGERY			
Radical cystectomy	3		
Orchiectomy	1		
Testicular torsion	1		
Radical prostatectomy	1		
TURBT	1		
TURP	1		
Radical nephrectomy	3		
Total	11		

[a] 10 carotid endartectomies, 4 cardiac cases
[b] 2 esophagectomies, 4 lung
[c] 20 laparoscopic, 8 open
[d] 25 laparoscopic, 6 open
[e] 7 performed as part of ovarian cancer staging
The total 1-year experience of the author's as 4th year surgical resident and his experience at Grants Pass, Oregon.

A fourth area of concern is the DOD, as mentioned in Part II of this manuscript. The wounds that are being treated by military surgeons are devastating wounds. Most involve the extremities, neck, and face. Body armor has been a godsend since it allows many of these soldiers to survive, but they still end up with very disabling injuries. Suicide bombers create a new threat: parts of the suicide bomber may penetrate the skin and thus lead to viral infection and transmission of disease. It is extremely difficult to train surgeons for our current conflicts. There have been many wars since World War I, but there are notable hiatuses between these conflicts and each generation has to learn from the previous generation. That includes avoiding some of the same mistakes. The DOD has also initiated a program where military surgeons spend a period of time in civilian trauma centers, but again, this is not quite as devastating as what they will be called upon to treat. DOD is also set up so that its hospitals have civilian trauma centers. Again, this does not mimic the types of wounds that it might see except in rare instances. An alternative solution that has been recommended is for DOD to fund a program where reserve surgeons could serve in civilian trauma centers on a regular basis but be subject to deployment as needed. This would mean that there would be an overage of personnel at times, and at other times, depending on the number deployed, there could be a shortage. The Air Force has a program already in place where it has reserve Air Force pilots working for commercial airlines and these individuals will do 3-month rotations to areas of conflict.

Another area of potential concern is the rise in the number of surgical hospitalists. This position is on the increase, but has yet to be fully defined. Ostensibly they are hired by the hospital to provide surgical coverage, usually on a 12-hour shift basis. Is this the same as emergency general surgery? Do all of these individuals have training in critical care? What is their incentive? Many are paid a flat salary and they are given an office (small) and their malpractice is paid for. This is attractive to many individuals, since they can have a professional career as a surgical hospitalist and yet have almost half of the month off to do other things. In many instances, these individuals are foreign medical graduates who have passed USMLE or have trained in this country.

Possibly the most contentious of the problem areas is in the area of trauma surgery. The future of trauma surgery could be very grim or it could be a time of opportunity. There are some problems that were outlined in Part II, not the least of which is the decrease in the number of open cases currently being done by trauma surgeons. Part of this is due to decreased penetrating trauma, and another is an improvement in diagnostic studies such as CT and MRI that allows one to avoid opening a body cavity. There is also the problem of competing with other specialists, particularly those in thoracic surgery and vascular surgery. This was not a problem 30 years ago, but in large academic centers, it is increasingly problematic. In my opinion, every trauma surgeon should be able to open a chest and be comfortable dealing with emergent problems. Similarly, many vascular cases do not lend themselves to endovascular arterial repairs and need to have open surgery. Who should do this when the patient arrives emergently? The trauma surgeon? The vascular surgeon? Another problem is the shift toward shift work. This creates problems in regards to continuity of care and dealing with the family. Many institutions have overlap of the shifts so that they can make rounds together, pass the baton, and discuss issues with the family. This still needs to be refined. There are also contentious areas with other specialties, including neurosurgery and orthopedics. How much should the trauma surgeon do, and when is the right time to call in a specialist? Should the trauma surgeon insert intracranial pressure monitoring devices or even intraventricular catheters? Should the trauma surgeon reduce fractures and do external fixation? There are certainly models around the world where this is done. The European model is particularly interesting, since in one instance you can train for 4 years as a general surgeon and then two or three additional years as an orthopedic surgeon, and then do both at a Level I center. In other parts of the world, such as Australia, Malaysia, and New Zealand, the general surgeon may have to do a decompressive burr hole or craniotomy because of the tyranny of distance. This is somewhat problematic in the Rocky Mountain West. In the near future, it would be optimal if trauma surgery leaders and leaders from other specialties would sit down and try to design a model that is best for the patient. This is problematic since there appears to be a shortage of specialists in the near future, such as in neurosurgery and orthopedics.

The last contentious problem that will have to be dealt with soon is the impact of health care reform on the trauma systems. I think it is fair to say that >90% of Level I trauma centers are in the traditional safety net hospitals. How will these safety net hospitals cope under health care reform? Health care reform did *not* solve all of the access problems, nor did it solve cost and quality problems. In fact, there are very few examples of systems of health care; however, trauma is probably a very notable exception. Similarly, transplantation and the STEMI program are models. Probably the biggest failure of health care reform is that there is no public option. Public option would be a clear advantage to the government and to patients if the government could contract to the safety net hospitals to provide all emergency care. In addition to these issues, health care reform has not addressed the deficiency in rehabilitation, and it certainly did not adequately address tort reform. It is the opinion of this author that we cannot wait for the next generation to solve these issues.

References

1. Majno G. *The Healing Hand: Man and Wound in the Ancient World.* Cambridge, MA: Harvard University Press; 1975.
2. Cannon WB. *Traumatic Shock.* New York: Appleton & Company; 1923.
3. Packard FR. *Life and Times of Ambroise Paré.* New York: Paule B. Hoeber; 1921.
4. Larrey DF. *Memoirs of Military Surgery and Campaigns of the French Armies.* Vol 1. Gryphon Editions. Birmingham, AL: Classics of Surgery Library; 1985.
5. Trunkey DD. Trauma. *Sci Am.* 1983;249:29–35.
6. Bazzoli GJ, Madura KJ, Cooper GF, et al. Progress in the development of trauma systems in the United States. *JAMA.* 1995; 273:395–401.
7. Bazzoli GJ. Community-based trauma system development: key barriers and facilitating factors. *J Trauma.* 1999;47(3 Suppl):322–324.
8. MacKenzie EJ, Rivara FP, Jurkovich GJ, et al. A national evaluation of the effect of trauma-center care on mortality. *N Engl J Med.* 2006; 354(4):366–78.
9. Papa L, Langland-Orban B, Flint L, et al. Assessing effectiveness of a mature trauma system: Association of trauma center presences with lower injury mortality rate. *J Trauma.* 2006;61(2):261–266; discussion 266–267.
10. Mackenzie EJ, Weir S, Rivara FP, et al. The value of trauma center care. *J Trauma.* 2010;69:1–10.
11. Carter D. The surgeon as a risk factor. *BMJ.* 2003;326:832.
12. Division of Advocacy and Health Policy. A growing crisis in patient access to emergency surgical care. *Bull Am Coll Surg.* 2006;91:9–18.
13. Esposito TJ, Maier RV, Rivara FP, et al. Why surgeons prefer not to care for trauma patients. *Arch Surg.* 1991;126:292–297.
14. The Lewin Group Analysis of AHA ED Hospital Capacity Survey, 2002. April 2001, 7–18. Available at http://www.aha.org/ahapolicyforum/resources/EDdiversionsurvey0404.html. Accessed April 4, 2006.
15. The Schumacher Group. *2005 Hospital Emergency Department Administration Survey.* Available at http://www.tsged.com/Survey2005.pdf.
16. *On-Call Specialist Coverage in U.S. Emergency Departments, American College of Emergency Physicians Survey of Emergency Department Directors.* April 2006. Available at http://www.acep.org/NR/rdonlyres/DF81A858-FD39-46F6-B46A-15DF99A45806/0/RWJ_OncallReport2006.pdf.
17. Cooper RA. Weighing the evidence for expanding physician supply. *Ann Intern Med.* 2004;141:705–714.
18. Cooper RA, Getzen TE, McKee HJ, et al. Economic and demographic trends signal an impending physician shortage. *Health Aff.* 2002;21:140–154.
19. Bland KI, Isaacs G. Contemporary trends in student selection of medical specialties: The potential impact on general surgery. *Arch Surg.* 2002;137:259–267.
20. Trunkey DD, Cahn RM, Lenfesty B, et al. Management of the geriatric trauma patient at risk of death. *Arch Surg.* 2000;135:34–38.
21. *Operation Desert Storm: Full Army Medical Capability not Achieved.* Washington, DC: U.S. General Accounting Office; 1992. GAO/NSAID–92–175.
22. *Operation Desert Storm: Improvements Required in the Navy's Wartime Medical Care Program.* Washington, DC: U.S. General Accounting Office; 1993. GAO/NSAID–93–189.
23. *Operation Desert Storm: Problems with Air Force Medical Readiness.* Washington, DC: U.S. General Accounting Office; 1993. GAO/NSIAD–94–58.
24. *Traumatic brain injury: Programs supporting long-term services in selected states.* Washington, DC: General Accounting Office; 1998. GAO/HEHS–98–55.
25. Trunkey D. Lessons learned. *Arch Surg.* 1993;128(3):261–264.

CHAPTER 21 ■ INITIAL EVALUATION OF THE TRAUMA PATIENT

LESLIE KOBAYASHI, RAUL COIMBRA AND DAVID B. HOYT

The assessment and management of the injured patient is a unique situation in which time and efficiency are of the essence. There is ample evidence in the literature that standardization of care improves outcomes and reduces morbidity and mortality in trauma patients.[1] Multiple trauma systems exist in the United States and throughout the world. However, one well-regarded and widely practiced system of trauma patient assessment and management has significantly shaped the care of the trauma patient in the last 25 years.

Advanced trauma life support (ATLS) is a course provided by the American College of Surgeons; it is meant to prepare a variety of clinicians to treat, triage, and transport the broad spectrum of trauma patients. Introduced in 1978 and rapidly adopted throughout the United States, it is now taught in more than 50 countries. Now in its eighth edition, it is the gold standard for trauma patient assessment and management. ATLS protocols are based on a comprehensive review of the international literature to date.[2]

In ATLS, the initial assessment of the trauma patient is broken down into many components including; triage, preparation, the primary and secondary surveys and their radiologic adjuncts, ongoing resuscitation, and transfer to definitive care.

The primary survey consists of the ABCDEs (airway, breathing, circulation, disability, and exposure/environment). Adjuncts to the primary survey include plain radiographs of the chest and pelvis, and the focused assessment with sonography for trauma (FAST). The secondary survey is a quick head-to-toe physical examination, the purpose of which is to rapidly identify critical injuries and determine if these injuries are going to require further imaging or necessitate transfer to another facility for definitive care. The secondary survey may include simple or advanced imaging such as extremity plain films or computed tomography (CT) scans.

Throughout the primary and secondary surveys, resuscitation of the patient must be ongoing and continually reassessed. Upon completion of the initial assessment and resuscitation of the patient to a stable or semi-stable state, a decision must be made regarding transfer to definitive care. Transfer to an appropriate setting (operating room, intensive care unit [ICU], interventional suite) or facility (tertiary care center, level I trauma center, burn center) should be initiated as soon as possible after completing the initial assessment.

With timely diagnosis and intervention being the driving force in trauma evaluation, we need to determine if our emphasis on speed is supported by the data. Much has been described regarding the Golden Hour of Trauma, the 1 hour following injury when lives may be lost or saved by proper medical attention, but is this truth or myth?

The classical trimodal distribution of trauma deaths was first described in the seminal article by Trunkey in 1983, in which he demonstrated that almost half of all trauma deaths occurred in the first hour after injury.[3] The other two peaks occurred within the next 1–4 hours and after the first week of injury. Trunkey considered many of the deaths occurring during the second peak (hours 1–4), as potentially preventable, and identification and treatment of these patients during the Golden Hour became the focus of the initial assessment. Great strides have been made in trauma systems management, prehospital emergency medical technology, resuscitation, and ICU care since this seminal paper. These advancements have resulted in more patients surviving to reach hospitals alive, and surviving after admission to the ICU, further emphasizing the need to concentrate on the early hours of trauma evaluation and resuscitation.[4,5] In a study by Bansal in a level I trauma center in San Diego, while the majority of deaths still occurred within the first hour, a second peak occurred within hours 1–3, and hemorrhage continued to contribute to deaths up to 6 hours post injury[4] (Fig. 21.1). A study by Demetriades et al.,[5] also in a mature level I trauma center in Los Angeles, revealed similar information, with the majority of deaths upon arrival and a second peak of trauma deaths between hours 1–6.[5] These studies also revealed that mechanism of injury (MOI) and body cavity involved affected time of death considerably.

TRIAGE

The concept of triage is an essential element in modern medical care where resources are nearly universally exceeded by demand, even in highly developed, technically advanced centers. The basic tenants of triage incorporate accurate assessment of victims, victim acuity and available resources, and quickly assign the proper resources to the proper patients.[6]

Many protocols exist for prehospital triage of victims, determining the optimal distribution of patients to hospitals in the area based on victim factors such as acuity and age, and the resources of the area such as number of, and distance to, specialty trauma or burn centers. The ACSCOT has a protocol for this in Resources for the Optimal Care of the Injured Patient 2006.[7]

Outside of mass casualty and disaster management situations, categorization of traumas is generally based on patient acuity. Prior to the patient's arrival, as much data from prehospital personnel should be gathered as possible. The components that determine level of acuity include clinical factors and MOI. Clinical indicators are subdivided into physiologic factors such as vital signs and level of consciousness, and anatomic factors such as body system involved—head, neck, thoracoabdominal, or isolated extremity trauma.

Trauma victims are generally classified into trauma team activations, urgent consults, or routine consults based on highest, medium, and lowest level of patient acuity and risk of substantial or operative injury. Trauma team activations (TTAs) are the highest level of trauma victims and generally require the presence of the most experienced trauma physician or surgeon, and the presence of the entire trauma team if one exists. Additional personnel who should be present at this level of acuity include an anesthesiologist or other airway specialist, radiology technologist, respiratory technologist, and trauma/emergency room/surgical ICU nurses. Additional personnel who may be helpful include a pharmacist, social worker, and ultrasonographer. Specific guideline for who must be present at TTAs for level I verification exist in the ACSCOT Resources for Optimal Care of the Injured Patient 2006.[7]

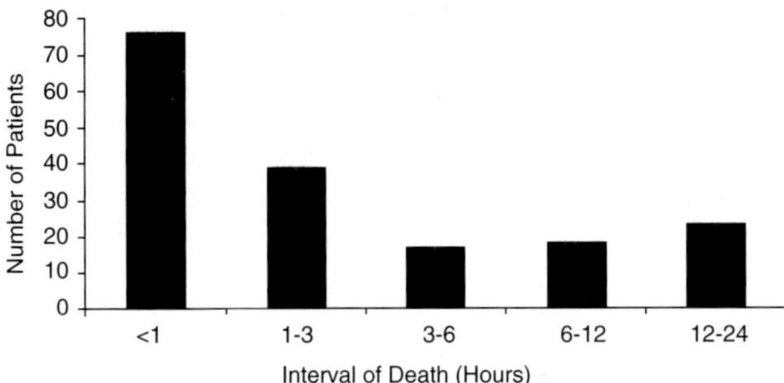

FIGURE 21.1. Distribution of in-hospital deaths over time for the first 24 hours after admission to trauma center (Data from Bansal V, Fortlage D, Lee JG, et al. Hemorrhage is more prevalent than brain injury in early trauma deaths: the Golden Six Hours. *Eur J Trauma Emerg Surg.* 2009;35:26–30.).

Many studies have validated this tiered system of trauma patient evaluation. A study by Petrie et al.[8] in 1996, comparing TTAs requiring the involvement of the trauma team in the patient's initial assessment and resuscitation to non-TTA trauma patients, revealed a notable improvement in the number of survivors compared to non-TTA patients per 100 population. This improvement in mortality occurred despite a considerably higher injury severity score (ISS). A similar study 10 years later by Cherry et al.,[9] in 2007, revealed similar results: TTA protocols correctly identified patients with higher ISS, and early (<4 weeks) mortality, and TTA patients had significantly improved survival compared to their less injured non-TTA counterparts.

Clinical Criteria

Clinical criteria for level of trauma acuity include physiologic derangements of heart rate, blood pressure, and level of consciousness. In most trauma centers, patients with significant tachycardia (heart rate ≥120), hypotension (systolic blood pressure <90), or depressed mental status (Glasgow Coma Scale (GCS) < 8) are classified as a TTA. Additionally, most patients who were intubated in the field or require assisted ventilation also meet TTA criteria.

Clinical criteria have been repeatedly validated as useful triage tools.[9–12] Although debate does exist in the literature as to specific cutoff values for triggering a TTA, several studies have confirmed hypotension with systolic blood pressure <90 as an excellent predictor of mortality and injury severity.[9–11] Tachycardia with heart rate >120 beats per minute is also a validated triage criteria, though it appears to be less specific than hypotension. Depressed mental status with GCS < 8 is also highly predictive of mortality.[9]

Mechanism Criteria

Penetrating mechanisms such as stab wounds and gunshot wounds to the trunk or neck should be considered high-level traumas. Blunt mechanisms that indicate significant force include falls over 15 feet, automobile versus pedestrian, and high-speed motor vehicle crashes. Additional factors denoting involvement of great forces in the trauma are accidents with fatalities at the scene, crashes with significant passenger space intrusion, steering column deformation, ejection of the victim from the vehicle or rollover of the vehicle.

It must be kept in mind that MOI criteria in isolation have a very low predictive value in identifying severely injured patients.[9–11] MOI criteria are most helpful when taken into account with additional patient variables such as heart rate, GCS, and anatomic area of injury. Some studies suggest that experienced EMTs are very helpful in improving the positive predictive value of MOI criteria by exercising proper discretion upon application of MOI criteria in stable and evaluable patients in the field.[10]

Age Criteria

In the Primary Survey chapter of ATLS 8th Edition, care is taken to emphasize the increased incidences of comorbidities and need for specialized resuscitation strategies for the elderly trauma patient.[13] While no specific age criteria for field triage currently exist in the ACSCOT guidelines, multiples studies confirm the unique characteristics of the elderly trauma patient.[14–18] The older trauma patient has less physiologic reserve and a much lower ability to respond to injury compared to younger patients. Elderly patients are at increased risk for substantial and more advanced comorbid conditions such as hypertension, diabetes, coronary or peripheral vascular disease, chronic obstructive pulmonary disease, and emphysema. Because of these comorbidities, the elderly are more likely to be on medications such as beta blockers, calcium channel blockers, and diuretics; these medications may mask tachycardia, worsen hypotension, and interfere with efforts at resuscitation. Additionally, elderly patients with significant injuries may not meet traditional hemodynamic criteria for a TTA. The hypertensive patients may have a normal appearing blood pressure, but compared to their baseline this may be relative hypotension; alternatively, if the patient is on a beta blocker, substantial hemorrhage may be ongoing but the compensatory tachycardic response may be blocked. Elderly patients are also more likely to be on medications such as antiplatelet agents or anticoagulants, which considerably increase their risk of bleeding. In addition, elderly patients may have a baseline alteration in mental status or dementia, or have hearing or visual deficits, making communication and evaluation more difficult.

Several studies have demonstrated increased mortality in the elderly trauma patients even after correcting for injury severity.[14,19–21] Additionally, analysis of mortality by age has identified 70 years or greater as the cutoff for considerably increased mortality.[14] Using an age of 70 years or greater alone as a TTA criteria has demonstrated improved outcomes in trauma patients.[19,20] In a series of studies by Demetriades et al., he noted that many patients 70 years or greater had severe injuries without meeting typical hemodynamic criteria for TTA (HR > 120, SBP < 90). The authors have also demonstrated improved survival in these patients after age alone was instituted as a TTA criteria.[19,20] An additional study by Scalea et al.[22] demonstrated that the elderly trauma patient had improved survival when early invasive monitoring was instituted.

Over and Undertriage

Because any triage system will not be perfect, they should be evaluated routinely to ensure over and undertriage rates are at acceptable levels. The ACSCOT has determined an acceptable under triage rate (seriously injured victims not taken to a trauma center) to be ≤5%, while the acceptable overtriage rate may vary from 25% to 50%. Because overtriage results primarily in overutilization of resources, while undertriage can result in missed injury, delay in treatment or death, there is a need to err toward overtriage rather than undertriage.

PREPARATION FOR PATIENT ARRIVAL

Given the importance of time in the initial assessment and management of the trauma patient, proper and thorough preparation prior to patient arrival is essential, and can prevent the loss of pivotal minutes in treatment after patient arrival. All monitoring devices, ECG leads, blood pressure cuffs in a variety of sizes, and pulse oximeter should be available. Warmed intravenous fluids, lactated ringers or normal saline should be available, as should blood products, O negative blood, and in some level I trauma centers, thawed universal donor plasma. Multiple intravenous access devices, angiocatheters in a variety of sizes, and central or intraosseous (IO) lines should be available, along with vacutainers for blood samples. Adjunctive devices such as suction canisters, laryngoscopes, masks and bags for ventilation, oral and nasal airways, urinary and nasogastric catheters, splinting or casting material, pelvic binders or sheets, and basic surgical instrument trays should also be available and kept stocked in standard locations that are easily and quickly accessible.

Prior to patient arrival, personal protective gear should be donned by all members of the assessment team. Universal precautions are necessary for all personnel coming into direct patient contact. Precautions should include occlusive gown, gloves, face shield or, at a minimum, eye protection, a mask and surgical cap if any sterile procedures are anticipated, and shoe covers. Protection is worn not only for the protection of the patient about to undergo sterile procedures, but for the protection of the staff from blood-borne infection. The incidence of blood-borne infections, most importantly HIV and Hepatitis C, vary in the literature, with recent studies revealing HIV in 1.4%–1.9% and Hepatitis C in 3%–8% of trauma patients.[23–25] However, a series of studies from John Hopkins University revealed much higher rates of infection among trauma patients, 26% for HIV and 33% for Hepatitis C.[26,27] The true incidence of HIV and hepatitis infection among trauma populations likely varies according to geography and type of hospital; however, full-barrier precautions should be universally employed.

PRIMARY SURVEY

The primary survey is a quick simple way to assess every trauma patient in a few minutes. Patients, upon arrival to the evaluation and resuscitation area, are visually surveyed for injuries; devices such as noninvasive blood pressure cuffs, pulse oximetry, and electrical cardiac monitors are used to obtain vital signs; large-bore intravenous access is established, and the patient is completely disrobed. The primary survey is performed by an experienced physician who should be designated prior to the patient's arrival, and is performed while simultaneously addressing any life-threatening situations in real time as they are identified.

The physical examination of the primary survey is broken down into five basic components, ABCDEs. The ABCDEs are a sequence of physical examinations that are taught in ATLS to occur in a specific sequence. This sequence has been derived to address the most quickly life-threatening injuries most rapidly; as such, airway obstruction, which can lead to death in 1–5 minutes, is first, while equally important but less rapidly lethal conditions such as hypoxia and hypotension are second and third, respectively. In reality, many of the components of the primary survey occur simultaneously; equally, many problems in one area of the primary survey impact on other areas of the primary survey. For example, a tension pneumothorax, primarily a breathing problem, may result in the appearance of airway obstruction as the patient demonstrates air hunger or inability to vocalize, and may also impact circulation by decreasing preload and resulting in hypotension. Because of this, while the protocol of the primary survey addressing ABCDE in a strict sequence is done for medical priority, the informed clinician must also be able to keep the big picture in mind. Although not part of the list of life-threatening conditions, hemorrhagic shock remains the most common cause of death following injury. However, it is unlikely that patients arriving alive to trauma centers will die of exsanguinating hemorrhage within the first few minutes after admission. These individuals may still be bleeding, but compensatory mechanisms such as vasoconstriction and tachycardia, in addition to clot formation, develop to slow down bleeding and maintain perfusion to vital organs.[6,28,29]

Adjuncts to the primary survey exist in each of the categories; in the past, these have focused primarily on plain x-rays of the cervical spine (cross-table lateral view), chest, and pelvis. In most level I trauma centers today, less emphasis is placed on plain radiography of the cervical spine during the initial assessment when protection of the cervical spine far outweighs the need to diagnose injury. The most important adjuncts of the primary survey today include a single anteroposterior view of the chest and pelvis, and ultrasonography or FAST, which includes views of the abdomen and pericardium.

During evaluation of the ABCDEs, resuscitation should be ongoing and titrated to improvements or deteriorations in vital signs. A type and screen for type-specific blood and plasma transfusion should be the first priority in obtaining blood samples. Blood should also be drawn to obtain hematologic, chemical, and coagulation profiles. Pregnancy tests should be done in all females. In addition, every effort should be made to obtain an arterial sample for the analysis of oxygenation, hypercapnia, and acid–base status.

It is important to keep in mind that the primary survey is applicable to all trauma patients; while the anatomic and physiologic responses to injury may vary, the priorities for pediatric, geriatric, and obstetric trauma patients are the same.

AIRWAY

Addressing the airway is the highest priority in the initial assessment because obstruction, occlusion, or loss of airway is the most rapidly lethal of all injuries. The clinician must assess if the airway is patent, if it is protected, and if there is an evolving injury that may impact the future patency of the airway.

The easiest way to rapidly assess for both patency and protection of the airway is to ask the patient a simple question—"are you ok?", "what is your name?" If the patient responds appropriately in a normal tone, timbre, and volume, you have assessed that they are conscious enough to protect their airway and that the airway is patent. The presence of hoarseness, weakness, or inability to speak in full sentences is an indication of impending airway compromise. Additionally, if there is gurgling, coughing, or obvious aspiration of material, this is definite evidence of obstruction. Lack of a verbal response, combativeness, or restlessness indicates inability of the patients to protect their airway. All of the above abnormalities require immediate intervention.

If airway compromise is diagnosed, the clinician should perform simple maneuvers such as the jaw thrust or chin lift, to bring the tongue and soft palate out of the oropharynx and provide high-flow supplemental oxygen by face mask. The oropharynx should be cleared with suctioning; care should be taken to avoid deep suctioning to prevent activating the gag reflex, causing vomiting and aspiration. Supplements to airway patency such as the nasal trumpet and oral airway can be considered. Care must be taken to use the oral airway only in completely obtunded patients again to avoid vomiting and aspiration. The oropharyngeal airway is placed with the aid of a tongue blade; in adults, it is inserted upside down, the end sliding along the palate, then rotated 180 degrees into proper position behind the base of the tongue; this is to avoid having the device push the tongue posteriorly during insertion and worsen obstruction. This maneuver is not used in children because of potential for injury to the palate. The nasal airway is generally well tolerated by conscious or semiconscious patients, and should be equivalent in length to the distance from the nares to the angle of the mandible. The nasopharyngeal airway should be lubricated, and then placed into one of the nares; however, it should not be used in the presence of obvious midface injury or possible facial fractures to avoid displacement of bone fragments or the device itself into the cranial vault (Fig. 21.2).

A more advanced temporary airway is the laryngeal mask airway (LMA). This soft plastic device, invented in 1983 by British anesthesiologist Archie Brain, comes in a variety of sizes and is meant to fit the posterior oropharynx. The LMA is placed in the supraglottic position and an inflatable cuff is deployed to seal the oropharynx for spontaneous or manual ventilation. A drawback of the LMA is that it does not fit into the trachea, so communication between the esophagus and trachea remains completely open and aspiration remains a significant risk. Some improvements in the design of the LMA have included esophageal drainage ports, and the ability to use the LMA to guide placement of an endotracheal tube (ETT). This last option may be attractive in patients with known or highly suspected cervical spine injuries where minimization of neck movement is of the utmost importance, and laryngoscopy may be difficult or impossible. However, optimal placement of the LMA, similar to intubation, often requires extension of the head on the neck, and, at a minimum, the jaw must be thrust forward for optimal placement. As with any airway maneuver, LMA placement is not risk free, and must be undertaken while simultaneously protecting the cervical spine with in-line traction.

Other supraglottic airways include the King Laryngeal tube and the esophageal/tracheal Combitube. These devices are meant to be inserted blindly or with the aid of a laryngoscope; they contain a large superior cuff to seal the supraglottic pharynx, and a smaller inferior cuff. In the case of the King Laryngeal tube, the smaller cuff is preferentially inserted into, and inflated in, the esophagus. Ventilation is achieved through port holes between the upper and lower cuffs in the supraglottic pharynx just above the trachea; the superior cuff prevents air leakage from the mouth and nose, and the inferior cuff prevents insufflation of the stomach and decreases risk of aspiration. The Combitube is also inserted blindly, and the superior cuff is inflated to prevent air leakage from the mouth and nose. However, the tube may be inserted into either the trachea or the esophagus; the distal portion of the tube enters the esophagus in over 90% of insertions.[30] Once the tube is placed, both cuffs are inflated. Once the cuffs are inflated, there are two ports to ventilate through—a distal port below the distal cuff can be used if the end of the Combitube is within the trachea—and ventilation proceeds as with any ETT. If, in contrast, the distal tube is in the esophagus, the patient is ventilated through proximal ports located between the superior and inferior cuffs, and ventilation proceeds through the supraglottic oropharynx, and the distal cuff prevents esophageal/stomach insufflation, as in the King Laryngeal tube. A comprehensive review of acute airway management is beyond the

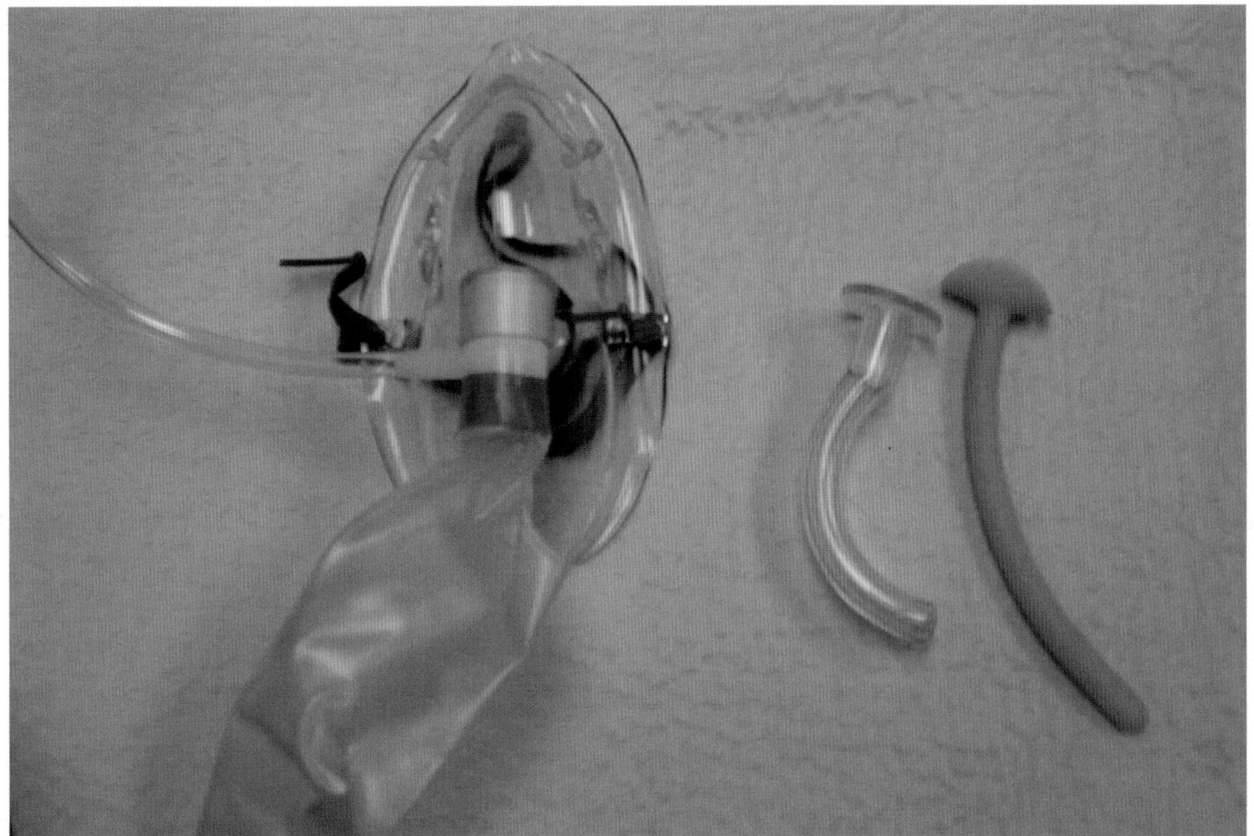

FIGURE 21.2. Basic airway adjuncts—mask with reservoir, oral and nasal airways.

scope of this chapter and can be found in the Airway Control Chapter 12 of Trauma 6th Edition.[31]

All above-mentioned maneuvers are temporizing and if the airway compromise does not resolve, a definitive airway is indicated. Strict indications for a definitive airway include obvious or impending airway obstruction, obtundation with GCS < 9, and respiratory insufficiency (hypoxia, hypercarbia, apnea). Definitive airways include orotracheal or nasotracheal intubation and surgical airways—cricothyroidotomy and tracheostomy.[32]

Placement of a definitive airway in the comatose patient can generally be accomplished without sedating or paralyzing medications, which has the benefit of avoiding pharmacologic interference with neurologic examination and possible hemodynamic compromise that is a side effect of many such agents. Additionally, the use of a paralyzing agent can often turn an urgent airway situation into an emergent airway; loss of the small amount of muscular tone in the pharynx can cause partial obstruction to turn into complete obstruction, making bag-mask-valve ventilation impossible. Occasionally, in the comatose patient, increased muscular tone and biting in the semiconscious patient make sedating and paralytic agents a necessity, as does intubation of the conscious patient. If the clinician tests jaw rigidity by performing a jaw thrust or attempts to gently open the jaws with the scissor technique and meets resistance, a sedative and paralytic should be used prior to any attempt at obtaining a definitive airway. Rapid sequence intubation is a technique of administering bolus doses of a sedative and paralytic simultaneously while using cricoid pressure (the Sellick maneuver) to prevent aspiration and the use of minimal or no preoxygenation to prevent gastric insufflation and minimize aspiration risk. One common agent used, Etomidate, is a short-acting sedative with relatively minimal cardiodepressive effects; the dosage is 0.3 mg/kg and induction occurs in 30–60 seconds. There is some suggestion in the literature that Etomidate may result in adrenal suppression and relative adrenal insufficiency, but this is still an area of active research. Some alternative sedatives include Propofol, which is also very rapid in onset, and short acting, or benzodiazepines. However, both may result in significant cardiac depression and hypotension. A popular paralytic agent is Succinylcholine, which has a rapid onset and brief duration of action. The induction dosage is 0.6 mg/kg, and the onset of action is typically within 60 seconds with a duration of 2–3 minutes. Succinylcholine is a depolarizing agent, and may result in malignant hyperthermia, and can cause cardiac arrest due to severe hyperkalemia in certain patients, including victims of burns, drowning, spinal cord transaction, and severe crush injury. In such patients, a non-depolarizing agent such as Vecuronium or Rocuronium should be considered; although the onset of action of these agents is slightly slower, their duration of action can persist much longer than with Succinylcholine, which may interfere with future neurologic examinations. If paralytic agents are used, it is important to obtain a very quick neurologic assessment prior to their administration. If 5–10 seconds can be spared, an assistant should ask the awake patient to move his or her arms/legs and briefly assess sensation, and perform a pupillary exam. In the comatose patient, painful stimuli should be applied to the arms/legs to see if any movement is elicited.

Once the patient is properly anesthetized, the preferred definitive airway is orotracheal intubation. It provides a rapid definitive airway, and the materials required to accomplish it are readily available in most health care settings. Preparation is the key in the successful intubation of a trauma patient. The most experienced physician should be utilized, and several well-trained assistants should be used to bag the patient, provide requested supplies, and maintain in-line cervical spine stabilization in addition to cricoid pressure. Equipment should include a laryngoscope with several types and sizes of blades and the light bulb should be checked for function prior to patient arrival. Other equipment includes several sizes of ETT, a stylet, equipment to suction the oropharynx, and a syringe for inflating the cuff. A minimum of three people should be involved in the intubation of the trauma patient, if at all possible. The most experienced person should be located at the head of the bed in position to intubate, the second most experienced should be in position below and to the side of the head of the bed to maintain the cervical spine in neutral position, and a third should be to the side of the bed to apply cricoid pressure if necessary and hand equipment to the person performing the intubation. All extraneous material should be removed from the patient's head and neck; the anterior portion of the C-collar be removed. The assistant maintaining cervical spine precautions must ensure that the head is maintained in line, and that the head is not extended during intubation.

Once intubation is accomplished, appropriate positioning of the ETT should be confirmed, clinically by observation of chest movements and auscultation, with a carbon dioxide detector, and radiographically. Clinical confirmation of placement is notoriously unreliable, and such markers as equal chest rise, symmetric bilateral breath sounds, and condensation on the ETT cannot be used alone for confirmation.[33] Capnography is most reliable for confirmation that the ETT is in the airway; if this is not available, colorimetric carbon dioxide detectors can be used. False-positive color change can occur with gastric intubation, but will generally fade after the first few breaths. False-negative color change can occur in patients in cardiac arrest as carbon dioxide production may be below threshold levels for detection. These instances all make continuous capnography much preferable to colorimetric detectors. Lastly, once the primary survey is completed and the patient is stable or semi-stable, a chest x-ray can confirm placement of the ETT in the trachea. Care should be taken to ensure it is not in one of the mainstem bronchi and that both lungs are equivalently inflated. Once successful tracheal intubation is confirmed, the rigid cervical collar should be reapplied. It is important that all personnel involved in the intubation remember that protection of the cervical spine is necessary at all times. Other devices such as the long backboard, sandbags, and struts with binding tape can also be used to immobilize the cervical spine.

Even after the placement of the ETT has been confirmed and it has been secured in place, care must be taken to repeatedly check that it has not been dislodged or become obstructed. Particular care must be taken to inspect for proper placement of the ETT after the patient has been moved or repositioned.

In some cases, traditional orotracheal intubation can be difficult or impossible; some high-risk situations include the obese patient, patients with substantial oromaxillofacial trauma or blood loss, mucus or emesis in the airway, patients with facial burns or inhalation injury, and patients with trauma to the neck. If available, every effort should be made to involve a clinician with advanced airway training such as the trauma surgeon, anesthesiologist, or otolaryngologist. In high-risk cases, the tools for a surgical airway should be immediately available and consideration should be given to using advanced airway adjuncts. Advanced airway tools include the bougie, Glide scope, fiberoptic intubation, and retrograde intubation (Fig. 21.3).

The bougie is a semirigid, long plastic tube with an upward angled tip; it can be passed blindly, or with laryngoscopic guidance, the upward angle preferentially directs it toward the tracheal aperture and away from the esophagus, as does the presence of cricoid pressure. The physician should be able to feel the tip pass the tracheal rings as bumps, then stop advancing when it encounters the carina, and in most cases, turn sharply right following the right mainstem bronchus. The bougie can then be used as a guide for placement of the ETT in a Seldinger-type technique.

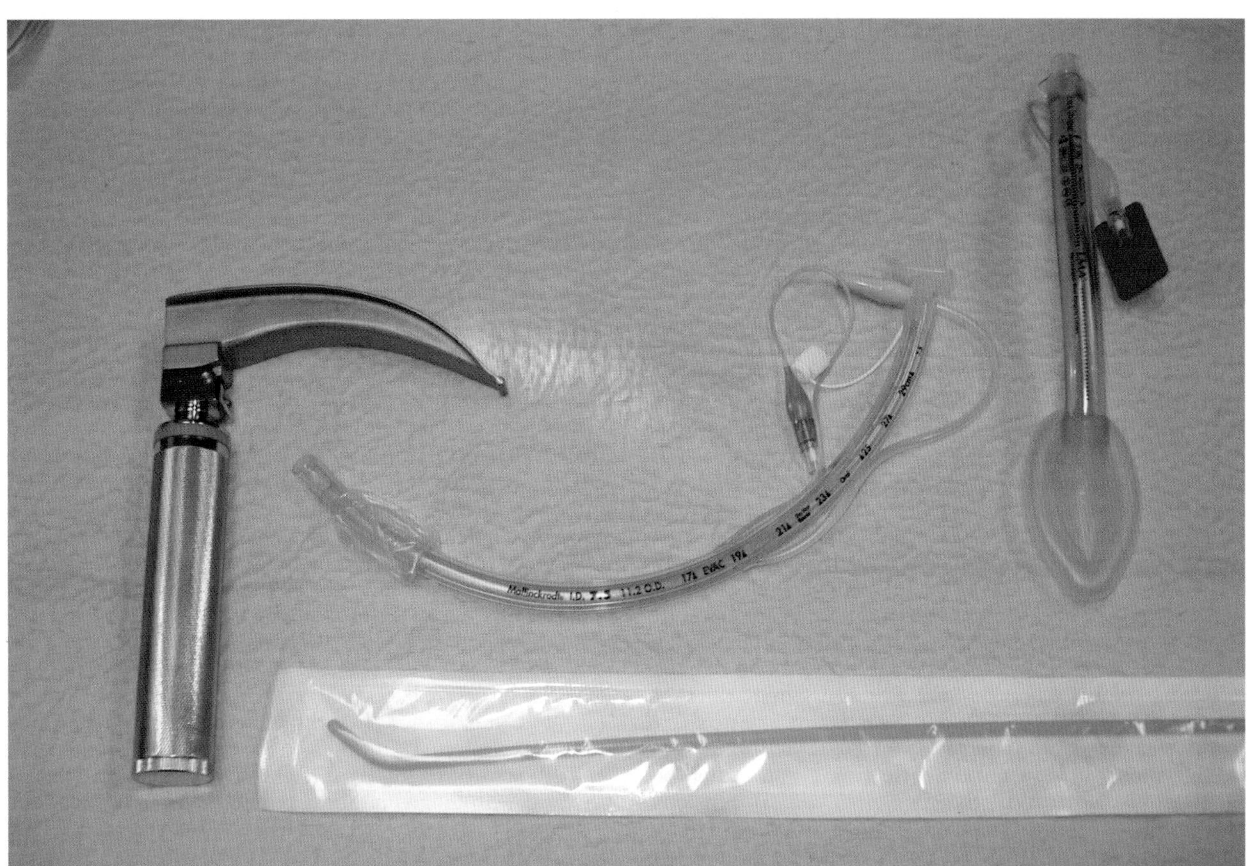

FIGURE 21.3. Definitive airway devices—ETT, LMA, bougie.

Other advanced airway techniques include use of a Glide scope, fiberoptic intubation, and retrograde intubation. The Glide scope is a laryngoscope with a camera located on the end of the laryngoscope blade. The image is sent to an attached video screen, allowing the clinician to more easily visualize the vocal cords, especially in a very anterior airway. It also allows for successful intubation with less risk of hyperextension of the neck in patients with possible cervical spine injury. Fiberoptic intubation is also an option in the potentially challenging airway. However, because fiberoptic intubation requires specialized equipment and training, it is not recommended for emergency airways, rather it is more suited to the semi-elective situation. It is particularly useful in patients that are stable or semi-stable but have injuries that make impending airway loss a high risk, such as burn patients without immediate airway compromise, patients with neck injury with possibility of expanding hematoma, or stable patients with oromaxillofacial trauma. Fiberoptic intubation ideally should take place in the operating room with surgical airway tools available should it fail. Another advanced airway technique is retrograde intubation, which is a hybrid between orotracheal intubation and surgical cricothyroidotomy. The airway is accessed via the cricothyroid membrane as in cricothyroidotomy, a wire is passed through the membrane and retrieved from the oropharynx with Magill forceps, the wire is held taught with clamps on either end and Seldinger technique is used to pass an ETT over the wire into the airway in a blind fashion.[34–36]

If the airway cannot be secured using the above techniques, or in cases where airway injury is suspected and attempts at intubation risk further injury, the goal should be to obtain a surgical airway immediately. Definitive surgical airways include cricothyroidotomy and tracheostomy. In the case of suspected or known laryngeal injury, a cricothyroidotomy would be above the level of the injury and in this case, emergent tracheostomy is the preferred airway. In all other cases, cricothyroidotomy is the preferred surgical airway. Cricothyroidotomy can be performed with percutaneous or open technique. In the traditional open technique, very few pieces of specialized equipment are necessary; a scalpel, small retractors, a Kelly, and ETT or tracheostomy tube are the only essential items. The patient's neck is exposed, again, an assistant is used to maintain strict cervical spine immobilization, the cricothyroid membrane is palpated between the thyroid and cricoid cartilages, a vertical midline incision is made in the skin, the membrane is exposed and divided in the transverse direction to avoid injury to the overlying vocal cords, and the ETT or tracheostomy tube is placed into the airway. Clinical exam and capnography are then used to confirm placement into the airway. In the obese patient or the patient with significant soft tissue injury that distorts the traditional landmarks, the cricoid cartilage can be located by placing the smallest finger of the clinician's right hand into the sternal notch; the index finger is then located immediately above the cricothyroid membrane. Many companies manufacture kits for percutaneous cricothyroidotomy. The kits will generally include a scalpel to create the incision, a large-bore needle for accessing the airway through the membrane, a wire to pass through the needle, a plastic dilator to create a passage, and a small rigid tube similar to a tracheostomy tube for ventilation.

There is some debate as to whether or not cricothyroidotomy tubes need to be replaced with a formal surgical tracheostomy for long-term ventilation. Traditionally, all cricothyroidotomies were converted electively to tracheostomies for fear of subglottic stenosis caused by irritation of the airway.

However, recent studies in trauma and ICU populations have demonstrated no increased risk of stenosis compared to tracheostomies.[37–40] These studies reveal that the rates of tracheal stenosis up to 60 months following decannulation are lower than previously thought (overall <3%), and are comparable to rates of stenosis following tracheostomy.[39] They additionally show equivalent rates of successful decannulation, and some reveal a significantly higher rate of complications associated with conversion to tracheostomy.[37,40] Although long-term use of cricothyroidotomy is still an area of controversy, its routine conversion to tracheostomy should be questioned.

In certain patients, the airway may be patent and protected upon initial inspection but may be in danger of rapidly becoming compromised. These high-risk patients benefit from elective placement of a definitive airway in a controlled fashion prior to the development of symptoms or frank airway compromise. Elective intubation to secure a definitive airway is particularly important if the patient will require transport to another location for definitive care, or if prolonged diagnostic studies are planned. Such situations include patients with significant burns, especially if the burn involves the face, or if there is evidence of inhalational injury, patients with substantial oromaxillofacial or neck trauma, where subsequent soft tissue swelling or copious bleeding or secretions may rapidly obstruct the airway, and patients with significant traumatic brain injury where declining or waxing and waning GCS may lead to inability to protect the airway. Finally, agitated and combative patients or those with acute alcohol or drug intoxication may be unable to protect their airway and should be promptly intubated as well.

Pediatric Airway

Intubation of the pediatric trauma victim requires knowledge of the anatomic and physiologic differences in pediatric patients. Children are obligate nasal breathers, so keeping the nasopharynx clear of obstruction, mucus, and blood is of paramount importance. Supplemental oxygen must be directed toward nasal breathing. If definitive airway is indicated, orotracheal intubation is again the preferred route, but it may be more challenging, especially to the inexperienced clinician. In particular, the pediatric airway is more challenging not simply due to smaller size but also because the epiglottis is proportionally larger and more floppy in children than adults and more difficult to maneuver around. Additionally, the airway is higher and more anterior, making visualization during direct laryngoscopy more difficult. Because of these anatomic features, intubation may be easier with the use of a straight or Miller blade, which can be used to directly lift up the epiglottis, allowing visualization of the true vocal cords. Lastly, the airway is proportionally shorter in children, this coupled with their smaller stature overall makes bronchial intubation a much higher risk in children. Outside of the airway itself, children have a more pronounced vagal response and may develop considerable bradycardia, which is also more likely to be severe and rapid in onset in response to hypoxia. Because cardiac output is primarily determined by heart rate in children, bradycardia will result in notable hypotension and hypoperfusion. Therefore, atropine should, at a minimum, be available during any airway maneuver, and prophylactic administration prior to laryngoscopy is widely practiced.

Proper sizing of the ETT can be determined by three general methods. First, the Broselow tape can be used to estimate the patient's weight and all equipment and drug dosages required for intubation; second, the patient's small finger is a rough estimate of the external diameter of the ETT; lastly, the modified Cole formula can be used. The (childs age + 4)/4 will give the optimal internal diameter of the ETT. The ETT should be inserted to a depth of three times the internal diameter of the ETT used. Again, care must be taken to confirm appropriate position of the ETT after intubation, keeping in mind the much higher risk of bronchial intubation. Tracheal placement can be confirmed with auscultation of symmetric breath sounds over both lateral lung fields, equivalent chest rise bilaterally, return of carbon dioxide on capnography or colorimetry, and lastly, with radiographic evaluation.

One area of controversy is the use of cuffed versus uncuffed ETTs in the pediatric population. Traditionally, it has been taught that all children <8 years of age should be intubated with an uncuffed ETT, to avoid compression of the tracheal mucosa against the nondistensible cricoid ring, which in children is the narrowest portion of the airway. This was thought to prevent post-extubation stridor and tracheal stenosis. However, there has been little in the literature to support such claims of damage. Additionally, ETTs today are technically advanced over earlier models and the low-pressure, high-volume cuffs much less damaging. Recent changes in pediatric guidelines from the American Heart Association in 2005 and the Resuscitation Council of the United Kingdom in 2005 regarding CPR in pediatric and neonatal patients state that cuffed ETTs may be used in infants and children (except newborns), and that provided proper cuff pressures (<20 cm water) are used, they are as safe as uncuffed ETT.[41,42] Additionally, rather than age, the primary determinants for use of cuffed or uncuffed ETT in children should be the underlying reason for intubation and suspected duration of intubation.[42–46] In particular, patients with burns or severe pulmonary injuries that are likely to require prolonged intubation with higher levels of ventilatory support will likely benefit from the use of cuffed ETT.[44,45] In these patients, the use of cuffed tubes will aid in the delivery of adequate ventilation at higher pressures, and prevent the need for dangerous ETT exchanges due to air leaks, which occur frequently in this population.[44,45] Even in the elective surgical population, there is level I evidence that the use of a cuffed ETT decreases the number of re-intubations or ETT exchanges due to sizing or air leak without any increase in unsuccessful extubations or post-extubation stridor in patients younger than 5 years.[46] While these studies apply primarily to the in-hospital population, there is a growing body of evidence to support the use of uncuffed ETT in the prehospital setting as well, though further studies are required before this can be recommended.[43]

If orotracheal intubation is unsuccessful, a surgical airway is indicated as in adults. However, cricothyroidotomy is not recommended for pediatric patients under 12 years of age. Instead, the airway is accessed with percutaneous placement of a large-bore needle into the cricothyroid membrane and jet insufflation is used to temporarily oxygenate the patient. Air is insufflated at high pressures using jet insufflation in order to overcome the high resistance of the long, narrow catheter. Insufflation is performed for 1 second with intervening 4-second intervals to allow passive release of carbon dioxide. Ventilation is necessarily restricted and carbon dioxide levels will predictably rise over time. Conversion to a tracheostomy or repeated attempt at intubation with advanced airway adjuncts or more experienced personnel must be performed within the next 45 minutes once oxygenation is improved to prevent the accumulation of unacceptable levels of carbon dioxide.[47]

BREATHING

Once the airway has been assessed as patent or a definitive airway has been secured, the primary survey moves on to breathing. Breathing encompasses a brief inspection of the chest and assessment of the adequacy of oxygenation and ventilation. Conditions in this realm that should be diagnosed in the primary survey include tension pneumothorax, open pneumothorax (or sucking chest wound), massive hemothorax, and flail chest.

Assessment begins with visual inspection of the thorax, all clothing must be removed and the anterior and posterior chest and axillae should be inspected for lacerations, ecchymoses, open wounds, air bubbling from wounds, symmetry of chest rise, paradoxical motion of any portion of the chest, and the use of accessory muscle for respiration. Pulse oximetry should be applied as soon as the patient arrives, and continuously reassessed for sufficiency. The chest should be palpated for crepitus, tenderness, and instability of the sternum or ribs. The chest should be auscultated for the presence and symmetry of breath sounds, and dullness of cardiac or breath sounds. Lastly, a chest x-ray should be performed as soon as is feasible to radiographically evaluate the soft tissues, bones, lung parenchyma, and thoracic cavities. Throughout the assessment, high-flow oxygen should be administered to the patient.

Tension pneumothorax is the most rapidly life-threatening of all breathing problems. It occurs when air continuously enters the thoracic cavity from the lung, airway, or atmosphere and cannot escape. The pressure causes collapse of the lungs, preventing oxygenation and ventilation on the ipsilateral side, and eventually causes deviation of the mediastinum away from the tension pneumothorax. This causes compression of the superior and inferior vena cava, decreasing preload to the heart and resulting in hypotension. Tension pneumothorax should be recognized immediately by air hunger, hypoxia, tachypnea, hyperresonance, unilateral absence of breath sounds, deviation of the trachea away from the affected side, distended neck veins, hypotension, and tachycardia. Crepitus may be felt as well, but is nonspecific. The tracheal deviation may be difficult to visualize with a rigid cervical collar in place, and may be prevented from occurring if the patient is intubated as a greater pressure is required to deform the more rigid plastic ETT. Additionally, distended neck veins may not be present if the patient has concomitant hypovolemia. Lastly, tension pneumothorax may be confused with pericardial tamponade as both result in distended neck veins, a feeling of impending doom or restlessness, and hypotension. However, tamponade will result in muffled heart sounds and does not cause tracheal deviation or asymmetrical breath sounds. If tension pneumothorax is suspected, emergent decompression must be performed. ATLS recommends needle decompression with large-bore needles or angiocatheters placed in the second intercostal space in the midclavicular line. If the needle is properly placed, a rush of air should be observed with an immediate improvement in vital signs, as the tension pneumothorax is converted to a simple pneumothorax. This should then be followed by the placement of a chest tube for more permanent decompression of the affected hemithorax, and drainage of any blood that may be associated with the tension pneumothorax.

If no air is noted, the needle may be in the subcutaneous tissue, there may be no pneumothorax, or the wrong side may have been accessed. A second decompression of the contralateral chest should be undertaken; if no rush of air is again noted, tension pneumothorax is unlikely and cardiac tamponade should be considered, and rapid FAST should be performed to assess for pericardial fluid. Occasionally, in the obese patient or in patients with significant soft tissue edema/hematomas, needle decompression may not be possible as the device may not be long enough to reach the thoracic cavity in this situation, or if the clinician is very comfortable with chest tube placement, needle decompression may be skipped in favor of immediate chest tube placement.

Chest tubes in experienced hands can be placed in <60 seconds. The most important step is the entry of the thoracic cavity to allow escape of the air trapped there, which is accomplished even more rapidly and occurs once the thorax has been entered by blunt dissection. The chest tube should be placed in the midaxillary line in the fourth or fifth interspace at the level of the nipple in males, and the inframammary fold in females. A small incision, approximately 1.5–2 cm in length, is made with a scalpel, a clamp is used to bluntly dissect the subcutaneous tissue until the bony rib is felt. The clamp is then used to bluntly enter the thoracic cavity immediately over the top of the rib to avoid injury to the neurovascular bundle located beneath each rib. Significant force may be required to create this entry. A rush of air or blood should be observed upon entry into the pleural cavity, immediately relieving intrathoracic tension and improving the patient's vital signs. The clamp is then used to bluntly spread the soft tissues, creating an opening in the intercostal tissue to accommodate a 36 French chest tube. Digital manipulation should be used to guide the tube posteriorly and cephalad to drain the thorax. In most adults, insertion of 10–12 cm of the tube should be adequate to ensure the last side port is within the chest cavity. In all cases, further advancement of the tube should be stopped as soon as resistance is felt. The tube is then secured in place with a suture and the insertion site dressed with an occlusive dressing. The end of the tube should then be connected to a closed drainage system. In all trauma patients, this collection system should be prepared sterilely with citrate, an anticoagulant, so that any collected blood can be autotransfused back into the patient if desired.

In cases where the tension pneumothorax has been converted to simple pneumothorax by needle decompression or in cases of simple pneumothorax or simple hemothorax, care should be taken during placement of chest tubes to maintain sterility. A cap, mask, gown, and sterile gloves should be worn by the clinician and a cap and mask should be worn by everyone in the room. Chlorhexidine preparations are preferred over povidone antiseptics as they have a decreased risk of surgical site infections. The site should be properly cleansed and anesthetized and completely draped to avoid contamination of the site, instruments, or chest tube. A single dose of preprocedure antibiotics with gram-positive coverage has proven as effective as a 24-hour course of periprocedure antibiotic prophylaxis. Antibiotic prophylaxis longer than 24 hours is not effective in preventing infection or empyema and is not recommended.

Massive hemothorax may also present with tension physiology. Hypotension may be a result of decreased preload from tension physiology as well as from massive blood loss. Treatment is immediate placement of a chest tube to the affected side. In contrast to tension pneumothorax, massive hemothorax rarely results in distended neck veins because of associated hypovolemia. Blood loss of >1,500 mL defines a massive hemothorax and is an indication for operative exploration. Additional indications for thoracotomy include massive continuous air leak, which may indicate massive parenchymal lung injury or injury to a major airway, and blood loss of 200 mL an hour for >4 hours. Again, every effort should be made to collect shed blood in a sterile fashion so that it may be autotransfused. Anticoagulation can be accomplished by the addition of citrate, in a 1:7 ratio, to the blood being transfused. After the addition of citrate, the blood can be immediately transfused back into the patient with the use of a standard blood filter and tubing. Many studies have demonstrated the safety of autotransfusion of blood collected from traumatic hemothorax.[48,49] Though the character of the autotransfused blood has not been extensively studied, available data would suggest that this blood is inherently depleted of coagulation factors, particularly Factor VIII and fibrinogen, as well as platelets; however, studies of circulating blood after autotransfusion show only mild increases in PT/aPTT, and a moderate decrease in circulating platelets.[50,51]Consideration should be given to additional transfusion of platelets when massive autotransfusion occurs.

TRAUMA

Open pneumothorax, or sucking chest wounds occur when a defect in the chest wall is full thickness and large enough for air to communicate between the thoracic cavity and the environment. During inspiration, negative pressure in the thoracic cavity sucks air into the hemithorax, preferentially over the lungs, resulting in hypoxia. The wound should be grossly decontaminated by removal of metal, dirt, and other visible objects, and an occlusive dressing should be applied and secured on three sides. This prevents air from being sucked into the thoracic cavity, but if intrathoracic pressure builds, it may escape from under the fourth side, preventing tension physiology from developing. A chest tube should be placed to relieve the pneumothorax as soon as possible. When the initial assessment is completed and the patient is stable, the wound should be cleansed, debrided, and closed in the operating room.

A flail chest occurs when three or more contiguous ribs are broken in two places, creating a segment of bone and muscle that can move independently of the thoracic wall (Fig. 21.4). This independent segment will move paradoxically with spontaneous respirations, pulling inward with inspiration secondary to negative intrathoracic pressure. This paradoxical motion can cause significant pain to the patient as the broken ribs grate upon one another, resulting in desire to take rapid shallow breaths, causing atelectasis and hypoxia. Additionally, the force required to create a flail segment is excessive and usually also results in significant underlying pulmonary contusion further increasing hypoxia. Lastly, the flail segment may be associated with a hemothorax or pneumothorax. These are treated with a chest tube as previously described. Treatment of the flail segment varies according to patient presentation. If stable, supplemental oxygen, aggressive pulmonary toilet, and adequate analgesia are suitable. Pain can be controlled with oral medications, intravenous medications, patient-controlled analgesia, local anesthetic with rib blocks, or catheters that deliver a continuous stream of local anesthetic, or with epidural anesthesia. There is evidence that epidural pain control is superior to other methods.[52,53] In unstable or semi-stable patients, intubation and positive pressure ventilation are the best treatments. The intubation allows more aggressive pain management and sedation; the positive pressure ventilation can be used to recruit atelectatic lung, and support contused lung to improve oxygenation. Additionally, the positive pressure ventilation splints the flail segment so that the paradoxical motion is halted and the entirety of the thoracic wall can move in synchrony, relieving pain and allowing healing of the soft tissue and bones. The elderly patient is particularly susceptible to deterioration after chest trauma, and pain management and pulmonary toilet should be very aggressive, with a low threshold for intubation. Avoidance of fluid overload in patients with flail chest and large pulmonary contusions is also advisable.

Once the most immediately life-threatening injuries have been addressed, adjuncts to the breathing assessment such as arterial blood gas and plain radiographs can be obtained. Arterial blood gas is especially important in the head-injured and comatose patient as significant hypercapnea may be present and is difficult or impossible to assess clinically. The ability to

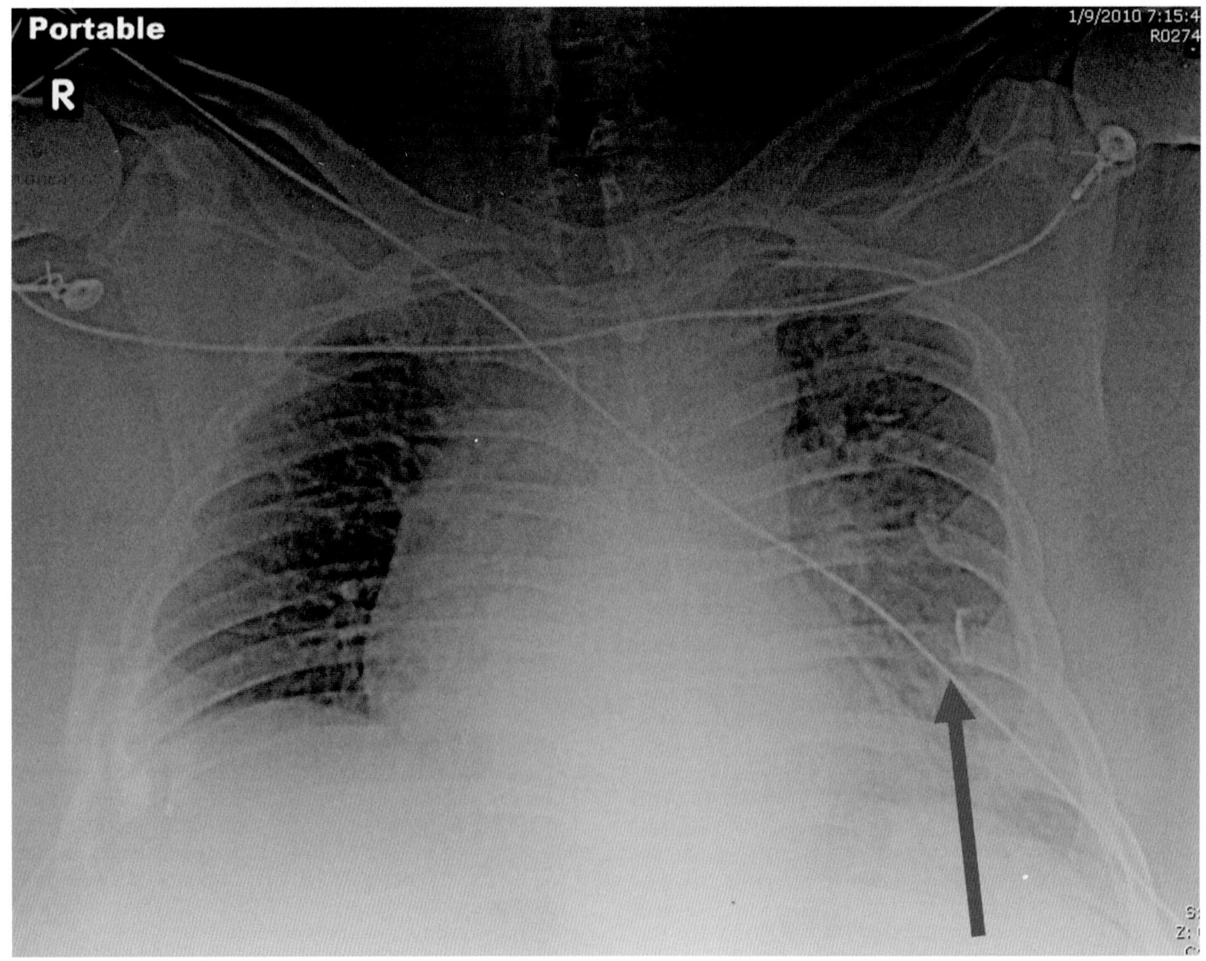

FIGURE 21.4. Chest x-ray showing multiple left-side rib fractures (flail chest).

monitor capnography in the trauma or resuscitation bay will help with the diagnosis of hypercapnea, although a baseline correlation with an arterial blood sample is recommended. Arterial blood gas can also be helpful in assessing oxygenation in patients in whom pulse oximetry may be unreliable such as very cold patients, patients who are very anemic, patients with significant soft tissue injury, making placement of the monitor difficult, patients with hypotension in whom peripheral vasoconstriction makes measurements unreliable, and burn patients. Burn patients also benefit from co-oximetry of arterial samples to detect carbon monoxide. Chest x-ray is an essential adjunct to the primary survey and can aid in diagnosis and guide treatment for both airway and breathing problems. It can be used to assess correct positioning of definitive airways and chest tubes, detect pneumothorax, hemothorax, pulmonary contusion, and broken ribs. Chest x-ray can also reveal a widened mediastinum, which can indicate thoracic aortic injury or thoracic spinal fracture, and enlarged cardiac silhouette that might indicate the presence of pericardial fluid.[54] Chest x-ray is quickly obtained, results in minimal exposure to ionizing radiation, and is easily repeatable. Additionally, the FAST can be extended to examine the thorax in the FASTER (FAST + extremities + respiratory) exam. In the FASTER exam, the ultrasound is used to look for sliding of the parietal pleura over the visceral pleura; absence of this sign indicates a pneumothorax. Several studies have shown the FASTER exam can be easily performed and is repeatable with excellent sensitivity.[55,56]

CIRCULATION

After securing the airway and restoring oxygenation and ventilation, attention can be turned to the circulation. Assessment of circulation is primarily an assessment of the presence or absence of shock. Shock is the inability of the body to maintain end-organ perfusion. The types of shock include cardiogenic, redistributive, and hypovolemic. Hypovolemic shock due to blood loss is the most common of the three, and should be assumed to be the cause of hypotension in all trauma patients until all obvious and occult blood loss has been completely ruled out.

Cardiogenic shock results from abnormalities of conduction or myocardial function with subsequent decrease in cardiac output. In trauma, blunt cardiac injury may rarely result in myocardial depression to the point of cardiogenic shock. However, this is extremely rare. Additional cardiac sources of hypotension in trauma patients include cardiac tamponade and tension pneumothorax. With cardiac tamponade, external compression of the heart, as well as decreased preload due to pericardial fluid result in hypotension. Clinical indications of tamponade include a feeling of restlessness and impending doom, inability of the patient to lie supine, distended neck veins, muffled heart sounds, and pulsus paradoxus. Diagnosis can be confirmed with pericardial FAST, which is highly sensitive and specific, nearing 100% in most studies.[57–60] If tamponade is confirmed, treatment is median sternotomy in the stable or semi-stable patient, and resuscitative thoracotomy in the Emergency Room in the unstable patient.[61] If no surgeon is present, pericardiocentesis via the subxiphoid window can be used to temporize the patient until surgical capabilities exist. Additionally, these patients should be given large volumes of fluids to increase preload and assist cardiac output.

Redistributive shock occurs as a result of increased vascular capacitance and occurs with sepsis and in neurogenic shock after high spinal cord injury where sympathectomy results in massive vasodilation. Neurogenic shock primarily occurs after cervical or high thoracic spinal cord transection. It is characterized by hypotension without evidence of blood loss, and if the transection occurs in the mid- or high cervical spine, it is often associated with inappropriate bradycardia due to unopposed vagal tone on the heart. Neurogenic shock is treated with volume expansion with crystalloids and, if necessary, vasopressors or inotropes. It is a diagnosis of exclusion in trauma patients and should not be considered the definite etiology of hypotension until hemorrhagic shock is exhaustively ruled out. Signs of neurogenic shock include evidence of spinal cord injury such as quadriplegia and apnea; occasionally, evidence of peripheral vasodilation can be seen with the lower half of the body becoming hyperemic with a linear demarcation at the level of cord injury.

By far the most common type of shock encountered in trauma is hemorrhagic shock. Hemorrhagic shock is classified according to severity, with class I shock being minor and generally asymptomatic, and class IV shock being severe, with loss of over 40% of circulating blood volume or 1,500 mL, and results in multisystem organ failure[6,28,29,61] (Table 21.1).

The clinical examination consists of measurement of heart rate, blood pressure, palpation of pulses in all extremities, and localization of blood loss. Indicators of shock include cool clammy extremities, pale skin, increased skin turgor, low urine output, dry mucus membranes, and alterations in mental status. In certain patients, the clinician must keep in mind that significant blood loss can occur, or be ongoing, with little derangement of heart rate and blood pressure. In particular, pediatric patients and young healthy athletes have excellent cardiovascular reserve and compliant vessels that are able to vasoconstrict considerably to prevent drop in blood pressure even in the presence of a great volume of blood loss. In these patients, often the first sign of hemorrhage is a narrowed pulse pressure as the body responds to blood loss with peripheral vasoconstriction, raising diastolic pressure, while maintaining normal systolic pressures. Narrowing pulse pressure may then be a sign of imminent cardiovascular collapse. Additionally,

TABLE 21.1

CLASSES OF HEMORRHAGIC SHOCK

	CLASS I	CLASS II	CLASS III	CLASS IV
EBL	<15% 500–750 mL	15%–30% 750–1,000 mL	30%–40% 1,000–1,500 mL	>40% >1,500 mL
HR	Normal	100–120	120–140	>140
BP	Normal	Decreased pulse pressure	Decreased SBP	Severe hypotension
Mental status	Anxious	Confused	Very confused	Obtunded
UOP	Normal	Normal	Decreased	Severely decreased or anuric

elderly patients often lack the intrinsic ability to mount a tachycardic response to hemorrhage, and may also be on beta blockers. The elderly often also have underlying hypertension and present with apparently normal blood pressure, which for them is relatively hypotensive. The lack of physiologic reserve in the elderly often results in patients presenting initially with apparently normal vital signs, then rapidly decompensating with complete cardiovascular collapse.

Resuscitation

Concomitant with examination to localize and control sources of blood loss, resuscitation should be ongoing. Resuscitation begins with placement of two large-bore intravenous lines or placement of an IO or central line if peripheral venous access is not possible secondary to peripheral vasoconstriction, or extremity trauma. IO lines can be placed into several areas, including the tibia, humerus, sternum, and clavicle. Traditionally, IO lines were only used for pediatric patients, but newer electric drills and increasing experience in both military and civilian populations have shown excellent results in adult populations.[62–68] Compared to peripheral and central venous access in a challenging multi-trauma patient, especially in combat, or transport settings, or if the treating team must wear protective (radiation, toxin, biological) gear, IO access is quicker and easier and may result in fewer exposures of staff to blood-borne infections.[65,66] The rate of infusion of crystalloid and blood products, and the range of medications that can be infused through an IO line are excellent and comparable to peripheral venous access.[62,66] Recent guidelines by the Eastern Association for the Surgery of Trauma (EAST) in 2009 recommend IO access in the prehospital setting if peripheral intravenous access is difficult or impossible.[69] As with any invasive procedure, complications from IO insertion do occur, such as compartment syndrome, osteomyelitis, and fracture; however, in most studies, the complication rate is very low.[62–68] The more traditional central venous catheter is also an option in patients in whom peripheral access is difficult or has failed. Locations for central lines include jugular, subclavian, and femoral. The choice of location should depend on the clinician's level of comfort and experience with each site, and location of injuries. Care should be taken to avoid placement of central lines when significant vascular injury proximal to the access site is suspected. The femoral sites and subclavian sites are easily accessible, while the jugular site tends to be less accessible due to the presence of cervical immobilization devices and need for access to the head for airway control. Other choices for venous access include saphenous vein cutdown at the ankle or groin, or cutdown to the cephalic or basilic vein in the antecubital fossa.

Once access has been obtained, resuscitation should begin with warmed fluids. Traditional teaching, including ATLS, suggests immediate infusion of 2 L of warmed crystalloid if hypotension is present. If the systolic blood pressure fails to improve to over 90 mm Hg with crystalloid bolus, O negative, or type-specific, (if available) packed red blood cells (PRBCs) should be transfused. However, there is data to suggest that in penetrating torso trauma, a strategy of permissive hypotension may be beneficial until patients can reach a location where definitive hemostasis can be achieved.[70] A study of penetrating torso trauma in which patients were randomized to traditional fluid resuscitation protocols, or delayed resuscitation receiving no more than 100 mL of fluid prior to arrival in the operating room, revealed a significant survival benefit in patients with delayed fluid resuscitation, as well as fewer complications and shorter hospital lengths of stay.[70] Proponents of permissive hypotension, including the military,[71] suggest that administration of crystalloid may aggravate the inflammatory response, dilute clotting factors, induce hypothermia, and increase blood pressures, resulting in higher levels of blood loss prior to definitive hemostasis, and result in increased transfusion requirements and worse outcomes. Opponents suggest that untreated hypoperfusion causes more tissue ischemia and resultant inflammation and reperfusion injury, and may increase secondary injury in patients with traumatic brain injury.[72] Additionally, few studies have been able to replicate the positive effects of delayed resuscitation.[73,74] At this time, there is still active debate as to the benefit of permissive hypotension and its application to any group other than penetrating torso trauma victims. The mainstay of the treatment of hemorrhagic shock continues to be active fluid resuscitation with warmed crystalloid followed by warmed blood and immediate localization and source control of bleeding.[6,29,75]

Once blood transfusion has begun, another area of controversy is the optimum ratio of red cells to fresh frozen plasma (FFP) and platelets in patients requiring ongoing massive transfusion. Massive transfusion is variably defined in the literature but is generally accepted for any patient requiring >10 units of PRBCs within the first 24 hours of hospitalization.[76] At this level of transfusion, hemodilution of fibrinogen, platelets, and clotting factors can occur as whole blood continues to be lost, and is replaced with only PRBCs. The goal of massive transfusion protocols (MTPs) is to standardize the replacement of platelets and clotting factors in the optimum ratio to red cells to prevent coagulopathy, but avoid increased risks of multisystem organ dysfunction and increase efficiency of transfusion.[77,78] Traditionally, MTPs have focused primarily on early and aggressive transfusion of PRBCs;[76] however, recent experience in both military and civilian settings have suggested that earlier aggressive transfusion of platelets and FFP can result in decreased mortality.[76,79–83] Two studies from the military revealed decreased mortality in a step-wise fashion with increasing plasma to red cell ratio, with optimal results approaching a ratio of one to one.[79,82] Civilian literature has also reflected improved mortality with a FFP:PRBC ratio approaching 1:1.3 to 1:1.5.[80,83,84] In addition to supporting a higher FFP:PRBC ratio, these studies found that the impact on mortality was most prominent in early and operative deaths, suggesting that the immediate replacement of clotting factors and the prevention of coagulopathy are most important in preventing deaths due to traumatic hemorrhage. Additionally, a study from Spain et al. found that while the institution of a MTP in their institution did not change the FFP:PRBC ratio, already high at 1:1.8, the protocol did result in faster times to transfusion of first blood products and decreased mortality.[81]

Another adjunct to balanced transfusion strategies is the use of pharmacologic agents to treat and prevent coagulopathy. One such agent undergoing scrutiny is recombinant human Factor VIIa. This agent was originally developed for the treatment of hemophilia. It has since enjoyed off-label use in a number of clinical scenarios, including treatment of coagulopathy in trauma and reversal of anticoagulation in patients with traumatic brain injury. A randomized controlled trial of recombinant Factor VIIa demonstrated a decrease in PRBC transfusion requirements and a reduced need for massive transfusion in blunt trauma patients, without an increase in complications compared to placebo.[85] A follow-up study from the same group confirmed the benefit of decreased transfusion requirements, and additionally demonstrated lower rates of multisystem organ failure and ARDS with the use of activated Factor VIIa.[86] However, no mortality benefit has been found in trauma patients, and concerns regarding increased thromboembolic complications exist. Equally effective is prothrombin complex, which has all four vitamin K-dependent coagulation factors: II, VII, IX, X.[76]

Other adjuncts to balanced transfusion include resuscitation with alternative crystalloid solutions, one of the most well studied being hypertonic saline. There is experimental evidence that hypertonic saline has anti-inflammatory effects in both humans and animal models, when compared to isotonic crystalloids.[87–93] Those data also demonstrate decreased lung and intestinal injury from hypoperfusion with hypertonic saline resuscitation.[88–90,93] There is also good clinical evidence to suggest that hypertonic saline resuscitation in trauma patients may improve survival compared to traditional resuscitation fluids, especially in the presence of hemorrhage requiring massive transfusion, surgical intervention, or depressed GCS.[94–97] It has additional benefits for patients with traumatic brain injury as it acts as an osmotic agent to decrease cerebral edema.[98–100] Hypertonic solutions also create more intravascular volume expansion than isotonic fluid on a volume-by-volume basis, making it an ideal resuscitation fluid for the military where portability and limited storage capacity must factor into all clinical decision making.[101,102]

Localizing Blood Loss

Areas where significant blood loss can occur include external loss onto the gurney or at the scene from open wounds, into the chest, into the abdomen, into the pelvis or retroperitoneum, and into the extremities.

Wounds

Open wounds and lacerations should be inspected for arterial or high-volume bleeding. Active bleeding should be addressed as soon as possible in the operating room or trauma bay. Temporizing measures in areas without surgical capabilities include application of pressure, manual compression dressings, tourniquets, or application of advanced local hemostatic agents. Hemostatic agents fall into a number of broad categories including cellulose based, desiccating agents (zeolite, chitan), collagen- and fibrin/thrombin-based products. A number of promising studies have arisen from military experience with application of tourniquets and advanced local hemostatic agents including chitan and xeolite based agents.[103–105] More superficial lacerations, especially if located on the scalp, should be closed with staples or sutures to tamponade bleeding as soon as is feasible.

Thoracic Cavity

Bleeding into the chest can be clinically apparent if massive hemothorax with tension physiology occurs, or if chest tubes are placed. More frequent bleeding into the thoracic cavity is clinically occult, with evidence of shock, but no obvious signs of thoracic source on clinical exam. Some subtle signs may be decreased breath sounds on auscultation on the ipsilateral hemithorax, and external evidence of trauma to the chest wall. In patients *in extremis*, bilateral chest tubes should be placed immediately to assess for thoracic source of bleeding.[61] The primary method of diagnosing a thoracic source of blood loss in stable patients is with chest x-ray. Pleural effusion, appearance of elevated hemidiaphragm, and "white-out" of the affected lung field are all indications of hemothorax and should be treated with immediate placement of a thoracostomy tube (Fig. 21.5). As stated previously, the collection

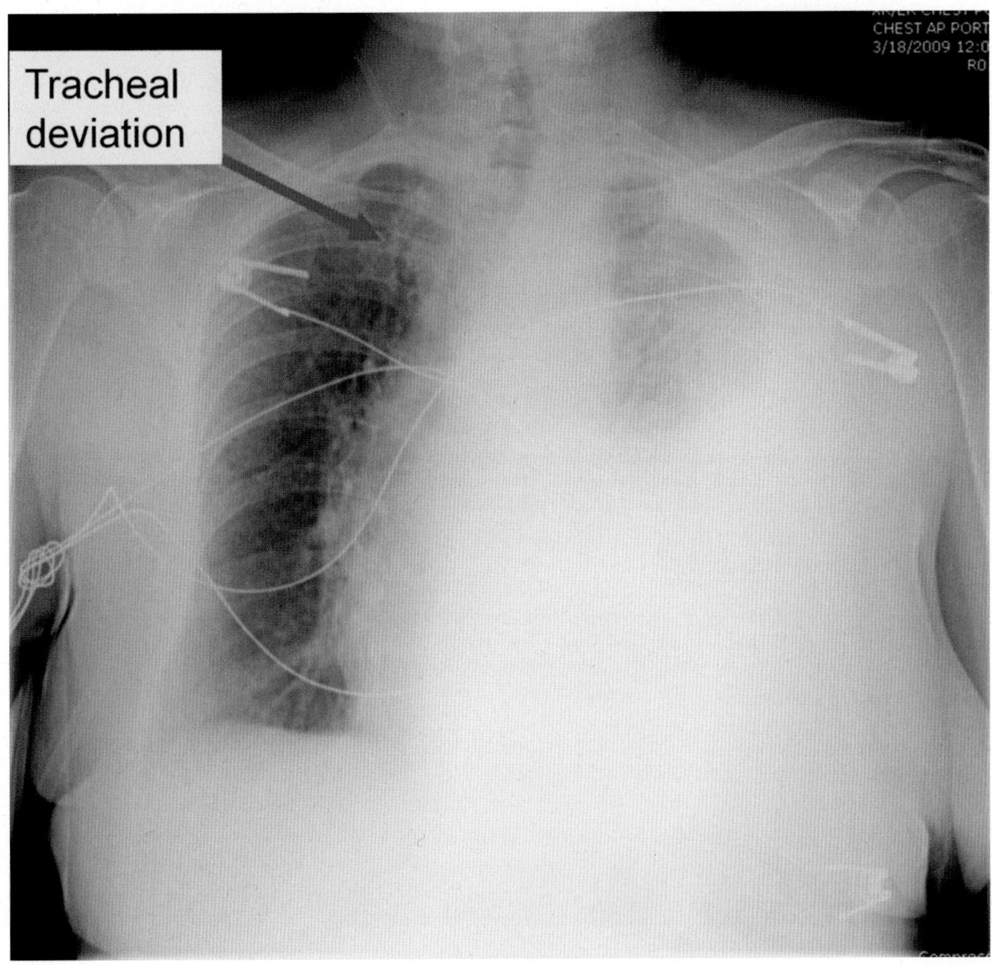

FIGURE 21.5. Massive hemothorax left chest, with tracheal deviation to the right side.

TRAUMA

system should be prepared for autotransfusion, and collected blood should be returned to the patient.

Abdomen

The evidence of significant abdominal trauma on physical exam includes seat belt signs, abdominal wall hematomas or lacerations, or abdominal distension.[106] Hemoperitoneum may also cause peritonitis and significant abdominal pain. Patients with peritonitis should be taken emergently for laparotomy regardless of hemodynamic status. Traditional teaching held that blood did not result in peritonitis and that significant abdominal pain signified hollow viscus injury rather than intra-abdominal bleeding. However, research done by Brown et al. revealed that in patients who are hemodynamically stable upon presentation following trauma and undergo laparotomy secondary to peritonitis alone, a large number had hemoperitoneum without hollow viscus injury and developed hypotension or required blood transfusion intraoperatively. A considerable minority also had major abdominal vascular injury.[107]

In patients without peritonitis, especially in the presence of hypotension, FAST should be performed immediately. FAST consists of four ultrasonographic views; the pericardium (subxiphoid or parasternal), hepatorenal fossa, splenorenal fossa, and pelvis around the bladder. The ultrasound is able to distinguish fluid in each of these potential spaces, indicating pericardial fluid, or hemoperitoneum. FAST is easily accessible, can be performed in <2 minutes by most clinicians in any setting, is portable, easily repeatable, inexpensive, and noninvasive. As discussed previously, the specificity and sensitivity for pericardial fluid is excellent;[57–60] however, sensitivity is significantly lower in the abdominal views, 20%–60%.[108,109] In the abdomen, results of ultrasonography appear to be much more operator dependent. Additionally, there appear to be inherent limitations to the sensitivity of the exam. Some studies with experienced ultrasonographers reveal a reliable detection rate with intraperitoneal volumes of 130–150 mL;[110] however, a study of emergency medicine, radiology, and surgery attendings and residents found that only 10% of participants were able to detect <400 mL, and the mean volume of fluid required for detection on FAST was 619 mL regardless of operator experience, and the volume required to achieve a sensitivity of 97% was 1 L.[111] A positive finding is reliable with specificity of 96%–100%.[59,108,109] The presence of a positive FAST in a hypotensive patient is an indication for immediate laparotomy (Fig. 21.6). However, an equivocal or negative FAST, especially in the hypotensive patient, cannot reliably rule out intra-abdominal bleeding as the source.

In the unstable patient, if the FAST is negative or equivocal, diagnostic peritoneal aspiration (DPA) should be performed. A small incision is made in the infraumbilical region and a large-bore needle is inserted into the abdominal cavity; aspiration of blood indicates a positive finding and need for surgical exploration. If no blood is aspirated, a wire can

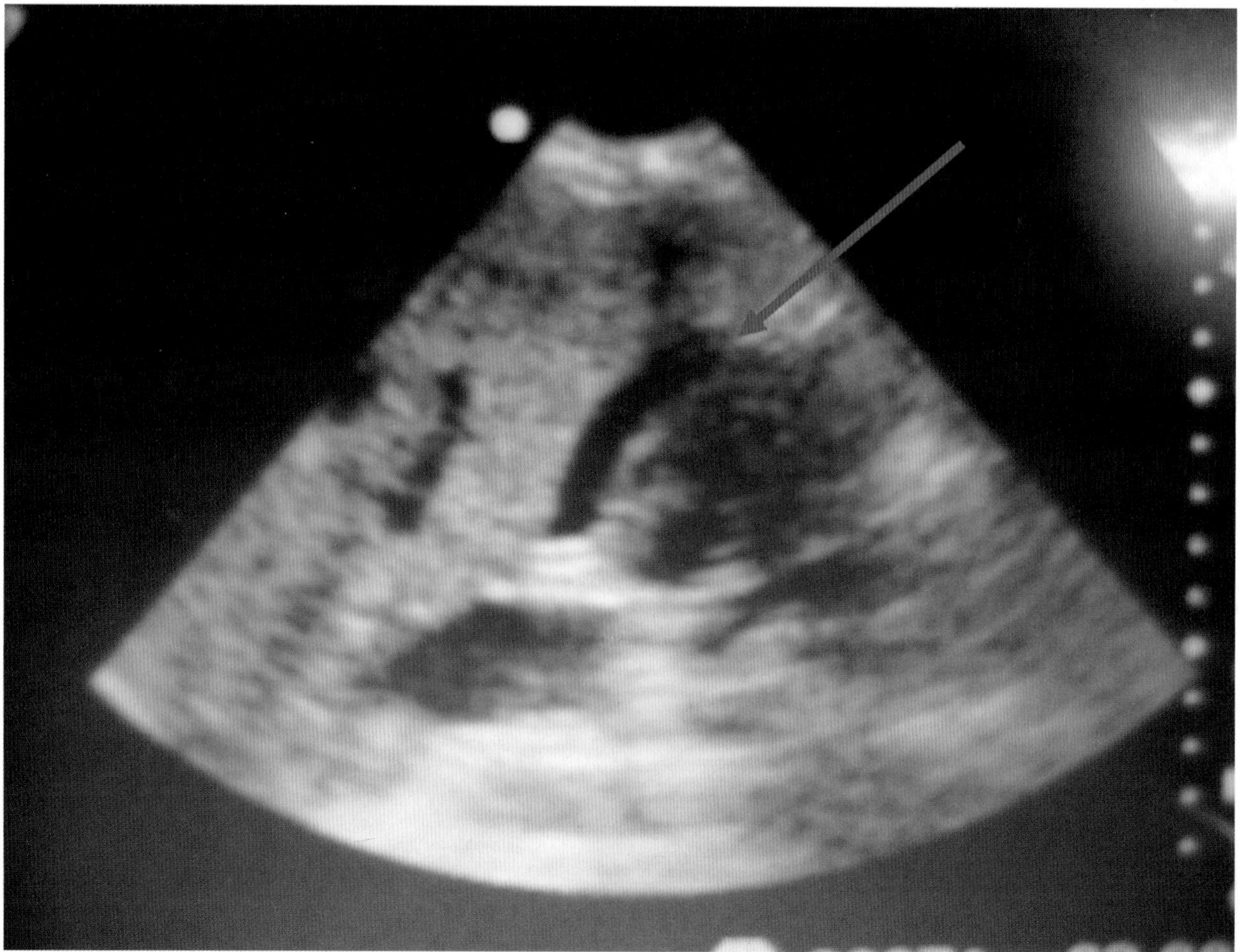

FIGURE 21.6. FAST demonstrating fluid stripe.

be passed through the needle and a multichannel soft plastic catheter is inserted using Seldinger technique. The catheter is also aspirated; if blood returns, this is also a positive DPA, and is an indication for immediate laparotomy. If again no blood returns, consideration can be given to diagnostic peritoneal lavage (DPL), during which 1 L of saline or 10 mL/kg of saline in pediatric patients is administered through the catheter, then allowed to return via the catheter into a bag placed to gravity drainage. If gross blood or mucus is noted, this is a positive finding and immediate laparotomy is indicated. If at least 75% of the infusate is returned but grossly negative for blood, bile, or mucus, microscopic examination can be undertaken. If >100,000 RBC/mm^3 (blunt) or 1,000 RBC/mm^3 (penetrating), >500 WBC/mm^3, or food particles are found, this is also considered a positive finding, necessitating laparotomy. In practice, if the DPA is negative, it is unlikely that intra-abdominal bleeding is the source, and DPL is a cumbersome and technically difficult exam to perform. Waiting for microscopic examination of infusate is impractical in the hypotensive patient, and the infusion of large volumes of fluid into the peritoneal cavity may make interpretation of future radiographic investigations (FAST, CT scan) difficult.

Pelvis

If FAST and DPA are negative in patients with abdominal trauma, retroperitoneal and pelvic bleeding are potential sources of hemorrhage. Retroperitoneal hemorrhage can occur with renal injury, injury to the great vessels of the abdomen (IVC, aorta, iliac arteries and veins), or with pelvic fractures. Clinical indications of retroperitoneal bleeding are rare, but can include hematomas of the flank and back, back pain, and hematuria with renal injury. Pelvic hematomas can also be a cause of hypotension and occur with pelvic fracture. Clinical examination includes palpation of the pelvis for lateral and anterior–posterior stability and bilateral hip range of motion. A stable pelvis on examination with full active range of motion of both hips nearly excludes significant pelvic fracture. In comatose patients, this may not be possible, and the mainstay of diagnosis is plain film of the pelvis (PXR). If pelvic fracture is diagnosed on clinical exam or PXR and hypotension is present, the pelvic ring should be reapproximated using an external compression device. Devices for pelvic stabilization and compression include pelvic binders, external fixators, and sheets. Pelvic binders come in a range of sizes and models, but consist of a padded firm girdle, which is fitted over the anterior–superior iliac spines superiorly, and the femoral heads inferiorly. The binder is then tightened with ties, Velcro, or buckles. If no commercially made binders are available, a plain bed sheet can be folded lengthwise into a long strip approximately 12 inches wide; the sheet is wrapped around the patient's pelvis in the same position as a binder and the ends twisted tightly and fixed with clamps. If orthopedic surgeons are available, an external fixation device can be placed quickly in the evaluation area and tightened to reapproximate the pelvic ring. The placement of stabilization devices closes the pelvic ring, decreasing pelvic volume to encourage tamponade of bleeding. They also help stabilize the broken ends of bone, preventing further laceration of nearby tissues and vessels, and decrease pain with repositioning and transport.

Hemorrhage associated with pelvic fracture can cause substantial hypotension, and severe pelvic fractures alone carry a high mortality.[112] The majority of bleeding in these patients is from the rich sacral venous plexus. Occasionally, bleeding may be from an arterial source. In stable or semi-stable patients with isolated pelvic hemorrhage, angiography should be considered for diagnostic and therapeutic purposes. If considerable arterial bleeding is found, selective embolization can be performed. If no arterial bleeding is found, bilateral internal iliac artery embolization with gelfoam or other temporary agent, or even permanent coil embolization can be performed to decrease pelvic vascular inflow, and allow venous injury to tamponade. The rich collateral circulation in the pelvis prevents ischemic complications in most patients. Very rarely, complications such as necrosis of pelvic organs or gluteal compartment syndrome can occur. In a series of patients undergoing bilateral internal iliac artery embolization, short- and long-term complications were identical to those found in patients with similar fractures not undergoing embolization.[113,114] In patients who are unstable and have suspicion for intra-abdominal injury, laparotomy should be performed. If a pelvic hematoma is found, consideration can be given to bilateral internal iliac artery ligation.[115,116] This performs the same function as angioembolization, with reduction in pelvic vascular inflow. If no intra-abdominal injury is suspected, operative pre-peritoneal packing can be performed. In this procedure, a midline laparotomy incision is made to the level of the anterior rectus sheath, the incision is stopped prior to entry into the abdominal cavity, and the preperitoneal space is dissected toward the sacral venous plexus and packed with sponges. Excellent results have been seen with this technique;[117] however, its use is not yet widespread, and it is difficult in the hypotensive patient with abdomino-pelvic trauma to definitively rule out intra-abdominal source of bleeding, even with FAST and CT scan.

Extremities

After eliminating the scene, chest, abdomen and pelvis as sources of bleeding, attention can be turned to the extremities. In the primary survey, extremity exam is brief, only to diagnose gross deformity or instability of the major long bones (humerus, femur, tibia), actively bleeding wounds, or hard signs of vascular injury including unexplained hypotension or anemia with extremity injury, arterial bleeding, pulsatile or expanding hematoma, lack of pulses distal to the site of injury, and bruit or thrill. Hard signs of vascular injury require immediate operative intervention. If surgical capabilities are lacking, the injured extremity should be reduced and splinted. If there is expanding hematoma or active bleeding, local pressure should be applied. In some cases, tourniquets can be considered. Recent experience from the military has shown that the proper application of tourniquets and their swift removal once definitive hemostasis is achieved can result in excellent survival.[118,119] If no hard signs of injury are present, the injured extremity should be reduced and splinted to prevent further injury and decrease pain and blood loss.

DISABILITY

After securing the airway and restoring oxygenation, ventilation, and adequate circulation, the patient's neurologic status should be ascertained. Within the primary survey, this consists of the Glasgow Coma Scale (GCS) (Table 21.2), pupillary exam, and gross determination of movement and sensation. With the exception of a very brief determination of motor response prior to administration of paralytic agents for airway control, the neurologic examination should be deferred until restoration of adequate oxygenation, ventilation, and circulation as any derangements can render the exam inaccurate. Additionally, hypoxia, hypercarbia, and hypotension all considerably increase secondary brain injury, with a single episode of hypotension or hypoxia resulting in doubled mortality.[120] Other factors that may alter the GCS and pupillary exam include intoxication with drugs or alcohol, hypothermia, and

TABLE 21.2

GLASGOW COMA SCALE

Eyes (E)		
	Open eyes spontaneously	4
	To verbal command	3
	To pain	2
	No Response	1
Verbal response (V)		
	Oriented & converses	5
	Disoriented & converses	4
	Inappropriate words	3
	Incomprehensible sounds	2
	No response	1
Motor response (M)		
	Obeys commands	6
	Localizes pain	5
To painful stimuli	Flexion-withdrawal	4
	Decorticate posturing	3
	Decerebrate posturing	2
	No response	1
	Total:	3–15

hypoglycemia. After restoration of oxygenation and circulation, any pupillary abnormalities or alterations in GCS should be presumed to be due to traumatic brain injury until advanced imaging has definitively ruled it out. Urine or plasma toxicology screens and alcohol levels can be drawn, and serum glucose level should be rapidly assessed; however, they should not be assumed to be the primary cause of altered GCS. Any patients with presumed brain injury should undergo CT scan as soon as possible after the primary survey is completed. Patients with a GCS of 8 or less, and two of the following; age >40, hypotension, or lateralizing signs are at significantly increased risk of intracranial hypertension, and should undergo placement of an intracranial pressure monitoring device regardless of CT findings.[120]

Patients with suspicion of intracranial hypertension, or definite clinical evidence of herniation such as unilateral pupillary dilation, bradycardia, hypertension, and irregular respirations (Cushings Triad) should be treated immediately with maneuvers to decrease intracranial pressure (ICP). These maneuvers include elevation of the head of the bed if spinal fracture is not a concern, removal of all tight or binding materials from around the neck to encourage venous drainage from the cranium, mild hyperventilation with goal carbon dioxide 32–35 mmHg, adequate sedation and pain control, and administration of osmotic agents such as Mannitol and hypertonic saline, or diuretic such as Lasix. However, in the trauma patient, the administration of Mannitol and Lasix may cause or worsen existing hypotension. An attractive alternative is hypertonic saline, which is an osmotic agent that will decrease brain edema by drawing fluid back into the intravascular space without causing hypovolemia/hypotension. Multiple studies have proven its effectiveness in decreasing ICP, and it appears to be equally, if not more effective than Mannitol.[95,99,100,121]

The other half of the disability exam in the primary survey is the assessment of spinal cord injury. Patients should be examined for motor and/or sensory deficit; in comatose or semiconscious patients, this may be challenging. If there is concern for, or definite evidence of spinal cord injury, full spinal precautions must be maintained with protection and immobilization of the entire spine. Previously, in patients with definite evidence of blunt spinal cord injury, steroid bolus followed by continuous infusion for 24–48 hours was recommended. However, a growing concern over limitations of the studies these guidelines were based on, and failure of subsequent studies to demonstrate a definite benefit to steroid administration have led ATLS to remove recommendations for the use of steroids in spinal cord injury from the 8th edition.[2] Steroids should now only be administered under strict guidance from a neurosurgeon or orthopedic spine surgeon on a case-by-case basis.

As with any portion of the primary survey, the GCS and pupillary exam should be repeated continuously to assess for improvement or deterioration; however, special consideration should be given to the anticoagulated trauma patient. Patients on antiplatelet agents or anticoagulants should all be imaged with CT scan given their high risk for intracranial hemorrhage even following minor head trauma. Patients on anticoagulation are also at risk for delayed hemorrhage, and consideration for routine repeat imaging with CT scan of the head, in addition to repeated physical examination, should be given to all such patients regardless of clinical appearance.

If intracranial hemorrhage is found, anticoagulation should be reversed with FFP, recombinant Factor VIIa, or prothrombin complex to prevent progression of hemorrhage and speed time to surgical intervention if necessary. While a recent Cochrane review reported no reliable evidence that the use of Factor VIIa decreased mortality or disability,[122] several studies have demonstrated benefits from Factor VIIa administration, including decreased hematoma progression, decreased transfusion requirements, decreased time to surgical intervention, and decreased cost.[123–127]

EXPOSURE

In order to complete the primary survey, the patient must be fully disrobed to reveal all injuries, and log rolled maintaining full spinal precautions to assess the back and perineum for injury or deformity. Generally, the patients' clothes are removed as soon as they enter the evaluation area by assistants while the primary clinician proceeds with the assessment of ABC and D. If only one person is available to perform the primary survey, the patient should be completely undressed at this point if any remaining clothing articles remain.

After complete visual inspection, the patient should be covered as quickly as possible with warm blankets, as thermal homeostasis is often disrupted in trauma patients and hypothermia can set in quickly. Hypothermia is a particular risk in pediatric patients with a much larger surface area to mass ratio and decreased ability to maintain normothermia. Hypothermia if allowed to occur can interfere with the neurologic examination, alter drug metabolism, and most importantly, worsen coagulopathy in the bleeding patient.

Interestingly, several studies of victims of nontraumatic cardiac arrest and patients undergoing cardiac or neurologic procedures have shown notable improvements in outcome with induction of mild–moderate hypothermia with core temperatures of 32–34 degrees centigrade.[128,129] Other patients who may benefit from therapeutic hypothermia include stroke victims and victims of drowning.[129] This has led to a reexamination of hypothermia in trauma patients; however, the results are less encouraging. In a multicenter, prospective, observational study of trauma patients, hypothermia was seen in 43% of patients and was associated with a significantly higher rate of multisystem organ dysfunction.[130] In another study of injured trauma patients undergoing cavitary surgery, hypothermia immediately after surgery was found to be an independent predictor of mortality with an odds ratio for death of 3.2 (95% CI 1.9–5.3, $p < 0.001$).[131] Traumatic brain injury, in particular, has also been well studied. In the largest multicenter, randomized, prospective trial of hypothermia in traumatic brain injury, there was no benefit in survival or neurologic outcome with therapeutic hypothermia.[132] Multiple studies of hypothermia in children for elective surgical procedures as well as traumatic brain injury show no benefit, and may even demonstrate an increase in mortality.[133,134] At this time, hypothermia should still be considered detrimental in both the adult and pediatric trauma population.

COMPLETION OF THE PRIMARY SURVEY

Once Airway, Breathing, Circulation, Disability, and Exposure have all been assessed and all life-threatening injuries have been addressed or stabilized, the entire primary survey should be repeated to ensure nothing has changed since the beginning of the evaluation. If the patient remains stable, the bladder and stomach should be decompressed. Continuous urine output monitoring is a helpful tool in gauging response to resuscitative efforts, and is a necessity in comatose or paralyzed patients. Gastric decompression aids in the prevention of aspiration, especially in the intubated patient. Care should be taken that the nasogastric route is avoided in patients with potential facial fractures to avoid insertion into the cranium. At this time, results of all laboratory and radiologic adjuncts to the primary survey should be reviewed and the clinician should determine if definitive care can be delivered locally, or if transfer to higher level of care is likely to be required. If transfer to another facility is definite, contact with the accepting facility should be initiated.

SECONDARY SURVEY

Upon completion of the primary survey, the secondary survey can be started. The secondary survey consists of a brief directed history and complete physical exam. The history should follow the AMPLE model of Allergies, Medications, Past illnesses/operations, Last meal, and Events/Environment related to injury. The history should be directed at detection of preexisting conditions, or medications that may alter management of life-threatening injuries. Physical examination should include brief inspection from head to toe, ensuring that full spinal precautions are kept during the evaluation.

The head and neck exam should include visual inspection and palpation to detect lacerations, hematomas, fractures and tenderness, otoscopic evaluation to detect hemotympanum, a sign of temporal bone fracture, and assessment of all cranial nerves in the conscious patient. The primary adjuncts to the head and neck assessment are CT scans of the head, face, and neck. CT scan of the head will reliably detect intracranial hemorrhage and skull fracture. CT scan of the neck is the screening exam of choice to detect cervical spine fractures, and has largely replaced plain films that have a notoriously low sensitivity, and are often inadequate. CT of the neck can also be performed with intravenous contrast to assess the soft tissues and CT angiography can be used to detect vascular injury to the carotid or vertebral arteries or jugular veins with high sensitivity.

The majority of the thoracic exam is undertaken in the primary survey, where physical exam, chest x-ray, and FASTER will detect most injuries. The two major exceptions are thoracic aortic injury and thoracic spine fracture.[54] Both may present with widened mediastinum, and back pain. Any patient with significant external evidence of thoracic trauma or with a widened mediastinum on chest x-ray or with midline thoracic spinal tenderness should undergo CT scan of the chest with intravenous contrast. The CT scan of the chest will reliably diagnose spinal fracture, give additional information on parenchymal lung injury (contusion, laceration, occult pneumothorax), and is now the screening exam of choice for thoracic aortic injury. Compared to angiography, the traditional gold standard, CT scan of the chest is faster, easier to obtain, requires less technical expertise, requires a lower contrast load, does not require arterial puncture, and has equivalent, possibly improved sensitivity and specificity.[135–137]

As with the chest, the majority of the abdominal and pelvic exam is performed during the primary survey. An adjunct to the secondary survey is a CT scan of the abdomen and pelvis. All stable patients who are unevaluable due to intoxication or depressed GCS should undergo CT scan of the abdomen and pelvis with intravenous contrast to detect fractures of the thoracolumbar spine, and be assessed for solid organ injury and pelvic fracture. Additionally, in the presence of concerning pelvic fractures, or gross hematuria, delayed phase images can be obtained. These images can detect contrast extravasation from the urinary collecting system and diagnose bladder and ureteral injuries. CT scan of the abdomen and pelvis cannot be relied upon to detect hollow viscus injury. Some signs of hollow viscus injury on CT scan include free fluid without solid organ injury, focally thickened bowel wall, and free intraperitoneal gas; however, these signs are neither sensitive nor specific. The gold standard for detection of hollow viscus injury remains serial observation and laparotomy.

A complete musculoskeletal survey should also be performed during the secondary survey, all joints should be assessed for passive and active range of motion, long bones should be assessed for instability, the limbs should be examined for external signs of trauma or violation of the joints, and a sensory examination of all dermatomes should be performed to assess for peripheral nerve injury. A complete assessment of all peripheral pulses should also be performed. If any asymmetry is noted, and in cases of obvious fracture or deformity even if pulses are present in the affected limb, an ankle–brachial index (ABI) or brachial–brachial index (BBI) should be performed after reduction of fractures to rule out occult vascular injury. The blood pressure should be taken below the level of injury. If the ABI or BBI is >0.9, occult arterial injury is unlikely, and if it is <0.9, further imaging should be obtained.[138,139] Ultrasound is an excellent option in the lower extremity below the inguinal ligament and in the upper extremity below the shoulder; however, the examination can be limited in the presence of soft tissue injury, is operator dependent, and can be difficult to obtain after hours. An alternative is CT angiography, which has excellent sensitivity and specificity.[140–142] CT angiography has the benefits discussed above over traditional angiography. Additionally, examination of both limbs can be performed simultaneously with the same contrast load. CT angiography is more reliable for proximal vessels such as the subclavian and iliac arteries than ultrasound, and has the added benefit of giving information on the associated soft tissue and bony injuries. Another adjunct in the secondary survey is the extremity portion of the FASTER exam. Ultrasound is used to detect cortical defects, ligamentous injuries, and soft tissue edema. A study of FASTER in nonphysicians with brief training revealed excellent sensitivity in detecting fractures and ligamentous injury.[143]

Extremities must be monitored frequently for the development of compartment syndrome. Compartment pressures should be measured if any symptoms such as pain out of proportion to exam or with passive range of motion, or signs such as edema or tense compartments develop. Elevated compartment pressures are an indication for emergent fasciotomy.

Musculoskeletal injuries are the most likely to be missed or delayed in diagnosis. Many facilities have instituted the tertiary survey, a complete physical examination performed after the initial assessment and resuscitation are completed to reduce the frequency of missed injuries.

COMPLETION OF THE SECONDARY SURVEY

Once the secondary survey has been completed, if the decision to transfer the patient to another facility has been made, transfer should not be delayed for adjunctive imaging, and appropriate level of transport care should be determined and arranged. All necessary interventions should be completed, with consideration to prophylactic intubation, or placement of chest tubes in anticipation of worsening hemothoraces or pneumothoraces. The stomach and bladder should be decompressed, and if the need is anticipated, warmed fluid and blood products should be provided. The patient should be attached to portable monitors and results of tests and hospital records readied for transfer.

References

1. Olson CJ, Arthur M, Mullins RJ, et al. Influence of trauma system implementation on process of care delivered to seriously injured patients in rural trauma centers. *Surgery*. 2001;130(2):273-279.
2. Kortbeek JB, Al Turki SA, Ali J, et al. Advanced trauma life support, 8th edition, the evidence for change. *J Trauma*. 2008;64(6):1638-1650.
3. Trunkey DD. Trauma. Accidental and intentional injuries account for more years of life lost in the U.S. than cancer and heart disease. Among the prescribed remedies are improved preventive efforts, speedier surgery and further research. *Sci Am* 1983;249(2):28-35.
4. Bansal V, Fortlage D, Lee JG, et al. Hemorrhage is more prevalent than brain injury in early trauma deaths: the Golden Six Hours. *Eur J Trauma Emerg Surg*. 2009;35:26-30.
5. Demetriades D, Murray J, Charalambides K, et al. Trauma fatalities: time and location of hospital deaths. *J Am Coll Surg* 2004;198(1):20-26.
6. Wilson M, Davis DP, Coimbra R. Diagnosis and monitoring of hemorrhagic shock during the initial resuscitation of multiple trauma patients: a review. *J Emerg Med* 2003;24(4):413-422.
7. Coscia R MJ. American College of Surgeons Committee on Trauma. *Resources for the Optimal Care of the Injured Patient*. 2006:142.
8. Petrie D, Lane P, Stewart TC. An evaluation of patient outcomes comparing trauma team activated versus trauma team not activated using TRISS analysis. Trauma and Injury Severity Score. *J Trauma*. 1996;41(5):870-873; discussion 873-875.
9. Cherry RA, King TS, Carney DE, et al. Trauma team activation and the impact on mortality. *J Trauma*. 2007;63(2):326-330.
10. Cox S, Smith K, Currell A, et al. Differentiation of confirmed major trauma patients and potential major trauma patients using pre-hospital trauma triage criteria. *Injury*. 2011;42:889-895.
11. Larsen KT, Uleberg O, Skogvoll E. Differences in trauma team activation criteria among Norwegian hospitals. *Scand J Trauma Resusc Emerg Med*. 2010;18:21.
12. Purtill MA, Benedict K, Hernandez-Boussard T, et al. Validation of a prehospital trauma triage tool: a 10-year perspective. *J Trauma*. 2008;;65(6):1253-1257.
13. *Anonymous ATLS Student Course Manual Eighth Edition*. Chicago, IL: American College of Surgeons Committee on Trauma.; 2008.
14. Caterino JM, Valasek T, Werman HA. Identification of an age cutoff for increased mortality in patients with elderly trauma. *Am J Emerg Med*. 2010;28(2):151-158.
15. Morris JA Jr, MacKenzie EJ, Damiano AM, et al. Mortality in trauma patients: the interaction between host factors and severity. *J Trauma*. 1990;30(12):1476-1482.
16. Pellicane JV, Byrne K, DeMaria EJ. Preventable complications and death from multiple organ failure among geriatric trauma victims. *J Trauma*. 1992;33(3):440-444.
17. Perdue PW, Watts DD, Kaufmann CR, et al. Differences in mortality between elderly and younger adult trauma patients: geriatric status increases risk of delayed death. *J Trauma*. 1998;45(4):805-810.
18. Richmond TS, Kauder D, Strumpf N, et al. Characteristics and outcomes of serious traumatic injury in older adults. *J Am Geriatr Soc*. 2002;50(2):215-222.
19. Demetriades D, Karaiskakis M, Velmahos G, et al. Effect on outcome of early intensive management of geriatric trauma patients. *Br J Surg*. 2002;89(10):1319-1322.
20. Demetriades D, Sava J, Alo K, et al. Old age as a criterion for trauma team activation. *J Trauma* 2001;51(4):754-756; discussion 756-757.
21. Schwab CW, Kauder DR: Trauma in the geriatric patient. *Arch Surg*. 1992;127(6):701-706.
22. Scalea TM, Simon HM, Duncan AO, et al. Geriatric blunt multiple trauma: improved survival with early invasive monitoring. *J Trauma*. 1990;30(2):129-134; discussion 134-136.
23. Bochicchio GV, Joshi M, Bochicchio K, et al. Incidence and impact of risk factors in critically ill trauma patients. *World J Surg*. 2006;30(1): 114-118.
24. Brady KA, Weiner M, Turner BJ. Undiagnosed hepatitis C on the general medicine and trauma services of two urban hospitals. *J Infect*. 2009;59(1):62-69.
25. Xeroulis G, Inaba K, Stewart TC, et al. Human immunodeficiency virus, hepatitis B, and hepatitis C seroprevalence in a Canadian trauma population. *J Trauma*. 2005;59(1):105-108.
26. Weiss ES, Cornwell EE III, Wang T, et al. Human immunodeficiency virus and hepatitis testing and prevalence among surgical patients in an urban university hospital. *Am J Surg*. 2007;193(1):55-60.
27. Weiss ES, Makary MA, Wang T, et al. Prevalence of blood-borne pathogens in an urban, university-based general surgical practice. *Ann Surg*. 2005;241(5):803-807; discussion 807-809.
28. Hoyt D, Coimbra R. General considerations in trauma. In: Mulholland MW, Lilliemoe KD, Doherty GM, et al. *Greenfield's Surgery: Scientific Principles and Practice*. 4th ed. Philadelphia, PA: Lippincott, Williams and Wilkins; 2005:344.
29. Hoyt D, Coimbra R. Initial care, operative care, and postoperative priorities. In: Rich NM, Mattox K, Hirschberg A. *Vascular Trauma*. 2nd ed. Edited by Philadelphia, PA: Elsevier-Saunders; 2004.
30. Langeron O, Birenbaum A, Amour J. Airway management in trauma. *Minerva Anestesiol*. 2009, 75(5):307-311.
31. Feliciano DV, Mattox KL, Moore EE. *Trauma:* 6th ed. New York: McGraw Hill; 2008.
32. Coimbra R, Davis DP, Hoyt DB. Pre-hospital airway management. In: Ascensio JA, Trunkey DD. *Current Therapy of Trauma and Surgical Critical Care.*. Philadelphia, PA: Mosby Elsevier; 2008:58.
33. Knapp S, Kofler J, Stoiser B, et al. The assessment of four different methods to verify tracheal tube placement in the critical care setting. *Anesth Analg*. 1999, 88(4):766-770.
34. Butler FS, Cirillo AA. Retrograde tracheal intubation. *Anesth Analg*. 1960;39:333-338.
35. Lehavi A, Weisman A, Katz Y. Retrograde tracheal intubation—an alternative in difficult airway management. *Harefuah*. 2008, 147(1):59-64, 93.
36. Marciniak D, Smith CE. Emergent retrograde tracheal intubation with a gum-elastic bougie in a trauma patient. *Anesth Analg*. 2007, 105(6):1720-1721, table of contents.
37. Altman KW, Waltonen JD, Kern RC. Urgent surgical airway intervention: a 3 year county hospital experience. *Laryngoscope*. 2005;115(12):2101-2104.
38. Francois B, Clavel M, Desachy A, et al. Complications of tracheostomy performed in the ICU: subthyroid tracheostomy vs surgical cricothyroidotomy. *Chest*. 2003;123(1):151-158.
39. Talving P, DuBose J, Inaba K, et al. Conversion of emergent cricothyrotomy to tracheotomy in trauma patients. *Arch Surg*. 2010;145(1):87-91.
40. Wright MJ, Greenberg DE, Hunt JP, et al. Surgical cricothyroidotomy in trauma patients. *South Med J*. 2003;96(5):465-467.
41. [http://www.resus.org.uk/pages/pals/pdf]
42. American Heart Association. 2005 American Heart Association (AHA) guidelines for cardiopulmonary resuscitation (CPR) and emergency cardiovascular care (ECC) of pediatric and neonatal patients: pediatric basic life support. *Pediatrics*. 2006;117(5):e989-1004.
43. Clements RS, Steel AG, Bates AT, et al. Cuffed endotracheal tube use in paediatric prehospital intubation: challenging the doctrine? *Emerg Med J*. 2007;24(1):57-58.
44. Newth CJ, Rachman B, Patel N, et al. The use of cuffed versus uncuffed endotracheal tubes in pediatric intensive care. *J Pediatr*. 2004;144(3):333-337.
45. Sheridan RL. Uncuffed endotracheal tubes should not be used in seriously burned children. *Pediatr Crit Care Med*. 2006;7(3):258-259.
46. Weiss M, Dullenkopf A, Fischer JE, et al.; European Paediatric Endotracheal Intubation Study Group. Prospective randomized controlled multicentre trial of cuffed or uncuffed endotracheal tubes in small children. *Br J Anaesth*. 2009;103(6):867-873.
47. Jorden RC, Moore EE, Marx JA, et al. A comparison of PTV and endotracheal ventilation in an acute trauma model. *J Trauma* 1985;25(10):978-983.
48. Ozmen V, McSwain NE Jr, Nichols RL, et al. Autotransfusion of potentially culture-positive blood (CPB) in abdominal trauma: preliminary data from a prospective study. *J Trauma*. 1992;32(1):36-39.
49. Sinclair A, Jacobs LM,Jr: Emergency department autotransfusion for trauma victims. *Med Instrum* 1982, 16(6):283-286.
50. Broadie TA, Glover JL, Bang N, et al. Clotting competence of intracavitary blood in trauma victims. *Ann Emerg Med*. 1981;10(3):127-130.

51. Napoli VM, Symbas PJ, Vroon DH, et al. Autotransfusion from experimental hemothorax: levels of coagulation factors. *J Trauma* 1987, 27(3):296-300.
52. Azad SC, Groh J, Beyer A, et al. Continuous peridural analgesia vs patient—controlled intravenous analgesia for pain therapy after thoracotomy. *Anaesthesist* 2000;49(1):9-17.
53. Mackersie RC, Karagianes TG, Hoyt DB, et al. Prospective evaluation of epidural and intravenous administration of fentanyl for pain control and restoration of ventilatory function following multiple rib fractures. *J Trauma*. 1991, 31(4):443-449; discussion 449-451.
54. Bansal V, Lee J, Coimbra R. Current diagnosis and management of blunt traumatic rupture of the thoracic aorta. *J Vasc Bras*. 2007;6:64.
55. Brook OR, Beck-Razi N, Abadi S, et al. Sonographic detection of pneumothorax by radiology residents as part of extended focused assessment with sonography for trauma. *J Ultrasound Med*. 2009;28(6):749-755.
56. Nandipati KC, Allamaneni S, Kakarla R, et al. Extended focused assessment with sonography for trauma (EFAST) in the diagnosis of pneumothorax: experience at a community based level I trauma center. *Injury*. 2011;42:511-514.
57. Ball CG, Williams BH, Wyrzykowski AD, et al. A caveat to the performance of pericardial ultrasound in patients with penetrating cardiac wounds. *J Trauma*. 2009;67(5):1123-1124.
58. Boulanger BR, Kearney PA, Tsuei B, et al. The routine use of sonography in penetrating torso injury is beneficial. *J Trauma*. 2001;51(2):320-325.
59. Rozycki GS, Feliciano DV, Ochsner MG, et al. The role of ultrasound in patients with possible penetrating cardiac wounds: a prospective multicenter study. *J Trauma*. 1999;46(4):543-551; discussion 551-552.
60. Rozycki GS, Feliciano DV, Schmidt JA, et al. The role of surgeon-performed ultrasound in patients with possible cardiac wounds. *Ann Surg*. 1996;223(6):737-744; discussion 744-746.
61. Farrier JM, Lall R, Coimbra R. Resuscitative Thoracotomy. In: Wilson WC, Grande CM, Hoyt DB. *Trauma: Emergency Resuscitation, Perioperative Anesthesia, and Surgical Management*. Vol 1. New York, NY: Informa-Healthcare USA, Inc; 2007:247.
62. Buck ML, Wiggins BS, Sesler JM. Intraosseous drug administration in children and adults during cardiopulmonary resuscitation. *Ann Pharmacother*. 2007;41(10):1679-1686.
63. Cooper BR, Mahoney PF, Hodgetts TJ, et al. Intra-osseous access (EZ-IO) for resuscitation: UK military combat experience. *J R Army Med Corps* 2007;153(4):314-316.
64. Gerritse BM, Scheffer GJ, Draaisma JM. Prehospital intraosseus access with the bone injection gun by a helicopter-transported emergency medical team. *J Trauma* 2009, 66(6):1739-1741.
65. Lamhaut L, Dagron C, Apriotesei R, et al. Comparison of intravenous and intraosseous access by pre-hospital medical emergency personnel with and without CBRN protective equipment. *Resuscitation* 2010;81(1):65-68.
66. Leidel BA, Kirchhoff C, Bogner V, et al. Is the intraosseous access route fast and efficacious compared to conventional central venous catheterization in adult patients under resuscitation in the emergency department? A prospective observational pilot study. *Patient Saf Surg* 2009;3(1):24.
67. Leidel BA, Kirchhoff C, Braunstein V, et al. Comparison of two intraosseous access devices in adult patients under resuscitation in the emergency department: A prospective, randomized study. *Resuscitation*. 2010;81:994-999.
68. Schwartz D, Amir L, Dichter R, et al. The use of a powered device for intraosseous drug and fluid administration in a national EMS: a 4-year experience. *J Trauma*. 2008;64(3):650-654; discussion 654-655.
69. [http://www.east.org/tpg/FluidResus.pdf]
70. Bickell WH, Wall MJ Jr, Pepe PE, et al. Immediate versus delayed fluid resuscitation for hypotensive patients with penetrating torso injuries. *N Engl J Med*. 1994;331(17):1105-1109.
71. Holcomb JB. The 2004 Fitts Lecture: current perspective on combat casualty care. *J Trauma*. 2005;59(4):990-1002.
72. Stahel PF, Smith WR, Moore EE. Current trends in resuscitation strategy for the multiply injured patient. *Injury*. 2009;40(Suppl 4):S27-S35.
73. Tien H, Nascimento B Jr, Callum J, et al. An approach to transfusion and hemorrhage in trauma: current perspectives on restrictive transfusion strategies. *Can J Surg*. 2007;50(3):202-209.
74. Yaghoubian A, Lewis RJ, Putnam B, et al. Reanalysis of prehospital intravenous fluid administration in patients with penetrating truncal injury and field hypotension. *Am Surg*. 2007;73(10):1027-1030.
75. Coimbra R, Hoyt D: Vascular Trauma: Epidemiology and natural history. In: Cronenwett J and Johnston KW. *Rutherford's Vascular Surgery*. 7th ed. Philadelphia, PA: Saunders Elsevier; 2010:2312.
76. Fraga GP, Bansal V, Coimbra R. Transfusion of blood products in trauma: an update. *J Emerg Med*. 2010;39:253-260.
77. Khan H, Belsher J, Yilmaz M, et al. Fresh-frozen plasma and platelet transfusions are associated with development of acute lung injury in critically ill medical patients. *Chest*. 2007;131(5):1308-1314.
78. Watson GA, Sperry JL, Rosengart MR, et al. Inflammation and Host Response to Injury Investigators: fresh frozen plasma is independently associated with a higher risk of multiple organ failure and acute respiratory distress syndrome. *J Trauma*. 2009, 67(2):221-227; discussion 228-230.
79. Borgman MA, Spinella PC, Perkins JG, et al. The ratio of blood products transfused affects mortality in patients receiving massive transfusions at a combat support hospital. *J Trauma*. 2007;63(4):805-813.
80. Duchesne JC, Islam TM, Stuke L, et al. Hemostatic resuscitation during surgery improves survival in patients with traumatic-induced coagulopathy. *J Trauma* 2009, 67(1):33-37; discussion 37-39.
81. Riskin DJ, Tsai TC, Riskin L, et al. Massive transfusion protocols: the role of aggressive resuscitation versus product ratio in mortality reduction. *J Am Coll Surg*. 2009, 209(2):198-205.
82. Spinella PC, Perkins JG, Grathwohl KW, et al. Effect of plasma and red blood cell transfusions on survival in patients with combat related traumatic injuries. *J Trauma*. 2008, 64(2 Suppl):S69-S77; discussion S77-S78.
83. Teixeira PG, Inaba K, Shulman I, et al. Impact of plasma transfusion in massively transfused trauma patients. *J Trauma*. 2009;66(3):693-697.
84. Sperry JL, Ochoa JB, Gunn SR, et al. Inflammation the Host Response to Injury Investigators: an FFP:PRBC transfusion ratio >/=1:1.5 is associated with a lower risk of mortality after massive transfusion. *J Trauma*. 2008;65(5):986-993.
85. Boffard KD, Riou B, Warren B, et al.; NovoSeven Trauma Study Group. Recombinant factor VIIa as adjunctive therapy for bleeding control in severely injured trauma patients: two parallel randomized, placebo-controlled, double-blind clinical trials. *J Trauma*. 2005;59(1):8-15; discussion 15-18.
86. Rizoli SB, Boffard KD, Riou B, et al.; NovoSeven Trauma Study Group. Recombinant activated factor VII as an adjunctive therapy for bleeding control in severe trauma patients with coagulopathy: subgroup analysis from two randomized trials. *Crit Care*. 2006;10(6):R178.
87. Deitch EA, Shi HP, Feketeova E, et al. Hypertonic saline resuscitation limits neutrophil activation after trauma-hemorrhagic shock. *Shock* 2003;19(4):328-333.
88. Deree J, de Campos T, Shenvi E, et al. Hypertonic saline and pentoxifylline attenuates gut injury after hemorrhagic shock: the kinder, gentler resuscitation. *J Trauma*. 2007;62(4):818-827; discussion 827-828.
89. Deree J, Loomis WH, Wolf P, et al. Hepatic transcription factor activation and proinflammatory mediator production is attenuated by hypertonic saline and pentoxifylline resuscitation after hemorrhagic shock. *J Trauma*. 2008;64(5):1230-1238; discussion 1238-1239.
90. Deree J, Martins JO, Leedom A, et al. Hypertonic saline and pentoxifylline reduces hemorrhagic shock resuscitation-induced pulmonary inflammation through attenuation of neutrophil degranulation and proinflammatory mediator synthesis. *J Trauma*. 2007;62(1):104-111.
91. Junger WG, Coimbra R, Liu FC, et al. Hypertonic saline resuscitation: a tool to modulate immune function in trauma patients? *Shock*. 1997;8(4):235-241.
92. Rizoli SB, Rhind SG, Shek PN, et al. The immunomodulatory effects of hypertonic saline resuscitation in patients sustaining traumatic hemorrhagic shock: a randomized, controlled, double-blinded trial. *Ann Surg*. 2006;243(1):47-57.
93. Yada-Langui MM, Coimbra R, Lancellotti C, et al. Hypertonic saline and pentoxifylline prevent lung injury and bacterial translocation after hemorrhagic shock. *Shock*. 2000;14(6):594-598.
94. Bulger EM, Jurkovich GJ, Nathens AB, et al. Hypertonic resuscitation of hypovolemic shock after blunt trauma: a randomized controlled trial. *Arch Surg*. 2008;143(2):139-148; discussion 149.
95. Coimbra R. Salt in the vein, good for the brain.. *Crit Care Med*. 2007;35(2):659-660.
96. Mattox KL, Maningas PA, Moore EE, et al. Prehospital hypertonic saline/dextran infusion for post-traumatic hypotension. The U.S.A. Multicenter Trial. *Ann Surg*. 1991;213(5):482-491.
97. Vassar MJ, Fischer RP, O'Brien PE, et al. A multicenter trial for resuscitation of injured patients with 7.5% sodium chloride. The effect of added dextran 70. The Multicenter Group for the Study of Hypertonic Saline in Trauma Patients. *Arch Surg*. 1993;128(9):1003-1011; discussion 1011-1013.
98. Coimbra R, Doucet JJ, Bansal V. Resuscitation strategies in hemorrhagic shock-Hypertonic saline revisted. In: McKenna J, Hughes T, Brewerton A, et al. *Emergency Medicine and Critical Care Review 2007*. London, UK: Touch Briefings; 2008:R1.
99. Himmelseher S. Hypertonic saline solutions for treatment of intracranial hypertension. *Curr Opin Anaesthesiol*. 2007;20(5):414-426.
100. Tyagi R, Donaldson K, Loftus CM, et al. Hypertonic saline: a clinical review. *Neurosurg Rev*. 2007;30(4):277-289; discussion 289-290.
101. Galarneau MR, Woodruff SI, Dye JL, et al. Traumatic brain injury during Operation Iraqi Freedom: findings from the United States Navy-Marine Corps Combat Trauma Registry. *J Neurosurg*. 2008;108(5):950-957.
102. Martin EM, Lu WC, Helmick K, et al. Traumatic brain injuries sustained in the Afghanistan and Iraq wars. *J Trauma Nurs*. 2008;15(3):94-99; quiz 100-101.
103. Gabay M. Absorbable hemostatic agents. *Am J Health Syst Pharm*. 2006;63(13):1244-1253.
104. Rhee P, Brown C, Martin M, et al. QuikClot use in trauma for hemorrhage control: case series of 103 documented uses. *J Trauma*. 2008;64(4):1093-1099.
105. Seyednejad H, Imani M, Jamieson T, et al. Topical haemostatic agents. *Br J Surg*. 2008;95(10):1197-1225.
106. Bansal V, Conroy C, Tominaga GT, et al. The utility of seat belt signs to predict intra-abdominal injury following motor vehicle crashes. *Traffic Inj Prev*. 2009;10(6):567-572.
107. Brown CV, Velmahos GC, Neville AL, et al. Hemodynamically "stable" patients with peritonitis after penetrating abdominal trauma: identifying those who are bleeding. *Arch Surg*. 2005;140(8):767-772.

108. Friese RS, Malekzadeh S, Shafi S, et al. Abdominal ultrasound is an unreliable modality for the detection of hemoperitoneum in patients with pelvic fracture. *J Trauma.* 2007;63(1):97-102.
109. Gaarder C, Kroepelien CF, Loekke R, et al. Ultrasound performed by radiologists-confirming the truth about FAST in trauma. *J Trauma.* 2009;67(2):323-327; discussion 328-329.
110. Von Kuenssberg Jehle D, Stiller G, Wagner D. Sensitivity in detecting free intraperitoneal fluid with the pelvic views of the FAST exam. *Am J Emerg Med.* 2003;21(6):476-478.
111. Branney SW, Wolfe RE, Moore EE, et al. Quantitative sensitivity of ultrasound in detecting free intraperitoneal fluid. *J Trauma.* 1995;39(2): 375-380.
112. Gustavo Parreira J, Coimbra R, Rasslan S, et al. The role of associated injuries on outcome of blunt trauma patients sustaining pelvic fractures. *Injury.* 2000;31(9):677-682.
113. Ramirez JI, Velmahos GC, Best CR, et al. Male sexual function after bilateral internal iliac artery embolization for pelvic fracture. *J Trauma.* 2004;56(4):734-739; discussion 739-741.
114. Velmahos GC, Chahwan S, Hanks SE, et al. Angiographic embolization of bilateral internal iliac arteries to control life-threatening hemorrhage after blunt trauma to the pelvis. *Am Surg.* 2000;66(9):858-862.
115. Dubose J, Inaba K, Barmparas G, et al. Bilateral internal iliac artery ligation as a damage control approach in massive retroperitoneal bleeding after pelvic fracture. *J Trauma.* 2010;69:1507-1514.
116. Yang J, Gao JM, Hu P, et al. Application of damage control orthopedics in 41 patients with severe multiple injuries. *Chin J Traumatol.* 2008;11(3):157-160.
117. Cothren CC, Osborn PM, Moore EE, et al. Preperitonal pelvic packing for hemodynamically unstable pelvic fractures: a paradigm shift. *J Trauma.* 2007;62(4):834-839; discussion 839-842.
118. Kragh JF Jr, Walters TJ, Baer DG, et al. Survival with emergency tourniquet use to stop bleeding in major limb trauma. *Ann Surg.* 2009;249(1):1-7.
119. Swan KG Jr, Wright DS, Barbagiovanni SS, et al. Tourniquets revisited. *J Trauma.* 2009;66(3):672-675.
120. Brain Trauma Foundation, American Association of Neurological Surgeons, Congress of Neurological Surgeons, Joint Section on Neurotrauma and Critical Care, AANS/CNS, Bratton SL, Chestnut RM, Ghajar J, McConnell Hammond FF, Harris OA, Hartl R, Manley GT, Nemecek A, Newell DW, Rosenthal G, Schouten J, Shutter L, Timmons SD, Ullman JS, Videtta W, Wilberger JE, Wright DW: Guidelines for the management of severe traumatic brain injury. I. Blood pressure and oxygenation. *J Neurotrauma.* 2007;24(Suppl 1):S7-S13.
121. Pascual JL, Maloney-Wilensky E, et al. Resuscitation of hypotensive head-injured patients: is hypertonic saline the answer? *Am Surg.* 2008;74(3):253-259.
122. Perel P, Roberts I, Shakur H, et al. Haemostatic drugs for traumatic brain injury. *Cochrane Database Syst Rev.* 2010;(1):CD007877.
123. Brown CV, Foulkrod KH, Lopez D, et al. Recombinant factor VIIa for the correction of coagulopathy before emergent craniotomy in blunt trauma patients. *J Trauma.* 2010;68(2):348-352.
124. Narayan RK, Maas AI, Marshall LF, et al.; rFVIIa Traumatic ICH Study Group. Recombinant factor VIIA in traumatic intracerebral hemorrhage: results of a dose-escalation clinical trial. *Neurosurgery.* 2008;62(4):776-786; discussion 786-788.
125. Stein DM, Dutton RP, Alexander C, Miller J, Scalea TM: Use of recombinant factor VIIa to facilitate organ donation in trauma patients with devastating neurologic injury. *J Am Coll Surg.* 2009;208(1): 120-125.
126. Stein DM, Dutton RP, Kramer ME, et al. Recombinant factor VIIa: decreasing time to intervention in coagulopathic patients with severe traumatic brain injury. *J Trauma.* 2008;64(3):620-627; discussion 627-628.
127. Stein DM, Dutton RP, Kramer ME, et al. Reversal of coagulopathy in critically ill patients with traumatic brain injury: recombinant factor VIIa is more cost-effective than plasma. *J Trauma.* 2009;66(1):63-72; discussion 73-75.
128. Bernard SA, Gray TW, Buist MD, et al. Treatment of comatose survivors of out-of-hospital cardiac arrest with induced hypothermia. *N Engl J Med.* 2002;346(8):557-563.
129. Varon J, Acosta P. Therapeutic hypothermia: past, present, and future. *Chest.* 2008;133(5):1267-1274.
130. Beilman GJ, Blondet JJ, Nelson TR, et al. Early hypothermia in severely injured trauma patients is a significant risk factor for multiple organ dysfunction syndrome but not mortality. *Ann Surg.* 2009;249(5):845-850.
131. Inaba K, Teixeira PG, Rhee P, et al. Mortality impact of hypothermia after cavitary explorations in trauma. *World J Surg.* 2009;33(4):864-869.
132. Clifton GL, Miller ER, Choi SC, et al. Lack of effect of induction of hypothermia after acute brain injury. *N Engl J Med.* 2001;344(8):556-563.
133. Goldberg CS, Bove EL, Devaney EJ, et al. A randomized clinical trial of regional cerebral perfusion versus deep hypothermic circulatory arrest: outcomes for infants with functional single ventricle. *J Thorac Cardiovasc Surg.* 2007;133(4):880-887.
134. Hutchison JS, Ward RE, Lacroix J, et al. Hypothermia Pediatric Head Injury Trial Investigators and the Canadian Critical Care Trials Group: Hypothermia therapy after traumatic brain injury in children. *N Engl J Med.* 2008;358(23):2447-2456.
135. Bruckner BA, DiBardino DJ, Cumbie TC, et al. Critical evaluation of chest computed tomography scans for blunt descending thoracic aortic injury. *Ann Thorac Surg.* 2006;81(4):1339-1346.
136. Cleverley JR, Barrie JR, Raymond GS, et al. Direct findings of aortic injury on contrast-enhanced CT in surgically proven traumatic aortic injury: a multi-centre review. *Clin Radiol.* 2002;57(4):281-286.
137. Fabian TC, Davis KA, Gavant ML, et al. Prospective study of blunt aortic injury: helical CT is diagnostic and antihypertensive therapy reduces rupture. *Ann Surg.* 1998;227(5):666-676; discussion 676-677.
138. Modrall JG, Weaver FA, Yellin AE. Diagnosis and management of penetrating vascular trauma and the injured extremity. *Emerg Med Clin North Am.* 1998;16(1):129-144.
139. Rowe VL, Lee W, Weaver FA. Acute arterial occlusion secondary to trauma. *Semin Vasc Surg.* 2009;22(1):25-28.
140. Inaba K, Potzman J, Munera F, et al. Multi-slice CT angiography for arterial evaluation in the injured lower extremity. *J Trauma.* 2006, 60(3):502-506; discussion 506-507.
141. Peng PD, Spain DA, Tataria M, et al. CT angiography effectively evaluates extremity vascular trauma. *Am Surg.* 2008;74(2):103-107.
142. Pieroni S, Foster BR, Anderson SW, et al. Use of 64-row multidetector CT angiography in blunt and penetrating trauma of the upper and lower extremities. *Radiographics.* 2009;29(3):863-876.
143. Dulchavsky SA, Henry SE, Moed BR, et al. Advanced ultrasonic diagnosis of extremity trauma: the FASTER examination. *J Trauma.* 2002;53(1):28-32.

CHAPTER 22 ■ TRAUMATIC BRAIN INJURY

PETER B. LETARTE

The acute care surgeon is certain to encounter neurologic disease while treating the acutely ill patient. Trauma will clearly be the source of most neurologic pathology encountered by the acute care surgeon. The serious nature of many neurologic emergencies, their dramatic forms of presentation, and their complexity can distract providers in the early stages of resuscitation. A preplanned, methodical, but efficient approach to these patients provides the best hope for a quality outcome.

INITIAL DECISIONS—EMERGENCY DEPARTMENT MANAGEMENT

The Advance Trauma Life Support Course has ensured that adequate resuscitation is provided to the victims of trauma. It is important to remember that other neurologic emergencies also require prompt primary resuscitation. In the case of trauma, management of airway, breathing, and life-threatening bleeding is essential.

Airway and Breathing

Epidemiology has demonstrated that patients with traumatic brain injury (TBI) who are allowed oxygen saturations <90% have poorer outcomes. Work with brain tissue monitors has demonstrated that hypoxic insults are additive. This means that multiple brief hypoxic insults add up to a total time of hypoxic insult. Studies have shown that a total of 30 minutes of hypoxia time can result in significantly poorer outcomes.[1-3]

It would seem that limiting such small insults via a well-secured airway would be best for the brain-injured patient. For this reason, orotracheal intubation has been advocated as part of prehospital care for all patients with a Glasgow Coma Score (GCS) < 9. Interestingly, when the impact of prehospital intubation on patients with severe head injuries was studied, patients who were intubated actually had worse outcomes.[4,5]

The factors contributing the increased morbidity in patients intubated in the field appear to be hyperventilation and poorly performed intubation. Hyperventilation has been implicated for some time as a source of secondary brain injury due to its capacity to cause cerebral vasoconstriction and cerebral ischemia.[6] Work in the last few years has demonstrated the tendency for patients intubated in the field to be hyperventilated and has demonstrated inferior outcomes in this same patient group. However, hypoventilated patients also appear to have inferior outcomes. Further complicating the issue of airway management in patients with TBI are concerns about the increased morbidity of poorly performed intubation. Many of the early providers of care to severely brain-injured patients will have poor intubation skills, only performing intubations on patients one to two times in 1–2 years.

Optimum care appears to be intubation at the earliest, safest time. This involves balancing the skill of the intubator with the time to intubation. In an urban setting, this might mean delaying intubation for the 10 minutes required to transport to an emergency department (ED) with an anesthesiologist available, while in a rural setting immediate intubation by a less skilled provider might be required.

Once intubated, pCO_2 should be maintained in the 35–40 mm Hg range per the Brain Trauma Foundation Guidelines, thereby avoiding both hypoventilation and hyperventilation. Recent data suggest that best outcomes may result from slightly lower levels, in the 30–35 mm Hg range, but this will require further validation prior to changing the recommendation.[7,8]

There should be no confusion that hyperventilation in the presence of signs of herniation is appropriate. In the prehospital or ED environments, before intracranial pressure (ICP) monitoring has been instituted, patients who manifest clinical signs of herniation such as a unilaterally dilated pupil, an asymmetric motor examination, or a declining GCS should be hyperventilated in an attempt to blunt the impact of herniation. What is to be avoided is prophylactic or inadvertent hyperventilation.

While end-tidal CO_2 ($ETCO_2$) has many uses in the early management of injured patients, it lacks the accuracy, sensitivity, and specificity to manage the pCO_2 parameters for ventilation in TBI. This is because concurrent conditions such as hypotension, cardiac failure, pulmonary contusion, and even frequent patient movement severely confound the correlation between Arterial and $ETCO_2$. A recent study confirmed this poor correlation and found that patients presenting with $ETCO_2$ in the 35–40 mm Hg range were likely to be underventilated (pCO_2 > 40 mm Hg) 80% of the time and severely underventilated (pCO_2 > 50 mm Hg) 30% of the time.[9]

Circulation

Even a single episode of systolic blood pressure below 90 mm Hg can result in poor outcomes for the victims of TBI.[3,10] For this reason, victims of TBI require vigorous resuscitation of their systolic blood pressure to >90 mm Hg. Ninety millimeters of mercury has traditionally been the threshold used in studies of outcome after head injury. Its basis lies in historical precedent, and it may be that sharp changes in mortality are actually observed at a different threshold.[11]

There is a trend in trauma surgery to set lower resuscitation thresholds and to limit crystalloid resuscitation, especially in penetrating abdominal trauma, to prevent exacerbation of physiologically staunched severe bleeding and to prevent dilution of oxygen carrying capacity. Both of these concerns argue that lower systolic blood pressure resuscitation end points may be appropriate. Without denying the validity of either argument, the fact remains that epidemiologically, TBI patients with systolic blood pressure <90 have poorer outcomes. While further research is needed to determine if another cutoff might make more sense from a physiologic, mortality, or outcome point of view, for now the data support resuscitation of patients with suspected brain injury to 90 mm Hg and all efforts should be expended to assure that patient's systolic blood pressures are kept at this level.

Neurologic Assessment

Pupillary Response. Pupillary asymmetry, the clinical manifestation of temporal lobe herniation, has high diagnostic and prognostic utility. Pupillary asymmetry is defined as a difference of >1 mm between pupils. A dilated pupil is >4 mm. A fixed pupil shows no response to bright light. Pupillary asymmetry and its duration should be carefully documented.

It should be remembered that multiple factors can create this finding. Hypotension, hypoxia, and direct orbital trauma are common causes of pupillary dilation. One iatrogenic cause is the belladonna alkaloids commonly used by ophthalmologists for detailed ophthalmologic examinations. Hypoxia and hypotension should be corrected as herniation is being excluded as the cause for pupillary dilatation. Orbital trauma can be excluded using a swinging light test that assesses the direct and consensual response of each pupil.

Until mass effect has been ruled out, pupillary dilatation should be assumed to be due to mass effect.

Glasgow Coma Score. An important part of the primary survey is to obtain an accurate GCS. The GCS[12] is critical in classifying the severity of head injury and determining its subsequent management. Patients with a GCS of 14–15 are classified as having mild head injury; they have a 2% chance of elevated ICP, a 2% chance of any lesion on computed tomography (CT), and <0.1% chance of that lesion being surgically significant. Moderate head injuries have a GCS of 9–13, a 20% chance of elevated ICP, and an approximately 10% chance of having a lesion on CT scan. Severe head injuries need to be intubated and have an approximately 50% chance of having elevated ICP. Severely head-injured patients with a normal head CT do not need ICP monitoring unless they are in a high-risk group defined as having two of the following three characteristics: age >40, a history of hypotension (systolic blood pressure <90), or unilateral or bilateral motor posturing. Severe head injuries have a GCS of 3–8.[12-14] Unfortunately, in as many as 44% of patients, a full GCS cannot be obtained, especially early in the course of care. Patients who are hypoxic, hypotensive, hypothermic, or hypoglycemic have depressed mental status due to a poor environment for the brain and not due to brain pathology. These conditions should be corrected prior to relying on the GCS for management decisions. Similarly, the common use of paralytics and sedatives in rapid sequence intubation introduces confounding factors that must clear prior to relying on the GCS.

Recent work has questioned the utility of the GCS for certain applications, suggesting other methods for classifying TBI. There also continues to be discussion about whether patients with GCS 13 should be treated as mild or moderate head injuries. It is the author's practice to treat them as moderate.[15]

Penetrating Injuries

Penetrating Brain Injuries (PBI) to the head, particularly gunshot wounds to the head, can carry as high as 90% mortality. Decisions on who should be resuscitated can often be particularly difficult.

Important factors to assess in making this decision are the age of the patient, the circumstance of the injury, and the caliber of weapon. In addition, it is useful to classify Penetrating Brain Injury (PBI) as tangential, penetrating, or perforating injuries. Tangential injuries, which strike but do not enter the calvarium, have a lower mortality rate.[16] A penetrating injury occurs when the projectile enters the calvarium, often driving bone before it into the brain, but remains lodged within the calvarium. A perforating injury occurs when the projectile also exits the brain, creating a tract completely across the head. Traditional PBI teaching has been that injuries that cross the midline are the most lethal, and some class III data support this.[16,17]

Victims of penetrating head trauma who present with a GCS of 3–5 have only a small chance of an acceptable outcome. At the same time, several studies have shown a reasonable prognosis for patients with PBI and GCS 13–15.[16,18-20] It should be remembered that these assumptions are based on postresuscitation GCS.

Patients with a depressed respiratory rate or hypotension on presentation after penetrating trauma are likely near death and are at greater risk for a poorer outcome.

DETERMINING THE NEED FOR EMERGENCY SURGERY

Emergency Radiologic Studies

Cervical Spine Management. Patient who have sustained TBI are at a higher risk for cervical spine injury. Identification of patients who have sustained cervical trauma is crucial since they are at a greater risk of further, possibly, catastrophic injury. Conversely, the morbidity of a prolonged time in a cervical collar, such as decubiti and infection, and the impediments to care created by cervical collars make identification of patients who are at acceptable low risk for further injury to the cervical spine also important, since in these patients the collar can be removed. The goal is to have a process that is very sensitive to detecting high-risk cervical spine injuries and very specific, able to exclude patients who are not at high risk for a major cervical spine injury.

Traditionally, screening was done via imaging. The plain cervical x-rays have been estimated to be 92%–96% sensitive and 78%–97% specific, with some estimates running lower.[21] CT has been estimated to be 96%–100% sensitive and 90%–100% specific for anatomical abnormalities.[21,22] Imaging modalities, however, detect anatomical abnormalities. Judgment is still required to determine which of these abnormalities are substantive or constitute an increased risk to the patient. Judgment is required to determine which patients have an acceptable risk, that is, which patients are "cleared."

Criteria other than imaging have been developed to identify low-risk patients. The National Emergency X-Radiography Utilization Study (NEXUS) criteria use characteristics of the history and physical to screen for low-risk patients. Per the NEXUS criteria, patients who can reliably answer questions and who are neurologically intact, without pain at rest, without pain with palpation of the neck and without pain or other symptoms with motion of the neck have a 99.8% chance of being free of cervical injury (negative predictive value) and may have their collar removed without imaging.[23] Unfortunately, only 12% of presenting patients meet these criteria.

The Canadian C-Spine Rule adds features of the mechanism of injury to the examination and history to screen for high-risk patients. The Canadian C-Spine Rule has a 100% negative predictive value.[24]

The goal of all these techniques is to identify to the practitioner both patients at an acceptably low risk for further neurologic injury, that is, those who are "cleared," and those who remain at increased risk and who warrant further protection and management of their cervical spine. Until this determination is made, all victims of TBI should have their cervical spine protected in a rigid cervical collar.

Computed Tomography of the Head

MILD HEAD INJURY

Since the overwhelming majority of head injuries that present are mild and insignificant, multiple organizations have released guidelines on which brain injury patients should undergo CT scanning, in an effort to limit its unnecessary utilization. The summary of these guidelines is that it is not necessary to obtain a head CT in patients who have no loss of consciousness and are neurologically normal. Problems arise, however, in defining what is meant by "neurologically normal." All guidelines define this as the absence of posttraumatic amnesia (PTA), confusion, or impaired alertness.[25-27] Some of these features may be present with a GCS of 15, depending on the method used for obtaining the GCS. While tests for PTA and screening tests for mild head injury are available, they are not in wide use in emergency rooms today and their utility in this busy environment is questionable.[28] It is therefore difficult to reliably identify and document patients who may not require CT scanning. While it is possible to omit CT scanning in some patients, in most cases, it appears to be cost-effective and safer to triage head-injury patients, including mild head-injury patients, with CT.

TIMING OF CT

CT scanning should be obtained as early as is safely possible in the patient's care. Patients should be adequately resuscitated prior to being taken to the CT scanner.[26] In many urban trauma centers, CT scans can often be obtained within minutes of arrival in the ED, indeed within minutes of the injury. These "ultra early" CT scans can be obtained prior to substantial accumulation of intracranial blood or swelling. Note should be made of patients who receive "ultra early" scanning and subsequently decline in mental status. Such patients may warrant repeat scanning.

FEATURES ON CT

The focus of the CT examination is to identify intracranial hematomas. There are several other features of the scan that are important.

Compression of the basal cisterns is important to note. Basal cistern effacement is the anatomic correlate for progressing temporal lobe herniation. Effaced or compressed basal cisterns are a warning of progressing herniation. Absent basal cisterns are a grim marker of well-advanced herniation.

Midline shift is also important; its use as a criterion for removal of various hematomas is discussed elsewhere. It is important to note that midline shift is caused not only by hematomas but also by cerebral edema.

Traumatic subarachnoid blood is, in fact. While tSAH does not create significant mass effect, it is a prognostic marker for increased ICP and poorer outcome.[136]

CT scanning also allows good imaging of the skull and the skull base. Many fractures can be identified on CT. Particular attention should be paid to skull fractures in "ultra early" scans since they may portend delayed development of a hematoma.[29]

In penetrating head injury, perforating lesions carry a higher mortality with perforating lesions that cross the midline being the most lethal; these lesions can be seen on CT. One exception worth noting is bilateral frontal lobe involvement. Kaufman noted a mortality rate of 12% in this group and good outcomes in 30%, considerably better than the outcomes for bihemispheric lesions in general.[30] Conversely, if the tract is further posterior in the brain, more critical structures will be damaged. Such a posterior tract is likely to traverse the ventricles and ventricular penetration by the tract has been shown to have a strong association with increased mortality.[18,31,32]

Because of the great reliance on CT scanning by many therapies for TBI, comparison of various therapies during research trials requires a standardized description of CT scans to allow classification and comparison of these scans. Marshall proposed such a classification in 1991.[33]

CT findings were divided into mass lesions and diffuse injuries. Mass lesions were further divided into evacuated (any lesion surgically evacuated) and not evacuated (high or mixed density lesion >25cc; not surgically evacuated).

Diffuse injury II, cisterns present with midline shift of 0-5 mm and no high or mixed density lesions >25cc but may include bone fragments and foreign bodies; Diffuse injury III, cisterns compressed or absent with midline shift of 0-5 mm and no high or mixed density lesions >25cc; Diffuse injury IV, midline shift >5 mm; no high or mixed density lesion >25cc.

The Marshall Scale has become a standard for classifying CT scans for research and clinical work. In addition, it has also been used as a tool to study the prognostic value of CT scans. This concept of performing risk analysis of various CT findings has been carried forward by several researchers.[34] Knowledge of a particular injuries natural history via quantitative risk analysis provides a more precise tool for determining who might require surgery for mass lesion evacuation, ICP monitoring or other interventions.

Magnetic Resonance Imaging. As new magnetic resonance imaging (MRI) technologies evolve, the role of MRI in the evaluation of the head-injured patient is changing. While there is much interesting research in this area, there is little that is ready for routine clinical use.

SURGICAL MANAGEMENT

Removal of Mass Lesions

After resuscitation, the most important decision is that of surgical management. One important factor in patients with some form of intracranial bleeding is the volume of the hematoma. Many CT scanners will estimate the hematoma volume. If such an estimate is not available, hematoma volume can be estimated by a technique described by Kothari.[35]

Acute Epidural Hematoma. All epidural hematomas with a volume >30 cm^2 need to be evacuated, regardless of the patient's GCS. The criteria for nonoperative management are a volume on CT < 30 cm^2, a thickness of <15 mm, and a midline shift <0.5 mm in a patient with a GCS > 8 and no focal deficit. All of these criteria should be met for the patient to be managed nonoperatively.[36]

Patients with an acute epidural hematoma, anisocoria, and a GCS < 9 should undergo craniotomy as soon as possible, regardless of the size of the hematoma.[36]

Acute Subdural Hematomas. For subdural hematomas, those with a thickness >10 mm or a midline shift >5 mm should be evacuated regardless of the patient's GCS. A patient with an acute subdural hematoma that is <10 mm thick and midline shift <5 mm but with fixed and dilated or asymmetric pupils, an ICP > 20 mmHg, or a decline in GCS of 2 or more points from the time of injury to hospital admission should also have their hematoma removed. Patients with acute subdural hematomas also need to have their clots removed as soon as possible.37 Subdural hematomas should be removed using craniotomy. All patients with a GCS < 9 and an acute subdural hematoma should be monitored with an ICP monitor.37

Parenchymal Lesions. Parenchymal lesions consist of intraparenchymal clots and contusions. Their management has always been less clearly defined than the management of epidural and subdural hematomas

Focal parenchymal lesions should be removed in three circumstances. Any patient with a parenchymal mass lesion and signs of progressive neurologic deterioration due to the lesion, medically refractory intracranial hypertension, or signs of mass effect on CT scan should be treated operatively. Any patient with any lesion >50 cm^3 in volume should be treated operatively. Patients with GCS scores of 6–8 with frontal or temporal contusions >20 cm^3 in volume with midline shift of at least 5 mm and/or cisternal compression on CT scan should be treated operatively.[38] Craniotomy with evacuation of mass lesion is recommended for these patients.[38]

Patients with parenchymal mass lesions who do not show evidence for neurologic compromise, have controlled ICP, and have no major signs of mass effect on CT scan may be managed nonoperatively with intensive monitoring and serial imaging.[38]

Posterior Fossa Lesions. Posterior fossa lesions are particularly dangerous. These lesions often do not manifest their mass effect by mental status change but rather by vital sign changes. These changes are often subtle and missed, with the ensuing tonsillar herniation often presenting as cardiopulmonary collapse.

Patients with mass effect on CT scan or with neurologic dysfunction or deterioration referable to the lesion should undergo operative intervention. Mass effect on CT scan is defined as distortion, dislocation, or obliteration of the fourth ventricle; compression or loss of visualization of the basal cisterns; or the presence of obstructive hydrocephalus. The operation should take place as soon as possible. A suboccipital craniectomy is the procedure most commonly performed.[39]

Patients with lesions and no major mass effect on CT scan and without signs of neurologic dysfunction may be managed by close observation and serial imaging.[39]

Surgical Management of Diffuse Brain Swelling—Decompressive Craniectomy

As with many techniques, the term decompressive craniectomy has been used by authors to refer to several different operations. A wide hemispheric craniectomy and bifrontal craniectomy with several different methods of dural opening have all been described.[40-42] Clinical experience has created the impression that decompressive craniectomy can have significant clinical value. Its true clinical efficacy is awaiting the outcome of multiple current ongoing studies (ClinicalTrials.gov identifier NCT00155987).

The quandary in decompressive craniectomy is its use in treating isolated diffuse cerebral swelling. Decompressive craniectomy may be done incidental to a craniotomy for removal of hematoma, but the decision making in this case is driven by the need to remove the hematoma. The more difficult problem is the decision and timing of surgery where the only indication is diffuse cerebral swelling.

Currently, it is felt that decompressive craniectomy should not be a "last-ditch," salvage procedure; rather, it should be a deliberate part of the treatment protocol that is aggressively invoked early in the patient's care when lower-tier therapies fail. Expert guidelines suggest that for patients with diffuse cerebral swelling, bifrontal decompressive craniectomy within 48 hours of injury is a treatment option. These patients should have diffuse, medically refractory posttraumatic cerebral edema and resultant intracranial hypertension.[38] In addition to bifrontal decompressive craniectomy, other decompressive procedures, including subtemporal decompression, temporal lobectomy, and hemispheric decompressive craniectomy, are treatment options for patients with refractory intracranial hypertension and diffuse parenchymal injury with clinical and radiographic evidence for impending transtentorial herniation.[38]

Depressed Skull Fractures

Patients with open (compound) depressed cranial fractures should undergo operative intervention to prevent infection and decompress the brain if clinical or radiographic evidence of dural penetration, major intracranial hematoma, bone depression >1 cm, frontal sinus involvement, gross cosmetic deformity, wound infection, pneumocephalus, or gross wound contamination is present. Nonoperative management is appropriate for patients without any of these findings.

Elevation of the fracture and debridement of the skull, scalp, and brain followed by closure of the dura is the surgical method of choice. Replacement of the bone at the time of surgery is appropriate, although the risk of infection must be considered when one is replacing bone fragments associated with an open wound. However, such replacement can be safe if thorough irrigation and debridement have been utilized. Antibiotics can be started on all patients with open (compound) depressed fractures.[43] Early operation is recommended to reduce the incidence of infection.

Closed (simple) depressed cranial fractures that are less than the width of the skull deep may be treated nonoperatively.[43]

In children, ping-pong fractures, or large depressions on the convexity of the skull reminiscent of the depressions commonly seen on old ping-pong (table tennis) balls, sometimes require elevation if the depression is deeper than the thickness of the skull. These fractures may be elevated by simply drilling an adjacent burr hole, carefully sliding a stout instrument underneath the fracture, and levering the fragments outward.

Fractures at the base of the skull, which involve the frontal sinuses or ethmoid sinuses, are more complex to manage and often require a collaborative approach with otolaryngology, plastics, or oromaxillofacial surgery.

Penetrating Injuries

The goals of surgery for the victim of PBI are to remove mass effect, control bleeding, control infection, to prevent cerebrospinal fluid (CSF) leak and to close the scalp. Although advocated in the past, aggressive removal of all bone and bullet fragments is no longer a goal for this surgery.[44-48]

Retained bullet and bone fragments do not have a large impact on the post-PBI infection rates, but CSF leakage does.[44,46] Tight dural closure is a mainstay of surgery for PBI. Scalp lacerations that result from PBI are often complex. Scalp incisions for PBI operations should be planned to allow for complex scalp repair at the end of the case.

Cerebrovascular Injury

Patients who present with arterial hemorrhage from mouth, nose, ears, or wounds, expanding cervical hematomas, cervical bruit in patients younger than 50 years old, or incongruous lateralizing neurologic deficit not explained by CT or other findings should have carotid dissection considered in their diagnosis. In addition, trauma patients who present with evidence of cerebral infarction should have carotid as well as vertebral artery injury considered in the diagnosis, although like contusion, infarction does not present on CT for 12–24 hours after the infarction. Patients suspected of harboring a carotid injury should undergo angiography on an emergent basis if they are otherwise stable. Coordination of the appropriate management for both the vascular and the intracranial injuries requires a well-coordinated multispecialty approach.[49]

INTENSIVE CARE UNIT MANAGEMENT

Intracranial Pressure

Early workers in TBI used ICP upper limits ranging from 20–30 mm Hg as the intraventricular pressure threshold for the treatment of ICP.[14,50-52] Analyzing data from the National Trauma Coma Data Bank (NTCDB), Marmarou found 20 mm Hg to be the critical cutoff identified by regression analysis.[53] Current guidelines recommend keeping the ICP below 20–25 mm Hg water.[54]

Placement of an intraventricular catheter, however, requires a certain level of skill and practice. Placement cannot always be achieved. They can require a high level of maintenance and they carry an approximately 2% infection rate. A common alternative is the intraparenchymal/intraventricular fiber-optic or microsensor ICP monitor. These are easier to place and have a lower infection rate. Their use can be coupled with a ventriculostomy.

Hyperosmolar Therapy. Hyperosmolar therapy for cerebral edema and elevated ICP has been in use since the 1950s. The first agent was urea, which was then superseded by Mannitol. More recently, hypertonic saline has been used as a hyperosmolar agent for TBI. Mannitol has long been accepted as an effective tool for reducing ICP.[55-59] Numerous mechanistic laboratory studies support this conclusion. Its impact on outcome has never, however, been directly demonstrated via a class I trial testing mannitol against placebo.

There is a commonly held belief that mannitol administration can cause or exacerbate hypotension in the early resuscitation of trauma victims. There are class III data that show infusion of mannitol at rates of 0.2–0.8 g/kg/min can lead to transient drops in blood pressure.[60-62] From these observations, a rate of no higher than 0.1 g/kg/min or 1 g/kg delivered over 10 minutes or more is recommended.[63] Careful monitoring of urine output with aggressive replacement of this fluid loss is also recommended to prevent hypotension associated with the use of mannitol.

Mannitol and other osmotics are known to be able to briefly open the blood brain barrier. Furthermore, at rates of administration that exceed the rate of excretion of mannitol, mannitol can accumulate in the extracellular space. These factors lead to the accumulation of mannitol in extracellular spaces and a reverse osmotic gradient that can lead to a "rebound effect" or movement of water into the brain. Class III data suggest that this effect is more likely with continuous infusion of mannitol, as opposed to bolus administration.[64-66]

Class II and III data have shown that doses of 0.25–1.0 g/kg of mannitol may be needed to achieve a reduction in ICP. This required dose varies from patient to patient and even may vary from time to time in the same patient.[29,57,65,67]

Hypertonic Saline. Hypertonic saline offers an attractive alternative to mannitol as a therapy for elevated ICP. Its ability to reduce elevated ICP has been demonstrated with class II and III data in the intensive care unit (ICU) and in the operating room.[68-71]

Hypertonic saline has been used in two very different ways in the resuscitation of trauma victims. In addition to being proposed as a hyperosmolar agent for the management of elevated ICP, it is also advocated as a low-volume resuscitation fluid. While the qualities that make it useful both as a low-volume resuscitation fluid and as a brain-targeted therapy are related, its efficacy in one role does not guarantee its efficacy in the other. Each therapeutic endpoint must be analyzed independently.

Previously, there had been no consensus on what was meant by "hypertonic saline." Concentrations of 3%, 7.2%, 7.5%, 10%, and 23.4% have all been used and described in the literature. Many current clinical trials have used 7.5% saline.[68-70,72]

In addition, hypertonic saline is described in the literature as being administered in a variety of different ways, the two principle ones being as a bolus or as a continuous drip.

When hypertonic saline is given as an infusion, the goal of the therapy is to elevate serum sodium to 155–160 mEq/L, although some investigators have gone as high as 180 mEq/L. This elevated serum sodium is thought to help stabilize ICP and reduce the therapeutic intensity required to manage elevated ICP.[73,74]

The more common route of administration, especially in early resuscitation, is to use hypertonic saline as a bolus to achieve an immediate reduction in ICP. This method takes advantage of the rapid rheologic improvement and improved cerebral blood flow (CBF) that, like mannitol, hypertonic saline can create.

Multiple animal studies and several human studies have demonstrated that hypertonic saline, as a bolus, can reduce ICP in a monitored environment such as the operating room or ICU where ICP monitoring is present.[75-77]

In two prospective clinical trials, however, hypertonic saline did not demonstrate any advantage over normal saline on neurologic outcome when given as a prehospital resuscitation fluid.[78,79] Further trials are continuing.

Hyperventilation. Hyperventilation has been used since the earliest days of ICP management to limit ICP by cerebral vasoconstriction. The cost of this intervention is the ischemia induced by this same vasoconstriction. Hyperventilation is considered mild when the arterial pCO_2 is kept between 30–35 mm Hg. Severe hyperventilation occurs when the arterial pCO_2 is below 30 mm Hg.

The only study of hyperventilation's impact on outcome demonstrated that at 12 months there was no difference between patients who were hyperventilated and those who were not. However, at 3 and 6 months, patients who were hyperventilated had poorer outcomes.[6]

The outcome data, combined with a body of data concerning the low blood flow and the near-ischemic conditions found in newly injured brains, raise concern about hyperventilation's ischemic potential.[80-82] In the 1990s, published guidelines discouraged hyperventilation except in the presence of impending herniation, as manifest by elevated ICP or clinical signs of herniation. This position has remained the therapeutic recommendation since. Recent work has shown the best outcomes for patients reliably kept in the 30–39 mm Hg range during the ED phases of their resuscitation.[83] In the prehospital environment, best outcomes are seen in the 30–35 mm Hg range.[7]

Hyperventilation is an acceptable modality in the presence of impending herniation for short periods of time or in the presence of elevated ICP refractory to sedation, paralysis, CSF drainage, or osmotic diuresis.[84]

Barbiturate Therapy. Barbiturate therapy or barbiturate "coma" can be used as a third-tier therapy for elevated ICP when other more standard therapies have failed. It has been demonstrated to be effective in reducing ICP.[85]

Barbiturate therapy also carries with it a high morbidity.[86] Barbiturates affect the function of not only the brain but also the heart and kidneys, among other organs. Substantial declines in the functioning of both of these organ systems can occur during therapy. For this reason, barbiturate coma should not be initiated if the victim of malignant ICP is also hemodynamically unstable. Patients should be carefully monitored to assure maintenance of hemodynamic stability during therapy.

Hypothermia. Hypothermia has been shown to reduce elevated ICP.[87-90] There are also some clinical data that demonstrate that hypothermia has a beneficial effect on the outcome from TBI.[87,91,92]

The National Acute Brain Injury Study: Hypothermia (NABISH) study was a large randomized prospective clinical trial designed to demonstrate this beneficial effect for hypothermia on the outcome from TBI. It failed to do so.[93]

Although the NABISH study failed to demonstrate the efficacy of hypothermia, many still believe that it has potential value as a therapy. Multiple clinical trials are in progress to explore its utility.

Therapeutic hypothermia for TBI is considered to be the rapid reduction and maintenance of a core body temperature to 32°C–35°C for 48 hours or less. The decision to induce the hypothermia must be made almost immediately upon presentation, and the patient must have the hypothermia induced and reach target temperature within 60 or perhaps even 30 minutes of presentation.[94] The therapy has not demonstrated efficacy as a third-tier therapy and should not be instituted several days into treatment as other therapies fail.[94]

Hypothermia is a complex therapy, which should only be performed at centers that are willing to make the substantial commitment to doing it correctly. It appears that marginal or inept application of this therapy at best will do no good and at worst will harm the patients.[95]

It has been shown that hyperthermia results in a poorer outcome from TBI.[96] Efforts to prevent excessive temperatures in the victims of TBI are appropriate.

Cerebral Perfusion Pressure

Cerebral perfusion pressure (CPP) is the difference between the mean arterial pressure and the ICP (CPP = MAP − ICP). The role of CPP in TBI is complex and our understanding of it is incomplete and controversial. Establishing what the correct CPP should be is therefore difficult.

There are actually many reasons cited to maintain an adequate CPP.[97] The most common is to reduce the incidence of secondary insults to the injured brain. This approach focuses on inadvertent hypotension to the brain and reduces the number of secondary insults, that is, the numbers of hypotensive episodes. A second reason to maintain adequate CPP is to assure that the brain is functioning within the autoregulatory limits. The third reason to maintain adequate CPP is to assure adequate oxygen delivery to the brain, the $PbrO_2$. In these studies, above a certain CPP threshold, $PbrO_2$ is no longer dependent on CPP. This number is commonly thought to be 60 mm Hg.

Robertson et al. examined some of these issues in a study published in 1999. In this class I study, patients were randomized to either a CBF-targeted therapy or an ICP-targeted therapy.[98] While the CBF-targeted group in this study showed better performance for many of the surrogate markers for CPP success, the study failed to show any improvement in outcome for CBF-directed therapy over ICP-focused therapy. Further, the study showed that patients with CPP of 70 mm Hg had a higher incidence of acute respiratory distress syndrome.[98]

The current synthesis of the data is that, except in cases of regional ischemia, a CPP of 60 mmHg is adequate and no benefit and some harm may come from elevating CPP to 70 mm Hg.[99]

Advanced Cerebral Monitoring

Oxygen delivery to the brain is traditionally monitored via pulse oximetry. However, knowing that blood oxygen saturation is >90% is not sufficient to determine if oxygen delivery to the brain is adequate.

Several methods for measuring oxygen delivery to the brain are available. One method is to measure the arterial-venous oxygen difference across the brain, the AVO_2: This value requires a sensor or sampling catheter high in the jugular vein.

Estimates of the adequacy of oxygen delivery to the brain can also be made by measuring the saturation of blood leaving the brain in the jugular bulb, the $SjvO_2$. This is most commonly done via a jugular bulb catheter. Most patients have an $SjvO_2$ of 55%–69% in the blood leaving the brain.

$SjvO_2$ appears to adequately reflect the status of oxygen delivery to the brain. While it has never been shown that maintaining $SjvO_2$ in the normal range improves outcome, multiple studies have shown that patients with increased numbers of episodes of $SjvO_2$ desaturation <50% have worse outcomes.[100-104]

A more direct approach is to measure cerebral tissue oxygen tension. This can be measured via cerebral tissue oxygen monitoring. Normal cerebral tissue oxygen pressures, $PbrO_2$, are approximately 32 mm Hg. Studies have shown that patients whose $PbrO_2$ is allowed to dip to 15 or lower have poorer outcomes.[101,105,106]

It appears that active management of cerebral oxygen delivery has the potential to improve outcomes from TBI. Applying technologies that allow the $SjvO_2$ to be kept above 50% and the $PbrO_2$ above 15 mm Hg is now a reasonable option to pursue in the management of TBI

Penetrating Injury

PBI can lead to delayed posttraumatic cerebral aneurysms. Between 3% and 33% of all victims of PBI may have a posttraumatic aneurysm.[107,108] Such aneurysms can develop as late as 2 weeks after the injury, and an early negative cerebral angiogram does not exclude an aneurysm later in the patient's course. Any patient who develops delayed or unexplained subarachnoid hemorrhage or other delayed bleeding should be suspected of harboring a posttraumatic aneurysm and should undergo cerebral angiography.

CSF leaks and subsequent infections are an important source of morbidity and mortality in the victims of PBI. Half of all CSF leaks may occur at sites remote from the entry or exit sites in the calvarium. These CSF leaks will not be apparent at surgery and will manifest after surgery. Seventy-two percent of these leaks will appear within 2 weeks of surgery and forty-four percent will seal spontaneously.[109]

Current infection rates for PBI in a military setting are 4%–11%. Current civilian rates are at 1%–5%.[110] Half (55%) of all intracranial infections occur within 3 weeks of the injury and 90% occur within 6 weeks.[110] Factors affecting infection risk are CSF leaks, air sinus wounds, and wound dehiscence. Because of the high infection rates with this injury, long-term antibiotics are commonly used.

In PBI, 30%–50% of victims develop posttraumatic epilepsy PTE.[48,111] This is slightly higher than the estimates of 4%–42% for nonpenetrating TBI.[112-114] Early seizures in the TBI literature are defined as seizures in the first 7 days after injury, when the vast majority of early seizures occur.[114] Current guidelines for antiepileptic therapy after PBI are the same as after TBI.[115]

The risk of PTE after PBI appears to decline with time. While 18% of victims may not have their first seizure until 5 or more years after the injury, 80% will have their first seizure within 2 years of the injury and 95% of patients who remain seizure free for 3 years following injury will remain seizure free.[48,111] Followed out to 15 years, 50% of patients who do develop PTE will stop having seizures.[48]

Systemic Management

The management of systemic parameters in head-injured patients is similar to the management of other trauma patients. Cardiovascular, pulmonary, renal, and other organ systems must be watched closely and supported as necessary with the goal of preventing secondary cerebral insults. There are some unique aspects of critical care management for brain-injured patients that should be highlighted.

Hypoglycemia and Hyperglycemia. Both elevations (hyperglycemia) and decreases (hypoglycemia) in blood sugar jeopardize ischemic brain tissue. The disastrous impact of significant hypoglycemia on the nervous system, during injury and at other times, is well known. In the absence of glucose, ischemic neurons can be permanently damaged. However, it is also true that prolonged serum glucose of >150 and perhaps >200 mg/dL may be harmful to the injured brain and should be avoided.[116,117]

Steroids. Although steroids were commonly administered to head-injured patients in the past, multiple studies have failed to show any benefit to mortality or outcome for steroid administration. The largest study to date, the CRASH trial, was terminated early after accrual of 10,008 patients when analysis showed a substantially increased risk of death for the head injury population receiving steroids.[118] There is currently no known benefit to administering steroids to brain-injured patients for the purpose of neuroprotection or ICP control.

Anticonvulsants. Current guidelines for antiepileptic therapy after TBI distinguish between two uses for antiepileptic drugs post injury, treatment and prophylaxis. Antiepileptic drugs do appear to be effective in treating an established posttraumatic seizure disorder and in preventing immediate postinjury seizures in the first week after injury. They do not appear to be effective in reducing the incidence of posttraumatic epilepsy. Maintenance of TBI victims on prophylactic doses of anticonvulsant medications beyond the first week of therapy does not appear to reduce the incidence of posttraumatic seizures. The recommendation for TBI is to treat the patient with anticonvulsants for 7 days and then discontinue the medication, only restarting it if seizures develop.[95,115]

Prevention and Management of Complications

Coagulopathy. Unlike most critically injured trauma patients, who tend to have low plasma antithrombin (AT) activity, those with closed head injury tend to have supranormal plasma AT activity, perhaps explaining in part the frequent occurrence of coagulopathy after TBI.[119] DIC is often associated with the development of potentially dangerous delayed or recurrent intracranial hematomas in head-injured patients and can cause expansion of otherwise small hematomas and contusions.[120]

In addition, the increasing use of anticoagulants in treating various cardiac, vascular, and neurologic conditions has resulted in an increasing older population of patients with iatrogenic coagulopathy. These patients are also at risk for expansion of seemingly insignificant clots into life-threatening masses. Special caution should be observed in the elderly if the initial CT scan is a "hyperacute" scan, that is, one obtained very soon after the precipitating trauma.

Fresh-frozen plasma is a commonly used and effective empiric treatment for patients with coagulation defects. Unfortunately, reduction of an elevated INR to acceptable levels for surgery can sometimes take several hours. The decision to operate in the face of significantly elevated INR can easily lead to surgical disaster.

Recombinant factor VIIa offers a potential solution to this dilemma, with the ability to rapidly reverse an elevated INR and allow almost immediate surgery.[121-123] This use of factor VIIa is currently an off-label indication, and work is ongoing to investigate the safety and efficacy of this drug in the treatment of the victims of TBI.[124]

Thromboembolic Events. Head-injured patients are at increased risk of deep venous thrombosis (DVT) and pulmonary embolism (PE). In a large series of trauma patients, 4.3% of those with head injury were diagnosed with DVT, twice the rate seen in patients without neurologic injury.[125]

Neurosurgeons are concerned about potentially catastrophic postoperative hemorrhagic complications and prefer DVT prophylaxis techniques that avoid compromise of the clotting cascade.

Pneumatic compression stockings are one such technique. In several clinical series of patients with various types of neurosurgical disease, such devices were associated with an incidence of DVT of 1.7%–2.3% and PE of 1.5%–1.8%.[126,127] These results have not been uniformly demonstrated by all studies, but pneumatic stockings are a mainstay of DVT prophylaxis.

Experience with low-molecular-weight heparin used in conjunction with pneumatic compression suggests that this regimen is even more effective than pneumatic compression alone in general neurosurgery patients[127] and is safe and effective in trauma patients (including those with head injury).[128]

Treatment of thromboembolic events in head-injured patients must weigh the dangers of PE with the risk of bleeding. There are scant data relating the risk of bleeding to time after injury. Anticoagulation may be deferred from 72 hours to as long as 6 weeks after injury in an attempt to prevent recurrent bleeding, depending on local custom.

Thromboembolic events within this window are usually best treated by insertion of an inferior vena cava filter (IVCF). Prophylactic use of IVCFs in all high-risk patients is controversial.

OUTCOME

Of the patients who survive to reach the Emergency department, 80% have mild injuries. Moderate and severe injuries each account for 10% of the total. Survivors of TBI are often left with varying degrees of disability, which occur in roughly 10% of mild, 50%–67% of moderate, and >95% of severe closed TBI survivors.[129] The most widely used tool for assessing outcome after TBI is the Glasgow Outcome Scale,[130] although more refined assessment tools are constantly being sought.

Outcome Prediction

Many prediction models have been developed over the years. Different indicators of outcome have different significance and different precedence depending on the population to which they are applied. A grim prognostic indicator in the elderly might have much less dire implications for a younger patient. As a result, generalization of findings from a specific population and prediction model to the general population is often inappropriate.[131,132] Care needs to be used when applying prediction models in everyday practice.

Although very good and very bad outcomes can usually be predicted with a high degree of confidence early after injury, it is much harder to prognosticate about patients in intermediate categories. Studies have shown that even with the diligent application of known indicators, physicians tend to overestimate the likelihood of poor outcome and underestimate the likelihood of good outcome early in the care of head-injured patients. In one study, physician's predictive accuracy was only 56%.[133] This "false pessimism" phenomenon takes on greater significance when combined with work demonstrating that providers will alter their care based on these predictions, increasing the use of therapies considered beneficial for those thought to have a good outcome and decreasing it for those felt not to have a good prognosis.[134] Care should therefore be exerted when offering predictions or withholding care of the brain-injured patient early in the course of their treatment.

BRAIN DEATH AND ORGAN DONATION

The diagnosis of brain death is made when there is no clinical evidence of neurologic function in a patient whose core temperature is >32.8°C, whose mental status is not impacted by sedating or paralyzing medications, who is completely resuscitated with a systolic blood pressure >90 mm Hg and whose oxygen saturations are >90%.[135]

The absence of neurologic function must be scrupulously established and documented. Most errors in declaring brain death are the result of poorly performed neurologic examinations. Nationally recognized standards for examination can be found in the references.[135]

Many clinical protocols and some state statutes also require that brain death be confirmed by further neurologic tests, an ancillary test such as radionucleotide CBF studies or EEG.[135]

The physiologic definition of brain death described above is the one commonly used in the United States. Various hospitals and systems will have differing methods for declaring brain death and the states have varying legal statute on who may declare death and brain death and how it is to be declared. Those interested should ask within their local system.

References

1. Bardt TF, Unterberg AW, Hartl R, et al. Monitoring of brain tissue PO_2 in traumatic brain injury: effect of cerebral hypoxia on outcome. *Acta Neurochir Suppl*. 1998;71:153-156.
2. Bardt TF, Unterberg AW, Kiening KL, et al. Multimodal cerebral monitoring in comatose head-injured patients. *Acta Neurochir*. 1998;140:357-365.
3. Chestnut RM, Marshall LF, Klauber MR, et al. The role of secondary brain injury in determining outcome from severe head injury. *J Trauma*. 1993;34:216-222.
4. Davis DP, Dunford JV, Poste JC, et al. The impact of hypoxia and hyperventilation on outcome after paramedic rapid sequence intubation of severely head-injured patients. *J Trauma*. 2004;57:1-8.
5. Davis DP, Hoyt DB, Ochs M, et al. The effect of paramedic rapid sequence intubation on outcome in patients with severe traumatic brain injury. *J Trauma*. 2003;54:444-453.
6. Muizelaar JP, Marmarou A, Ward JD, et al. Adverse effects of prolonged hyperventilation in patients with severe head injury: a randomized clinical trial. *J Neurosurg*. 1991;75:731-739.
7. Warner KJ, Cuschieri J, Copass MK, et al. The impact of prehospital ventilation on outcome after severe traumatic brain injury. *J Trauma*. 2007;62:1330-1336.
8. Warner KJ, Cuschieri J, Copass MK, et al. Emergency department ventilation effects outcome in severe traumatic brain injury. *J Trauma*. 2008;64:341-347.
9. Warner KJ, Cuschieri J, Garland B, et al. The utility of early end-tidal capnography in monitoring ventilation status after severe injury. *J Trauma*. 2009;66:26-31.
10. Marmarou A, Anderson RL, Ward JL, et al. Impact of ICP instability and hypotension on outcome in patients with severe head trauma. *J Neurosurg*. 1991;75:S59-S66.
11. Eastridge BJ, Salinas J, McManus JG, et al. Hypotension begins at 110 mm Hg: redefining "hypotension" with data. [Erratum appears in *J Trauma*. 2008;65(2):501. Note: Concertino, Victor A [corrected to Convertino, Victor A]]. *J Trauma*. 2007;63:291-297.
12. Teasdale G, Jennett B. Assessment of coma and impaired consciousness: a practical scale. *Lancet*. 1974;2:81.
13. Narayan RK, Greenberg RP, Miller JD. Improved confidence of outcome prediction in severe head injury: a comparative analysis of the clinical examination, multimodality evoked potentials, CT scanning, and intracranial pressure. *J Neurosurg*. 1981;54:751-762.
14. Narayan RK, Kishore PR, Becker DP. Intracranial pressure: to monitor or not to monitor? A review of our experience with severe head injury. *J Neurosurg*. 1982;56:650-659.
15. Saatman KE, Duhaime AC, Bullock R, et al. Classification of traumatic brain injury for targeted therapies. *J Neurotrauma*. 2008;25:719-738.
16. Arabi B. Surgical outcome in 435 patients who sustained missile head wounds during the Iran-Iraq War. *Neurosurg*. 1990;27:692-695.
17. Part 2: prognosis in penetrating brain injury [Review]. *J Trauma*. 2001;51:S44-S86.
18. Brandvold B, Levi L, Feinsod M, et al. Penetrating craniocerebral injuries in the Israeli involvement in the Lebanese conflict, 1982-1985. Analysis of a less aggressive surgical approach [Review]. *J Neurosurg*. 1990;72:15-21.
19. Grahm TW, Williams FC Jr, Harrington T, et al. Civilian gunshot wounds to the head: a prospective study [see comment]. *Neurosurgery*. 1990;27:696-700.
20. Kaufman HH, Makela ME, Lee KF, et al. Gunshot wounds to the head: a perspective. *Neurosurgery*. 1986;18:689-695.
21. Blackmore CC, Ramsey SD, Mann FA, et al. Cervical spine screening with CT in trauma patients: a cost-effectiveness analysis. *Radiology*. 1999;212:117-125.
22. Hennessy D, Widder S, Zygun D, et al. Cervical spine clearance in obtunded blunt trauma patients: a prospective study. *J Trauma*. 2010;68:576-582.
23. Hoffman JR, Mower WR, Wolfson AB, et al. Validity of a set of clinical criteria to rule out injury to the cervical spine in patients with blunt trauma. National Emergency X-Radiography Utilization Study Group. [Erratum appears in *N Engl J Med*. 2001;344(6):464]. *N Engl J Med*. 2000;343:94-99.
24. Stiell IG, Clement CM, McKnight RD, et al. The Canadian C-spine rule versus the NEXUS low-risk criteria in patients with trauma. *N Engl J Med*. 2003;349:2510-2518.
25. The management of minor closed head injury in children. Committee on Quality Improvement, American Academy of Pediatrics. Commission on Clinical Policies and Research, American Academy of Family Physicians [see comment] [Review]. *Pediatrics*. 1999;104:1407-1415.
26. ACR Appropriateness Criteria Expert Panel on Neurologic Imaging. Head Trauma. *American College of Radiology* [serial online] 2006.
27. The East Practice Management Guidelines Work Group. Practice Management Guidelines for the Management of Mild Traumatic Brain Injury. *Eastern Association for the Surgery of Trauma* [serial online] 2001; Available from: Eastern Association for the Surgery of Trauma.
28. McCrea M, Kelly JP, Kluge J, et al. Standardized assessment of concussion in football players. *Neurology*. 1997;48:586-588.
29. CT Scan Features. *Management and Prognosis of Severe Traumatic Brain Injury*. 2nd ed. Brain Trauma Foundation; 2000:65-116.
30. Kaufman HH, Levy ML, Stone JL, et al. Patients with Glasgow Coma Scale scores 3, 4, 5 after gunshot wounds to the brain [Review]. *Neurosurg Clin North Am*. 1995;6:701-714.
31. Clark WC, Muhlbauer MS, Watridge CB, et al. Analysis of 76 civilian craniocerebral gunshot wounds. *J Neurosurg*. 1986;65:9-14.
32. Shaffrey ME, Polin RS, Phillips CD, et al. Classification of civilian craniocerebral gunshot wounds: a multivariate analysis predictive of mortality. *J Neurotrauma*. 1992;9(suppl 1):S279-S285.
33. Marshall LF, Marshall SB, Klauber MR. A new classification of head injury based on computerized tomography. *J Neurosurg*. 1991;75:S14-S20.
34. Maas AI, Marmarou A, Murray GD, et al. Prognosis and clinical trial design in traumatic brain injury: the IMPACT study [Review]. *J Neurotrauma*. 2007;24:232-238.
35. Kothari RU, Brott T, Broderick JP, et al. The ABCs of measuring intracerebral hemorrhage volumes. *Stroke*. 1996;27:1304-1305.
36. Bullock MR, Chesnut R, Ghajar J, et al. Surgical management of acute epidural hematomas. *Neurosurgery*. 2006;58:S2-7-S2-15.
37. Bullock MR, Chesnut R, Ghajar J, et al. Surgical Management of acute subdural hematomas. *Neurosurgery*. 2006;58:S2-16-S2-24.
38. Bullock MR, Chesnut R, Ghajar J, et al. Surgical management of traumatic parenchymal lesions. *Neurosurgery*. 2006;58:S25-S46.
39. Bullock MR, Chesnut R, Ghajar J, et al. Surgical management of posterior fossa mass lesions. *Neurosurgery*. 2006;58:S47-S55.
40. Aarabi B, Hesdorffer DC, Ahn ES, et al. Outcome following decompressive craniectomy for malignant swelling due to severe head injury [see comment]. *J Neurosurg*. 2006;104:469-479.
41. Hejazi N, Witzmann A, Fae P. Unilateral decompressive craniectomy for children with severe brain injury. Report of seven cases and review of the relevant literature [Review]. *Eur J Pediatr*. 2002;161:99-104.
42. Polin RS, Shaffrey ME, Bogaev CA, et al. Decompressive bifrontal craniectomy in the treatment of severe refractory posttraumatic cerebral edema. *Neurosurgery*. 1997;41:84-92.
43. Bullock MR, Chesnut R, Ghajar J, et al. Surgical management of depressed cranial fractures. *Neurosurgery*. 2006;58:S56-S60.
44. Carey ME, Young HF, Rish BL, et al. Follow-up study of 103 American soldiers who sustained a brain wound in Vietnam. *J Neurosurg*. 1974;41:542-549.

45. Chaudhri KA, Choudhury AR, al Moutaery KR, et al. Penetrating craniocerebral shrapnel injuries during "Operation Desert Storm": early results of a conservative surgical treatment. *Acta Neurochir (Wien)*. 1994;126:120-123.
46. Gonul E, Baysefer A, Kahraman S, et al. Causes of infections and management results in penetrating craniocerebral injuries. *Neurosurg Rev*. 1997;20:177-181.
47. Hammon WM. Analysis of 2187 consecutive penetrating wounds of the brain from Vietnam. *J Neurosurg*. 1971;34:127-131.
48. Salazar AM, Jabbari B, Vance SC, et al. Epilepsy after penetrating head injury. I. Clinical correlates: a report of the Vietnam Head Injury Study. *Neurology*. 1985;35:1406-1414.
49. Biffl WL, Cothren CC, Moore EE, et al. Western Trauma Association critical decisions in trauma: screening for and treatment of blunt cerebrovascular injuries [Review]. *J Trauma*. 2009;67:1150-1153.
50. Becker DP, Miller JD, Ward JD, et al. The outcome from severe head injury with early diagnosis and intensive management. *J Neurosurg*. 1977;47:491-502.
51. Marshall LF, Smith RW, Shapiro HM. The outcome with aggressive treatment in severe head injuries. Part I: the significance of intracranial pressure monitoring. *J Neurosurg*. 1979;50:20-25.
52. Saul TG, Ducker TB. Effect of intracranial pressure monitoring and aggressive treatment on mortality in severe head injury. *J Neurosurg*. 1982;56:498-503.
53. Marmarou A, Anderson RL, Ward JD. Impact of ICP instability and hypotension on outcome in patients with severe head trauma. *J Neurosurg*. 1991;75:S159-S166.
54. Intracranial Pressure Treatment Threshold. *Management and Prognosis of Severe Traumatic Brain Injury*. 2nd ed. Brain Trauma Foundation; 2000:71-74.
55. Becker DP, Vries JK. *The Alleviation of Increased Intracranial Pressure by the Chronic Administration of Osmotic Agents*. Springer; 1972.
56. Eisenberg HM, Frankowski RF, Contant CF. High-dose barbiturate control of elevated intracranial pressure in patients with severe head injury. *J Neurosurg*. 1988;69:15-23.
57. James HE. Methodology for the control of intracranial pressure with hypertonic mannitol. *Acta Neurochir (Wein)* 1980;51:161-172.
58. Schwartz ML, Tator CH, Rowed DW. The University of Toronto Head Injury Treatment Study: a prospective, randomized comparison of pentobarbitol and mannitol. *J Neurol Sci*. 1984;11:434-440.
59. Smith HP, Kelly DL Jr, McWhorter JM, et al. Comparison of mannitol regimens in patients with severe head injury undergoing intracranial monitoring. *J Neurosurg*. 1986;65:820-824.
60. Cote CJ, Greenhow DE, Marshall BE. The hypotensive response to rapid intravenous administration of hypertonic solutions in man and in the rabbit. *Anesthesiology*. 1979;50:30-35.
61. Domaingue CM, Nye DH. Hypotensive effect of mannitol administered rapidly. *Anaesth Intensive Care*. 1985;13:134-136.
62. Ravussin P, Archer DP, Tyler JL. Effects of rapid mannitol infusion on cerebral blood volume: a positron emission tomographic study in dogs and man. *J Neurosurg*. 1986;64:104-113.
63. Schrot RJ, Muizelaar JP. Is there a "best" way to give Mannitol? In: Valadka AB, Andrews BT, eds. *Neurotrauma*. 1st ed. New York: Thieme; 2005:142-147.
64. Kaufmann AM, Cardoso ER. Aggravation of vasogenic cerebral edema by multiple-dose mannitol. *J Neurosurg*. 1992;77:584-589.
65. McGraw CP, Alexander E, Howard G. Effect of dose and dose schedule on the response of intracranial pressure to mannitol. *Surg Neurol*. 1978;10:127-130.
66. Pupillary Diameter and Light Reflex. *Management and Prognosis of Severe Traumatic Brain Injury*. 2nd ed. Brain Trauma Foundation; 2000.
67. Marshall LF, SMith RW, Rauscher LA, et al. Mannitol dose requirements in brain-injured patients. *J Neurosurg*. 1978;48:169-172.
68. DeVivo P, Del Gaudio A, Ciritella P. Hypertonic saline solution: a safe alternative to mannitol 18% in neurosurgery. *Minerva Anestesiol*. 2001;67:603-611.
69. Gemma M, Cozzi S, Tommasino C. 7.5% hypertonic saline versus 20% mannitol during elective neurosurgical supratentorial procedures. *J Neurosurg Anesthesiol*. 1997;9:329-334.
70. Munar F, Ferrer AM, de Nadal M. Cerebral hemodynamic effects of 7.2% hypertonic saline in patients with head injury and raised intracranial pressure. *J Neurotrauma*. 2000;17:41-51.
71. Peterson B, Khanna S, Fisher B, et al. Prolonged hypernatremia controls elevated intracranial pressure in head-injured pediatric patients [see comment]. *Crit Care Med*. 2000;28:1136-1143.
72. Suarez JI, Qureshi AI, Bhardwaj A. Treatment of refractory intracranial hypertension with 23.4% saline. *Crit Care Med*. 1998;26:1118-1122.
73. Peterson B, Khanna S, Fisher B, et al. Prolonged hypernatremia controls elevated intracranial pressure in head-injured pediatric patients [see comment]. *Crit Care Med*. 2000;28:1136-1143.
74. Qureshi AI, Wilson DA, Traystman RJ. Treatment of elevated intracranial pressure in experimental intracerebral hemorrhage: comparison between mannitol and hypertonic saline. *Neurosurgery*. 1999;44:1055-1063.
75. Doyle JA, Davis DP, Hoyt DB. The use of hypertonic saline in the treatment of traumatic brain injury [Review]. *J Trauma*. 2001;50:367-383.
76. Schatzmann C, Heissler HE, Konig K, et al. Treatment of elevated intracranial pressure by infusions of 10% saline in severely head injured patients. *Acta Neurochir Suppl*. 1998;71:31-33.
77. Shackford SR. Effect of small-volume resuscitation on intracranial pressure and related cerebral variables. *J Trauma*. 1997;42:S48-S53.
78. Bulger EM, May S, Brasel KJ, et al. Out-of-hospital hypertonic resuscitation following severe traumatic brain injury: a randomized controlled trial. *JAMA*. 2010;304:1455-1464.
79. Cooper DJ, Myles PS, McDermott FT. Prehospital hypertonic saline resuscitation of patients with hypotension and severe traumatic brain injury: a randomized controlled trial. *JAMA*. 2004;291:1350.
80. Bouma GJ, Levasseur JE, Muizelaar JP, et al. Description of a closed window technique for in vivo study of the feline basilar artery. *Stroke*. 1991;22:522-526.
81. Bouma GJ, Muizelaar JP, Choi SC, et al. Cerebral circulation and metabolism after severe traumatic brain injury: the elusive role of ischemia. *J Neurosurg*. 1991;75:685-693.
82. Jaggi JL, Obrist WD, Gennarelli TA, et al. Relationship of early cerebral blood flow and metabolism to outcome in acute head injury. *J Neurosurg*. 1990;72:176-182.
83. Warner KJ, Cuschieri J, Copass MK, et al. Emergency department ventilation effects outcome in severe traumatic brain injury. *J Trauma*. 2008;64:341-347.
84. Hyperventilation. *Management and Prognosis of Severe Traumatic Brain Injury*. 2nd ed. Brain Trauma Foundation; 2000:101-114.
85. Eisenberg HM, Frankowski RF, Contant CF, et al. High-dose barbiturate control of elevated intracranial pressure in patients with severe head injury. *J Neurosurg*. 1988;69:15-23.
86. Ward JD, Becker DP, Miller JD, et al. Failure of prophylactic barbiturate coma in the treatment of severe head injury. *J Neurosurg*. 1985;62:383-388.
87. Marion DW, Penrod LE, Kelsey SF, et al. Treatment of traumatic brain injury with moderate hypothermia. *N Engl J Med*. 1997;336:540-546.
88. Shiozaki T, Hayakata T, Taneda M, et al. A multicenter prospective randomized controlled trial of the efficacy of mild hypothermia for severely head injured patients with low intracranial pressure. Mild Hypothermia Study Group in Japan. *J Neurosurg*. 2001;94:50-54.
89. Shiozaki T, Sugimoto H, Taneda M, et al. Selection of severely head injured patients for mild hypothermia therapy [see comment]. *J Neurosurg*. 1998;89:206-211.
90. Shiozaki T, Sugimoto H, Taneda M, et al. Effect of mild hypothermia on uncontrollable intracranial hypertension after severe head injury [see comment]. *J Neurosurg*. 1993;79:363-368.
91. Marion DW, Obrist WD, Carlier PM, et al. The use of moderate therapeutic hypothermia for patients with severe head injuries: a preliminary report [see comment]. *J Neurosurg*. 1993;79:354-362.
92. Zhi D, Zhang S, Lin X. Study on therapeutic mechanism and clinical effect of mild hypothermia in patients with severe head injury. *Surg Neurol*. 2003;59:381-385.
93. Clifton GL, Miller ER, Choi SC, et al. Lack of effect of induction of hypothermia after acute brain injury [see comment]. *N Engl J Med*. 2001;344:556-563.
94. Markgraf CG, Clifton GL, Moody MR. Treatment window for hypothermia in brain injury. *J Neurosurg*. 2001;95:979-983.
95. Brain Trauma Foundation, American Association of Neurological Surgeons, Congress of Neurological Surgeons. Guidelines for the management of severe traumatic brain injury [Erratum appears in *J Neurotrauma*. 2008;25(3):276-278]. *J Neurotrauma*. 2007;24(suppl):106.
96. Diringer MN, Reaven NL, Funk SE, et al. Elevated body temperature independently contributes to increased length of stay in neurologic intensive care unit patients [see comment] [Erratum appears in *Crit Care Med*. 2004;32(10):2170]. *Crit Care Med*. 2004;32:1489-1495.
97. Robertson CS. Management of cerebral perfusion pressure after traumatic brain injury [Review]. *Anesthesiology*. 2001;95:1513-1517.
98. Robertson CS, Valadka AB, Hannay HJ, et al. Prevention of secondary ischemic insults after severe head injury. *Crit Care Med*. 1999;27:2086-2095.
99. Hlatky R, Robertson C. Does raising cerebral perfusion pressure help head injured patients? In: Valadka AB, Andrews BT, eds. *Neurotrauma*. 1st ed. New York: Thieme; 2005:75-82.
100. Gopinath SP, Robertson CS, Contant CF, et al. Jugular venous desaturation and outcome after head injury. *J Neurol Neurosurg Psychiatry*. 1994;57:717-723.
101. Gopinath SP, Valadka AB, Uzura M, et al. Comparison of jugular venous oxygen saturation and brain tissue PO_2 as monitors of cerebral ischemia after head injury [see comment]. *Crit Care Med*. 1999;27:2337-2345.
102. Obrist WD, Langfitt TW, Jaggi JL, et al. Cerebral blood flow and metabolism in comatose patients with acute head injury. Relationship to intracranial hypertension. *J Neurosurg*. 1984;61:241-253.
103. Robertson C. Desaturation episodes after severe head injury: influence on outcome. *Acta Neurochir Suppl (Wien)*. 1993;59:98-101.
104. Robertson CS, Narayan RK, Gokaslan ZL, et al. Cerebral arteriovenous oxygen difference as an estimate of cerebral blood flow in comatose patients [see comment]. *J Neurosurg*. 1989;70:222-230.
105. Kiening KL, Hartl R, Unterberg AW, et al. Brain tissue PO_2-monitoring in comatose patients: implications for therapy. *Neurol Res*. 1997;19:233-240.

106. Stiefel MF, Spiotta A, Gracias VH, et al. Reduced mortality rate in patients with severe traumatic brain injury treated with brain tissue oxygen monitoring. *J Neurosurg*. 2005;103:805-811.
107. Aarabi B. Traumatic aneurysms of brain due to high velocity missile head wounds. *Neurosurgery*. 1988;22:1056-1063.
108. Aarabi B. Management of traumatic aneurysms caused by high-velocity missile head wounds [Review]. *Neurosurg Clin North Am*. 1995;6:775-797.
109. Meirowsky AM, Caveness WF, Dillon JD, et al. Cerebrospinal fluid fistulas complicating missile wounds of the brain. *J Neurosurg*. 1981;54:44-48.
110. Antibiotic prophylaxis for penetrating brain injury [Review]. *J Trauma*. 2001;51:S34-S40.
111. Caveness WF, Meirowsky AM, Rish BL, et al. The nature of posttraumatic epilepsy. *J Neurosurg*. 1979;50:545-553.
112. Antiseizure prophylaxis for penetrating brain injury [Review]. *J Trauma*. 2001;51:S41-S43.
113. Annegers JF, Hauser WA, Coan SP, et al. A population-based study of seizures after traumatic brain injuries. *N Engl J Med*. 1998;338:20-24.
114. Temkin NR, Dikmen SS, Wilensky AJ, et al. A randomized, double-blind study of phenytoin for the prevention of post-traumatic seizures [see comment]. *N Engl J Med*. 1990;323:497-502.
115. Bullock R, Chesnut RM, Clifton G, et al. Guidelines for the management of severe head injury. Brain Trauma Foundation [Review]. *Eur J Emerg Med*. 1996;3:109-127.
116. Lam AM, Winn HR, Cullen BF, et al. Hyperglycemia and neurological outcome in patients with head injury. *J Neurosurg*. 1991;75:545-551.
117. Young B, Ott L, Dempsey R, et al. Relationship between admission hyperglycemia and neurologic outcome of severely brain-injured patients. *Ann Surg*. 1989;210:466-472.
118. Roberts I, Yates D, Sandercock P, et al. Effect of intravenous corticosteroids on death within 14 days in 10008 adults with clinically significant head injury (MRC CRASH trial): randomised placebo-controlled trial [see comment]. *Lancet*. 2004;364:1321-1328.
119. Owings JT, Bagley M, Gosselin R, et al. Effect of critical injury on plasma antithrombin activity: low antithrombin levels are associated with thromboembolic complications. *J Trauma*. 1996;41:396-405.
120. Kaufman HH, Moake JL, Olson JD, et al. Delayed and recurrent intracranial hematomas related to disseminated intravascular clotting and fibrinolysis in head injury. *Neurosurgery*. 1980;7:445-449.
121. Boffard KD, Riou B, Warren B, et al. Recombinant factor VIIa as adjunctive therapy for bleeding control in severely injured trauma patients: two parallel randomized, placebo-controlled, double-blind clinical trials [see comment]. *J Trauma*. 2005;59:8-15.
122. Mayer SA, Brun NC, Begtrup K, et al. Recombinant activated factor VII for acute intracerebral hemorrhage [see comment]. *N Engl J Med*. 2005;352:777-785.
123. Stein DM, Dutton RP, Kramer ME, et al. Recombinant factor VIIa: decreasing time to intervention in coagulopathic patients with severe traumatic brain injury. *J Trauma*. 2008;64:620-627.
124. O'Connell KA, Wood JJ, Wise RP, et al. Thromboembolic adverse events after use of recombinant human coagulation factor VIIa [see comment]. *JAMA*. 2006;295:293-298.
125. Dennis JW, Menawat S, Von Thron J, et al. Efficacy of deep venous thrombosis prophylaxis in trauma patients and identification of high-risk groups. *J Trauma*. 1993;35:132-138.
126. Black PM, Baker MF, Snook CP. Experience with external pneumatic calf compression in neurology and neurosurgery. *Neurosurgery*. 1986;18:440-444.
127. Frim DM, Barker FG, Poletti CE, et al. Postoperative low-dose heparin decreases thromboembolic complications in neurosurgical patients. *Neurosurgery*. 1992;30:830-832.
128. Knudson MM, Morabito D, Paiement GD, et al. Use of low molecular weight heparin in preventing thromboembolism in trauma patients. *J Trauma*. 1996;41:446-459.
129. Kraus JF. Epidemiology of head injury. In: Cooper PR, ed. *Head Injury*. 3rd ed. Baltimore, MD: Williams & Wilkins; 1993:1-25.
130. Jennett B, Bond M. Assessment of outcome after severe brain damage. *Lancet*. 1975;1:480-484.
131. Early Indicators of Prognosis in Severe Traumatic Brain Injury. *Management and Prognosis of Severe Traumatic Brain Injury*. 2nd ed. Brain Trauma Foundation; 2000:1-116.
132. Choi SC, Muizelaar JP, Barnes TY, et al. Prediction tree for severely head-injured patients [see comment]. *J Neurosurg*. 1991;75:251-255.
133. Kaufmann MA, Buchmann B, Scheidegger D, et al. Severe head injury: should expected outcome influence resuscitation and first-day decisions? *Resuscitation*. 1992;23:199-206.
134. Murray LS, Teasdale GM, Murray GD, et al. Does prediction of outcome alter patient management? [see comment]. *Lancet*. 1993;341:1487-1491.
135. Guidelines for the determination of death. Report of the medical consultants on the diagnosis of death to the President's Commission for the Study of Ethical Problems in Medicine and Biomedical and Behavioral Research. *JAMA*. 1981;246:2184-2186.
136. Mass AI, Steyerberg EW, Butcher I et al. Prognostic value of computerized tomography scan characteristics in traumatic brain injury: results from the IMPACT stydy. *Journal of Neurotrauma* 2007;24:303-314.

CHAPTER 23 ■ MAXILLOFACIAL INJURIES

NATHANIEL McQUAY Jr AND DANIEL LADER

Maxillofacial trauma encompasses injuries to the soft tissue and skeletal and visceral organs of the face. Fractures occur when forces that exceed their tolerance are applied. Although facial injuries are often not life threatening, their significance cannot be understated. Facial injuries may interfere with nasal, auditory, mandibular, or ocular function. The potential for postinjury disfigurement and disability can be associated with long-term physical and psychological sequela.

The management of maxillofacial trauma can be traced back to ancient times. The Edwin Smith papyrus (1550 BC), the oldest known medical papyrus, contains detailed descriptions of the surgical management of facial skeletal and soft tissue injuries. Hippocrates described the timeless methods of closed reduction of mandible dislocations, wiring of teeth and jaw immobilization of mandible fractures, and closed reduction of nasal fractures.[1] The management of these injuries in isolation is straightforward. However, facial trauma is often associated with other injuries that may be life threatening, requiring immediate attention. So when does one begin to address the maxillofacial injuries in the multiply injured patient? It is the purpose of this chapter to review the mechanisms of injury, clinical presentation, diagnostic modalities, and the initial management of the wide spectrum of maxillofacial injuries. The priority-based approach to the polytrauma patent is reviewed as pertains to the patient with facial trauma.

INITIAL ASSESSMENT

Airway

The initial assessment of the acutely injured patient, irrespective of the injury complex, remains unchanged. The Adult Trauma Life Support® (ATLS) program provides a standard prioritized approach to the initial evaluation and management of the trauma patient.[2] The first priority is that of the airway. In the patient with maxillofacial trauma, the airway may be compromised by lack of support from the tongue, unstable skeletal support, or obstruction of the airway due to foreign bodies or bloody secretions. An organized approach should be utilized in managing the airway to optimize patient outcome (Algorithm. 23.1). The oral cavity should be first cleared of secretions, supplemental oxygen given, an oral airway placed, and the jaw thrust maneuver applied to assist with the opening of the posterior pharynx. The cervical spine is immobilized assuming the presence of a cervical spine injury, which occurs in approximately 1%–5% of patients with facial fractures.[3–6] Immobilization is maintained until the cervical spine is both radiographically and clinically evaluated to exclude an acute fracture. Patients with immediate or persistent airway problems require placement of a definitive airway defined as a cuffed tube within the trachea. The definitive airway of choice is a translaryngeal endotracheal tube.[2] Care should be taken to avoid iatrogenic injury to the maxillary central incisors during intubation. Nasally placed tubes (nasotracheal, nasogastric) should be avoided in the setting of facial trauma as central bony fractures may be present allowing passage into the cranial vault. When the difficult airway is encountered, a surgical airway, cricothyroidotomy, is the definitive airway of choice.[2]

Breathing

Patients with facial trauma may present with oxygenation and ventilatory difficulties. Although airway compromise is often assumed, a respiratory etiology must also be sought. Penetrating injuries should be assessed for trajectory as missiles may be present in the neck or thoracic cavity. The presence of subcutaneous emphysema should prompt further investigation to rule out injury to the upper airway, aerodigestive tract, or tracheobronchial tree. A supine portable CXR serves as the initial adjunct study for further assessment of the hypoxic patient. Clinical findings consistent with a tension pneumothorax (absent breath sound, tracheal deviation, hypoxemia, and hemodynamic lability) require immediate needle decompression with subsequent thoracostomy tube placement. Hypoxemia in the stable patient with evidence of a pneumothorax or hemothorax is managed with placement of a thoracostomy tube.

Circulation

Acute hemorrhage continues to be the second most common cause of death in the trauma population.[7] Fatal traumatic hemorrhage accounts for a large portion of early deaths, with the majority of exsanguinations occurring within the first 48 hours.[8,9] Following stabilization of the airway and breathing, circulation with hemorrhage control is the next priority in assessing acutely injured patients. The vascular supply to the face is vast and in the setting of diffuse soft tissue injury may serve as a source of considerable blood loss. The best way to control hemorrhage in the acute setting is with well-placed direct pressure. This concept is central even in the setting of oral and maxillofacial injuries. Following placement of intravenous access, the site of hemorrhage is assessed to determine the method of pressure to be applied. Nasal fractures are often associated with bleeding. Direct pressure on the nares often controls epistaxis from an anterior source. Substantial bleeding from a posterior source may require nasal packing, balloon compression, or both to obtain hemostasis (Fig. 23.1). Patients with complex facial fractures due to either blunt or penetrating trauma have multiple sites of bleeding that may prove difficult to control. Encompassing the concept of direct pressure, facial packing and compressive dressings techniques have been described to achieve hemostasis.[10] Packing of the oropharynx following airway control is in essence similar to the four-quadrant packing of the abdomen in an attempt to obtain hemorrhage control.[11–14] When bleeding is refractory to compressive methods, angioembolization is employed for definitive control (Algorithm. 23.2).

DEFICIT AND ENVIRONMENT

The initial neurological evaluation includes the assessment of the pupillary response and the computation of the Glasgow Coma Score (GCS).[15] Abnormal pupillary response and/or a low GCS score indicate the presence of a traumatic brain injury (TBI) requiring computed tomography (CT) scan of the brain

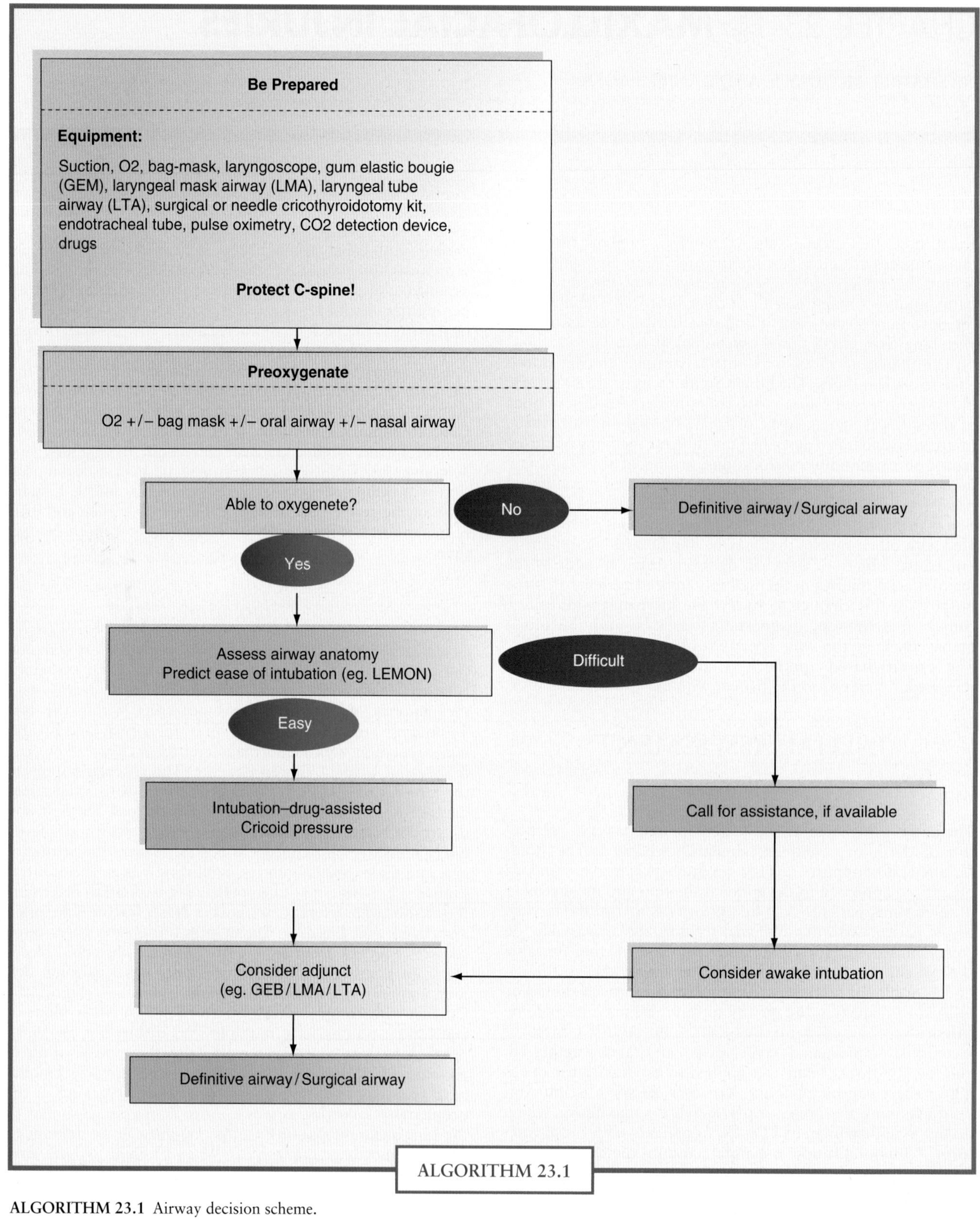

ALGORITHM 23.1 Airway decision scheme.

for further assessment. Certain facial fractures, are often associated with an intracranial injury. When a TBI is diagnosed, prompt neurosurgical consult should ensue. Exposure of the patient by removing all clothing allows for unobstructed evaluation of associated injuries. During the initial evaluation, the environment should be controlled. Warm fluids and external warming methods are used to prevent hypothermia as it may contribute to the development of coagulopathy.

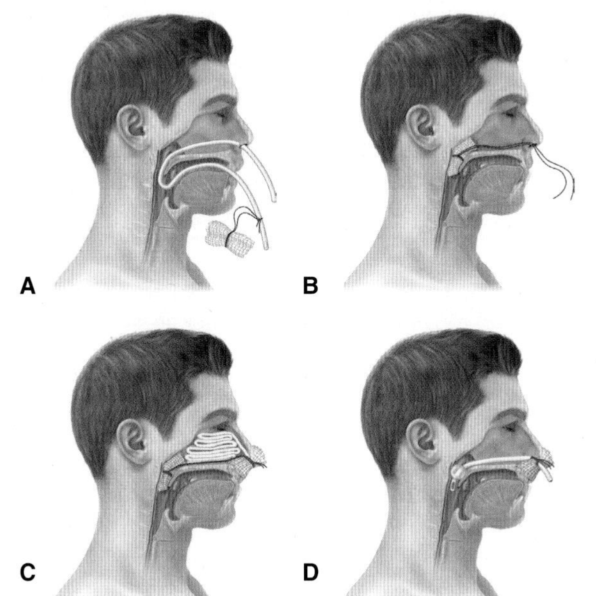

FIGURE 23.1. Nasal packing: packing to control bleeding from the posterior nose, (**A**) catheter inserted and packing attached; (**B**) packing drawn into position as catheter is removed; (**C**) strip tied over bolster to hold packing in place with anterior pack installed "accordion pleat" style; (**D**) alternative method, using balloon catheter instead of gauze packing.

SECONDARY SURVEY

Only upon stabilization of the patient and completion of the primary survey can one proceed with the secondary assessment. Potential life-threatening injuries are assessed and managed during this stage of the evaluation. A history and complete "head-to-toe" physical examination should be performed. The information provided by the prehospital personnel about the mechanism of injury and surrounding events guides the astute provider in the assessment for possible associated injuries. Patients with facial injuries due to a blunt mechanism (MVC, falls, assaults), often have associated injuries. Once the less life-threatening injuries have been excluded, then evaluation of the maxillofacial region can begin. The approach to the maxillofacial examination should include evaluation of the soft tissues, skeleton, dentition, and nerves. In the awake patient, focused questioning can provide clues to the presence of underlying skeletal fractures (Table 23.1). The physical examination must be organized and methodical to minimize missed injuries. Inspection and palpation serves as the basis for the maxillofacial examination. Drainage from the nose, rhinorrhea, or the external auditory canal, otorrhea, should be carefully inspected for the presence of cerebral spinal fluid (CSF). Clinically the diagnosis is made upon observing the "double ring" sign (small central blood ring surrounded by a larger peripheral clear ring) that is produced when the fluid is placed on a paper towel. If there is a high index of suspicion of CSF leak, the fluid should be sent to the laboratory for a β_2-transferrin (which is present only in CSF) or a quantitative glucose analysis. The presence of β_2-transferrin or a glucose level >30 mg/100 mL is consistent with the presence of CSF. The oral cavity is then inspected for lacerations, soft tissue injuries, abnormal dentition, and bleeding. The tongue is often a source of non–life-threatening bleeding, but may require suture placement for hemostasis. Lacerations of the soft tissue and gingival, bony irregularities, tenderness, and numbness must be adequately evaluated to diagnose an underlying skeletal fracture. The presence of numbness is due to the involvement of the sensory branch of the trigeminal nerve and, in mandible fractures, the inferior alveolar nerve. Avulsed dentition may serve as a possible source of airway obstruction when aspirated; therefore, a CXR should be obtained. Once the examination is completed, appropriate imaging studies, (CT scan, panorex) are performed. Complete CT scans of the face with coronal views aid in the diagnosis of facial fractures and planning of operative intervention if required.

Soft Tissue Injuries

Soft tissue injuries to the maxillofacial region present a considerable challenge in management as there can be untoward cosmetic and functional deficits if not addressed in an appropriate manner. Complex facial lacerations can cause substantial bleeding as the face is very well vascularized with the terminal branches of the external carotid artery as its main supply. This vast vascular supply also allows for lacerated tissues with small pedicles to survive if managed carefully.[16,17] Therefore the initial approach to soft tissue injuries includes copious irrigation, appropriate antibiotics, and limited debridement. Primary closure of facial wounds, for up to 24 hours postinjury, is employed when adequate tissue is present. Good cosmesis is generally achieved due to an abundant blood supply and repeatable patterns of soft tissue injury.[18] Proper suturing technique is essential to minimize potential disfigurement. Layered closure with approximation of deep layers using braided absorbable sutures to eliminate potential dead space and fine monofilament sutures for skin closure that is tension-free minimizes scarring. Skin sutures should be removed in 3–5 days as this also minimizes scarring. The patient should be advised to apply sunscreen to the affected area during the first year of healing to prevent discoloration of the scar.

Lip laceration repair requires careful attention. Wound management follows the general principle of soft tissue management of the face. Thorough irrigation should be used prior to closure and antibiotics that cover gram-negative anaerobes should be considered. The wound is inspected for the presence of foreign body and tooth fragments from associated dentoalveolar injuries. Wound depth evaluation is crucial as unrecognized penetration through the oral mucosa may allow salivary contamination. The oral mucosa should be approximated to prevent salivary contamination. The muscle fibers of the orbicularis oris run in a transverse manner and tend to pull the wound edges apart, giving the appearance of an avulsive tissue loss, which is rarely the case. Alignment of the vermilion border is central in the closure technique to obtain a good cosmetic result.[19] When it is properly performed, cosmetic results are maximized, and scarring is minimal.

Avulsive maxillofacial injuries are typically the result of an impact with high kinetic energy. Close-range gunshot wounds (GSW) and high-speed MVC impact can lead to large full-thickness soft tissue loss. These wounds are frequently associated with other life-threatening conditions such as hypovolemic shock and airway embarrassment. Soft tissue injury management is best performed with serial dressing changes of saline-soaked gauze in the multi-injured patient. Once stabilized, extensive reconstructive procedures are often required to address large soft tissue loss. Injured soft tissue surrounding the area of initial trauma progresses to an evolving pattern of tissue loss and necrosis requiring serial debridements. Once all devitalized tissue is removed, a variety of tissue transfer techniques (local, regional, free flap) can be employed to obtain skeletal coverage.[20–24] Early reconstruction provides better cosmetic and functional results as compared to delayed secondary repair.[20,25]

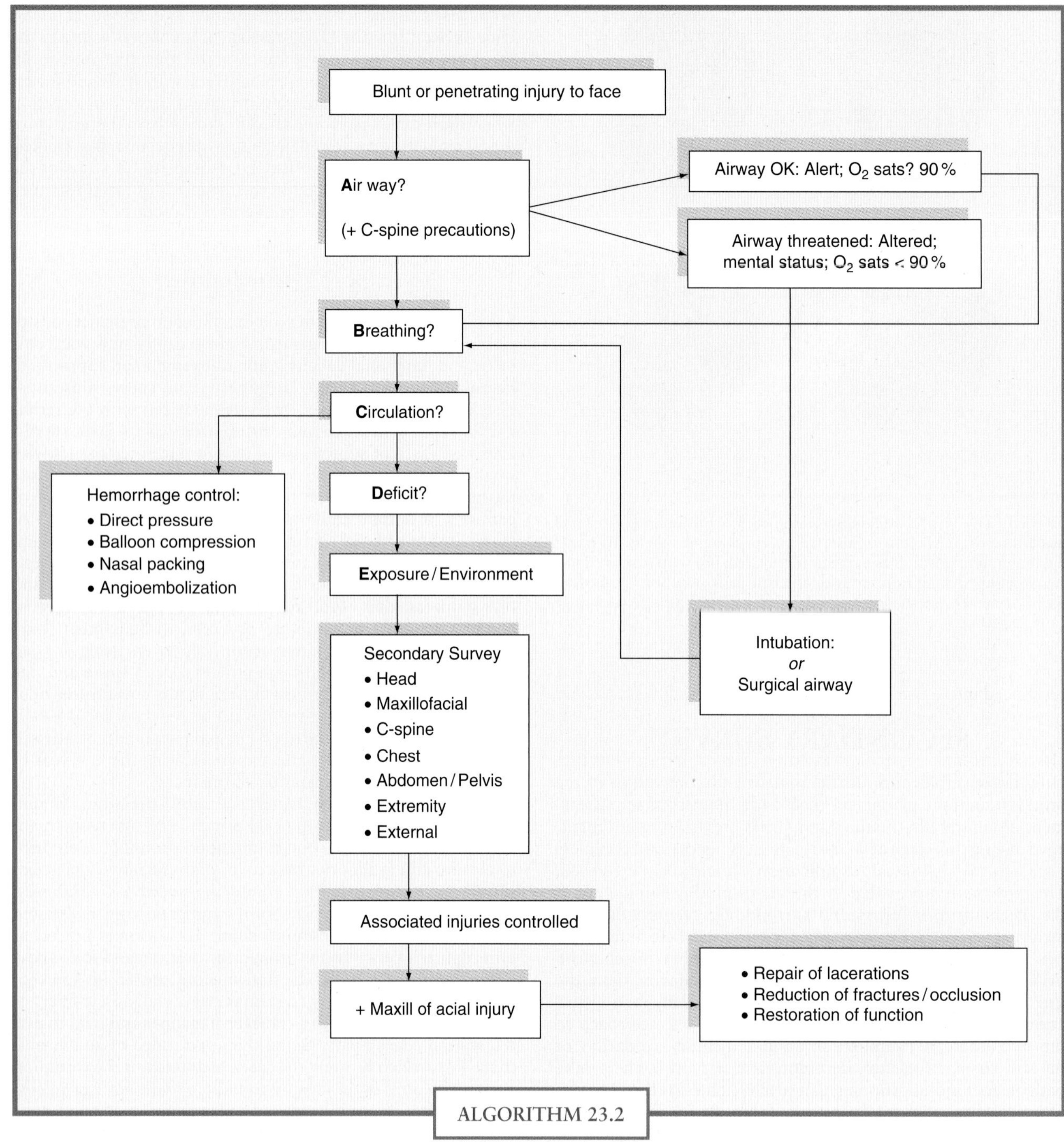

ALGORITHM 23.2 Facial trauma management algorithm.

TABLE 23.1

SCREENING QUESTIONS FOR EVALUATION OF CRANIOFACIAL TRAUMA

1. Where does it hurt?
2. Do you see double?
3. Do you feel numbness? Where?
4. Does it hurt when you open your mouth?
5. Do your teeth come together normally?

Dentoalveolar Injuries

Traumatic facial injuries frequently involve the dentition and dentoalveolar structures. Common causes of dentoalveolar trauma include MVC, falls, sports injuries, and assaults. Involvement of the maxillary incisors due to their prominent position in the mouth is common. Injury patterns range from various fractures of the teeth to fractures involving the supporting bony alveolus (Fig. 23.2). Lacerations of the lips and gingiva are frequently associated with dentoalveolar trauma and can complicate their management. Prompt diagnosis and treatment of these injuries are important when

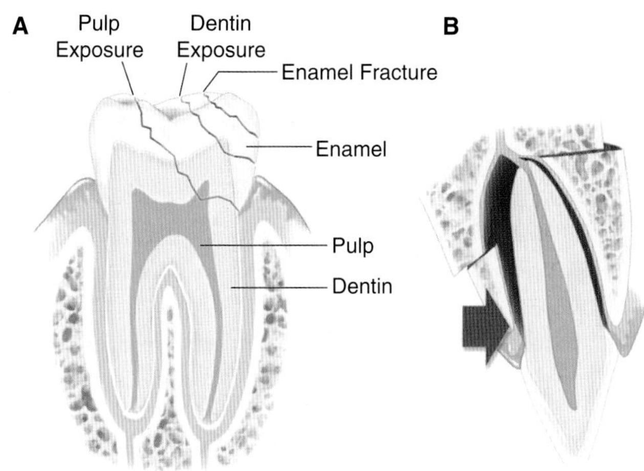

FIGURE 23.2. **A:** Level of tooth fractures. **B:** Dentoalveolar fracture.

one considers the esthetic implications of tooth loss, especially since these injuries tend to occur in children and young adults.

A complete physical exam of the maxillofacial region should be performed when assessing dentoalveolar injuries to rule out associated injuries. The Universal Tooth Designation System is most commonly used in the United States as a standard in tooth identification (Fig. 23.3). It is important to take note of any missing teeth as they may have been aspirated or displaced into other structures such as the facial soft tissues or nasal cavity. In the severely injured or obtunded patient, imaging of the chest should be included to locate aspirated teeth. Timely diagnosis is critical as tooth reimplantation and fracture reduction should ideally be performed within 1 hour of injury to minimize delayed loss of teeth. Injuries to the coronal portion of teeth can result in fractures of the crown that may be limited to the enamel or involve the innervated dentin and pulp. Fractures limited to the enamel are not emergent and can be treated at a later time. Injuries with exposed dentin or pulp are quite uncomfortable and require more immediate attention and restoration. Tooth injury with associated loss of the crown at or below the gingiva or a fracture involving the tooth root may not be amenable to restoration. Complete tooth avulsion requires immediate attention as successful reimplantation is a time-sensitive process. Reimplantation rate decreases as the periodontal tissues attached to the tooth desiccate and become nonviable. Teeth can be reimplanted within 20 minutes if not placed in a suitable transport medium verses up to 3 hours when immediately placed in an appropriate solution such as milk, or Hank's balanced salt solution found in Save-A-Tooth kits (3M Health Care, St. Paul MN).[26,27] Once the tooth is reimplanted, it must be stabilized with either a splint or an arch bar for several weeks. Fractures of the supporting alveolar bone and subluxation tend to involve prominent anterior teeth and require reduction of the subluxed tooth or entire alveolar segment. This can usually be performed with local anesthesia; however, more severe injuries or uncooperative patients may require conscious sedation or general anesthesia in the operating room. Treatment involves adequate reduction to re-establish the dental occlusion and placement of either a splint or an arch bar for 4–6 weeks.

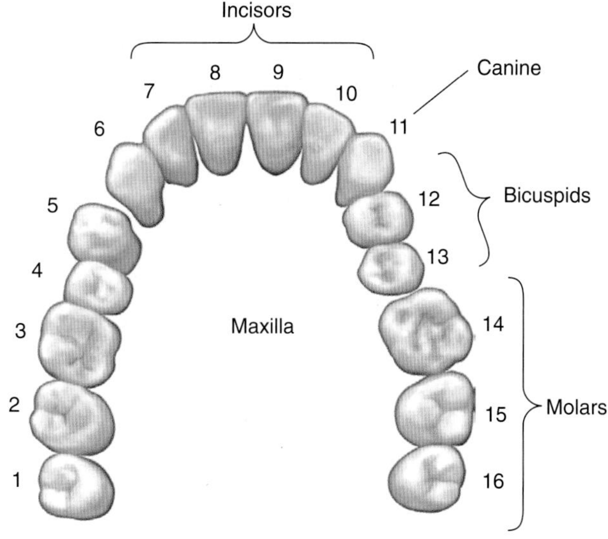

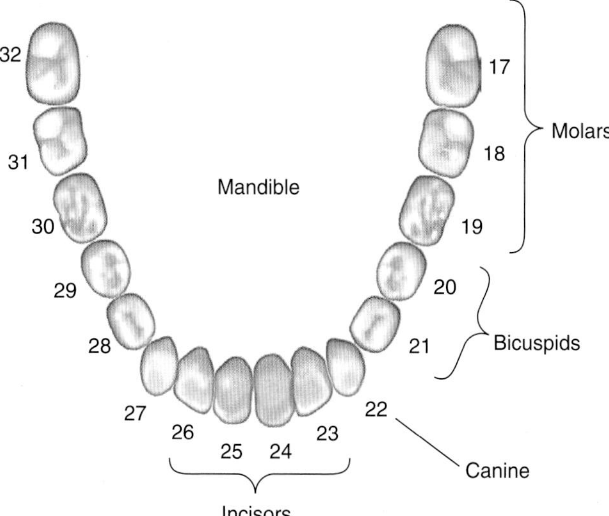

FIGURE 23.3. The universal tooth designation system. A drawing of the occlusal and incisal surfaces of the maxillary and mandibular adult dentition. The numerals 1 to 32 give the Universal numbering code commonly used for record keeping.

Orbital Fractures

Blunt trauma (MVC, Assault, Sports injuries) accounts for the majority of isolated orbital fractures. The force of impact is transferred to the thin orbital bones, which fracture in a "blow-out" fashion. This repeatable pattern of injury most likely serves as a protective mechanism against globe injuries. Both the orbital floor and medial wall of the orbit are often fractured, with the former occurring more commonly. The orbital floor also functions as the roof of the maxillary sinus, and this injury typically leads to air emphysema. Due to the proximity of the inferior rectus and the inferior oblique muscles to the orbital floor, muscle entrapment may occur. Findings on physical examination include diplopia and restriction of the upward gaze in the ipsilateral eye. A forced duction test is recommended to differentiate muscle entrapment from other muscle or nerve complications. As with other facial fractures, orbital fractures warrant a thorough ophthalmologic evaluation as associated globe injuries (corneal abrasion, hyphema, globe rupture) occur. Exophthalmos and epistaxis are often present initially. As the edema resolves, enophthalmos develops due to retraction of the eye into the ocular cavity. Radiological evaluation of orbital fractures with coronal CT is useful in evaluating orbital injuries and soft tissue details. Findings include disruption of one or more of the orbital walls, air fluid level in the maxillary sinus, and herniation of periorbital fat into the sinus.

Indications for surgical intervention include muscle entrapment, enophthalmos, positive force duction test and globe malposition. Symptoms of concomitant oculocardiac reflex (bradycardia, heart block, nausea, vomiting, or syncope) warrant immediate surgical intervention as they may be fatal.[28] Surgical repair of the orbital floor may be delayed until swelling subsides as this allows for better incision placement and improved cosmesis. Proper reconstruction is essential to prevent cosmetic deformity, delayed enophthalmos, or persistent diplopia. Small or nondisplaced fractures are often amendable to nonoperative management.

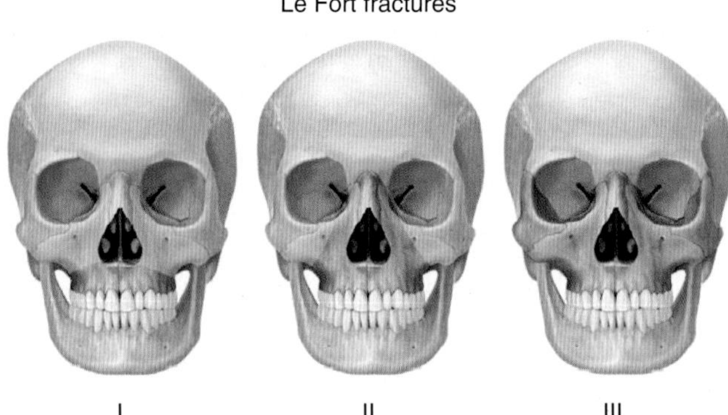

FIGURE 23.5. Lefort classification of midfacial fractures.

Maxillary Fractures

Trauma to the midface can result in a fracture of the maxilla (Fig. 23.4). Maxillary fractures usually involve the teeth-bearing segments and follow certain fracture patterns (Fig. 23.5). The Lefort classification is widely used to describe fracture patterns of the maxilla and midface.[29] A Lefort I fracture represents a *horizontal* fracture located above the roots of the teeth. Clinically the maxillary fragment is mobile due to the separation of the upper jaw from the cranial base. Lefort II fracture follows a *pyramidal* outline and involves the nasal bones. Lefort III fracture results in complete *craniofacial separation* in which the entire midface is separated from the cranial base.

Traumatic midfacial injuries can present with substantial bleeding from the nose and oral cavity. This may require the use of nasal packing, balloon compression, or angioembolization to control associated hemorrhage. The use of nasogastric tubes in patients with midfacial injuries is contraindicated as passage through a fractured cribiform plate and into the cranial vault is known to occur. Patients sustaining midfacial injuries are usually subject to considerable blunt force trauma and often have associated injuries. As with other facial fractures, paresthesia in the distribution of adjacent nerves is present. In addition to various fracture combinations, substantial malocclusion can occur and the upper jaw can appear to be freely mobile. CT is the most appropriate imaging modality in evaluating midfacial injuries. Definitive treatment usually requires some form of open reduction and internal fixation for displaced fractures.

Mandible Fractures

Mandible fractures are the second the most commonly encountered facial skeletal injuries. As with most facial injuries, the severity of the fracture is proportional to the location and force of impact. Fractures tend to occur at the local site of impact and in areas of weakness. The weak points of the mandible include the condyle, angle, and symphysis regions at which mandibular fractures commonly occur (Fig. 23.6). Depending on the location, mandible fractures may serve as a source of airway compromise due to posterior displacement of the tongue into the oropharynx. Substantial bleeding from mandible fractures is rare; however, when this is present, fracture reduction and stabilization usually achieves hemostasis.

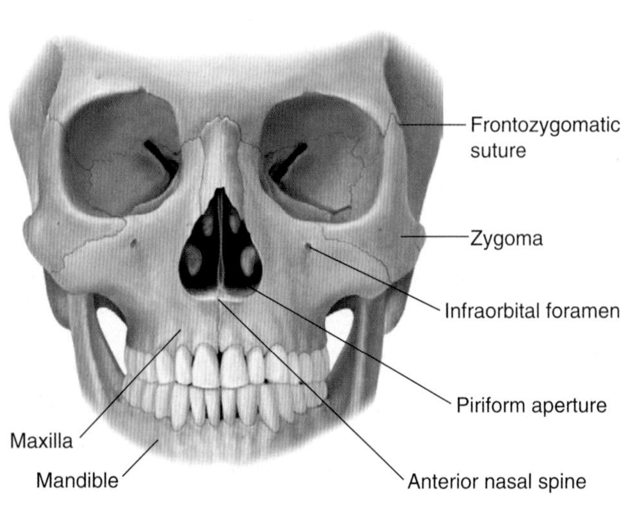

FIGURE 23.4. Midfacial anatomy.

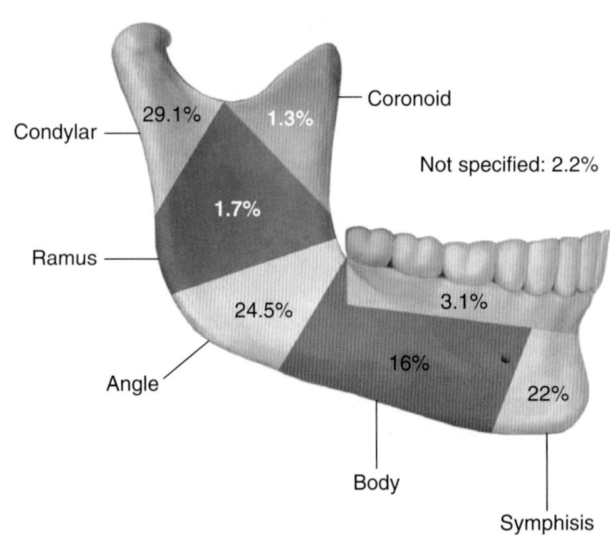

FIGURE 23.6. Mandibular fracture sites.

There is also a 10% incidence of an associated cervical spine injury and head injuries that must be considered when managing mandibular injuries.[4,5]

There are several important factors regarding the diagnosis and treatment of mandibular fractures relative to the anatomy of the mandible. The mandible has a dual articulation with the base of the skull at the glenoid fossae commonly referred to as the temporomandibular joints. Multiple muscles (masseter, medial and lateral pterygoids) insert into the mandible where they tend to distract fractured segments along the vector of contraction. The inferior alveolar nerve, which represents the third division of the trigeminal nerve, enters the mandibular ramus along its medial aspect and courses through a bony canal within the mandibular body and exits via the mental foramen. This nerve is frequently injured in mandibular fractures and can lead to a subsequent paresthesia along its distribution.

Patients who present with mandibular fractures will typically demonstrate several key clinical findings. The inability to bring the teeth into proper occlusion (malocclusion) or restriction of mouth opening (trismus) assists with identifying mandible fracture location. Dental injuries can accompany mandible fractures and may serve as a source of intraoral bleeding. In addition, there may be sublingual hematoma formation resulting in elevation of the tongue. Facial lacerations may also be present resulting in an open or compound fracture. Several imaging modalities are utilized in diagnosing mandibular fractures. The panoramic radiograph gives an excellent view of the entire mandible, the joints, and dentition. However, its use may be limited by availability or contraindications secondary to patient factors. If a panoramic radiograph is unavailable or contraindicated, a series of radiographs (lateral oblique, posteroanterior, and a reverse Towne's view) have been used to diagnose skeletal fractures. These are often not applicable in the trauma patient as they require cervical spine clearance for head manipulation. CT scanning has mostly replaced plain film evaluation of the mandible. CT images offer better views of fracture lines and segments. Three-dimensional reconstruction allows for a fracture to be viewed from multiple planes, thereby providing a more detailed preoperative model facilitating surgical planning.

Nasal Fractures

Nasal fractures are the most common facial fracture due to the prominent position of the nose on the face. Nasal bones are relatively thin and tend to fracture with little force. Laterally displaced fractures of the bony skeleton often produce a nasal deformity as well as impairment of inspiration secondary to deviation of the nasal septum. In more severe fractures (naso-orbitethmoid fracture), extension to the frontal and ethmoid bones frequently occurs, resulting in posterior displacement of the bony structures. Clinically, facial edema, ecchymosis, nasal deformity, bony crepitus, and epistaxis are the usual findings. The mucosal lining of the nasal cavity is well vascularized, which may serve as a substantial source of hemorrhage. A nasal speculum should be used to look for evidence of septal deviation and hematomas. Septal hematomas should be promptly drained to prevent complications including perforation, septal necrosis, abscess formation, and the development of a saddle nose deformity.[30] Epistaxis may require the use of a nasal packing, balloon compression, local anesthesia with a vasoconstrictor, or a combination of the above to obtain hemorrhage control.

Although the diagnosis of nasal fractures is mainly clinical, CT scanning is the imaging modality of choice. Facial CT tends to better define the anatomy and severity of the fracture assisting in treatment planning. Closed reduction under local anesthesia with or without mild sedation is usually adequate to address simple nasal and septal injuries. In the setting of a severely displaced fracture, nasal retrusion, open fractures, or persistent postreduction deformity, open reduction under general anesthesia is performed.

Zygoma Fractures

The zygoma is a prominent bone and provides contour to the lateral aspect of the midface. The body of the zygoma is relatively thick in comparison to its articulations and tends to fracture with a distinct "tripod" pattern involving the zygomaticomaxillary complex (ZMC). A fracture of the ZMC will typically occur at the zygomatic arch, frontal bone articulation, and along the anterior wall of the maxillary sinus extending through the inferior orbital rim and orbital floor. Frequently the infraorbital nerve is affected, leading to paresthesia along its distribution of the ipsilateral cheek. Appreciable facial emphysema secondary to the disruption of the maxillary sinus wall is commonly present on initial presentation. Often, patients report that after sustaining facial trauma they blow their nose, and there is immediate profound swelling that prompts them to seek care. Other common presenting symptoms are periorbital ecchymosis and edema. After the initial edema subsides, there can be substantial loss of soft tissue support and flattening of the malar prominence. Trismus may be present if the depressed zygoma leads to mechanical impingement of the underlying coronoid process of the mandible. Palpable bone step deformities may be present along the zygomaticofrontal suture, zygomatic arch, and inferior orbital rim. CT scan is the imaging study of choice for ZMC fractures. Typical findings include soft tissue air emphysema, layering of blood in the maxillary sinus, and the "tripod" fracture pattern. Additional involvement of the sphenoid interface is described as the "quadramalar" fracture pattern. Associated globe injuries are common for which some authors recommend routine ophthalmologic examination prior to surgical repair.[31] Open reduction with internal fixation of displaced fractures is the surgical technique often applied. Nondisplaced fractures may be treated nonoperatively as the zygoma is not a load-bearing bone.

Ocular Injuries

Eye injuries are the leading cause of monocular blindness in the United States.[32] Sources of injuries include blunt objects, penetrating injuries, impalements, and MVC with airbag deployment. Orbital fractures are often associated with ocular and periocular injuries. Although ocular injuries may be obvious when caused by penetrating trauma, those caused by blunt trauma are sometimes difficult to detect as serious and potentially blinding injuries may go unnoticed. Routine ophthalmological evaluation in all patients with orbital fractures to address delay in diagnosis and management of serious injuries has been proposed.[31] Careful history and physical examination play an important role in decreasing the time to diagnosis especially in the multiple injured or comatose patients. Inquisition about the wearing of eyeglasses or contacts, preexisting ocular conditions, as well as the circumstances surrounding the injury event should occur. Physical findings of orbital pain, visual changes, eno- or exopthalmos, hyphema, or decreased extraocular motor activity should lead one to evaluate not only for an ocular injury but also an associated orbital fracture. Visual acuity is the first step in the evaluation of ocular trauma. Documentation of light perception and projection should be performed in the injured globe and compared to the uninjured globe. Initial gross examination should be performed without placing pressure and ocular injuries classified.[33] Upon completion of the physical exam, CT scan is often obtained to further assess soft tissue injury and rule out orbital fractures, retained foreign bodies, or a ruptured globe.

Early ophthalmology consult is indicated in penetrating injuries or decreased visual acuity. A ruptured globe is the most serious injury requiring early evaluation. The involved globe should be protected with an eye shield, and precautions to reduce intraocular pressure are instituted.[34] Signs and symptoms of a possible globe rupture include loss of vision, traumatic hyphema, hemorrhagic chemosis, or a displaced lens. During the ocular exam, refrain from applying pressure to the globe as this may cause extravasation of intraocular contents. Intravenous prophylactic antibiotics are administered, as topical eye drops should be avoided. Operative intervention should include primary repair when possible. Enucleation is sometimes required when loss of vision in the injured eye is irreversible and to prevent the development of sympathetic ophthalmia in the uninjured eye.

Parotid

Parotid gland injuries are relatively uncommon, but when present must be appropriately addressed to prevent long-term complications. The identification and definitive management of a parotid duct injury is crucial in order to prevent formation of a sialocele or a salivary fistula. The parotid duct, or Stenson duct, measures approximately 7 cm in length coursing the middle third of a line drawn between the tragus of the ear and the middle of the upper lip. For any facial injury that crosses this line, parotid duct involvement is assumed until proven otherwise. Injury to the duct is often associated with injury to the buccal branch of the facial nerve due to its close proximity. Parotid duct injury identification is facilitated by gentle message of the gland inducing saliva secretion or by cannulation of the intraoral papilla located opposite the upper second molar. Several operative techniques, primary anastamosis[35,36], duct ligation, and duct fistulization into the oral cavity have been described.[37] The operative technique most often utilized is primary anastamosis. The injury is repaired over a stent with fine absorbable sutures. Instances in which there is extensive tissue damage precluding primary repair, duct ligation is often performed.

Nerve

The trigeminal and facial nerves serve as the main source of sensory and motor innervation to the face respectively. During the physical examination of the patient with facial trauma, the identification of the nerve branches for primary repair is not necessary as in other anatomic regions. This is due to the lack of severe disfigurement and minimal functional loss. Injury to the branches medial to the lateral canthus of the eyes need not be repaired as with good skin approximation, nerve regeneration is accomplished via neurotization of muscle. Sensation in the involved area usually returns within a year. Nerve lacerations laterally located require primary anastomosis, ideally at the time of initial operation. When segmental loss of nerve tissue exists, interposition grafting using either the auricular or the sural nerves is used.[38–40]

Antibiotics for Facial Fractures

The role of antibiotic therapy has been one of great debate for many years.[41,42] Andreasen et al.'s[43] evidence-based analysis of the use of prophylactic antibiotics in relation to surgical management of mandibular injuries is informative. The authors' review of four randomized control trials[44–47] revealed a significant decrease in infections when comparing the antibiotic group to the control group (Table 23.2) This benefit was also noted to be procedure specific when open versus closed reduction procedures were compared.[41] In the open reduction group,

TABLE 23.2

COMPARISON OF POSTOPERATIVE INFECTION RATES RELATED TO THE USE OR NOT OF ANTIBIOTICS

		CONTROL GROUP			TEST GROUP			
		NO ANTIBIOTICS			ANTIBIOTICS			
STUDY	ADMINISTRATION	NO.	X	%	NO.	X	%	PROBABILITY LEVEL
Zallen and Curry (1975)		30	16	53	32	2	6	0.001
Aderhold et al. (1983)	Control	40	8	20				
	≤48 h				40	2	5	0.06
	>48 h				40	4	10	
Gerlach and Pape (1988)	Control	49	11	22				0.001
	1 d				50	1	2	
	1 shot				50	3	6	
	3 d				51	4	8	
Chole and Yee (1987)		42	18	62	37	5	14	0.01

x, Number of infections.

From Andreasen JO, Jensen SS, Schwartz O, et al. A systematic review of prophylactic antibiotics in the surgical treatment of maxillofacial fractures. *J Oral Maxillofac Surg*. 2006;64(11):1664–1668.

prophylactic antibiotic administration resulted in a decrease in infections (8% antibiotic group vs. 62% no antibiotics). Antibiotic prophylaxis was not beneficial in the closed reduction group as the infection rates were similar whether given or not (23% antibiotic group vs. 28% no antibiotic group). While some may argue that these studies are too heterogenous to make definitive conclusions regarding the use of antibiotics in facial fractures, our practice is to use antibiotic prophylaxis for mandible fractures without condylar involvement, for open fractures, and when open reduction is the operative procedure to be performed.

Chemoprophylaxis with antibiotics in head trauma to prevent posttraumatic meningitis is another area where variation of practice is controversial. Patients with basilar skull fractures (BSF) and possible CSF leak are often thought to be at increase risk of developing posttraumatic meningitis. The prevention of possible serious complications has served as the basis for administering prophylactic antibiotics with little evidence of efficacy. Ratilal et al.[48] have recently performed a systematic review of the best evidence on the efficacy of prophylactic antibiotics for the prevention of posttraumatic meningitis. Their review found no significant differences in the frequency of meningitis or all-cause or meningitis-related mortality between the treatment and control groups. The presence or absence of CSF in subgroup analysis revealed similar findings.

In conclusion, the management of maxillofacial trauma requires a multidisciplinary approach. Injury priority based on the standardized ATLS approach is paramount to optimize outcomes. Upon stabilization and addressing life-threatening injuries, the clinical assessment and diagnostic evaluation of potential facial injuries may commence. Injury-specific management is carried out by the surgical specialist (plastic surgery, oral and maxillofacial surgery, ophthalmology) with the goal of restoring function with good cosmesis.

References

1. Gahhos F, Ariyan S. Facial fractures: hippocratic management. *Head Neck Surg.* 1984;6(6):1007–1013.
2. Rosen P. *ATLS. Emergency Medicine: Concepts and Clinical Practice.* 4th ed. St. Louis, MO: Mosby; 1998.
3. Gwyn PP, et al. Facial fractures—associated injuries and complications. *Plast Reconstr Surg.* 1971;47(3):225–230.
4. Davidson JS, Birdsell DC. Cervical spine injury in patients with facial skeletal trauma. *J Trauma.* 1989;29(9):1276–1278.
5. Hackl W, et al. The incidence of combined facial and cervical spine injuries. *J Trauma.* 2001;50(1):41–45.
6. Luce EA, Tubb TD, Moore AM. Review of 1,000 major facial fractures and associated injuries. *Plast Reconstr Surg.* 1979;63(1):26–30.
7. Sauaia A, et al. Epidemiology of trauma deaths: a reassessment. *J Trauma.* 1995;38(2):185–193
8. Acosta JA, et al. Lethal injuries and time to death in a level I trauma center. *J Am Coll Surg.* 1998;186(5):528–533.
9. Hoyt DB, et al. Death in the operating room: an analysis of a multi-center experience. *J Trauma.* 1994;37(3):426–432.
10. Naimer SA, et al. Control of massive bleeding from facial gunshot wound with a compact elastic adhesive compression dressing. *Am J Emerg Med.* 2004;22(7):586–588.
11. Calne RY, McMaster P, Pentlow BD. The treatment of major liver trauma by primary packing with transfer of the patient for definitive treatment. *Br J Surg.* 1979;66(5):338–339.
12. Carmona RH, Peck DZ, Lim Jr, RC. *The role of packing and planned reoperation in severe hepatic trauma. J Trauma.* 1984;24(9):779–784.
13. Feliciano DV, et al. Packing for control of hepatic hemorrhage. *J Trauma.* 1986;26(8):738–743.
14. Svoboda JA, et al. Severe liver trauma in the face of coagulopathy. A case for temporary packing and early reexploration. *Am J Surg.* 1982;144(6):717–721.
15. Teasdale G, Jennett B. Assessment of coma and impaired consciousness. A practical scale. *Lancet.* 1974;2(7872):81–84.
16. Holt GR. Concepts of soft-tissue trauma repair. *Otolaryngol Clin North Am.* 1990;23(5):1019–1030.
17. Leach J. Proper handling of soft tissue in the acute phase. *Facial Plast Surg.* 2001;17(4):227–238.
18. Lee RH, et al. Patterns of facial laceration from blunt trauma. *Plast Reconstr Surg.* 1997;99(6):1544–1554.
19. Trott A. *Special Problems and Anatomic Concerns. Principles and Techniques of Minor Wound Care.* Hyde Park, NY: Medical Examination Publishing; 1985.
20. Clark N, et al. High-energy ballistic and avulsive facial injuries: classification, patterns, and an algorithm for primary reconstruction. *Plast Reconstr Surg.* 1996;98(4):583–601.
21. Endo T, et al. Facial contour reconstruction in lipodystrophy using a double paddle dermis-fat radial forearm free flap. *Ann Plast Surg.* 1994;32(1):93–96.
22. Jurkiewicz MJ, Nahai F. The omentum: its use as a free vascularized graft for reconstruction of the head and neck. *Ann Surg.* 1982;195(6):756–765.
23. Landra AP. One-stage reconstruction of a massive gun-shot wound of the lower face with a local compound osteo-musculocutaneous flap. *Br J Plast Surg.* 1981;34(4):395–397.
24. Williams CN, Cohen M, Schultz RC. Immediate and long-term management of gunshot wounds to the lower face. *Plast Reconstr Surg.* 1988;82(3):433–439.
25. Yuksel F, et al. Management of maxillofacial problems in self-inflicted rifle wounds. *Ann Plast Surg.* 2004;53(2):111–117.
26. Huang S, Remeikis N, Daniel J. Effect of long-term exposure of human periodontal ligament cells to milk and other solutions. *J Endod.* 1996;22(30).
27. Olson B, Mailhot J, Anderson R, et al. Comparison of various transport media on human periodontal ligament cell viability. *J Endod.* 1997;23(676).
28. Sires BS, Stanley RB Jr, Levine LM. Oculocardiac reflex caused by orbital floor trapdoor fracture: an indication for urgent repair. *Arch Ophthalmol.* 1998;116(7):955–956.
29. LeFort R. Etude experimental sur les fractures de la machoire superieuse. *Rev de Chir.* 1901;23:208–227.
30. Savage RR, Valvich C. Hematoma of the nasal septum. *Pediatr Rev.* 2006;27(12): 478–479.
31. Cook T. Ocular and periocular injuries from orbital fractures. *J Am Coll Surg.* 2002;195(6):831–834.
32. *United States Eye Injury Registry.* http://www.useironline.org/
33. Kuhn F, Morris R, Witherspoon, et al. A standard classification of ocular trauma. *Ophthalmology.* 1996;103(240).
34. Hamill M. Clinical evaluation. In: Shingleton BJ, Hersh PS, Kenyon KR, eds. *Eye Trauma.* St. Louis, MO: Mosby-Year Book;1991.
35. Nicoladoni. Ueber Fisteln des Ductus Stenonianus. *Verh Dtsch Ges Chir.* 1896;81.
36. Sparkman RS. Primary repair of severed parotid duct: review of literature and report of three cases. *Ann Surg.* 1949;129(5):652–660.
37. Morestin H. Contribution a l'etude du traitement des fistules salivaraires consecutives aux blessures de guerre. *Bull Soc Chir.* 1917;43:845.
38. Adkins WY, Osguthorpe JD. Management of trauma of the facial nerve. *Otolaryngol Clin North Am.* 1991;24(3):587–611.
39. Baker DC, Conley J. Facial nerve grafting: a thirty year retrospective review. *Clin Plast Surg.* 1979;6(3):343–360.
40. Fisch U, Lanser MJ. Facial nerve grafting. *Otolaryngol Clin North Am.* 1991;24(3):691–708.
41. Haug RH, Assael L. *Infection in the Maxillofacial Trauma Patient.* 4 ed. Oral and Maxillofacial Infections, Philadelphia, PA: Saunders; 2002.
42. Kaiser AB. Antimicrobial prophylaxis in surgery. *N Engl J Med.* 1986;315(18):1129–1138.
43. Andreasen JO, et al. A systematic review of prophylactic antibiotics in the surgical treatment of maxillofacial fractures. *J Oral Maxillofac Surg.* 2006;64(11):1664–1668.
44. Aderhold L, Jung H, Frenkel G. Untersuchungen uber den wert einer Antibiotika Prophylaxe bei Kiefer-Gesichtsverletzungen—eine prospective Studie. *Dtsch Zahnarztl Z.* 1983;38(402).
45. Chole RA, Yee J. Antibiotic prophylaxis for facial fractures. A prospective, randomized clinical trial. *Arch Otolaryngol Head Neck Surg.* 1987;113(10):1055–1057.
46. Gerlach KL, Pape H-D, Untersuchengen zur Antibiotikaprophylaxe bei der operativen Behandlung von Unterkieferfrakturen. *Dtsch Z Mund Kiefer Gesichts Chir* 1988;12(497).
47. Zallen RD, Curry JT. A study of antibiotic usage in compound mandibular fractures. *J Oral Surg.* 1975;33(6):431–434.
48. Ratilal B, Costa J, Sampaio C. Antibiotic prophylaxis for preventing meningitis in patients with basilar skull fractures. *Cochrane Database Syst Rev* 2006(1):CD004884.

TRAUMA

CHAPTER 24 ■ SPINAL COLUMN AND SPINAL CORD INJURY

KHALID M. ABBED AND KIMBERLY A. DAVIS

Injuries to the spine, including injuries to the vertebral column, ligaments, and cord, are common. Spine injuries occurred in 106,762 patients in 2008, representing 17% of the population of patients reported to the National Trauma Data Bank.[1] According to the Foundation for Spinal Cord Injury Prevention, Care and Cure, the incidence of spinal cord injury, excluding those who die at the scene, is approximately 40 cases per million population in the United States, or approximately 12,000 new cases per year.[2]

Spinal cord injury is a disease of young male adults. The average age at injury during the 1970s was approximately 28 years with most injuries ranging between the ages of 16 and 30. However, as the median age of the population has increased, the average age at injury has also steadily increased to approximately 42 years in 2005. Spinal cord injury affects males more commonly than females, with a ratio of 4 to 1. The most common etiology of spinal cord injury in the United States is motor vehicle crashes (42.1%) followed by falls and acts of violence (primarily gunshot wounds). The proportion of injuries due to sports has decreased over time.[2]

Injuries to the spinal cord are devastating: 30% of patients have incomplete tetraplegia, 25% have complete paraplegia, 20% have complete tetraplegia, and 18.5% have incomplete paraplegia. Less than 1% of patients experience functional neurologic recovery by the time of hospital discharge. The median hospital length of stay in an acute care hospital has declined over the last three decades, averaging 12 days in the years 2005-2008. Similar downtrends are noted for days in rehabilitation, averaging 37 days in the years 2005-2008. Overall median hospitalized days including acute care and rehabilitation were greater for neurologically complete injuries.[2]

Spinal cord injuries represent a major societal economic burden. Although more than half of patients with spinal cord injury (57.5%) report being employed at the time of their injury, this drops significantly to 11.5% at 1 year postinjury. Additionally, in 2008 dollars, the average first year postinjury costs range from $236,109 to $801,161 with each subsequent year's cost ranging from $16,547 for incomplete motor function at any level to $143,507 for a patient with high tetraplegia (C1-C4). These costs noted are only direct costs and do not acknowledge the indirect costs, including loss of future wages, fringe benefits, and productivity. As >95% of patients survive their initial hospitalization, the lifetime costs of injury in a young spinal cord injury patient with a high cervical spine injury (C1-C4) are in excess of $3,160,000. Indirect costs have been estimated at approximately $64,443 per year in December of 2008.[2]

Spine injuries occur in mobile spinal segments: the cervical spine and the thoracolumbar spine. In the cervical spine, 25% of all injuries occur in the upper cervical spine, while 75% occur between C3 and C7. Multiple-level spine injuries have been estimated to occur in 4%-20% of all cases. In the thoracolumbar spine, the anatomic distribution of injury is most common around the thoracolumbar junction.

The most common spine fracture is a vertebral body compression fracture. Anterior column wedge fractures are the most common type of compression fractures and are the typical compression fractures seen in osteoporotic patients. Fractures occurring from major flexion and distraction forces often disrupt the posterior ligamentous complex causing these fractures to be relatively unstable. These fractures are often caused by lap belts in motor vehicle accidents. High-energy axial loads to the spine may cause compression fractures with retropulsion of bone fragments into the canal. These fractures are called burst fractures, which have a higher risk of causing neurologic deficit and instability. A combination of compression, tension, rotation, and/or shear forces causes fracture dislocation injuries that disrupt all three columns of the spine. Fracture dislocations are the most unstable type of spinal fracture.

Cervical spine injuries occur in a bimodal fashion, involving either the young (age 15-45 years) or elderly (age 65-85 years).[3] While cervical spine injury is more common in younger patients, the elderly (age 50-80) are more likely to sustain thoracolumbar fractures.[4]

The main tenet of prehospital care for spinal cord injury is effective spinal immobilization to prevent further injury. It is estimated that 3%-25% of spinal cord injuries occur after the initial trauma, either during transport or in the initial phases of evaluation and treatment. Effective spine immobilization includes the use of a rigid cervical collar and a backboard, with the head of the patient secured to the backboard with head blocks and straps. The practice of immobilization with sandbags and tape is not recommended.[5,6]

BONY AND LIGAMENTOUS ANATOMY OF THE VERTEBRAL COLUMN

The vertebral column, which along with the skull and rib cage comprises the axial skeleton, provides support and protects neural elements. It consists of 33 vertebrae, 24 of which are mobile and 9 immobile. The mobile vertebrae include 7 cervical, 12 thoracic, and 5 lumbar vertebrae. The immobile vertebrae include 5 sacral and 4 coccygeal vertebrae, which are fused to form the sacrum and coccyx, the caudal-most portion of the vertebral column.

The adult spine has natural curves in the sagittal plane that form an S-shape. This S-shape is formed by lordosis in the cervical and lumbar regions and kyphosis in the thoracic region. This natural curvature of the spine allows for shock absorption, maintenance of balance, and body movement. The basic motion segment is comprised of two adjacent vertebral bodies, intervening disc, facet joints, and the stabilizing ligaments. These spinal motion segments allow flexibility and motion while maintaining stability.

Because of anatomic and kinematic differences, the cervical spine is often differentiated into upper (C1-C2) and lower (C3-C7) regions. The pedicles of C2 are a transition zone between the upper and subaxial spine and are oblique in order to connect the anterior C1 facets to the posterior

C3 facets. The occiput and the upper cervical spine form a complex and highly mobile unit. C1 articulates with the occipital condyles as well as the dens and facets of C2. The occiput–C1 articulation allows for flexion–extension and lateral bending. C2, also known as the axis, has a distinctive odontoid process that articulates with the anterior arch of C1 and is stabilized by the transverse ligament. The C1-C2 (atlantoaxial) articulation allows for 50% of head rotation. The vertebrae of C3-C7, also known as the subaxial cervical spine, are more uniform and, because of the shingle-like orientation of the facets, allow primarily flexion and extension in this region.

The 12 vertebrae of the thoracic spine form a long, rigid column with limited motion due to their attachments to the rib cage and sternum. The thoracolumbar junction is a transition zone from the rigid thoracic spine to the mobile lumbar spine. In this region, the facet joints gradually change from a more coronal orientation to a sagittal orientation. The five lumbar vertebrae are the largest vertebrae in the spine. The facets of the lumbar spine are oriented at 45 degrees of sagittal angulation allowing flexion–extension, rotation, and lateral bending. The lumbosacral junction is another transition zone between mobile and rigid segments that has significance when surgical stabilization procedures are being considered.

Spinal ligaments and intervening discs stabilize the mobile segments of the vertebral column. In the cervical spine, the intervertebral discs and the anterior and posterior longitudinal ligaments stabilize the anterior column. The posterior column is stabilized by the facet capsules, ligamentum flavum, interspinal and supraspinal ligaments, and the ligamentum nuchae. The odontoid process of C2 is stabilized by the alar, transverse, and apical ligaments.

First described by Denis, the spine can be divided into three longitudinally oriented columns.[7] The anterior column includes the anterior longitudinal ligament, the anterior annulus, and the anterior half of the vertebral body. The middle column includes the posterior longitudinal ligament, posterior annulus, and the posterior half of the vertebral body. The posterior column is comprised of the pedicles, facets, laminae, and posterior ligamentous complex (Fig. 24.1).

ANATOMY AND PHYSIOLOGY OF THE SPINAL CORD

The spinal cord is an extension of the brainstem that begins at the foramen magnum and continues down through the vertebral canal to the first lumbar vertebra, where the spinal cord tapers to form the conus medullaris. A cluster of lumbosacral nerve roots below the conus medullaris forms the cauda equina. Along the length of the spinal cord, ventral and dorsal nerve roots emerge together bilaterally to form spinal nerve roots, exiting through the neural foramen at each intervertebral space.

The spinal cord is held in position at its inferior end by the filum terminale, an extension of the pia mater that attaches to the coccyx. Along its length, the spinal cord is held within the vertebral canal by denticulate ligaments that are lateral extensions of the pia mater attaching to the dural sheath. The subarachnoid space between the spinal cord and dura is an extension of, and communicates directly with, the subarachnoid space around the brain, containing cerebrospinal fluid (CSF) that acts as a shock absorber.

The spinal cord has variable diameters along its length. In the upper spinal cord, between C4 and T1, the spinal cord widens as the cervical enlargement, which is where spinal nerves innervating the upper extremities originate and terminate. The lumbar enlargement, between T9 and T12, is a widening in the lower part of the spinal cord where spinal nerves innervating the lower extremities originate and terminate.

The cross-sectional anatomy of the spinal cord consists of white matter located on the periphery and gray matter located centrally. The white matter contains myelinated axons that form the ascending and descending spinal tracts. The gray matter contains primarily neurons and unmyelinated axons and is divided into three "horns": anterior, posterior, and intermediate. The anterior horns contain lower motor neurons that innervate the muscles of the neck, trunk, and extremities. The upper motor neurons that synapse with these lower motor neurons originate in the contralateral cerebral cortex or brain stem and descend as the lateral and anterior corticospinal tracts prior to synapsing in the anterior horn. The posterior horns contain neurons that synapse with afferent

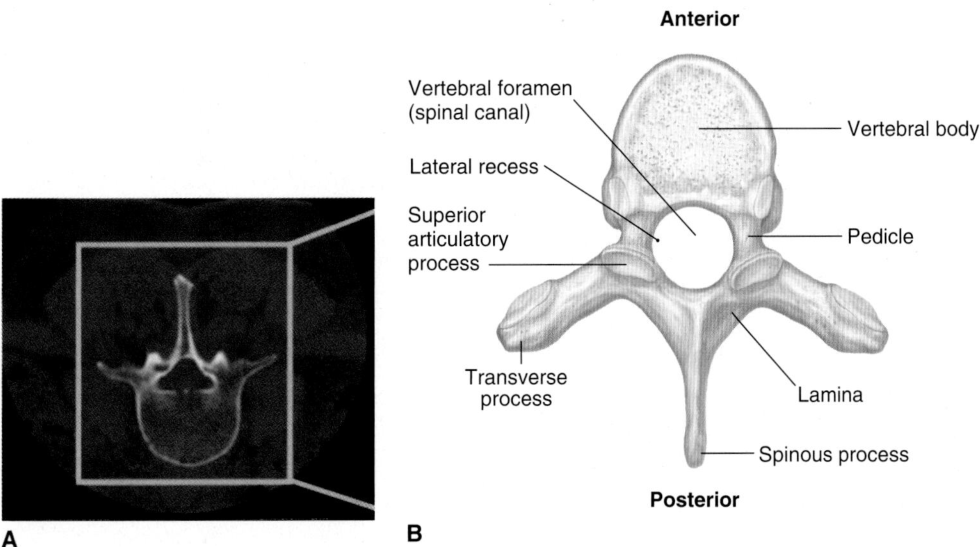

FIGURE 24.1 A: Noncontrast axial CT and (B) schematic representation of a vertebral body highlighting the relevant anatomy (Reprinted with permission from Blumenfeld H. *Neuroanatomy through Clinical Cases*. Sinauer Associates; 2002).

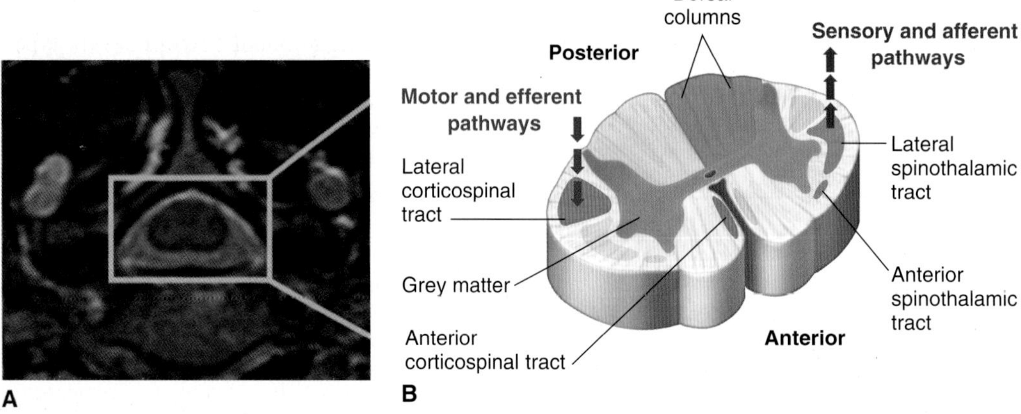

FIGURE 24.2 **A:** Noncontrast axial MRI and (**B**) schematic representation of the spinal cord highlighting the major anatomic tracts.

sensory axons. The intermediate horns contain the preganglionic autonomic sympathetic neurons between T1 and L3 and the parasympathetic neurons between S2 and S4 (Fig. 24.2).

Sensory signals originate in somatic or visceral receptors and are transmitted via axons to the dorsal root ganglion. From there, sensory afferent axons enter the posterior horns of the gray matter and travel within varied regions of spinal cord white matter toward sensory regions of the brain. Pain and temperature signals cross immediately and ascend in the contralateral lateral spinothalamic tract. Touch also crosses immediately and ascends mainly in the anterior spinothalamic tract. Proprioception and vibration ascend in the ipsilateral dorsal column and cross in the brainstem. The dorsal columns are divided into the fasciculus gracilis and the fasciculus cuneatus. The fasciculus gracilis is located medially and carries sensory signals from the lower extremities, whereas the fasciculus cuneatus is located laterally and carries sensory signals from the upper extremities.

ACUTE VERTEBRAL COLUMN INJURIES

Spinal Instability

The determination of spinal instability is a complex and controversial subject, and spinal instability is often difficult to precisely ascertain. A widely accepted definition of clinical instability is the loss of the ability of the spine, under physiologic loads, to maintain its pattern of displacement so that there is no initial or additional neurologic deficit, no major deformity, or no incapacitating pain.[8] Although many theories of spinal instability have been proposed, Denis' previously described three-column theory is most widely accepted.[7] The integrity of the middle column is of the utmost importance as an injury to two adjoining columns defines an unstable fracture. Punjabi and colleagues have validated the three-column theory of instability using high-speed trauma models of thoracolumbar spinal fractures and demonstrated that the integrity of the middle column correlated best with eight of nine flexibility parameters.[9]

Occipitoatlantal Dislocation

Among traumatic injuries to the cervical spine and causes for occipital–cervical instability, occipitoatlantal dislocation (OAD) is one of the most severe. A hyperflexion–distraction injury resulting in ligamentous disconnection of the skull from the cervical spine, OAD is often immediately fatal because of associated neurologic and vascular injuries. Any high-impact injury should arouse suspicion of OAD. Although plain radiographs of the cervical spine may reveal prevertebral soft tissue swelling and an increase in the basion–dens interval, which should measure 12 mm or less, more definitive diagnosis is made with reconstructed computed tomography (CT) images of the craniocervical junction. Magnetic resonance imaging (MRI) and CT are comparable in terms of diagnosing OAD, but MRI identifies the specific ligaments injured. OAD injuries can be defined in three broad categories. Type I injuries are characterized by anterior displacement of the occipital condyles on the C1 lateral masses; Type II injuries are characterized by displacement of the occiput and C1 in the vertical plane, and Type III injuries are marked by posterior displacement of occipital condyles compared to C1. These injuries are rare and usually fatal. If the patient survives and there are no contraindications, posterior occipital–cervical stabilization and fusion are required.

Occipital Condyle Fractures

The Anderson and Montesano scheme classifies occipital condyle fractures into three main types.[10] These fractures are seen in 1%-3% of blunt trauma to the craniocervical region. Type 1 fractures are comminuted, and result from axial loading injuries. Type II fractures are linear fractures that originate in the squama of the occipital bone and extend into the condyle. Type III fractures are avulsion fractures of the condyles and are most prone to instability and OAD. While types I and II fractures are generally stable, type III fractures are potentially unstable. Stable fractures can be treated in a cervicothoracic brace; however, unstable fractures mandate stabilization and fusion.

BONY AND LIGAMENTOUS INJURIES TO THE CERVICAL SPINE

C1 Fractures and Transverse Ligament Injuries

Fractures of the atlas are usually defined in relation to the lateral masses and extent of arch involvement.[11] They can involve any parts of the ring in isolation or in combination, ranging from single unilateral fractures to burst-type fractures involving all aspects, also known as a Jefferson fracture. Since isolated atlas fractures without ligamentous injury are stable and heal with simple immobilization, clinical decision making is based on the identification of injuries to the transverse ligament, the vertebral artery, and other associated spinal fractures. The most commonly cited radiographic criteria indicating unstable disruption of the transverse ligament include the rule of Spence (lateral displacement of C1 lateral masses over C2 > 6.9 mm) and the atlantodental interval > 3 mm.[12,79] However, when feasible, this author prefers MRI evaluation of all atlas fractures to assess for concomitant ligamentous injury, which is an indication for surgical fixation.

Atlantoaxial Joint Injuries

Atlantoaxial subluxation occurs when the transverse ligament is disrupted. This is an extremely unstable injury with a high risk for neurologic deficit. Traction may be appropriate initially to achieve reduction. Definitive treatment mandates posterior cervical fusion of C1-C2.

C2 Fractures

Odontoid process fractures commonly affect the elderly. The most common classification scheme for fractures of C2, the Anderson and D'Alonzo scheme, relies on the location of the fracture line within the odontoid process or body of C2.[13] In this scheme, type I fractures involve the tip of the dens, type II fractures run through the junction of the dens and the body of C2, and type III fractures course through the vertebral body of C2 (Figs. 24.3 and 24.4).

Management of C2 fractures is determined by type. Type I fractures are an avulsion of the alar ligament and are usually stable. Cervical collar immobilization for symptomatic management is usually sufficient. Type II fractures are the most common type of dens fracture and are more often subject to nonunion, especially in patients older than 50 years of age and those with displacement >5 mm. When choosing treatment strategies for type II fractures, the integrity of the transverse ligament, age and orientation of the fracture, displacement and/or angulation of the fractured process, and patient-specific factors such as medical comorbidities, and body habitus should be considered. Type III fractures extend into the C2 vertebral body. This fracture type can be mechanically unstable but generally heals well with immobilization. As such, treatment usually entails cervical immobilization in either a rigid cervical orthosis or a halo vest for 12 weeks.

Fractures of the C2 pedicles (also known as traumatic spondylolisthesis or hangman's fractures) are often classified based on the mechanism of injury, where flexion (type III) and flexion–distraction (type IIa) are often unstable and require surgical fixation, especially type IIa injuries with >4 mm distraction and/or >11 degrees of angulation.[15,76] Other fractures of the axis can include isolated fractures of the C2 vertebral body or fractures of the C2 spinous process or lamina, which are usually stable and can achieve good union with nonoperative immobilization.

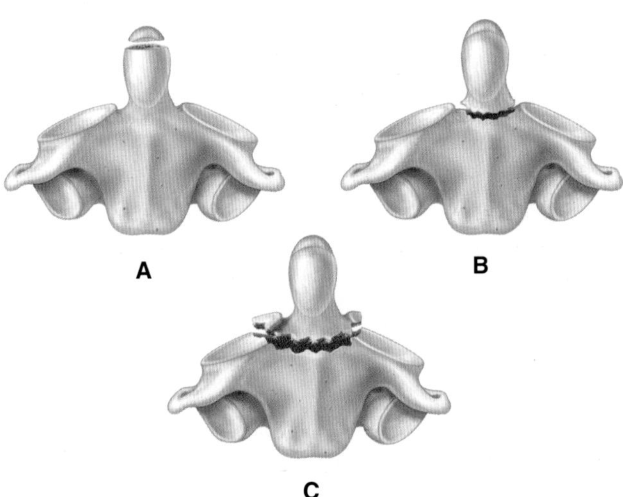

FIGURE 24.3 Schematic representation of the three types of odontoid fractures: (A) type 1, (B) type 2, and (C) type 3.

Injuries of the Subaxial Cervical Spine (C3-C7)

Subaxial cervical spine injuries include fractures, dislocations, subluxations, and a combination of these injuries. Unilateral facet injuries can cause nerve root irritation and radiculopathy, whereas bilateral facet injuries frequently cause spinal cord compromise. Both unilateral and bilateral facet disruptions are treated initially with closed reduction with traction. If this reduction can be maintained, unilateral injuries can be definitively treated with halo immobilization. Bilateral facet injuries, however, are grossly unstable and require surgical fusion for definitive treatment.

Compression Fractures. Compression fractures are anterior column injuries with wedging of the anterior portion of vertebral body. The posterior portion of the vertebral body and the spinal canal remain intact. As a result, neurologic compromise is rare. These are generally stable injuries, but if angulation exceeds 11 degrees, wedge compression exceeds 25% of the anterior vertebral body, or translation exceeds 2.5 mm, brace immobilization may not be sufficient. If the anterior vertebral body wedge compression exceeds 50%, there is a greater likelihood that the posterior ligamentous complex has been disrupted. This unstable form of compression injury requires surgical stabilization.

Burst Fractures. Burst fractures are characterized by disruption of both the anterior and middle columns, have some degree of spinal canal compromise, and are commonly associated with neurologic deficit and instability. These injuries are caused by a large axial load applied to a cervical spine while in a straight position. If there is no neurologic deficit or malalignment, halo immobilization may be an acceptable treatment. If, however, neurologic deficit is present and/or reduction cannot be achieved, anterior decompression and fusion is indicated. Anterior and posterior stabilization may be required if there is associated posterior ligamentous injury.

Other Cervical Fractures. Other common cervical injuries include lateral mass fractures, laminar fractures, spinous process fractures, flexion tear drop fractures (Fig. 24.5), extension tear drop fractures, and ligamentous injuries. These are generally stable injuries except for flexion tear drop fractures, which result from a flexion–compression mechanism. In this very unstable fracture, all three columns are involved, and there is a high incidence of neurologic compromise. In contrast, extension tear drop fractures are a stable avulsion injury involving only the anterior column.

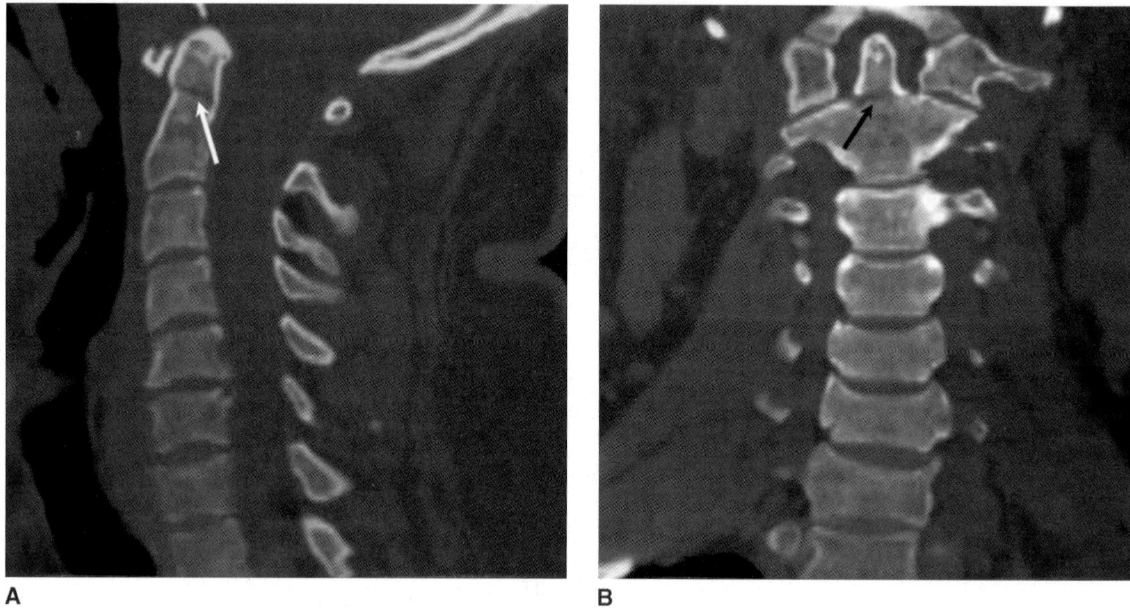

FIGURE 24.4 Noncontrast sagittal (A) and coronal (B) CTs demonstrate a type 2 odontoid fracture (*arrows*).

Injuries to the Thoracic Spine

Unlike the cervical and lumbar spine, the thoracic spine is inherently stable. As a result, thoracic spine fractures are usually caused by high-energy mechanisms, and associated injuries occur in about 75% of patients. Stable thoracic spine fractures without neurologic deficit can often be treated nonsurgically with bracing or vertebroplasty/kyphoplasty (Fig. 24.6). Unstable thoracic spine fractures are usually associated with neurologic deficit and malalignment and require surgical reduction and stabilization (Fig. 24.7).

Injuries to the Thoracolumbar Spine

Thoracolumbar spine fractures are extremely common due to the relatively mobile characteristics of this region compared to the adjacent rigid thoracic spine and sacrum. Fractures in this location include compression fractures, burst fractures, fracture–distraction injuries, and fracture dislocation injuries. Flexion–distraction injuries consist of both bony and ligamentous disruption without loss of vertebral height. Most of these injuries are treated surgically, especially if there is substantial disc or ligamentous involvement. Fracture dislocations consist

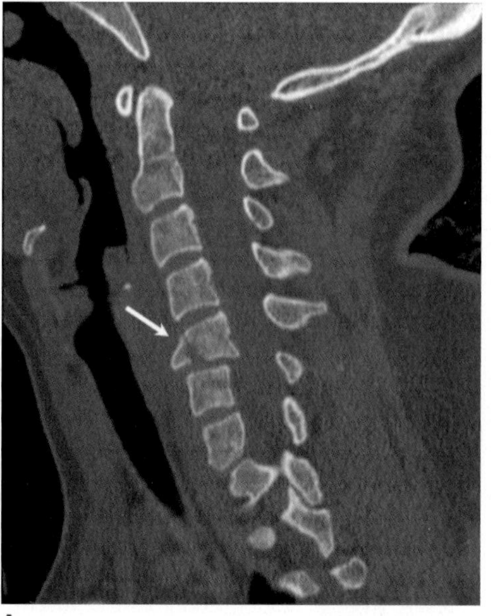

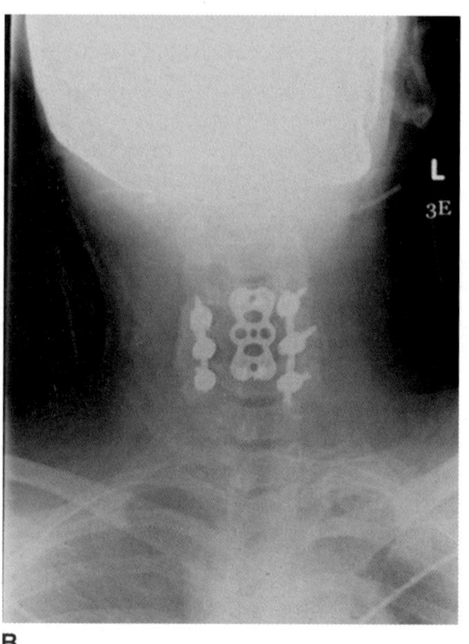

FIGURE 24.5 Noncontrast sagittal CT (A) demonstrates a C5 tear drop fracture (*arrow*). Postoperative AP radiograph of the cervical spine (B) with anterior and posterior fixation hardware in place.

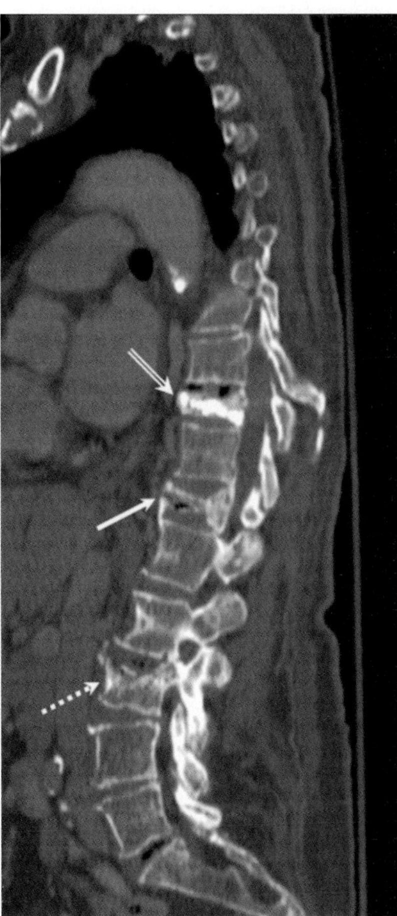

FIGURE 24.6 Noncontrast sagittal CT demonstrates a chronic T10 compression fracture, status postkyphoplasty (*double arrow*), as well as acute compression fractures at T12 (*single arrow*) and L3 (*dashed arrow*).

of varying degrees of rotation, flexion, and translation and are extremely unstable injuries. The majority of these injuries are associated with neurologic deficit, and require surgical decompression and stabilization (Fig. 24.8).

ACUTE SPINAL CORD INJURY

Mechanism of Injury

Based on the mechanism of injury, spinal cord injury can be categorized as direct/penetrating or indirect/blunt injuries. The direct or penetrating injuries are caused by a space-occupying lesion as a result of a focal injury to the neural elements at the site of impact (Figs. 24.9 and 24.10). These are most often caused by a gunshot wound or a knife laceration and most often result in complete neurologic deficit. The indirect or blunt injuries are caused by stretching, shearing, or compressive forces on the spinal cord (Fig. 24.11). These often occur in the setting of a motor vehicle accident, fall, or sport-related activity and are the most frequent type of spinal cord injury encountered in clinical practice.

Morphologic and Functional Changes

Spinal cord injuries can be further subclassified as primary or secondary injuries. Primary traumatic lesions are due to direct mechanical disruption of the cord parenchyma, typically occurring at the time of the injury. Secondary traumatic lesions evolve as a consequence of injury-related factors such as edema, ischemia, or mechanical injury from persistent pressure on the cord or improper immobilization. Although structural damage of neural tissue is irreversible, the prevention of secondary spinal cord injury is the major goal for early intervention in spinal cord injury.

The secondary events, triggered by the mechanical injury to the neural tissue, are a complex cascade of biomechanical and

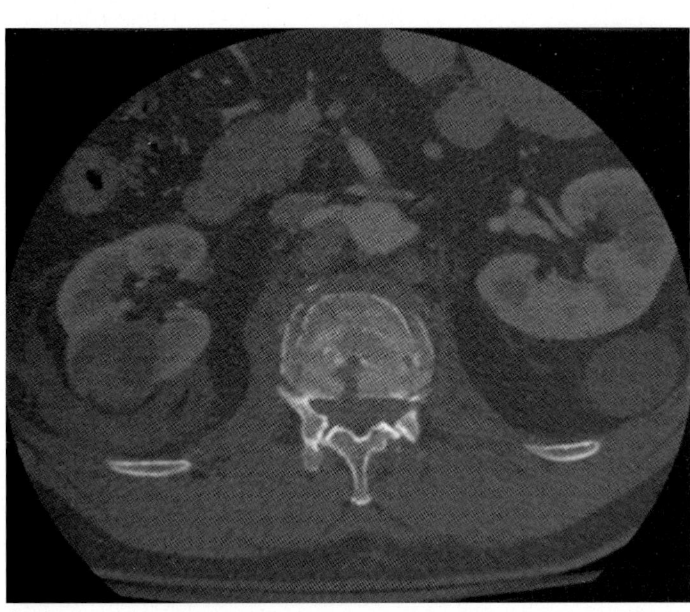

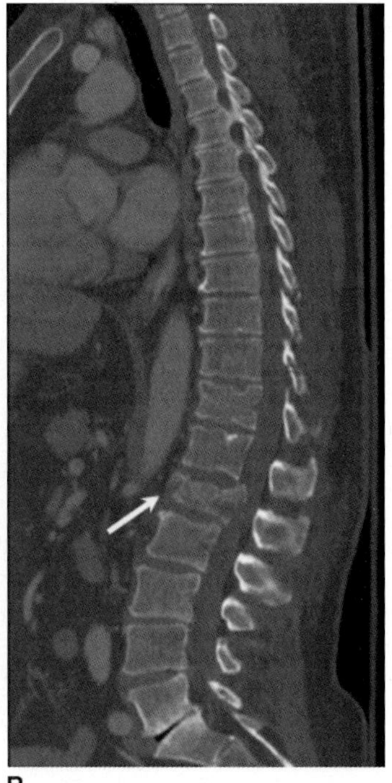

A B

FIGURE 24.7 Noncontrast axial (**A**) and sagittal (**B**) CTs demonstrate an L1 burst fracture with retropulsion of bone fragments into the spinal canal.

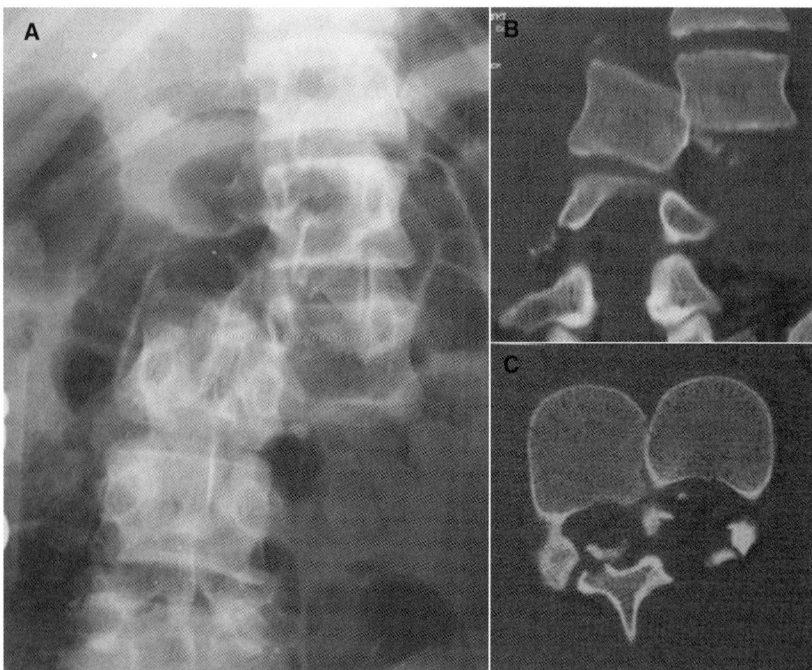

FIGURE 24.8 Lumbar AP radiograph (**A**) and noncontrast coronal (**B**) and axial (**C**) CTs demonstrate an L2–L3 fracture dislocation with malalignment of the vertebral column (Reprinted with permission from: Loftus CM, Macias MY, Wolfla CE. *Neurosurgical Emergencies*. Thieme Medical Publishers; 2008).

cellular processes that are poorly understood. Several theories have been proposed to explain the pathophysiologic events of secondary injury such as the neurotransmitter theory (which implicates increased levels of the excitatory amino acids, glutamate and aspartate), free-radical theory (which implicates free radical accumulation), calcium ion theory (which implicates the influx of extracellular calcium ions), the inflammation theory (which implicates the accumulation of inflammatory mediators such as prostaglandins and leukotrienes), and others; in reality, the synergistic effect of all of these events most likely occurs.[16-19]

The gray matter, within the central substance of the spinal cord, is most susceptible to direct injury, due to the higher metabolic rate of gray matter and the presence of neurons, which are responsible for repair, existing within the site of injury. In contrast, the neuronal cell bodies of white matter are located at a remote site.[20]

Similar to the ischemic penumbra seen in strokes and closed head injuries, spinal cord tissue adjacent to the site of injury is at risk. Following initial injury, inflammation spreads throughout the adjacent areas of the cord, and neurogenic shock, manifesting as autonomic dysfunction, hypotension, and bradycardia, can develop further impairing spinal cord perfusion and increasing ischemia. Management strategies for neurogenic shock include resuscitation from hypovolemia as appropriate with crystalloids and blood or blood products, although the often profound hypotension of neurogenic shock may be refractory to fluid resuscitation alone. Therefore, the administration of pressors may be required with the goal of maintaining mean arterial pressure of 85-90 mm Hg for the first week after injury to improve spinal cord perfusion and prevent secondary injury. Pressors with intrinsic β1 agonist and chronotropic activity, including dopamine and dobutamine, may be particularly useful as they address not only the vasomotor component of neurogenic shock but also

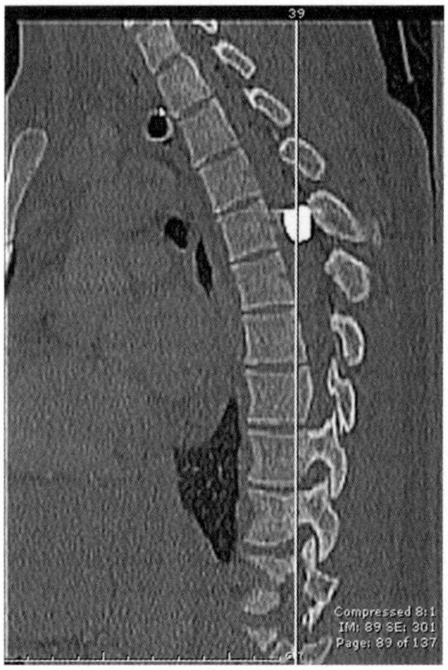

FIGURE 24.9 Gunshot wound with bullet in thoracic spinal canal at T4–T5 (Sagittal CT reconstruction).

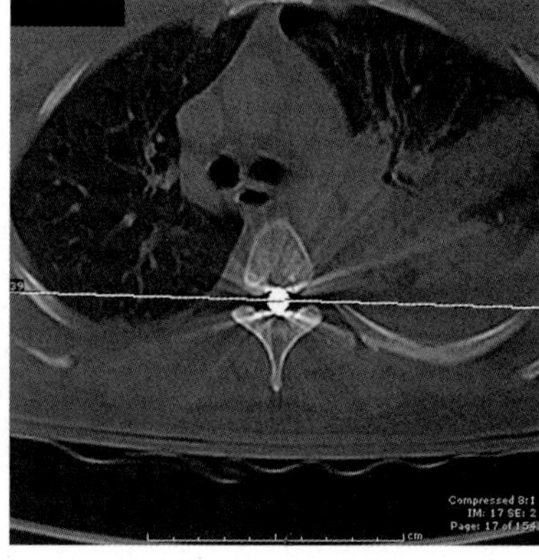

FIGURE 24.10 Gunshot wound with bullet in thoracic spinal canal at T4–T5 (Axial CT).

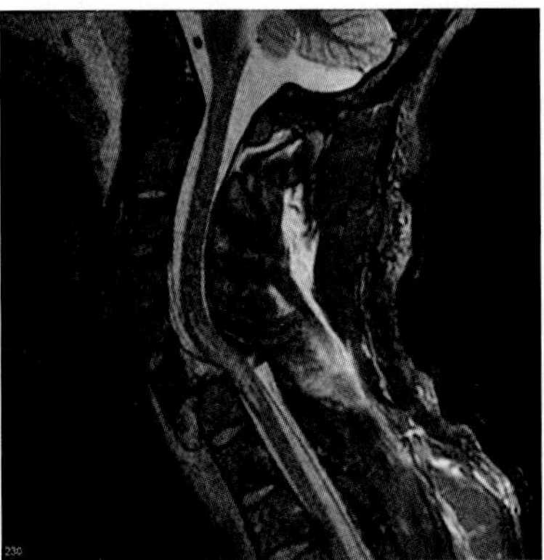

FIGURE 24.11 Fracture dislocation at C6–C7 with spinal cord compression and instability.

the cardiogenic component. However, current recommendations are the use of neosynephrine in the management of these patients. Duration of pressor requirement in these patients is generally between 3 and 7 days but can extend as long as 14 days, and patients should be carefully monitored in an intensive care unit or other monitored setting until their hemodynamic status normalizes.[21]

Clinical Presentation

Presenting signs and symptoms vary depending on whether upper or lower motor neuron function is impaired. Patients with spinal cord injury often have symptoms of lower motor neuron injury at the level of the injured segment and upper motor neuron symptoms to all segments below the level of injury. Upper motor neuron signs and symptoms, such as spastic paralysis with inability for voluntary movement, increased deep tendon reflexes, loss of superficial reflexes, and positive Babinski sign and clonus, can occur from injury to white matter tracts within the spinal cord. Lower motor neuron signs and symptoms, such as flaccid paralysis with inability for voluntary movement, loss of all reflexes, and atrophy of muscles, can occur from injury to peripheral nerves and anterior horns of the spinal cord gray matter. Spinal shock, unlike neurogenic shock, is a transient state of physiologic reflex depression of cord function below the level of injury with an associated loss of sensory and motor function. Hallmarks of spinal shock include flaccid paralysis, bladder dysfunction, and occasionally sustained priapism. These findings can last from hours to days following injury until the reflex arcs below the level of injury resume function. Following spinal cord trauma, the presence or absence of the bulbocavernosus reflex, referring to anal sphincter contraction in response to squeezing of the glans of the penis or tugging on the Foley catheter, carries prognostic significance. Return of the bulbocavernosus reflex represents sacral sparing and may portend an improved outcome.

Severity/Grading of Spinal Cord Injuries

Numerous classification schemes have been devised to describe patients with spinal cord injury over the years. The first standardized neurologic assessment scale for spinal injury was proposed by Frankel and associates in 1969.[22] In this classification scheme, a five-grade scale ranging from A to E is used to grade spinal cord injury patients based on the degree of motor and sensory function preserved after injury. Frankel grade A patients have complete motor and sensory lesions with no preserved function. Grade B patients have preserved sensory but no motor function below the level of injury. Grade C patients have some nonfunctional motor and some preserved sensory function. Grade D patients have functional, but not normal, motor function below the level of injury. Lastly, grade E patients have completely normal motor and sensory function. The Frankel scale provided an excellent framework from which several classification schemes have been derived. The main deficiencies of this scale were the difficulty in discerning grade C from grade D and relatively poor interobserver reliability. The American Spinal Injury Association (ASIA) Impairment Scale (Fig. 24.12) is one of the most studied and useful spinal cord injury neurologic classification schemes. It is a permutation of the original Frankel scale that provides objective parameters to better assess the significance of the preserved motor function.

Spinal Cord Syndromes

Central Cord Syndrome. Central cord syndrome is a common pattern of spinal cord injury occurring in older patients with preexisting cervical spondylosis who sustained a hyperextension injury. This injury involves the central portion of the spinal cord resulting in upper extremity greater than lower extremity motor and sensory deficit, due to the more central positioning of the upper extremity axons within the tracts of the spinal cord. The prognosis for recovery from central cord syndrome is fair, but patients may have some limited return of upper extremity function.[23]

Anterior Cord Syndrome. Anterior cord syndrome is caused by injury to the anterior two-thirds of the spinal cord. The mechanism of injury is usually a compression- or flexion-type injury that causes vascular injury. Patients present with complete loss of motor function and loss of sharp pain and temperature sensation but retain proprioception, vibration, and deep pressure sense. The prognosis for recovery is very poor.[24]

Brown-Sequard Syndrome. Brown-Sequard syndrome results from transection of one side of the spinal cord resulting in unilateral damage to the corticospinal and spinothalamic tracts. Patients present with loss of ipsilateral motor and dorsal column function, and contralateral pain and temperature sensation. Considerable improvement may occur with this syndrome.[25]

Posterior Cord Syndrome. Posterior cord syndrome involves the dorsal columns and is rare. It leads to loss of proprioception and vibration with preserved motor function. The prognosis is generally good.

Conus Medullaris Syndrome. The conus is usually located around the T11-L1 vertebral levels. Injury to the conus can result in a clinical picture with mixed upper and lower motor neuron symptoms. Injury in this region can also cause loss of bowel and bladder control. The prognosis for recovery is very poor.

Cauda Equina Syndrome. The cauda equina is composed of lumbar and sacral nerve roots. Injury to these nerve roots results in lower motor neuron symptoms with variable motor and sensory loss. Patients may also present with bowel and/or bladder dysfunction. The prognosis for motor recovery is good.

Clearing the Spine

Clearance of the cervical spine is a matter of some controversy, which has been addressed on three occasions by the Eastern

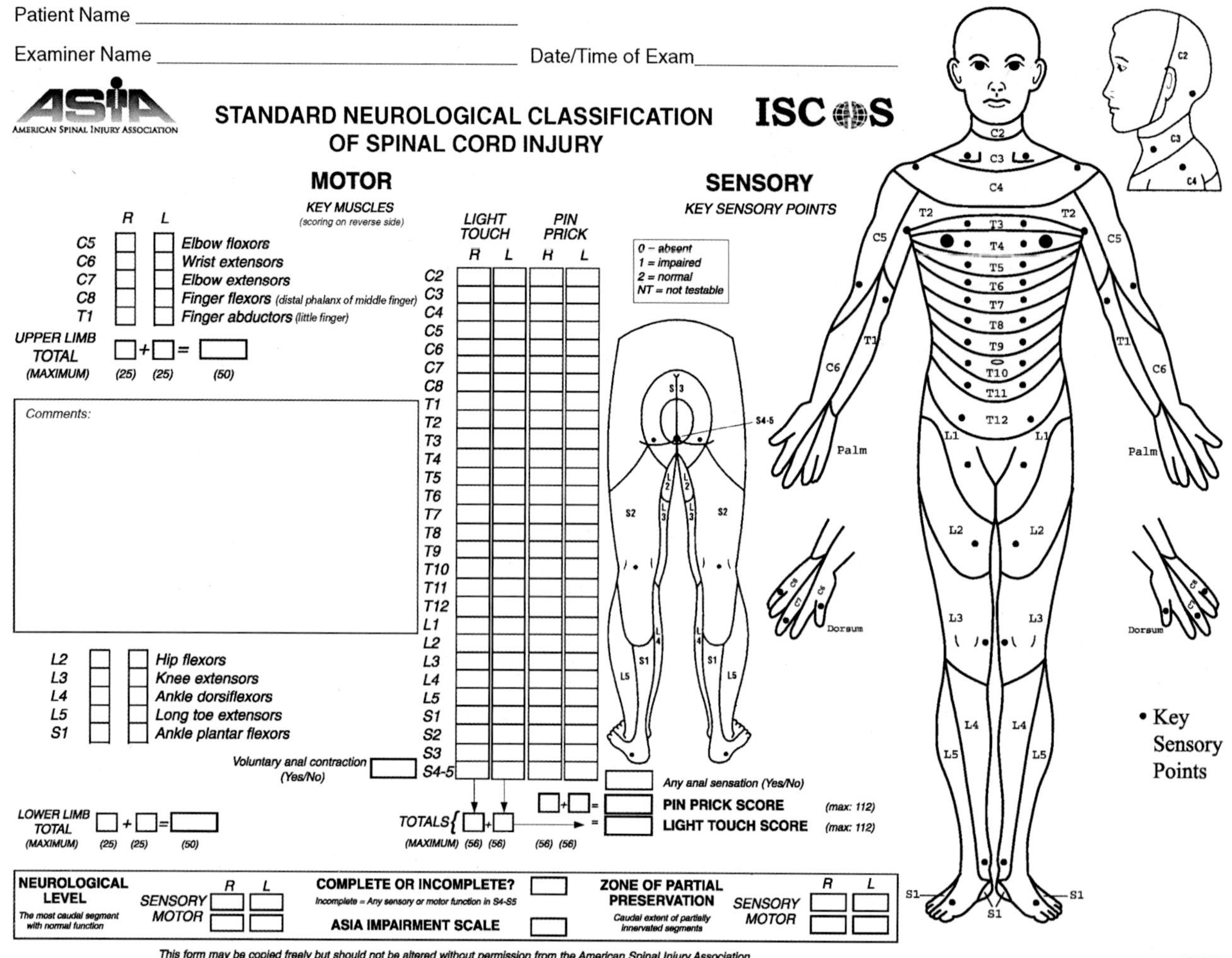

Patient Name ______________________

Examiner Name ______________________ Date/Time of Exam ______________________

ASIA AMERICAN SPINAL INJURY ASSOCIATION

STANDARD NEUROLOGICAL CLASSIFICATION OF SPINAL CORD INJURY

ISCoS

MOTOR

KEY MUSCLES (scoring on reverse side)

	R	L	
C5			Elbow flexors
C6			Wrist extensors
C7			Elbow extensors
C8			Finger flexors (distal phalanx of middle finger)
T1			Finger abductors (little finger)

UPPER LIMB TOTAL (MAXIMUM) □ + □ = □ (25) (25) (50)

Comments:

	R	L	
L2			Hip flexors
L3			Knee extensors
L4			Ankle dorsiflexors
L5			Long toe extensors
S1			Ankle plantar flexors

Voluntary anal contraction (Yes/No) □

LOWER LIMB TOTAL (MAXIMUM) □ + □ = □ (25) (25) (50)

SENSORY

KEY SENSORY POINTS

	LIGHT TOUCH R	LIGHT TOUCH L	PIN PRICK R	PIN PRICK L
C2				
C3				
C4				
C5				
C6				
C7				
C8				
T1				
T2				
T3				
T4				
T5				
T6				
T7				
T8				
T9				
T10				
T11				
T12				
L1				
L2				
L3				
L4				
L5				
S1				
S2				
S3				
S4-5				

0 = absent
1 = impaired
2 = normal
NT = not testable

Any anal sensation (Yes/No) □

TOTALS □ + □ = □ PIN PRICK SCORE (max: 112)
□ + □ = □ LIGHT TOUCH SCORE (max: 112)
(MAXIMUM) (56) (56) (56) (56)

NEUROLOGICAL LEVEL (The most caudal segment with normal function) SENSORY R □ L □ MOTOR R □ L □

COMPLETE OR INCOMPLETE? □ (Incomplete = Any sensory or motor function in S4-S5)

ASIA IMPAIRMENT SCALE □

ZONE OF PARTIAL PRESERVATION (Caudal extent of partially innervated segments) SENSORY R □ L □ MOTOR R □ L □

This form may be copied freely but should not be altered without permission from the American Spinal Injury Association.

REV 03/06

FIGURE 24.12 ASIA Standard Neurological Classification of Spinal Cord Injury worksheet. Reprinted with permission from American Spinal Injury Association: International Standards for Neurological Classification of Spinal Cord Injury, reprint 2008; Chicago, IL.

Association for the Surgery of Trauma Practice Management Guidelines committee, most recently in September 2009.[26] Removal of cervical collars should be accomplished as soon as feasible after trauma, to avoid the development of device-related complications. While all patients with blunt trauma should have a cervical collar placed prior to transport, in the patient with penetrating trauma to the brain, immobilization of the cervical spine is not necessary unless the trajectory suggests direct injury to the cervical spine. In fact, placement of collars following penetrating trauma has been associated with adverse outcomes in a number of studies.[27]

In the awake, alert trauma patients without neurologic deficit or distracting injury who have no neck pain or tenderness with full range of motion of the cervical spine, imaging is not necessary, and the cervical collar may be removed ("clinical clearance"). All other patients in whom cervical spine injury is suspected should have radiographic evaluation, including those with pain or tenderness, neurologic deficit, altered mental status, and distracting injuries. In a change from prior practice management guidelines, the primary screening modality in the multiply injured trauma patient has become axial CT from the occiput to T1 with sagittal and coronal reconstructions in place of plain radiographs. Formal spine consultation should be obtained for patients with identified fractures and patients with a neurologic injury attributable to the cervical spine. In the latter group, MRI is also recommended.[26]

Controversy persists regarding the management of the neurologically intact awake and alert patient complaining of neck pain with a negative CT examination. Options for further evaluation include imaging with MRI or adequate active flexion–extension films. For the obtunded patient with a negative CT and gross motor function of extremities, passive flexion/extension radiography should not be performed. Options for management in this patient population vary by institutional preference but include early MRI imaging, continued cervical spine immobilization until a clinical examination can be obtained, or removal of the cervical collar on the basis of the CT results only, recognizing a small risk of potentially unstable undiagnosed ligamentous injury may exist. A recent meta-analysis comparing CT alone to CT and MRI in the obtunded patient demonstrated that the addition of MRI identified injuries in 12% of patients, and changed management in 6% of patients.[12] If MRI is chosen as the management strategy, the collar may be safely removed if the MRI is negative.[26] A suggested algorithm for spine clearance can be found in Algorithm 24.1.

Clearance of the thoracic and lumbar spine follows similar guidelines. In the awake, alert trauma patients without neurologic deficit or distracting injury who have no back pain, tenderness or palpable step-off, imaging is not necessary, and the backboard may be removed. All other patients in whom thoracic or lumbar spine injury is suspected should have

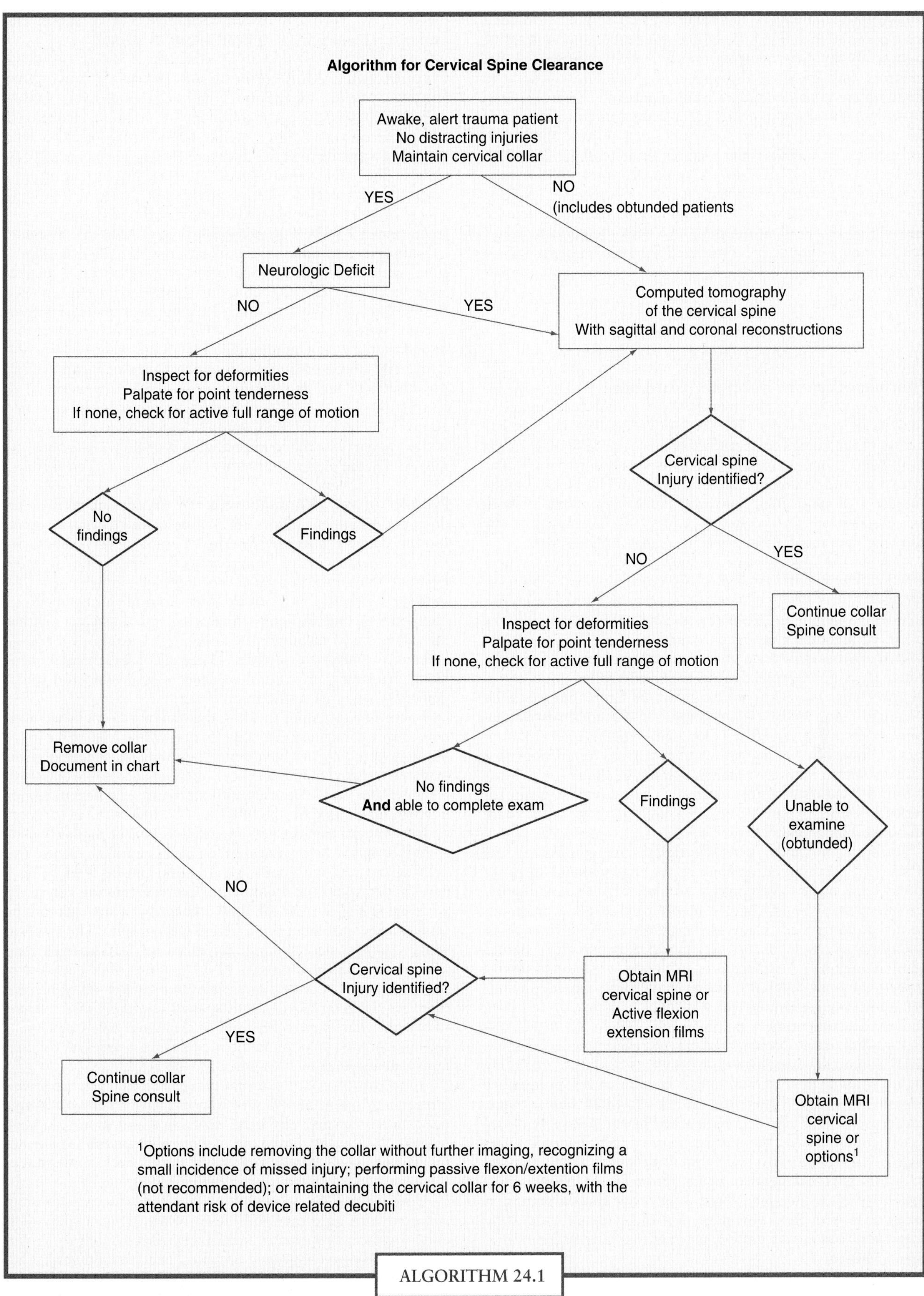

ALGORITHM 24.1 Spine clearance algorithm.

radiographic evaluation, including those with pain or tenderness, neurologic deficit, altered mental status, and distracting injuries. Plain anteroposterior and lateral radiographs are adequate for clearance of the spine, but are often difficult to obtain in the multiply injured trauma patient. Therefore, axial CT with sagittal and coronal reconstructions from images of the thoracic and lumbar spine obtained during abdominal and pelvic CT scanning has become an increasingly common method of thoracic and lumbar spine clearance.[28,29] All areas of bony abnormality identified on either plain or CT imaging studies should undergo further evaluation with dedicated CT imaging of the level in question. As with the cervical spine, MRI imaging should be considered in those patients with a neurologic injury attributable to their thoracic and lumbar spine.

Therapeutic Interventions

Pharmacotherapy in Spinal Cord Injury. The role for pharmacotherapy in the treatment of spinal cord injury is an area of controversy. The concept of neuroprotection has recently been coined to characterize those measures that might be utilized to attenuate the extent of spinal cord injury. The theory behind neuroprotective intervention is based on the premise that neurologic outcome can be improved by both the elimination of secondary injury mechanisms and by allowing damaged neural tissue to recover functionally.

One of the classes of drugs most heavily studied as neuroprotective agents is high-dose corticosteroids. Steroids effectively limit both cellular and molecular events of injury-induced inflammation, thereby theoretically decreasing the extent of secondary injury on neural tissue.[30] To date, high-dose methylprednisolone is the only steroid that has been tested as a neuroprotective agent in controlled multicenter clinical trials. The National Acute Spinal Cord Injury Studies (NASCIS-2 and NASCIS-3) recommend that methylprednisolone should be given as a bolus of 30 mg/kg over 15 minutes, followed by 5.4 mg/kg/h, and continued for 24 hours for patients within 3 hours of injury, and for 48 hours for patients within 3-8 hours of injury. Steroids should not be given for patients with penetrating injuries and patients who arrive >8 hours after injury.[31-36]

Recently, however, several studies have questioned the efficacy of methylprednisolone in the management of acute spinal cord injury. Although a number of retrospective trials questioned the efficacy of methylprednisolone, one randomized controlled study demonstrated no difference in functional recovery as defined by ASIA score with steroid administration.[37] Furthermore, concerns regarding several aspects of both NASCIS studies have been raised, including questions regarding the statistical analysis of the data and the documentation of the results.[38,39] In addition, several studies have documented an increase in complication rates in patients treated with methylprednisolone, including higher rates of pneumonia, longer hospital stays, pulmonary embolism, wound infection, gastrointestinal hemorrhage, and sepsis.[32,34,40,41] As a consequence of the above findings, recent guidelines for the management of spinal cord injuries states, "treatment with methylprednisolone for either 24 or 48 hours is recommended as an option in the treatment of patients with acute spinal cord injury that should be undertaken only with the knowledge that the evidence suggesting harmful side effects is more consistent than any suggestion of clinical benefit."[42]

Other neuroprotective agents have been tried with limited success, demonstrating only modest improvement in neurologic recovery following spinal cord injury.[43-45,77] For monosialotetrahexosylganglioside (GM-1) gangliosides,[19,20,46,78] tirilazad mesylate,[33,47] naloxone[44] and nimodipine,[48] more substantial evidence regarding their clinical efficacy is needed.

Hypothermic Management of Acute Spinal Cord Injury. Systemic hypothermia has been extensively studies as a neuroprotective agent following brain injury, stroke, and cardiac arrest. Local and systemic hypothermia has also been used as a spinal protective measure during aortic revascularization and replacement surgeries. Recently, attention was directed toward this novel management strategy following its use in a professional football player who sustained a C3/4 fracture dislocation with complete injury (ASIA A). Systemic hypothermia was utilized in association with early decompression, with subsequent considerable improvement in neurologic function (ASIA D).[49] Similar results have been reported by the Miami Project to Cure Paralysis at the University of Miami. Systemic hypothermia, with intravascular cooling to a temperature of 33°C maintained for 48 hours, in conjunction with early decompression and maintenance of mean arterial pressures >90 mm Hg, resulted in a 42.7% improvement in neurologic outcomes as compared to age- and injury-matched controls.[50] The safety demonstrated in this initial phase 1 trial, with apparent associated improvements in neurologic outcome may justify the pursuit of further phase 2 and 3 clinical trials.

Nonoperative Management of Spine Injuries. No definitive treatment algorithm has been universally accepted for the determination of whether a spinal injury should be treated operatively or nonoperatively. The surgeon must examine the injury in relation to neurologic impairment and structural integrity of both the osseous and the ligamentous components. One difficulty in treating spinal fractures is that the definition of instability is ambiguous because of the large spectrum of spinal disorders. The goal of treatment is neurologic recovery, prevention of neurologic decline and spinal deformity, and maximizing pain relief.

For most acute spine injuries, this can be accomplished nonoperatively, which usually consists of external immobilization. As most bony injuries have potential to heal with immobilization, nonsurgical management is often an acceptable definitive treatment for stable injuries without neurologic deficit. Major ligamentous injury, on the other hand, often requires surgery.

Cervical traction is often an initial treatment modality used to reduce spinal deformities, decompress neural elements, and provide cervical spine stability. Traction can be done using a head halter, tongs, or a halo ring. Cervical traction can begin with an initial weight of 10-15 pounds, which should be immediately evaluated with lateral radiographs. The traction weight is then incrementally increased by 5-10 pounds with lateral radiographs obtained 10-15 minutes after each incremental weight increase. Analgesia and muscle relaxants are often required to relieve muscle spasm. The maximum amount of weight that should be used is controversial; Crutchfield recommended a maximum of 5 pounds per level of cervical injury, in addition to 10 pounds for the head.[51]

Spinal orthoses are external braces that can restrict spinal motion and are a mainstay of nonoperative treatment of spinal trauma. Bracing of the cervical spine and thoracolumbar spine is challenging due to the considerable amount of normal movement. The inherent rigidity of the thoracic spine makes this region more amenable to bracing.

Conservative management of cervical injuries is usually achieved with rigid immobilization of the cervical spine with either rigid cervical collars, such as the Aspen collar or Miami J collar, and cervicothoracic orthoses, or with halo vests. Cervical collars provide good sagittal motion restriction in the upper cervical and subaxial spine. However, they are easy to remove and have variable rates of user adherence. Halo vests provide good upper cervical and subaxial sagittal motion restriction. They also provide superior axial plane motion restriction compared to cervical collars. In addition, halo vests are secured to the skull and cannot be easily removed by users. Halo vests are associated with a higher morbidity and mortality rate, especially for elderly patients. For these reasons, halo vest use in the aging population, while sometimes unavoidable, should be approached with caution.

Adequate stabilization of the thoracolumbar and lumbar spine often requires extension of the brace to include as much as four or five levels proximal and distal to the unstable segment. Available thoracolumbar and lumbar orthoses include lumbosacral corsets, Jewett braces, and full-contact, custom-molded orthoses.

Surgical Management of Spinal Injuries. Unstable injuries, with or without neurologic deficit, requires surgical treatment. The goals of surgery include reduction of spinal deformity, restoration of stability, and decompression of neural elements. With modern-day techniques and technologies, spine surgeons can now approach the spine from nearly any direction: anterior, direct lateral, posterolateral, posterior, or any combination of these approaches. Posterior reduction and stabilization is the most frequently utilized approach for thoracolumbar spine fractures. The injury type and the time to surgical intervention determine the most appropriate approach.

The optimal timing of surgery following spinal injury is controversial. Progressive neurologic deterioration and unstable fractures with incomplete or no neurologic deficit are indications for immediate surgery. Early stabilization and mobilization of spinal patients has reduced the incidence of complications such as acute respiratory distress syndrome and deep venous thrombosis.[52]

PENETRATING SPINE TRAUMA

Thirteen percent of all spinal column are a result of gunshot wounds, the third most common mechanism of injury following motor vehicle crashes and falls. However, gunshot wounds are responsible for 25% of injuries to the spinal cord, second only to motor vehicle crashes.[53] Gunshot wounds can be devastating injures due to the high kinetic energy of the missile, and the cavitation that the missile creates during its passage through tissue. Neurologic injury results not only from the immediate trajectory of the bullet but also the concussive effects of the bullet's cavitating effects.[54]

The evaluation of any gunshot wound victim requires attention to the tenets of ATLS.[5] After stabilization and resuscitation, a detailed neurologic examination should be performed to determine the neurologic status of the patient as defined by ASIA Scale (Fig. 24.12). Concomitant injuries should be considered, particularly those of a vascular nature. Evaluation of the spine can be performed with either plain films or CT scan, or both depending on local practice paradigms. MRI is contraindicated due to the artifacts created by the missile fragment as well as their ferromagnetism.[55] Although most gunshot injuries to the spine are considered inherently stable, recent literature suggests that this may not be true, particularly for injuries to the cervical spine.[56] Postinjury administration of either steroids or prophylactic antibiotics is controversial, but neither is likely indicated, although consideration should be given to the administration of antibiotics in those patients in whom the bullet penetrates the gastrointestinal tract prior to injuring the spine.[57] Spinal cord decompression for neurologic deficit may be indicated only in the face of progressive neurologic deterioration, and is often complicated by an increased incidence of infection and cerebral spinal fluid fistula.[58]

COMPLICATIONS FOLLOWING SPINAL CORD INJURY

In discussing complications associated with spinal cord injury, it is important to differentiate between those that are related to the management of the injury and those that are systemic in nature. Acute complications, defined as those occurring within the initial hospitalization, range from hemodynamic instability to infections including pneumonia, urinary tract infections, and sepsis, as well as thromboembolic phenomenon. Many of these complications require preventive and/or prophylactic measures in order to reduce their occurrence in both the inpatient and outpatient settings.

Complications of spinal cord therapy have also been frequently reported. Most complications are a result of failure to achieve and maintain adequate reduction due to either poor bone quality or failures of instrumentation. Postoperative wound infections are also common after spinal surgery with a risk ranging between 1% and 6%. However, the most devastating complication is neurologic progression of the injury. This may be caused by several factors including direct neural injury during surgical repair or the development of a postoperative expanding epidural hematoma. Finally, cerebral spinal fluid leakage may complicate spine trauma surgery. This can be caused either by the initial injury or by iatrogenic laceration of the dura. Any injury identified intraoperatively should be repaired at the time of surgery. If the CSF leakage is identified postoperatively, treatment options include reoperation and repair, recumbency, and lumbar drains.

Systemic complications are also common after spinal cord injury. Pulmonary complications represent a significant cause of morbidity and mortality in both the acute and chronic setting. The majority of patients with high cervical spine injury will require prolonged mechanical ventilation and often necessitate tracheostomy. This is due to a lack of function of the ipsilateral phrenic nerve. Injuries of the lower cervical spine and upper thoracic spine similarly may cause respiratory failure due to a lack of innervation of the intercostal musculature, resulting in reduced lung volumes, intrapulmonary shunting, and decreased oxygen saturation.[59] The excessive use of analgesia and sedation can further depress respiratory function. In order to decrease the incidence of respiratory failure and subsequent pneumonia, early aggressive pulmonary toilet regimes should be implemented. Additionally early mobilization, if possible, serves to improve overall pulmonary function.

Another common systemic complication after spinal cord injury is venous thromboembolic phenomenon including deep venous thrombosis and pulmonary embolism. In the immediate postinjury population, there is a 500-fold increase in the risk of dying from a pulmonary embolism in the first month following injury when compared to both age and gender match controls.[60] Although this risk of venous thrombolic disease declines proportionally from time of injury, those with complete injury have a perpetually elevated risk due to immobility. For this reason, prophylaxis for at least 3 months following injury has been suggested as a standard of care in spinal cord injury patients.[61] The use of prophylactic regimens has been shown to reduce the risk of DVT following spinal cord injury. In the event that patients have contraindication to anticoagulation, inferior vena cava filters are recommended.

Spinal cord injury results in genitourinary complications. Alterations in detrusor motor functions and bladder sensation as well as compromised sphincter activity all play a role in incomplete bladder emptying. This results in the development of infection and elevated bladder pressures and contributes to the development of bladder and renal calculi. In order to limit these complications, a strict bladder regimen is recommended. While Foley catheters are recommended during the intensive care unit course, intermittent clean catheterization is recommended every 4-6 hours with the goal of maintaining bladder volumes of <500 mL. Prophylactic antibiotics are not recommended. However, any suspected urinary tract infection should be treated.

As with all critically injured patients, stress ulcer prophylaxis to prevent the development of gastrointestinal hemorrhage is recommended. Standard prophylaxis with histamine-2 (H2) blockers or proton pump inhibitors (PPI) until gastric feeds have been initiated remains the standard of care. In the event that patients are fed directly into the small bowel, it is recommended that gastric prophylaxis with either an H2 blocker or a PPI continue. Development of an adynamic ileus is also common. Patients often require aggressive bowel regime including a combination of stool softeners, a high-fiber diet, intermittent digital stimulations, suppositories, and intermittent disimpaction.

In areas of bony prominence, in the setting of neurologic injury, the development of pressure ulcers is a major source of discomfort and a potential route of significant morbidity and mortality due to infection-related complications. The incidence of ulcerations requiring surgical debridement within two years of spinal cord injury is approximately 4%.[62] Early mobilization, protective devices including specialized mattresses, and frequent skin inspection are preventive measures for the development of decubiti.

Mortality following spinal cord injury can be divided into the acute and chronic phases. Despite advances in medical management, approximately 10%-20% of acute spinal cord injuries do not survive their initial hospitalization.[60] For those who do survive their acute hospitalization, the major cause of mortality is infection, often pulmonary in nature. Suicide is also a frequent cause of death in paraplegics, with higher rates in patients under the age of 25 at the time of injury. Spinal cord injury lowers patients' life expectancy with the average patient surviving only 30-40 years, depending on the level of injury.[63]

Novel Therapies for Spinal Cord Injury. Current strategies to restore motor functions after spinal cord injury include prevention of secondary damage, promotion of axonal regeneration, replacement of lost cells, training of central patterns generators (CPGs), and reduction in spasticity. Secondary lesional processes induce further death of neurons and myelinating oligodendrocytes.[64] Neurotropic/growth factors like brain-derived neurotrophic factor or neurotrophin-3 have neuroprotective properties and can limit secondary damage.[80] Riluzole, which reduces glutamatergic neurotoxicity, markedly enhances the survival of injured motor neurons, even after treatment delays.[65]

After incomplete lesions, progressive partial restoration of motor control can occur due to axonal sprouting.[66] The glial scar at the lesion site forms a physical barrier for regenerating axons, producing chondroitin sulfate proteoglycans that further inhibit axonal growth. Administration of chondroitinase ABC can promote plasticity and long-distance axonal regeneration of injured fibers, improving functional recovery after partial spinal cord injury in primates.[67] Elevation of intracellular levels of cAMP in adult neurons, by means of db-cAMP and/or rolipram, is neuroprotective, promotes axonal regeneration, and improves functional recovery.[68] Finally, some endogenous metalloproteinases seem to promote angiogenesis, neuroprotection, neurogenesis, and remyelination.[69]

The previously described strategies work only when the two ends of the spinal cord remain in proximity with one another. For larger defects, the gap may be bridged using peripheral nerve segments, or Schwann cell transplants, which can also facilitate remyelination of injured axons.[70] Cell replacement strategies also exist. Transplantation of human spinal cord stem cells into the rat spinal cord after injury following directed differentiation to oligodendrocyte lineage prior to transplantation increases remyelination.[71] Adult autologous bone marrow stromal cells, transdifferentiated prior to transplant, will migrate to the site of spinal cord injury after systemic injection, and promote axonal regeneration.[72]

Stimulation of the neuronal network responsible for the rhythmic movements underlying locomotion (the central pattern generator) with pharmacologic or electrical stimulation and locomotor training has shown promise. Serotonin pathways have shown particular promise in this area and may be capable of reactivating the CPG.[73] Training, using manually assisted stepping by therapists or robotic devices, is also effective in humans with clinically complete spinal cold injury, resulting in increased electromyography (EMG) activity in the ankle extensor muscles and increased weight-bearing function.[14] Restoration of postural control is also extremely important for recovery of locomotor function after spinal cord injury. Postural corrective movements are typically absent when the ventral cord is injured, but recover within 2 weeks if the dorsal cord is injured. Tilt table training, with or without the intrathecal administration of serotonin at the lumbar level, increases correctly phased EMG responses.[74]

Combinations of the above strategies have resulted in clinical improvement in spinal cord–injured patients. There is at least one report in the literature documenting improvements from an ASIA A to an ASIA D classification, resulting in the ability of patients with spinal cord injury to stand up and walk with varying degrees of effectiveness.[75]

References

1. Committee on Trauma, American College of Surgeons, National Trauma Data Bank Annual Report 2009, http://www.facs.org/trauma/ntdb/docpub.html, Accessed December 14, 2009.
2. Foundation for spinal cord injury prevention, care and cure, Spinal Cord Injury Statistics, updated June 2009, http://www.fscip.org/fact.htm, Accessed December 14, 2009.
3. Lowery DW, Wald MM, Browne BJ, et al. Epidemiology of cervical spine injury victims. *Ann Emerg Med.* 2001;38:12.
4. Holmes J, Miller P, Panacek E, et al. Epidemiology of thoracolumbar spine injury in blunt trauma. *Acad Emerg Med.* 2001;8:866.
5. American College of Surgeons. *Advanced Trauma Life Support.* 8th ed.; 2008.
6. Cervical spine immobilization before admission to the hospital. *Neurosurgery.* 2002;50(3 suppl):S7-S17.
7. Denis F. The three-column spine and its significance in the classification of acute thoracolumbar spinal injuries. *Spine.* 1984;8:817.
8. White AA, Johnson RM, Panjabi MM, et al. Biomechanical analysis of clinical instability in the cervical spine. *Clin Orthop Relat Res.* 1975;109:85.
9. Punjabi MM, Oxland TR, Kifune M, et al. Validity of the three column theory of thoracolumbar fractures: a biomechanical investigation. *Spine.* 1995;15:1122.
10. Anderson PA, Montesano PX. Morphology and treatment of occipital condyle fractures. *Spine.* 1988;13:731-736.
11. Landells CD, Van Peteghem PK. Fractures of the atlas: classification, treatment and morbidity. *Spine.* 1988;13:450-452.
12. Schoenfeld AJ, Bono CM, McGuire KJ, et al. Computed tomography alone versus computed tomography and magnetic resonance imaging in the identification of occult injuries to the cervical spine: a meta-analysis. *J Trauma.* 2010;68:109-114.
13. Anderson LD, D'Alonzo RT. Fractures of the odontoid process of the axis. *J Bone Joint Surg Am.* 1974;56:1663-1674.
14. Edgerton VR, Roy RR. Robotic training and spinal cord plasticity. *Brain Res Bull.* 2009;78:4-12.
15. Levine AM, Edwards CC. The management of traumatic spondylolisthesis of the axis. *J Bone Joint Surg Am.* 1985;67:217-226.
16. Anderson DK, Hall ED. Pathophysiology of spinal cord trauma. *Ann Emerg Med.* 1993;22:987.
17. Hall ED, Springer JE. Neuroprotection and acute spinal cord injury: a reappraisal. *NeuroRx.* 2004;1:80.
18. Panter SC, Yum SW, Faden AI. Alteration in extracellular amino acids after traumatic spinal cord injury. *Ann Neurol.* 1990;27:96.
19. Young W, Koren I. Potassium and calcium changes in injures spinal cords. *Brain Res.* 1986;365:42.
20. Geisler FH. GM-1 ganglioside and motor recovery following human spinal cord injury. *J Emerg Med.* 1993;11:49-55.

21. Management of acute spinal cord injuries in the intensive care unit or other monitored setting, *Neurosurgery*. 2002;50:S51-S57.
22. Frankel HL, Hancock DO, Hyslop G, et al. The value of postural reduction in the initial management of closed injuries of the spine with paraplegia and tetraplegia. *Paraplegia*. 1969;7:179-192.
23. Bosch A, Stauffer ES, Nickel VL. Incomplete traumatic quadriplegia: a ten year review. *JAMA*. 1971;216:473.
24. Stauffer ES. Neurologic recovery following injuries to the cervical spinal cord and nerve roots. *Spine*. 1984;9:532.
25. Little JN, Halar E. Temporal course of motor recovery after Brown-Sequard spinal cord injuries. *Paraplegia*. 1985;23:39.
26. Como JJ, Diaz JJ, Dunham CM, et al. Practice management guidelines for identification of cervical spine injuries following trauma: update from the Eastern Association for the Surgery of Trauma Practice Management Guidelines Committee. *J Trauma*. 2009;67:651-659.
27. Medzon R, Rothenhaus T, Bono CM, et al. Stability of cervical spine fractures after gunshot wounds to the head and neck. *Spine*. 2005;30(20):2274-2279.
28. Howes MC, Pearce AP. State of play: clearing the thoracolumbar spine in blunt trauma victims. *Emerg Med Australas*. 2006;18:471-477.
29. Inaba K, Munera F, McKenney M. Visceral torso computed tomography for clearance of the thoracolumbar spine in trauma: a review of the literature. *J Trauma*. 2006;60:915-920.
30. Amar AP, Levy MP. Pathogenesis and pharmacological strategies for mitigating secondary damage in acute spinal cord injury. *Neurosurgery*. 1999;44:1027-1039.
31. Bracken MB, Holford TR. Effects of timing of methylprednisolone or naloxone administration on recovery of segmental and long-tract neurological function in NASCIS-2. *J Neurosurg*. 1993;79:500-507.
32. Bracken MB, Shepard MJ, Collins WF, et al. Methylprednisolone or naloxone treatment after acute spinal cord injury: results of Second National Spinal Cord Injury Study. *N Engl J Med*. 1990;322:1405-1411.
33. Bracken MB, Shepard MJ, Collins WF, et al. Methylprednisolone or naloxone treatment after acute spinal cord injury: 1-year follow-up. Results of the Second National Acute Spinal Cord Injury Study. *J Neurosurg*. 1992;76:23-31.
34. Bracken MB, Shepard MJ, Collins WF, et al. Methylprednisolone or naloxone treatment after acute spinal cord injury: 1-year follow-up. Results of the Second National Acute Spinal Cord Injury Study. *J Neurosurg*. 1992;76:23-31.
35. Bracken MB, Shepard MJ, Holford TR, et al. Administration of methylprednisolone for 24 or 48 hours or tirilazade mesylate for 48 hours in the treatment of acute spinal cord injury. Results of the Second National Acute Spinal Cord Injury Trial. National Acute Spinal Cord Injury Study. *JAMA*. 1997;277:1597-1604.
36. Bracken MB, Shepard MJ, Holford TR, et al., Methylprednisolone or tirilazade mesylate administration after acute spinal cord injury: 1-year follow-up data: results of the third National Acute Spinal Cord Injury randomized controlled trial. *J Neurosurg*. 1998;89:699-706.
37. Pointillart V, Petitjean ME, Wart L, et al. Pharmacological therapy of spinal cord injury during the acute phase. *Spinal Cord*. 2000;39:71-76.
38. Coleman WP, Benzel D, Cahill DW, et al. A critical appraisal of the reporting of the National Acute Spinal Cord Injuries Studies (II and II) of methylprednisolone in acute spinal cord injury. *J Spinal Disord*. 2000;13:185-199.
39. Hurlbert RJ. Methylprednisolone for acute spinal cord injury: an inappropriate standard of care. *J Neurosurg*. 2000;93:1-7.
40. Galandiuk S, Raque G, Appel S, et al. The two-edged sword of large-dose steroids for spinal cold trauma. *Ann Surg*. 1993;218:419-425; discussion 425-427.
41. Gerndt SJ, Rodriguez JL, Pawlik JW, et al. Consequences of high-dose steroid therapy for acute spinal cord injury. *J Trauma*. 1997;42:279-284.
42. Hadley MN, Walters BC, Grabb PA, et al. Guidelines for the management of acute cervical spine and spinal cord injuries. *Clin Neurosurg*. 2002;93:175-179.
43. Geisler FH, Dorsey FC, Coleman WP. Past and current clinical studies with GM-1 ganglioside in acute spinal cord injury, *Ann Emerg Med*. 1993;22:1041-1047.
44. Olsson Y, Sharma HS, Nyberg F, et al. The opioid receptor antagonist naloxone influences the pathophysiology of spinal cord injury, *Prog Brain Res*. 1995;104:381-399.
45. Zeidman SM, Ling GS, Ducker TB, et al. Clinical applications of pharmacologic therapies for spinal cord injury: past and current clinical studies with GM-1 ganglioside in acute spinal cord injury. *J Spinal Disord*.1996;9:367-380.
46. Geisler FH, Dorsey FC, Coleman WP. Recovery of motor function after spinal cord injury: a randomized, placebo-controlled trial with GM-1 ganglioside. *N Engl J Med*. 1991;324:1829-1839.
47. Clark WM, Hazel JS, Coull BM. Lazaroids: CNS pharmacology and current research. *Drugs*. 1995;50:971-983.
48. Petitjean ME, Pointillart V, Dixmerias F et al. Traitement medicamenteux de la lesion medullaire traumatique au stade aigu. *Ann Fr Anesth Reanim*. 1998;17:114-122.
49. Cappuccino A, Bisson LJ, Carpenter B, et al. The use of systemic hypothermia for the treatment of an acute cervical spinal cord injury in a professional football player. *Spine*. 2010;35:E57-E62.
50. Levi AD, Casella G, Green BA, et al. Clinical outcomes using modest intravascular hypothermia after acute cervical spinal cord injury. *Neurosurgery*. 2010;66:670-677.
51. Crutchfield WG. Skeletal traction in treatment of injuries to the skeletal spine. *JAMA*. 1954;1:29.
52. Brazinski M, Yoo JU. Review of pulmonary complications associated with early versus late stabilization of thoracic and lumbar fractures. Proceedings of the 12th Annual Meeting of the Orthopedic Trauma Association, 1996.
53. Yoshida GM, Garland D, Waters RL. Gunshot wounds to the spine. *Orthop Clin North Am*. 1995l;26:109.
54. Demuth WE. Bullet velocity as applied to military rifle wounding capacity. *J Trauma*. 1969;9:27.
55. Teitelbaum GP, Yee CA, Van Horn DD, et al. Metallic ballistic fragments: MR imaging safety and artifacts. *Radiology*. 1990;175:855.
56. Isiklar ZU, Lindsey RW. Low velocity civilian gunshot wounds of the spine. *Orthopedics*. 1997;20:967.
57. Roffl RP, Waters RL, Adkins RH. Gunshot wounds to the spine associated with a perforated viscus. *Spine*. 1989;14:808.
58. Stauffer ES, Wood RW, Kelly EG. Gunshot wounds of the spine: the effects of laminectomy. *J Bone Joint Surg*. 1979;61A:389.
59. Ledsom JR, Sharp JM. Pulmonary function in acute cervical cord injury, *Am Rev Respir Dis*. 1981;124:41-44.
60. DeVivo MJ, Kartus PL, Stover SL, et al. Cause of death for patients with spinal cord injury. *Arch Intern Med*. 1989;149:1761-1766.
61. Deep venous thrombosis and thromboembolism in patients with cervical spinal cord injuries. Neurosurgery. 2002;50:S73-S80.
62. Rimoldi, RL, Zigler JE. Immediate post operative care. In: Levine AM, Garfin SR, Eismont FJ, et al., eds. *Spine Trauma*. Philadelphia, PA: WB Saunders; 1998:562-566.
63. Tasjian VS, Gonzalez NR, Khoolt LT. Spine: spinal cord injury blunt and penetrating, neurogenic and spinal shock. In: Ascensio JA, Trunkey DD, eds. *Current Therapy of Trauma in Surgical Critical Care*. Philadelphia, PA: Saunders/Elsevier; 2009160-173.
64. Kwon BK, Tetzlaff W, Grauer JN, et al. Pathophysiology and pharmacologic treatment of acute spinal cord injury. *Spine J*. 2004;4:451-464.
65. Hawryluk GW, Rowland J, Kwon BK, et al. Protection and repair of the injured spinal cord: a review of completed, ongoing and planned clinical trials for acute spinal cord injury. *Neurosurg Focus*. 2008;25:E14
66. Weidner N, Ner A, Salimi H, et al. Spontaneous corticospinal axonal plasticity and functional recovery after adult central nervous system injury. *Proc Natl Acad Sci U S A*. 2001;98:3513-3518.
67. Kwok JC, Afshari F, Garcia-Alias F, et al. Proteoglycans in the central nervous system: plasticity, regeneration and their stimulation with chondroitinase ABC. *Restor Neurol Neurosci*. 2008;26:131-145.
68. Hannila SS, Filbin MT. The role of cyclic AMP signaling in promoting axonal regeneration after spinal cord injury. *Exp Neurol*. 2008;209:321-332.
69. Hsu JY, MeKeon R, Goussev S, et al. Matrix metalloproteinase-2 facilitates wound healing events that promote functional recovery after spinal cord injury. *J Neurosci*. 2006;26:9841-9850.
70. Pearse DD, Sanchez AR, Pereira FC, et al. Transplantation of Schwann cells and/or olfactory ensheathing glia into the contused spinal cord: survival, migration, axon association and functional recovery. *Glia*. 2007;55:976-1000.
71. Keirstead HS, Nistor G, Bernal G, et al. Human embryonic stem cell-derived oligodendrocyte progenitor cell transplants remyelinate and restore locomotion after spinal cord injury. *J Neurosci*. 2005;25:4694-4705.
72. Sykova E, Jendelova P. Migration, fate and *in vivo* imaging of adult stem cells in the CNS. *Cell Death Differ*. 2007;14:1336-1342
73. Landry ES, Lapointe NP, Rouillard C, et al. Contribution of spinal 5-HT1A and 5-HT7 receptors to locomotor-like movement induced by 8-OH-DPAT in spinal cord-transected mice. *Eur J Neurosci*. 2006:24:535-546
74. Lyalka VF, Musienko PE, Orlovsky GN, et al. Effect of intrathecal administration of serotoninergic and noradrenergic drugs on postural performance in rabbits with spinal cord lesions. *J Neurophysiol*. 2008;100:723-732
75. Moviglia FA, Varela G, Brizuela JA, et al. Case report on the clinical results of a combined cellular therapy for chronic spinal cord injured patients. *Spinal Cord*. 2009;47:499-503
76. Effendi B, Roy D, Cornish B, et al. Fractures of the ring of the axis. A classification based on the analysis of 131 cases. *J Bone Joint Surg Br*. 1981;63:319-327.
77. Geisler FH. Clinical trials of pharmacotherapy for spinal cord injury. *Ann N Y Acad Sci*. 1998;845:374-381.
78. Geisler FH: GM-1 ganglioside and motor recovery following human spinal cord injury. *J Emerg Med*. 1993;11:49.
79. Spence KF Jr, Decker S, Sell KW. Bursting atlantal fracture associated with rupture of the transverse ligament. *J Bone Joint Surg Am*. 1970;52:543-549.
80. Tobias CA, Shumsky JA, Shibata M, et al. Delayed grafting of BDNF and NT-3 producing fibroblasts into the injured spinal cord stimulates sprouting, partially rescues axotomized red nucleus neurons from loss and atrophy, and provides limited regeneration. *Exp Neurol*. 2003;184:97-113

CHAPTER 25 ■ OPHTHALMIC INJURY

FRANCIS L. COUNSELMAN AND SHANNON M. McCOLE

Hippocrates was the first person to record the association between facial trauma and blindness.[1] Trauma is responsible for bilateral blindness in more than one million people worldwide; unilateral blinding injuries have an estimated incidence of 500,000 cases each year.[2] It is estimated that ocular trauma represents 3% of all emergency department visits in the United States.[3] In the United States alone, there are approximately 900,000 cases of occupation-related eye injury each year.[4] The majority of patients are male (75%–83%) and young (median age of 27–31-years old)[5–7] The most common cause of orbital fractures is motor vehicle accidents and assaults. Sports-related injury, especially basketball and baseball, is also a common cause of ocular trauma.[8] While many eye injuries are minor in nature, some require urgent evaluation and management and even immediate surgical intervention to preserve sight (Table 25.1).

HISTORY

A thorough history should be obtained, including the timing and specific events surrounding the injury. A history of grinding or hammering raises the risk for the presence of a foreign body. Important questions regarding ocular history include past visual acuity, need for corrective glasses or contact lenses, and history of glaucoma or cataracts. Specifically inquire about visual symptoms, including change in vision, floaters, flashing lights, pain, discharge, or diplopia.[3] Previous ophthalmic surgery (i.e., radial keratotomy and lens implant) may make the eye more susceptible to injury. A past medical history of hematologic disorders (i.e., sickle-cell disease or trait), coagulopathy or use of anticoagulation medications (i.e., warfarin and enoxaparin) increases the risk of bleeding complications, especially in hyphema and retrobulbar hemorrhage. Tetanus immunization status and medication allergies should be elicited.

PHYSICAL EXAMINATION

External Exam and Motility Exam

A general observation should be made for overt abnormalities or defects of the periorbital region and lids. Any evidence of enophthalmos (one eye appearing further back than the other) or proptosis (one eye more anterior than the other) should be noted, as this may indicate damage to the bony orbits. Eyelid position and function, along with any evidence of damage such as lacerations, contusions, or edema should be noted. Pay special attention to any injury that may involve the canalicular region (medially). An observation of the entire ocular surface can be performed by holding the lids open while asking the patient to look up, down, left, and right. The bony structures should be palpated to help identify fractures. Examine for any sign of hemorrhage or foreign body on the surface of the globe. Do not place pressure on the globe if a perforating injury is suspected (see Fig. 25.1).

Assess extraocular movements by having the patient look in all eight cardinal positions, noting eye alignment and smoothness of pursuit, while asking the patient to report any diplopia or pain. Abnormalities may be indicative of muscle entrapment or orbital hemorrhage, which may require urgent intervention.

Visual Acuity

The traditional way to test visual acuity is to have the patient read the Snellen chart at 20 feet. Each eye should be tested individually and then together. If eye pain is present, placing a drop or two of topical ophthalmic anesthetic can greatly facilitate obtaining an accurate visual acuity. See Table 25.2 for the list of medications. Each eye is then assigned a two-digit score (i.e., 20/50).[9] The first number is the distance between the patient and the chart; the second number refers to the smallest line the patient is able to read. If the patient wears corrective lenses, they should be allowed to use them (but document it). For patients who do not have their corrective lenses or their vision is altered, visual acuity should be tested using a pinhole. A pinhole corrects for most refractive errors by ensuring that only light striking the lens perpendicularly reaches the retina.[10] If the visual acuity corrects with a pinhole, the problem is likely due to refractive error. If it does not correct, the problem is usually more serious.[10]

For patients who cannot read English, a tumbling E chart may be used, in which the patient identifies the orientation of the letter E (i.e., facing right, facing up).[9] For patients confined to the supine position, a near-vision card can be used, held 14 inches from the patient's face.[9] For patients who cannot read the Snellen chart or near-vision card, the patient should be asked to count the examiner's fingers at a distance of 2 feet. If the patient is unable to count fingers, assess the patient's ability to detect hand motion from a distance of 1–2 feet. Finally, if unable to detect hand motion, test for light perception. Turn off all lights in the room, completely cover the eye, and test for light perception.[9,11] If the patient is unable to detect light, then that eye is considered completely blind.

Pupils

First, perform a general observation of the pupils in ambient room light, noting the shape and size of each pupil while having the patient focus on a distant target. With room lights dim, re-examine the pupils using as little light as possible, noting: shape, size, symmetry, and direct and consensual reaction to light. A relative afferent pupillary defect (RAPD) can be assessed with a rapid swinging light technique while observing the pupils. If the lids are swollen, it may be necessary to have an assistant gently hold the lids open to assist in the examination. A RAPD indicates damage to the anterior visual pathways (optic nerve or retina).

Slit Lamp Examination

The slit lamp is a three-part machine, consisting of a table-mounted binocular microscope with an attached special adjustable light source and a patient headrest.[12] Magnification can be adjusted from 6× to 16×. For the examination,

TABLE 25.1

EMERGENT AND URGENT OPHTHALMOLOGIC INJURIES

Ophthalmic conditions requiring immediate surgical intervention
Corneal laceration
Suspected open globe
Intraocular foreign body
Conditions requiring urgent evaluation and treatment
Chemical burn
Hyphema
Retrobulbar hemmorrhage
Sudden decreased vision

the patient is seated, and the chin is placed on a padded rest with the forehead pressed firmly against the forehead bar. The chin rest should be adjusted, so that the patient's eyes rest at the level of the marker on the vertical poles of the slit lamp.[10] The height of the slit lamp is adjusted, so that the light beam is centered on the patient's eyes. The light source has several adjustments, which allow the beam to be varied from a narrow slit to a wide beam, from short to long, and from dim to bright.[12] Most slit lamps allow for changing the filter on the beam, from neutral to cobalt blue (for evaluation of flourescein staining) and red free.[10]

The examiner should adjust the diopter rings on the ocular piece to account for their individual refractive error and accomodation.[10] It is the examiner's choice to wear their corrective lenses. The patient should be asked to focus on a fixed object (i.e., examiner's ear). The light beam should be at 45 degree from the patient–clinician axis, using a low-voltage, wide beam. Using the lowest magnification level, the joystick is used to move the device on the chassis until focused.[10] Once the eye is in focus, the examiner should conduct a systematic examination of the individual structures. Typically, start with the most external structures (i.e., eyelids and eyelashes) and work deeper, culminating in examination of the anterior chamber (looking for blood, cells, flare, etc.). Magnification can be modified as needed.

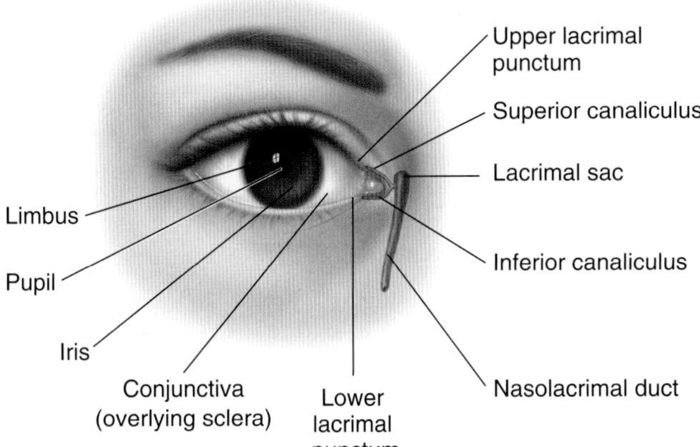

FIGURE 25.1. Ocular anatomy as seen when examining a patient.

TABLE 25.2

COMMONLY USED MEDICATION IN OPHTHALMOLOGY

I. Topical local anesthetics/white caps
- 1. Proparacaine 0.5% solution
  - One drop; rapid onset; 10–20-min duration
- 2. Tetracaine 0.5%
  - One drop; rapid onset

II. Mydriatic and cycloplegic agents (for dilation)/red caps
- 1. Phenylephrine 2.5% and 10%
  - One drop; max effect 20 min; 3-h duration
- 2. Tropicamide 0.5% and 1%
  - One drop; max effect 20–30 min; 3–6-h duration
- 3. Homatropine 2% and 5%
  - one drop; max effect 20–90 min; 2–3-d duration
- 4. Atropine 0.5%, 1%, and 2%
  - One drop; max effect 30–40 min; 1–2-wk duration

III. Antibacterial agents/tan cap
- A. Sulfonamides
  - 1. Sulfacetamide 1%, 10%, and 30%; ointment 10%
    - Dose q3–4 h
- B. Fluoroquinolones
  - 1. Ciprofloxacin 0.3%; ointment 0.3%
    - Dose at least QID
  - 2. Ofloxacin 0.3%
  - 3. Levofloxacin 0.5%
  - 4. Gatifloxacin 0.3%
  - 5. Moxifloxacin 0.5%
    - Dose up to 6/d
- C. Aminoglycoides (for pseudomonas)
  - 1. Tobramycin 0.3%
  - 2. Gentamicin 0.3%
- D. Others
  - 1. Erythromycin 0.5%
  - 2. Polymyxin B/trimethoprim
    - Dose up to 6/d

IV. Nonsteroidal anti-inflammatory agents
- 1. Diclofenac 0.1%
  - Dose QID
- 2. Ketorolac 0.5%
  - Dose QID

V. Treatment for increased IOP
- A. Alpha agonists
  - 1. Apraclonidine 0.5% and 1%
    - Dose TID
  - 2. Brimonidine tartrate 0.15%
    - Dose TID
- B. Beta-adrenegic antagonists
  - 1. Timolol maleate 0.25% and 0.5%
    - Dose BID
  - 2. Timolol hemihydrate 0.25% and 0.5%
    - Dose BID
  - 3. Betaxolol 0.5%
    - Dose BID
- C. Miotics/green tops
  - 1. Physostigmine 0.25% and 0.5%
  - 2. Pilocarpine hydrochloride 0.25%

VI. Corticosteroids
- 1. Prednisolone acetate 0.12%, 0.125%, or 1%

Adapted from Ehlers JP, Shah CP, Fenton GL, et al. *The Wills Eye Manual: Office and Emergency Room Diagnosis and Treatment of Eye Disease.* 5th ed. Philadelphia, PA: Lippincott Williams & Wilkins; 2008 with permission

Flourescein Staining

Flourescein staining should be performed in all patients with ocular trauma. The only absolute contraindication is flourescein allergy.[10] To do this, the eye should be anesthetized first, and then a few drops of sterile saline placed in the eye to moisten it. The fluorescein strip is then placed on the conjunctiva of the eye, and the patient is asked to blink several times to distribute the dye in a thin film over the entire eye.[10] The lights should be turned low/off, and the eye examined with a cobalt blue light (i.e., hand-held, Wood's lamp, or using the slit-lamp). Injured epithelium (i.e., abrasion) will appear yellow green. The location of the abrasion should be documented, normally using the clock method (i.e., 3-mm linear abrasion at 7 O'clock). A variation of this, called the Seidel test, can be performed when a full thickness corneal disruption or open-globe injury is suspected. For this test, a large amount of flourescein dye is placed on the eye, causing the entire eye to appear orange. Then, with the lights out, the globe is examined for a dark stream interrupting the flourescein, indicating leakage of aqueous humor and a globe rupture.[10]

For this to be best observed, the patient needs to be in an upright (i.e., seated) position (see Fig. 25.2).

Tonometry

Tonometry is the measurement of intraocular pressure (IOP). Normal IOP is between 10 and 20 mm Hg. The most common condition for low IOP in the setting of trauma is perforating globe injury with loss of aqueous fluid. However, if a perforated globe is suspected, tonometry should not be performed because of the possibility of causing further extrusion of intraocular contents. High IOP (i.e., >30 mm Hg) in the setting of orbital trauma is commonly observed in hyphema, anterior lens dislocation, or retrobulbar hemorrhage. A baseline IOP should be measured in all patients with blunt orbital trauma, except in the case of suspected globe rupture or perforating globe injury.

The most common tools used for performing tonometry are a portable hand-held device (i.e., Tonopen) or the older Schiotz tonometer. The hand-held device is digital, has good interexaminer reliability, and can be used with the patient in any position. The Schiotz tonometer requires the patient to be in the supine position. Both methods determine IOP by measuring the amount of corneal indentation produced by a certain amount of force. Both methods also require the eye to be anesthetized and the patient cooperative. It is best to repeat measurements several times in order to obtain a reliable reading.

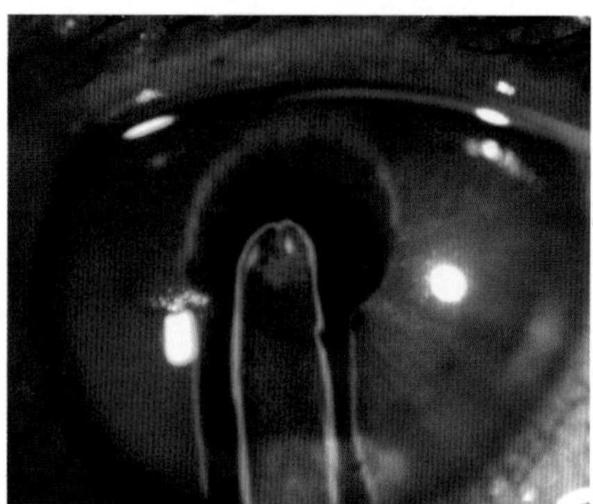

FIGURE 25.2. A positive Seidel test in a patient with a full-thickness corneal laceration. Note the downward streaming of aqueous humor. (Reprinted with permission from Ehlers JP, Shah CP, Fenton GL, et al. *The Wills Eye Manual: Office and Emergency Room Diagnosis and Treatment of Eye Disease.* 5th ed. Philadelphia, PA: Lippincot Williams & Wilkins; 2008.)

Direct Fundoscopic Exam

The direct ophthalmoscope allows a fundoscopic examination with approximately 15× magnification. Since the examiner performs the exam using only one eye, the view is not stereoscopic. Although a view may be obtained through a small pupil, pharmacologic dilation will enhance the view. The instrument field of view is limited to about the equator, making it inappropriate for a full peripheral funduscopic examination. The examination is performed with the eye that corresponds to the eye being examined. The focusing lens is rotated to the examiner's refractive error or starting at zero and rotating until fundus details come into view. Focus first on a blood vessel and then trace it back to the optic nerve, noting color, clarity of disc margins, and cup to disc ratio. Note any abnormalities such as hemorrhages, exudates, or pigment changes.

IMAGING IN OCULAR TRAUMA

The decision for imaging patients with suspected ocular trauma should be guided by the mechanism of injury, clinical presentation, and physical examination. Frequently, the history and physical exam may be limited due to the severity of the injury, associated injuries, and/or facial swelling. The decision on which imaging study to order will depend on resource availability, local practice and custom, and the type of injury suspected. That said, computed tomography (CT) is considered the imaging study of choice in the evaluation of orbital trauma.[3,13]

Radiographs

Radiographs are being used less frequently. While the sensitivity of radiographs for detecting fractures is 64%–78%, it is very poor in identifying orbital content injuries.[14] Radiographic findings suggesting fracture include an air-fluid level in, or opacification of, the maxillary sinus (from bleeding secondary to an orbital floor fracture) and the tear drop sign (orbital contents herniating into the maxillary sinus due to an orbital floor fracture). If there is a low suspicion for metallic orbital or intraocular foreign body (IOFB), a Water's view x-ray may be a cost-effective test. However, if the pretest probability is high or the suspected foreign body is nonmetallic, radiographs play no role.

Ultrasound

Ultrasound has been used in the evaluation of the multitrauma patient for some time. It is now being increasingly used for the evaluation of ocular trauma. Ultrasound can be performed directly at the bedside and is fast, safe, noninvasive, and avoids the use of ionizing radiation. Ocular sonography has been shown to be used successfully by nonradiology and nonopthalmology physicians.[15]

A high-resolution linear array 10 MHz transducer (or vascular probe) should be used. The output and gain should be minimized to prevent image distortion by eyelid echos and to maximize image quality.[16] The eye should be closed, ultrasound gel applied, and scanned in the sagittal and transverse plains. Injuries identified by ultrasound include retrobulbar hemorrhage (hypoechoic lucency deep to the retina), lens dislocation (abnormal position of the lens within the globe), vitreous hemorrhage (echogenic material within the vitreous body), IOFB (echogenic foreign body visualized within the globe), and globe rupture (difference in globe size between the eyes).[16] There is some controversy regarding the role of ultrasound in evaluating suspected globe rupture. It appears that the majority of experts feel that ultrasound is contraindicated in suspected globe rupture due to potentially causing extrusion of intraocular contents.[3,13,17] Those in favor of ultrasound recommend placing a large amount of ultrasound gel over the closed eye, so that the probe never actually exerts pressure on the eye.[16] Regardless, if there is an obvious anterior perforation, ultrasound should not be performed.

Computed Tomography

CT is considered the standard imaging modality in the evaluation of mid-face fractures and orbital trauma.[3] Typically, thin slices (i.e., 1 mm) with multiplanar reformation has the best results.[11,13] The sensitivity of CT for orbital fractures is 79%–96%, with a lower sensitivity for infraorbital rim injury.[18] CT identifies open-globe injuries with a sensitivity of approximately 71%.[19] Findings suggesting open-globe injury on CT include a change in globe contour, an obvious loss of volume, a deep anterior chamber, scleral discontinuity, and intraocular air.[13] The sensitivity of CT for detecting clinically occult open-globe injuries is slightly less, varying from 56% to 68%.[13] When an IOFB is suspected, CT is usually the study of choice. It can demonstrate metal fragments <1 mm in size.[13] It is also the best study for detecting glass, compared to US and magnetic reasonance imaging (MRI). Glass fragments of at least 1.5 mm diameter are detected 96% of the time and 48% for glass fragments 0.5 mm in size.[20] Other injuries detected by CT include corneal laceration (decreased volume of the anterior chamber with decreased anterior–posterior dimension compared to normal globe) and lens displacement/dislocation (abnormal lens position).

Magnetic Resonance Imaging

Given the limitations of MRI, including availability, contraindications (i.e., presence of metal), and length of imaging time, MRI is not recommended as the initial imaging modality in orbital trauma. Currently, it is most useful in identifying intraorbital wood or organic material when CT results are either negative or equivocal.[3,13]

CORNEAL ABRASION

Patients will present with pain, foreign body sensation, photophobia, and tearing. Frequently, there is a history of trauma, but sometimes the patient does not recall any specific event. Placing a drop of topical ophthalmic anesthetic in the affected eye will allow for a more efficient history and physical examination. The immediate pain relief following placement is characteristic of corneal abrasion. Physical exam reveals conjunctival injection, tearing, and decreased visual acuity if the abrasion is large or lies within the visual axis. Fluorescein staining and examination under the slit lamp or use of a cobalt-blue light will reveal fluorescein uptake if there is an epithelial defect. The size and location should be documented. The anterior chamber should be examined for cells, flare, and blood. Always examine the eye carefully for the presence of foreign bodies, including everting the upper and lower eyelids. Treatment includes the use of cycloplegics to decrease ciliary spasm (and pain), topical ophthalmic antibiotic ointment, and analgesia (see Table 25.2). Pain may be managed with topical or po nonsteroidal anti-inflammatory medications or a short course of po narcotics. Patching the eye has been shown to offer no benefit for simple corneal abrasions and should not be used.[21] Never give or prescribe the patient topical anesthetic agents, as their repetitive use will cause ocular toxicity. Because contact lens wearers are at risk for pseudomonas infection, topical ophthalmic tobramycin ointment should be used in these patients. Patients with corneal abrasions should be instructed not to wear their contact lenses until the abrasion is completely healed. All patients should be re-examined within 24 hours.

CORNEAL FOREIGN BODY

For a corneal foreign body, the presentation, evaluation, and management (after foreign body removal) are similar to corneal abrasion. Patients complain of foreign body sensation, pain, photophobia, and tearing. Vision may be affected if the foreign body is large or within the visual axis. Similar to corneal abrasion, placement of a drop or two of topical ophthalmic anesthetic will facilitate the history and physical examination. Foreign bodies are frequently visible without magnification; however, if available, a slit lamp exam should be performed. Examine the eye closely for any other injuries. Make sure to evert the lids to inspect for foreign bodies. The majority of corneal foreign bodies are superficial and can be safely removed in the ED. Full thickness corneal foreign bodies require ophthalmology consultation. Foreign bodies are best removed under slit lamp magnification. A 27-gauge needle on the end of a tuberculin syringe or a moistened Q-tip will usually work well in removing the foreign body. Both eyes should be anesthetized to decrease reflex blinking. During removal, the patient's forehead should be pressed firmly against the slit lamp, the lids held open with the physician's nondominant hand, and the dominant hand (holding needle or Q-tip) should rest against the bar of the slit lamp machine to stabilize it. Using the bevel of the needle, the motion should be a gentle scraping motion, away from the patient, and parallel to the eye.

Corneal rust rings are a complication of metallic foreign bodies. If the rust ring is superficial, not over the visual axis, and an ophthalmic burr is available, removal can be attempted. All patients should be referred for ophthalmologic follow-up within 24 hours. Rust ring removal is actually easier the following day due to corneal edema and anterior displacement of the foreign material.

Postremoval treatment includes cycloplegics, ophthalmic antibiotic ointment, and analgesia, as in corneal abrasion. If the foreign body is organic (i.e., plant or vegetable material), a topical ophthalmic fluoroquinolone should be used (see Table 25.2).

CHEMICAL INJURIES

The spectrum of injuries to the eye caused by exposure to chemicals varies from mild to very severe with potential blindness. The most common agents include alkalis (i.e., lye, plaster, cement, airbag powder or agents containing ammonia, sodium hydroxide, or lime), acids (sulfuric, sulphurous, hydrofluoric, acetic, chromic, and hydrochloric), solvents and detergents, and cyanoacrylate (superglue).[22] We will discuss cyanoacrylate injury separately.

The severity of the chemical injury is related to the properties of the chemical, the duration and extent of exposure, and other concomitant injuries to the eye, including thermal exposure. In general, alkali injury is more severe than acid. Alkali injuries are especially damaging due to rapid, deep tissue penetration; complete corneal opacification and melting can occur. Acid burns cause denaturation of tissue proteins, which then acts as a barrier to further penetration, thus limiting their damage.[23] Solvents and detergents typically result in chemical conjunctivitis.

Conjunctival and eyelid hyperemia, chemosis (conjunctival swelling/edema), and corneal punctuate epithelial defects are frequently observed in mild injuries. Conjunctival hyperemia or blanching (due to limbal ischemia), corneal haze, or opacification can be observed in severe cases.

Treatment should be instituted immediately and without delay, even before obtaining a visual acuity or pH testing. The only exception is in the case of a suspected open-globe injury, in which further damage may be caused by the force of irrigation.

A topical anesthetic should be placed into the eye along with an eyelid speculum. The treatment involves copious irrigation of the corneal surface with normal saline or Ringer's lactate (preferred) for at least 30 minutes. This can be performed by attaching IV tubing to the irrigation solution and directing the flow of fluid into the eye. Tap water irrigation can be used if these solutions are unavailable. The upper and lower lids should be everted and inspected for retained particulate, which should be removed if present and then copiously irrigated. After 30 minutes of irrigation, wait 5–10 minutes and then check the pH by placing litmus paper in the inferior fornix. Irrigation should then continue until a neutral pH of 7.0 is reached. The volume of irrigation fluid and time needed to reach neutral pH varies widely and may involve as much as 8–10 L of irrigation.[24]

Cyanoacrylate (i.e., Super Glue and Krazy Glue) in the eye is managed differently. The most common injury following cyanoacrylate administration into the eye is a corneal and/or conjunctival abrasion. Cyanoacrylate bonds only with dry surfaces; therefore, fusion of the upper and lower lids occurs predominantly through bonding of the eyelashes.[25] Collections of hardened glue particulate will tend to occur in the inferior fornix. Periocular skin irritation and dermatitis can also occur.

Initial management includes attempting to remove any loose glue stuck to the lashes and to gently open the eye. The use of ophthalmic ointment gently rubbed into the lashes may facilitate glue removal, especially if it is allowed to penetrate before attempting to mechanically remove loose glue. Avoid use of alcohol or other solvents. Cutting of the lashes may be necessary to open the eye. The eye should then be irrigated with normal saline or Ringer's lactate for at least 15 minutes. Topical anesthetic and fluroscein should be used to aid in inspection of the cornea for any abrasions or glue debris, which should be removed. The upper and lower fornicies should be inspected for retained glue particulate. Any associated corneal abrasion or persistant glue on the lashes can be treated with ophthalmic antibiotic ointment. Most reported cases suggest spontaneous separation of the upper and lower lids will occur within 1 week from initial application of cyanoacrylate.[25] Associated dermatitis can be treated with periocular skin lubrication, such as ophthalmic ointment. Cycloplegic agents may be used to increase patient comfort in the case of associated ciliary spasm or photophobia. Patients with corneal involvement should have ophthalmic follow up within 24 hours.

CONJUNCTIVAL LACERATIONS

Lacerations of the conjunctiva are usually associated with intraocular foreign bodies or scleral perforation.[3] For these reasons, it is important to exclude a ruptured globe. Conjunctival lacerations may appear as a conjunctival defect or presence of fat. Slit lamp examination will usually be necessary to differentiate superficial from deep lacerations. Superficial lacerations <1 cm in length do not usually require repair and will normally heal quickly.[3] Lacerations >1 cm should be repaired by ophthalmology, normally using 6–0 to 8–0 absorbable sutures. All patients should be treated with prophylactic antibiotic ointment or drops.[3]

LID LACERATIONS

The upper and lower eyelid skin is very thin, with minimal dermal tissue. Directly under the skin and dermis is the orbicularis muscle, responsible for eyelid closure. The muscle completely surrounds the lid fissure and is attached medially and laterally by the medial and lateral canthal tendons, which are adherent to the orbital rim. The orbital septum extends from the orbital rim and attaches superiorly to the levator aponeurosis and inferiorly to the lower lid retractors. The orbital septum separates the lid from the underlying orbital fat. The tarsus is the dense connective tissue deep to the orbicularis muscle, which gives the lid rigidity. Conjunctiva lines the lids and lid fissures and is continuous over the surface of the globe (see Fig. 25.1).

Multiple mechanisms of injury may result in laceration of the eyelid. It is critical that the patient presenting with a lid laceration be meticulously examined for the possibility of concurrent injuries such as canalicular lacerations, corneal or sclera lacerations, orbital wall fractures, an intraocular or embedded foreign body or injury to the extraocular muscles. Beginning with the external examination, an attempt should be made to ascertain the depth of the injury. If orbital fat is prolapsed through the wound, the orbital septum has been violated, and the fat will require repositioning. The presence of orbital fat at the wound should alert the practitioner to the possibility of deeper injuries involving the globe. In cases of possible high-velocity fragment injury, one should suspect penetration into the eye or perforation into the globe and obtain CT imaging. A foreign body should only be removed if there is no evidence of deeper extension into the globe or orbit.

Avulsion of the canalicular apparatus, which is medial, can occur with lateral traction injuries to the eyelid; this can commonly be seen in assault and dog-bite injuries. These injuries will require specialized surgical intervention to repair the lacrimal drainage system and prevent chronic tearing and lid malposition.

The presence of ptosis in a patient presenting with a lid laceration may indicate injury to the underlying levator muscle. Such injuries may require subsequent surgical intervention following initial repair in order to restore lid function. Cleansing of lid wounds should be performed using povidone–iodine 5% solution, only after the integrity of the globe has been established.

In extensive lid injuries in which closure of the eye is affected or when surgical repair needs to be delayed, saline-soaked dressings should be applied to the area to promote viability of the tissue.

For repair of lid lacerations, general anesthesia is used in children and in uncooperative adults. Otherwise, local anesthesia is used in adults (2% xylocaine with epineherine 1:100,000). Because direct injection of local anesthetic causes tissue distortion and bleeding, use the minimal amount of anesthetic necessary to obtain adequate pain control. Make sure that there is no injury to the globe before attempting eyelid repair. Place a drop of topical anesthetic into the eye to facilitate patient comfort. The wound should be irrigated thoroughly with normal saline or Ringer's lactate.

Use toothed forceps or cotton-tipped applicators to gently open the edge of the wound to determine depth of penetration. The lid tissue should be realigned and repaired in layers. Any injury involving the lid margin or canalicular region will require specialized repair by an ophthalmologist or surgeon specialized in lid anatomy and surgical procedures. Lid margin injuries require precise apposition of tissue to prevent lid notching. If the tarsus is involved, use 5–0 absorbable sutures.[26] Extreme care must be taken to avoid injury to the underlying globe. A corneal shield can be placed to avoid such injury, although it can make the repair more difficult due to its bulk and distortion of tissue. The orbicularis/deeper tissue can be repaired using 6–0 interrupted vicryl sutures, and the skin closed using 6–0 interrupted silk or nylon sutures. Care should be taken to evert the wound margin to avoid depressed scars. In some cases, where patient follow up may be limited, or in the case of children when it may be desirable to avoid suture removal, the skin may be closed with 6–0 fast absorbing gut or vicryl suture. Topical ophthalmic antibiotic ointment is applied to the wound. Generally, silk or nylon sutures are removed within 5–7 days. Contaminated injuries should be treated with systemic antibiotics: dicloxacillin or cephalexin, 250–500 mg PO QID in adults and 25–50 mg/kg/d divided into four doses for pediatric patients.[26] In animal bite injuries, infection and rabies prophylaxis require consideration.

TRAUMATIC HYPHEMA

Hyphema is defined as blood in the anterior chamber. In urban settings, two-thirds of traumatic hyphema are due to blunt ocular trauma and one-third due to traumatic globe rupture.[27] The source of bleeding is usually from the iris or ciliary body. The amount of blood present in the anterior chamber determines the grade of the hyphema: grade 0—microhyphema with red blood cells detected only by slit-lamp examination; grade 1—blood occupying less than one-third of the anterior chamber; grade 2—blood filling one-third to one half; grade 3—one half to less than total; and grade 4—chamber filled completely with blood (also known as an eight ball).[3] The majority of hyphemas are grade 1 (see Fig. 25.3).

Patients will present with complaints of pain, photophobia, and decreased visual acuity. The hyphema is usually visible as a meniscus in the anterior chamber (with the patient's head upright) on gross exam. If possible, however, all patients should undergo slit-lamp examination to evaluate for other possible injuries (i.e., globe rupture) and to better estimate the size of the hyphema. The following factors are associated with a good prognosis: small size (i.e., height < 4 mm, measured from the inferior 6 O'clock limbus), light red color of the blood, and normal IOP.[28]

Recurrent bleeding and elevated IOP are the two most serious complications of hyphema. Frequently, there is a moderate elevation (<24 mm Hg) in IOP after the injury due to mechanical obstruction of the trabecular meshwork from blood.[28] Recurrence of hemorrhage usually occurs between the 3rd and 5th day postinjury and is secondary to normal blood clot dissolution. The incidence of rebleeding is variable (0.4%–38%).[28] Risk factors for rebleeding include large hyphemas (greater than one-third of the anterior chamber), sickle-cell disease/trait, anticoagulant medication, and elevated IOP on initial exam.[28,29] Management involves elevating the patient's head, placing a metal shield over the eye (not patch), topical ophthalmic atropine 1% one drop tid to the affected eye and ophthalmic prednisolone acetate 1% one drop QID.[11] If increased IOP is present (i.e., >30 mm Hg), administer a topical beta-blocker (i.e., timolol 0.5% one drop). If the IOP remains elevated, give 1 g/kg mannitol IV and po or IV acetazolamide 500 mg. However, if the patient has sickle-cell disease/trait, acetazolamide is contraindicated. Patients with small hyphemas (less than one-third of the anterior chamber) and normal IOP may be treated as an outpatient with close and reliable follow-up; all others should be admitted. Avoid aspirin and nonsteroidal anti-inflammatory drugs for pain control because of their antiplatelet effect, which can increase the incidence of rebleeding.

LENS SUBLUXATION/ DISLOCATION

The lens is a convex, transparent structure held in place behind the iris by the zonule fibers, which connect to the ciliary body[9] (see Fig. 25.4). Blunt trauma can cause damage to these zonule fibers, resulting in lens subluxation or dislocation. Incomplete disruption of the lens zonule fibers results in subluxation.[29] If complete disruption occurs, the lens is displaced posteriorly

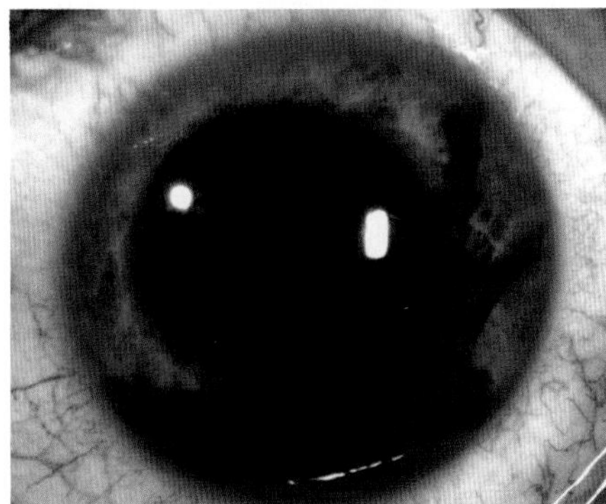

FIGURE 25.3. Grade 1 hyphema in a patient struck in the eye with a ball. (Reprinted with permission from Ehlers JP, Shah CP, Fenton GL, et al. *The Wills Eye Manual: Office and Emergency Room Diagnosis and Treatment of Eye Disease*. 5th ed. Philadelphia, PA: Lippincott Williams & Wilkins; 2008.)

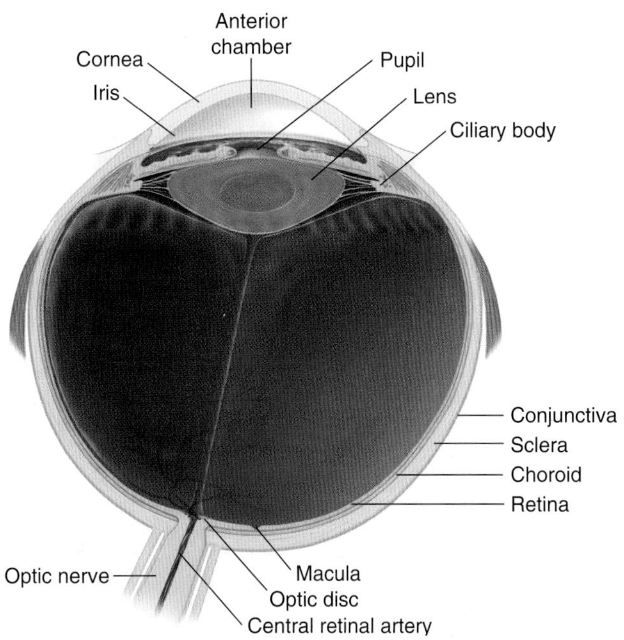

FIGURE 25.4. Ocular anatomy, horizontal section.

(most common) or anteriorly into the anterior chamber. Patients will present with fluctuating vision, blurred vision, or monocular diplopia with subluxation if the lens remains in the visual axis.[3,29] Visual acuity testing will reveal decreased vision, ranging from mild (subluxation) to marked (dislocation). If displaced anteriorly, the lens may be visualized on gross or slit-lamp examination. Dilation of the pupil is usually necessary to observe the lens if dislocated posteriorly.[3] Another helpful finding is iridodonesis, a tremor of the iris after rapid eye movement observed in posterior lens dislocation.[3] If the lens is dislocated anteriorly, then IOP should be measured, as the dislocated lens can obstruct the outflow of aqueous humor and cause acute angle closure glaucoma and elevated IOP. The management of lens subluxation and dislocation will frequently involve surgical repair. In the case of an anterior lens dislocation causing increased IOP, repair should be performed emergently.

TRAUMATIC IRIDOCYCLITIS

Traumatic iridocyclitis results from blunt trauma to the globe. This causes inflammation of the iris and ciliary body and resulting ciliary spasm. Patients typically complain of pain, photophobia, and blurred vision. Visual acuity may or may not be affected. Conjunctival injection and a small, poorly dilating pupil can be observed.[3] The slit-lamp examination will reveal the presence of cells (small, floating particulate matter within the aqueous humor) and flare (scattered light caused by the presence of inflammatory proteins in the aqueous humor) in the anterior chamber.[10] The condition is self-limited and the management symptomatic. A topical cycloplegic agent will usually be enough. One may consider a topical ophthalmic steroid to decrease inflammation. However, if a corneal epithelial defect (i.e., abrasion) exists, its use is contraindicated.

ORBITAL WALL FRACTURES

Orbital wall fractures can be classified as either blow-out or blow-in. Typically, blow-out fractures involve either the orbital floor and/or medial wall. Blow-in fractures are usually either superior or inferior. Each will be discussed separately.

Blow-out fractures occur in response to blunt force to the eye. They account for approximately 11% of fractures involving the orbit.[30] The orbital rim may or may not be involved. The most common location for a blow-out fracture is the middle one-third of the orbital floor. The second most common location is the medial wall. Medial wall fractures may either occur in combination with orbital floor fractures (most common) or as an isolated fracture.

While most patients with a blow-out fracture will have some complaint other than pain, on rare occasion, they can be otherwise asymptomatic. A common complaint in orbital floor fractures is diplopia, which is often vertical and worse with attempted upward or downward gaze. Patients may also complain of numbness of the cheek and gum on the injured side, due to infraorbital nerve injury. Visual acuity may be normal or decreased. Physical examination can reveal periorbital swelling and ecchymoses. Enophthalmos (sunken eye) may be present if the orbital contents have prolapsed into the maxillary sinus. Similarly, there may be limitations of vertical eye movement if there is entrapment of the inferior rectus muscle within the fracture. Decreased sensation in the distribution of the infraorbital nerve (i.e., cheek and upper gum) will be present on exam if the nerve is trapped in the fracture site or contused.

For medial wall fractures, epistaxis and subcutaneous emphysema (due to communication with the ethmoid sinus) are common. Diplopia can be present, but with medial and lateral gaze. Patients may complain of increased periorbital swelling with noseblowing (i.e., due to increased subcutaneous emphysema).

The eye should be thoroughly examined for associated injuries, which may occur in 10%–25% of patients with orbital floor fractures.[30] Globe rupture, hyphema, iridodialysis, lens dislocation/subluxation, and retinal injuries can all be found in association with orbital wall fractures. It is extremely important to examine the full range of extraocular muscles, looking specifically for any limitations.

Findings of orbital wall fracture on x-ray include the tear drop sign or the presence of air fluid levels or opacification of the sinuses. CT scan of the face or orbits, with 1.5 mm cuts, is the best imaging study for identifying the fracture, complications of the fracture (i.e., inferior rectus muscle entrapment, etc.), and associated injuries (i.e., globe rupture; see Fig. 25.5).

Blow-in fractures also occur secondary to blunt trauma, but with the force directed primarily against the frontal bone or maxilla. Blunt trauma against the frontal bone can result in an orbital roof fracture, with displacement into the orbital space. This can result in injury to the optic nerve or compression of the superior rectus and levator palpebrae muscles. If the force is directed primarily against the maxilla, an inferior blow-in fracture of the orbital floor can occur. Similar to blow-out fractures, the inferior rectus and inferior oblique muscles can be entrapped in fracture fragments. Assume a high index of suspicion for an associated globe injury for both blow-in and blow-out fractures.

Management for both types of fractures is emergent in the case of visual impairment, entrapped muscle(s), or globe rupture. If none of these are present, patients can be treated as outpatients with instructions to apply ice and avoid noseblowing, valsalva maneuver, and nasal decongestant sprays. Broad spectrum antibiotic prescription is controversial; if adjacent sinusitis is present, however, they should be used.

PERFORATING INJURIES OF THE CORNEA OR SCLERA/OPEN GLOBE

Blunt or sharp trauma to the eye may result in a corneal or scleral laceration. Symptoms include pain, decreased vision, and tearing, or "loss of fluid" from the eye. The patient should be examined using a penlight and avoid placing pressure on the

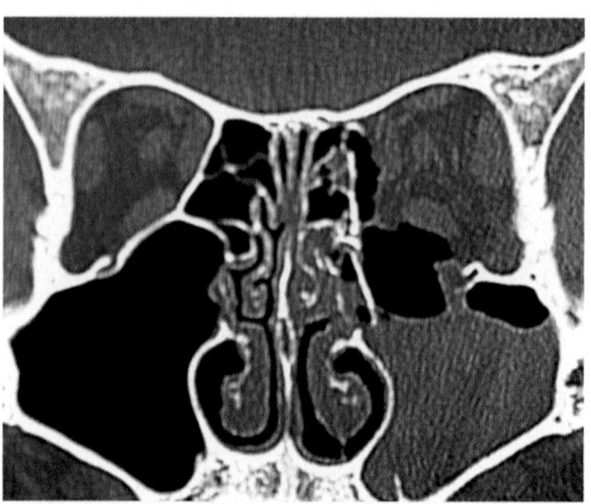

FIGURE 25.5. CT scan of orbital blow-out fracture. Note disruption of the orbital floor and blood in the maxillary sinus. (Reprinted with permission from Ehlers JP, Shah CP, Fenton GL, et al. *The Wills Eye Manual: Office and Emergency Room Diagnosis and Treatment of Eye Disease.* 5th ed. Philadelphia, PA: Lippincott Williams & Wilkins; 2008.)

eye. Physical findings, which can sometimes be subtle, include a flat anterior chamber (compared to the unaffected eye), extension of the iris to the corneal wound, pupil irregularity, severe subconjunctival hemorrhage or hematoma, or evidence of pigmented tissue (uvea) on the surface of the sclera. Suspicion for an open-globe injury should be high in cases of lid laceration or extensive subconjunctival hemorrhage. Intraocular contents, including the lens, may have exited the wound or be displaced into the anterior chamber or vitreous. Blood within the anterior chamber or in the vitreous may be present. Posterior eye findings such as retinal swelling, tears, or detachment may not be visible if there is major hemorrhage within the anterior chamber or vitreous.

Gentle ultrasound may be needed to localize a posterior rupture site or to rule out intraocular foreign bodies not visible on CT scan (i.e., nonmetallic and wood). Ultrasound should not be performed if an obvious anterior rupture is present.

At times, the depth of a deep corneal injury may be uncertain; however, all suspected cases of a full thickness eye injury should be approached as an open globe until proven otherwise. The patient should be kept still and quiet and should not bend, strain, or apply pressure around the orbit. The Seidel test can be performed to help determine if a full-thickness corneal wound is present.

Once the diagnosis of a possible or probable ruptured globe is made, further examination should be deferred until the time of surgical repair by an ophthalmologist in the operating room. This is to prevent extrusion of intraocular contents. A hard plastic shield (or paper cup if shield in unavailable) should be placed over the eye, with great care taken to avoid any pressure to the eye or periorbit. Obtain a CT scan of the brain and orbits with fine 1 mm axial and coronal sections to rule out IOFB.[31] The patient should be admitted and maintained NPO for surgery and should avoid valsalva maneuvers. Administration of antiemetics should be considered to avoid vomiting. Although randomized, prospective studies of open-globe injuries treated with or without systemic antibiotics are not available, systemic antibiotics are generally administered within 6 hours of injury. For adults, consider cefazolin 1 g IV q8h or vancomycin 1 g IV q12h. The addition of systemic fluroquinolone therapy (i.e., ciprofloxacin 400 mg p.o./i.v. b.i.d, gatifloxacin 400 mg daily, or moxifloxacin 400 mg daily) is beneficial for antimicrobial activity against *Bacillus* and for good vitreous penetration.[32] For children, consider cefazolin 25–50 mg/kg/day IV in three divided doses and gentamicin 2 mg/kg IV q8h.[31] Surgical repair by an experienced eye surgeon should be performed as soon as possible.

INTRAOCULAR FOREIGN BODY

Injuries that result in an IOFB, whether in the anterior chamber or in the posterior segment, are considered ophthalmic emergencies. Prompt evaluation and surgical intervention are necessary. An IOFB enters the eye through a break in the cornea or sclera. These injuries are most common with small particulate, high-velocity perforating trauma, such as occurs with hammering on metal, grinding accidents, or shrapnel such as glass in a motor vehicle crash. The entry site may be small and difficult to see on examination and may even be self-sealing. A history consistent with possible ocular perforation should raise the clinician's index of suspicion for a foreign body. If there is an obvious perforation site, the remainder of the examination may be deferred until the time of surgery. Signs and symptoms include decreased vision, pain, a visible entrance site, or visualization of foreign material anteriorly on slit-lamp examination, or posteriorly on funduscopic examination. These open-globe injuries have a much higher incidence of endophthalmitis and ocular demise. Rates of endophthalmitis following globe perforation are reported to be 3%–17%. A recent study showed that eyes with an IOFB had a higher percentage of endophthalmitis than those without.[33]

A CT scan of the brain and orbits should be obtained to evaluate the position and extent of foreign material within the eye and the orbit (coronal and axial views with 1-mm sections through the orbit). MRI is contraindicated in case of metallic foreign body.

Management of patients with IOFB includes hospitalization, made NPO for surgery, and an eye shield placed to protect the globe from external pressure. Intravenous antibiotics should be administered; accepted regimen include vancomycin 1 g IV q12h or ceftazidime 1 g IV q12h or ciprofloxacin 400 mg IV q12h or moxifloxacin 400 mg IV daily or gatifloxacin 400 mg IV daily.[34] Surgical repair of the globe and removal of intraocular foreign bodies requires the expertise of ophthalmologists and vitreoretinal specialists with extensive experience in such cases.

RETINAL INJURY AND VITREOUS HEMORRAGE

Blunt trauma can damage the retina, vitreous, and other intraocular layers in various ways. Blunt trauma to the eye can result in a retinal tear, especially in patients who are myopic or who have a history or family history of retinal holes, tears, or detachments. The patient may present with varying degrees of decreased vision, dependent upon the location and extent of the injury, or may experience a defect in vision affecting a specific part of the visual field. Some may report seeing flashes of light or floaters.

Retinal Commotio

One of the milder forms of injury to the retina is retinal edema, or commotio, caused presumably by a disruption in the photoreceptor outer segments and decreased function of the retinal pigment epithelium.[35] Retinal commotio appears as retinal whitening ophthalmoscopically and, depending upon its location, can result in substantial decreased vision. In general, the vision will improve as the swelling decreases over several weeks.

A careful ophthalmoscopic examination is necessary to rule out the possibility of associated retinal holes, tears, or even retinal detachment.

Retinal Holes/Tears/Detachment

Blunt trauma can lead to retinal or macular holes. The mechanism of injury involves rapid displacement of the vitreous causing vitreoretinal traction with resultant retinal hole formation. The most common area of retinal break in trauma is the superonasal or infratemporal quadrant.[35] Retinal breaks are usually treated using cryotherapy or laser photocoagulation by a qualified ophthalmologist to decrease the possibility of subsequent retinal detachment. Retinal detachment occurs when liquefied vitreous passes through a retinal hole, detaching the retina from the globe. Since most trauma patients are young, with firm, nonliquefied vitreous, retinal detachment is not a common presentation at time of trauma. However, large retinal tears (>3 clock hours) or macular holes may lead to traumatic retinal detachments presenting at the time of injury[35] (see Figs. 25.6 and 25.7).

Such detachments are treated by vitreoretinal specialists using an encircling element "scleral buckle" along with

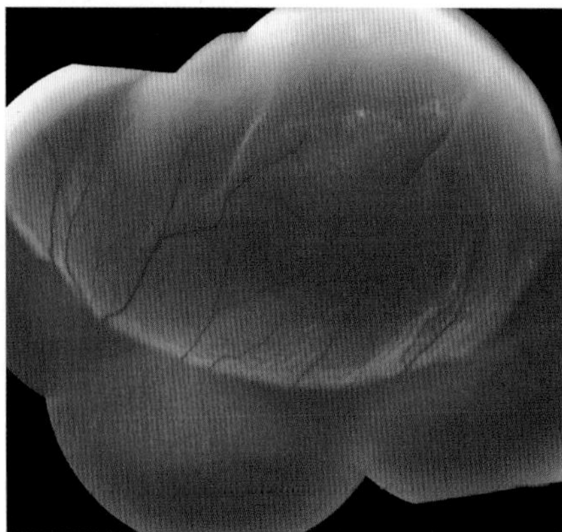

FIGURE 25.6. Large retinal detachment. (Reprinted with permission from Ehlers JP, Shah CP, Fenton GL, et al. *The Wills Eye Manual: Office and Emergency Room Diagnosis and Treatment of Eye Disease.* 5th ed. Philadelphia, PA: Lippincott Williams & Wilkins; 2008.)

advanced vitreous surgery to remove any tractional component on the retina. In addition, a variety of intraocular gases or fluids can be used to flatten the retina and tamponade the break in the hope of reattaching the retina. Resultant visual acuity is dependent upon a number of factors including location of the detachment, amount of time prior to surgical intervention, other confounding ophthalmic conditions, tissue integrity, and surgical technique.

Vitreous Hemorrhage

The vitreous is the gelatinous substance that fills the globe posterior to the lens and provides structural integrity. It is most adherent to the retina at the most anterior portion of the retina, the optic disc, and along the retinal vessels. The composition tends to change with age from a more firm gelatinous substance to a more liquid form. As this change occurs, the vitreous may detach from the retina which may be an asymptomatic event or may be accompanied by "photopsias" or visual images such as flashes of light or lines. Photopsias indicate tension on the retina. In trauma, rapid displacement of the vitreous may cause substantive tension on the retina and retinal vessels and produce vitreous hemorrhage. The patient presents with varying degrees of decreased vision or clouding of vision and may also experience photopsias. Fundus examination through a dilated pupil will reveal varying loss of fundus detail, blood obscuring the view of the posterior pole or retina, or red "debris" seen within the vitreous. All trauma patients with vitreous hemorrhage require a careful bilateral ophthalmologic examination for retinal holes, tears, or detachment by an ophthalmologist.

If the view of the retina is obscured by blood, ultrasound should be performed to assess for underlying retinal detachment. Experienced practitioners can differentiate between vitreous hemorrhage, vitreous detachment, and retinal detachment using ultrasound.

Underlying diseases that increase risk of vitreous hemorrhage include diabetes, sickle-cell disease (especially SC disease), clotting disorders, and hypertension.

Treatment of associated retinal pathology is performed by an ophthalmologist. If the patient has no retinal tears, treatment is activity restriction, avoidance of aspirin containing medications or nonsteroidal anti-inflammatory medication, and maintaining head-up positioning to promote inferior settling of the blood. The patient is followed closely for any retinal pathology as the hemorrhage clears and view of the fundus improves.

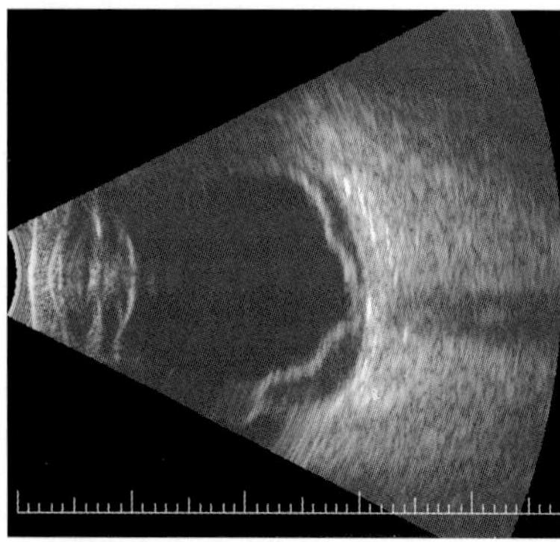

FIGURE 25.7. Ultrasound demonstrating retinal detachment. (Reprinted with permission from Ehlers JP, Shah CP, Fenton GL, et al. *The Wills Eye Manual: Office and Emergency Room Diagnosis and Treatment of Eye Disease.* 5th ed. Philadelphia, PA: Lippincoti Williams & Wilkins; 2008.)

TRAUMATIC RETROBULBAR HEMORRHAGE

Following blunt trauma to the periorbit, bleeding behind the globe may result in retrobulbar hemorrhage with resultant decreased ability to move the eye and the risk of optic nerve damage due to compressive optic neuropathy. Symptoms include pain, decreased vision, diplopia, and an inability to open the eye in the case of severe swelling. The patient is typically proptotic with major subconjunctival hemorrhage and chemosis. Pressure upon the globe reveals resistance to retopulsion. Ominous signs include an afferent pupillary defect, increased IOP, and vision loss. Prolonged intraorbital hemorrhage with excessive congestion may result in vascular occlusion and permanent damage to the optic nerve.

Funduscopic examination should be performed to assess for any vascular congestion or optic nerve edema. A CT scan of the orbit should be obtained to visualize retrobulbar hemorrhage, which usually appears as a diffuse increased reticular pattern seen within the orbital fat. The degree of proptosis and evidence of tension on the optic nerve should also be assessed. Optic nerve straightening may be seen, and, in severe cases, "tenting" of the globe may be evident. It should be noted that CT scan examination should be deferred if the vision is threatened, and attention should first be directed toward decreasing orbital pressure.

The treatment of retrobulbar hemorrhage is aimed at timely decompression of the orbit. If there is evidence of optic neuropathy (i.e., progressive visual loss, afferent pupillary defect, or retinal vessel and disc congestion), emergent decompression is necessary. This is accomplished at the bedside by lateral canthotomy and cantholysis. The goal of the procedure is to allow soft tissue decompression via disinsertion of the lateral canthal tendon, which adheres the lower lid to the periosteum.

In order to perform a lateral canthotomy, one needs blunt tip (i.e., Westcott) scissors, hemostat, and toothed forceps. Anesthetize the lateral canthal region using lidocaine 2% with epinephrine. Place a hemostat horizontally at the full thickness of the lateral canthus from conjunctiva to the skin. Clamp for approximately 1 minute to compress the tissue and reduce bleeding. Use the scissors to perform a full thickness canthotomy, approximately 1 cm in length. In order to obtain adequate decompression, a cantholysis must then be performed to cut the inferior crus of the lateral canthal tendon. This procedure is performed by locating the tendon by feel with one blade of the scissors and excising the tissue. When the canthal tendon is cut, the eye should further proptose, and the lid should no longer be apposed to the globe (see Fig. 25.8).

Pressure on the incision site should be adequate to control hemostasis. If the procedure is successful, the IOP should begin to decrease and retinal perfusion be re-established within approximately 15 minutes.[36] The vision may or may not improve at this point. If the procedure is unsuccessful, the patient should have orbital decompression into the sinus by an experienced surgeon.

If there is no evidence of compressive optic neuropathy (i.e., no afferent pupillary defect, vascular compromise, or decreased vision), but the IOP is elevated, the patient can be first treated with glaucoma drops such as a topical beta blocker, an alpha agonist, or, in more severe cases, a hyperosmotic agent (i.e., mannitol 1–2 g/kg IV over 45 minutes).[36] Topical drops may require repeat administration every 30 minutes. The patient should be monitored closely for the evidence of evolving optic nerve compromise (i.e., check vision and IOP frequently) and treated as outlined earlier if their condition deteriorates. Cool compresses or ice packs should be used to decrease swelling.

TRAUMATIC OPTIC NEUROPATHY

Traumatic injury to the optic nerve may occur with blunt or penetrating head trauma. The optic nerve injury may be accompanied by any number of ocular or periocular injuries, but can also present without evidence of external injury, such

TRAUMA

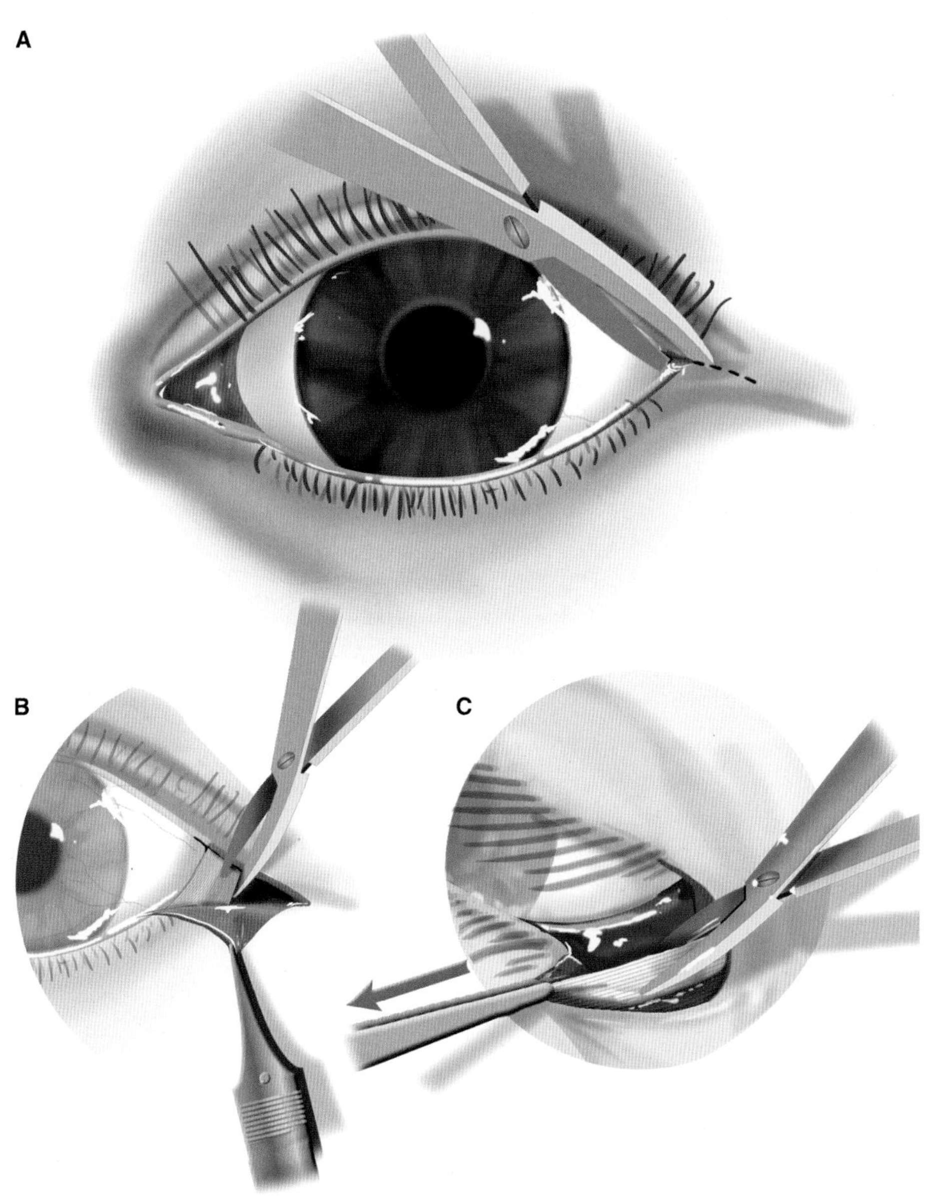

FIGURE 25.8. **A:** Lateral canthotomy. **B:** Pull the lower lid inferiorly and then anteriorly. **C:** Cut the lateral canthal tendon. (Reprinted with permission from Ehlers JP, Shah CP, Fenton GL, et al. *The Wills Eye Manual: Office and Emergency Room Diagnosis and Treatment of Eye Disease.* 5th ed. Philadelphia, PA: Lippincott Williams & Wilkins; 2008.)

as in the case of a whiplash type injury. Following injury to the nerve, edema may cause further damage and result in traumatic optic neuropathy (TON) with severe visual loss. TON should be suspected in the case of a patient presenting with decreased vision following trauma, but without evidence of anterior segment or retinal pathology to explain the deficit.

The patient should have a complete ocular examination including assessment of visual acuity and a careful pupillary examination. Visual fields can be tested by confrontation. If possible, color vision testing can be very helpful (i.e., if one eye reveals a relative decrease) in detecting optic nerve compromise. Fundus examination may reveal evidence of acute optic nerve swelling, optic nerve pallor, or even an optic nerve avulsion. Frequently, the optic nerve appears normal in the acute stage.

A CT scan of the orbit with attention to the optic canals (1 mm axial and coronal cuts at the canals) should be obtained to rule out the possibility of an impending fracture or foreign body causing pressure on the optic nerve.

Treatment is aimed at the causative mechanism of the TON. In the case of a traumatic retrobulbar hemorrhage, lateral canthotomy and cantholysis may be necessary. Evacuation of an orbital foreign body or optic sheath hematoma may be necessary. Optic canal decompression surgery may be required by an experienced oculoplastic surgeon. There is no effective treatment for an optic nerve laceration or optic nerve head avulsion.

Historically, the use of high-dose corticosteroids in TON has been common. Despite this practice, the majority of clinical and experimental evidence shows no support for this treatment.[37] Steroids have actually been shown to result in poorer outcomes if administered >8 hours postinjury.[37]

References

1. Chadwick J, Mann W. *The Medical Works of Hippocrates*. London, UK: Blackwell Scientific; 1950.
2. Perry M, Dancey A, Mireskandari K, et al. Emergency care in facial trauma—a maxillofacial and ophthalmic perspective. *Injury, Int J Care Injured*. 2005;36:875-896.
3. Bord SP, Linden J. Trauma to the globe and orbit. *Emerg Med Clin North Am*. 2008;28:97-123.
4. Leads from MMWR: leading work-related diseases and injuries—United States. *JAMA*. 1990;251:2503-2504.
5. Katz J, Tielsch JM. Lifetime prevalence of ocular injuries from the Baltimore Eye Survey. *Arch Ophthalmol*. 1993;111:1564-1568.
6. Guly CM, Guly HR, Bouamra O, et al. Ocular injuries in patients with major trauma. *Emerg Med J*. 2006;23:915-917.
7. Ansari MH. Blindness after facial fractures: a 19-year retrospective study. *J Oral Maxillofac Surg*. 2005;63:229-237.
8. Heimmel MR, Murphy MA. Ocular injuries in basketball and baseball: what are the risks and how can we prevent them? *Curr Sports Med Rep*. 2008;7:284-288.
9. Robinett DA, Kahn JH. The physical examination of the eye. *Emerg Med Clin North Am*. 2008;26:1-16.
10. Babineau MR, Sanchez LD. Ophthalmologic procedures in the emergency department. *Emerg Clin North Am*. 2008;26:17-34.
11. Mitchell JD. Ocular emergencies. In: Tintinalli JE, et al., eds. *Emergency Medicine—A Comprehensive Study Guide*. 6th ed. New York: McGraw-Hill; 2004:1449-1464.
12. Crown LA. Introduction to slit lamp biomicroscopy: a how to guide for non-ophthalmologists. *Am J Clin Med*. 2006;3:12-16.
13. Kubal WS. Imaging of orbital trauma. *RadioGraphics*. 2008;28:1729-1739.
14. Iinuma T, Hirota Y, Ishio K. Orbital wall fractures: conventional views and CT. *Rhinology*. 1994;32:81-83.
15. Blaivas M, Theodoro D, Sierzenski PR. A study of bedside ocular ultrasonography in the emergency department. *Acad Emerg Med*. 2002;9:791-799.
16. Legome E, Pancu D. Future applications for emergency ultrasound. *Emerg Med Clin North Am*. 2004;22:817-827.
17. Khare GD, Symons RD, Do DV. Common ophthalmic emergencies. *Int J Clin Pract*. 2008;62:1776-1784.
18. Jank S, Deibl M, Strobl H, et al. Intrarater reliability in the ultrasound diagnosis of medial and lateral orbital wall fractures with a cured array transducer. *J Oral Maxillofac Surg*. 2006;64:68-73.
19. Arey ML, Mootha W, Whittemore AR, et al. Computed tomography in the diagnosis of occult open globe injuries. *Ophthalmology*. 2007;114:1448-1452.
20. Gor DM, Kirsch CF, Leen J, et al. Radiologic differentiation of intraocular glass: evaluation of imaging techniques, glass types, size and effect of intraocular hemorrhage. *AJR Am J Roentgenol*. 2001;177:1199-1203.
21. Turner A, Rabiu M. Patching for corneal abrasion. *Cochrane Database Syst Rev* 2007;4:Art No: CD004764.
22. Kanski J. *Clinical Ophthalmology, A Systematic Approach*. 5th ed. London, UK: Butterworth Heinemann; 2003:677-680.
23. Wilson F. *Practical Ophthalmology*. 5th ed. San Francisco, CA: American Academy of Ophthalmology; 2005:350-351.
24. Ehlers JP, Shah CP, eds. *The Wills Eye Manual*. 5th ed. Philadelphia, PA: Lippincott Williams and Wilkins; 2008:12-13.
25. McClean CJ. Ocular superglue injury. *J Acad Emerg Med*. 1997;14:40-41.
26. Ehlers JP, Shah CP, eds. *The Wills Eye Manual*. 5th ed. Philadelphia, PA: Lippicott Williams and Wilkins; 2008:24-28.
27. Walton W, Von Hagen S, Grigorian R, et al. Management of traumatic hyphema. *Surv Ophthalmol*. 2002;47:297-334.
28. Papaconstantinou D, Georgalas I, Kourtis N, et al. Contemporary aspects in the prognosis of traumatic hyphemas. *Clin Ophthalmol*. 2009;3:287-290.
29. Brunette DD. Ophthalmology. In: Marx JA, et al., eds. *Rosen's Emergency Medicine—Concepts and Clinical Practice*. 6th ed. Philadelphia, PA: Mosby Elsevier; 2006:1044-1065.
30. He D, Blomquist P, Ellis E. Association between ocular injuries and internal orbital fractures. *J Oral Maxillofac Surg*. 2007;65:713-720.
31. Ehlers JP, Shah CP, eds. *The Wills Eye Manual*. 5th ed. Philadelphia, PA: Lippincott Williams & Wilkins; 2008:39-41.
32. Cebulla CM, Flynn HW. Endophthalmitis after open globe injuries. *Am J Ophthalmol*. 2009;147:567.
33. Andreoli CM, Andreoli MT, Kloek CE, et al. Low rate of endophthalmitis in a large series of open globe injuries. *Am J Ophthalmol*. 2009;147:601-608.
34. Ehlers JP, Shah CP, eds. *The Wills Eye Manual*. 5th ed. Philadelphia, PA: Lippincott Williams and Wilkins; 2008:41-42.
35. Ryan SJ, Hinton DR, Schachat AP, et al., eds. *Retina*. 4th ed. Philadelphia, PA: Elsevier Mosby; 2006:2383-2384.
36. Ehlers JP, Shah CP, eds. *The Wills Eye Manual*. 5th ed. Baltimore, MD: Lippincott Williams and Wilkins; 2008:30-34.
37. Steinspar K. Treatment of traumatic optic neuropathy with high-dose corticosteroids. *J Neuro Ophthalmol*. 2006; 26:65-67.

CHAPTER 26 ■ BLUNT AND PENETRATING NECK INJURY

JOSEPH DUBOSE AND THOMAS M. SCALEA

The complex anatomical relationships within a small area make the diagnosis and management of both penetrating neck injuries (PNI) and blunt neck injuries (BNI) challenging. Radiographic evaluation continues to evolve, with a shift from invasive to noninvasive diagnostics. Despite advances in both diagnosis and therapeutics, the optimal management of neck injuries remains a matter of active investigation.

PENETRATING INJURIES

Epidemiology

Firearms are responsible for approximately 43%, stab wounds for 40%, shotguns for 4%, and other weapons for 12% of all PNI.[1] Overall, about 35% of all gunshot wounds (GSW) and 20% of stab wounds (SW) to the neck cause major injuries, but only 16% of GSW and 10% SW require surgical therapy. Even though transcervical GSWs cause major injuries in 73% of victims, only 21% require surgery.[2] The most common injury after PNI is vascular.[1,3] Spinal cord injuries and injuries to the aerodigestive tracts and various nerves are also common.[1]

Anatomical Zones

The neck can be divided into three anatomical zones for evaluation and therapeutic strategy purposes (Fig. 26.1). Zone I comprises the area between the clavicles and the cricoid cartilage. Criticial structures include the innominate vessels, the origin of the common carotid artery, the subclavian vessels and the vertebral artery, the brachial plexus, the trachea, the esophagus, the apex of the lung, and the thoracic duct. Surgical exposure in zone I can be difficult because of the presence of the clavicle and bony structures of the thoracic inlet. Zone II comprises the area between the cricoid cartilage and the angle of the mandible and contains the carotid and vertebral arteries, the internal jugular veins, trachea, and esophagus. This zone is more accessible to clinical exam and surgical exploration than the other zones. Zone III extends between the angle of the mandible and the base of the skull and includes the distal carotid and vertebral arteries and the pharynx. The proximity to the skull base makes zone III structures less amenable to physical exam and difficult to explore. Overall, zone II is the most commonly injured area (47%) after PNI, followed by zone III (19%) and I (18%).[4] In 16%, injuries will involve more than one zone.[1]

Airway Management

Approximately 8%–10% of patients with PNI present with airway compromise.[2,5–7] In patients with laryngotracheal injuries, about 30% require the establishment of a secure airway in the ED.[7] Airway compromise may be due to direct trauma, airway edema, or from external compression by a large hematoma. Small penetrating airway injuries by knife or low-velocity bullets are less likely to result in respiratory problems than laryngotracheal transections or high-velocity GSW.[1]

Air bubbling through a neck wound is pathognomonic of airway injury. Firm manual compression over the wound reduces the air leak and will usually improve oxygenation. Orotracheal intubation in the ED after PNI should be performed by the most experienced provider, recognizing the potential need for emergent surgical airway. The severity of respiratory distress, hemodynamics, the size and site of hematoma, presence of a large air leak, and the experience of the trauma team will determine the best technique. For patients with large neck hematomas who are not in respiratory distress, fibreoptic intubation may be safe. However, this procedure requires experience and skill and can be performed only semielectively; there is a reported failure rate of approximately 25%.[7]

The use of neuromuscular paralysis during intubation in the ED after PNI remains controversial. Orotracheal intubation without neuromuscular paralysis increases difficulty. Coughing or gagging worsens bleeding. However, pharmacologic paralysis may prove dangerous if the cords cannot be visualized secondary to distorted anatomy from a compressing hematoma or edema. Loss of the muscle tone after paralysis may further displace the airway, leading to total obstruction. In a recent review of PNIs, 21% required ED airway. In 12% of patients, orotracheal intubation failed, requiring emergent cricothyroidotomy.[8]

In the presence of large midline hematomas, cricothyroidotomy is difficult and may be associated with severe bleeding. Large laryngotracheal wounds can be intubated under direct view into the distal transected segment through the neck wound itself. The distal airway should be grasped with forceps before insertion of the tube to avoid complete tracheal transection or retraction into the mediastinum.

Initial Control of Hemorrhage

External bleeding due to PNI is controlled by direct pressure in most cases. However, bleeding from behind the clavicle, near the base of the skull, or from the vertebral artery is often difficult to control by external pressure. Digital compression with an index finger through the wound can help. Ballon tamponade techniques may also help.[2,9] A Foley catheter is inserted into the wound and advanced as far as possible without resistance. The balloon is then inflated until the bleeding stops or moderate resistance is felt. If the bleeding continues, the balloon is deflated, and the catheter is slightly withdrawn and reinflated. Substantial bleeding through the catheter is suggestive of distal bleeding and indicates the need for repositioning.

With periclavicular injuries, bleeding can occur into the thorax. In these cases, the Foley catheter is advanced into the chest through the wound, the balloon inflated, and the catheter pulled back until resistance is felt, compressing the bleeding vessels against the first rib or the clavicle. Traction is maintained with a clamp placed on the catheter just above the skin until operative exposure is obtained.[9] Blind clamping of bleeding is rarely successful and may cause vascular or nerve damage.

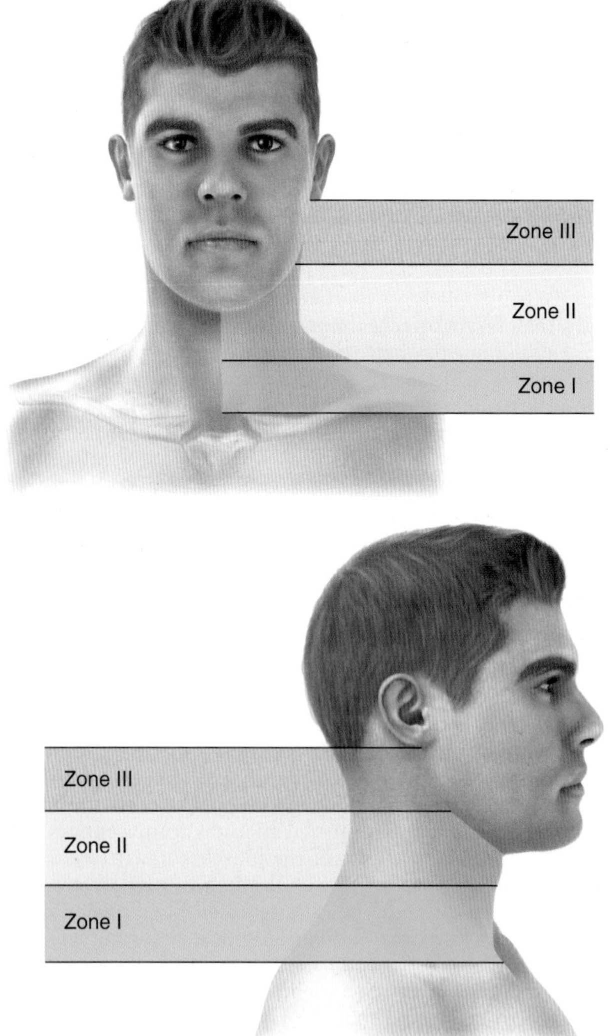

FIGURE 26.1. Surgical zones of the neck: zone I is between the clavicle and the cricoid, zone II between the cricoid and the angle of the mandible, and zone III is between the angle of the mandible and the base of the skull.

Initial Evaluation

Physical examination, preferably according to a written protocol (Algorithm. 26.1; Table 26.1), remains the most reliable initial diagnostic tool. Physical exam should be systematic and specifically directed to look for signs or symptoms of injuries to the vital structures. Signs can be classified into "hard" signs, which are pathognomonic of injury, and "soft" signs, which are suspicious but not diagnostic of injury[1,10] (Table 26.2). In GSW, the most common sign is a moderate or large hematoma (20.6%). Following SW, painful swallowing (14.3%) and hemo/pneumothorax (13.5%) are most common.[1] Subcutaneous emphysema occurs in about 7% of PNIs.[1] This may be secondary to laryngotracheal or esophageal injury or an associated pneumothorax. Only about 15% of patients with soft signs have substantive laryngotracheal injury.[1]

In one of the largest series of patients with PNI, patients with hard signs of vascular injury required operation as compared to about 3% with soft signs.[1] Of the patients with soft signs who underwent angiographic evaluation, 23.5% had an angiographic abnormality, but only 3% required operation.[1]

Evaluation for Nervous System Injuries

Although the diagnosis and management of spinal cord injuries are covered elsewhere in this text, the initial evaluation warrants mention. The clinical examination after PNI should include assessment of the Glasgow Coma Scale (GCS) score, localizing signs, pupils, cranial nerves (VII, IX-XII), spinal cord, brachial plexus (median, ulnar, radial, axillary, and musculocutaneous nerves), the phrenic nerve, and the sympathetic chain (Horner's syndrome). The GCS may be abnormal from ischemia secondary to a carotid injury or associated intracranial missile injury.

The Value of a Protocolized Approach to Physical Exam

A protocolized exam provides reliable identification of the majority of major injuries requiring therapeutic intervention.[1,4] In one large prospective study with predominantly SW to the neck, 80% was found to have no symptoms or signs suggestive of vascular or aerodigestive injuries and were selected for nonoperative management. Only two of the observed patients (0.7%) required semielective operation for vascular injuries. In both cases, a bruit was detected the day after admission, and angiography demonstrated an arteriovenous fistula.[4]

In another prospective study of predominantly GSW, 71.7% had no clinical signs suggestive of vascular injury. None of these patients required operation or other form of therapeutic treatment (negative predictive value [NPV] 100%). Angiography was performed on 127 of the asymptomatic patients from this series, revealing 11 vascular injuries (8.3%), but none required intervention. None of the patients without signs or symptoms of aerodigestive injuries had an injury requiring operation (NPV 100%).

For patients with soft signs of injury, including concerning wound proximity, additional investigations are warranted. The specific protocol will vary based on institutional capabilities. The utility and limitations of the respective possible investigations following PNI are outlined in the following sections.

INVESTIGATIONS

Plain Chest and Neck Films

Chest films should be obtained in all stable patients with penetrating injuries in zone I or any other wounds that might have violated the chest cavity. Approximately 16% of GSWs and 14% of stab wounds to the neck have an associated hemo/pneumothorax.[1] Other important radiological findings include a widened upper mediastinum suspicious for thoracic inlet vascular injury, subcutaneous emphysema, fractures, and missiles.

Angiography

Angiographic evaluation of the neck vessels following PNI once was standard.[10–12] However, angiography in asymptomatic patients is low yield and offers no benefit over physical exam combined with noninvasive investigations.[1,2,4,6,13–18] In a prospective study, asymptomatic patients were evaluated

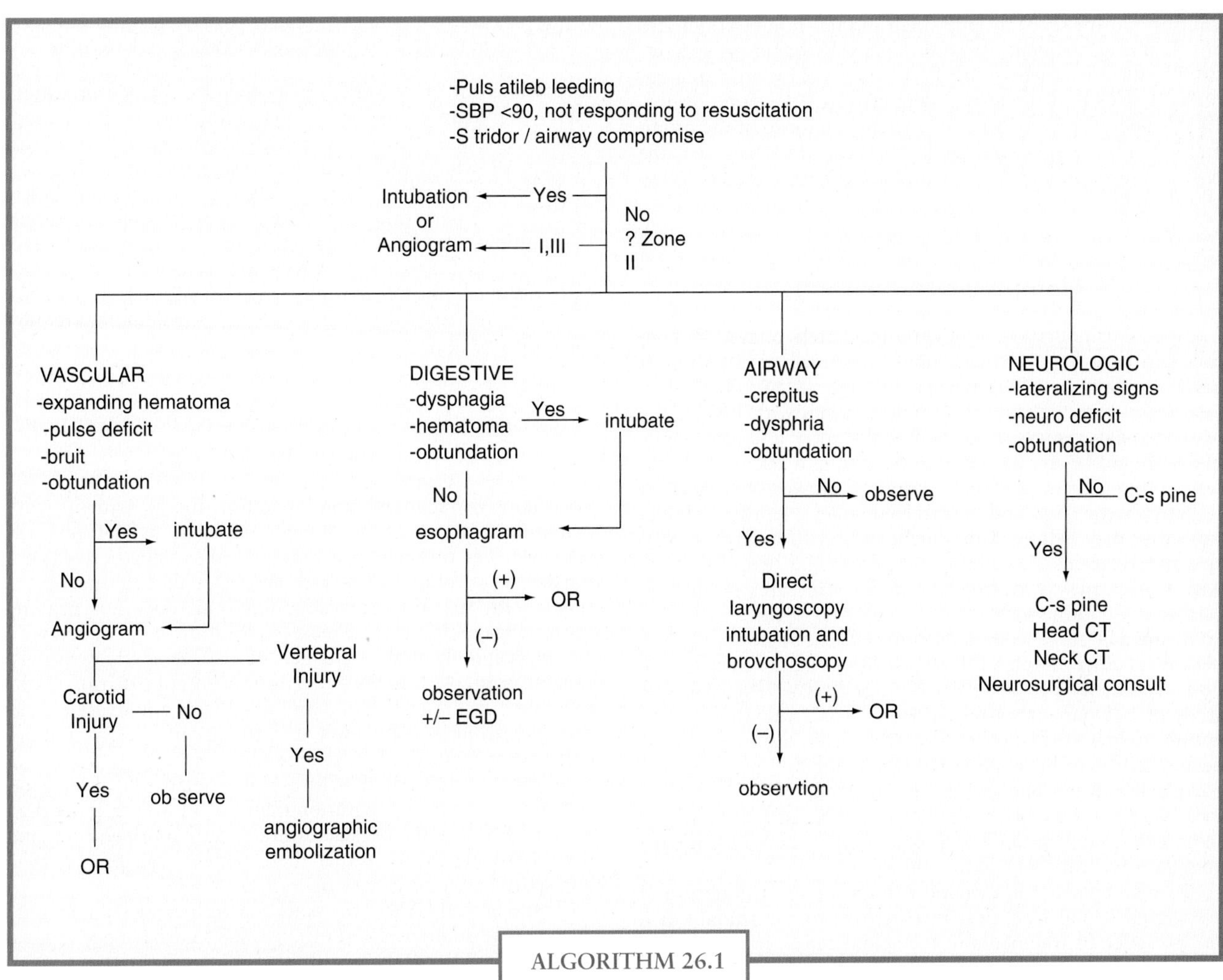

ALGORITHM 26.1 Protocol of examination and initial evaluation of penetrating neck injuries. (Modified from Demetriades D, Salim A, Brown C, et al. Neck injuries. *Curr Probl Surg*. 2007;44(1):13–85 with permission.)

angiographically at a cost of $254,000 and 11 vascular injuries not requiring treatment were identified. Additionally, the combination of clinical examination and Color Flow Doppler (CFD) in this series diagnosed all vascular injuries.[1] In another prospective study, 80% were selected for nonoperative management. Angiography was performed on only seven patients. There were no deaths or substantial complications. Early and late follow up demonstrated no substantial missed vascular injuries.[4]

TABLE 26.1

HARD AND SOFT SIGNS OF INJURY AFTER PENETRATING NECK TRAUMA

HARD SIGNS OF INJURY	SOFT SIGNS OF INJURY
Active arterial hemorrhage	Stable hematoma
Absent peripheral pulse on affected side	Trajectory
Expanding hematoma	Dysphagia
Air or saliva from wound	Pulse abnormality on affected side
Bruit	Nerve deficit
Hemoptysis	

Some studies have suggested that clinically occult, angiographically identified injuries have a benign prognosis and require no treatment.[19,20] There is, however, concern regarding the natural history of such lesions and adequacy of physical exam for their detection. Although the absence of hard clinical signs reliably excludes substantial injuries requiring treatment, the presence of soft signs of vascular injury does not reliably differentiate patients who require operation.[1,15] In one study, a subgroup of 34 patients with soft signs of vascular injury had angiography.[1] Eight (23.5%) had vascular injuries but only one (3%) needed intervention. Some form of imaging is needed to follow identified injuries. Several noninvasive modalities are alternatives.

Color Flow Doppler

CFD has been suggested as a reliable alternative to angiography in the evaluation for vascular injuries following PNI.[1,2,15,21–25] In a prospective study conducted by Demetriades et al., CFD diagnosed 10 of 11 angiographically detected injuries and missed only one small intimal injury, which did not require subsequent operation. In a subsequent prospective study with 25 patients with PNI evaluated by both angiography and CFD, Corr et al.[22] demonstrated the same results. CFD is operator-dependent and may miss injuries of the proximal left subclavian artery, the internal carotid artery near the base of the skull, and the vertebral artery under the bony vertebral canal.

Computed Tomography

Computed tomography (CT) with adequately phased IV contrast protocols has become a useful tool in the evaluation of PNI, especially in GSW, and has become the first line investigation in hemodynamically stable patients with PNI to the neck in many centers. Prior to CT, the entry and exit of the bullet should be marked with radioopaque markers. In addition, 3-mm CT cuts should be obtained between the markers or between the entry and the retained bullet. Identifying bullet trajectory may help in determining the need for further invasive investigations, such as angiography or endoscopy. Patients with trajectories away from the major structures require no further evaluation.[16,26–29]

Munera et al.[27,28] compared conventional angiography and helical CT angiography. CT angiography had a sensitivity of 90%, specificity 100%, PPV 100%, and NPV 98%. Another study of 175 patients also suggested CT is a valuable investigation for the evaluation of suspected arterial injuries of the neck.[28] CT may have some important limitations, however, particularly when images are obscured due to artifact from metallic fragments or excessive air in the soft tissues.[29] In these cases, conventional angiography may be necessary for adequate exclusion of vascular injury.

CT also provides information about the site and nature of associated spinal fractures, involvement of the spinal cord, the presence of fragments in the spinal canal, or hematoma compressing the cord. A brain CT scan is also indicated for patients with PNI and unexplained central neurological deficits. In these instances, CT should be used to evaluate for possible anemic infarction secondary to a carotid artery injury or an associated direct brain injury due to a missile fragment.

Esophageal Studies

Esophageal studies are indicated in stable patients with soft signs and in cases with a CT scan bullet trajectory near the esophagus. Contrast esophagography is commonly used but may miss small injuries. Armstrong et al.[30] reported that contrast esophagography diagnosed only 62% of perforations, compared to100% with rigid esophagoscopy. The technique of esophagography may be important to minimize false-negative studies. Esophagography should first be performed with a water-soluble contrast, such a gastrographin. If no leak is identified, the study is repeated with thin barium, as gastrographin alone may miss small injuries.[31]

Esophagoscopy, if performed by an experienced endoscopist, may also be useful. Flexible endoscopy has been shown to have a NPV of 100% but a positive predictive value of only 33%.[32,33] This is the study of choice in many centers for patients who cannot undergo esophagogram because of a depressed level of consciousness or during intraoperative evaluations. Rigid esophagoscopy may be superior to flexible endoscopy in the evaluation of the upper esophagus, but requires general anesthesia, and many surgeons are not experienced with the technique.[34]

Studies for Laryngotracheal Evaluation

Indications for laryngotracheal evaluation include proximity injury, soft signs suspicious of airway injuries (minor hemoptysis, hoarseness, and subcutaneous emphysema) or CT scan findings showing a bullet tract near the larynx or trachea.

Flexible fibreoptic endoscopy is the investigation of choice, and it can be performed in the ED. The most common abnormal findings are blood or edema in the laryngotracheal tract and vocal cord dyskinesia.[1] GSWs are more likely to be associated with abnormal findings than SW (24.6% vs. 8.5%). However, only 20% of patients with abnormal findings require operation.[1,34]

Operative versus Nonoperative Management of Penetrating Injuries

For many years, mandatory operation for all patients with penetrating injuries of the neck that violated the platysma was standard. The rationale was that clinical examination was not reliable. In addition, it has been suggested that routine operation avoids expensive investigations and does not prolong hospital stay.[35] Routine surgical exploration is associated with an unacceptably high incidence of unnecessary operations, ranging from 30% to 89%.[35,36] Improved appreciation of the reliability of physical exam, combined with noninvasive diagnostic capabilities, has resulted in the use of selective nonoperative management at most centers.[1,4,14,15,19,37,38]

GSWs are associated with a higher incidence of substantial injuries requiring operation than SW. However, more than 80% of GSW to the neck does not require an operation, and there is strong evidence that these patients can be identified and spared an unnecessary operation.[1,4,6,15,39,40]

Transcervical GSWs are associated with a much higher incidence of substantial injuries than GSW that have not crossed the midline (73% vs. 31%).[15] It has been suggested that all such patients undergo exploration, irrespective of clinical exam.[41] However, many of these injuries, such as spinal cord or nerve injuries, do not require operation. In one prospective study of transcervical GSW, 73% of patients had injuries to vital structures, but only 21% required operation.[15,34] Several studies have demonstrated that CT angio with thin cuts can reliably identify those patients who do not need further investigation or those who might benefit from specific studies.[16,17,29–32,42]

BLUNT INJURIES

Although physical exam and initial management priorities for BNI are much the same as for penetrating injuries, a knowledge of the differences in injury patterns is essential for prompt diagnosis and management. We will focus on BNI causing laryngotracheal, pharyngoesophageal, and vascular trauma.

Epidemiology

Although BNI is common, when cervical spine injuries are excluded, injuries to the remaining structures are rare. Injuries to the aerodigestive tract are typically from direct force to the anterior neck.[43,44] Both laryngotracheal and pharyngoesophageal are rare after BNI, occurring in 0.04%–0.3% of patients.[45,46] Similarly uncommon, but far more lethal, are blunt cerebrovacsular injuries, including injury to the vertebral and carotid arteries. With increased appreciation and availability of noninvasive diagnostics, the rates of these injuries are now between 1.0% and 2.0%.[47–54]

INVESTIGATIONS

Plain Radiographs

Plain x-rays of the neck and chest are a rapid noninvasive method of evaluating patients with suspected BNI. Cervical or mediastinal emphysema has been reported in as many as 95% of aerodigestive injuries. Cervical spine fractures are a risk factor for blunt cervical vascular injury.[47,50] In particular, vertebral artery injuries are associated with complex cervical spine fractures with subluxation, extension into the foramen transversarium, or fractures to the higher cervical vertebrae.[48]

CT and Oral Contrast Studies

CT is the cornerstone of initial imaging for blunt trauma patients. Though aerodigestive injuries are best visualized with panendoscopy, CT and contrast studies may help patients with a high suspicion of injury. For laryngotracheal injuries, CT is more sensitive than plain radiographs in identifying cervical emphysema. CT also identifies small amounts of cervical air or contained leak after pharyngoesophageal injury. Gastrograffin or barium swallow will reveal an abnormality in 75%–100% of cases of cervical esophageal perforation.[55]

At many trauma centers, CT angiography has emerged as the initial screening test of choice for blunt carotid and vertebral injuries.[53,56–61] However, there remain conflicting results as to the utility of CT angiography after BNI. Berne et al.[59] found CT angiography to have a sensitivity of 100% and specificity of 94% when screening patients for blunt cerebrovascular injuries (BCVIs). In contrast, Biffl et al.[51] found the sensitivity and specificity for CT angiography to be 68% and 67%, respectively. Further studies are needed directly comparing conventional angiography and CT angiography.

Color Flow Doppler

CFD after BNI may help identify dissections, thrombosis, or pseudoaneurysms of the carotid and vertebral arteries. Its limited visualization of the distal carotid arteries and the portions of the vertebral arteries protected by the cervical spine can be a problem. In a multicenter trial, Cogbill et al.[62] demonsrated that duplex was able to identify 86% of injuries.Likewise, both Fry et al.[21] and DiPerna et al.[63] found that CFD did not miss a substantial carotid injury in patients with BNI. Both these studies, however, consisted of a limited number of patients.

Angiography

In the past, four-vessel angiography was the mainstay of diagnosis of vascular injuries in the neck. The indications remain controversial. Cothren et al.[47] recommend four-vessel angiography for all patients with signs or symptoms of cerebrovascular injury on clinical exam as well as high-risk mechanisms and any of the following: severe facial or cervical spine fracture, basilar skull fracture with carotid canal involvement, near-hanging injury with anoxia, and diffuse axonal injury with depressed mental status.

Endoscopy

Endoscopy is useful to evaluate suspected aerodigestive injury after BNI. Though both rigid and flexible endoscopies are options, flexible endoscopy does not require general anesthesia and can be performed while maintaining cervical spine immobilization in a collar. For laryngotracheal injuries, the combination of flexible laryngoscopy and bronchoscopy can be used to rule out an airway injury. Injuries to the pharynx and cervical esophagus may be difficult to visualize due to blood in the pharyngeal space. If the area of interest cannot be visualized clearly or if there is any suspicion of an esophageal injury, the patient should have a contrast swallow.

SPECIFIC NECK INJURIES

Cerebrovascular Injuries

BCVIs were previously thought to be rare. Increased screening has revealed an incidence ranging from 1% to 2% after trauma.[47,49,50,56,57] While controversy remains regarding patients at risk, failure to identify and treat these lesions may result in mortality between 25% and 59% of patients.[50,51,62,64,65]

Clinical Presentation

Many patients die before reaching a hospital or present to the ED in cardiac arrest. Those surviving to reach the hospital may be completely asymptomatic have subtle findings or active arterial hemorrhage, neck hematoma, and hemodynamic instability. Associated injuries may mask BCVI, but they should be suspected in any patient with a suspicious exam (such as the seatbelt sign; Fig. 26.2), concerning mechanism, or neurologic deficits or deterioration not explained by head CT.

Many patients initially with vascular injury are asymptomatic only to develop symptoms hours to days later, missing the window for intervention. In 1996, Fabian et al.[65] found an average time to diagnosis of 53 hours, with a range of 2–672 hours. The majority (78%) developed neurologic deficits prior to diagnosis. After initiating screening criteria, they demonstrated reduced the mean time to diagnosis of 20 hours, with 38% of injuries diagnosed based on the screening criteria alone. Only 34% of patients developed ischemic symptoms before diagnosis.[66]

Management of Cerebrovacular Injuries

Carotid repair and/or reconstruction is indicated for most patients with PNI. Optimal treatment of patients with coma or dense contralateral neurologic deficits is less clear. While some earlier reports warned against revascularization in the presence of neurologic deficits due to the concern of converting an ischemic infarct to a hemorrhagic infarct,[67] subsequent studies support that the best chance for neurologic improvement is early revascularization.[68] However, patients with coma (>4 hours) have an extremely poor prognosis regardless of treatment, and revascularization often exacerbates cerebral edema and intracranial hypertension.[69,70] In these patients, one should procede with revascularization only if there is no infarct present on CT.[71]

Most blunt carotid injuries occur at the base of the skull, making them inaccessible by standard neck incision. Options include observation, anticoagulation, antiplatelet therapy, endovascular stenting and operation. Biffl et al.[51,52] developed a widely used grading scale that can be used to make treatment decisions (Algorithm. 26.2). These investigators found that grade I injuries healed in the majority of cases with or without anticoagulation. Only 10% of grade II injuries healed with anticoagulation, with the majority (60%) progressing to grade III lesions (pseudoaneurysms) on repeat angiography. Almost all grade III lesions (85%) remained unchanged, with 1 of 13 healing with the use of IV heparin. No grade III lesion healed without treatment.

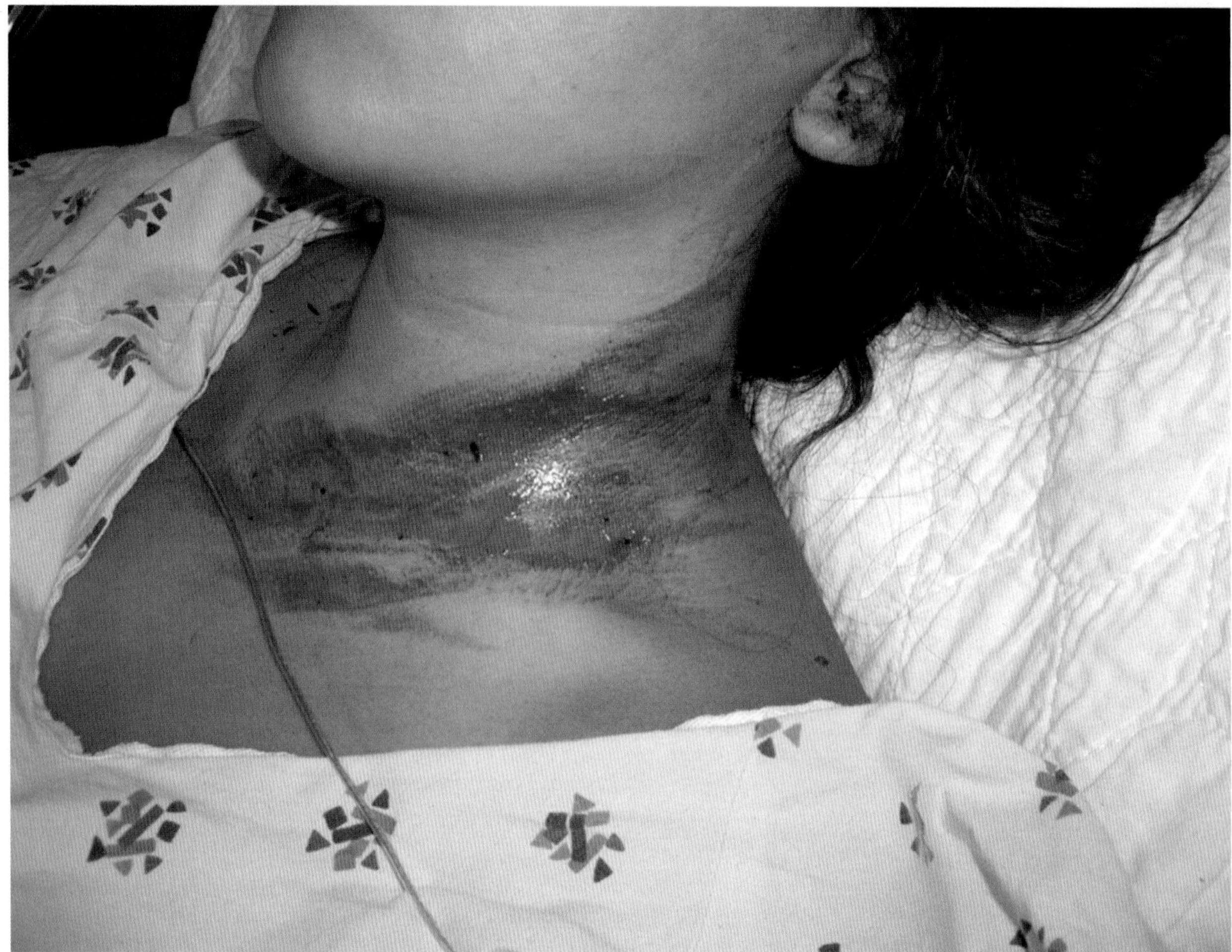

FIGURE 26.2. "Seatbelt Sign" after motor vehicle accident.

Endovascular stents were used to treat the majority of persistent grade III lesions, with an 89% initial success rate. Grade IV injuries (occlusion) remained unchanged despite anticoagulation but none of the patients treated with heparin developed a stroke. Grade V injuries were uniformly fatal in this series, despite attempts at angiographic embolization in two of the four patients. The authors also suggested categorizing arteriovenous or carotid-cavernous fistulae as grade II or grade.

Angiographic embolization, balloon occlusion or angioplasty, or stents may be used as a temporizing bridge to surgical repair for definitive treatment. Angiography with possible endovascular intervention should be considered in (1) hemodynamically stable patients with either physical exam or radiographic evidence of a distal internal carotid artery injury, (2) stable patients with evidence of an arteriovenous or carotid–cavernous sinus fistula, (3) ongoing facial or intraoral hemorrhage from external carotid branches, and (4) small intimal defects or pseudoaneuryms in surgically inaccessible locations or high-risk surgical candidates. Stents/grafts may be particularly useful for patients with post-traumatic false aneurysms, arteriovenous fistulae, or arterial stenosis. Expanding experience with the use of interventional techniques for arterial injury is likely to better elucidate the optimal indications, timing, techniques, and outcomes.[72]

There is class III evidence that systemic anticoagulation or antiplatelet therapy improves survival and neurological outcome after blunt carotid injury.[65,66] Although anticoagulation may be more effective in carotid dissection than pseudoaneurysms.[73] Some studies, however, failed to show any obvious benefit from systemic heparin.[74]

A recent study conducted at our own institution by Stein et al.[49] highlighted the difficulties with any approach to therapy for BCVI as nearly one-third of patients were not candidates for therapy. While treatment reduced the risk of infarction, strokes that did occur were not preventable. In the absence of prospective, randomized data regarding treatment, management decisions must be based on the injury pattern, associated injuries, clinical condition of the patient, and the currently available literature. The algorithm for our present management approach of BCVI at R Adams Cowley Shock Trauma Center is shown in Figure 26.3 and Algorithm 26.2.

Operative Management—Carotid Injuries

The patient is placed in slight Trendelenburg with neck extended and the head rotated away from the side of injury. The patient should be prepped from the chin down to the knees in anticipating the need for a thoracic incision or saphenous vein harvest.

The most common incision for exposure of the unilateral carotid artery is a vertical oblique incision made over the anterior border of the sternocleidomastoid muscle (SCM), from the angle of the mandible to the sternoclavicular joint. Retracting the SCM laterally will expose the internal jugular vein, with the carotid artery lying medial and deep to the vein. The vagus nerve is located in the posterior carotid sheath. Division of the facial vein exposes the carotid bifurcation and allows mobilization and control of the internal and external carotids. Simple lacerations of the internal jugular vein or external carotid artery may be repaired, but, in most cases, veins can be ligated without sequla.

Cerebrovascular Injury Grades

Grade I	Luminal irregularity or dissection / intraluminal hematoma with <25% luminal narrowing
Grade II	Dissection or intraluminal hematoma of ≥ 25% of the lumen
Grade IIa	Dissection or intraluminal hematoma of 25-50% of the lumen
Grade IIb	Dissection or intraluminal hematoma of ≥ 50% of the lumen or intimal flap
Grade III	Pseudoaneurysm
Grade IV	Vessel occlusion
Grade V	Vessel transection

FIGURE 26.3. Grading scale for cerebrovascular injuries.

Some zone I injuries may be controlled and repaired through a cervical incision, but proximal zone I injuries may require extension inferiorly into a median sternotomy. Mobilization and superior retraction of the brachiocephalic veins will expose the aortic arch, brachiocephalic artery, and proximal common carotid arteries. Care should be taken to avoid the recurrent laryngeal nerves ascending posterior to the vessels.

Zone III carotid injuries are the most difficult to expose and get distal control. The cervical incision should be extended superiorly into the posterior auricular area and the digastric muscle divided, avoiding injury to the hypoglossal, glossopharyngeal, and facial nerves. Anterior subluxation of the mandible, further improved by mandibular osteotomy, excision of the styloid process, and removal of the anterior clinoid process improve exposure (Fig. 26.4). Temporary control of uncontrolled zone I or III hemorrhage may be obtained by insertion of an embolectomy catheter through the arterial defect or an arteriotomy and inflation of the balloon.

Most external carotid injuries may be ligated without consequence. Ligation of the common or internal carotid artery can result in devastating neurologic sequelae if collaterals are inadequate. Carotid ligation should be reserved for patients in whom repair is not technically possible, such as injuries at the base of the skull or patients with an established anemic cerebral infarction. In unstable patients, placement of a temporary intraluminal shunt and delayed reconstruction is an option.

Intravenous heparin should be administered if there are no other sites of hemorrhage or intracranial injury, preferably before clamping the artery. Alternatively, local administration of heparin at the site of injury may be used. Adequate collateral flow may not be present. Use of an intraluminal shunt to provide antegrade flow in complex repairs requiring a graft may be wise. Small lacerations may be primarily repaired using an interrupted or running suture after adequate debridement of wound edges. If primary repair is not possible, then a vein or prosthetic patch plasty of the defect is performed. Clean transections, such as stab wounds, may be repaired by mobilization of the proximal and distal artery and primary end-to-end anastomosis if this can be achieved without stenosis or tension.

Many carotid injuries, particularly from GSW, are not amenable to primary repair or anastomosis after debridement. Reconstruction with either a vein or prosthetic interposition graft is needed. Saphenous vein is preferred for internal carotid artery reconstruction, with some evidence of improved patency and lower infection rates compared to prosthetic graft.[75,76] Alternatively, reconstruction of the proximal internal carotid may be performed by transecting the proximal external carotid artery and transposing it to the distal transected internal carotid (Fig. 26.5).

Common carotid artery injuries are best repaired using a thin-walled polytetrafluoroethylene graft, which has a better size match with the native artery and excellent long-term patency. An intraluminal shunt may be used here as well. If associated injuries to the aerodigestive tract have been repaired, well-vascularized tissue such as a SCM flap should be placed between the repairs.[77]

If the injury or dissection extends into the distal internal carotid artery (zone III), exposure and repair are substantially more difficult. Ligation or catheter-assisted thrombosis of the injured vessel should be considered in the asymptomatic patient or if the appropriate expertise is not available to perform distal revascularization. Extra-cranial to intracranial carotid bypass may be performed, but requires substantial exposure of the intracranial carotid artery. Alternatively, saphenous vein bypass from the proximal internal carotid to the petrous carotid artery or middle cerebral artery has been reported. This technique avoids intracranial dissection of the carotid artery and has been associated with excellent associated long-term outcome and graft patency.[75,78]

Operative Management—Vertebral Arteries

Operative management is almost always necessary when there is severe active bleeding from the vertebral artery. The head is turned away from the injured site and the neck is slightly extended. A generous incision is made on the anterior border of the SCM. The fascia is incised and the SCM retracted laterally. The omohyoid muscle is divided, and the carotid sheath is exposed and retracted while the midline structures are retracted medially. A tissue plane anterior to the prevertebral muscles is opened, taking care to avoid the ganglia of the cervical sympathetic chain. Next the anterior longitudinal ligament is incised longitudinally. The transverse processes are palpated, and the overlying longus coli and the longissiuns capitis muscle should be mobilized laterally with a periosteal elevator (Fig. 26.6). The anterior aspect of the vertebral foramen is then best removed with rongeurs to expose the underlying vertebral artery. The artery can then be ligated. The cervical roots are just behind the artery, and care should be taken not to injure them. Blind clamping or clipping should be avoided. Although the artery can be identified between the transverse processes, this is technically challenging. In addition, the venous plexuses can be troublesome.

Another option for rapid control of the proximal vertebral artery is to approach it at the base of the neck where it comes off the subclavian artery. One method is to extend the incision toward the clavicle and transect the SCM off the clavicle, retract the subclavian vein caudal, and transect or retract the anterior scalene muscle laterally. The first portion of the subclavian artery is medial, and it gives off the vertebral artery, the thyrocervical trunk, and the internal mammary muscle.

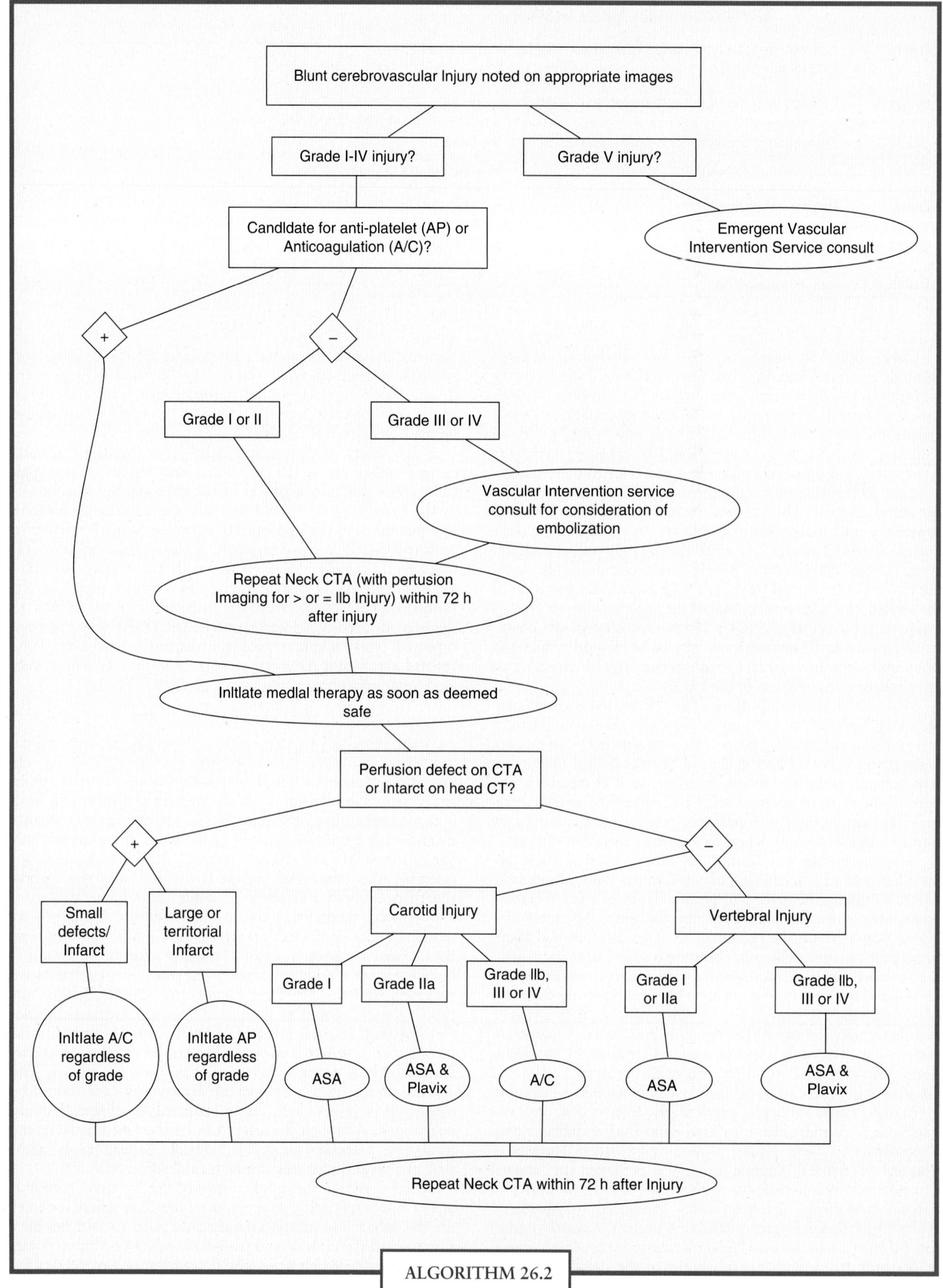

ALGORITHM 26.2 Initial management algorithm for blunt cerebrovascular injury at R Adams Cowley Shock Trauma Center.

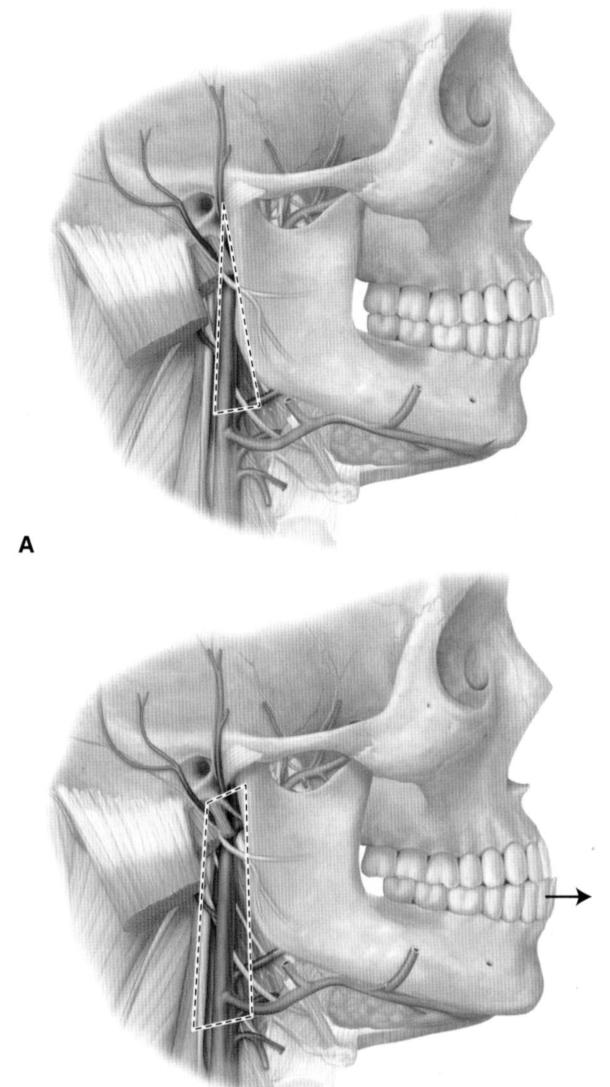

FIGURE 26.4. Exposure of Zone III carotid injuries.

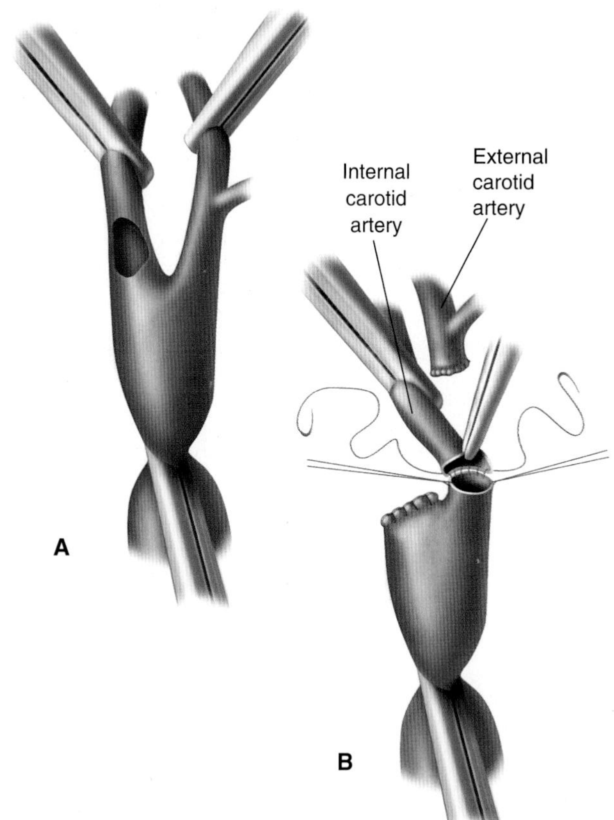

FIGURE 26.5. Reconstruction of the proximal internal carotid by transecting the proximal external carotid artery and transposing it to the distal transected internal carotid.

The vertebral artery comes off the dorsosuperior aspect of the ascending subclavian artery. When approaching the left vertebral artery, care should be taken not to injure the thoracic duct. The second method is to cut down directly on the clavicle and open the periostium. The clavicle can be disarticulated at the sternal boarder and resected with towel clamps as a handle. This can be a rapid way of identifying the artery. Repair of the vertebral artery is extremely difficult and is not usually attempted. The collaterals are usually sufficient to not cause an ischemic stroke. When dealing with an active bleeding vertebral artery and obtaining vascular control is difficult, packing is an option if bleeding can be controlled in this manner.[79]

LARYNGOTRACHEAL INJURIES

Injuries to the larynx and trachea are uncommon. The risk of airway compromise makes prompt diagnosis and intervention mandatory. Although certain injuries to the larynx and trachea may be managed nonoperatively, most require early operation.

Epidemiology

Laryngotracheal injuries account for 1 in 30,000 ED visits.[80] The incidence varies between 2% and 4% in patients with PNI. Blunt trauma to the neck is an uncommon cause of laryngotracheal injury, accounting for <1% of blunt trauma admissions.[46] In a large review, laryngotracheal injuries were found in only 0.34% patients.[34] Direct blows to the anterior neck, decelereation injuries such as in high-speed traffic accidents, and anteroposterior crushing injuries to the chest with in a sudden increase of the intratracheal pressure against a closed glottis can also cause these injuries.

Clinical Presentation

Laryngotracheal injuries vary from subtle disorders of the vocal cord to lacerations and fractures of the larygotracheal skeleton. Presentation varies from dysphonia to stridor and impending airway obstruction. In awake patients, careful clinical examination can reliably diagnose or exclude injuries. In the absence of any suspicious clinical findings, it is unlikely that a substantial injury exists. In a prospective study of 223 patients with penetrating trauma, 152 patients were awake, alert, and had no symptoms of aerodigestive tract injuries. None of these patients had injury requiring treatment.[1]

Air bubbling through a penetrating neck wound is the only hard sign diagnostic of laryngotracheal trauma. This finding is confirmed by asking the patient to cough. Other signs

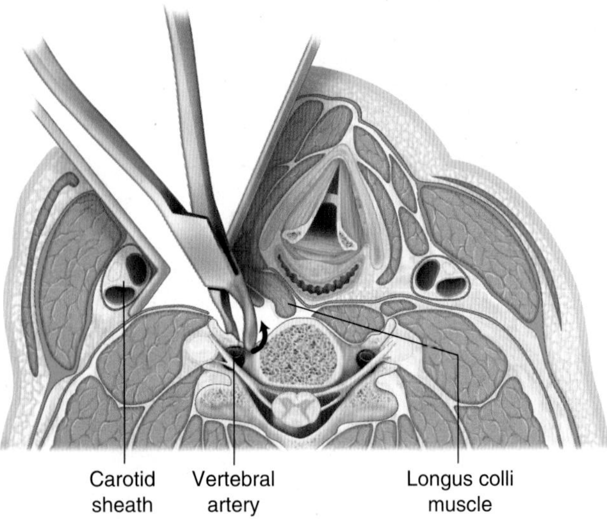

FIGURE 26.6. Vertebral artery exposure.

and symptoms seen with both blunt and penetrating injuries include subcutaneous emphysema, hemoptysis, odynophagia, hoarseness, and dyspnea.[34,46,80] Tenderness on palpation, cervical ecchymosis, or hematoma suggests laryngotracheal injury in BNI.[43] Though rare, cricotracheal separation may present with a triad of cervical ecchymosis, aphonia, and subcutaneous emphysema.[44]

MANAGEMENT

Nonoperative Management

Patients with minimal intralaryngeal injuries, nondisplaced fractures of the laryngotracheal skeleton, minor mucosal lacerations, and lacerations of the trachea less than one-third the circumference can safely be managed nonoperatively.[34,44] In penetrating trauma, small tracheal wounds with no tissue loss and well opposed edges on endoscopy can be safely observed.[81] In one prospective study, 80% of patients with abnormal endoscopic findings were successfully managed nonoperatively.[1]

Nonoperative management requires close observation and serial endoscopies. The role of steroids or prophylactic antibiotics is controversial, as is the use of prophylactic antibiotics. With nonoperative management of appropriate injuries, good results in terms of voice quality and airway patency are expected.

Operative Management

A collar incision, approximately 2 cm above the sternal notch, gives the best exposure to the larynx. Patients with substantial endolaryngeal injuries require a midline thyrotomy. For patients with proximal tracheal injuries, a transverse collar or an anterior sternocleidomastoid incision is appropriate. For more distal tracheal injuries, a partial sternal split exposes virtually all injuries not requiring a thoracic approach. For injuries in the distal third of the trachea, or injuries at the carina, a right posterolateral thoracotomy is preferred. Small tracheal wounds are primarily repaired with interrupted 3–0 synthetic absorbable sutures. Prophylactic tracheostomy in these simple repairs is generally not necesary and may increase infection-related morbidity.[82]

More complex and extensive tracheal injuries require individualized surgical technique. It is essential to achieve a tension-free, well-vascularized, mucosa-to-mucosa anastamosis. The blood supply to the trachea runs in the lateral aspects, so that mobilization should be performed by anterior and/or posterior dissection. If the total length of damaged or debrided trachea is less than 2 or 3 cm, reapproximation of the free edges with interrupted absorbable suture without tension is feasible. For larger defects, more complicated release maneuvers may be necessary. Thyroid or suprahyoid release, with flexion of the neck, can provide up to 6 cm of further mobilization. Flexion of the neck is then maintained for 1 week postoperatively by securing the chin to the presternal skin. Retention submucosal sutures can also reduce anastomotic tension. When wound closure cannot be achieved because of extensive defects, musculofascial flaps or synthetic material can be used. Tracheostomy alone is reserved for large anterior wounds or in cases in which instability prohibits prolonged surgical explorations, and tracheal reconstruction is postponed for a later time.

PHARYNGOESOPHAGEAL INJURIES

Pharyngoesophageal injuries are rare. A multicenter study involving 34 trauma centers over a 10.5-year period only identified 229 patients with cervical esophageal injuries.[83] Pharyngoesophageal injuries are not immediately life threatening, and so associated injuries often take higher priority. The first and most urgent priority is to ensure adequate airway. While there are no "hard" signs, diagnostic of pharyngoesophageal injuries, "soft" signs include odynophagia, subcutaneous emphysema, or hematemesis or hemoptysis. These symptoms are present in about 23% of patients PNI, and they are not specific.[34] Only about 18% of patients with these findings have pharyngoesophageal injury.[1] Absence of these findings, combined with the absence of subcutaneous emphysema on radiologic evaluation, makes it highly unlikely that the patient has an injury requiring treatment.

Operative Management

Early surgical repair of esophageal injuries reduces septic complications and leaks. Velmahos et al.[84] showed no deaths occurred among patients treated within 24 hours, whereas with delayed (more than 24 hours) treatment, 36% died due to uncontrollable sepsis. Others have also reported that deaths were all associated with delayed repair.[85]

A sternomastoid or transverse incision provides good exposure to the pharynx and cervical esophagus. The SCM retracted laterally, and the omohyoid muscle either retracted or divided. The carotid sheath is retracted laterally while the trachea and thyroid are retracted medially. The inferior thyroid artery and middle thyroid vein may be divided. Care should be taken to avoid injury to the recurrent laryngeal nerves located in the tracheoesophageal groove. Identification of this nerve is important if circumferential mobilization of the esophagus is needed.

A nasogastric tube or foley catheter inserted into the posterior pharynx can be insufflated with air to look for bubbling to identify small injuries. An alternative is to infuse fluid such as methylene blue but this risks aspiration even with the endotracheal tube in place. During the insufflation, the distal esophagus should be manually compressed. Injuries can be repaired in one layer with absorbable suture or two layers with absorable sutures followed by a nonabsorbable layer. For SW, debridement is usually not necessary but it usually is for GSW. The strap muscles are placed between the trachea and vascular injuries if possible. The wound is closed over a drain.

In neglected injuries requiring debridement, T-tube drainage is an option.[86,87] This converts the injury to a controlled fistula. Esophagectomy in the acute setting is rare, and external diversion or exclusion is usually reserved for injuries with infection and abscess due to late presentation.

References

1. Demetriades D, Theodorou D, Cornwell E, et al. Evaluation of penetrating injuries of the neck: Prospective study of 223 patients. *World J Surg.* 1997;21(1):41-47; discussion 47-48.
2. Demetriades D, Theodorou D, Cornwell E, et al. Transcervical gunshot injuries: Mandatory operation is not necessary. *J Trauma* 1996;40(5):758-760.
3. Danic D, Prgomet D, Milicic D, Leovic D, Puntaric D. War injuries to the head and neck. *Mil Med.* 1998;163(2):117-119.
4. Demetriades D, Charalambides D, Lakhoo M. Physical examination and selective conservative management in patients with penetrating injuries of the neck. *Br J Surg.* 1993;80(12):1534-1536.
5. Pate JW. Tracheobronchial and esophageal injuries. *Surg Clin North Am.* 1989;69(1):111-123.
6. Demetriades D, Asensio JA, Velmahos G, et al. Complex problems in penetrating neck trauma. *Surg Clin North Am.* 1996;76(4):661-683.
7. Mandavia DP, Qualls S, Rokos I. Emergency airway management in penetrating neck injury. *Ann Emerg Med.* 2000;35(3):221-225.
8. Vassiliu P, Baker J, Henderson S, et al. Aerodigestive injuries of the neck. *Am Surg.* 2001;67(1):75-79.
9. Gilroy D, Lakhoo M, Charalambides D, et al. Control of life-threatening haemorrhage from the neck: a new indication for balloon tamponade. *Injury.* 1992;23(8):557-559.
10. Sclafani SJ, Cavaliere G, Atweh N, et al. The role of angiography in penetrating neck trauma. *J Trauma.* 1991;31(4):557-562; discussion 562-563.
11. Hiatt JR, Busuttil RW, Wilson SE. Impact of routine arteriography on management of penetrating neck injuries. *J Vasc Surg.* 1984;1(6):860-866.
12. Weigelt JA, Thal ER, Snyder WH III, et al. Diagnosis of penetrating cervical esophageal injuries. *Am J Surg.* 1987;154(6):619-622.
13. Beitsch P, Weigelt JA, Flynn E, et al. Physical examination and arteriography in patients with penetrating zone II neck wounds. *Arch Surg.* 1994;129(6):577-581.
14. Eddy VA. Is routine arteriography mandatory for penetrating injury to zone 1 of the neck? Zone 1 penetrating neck injury study group. *J Trauma.* 2000;48(2):208-213; discussion 213-214.
15. Demetriades D, Theodorou D, Cornwell E III, et al. Penetrating injuries of the neck in patients in stable condition. Physical examination, angiography, or color flow doppler imaging. *Arch Surg.* 1995;130(9):971-975.
16. Inaba K, Munera F, McKenney M, et al. Prospective evaluation of screening multislice helical computed tomographic angiography in the initial evaluation of penetrating neck injuries. *J Trauma.* 2006;61(1):144-149.
17. Osborn TM, Bell RB, Qaisi W, et al. Computed tomographic angiography as an aid to clinical decision making in the selective management of penetrating injuries to the neck: a reduction in the need for operative exploration. *J Trauma* 2008;64(6):1466-1471.
18. Schroeder JW, Baskaran V, Aygun N. Imaging of traumatic arterial injuries in the neck with an emphasis on CTA. *Emergy Radiol.* 2010;17:109-122.
19. Stain SC, Yellin AE, Weaver FA, Pentecost MJ. Selective management of nonocclusive arterial injuries. *Arch Surg.* 1989;124(10):1136-1140; discussion 1140-1141.
20. Frykberg ER, Crump JM, Vines FS, et al. A reassessment of the role of arteriography in penetrating proximity extremity trauma: a prospective study. *J Trauma.* 1989;29(8):1041-1050; discussion 1050-1052.
21. Fry WR, Dort JA, Smith RS, et al. Duplex scanning replaces arteriography and operative exploration in the diagnosis of potential cervical vascular injury. *Am J Surg.* 1994;168(6):693-695; discussion 695-696.
22. Corr P, Abdool Carrim AT, Robbs J. Colour-flow ultrasound in the detection of penetrating vascular injuries of the neck. *S Afr Med J.* 1999;89(6):644-646.
23. Montalvo BM, LeBlang SD, Nunez DB Jr, et al. Color Doppler sonography in penetrating injuries of the neck. *AJNR Am J Neuroradiol.* 1996;17(5):943-951.
24. Ginzburg E, Montalvo B, LeBlang S, et al. The use of duplex ultrasonography in penetrating neck trauma. *Arch Surg.* 1996;131(7):691-693.
25. Kuzniec S, Kauffman P, Molnar LJ, et al. Diagnosis of limbs and neck arterial trauma using duplex ultrasonography. *Cardiovasc Surg.* 1998;6(4):358-366.
26. Gracias VH, Reilly PM, Philpott J, et al. Computed tomography in the evaluation of penetrating neck trauma: a preliminary study. *Arch Surg.* 2001;136(11):1231-1235.
27. Munera F, Soto JA, Palacio D, et al. Diagnosis of arterial injuries caused by penetrating trauma to the neck: comparison of helical CT angiography and conventional angiography. *Radiology.* 2000;216(2):356-362.
28. Munera F, Soto JA, Palacio DM, et al. Penetrating neck injuries: helical CT angiography for initial evaluation. *Radiology.* 2002;224(2):366-372.
29. Nunez DB Jr, Torres-Leon M, Munera F. Vascular injuries of the neck and thoracic inlet: Helical CT-angiographic correlation. *Radiographics.* 2004;24(4):1087-1098; discussion 1099-1100.
30. Armstrong WB, Detar TR, Stanley RB. Diagnosis and management of external penetrating cervical esophageal injuries. *Ann Otol Rhinol Laryngol.* 1994;103(11):863-871.
31. Fan ST, Lau WY, Yip WC, et al. Limitations and dangers of gastrografin swallow after esophageal and upper gastric operations. *Am J Surg.* 1988;155(3):495-497.
32. Srinivasan R, Haywood T, Horwitz B, et al. Role of flexible endoscopy in the evaluation of possible esophageal trauma after penetrating injuries. *Am J Gastroenterol.* 2000;95(7):1725-1729.
33. Flowers JL, Graham SM, Ugarte MA, et al. Flexible endoscopy for the diagnosis of esophageal trauma. *J Trauma.* 1996;40(2):261-265; discussion 265-266.
34. Demetriades D, Velmahos GG, Asensio JA. Cervical pharyngoesophageal and laryngotracheal injuries. *World J Surg.* 2001;25(8):1044-1048.
35. Apffelstaedt JP, Muller R. Results of mandatory exploration for penetrating neck trauma. *World J Surg.* 1994;18(6):917-919; discussion 920.
36. Meyer JP, Barrett JA, Schuler JJ, et al. Mandatory vs selective exploration for penetrating neck trauma. A prospective assessment. *Arch Surg.* 1987;122(5):592-597.
37. Azuaje RE, Jacobson LE, Glover J, et al. Reliability of physical examination as a predictor of vascular injury after penetrating neck trauma. *Am Surg.* 2003;69(9):804-807.
38. Sekharan J, Dennis JW, Veldenz HC, et al. Continued experience with physical examination alone for evaluation and management of penetrating zone 2 neck injuries: results of 145 cases. *J Vasc Surg.* 2000;32(3):483-489.
39. Ordog GJ, Albin D, Wasserberger J, et al. 110 bullet wounds to the neck. *J Trauma.* 1985;25(3):238-246.
40. van As AB, van Deurzen DF, Verleisdonk EJ. Gunshots to the neck: selective angiography as part of conservative management. *Injury.* 2002;33(5):453-456.
41. Hirshberg A, Wall MJ, Johnston RH Jr, et al. Transcervical gunshot injuries. *Am J Surg.* 1994;167(3):309-312.
42. Brywczynski JJ, Barrett TW, Lyon JA, et al. Management of penetrating neck injury in the emergency department: a structured literature review. *Emerg Med J.* 2008;25(11):711-715.
43. Yen PT, Lee HY, Tsai MH, et al. Clinical analysis of external laryngeal trauma. *J Laryngol Otol.* 1994;108(3):221-225.
44. Chagnon FP, Mulder DS. Laryngotracheal trauma. *Chest Surg Clin N Am.* 1996;6(4):733-748.
45. Gussack GS, Jurkovich GJ, Luterman A. Laryngotracheal trauma: a protocol approach to a rare injury. *Laryngoscope.* 1986;96(6):660-665.
46. Minard G, Kudsk KA, Croce MA, et al. Laryngotracheal trauma. *Am Surg.* 1992;58(3):181-187.
47. Cothren CC, Moore EE, Biffl WL, et al. Anticoagulation is the gold standard therapy for blunt carotid injuries to reduce stroke rate. *Arch Surg.* 2004;139(5):540-545; discussion 545-546.
48. Cothren CC, Moore EE, Biffl WL, et al. Cervical spine fracture patterns predictive of blunt vertebral artery injury. *J Trauma* 2003;55(5):811-813.
49. Stein DM, Boswell S, Sliker CW, et al. Blunt cerebrovascular injuries: does treatment always matter? *J Trauma* 2009;66(1):132-143; discussion 143-144.
50. Miller PR, Fabian TC, Croce MA, et al. Prospective screening for blunt cerebrovascular injuries: Analysis of diagnostic modalities and outcomes. *Ann Surg.* 2002;236(3):386-393; discussion 393-395.
51. Biffl WL, Ray CE Jr, Moore EE, et al. Treatment-related outcomes from blunt cerebrovascular injuries: importance of routine follow-up arteriography. *Ann Surg.* 2002;235(5):699-706; discussion 706-707.
52. Biffl WL, Moore EE, Offner PJ, et al. Optimizing screening for blunt cerebrovascular injuries. *Am J Surg.* 1999;178(6):517-522.
53. Berne JD, Reuland KS, Villarreal DH, et al. Sixteen-slice multi-detector computed tomographic angiography improves the accuracy of screening for blunt cerebrovascular injury. *J Trauma.* 2006;60(6):1204-1209; discussion 1209-1210.
54. Mayberry JC, Brown CV, Mullins RJ, et al. Blunt carotid artery injury: the futility of aggressive screening and diagnosis. *Arch Surg.* 2004;139(6):609-612; discussion 612-613.
55. Goudy SL, Miller FB, Bumpous JM. Neck crepitance: evaluation and management of suspected upper aerodigestive tract injury. *Laryngoscope.* 2002;112(5):791-795.
56. Schneidereit NP, Simons R, Nicolaou S, et al. Utility of screening for blunt vascular neck injuries with computed tomographic angiography. *J Trauma.* 2006;60(1):209-215; discussion 215-216.
57. Utter GH, Hollingworth W, Hallam DK, et al. Sixteen-slice CT angiography in patients with suspected blunt carotid and vertebral artery injuries. *J Am Coll Surg.* 2006;203(6):838-848.
58. Mutze S, Rademacher G, Matthes G, et al. Blunt cerebrovascular injury in patients with blunt multiple trauma: diagnostic accuracy of duplex doppler US and early CT angiography. *Radiology.* 2005;237(3):884-892.

59. Berne JD, Norwood SH, McAuley CE, et al. Helical computed tomographic angiography: an excellent screening test for blunt cerebrovascular injury. *J Trauma.* 2004;57(1):11-17; discussion 17-19.
60. Rogers FB, Baker EF, Osler TM, et al. Computed tomographic angiography as a screening modality for blunt cervical arterial injuries: preliminary results. *J Trauma.* 1999;46(3):380-385.
61. Stuhlfaut JW, Barest G, Sakai O, et al. Impact of MDCT angiography on the use of catheter angiography for the assessment of cervical arterial injury after blunt or penetrating trauma. *AJR Am J Roentgenol.* 2005;185(4):1063-1068.
62. Cogbill TH, Moore EE, Meissner M, et al. The spectrum of blunt injury to the carotid artery: a multicenter perspective. *J Trauma.* 1994;37(3):473-479.
63. DiPerna CA, Rowe VL, Terramani TT, et al. Clinical importance of the "seat belt sign" in blunt trauma to the neck. *Am Surg.* 2002;68(5):441-445.
64. Berne JD, Norwood SH, McAuley CE, et al. The high morbidity of blunt cerebrovascular injury in an unscreened population: more evidence of the need for mandatory screening protocols. *J Am Coll Surg.* 2001;192(3):314-321.
65. Fabian TC, Patton JH Jr, Croce MA, et al. Blunt carotid injury. Importance of early diagnosis and anticoagulant therapy. *Ann Surg.* 1996;223(5):513-522; discussion 522-525.
66. Miller PR, Fabian TC, Bee TK, et al. Blunt cerebrovascular injuries: diagnosis and treatment. *J Trauma.* 2001;51(2):279-285; discussion 285-286.
67. Thal ER, Snyder WH III, Hays RJ, et al. Management of carotid artery injuries. *Surgery.* 1974;76(6):955-962.
68. Ramadan F, Rutledge R, Oller D, et al. Carotid artery trauma: a review of contemporary trauma center experiences. *J Vasc Surg.* 1995;21(1):46-55; discussion 55-56.
69. Bowley DM, Degiannis E, Goosen J, et al. Penetrating vascular trauma in Johannesburg, South Africa. *Surg Clin North Am.* 2002;82(1):221-235.
70. Teehan EP, Padberg FT Jr, Thompson PN, et al. Carotid arterial trauma: assessment with the Glasgow Coma Scale (GCS) as a guide to surgical management. *Cardiovasc Surg.* 1997;5(2):196-200.
71. Murray JA, Demetriades D, Asensio JA. Carotid injury: postrevascularization hemorrhagic infarction. *J Trauma.* 1996;41(4):760-762.
72. DuBose J, Recinos G, Teixeira PG, et al. Endovascular stenting for the treatment of traumatic internal carotid injuries: expanding experience. *J Trauma* 2008;65(6):1561-1566.
73. Biffl WL, Moore EE, Ryu RK, et al. The unrecognized epidemic of blunt carotid arterial injuries: early diagnosis improves neurologic outcome. *Ann Surg.* 1998;228(4):462-470.
74. Eachempati SR, Vaslef SN, Sebastian MW, et al. Blunt vascular injuries of the head and neck: is heparinization necessary? *J Trauma.* 1998;45(6):997-1004.
75. Vishteh AG, Marciano FF, David CA, et al. Long-term graft patency rates and clinical outcomes after revascularization for symptomatic traumatic internal carotid artery dissection. *Neurosurgery.* 1998;43(4):761-767; discussion 767-768.
76. Becquemin JP, Cavillon A, Brunel M, et al. Polytetrafluoroethylene grafts for carotid repair. *Cardiovasc Surg.* 1996;4(6):740-745.
77. Losken A, Rozycki GS, Feliciano DV. The use of the sternocleidomastoid muscle flap in combined injuries to the esophagus and carotid artery or trachea. *J Trauma.* 2000;49(5):815-817.
78. Rostomily RC, Newell DW, Grady MS, et al. Gunshot wounds of the internal carotid artery at the skull base: management with vein bypass grafts and a review of the literature. *J Trauma.* 1997;42(1):123-132.
79. Firoozmand E, Velmahos GC. Extending damage-control principles to the neck. *J Trauma.* 2000;48(3):541-543.
80. Schaefer SD. The acute management of external laryngeal trauma. A 27-year experience. *Arch Otolaryngol Head Neck Surg.* 1992;118(6):598-604.
81. Ngakane H, Muckart DJ, Luvuno FM. Penetrating visceral injuries of the neck: results of a conservative management policy. *Br J Surg.* 1990;77(8):908-910.
82. Feliciano DV, Bitondo CG, Mattox KL, et al. Combined tracheoesophageal injuries. *Am J Surg.* 1985;150(6):710-715.
83. Asensio JA, Chahwan S, Forno W, et al. Penetrating esophageal injuries: Multicenter study of the american association for the surgery of trauma. *J Trauma* 2001;50(2):289-296.
84. Velmahos GC, Souter I, Degiannis E, Mokoena T, Saadia R. Selective surgical management in penetrating neck injuries. *Can J Surg.* 1994;37(6):487-491.
85. Sheely CH II, Mattox KL, Beall AC Jr, et al. Penetrating wounds of the cervical esophagus. *Am J Surg.* 1975;130(6):707-711.
86. Naylor AR, Walker WS, Dark J, et al. T tube intubation in the management of seriously ill patients with oesophagopleural fistulae. *Br J Surg.* 1990;77(1):40-42.
87. Andrade-Alegre R. T-tube intubation in the management of late traumatic esophageal perforations: case report. *J Trauma* 1994;37(1):131-132.

CHAPTER 27 ■ **CHEST INJURY**

AMY N. HILDRETH AND J. WAYNE MEREDITH

Chest trauma is a significant contributor to patient morbidity and mortality. Thoracic injuries are often accompanied by substantial injuries to other regions. These injuries contribute to approximately 50% of all trauma-related deaths in this country and are the leading cause of death in those under 40-years-old.[1–3] Fortunately, most of these injuries can be managed with skills easily acquired by physicians involved in the initial care of the trauma patient. Only 10%-15% will require operative intervention for life-threatening thoracic injuries. The skill set involved in treatment of these severe thoracic injuries is complex and requires a thorough knowledge of thoracic anatomy and cardiopulmonary physiology. This chapter will discuss the diagnosis and management of the spectrum of thoracic injuries as well as indications for intervention.

INITIAL ASSESSMENT

Initial evaluation of the trauma patient follows the guidelines common to evaluation of any patient suspected to have multitrauma. The evaluation begins with a rapid assessment of the elements of the primary survey to evaluate and quickly treat any immediate life-threatening problems. The primary survey is discussed elsewhere in this text, but the specifics of this survey as they relate to thoracic trauma deserve mention here. Injuries that should be identified during the primary survey include tension and open pneumothorax, massive hemothorax, flail chest, and cardiac tamponade. The specifics of treating these injuries will be discussed later in the chapter.

Establishment of an adequate airway is the first priority during this survey. Severely injured patients will require nasotracheal or orotracheal intubation. Some patients with extensive maxillofacial trauma may require cricothyroidotomy or tracheostomy. Once the airway is deemed intact, the next priority is determining the adequacy of ventilation. If the patient is not breathing, endotracheal intubation is indicated immediately. Other sources of ventilatory insufficiency include the presence of open or tension pneumothorax. These injuries must be promptly addressed as soon as they are recognized.

The next priority is hemorrhage control and restoration of adequate circulation. External hemorrhage is best controlled with direct pressure. Inadequate perfusion is most often a result of either hypovolemia or an inadequate pump. Ongoing internal hemorrhage contributing to hypovolemia must be addressed operatively. Distended neck veins signal one of four common traumatic causes of pump failure: tension pneumothorax, pericardial tamponade, coronary air embolism, or cardiac contusion/myocardial infarction. One must rapidly undertake treatment of these problems to restore circulation.

SECONDARY SURVEY AND RADIOLOGIC ADJUNCTS

If there are no immediately life-threatening injuries identified during the primary survey, the trauma team can progress to a more thorough evaluation and physical examination. Secondary survey of the thorax should focus on identification of potentially life-threatening injuries not identified in the primary survey and discovery of other thoracic injuries. Important injuries to recognize during the secondary survey include simple pneumothorax, hemothorax, pulmonary contusion, tracheobronchial injury, blunt cardiac injury, aortic transection, and diaphragmatic injury. Pain from clinically relevant rib fractures will be evident upon palpation of the chest wall. Pneumothorax and hemothorax may become evident at this stage of evaluation if they were not discovered on primary survey. Visualization of chest wall movement during spontaneous respiration can diagnose flail chest.

Important adjuncts to the secondary survey include the portable chest radiograph, the standard and extended Focused Assessment with Sonography for Trauma (FAST) exam, formal echocardiography, and CT angiography. Chest radiography remains a vital first imaging step in the injured trauma patient. Pneumothorax, hemothorax, rib fractures, and mediastinal abnormalities may be identified on a chest radiograph. Extended FAST is useful in rapid diagnosis of pneumothorax and may also assist in diagnosis of pulmonary contusion.[4–6] FAST also has an excellent ability to evaluate for hemopericardium with reported sensitivities of 96%-100% and a specificity of 100%.[7] The accuracy of these examinations is significantly operator-dependent. Formal echocardiography may be used in later stages of evaluation to assess cardiac function, but it is time consuming and requires appropriately trained personnel. CT angiography is recommended in stable patients with evidence of blunt multisystem trauma, even among those without obvious signs of injury as a substantial number of patients with a normal chest radiograph will have findings of thoracic injury on CT scan.[8,9]

INDICATIONS FOR OPERATION

Emergency Department Resuscitative Thoracotomy

Emergency department resuscitative thoracotomy (ED-RT) is a drastic measure employed only in patients in extremis after penetrating and, to a lesser extent, blunt trauma. The purpose of this procedure is to attempt to stabilize the patient for transport to the operating room for definitive repair of their injuries. For this reason, the ED-RT must be performed expediently and with clear goals in mind. These goals include relief of cardiac tamponade if present, control of hemorrhage, effective cardiac compression, cross-clamping of the pulmonary hilum in the presence of major lung hemorrhage, air embolism, or massive broncho-pleural fistula, and cross-clamping of the descending aorta for lower torso hemorrhage control. The average survival rate to discharge following this procedure is approximately 7%.[10–12]

RT has the best chance of success when reserved for those who arrive at the ED and subsequently deteriorate or those who suffered cardiac arrest just prior to arrival. RT should not be performed in those who have had prehospital CPR for longer than 10 minutes in the setting of blunt trauma and 15 minutes in the setting of penetrating trauma or when the initial presenting rhythm is asystole. The survival rate for patients injured by blunt mechanism undergoing ED thoracotomy is reported to be around 1%.[12] Survival rates are significantly better for those undergoing this procedure following penetrating trauma; survival to discharge rates of 16%-57% have been reported.[10–14] Better outcomes are seen when ED thoracotomy is performed for stab wounds than for gunshot wounds. Worse outcomes are described when ED thoracotomy is performed following multiple gunshot wounds.[13]

To perform ED thoracotomy, a left anterolateral thoracotomy incision is used to enter the chest. Attention is directed first to the injury. If there is exsanguination from a great vessel, the hemorrhage is controlled with pressure. If air embolism is the cause of the arrest, the hilum is clamped, and air evacuated from the left cardiac chambers. Otherwise, the pericardium is opened anterior and parallel to the phrenic nerve. The hemopericardium is evacuated, the cardiac injury is controlled with digital pressure, and a temporary repair is performed. After the cause of the arrest has been addressed, the descending thoracic aorta is occluded with a vascular clamp or digital pressure, and intrathoracic cardiac compression is initiated. The patient's intravascular volume is restored, and electrolyte imbalances are corrected. If the patient can be saved, he or she is transported to the OR for definitive repair and closure.

URGENT THORACOTOMY

Urgent thoracotomy in the trauma patient is indicated for suspicion of life-threatening injuries that may require surgical repair. Indications for operative treatment of thoracic injuries fall into four broad categories: (1) hemorrhage, (2) major airway disruption, (3) cardiac and vascular injuries, and (4) esophageal disruption. For hemorrhage, operative intervention is indicated by the volume of chest tube output in combination with the hemodynamic profile of the patient. In general, thoracotomy is indicated when chest tube output initially exceeds 1,500 mL initially or if ongoing bleeding exceeds 300 mL per hour for 3 hours. There are, however, pitfalls inherent in this method of determining need for operation. A caveat to chest tube output as an indication for thoracotomy is chest trauma with a delayed presentation and the presence of a coagulopathy. Patients presenting with chest trauma in a delayed fashion may have a substantial hemothorax that has accumulated in the time it has taken the patient to arrive in the ED. Furthermore, in some instances, a tube thoracostomy is malpositioned, kinked, or clotted, allowing accumulation of a hemothorax prior to arrival. In these situations, placement of a second chest tube and/or evidence of ongoing bleeding rather than an absolute amount may be a more reliable indicator of the need for thoracic operation.[15] In addition to chest tube output, patient physiology suggestive of ongoing hemorrhage should play a role in the decision for operative intervention. Low-tube thoracostomy output due to a malpositioned tube may also be misleading. As a result, a chest radiograph should be obtained following tube placement to determine whether the hemothorax has been adequately evacuated. Complete lung re-expansion should also be confirmed on this film, as hemostasis in the chest often will not occur until expansion is complete. Massive air leak after chest tube placement or the presence of gastric or esophageal contents in the chest tube effluent are also indications for operation.

The order of an exploratory thoracotomy should proceed in a logical and orderly fashion. If the diagnosis is uncertain, a posterolateral thoracotomy is the incision of choice. With a known diagnosis, the incision should be chosen to provide optimal exposure of the injury. First, the remaining hemothorax should be evacuated. The lung is then packed out of the field; this procedure may be facilitated by the division of the inferior pulmonary ligament. The mediastinum and pericardium should be evaluated carefully for bleeding. It is difficult to detect the presence of blood in the pericardium by simple visual inspection. A small (5 mm) pericardotomy that can be expanded as necessary is useful to confirm or exclude the presence of hemopericardium. The presence of clear fluid in the pericardium precludes the need for creating a larger pericardial incision. Major vascular injuries are isolated using proximal and distal control; hilar control can be used in cases of pulmonary parenchymal bleeding. Formal repair of injuries may then proceed. The use of a double lumen endotracheal tube or bronchial blocker may be useful and should be considered when patient physiology and injury pattern permit.

INCISION CHOICE

Appropriate incision choice is essential for obtaining adequate exposure of thoracic injuries requiring operative intervention. The choice of incision varies according to several factors, including suspected site of injury and the indication for operation, the urgency of the situation, the presence of associated injuries, the mechanism of injury, and the results of preoperative studies. For injuries that are suspected or diagnosed preoperatively, the choice of approach to the affected structure is greatly simplified (Table 27.1). Preoperative imaging using CTA in the stable patient, even with penetrating mechanism, can assist with the identification of specific injuries and operative planning.[16]

A median sternotomy is one of the more versatile thoracic incisions. It can be opened and closed more quickly than a thoracotomy, is associated with less postoperative pain, and may be less likely to result in contamination of the dependent hemithorax, which may occur with the patient in a lateral position during thoracotomy. In general, a median sternotomy provides the best exposure of the right-side cardiac chambers, the ascending aorta, the aortic arch, and the arch vessels (excluding the left subclavian artery), and it provides adequate exposure of the right lung and hemidiaphragm. A sternotomy may be extended into the neck or supraclavicular fossa to enhance exposure of the great vessels. The main limitation of this incision is that it does not provide exposure of the posterior mediastinal structures (Fig. 27.1).

For the exploration of lateral stab or gunshot wounds or massive hemothorax, a posterolateral thoracotomy on the side of the injury is the incision of choice. The fifth interspace thoracotomy is the most versatile approach to ipsilateral pulmonary and mediastinal pathologic states. Exposure can be markedly enhanced by the removal of the fifth rib. Right thoracotomy is an excellent approach for right lung, tracheal, and proximal left mainstem bronchial injuries. Most injuries of the thoracic esophagus can also be accessed in this manner, except in the case of distal esophageal injuries, which are best approached via left thoracotomy. The right atrium and ventricle are easily exposed by a right thoracotomy as well. Left thoracotomy is ideal for the exposure of the left lung, left pulmonary hilum, aorta, proximal left subclavian artery, left heart chambers, distal esophagus, and distal left mainstem bronchus (Fig. 27.2). In urgent/emergent situations, a clamshell incision, formed by extending a left anterolateral thoracotomy incision transversely across the sternum, provides access but only suboptimal exposure of intrathoracic and mediastinal structures except the right ventricle and atrium (Fig. 27.3).

THORACIC DAMAGE CONTROL

While damage control is critically important in abdominal trauma, it is less frequently needed in thoracic trauma. In most instances, serious bleeding from thoracic structures is unlikely to be controlled with packing; however, severe coagulopathy

TABLE 27.1

SURGICAL APPROACHES FOR TRAUMATIC INJURIES TO THORACIC VESSELS

SITE	STERNOTOMY	RIGHT THORACOTOMY	LEFT THORACOTOMY
R Atrium	+++	++	0
R Ventricle	+++	+	+
L Atrium	+++	+	+
L Ventricle	++	0	+++
SCV	+++	++	0
Azygos Vein	++	+++	0
IVC	+++	++	0
Aortic Root	+++	+	0
Aortic Arch	+++	0	++
R Subclavian	++	++	0
Proximal R Carotid	+++	+	0
Innominate	+++	++	0
L Subclavian	+	0	+++
Proximal L Carotid	++	0	++
Descending Aorta	0	+	+++
Main PA	+++	0	++
R PA	++	+++	0
L PA	++	0	+++
RUL	++	+++	0
RML	++	+++	0
RLL	+	+++	0
LUL	+	0	+++
LLL	0	0	+++
R Hilum	++	+++	0
L Hilum	++	0	+++
Pericardium	+++	++	++
P IMA	++	+++	0
L IMA	++	0	+++
Proximal Esophagus	0	+++	0
Distal Esophagus	0	++	+++
Proximal Trachea	++	+	+
Carina	0	+++	+
R Mainstem	0	+++	0
L Mainstem	0	++	++
R Hemidiaphragm	+	+++	0
L Hemidiaphragm	+	0	+++
CPB	+++	++	++

CPB, cardiopulmonary bypass; IMA, internal mammary artery; IVC, inferior vena cava; LL, lower lobe; ML, middle lobe; PA, pulmonary artery; SVC, superior vena cava; UL, upper lobe.
+++, preferred; ++, acceptable; +, with difficulty; 0, not acceptable.

TRAUMA

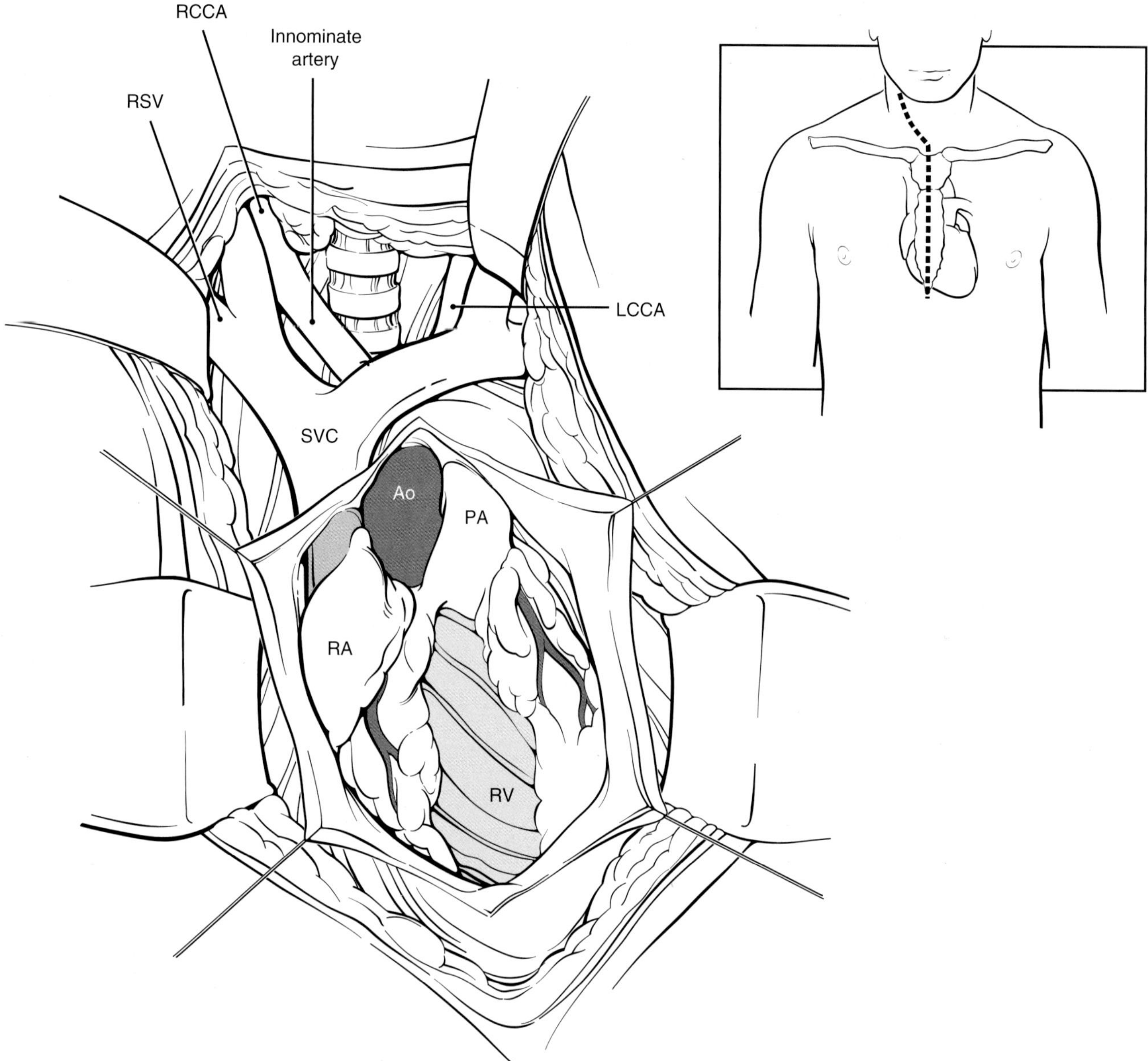

FIGURE 27.1. Median sternotomy with optimal extension. A median sternotomy provides excellent exposure for the right atrium and ventricle, the superior vena cava, atrial appendage, right pulmonary artery, and lung. If necessary, the incision may be extended into the neck or supraclavicular fossa (**inset**) to enhance exposure of the great vessels. Ao, aorta; LCCA, left common carotid artery; PA, pulmonary artery; RA, right atrium; RCCA, right common carotid artery; RSV, right subclavian vein; RV, right ventricle; SVC, superior vena cava.

occasionally prevents definitive repair and necessitates abbreviation of surgery and temporary closure of the chest by suturing or stapling the skin incision only.[17] The two most common locations of injury in these scenarios are the lung and the chest wall. Hemorrhage from lung lacerations in patients with metabolic exhaustion generally should not be treated with formal anatomic resection: stapled wedge resection, tractotomy, or simple suture repair is more appropriate. In patients with persistent chest wall bleeding that is not associated with a major vessel, treatment with lung re-expansion for local tamponade and correction of coagulopathy usually suffices. Patients who have air embolus or massive bronchopleural fistula will require temporary clamping or twisting of the pulmonary hilum on the affected side, so that the patient may be stabilized prior to proceeding with definitive operation. In rare circumstances, complex esophageal injuries may be associated with extensive loss of tissue, necessitating rapid exclusion and proximal diversion. In most patients with any chance of survival, however, the surgeon should attempt primary closure of the injury, buttressing the repair with autologous tissue, and employing wide drainage. Even with large defects, this approach has a surprisingly high rate of ultimate success. The VAC dressing may be employed for temporary closure when definitive closure of the thorax is not possible.

INDICATIONS FOR DELAYED THORACOTOMY

Indications for delayed thoracotomy include missed tracheobronchial injuries, traumatic aortic rupture, intracardiac injuries, retained hemothorax, and posttraumatic empyema. Specifics of intervention for these injuries will be discussed in the ensuing sections.

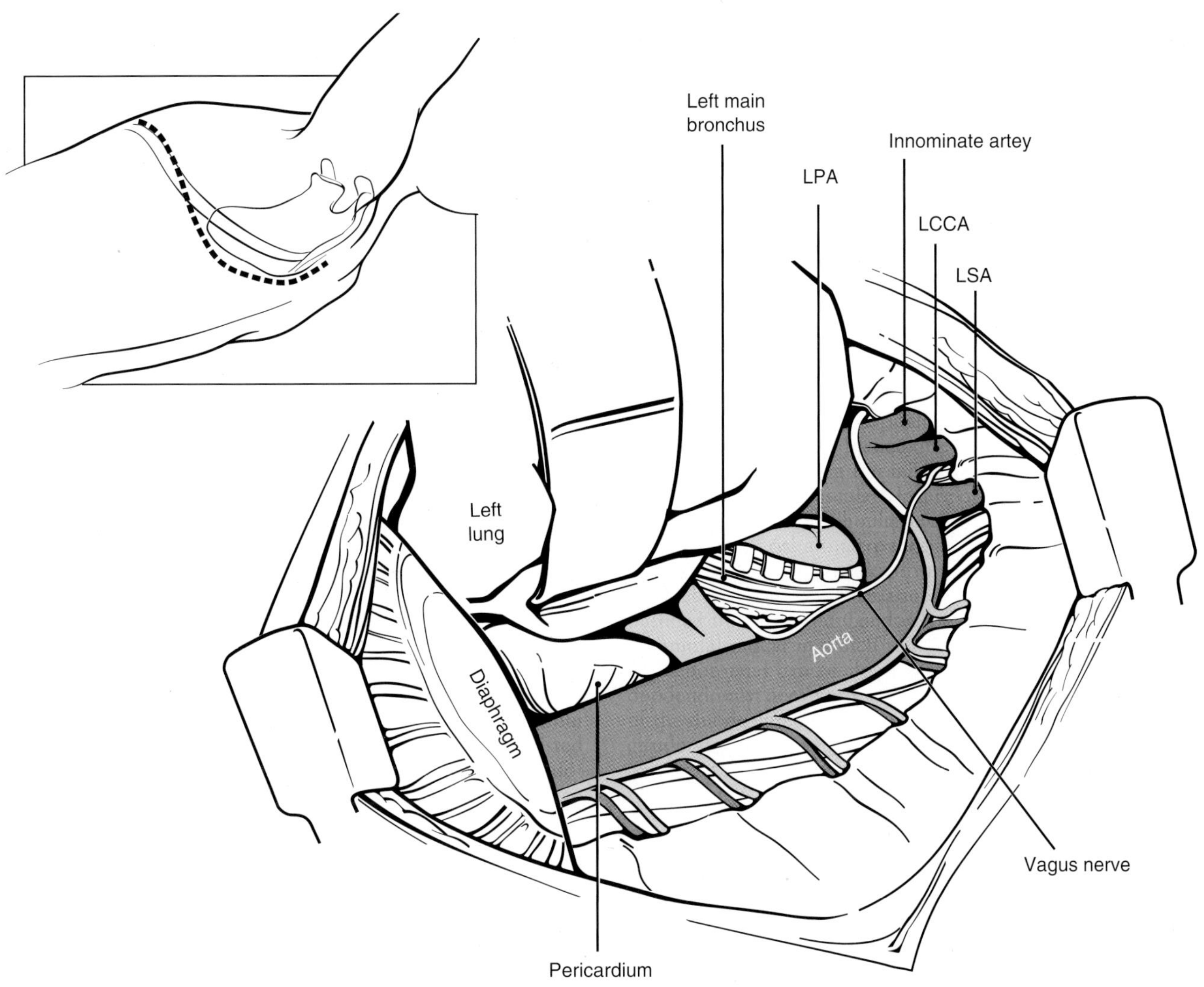

FIGURE 27.2. Left posterolateral thoracotomy. A left posterolateral thoracotomy (**inset**) provides excellent exposure of the left pulmonary hilum, left lung, proximal left subclavian artery, descending aorta, distal esophagus, and left diaphragm. LCCA, left common carotid artery; LPA, left pulmonary artery; LSA, left subclavian artery.

MANAGEMENT OF SPECIFIC INJURIES

Chest Wall Injuries

Rib Fractures. Rib fractures are quite common following blunt trauma and can be present in as many as 10% of total trauma admissions. These injuries rarely require operative stabilization, but they do contribute significantly to patient morbidity and mortality. Rib fractures carry a risk of 12% for mortality and 33% for pulmonary complications.[18] Rib fractures in the elderly are associated with especially high morbidity and mortality. The mortality associated with rib fractures is twice as high in patients older than 65 years than in younger patients, and the relative increase in the incidence of pneumonia in older patients is even higher, even after patient comorbidities are considered.[19,20]

The main pathophysiologic consequences of rib fractures are pain, splinting, and prevention of adequate cough, impeding pulmonary toilet. The diagnosis should be suspected if pain or splinting occurs on deep inspiration, and it is confirmed by careful physical examination, consisting of anterior–posterior and lateral–lateral manual compression. If an alert patient feels no pain with these maneuvers, clinically important rib fractures can be excluded. Although rib fractures are often identified on routine chest radiographs, they are more likely to be detected on rib-detail films, which are rarely clinically indicated. A variant of rib fracture that falls into the same physiologic category is costochondral or costosternal separation. This condition is usually detected during physical examination or on CT scan of the thorax but is not seen on routine chest radiographs.

Pain from isolated rib fractures can usually be adequately managed with oral or parenteral analgesics, encouraging good pulmonary toilet, and use of thoracic epidural anesthesia (discussed below) in select patients. We mention chest wall strapping, taping, and bracing only to condemn these practices. Binding devices generally restrict tidal volume and thus promote rather than prevent atelectasis and pulmonary complications. Increasingly, reports have demonstrated the feasibility of rib fracture repair using a variety of different methods including wire sutures, intramedullary wires, staples, and various plating systems.[21] Potential indications for operative repair

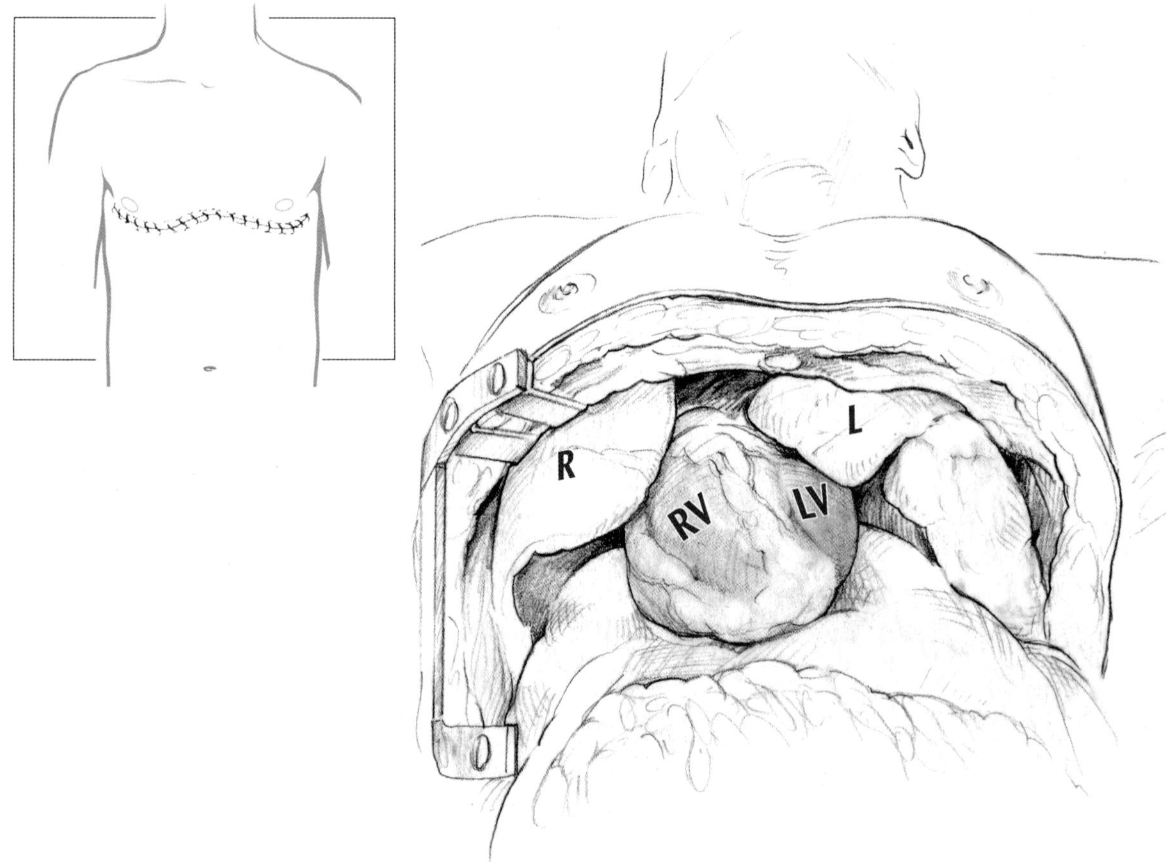

FIGURE 27.3. Clamshell extension of left anterolateral thoracotomy. In urgent/emergent situations, a clamshell incision, formed by extending a left anterolateral thoracotomy incision, transversely across the sternum, provides access but only suboptimal exposure of intrathoracic and mediastinal structures except the right ventricle and atrium. R, right lung; RV, right ventricle; LV, left ventricle; L, left lung.

of rib fractures include flail chest, painful, and mobile rib fractures, which are refractory to conventional management, chest wall deformity/defect, rib fracture nonunion, and during thoracotomy for other indications. In isolated reports, clinical outcomes have been excellent when repair is undertaken. However, there is a need for clinical trials documenting the superiority of rib fracture repair versus conventional management in select patient populations and defining indications for repair.[22,23]

Sternal Fractures. Sternal fractures commonly result from motor vehicle collisions and are associated with the use of three-point restraints. Isolated sternal fractures are relatively benign, having a low incidence of associated cardiac, great vessel, and pulmonary injuries. Sternal fractures in unrestrained occupants and victims of crush injuries, however, are commonly associated with underlying visceral injuries, which must be excluded.[17,24]

The diagnosis of sternal fracture is based on the presence of severe pain, often associated with instability on sternal palpation. In many cases, physical examination can clarify the nature of the fracture. Sternal fractures are almost invariably transverse, with the majority occurring at the sternomanubrial joint or in the midbody of the sternum. They may be characterized as simple (two fragments) or comminuted (multiple fragments), as displaced or aligned, or as stable or unstable. The fragments of an unstable fracture move substantially with activity.

Initial management of a sternal fracture is directed toward resuscitation and identification or exclusion of other life-threatening injuries. In patients with isolated sternal fractures, a normal electrocardiogram and a normal chest radiograph suggest that associated serious injuries are unlikely. If the pain is controlled with oral analgesics, these fractures can usually be managed on an outpatient basis. Displaced fractures may be reduced by the simple (albeit painful) maneuver of having the patient simultaneously raise his or her head and legs from the bed. Such a position requires contraction of the rectus abdominis, which distracts the caudad segment inferiorly, and the sternocleidomastoid muscles, which retract the cephalad segments superiorly. The physician can then depress the anterior segment and allow the patient to relax. This measure often suffices for alleviation of subsequent pain and sometimes constitutes adequate long-term treatment.

The vast majority of sternal fractures heal without repair. Those that are unstable or are displaced by more than 1 cm of overlap are more likely to exhibit malunion or nonunion and subsequent chronic pain; they may require open reduction and internal fixation. Occasionally, a patient with a clinically stable, minimally displaced sternal fracture associated with lower extremity injuries who requires crutches for ambulation, experiences such disabling sternal pain during ambulation that fracture repair is necessary. Sternal fractures may be repaired with either of two operative techniques. In both, the sternum is approached via either a vertical midline incision or a sweeping transverse inframammary incision similar to that used for repair of pectus excavatum. The fracture is exposed, and the ends are mobilized and fixed with either reconstruction plates or No. 6 sternal wires. Both wire fixation and plate fixation are well tolerated and are appropriate for properly selected patients.

Flail Chest. Flail chest is defined as the presence of two or more ribs fractured in two or more places, resulting in paradoxical movement of a section of the chest wall. It is the most serious of the chest wall injuries caused by blunt trauma. Although flail chest may present as an isolated injury, it is much more commonly associated with other injuries.[25] The diagnosis may be suspected based on radiologic findings and confirmed by examination of the spontaneously breathing patient. The flail segment may be overlooked in the patient receiving mechanical ventilation because of the absence of paradoxical movement.

There are three important pathophysiologic components that contribute to the severity of flail chest. The first is the alteration in chest wall mechanics secondary to the flail segment. Although this is usually not the most clinically important abnormality, the paradoxical motion of a large flail segment occasionally impairs the patient's ability to achieve an adequate tidal volume or an effective cough. The second important pathophysiologic component is underlying pulmonary contusion. In the vast majority of serious flail chest injuries, this is the most important physiologic aberration.[26] In the contused portion of the lung, there is extravasation and accumulation of blood and fluid in the alveolar air space, which results in sufficient shunting to produce hypoxemia. The third factor is the pain of multiple rib fractures, leading to splinting and diminution of tidal volumes; it prevents adequate coughing and pulmonary toilet. The combination of depressed tidal volume and inadequate cough leads to hypoventilation, atelectasis, and often pneumonia.

Central to management of the flail chest is the concept that the injury is not static but is in constant evolution. Frequent reevaluation is essential; prompt intervention should be undertaken when patient physiology changes. All awake and alert patients with adequate oxygenation and ventilation deserve a trial of management without intubation.[27] Pain cannot be eliminated entirely, but it usually can be diminished sufficiently to allow an adequate tidal volume and a forceful cough. Oral analgesics rarely suffice for patients with even a small flail segment; stronger agents are required for all but the most stoic of patients. Parenteral narcotics are effective, especially when administered in a patient-controlled analgesia (PCA) device. Potential disadvantages of parenteral narcotics include excess sedation, cough suppression, and respiratory depression.

When PCA analgesia is not adequate or is contraindicated, other modalities of analgesia may be considered. These methods include epidural analgesia, intercostal nerve block, intrapleural anesthesia, and thoracic paravertebral block. Each of these modalities has inherent risks and benefits, and choice of analgesia should be based on patient physiology, injuries, and medical history.

Epidural analgesia is the most common method used for the treatment of chest wall pain. It consists of insertion of a catheter into the thoracic or lumbar epidural space with infusion of a narcotic, a local anesthetic, or most commonly, a combination of the two medications. Purported benefits include improved analgesia as well as improvement in respiratory mechanics and decrease in proinflammatory cytokines.[28,29] The benefits of epidural analgesia may translate into decrease in ventilator days, decrease in pulmonary complications, and lower mortality.[19,30] Disadvantages include the potential for epidural infection and hematoma as well as direct spinal cord trauma. Hypotension (when local anesthetic agents are used), peripheral neurologic effects, and pruritus are also potential side effects.

The Eastern Association for the Surgery of Trauma (EAST) has published recent guidelines regarding the use of analgesic adjuncts. These guidelines state that epidural analgesia is the preferred method of pain relief for blunt chest wall injury. They recommend epidural analgesia for patients who are ≥65-years-old if there is no contraindication, and they state that it may be considered for those under 65 years as well.[31] When epidural analgesia is contraindicated, another regional anesthetic technique may be considered. These other techniques, including intercostal nerve block, intrapleural analgesia, and paravertebral block, are relatively safe but have not been studied extensively in the trauma population.

The decision-making process for the management of flail chest should begin with the assessment of the patient's ability to cough. If the patient is able to clear tracheal secretions, then observation in an acute care setting with small, infrequent doses of narcotics, is appropriate. If the patient has no cough or has a very truncated cough that moves secretions but does not propel them into the oropharynx, an aggressive program to promote pulmonary toilet should be instituted. If a sufficiently vigorous cough cannot be achieved and there is no specific contraindication, an epidural catheter is considered, and the patient is followed closely with frequent physical examinations in the intensive care unit. Ambulation is encouraged, and frequent coughing is required. It is important that management decisions be made early, so that effective therapy can be started expeditiously. There is no role for antibiotic prophylaxis or steroid use in the management of patients with flail chest or pulmonary contusion.

Any patient with flail chest demonstrates that further deterioration of pulmonary function as evidenced by worsening hypoxia or hypercarbia should undergo endotracheal intubation and mechanical ventilation. Goals of mechanical ventilation include the establishment of tidal volume adequate for normal chest wall excursion and maintenance of normocarbia through an adequate respiratory rate. Hypoxia is managed by increasing the fraction of inspired oxygen (FiO_2) and applying sufficient positive end-expiratory pressure to achieve adequate oxygenation (usually defined as arterial oxygen saturation >90%) with nontoxic levels of FiO_2.

A few patients with severe disruption of chest wall mechanics as a result of flail chest continue to require positive pressure ventilation even though adequate pain control has been achieved, and the pulmonary contusions are beginning to resolve. Some of these patients may benefit from internal fixation of the multiple rib fractures, which restores chest wall stability and eliminates much of the fracture-related pain. A variety of methods have been described to stabilize the ribs and obtain compression osteosynthesis of each fracture site. Two single institutional series describe the efficacy of this procedure in patients with flail chest.[32,33] Further clinical trials are needed to better define indications for fracture repair.

Penetrating Chest Wall Injury

In most cases of penetrating thoracic trauma, the injury to the chest wall is vastly overshadowed by the injury, or potential for injury, to the intrathoracic structures. The notable exceptions to this general rule are hemorrhage and open chest wounds.

Hemorrhage. Stab wounds and low-caliber gunshot wounds to the anterior chest are common in urban areas. Once serious injury to intrathoracic organs has been excluded, such injuries often can be managed with tube thoracostomy or observation alone. Indications for urgent thoracotomy have been discussed previously.

In patients with persistent hemorrhage from chest tubes who require thoracotomy, the most common source of the bleeding is a lacerated internal mammary or intercostal artery. Attempts to control bleeding from these vessels nonoperatively usually fail. Angiography to localize the bleeding vessel is unnecessary and delays definitive care; coupled with embolization of the lacerated vessel, it is more time-consuming than surgical intervention and does not address associated injuries and hemothorax.

Penetrating wounds to the midportion of the pectoral muscle occur with surprising frequency, possibly as a result of an assailant's erroneous conception of the location of the heart. Such injuries often lacerate the pectoral branch of the thoracoacromial artery, which courses along the posterior surface of the pectoral muscle. Control of this troublesome bleeding is extremely difficult to achieve if exploration is attempted directly through an extension of the entrance wound. Exposure is much improved if exploration is attempted through an oblique wound along the lateral pectoral margin after entry into the subpectoral plane.

Open Chest Wounds. The diagnosis of an open chest wound is usually obvious, and treatment of this wound depends on the size of the wound the chest wall defect. Most small open pneumothoraces can be managed initially with occlusive dressings, but there is usually an underlying pulmonary injury with air leakage, which necessitates early tube thoracostomy to prevent tension pneumothorax. Once the patient's condition is stable, the wound can be débrided and closed. Occasionally, primary skin closure must be delayed.

Larger chest wall defects pose a challenging therapeutic problem. Such wounds usually result from high-velocity missiles or shotguns fired at close range. Initial management is directed toward restoration of respiratory mechanics with early intubation and mechanical ventilation.

The next priority is to address any underlying intrathoracic injuries, which may range from mild pulmonary contusion to massive hemorrhage in conjunction with severe lung or hollow viscus injury. When associated intrathoracic injuries are present, the first step in the closure of the defect is to select an appropriate operative approach. Although the primary objective in this situation is to provide adequate exposure for repair of what may be life-threatening injuries, whenever possible, the thoracotomy should be performed in such a way as to preserve the blood supply and muscle mass of the chest wall adjacent to the defect.

After definitive repair of intrathoracic injuries and debridement of devitalized chest wall tissue, planning begins for wound closure. Such planning requires a degree of familiarity with current and developing techniques and an understanding of pleural drainage, respiratory mechanics, and techniques of tissue transfer. Collaboration with plastic and thoracic surgeons is often helpful. Most chest wall defects can be closed with viable autogenous tissue, usually through rotation of local myocutaneous or myofascial flaps of the pectoral muscle, the latissimus dorsi, or the rectus abdominis.

Pleura and Lungs

Pneumothorax. Pneumothorax occurs when there is injury to the lung and/or tracheobronchial tree, resulting in air in the pleural space. A simple pneumothorax requires tube thoracostomy when it is large enough to be seen on plain chest radiograph. With the advent of modern imaging techniques, even clinically insignificant pneumothoraces may be identified during evaluation of the patient. If a pneumothorax is seen on thoracic CT but not on plain chest radiograph, it is known as an occult pneumothorax. Studies have examined the need for tube thoracostomy in these cases. The majority of evidence indicates that asymptomatic occult pneumothoraces may be observed, regardless of the need for positive pressure ventilation.[34–38] Patients with occult pneumothoraces who are treated without tube thoracostomy should be observed for at least 24 hours with repeat chest radiography to ensure the pneumothorax has not enlarged.

Progression of simple pneumothorax leads to tension pneumothorax, a life-threatening injury that should be recognized on primary survey. Air released from the lung parenchyma and tracheobronchial tree continues to accumulate in the pleural space, leading to an increased intrapleural pressure. This pressure is transmitted to the cardiac chambers and vena cava, impeding venous return to the heart and ultimately resulting in cardiovascular collapse. This entity may be recognized by unilateral decreased breath sounds, tympany on the affected side, tracheal deviation, and distension of neck veins. However, these signs may be absent or go unrecognized in a busy ED. The diagnosis is often suggested by the presence of shock accompanied by the evidence of inadequate venous filling on physical examination as well as recognition of asymmetric chest wall motion.

Radiographic evaluation should not delay treatment of a suspected tension pneumothorax with tube thoracostomy in patients with hemodynamic compromise.

Hemothorax. Hemothorax may occur in isolation or present in combination with pneumothorax. Hemothorax may be recognized on plain chest radiography as well as on thoracic CT. If the volume of hemothorax is great enough (massive hemothorax), physiologic compromise occurs in a manner similar to that of tension pneumothorax. Initial treatment of hemothorax is similar to the treatment of pneumothorax. After placement of tube thoracostomy, initial tube output as well as ongoing output should be carefully monitored. Indications for urgent thoracotomy based on tube thoracostomy output have been previously outlined.

The goal of treatment with tube thoracostomy is complete removal of blood. Prophylactic antibiotics for tube thoracostomy placement are not currently indicated.[39] Complications such as atelectasis and empyema after chest trauma are clearly related to the presence of residual blood, fluid, and air, as can occur secondary to improper positioning (i.e., within a fissure) or obstruction of the tube. A retained hemothorax is suggested by the presence of a persistent opacification in the pleural space in a patient with a known previous hemothorax. However, plain chest radiography can be misleading and often underestimates the amount of fluid in the chest. The radiodensity seen can be confused with adjacent pulmonary contusion or atelectasis. Thoracic CT confirms the diagnosis, providing information about the size and location of the hemothorax that can be used intraoperatively to make the appropriate incision. Evacuation of hemothorax is indicated, as blood can serve as a nidus for infection.[40] If the hemothorax is incompletely evacuated using a functional single tube, placement of a second tube is unlikely to be helpful in removing clotted blood and may likely increase the risk of infection.[41]

Thus, an operative approach is needed. When used early (<5 days after injury), video-assisted thoracic surgery (VATS) has been shown to be cost-effective method for managing clotted hemothoraces and free-flowing blood in patients who ideally can tolerate single-lung ventilation. However, VATS reduces the surgeon's ability to control bleeding and perform definitive repair of injuries; thus, in patients who have ongoing bleeding, posterolateral thoracotomy is required.[42–44] It is our practice to routinely obtain chest CT when patients have persistent pleural effusion after tube thoracostomy on chest radiograph within 48 hours of injury. In patients confirmed to have a persistent pleural effusion, we proceed directly to VATS as it is well documented that delaying the operation increases the technical difficulty of the procedure and rate of conversion to thoracotomy.[45,46]

Empyema Thoracis. Empyema thoracis is a troublesome complication after chest trauma, occurring in approximately 1.5%-5% of patients.[39,40,47,48] Possible causes include retained hemothorax, pneumonia with parapneumonic effusion, persistent foreign body, ruptured pulmonary abscess, bronchopleural fistula, esophageal leakage, and tracking through the intact or injured diaphragm from an abdominal source. Empyema may be difficult to diagnose in the posttraumatic setting and must be differentiated from pleural thickening, pulmonary contusion, or uninfected effusion. Thoracic CT with intravenous contrast usually demonstrates a fluid collection with loculations or an enhancing rim. Such findings, coupled with a clinical scenario of low-grade sepsis, worsening respiratory function, or failure to thrive, are diagnostic. Analysis and culture of fluid obtained at thoracocentesis or chest tube placement typically confirm the diagnosis, but the fluid may be sterile if the patient is already receiving antibiotics.

Antibiotic therapy, either broad-spectrum or specifically directed against cultured organisms (usually gram-positive pathogens), is certainly an important component of therapy for empyema thoracis, but the primary goal is the removal of the infection while the fluid is still thin. When this goal is met, a more modest therapeutic procedure can be performed, there is less risk that a restrictive pulmonary peel will develop, and the injured patient recovers faster overall. Rarely, in the early stages, tube thoracostomy may suffice for treatment; more commonly, the infected pleural process cannot be completely evacuated via chest tube because of thicker fluid, loculations, or pleural adhesions. In these cases, VATS or a formal thoracotomy with decortication is generally required.

Decortication is the cornerstone of effective therapy for posttraumatic empyema. Emphasis should be placed on completely removing the visceral pleural peel to allow complete lung expansion postoperatively. Decortication should not be undertaken in the face of severe sepsis. Instead, antibiotics and drainage (via tube thoracostomy, CT-directed catheter placement, or open rib resection) should be employed until the sepsis is controlled. Once the patient's condition has stabilized, decortication may be performed. In cases of early empyema, VATS has been successfully used for lysis of adhesions and removal of fluid.[48,49] Because of the limited capacity for performing pleurectomy with this procedure, VATS should not be used when thick peel or a trapped lung is present.

Pulmonary Contusion. Pulmonary contusions are bruises to the lung that are caused by either blunt or penetrating trauma. The contused segment of the lung has a profound ventilation–perfusion mismatch, which produces an intrapulmonary right-to-left shunt and hypoxia. The clinical sequelae of lung contusion vary from simple shortness of breath to respiratory failure requiring mechanical ventilation. Lung contusion results in systemic activation of the innate immune system as evidenced by local and systemic production of various inflammatory mediators such as the interleukins, prostaglandins, and chemokines. This resultant inflammatory response contributes to the evolution of pulmonary and remote organ dysfunction.[50] The contusion is usually not fully evident on plain chest radiograph but is better imaged with thoracic CT. The size of the contusion has been found to be directly proportional to the risk of developing acute respiratory distress syndrome.[51] Lung contusion is a well-established risk factor for pneumonia, and the bruised lung also may serve later as a source of sepsis.

Most pulmonary contusions that are not complicated by excessive attempts at resuscitation or by superinfection resolve over 3–5 days. Cardiovascular and ventilatory support is provided. In general, pulmonary contusion is treated in much the same fashion as flail chest. Patients with rib fractures and painful chest wall excursions must be given sufficient analgesic support to allow them to produce a forceful cough. Intubated patients should undergo suctioning frequently. Patients with pulmonary contusions who require substantial volume resuscitation should be considered for pulmonary arterial catheter monitoring. Steroids are not indicated, because they have no effect on the development or resolution of the contusion and because they set the stage for subsequent infection. Diuretics and prophylactic antibiotics are also unnecessary.

Pulmonary Lacerations. Bleeding pulmonary lacerations can be oversewn, resected, or explored via pulmonary tractotomy. Bleeding from small or shallow lacerations can be controlled with a continuous monofilament suture. Bleeding from deeper lacerations is controlled with resection or tractotomy. Most pulmonary resections for trauma should be stapled, nonanatomic resections. However, anatomic lung resection is required in rare instances, and trauma surgeons should remain familiar with the technical aspects of this procedure. Mortality is proportional to the amount of lung tissue resected: with suture repair alone, mortality is 9%; with tractotomy, 13%; with wedge resection, 30%; with lobectomy, 43%; and with pneumonectomy, 50%.[52,53]

Tractotomy is especially useful for deep through-and-through injuries that do not involve the hilum.[54] In this technique, the injury tract is opened with a linear stapler or between two aortic clamps. If clamps are used, the cut lung edges are oversewn and the tract left open (Fig. 27.4). Tractotomy exposes bleeding vessels and air leaks inside the tract and permits selective ligation. Occasionally, it exposes an injury to a major vascular or airway structure that must be treated with a formal resection. Because of the risk of exsanguination or excessive devitalization of lung tissue, tractotomy is not indicated when the injury traverses the hilum or when the entire thickness of a lobe will be cut.

Central lung injuries often cause massive hemorrhage. In addition, they may be sources of pulmonary venous air emboli when both a major pulmonary vein and a large airway are disrupted. A common scenario involves an intubated patient who exhibits sudden deterioration of central nervous system (CNS) and cardiac status shortly after being placed on positive pressure ventilation. Emergency thoracotomy must be performed and the pulmonary hilum clamped or twisted. The diagnosis is confirmed by visualizing air in the epicardial coronary arteries. Aspiration of air from the left-side cardiac chambers and elevation of central blood pressure are useful maneuvers. Most central lung injuries are associated with extensive parenchymal injury in gravely ill patients. Selective repair of hilar structures is usually impractical in this setting, and lobectomy or pneumonectomy is the salvage procedure of choice.

Tracheobronchial Injuries

Although tracheobronchial injuries are often lethal, a high index of suspicion for the existence of the injury, a timely diagnosis, and appropriate intervention can improve the chances of a successful outcome. The reported incidence of tracheobronchial injury in blunt chest trauma patients ranges from 0.2% to 8%.[55-57] Concomitant injury is the rule rather than the exception, but the patterns of associated injury vary widely. More than 80% of tracheobronchial ruptures occur within 2.5 cm of the carina.[58]

Clinical presentation of injury to the tracheobronchial tree is dependent upon severity and location of injury. In the neck, airway involvement may create severe respiratory distress that results in death before emergency care can be given. Alternatively, patients with cervical tracheal injuries may present with stridor, hoarseness, hemoptysis, or cervical subcutaneous emphysema. The presentation of thoracic tracheobronchial injury depends on whether the injury is confined to the mediastinum or communicates with the pleural space. Injuries confined to the mediastinum usually present with massive pneumomediastinum. Injuries that extend to the pleural space create an ipsilateral pneumothorax that may or may not be under tension. A pneumothorax that persists despite adequate placement of a thoracostomy tube with a continuous air leak is suggestive of tracheobronchial tree injury and bronchopleural fistula. Dyspnea may actually worsen after insertion of the chest tube because of the loss of tidal volume via the tube. Of note, these injuries are rare, and most pneumothoraces that do not resolve with multiple tube thoracostomies do not represent tracheobronchial injury; malpositioned or clotted tubes are a much more likely culprit.

The diagnosis is typically suspected on the basis of the clinical history and the characteristic signs and symptoms. The advent of spiral CT with multiplanar reconstruction has led to increased use of this modality to evaluate tracheobronchial injury. There are an increasing number of reports demonstrating the utility of CT technology in diagnosing tracheobronchial injuries with a sensitivity approaching 100%.[59,60] Because of its excellent negative predictive value, CT may be employed as a screening tool to look for these injuries in stable patients; however, at present, diagnostic bronchoscopy remains necessary to reliably exclude the diagnosis of tracheobronchial injury. In stable patients with transmediastinal

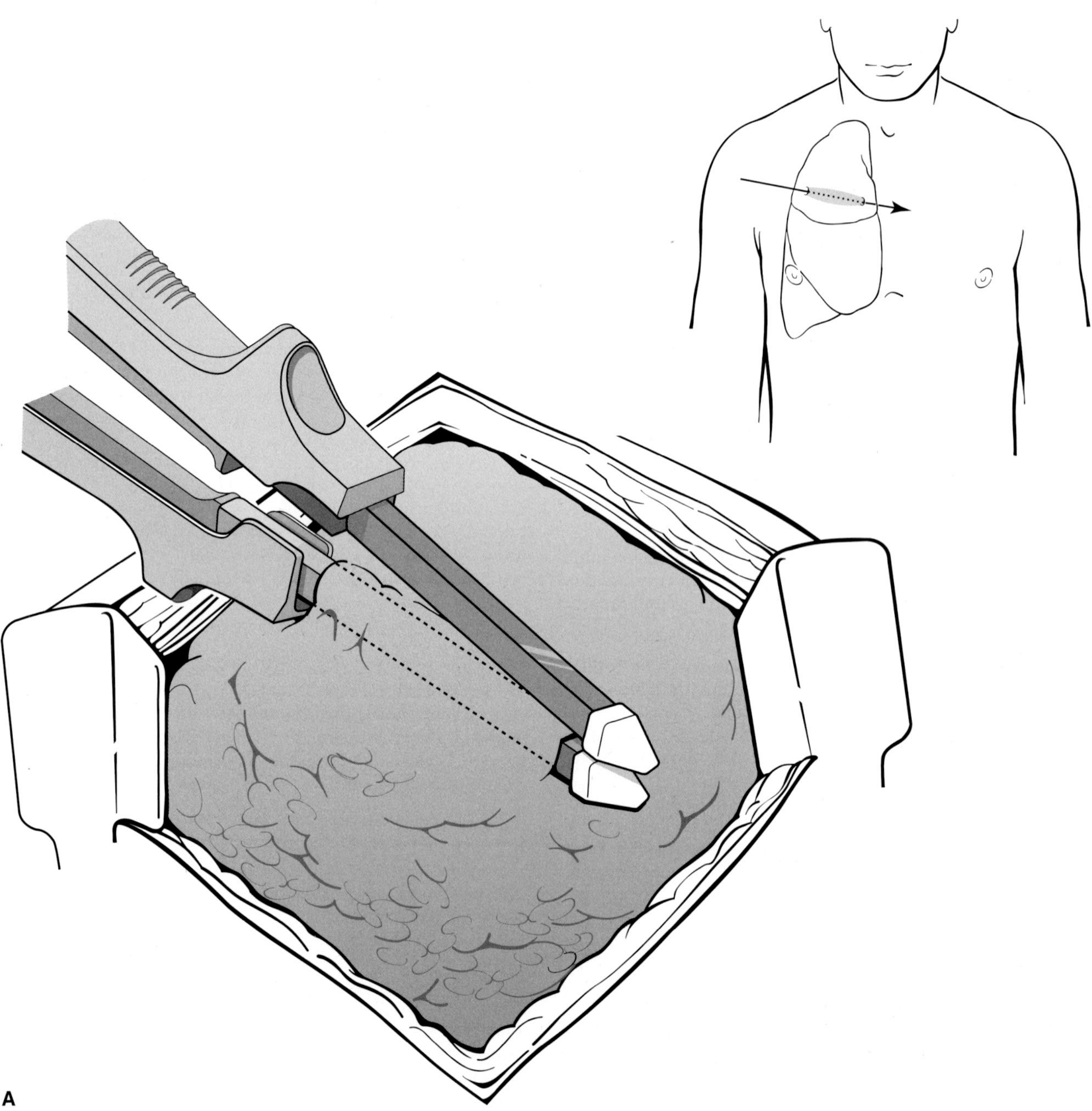

FIGURE 27.4. Tractotomy for nonhilar pulmonary injuries. **A:** The principle is to open the tract of the bullet or knife wound (**inset**), so that larger interior vessels may be identified and ligated individually.

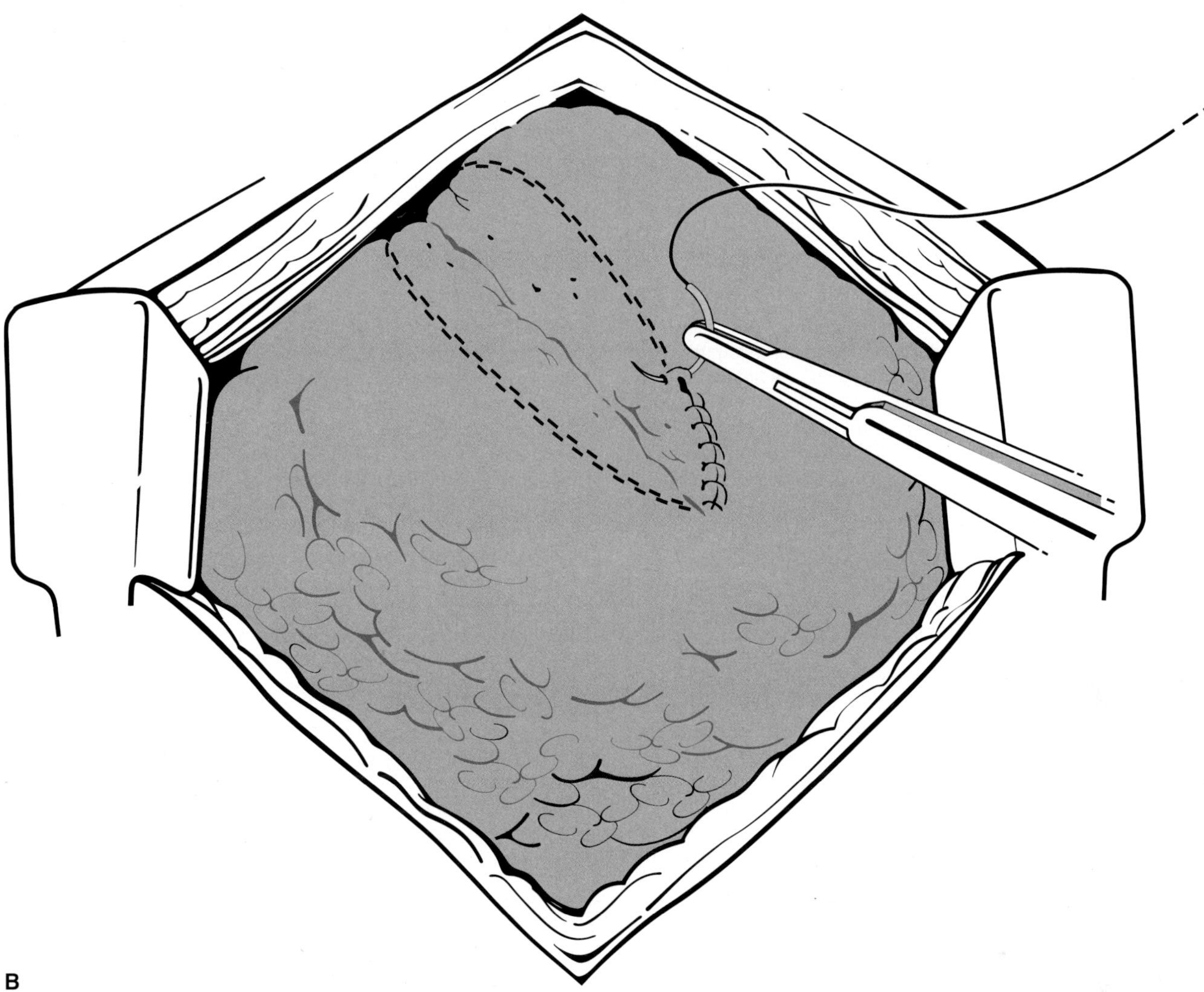

FIGURE 27.4. *(Continued)* B: 3-0 polypropylene suture may be used to individually ligate the vessels or may be run along the length of the tractotomy.

gunshot wounds, thoracic CT may be employed to detect proximity of the missile tract to mediastinal structures, directing subsequent evaluation.[61] Indications for bronchoscopy in this setting include a large pneumomediastinum, a refractory pneumothorax, a large air leak, persistent atelectasis, and possibly marked subcutaneous emphysema.[62]

The first priority in the treatment of tracheobronchial injury is airway management. If the patient is maintaining his or her own airway and is adequately ventilated, a cautious noninterventional approach is probably the best choice until further diagnostic workup is performed or other life-threatening injuries are stabilized. Careless handling of the airway can be disastrous and may compound the injury. The best method to secure an airway in a patient with neck trauma, and possible tracheal injury is a matter of debate. With blind endotracheal intubation, the path of the tube distal to the larynx is unknown, and it is possible to lose the lumen or create a false passage. With intubation over a flexible bronchoscope, the tube can be visualized as it passes beyond the site of injury, and some of the dangers of blind intubation are thereby mitigated. However, some degree of sedation is usually required, and if the patient is oversedated, the airway that was being spontaneously protected may be lost. For this reason, paralytic medications should generally be avoided in this setting. Urgent tracheostomy, performed in the OR, is advocated by many as the safest and most secure way of obtaining airway control. If the trachea is completely transected, the distal trachea can usually be found in the superior mediastinum and grasped for insertion of a cuffed tube. The approach taken to airway control must vary with the resources and expertise available at each institution. One must also keep in mind that even after the airway is secured, it may still be possible to exacerbate the injury by means of aggressive ventilation with high airway pressures. Tube thoracostomies should be appropriately placed at this time and connected to suction, even though dyspnea may worsen. Once the airway is controlled, there is time for orderly identification of concurrent injuries, esophagoscopy, laryngoscopy, arteriography, transport to definitive care areas, and, if necessary, celiotomy.

Selected tracheobronchial tears may be managed nonoperatively. Lesions suitable for observation must involve less than one third of the circumference of the tracheobronchial tree. The lungs must be fully re-expanded with tube thoracostomy. Prophylactic antibiotics, humidified oxygen, voice rest, frequent suctioning, and close observation for sepsis and airway obstruction are required. Small penetrating wounds with well-opposed edges and no evidence of loss or devitalization of tracheal tissue may be effectively treated with temporary endotracheal intubation.[58] The cuff of the endotracheal tube should be inflated below the level of injury and left undisturbed for 24–48 hours while the wound seals. If a conservatively managed patient's clinical condition deteriorates, bronchoscopy should be liberally repeated.

More commonly, operative repair is required. Intrathoracic tracheal, right bronchial- and proximal left mainstem bronchus injuries are best repaired through a right posterolateral thoracotomy at the fourth or fifth intercostal space, because this approach avoids the heart and the aortic arch. Distal left bronchial injuries more than 3 cm from the carina are approached through a left posterolateral thoracotomy in the fifth intercostal space. Optimal repair includes adequate débridement of devitalized tissue (including cartilage) and primary end-to-end anastomosis of the clean tracheal or bronchial ends. The anastomosis can be accomplished without tension by mobilizing the structures anteriorly and posteriorly, thereby preserving the lateral blood supply. Tension may also be released with cervical flexion, which can be maintained postoperatively by securing the chin to the chest with a suture. The repair may be buttressed with pleura, pericardium, or an intercostal muscle flap.

Esophageal Injury

Injury to the esophagus, though relatively rare, poses particular problems for the treating physician because of the complexity of the presentation, the workup, and the treatment options. Despite diagnostic and therapeutic advances, the morbidity and mortality associated with esophageal injury remain high. Most esophageal injuries result from penetrating trauma. If surgical exploration is performed for all penetrating cervical wounds that violate the platysma, the esophagus is found to be injured approximately 12% of the time. Penetrating intrathoracic esophageal injuries are less common, however, occurring in about 0.7% of all penetrating chest wounds.[63]

Signs and symptoms of esophageal injury include odynophagia, dysphagia, hematemesis, oropharyngeal blood, cervical crepitus, pain and tenderness in the neck or chest, resistance to passive motion, dyspnea, hoarseness, bleeding, cough, and stridor. Fever, subcutaneous emphysema, abdominal tenderness, and mediastinal crunching sounds (Hamman's sign) may be observed. Pain is the most common presenting symptom (71% of patients), followed by fever (51%), dyspnea (24%), and crepitus (22%).[64] Overall, the signs and symptoms associated with esophageal injury are fairly nonspecific, and a high index of suspicion must be maintained to make the diagnosis.

Evaluation of potential esophageal injuries due to penetrating trauma is usually performed surgically: either the tract is found to be inconsistent with esophageal injury or direct inspection of the esophagus reveals it to be uninjured. If neither option is feasible, diagnostic testing is necessary. Plain radiographs, CT scans, and contrast esophagrams are all commonly used imaging modalities with varying sensitivities and specificities. Endoscopy may add to the diagnosis, but the results depend on the operator's technique and experience, and there is a risk that it may exacerbate an esophageal tear or further injure an unstable cervical spine. In an otherwise asymptomatic patient who is awake, alert, and able to cooperate, a simple contrast swallow is usually sufficient to exclude injury. Injuries resulting from low-velocity projectiles and stab wounds do not cause large tissue defects; for these injuries, barium gives superior anatomic detail and is the agent of choice. Injuries from large-caliber or high-velocity projectiles usually cause more damage, and, thus, the contrast agent tends to spread more widely throughout the mediastinum during a diagnostic swallow. If contrast studies are indicated in this setting, a water-soluble agent may be used first. Such agents cause pulmonary damage when aspirated, however, and should not be used if tracheoesophageal fistula is suspected.

In cases of blunt trauma, determining when further study is needed is a vexing task. In general, whenever a patient has pneumomediastinum that is extensive or is associated with any of the symptoms of esophageal injury, the esophagus should be evaluated. Simple pneumomediastinum seen on thoracic CT without other indication of aerodigestive injury rarely warrants evaluation of the esophagus.[65] Regardless of the diagnostic studies obtained, evaluation must be carried out expeditiously. Considerable delays in management can increase the incidence of esophageal injury-related morbidity by as much as a factor of two.[66]

Injuries to the distal third of the thoracic esophagus are most easily approached via the left chest. More proximal injuries are best approached through the right chest or via a combination of chest and cervical incisions. The incision should be made so as to facilitate subsequent buttressing of the repair (e.g., with a pedicle from an intercostal muscle or the latissimus dorsi). Surgical repair entails local débridement, wide drainage, primary repair of the perforation with absorbable suture, and buttressing of the repair with a viable muscle flap. Primary repair can usually be accomplished when the perforation is repaired within 24 hours of occurrence. Placement of a gastrostomy tube for gastric drainage and jejunal feeding tube for enteral feeding access should be considered in all these patients. In the absence of distal obstruction, almost all late-presenting esophageal perforations heal after primary repair and tissue flap coverage. Generally speaking, techniques such as esophageal exclusion, diversion, and resection should be needed only when perforation occurs in the setting of a primary esophageal pathologic condition (e.g., cancer); esophageal perforation in this setting is rarely managed by trauma surgeons.

Thoracic Duct Injuries

Chylothorax after blunt or penetrating chest trauma is rare: only case reports and small case series are found in the literature. Much of the management of this condition is extrapolated from management of iatrogenic thoracic duct injuries, which are much more common. Most patients with traumatic chylothorax show evidence of other axial injuries to the chest, especially spine fractures.[67] The diagnosis is made by finding chylomicrons and high levels of triglycerides in a typically large pleural effusion of milky appearance. Drainage of as much as 1,000 mL per day is not unusual and results in severe nutritional and immunologic derangements, which are the main causes of the high mortality associated with this condition.

Treatment usually begins with limiting oral intake of short- and long-chain triglycerides, which cause increased flow of chyle. Diets high in medium-chain triglycerides must often be given enterally, because they are not palatable. Some clinicians recommend instituting total parenteral nutrition with complete abstinence from oral intake. Administration of octreotide may also help decrease chyle production.[68] These treatments, in conjunction with adequate pleural drainage and lung expansion, are successful in approximately 50% of cases after 2–6 weeks.

Operative strategies for managing thoracic duct injuries are generally undertaken only after conservative measures fail. Preoperatively, patients are fed cream, with or without dyes such as Sudan black, to increase chyle flow and enhance visualization of the site of injury. The thoracic duct is then ligated above and below the injury; this may be performed by means of VATS on the hemithorax ipsilateral to the effusion.[57] Fibrin glue and talc pleurodesis may be used as adjuncts to ligation. Because there are usually multiple areas of injury and because the thoracic duct is friable by nature, surgical treatment is not always successful. Continued nutritional management and reoperation may be required.

Cardiac Injury

Cardiac injuries may result from either blunt or penetrating trauma and involve the myocardium, coronary arteries, valves, or septum. Mortality rates range from 10% to 70% depending on presentation and mechanism of injury.[69–71]

Penetrating. Patients with penetrating cardiac injuries generally present in one of three ways. In approximately 20% of patients, the injury is clinically silent, at least initially, and is subsequently diagnosed at operation or on diagnostic imaging. In approximately 50%, there is evidence of pericardial tamponade, including one or more of the signs in Beck's triad (hypotension, distended neck veins, and muffled heart sounds). In the remaining patients, hemorrhagic shock develops after free bleeding from an atrial or ventricular wound into one or both hemithoraces.

Diagnosis of penetrating injuries to the heart often requires a high index of suspicion. The locations of entrance and exit wounds, the trajectory and path of the wounding object, and the locations of any retained missiles on radiographs are helpful in predicting heart injuries. Proximity wounds to the heart are defined as those that penetrate the chest wall in the area bounded superiorly by the clavicles, laterally by the midclavicular lines, and inferiorly by the costal margins. Any crossing of the anterior mediastinum by a missile or an instrument is also considered a proximity wound. Because cardiac injuries are present in 15%-20% of patients who present with proximity wounds, these injuries must be definitively excluded.

Physical examination is often unreliable in detecting pericardial tamponade. It is rare for all three signs in Beck's triad to be found; in fact, only about half of patients with tamponade show even two of the three. Moreover, detection of muffled heart sounds and distended neck veins amid the commotion typical of the trauma bay can be extremely difficult. Imaging studies may be helpful in this scenario.

As surgeons become more familiar with the use of ultrasonography in the trauma setting, two-dimensional surface echocardiography is gaining acceptance as a means of diagnosing cardiac injuries. When performed by appropriately trained surgeons, FAST detects blood within the pericardial sac with a sensitivity of 96%-100% and a specificity of 100%—results essentially equivalent to those achieved with a pericardial window.[7] In cases of concurrent laceration of the pericardial sac, pericardial ultrasound may not detect a cardiac injury because of associated decompression into the thoracic cavity.[72] If hemothorax is present, other diagnostic methods such as pericardial window are recommended.

The subxiphoid pericardial window remains the gold standard for diagnosis of cardiac injury. For otherwise stable patients with proximity wounds or suggestive signs and symptoms, a pericardial window should be considered when ultrasonographic findings are equivocal or when ultrasonography is unavailable. This procedure is usually performed in the OR with the patient under general anesthesia, often in combination with abdominal exploration (Fig. 27.5).

Some authorities advocate using pericardiocentesis to detect cardiac injuries, especially when rapid access to the OR, trauma surgeons, and anesthesiologists is not available. Drawbacks to this approach include the high rate of false positives and false negatives and the potential for iatrogenic cardiac injury. Furthermore, pericardiocentesis is of limited use in treating tamponade, because blood within the pericardial sac often is clotted and is not amenable to removal through a needle.

Surgical approach to penetrating cardiac injuries varies with mechanism of injury, patient physiology, and injury pattern. A median sternotomy is a logical extension of a subxiphoid pericardial window and provides access to all four chambers of the heart. It is appropriate for most precordial stab wounds and some low-caliber gunshot wounds. Its main limitations are that it does not allow repair or cross-clamping of the descending aorta or examination or repair of the esophagus and bronchi. It also provides only limited exposure of the lower lobes of the lungs and the hemidiaphragms. A left thoracotomy is appropriate for patients who may require cross-clamping of the thoracic aorta and for those with suspected cardiac injuries in conjunction with other complex thoracic visceral injuries. Only occasionally is a right thoracotomy required; this incision generally does not provide adequate exposure of the heart.

Atrial wounds are generally amenable to early control by finger pressure or by exclusion with a vascular clamp and simple oversewing. Right or left ventricular free wall injuries away from the coronary arteries may be treated by applying digital pressure over the entrance wound for hemostasis, then placing horizontal mattress sutures under the wound, reinforced with an epicardial continuous suture along the site of injury. All left ventricular wounds should be repaired with felt-pledgetted or pericardial-pledgetted sutures. Many right ventricular stab wounds can be closed primarily without pledgets if the sutures are tied accurately.

Injuries near coronary arteries must be closed without incorporating the coronary artery in the suture. This can be accomplished by placing horizontal mattress sutures lateral and deep to the coronary artery across the cardiac laceration. If the sutures are tied with careful attention to the function of the myocardium distal to the injury and equally careful attention to the electrocardiogram, the laceration can be closed without coronary artery occlusion and subsequent ischemia. With all penetrating cardiac wounds, it is important to recognize the possibility of associated intracardiac injuries.

Blunt. Blunt cardiac injuries range from disruption of myocardium, septa, or valvular structures to cardiac contusion. Both cardiac disruption (also known as cardiorrhexis) and cardiac contusion are common; the former is seen most often in patients who die at the scene, the latter in those who survive to reach the hospital. Blunt cardiac injury typically involves a direct blow to the chest, usually sustained in a motor vehicle collision or a fall. Cardiac injuries generally are associated with sternal or rib fractures, though they may occur in the absence of any chest wall fracture; sternal fractures do not predict the presence of blunt cardiac injury.

The diagnosis of myocardial contusion is elusive. Many tests have been proposed, but none have proved definitive, except for direct visualization of the heart at surgery or autopsy. For practical purposes, the clinically important sequelae of myocardial contusion are myocardial dysrhythmias and pump failure. Guidelines have been proposed that may facilitate the workup of this condition.

The EAST guidelines recommend 12-lead EKG as an initial screening test in those with mechanism for and suspicion of blunt cardiac injury. If this screening EKG is normal, no further workup is required. If the admission EKG is abnormal, the patient should be admitted for continuous EKG monitoring for 24–48 hours. If a patient is hemodynamically unstable or abnormal, echocardiography should be obtained (transthoracic echocardiography or transesophageal if transthoracic is suboptimal). There is no role for cardiac enzyme analysis or cardiac troponin assay in the setting of blunt cardiac injury. The latter test may detect myocardial injury, but this information does not complement ECG and echocardiographic findings and has no clinical utility. Similarly, there is no role for nuclear medicine studies.[73]

Pump failure associated with blunt cardiac injury is usually the result of right heart failure, because most hemodynamically

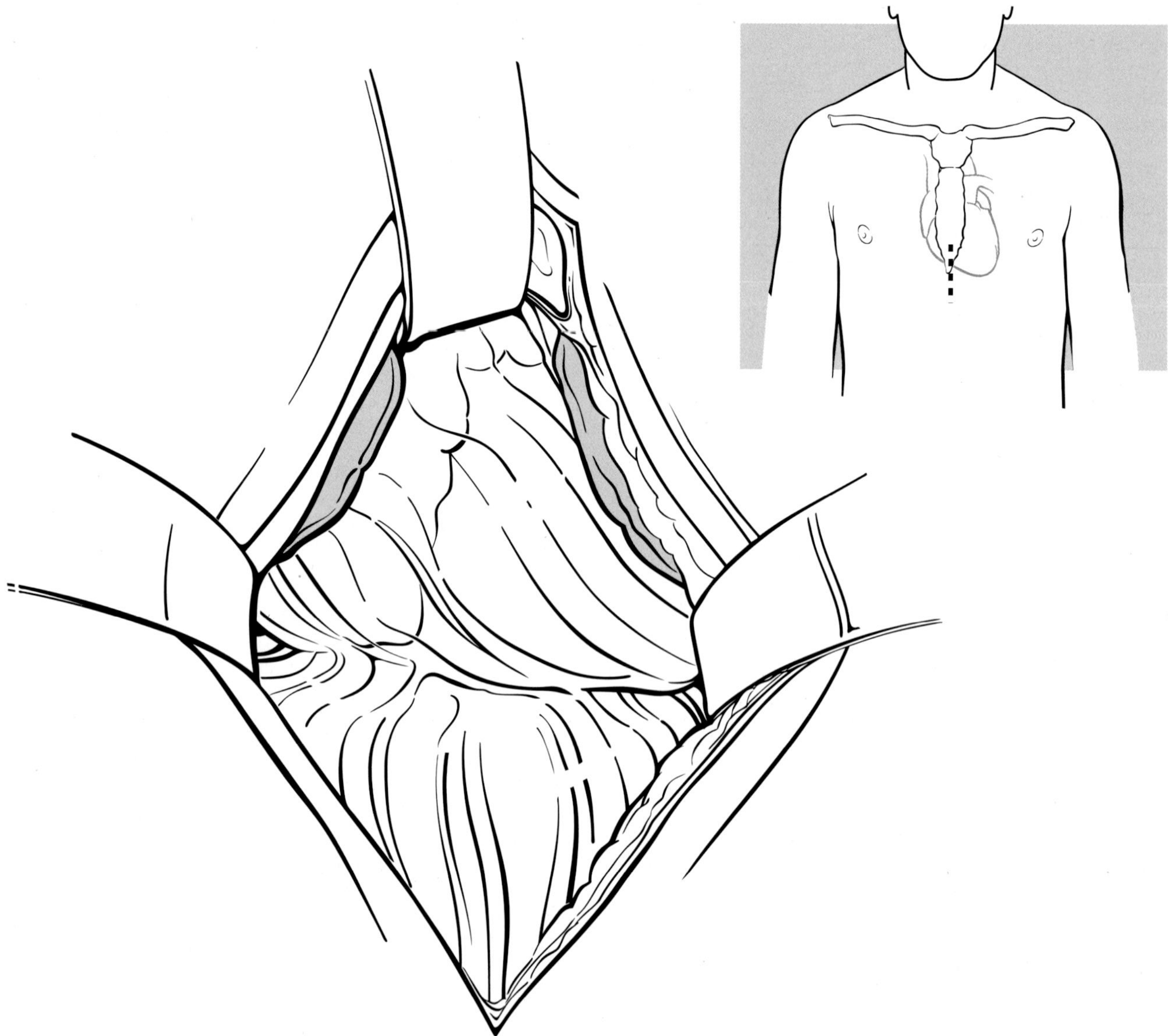

FIGURE 27.5. Subxiphoid pericardial window. The subxiphoid pericardial window remains the gold standard for diagnosis of cardiac injury.

major blunt cardiac injuries are caused by injury to the anterior right ventricular free wall. Treatment of right heart failure from blunt cardiac injury consists of inotropic support and reduction of right ventricular afterload. Dysrhythmias secondary to blunt cardiac injuries are treated in the same manner as dysrhythmias of any other etiology.

In the rare patient with cardiorrhexis who presents to the hospital with signs of life, the most common injury is right atrial perforation. Other lesions seen in patients with vital signs, in order of decreasing incidence, are left atrial perforation, right ventricular perforation, atrial septal perforation, ventricular septal perforation, coronary artery thrombosis, and valvular insufficiency (most commonly involving the tricuspid and mitral valves).[70,74,75] Principles of operative repair do not differ from those of penetrating cardiac trauma.

Blunt Aortic Injuries

Traumatic rupture of the aorta may account for as many as 10%-15% of all traffic fatalities, and the majority of such injuries are fatal at the scene. Traumatic disruption of the thoracic aorta results from rapid deceleration and is produced by a shearing effect caused by differences in the mobility of the aorta above and below a point where the vessel is fixed. Most thoracic aortic disruptions in survivors occur at the aortic isthmus just distal to the origin of the left subclavian artery, where the aorta is fixed to a substantial degree by the ligamentum arteriosum. Autopsy series reveal that as many as 40% of aortic injuries in nonsurvivors are not located at the isthmus, and the injuries tend to be complex.[76]

Suspicion of an aortic injury is most often triggered by abnormal findings on a chest radiograph in a patient with a high-speed mechanism of injury and multiple other injuries. Most patients show no signs or symptoms on physical examination, but some complain of interscapular pain or hoarseness. Others may exhibit a difference in blood pressure or pulse fullness between the upper and lower extremities or between the right and left upper extremities. Accordingly, the diagnosis is usually made radiographically.

Numerous radiographic signs of thoracic aortic disruption have been described, all representing hemorrhage within the mediastinum that alters or obliterates the shadows seen on a normal chest radiograph. Mediastinal widening is the most frequent indicator. Other important signs are obscuration of the contour of the aortic knob, opacification of the aortopulmonary window, depression of the left mainstem bronchus, apical capping, deviation of the nasogastric tube, and displacement of the esophagus to the right. These signs may be present in any combination or may be entirely absent. Currently, thoracic CT is used liberally for diagnosis of thoracic vascular injuries. CT is used in virtually all patients with abnormal chest radiographs and in many patients with normal chest radiographs with a mechanism involving a high degree of energy transfer. CT findings that are suggestive of aortic injury include mediastinal hematoma, periaortic hematoma, intraluminal irregularity (intimal flap), acute coarctation, and abnormal aortic contour. Depending on the experience of the interpreting clinician, aortography may be eliminated in most of these patients before surgical repair; the sensitivity and specificity of CT in this setting approach 100%.[77–79] Aortography should continue to be used for equivocal cases or cases in which spiral CT is not available.

Essentially all aortic injuries associated with mediastinal hematomas should be repaired. Repair of these injuries, however, is less urgent than attainment of an adequate airway, control of external or cavitary hemorrhage, and evacuation of intracranial mass lesions. If there is active bleeding from a blunt aortic injury, it will be massive and the need for exigent and primary attention should be apparent; lesser amounts of bleeding from a chest tube often derive from associated injuries. If intra-abdominal bleeding is present, laparotomy is indicated before repair of the contained thoracic aortic injury and before aortography. Similarly, in patients with intracranial hemorrhage that necessitates operative evacuation, craniotomy should take precedence over repair of the contained thoracic aortic injury.

While one is temporizing, stringent efforts must be made to prevent hypertension and reduce shear forces across the injury, ideally by means of intravenous beta blockade. Esmolol, because of its short half-life, is the best agent to use in these patients, who are at risk for sudden hypovolemic episodes of hypotension. The goals of medical therapy are a heart rate lower than 100 beats per minute and a systolic blood pressure of approximately 100 mm Hg (in young and middle-aged patients) or 110–120 mm Hg (in elderly patients). With careful delayed operative management of aortic injuries, the risk of rupture is low but is not completely eliminated.[80,81]

Traditional repair techniques include exposure of the injury via left thoracotomy with direct repair or interposition graft placement. Although excellent results have been obtained with so-called clamp-and-sew techniques, most guidelines recommend use of some form of distal aortic perfusion using either left atrial–distal aortic bypass or partial cardiopulmonary bypass with femoral cannulation. With distal aortic perfusion, the risk of paraplegia is approximately 5% and is independent of clamp time; without distal aortic perfusion, ischemic times longer than 30 minutes are associated with an exponential rise in the incidence of spinal cord injury.

The use of endovascular stent grafting for repair of blunt aortic injury is increasing rapidly. Several reports have demonstrated success in the use of this technique.[82–84] Initial reports regarding the use of this technology report that advantages include a lower incidence of paraplegia, fewer respiratory complications, and lower mortality than the open approach to repair.[85–87] However, most studies examining this technique are single-institution and retrospective without long-term outcome data, and so interpretation of results should be approached with caution. There are limitations with the current level of stent graft technology, and device-related complications have been reported. However, the field of endovascular intervention is expanding rapidly, and indications for endovascular repair of blunt aortic injury are in evolution.

Great Vessel Injuries

Except for tears in the descending aorta, injuries to the thoracic great vessels, by any mechanism, are rarely seen in clinical practice; the best descriptions come from wartime and autopsy series. Diagnosis and management of these injuries cover a wide spectrum of possibilities, depending on mechanism of injury, presenting features, and associated injuries.

Penetrating Injuries. Penetrating thoracic great vessel injuries are usually obvious. The presence of an entrance wound at the base of the neck or in the chest should alert the clinician to this possibility. If the patient is in shock, urgent operation is required. If the patient's condition stabilizes with resuscitation, an arteriogram should be performed to localize the injury. Reports are emerging that Computed Tomography Angiography (CTA) may also be useful for delineation of these injuries.[16]

Exposure is most often obtained via a median sternotomy, with or without neck extension as needed for innominate, right subclavian, or carotid arterial injuries. Exposure of the left subclavian artery can be more difficult, even through a sternotomy with a trap-door extension. For isolated injuries to the proximal subclavian artery, a fourth-interspace left posterolateral thoracotomy is most useful. For injuries to the middle and distal thirds, supraclavicular incisions or deltopectoral incisions—or, occasionally, a combination thereof—are appropriate, provided that inflow control can be achieved. When inflow control is not attainable, as in cases involving injury at the thoracic outlet or the presence of a large hematoma, endovascular control of the proximal subclavian artery by means of a balloon catheter may be necessary. Moreover, there is a growing body of literature supporting endovascular management of great vessel injuries.[84,88–91] Endovascular repair may be considered in stable patients with arteriovenous fistula or pseudoaneurysm. Concerns with this modality primarily center on lack of data on long-term outcomes in a typically young patient population.

Most penetrating wounds of the middle and distal segments of the great vessels are amenable to lateral repair or end-to-end anastomosis; injuries involving greater tissue destruction usually prove fatal before the patient arrives at the hospital. The subclavian artery is a notable exception to this general rule, because the lack of elastic fibers in its tunica media makes it extremely friable. End-to-end anastomosis of an injured subclavian artery under any tension is doomed to failure. Accordingly, many subclavian injuries should be repaired with an interposition graft. Proximal injuries to the great vessels are best repaired by exclusion and bypass grafting with prosthetic material from the ascending aorta. Because bleeding is usually active, there is rarely enough time to arrange for cardiopulmonary bypass. Bypass is generally unnecessary, except in rare cases of associated ascending or aortic arch injury.

Blunt Injuries. Blunt injuries of the great vessels are typically the result of high speed and rapid deceleration. In postmortem examinations, pedestrians struck by motor vehicles have the highest rate of great vessel injuries. Patients with such injuries are rarely seen in the ED with signs of life.[88] Superior mediastinal hematoma is the most common finding during workup; its presence is an indication for further imaging with thoracic CT or angiography. Other presentations of blunt thoracic great vessel injury include dissection and thrombosis, which may be asymptomatic if localized to the proximal segments. Central neurologic injury may also be present, especially with carotid dissection. Associated stretch injury of the brachial plexus or the cervical nerve roots is common with subclavian artery injuries.

Once the diagnosis is made, all great vessel injuries require intervention, typically surgical therapy. However, there are increasing numbers of reports describing successful endovascular treatment of these injuries in select patients. Small intimal defects found incidentally can sometimes be managed nonoperatively with repeat imaging and antiplatelet therapy. Surgery is contraindicated if neurologic injury is present, the injury is deemed nonsurvivable, or a common carotid dissection has extended into the distal internal carotid artery. As with blunt aortic injuries, the timing of surgery should be tailored to the treatment priorities mandated by the associated injuries. When time permits, proximal lesions are best managed with cardiopulmonary bypass and hypothermic circulatory arrest. Arranging for these techniques is mandatory with injuries involving the ascending aorta and the arch. Associated venous injuries are commonly encountered during exploration for great vessel arterial injury. If possible, they should be treated with lateral repair or patch venorrhaphy with pericardium or saphenous vein. However, ligation of these veins sometimes proves necessary and is generally well tolerated.

CONCLUSION

Thoracic trauma is a contributing factor in a majority of trauma-related deaths. With thorough physical examination and appropriate radiographic evaluation, the majority of these injuries can be identified and treated promptly. Most thoracic injuries do not require operative intervention; many may be treated with simple life-saving bedside procedures. However, when considering surgical intervention, many variables must be considered in this decision process, and each injury has unique issues to be addressed. Once the need for intervention is apparent, the critical decision for an appropriate surgical approach is based on a complete understanding of the location and nature of the injury.

References

1. Kemmerer WT, Eckert WG, Gathright JB, et al. Patterns of thoracic injuries in fatal traffic accidents. *J Trauma*. 1961;1:595-599.
2. Blansfield JS. The origins of casualty evacuation and echelons of care: lessons learned from the American Civil War. *Int J Trauma Nurs*. 1999;5(1):5-9.
3. LoCicero J III, Mattox KL. Epidemiology of chest trauma. *Surg Clin North Am*. 1989;69(1):15-19.
4. Soldati G, Testa A, Pignataro G, et al. The ultrasonographic deep sulcus sign in traumatic pneumothorax. *Ultrasound Med Biol*. 2006;32(8):1157-1163.
5. Soldati G, Testa A, Sher S, et al. Occult traumatic pneumothorax: diagnostic accuracy of lung ultrasonography in the emergency department. *Chest*. 2008;133(1):204-211.
6. Rocco M, Carbone I, Morelli A, et al. Diagnostic accuracy of bedside ultrasonography in the ICU: feasibility of detecting pulmonary effusion and lung contusion in patients on respiratory support after severe blunt thoracic trauma. *Acta Anaesthesiol Scand*. 2008;52(6):776-784.
7. Rozycki GS, Feliciano DV, Ochsner MG, et al. The role of ultrasound in patients with possible penetrating cardiac wounds: a prospective multicenter study. *J Trauma*. 1999;46(4):543-551; discussion 551-542.
8. Exadaktylos AK, Sclabas G, Schmid SW, et al. Do we really need routine computed tomographic scanning in the primary evaluation of blunt chest trauma in patients with "normal" chest radiograph? *J Trauma*. 2001;51(6):1173-1176.
9. Salim A, Sangthong B, Martin M, et al. Whole body imaging in blunt multisystem trauma patients without obvious signs of injury: results of a prospective study. *Arch Surg*. 2006;141(5):468-473; discussion 473-465.
10. Bleetman A, Kasem H, Crawford R. Review of emergency thoracotomy for chest injuries in patients attending a UK Accident and Emergency department. *Injury*. 1996;27(2):129-132.
11. Ivatury RR, Kazigo J, Rohman M, et al. "Directed" emergency room thoracotomy: a prognostic prerequisite for survival. *J Trauma*. 1991;31(8):1076-1081; discussion 1081-1072.
12. Rhee PM, Acosta J, Bridgeman A, et al. Survival after emergency department thoracotomy: review of published data from the past 25 years. *J Am Coll Surg*. 2000;190(3):288-298.
13. Seamon MJ, Shiroff AM, Franco M, et al. Emergency department thoracotomy for penetrating injuries of the heart and great vessels: an appraisal of 283 consecutive cases from two urban trauma centers. *J Trauma*. 2009;67(6):1250-1257; discussion 1257-1258.
14. Feliciano DV, Bitondo CG, Cruse PA, et al. Liberal use of emergency center thoracotomy. *Am J Surg*. 1986;152(6):654-659.
15. Karmy-Jones R, Jurkovich GJ, Nathens AB, et al. Timing of urgent thoracotomy for hemorrhage after trauma: a multicenter study. *Arch Surg*. 2001;136(5):513-518.
16. O'Connor JV, Scalea TM. Penetrating thoracic great vessel injury: impact of admission hemodynamics and preoperative imaging. *J Trauma*. 2010;68(4):834-837.
17. Brookes JG, Dunn RJ, Rogers IR. Sternal fractures: a retrospective analysis of 272 cases. *J Trauma*. 1993;35(1):46-54.
18. Ziegler DW, Agarwal NN. The morbidity and mortality of rib fractures. *J Trauma*. 1994;37(6):975-979.
19. Bulger EM, Arneson MA, Mock CN, et al. Rib fractures in the elderly. *J Trauma*. 2000;48(6):1040-1046; discussion 1046-1047.
20. Bergeron E, Lavoie A, Clas D, et al. Elderly trauma patients with rib fractures are at greater risk of death and pneumonia. *J Trauma*. 2003;54(3):478-485.
21. Nirula R, Diaz JJ Jr, Trunkey DD, et al. Rib fracture repair: indications, technical issues, and future directions. *World J Surg*. 2009;33(1):14-22.
22. Mayberry JC, Ham LB, Schipper PH, et al. Surveyed opinion of American trauma, orthopedic, and thoracic surgeons on rib and sternal fracture repair. *J Trauma*. 2009;66(3):875-879.
23. Richardson JD, Franklin GA, Heffley S, et al. Operative fixation of chest wall fractures: an underused procedure? *Am Surg*. 2007;73(6):591-596; discussion 596-597.
24. Recinos G, Inaba K, Dubose J, et al. Epidemiology of sternal fractures. *Am Surg*. 2009;75(5):401-404.
25. Ciraulo DL, Elliott D, Mitchell KA, et al. Flail chest as a marker for significant injuries. *J Am Coll Surg*. 1994;178(5):466-470.
26. Craven KD, Oppenheimer L, Wood LD. Effects of contusion and flail chest on pulmonary perfusion and oxygen exchange. *J Appl Physiol*. 1979;47(4):729-737.
27. Richardson JD, Adams L, Flint LM. Selective management of flail chest and pulmonary contusion. *Ann Surg*. 1982;196(4):481-487.
28. Moon MR, Luchette FA, Gibson SW, et al. Prospective, randomized comparison of epidural versus parenteral opioid analgesia in thoracic trauma. *Ann Surg*. 1999;229(5):684-691; discussion 691-682.
29. Mackersie RC, Karagianes TG, Hoyt DB, et al. Prospective evaluation of epidural and intravenous administration of fentanyl for pain control and restoration of ventilatory function following multiple rib fractures. *J Trauma*. 1991;31(4):443-449; discussion 449-451.
30. Bulger EM, Edwards T, Klotz P, et al. Epidural analgesia improves outcome after multiple rib fractures. *Surgery*. 2004;136(2):426-430.
31. Simon BJ, Cushman J, Barraco R, et al. Pain management guidelines for blunt thoracic trauma. *J Trauma*. 2005;59(5):1256-1267.
32. Tanaka H, Yukioka T, Yamaguti Y, et al. Surgical stabilization of internal pneumatic stabilization? A prospective randomized study of management of severe flail chest patients. *J Trauma*. 2002;52(4):727-732; discussion 732.
33. Granetzny A, Abd El-Aal M, Emam E, et al. Surgical versus conservative treatment of flail chest. Evaluation of the pulmonary status. *Interact Cardiovasc Thorac Surg*. 2005;4(6):583-587.
34. Garramone RR Jr, Jacobs LM, Sahdev P. An objective method to measure and manage occult pneumothorax. *Surg Gynecol Obstet*. 1991;173(4):257-261.
35. Collins JC, Levine G, Waxman K. Occult traumatic pneumothorax: immediate tube thoracostomy versus expectant management. *Am Surg*. 1992;58(12):743-746.
36. Ball CG, Kirkpatrick AW, Laupland KB, et al. Incidence, risk factors, and outcomes for occult pneumothoraces in victims of major trauma. *J Trauma*. 2005;59(4):917-924; discussion 924-915.
37. Brasel KJ, Stafford RE, Weigelt JA, et al. Treatment of occult pneumothoraces from blunt trauma. *J Trauma*. 1999;46(6):987-991.
38. Enderson BL, Abdalla R, Frame SB, et al. Tube thoracostomy for occult pneumothorax: a prospective randomized study of its use. *J Trauma*. 1993;35(5):726-729; discussion 729-730.
39. Maxwell RA, Campbell DJ, Fabian TC, et al. Use of presumptive antibiotics following tube thoracostomy for traumatic hemopneumothorax in the prevention of empyema and pneumonia-a multi-center trial. *J Trauma*. 2004;57(4):742-748; discussion 748-749.
40. Aguilar MM, Battistella FD, Owings JT, et al. Posttraumatic empyema. Risk factor analysis. *Arch Surg*. 1997;132(6):647-650; discussion 650-641.
41. Karmy-Jones R, Holevar M, Sullivan RJ, et al. Residual hemothorax after chest tube placement correlates with increased risk of empyema following traumatic injury. *Can Respir J*. 2008;15(5):255-258.
42. Meyer DM, Jessen ME, Wait MA, et al. Early evacuation of traumatic retained hemothoraces using thoracoscopy: a prospective, randomized trial. *Ann Thorac Surg*. 1997;64(5):1396-1400; discussion 1400-1391.
43. Carrillo EH, Richardson JD. Thoracoscopy in the management of hemothorax and retained blood after trauma. *Curr Opin Pulm Med*. 1998;4(4):243-246.
44. Carrillo EH, Richardson JD. Thoracoscopy for the acutely injured patient. *Am J Surg*. 2005;190(2):234-238.
45. Heniford BT, Carrillo EH, Spain DA, et al. The role of thoracoscopy in the management of retained thoracic collections after trauma. *Ann Thorac Surg*. 1997;63(4):940-943.

46. Morales Uribe CH, Villegas Lanau MI, Petro Sánchez RD. Best timing for thoracoscopic evacuation of retained post-traumatic hemothorax. *Surg Endosc*. 2008;22(1):91-95.
47. Mandal AK, Thadepalli H, Chettipalli U. Posttraumatic empyema thoracis: a 24-year experience at a major trauma center. *J Trauma*. 1997;43(5):764-771.
48. Scherer LA, Battistella FD, Owings JT, et al. Video-assisted thoracic surgery in the treatment of posttraumatic empyema. *Arch Surg*. 1998;133(6):637-642.
49. O'Brien J, Cohen M, Solit R, et al. Thoracoscopic drainage and decortication as definitive treatment for empyema thoracis following penetrating chest injury. *J Trauma*. 1994;36(4):536-539; discussion 539-540.
50. Hoth JJ, Hudson WP, Brownlee NA, et al. Toll-like receptor 2 participates in the response to lung injury in a murine model of pulmonary contusion. *Shock*. 2007;28(4):447-452.
51. Miller PR, Croce MA, Bee TK, et al. ARDS after pulmonary contusion: accurate measurement of contusion volume identifies high-risk patients. *J Trauma*. 2001;51(2):223-228; discussion 229-230.
52. Karmy-Jones R, Jurkovich GJ, Shatz DV, et al. Management of traumatic lung injury: a Western Trauma Association Multicenter review. *J Trauma*. 2001;51(6):1049-1053.
53. Cothren C, Moore EE, Biffl WL, et al. Lung-sparing techniques are associated with improved outcome compared with anatomic resection for severe lung injuries. *J Trauma*. 2002;53(3):483-487.
54. Wall MJ Jr, Hirshberg A, Mattox KL. Pulmonary tractotomy with selective vascular ligation for penetrating injuries to the lung. *Am J Surg*. 1994;168(6):665-669.
55. Barmada H, Gibbons JR. Tracheobronchial injury in blunt and penetrating chest trauma. *Chest*. 1994;106(1):74-78.
56. Baumgartner F, Sheppard B, de Virgilio C, et al. Tracheal and main bronchial disruptions after blunt chest trauma: presentation and management. *Ann Thorac Surg*. 1990;50(4):569-574.
57. Campbell DB. Trauma to the chest wall, lung, and major airways. *Semin Thorac Cardiovasc Surg*. 1992;4(3):234-240.
58. Symbas PN, Justicz AG, Ricketts RR. Rupture of the airways from blunt trauma: treatment of complex injuries. *Ann Thorac Surg*. 1992;54(1):177-183.
59. Faure A, Floccard B, Pilleul F, et al. Multiplanar reconstruction: a new method for the diagnosis of tracheobronchial rupture? *Intensive Care Med*. 2007;33(12):2173-2178.
60. Scaglione M, Romano S, Pinto A, et al. Acute tracheobronchial injuries: impact of imaging on diagnosis and management implications. *Eur J Radiol*. 2006;59(3):336-343.
61. Stassen NA, Lukan JK, Spain DA, et al. Reevaluation of diagnostic procedures for transmediastinal gunshot wounds. *J Trauma*. 2002;53(4):635-638; discussion 638.
62. Flynn AE, Thomas AN, Schecter WP. Acute tracheobronchial injury. *J Trauma*. 1989;29(10):1326-1330.
63. Cornwell EE III, Kennedy F, Ayad IA, et al. Transmediastinal gunshot wounds. A reconsideration of the role of aortography. *Arch Surg*. 1996;131(9):949-952; discussion 952-943.
64. Nesbitt JC, Sawyers JL. Surgical management of esophageal perforation. *Am Surg*. 1987;53(4):183-191.
65. Dissanaike S, Shalhub S, Jurkovich GJ. The evaluation of pneumomediastinum in blunt trauma patients. *J Trauma*. 2008;65(6):1340-1345.
66. Asensio JA, Chahwan S, Forno W, et al. Penetrating esophageal injuries: multicenter study of the American Association for the Surgery of Trauma. *J Trauma*. 2001;50(2):289-296.
67. Silen ML, Weber TR. Management of thoracic duct injury associated with fracture-dislocation of the spine following blunt trauma. *J Trauma*. 1995;39(6):1185-1187.
68. Markham KM, Glover JL, Welsh RJ, et al. Octreotide in the treatment of thoracic duct injuries. *Am Surg*. 2000;66(12):1165-1167.
69. Demetriades D. Cardiac wounds. Experience with 70 patients. *Ann Surg*. 1986;203(3):315-317.
70. Henderson VJ, Smith RS, Fry WR, et al. Cardiac injuries: analysis of an unselected series of 251 cases. *J Trauma*. 1994;36(3):341-348.
71. Arreola-Risa C, Rhee P, Boyle EM, et al. Factors influencing outcome in stab wounds of the heart. *Am J Surg*. 1995;169(5):553-556.
72. Ball CG, Williams BH, Wyrzykowski AD, et al. A caveat to the performance of pericardial ultrasound in patients with penetrating cardiac wounds. *J Trauma*. 2009;67(5):1123-1124.
73. Pasquale M, Fabian TC. Practice management guidelines for trauma from the Eastern Association for the Surgery of Trauma. *J Trauma*. 1998;44(6):941-956; discussion 956-947.
74. Lancey RA, Monahan TS. Correlation of clinical characteristics and outcomes with injury scoring in blunt cardiac trauma. *J Trauma*. 2003;54(3):509-515.
75. Fulda G, Brathwaite CE, Rodriguez A, et al. Blunt traumatic rupture of the heart and pericardium: a ten-year experience (1979–1989). *J Trauma*. 1991;31(2):167-172; discussion 172-163.
76. Burkhart HM, Gomez GA, Jacobson LE, et al. Fatal blunt aortic injuries: a review of 242 autopsy cases. *J Trauma*. Jan 2001;50(1):113-115.
77. Melton SM, Kerby JD, McGiffin D, et al. The evolution of chest computed tomography for the definitive diagnosis of blunt aortic injury: a single-center experience. *J Trauma*. 2004;56(2):243-250.
78. Dyer DS, Moore EE, Ilke DN, et al. Thoracic aortic injury: how predictive is mechanism and is chest computed tomography a reliable screening tool? A prospective study of 1,561 patients. *J Trauma*. 2000;48(4):673-682; discussion 682-673.
79. Fabian TC, Richardson JD, Croce MA, et al. Prospective study of blunt aortic injury: multicenter Trial of the American Association for the Surgery of Trauma. *J Trauma*. 1997;42(3):374-380; discussion 380-373.
80. Hemmila MR, Arbabi S, Rowe SA, et al. Delayed repair for blunt thoracic aortic injury: is it really equivalent to early repair? *J Trauma*. 2004;56(1):13-23.
81. Fabian TC, Davis KA, Gavant ML, et al. Prospective study of blunt aortic injury: helical CT is diagnostic and antihypertensive therapy reduces rupture. *Ann Surg*. 1998;227(5):666-676; discussion 676-667.
82. Kasirajan K, Heffernan D, Langsfeld M. Acute thoracic aortic trauma: a comparison of endoluminal stent grafts with open repair and nonoperative management. *Ann Vasc Surg*. 2003;17(6):589-595.
83. Amabile P, Collart F, Gariboldi V, et al. Surgical versus endovascular treatment of traumatic thoracic aortic rupture. *J Vasc Surg*. 2004;40(5):873-879.
84. Schonholz CJ, Uflacker R, De Gregorio MA, et al. Stent-graft treatment of trauma to the supra-aortic arteries. A review. *J Cardiovasc Surg (Torino)*. 2007;48(5):537-549.
85. Ott MC, Stewart TC, Lawlor DK, et al. Management of blunt thoracic aortic injuries: endovascular stents versus open repair. *J Trauma*. 2004;56(3):565-570.
86. Xenos ES, Abedi NN, Davenport DL, et al. Meta-analysis of endovascular vs open repair for traumatic descending thoracic aortic rupture. *J Vasc Surg*. 2008;48(5):1343-1351.
87. Jonker FH, Giacovelli JK, Muhs BE, et al. Trends and outcomes of endovascular and open treatment for traumatic thoracic aortic injury. *J Vasc Surg*. 2010;51(3):565-71.
88. Althaus SJ, Keskey TS, Harker CP, et al. Percutaneous placement of self-expanding stent for acute traumatic arterial injury. *J Trauma*. 1996;41(1):145-148.
89. Carrick MM, Morrison CA, Pham HQ, et al. Modern management of traumatic subclavian artery injuries: a single institution's experience in the evolution of endovascular repair. *Am J Surg*. 2010;199(1):28-34.
90. du Toit DF, Odendaal W, Lambrechts A, et al. Surgical and endovascular management of penetrating innominate artery injuries. *Eur J Vasc Endovasc Surg*. 2008;36(1):56-62.
91. du Toit DF, Lambrechts AV, Stark H, et al. Long-term results of stent graft treatment of subclavian artery injuries: management of choice for stable patients? *J Vasc Surg*. 2008;47(4):739-743.

CHAPTER 28 ■ ABDOMINAL TRAUMA

JUAN ASENSIO, AURELIO RODRIGUEZ, GRACIELA BAUZA, T. VU, F. MAZZINI, F. HERRERIAS, AND ANDREW B. PEITZMAN

Evaluation and management of complex abdominal injury can challenge even the most seasoned surgeon, and missed abdominal injury remains a common cause of preventable morbidity and mortality. In the trauma patient, the abdomen is defined as the area between the nipples and the symphysis pubis. Because of the wide excursion of the diaphragm, penetrating injury at or below the nipple line (4th intercostal space) may involve the abdominal viscera. Understanding injury patterns increases the likelihood of timely diagnosis and treatment of injuries. The broad categories of abdominal injury are blunt injury and penetrating injury, with different injury patterns and different management and treatment. The paradigm shift to nonoperative management for blunt abdominal injury, and occasionally penetrating injury, has been made possible by the wide availability of computed tomography (CT) and a better understanding of the natural history of injury to the solid organs; spleen, liver, and kidney, specifically.[1]

INITIAL ASSESSMENT

The initial assessment of the trauma patient begins with the assessment of airway, breathing, and circulation. Based upon patient physiology on emergency department presentation, different levels of detailed examination and attention to life-threatening and non-life-threatening injuries may have occurred. Initial resuscitation of the trauma patient is discussed in Chapter 21, but for the purpose of this chapter, it is imperative to know that in a patient with potential abdominal injury, intravenous access should be supradiaphragmatic (i.e., subclavian, internal jugular, or antecubital fossa). In the patient with femoral intravenous access, potential abdominal vascular injuries such as liver, inferior vena cava (IVC), iliac arteries/veins, or aorta will result in fluid/colloid infusion into the abdominal compartment, creating further complications and ineffective resuscitation. In the patient with multiple gunshot wound (GSW) or stab wound (SWs) injuries, and high likelihood of both chest and abdominal injuries, intravenous access must be secured above and below the diaphragm.

Critically ill trauma patients are typically cold, coagulopathic, and acidotic; a lethal state referred to as the **triad of death**. Remember that trauma patients die from abnormal physiology. Do not focus on defining every anatomic injury in a critically ill trauma patient; the critical determination is the need for laparotomy.

BLUNT TRAUMA

Blunt mechanisms of injury include motor vehicle collision (MVC), motorcycle collision, pedestrians being struck, blast and crush injury, and fall from a height. Intra-abdominal injury in these scenarios results from compression and shearing forces on the tissues. Solid organ injury is most common: liver, spleen, kidney, or mesentery. Remember that seat belts not only save lives, but change injury patterns. Intestinal perforation or mesenteric injury is common in the restrained victim of MVC; present in 25% of patients with a lap belt mark.

The trauma patient is initially triaged by EMS along with a physician by protocol or over radio communication, which then alerts the trauma team of the mechanism and suspected injuries. The trauma team prepares accordingly to perform a number of procedures starting always with the ABCs. In hemodynamically unstable patients, focused abdominal sonography for trauma (FAST) is utilized in the trauma bay to detect hemoperitoneum (Fig. 28.1). A positive initial FAST (~80% accuracy) in an unstable patient mandates immediate exploration. Diagnostic peritoneal lavage (DPL) has largely been supplanted by FAST and CT due to its invasive nature and lack of specificity for organ injury. However, DPL is sensitive for hemoperitoneum and may be appropriate in the unstable patient with a negative or nondiagnostic FAST. Depending on the injuries suspected or identified, the disposition of the patient will be to the radiology suite for further imaging, the operating room (OR) for definitive repairs, or the ICU for further resuscitation and monitoring. Many hemodynamically normal patients following substantial blunt injury will complete CT from head to midthigh, including the neck, chest, abdomen, and pelvis, although individual institutions and patient management algorithms exist on imaging strategies. Imaging of the abdominal and pelvic cavities has multiple goals: identify solid organ injury and severity, active arterial extravasation, vascular injury, and the presence of free air or free fluid in the pelvis. For these reasons, CT is obtained in an arterial phase and a venous phase.

Abdominal solid organs include the liver, spleen, pancreas, and kidneys. Over the last two decades, a marked paradigm shift toward nonoperative management of most solid organ injuries in hemodynamically stable patients has occurred (with the pancreas as the major exception).[2] Nonoperative management of solid organ injury at a minimum involves observation with frequent abdominal exams and serial hemoglobin checks. A major reason for the success of nonoperative management of blunt solid organ injury is the infrequent occurrence of hollow viscus injury. The Eastern Association for the Surgery of Trauma (EAST) multicenter study documented small bowel injury in only 0.3% of 275,000 patients.[3,4] On the other hand, the authors also documented that delay of only 8 hours in the treatment of an intestinal perforation increased mortality fourfold (from 2% to 9%).[3,4] Thus, we must be aware of clinical situations in which hollow viscus injury is likely, as its diagnosis remains difficult. Associated injuries on physical exam include seat belt or tire marks across the chest or abdomen, abdominal wall contusion, or truncal degloving injury. A Chance fracture (lumbar flexion/compression fracture) secondary to a lap belt has associated intestinal injury in as many as 25%-30% of patients. CT (with or without oral contrast) is a poor predictor of small bowel injury with a false-negative rate of 15%-30%. Findings suggestive of small bowel injury on CT include free fluid, free air, and bowel wall thickening. Eighty-four percent of patients with free fluid in the abdomen after blunt trauma on CT without solid organ injury have an intestinal injury or mesenteric injury, but only 30% of those have full thickness perforation. Moreover, a negative CT scan does not exclude intestinal perforation. Thus, when there is free fluid in the abdomen without solid organ injury, intestinal/mesenteric injury is present until proven otherwise by surgical exploration. Nance et al.[5] demonstrated that increasing number of

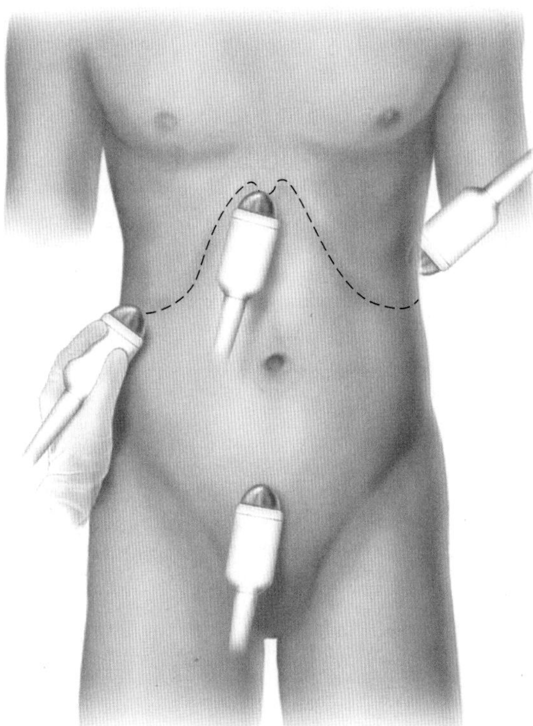

FIGURE 28.1. Focused abdominal sonography for trauma. (Redrawn from Rozycki GS, Ochsner MG, Schmidt JA, et al. A prospective study of surgeon-performed ultrasound as the primary adjuvant modality for injured patient assessment. *J Trauma.* 1995;39:493.)

solid organ injuries increased the likelihood of hollow viscus injury (most commonly small intestine). A single solid organ injury (spleen, liver, pancreas, or kidney) seen on CT had an associated hollow viscus injury in 7.3%, irrespective of the grade of solid organ injury. With additive solid organ injury, the incidence of hollow viscus injury increased; 15.4% with two solid organ injuries and 34.4% with three solid organ injuries. As mentioned, delay to operative intervention for hollow viscus perforation leads to greater mortality, sepsis, and wound dehiscence. Early exploration with control of intestinal contamination reduces morbidity and mortality considerably. The stomach and colon/rectum are injured less commonly than small bowel in blunt trauma, but require prompt diagnosis and exploration as well.

PENETRATING TRAUMA

Penetrating trauma mechanisms include GSWs, knife or SWs, and less commonly, impalement. The likelihood of injury requiring operative repair is higher for abdominal GSW (80%-95%) than for SWs (25%-33%), and the management algorithms differ. Abdominal organs commonly injured with penetrating wounds include the small bowel, liver, stomach, colon, and vascular structures. Any penetrating wound from the nipple line anteriorly (4th intercostal space) or scapular tip posteriorly to the buttocks inferiorly can produce an intraperitoneal injury.

GUNSHOT WOUNDS

In most instances, patients sustaining GSWs to the abdomen require laparotomy as their diagnostic and therapeutic modality, because of the high incidence of injury requiring repair.

PHYSICAL EXAMINATION

Carefully inspect the patient to avoid missing wounds. Bullets that do not strike bone or other solid objects generally travel in a straight line. Trajectory determination is the key to injury identification. Based on your estimate of the path of the bullet(s), determine which body cavities were violated and if so, which structures are at greatest risk of injury. With multiple GSWs, multiple cavity violation, this may be difficult. Nonetheless, hemodynamically unstable patients with abdominal GSWs should not have extensive evaluation before laparotomy. Carefully examine the patient, paying special attention to the body creases, perineum, ears, eyes, and rectum. Bullet wounds should be counted and assessed. An odd number of wounds suggests a retained bullet; elongated wounds without penetration typify graze injuries. Do not describe bullet wounds as entry or exit wounds; physical examination findings are unreliable in this regard. Describe in detail all missile wounds: site, size and configuration, presence of stippling or powder burns. Palpate the abdomen for signs of tenderness. A neurologic examination should be performed to exclude spinal cord injury.

Plain radiographs are essential in the determination of bullet trajectory. This is facilitated by marking cutaneous bullet wounds with radiopaque markers. In addition, pneumoperitoneum, spinal fractures, pneumothorax, or hemothorax may be found. CT has a limited role in the evaluation of patients with abdominal GSW. However, in hemodynamically stable patients in whom peritoneal penetration is questioned, the extraperitoneal path may be documented on CT. On the other hand, high-velocity weapons can produce full-thickness bowel perforation or thrombosis of major vessels without peritoneal penetration. If any doubt exists, laparotomy is mandatory. In addition, selected patients with right upper quadrant GSW isolated to the liver may be candidates for nonoperative management. Similarly, FAST has a limited role in the evaluation of patients with abdominal GSW. It may be useful in operative planning of hypotensive patients with multi-cavity wounds or documenting cardiac effusion/tamponade. Laparoscopy can be useful in the assessment of peritoneal violation or diaphragmatic injury in hemodynamically stable patients with tangential GSW, particularly in the left upper abdomen.

STAB WOUNDS

Indications for immediate exploration of abdominal SWs include hypotension, peritoneal signs, and evisceration. If these signs are not present, a selective management approach is justified. Although several articles have advocated observation of the stable patient with omental evisceration after a SW, we believe the incidence of visceral injury makes routine exploration the safest approach in these patients as well.[6,7] Anterior SWs refer to those in front of the anterior axillary line. One-third of SWs fail to violate the peritoneal cavity. Thus, two-thirds of anterior SWs enter the peritoneal cavity. Of these, less than half produce visceral injury, which requires operative repair. Thus, of patients with anterior SWs, only one-fourth to one-third require laparotomy. The clinical challenge is to safely select patients who require laparotomy and avoid nontherapeutic laparotomy in patients without major injury. Abdominal organs are at risk with thoracic wounds inferior to the nipple line anteriorly (4th intercostal space) and scapular tip posteriorly (Fig. 28.2). Flank SWs lie between the anterior and posterior axillary lines from the scapular tip to the iliac crest (Fig. 28.2b). Back (posterior) SWs are posterior to the posterior axillary line. Flank and posterior SWs have a lower incidence of visceral injury than anterior SWs (Fig. 28.2a).

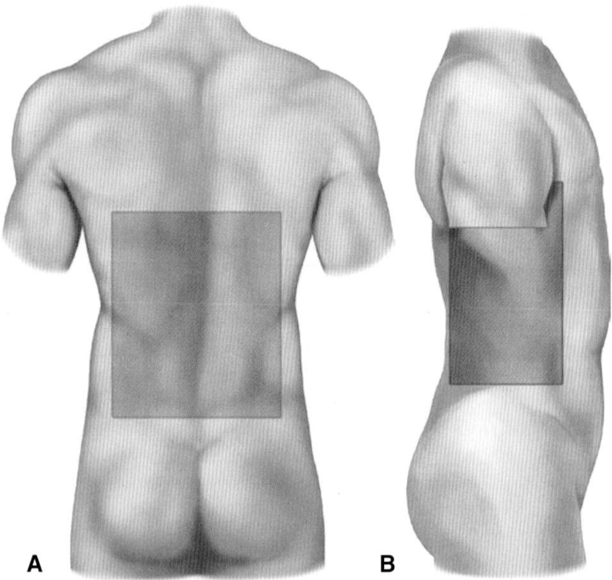

FIGURE 28.2. **A.** The posterior zone is from scapular tip to iliac crest and between each posterior axillary line. **B.** The flank zone is from 4th intercostal space to iliac crest between anterior and posterior axillary lines. (Redrawn from Boyle EM Jr, Maier RV, Salazar JD, et al. Diagnosis of injuries after stab wounds to the back and flank. *J Trauma.* 1997;42:261.)

Selective management (serial examination) can be used to detect the development of peritoneal signs in a hemodynamically stable patient. The same surgeon should repeat abdominal examinations documenting subtle change in abdominal findings, temperature, pulse rate, and white blood count. With this evaluation method, the delayed laparotomy rate is 40% with <3% mortality.[6-9]

Local wound exploration can be performed in the trauma resuscitation area on patients without indications for operation after anterior abdominal stab. The skin is prepared and anesthetized and the original wound is enlarged. Exploration is considered positive if fascial penetration is found. Most series define this as violation of the anterior fascia, as assessment of posterior fascial penetration is more difficult and less reliable.[8,9] Patients with positive local wound exploration progress to laparotomy.

CT scan with triple contrast (oral, IV, and rectal) can be used to evaluate back and flank SW. Although a popular tool in the past, triple-contrast CT is not often utilized nowadays. CT is not helpful in the evaluation of anterior abdominal SWs, especially in thin patients with slight abdominal musculature.

DPL has been used to evaluate abdominal SWs. The criteria for red blood cell (RBC) counts are generally lower than that for patients with blunt injury, but the range for positive results is from 1,000 to 100,000/mm^3.[10,11] Lower threshold values will improve the sensitivity of the modality, but increase the negative or nontherapeutic laparotomy rate.

Shotgun wounds. Close-range shotgun wounds are high-energy injuries. As such, they can result in blast and penetrating abdominal wounds. Shotgun wounds with peritoneal penetration mandate laparotomy. Those delivered from a distance, and thus lower velocity injury, can be evaluated with CT to determine peritoneal penetration by the pellets. The wider the area of scatter by the pellets, the greater the distance from the shotgun to the victim, with less tissue penetration.

Impalement injury. The impaled object is secured in place and removed in the OR under direct visualization with the abdomen open.

THE EXPLORATORY LAPAROTOMY

Refinements in diagnostic capabilities have allowed a more selective application of laparotomy, reducing the number of nontherapeutic laparotomies.

Indications for Exploratory Laparotomy

Laparotomy for trauma is performed on the basis of physical examination findings alone or on the basis of results of further diagnostic tests. Remember that physical examination alone with blunt injury will miss up to 45% of abdominal injuries, generally in patients with altered mental status or distracting injuries. Indications for laparotomy based on physical finding include obvious peritoneal signs on physical examination, hypotension with a distended abdomen on physical examination, abdominal GSW with peritoneal penetration, or abdominal SW with evisceration, hypotension, or peritonitis.

Findings on diagnostic tests, which mandate laparotomy include positive FAST (in the unstable patient), grossly positive DPL or peritoneal aspiration, or findings with any other diagnostic intervention (e.g., chest x-ray with ruptured diaphragm or pneumoperitoneum, abdominal CT, or laparoscopy suggestive of an intra-abdominal injury requiring repair).

An OR appropriately stocked with appropriate anesthetics and nursing and support should be immediately available 24 hours a day. Once the decision is made to operate, the patient must be rapidly transported directly to the OR with appropriate airway support personnel and the trauma team in attendance. Informed consent is obtained from the patient or relative before laparotomy if possible. This is not always possible or practical, depending on the injuries involved and the clinical state of the patient. In such cases, the operation should proceed without delay to obtain consent.

The patient should already have at least two large-bore intravenous lines placed; other intravenous and arterial access can be placed as necessary in the OR. Control of cavitary bleeding should not be delayed by fluid resuscitation; *the primary goal in the hemorrhaging patient is control of the bleeding.* Administer broad-spectrum, gram-negative, and anaerobic antibiotic coverage (e.g., an extended-spectrum penicillin or a third-generation cephalosporin). Attach chest tubes to underwater seal, do not clamp them, during transport and immediately to suction drainage on arrival in the OR. Make certain that anesthesia and the operating team can visualize the drainage systems of the chest tubes to monitor output during the operation.

Place nasogastric or orogastric tubes and a bladder catheter before laparotomy. However, no procedure should be performed in such a way, which delays control of bleeding and contamination. Sequential compression devices can be used for hemodynamically stable patients. Move the patient onto the operating table with appropriate cervical spine and thoracolumbar spine precautions. If the patient is still immobilized on a backboard, log roll the patient and remove the board before beginning the operation. Occult penetrating wounds must be sought before beginning laparotomy. Be certain to check all creases and folds where penetrating injury is likely to be missed.

Prime the infusion system to infuse blood products and "cell-saved blood" quickly via large-bore lines before the incision releases the tamponade. Ascertain that packed RBCs are in the OR and plasma and platelets are available for the patient with active hemorrhage. Activate the massive transfusion protocol if indicated.

Preparation of the Patient

The patient is shaved only if time allows. The entire anterolateral neck (remove anterior portion of cervical collar and then sandbag to maintain cervical spine immobilization), chest to the table bilaterally, abdomen, groin, and thigh regions (to the knees bilaterally) are prepared and draped in sterile fashion (Fig. 28.3).

CONDUCT OF THE TRAUMA LAPAROTOMY

Initial Goals

Stop bleeding and control gastrointestinal contamination. The exploratory laparotomy for trauma is a sequential, consistently conducted, operation. For urgent laparotomy, a generous midline incision is made. Adequate exposure is critical. Self-retaining retractor systems and headlights are useful. Control active bleeding first. Scoop free blood and rapidly pack all four quadrants to control bleeding as a first step. With blunt injury, the likely sources of bleeding are the liver, spleen, and mesentery. Pack the liver and spleen, and quickly clamp the mesenteric bleeders. With penetrating injury, the likely sources of bleeding are the liver, retroperitoneal vascular structures, and mesentery. Pack the liver and retroperitoneum, and quickly clamp bleeding mesenteric vessels. If packing does not control a bleeding site, this source of hemorrhage must be controlled as the first priority.

Once active bleeding is stopped, control of gastrointestinal contamination must be achieved next. Quickly control bowel content spillage using Babcock clamps, Allis clamps, a stapler, rapid temporary sutures, or ligatures. Only when hemorrhage and GI contamination are controlled, should the surgeon proceed to full exploration of the abdomen. Systematically explore the entire abdomen, giving priority to areas of ongoing hemorrhage to definitively control bleeding: liver, spleen, stomach, right colon, transverse colon, descending colon, sigmoid colon, rectum, and small bowel, from ligament of Treitz to terminal ileum, carefully inspecting the entire bowel wall and the mesentery. Next, open the lesser sac and explore the pancreas (visualize and palpate). A Kocher maneuver may be needed to visualize the duodenum, with evidence of possible injury. Finally, inspect the left and right hemidiaphragms and retroperitoneum, pelvic structures, including the bladder and rectum. Note the size of any retroperitoneal hematoma. With penetrating injury, exploration should focus on following the path of the weapon or missile. Retroperitoneal violation by a penetrating wound requires exploration of the retroperitoneum. The abdomen may be closed with running nonabsorbable or absorbable monofilament suture (e.g., No. 1 nylon or No. 1 looped slowly absorbable suture). Leave skin open with delayed secondary closure if there is contamination or prolonged hypoperfusion. If gross edema of abdominal contents precludes closure, absorbable mesh, sterile intravenous bags (Bogota bag), or intestinal bags can be used with moist gauze and an impermeable dressing, or a vacuum-assisted closure (VAC) dressing to prevent possible abdominal compartment syndrome (ACS) (see Chapter 6). Recognize the combination of complex injuries and physiologic signs (hypothermia, acidosis, and coagulopathy) that dictate abbreviated laparotomy (damage control).

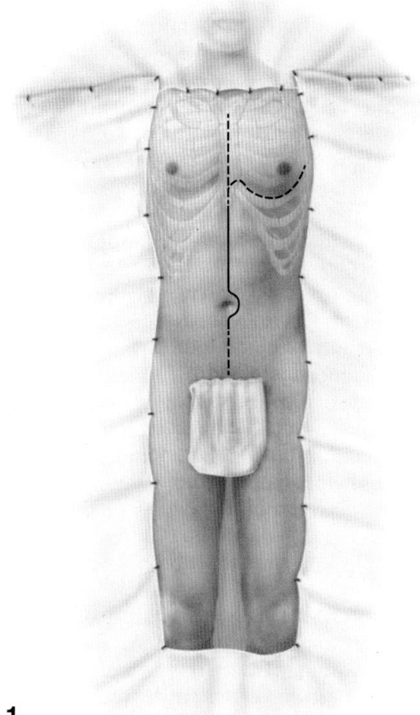

FIGURE 28.3. Full prep of the trauma patient for laparotomy. (Redrawn from Champion HR, Robbs JV, Trunkey DD. Trauma surgery. In: Dudley H, Carter D, Russell RCG, eds. *Rob and Smith's Operative Surgery*. Boston, MA: Butterworth; 1989:540, Figure 1).

SPECIFIC ORGAN INJURY

Diaphragmatic Injury

Anatomy and Physiology. The diaphragm is an arched muscular tendinous structure that separates the thorax from the abdomen. It is formed of a central tendon, which receives muscle fibers in a radial fashion. These fibers originate from the xiphoid and sternum anteriorly, the inferior border of the cartilage of the 9th-10th rib, and portions of the tips of the 11th and 12th ribs. Posteriorly, the diaphragm originates from the first and second lumbar vertebrae.

The aorta, thoracic duct, and azygos vein course through the aortic hiatus at the level of the 12th thoracic vertebra. The esophagus and the vagus nerves course through the esophageal hiatus at the level of the tenth thoracic vertebra and the vena cava is the only anatomic structure coursing through the caval hiatus, at the level of the eighth thoracic vertebra (Fig. 28.4).

The diaphragm has a fundamental function in the respiratory process, when it flattens, increasing the size of the thoracic cavity, thus creating a tidal volume. To accomplish this function, the diaphragm moves 3–5 cm in either direction. The simultaneous contraction of the abdominal muscles creates a gradient between the abdominal and thoracic cavity. When the patient is in the supine position, the gradient between the abdominal and thoracic pleural cavity fluctuates from 7 to 20 cm of water. During maximal inspiration, this gradient can be higher than 100 cm of water. It has been postulated, that

TRAUMA

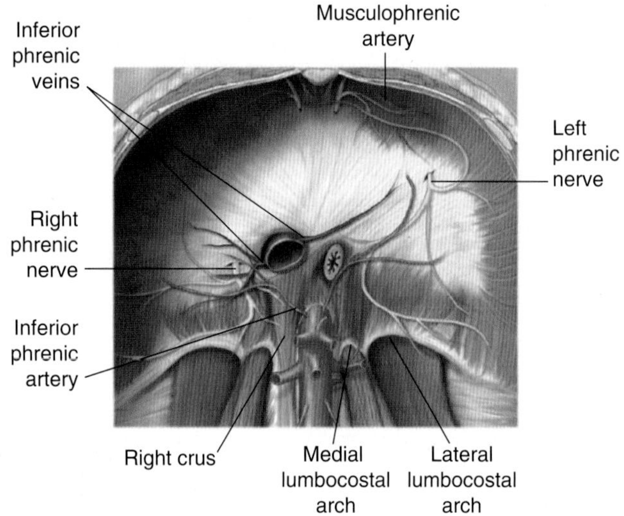

FIGURE 28.4. The origins and neurovascular supply of the diaphragm. (From Valentine RJ, Wind SS. Anatomic exposures in vascular surgery. Philadelphia, PA: Lippincott Williams and Wilkins; 2003:236, Figure 9-7).

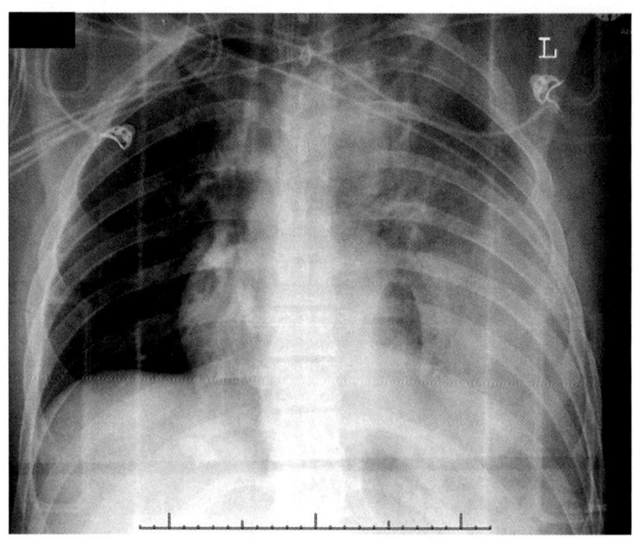

FIGURE 28.5. Chest radiograph of a patient with a ruptured left hemidiaphragm following a motor vehicle crash. A hemothorax is present and a hollow viscus as a result of the diaphragmatic tear is clearly seen in the chest.

the sudden increase of the intra-abdominal pressure (IAP), as in the case of blunt compressive mechanisms, elevates the gradient to levels responsible for the disruption of the diaphragm. Furthermore, this increase in the thoracoabdominal gradient may facilitate the migration of abdominal organs into the thoracic cavity.

Incidence. From the National Trauma Data Base, the incidence of diaphragmatic injury is 35% for blunt trauma and 65% for penetrating injury.[12] The most common location of diaphragmatic injury is the left side; in blunt trauma, 80% on the left and 20% on the right.[13] In penetrating trauma, diaphragmatic injury is more common on the left due to the preponderance of right hand-handed assailants and the fact that the liver protects the right hemidiaphragm, preventing abdominal viscera from herniation into the thoracic cavity. The organs more frequently involved in herniation in order of frequency are the stomach, colon, spleen, and small bowel.

Diagnosis. The high incidence of associated injuries can overshadow the diagnosis of diaphragmatic injury in the acute phase. High index of suspicion should be exercised when a penetrating wound of the left chest occurs below the 4th interspace and in blunt trauma when there is a simultaneous hemoperitoneum and left hemopneumothorax. The clinician should also be cognizant of the location and trajectory of the penetrating object and the possibility of diaphragmatic involvement. Most diaphragmatic injuries from penetrating trauma are diagnosed intraoperatively. Blunt diaphragmatic injury is generally a larger tear. During the laparotomy, the diaphragm should be inspected carefully with the help of a good headlamp illumination and an extension of your hand using a sponge stick, which allows spreading this floppy muscular organ, to avoid missing other rents. Injury to the diaphragm may be missed at laparotomy (5%), usually a posterior laceration.

The symptoms and signs of diaphragmatic injury range from minimal dyspnea, chest pain, shoulder pain, bowel sounds in the chest, to severe respiratory distress and shock, when associated with massive viscus herniation or associated thoracoabdominal injuries. On occasion, a scaphoid abdomen is seen on physical examination, with extensive herniation of abdominal contents into the chest.

The chest radiograph is the best screening modality in the diagnosis of diaphragmatic rupture, and any lack of delineation of this organ, particularly if it is associated with pleural effusion, should raise the suspicion of diaphragmatic injury. The chest radiograph will be diagnostic for diaphragmatic rupture in 25% of cases with abdominal viscera (usually stomach or small bowel) seen in the chest and normal in 25% of cases of blunt diaphragmatic injury. In 50% of cases, the chest radiograph is abnormal but not diagnostic (Fig. 28.5). Findings include elevation of a hemidiaphragm, obscuring of the diaphragmatic border, loss of the costophrenic angles, or lower lobe collapse.

Both DPL and FAST (focused assessment sonographic for trauma) will miss diaphragmatic injury.[13] CT has become the most used tool in the evaluation of abdominal injury in the last two decades. Initially, CT reported a sensitivity of 14%--61% and a specificity of 76%-99% in the diagnosis of diaphragmatic rupture. More modern CT technology has improved the accuracy to 80%--100%.[14,15] Magnetic resonance imaging may also be useful, particularly in cases of questionable CT or delayed diagnosis of diaphragmatic injury.[16]

Laparoscopy and thoracoscopy have become useful adjuncts in the diagnosis of diaphragmatic rupture.[17] Laparoscopy perhaps is more useful in patients without other indication for laparotomy, and thoracoscopy in a subacute situation of diagnostic dilemma. Laparoscopy is ideal with penetrating thoracoabdominal wounds on the left side, where the presence of diaphragmatic or abdominal injury is unclear. Laparoscopy may be used as a therapeutic tool in this setting, allowing repair of the diaphragm.

Surgical Management of Acute Diaphragmatic Rupture. The surgical management of acute diaphragmatic rupture, once the abdominal cavity is open, should not preclude the meticulous inspection of the entire abdominal cavity and its contents (Table 28.1). Once other priorities such as control of bleeding and contamination are accomplished, the attention should be focused on the diaphragm. With herniation of abdominal structures, these organs should be carefully retracted back to the abdomen. Good illumination with head lamps, and good exposure, with the transection of the triangular and falciform ligaments if necessary, will provide excellent

TABLE 28.1

DIAPHRAGM INJURY SCALE

GRADE[a]	DESCRIPTION OF INJURY	AIS-90
I	Contusion	2
II	Laceration <2 cm	3
III	Laceration 2–10 cm	3
IV	Laceration >10 cm with tissue loss ≤25 cm^2	3
V	Laceration with tissue loss >25 cm^2	3

[a]Advance one grade for bilateral injuries up to grade III.
AIS, abbreviated injury score.
From Moore EE, Malangoni MA, Cogbill TH, et al. Organ injury scaling IV: thoracic vascular, lung, cardiac and diaphragm. *J Trauma*. 1994;36:229–300.

visualization of the area. Careful downward traction of the spleen and stomach on the left side and the liver on the right will allow inspection of the diaphragms.

The edges of the diaphragmatic tear should be grasped with long Allis clamps and then proceed with a careful inspection of any lesion in the intrathoracic organs, if the rent is big enough. If there is evidence of contamination of the pleural cavity, with gastroenteric contamination, extensive irrigation of the thoracic cavity should be performed at this time. If the irrigation of the thoracic cavity is considered inadequate, a subsequent thoracotomy, according to some authors,[18] or a video-assisted thoracoscopy are options after completion of the laparotomy. In either case, large chest tubes should be placed as part of the procedure.

Multiple techniques are appropriate to suture the torn diaphragm. The diaphragm should be repaired with monofilament 0 or 1 (polypropylene) nonabsorbable material, with a one-layer or two-layer closure. Horizontal mattress sutures may serve as definitive closure or as the first of two layers of closure. This may be followed by a second layer of a running interlocking suture of the same material, superficial to the first layer. The function of this layer is, in theory, to prevent postoperative bleeding from the edges of this extremely vascularized structure. Central/pericardial tears occur in 5% of cases. The heart must be carefully inspected as well. With lacerations that extend to the esophageal hiatus, be certain not to compromise the orifice when closing; a large bougie may be helpful in this setting. On rare occasion, a detachment of lower insertion of the diaphragmatic fibers with reattachment of the diaphragm in a more cephalad manner is necessary. Mesh is rarely necessary in the acute phase. Diaphragmatic rupture has also been repaired successfully laparoscopically and thoracoscopically.

As a principle, an acute diaphragmatic disruption should be repaired through the abdomen, to address other intra-abdominal injury, which will be present in the majority of patients. In cases of subacute or delayed diagnosis of diaphragmatic injury, a thoracic approach may be easier, avoiding adhesions within the abdomen.

Stomach and Small Bowel Injury

Injury to the stomach or small intestine is more common after penetrating than blunt abdominal trauma. GSWs that violate the peritoneal cavity have a higher incidence of hollow viscus injury (70%) compared to SWs (30%). Thus, we have different strategies for the management of GSW versus SW of the abdomen; mandatory surgery for the GSWs and the possibility of a selective approach for the SWs. Blunt injuries of the stomach and small bowel are uncommon. The incidence found in a multicenter study of 275,000 blunt trauma victims by the EAST was 0.3%.[3,4] In patients with any blunt abdominal injury, 4%–7% will have hollow viscus injury. The finding of solid organ injuries increases the likelihood of hollow viscus injury.[5]

Anatomy. The empty stomach is essentially intrathoracic and protected by the ribcage. When distended, the stomach is at risk for rupture because of direct compression or acute increase in intraluminal pressure. The arterial blood supply of the stomach is the left gastric artery, right gastric artery, left and right gastroepiploic arteries, and the short gastric arteries.

The small intestine distal to the ligament of Treitz is 5–6 m. The small intestine is suspended on its mesentery, with its blood supply originating from the superior mesenteric artery (SMA). The arterial supply to the small intestine has multiple arcades and thus is a well-vascularized structure.

Pathophysiology. Blunt trauma usually produces contusions and intramural hematomas on the stomach and small bowel; more serious injuries such as perforations and mesenteric avulsions are less common.[19-21] Localized blows to the abdomen, by farm animals or handlebar injuries have been replaced by automobile crashes and sports injuries such as lacrosse sticks slashes to the abdomen, or football helmet collisions against the unprotected torso. Furthermore, the mandatory use of the seat belt has saved many lives but has increased the incidence of small bowel injury. The incidence of injury to the small intestine with the use of the three-point lap and shoulder restrain is increased 4.3-fold and increased 10-fold with the lap belt-only restraint, compared to the unrestrained victim.[3] The association of small bowel perforation or mesenteric injury with Chance fractures of the lumbar spine, associated with the seat belt, has been emphasized earlier.

Blast injury presents different complexes of injury from contusions to perforation, depending whether from primary blast effect and depending on proximity of the patient to the center of the explosion. Secondary blast effect is caused by projectiles from the explosion, with a penetrating component. Tertiary and quaternary injuries are caused by the generation of "blast winds" and fire, respectively. The more serious concern with blast injuries is the possibility of delayed clinical presentation with serious adverse consequences.

Diagnosis. An accurate history of the mechanism of injury, penetrating or blunt, is essential. The location of entrance and trajectory of the penetrating weapons: thoracic–abdominal wall or anterior abdomen should raise the suspicion of gastric or small bowel injury.

The initial laboratory studies: hemoglobin, hematocrit, serum amylase, and white blood cell count are of little value in the initial diagnosis of gastric or small bowel injury. However, fever, leukocytosis, increase in the serum amylase, and metabolic acidosis in the next 24 hours postadmission may be the first sign of a missed hollow viscus injury

DPL has been supplanted by FAST and CT. However, DPL has its value in the detection of hemoperitoneum. In addition, when the white cell count in the DPL effluent is more than 500 per mm^3, it may be considered positive for bowel injury. Nevertheless, Jacobs et al.[22] demonstrated that even using an elevation of over 500 per mm^3 white cells in the lavage, it should not be used a sole criterion in the diagnosis of bowel perforation. Elevation of the alkaline phosphatase >10 units in the DPL effluent or an elevation of the amylase >20 IU/L suggests bowel injury. More recently, authors[23] have used ratios of red cells/white cells in the DPL effluent to make a more accurate diagnosis of bowel lesions, avoiding the "lag period" of appearance of the white cells after the injury occurs.

Despite its sensitivity of 84% and the specificity of 99% for detection of hemoperitoneum, Focused assessment by sonography for trauma (FAST) is unreliable in the diagnosis of bowel injury. CT findings of free intraperitoneal air, free peritoneal fluid, thickening of the bowel wall, and mesenteric fat streaking are important predictors of injury. The Elvis Presley trauma center[23] found that the overall sensitivity and specificity of CT for bowel injury was 88.3% and 99.4%, respectively. The authors go further to recommend DPL if a single abnormal finding is found at CT and laparotomy or if several signs are found in the same diagnostic modality. The presence of intraperitoneal fluid on CT has different discriminatory values for different studies. Fakhry directed a multi-institutional study for EAST in 95 trauma centers and found that only 29% of patients with free fluid had full-thickness bowel injury. In the same series, 38% of patients with free fluid without solid viscus injury had bowel injury.[3,4] Despite a plethora of publications on the subject, there is no consensus in regard to the best management of the patient with free abdominal fluid in the absence of solid viscus injury; DPL, serial abdominal physical examinations; "diet trials" in the absence of abdominal pain or diagnostic laparoscopy have been proposed. The EAST trial noted that 12% of patients with normal CT had bowel injury.[3,4] Therefore, a prudent decision could be to keep the patient for observation.

Laparoscopy has been used for diagnosis and treatment of penetrating injury to the thoracoabdominal torso, to exclude penetration of the peritoneum and to assist in the diagnosis of diaphragmatic injuries. Its use in the diagnosis of gastric or small bowel lesions is limited at this point in time. However, it may have a role in the patient about whom there is a low level of suspicion to exclude bowel injury in the presence of fluid without a solid viscus injury.

TABLE 28.2

STOMACH INJURY SCALE

GRADE[a]	DESCRIPTION OF INJURY	AIS-90
I	Contusion or hematoma	2
	Partial thickness laceration	2
II	Laceration in GE junction or pylorus <2 cm	3
	In proximal one-third of stomach <5 cm	3
	In distal two-thirds of stomach <10 cm	3
III	Laceration >2 cm in GE junction or pylorus	3
	In proximal one-third of stomach ≥5 cm	3
	In distal two-thirds of stomach ≥10 cm	3
IV	Tissue loss or devascularization less than two-thirds of stomach	4
V	Tissue loss or devascularization greater than two-thirds of stomach	4

[a]Advance one grade for multiple lesions up to grade III.
GE, gastroesophageal.
From Moore EE, Jurkovich GJ, Knudson MM, et al. Organ injury scaling VI: extrahepatic biliary, esophagus, stomach, vulva, vagina, uterus, fallopian tube, ovary. *J Trauma*. 1995;39:1069–1070.

Management of Gastric Injuries. Gastric injuries are managed with the help of a good illumination (head lights) and good exposure (Table 28.2). The gastroesophageal junction may be difficult to visualize. This area can be exposed better with the division of the left triangular ligament of the left lobe of the liver and reverse Trendelenburg maneuver. The posterior wall of the stomach should always be inspected, particularly in the presence of penetrating injuries of this organ, which have involved the anterior wall. The gastrocolic ligament should be opened carefully, trying to avoid injury to the middle colic artery.

The surgical repair of the stomach wall is according the grade of severity.[19] Most grade I injuries, such as gastric wall hematomas, can be treated with evacuation of the hematoma if considered necessary, and the use of interrupted Lembert sutures. Small perforations can be treated with one- or two-layer closure. Larger perforations should be closed in two layers: a running suture of absorbable material is used for the inner layer and interrupted seromuscular silk stitches for the outer layer. Grade III gastric injury with major involvement of the greater curvature can be repaired with the assistance of GIA stapler, being certain to avoid unacceptable narrowing of the stomach lumen. The management of grade IV stomach injuries may require the use of a Bilroth 1 or a Bilroth 2 anastomosis for the repair. Grade V gastric injuries are rare; massive destruction of the organ, which could require a total gastrectomy and the use of a Roux-en-Y, with an esophagojejunostomy.

Surgical Management of Injuries of the Small Bowel. The evaluation of the bowel at the beginning of the laparotomy is fundamental. Systematic inspection of every loop of small bowel, starting from the ligament of Treitz, is better performed with the attentive help of the assistant surgeon for visualization of the bowel (Table 28.3). It is preferable to initially control a bowel injury, secondary to a penetrating injury and continue the "running of the bowel" to make a total assessment of the injuries and plan the surgical therapy. Grade I bowel injury can be treated by inversion with seromuscular sutures. Grade II bowel injury can be treated with debridement if necessary and with single- or double-layer closure, using absorbable and nonabsorbable material. Grade III or IV injury, more likely, will require bowel resection and anastomosis, unless the transverse closure will not produce a narrowing of the lumen of more than 30%.[20]

The anastomoses can be handsewn in one or two layers, or stapled. However, remember that the stapling devices are designed for normal thickness intestine. Stapled anastomosis should be avoided if possible, in the presence of edematous bowel, unless a new type of staplers with longer staple length can be obtained. Although the literature is inconclusive, several studies have suggested higher leak rates for stapled anastomoses versus handsewn anastomoses in the trauma patient.[24,25] Grade V bowel injury is associated with devascularization of the intestine requiring resection. In the presence of doubt regarding bowel viability, a 24-hour "second look" reexploration is necessary.

Colon and Rectal Injury. Management of colorectal injury has evolved over the past 40 years with the acceptance of evidence-based guidelines generated by civilian trauma centers, overriding the prior approach championed by military surgeons based on the application of lessons learned from battlefield injuries.[26-28] During the World War II, influenced by Ogilvie,[27] the Office of the Surgeon General of the United States mandated colostomy for all colonic injuries. This declaration made colostomy or exteriorization the standard of care for injury of the large bowel for 40 years. Woodhall and Oschner in 1951 pioneered the use of primary repair in the civilian injuries.[28] However, it was not until 1979 when Stone

TABLE 28.3

SMALL BOWEL INJURY SCALE

GRADE[a]	TYPE OF INJURY	DESCRIPTION OF INJURY	AIS-90
I	Hematoma	Contusion or hematoma without devascularization	2
	Laceration	Partial thickness, no perforation	2
II	Laceration	Laceration <50% of circumference	3
III	Laceration	Laceration ≥50% of circumference without transection	3
IV	Laceration	Transection of the small bowel	4
V	Laceration	Transection of the small bowel with segmental tissue loss	4
	Vascular	Devascularized segment	4

[a]Advance one grade for multiple injuries up to grade III.
AIS, abbreviated injury score.
From Moore EE, Cogbill TH, Malangoni MA, et al. Organ injury scaling II: pancreas, duodenum, small bowel, colon, and rectum. *J Trauma*. 1990;30:1427–1429.

and Fabian[29] in the United States and Demetriades[30] in South Africa produced seminal reports, confronting the dogma of "mandatory colostomy." Nevertheless, this was a select population of patients, without hypotension or associated injuries. Chaping et al.[31] in a prospective, randomized study of 59 patients concluded that irrespective of risk factors, primary repair does not increase the incidence of complications and should be recommended for any type of colonic lesion. A meta-analysis of five prospective studies[32] showed no difference in mortality between primary repair and colostomy for colonic injury. Blunt trauma is responsible for only 5% of the colonic injuries, and in nonurban settings, is most often caused by motor vehicle accidents, and results in sheering damage, due to acute increase in intraluminal pressure causing blowout, or avulsion/crush injury to the mesocolon. The colon is injured in 25% of GSW and 5% of SWs. Other injuries to the colon can be caused iatrogenically during colonoscopy, or can be the result of swallowed objects or objects inserted rectally. Injuries to the rectum are most often caused by penetrating objects, either to the abdomen or to the buttocks.

Anatomy. The colon begins at the ileocecal valve and ends at the rectosigmoid junction at the sacral promontory where the three taenia coli begin to diverge, and the epiploic appendages and mesentery stop. The rectum continues from the rectosigmoid junction and remains intraperitoneal for approximately 8 cm to the middle transverse fold, at which point the peritoneal reflection ends and the rectum becomes extraperitoneal. It extends for an additional 8 cm until the anorectal ring, demarcated by the dentate line.

The ascending colon is supplied by the ileocolic and right colic arteries from the SMA. The splenic flexure and proximal transverse colon are supplied by the middle colic artery, also from the SMA. The hepatic flexure is supplied by the marginal artery, formed by the anastomosis of the arcades from the middle colic and left colic arteries. The descending colon is supplied by the left colic artery from the inferior mesenteric artery (IMA). The sigmoid colon is supplied by the sigmoid artery, also from the IMA. The proximal rectum is supplied by the terminal branch of the IMA, the superior rectal artery. Finally, the distal two-thirds of the rectum is supplied by the middle and inferior rectal arteries from the internal iliac and internal pudendal arteries.

Diagnosis. The single most important method for diagnosis of colonic injury is serial examinations by a single examiner to allow assessment of the relative stability of the patient and subtle changes in physical examination. In trauma patients with obvious peritoneal signs (rebound, distension, guarding), an exploratory laparotomy is warranted without the need for further evaluation. Several studies[33] have shown that selective management, based on serial physical examinations of the patient, is safe, cost-effective, and avoids unnecessary laparotomy.

The presence of extraluminal air, contrast extravasation, colonic wall thickness, and stranding of the mesentery are suggestive of colon injury on CT or plain radiograph. Even though many trauma centers perform triple contrast CT (oral, IV, and rectal contrast) in the presence of penetrating trauma of the flank or back to exclude colonic injury, others believe that is unnecessary[34] in the diagnosis and management of colon injury.

Patients who have a penetrating injury to the abdomen, disruption of the bony pelvis, history of anal trauma, or pain in the buttock region should be suspected of harboring rectal injury. Any patient with suspected rectal injury must undergo rigid sigmoidoscopy, even if an exploratory laparotomy is already planned. Hematoma, perforation, and intraluminal blood are indicators of rectal injury. Transabdominal examination of the lower rectum is not recommended and provides no diagnostic benefit while subjecting the patient to increased risk of iatrogenic injury (Tables 28.4 and 28.5).

Management. When the decision is made to take a patient to the OR, a preoperative dose of broad spectrum antibiotics that cover aerobes and anaerobes, especially gram-negative rods should be given. Second-generation cephalosporin, ampicillin/sulbactan, or piperacillin is as effective as multiple antibiotics.[35] In addition, several studies have demonstrated the value of only 24 hours antibiotic coverage versus 5 days.[36]

Most colonic injuries are identified as part of a trauma laparotomy for penetrating abdominal trauma. Once bleeding and active GI soilage are controlled, the colon is mobilized by incising the white line of Toldt, the avascular plane between the omentum and transverse colon, and the splenocolic ligament. As mentioned above, operative management of colon injury has undergone a major shift toward primary repair and avoidance of colostomy.[37] The guidelines for primary repair,

TABLE 28.4

COLON INJURY SCALE

GRADE[a]	TYPE OF INJURY	DESCRIPTION OF INJURY	AIS-90
I	Hematoma	Contusion or hematoma without devascularization	2
	Laceration	Partial thickness, no perforation	2
II	Laceration	Laceration <50% of circumference	3
III	Laceration	Laceration ≥50% of circumference without transection	3
IV	Laceration	Transection of the colon	4
V	Laceration	Transection of the colon with segmental tissue loss	4

[a]Advance one grade for multiple injuries up to grade III.
AIS, abbreviated injury score.
From Moore EE, Cogbill TH, Malangoni MA, et al. Organ injury scaling II: pancreas, duodenum, small bowel, colon, and rectum. *J Trauma.* 1990;30:1427–1429.

even including colon injury which requires resection, include minimal stool contamination, no hypotension/shock, <1 L blood loss, <8 hour delay to operation, and minimal associated intra-abdominal injury. If primary repair cannot be safely performed due to patient instability or edematous or ischemic intestine, colostomy may be a safer option.

Areas of controversy include the use of GI staplers versus hand-sewn anastomoses and the use of one versus two layers of repair. Either technique can be used[37-39] and the decision should be guided by the surgeon experience and preference. If the patient is hemodynamically unstable, a damage control approach is necessary. Bleeding cessation and fecal contamination control should be the priority.

Inappropriately worn lap belts can cause a deserosalization type injury to the colon. This results in an intact mucosal tube exposed by a 360-degree tear of the muscular and serosal layers and tear of the mesentery. This injury is repaired by telescoping the mucosa on itself and suturing the muscular and serosal layers.

Proximal rectal injuries (intraperitoneal) are treated with a similar approach to colon injuries. The extraperitoneal colon injuries, if they are located distally near the anus, at times can be repaired transanally. However, in general, the rectal injury per se, is not repaired. More generally, middle and lower third rectal injuries are managed primarily by proximal diversion. Currently, there is no role for rectal washout.[40] The use of presacral drainage is also controversial, due to the complications and discomfort for the patient.[41] Presacral drainage should be considered only for lower one-third injury, essentially anal canal.

Special Considerations. For patients who undergo a colostomy, the timing of the takedown is still debated.[42] Current recommendations vary from performing the takedown within 14 days of the placement to waiting 9 months. Since most injuries heal within 10 days, there is no necessity to delay the takedown beyond 2 weeks in the patient who is stable and fully recovered otherwise.

TABLE 28.5

RECTUM INJURY SCALE

GRADE[a]	TYPE OF INJURY	DESCRIPTION OF INJURY	AIS-90
I	Hematoma	Contusion or hematoma without devascularization	2
	Laceration	Partial-thickness laceration	2
II	Laceration	Laceration <50% of circumference	3
III	Laceration	Laceration ≥50% of circumference	4
IV	Laceration	Full-thickness laceration with extension into the perineum	5
V	Vascular	Devascularized segment	5

[a]Advance one grade for multiple injuries up to grade III.
AIS, abbreviated injury score.
From Moore EE, Cogbill TH, Malangoni MA, et al. Organ injury scaling II: pancreas, duodenum, small bowel, colon, and rectum. *J Trauma.* 1990;30:1427–1429.

Duodenal Injury

Anatomy. The anatomy of the structures in the right upper quadrant of the abdomen is complex. The duodenum constitutes the beginning of the small bowel and measures approximately 21 cm.[43] It is divided into four portions: the first (superior), second (descending), third (transverse), and fourth (ascending) portions. The first portion of the duodenum ranges from the pyloric muscle to the common bile duct superiorly and the gastroduodenal artery inferiorly. Its origin is marked by the pyloric vein of Mayo. The second portion extends from the common bile duct and the gastroduodenal artery to the ampulla of Vater. The third portion extends from the ampulla of Vater to the mesenteric vessels (SMA and vein), which cross anteriorly over the junction of the third and fourth portions as they emerge from the inferior border of the neck of the pancreas. The fourth portion extends from these vessels to the point at which the duodenum emerges from the retroperitoneum to join the jejunum just to the left of the second lumbar vertebra. The entry to the duodenum is closed by the pyloric sphincter, and its exit is suspended by the fibromuscular ligament of Treitz. The duodenum is mobile at the pylorus and its fourth portion but remains fixed at other points.[44,45]

The duodenum is, for all practical purposes, a retroperitoneal organ, except for the anterior half of the circumference of its first portion. The first portion, the distal half of the third portion, and the fourth portion in its entirety lie directly over the vertebral column, which, coupled with the psoas muscles, aorta, IVC, and right kidney, form its posterior boundaries.

The duodenum shares its blood supply with the pancreas (Fig. 28.6). Vessels, which supply the duodenum include the gastroduodenal artery and its branches, the retroduodenal artery, the supraduodenal artery of Wilkie, the superior pancreaticoduodenal artery, and the SMA and its first branch, the inferior pancreaticoduodenal artery. The gastroduodenal artery courses from its hepatic origin at the superior surface of the duodenum under its second portion and enters the pancreas just below and opposite the common bile duct above the duodenum. The dorsal and ventral pancreaticoduodenal arcades are formed by the anastomosis of the superior and inferior pancreatic duodenal arteries and supply numerous branches to the pancreas and the duodenum.[46-50] The common bile duct enters the posterior substance of the head of the pancreas in 83% of patients after it passes under the duodenum.[51,52]

After piercing the capsule of the pancreas posteriorly, the duct courses down within the pancreatic substance a few centimeters from the curve of the duodenum, entering the duodenal lumen at the junction between the second and third portion of the duodenum approximately 2.0–2.5 cm from the pylorus.[53] Three main variations exist with regard to how both the common bile duct and pancreatic duct enter the duodenum. In 85% of individuals, both ducts enter through a common channel at the ampulla of Vater; in 5% both ducts enter the duodenum on the same ampulla but through separate channels.[47] In the remaining 10% of individuals, each duct enters the duodenum separately.

The duodenum serves as the mixing point for the partially digested chyle from the stomach and the proteolytic and lipolytic secretions of the biliary tract and pancreas. As such, it commonly contains not only food but powerful activated digestive enzymes, including lipase, trypsin, amylase, elastase, and peptidases, among others.[54]

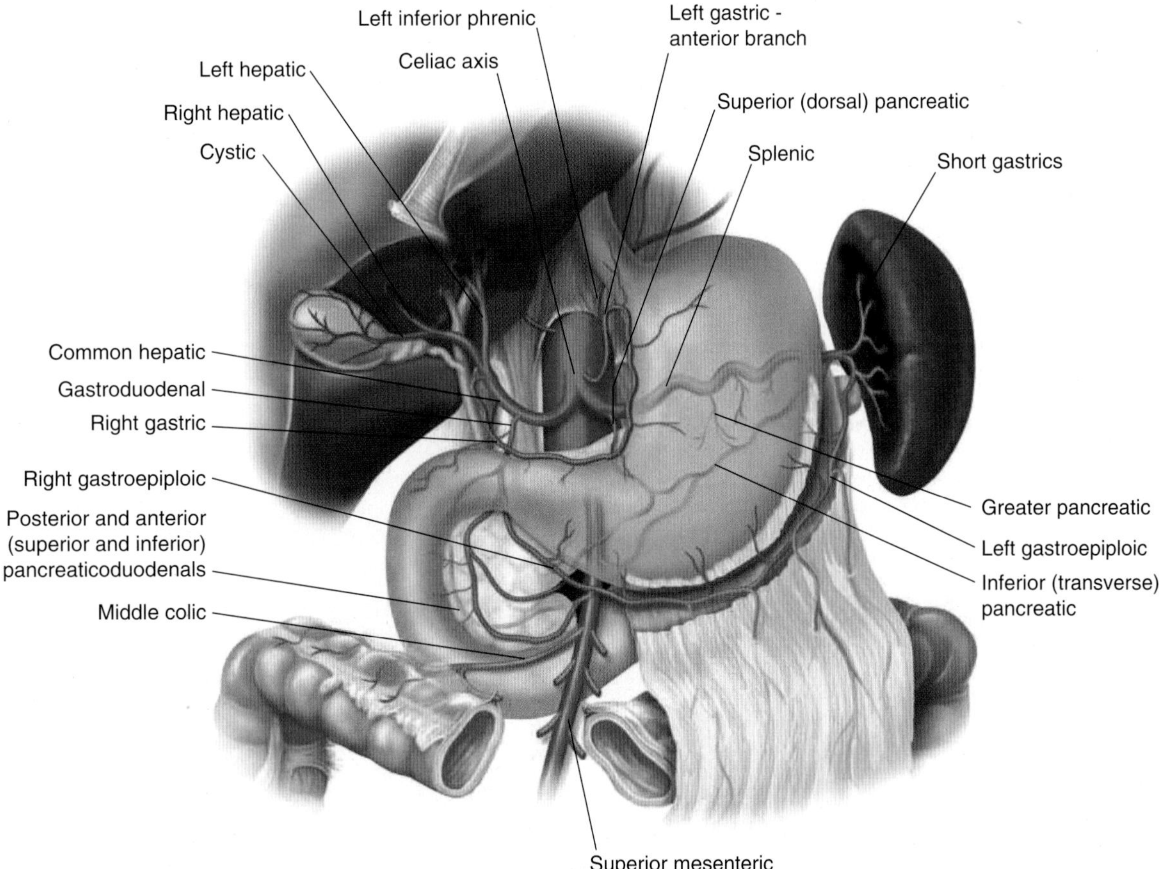

FIGURE 28.6. Relationship and shared vascular supply of the duodenum and pancreas. (Redrawn from Zollinger RM Jr, Ellison EC. *Zollinger's Atlas of Surgical Operations*. New York: McGraw Hill;2011: 19, Plate 1.)

Mechanism of Injury. The true incidence of duodenal injury is difficult to determine.[48,55-69] As best estimated, duodenal injuries occur in approximately 4.3% of patients with abdominal injuries. The anatomic location of the duodenum protects it from injury. Overall, penetrating injury is the most common cause of duodenal trauma. In a review of the literature encompassing 17 series published during the last 22 years, 1,513 cases of duodenal injuries were identified; 77.7% occurred as the result of penetrating trauma, whereas 22.3% occurred as the result of blunt trauma.[67-159] Blunt injury may cause wall disruption from crushing, shearing, or bursting. A good example of crush injury occurs when the steering wheel impacts on the midepigastrium.

Associated Injuries. The duodenum, by virtue of its anatomic proximity to other important organs, is rarely injured alone; multiple associated injuries are the rule rather than the exception. This is particularly true with penetrating trauma, but it also occurs with blunt trauma. Isolated duodenal injury usually occurs in the form of duodenal hematoma. In the study by Stone and Fabian,[75] of the 321 patients reviewed, 91.5% had associated injuries, with a total of 1,143 associated injuries in these patients. The liver was the most commonly injured organ (16.9%). Other commonly injured organs included the pancreas (11.6%); small bowel (11.6%); colon (11.5%); and genitourinary in 6.6%.[68-79] Major abdominal venous injuries occurred in 9.8%; the IVC accounted for most of these injuries. Arterial injuries occurred in 6.6%, with the aorta most commonly. Miscellaneous injuries, mostly extra-abdominal, accounted for 253 injuries (8.3%). The lung was the most frequently injured extra-abdominal organ.[75]

Anatomic Location of Injury. The most frequent site of duodenal injury was the second portion, 33.0% in review of 1,033 cases.[67,71,72,75-80] The third and fourth portions sustained injury in 19.4% and 19.0%, respectively. The least frequently injured portion of the duodenum was the first (14.4%). However, with penetrating trauma, injuries were distributed throughout the anatomic course of the duodenum, whereas in blunt trauma most injuries remained confined to the second portion of the duodenum, usually its posterior surface.[76]

Diagnosis. Delay in the diagnosis and management of duodenal injury results in significant morbidity and mortality. Patients involved in head-on collision or force impacts from the right, who have struck the steering wheel, or required extrication should be suspected as harboring duodenal injuries. Patients who have sustained blows to the midepigastrium must always be evaluated thoroughly. Finally, patients who have fallen from great heights are subject to deceleration injuries of the duodenum.

When examining the patient, remember that the retroperitoneal location of the duodenum may preclude early manifestation of injury on physical examination. Abdominal discomfort may be out of proportion to the physical findings, and peritoneal irritation may occur late and become apparent only when blood, enteric contents, or enzymes that were initially contained retroperitoneally enter the peritoneal cavity. Physical examination may be characterized by minimal findings. Any tenderness over the right upper quadrant or midepigastrium must raise the suspicion of duodenal injury. Signs of rebound tenderness, abdominal rigidity, or absence of bowel sounds indicate intra-abdominal injury and should prompt early surgical intervention. Laboratory tests are of little help in the early diagnosis of duodenal injury.

Plain films of the abdomen are useful only if they are positive. Positive findings include the presence of air collections outlining the right kidney with extraperitoneal rupture of the duodenum, presence of gas around the right psoas muscle and in the retrocecal region, but these findings are rare.

CT with oral and intravenous contrast is the diagnostic method of choice in hemodynamically stable patients with suspected duodenal injury who have sustained blunt abdominal trauma.[84-90] If the CT identifies extravasation of oral contrast from the duodenum associated with a retroperitoneal hematoma, no further studies are needed. However, if the CT scan is inconclusive, we recommend an upper gastrointestinal series with Gastrografin and fluoroscopic visualization of duodenal peristalsis to confirm extravasation of contrast from the duodenum. If no extravasation is identified, thin barium is then administered, which can provide better delineation of duodenal anatomy and thus establish the presence of duodenal hematoma. Additionally, in patients with high concern for duodenal injury in whom no conclusion could be reached from both the contrast and the CT scan studies, exploratory laparotomy and retroperitoneal exploration of the duodenum should be considered to exclude duodenal injury. DPL may be unreliable in evaluation of injury to the retroperitoneal organs.[69,73,91]

Surgical Management of Duodenal Injury. Proven or suspected duodenal injury, coupled with the classic findings of intra-abdominal injury (i.e., abdominal tenderness, guarding, rebound tenderness, or decreased bowel sounds), mandates immediate exploratory laparotomy. Broad-spectrum antibiotics are administered before the abdominal incision.[92,93]

The duodenum must be thoroughly explored with all four portions visualized directly. Findings that should increase suspicion of a duodenal injury include crepitation along the duodenal sweep, bile staining of paraduodenal tissue or a documented bile leak, or the presence of a right-sided retroperitoneal hematoma or perirenal hematoma. The duodenum should then be mobilized by a Kocher maneuver, a Cattell and Braasch maneuver, or both[94] (Fig. 28.7). These maneuvers should provide full visualization of the anterior and posterior walls of all portions of the duodenum. The nasogastric tube should be advanced through the pylorus and palpated digitally while the surgeon performs the dissection. This provides a guide to identify the duodenum in the midst of a large retroperitoneal hematoma and will thus avoid iatrogenic laceration

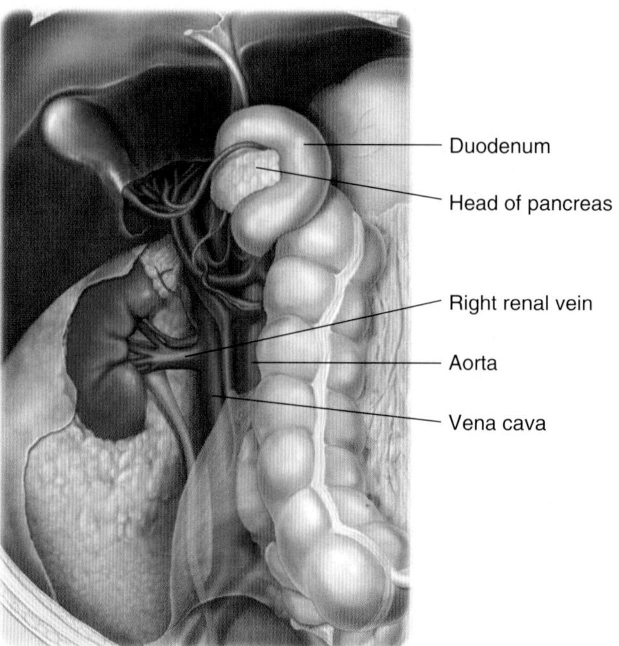

FIGURE 28.7. Right medial visceral rotation. (Redrawn from Singh N. Major abdominal vascular trauma. In: Martin MJ, Beekley AC, eds. *Front Line Surgery*. New York: Springer, 2010:148, Figure 11.4.)

to the duodenal wall during dissection. Inspection of the third portion of the duodenum requires mobilization of the hepatic flexure of the colon according to the method described by Cattell and Braasch.[94] The retroperitoneal attachments of the small bowel are incised sharply from the right lower quadrant to the duodenojejunal junction, and the small bowel is reflected in its entirety out of the abdominal cavity. This maneuver is often unnecessary, and its performance in the presence of a large retroperitoneal hematoma, especially those caused by pelvic fractures, may lead to exsanguination. The fourth portion of the duodenum can be visualized by transecting the ligament of Treitz while avoiding injury to the inferior mesenteric vein or, again, by performing the Cattell and Braasch maneuver.[94]

Duodenal injury can easily be missed, with disastrous consequences. Massive injury, such as may occur with associated vascular injuries to the aorta or vena cava, may divert the surgeon's attention from the duodenum. If findings such as minimal hematoma or insignificant edema are deemed trivial and disregarded, a duodenal injury may be missed.

After a duodenal injury is identified, its extent should be defined. Factors which have a role in its management include the number of associated injuries, especially to the pancreas and biliary tree, and the period of time which has elapsed from identification to treatment. Snyder et al.[77] identified several important factors of value in evaluation of the severity of duodenal injury; agent of entry, the size and site of injury, the interval from injury to repair (in hours), and an associated injury to the common bile duct. Injuries were classified as mild on the basis of the following: (1) the agent of entry consisted of a SW; (2) the size of injury encompassed <75% of the duodenal wall; (3) the site of injury was located in the third or fourth portion of the duodenum; (4) the injury repair interval was <24 hours; and (5) no associated injury to the common bile duct. Injuries were classified as severe on the basis of the following: (1) the agent of entry was blunt trauma or a missile; (2) the size of injury encompassed more than 75% of the duodenal wall; (3) the site of injury was located in the first or second portion of the duodenum; (4) the repair interval was >24 hours; and (5) an associated injury to the common bile duct. Most authors have reported the presence of associated pancreatic injury to be predictive of increased morbidity and mortality.[21,73,95,96]

Cogbill et al.[82] used American Association for the Surgery of Trauma organ injury scale (AAST-OIS) for duodenum in a cooperative multicenter trial in which they graded 164 duodenal injuries (Table 28.6). Mortality rates for grade I-V duodenal injuries were 8%, 19%, 21%, 75%, and 25%, respectively. The authors found that mortality did not correlate well with the severity of duodenal injury and concluded that anatomic features of duodenal injury represent only a part of the risk of morbidity and mortality.

Approximately 75%-85% of all duodenal injuries can be repaired safely using simple surgical techniques. Basic surgical principles, such as debridement of the duodenal injuries to viable tissues and a meticulous double-layer technique for closure, approximating the inner layer using fine absorbable sutures and a seromuscular closure of interrupted nonabsorbable Lembert sutures, should be used. Duodenorrhaphy alone carries a small risk of narrowing the duodenal lumen. Several technical points must be kept in mind to avoid this problem when closing duodenal lacerations. These technical points were outlined by Kraus and Condon[97] on the basis of the results of an animal model in which they established that longitudinal duodenotomies can be closed transversely if the length of the duodenotomy does not exceed one half of the circumference of the duodenum. These investigators recommended that longitudinal closures be performed if the duodenotomy exceeds one-half of the circumference of the duodenum. In neither of these closures was the duodenal lumen narrowed.

We recommend that drains be used routinely, but emphasize that this drain system should be of the closed-suction type and should not be placed directly against the suture line to avoid duodenal fistula formation. Other points to be considered for penetrating injuries include the potential for blast effect. For blunt injuries, the degree of associated retroperitoneal and

TRAUMA

TABLE 28.6

DUODENUM INJURY SCALE

GRADE[a]	TYPE OF INJURY	DESCRIPTION OF INJURY	AIS-90
I	Hematoma	Involving single portion of duodenum	2
	Laceration	Partial thickness, no perforation	3
II	Hematoma	Involving more than one portion	2
	Laceration	Disruption <50% of circumference	4
III	Laceration	Disruption 50%-75% of circumference of D2	4
		Disruption 50%-100% of circumference of D1, D3, D4	4
IV	Laceration	Disruption >75% of circumference of D2	5
		Involving ampulla or distal common bile duct	5
V	Laceration	Massive disruption of duodenopancreatic complex	5
	Vascular	Devascularization of duodenum	5

[a]Advance one grade for multiple injuries up to grade III.
D1, first portion of duodenum; D2, second portion of duodenum; D3 third portion of duodenum; D4, fourth portion of duodenum; AIS, abbreviated injury score.
From Moore EE, Cogbill TH, Malangoni MA, et al. Organ injury scaling II: pancreas, duodenum, small bowel, colon, and rectum. *J Trauma*. 1990;30:1427–1429.

periduodenal inflammatory processes resulting from extruded duodenal contents should be assessed. After evaluation of these factors, the surgeon can choose the procedures that are needed to repair or decompress the duodenum, resect devitalized areas, buttress the repair, or exclude the duodenum from the passage of gastric contents.

In the past, adjunct maneuvers were used to safeguard the duodenal closure. One of these maneuvers is tube duodenostomy, of which the following three types exist: (1) primary, in which the tube is placed through a separate SW in the duodenum (the authors do not support this method); (2) antegrade, in which the duodenum is decompressed by way of the passage of a tube through the pylorus; or (3) retrograde, in which the tube is passed through a jejunostomy site. However, these techniques now are used much less commonly.

The addition of tube decompression for duodenal repair is controversial; opinions are strongly divided between those who staunchly support its routine use, such as Corley et al.,[72] Stone and Fabian,[75] and Hasson et al.,[99] and those who advocate against its use, including Ivatury et al.[80] and Kashuk et al.[101] Stone and Fabian[75] reported a high rate of duodenal complications in 8 of 44 duodenal wounds closed without tube decompression, with three subsequent deaths attributed to duodenal complications before the routine use of decompressive techniques. These investigators reported only one duodenal fistula in 237 patients after the routine use of decompression began.

Hasson et al.[99] reviewed several series of duodenal injuries and found a 2.3% rate of fistula formation in decompressed repairs versus an 11.8% rate in patients without decompression. Contrasting data are presented by Ivatury[80,100] in two separate studies in which they evaluated patients who sustained duodenal injuries and associated injuries of comparable severity. These investigators found consistently higher duodenal morbidity rates in the form of duodenal fistulas and abdominal sepsis as well as higher mortality rates in the group treated with duodenal repair and decompression. Most other series in the literature advocate the use of decompression in a selective fashion.[69,76-78] We advocate individualization of treatment with regard to decompressive techniques and agree with Kelly that "treatment of duodenal injuries, perhaps more than any other bowel trauma, must be individualized."[68]

In some cases, either the injury itself or debridement necessary to remove devitalized tissue may leave a defect in the duodenal wall that, if repaired primarily, might narrow the duodenal lumen or subject the suture line to undue tension and possible breakdown. The reasons cited for disruption of duodenal closures after tissue loss are high intraluminal pressure, tendency of duodenal mucosa to extrude through closure leading to the leakage, and breakdown from autodigestive enzymes of the pancreas and bile. In these cases, a jejunal serosal patch may be used to effect a safe closure.[102-106] An on-lay Roux en Y duodenojejunostomy may be utilized to close large duodenal defects. For larger defects, the ingenious techniques of a jejunal mucosal patch were described by Jones and Joergenson[106] and later modified to include a fairly large pedicle graft by DeShazo et al.[107] This patch can be constructed by using a proximal segment of jejunum, which can be carried up in a retrocolic location on its vascular pedicle. The antimesenteric border of the jejunum can then be split longitudinally and anastomosed using a double-layer technique to the duodenum to close the defect. This technique has also been used successfully by others.[102,108]

If the entire circumference of the duodenum has been devitalized, a segmental resection and end-to-end duodenoduodenostomy may be performed. Resections of segments of the first, third, and fourth portions of the duodenum, although technically challenging, are not associated with the high risk of vascular compromise during mobilization of the second portion. The rate-limiting step in mobilization of the second portion of the duodenum is the shared blood supply with the pancreas. Nevertheless, segmental resection and primary end-to-end duodenoduodenostomy are possible in the second portion. In cases where the duodenal wound is immediately adjacent to the ampulla of Vater, extreme caution must be exercised to preserve the integrity of this structure. In such cases, a choledochostomy may be necessary, with the passage of a probe to identify the ampulla and keep it in view during the creation of the anastomosis. Avulsions of the ampulla of Vater have been treated successfully by duodenorrhaphy and implantation of the ampulla into a Roux-en-Y limb of jejunum.[109] Similarly, avulsions of the common bile duct resulting from lacerations of the second portion of the duodenum have been repaired successfully with common bile duct reimplantation.[103] If an end-to-end anastomosis of the duodenum cannot be performed without tension, a Roux-en-Y duodenojejunostomy may be performed and the distal portion of the duodenum oversewn.

Patients sustaining severe duodenal injury may be considered as candidates for more complex duodenal repairs such as pyloric exclusion.[109,110] Such injuries include those caused by blunt trauma or missiles, those involving more than 75% of the wall, those involving the first and second portions of the duodenum, those associated with a delay in repair of more than 24 hours, and those with associated injuries to the pancreas, common bile duct, or both. Injuries described as grades III and IV of the AAST-OIS duodenum organ injury scale[20] can also be considered for these repairs (see Table 28.6). Other criteria that may lead the surgeon to consider these more complex surgical procedures include compromised blood supply to the duodenum and associated injury to the head of the pancreas without disruption of the main pancreatic duct. We consider injuries involving more than 50% of the circumference of the duodenal wall, whether associated with pancreatic injuries or not, to be high-risk. The main purpose of these procedures is to exclude the duodenum from the passage of gastric contents to allow time for the duodenal repair to heal and to prevent suture line dehiscence.

Pyloric exclusion entails duodenorrhaphy plus a gastrotomy in the most dependent portion of the greater curvature of the stomach. The pylorus is identified through the gastrotomy and occluded using a running suture of nonabsorbable monofilament polypropylene sutures or absorbable polyglycolic acid sutures. Care must be taken to avoid exclusion of antral tissue from the gastric lumen. A gastrojejunostomy is then performed through the previously created gastrotomy to achieve complete pyloric occlusion and diversion of gastric contents. Vagotomy is not a part of this surgical procedure. Gastrojejunostomy without a vagotomy is suspected as being an ulcerogenic procedure by many surgeons. Patients in whom the pyloric exclusion procedure was performed by upper gastrointestinal studies after periods ranging from 2 months to 3 years after the operations demonstrated a functioning pylorus with passage of contents into the duodenum (Fig. 28.8).

An alternate method for achieving pyloric exclusion is using a stapling device placed across the pylorus. This procedure was popularized by Kelly et al.[68]; however, it should not be employed and has been largely abandoned as it generally fails to reopen. Martin[112] reported a follow-up study describing an expanded experience with pyloric exclusion in which 128 of 313 patients (41%) who sustained duodenal injuries were treated with this procedure; a 5.5% duodenal fistula rate was seen. In this study, 42 patients underwent upper gastrointestinal tract examination after their operations. In patients examined 21 days or more after their operations, 94% had a patent pylorus. Marginal ulceration was infrequent and reported in only four of these patients, thus confirming the efficacy of this surgical procedure.

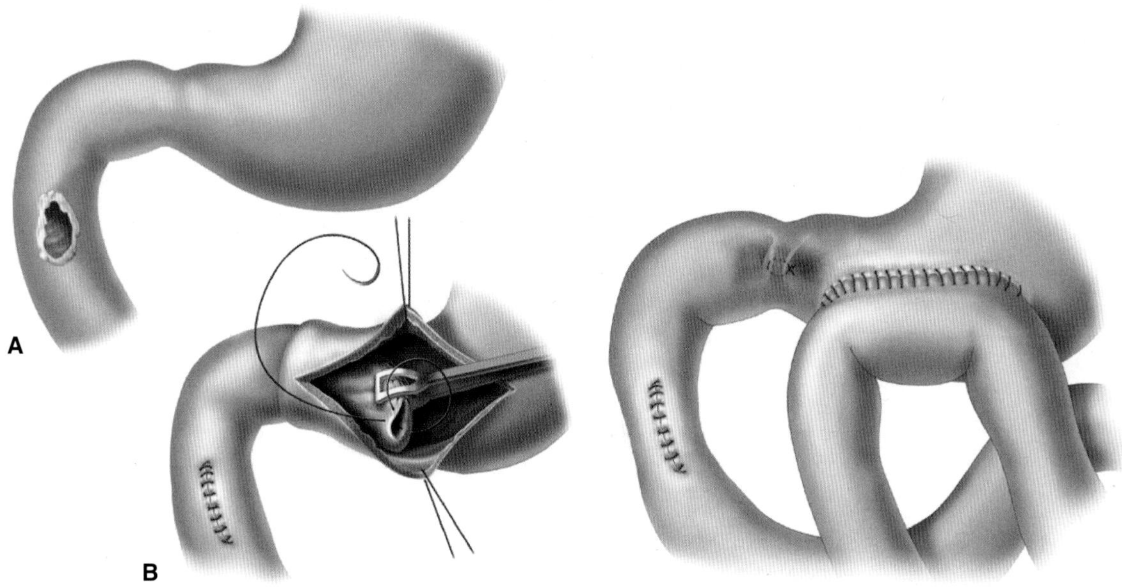

FIGURE 28.8. A: Pyloric exclusion. The duodenal injury is repaired. A gastrotomy is made on a dependent portion of the stomach and the pylorus oversewn from within using a nylon suture. (Redrawn from Frey C, Araida T. Trauma to the pancreas and duodenum. In: Blaisdell FW, Trunkey DD, eds. *Abdominal Trauma*. New York: Thieme; 1993:145, Figure 9–10A,B.) B: Pyloric exclusion. The pyloric exclusion is completed with the gastrojejunostomy. (Redrawn from Frey C, Araida T. Trauma to the pancreas and duodenum. In: Blaisdell FW, Trunkey DD, eds. *Abdominal Trauma*. New York,: Thieme; 1993:146, Figure 9–10C.)

Monsour et al.[113] and Flynn et al.[114] reported their experiences in the management of pancreaticoduodenal injuries. These investigators concluded that well-defined protocols, with careful selection of surgical procedures according to the grade of injury, yield better outcomes. They also concluded that techniques such as pyloric exclusion should be reserved for the infrequent complex injuries that involve both the pancreas and duodenum.[111] As previously shown, between 75% and 85% of duodenal injuries are amenable to repair by duodenorrhaphy. Pyloric exclusion should be performed for complex duodenal injuries AAST-OIS grades III-IV, which are amenable to primary repair and associated with a pancreatic injury AAST-OIS grades II-III. A variation of the duodenal diverticularization procedure as originally described by Berne should be employed when there are destructive injuries of the first portion of the duodenum with associated antral injuries requiring resection and reconstruction with a gastrojejunostomy also in the presence of a pancreatic injury.[115]

Pancreaticoduodenectomy is a formidable procedure in critically ill patients. Combined destructive injury to both the head of the pancreas and the duodenum is the major indication. In essence, pancreaticoduodenectomy is indicated when the injury has necessitated the operation, which then is completing the resection. A review of 70 series[69,70,116-155] reported in the literature from 1964 to 2008 yielded a total of 255 patients who underwent pancreaticoduodenectomy. The tabulated mortality rate for all the series reviewed was 31%.

Mortality. Duodenal injuries, as a whole, carry a considerable mortality rate ranging from 5.3% to 30%; with calculated average mortality rate of 17%.[67-83] Several authors reported early mortality rates associated with shock, prolonged bleeding, and the sequelae of massive blood replacement ranging from 35.7% to 73%, with an average of 52.9%.[55,67,76] The figures on late mortality can be attributed exclusively to the end results of the duodenal injury and associated complications which include sepsis, duodenal fistula formation, and multiple organ failure. Thus, early deaths are from hemorrhage due to associated vascular injury and late deaths are attributable to sepsis from the duodenal injury.

Factors known to increase mortality rates include the presence of associated pancreatic[67,68,70,75] and common bile duct injury.[77] Perhaps, the most important associated factor in determination of the mortality associated with duodenal injury is the delay in time from recognition to definitive repair.

Morbidity. Duodenal injuries are associated with high rates of morbidity, averaging 63.7%. Duodenal morbidity is represented primarily by duodenal fistula formation resulting from failure of surgical repair because of suture line dehiscence and is represented occasionally by duodenal obstruction. Duodenal fistula rates ranged from 0% to 16.2%, with an average of 6.6%.[65,69,72,75-77] Other important complications caused by associated injuries include intra-abdominal abscess, 10.9%-18.4%; recurrent pancreatitis, 2.5%-14.9%; and bile duct fistula, 1.3%.[65,69,75,77]

Blunt Duodenal Rupture. Diagnosis of blunt injury of the duodenum is difficult. All sizable series of blunt duodenal injuries include multiple instances in which this diagnosis was delayed.[44,69,73-83] Delay in diagnosis and treatment of blunt duodenal rupture more than 24 hours increases mortality several-fold. These findings support the concept that early surgical intervention improves outcome and demonstrates that the critical delay period is less than the classically reported 24 hours. The frequent difficulty with diagnosis of blunt rupture of the duodenum and the danger posed by the delayed recognition merit special discussions of the diagnostic features of these injuries. The most common cause of blunt rupture of the duodenum is impact of the epigastrium of an unrestrained driver against the steering wheel of an automobile. A variety of other blows to the abdomen may also cause this injury; it has occurred as a result of punches, kicks, falls, deceleration, and handlebar injuries. With the advent of high-resolution multi-slice CT, the delayed detection of blunt duodenal injuries has been reduced.

The ultimate diagnostic test in blunt abdominal trauma remains the exploratory laparotomy. Because no noninvasive test is completely accurate, patients having met the clinical profile described previously and who have persistent or increasing abdominal pain 6 hours after injury, especially if accompanied by increased abdominal tenderness or rising white blood cell count or serum amylase level, should be considered candidates for exploratory laparotomy.

The devastating consequences of duodenal rupture, coupled with mortality rates ranging from 40% to 71%[44,69,75,77] and the high incidence of fistula formation in survivors as high as 50%,[44] warrant an aggressive diagnostic approach in establishment of this diagnosis and institution of early surgical treatment. The surgeon must also be aware that retroperitoneal rupture of the duodenum may be overlooked at operation.[67,70]

Intramural Duodenal Hematoma. The management of intramural duodenal hematoma remains controversial. Intramural duodenal hematomas are usually caused by blunt abdominal trauma and can occur in any part of the duodenum. Although most cases have been documented in normal persons (including many children), their occurrence has been associated with clotting disorders, anticoagulant therapy, and alcoholism.[160-173] Intramural hematomas of the duodenum are believed to be the result of shearing forces that rupture vessels within the duodenal wall.[161-165] They are most often submucosal, but subserosal and intramuscular hematomas have also been reported. Duodenal hematomas are usually manifested by signs of upper gastrointestinal obstruction after trauma. Copious bilious vomiting after blunt abdominal trauma should raise the suspicion of the evaluating physician. Often, a symptom-free interval of several hours is described. Physical examination usually discloses mild epigastric tenderness. A history of trauma may not be obtainable. An abdominal mass is rarely palpable. Laboratory values may show a mild elevation in the white blood cell count and, occasionally, an elevation of the serum bilirubin or amylase level. Profound fluid and electrolyte disturbances may be present if the obstruction has been long-standing, but this is rare. The basic findings on plain films of the abdomen are gastric distention, sometimes dilation of the proximal duodenum, an air fluid level in the duodenum, and absence of the right psoas shadow. The diagnostic test of choice has been an upper gastrointestinal series using water-soluble contrast material. This technique may demonstrate the classic "coiled spring" deformity of the duodenal mucosa known as Felson's sign[166] or the "stacked coin" sign. This radiographic finding reflects mucosal dissection of the hematoma. The obstruction is usually partial. If no duodenal perforation is observed, superior detail may be seen by repeating the upper gastrointestinal series using thin barium. Evidence of duodenal perforation must be sought diligently. If the serum amylase level is elevated, it is wise to obtain an abdominal CT to look for an associated pancreatic injury. The CT scan may also detect peritoneal air or extravasated contrast material in occult perforations.

Although some authors recommend operative intervention for duodenal hematoma,[161-168] consensus generally is to avoid surgical intervention, as most patients can be treated successfully without operation.[169-172] Nasogastric suction and parenteral feeding or hyperalimentation should be instituted. Careful attention should be paid to fluid and electrolyte balance. If the patient exhibits no sign of increase in abdominal pain or tenderness, then nonoperative management should be continued until the obstruction resolves. In most cases, this resolution occurs within 1 week; however, duodenal obstruction has persisted up to 38 days.[172] Patients with a diagnosis of duodenal hematoma must be observed carefully as a small number may harbor an occult duodenal perforation. The appearance of increased abdominal pain or tenderness on clinical examination, or retroperitoneal air on follow-up of plain abdominal films, mandates immediate surgical intervention. Approximately 3% of the patients with duodenal hematoma have occult duodenal perforations.[160] Some authors have recommended that an obstructing duodenal hematoma be evacuated through a seromuscular incision if discovered at the time of laparotomy for trauma.[161-168] If this evacuation cannot be accomplished, performance of a gastrojejunostomy has been recommended.[14] However, most authors would leave the duodenal hematoma undisturbed and allow 2–4 weeks for its resolution.[169-172] After this time has elapsed, and if the duodenal hematoma is not resolved, surgical intervention is then recommended for evacuation. Evacuation after this time may be technically easier. The evacuation is carried out by way of a seromuscular incision, avoiding penetration into the duodenal lumen. The seromuscular layer is then approximated with Lembert sutures of nonabsorbable materials.

Jewett et al.[173] recommended conservative management as the treatment of choice in the uncomplicated case in the pediatric population because obstruction is relieved in almost all patients. In contrast, the surgical approach carries a higher complication rate and results in an appreciably longer hospital stay. These authors recommended that surgery should be reserved for those cases complicated by perforation or a severely damaged duodenum. They also recommended hematoma evacuation, rather than bypass operations, for those few cases in which perforation or severe injury to the duodenum occurred.

PANCREATIC INJURY

Anatomy. The pancreas lies transversely in the retroperitoneal sac across the upper abdomen. It measures 15–20 cm in length, 3 cm in width, and 1–1.5 cm in thickness. Its average weight is approximately 90 g, ranging from 40 to 180 g. It is almost triangular in shape and is related to the omental bursa superiorly, the transverse mesocolon anteriorly, and the greater abdominal cavity inferiorly. Its motion is relatively limited, and for all practical purposes it is a fixed organ. The SMA and vein course posterior to the neck of the pancreas and are closely attached to the uncinate process, with this process wrapping around the posterolateral aspect of the vein (see Fig. 28.6).

The head of the pancreas lies within the concave sweep of the duodenum with the body crossing the spine and angled superiorly and toward the left shoulder, and the tail is in close proximity to the hilum of the spleen. Because of these relationships, the potential for associated injuries with injury to the pancreas is obvious; pancreatic injuries are uncommonly isolated.

The pancreas is arbitrarily divided into five parts: the head, uncinate process, neck, body, and tail. The head of the pancreas is defined as the portion lying to the right of the SMA and vein. It is located at the level of the second lumbar vertebra in the midline or slightly to the right of it. The head of the pancreas, which lies nestled in the C-loop of the duodenum and in conjunction with it, is suspended from the liver by the hepatoduodenal ligament. The head is firmly fixed to the medial aspect of the second and third portions of the duodenum. The division between the head and the neck is marked anteriorly by a line originating from the portal vein (PV) superiorly to the superior mesenteric vein (SMV) inferiorly.

The anterior pancreaticoduodenal arcade parallels the duodenal curvature but is related to the anterior pancreatic surface rather than to the duodenum. Similarly, the posterior surface of the head of the pancreas is related to the hilum and medial border of the right kidney, the right renovascular pedicle, the IVC, and ostium of the left renal vein (RV), the right crus of the diaphragm, the posterior pancreaticoduodenal arcade, and the right gonadal vein.

The uncinate process is an extension of the lower left part of the posterior surface of the head, usually passing behind the PV and the superior mesenteric vessels just anterior to the aorta and IVC. The morphologic features of the uncinate process are variable. It may be entirely absent, or it may completely encircle the superior mesenteric vessels. In the presence of an uncinate process, 65% of the pancreas lies to the left of the superior mesenteric vessels. However, in its absence, 80% of the mass of the gland lies to the left of the superior mesenteric vessels. This is an important surgical consideration when planning distal pancreatectomy.

The neck of the pancreas measures approximately 1.5–2 cm in length and lies at the level of the first lumbar vertebra. It is defined as the portion that overlies the superior mesenteric vessels and is fixed between the celiac trunk superiorly and the superior mesenteric vessels inferiorly. Anteriorly, the neck is partially covered by the pylorus. To the right, the gastroduodenal artery gives rise to the superior pancreaticoduodenal artery. Posteriorly, the PV is formed by the union of the superior mesenteric and splenic veins (SV). In general, there are no anterior tributaries to these vessels. On occasion, however, one or two small veins may enter the PV and four to five may enter the SMV. Making contributions to the PV from the right are a few short lateral veins, and entering the PV from the left are both the left gastric and SV and, rarely, the inferior mesenteric vein.

The body of the pancreas lies at the level of the first lumbar vertebra and is technically defined as that portion of the pancreas that lies to the left of the superior mesenteric vessels. It is triangularly shaped and is related to the fourth portion of the duodenum and the ligament of Treitz. Both superior mesenteric vessels emerge from under the inferior border of the body and pass over the uncinate process of the head of the pancreas.

The splenic artery and vein course along the superior border of the pancreas. The anterior surface of the body of the pancreas is covered by the posterior wall of the omental bursa that separates the pancreas from the stomach. The pancreas is also related to the transverse mesocolon, which separates into two layers, one leaf covering the anterior and one leaf covering the inferior surface of the pancreas. The middle colic artery emerges from beneath the inferior border of the pancreas to course between the two leaves of the mesocolon. The inferior mesenteric vein passes posterior to the pancreas at the distal inferior margin of the body.

The tail of the pancreas rises to the level of the 12th thoracic vertebra. It is more mobile than the proximal pancreas. The tip is closely related to the hilum of the spleen and, along with the splenic vessels, is covered by the two leaves of the splenorenal ligament. There is no true anatomic division between the body and the tail of the pancreas.

The main pancreatic duct of Wirsung originates in the tail of the pancreas. According to Anacker,[174] two small ducts arise infrequently to form the main duct. Throughout its course in the tail and body, the duct lies midway between the superior and inferior margins and slightly more posterior than anterior. The duct of Wirsung and the accessory duct of Santorini lie anterior to the major pancreatic vessels.

The duct of Wirsung crosses the spinal column between the 12th thoracic and the 2nd lumbar vertebra.[175,176] In the body and tail, 15–20 short tributaries enter the duct at almost right angles.[174]. The superior and inferior tributaries tend to alternate with one another. In addition, the duct of Wirsung may receive a longer tributary draining the uncinate process. In some patients, the duct of Santorini in the head empties into the main duct. Multiple small tributary ducts in the head may open directly into the intrapancreatic portion of the common bile duct or empty directly into the duodenum.[177] This is often cited as the reason for draining all pancreatic injuries postoperatively.

The arterial blood supply of the pancreas originates from both the celiac trunk and the SMA. Anatomic proximity and shared blood supply commonly result in both pancreatic and duodenal injuries. The duodenum and head of the pancreas are supplied by paired pancreaticoduodenal arterial arcades that are always present. They are formed by a pair of superior and inferior pancreaticoduodenal arteries, each bifurcating into anterior and posterior branches to form these arcades. These arcades lie within the pancreas and also supply the duodenum. They constitute the chief obstacles to complete pancreatectomy. All major arteries lie posterior to the ducts.

The gastroduodenal artery arises as the first major branch from the common hepatic artery approximately 1 cm after the common hepatic originates from the celiac trunk. It gives off the right gastroepiploic and, subsequently, the superior pancreaticoduodenal artery, which bifurcates into the anterior superior and posterior superior pancreaticoduodenal arteries. The anterior superior pancreaticoduodenal artery lies on the surface of the pancreas and gives off 8–10 branches to the anterior surface of the duodenum, 1–3 branches to the proximal jejunum, and numerous branches to the pancreas. During pancreatic resection, the duodenal branches may be ligated, but the jejunal branches must be preserved. The anterior superior pancreaticoduodenal artery enters the substance of the pancreas and passes posteroinferiorly to anastomose with the anterior inferior pancreaticoduodenal artery, a branch of the inferior pancreaticoduodenal artery arising from the SMA. The posterior superior pancreaticoduodenal artery can only be seen when the pancreas is mobilized in a cephalad direction to expose its posterior surface. The posterior superior pancreaticoduodenal artery then joins the posterior inferior pancreaticoduodenal artery from the inferior pancreaticoduodenal artery to form the posterior arcade. The dorsal pancreatic artery lies posterior to the neck of the pancreas and the SV and measures 1.5 mm in diameter.

The splenic artery is located on the posterosuperior aspect of the body and tail of the pancreas and follows a tortuous course along the superior margin of the pancreas. There are 2–10 branches of the splenic artery that supply the body and tail of the pancreas. Many of these branches anastomose with the transverse pancreatic artery. There are three possible configurations of the blood supply to the body and tail of the pancreas: type 1, the blood supply is from the splenic artery alone (22%); type 2, the blood supply is from the splenic and transverse pancreatic arteries with anastomosis in the tail of the pancreas (53%); and type 3, the blood supply is from the splenic and transverse pancreatic arteries without distal anastomosis (25%).

The pancreatica magna arises from the distal one-third of the splenic artery and quickly gives off numerous branches to the tail of the pancreas, several of which anastomose with the transverse pancreatic artery. The final contribution to pancreatic perfusion is the caudal pancreatic artery, which arises from the left gastroepiploic artery or from a splenic hilar branch. It anastomoses with branches of the pancreatica magna. The venous drainage of the pancreas in general parallels the arteries and lies superficial to them. Similar to the arteries, the veins are posterior to the ducts. The venous drainage of the pancreas is to the PV, the SV, and the superior and inferior mesenteric veins. Four pancreaticoduodenal veins form venous arcades that drain the head of the pancreas and the duodenum. The SV receives 3–13 short pancreatic tributaries.

The PV arises from the confluence of the superior mesenteric and SV behind the neck of the pancreas. Rarely, the inferior mesenteric vein can also enter at this junction. The PV lies behind the pancreas and in front of the IVC and can be separated easily from the posterior surface of the pancreas.

Physiology. The pancreas is a compound tubuloalveolar gland with both endocrine and exocrine cells. The endocrine cells are separated histologically into nests of cells known as the islets of Langerhans. The proportion of the islet population in the tail is considerably greater than in the body and head.[178] There are three dominant types of islet cells: the alpha cells produce glucagon, the beta cells produce insulin, and the delta cells produce somatostatin. Insulin and glucagon secretion are both strictly regulated by blood sugar levels. A decrease in blood sugar triggers glucagon secretion, and the subsequent increase in blood sugar fosters insulin secretion.

The high concentration of islet cells in the tail of the pancreas suggests that distal pancreatectomy would be tolerated poorly in terms of the endocrine secretion of the gland. However, excision of more than 90% of the substance of the pancreas is required to produce endocrine deficiency, provided that the pancreas is otherwise normal. Partial resection induces hypertrophy and an increase in the physiologic activity of the remaining islets as a compensatory mechanism. A 90%-95% pancreatic resection performed for trauma will produce diabetes, but the digestion and absorption of food may not be disturbed. However, after total pancreatectomy, both enzymatic and hormonal replacement must be administered.

The exocrine secretion of the pancreas contains two components. The first component is an aqueous secretion of variable volume that is remarkable for its high concentration of bicarbonate. The other component is a solution of small volume containing digestive enzyme precursors that are synthesized and secreted by the acinar cells of the pancreas. A leak of pancreatic secretions from a duodenal repair or from a pancreaticojejunostomy will easily digest any suture line in close proximity, whether gastrointestinal or vascular.

Mechanism of Injury. Pancreatic injury is uncommon, 3.8% of all patients sustaining abdominal injuries.[179-184] The retroperitoneal location of the pancreas protects it from injury. Penetrating injuries include GSWs, SWs, shotgun wounds, and, during wartime, fragment injuries from grenades or shrapnel. Most blunt injuries occur as a result of motor vehicular crashes or assaults.

Penetrating injury is the most common cause of pancreatic trauma. In a review of the literature encompassing 76 series published during the last 44 years, 4,982 cases of pancreatic injury were identified. Seventy percent occurred as a result of penetrating trauma; 30% as a result of blunt trauma. Among the penetrating injuries 72.3% were by gunshots; 23.1% were stabbings, and 4.3% were shotgun blasts. Among blunt injuries, 85.5% were caused by motor vehicular crashes and 14.5% were caused by assault or miscellaneous injuries.[185-206]

The pancreas is a retroperitoneal organ that lies against a rigid vertebral column. Unlike the somewhat mobile duodenum, the pancreas is fixed in position and therefore prone to crush injury. Crushing injuries usually occur when a direct force is applied to the abdominal wall and transmitted to the pancreas, which is then compressed posteriorly against the rigid, unyielding vertebral column. A classic example of crush injury occurs when the steering wheel or bicycle handbar impacts the midepigastrium. Forces applied to the right upper quadrant can be expected to cause injuries to the head of the pancreas, whereas direct impacts on the midepigastrium usually fracture the neck of the pancreas. Forces applied to the left upper quadrant often cause injury to the tail of the pancreas.

Associated Injuries. The pancreas, by virtue of its anatomic proximity to other important organs, is rarely injured alone; multiple associated injuries are the rule. Isolated pancreatic injury is usually seen in the form of blunt pancreatic transection, generally at the neck of the gland. A review of 50 series published during the last 45 years identified a total of 3,465 cases of pancreatic injury. These patients sustained a total of 7,526 associated injuries. The liver was the most commonly injured organ (19.3%). Other commonly injured organs included the stomach (16%); spleen (11%); colon (8%); and duodenum (7.8%).

Major abdominal venous injuries occurred in 5.5%; IVC, PV, and SMV most commonly. Arterial injuries occurred in 4.5%, with the aorta and SMA most frequently. Two hundred sixty-eight unspecified major vascular injuries could not be classified; thus, major vascular injuries in 13.7% overall. Vascular injuries were therefore the third most frequent injuries encountered with pancreatic injury.

Anatomic Location of Injury. To identify the anatomic location of pancreatic injuries, we reviewed 12 series published during the last 40 years. The most frequent site of injury was the pancreatic head and neck (37%). The pancreatic body was injured in 36%, and the pancreatic tail in 26%. Multiple sites of injury occurred in 3%. The distribution of injuries differs for penetrating and blunt trauma. Whereas penetrating trauma injuries are distributed throughout the anatomic course of the pancreas, in blunt trauma most injuries occur at the neck of the gland.

Diagnosis. The diagnosis of pancreatic injury requires a high index of suspicion. Delay in diagnosis and management of pancreatic injury will be accompanied by substantially increased morbidity and mortality rates. For example, patients involved in head-on collisions and patients who have sustained steering wheel damage or required extrication, particularly when they have been trapped against the steering wheel, may harbor pancreatic injury. Patients who have sustained blows to the midepigastrium should also be evaluated carefully.

Retroperitoneal location of the pancreas usually precludes early detection of injury by physical examination. Abdominal discomfort and pain may be out of proportion to the physical examination findings because peritoneal irritation may occur late and become apparent only when blood or pancreatic enzymes, initially contained within the retroperitoneum, extravasate into the peritoneal cavity. The physical examination is usually characterized by few, if any, findings. Any tenderness over the right upper quadrant or midepigastrium should always be evaluated with a suspicion for an underlying pancreatic injury. Obviously, signs of rebound tenderness, abdominal rigidity, or the absence of bowel sounds indicate intra-abdominal injury; although nonspecific findings, they should prompt immediate surgical intervention.

Laboratory tests provide little help in the early diagnosis of pancreatic injuries. The serum amylase level has long been considered as a diagnostic test for pancreatic injury. However, a wide range of elevations in the serum amylase level has been reported in 10%-91% of patients who had serum amylase determinations obtained preoperatively.[186-189] Amylase determinations are neither sensitive nor specific for pancreatic injury.[186-206] Serum amylase isoenzymes are not considerably more accurate than conventional serum amylase levels.[192-196]

Currently, CT is the imaging method of choice for the diagnosis of acute pancreatic injury. On the other hand, the findings of pancreatic injury may be subtle, especially soon after injury. Unexplained thickening of the anterior renal fascia suggests pancreatic injury and should prompt further evaluation of the pancreas by other methods.[194-213] Recently, Lane et al.[211] summarized the positive CT findings in pancreatic injury, including "direct visualization of a parenchymal fracture or hematoma, intraperitoneal and extraperitoneal fluid, fluid separating the SV and pancreatic body, thickened left anterior renal fascia, focal fluid at the sight of fracture, and retroperitoneal hematoma." A recent multicenter from AAST comparing 16-slice to 64-slice CT demonstrated that even new technology CT commonly misses pancreatic injury.[214] The sensitivity for diagnosis of any pancreatic injury was 60% for 16-slice CT and 47% for 64-slice CT. The sensitivity for diagnosis of pancreatic duct injury was 54% for 16-slice CT and 52% for 64-slice CT.

Hayward et al.[215] in 1989 proposed the routine use of ERCP preoperatively as a valuable tool for excluding pancreatic injury. Whittwell et al.[216] further validated the role of early ERCP in the evaluation of patients with blunt pancreatic trauma.

In addition to diagnosis, ERCP has been used as an interventional modality for ductal disruptions.[217,218] Duchesne used ERCP to stage patients in the initial evaluation of possible pancreatic injury. This preoperative evaluation confirmed ductal injury in patients who then underwent laparotomy and avoided operation in those patients with an intact pancreatic duct. He also cited the opportunity to intervene with ERCP, with placement of a stent.[219]

Surgical Management of Pancreatic Injury. Proven or suspected pancreatic injury, coupled with the classic findings of intra-abdominal injury (i.e., abdominal tenderness, guarding, or rebound tenderness), mandates immediate exploratory laparotomy. Broad-spectrum antibiotics are administered before the abdominal incision. We prefer the use of a second-generation cephalosporin and agree with Jones[220] and Nichols et al.[221] that cefoxitin provides ample coverage initially.

Abdominal injuries should be explored through a midline incision extending from xiphoid to pubis. The goals in the operative management of pancreatic injury have changed little since Stone's classic report in 1981. "Proper management of pancreatic wounds is based on three essentials: (1) arrest of hemorrhage, (2) selective debridement, and (3) control of pancreatic secretions. Failure to satisfy these tenets routinely leads to the development of serious and often lethal complications."[189] Immediate control of life-threatening hemorrhage from vascular or solid organs such as the liver or spleen should be the first goal of the operation, followed by immediate control of any sources of gastrointestinal spillage. The next step in the management of abdominal trauma should consist of a thorough exploration of the abdominal cavity. The pancreas should be explored carefully, and the pancreatic head, neck, body, and tail should be visualized directly. Intraoperative findings that should increase the suspicion of a pancreatic injury include the presence of a central retroperitoneal hematoma, proximity injuries, bile staining of the retroperitoneum, and edema surrounding the pancreas and lesser sac.

Exsanguinating injuries posing an immediate threat to life may divert the trauma surgeon's attention from detection of a pancreatic injury. The goal of a thorough and meticulous exploration of all pancreatic injuries is to establish the presence or absence of a major pancreatic ductal injury. The presence of ductal disruption is the "sine qua non" of a major pancreatic injury, and a major determinant in morbidity. A complete exploration and visualization of the entire pancreas and duodenum requires multiple approaches, including a thorough and extensive retroperitoneal exploration with the use of several maneuvers.

Recently, Asensio et al.[222] described a unified approach for the surgical exposure of pancreatic injuries. These maneuvers provide full visualization of the anterior and posterior walls of the entire pancreatic gland. A Kocher maneuver should first be performed by incising the lateral peritoneal attachments of the duodenum and sweeping the second and third portions medially with the use of a combination of sharp and blunt dissection. When a large retroperitoneal hematoma is encountered, the nasogastric tube should be advanced through the pylorus and palpated digitally to serve as a guide and to avoid iatrogenic laceration of the duodenal wall during dissection. This mobilization should be extensive enough that the surgeon can palpate the entire head of the pancreas to the level of the superior mesenteric vessels. This maneuver will allow the surgeon to visualize the anterior and posterior aspects of the second and third portions of the duodenum and will also permit exposure of the head and uncinate process of the pancreas and IVC. If the pericaval tissues are dissected cephalad, the suprarenal IVC can also be exposed. The uncinate process is absent in 15% of patients. When the trauma surgeon considers performing a distal pancreatectomy, the determination should be whether the patient possesses an uncinate process. Normally, a resection to the left of the superior mesenteric vessels extirpates approximately 65% of the gland. Although this is an extensive resection, pancreatic exocrine or endocrine insufficiency generally does not result. However, when the uncinate process is absent, a resection to the left of the superior mesenteric vessels may result in pancreatic insufficiency and the need for insulin replacement.

The next maneuver to be performed in the exposure of the pancreas consists of division of the gastrohepatic ligament to gain access to the lesser sac. This facilitates inspection of the superior border of the pancreas including the head and body and the splenic artery and vein as they course along the superior border of the pancreas. Division of the gastrocolic ligament permits full inspection of the anterior aspect and inferior border of the gland along its entire length.

On occasion, an associated splenic injury is found with a hematoma that obscures the splenic hilum and tail of the pancreas. Aird and Helman[223] described a maneuver to expose the splenic hilum by mobilizing the splenic flexure of the colon and the lienosplenic, splenocolic, and splenorenal ligaments to mobilize the spleen from a lateral to medial position. In addition to excellent exposure of the spleen and its vascular supply, this allows visualization of the posterior aspect of the tail of the pancreas.

When an injury penetrates the anterior surface of the pancreas, the surgeon must ascertain whether the integrity of the main pancreatic duct has been violated. This requires exposure of the posterior aspect of the body and tail of the pancreas. This may be accomplished by transecting the retroperitoneal attachments of the inferior border of the pancreas while elevating the pancreas cephalad to allow inspection of the posterior surface of the gland followed by bimanual palpation. This maneuver is technically challenging and should be performed with meticulous precision to prevent iatrogenic injury to the superior mesenteric vessels. These maneuvers provide accurate intraoperative assessment of both glandular and ductal integrity. Thus, thorough assessment of the pancreas intraoperatively requires both **visual inspection** of the entire gland and **bimanual palpation** of the pancreas.

In the assessment of pancreatic injuries, it is important to recognize any major ductal injury. The use of intraoperative observations such as direct visualization of ductal violation, complete transection of the pancreas, free escape of pancreatic fluid, laceration of more than one-half of the diameter of the gland, central perforation, and severe laceration with or without massive tissue disruption predict the presence of a major ductal injury with a high degree of accuracy. However, there are circumstances in which the assessment of ductal integrity cannot be made. In these uncommon cases, intraoperative pancreatography has been recommended as a technique for the visualization of the main pancreatic duct. In our opinion, intraoperative pancreatography has a limited role and should be reserved for the assessment of ductal integrity when injuries have occurred at the head of the pancreas and when the trauma surgeon considers vital the determination of whether there is extensive damage to the major duct in the head (i.e., as a criterion for selection of a complex procedure such as pancreaticoduodenectomy).

After a pancreatic injury is identified, its extent should be defined. Factors that play a role in its management include the number of associated injuries and their acuity. Risk factors defined by Asensio et al.[224] known to increase mortality rates in patients with pancreatic injury include the presence of associated duodenal and common bile duct injuries because their management must be taken into account in the operative procedure selected to treat the pancreatic injury. We recommend that all pancreatic injuries be staged according to the AAST-OIS for duodenum[20] (Table 28.7).

Many different surgical techniques for the treatment of pancreatic injuries have been described. Approximately 60% of all pancreatic injuries can be treated by external drainage alone. Closed-suction systems with wide drainage of the pancreas are critical in the management. Fabian[119] reported the superiority of closed-suction drainage for pancreatic trauma in a randomized prospective study, with septic complications after pancreatic injury considerably reduced by closed-suction drainage. The authors postulated that bacterial contamination through sump catheters is a major source for intra-abdominal infections after pancreatic trauma. There is no consensus about the length of time that drains must remain in place. We recommend leaving the drains in place for a minimum of 10–14 days and certainly until after the patient resumes oral intake.

The trauma surgeon should decide early whether damage control is needed according to the patient's physiologic state. Subsequently, the trauma surgeon can choose the procedures that are needed to repair the pancreatic injury definitively. Grade I and grade II injuries occur with a frequency of 60% and 20%, respectively.[11] Grade III injuries represent 15% of all pancreatic injuries, whereas grades IV and V injuries are uncommon, occurring with a frequency of only 5%. It is for this higher grade of injury that the more complex surgical techniques should be reserved.

We advocate that all pancreatic contusions and shallow capsular tears or lacerations be managed by simple external drainage with closed-suction systems. The capsule of the pancreas should not be closed by itself, because this has been known to lead to the formation of pancreatic pseudocyst. Any injury that violates the pancreatic parenchyma should be examined meticulously to determine whether there is ductal involvement.

At times it may be quite difficult for the surgeon to establish the involvement of the major ductal system. This presents a dilemma for the trauma surgeon. Performing a pancreatorrhaphy in this scenario will not only miss, but undertreat a major ductal injury, thereby increasing the possibility for the development of severe postoperative complications. In this situation, we assume a ductal injury and upgrade the injury to select a more appropriate treatment, which, in this case, would be pancreatic resection. This decision is straightforward if the injury lies to the left of the superior mesenteric vessels where distal resection, although challenging, does not approach the degree of complexity of a resection to the right of the superior mesenteric vessels. If the injury is to the right of the superior mesenteric vessels, the surgeon must consider either draining extensively and accepting the potential development of a pancreatic fistula with its attendant morbidity or performing an extended resection to the right of the superior mesenteric vessels.[225-229] Patton et al.[230] addressed intraoperative assessment and management of pancreatic injury in 134 patients. Thirty percent of injuries were to the right of the superior mesenteric vessels (proximal) and 70% were distal. All proximal pancreatic injuries were managed by drainage without resection. Two-thirds of distal pancreatic injuries underwent distal pancreatectomy based on high suspicion of ductal injury. In the subgroup of patients with distal pancreatic injury and indeterminate ductal integrity, the complication rate was similar whether managed by drainage alone (27%) or distal resection (33%). The incidence of pancreatic fistula in this series of pancreatic injuries was 15%, nearly all of which closed spontaneously. Thus, this paper suggests that the vast majority of proximal pancreatic injuries can be treated by drainage alone. The rare, devastating combined pancreatic and duodenal injury may require pancreaticoduodenectomy.

In 1961, Fogelman[231] reported the first series of many from Parkland Memorial Hospital in Dallas. The author clearly outlined some of the basic surgical principles in use today for the management of pancreatic injuries. He recommended the use of pancreatorrhaphy with nonabsorbable suture to repair pancreatic parenchymal lacerations, adding the caveat that the

TABLE 28.7

PANCREAS INJURY SCALE

GRADE[a]	TYPE OF INJURY	DESCRIPTION OF INJURY	AIS-90
I	Hematoma	Minor contusion without duct injury	2
	Laceration	Superficial laceration without duct injury	2
II	Hematoma	Major contusion without duct injury or tissue loss	2
	Laceration	Major laceration without duct injury or tissue loss	3
III	Laceration	Distal transection or parenchymal injury with duct injury	3
IV	Laceration	Proximal transection or parenchymal injury involving ampulla[b]	4
V	Laceration	Massive disruption of pancreatic head	5

[a]Advance one grade for multiple injuries up to grade III.
[b]Proximal pancreas is to the patient's right of the SMV.
AIS, abbreviated injury score.
From Moore EE, Cogbill TH, Malangoni MA, et al. Organ injury scaling II: pancreas, duodenum, small bowel, colon, and rectum. *J Trauma*. 1990;30:1427–1429.

pancreatorrhaphy should not be performed until the continuity of the main pancreatic duct has been evaluated. He recommended obligatory drainage of pancreatic injuries and outlined reasons such as the technical impossibility of completely closing disrupted pancreatic tissue and the high frequency of secondary pancreatic breakdown resulting in enzyme spillage and lesser sac chemical and bacterial phlegmon formation. He also strongly advocated pancreatic resection as the most reliable method for treating pancreatic injuries.

Kerry and Glass[232] in 1962 were the first to report pancreaticoduodenal injuries as an entity and described an approach to their management that included resection of the traumatized pancreas whenever possible, wide debridement of the duodenum, and diversion of gastrointestinal secretions from the injured area. They recommended early diagnosis and prompt, aggressive surgical management. This publication set in motion the ideas that would later crystallize with the development of duodenal diverticularization and pyloric exclusion procedures.

Stone et al.[233] in 1962 outlined the evolution of principles for the care of pancreatic injuries. Reporting his own experience with 62 cases of pancreatic injuries, the author recommended a step-by-step approach to management consisting of hemostasis, conservative debridement, and control of pancreatic secretions. He condemned reanastomosis of the ductal system of the pancreas and advocated ligation of the end of the severed major duct and proposed pancreatectomy as the mainstay of management of pancreatic injury. Similarly, he recommended that pancreaticojejunostomy should be used infrequently and only when conservation of pancreatic tissue is of the utmost necessity.

Pancreaticoduodenectomy was suggested by Thal and Wilson[234] in 1964 as a treatment for patients who sustained severe blunt trauma to the head of the pancreas. Thal and others have recommended that pancreaticoduodenectomy should be limited to patients with massive pancreaticoduodenal injuries.[222,234-237]

In 1979, Pachter et al.[238] reported the use of a stapling device to perform distal pancreatectomy. In 1982, Robey et al.[239] reported four cases of distal pancreatectomy with splenic salvage for blunt traumatic injuries. In 1989, Pachter et al.[240] reported the nine patients treated with distal pancreatectomy with splenic preservation, and refuted the surgical dogma that splenic preservation is more time-consuming than distal pancreatectomy and splenectomy.

In 1991, Gentilello et al.[241] reported pancreatic ductal ligation as a safe alternative to pancreaticojejunostomy after pancreaticoduodenectomy in hemodynamically unstable patients. When comparing pancreatic duct ligation to pancreaticojejunostomy, he found no statistical difference in either the mortality rate or pancreatic morbidity rate.

We reviewed 62 series that outlined the surgical methods used to treat pancreatic injury. Fifty-nine percent of the patients were treated with external drainage, and 28% were treated with distal pancreatectomy. A combination of distal pancreatectomy and pancreaticojejunostomy was used in only 2.5% of the cases. Pancreaticoduodenectomy is a formidable procedure in critically ill patients. A review of 80 series reported in the literature from 1964 to 2008 yielded a total of 255 patients who underwent pancreaticoduodenectomy. The tabulated mortality rate for all series reviewed was 31%, essentially unchanged for decades.[232-245]

Pancreaticoduodenal Injury. Severe pancreaticoduodenal injury is fortunately rare. The vast majority of these injuries are commonly caused by penetrating trauma and frequently associated with multiple injuries. Patients with higher pancreatic injury severity who have associated duodenal injuries should be considered candidates for more complex pancreaticoduodenal repairs such as pyloric exclusion. Candidates include patients with pancreatic injury grade II or above in association with injury to the common bile duct, involving more than 75% of the duodenal wall and involving the first and second portions of the duodenum or associated with delay in repair of more than 24 hours. Other criteria that may lead the surgeon to consider diverticularization or pyloric exclusion include compromised blood supply to the duodenum and associated injury to the head of the pancreas without disruption of the main pancreatic duct or pancreatic injury associated with a duodenal injury involving more than 50% of the circumference of the duodenum. The main purpose of these procedures is to exclude the duodenum from the passage of gastric contents and a suitable period of time for the duodenal repair to heal. In the presence of a pancreatic injury, these procedures can only be used if the duodenal injury is amenable to primary repair.

The original duodenal diverticularization was described by Berne et al.[115]; its main purpose was to decrease the high rate of morbidity and mortality in patients who incurred combined pancreaticoduodenal injuries. The original diverticularization procedure included antrectomy, debridement, and closure of the duodenum, tube duodenostomy, vagotomy, biliary tract drainage, and feeding jejunostomy. The classical duodenal diverticularization is a time-consuming and complicated surgical procedure that many critically injured patients can hardly withstand and has thus been abandoned.

An alternative method to achieve exclusion of the duodenal suture line and diversion of the gastric contents was devised by Vaughan et al.[245] This procedure entailed duodenorrhaphy plus a gastrotomy in the most dependent portion of the greater curvature of the stomach through which the pylorus is identified and occluded with a large, running, nonabsorbable suture. Care must be taken to avoid exclusion of antral tissue from the gastric lumen. A gastrojejunostomy is then performed through the previously created gastrotomy to achieve complete pyloric occlusion and diversion of the gastric contents, plus any pancreatic repair or resection, and external drainage (see Fig. 28.8). Graham et al.[246] reported 68 patients who sustained combined pancreaticoduodenal injuries, 32 of whom required pyloric exclusion (30 temporarily and 2 permanently) resulting from gastric antral wounds. No deaths occurred, and only two duodenal fistulas developed, for an incidence rate of 6.9%. Both fistulas healed successfully.

Mortality. Pancreatic injury carries a considerable mortality rate. A review of a total of 4,134 patients in the literature reveals a mean mortality of 19.1% (range 5%-54%). Associated injuries are responsible for the majority of the deaths in patients with pancreatic injury. Early deaths are from hemorrhage due to associated vascular, splenic, or hepatic injury. Shock is a strong predictor of mortality in the patient with pancreatic injury. Late deaths are due to infection, associated with pancreatic or hollow viscus injury.

The number of associated injuries is also an important determinant of the mortality rate, with increasing mortality as the number of associated injuries rises. In series totaling 712 patients, reported the mortality rate for patients with 0–1, 2–3, and 4 or more associated injuries was 2.5%, 13.6%, and 29.6%, respectively.[200,190,248]

The mechanism of injury is an important determinant of the mortality rate, with the highest mortality associated with close range shotgun injury (54%). Nineteen series presented a breakdown of mortality rates according to the mechanism of injury. The mean mortality rate for penetrating injury was 20% versus 19% for blunt trauma. Proximal pancreatic injuries are also related to increases in mortality rates.

Morbidity. Forty series in the literature encompassing 3,898 patients with pancreatic injury were reviewed, reporting an average morbidity of 36.6% (range 11%-62%).[102-150]

Pancreatic morbidity is represented primarily by fistulas, with an incidence of 14%. Pancreatic abscess was the second most frequent complication (8%), followed by posttraumatic pancreatitis (4%), pseudocyst (3%), and late hemorrhage (1%). Collected under the category of other complications that occurred in 4% is exocrine and endocrine insufficiency. Exocrine or endocrine insufficiency is unusual after pancreatic injuries. Distal pancreatectomy to the left of the superior mesenteric vessels should leave adequate functioning pancreatic tissue.[88,246,247,249]

The literature shows no uniformity in the definition of what constitutes a pancreatic fistula. In fact, prolonged pancreatic drainage is considered the rule with these injuries. Furthermore, a controlled pancreatic fistula may be simply an expected result of appropriate therapy. Our definition of a fistula is any drainage of >50 mL that persists longer than 2 weeks with objectively measured and elevated amylase and lipase levels. The majority of pancreatic fistulae will ultimately close without further operative intervention.

Fistulas may rarely result in death if they are associated with pancreatic abscess. Aggressive parenteral nutrition with absolute gastrointestinal tract rest is the standard method for the treatment of these fistulas. Enteral nutrition with an elemental diet provided with a distal feeding jejunostomy has been tried as an alternative, but the authors have observed in some cases that the fistula output has increased considerably in some patients whereas others tolerate enteral nutrition well and without any concomitant increase in the output.

More recently, the long-acting somatostatin analog, octreotide acetate, has been used to inhibit pancreatic exocrine secretion. This treatment was originally reported as a helpful adjunct in the management of postoperative complications after elective pancreatic procedures.[250] Good results were noted, with decreased time to closure of the postoperative fistula. The use of this synthetic analog has been extended to the treatment of posttraumatic pancreatic fistulas, but there are few data in the literature documenting its efficacy.

It is difficult to establish definitive guidelines for when operative intervention or ERCP with stent placement is required in the management of fistulae. However, reintervention should be considered for fistulae of >2 months duration with unrelenting production of high volumes. These fistulas can be managed either by pancreatic resection or resection with internal drainage.

Pancreatic abscess as a specific infectious complication of pancreatic injury is difficult to define, given the large number of associated injuries in pancreatic trauma. The association with either a colon or duodenal injury is known to result in a 60% rate of abscess formation versus a much lower rate of 10%-15% in patients without colonic or duodenal injuries. Similarly, Jones[247] reported that 60% of patients with colon injuries in his series experienced the development of intra-abdominal abscess, but few were related to the pancreatic injury.

Cogbill et al.[225] reported intra-abdominal abscess formation in 24 of 71 surviving patients, for an incidence of 34%. He established a correlation between abscess formation and large requirements for blood transfusions during the first 24 hours and also reported that these abscesses were found much more frequently in patients with associated hollow viscus injuries. Left upper quadrant abscesses are much more common after distal pancreatectomy than after distal pancreatectomy with splenic preservation. The mainstay of management consists of percutaneous CT-guided drainage. Cogbill et al.[225] reported a 79% success rate with this approach.

True pancreatic complex abscesses associated with pancreatic necrosis and infected peripancreatic fluid collections are generally not amenable to percutaneous CT-guided drainage. These abscesses often require surgical reintervention to debride necrotic pancreatic tissue and to establish generous drainage.

Posttraumatic pancreatitis has been defined by Cogbill et al.[225] as persistent serum amylase elevations persisting for more than 3 days. The vast majority of posttraumatic pancreatitis results from blunt abdominal trauma. A complication of posttraumatic pancreatitis is its evolution into hemorrhagic pancreatitis. This is usually manifested by bloody pancreatic drainage. This condition carries a high mortality rate.

Pancreatic pseudocysts generally result from overlooked blunt pancreatic injuries treated nonoperatively. In addition, pseudocyst formation is regarded as failure to establish adequate postoperative drainage for pancreatic secretions. The presence of a pseudocyst should be considered if there is prolonged elevation of the serum amylase postoperatively and should be pursued aggressively.

Posttraumatic pseudocysts should be investigated with ERCP, which will delineate the status of the pancreatic duct. This is important for selection of the method of treatment. If the ductal system is found to be intact, the pseudocyst can be managed with percutaneous drainage. If the pseudocyst is a result of a missed ductal injury, percutaneous drainage will not provide definitive therapy, and these patients are best treated by reexploration and pancreatectomy or internal drainage by a Roux-en-Y jejunal limb. In rare circumstances, endoscopic transpancreatic stenting of the pancreatic duct has been tried successfully.

Posttraumatic hemorrhage can be a lethal complication. Erosion of the vessels surrounding the pancreas may occur when there has been an inadequate debridement or external drainage and is unpredictable. The management consists of urgent return to the OR, but this carries a high mortality rate. Angiographic embolization has been used as a temporizing measure before return to the OR, or for definitive control.

Liver Injury

The liver is the most commonly injured intra-abdominal organ; injury occurs more often with penetrating trauma than in blunt trauma. The mortality rate for liver injury is 10%, higher for blunt than penetrating injury. Richardson[251,252] has documented this decrease in mortality from liver injury over the past several decades. As he outlined, the reasons for improved outcome include damage control and packing of liver injury, improved operative techniques, arteriography and embolization, and the nonoperative management of the majority of hepatic injuries.

Anatomy. An understanding of hepatic anatomy is essential to manage complex liver injuries.[253-255] A sagittal plane from the IVC to the gallbladder fossa separates the right and left lobes of the liver (Cantlie's line). The segmental anatomy of the liver is shown in Figure 28.9. The right and left hepatic veins have a short extrahepatic course before they empty directly into the IVC (Fig. 28.10).[253] The middle hepatic vein usually joins the left hepatic vein within the liver parenchyma. The retrohepatic IVC (8–10 cm in length) has multiple, small hepatic veins which enter the IVC directly; this area is difficult to access and control. The PV delivers 75% of the hepatic blood flow and 50% of the oxygenated blood. The right and left hepatic arteries generally arise from the common hepatic artery. Anomalies are frequent and include the right hepatic artery originating from the SMA (15%) and the left hepatic artery originating from the left gastric artery (12%).

Adequate mobilization of the liver requires division of the ligamentous attachments. The falciform ligament divides the left lateral segment of the liver from the medial segment of the left lobe. The coronary ligaments are the diaphragmatic attachments to the liver (anterior and posterior leaflets); they do not meet on the posterior surface of the liver (the bare area). The triangular ligaments (left and right) are the more

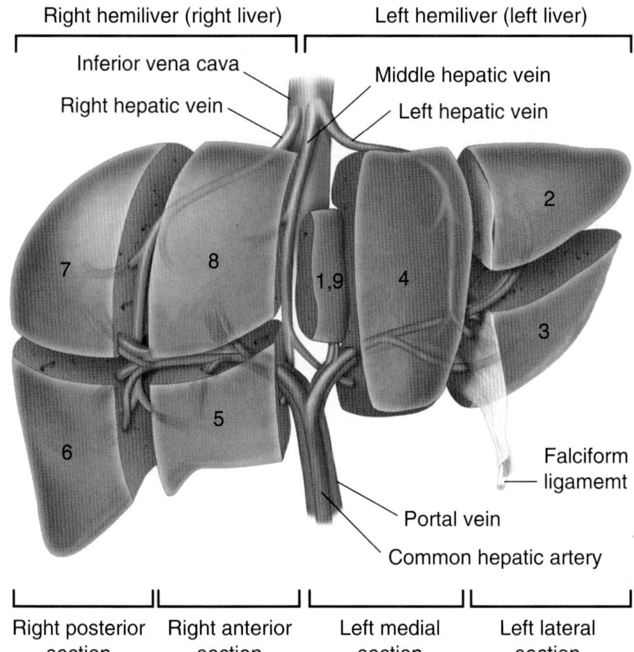

FIGURE 28.9. Hepatic anatomy. The liver is separated into nine anatomic segments. (Redrawn from Burlew CC, Moore EE. Injuries to the liver, biliary tract, spleen, and diaphragm. In: ACS Surgery: Principles and Practice. 2010 Decker Intellectual Properties. http://74.205.62.209/bcdecker/pdf/acs/part7_ch07.pdf., page 4, Figure 6.)

lateral extensions of the coronary ligaments. Injury to the diaphragm, phrenic veins, and hepatic veins must be avoided during mobilization of the liver.

Diagnosis. The appropriate diagnostic modality depends on the hemodynamic status of the patient on arrival in the trauma resuscitation area. If the patient is hemodynamically unstable due to liver injury, immediate laparotomy is required; these patients generally have grade IV or V hepatic injury. If the patient is hemodynamically stable with a blunt mechanism of injury, CT is the diagnostic test of choice. The key decision point in the management of the patient with liver injury is whether he/she is stable and can undergo CT. In essence, hemodynamically stable patients with liver injuries can be treated nonoperatively. FAST and DPL will document hemoperitoneum, but are not specific for liver injury. Of liver injuries, 70% are no longer bleeding at the time of laparotomy for a positive DPL.

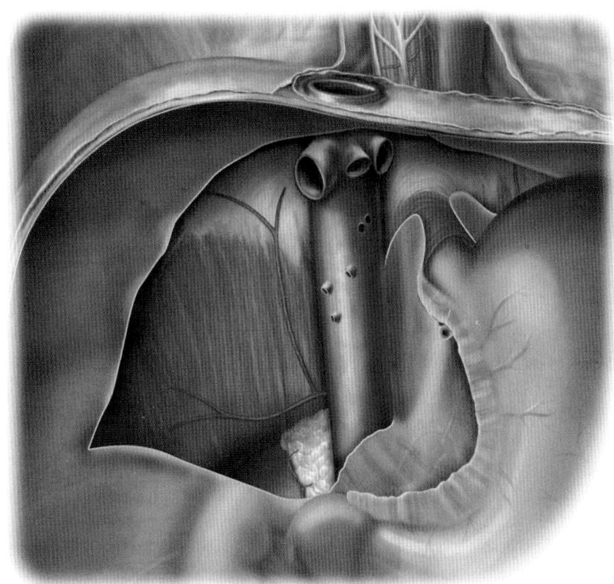

FIGURE 28.10. Anatomy of the retrohepatic IVC. (Redrawn from Buckman RF Jr, Miraliakbari R, Badellino MM. Juxtahepatic venous injuries: a critical review of reported management strategies. *J Trauma* 2000;48:979, Figure 1.)

Treatment. The management of blunt hepatic injury has evolved substantially in the past several years. The hemodynamically stable patient with blunt injury of the liver, without other intra-abdominal injury requiring laparotomy, can be treated nonoperatively, regardless of the grade of the liver injury.[252,253,255-260] This represents 60%-85% of patients with liver injury. The presence of hemoperitoneum on CT does not mandate laparotomy. Arterial blush or pooling of contrast on CT and high-grade (grade IV and V) hepatic injuries is most likely to fail nonoperative management. Nonetheless, embolization can circumvent the need for laparotomy; angioembolization has assumed an increasing role in the treatment of liver injury, both in nonoperative management and postoperatively after laparotomy.[261-264] If arterial bleeding is suspected intraoperatively, postoperative angiography/embolization may be necessary. Liver necrosis is not unexpected after substantial embolization. This may be complicated by abscess formation.

The criteria for nonoperative management of blunt liver injuries include hemodynamic stability, absence of peritoneal signs, lack of continued need for transfusion for the hepatic injury. Posterior right lobe injuries (even if extensive) and the split-liver type of injuries (extensive injury along the relatively avascular plane between the left and right lobes) can generally be managed successfully nonoperatively. The details of nonoperative management are institution-specific and provider-specific. Remember that as many as 26% of patients managed nonoperatively will require an intervention for a complication; only 15% will require an operation. Ninety percent of the patients with a complication requiring treatment have grade IV or V liver injury.[262] The complications generally are managed by ERCP and stent for bile duct leak, percutaneous drainage of an abscess or biloma, or arteriography/embolization for bleeding. Similarly, the need to re-image asymptomatic hepatic injuries by CT scan is not documented. Follow-up CT can be deferred, except to document healing (at ~8 weeks) in physically active patients (e.g., athletes) before resumption of normal activities.

Immediate laparotomy or angiographic intervention is required for those patients with hemodynamic instability, continued blood product requirement (<10%), or who fail nonoperative therapy by demonstrating enlarging lesions on CT scan.[258,265-268] The majority of patients requiring laparotomy for hepatic injury are hemodynamically unstable on arrival and have grade IV or V liver injury. The hemodynamically unstable patient requires immediate operative management. Management principles include availability of blood and a rapid infusion system through upper torso access. Exploration is through a long midline incision. In the past, extension to a median sternotomy or right thoracotomy was advocated for exposure of the liver injury. A right subcostal extension, (left or even bilateral subcostal extension) gives good exposure and nearly always avoids the thoracotomy or sternotomy (Fig. 28.11).[269] Use of a self-retaining retractor (Rochard, Thompson, or Upper Hand) to lift the upper edges of the wound cephalad and anteriorly facilitates exposure of the liver. Complete mobilization of the liver is performed, including division of the ligaments.[265-279]

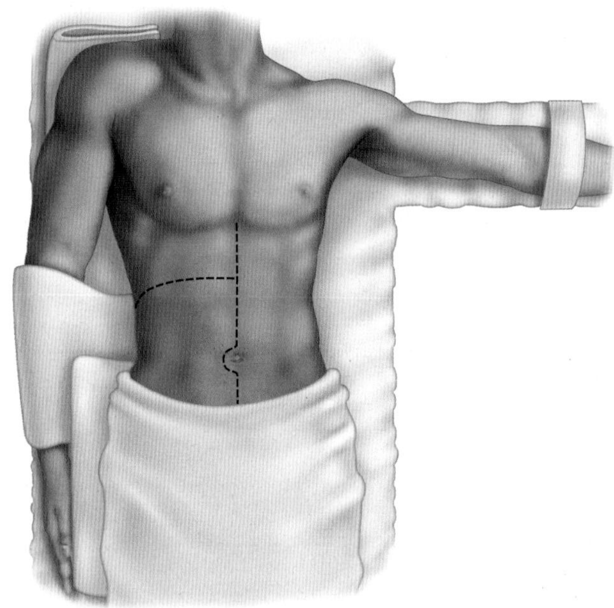

FIGURE 28.11. Combined midline–transverse incision for major hepatic injury. The patient is in the supine position with the right flank and shoulder slightly elevated. (Redrawn from Berney T, Morel P, Huber O, et al. Combined midline–transverse surgical approach for severe blunt injuries to the right liver. *J Trauma* 2000;48: 350, Figure 1.)

Most blunt and penetrating hepatic injuries are grades I-III (85%) and can be managed with simple techniques (e.g., electrocautery, simple suture, or hemostatic agents) (Table 28.8). Complex liver injuries can produce exsanguinating hemorrhage. Rapid, temporary tamponade of the bleeding by manual compression of the liver injury immediately after entering the abdomen allows the anesthesiologist to resuscitate the patient (Fig. 28.12A). After resuscitation, the liver injury can be repaired. Attempts to identify major hepatic injury prior to effective resuscitation will generally exacerbate the patient's bleeding and coagulopathy (Fig. 28.12B).

For complex hepatic injuries, occlude the portal triad with an atraumatic clamp or vessel loops (Pringle maneuver). This should reduce bleeding from the liver, except in the setting of retrohepatic venous injuries. Studies suggest that 60 minutes of warm hepatic ischemia can be tolerated. Especially in the hypotensive patient, we intermittently release the clamp to perfuse the liver, rather than allow continuous ischemia. Hepatorrhaphy with individual vessel ligation is recommended instead of large ischemia-producing mass parenchymal suturing. Glisson's capsule is incised with the electrocautery. The injury within the liver is approached by the finger fracture technique (Fig. 28.13) or by division of the liver tissue over a right-angled clamp with ligation of the hepatic tissue with 2-0 silk sutures, or more recently with the stapler. Use of the stapling devices has greatly facilitated management of elective and urgent liver surgery because of the speed added to the operation. With gentle traction on the liver edges, expose the injury site. Blood vessels and bile ducts are directly visualized and ligated or repaired. Nonviable liver tissue should be debrided. The defect in the liver can be packed with viable omentum. Use closed-suction drainage of grade III-V injuries. Drains are not necessary for grade I and II injuries if bleeding and bile leakage are controlled. Perform resectional debridement of nonviable tissue rather than formal anatomic resection. Perform perihepatic packing in cases of hemorrhage, hypothermia, and coagulopathy. Approximately 5% of patients with hepatic injury require perihepatic packing (damage control laparotomy).[253,265,266,272-282] Indications include coagulopathy, subcapsular hematomas, bilobar injuries, and hypothermia, or to allow transfer of the patient to a higher level of care.

Anatomic hepatic resection (segment or lobe) is not often required for liver injury; resectional debridement and direct suture control of the vessels and ducts can generally accomplish the same objectives, with lower mortality. Indications for formal hepatic resection include total destruction of a segment or lobe, an extensive injury that cannot be controlled with perihepatic packing and control of bleeding that can be achieved only by anatomic resection. Planned, delayed anatomic resection is also an approach for major hepatic injury, if packing sufficiently controls hemorrhage during the initial laparotomy.[265,272,275,278,281]

TABLE 28.8

LIVER INJURY SCALE (1994 REVISION)

GRADE[a]	TYPE OF INJURY	DESCRIPTION OF INJURY	AIS-90
I	Hematoma	Subcapsular, <10% surface area	2
	Laceration	Capsular tear, <1 cm parenchymal depth	2
II	Hematoma	Subcapsular, 10%-50% surface area; intraparenchymal <10 cm in diameter	2
	Laceration	Capsular tear 1–3 cm parenchymal depth, <10 cm in length	2
III	Hematoma	Subcapsular, >50% surface area or expanding; ruptured subcapsular or parenchymal hematoma; intraparenchymal hematoma >10 cm or expanding	3
	Laceration	Parenchymal depth >3 cm	3
IV	Laceration	Parenchymal disruption involving 25%-75% hepatic lobe or 1–3 Couinaud's segments	4
V	Laceration	Parenchymal disruption involving >75% of hepatic lobe or >3 Couinaud's segments within a single lobe	5
	Vascular	Juxtahepatic venous injuries (i.e., retrohepatic vena cava/central major hepatic veins)	5
VI	Vascular	Hepatic avulsion	6

[a]Advance one grade for multiple injuries up to grade III.
AIS, abbreviated injury score.
From Moore EE, Shackford SR, Pachter HL. Organ injury scaling: spleen, liver and kidney. *J Trauma*. 1995;38:323–324.

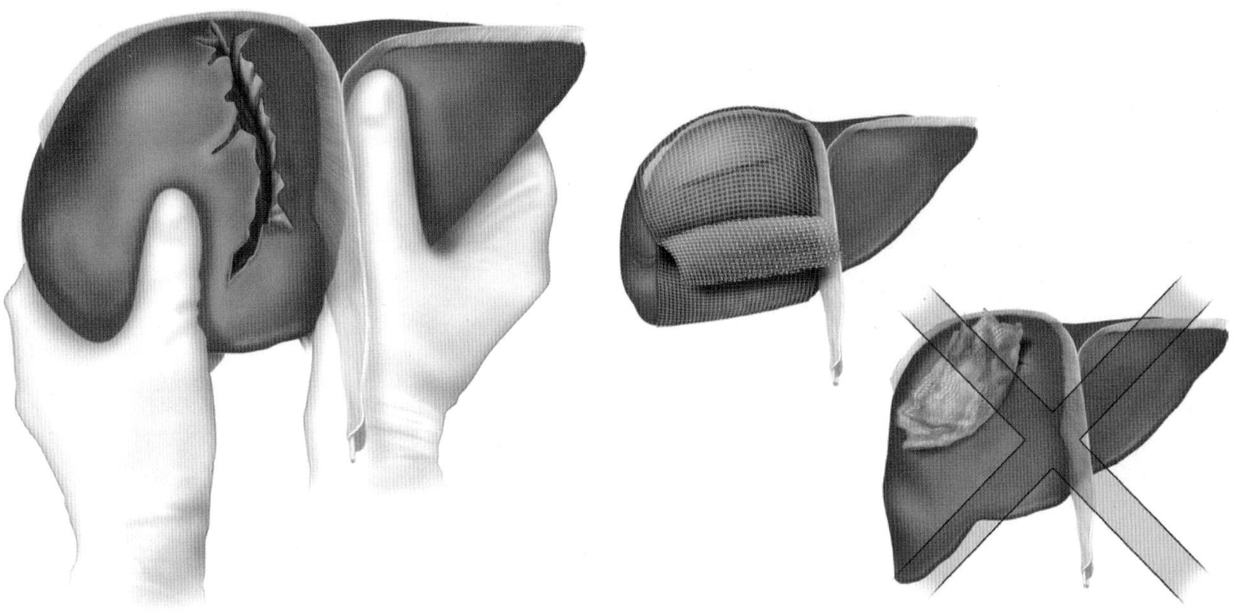

FIGURE 28.12. **A:** When compressing the liver to achieve tamponade, it is critical to realign the liver parenchyma back to its normal anatomic position. When compressing the left and right lobes back together, gently push the liver posteriorly and superiorly to compress any venous bleeding from behind the liver. (Redrawn from Badger SA, Barclay R, Campbell P, et al. Management of liver trauma. *World J Surg.* 2009;33:2528, Figure 5). **B:** The same principles of normal anatomic restorations are essential when packing the liver. Do so with the intent of realigning the liver to normal position. Forcing packs in a crack within the liver will worsen the injury and bleeding. (From Badger SA, Barclay R, Campbell P, et al. Management of liver trauma. *World J Surg* 2009;33:2529, Figure 7.)

Selective hepatic artery ligation has been reported in 1%-2% of hepatic injury cases. (We rarely use this technique.) The liver will generally tolerate this because of the oxygen content of portal blood. Direct suture control of bleeding within the liver is preferable to hepatic artery ligation. Nonetheless, patients with considerable central hepatic laceration who had damage control laparotomy may be candidates for arteriography with possible embolization postoperatively.

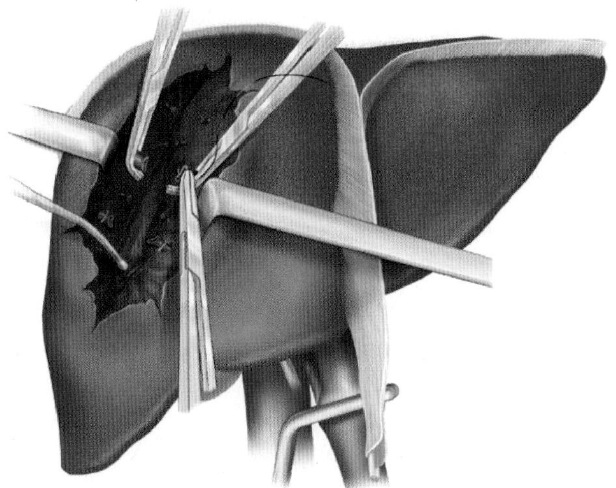

FIGURE 28.13. To gain control of bleeding from the liver, the liver injury is enlarged by hepatotomy and bleeding controlled by direct suture or ligation. Rapid access may be obtained by finger-fracture technique or the stapling devices. (Redrawn from Badger SA, Barclay R, Campbell P, et al. Management of liver trauma. *World J Surg.* 2009;33:2530, Figure 8.)

Cholecystectomy may be required secondary to ischemic complications from interruption of the right hepatic artery.

Hepatic vascular isolation with occlusion of the suprahepatic and infrahepatic venae cavae, as well as application of the Pringle maneuver, may be required for major retrohepatic venous injury. Atrial-caval shunts have been recommended by some for retrohepatic caval injury (not the authors). A 36F chest tube or 9-mm endotracheal tube, each with extra side holes, is inserted through the right atrial appendage. The side holes allow flow from the shunt into the right atrium. The distal end of the tube is at the level of the RV. Survival with this technique is dismal. Alternatively, complex retrohepatic vascular injury in which tamponade does not achieve hemostasis can be repaired in an avascular field on venovenous bypass with total hepatic vascular isolation. The hypovolemic trauma patient may not tolerate suprahepatic caval clamping for any period of time. Survival depends on prompt recognition of this anatomic site of injury. Our approach to retrohepatic venous injuries includes experienced help at the OR table, self-retaining retractors with anterior and cephalad pull on the costal margin for exposure, rapid and full mobilization of the liver, extension of the midline incision as discussed above, and direct exposure and repair of the venous injury.

Bleeding from penetrating wounds of the liver that are not easily accessed, at times, can be controlled with internal tamponade (Fig. 28.14). This is accomplished by using Penrose drains tied at each end (as a balloon) over a red rubber catheter. The end of the Penrose drain is brought through the skin.[279] Finally, in wounds where tamponade does not achieve hemostasis, consider repair under vascular isolation by experienced personnel.

Outcome. Mortality correlates with the degree of injury. Because most hepatic injuries are grades I-II, the overall mortality for liver injuries is 10%. However, the mortality for more severe liver injury is grade III, 25%; grade IV, 46%; and grade

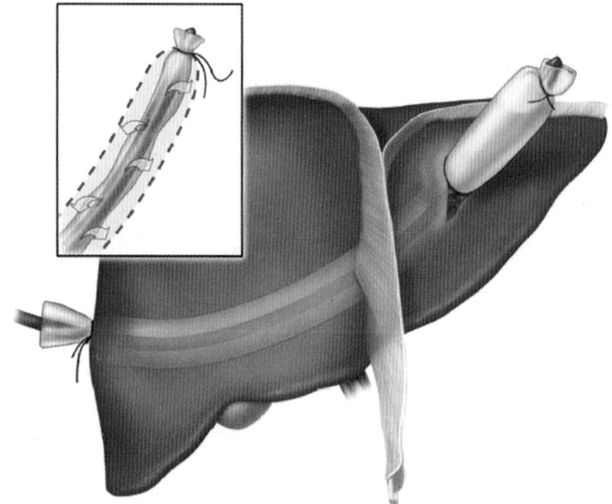

FIGURE 28.14. Balloon tamponade to control bleeding from a bullet tract through the liver, using a foley within a penrose drain. (Redrawn from Burlew CC, Moore EE. Injuries to the liver, biliary tract, spleen, and diaphragm. In: ACS Surgery: Principles and Practice. Decker Intellectual Properties; 2010. http://74.205.62.209/bcdecker/pdf/acs/part7_ch07.pdf., page 10, Figure 10.)

V, 50%-80%, in many series. Notably, Polanco et al. recently reported a liver-related mortality of 9% for high-grade liver injury.[259,267,271]

Complications. With recurrent bleeding (occurs in 2%-7% of patients), return the patient to the OR or, in selected patients, obtain an angiogram and perform embolization. Recurrent bleeding is generally caused by inadequate initial hemostasis. Hypothermia and coagulopathy must be corrected. Preparations to control retrohepatic hemorrhage (i.e., vascular bypass) should be made. Hemobilia is a rare complication of liver injury. The classic presentation is right upper quadrant pain, jaundice, and hemorrhage; one-third of patients have all three components of the triad. The patient may present with hemobilia days or weeks after injury. Treatment is angiogram and embolization.

Intrahepatic or perihepatic abscess or biloma (occurs in 7%-40% of patients) can generally be drained percutaneously. Meticulous control of bleeding and repair of bile ducts, adequate debridement, and closed-suction drainage are essential to avoid abscess formation. Biliary fistulas (>50 mL per day for >2 weeks) usually resolve nonoperatively if external drainage of the leak is adequate and distal obstruction is not present. If >300 mL of bile drains each day, further evaluation with a radionuclide scan, a fistulogram, ERCP, or a transhepatic cholangiogram may be necessary. Major ductal injury can be stented to facilitate healing of the injury or as a guide if operative repair is required. Endoscopic sphincterotomy or transampullary stenting may facilitate resolution of the biliary leak. *Extrahepatic biliary tract injury* is uncommon. The gallbladder is the most common site; cholecystectomy is the usual treatment. Injury to the extrahepatic bile ducts can be missed at laparotomy unless careful operative inspection of the porta hepatis is performed. A cholangiogram through the gallbladder or cystic duct stump defines the injury. The location and severity of the injury will dictate the appropriate treatment. Simple bile duct injury (<50% of the circumference) can be repaired with primary suture repair. Complex bile duct injury (>50% of the circumference) may require Roux-en-Y choledochojejunostomy or hepaticojejunostomy. Primary end-to-end anastomosis of the bile duct is not advised; the stricture rate approaches 50%.

Splenic Injury

The paradigm shift toward nonoperative management of blunt abdominal injury has been dramatic with injury to the spleen.[252,283-292] Several decades ago, the only therapy for blunt injury of the spleen, irrespective of magnitude, was splenectomy. Led by the pediatric surgeons who demonstrated that splenic injury could be observed and the awareness of overwhelming post-splenectomy infection (OPSI), the majority of blunt splenic injuries are observed currently.[285,293-303] Blunt splenic injury is produced by compression or deceleration force (e.g., from motor vehicle crashes, falls, or direct blows to the abdomen). Penetrating injury to the spleen is far less common.

Anatomy and Function. The spleen is bounded by the stomach, left hemidiaphragm, left kidney and adrenal gland, colon, and chest wall.[304] These relationships define the attachment of the spleen: gastrosplenic ligament, splenorenal ligament, splenophrenic ligament, splenocolic ligament, and pancreaticosplenic attachments. The spleen receives 5% of the cardiac output, primarily through the splenic artery. The splenic artery usually bifurcates into superior and inferior polar arteries. Further division of the blood supply is along transverse planes. The spleen has an open microcirculation without endothelium. The white pulp comprises 25% of splenic volume and is the lymphoid component of the spleen. The red blood is 75% of splenic volume and contains the splenic cords and sinuses. It filters blood-borne bacteria, particulate matter, and aged cells. The spleen produces antibodies, properdin, and tuftsin. In addition, the spleen comprises 25% of the lymphoid mass in humans.

Diagnosis. The patient may have signs of hypovolemia with tachycardia or hypotension, or complain of left upper quadrant tenderness or referred pain to the left shoulder (Kehr's sign). Physical examination is insensitive and nonspecific in the diagnosis of splenic injury. The patient may have signs of generalized peritoneal irritation or left upper quadrant tenderness or fullness. Twenty-five percent of patients with left lower rib fractures (ribs 9 through 12) will have splenic injury. In the unstable trauma patient, ultrasound or DPL provides the most rapid diagnosis of hemoperitoneum, the source of which is commonly the spleen. In the stable patient with blunt injury, CT of the abdomen provides delineation and grading of the splenic injury (Table 28.9).[260] The most common finding on CT in association with a splenic injury is hemoperitoneum. Interestingly, hemoperitoneum in children with blunt injury to the spleen is uncommon, thus making FAST unreliable in the pediatric population. The need and timing of follow-up CT remain controversial. Our practice is to obtain follow-up CT of blunt splenic injury at 48 hours. This is based on the data of Fabian's group,[305-307] demonstrating that serial CT documented early splenic artery pseudoaneurysms in 4% of patients and another 3% of splenic artery pseudoaneurysms were found only on the follow-up CT.

Angiography has been used as an adjunct in the management of splenic injury in highly selected patients, with therapeutic embolization of arterial bleeding. The role of angiography/embolization for splenic injury is still evolving and highly variable between hospitals.[305-323] The majority of the studies advocating liberal use of angiography/embolization utilize historical controls.[308-316] With the rapid evolution toward nonoperative management of blunt splenic injury, such comparisons are difficult to interpret. We use angiography/

TABLE 28.9

SPLEEN INJURY SCALE (1994 REVISION)

GRADE[a]	INJURY TYPE	DESCRIPTION OF INJURY	AIS-90
I	Hematoma	Subcapsular, <10% surface area	2
	Laceration	Capsular tear, <1 cm parenchymal depth	2
II	Hematoma	Subcapsular, 10%-50% surface area; intraparenchymal, <5 cm in diameter	2
	Laceration	Capsular tear, 1–3 cm parenchymal depth that does not involve a trabecular vessel	2
III	Hematoma	Subcapsular, >50% surface area or expanding; ruptured subcapsular or parenchymal hematoma; intraparenchymal hematoma ≥5 cm or expanding	3
	Laceration	Parenchymal depth >3 cm or involving trabecular vessels	3
IV	Laceration	Laceration involving segmental or hilar vessels producing major devascularization (>25% of spleen)	4
V	Laceration	Completely shattered spleen	5
	Vascular	Hilar vascular injury that devascularizes spleen	5

[a]Advance one grade for multiple injuries up to grade III.
AIS, abbreviated injury score.
From Moore EE, Shackford SR, Pachter HL. Organ injury scaling: spleen, liver and kidney. *J Trauma*. 1995;38:323–324.

embolization of splenic injury in the stable patient with an arterial blush.

The time course for healing of blunt splenic injuries treated nonoperatively has not been clearly delineated. What seems defined is that the higher the grade splenic injury, the longer the spleen takes to heal; time to radiographic evidence of healing of the spleen correlates with the grade of splenic injury. Second, more than 80% of splenic injuries will heal by 2–2½ months postinjury.[324,325]

Treatment. The availability of abdominal CT and an understanding of the importance of splenic function have resulted in the preservation of the majority of injured spleens, by nonoperative management. Safe management of splenic injury depends primarily on the hemodynamic stability of the patient on presentation. Unstable patients due to splenic injury, irrespective of the grade, should be in the OR. Other factors include the age of the patient, associated injuries (which are the rule in adults), and the grade of the splenic injury. Nonoperative management of splenic injury is successful in >90% of children, irrespective of the grade of splenic injury. Nonoperative management of blunt splenic injury in adults has become more routine; 65%-80% of adults ultimately managed nonoperatively for blunt injury to the spleen.[288,326] If hemodynamically stable, adult patients with grade I or II injury can generally be treated nonoperatively. Patients with grade IV or V splenic injuries are most often unstable. Grade III splenic injuries (certainly in children, and in selected adults) can be treated nonoperatively based on stability and reliable physical examination. The failure rate of nonoperative management of splenic injuries in adults is 5%-10% and increases with grade of splenic injury: grade I, 5%; grade II, 10%; grade III, 20%; grade IV, 33%; and grade V, 75%.[286,327,328] In two recent studies from the National Trauma Data Bank, failure rates for high-grade splenic injuries (grades IV and V) were 53% and 55%.[290,319] In the study by Watson et al., 60% of 3,085 adults with grade IV and V splenic injuries went directly to the OR. Of the 40% of high-grade splenic injuries which were admitted for observation, 55% failed. Thus, the majority (80%) of grade IV and V splenic injuries in adults ultimately underwent laparotomy. As mortality for failed nonoperative management increased from 0% to 15.7% over the period of the study, it suggests that many of these patients may have been better served by early splenectomy. The EAST multicenter study of failure of nonoperative management of blunt splenic injury corroborates the hypothesis that high-grade splenic injuries and hypotensive patients need to be in the OR.[327] The potential consequences of observation of the adult with blunt splenic injury, especially high-grade injuries or patients with hypotension, are that preventable deaths will occur. Fastidious judgment and patient selection are critical for safe nonoperative management of blunt splenic injury. In adults (but not in children), risk of failure of nonoperative management of blunt splenic injury correlates with grade of splenic injury and quantity of hemoperitoneum.

Sixty percent of failures occur within 24 hours of injury; 90% of failures occur within 72 hours of injury.[325-327] Patients with substantial splenic injuries managed nonoperatively should be observed in a monitored unit and have immediate access to CT, a surgeon, and an OR. Changes in physical examination, hemodynamic stability, ongoing blood or fluid requirements indicate the need for laparotomy.

If the patient is not hemodynamically stable, operative treatment is required. The operative therapy of choice is splenic conservation where possible to avoid the risk of death from OPSI. However, in the presence of multiple injuries or critical instability, splenectomy is most appropriate.

Exploration is through a long midline incision. The abdomen is packed and explored. Exsanguinating hemorrhage and gastrointestinal soilage are controlled first.

Mobilize the spleen to visualize the injury. The operator's nondominant hand will provide medial traction on the spleen to facilitate the operation. The splenocolic ligament can be vascular and require ligation. The splenorenal and splenophrenic ligaments are avascular and should be divided sharply; avoid injury to the splenic capsule as this is performed (Fig. 28.15). Further mobilize the spleen by bluntly freeing it from the retroperitoneum. It is important to stay in the plane posterior to the pancreas as the spleen and pancreas are mobilized. The hilum of the spleen can then be controlled with manual compression. The gastrosplenic ligament with the short gastric vessels is divided and ligated near the spleen to avoid injury or late necrosis of the gastric wall. Fully mobilize the spleen into the operative field. Splenectomy should be performed in unstable patients, and in those with associated life-threatening injury, or multiple sources for postoperative blood loss (pelvic fracture, multiple long bone fractures), and complex

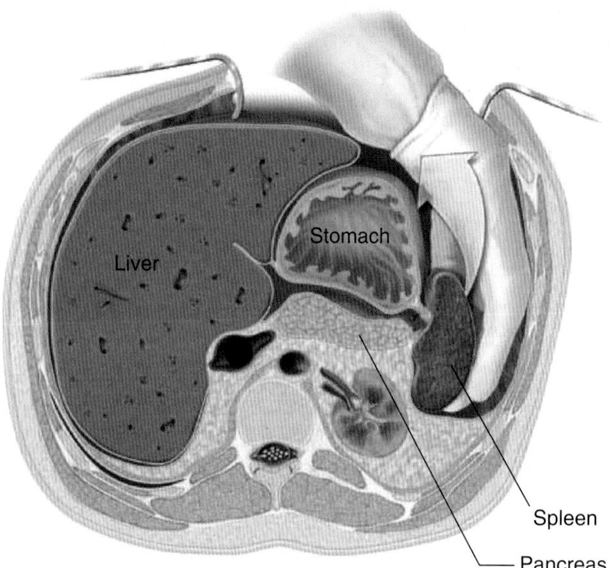

FIGURE 28.15. Mobilization of the spleen from the left upper quadrant to the midline. (Redrawn from Trunkey DD. Spleen. In: Blaisdell FW, Trunkey DD, eds. *Trauma Management: Abdominal Trauma*. New York, NY: Thime-Stratton; 1982:190, Figure 10.3.)

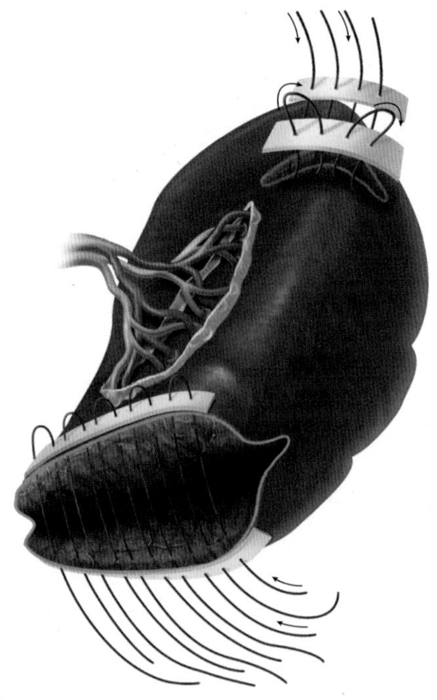

FIGURE 28.16. Splenic repair using pledgets after splenic resection. (Redrawn from Moore EE. Splenic injury. In: Dudley H, Carter D, Russell RCG, eds. *Rob and Smith's Operative Surgery*. Boston, MA: Butterworth; 1989:370, Figure 9.)

splenic injuries. Splenorrhaphy should be considered when circumstances permit. Because of the increased reliance on nonoperative management of splenic injury, the opportunity to attempt splenorrhaphy is uncommon. The technique is dictated by the magnitude of the splenic injury and the patient's hemodynamic status. Nonbleeding grade I splenic injury may require no treatment. Topical hemostatic agents, an argon beam coagulator, or electrocautery may suffice. Grade II-III splenic injuries may require the aforementioned interventions, suture repair, or mesh wrap of capsular defects. Suture repair in adults often requires Teflon pledgets to avoid tearing of the splenic capsule (Fig. 28.16). Grade IV and V splenic injuries may require anatomic resection, including ligation of the lobar artery. A small rim of capsule at the resection line may help reinforce the resection line. Pledgeted horizontal mattress sutures may also be necessary. Grade V splenic injury usually requires splenectomy. One-third of the splenic mass must be functional to maintain immunocompetence.[328] Thus, at least one-half of the spleen must be preserved to justify splenorrhaphy. Drainage of the splenic fossa is associated with an increased incidence of subphrenic abscess and should be avoided. The exception is when concern exists about injury to the tail of the pancreas.

Outcome. The outcome is generally good; rebleeding rates as low as 1% have been reported with splenorrhaphy. The failure rate of nonoperative therapy is 2% in children and generally 5%-10% in adults. It had been reported previously that adults >55 years of age are especially susceptible to failure of nonoperative therapy[329,330]; current data do not support this contention.[331,332] Although the failure of nonoperative management of blunt splenic injury is higher in the very old (>75 years), age alone does not mandate operation.[332]

Pulmonary complications, which are common in patients treated operatively and nonoperatively, include atelectasis, left pleural effusion, and pneumonia. Left subphrenic abscess occurs in 3%-13% of postoperative patients and may be more common with the use of drains or with concomitant bowel injury.

Thrombocytosis occurs in as many as 50% of patients after splenectomy; the platelet count usually peaks 2–10 days postoperatively. The elevated platelet count generally abates in several weeks. Treatment is usually not required.

The risk of OPSI is greater in children than in adults; the overall risk is <0.5%.[293,300-304] The mortality rate for OPSI approaches 50%. The common organisms are encapsulated organisms: meningococcus, *Haemophilus influenzae*, and *Streptococcus pneumoniae*, as well as *Staphylococcus aureus* and *Escherichia coli*. After splenectomy, pneumococcal (Pneumovax), *H. influenzae*, and meningococcal vaccines should be administered.[293-296,317,334] The timing of injection of the vaccine is controversial. Some authors recommend giving the vaccine 3–4 weeks postoperatively because the patient may be too immunosuppressed in the immediate postinjury period. We vaccinate the patient prior to discharge from the initial hospitalization. Current recommendation is to repeat the pneumococcal vaccination at 5 years. The patient should be discharged from the hospital with a clear understanding of the concerns about OPSI, should wear a tag alerting health care providers of his or her asplenic state, and should begin penicillin therapy with the development of even mild infections.

Abdominal Vascular Injury

Abdominal vascular injuries are among the most lethal injuries sustained by trauma patients. Similarly, these injuries are also among the most difficult and challenging injuries encountered by trauma surgeons. Generally, these patients arrive at trauma centers in profound shock secondary to massive blood loss, which is often unrelenting. Patients sustaining abdominal vascular injuries best exemplify the lethal vicious cycle of shock, acidosis, hypothermia, coagulopathy, and cardiac dysrhythmias.[335-340] Many of these patients present in cardiopulmonary arrest and require drastic life-saving measures, such as emergency department thoracotomy, aortic cross-clamping, and open cardiopulmonary resuscitation for any opportunity to reach the OR alive. To compound the problem, exposure of bleeding retroperitoneal vessels is difficult and requires extensive dissection and mobilization of intra-abdominal organs. These maneuvers are time-consuming and fraught with pitfalls, as rapid dissection through large retroperitoneal hematomas can lead to iatrogenic injury in patients who can ill afford further injury.[335-340]

Abdominal vascular injury rarely occurs as an isolated entity. In fact, multiple associated injuries are the rule rather than the exception, thus increasing not only injury severity but the time needed to repair many critical associated injuries. Abdominal vascular injuries are also characterized by massive blood losses requiring large quantities of crystalloid solution, blood and blood products for intravascular volume replacement. Coupled with the frequent need to cross-clamp the aorta or other major intra-abdominal vessels, this scenario predisposes these patients to the development of reperfusion injuries and if they survive, their sequelae.[6]

The concept of "bail out" later renamed as "damage control" is usually applied in patients sustaining abdominal vascular injuries. Similarly, these patients often demand temporary abdominal wall closure with prosthetic materials, which initiates a cycle of frequent surgical reinterventions, producing additive physiologic and immunologic insults to an already compromised patient.[338]

The classical dilemma encountered by trauma surgeons of how to repair vascular injuries in the midst of massive contamination while avoiding graft infections and vessel blowout remains a difficult problem. Septic processes and multiple system organ failure (MSOF) are frequent complications encountered by these patients, as profound shock, tissue hypoperfusion, massive blood volume replacement, generalized edema, and prolonged contamination places these patients at risk for these complications. All of these factors clearly conspire to produce high morbidity rates for patients sustaining these injuries. Improved outcomes are generally the result of expedient and precise surgical interventions by trauma surgeons with experience in the management of these injuries along with the vast surgical armamentarium needed to effectively deal with them.[339-342]

Anatomic Location of Injury. Abdominal vascular injury associated with blunt trauma most commonly occurs in upper abdominal vessels (Table 28.10).[335] However, penetrating injuries may occur in any of the retroperitoneal zones, as missile

TABLE 28.10

ABDOMINAL VASCULAR INJURY SCALE

GRADE[a]	DESCRIPTION OF INJURY	AIS-90
I	Non-named SMA or SMV branches	NS
	Non-named IMA or inferior mesenteric vein branches	NS
	Phrenic artery or vein	NS
	Lumbar artery or vein	NS
	Gonadal artery or vein	NS
	Ovarian artery or vein	NS
II	Right, left, or common hepatic artery	3
	Splenic artery or vein	3
	Right or left gastric arteries	3
	Gastroduodenal artery	3
	IMA, or inferior mesenteric vein, trunk	3
	Primary named branches of mesenteric artery (e.g., ileocolic artery) or mesenteric vein	3
	Other named abdominal vessels requiring ligation or repair	3
III	SMV, trunk	3
	Renal artery or vein	3
	Iliac artery or vein	3
	Hypogastric artery or vein	3
	Vena cava, infrarenal	3
IV	SMA, trunk	3
	Celiac axis proper	3
	Vena cava, suprarenal and infrahepatic	3
	Aorta, infrarenal	4
V	Portal vein	3
	Extraparenchymal hepatic vein	3/5
	Vena cava, retrohepatic or suprahepatic	5
	Aorta suprarenal, subdiaphragmatic	4

[a]This classification system is applicable to extraparenchymal vascular injuries. If the vessel injury is within 2 cm of the organ parenchyma, refer to specific organ injury scale. Increase one grade for multiple grade III or IV injuries involving >50% vessel circumference. Downgrade one grade if <25% vessel circumference laceration for grade IV or V.

NS, not scored; AIS, abbreviated injury score.

From Moore EE, Cogbill TH, Jurkovich GJ, et al. Organ injury scales III: chest wall, abdominal vascular, ureter, bladder and urethra. *J Trauma*. 1992;33:337–339.

trajectories are unpredictable, frequently injuring more than one vessel. The cumulative effect on mortality rises as multiple vessels are injured. Because of close proximity between abdominal arteries and veins, the potential for the development of arteriovenous fistulas exists either acutely or chronically; however, they are uncommon.[343-344]

The abdominal aorta may be injured at its suprarenal or infrarenal portions. The IVC may be injured at its suprarenal or infrarenal portions or its retrohepatic location, one of the most lethal injuries. The SMA may be injured in any of its four zones, just as the SMV may be injured at its infrapancreatic or retropancreatic location. The PV may be injured either at its origin at the confluence of the superior mesenteric and SV or it may be injured alone within the confines of the portal triad. The renal artery (RA) may be injured in one of its three portions whereas the RVs may be injured either at their confluence with the IVC or at the renal hilum.[343-344]

Operative Intervention. In the OR, the patient's entire torso from the neck to mid-thighs and table to table laterally is prepared and draped. The area to the mid-thighs is important should the necessity arise to obtain autogenous saphenous vein graft. The trauma surgeon must confirm that there are sufficient units of blood in the OR for immediate transfusion via rapid infusion technology. Maneuvers to prevent hypothermia include placement of a warming blanket on the operating table, covering the patient's lower extremities with a circulating warm air mattress, covering the head to prevent heat loss, increasing the ventilator cascade temperature to 42°C, and an ample supply of heated irrigation fluids. In addition, the availability of autotransfusion apparatus and cell-saving technology is of great value. Appropriate instruments and shunts must be available, including the Argon beam coagulator and newer hemostatic agents.[335,343]

Exposure and Incisions. Abdominal injuries should be explored through a midline incision extending from xiphoid to pubis. Immediate control of life-threatening hemorrhage followed by immediate control of sources of gastrointestinal spillage are early goals. The next step in the management of abdominal injuries consists of a thorough exploration of the abdominal cavity. Since the abdominal vasculature resides in the retroperitoneum, a thorough exploration of these structures must be performed utilizing a systematic approach of the anatomic zones of the retroperitoneum.

Surgical Technique. The first and most important goal in the management of abdominal vascular injuries is hemorrhage control. As in all vascular injuries, proximal and distal control of the bleeding vessel is required. However, in exsanguinating abdominal vascular injury, achieving this rapidly may be difficult. Unfortunately, a notable number of patients succumb without vascular control.[335-341,343,345]

Frequently, these patients experience severe and profound hypotension, therefore cross-clamping of the aorta is the first maneuver instituted to stop life-threatening hemorrhage. If the patient arrives profoundly hypotensive or experiences cardiopulmonary arrest in the OR, an immediate left anterolateral thoracotomy with aortic cross-clamping and open cardiopulmonary resuscitation should be performed prior to proceeding with the laparotomy.[335,336-340,343,345]

For patients who arrive with hemodynamic stability, but decompensate during laparotomy, the abdominal aorta can be controlled at the aortic hiatus, either digitally or by the use of an abdominal aortic root compressor, or by cross-clamping with a Crawford-DeBakey or other aortic clamps. Placement of a cross-clamp in this location is difficult, as the abdominal aorta is surrounded by the crura of the diaphragm, which often requires transection of the crus to reach a portion of the infradiaphragmatic aorta to place the aortic crossclamp.

Once the exsanguinating hemorrhage has been controlled, the trauma surgeon should classify the hemorrhage or hematoma into one of the three zones of the retroperitoneum. Zone I begins at the aortic hiatus and ends at the sacral promontory; it is located at the midline with the spinal column posteriorly. This zone is divided into supramesocolic and inframesocolic compartments. Zone II, right and left are located at the pericolic gutters. Zone III begins at the sacral promontory and contains the major pelvic blood vessels (Fig. 28.17).

Zone I supramesocolic contains the suprarenal abdominal aorta, the celiac axis (Tripod of Haller), and the first two parts of the SMA. The SMA is divided into four parts. Part 1 has its origin at the aorta and ends at the point where the inferior pancreaticoduodenal artery emerges; Part 2 from the origin of the inferior pancreaticoduodenal to the origin of the middle colic artery; Part 3 is the trunk distal to the middle colic artery; and Part 4 encompasses the origins of the segmental jejunal, ileal, or colic branches. Zone I supramesocolic also contains the infrahepatic suprarenal IVC, the infrarenal IVC as well as the proximal portion of the SMV.[345-349]

Zone I inframesocolic contains the last two portions of the SMA, the IMA, the infrarenal aorta and vena cava, as well as the distal SMV. Zone II is divided into right and left, each containing the renal vascular pedicle. Zone III contains the bifurcation of the aorta into the common iliac arteries and veins which further bifurcate into the internal and external iliac vessels. It also contains the retroperitoneal venous plexus of the Batson. The portal–retrohepatic area contains the PV, hepatic artery, and retrohepatic vena cava.[345-350]

Thus, the trauma surgeon first identifies the location of the hemorrhage or hematoma into one of the zones of the retroperitoneum. The surgeon must then approach this zone to obtain vascular control, expose the injured blood vessel, and attempt definitive repair and/or ligation. Each zone requires different and complex maneuvers for exposure of these vessels.

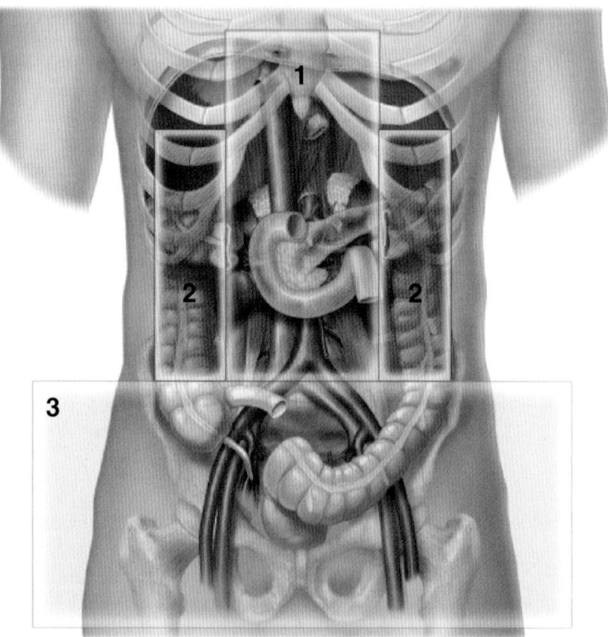

FIGURE 28.17. Retroperitoneal zones. (Redrawn from Kudsk KA, Sheldon GF. Retroperitoneal hematoma. In: Blaisdell FW, Trunkey DD, eds. *Trauma Management: Abdominal Trauma*. New York: Thime-Stratton; 1982:281, Figure 14-2.)

Zone I supramesocolic is generally approached utilizing a maneuver that rotates the left-sided viscera medially (left medial visceral rotation) (Fig. 28.18). This approach requires transection of the avascular line of Toldt of the left colon, along with incision of the lienosplenic ligament and rotation of the left colon, spleen, tail, and body of the pancreas as well as the stomach medially. This exposes the aorta from its entrance into the abdominal cavity via the aortic hiatus and includes exposure of the origin of the celiac axis,[348] the first two zones of SMA and the left renal vascular pedicle.[345-351] The left kidney can be mobilized medially, although this is generally not done.[351]

An alternative maneuver includes performing an extended Kocher maneuver along with transection of the avascular line of Toldt of the right colon, mobilizing medially the right colon, hepatic flexure, duodenum, and head of the pancreas to the level of the superior mesenteric vessels; elevating these structures in a cephalad direction and incising the loose retroperitoneal tissue to the left of the IVC (right medial visceral rotation) (see Fig. 28.7). This maneuver exposes the suprarenal abdominal aorta between the celiac axis and the SMA. This maneuver has a disadvantage in that the exposure obtained is below the level of any injury to the supraceliac aorta and the aorta at the hiatus.[335-341]

Maneuvers used to expose injuries in zone I inframesocolic include displacing the transverse colon and mesocolon cephalad, eviscerating the small bowel to the right, locating the ligament of Treitz, transecting it along with the loose retroperitoneal tissue alongside the left of the abdominal aorta until left RV is located. This exposes the infrarenal aorta. Meticulous attention must be directed to avoid iatrogenic injury to the IMV. To expose the infrarenal IVC, the avascular line of Toldt of the right colon is transected while performing an extensive Kocher maneuver sweeping the pancreas and duodenum to the left and incising the retroperitoneal tissues covering the IVC.

Exposure to right and left zone II depends as to whether the perirenal hematoma is actively bleeding and whether it is located laterally or medially. If active bleeding is found medially or if there is an expanding hematoma, vascular control of the RA and vein is required. Vessel loops should be used for control; alternatively, a Henley subclavian/renal clamp may also be used. On the right, this is achieved by mobilizing the right colon and hepatic flexure as well as performing a Kocher maneuver, exposing the IVC infrarenally and continuing the dissection cephalad by incising the tissues directly over the suprarenal infrahepatic IVC. This is continued until the right RV is encountered. Further dissection superiorly and posteriorly to the right RV will locate the right RA.[351]

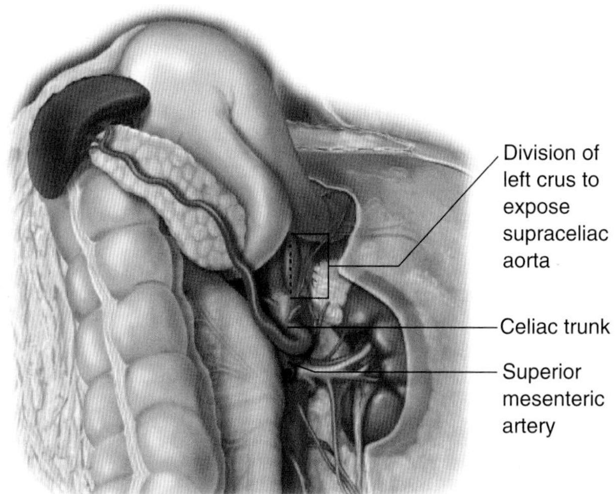

FIGURE 28.18. Left medial visceral rotation. (Redrawn from Singh N. Major abdominal vascular trauma. In: Martin MJ, Beekley Ac, eds. *Front Line Surgery*. New York, NY: Springer; 2010:145, Figure 11.2.)

On the left side, the left colon and splenic flexure are mobilized. The small bowel is then eviscerated to the right. The ligament of Treitz is located, and the transverse colon and mesocolon are displaced cephalad. This should expose the intrarenal abdominal aorta. Cephalad dissection will locate the left RV as it crosses over the abdominal aorta. The left RA will also be found superiorly and posteriorly to the left RV. Once mobilized and controlled and if uninjured, the renal vessels may be retracted with a vein retractor Alternatively, if a perirenal hematoma or active bleeding is found laterally with no extension into the hilum of the kidney, the lateral aspects of Gerota's fascia can be incised and the kidney elevated and displaced medially to locate the hemorrhage.

Exposure of the vessels in zone III can be achieved by transection of the avascular line of Toldt of both the right and left colons and displacing them medially. Utilizing a combination of blunt and sharp dissection, the common iliac vessels are located. Meticulous attention must be paid to locate and preserve the ureter as it crosses the common iliac artery. Avoid devascularization of the ureter's blood supply. A vessel loop should be passed around the ureter to retract it. Dissection is then extended in a caudad direction, opening the retroperitoneum over the vessels.[351]

Structures in the portal–retrohepatic area are difficult to expose and require extensive dissection. The PV is formed by the confluence of the SMV and the slightly smaller SV posterior to the neck of the pancreas.[349] This confluence is located just to the right of the body of the second lumbar vertebra (L2) and immediately anterior to the left border of the IVC. The inferior mesenteric vein (IMV) is the third major tributary to the IVC contributing its flow to the PV, by entering either the SV generally, or SMV in the immediate vicinity of the major confluence rarely. In as many as 30% of cases, the IMV enters at the angle of the major confluence. In contrast to the suprapancreatic PV, the retropancreatic confluence zone is not intimately related to the bile duct or hepatic artery.

Sound knowledge of the anatomy of the portal confluence is of utmost importance to trauma surgeons. From its origin, the valveless PV passes cephalad, inclining slightly rightward over its course of 7.5–10 cm to reach the hilum of the liver, where it divides extrahepatically into right and left branches. During its course, it passes in succession behind the upper pancreatic neck and the first portion of the duodenum. Then, upon entering the hepatoduodenal ligament, it forms a relationship with the hepatic artery and bile duct, lying behind these structures and forming the anterior border of the foramen of Winslow. Throughout its length, the PV lies immediately anterior to the suprarenal segment of the IVC. The PV receives, in addition to its main tributaries, the pyloric vein from the pancreas and duodenum, left gastric (coronary) vein, and the superior pancreaticoduodenal vein. A cystic vein, if present, also drains into the PV.

Wounds of the suprapancreatic PV can be exposed by an extensive Kocher maneuver, with mobilization and rotation of the hepatic flexure of the colon. Preliminary hepatic inflow occlusion and the division of the cystic duct facilitate the exposure. Retropancreatic wounds involving the portal confluence or its major tributaries and suprapancreatic wounds with suspected additional injury of the IVC or other vessels are exposed by a combination of an extensive Kocher maneuver and mobilization of the entire right colon and mesenteric base, from the cecum to the duodenojejunal flexure. This maneuver, when combined with leftward mobilization of hepatic flexure, provides access to the entire PV and the proximal portions of its major tributaries. It also exposes the entire infrahepatic vena cava and the aorta up to the origin of the SMA.[335-339,345-347]

Surgical transection of the neck of the pancreas can also be utilized to expose the retropancreatic PV. An avascular plane exists between the neck of the pancreas and the anterior surface of the PV, as there are no venous tributaries draining into the anterior surface of the PV. Transection of the neck of the pancreas can be achieved either with a GIA or TIA stapler. This maneuver is recommended when there is an associated pancreatic injury, which will mandate distal pancreatectomy, or as completion pancreatectomy for an almost totally transected pancreas at its neck. It may be utilized as the last ditch effort, if hemorrhage containment cannot be accomplished in any other way. All of these maneuvers as well as direct dissection of the portal triad will also expose the hepatic artery and its branches.

One of the most difficult vascular structures to expose is the retrohepatic vena cava. This segment of the IVC has unique anatomic features such as multiple tributaries draining anteriorly at the level of the caudate lobe. This portion of the vena cava measures approximately 7–12 cm in length and lies in a groove on the posterior aspect of the liver. The retrohepatic cava is joined by the major hepatic veins: the right, middle, and left hepatic veins. Frequently, the left and the middle hepatic veins join in a short 1–2 cm common trunk prior to entering the retrohepatic IVC. Similarly, other major accessory hepatic veins of different sizes may also drain into the retrohepatic IVC.[353-355]

Exposure of the retrohepatic IVC and the major hepatic veins is both difficult and fraught with pitfalls. Prior to any direct attempts at exposure, a wide right-sided visceral rotation is undertaken by transecting the avascular line of Toldt of the right colon and performing an extensive Kocher maneuver, thus exposing both infrarenal as well as the suprarenal infrahepatic IVC. Similarly, the falciform ligament is sharply transected toward its origin at the bare area of the liver where meticulous transection of the coronary ligaments will expose 1–2 cm of the retrohepatic IVC.

One of the ways to expose the retrohepatic IVC is by directly approaching it via an extensive hepatotomy through the interlobar plane at Cantlie's line; frequently, this is done as completion of a massive fracture. Alternatively, sharp transection of the right triangular ligament with extensive right to left mobilization of the right lobe of the liver will expose the right hepatic vein as well as the retrohepatic IVC. The left hepatic vein can be exposed by transecting the left triangular ligament and rotating laterally the lateral segment of the left lobe of the liver. Uncommonly, a median sternotomy is necessary to control the intrapericardial portion of the IVC.

Once exposure and proximal and distal control have been obtained, all abdominal vascular injuries should be graded utilizing the AAST-OIS for vascular injuries (Table 28.10).[335] Routine principles of vascular surgery apply to the management of abdominal vascular injuries. Adequate exposure, proximal and distal control, debridement of injured vessel wall, prevention of embolization of clot, debris or plaque, irrigation with heparinized saline, judicious use of Fogarty catheters, meticulous arteriorrhaphy or venorrhaphy with monofilament vascular sutures, avoidance of narrowing of the vessel during repair, insertion of an autogenous or prosthetic graft when applicable, and, rarely, intraoperative angiography when feasible are the mainstays of successful repair. Occasionally, the use of temporary vascular shunts as part of damage control may be required.

The management of vascular injuries in zone I supramesocolic will consist of primary arteriorrhaphy of the suprarenal abdominal aorta when feasible, and in rare occasions, the insertion of a Dacron or PTFE graft. Injuries to the celiac axis usually undergo primary repair if simple, or ligation if destructive. Management of injuries to the first two parts of the SMA should be dealt with by primary repair whenever possible. Intense vasoconstriction makes this difficult. These injuries can also be ligated, as theoretically there are sufficient collaterals to preserve the viability of the small and large bowel; however, profound vasospasm may lead to intense ischemia and bowel necrosis. The first two zones of the SMA can also be repaired either with an autogenous or prosthetic graft. Insertion of a shunt may be utilized as a temporary measure.

The management of injuries in zone I inframesocolic employs the same techniques as in zone I supramesocolic. Parts 3 and 4 of the SMA should also be repaired, although the main jejunal, ileal, and colic branches of Part 4 may be ligated.[12,13] The management of IMA injury is usually by ligation; it rarely requires reconstruction.[335,337-340,345-347] The management of injury to infrahepatic suprarenal IVC, as well as the infrarenal IVC will consist of lateral venorrhaphy whenever feasible. If through-and-through injuries are found in these vessels, both anterior and posterior aspects of the vessel must be repaired. This can prove quite challenging. Complex infrarenal IVC injuries not amenable to repair will require ligation.

Although the infrahepatic suprarenal IVC has no venous tributaries, it is very difficult to mobilize. In general, these repairs are accomplished by extension of the injury in the anterior wall and repair of the posterior wall from within.

With massive destruction of the infrahepatic suprarenal IVC, ligation can be considered; however, survival rates are low. Rarely, prosthetic grafts have been utilized in this position. The management of injuries to the infrarenal IVC generally consists of lateral venorrhaphy after placement of a partially occluding Satinsky or Derra vascular clamp. In the presence of through-and-through injuries, primary repair can be accomplished either by extending the laceration or rotating the vessel. However, this involves ligation of many of its lumbar veins which are quite fragile. We recommend performing the repair from within the vessel. The infrarenal IVC can be ligated in cases of massive destruction. Ligation is generally well tolerated. Injuries to the SMV should be primarily repaired although they can also be ligated; serious sequelae to the circulation of the small and large bowel may result.[349]

Injuries to either right or left zone II can be challenging. Injury to the RA can be either primarily repaired or resected and grafted utilizing either an autogenous or prosthetic graft.[351] Rarely, an aortorenal bypass can be performed utilizing a distal site in the anterior wall of the abdominal aorta. Primary repair of the renal arteries is difficult. Generally, ligation of the RA is performed with subsequent nephrectomy. Injury to the RVs can also be repaired with primary venorrhaphy or ligation. An injury to the right RV that cannot be successfully repaired requires ligation and will demand that a nephrectomy be performed secondary to the lack of venous collaterals. Ligation of the left RV is generally well tolerated provided that it is performed proximally and close to the IVC as the venous collaterals such as the gonadal, adrenal, and renolumbar veins handle the venous outflow.

Injury to zone III can also be challenging, often with associated colonic and genitourinary injuries resulting in considerable contamination. Injury to the common iliac arteries can be primarily repaired via arteriorrhaphy. Occasionally, resection and primary anastomosis can be performed. Prosthetic and rarely autogenous grafts can also be utilized to repair common iliac arteries. Internal iliac artery injuries are generally treated by ligation. Injury to the external iliac artery can be primarily repaired via arteriorrhaphy and occasionally by resection and primary anastomosis. Iliofemoral bypasses can be performed usually with prosthetic and rarely with autogenous grafts, as it is uncommon to find a saphenous vein of adequate size to perform an iliofemoral repair. In the presence of massive contamination, it is strongly recommended that all grafts, whether autogenous or prosthetic, be covered by reperitonealization with autogenous tissues to avoid grafts blowouts. Insertion of shunts may be utilized as a temporary measure in either the iliac artery or vein.

When there has been massive destruction of either the common or internal iliac artery, ligation may be needed. Arterial flow can be restored utilizing a crossover femoro-femoral or axillo-femoral bypass. These bypasses have the disadvantages of involving uninjured vessels and have a high incidence of thrombosis. Injury to the iliac veins, either common, external, or internal, can be dealt with by ligation, as this is frequently well tolerated, although they can also be dealt with by lateral venorrhaphy.

Injury to the PV should be primarily repaired whenever possible. Lateral venorrhaphy, although technically difficult, should be attempted even if the repair narrows the PV. Alternatively, if the patient is acidotic, hypothermic, and coagulopathic, the PV can be ligated. This frequently results in the splanchnic hypervolemia and systemic hypovolemia syndrome.[353-355] Other techniques that have been employed with rare success include resection of the damaged segment and primary end-to-end anastomosis, autogenous and prosthetic grafts, end-to-side portacaval shunts, and transposition of the SV to the SMV. Injury to the hepatic artery can be primarily repaired or ligated.

The management of injury to the retrohepatic IVC consists of primary venorrhaphy, as this represents the only chance for survival in these patients. Ligation is not an option as patients will not survive. In a few reported cases in the literature, the entire liver has been extirpated and a number 36 or 40 Fr chest tube has been placed in the retrohepatic IVC as a shunt in anticipation of a hepatic transplant. Injury to the hepatic veins should be primarily repaired; ligation will most often result in hepatic necrosis as there are no collateral venous channels between the hepatic lobes.

Whenever a trauma surgeon performs an abdominal vascular repair, serious consideration must be given to "second look" operation to assess for bowel viability. This is particularly important after repair of any part of the SMA and should be considered after repair or ligation of the PV or SMV. Contamination from gastrointestinal or genitourinary injuries pose great risks for the development of infection in prosthetic grafts inserted to bypass injured vessels. Whenever possible, all grafts, either autogenous or prosthetic, should be reperitonealized. Similarly, for all vascular repairs adjacent to gastrointestinal suture lines, an effort should be made to interpose viable tissue, generally omentum between the suture lines to prevent vascular-enteric fistula or anastomotic dehiscence.

Abdominal Compartment Syndrome

The World Society of the ACS has developed consensus definitions, diagnostic criteria, and treatment algorithms for intra-abdominal hypertension and ACS.[355-358] Normal IAP pressure represents pressure within the abdominal cavity (normal IAP is 5–7 mm Hg in the ICU population); intra-abdominal hypertension (IAH) is defined as IAP ≥ 12 mm Hg. ACS is sustained IAP > 20 mm Hg associated with new organ dysfunction/failure secondary to decreased end-organ perfusion. Intra-abdominal hypertension affects multiple systems in a vicious cycle, which will culminate in multiple system organ dysfunction if untreated.

ACS has been classified as primary, secondary, or recurrent.[355-357]) *Primary ACS* is associated with injury or pathology within the abdominal cavity: intra-abdominal hemorrhage, intra-abdominal sepsis, ischemic bowel, ileus, or severe pancreatitis. *Secondary ACS* is associated with conditions which do not originate in the abdominal cavity such as massive fluid resuscitation with the burn patient. *Recurrent ACS* occurs after surgical decompression, prior to or after definitive closure.

The common etiologies for ACS include major abdominal trauma, massive fluid resuscitation, burns, ruptured abdominal aortic aneurysm, intraperitoneal or retroperitoneal hemorrhage, pancreatitis, intestinal obstruction or ileus, and abdominal surgery. Risk factors for the development of ACS include abdominal surgery/trauma, fluid resuscitation >5 L per 24 hours, ileus, pulmonary/renal/liver dysfunction, hypothermia, acidosis, and anemia.

Clinical manifestations of ACS are seen in multiple organ systems. Direct end-organ compression combined with decreased cardiac output from ACS has a mortality >40% when diagnosed; 100% if left untreated. Physical examination of the abdomen is not sensitive in the diagnosis of IAH. Neurologic findings in IAH include potential increase in intracranial pressure secondary to decreased internal jugular venous drainage, important with closed head injury patients. Abdominal decompression has been reported as therapeutic treatment for elevated intracranial pressure.[358] Pulmonary effects include high peak airway pressures (>40 cm H_2O) and decreased functional residual capacity secondary to the elevated diaphragm with poor excursion. If untreated, ACS ultimately results in hypoxia, hypercapnia, and respiratory acidosis. Cardiovascular effects may be difficult to delineate as decreased venous return and falsely elevated filling pressures from abdominal hypertension and elevated intrathoracic pressure lead to decreased cardiac output and end-organ perfusion. These effects are exacerbated if the patient is hypovolemic. The kidney and intestine are most sensitive to IAH. IAH leads to splanchnic hypoperfusion, bowel ischemia, and potential bacterial translocation. Oliguria and decreased GFR secondary to renal compression and decreased cardiac output occur with minimal elevation in IAP (as low as 15–20 mm Hg); oliguria is one of the earliest signs of ACS.

Diagnosis. The standard method for diagnosis of IAH is the measurement of bladder pressure via an arterial line transducer. If IAH is suspected, serial bladder pressures are recommended. Bladder pressures >20–25 mm Hg, with the appropriate clinical signs, suggest ACS.[356-358]

Multiple strategies to decrease IAP involve medical and surgical approaches. Abdominal decompression is the only treatment for ACS once end-organ dysfunction is present. The intra-abdominal organs are allowed to eviscerate and a temporary closure device is placed on the abdomen (VAC, Bogota bag). *Reperfusion syndrome* is a postoperative complication with its effects ranging from hemodynamic instability to cardiac arrest. The administration of mannitol and bicarbonate prior to decompression may be of benefit. In extreme situations when patients cannot tolerate transport to the OR, the abdomen may be opened at the bedside in the ICU. Avoid doing this in cases where ACS is secondary to intra-abdominal hemorrhage. Keep in mind that as fluid resuscitation continues, recurrent ACS may occur even with temporary abdominal closure, or after definitive closure. Preemptive "open abdomen" is usually exercised in patients undergoing damage control surgery or in those at high risk for ACS at time of surgical exploration.

Aggressive intravenous resuscitation with isotonic fluids is a major cause of secondary ACS as a result of third-spacing and visceral edema. Restrictive fluid administration should be practiced in patients with IAH or at risk for ACS. Excess fluid removal is the key in the medical management of oliguric/anuric patients who may respond to diuretic therapy or continuous venovenous hemofiltration/ultrafiltration.

Additional medical management of IAH includes sedation, analgesia, pharmacologic paralysis, body positioning, intestinal decompression, and percutaneous decompression of the abdomen. Judicious use of neuromuscular blockade in conjunction with adequate sedation and analgesia may help IAH; however, the benefits must outweigh the risks. Ileus or bowel obstruction is not an uncommon occurrence in ICU patients at risk for ACS. Decompression of intraluminal intestinal contents via nasogastric or rectal tubes can also reduce IAP. Percutaneous drainage of intra-abdominal fluid may reduce IAP. Close monitoring of urine output and serial (q4–6h) bladder pressures along with these medical strategies may help prevent the transition from IAH without end-organ damage to ACS with renal dysfunction and intestinal ischemia.

Damage Control

Damage control is the global approach taken toward the patient in extremis (see Chapter 6). Life-threatening injuries are addressed first as dictated by the patient's physiologic reserve. Any operative procedure adds physiologic stress to an injured patient; the magnitude and duration of the operation dictate degree of additional physiologic insult. Damage control is not specific to abdominal catastrophe; it applies to the critically injured multitrauma patient. Injuries are prioritized and treatment is staged as dictated by physiologic state. Indications for a damage control approach include the multiply injured patient with intra-abdominal injury along with hemodynamic instability, acidosis, hypothermia, or nonsurgical bleeding (coagulopathy). It is critical that major bleeding (surgical bleeding) be controlled at the index operation. Common abdominal injuries where damage control is applied include vascular, major hepatic, or pelvic injury. The major goals of the trauma laparotomy are control of hemorrhage and contamination (intestinal contents, pus) by packing, temporary shunting of vessels, or bowel resection without anastomosis. The abdomen is left open for a second look in 24–48 hours or to prevent ACS in at-risk patients (e.g., >10 units PRBCs or 5 L crystalloid). Additional criteria which suggest the need for damage control include arterial pH ≤ 7.1, temperature $< 35°C$, or coagulopathy.

The laparotomy is then truncated and the patient transferred to the ICU. Aggressive resuscitation in ICU, correction of coagulopathy and acidosis and core rewarming. Most importantly in the ICU, is the prompt management of hypothermia, coagulopathy, and metabolic acidosis. Particularly in polytrauma patients with substantial hemorrhage, it is not uncommon to see continuous oozing from wounds or line sites. Nonsurgical bleeding (coagulopathy) must be addressed aggressively. Ongoing bleeding and failure to correct coagulopathy indicate need for return to the operating; 20% of damage control patients will require early return to the OR. With planned return to the OR, perform reexploration with more detailed look at injuries, definitive or partial repair of injuries (i.e., bowel anastomosis, pack removal, ligation/bypass), depending upon the patient's reserve, may take more than one trip to the OR. The abdomen may be left open or closed, depending upon the patient's status at the completion of definitive repair and degree of bowel edema.

Damage control decreases mortality in these severely injured patients, but adds real morbidity. The complications of damage control surgery include intra-abdominal abscess, anastomotic leak, an open abdomen, and gastrointestinal fistula.

The open abdomen is the by-product of damage control surgery and ACS. It refers to a patient whose abdominal fascia is left temporarily in discontinuity for the purpose of reexploration, prevention of ACS in patients who will require massive resuscitation, or as treatment of ACS. Temporary closure techniques aim to control third-spaced fluid and allow swelling of intestines during resuscitation. These devices usually consist of a nonadhesive barrier that covers the intestines while allowing excess fluid to be suctioned via superficial drains. Currently, the most common device is the VAC, which uses a sponge as means of suction to collect fluid and pull fascia and skin edges together. If tolerated, judicious fluid removal may decrease visceral edema and increase the likelihood of primary closure of the abdomen. If fascial closure is not possible, skin-only closure with future plans to repair ventral hernia is the next best option. Skin grafting and biologic meshes can be used for closure when fascial or skin-only closure is no longer an option. Subsequent fascial closure can be accomplished when the patient is completely recovered, months later.

Retroperitoneal Hematoma

Prior to widespread use of abdominal CT, preoperative diagnosis of retroperitoneal hematoma was an uncommon diagnosis. Its presence is usually associated with multiple injuries and consequently, with an increase in morbidity and mortality. The retroperitoneum is a protected space, located behind the posterior parietal peritoneum and anterior to the spine and associated muscles. This large and potentially expandable space may hold more than 3,000 mL of blood and be responsible for the presence of severe hemodynamic instability.

Mechanism of Injury and Clinical Presentation. Retroperitoneal hematoma is present in 15%-40% of patients admitted with blunt trauma.[360-362] The most common etiology of this injury is motor vehicle crash (32%-73%) followed by pedestrian struck by a car (12%-42%). We reported a mean Trauma Score and injury severity score of 10.6 and 40, respectively, in patients with retroperitoneal hematoma.[360] Furthermore, 20%-40% of patients with traumatic retroperitoneal hematoma arrive to the hospital in hypovolemic shock. In our series, transfusions during the first 24 hours postinjury were 3,532 mL. The association of extra-abdominal injuries is significant, as high as 74%.[360] Penetrating retroperitoneal hematoma is generally associated with multiple injuries and is more likely diagnosed intraoperatively.

Diagnosis. Prior to availability of CT, traumatic retroperitoneal hematomas were diagnosed at the time of laparotomy in 60%-70% of cases.[362-365] The introduction of CT has revolutionized the evaluation of the patient with abdominal trauma, including the patient with retroperitoneal hematoma. With the introduction of the DPL, a negative result was considered reliable to exclude significant intra-abdominal injury. In the presence of pelvic fractures, the DPL should be performed with a supra-umbilical technique to avoid false-positive results.

Retroperitoneal hematoma has been classified by Kudsk and Sheldon[363] (see Fig. 28.17), dividing the abdomen into three zones: zone 1 (central or medial hematoma), zone 2 (perirenal, flank hematoma), and zone 3 (pelvic hematoma). Henao and Aldrete added zone 4 for hematoma occupying two or more zones.[361] The most common location of the retroperitoneal hematoma is localized in zones 2 and 3.

Management of Traumatic Retroperitoneal Hematoma. Preoperative CT of the abdomen in the hemodynamically stable patient allows evaluation of solid and hollow organs and vessels of the retroperitoneal space, facilitating not only the decision-making processes but also the surgical strategy. On the other hand, intraoperative management of the retroperitoneal hematoma continues with few modifications for the last few decades.

Zone 1 (central hematoma) following blunt trauma[5] should be explored to exclude bleeding from a major vessel or branch thereof (aorta or vena cava) and allow inspection of the pancreas and duodenum; visceral injuries are found in two-thirds.[362] The IVC is the most common organ affected with an associated mortality of 43%. Pancreatic injury due to blunt trauma occurs in 1%-27% with a mortality of 17%-27%.[363-367] It is imperative to recognize these injuries at the time of laparotomy or with interpretation of preoperative CT.

The decision to explore zone 2 retroperitoneal hematomas from blunt injury is more complex. The indications for exploration are the presence of pulsatile or expanding hematoma, large extravasation of urine, or clinical or radiographic evidence of renovascular injury. In our series of blunt traumatic retroperitoneal hematomas, 41% of hematomas located in zone 2 were explored and in 49% of the cases, an organ injury was identified.[360] The kidney is the most common organ injured in this location; management of kidney injuries is discussed in Chapter 29.

Zone 3 (pelvic hematoma) blunt injury should not be explored routinely, unless in the presence of exsanguination, generally due to injury of the main iliac artery or vein which needs to be emergently controlled. Many of these hematomas in a hemodynamically stable patient can be controlled by angiographic embolization, or packing with some type of external abdominal compression.

The mortality of patients explored with hematomas in zone 3 ranges from 63% to 83%. Flint et al.[365] reported 66% mortality with hypogastric artery ligation, today rarely performed, and 50% with packing, today successful in penetrating trauma and damage control of this area. In our series, 12% of patients with blunt retroperitoneal hematoma were explored and 38% had iliac vein injury. The majority of zone 3 blunt retroperitoneal hematomas are associated with bony pelvic disruption.[361]

The management of retroperitoneal hemorrhage in zone 3 associated with pelvic fracture has evolved. In the past, the sequence was as follows: Resuscitation, DPL, external fixation, followed by angiographic embolization if more than six units of blood were required to keep the patient hemodynamically stable. Currently, the modern management scheme is resuscitation, temporary pelvic stabilization, with sheets or pelvic corset devices, FAST, less commonly DPL, followed by CT, and finally, angiographic embolization, if evidence of active bleeding (blush) in the CT or continued requirement of blood transfusions. The indications to go to the OR, at times for pelvic packing are presence of another organ injury requiring laparotomy or inability to control the bleeding angiographically.

The management of a retroperitoneal hematoma secondary to penetrating mechanism is more straightforward. Retroperitoneal hematomas secondary to penetrating trauma should all be explored, regardless of the location.

Morbidity and Mortality. The patients who survive more than 24 hours develop complications in 50%, generally associated with MSOF. Respiratory failure occurred in over 40%. Intra-abdominal abscesses occur with the similar frequency of 4.3% to that of blunt abdominal trauma more generally. The mortality from a traumatic retroperitoneal hematoma ranges from 18% to 40%.[360] The management of the patient with traumatic retroperitoneal hematoma should be multidisciplinary, often involving interventional radiology, orthopedic surgery, urology, in addition to the acute care surgeon.

References

1. Peitzman AB, et al. *The Trauma Manual: Trauma and Acute Care Surgery*. 3rd ed. Philadelphia, PA: Wolters Kluwer; 2008.
2. Peitzman AB, Richardson JD. Surgical treatment of injuries to the solid abdominal organs: a 50-year perspective from the journal of trauma. *J Trauma*. 2010;69:1011-1021.
3. Fakhry SM, et al. Current diagnostic approaches lack sensitivity in the diagnosis of perforated blunt small bowel injury: analysis from 275,557 trauma admissions from the EAST Multi-Institutional HVI Trial. *J Trauma*. 2003;54:295-306.
4. Fakhry SM, Brownstein M, Watts DD, et al. Relatively short diagnostic delays (<8 hours) produce morbidity and mortality in blunt small bowel injury. *J Trauma*. 2000;48:409-415.
5. Nance ML, Peden GW, Shapiro MB, et al. Solid viscus injury predicts major hollow viscus injury in blunt abdominal trauma. *J Trauma*. 1997;43:618-623.
6. Como JJ, Bokhari F, Chiu WC, et al. Practice management guidelines for selective management of penetrating abdominal trauma. *J Trauma*. 2010;68:721-733.
7. da Silva M, Navsaria PH, Edu S, et al. Evisceration following abdominal stab wounds: analysis of 66 cases. *World J Surg*. 2009;33:215-219.
8. Biffl WL, Kaups KL, Cothren CC, et al. Management of patients with anterior stab wounds: a Western Trauma Association Multicenter trial. *J Trauma*. 2009;66:1294-1301.
9. Plackett TP, Fleurat J, Putty B, et al. Selective nonoperative management of anterior abdominal stab wounds: 1992–2008. *J Trauma*. 2011;70:408-414.
10. Thacker LK, Parks J, Thal ER. Diagnostic peritoneal lavage: is 100,000 RBCs a valid figure for penetrating abdominal trauma? *J Trauma*. 2007;62:853-857.
11. Galbraith TA, Oreskovich MR, Heimbach DM, et al. The role of peritoneal lavage in the management of stab wounds to the abdomen. *Am J Surg*. 1980;140:60-64.
12. National Trauma Data Base (NTDB) American College of Surgeons Years 2000–2004.
13. Rodriguez-Morales G, Rodriguez A, Shatney CH. Acute rupture of the diaphragm in blunt trauma: analysis of 60 patients. *J Trauma*. 1986;26:438-444.
14. Larici AR, Gotway MB, Litt HI, et al. Helical CT with sagittal and coronal reconstructions accuracy for detection of diaphragmatic rupture. *Am J Radiol*. 2002;179:451-457.
15. Nchimi A, Szapiro D, Gharye B, et al. Helical CT of blunt diaphragmatic rupture. *Am J Radiol*. 2005;184:24-30.
16. Shanmuganathan K, Mirvis SE, White CS. MR imaging evaluation of hemidiaphragm in acute blunt trauma: experience in 16 patients. *AJR Am J Roentgenol*. 1996;167:397-402.
17. Ivatury RR, Simon RJ, Stahl WM. A critical evaluation of laparoscopy in penetrating abdominal trauma. *J Trauma*. 1993;34:822.
18. Moore EE, Malangoni MA, Cogbill TH, et al. Organ injury scaling IV: thoracic vascular, lung, cardiac and diaphragm. *J Trauma*. 1994;36:229-300.
19. Moore EE, Jurkovich GJ, Knudson MM, et al. Organ injury scaling VI: extrahepatic biliary, esophagus, stomach, vulva, vagina, uterus, fallopian tube, ovary. *J Trauma*. 1995;39:1069-1070.
20. Moore EE, Cogbill TH, Malangoni MA, et al. Organ injury scaling II: pancreas, duodenum, small bowel, colon, and rectum. *J Trauma*. 1990;30:1427-1429.
21. Anderson PA, Rivara FP, Maier RV, et al. The epidemiology of seatbelt associated injuries. *J Trauma*. 1991;31:60-67.
22. Jacobs DG, Angus L, Rodriguez A. Peritoneal lavage white counts: a reassessment. *J Trauma*. 1990;30:607-612.
23. Malhotra AK, Fabian TC, Katsis SB, et al. Blunt bowel and mesenteric injuries, the role of screening computerized tomography. *J Trauma*. 200;48:991-1000.
24. Brundage SI, Jurikovich CD, Hoyt DB, et al. Stapled versus sutured gastrointestinal anastomosis in trauma patients. *J Trauma*. 1999;47:500-508.
25. Brundage SI, Jurkovich GJ, Hoyt DB, et al. Stapled versus sutured anastomosis in the trauma patient: a multiple center trial. *J Trauma*. 2001;51:1054-1061.
26. Fabian TC. Infections in penetrating abdominal trauma: risk factors and preventive antibiotics. *Am Surg*. 2002;68:29-35.
27. Ogilvie WH. Abdominal wounds in the western desert. *Surg Gynecol Obstet*. 1944;78:225-238.
28. Woodhall JP, Ochsner A. The management of perforating injuries of the colon and rectum in civilian practice. *Surgery*. 1951;29:305-320.
29. Stone H, Fabian TC. Management of perforating colon trauma: randomization between primary closure and exteriorization. *Ann Surg*. 1979;1990:430-436.
30. Demetriades DD, Rabinowitz B, Sofianos C, et al. The management of colon injuries by primary repair or colostomy. *Br J Surg*. 1985;72:881-883.
31. Chaping CW, Fry DJ, Dietzen CD, et al. Management of penetrating colon injuries. A prospective randomized trial. *Ann Surg*. 1999;213:492-497.

32. Nelson R, Singer M. Primary repair for penetrating colon injuries. *Cochrane Database Syst Rev*. 2003;3:CD002247.
33. Velmahos GC, Demetriades D, Toutouzas KG. Selective non-operative management in 1,856 patients with abdominal gunshot wounds should laparotomy still be the standard of care? *Ann Surg*. 2001;234:395-403.
34. Velmahos GC, Constantinou C, Tillou A, et al. Computed tomographic scanning for patients with gunshot wounds of the abdomen selected for non-operative management. *J Trauma*. 2005;59:1155-1161.
35. Velmahos GC, Toutouzas KG, Sarskiyan G, et al. Severe trauma is not an excuse for prolonged antibiotic prophylaxis. *Arch Surg*. 2002;137:537-542.
36. Cayten CG, Fabian TC, Garcia VF, et al. *Patient Management Guidelines for Penetrating Colon Injuries. Trauma Practice Guidelines*. Eastern Association for the Surgery of Trauma; 1998. http://www.east.org.
37. Demetriades D, Murray JA, Chan LC, et al. Penetrating colon injuries requiring resection: diversion or primary anastomosis? An AAST Prospective Multicenter Study. *J Trauma*. 2001;50:765-775.
38. Eshrashi N, Mullins RJ, Mayberry JC. Surveyed opinion of American trauma surgeons in management of colon injuries. *J Trauma*. 1998;44:93-97.
39. Burch JM, Franciose RJ, Moore EE. Single-layer continuous versus two-layer interrupted intestinal anastomosis: a prospective randomized trial. *Ann Surg*. 2000;231:832-837.
40. Zmora D, Manhajna A, Bar-Zakai B, et al. Colon and rectal surgery without mechanical bowel preparation: a randomized prospective trial. *Ann Surg*. 2003;237:363-367.
41. Gonzalez RP, Faliminsky ME, Holevar MR. The role of presacral drainage in the management of penetrating rectal injuries. *J Trauma*. 1998;45:656-661.
42. Velmahos GG, Degiannis E, Wells M, et al. Early closure of colostomy in trauma patients: a prospective randomized trial. *Ann Surg*. 1995;118:815-820.
43. Hirsch JE, Arhens EH Jr, Blankehorn DH. Measurement of the human intestinal length *in vivo* and some causes of variation. *Gastroenterology*. 1956;31:274-284.
44. Cocke WM Jr, Meyer KK. Retroperitoneal duodenal rupture: proposed mechanism. Review of the literature and a report of a case. *Am J Surg*. 1964;108:834-839.
45. Haley JC, Peden JK. The suspensory muscle of the duodenum. *Am J Surg*. 1943;59:546-550.
46. Michaels NA. Variational anatomy of the hepatic, cystic and retroduodenal arteries. *Arch Surg*. 1953;66:20-32.
47. Michaels NA, ed. Blood supply to the pancreas and duodenum. In: *Blood Supply and Anatomy of the Upper Abdominal Organs with a Descriptive Atlas*. Philadelphia, PA: JB Lippincott, 1955:236-247. 1084 *Curr Probl Surg*. 1993.
48. Frey C. Trauma to the pancreas and duodenum. In: Blaisdell F, Trunkey DD, eds. *Trauma Management*. Vol. 1. *Abdominal Trauma*. New York: Thieme-Stratton, Inc; 1982:87-120.
49. Michaels NA. The hepatic, cystic and retroduodenal arteries and their relations to the biliary ducts. *Ann Surg*. 1951;133:503-524.
50. Thompson IM. On the arteries and ducts in the hepatic pedicle: a study in statistical human anatomy. *Univ CA Publ*. 1953;1:55-70.
51. Gray SW, Skandalakis JE. *Embryology for Surgeons*. Philadelphia, PA: WB Saunders Co; 1972.
52. Smanio T. Varying relations of the common bile duct with the posterior face of the pancreatic head in Negroes and white persons. *J Int Coll Surg*. 1954;22:150-173.
53. Skandalakis JE, Gray SW. Anatomical complications of pancreatic surgery. *Cont Surg*. 1979;1521-1550.
54. Davenport HW. *A Digest of Digestion: Functions of the Small Intestine*. Chicago, IL: Year Book Medical Publishers; 1978:75-83.
55. Thompson JC. The stomach and duodenum. In: Sabiston DC Jr, ed. *Textbook of Surgery: the Biological Basis of Modern Surgical Practice*. 13th ed. Philadelphia, PA: WB Saunders; 1986:810-853.
56. McClelland RN, Jones RC, Perry MO, et al. Trauma abdominal trauma. In: Schwartz SI, Shires CT, Spencer FC, et al., eds. *Principles of Surgery*. 3rd ed. New York: McGraw-Hill, 1979:119-203.
57. Jordan PH Jr. Stomach and duodenum. In: Hardy JD, ed. *Hardy's Textbook of Surgery*. 1st ed. Philadelphia, PA: JB Lippincott; 1983:497-521.
58. Rodkey GV, Welch CE. Injuries to the stomach and duodenum. In: Schwartz SI, Ellis H, eds. *Maingot's Abdominal Operations*. 8th ed. Norwalk, CT: Appleton-Century-Crofts; 1985:605-699.
59. Asensio JA, Buckman RF. Injuries of the duodenum: surgery of the alimentary tract. In: Shackelford RT, Zuidema GD, eds. *Duodenal Injuries*. Vol. 2. Philadelphia, PA: WI3 Saunders Co; 1981:219-243.
60. Zeppa R. Stomach and duodenum. In: Nora PF, ed. *Operative Surgery: Principles and Techniques*. 2nd ed. Philadelphia, PA: Lea & Febiger; 1980:371-380.
61. Jordan GL Jr. Injury to the pancreas and duodenum. In: Moore KL, Mattox EE, Feliciano DV, eds. *Trauma*. 2nd ed. East Norwalk, CT: Appleton and Lange; 1991:499-520.
62. Flint LM, Malangoni MA. Abdominal injuries. In: Richardson JD, Polk HC Jr, Flint LM, eds. *Trauma: Clinical Care and Pathophysiology*. 1st ed. Chicago, IL: Year Book Medical Publishers; 1987:353-396.
63. Anderson CB, Ballinger WF. Abdominal injuries. In: Zuidema GD, Rutherford RB, Ballinger WF, eds. *The Management of Trauma*. 4th ed. Philadelphia, PA: WB Saundem Co; 1985:449-504.
64. Weiner SL, Barrett J. Abdominal injuries. In: Weiner SL, Barrett J, eds. *Trauma Management for Civilian and Military Physicians*. 1st ed. Philadelphia, PA: WB Saunders Co; 1986:212-250.
65. Frey CF. Pancreas and duodenum. In: Trunkey, DD, Lewis FR, eds. *Current Therapy in Trauma*. 2nd ed. Toronto, Canada: BC Decker, Inc.; 1986:281-292.
66. Weigelt JA, Borman KR. Management of duodenal injuries. In: Maull KI, Cleveland HC, Strauch GO, et al., eds. *Advances in Trauma*. Vol. 3. Chicago, IL: Yearbook Medical Publishers; 1988:115-126.
67. Morton JR, Jordan GL. Traumatic duodenal injuries: review of 131 cases. *J Trauma*. 1968;8:127-139.
68. Kelly G, Norton L, Moore G, et al. The continuing challenge of duodenal injuries. *J Trauma*. 1978;18:160-165.
69. Levinson MA, Peterson SR, Sheldon GF, et al. Duodenal trauma: experience of a trauma center. *J Trauma*. 1982;24:475-480.
70. Smith AD, Woolverton WC, Weichert RF, et al. Operative management of pancreatic and duodenal injuries. *J Trauma*. 1971;14:570-579.
71. McInnis WD, Aust JB, Cruz AB, et al. Traumatic injuries of the duodenum: a comparison of 1′ closure and the jejunal patch. *J Trauma*. 1975;15: 847-853.
72. Corley RD, Norcross WJ, Shoemaker WC. Traumatic injuries to the duodenum: a report of 98 patients. *Ann Surg*. 1974;181:92-98.
73. Lucas CE, Ledgerwood AM. Factors influencing outcome after blunt duodenal injury. *J Trauma*. 1975;15:839-846.
74. Matolo NM, Colten SE, Fontanetta AP, et al. Traumatic duodenal injuries: an analysis of 32 cases. *Am Surg*. 1975;6:331-336.
75. Stone HH, Fabian TC. Management of duodenal wounds, *J Trauma*. 1973;19:334-339.
76. Flint LM Jr, McCoy M, Richardson JD, et al. Duodenal injury: analysis of common misconceptions in diagnosis and treatment. *Ann Surg*. 1979;191:697-702.
77. Snyder WH III, Weigelt JA, Watkins WL, et al. The surgical management of duodenal trauma. *Arch Surg*. 1980;115:422-429.
78. Adkins RB Jr, Keyser JE III. Recent experiences with duodenal trauma. *Am Surg*. 1984;5:121-131.
79. Fabian TC, Mangiante EC, Millis M. Duodenal rupture due to blunt trauma: a problem in diagnosis. *South Med J*. 1984;77:1078-1082.
80. Ivatury RR, Nallathambi M, Gaudino J, et al. Penetrating duodenal injuries: analysis of 100 consecutive cases. *Am Surg*. 1985;2:153-158.
81. Bostman L, Bostman O, Leppaniemi A, et al. Primary duodenorrhaphy and nasogastric decompression in the treatment of duodenal injury. *Acta Chir Stand*. 1989;155:333-335.
82. Cogbill TH, Moore EE, Feliciano DV, et al. Conservative management of duodenal trauma: a multicenter perspective. *J Trauma*. 1990;30:1469-1475.
83. Cuddington G, Rusnak CH, Cameron RDA, et al. Management of duodenal injuries. *Can J Surg*. 1990;33:41-44.
84. Donohue JH, Federle MP, Griffiths BG, et al. Computed tomography in the diagnosis of blunt intestinal and mesenteric injuries. *J Trauma*. 1987;27:11-17.
85. Donohue JH, Crass RA, Trunkey DD. The management of duodenal and other small intestinal trauma. *World J Surg*. 1985;9:904-913.
86. Federle MP, Goldberg HI, Kaiser JA, et al. Evaluation of abdominal trauma by computed tomography. *Radiology*. 1981;138:637-644.
87. Glazer GM, Buy JN, Moss AA, et al. CT detection of duodenal perforation. *Am J Radiol*. 1981;137:333-336.
88. Jeffrey RB Jr, Federle MP, Stein SM, et al. Intramural hematoma of the cecum following blunt trauma. *J Comput Assist Tomogr*. 1982;6:404-405.
89. Karnaze GC, Sheedy PF II, Stephens DH, et al. Computed tomography in duodenal rupture due to blunt abdominal trauma. *J Comput Assist Tomogr*. 1981;5:267-269.
90. Kaufman RA, Towbin R, Babcock DS, et al. Upper abdominal trauma in children: imaging evaluation. *Am J Radiol*. 1984;142:449-460.
91. Root HD, Hauser CW, McKiney CR, et al. Diagnostic peritoneal lavage. *Surgery*. 1965;57:633-637.
92. Jones JC, Thal ER, Johnson NA, et al. Evaluation of antibiotic therapy following penetrating abdominal trauma. *Ann Surg*. 1985;201:576-585.
93. Nichols RL, Smith JW, Klein DB, et al. Risk of infection after penetrating abdominal trauma. *N Engl J Med*. 1984;311:1065-1070.
94. Cattell RB, Braasch JW. A technique for exposure of the duodenum. *Surg Gynecol Obstet*. 1954;98:376-377.
95. Ananeh-Sefah J, Norton LW, Eisenman B. Operative choice and technique following pancreatic injury. *Arch Surg*. 1975;110:161-166.
96. Graham JM, Mattox KL, Vaughan GD III, et al. Combined pancreatoduodenal injuries. *J Trauma*. 1979;19:340-346.
97. Kraus M, Condon RE. Alternate techniques of duodenotomy. *Surg Gynecol Obstet*. 1974;139:417-419.
98. Stone HH, Garoni WJ. Experiences in the management of duodenal wounds. *South Med J*. 1966;59:864-867.
99. Hasson JE, Stern D, Mosds GS. Penetrating duodenal trauma. *J Trauma*. 1984;24:471-474.
100. Ivatury RR, Gaudino J, Aster E, et al. Treatment of penetrating duodenal injuries: primary repair vs repair with decompressive enterostomy/serosal patch. *J Trauma*. 1985;25:337-341.
101. Kashuk JL, Moore EE, Cogbill TH. Management of the intermediate severity duodenal injury. *Surgery*. 1982;92:758-764.
102. Walley DB, Goco I. Duodenal patch grafting. *Am J Surg*. 1980;140:706-708.
103. Kobbold EE, Thal AP. A simple method for the management of experimental wounds of the duodenum. *Surg Gynecol Obstet*. 1963;116:340-344.

104. Wynn M, Hill DM, Miller DR, et al. Management of pancreatic and duodenal trauma. *Am J Surg*. 1985;150:327-332.
105. Jones SA, Gazzaniga AB, Keller TB. The serosal patch: a surgical parachute. *Am J Surg*. 1973;126:188-196.
106. Jones SA, Joergenson EJ. Closure of duodenal wall defects. *Surgery*. 1963;53:438-442.
107. DeShazo CV, Snyder WH III, Daughtery CG, et al. Mucosal pedicle graft of jejunum for large gastrointestinal defects. *Am J Surg*. 1972;124:671-672.
108. McIlrath DC, Larson RH. Surgical management of large perforations of the duodenum. *Surg Clin North Am*. 1971;51:857-861.
109. Feliciano DV, Martin DT, Cruse PA, et al. Management of combined pancreatoduodenal injuries. *Ann Surg*. 1987;205:673-680.
110. Buck JR, Sorensen VJ, Fath JJ, et al. Severe pancreaticoduodenal injuries: the effectiveness of pyloric exclusion with vagotomy. *Am Surg*. 1992;58:557-561.
111. Moore EE, Cogbill TH, Malongoni MA, et al. Organ injury scaling. II. Pancreas, duodenum, small bowel, colon and rectum. *J Trauma*. 1990;30:1427-1429.
112. Martin TD, Feliciano DV, Mattox KL, et.al. Severe duodenal injuries treatment with pyloric exclusion and gastrojejunostomy. *Arch Surg*. 1983;116:631-635
113. Monsour MA, Moore JB, Moore FA. Conservative management of combined pancreatoduodenal injuries. *Am J Surg*. 1989;158:531-535.
114. Flynn WJ, Cryer HG, Richardson JP. Reappraisal of pancreatic and duodenal injury management based on injury severity. *Arch Surg*. 1990;125:1539-1541.
115. Berne CJ, Donovan AJ, White EJ, et al. Duodenal "diverticulization" for duodenal and pancreatic injury. *Am J Surg*. 1974;127:503-507.
116. Thal AP, Wilson RF. A pattern of severe blunt trauma to the region of the pancreas. *Surg Gynecol Obstet*. 1964;119:773-778.
117. Foley WJ, Gaines RD, Fry WJ. Pancreaticoduodenectomy for severe trauma to the head of the pancreas and associated structures. *Ann Surg*. 1969;170:759-765.
118. Walter RL, Gaspard DJ, Germann TD. Traumatic pancreatitis. *Am J Surg*. 1966;111:364-368.
119. Fabian TC, Kudsk KA, Crose MA, et.al. Superiority of closed suction drainage for pancreatic trauma *Ann Surg*. 1990;211:724-730
120. Salyer K, McClelland RN. Pancreatidoduodenectomy for trauma. *Arch Surg*. 1967;95:636-639.
121. Sawyers JL, Carlisle BB, Sawyers JE. Management of pancreatic injuries. *South Med J*. 1967;60:382-386.
122. Wilson RF, Tagett JP, Pucelik JP, et al. Pancreatic Trauma, *J Trauma*. 1967; 7:643-651.
123. Brawley RK, Cameron JL, Zuidema G. Severe upper abdominal injuries treated by pancreaticoduodenectomy. *Surg Gynecol Obstet*. 1968; 126:516-522.
124. Werschky LR, Jordan GL. Surgical management of traumatic injuries to the pancreas. *Am J Surg*. 1968;116:768-772.
125. Pantazelos HH, Kerhulas AA, Byrne JJ. Total pancreaticoduodenectomy for trauma. *Ann Surg*. 1969;170:1016-1020.
126. Gibbs BF, Crow JL, Rupnik EJ. Pancreaticoduodenectomy for blunt pancreaticoduodenal injury. *J Trauma*. 1971;10:702-705.
127. Bach RD, Frey CF. Diagnosis and treatment of pancreatic trauma. *Am J Surg*. 1971;121:20-29.
128. Nance FC, DeLoach DH. Pancreaticoduodenectomy following abdominal trauma. *J Trauma*. 1971;11:577-782.
129. Jones RC, Shires GT. Pancreatic trauma. *Arch Surg*. 1971;102:424-430.
130. Salam A, Warren WD, Kalser M, et al. Pancreaticoduodenectomy for trauma: clinical and metabolic studies. *Ann Surg*. 1972;175:663-672.
131. Owens MP, Wolfman EF. Pancreatic trauma: management and presentation of a new technique. *Surgery*. 1973;73:881-886.
132. Steele M, Sheldon GF, Blaisdell FW. Pancreatic injuries. *Arch Surg*. 1973;106:544-549.
133. Strum JT, Quattlebaum FW, Mowlem A, et al. Patterns of injury requiring pancreaticoduodenectomy. *Surg Gynecol Obstet*. 1973;132:629-632.
134. Yellin AE, Rosoff L. Pancreatoduodenectomy for combined pancreatoduodenal injuries. *Arch Surg*. 1975;110:1117-1183.
135. Chambers RT, Norton L, Hinchey EJ. Massive right upper quadrant intraabdominal injury requiring pancreaticoduodenectomy and partial hepatectomy. *J Trauma*. 1975;15:714-719.
136. Heitsch RC, Knutson CO, Fulton RL, et al. Delineation of critical factors in the treatment of pancreatic trauma surgery. *Surgery*. 1976;80: 523-529.
137. Lowe RJ, Saletta JD, Moss GD. Pancreaticoduodenectomy for penetrating pancreatic trauma. *J Trauma*. 1977;17(9):732-741.
138. Karl HW, Chandler JG. Mortality and morbidity of pancreatic injury. *Am J Surg*. 1977;134:549-554.
139. Hagan WV, Urdaneta LF, Stephenson SE. Pancreatic injury. *South Med J*. 1978;171:892-894.
140. Majeski JA, Tyler G. Pancreatic trauma. *Am Surg*. 1980;46:593-596.
141. Cogbill TH, Moore EE, Kashuk JL. Changing trends in the management of pancreatic trauma. *Arch Surg*. 1982;117:722-728.
142. Henarejos A, Cohen DM, Moosa AR. Management of pancreatic trauma. *Ann R Coll Surg Engl*. 1983;65:297-300.
143. Oreskovich MR, Carrico CJ. Pancreaticoduodenectomy for trauma: a viable option. *Am J Surg*. 1984;147:618-623.
144. Moore JB, Moore EE. Changing trends in the management of combined pancreatoduodenal injuries. *World J Surg*. 1984;8:77-97.
145. Jones RC. Management of pancreatic trauma. *Am J Surg*. 1985;150: 698-704.
146. Roman E, Sifva YJ, Lucas CE. Management of blunt duodenal injury. *Surg Gynecol Obstet*. 1971;132:7-14.
147. Sims EH, Mandal AU, Schlatter T, et al. Factors affecting outcomes in pancreatic trauma. *J Trauma*. 1984;24:125-128.
148. Smego DR, Richardson JD, Flint LM. Determinants of outcome in pancreatic trauma. *J Trauma*. 1985;25:771-775.
149. Wynn M, Hill DM, Miller DR, et al. Management of pancreatic and duodenal trauma. *Am J Surg*. 1985;150:327-332.
150. Walker ML. Management of pancreatic trauma: concepts and controversy. *J Nat Med Assoc*. 1986;78:1177-1183.
151. Melissas J, Baart GD, Mannell A. Pancreaticoduodenectomy for pancreatic trauma. *S Afr Med J*. 1987;71:323-324.
152. McKonek TK, Bursch LR, Scholten DJ. Pancreaticoduodenectomy for trauma: a life-saving procedure. *Am Surg*. 1988;54:361-364.
153. Eastlick L, Fogler RJ, Shaftan GW. Pancreaticoduodenectomy for trauma: delayed reconstruction [case report]. *J Trauma*. 1990;30:503-505.
154. Gentilello LM, Cortes V, Buechter K, et al. Whipple procedure for trauma: is duct ligation a safe alternative to pancreatico-jejunostomy? *J Trauma*. 1991;31:661-668.
155. Heimonsohn DA, Canal DF, McCarthy MC, et al. The role of pancreaticoduodenectomy in the management of trauma to the pancreas and duodenum. *Am Surg*. 1990;56:511-514.
156. Roman E, Silva YJ, Lucas C. Management of blunt duodenal injury. *Surg Gynecol Obstet*. 1971;132:7-14.
157. Kerry RL, Glas WW. Traumatic injuries of the pancreas and duodenum. *Arch Surg*. 1962;85:813-816.
158. Talbot WA, Shuck JM. Retroperitoneal duodenal injury due to blunt abdominal trauma. *Am J Surg*. 1975;130:659-666.
159. Welch CE, Rodkey GV. A method of management of the duodenal stump after gastrectomy. *Surg Gynecol Obstet*. 1954;98:376-379.
160. Janson KL, Stockinger F. Duodenal hematoma: critical analysis of recent treatment techniques. *Am J Surg*. 1975;129:304-308.
161. Devroede GJ, Tirol ET, Lo Russo VA, et al. Intramural hematoma of the duodenum and jejunum. *Am J Surg*. 1966;112:947-954.
162. Ferguson IA, Goade WJ. Intramural hematoma of the duodenum. *N Engl J Med*. 1959;260:1176-1177.
163. Freeark RJ, Corley RD, Norcross WJ, et al. Intramural hematoma of the duodenum. *Arch Surg*. 1966;92:463-475.
164. Ghosh S, Walker BQ, McKenna CM. Traumatic intramural hematoma of the duodenum. *Arch Surg*. 1968;96:959-962.
165. Jones WR, Hardin WJ, Davis JT, et al. Intramural hematoma of the duodenum: a review of the literature and case report. *Ann Surg*. 1971;173:534-544.
166. Felson B, Levin EJ. Intramural hematoma of the duodenum: a diagnostic roentgen sign. *Radiology*. 1954;63:823-831.
167. Moore SW, Erlandson ME. Intramural hematoma of the duodenum. *Ann Surg*. 1963;157:798-809.
168. Rowe EG, Baxter MR, Rowe CW. Intramural hematoma of the duodenum: report of a case with an unusual complication. *Arch Surg*. 1959;78:560-564.
169. Izant RJ, Drucker WR. Duodenal obstruction due to intramural hematoma in children. *J Trauma*. 1964;4:797-813.
170. Fullen WD, Selle JG, Whitely DH. Intramural duodenal hematoma. *Ann Surg*. 1974;179:549-556.
171. Woolley MM, Mahour GH, Sloan T. Duodenal hematoma in infancy and childhood: changing etiology and changing treatment. *Am J Surg*. 1978;136:8-14.
172. Touloukian RJ. Protocol for the nonoperative treatment of obstructing intramural duodenal hematoma during childhood. *Am J Surg*. 1983;145:330-334.
173. Jewett TC, Caldarola V, Karp MP, et al. Intra-mural hematoma of the duodenum. *Arch Surg*. 1988;123:54-58.
174. Anacker H. Radiological anatomy of the pancreas. In: Anacker H, ed. *Efficiency and Limits of Radiologic Examination of the Pancreas*. Thieme ed. Acton, MA: Publishing Sciences Group; 1975.
175. Classen M, Koch H, Ruskin H, et al. Pancreatitis after endoscopic retrograde pancreatography (ERCP). *Gut*. 1973;14:431.
176. Sivak MV, Sullivan BH. Endoscopic retrograde pancreatography: analysis of the normal pancreatogram. *Am J Dig Dis*. 1976;21:263.
177. Gross RE. Surgery of infancy and childhood. Philadelphia, PA: Saunders; 1972.
178. Wittingen J, Frey CE. Islet concentration in the head, body, tail and uncinate process of the pancreas. *Ann Surg*. 1974;179:412-414.
179. Culotta RJ, Howard JM, Jordan GL. Traumatic injuries of the pancreas. *Surgery*. 1956;40:320-327.
180. Medical Services Surgery of the War. *History of the Great War Based on Official Documents*. Vol I. London, UK: His Majesty's Stationery Office; 1922.
181. Jolly DW. *Field Surgery in Total War*. New York: Paul B. Hoeber; 1941.
182. Poole HL. Wounds of the pancreas. In: Coates JB Jr, DeBakey ME, eds. *Medical Department, United States Army, Surgery in World War H: General Surgery*. Vol. 2. Washington, DC: Office of Surgeon General; 1955:285.

183. Sako Y, Artz CP, Howard JM, et al. A survey of evacuation, resuscitation, and mortality in a forward surgical hospital. *Surgery*. 1955;37:602-611.
184. Asensio JA. Operative pancreatograms at 2 AM? In: Critical decision points in trauma care. Proceedings of post-graduate course No. 5. *Am Coil Surg*. 1992:55-57.
185. Nilson E, Norrby S, Skullman S, et al. Pancreatic trauma in a defined population. *Acta Chir Scan*. 1986;152:647-651.
186. Anderson CB, Connors JP, Mejia DC, et al. Drainage methods in the treatment of pancreatic injuries. *Surg Gynecol Obstet*. 1974;138:587-590.
187. Jones RC, Shires T. Pancreatic trauma. *Arch Surg*. 1971;102:424-430.
188. Cogbill TH, Moore EE, Kashuk JL. Changing trends in the management of pancreatic trauma. *Arch Surg*. 1982;117:722-758.
189. Stone HH, Fabian TC, Satiani B, et al. Experiences in the management of pancreatic trauma. *J Trauma*. 1981;21:257-262.
190. Balasegaram M. Surgical management of pancreatic trauma. *Curr Probl Surg*. 1979;16:1-59.
191. Moretz JA III, Campbell DP, Parker DE, et al. Significance of serum amylase level in evaluating pancreatic trauma. *Am J Surg*. 1975;130:739 741.
192. Bouwman DL, Weaver DW, Walt AJ. Serum amylase and isoenzimes: a clarification of their implications in trauma. *J Trauma*. 1984;24:573-577.
193. Greenlee T, Murphy K, Ram MD. Amylase isoenzime in the evaluation of trauma patients. *Am Surg*. 1984;50:637-640.
194. White PH, Benfield JR. Amylase in the management of pancreatic trauma. *Arch Surg*. 1972;105:158-162.
195. Block RS, Weaver DW, Bowman DL. Acute alcohol intoxication: significance of the amylase level. *Ann Emerg Med*. 1983;12:294-301.
196. Smego DR, Richardson JD, Flint LM. Determinants of outcome in pancreatic trauma. *J Trauma*. 1985;25:771-776.
197. Lucas CE. Diagnosis and treatment of pancreatic and duodenal injury. *Surg Clin N Am*. 1977;57:49-65.
198. Doubilet H, Mulholland JH. Surgical management of injury to the pancreas. *Ann Surg*. 1959;150:854-860.
199. Fabian TC, Kudsk KA, Croce MA, et al. Superiority of closed suction drainage for pancreatic trauma: a randomized prospective study. *Ann Surg*. 1990;211:724-730.
200. Graham JM, Mattox KL, Jordan GL. Traumatic injuries of the pancreas. *Am J Surg*. 1978;136:744-748.
201. Heitsch RC, Knutson CO, Fulton RL, et al. Delineation of critical factors in the treatment of pancreatic trauma. *Surgery*. 1976;80:523-529.
202. Leppaniemi A, Haapiainen R, Kiviluqto T, et al. Pancreatic trauma: acute and late manifestations. *Br J Surg*. 1988;75:165-167.
203. Wilson RH, Moorehead RJ. Current management of trauma to the pancreas. *Br J Surg*. 1991;78:1196-1202.
204. Asensio JA, Petrone P, Roldan G, et al. Pancreaticoduodenectomy: a rare procedure for the management of complex pancreaticoduodenal injuries. *J Am Coll Surg*. 2003;197:937-942.
205. Wisner D, Wold R, Frey C. Diagnosis and treatment of pancreatic injuries. *Arch Surg*. 1990;125:1109-1113.
206. Strax R, Sandier CM, Toombs BD. CT demonstration of pancreatic transections: a case report and comparison with other diagnostic modalities in the evaluation of blunt pancreatic trauma. *J Comput Tomogr*. 1980;4:319-322.
207. Baker LP, Wagner EJ, Brotman S, et al. Transection of the pancreas. *J Comput Assist Tomogr*. 1982;6:411-412.
208. Jeffrey RB, Federle MP, Crass RA. Computed tomography of pancreatic trauma. *Radiology*. 1983;147:491-494.
209. Cook DE, Waish JW, Vick CW, et al. Upper abdominal trauma: pitfalls in CT diagnosis. *Radiology*. 1986;159:65-69.
210. Peitzman AB, Makaroun MS, Slasky BS, et al. Prospective study of computed tomography in initial management of blunt abdominal trauma. *J Trauma*. 1986;26:585-592.
211. Lane M, Mindelzum R, Jeffrey B. Diagnosis of pancreatic injury after blunt abdominal trauma. *Semin Ultrasound CT MRI*. 1996;17:177-182.
212. Belohlavek D, Merkle P, Probst M. Identification of traumatic rupture of the pancreatic duct by endoscopic retrograde pancreatography. *Gastrointest Endosc*. 1978;24:255-266.
213. Taxier M, Sivak MV, Cooperman AM, et al. Endoscopic retrograde pancreatography in the evaluation of trauma to the pancreas. *Surg Gynecol Obstet*. 1980;150:65-68.
214. Phelan HA, Velmahos GC, Jurkovich GJ, et al. An evaluation of multidetector computer tomography in detecting pancreatic injury: results of a multicenter AAST study. *J Trauma*. 2009;66:641-646.
215. Hayward SR, Lucas C, Sugawa C, et al. Emergent endoscopic retrograde cholangiopancreatography: a highly specific test for acute pancreatic trauma. *Arch Surg*. 1989;124:745-746.
216. Whittwell AE, Gomez GA, Byers P, et al. Blunt pancreatic trauma: prospective evaluation of early endoscopic retrograde pancreatography. *South Med J*. 1989;85:586-591.
217. Kopelman D, Suissa A, Klein Y, et al. Pancreatic duct injury: intraoperative endoscopic transpancreatic drainage of parapancreatic abscess. *J Trauma*. 1998;44:555-557.
218. Huckfeldt R, Age C, Nichols K, et al. Nonoperative treatment of traumatic pancreatic duct disruption using an endoscopically placed stent. *J Trauma*. 1996;41:143.
219. Duchesne JC, Schmieg R, Islam S, et al. Selective nonoperative management of pancreatic injury: are we there yet? *J Trauma*. 2008;65:49-53.
220. Jones RC. Evaluation of antibiotic therapy following penetrating abdominal trauma. *Ann Surg*. 1985;201:576.
221. Nichols RL, Smith JW, Klein DB, et al. Risk of infection after penetrating abdominal trauma. *N Engl J Med*. 1984;311:1065.
222. Asensio J, Demetriades D, Berne J, et al. A unified approach to the surgical exposure of pancreatic and duodenal injuries. *Am J Surg*. 1997;174: 54-60.
223. Aird I, Helman E. Bilateral anterior transabdominal adrenalectomy. *BMJ* 1055;2:708-709.
224. Asensio J, Feliciano DV, Britt LD, et al. Management of duodenal injuries. *Curr Probl Surg*. 1993;11:1021-1100.
225. Cogbill TH, Moore EE, Morris JA, et al. Distal pancreatectomy for trauma: a multicenter experience. *J Trauma*. 1991;31:1600-1606.
226. Jones RC. Management of pancreatic trauma. *Ann Surg*. 1978;187:555-564.
227. Culotta RJ, Howard JM, Jordan GL. Traumatic injuries of the pancreas. *Surgery*. 1956;40:320-327.
228. Hannon DW, Spafka J. Resection for traumatic pancreatitis. *Ann Surg*. 1957;146:136-138.
229. Letton H, Wilson JP. Traumatic severance of pancreas treated by Roux-en-Y anastomosis. *Surg Gynecol Obstet*. 1959;109:473.
230. Patton J Jr, Lyden SP, Croce MA, et al. Pancreatic trauma: a simplified approach. *J Trauma*. 1997;43:234-241.
231. Fogelman MJ, Robinson LJ. Wounds of the pancreas, *Am J Surg*. 1961; 101:698-706.
232. Kerry RL, Glass WW. Traumatic injuries of the pancreas and duodenum. *Arch Surg*. 1962;85:133-136.
233. Stone HH, Stowers KB, Shippey SH. Injuries to the pancreas. *Arch Surg*. 1962;85:187-192.
234. Thal AP, Wilson RF. A pattern of severe blunt trauma to the region of the pancreas. *Surg Gynecol Obstet*. 1964;119:773-778.
235. Jones RC, Shires GT. The management of pancreatic injuries. *Arch Surg*. 1965;90:502-508.
236. Mule JE, Adaniel M. The management of trauma to the pancreas. *Surgery*. 1969;65:423.
237. Foley W J, Gaines RD, Fry WJ. Pancreatoduodenectomy for severe trauma to the head of the pancreas and the associated structures: report of three cases. *Ann Surg*. 1969;170:759-765.
238. Pachter HL, Pennington R, Chassin J, et al. Simplified distal pancreatectomy with auto suture stapler: preliminary clinical observations. *Surgery*. 1979;85:166-170.
239. Robey E, Mullen JT, Schwab CW. Blunt transection of the pancreas treated by distal pancreatectomy, splenic salvage and hyperalimentation. *Ann Surg*. 1982;196:695-699.
240. Pachter HL, Hofstetter SR, Liang HG, et al. Traumatic injuries to the pancreas: the role of distal pancreatectomy with splenic preservation. *J Trauma*. 1989;29:1352-1355.
241. Gentilello LM, Cortez V, Buechter K, et al. Whipple procedure for trauma: is duct ligation a safe alternative to pancreaticojejunostomy? *J Trauma*. 1991;31:661-668.
242. Yellin AE, Rossof L. Pancreatoduodenectomy for combined pancreatoduodenal injuries. *Arch Surg*. 1975;110:1117-1183.
243. Oreskovich MR, Carrico CJ. Pancreaticoduodenectomy for trauma: a viable option. *Am J Surg*. 1984;147:618-623.
244. Berne C J, Donovan AJ, Hagen WE. Combined duodenal pancreatic trauma. *Arch Surg*. 1968;96:712-722.
245. Vaughn GD III, Frazier OH, Graham DJ et al. The use of pyloric exclusion in the management of severe duodenal injuries. *Am J Surg*. 1977;134:785-790.
246. Graham JM, Mattox KL, Vaughan GD III, et al. Combined pancreatoduodenal injuries. *J Trauma*. 1979;19:340-346.
247. Jones RC. Management of pancreatic trauma. *Am J Surg*. 1985;150:698-704.
248. Werschky LR, Jordan GL. Surgical management of traumatic injuries to the pancreas. *Am J Surg*. 1968;116:768-772.
249. Balasegaram M. Surgical management of pancreatic trauma. *Am J Surg*. 1976;131:536-540.
250. Buchler M, Friess H, Klempa I, et al. Role of octreotide in the prevention of postoperative complications following pancreatic resection. *Am J Surg*. 1992;163:126-131.
251. Richardson JD, Franklin GA, Lukan JK, et al. Evolution in the management of hepatic trauma: a 25-year perspective. *Ann Surg*. 2000;232:324-330.
252. Richardson JD. Changes in the management of injuries to the liver and spleen. *J Am Coll Surg*. 2005;200:648-669.
253. Buckman RF Jr, Miraliakbari R, Badellino MM. Juxtahepatic venous injuries: a critical review of reported management strategies. *J Trauma*. 2000;48:978-984.
254. Skandalakis JE, Skandalakis LJ, Skandalakis PN, et al. Hepatic surgical anatomy. *Surg Clin N Am*. 2004;84:413-435.
255. Burlew CC, Moore EE. Injuries to the liver, biliary tract, spleen and diaphragm, In: *ACS Surgery: Principles and Practice*. 2010 Decker Intellectual Properties. http://74.205.62.209/bcdecker/pdf/acs/part7_ch07.pdf
256. Badger SA, Barclay R, Diamond T, et al. Management of liver trauma. *World J Surg*. 2009;33:2522-2537.
257. Kozar RA, Moore FA, Moore EE, et al. Western Trauma Association critical decisions in trauma: nonoperative management of blunt hepatic injury. *J Trauma*. 2009;67:1144-1149.

258. Fang JF, Wong YC, Lin BC, et al. The CT risk factors for the need of operative treatment in initially hemodynamically stable patients after blunt hepatic trauma. *J Trauma*. 2006;61(3):547-553; discussion 553-554.
259. Trunkey DD. Hepatic trauma: contemporary management. *Surg Clin N Am*. 2004;84:437-450.
260. Moore EE, Shackford SR, Pachter HL. Organ injury scaling: spleen, liver and kidney. *J Trauma*. 1995;38:323-324.
261. Misselbeck TS, Teicher EJ, Cipolle MD, et al. Hepatic angioembolization in trauma patients: indications and complications. *J Trauma*. 2009;67(4):769-773.
262. Carillo EH, Spain DA, Wohltmann CD, et al. Interventional techniques are useful adjuncts in nonoperative management of hepatic injuries. *J Trauma*. 1999;46:619-622.
263. Sclafani SJ, Shaftan GW, McAuley J, et al. Interventional radiology in the management of hepatic trauma. *J Trauma*. 1984;24:256.
264. Wahl WL, Ahrns KS, Brandt MM, et al. The need for early angiographic embolisation in blunt liver injuries. *J Trauma*. 2002;52:1097-1101.
265. Polanco P, Leon S, Pineda J, et al. Hepatic resection in the management of complex injury to the liver. *J Trauma*. 2008;65(6):1264-1269; discussion 1269-1270.
266. Kozar RA, Feliciano DV, Moore EE, et al. Western Trauma Association/critical decisions in trauma: operative management of adult blunt hepatic trauma. *J Trauma*. 2011;71:1-5.
267. Duane TM, Como JJ, Bochicchio GV, et al. Reevaluating the management and outcomes of severe blunt liver injury. *J Trauma*. 2004;57:494-500.
268. Asensio JA, Demetriades D, Chahwan S, et al. Approach to the management of complex hepatic injuries. *J Trauma*. 2000;48:66-69.
269. Berney T, Morel P, Huber O, et al. Combined midline-transverse surgical approach for severe blunt injuries to the liver. *J Trauma*. 2000;48:349-353.
270. Caruso DM, Battistella FD, Owings JT, et al. Perihepatic packing of major liver injuries. *Arch Surg*. 1999;134:958-963.
271. Beal SL. Fatal hepatic hemorrhage: an unresolved problem in the management of complex liver injuries. *J Trauma*. 1990;30(2):163-169.
272. Strong RW, Lynch SV, Wall DR, et al. Anatomic resection for severe liver trauma. *Surgery*. 1998;123:251-257.
273. Liau KH, Blumgart LH, DeMatteo RP. Segment-oriented approach to liver resection. *Surg Clin N Am*. 2004;84:543-561.
274. Abdalla EK, Noun R, Belghiti J. Hepatic vascular occlusion: which technique? *Surg Clin N Am*. 2004;84:563-585.
275. Tsugawa K, Koyanagi N, Hashizume M, et al. Anatomic resection for severe blunt liver injury in 100 patients: significant differences between young and elderly. *W J Surg*. 2002;26:544-549.
276. Pachter HL, Spencer FC, Hofstetter SR, et al. Significant trends in the treatment of hepatic injuries. Experience with 411 injuries. *Ann Surg*. 1992;215:492-500.
277. Menegaux F, Langlois P, Chigot J-P. Severe blunt trauma of the liver: study of mortality factors. *J Trauma*. 1993;35:865-869.
278. Poggetti RS, Moore EE, Moore FA, et al. Balloon tamponade for bilobar transfixing hepatic gunshot wounds. *J Trauma*. 1992;33:694-697.
279. Chen R-J, Fang J-F, Lin B-C, et al. Surgical management of juxtahepatic venous injuries in blunt hepatic trauma. *J Trauma*. 1995;38:886-890.
280. Chen R-J, Fang J-F, Lin B-C, et al. Factors determining operative mortality of Grade V blunt hepatic trauma. *J Trauma*. 2000;49:886-891.
281. Carillo EH, Spain DA, Miller FB, et al. Intrahepatic vascular clamping in complex hepatic vein injuries. *J Trauma*. 1997;43:131-133.
282. Sherman R. Perspectives in management of trauma to the spleen: 1979 Presidential Address, American Association for the Surgery of Trauma. *J Trauma*. 1980;20:1-13.
283. Peitzman AB, Ford HR, Harbrecht BG, et al. Injury to the spleen. *Curr Probl Surg*. 2001;38:923-1008.
284. Powell M, Courcoulas A, Gardner M, et al. Management of blunt splenic trauma: significant differences between adults and children. *Surgery*. 1997;122:654-660.
285. Clancy TV, Ramshaw DG, Maxwell JG, et al. Management outcomes in splenic injury: a statewide trauma center review. *Ann Surg*. 1997;226:17-24.
286. Peitzman AB, Heil B, Rivera L, et al. Blunt splenic injury in adults: multi-institutional study of the Eastern Association for the Surgery of Trauma. *J Trauma*. 2000;49:177-189.
287. Hartnett KL, Winchell RJ, Clark DE. Management of adult splenic injury: a 20-year perspective. *Am Surg*. 2003;69:608-611.
288. Harbrecht BG, Zenati MS, Ochoa JB, et al. Evaluation of a 15-year experience with splenic injuries in a state trauma system. *Surgery*. 2007;141:229-238.
289. Velmahos GC, Chan LS, Kamel E, et al. Nonoperative management of splenic injuries: have we gone too far? *Arch Surg*. 2000;135:674-681.
290. Watson GA, Rosengart MR, Zenati MS, et al. Nonoperative management of severe splenic injury: are we getting better? *J Trauma*. 2006;61:1113-1119.
291. Todd SR, Arthur M, Newgard C, et al. Hospital factors associated with splenectomy for splenic injury: a national perspective. *J Trauma*. 2004;57:1065-1071.
292. King H, Shumacker HB Jr. Splenic studies: susceptibility to infection after splenectomy performed in infancy. *Ann Surg*. 1952;136:239-242.
293. Falimirski M, Syed A, Prybilla D. Immunocompetence of the severely injured spleen verified by differential interference contrast microscopy: the red blood cell pit test. *J Trauma*. 2007;63:1087-1092.
294. Chalmoff C, Douer D, Pick IA, et al. Serum immunoglobulin changes after accidental splenectomy in adults. *Am J Surg*. 1978;136:332-333.
295. Shatz DV, Romero-Steiner S, Elie CM, et al. Antibody responses in postsplenectomy trauma patients receiving the 23-valent pneumococcal polysaccharide vaccine at 14 versus 28 days postoperatively. *J Trauma*. 2002;53:1037-1042.
296. Potoka DA, Schall LC, Ford HR. Risk factors for splenectomy in children with blunt splenic trauma. *J Pediatr Surg*. 2002;37:294-299.
297. Mooney DP, Rothstein DH, Forbes PW. Variation in the management of pediatric splenic injuries in the United States. *J Trauma*. 2006;61:330-333.
298. Sims CA, Wiebe DJ, Nance ML. Blunt solid organ injury: do adult and pediatric surgeons treat children differently? *J Trauma*. 2008;65:698-703.
299. Pate JW, Peters TG, Andrews CR. Postsplenectomy complications. *Am Surg*. 1985;51:437-441.
300. Bisharat N, Omari H, Lavi I, et al. Risk of infection and death among post-splenectomy patients. *J Infect*. 2001;43:182-186.
301. Ezstrud P, Kristensen B, Hensen JB, et al. Risk and patterns of bacteremia after splenectomy: a population-based study. *Scand J Infect Dis*. 2000;32:521-525.
302. Holdsworth RJ, Irving AD, Cuschieri A. Postsplenectomy sepsis and its mortality rate: actual versus perceived risks. *Br J Surg*. 1991;78:1031-1038.
303. Chadburn A. The spleen: anatomy and anatomical function. *Semin Hematol*. 2000;37(S1):13-21.
304. Schurr MJ, Fabian TC, Gavant M, et al. Management of blunt splenic trauma: computed tomographic contrast blush predicts failure of nonoperative management. *J Trauma*. 1995;39:507-513.
305. Davis KA, Fabian TC, Croce MA, et al. Improved success in nonoperative management of blunt splenic injuries: embolization of splenic artery pseudoaneurysms. *J Trauma*. 1998;44:1008-1015.
306. Weinberg JA, Magnotti LJ, Croce MA, et al. The utility of serial computed tomography imaging of blunt splenic injury: still worth a second look? *J Trauma*. 2007;62:1143-1148.
307. Sclafani SJA, Weisberg A, Scalea TM, et al. Blunt splenic injuries: nonsurgical treatment with CT, arteriography, and transcatheter arterial embolization of the splenic artery. *Radiology*. 1991;181:189-196.
308. Sclafani SJA, Shaftan GW, Scalea TM, et al. Nonoperative salvage of computed tomography-diagnosed splenic injuries: utilization of angiography for triage and embolization for hemostasis. *J Trauma*. 1995;39:818-827.
309. Shanmuganathan K, Mirvis SE, Boyd-Kranis R, et al. Nonsurgical management of blunt splenic injury: use of CT criteria to select patients for splenic arteriography and potential endovascular therapy. *Radiology*. 2000;217:75-82.
310. Haan J, Scott J, Boyd-Kranis RL, et al. Admission angiography for blunt splenic injury: advantages and pitfalls. *J Trauma*. 2001;51:1161-1165.
311. Wahl WL, Ahrns KS, Chen S, et al. Blunt splenic injury: operation versus angiographic embolization. *Surgery*. 2004;136:891-899.
312. Haan JM, Biffl W, Knudson MM, et al. Splenic embolization revisited: a multicenter review. *J Trauma*. 2004;56:542-547.
313. Haan JM, Bochicchio GV, Kramer N, et al. Nonoperative management of blunt splenic injury: a 5-year experience. *J Trauma*. 2005;58:492-498.
314. Wei B, Hemmila MR, Arbabi S, et al. Angioembolization reduces operative intervention for blunt splenic injury. *J Trauma*. 2008;64:1472-1477.
315. Sabe AA, Claridge JA, Rosenblum DI, et al. The effects of splenic artery embolization on nonoperative management of blunt splenic injury: a 16-year experience. *J Trauma*. 2009;67:565-572.
316. Nakae H, Shimazu T, Miyauchi H, et al. Does splenic preservation treatment (embolization, splenorrhaphy, and partial splenectomy) improve immunologic function and long-term prognosis after splenic injury? *J Trauma*. 2009;67:557-564.
317. Ekeh PA, McCarthy MC, Woods RJ, et al. Complications arising from splenic embolization after blunt splenic trauma. *Am J Surg*. 2005;189:335-339.
318. Cooney R, Ku J, Cherry R, et al. Limitations of splenic angioembolization in treating blunt splenic injury. *J Trauma*. 2005;59:926-932.
319. Smith HE, Biffl WL, Majercik SD, et al. Splenic artery embolization: have we gone too far? *J Trauma*. 2006;61:541-546.
320. Harbrecht BG, Ko SH, Watson GA, et al. Angiography for blunt splenic trauma does not improve the success rate of nonoperative management. *J Trauma*. 2007;63:44-49.
321. Velmahos GC, Zacharias N, Emhoff TA, et al. Management of the most severely injured spleen: a multicenter study of the Research Consortium of New England Centers for Trauma. *Arch Surg*. 2010;145:456-460.
322. Harbrecht BG, Zenati MS, Alarcon LH, et al. Is outcome after blunt splenic injury in adults better in high-volume trauma centers? *Am Surg*. 2005;71:942-949.
323. Lynch JM, Meza MP, Newman B, et al. Computed tomography grade of splenic injury is predictive of the time required for radiographic healing. *J Pediatr Surg*. 1997;32:1093-1095.
324. Savage SA, Zarzaur BL, Magnotti LJ, et al. The evolution of blunt splenic injury: resolution and progression. *J Trauma*. 2008;64:1085-1092.
325. Bee TK, Croce MA, Miller PR, et al. Failures of splenic nonoperative management: is the glass half empty or half full? *J Trauma*. 2001;50:230-236.
326. McIntyre LK, Schiff M, Jurkovich GJ. Failure of nonoperative management of splenic injuries: causes and consequences. *Arch Surg*. 2005;140:563-569.

327. Peitzman AB, Harbrecht BG, Rivera L, et al. Failure of observation of blunt splenic injury in adults: variability in practice and adverse consequences. *J Am Coll Surg*. 2005;201:179-187.
328. Resende V, Petroianu A. Functions of the splenic remnant after subtotal splenectomy for treatment of severe splenic injuries. *Am J Surg*. 2003;185:311-315.
329. Smith JS Jr, Wengrovitz MA, DeLong BS. Prospective validation of criteria, including age, for safe, non-surgical management of the ruptured spleen. *J Trauma*. 1992;33:363-369.
330. Godley CD, Warren RL, Sheridan RL, et al. Nonoperative management of blunt splenic injury in adults: age over 55 years as a powerful indicator for failure. *J Am Coll Surg*. 1996;183:133-139.
331. Cocanour CS, Moore FA, Ware DN, et al. Age should not be a consideration for nonoperative management of blunt splenic injury. *J Trauma*. 2000;48:606-612.
332. Harbrecht BG, Peitzman AB, Rivera L, et al. Contribution of age and gender to outcome of blunt splenic injury in adults: multicenter study of the Eastern Association for the Surgery of Trauma. *J Trauma*. 2001;51:887-895.
333. Shatz DV, Schinsky MF, Pais LB, et al. Immune responses of splenectomized trauma patients to the 23-valent pneumococcal polysaccharide vaccine at 1 versus 7 versus 14 days after splenectomy. *J Trauma*. 1998;44:760-766.
334. Asensio JA, Chahwan S, Hanpeter D, et al. Operative management and outcome of 302 abdominal vascular injuries. *Am J Surg*. 2000;180(6): 528-533; discussion 533-534.
335. Moore EE, Cogbill TH, Jurkovich GJ, et al. Organ injury scales III: chest wall, abdominal vascular, ureter, bladder and urethra. *J Trauma*. 1992;33:337-339.
336. Tyburski JG, Wilson RF, Dente C, et al. Factors affecting mortality rates in patients with abdominal vascular injuries. *J Trauma*. 2001;50(6):1020-1026.
337. Davis TP, Feliciano DV, Rozycki GS, et al. Results with abdominal vascular trauma in the modern era. *Am Surg*. 2001;67:565-571.
338. Asensio JA, McDuffie L, Petrone P, et al. Reliable variables in the exsanguinated patient which indicate damage control and predict outcome. *Am J Surg*. 2001;182(6):743-751.
339. Asensio JA, Soto SN, Forno W, et al. Abdominal vascular injuries: the trauma surgeon's challenge [Review]. *Surg Today*. 2001;31(11):949-957.
340. Paul JS, Webb TP, Aprahamian C, et al. Intraabdominal vascular injury: are we getting any better? *J Trauma*. 2010;69(6):1393-1397.
341. Cornwell EE 3rd, Velmahos GC, Berne TV, et al. Lethal abdominal gunshot wounds at a level I trauma center: analysis of TRISS (Revised Trauma Score and Injury Severity Score) fallouts. *J Am Coll Surg*. 1998;187(2):123-129.
342. Asensio JA, Forno W, Gambaro E, et al. Abdominal vascular injuries: the trauma surgeon's challenge. *Ann Chir Gynaecol*. 2000;89(1):71-78.
343. Velmahos GC, Demetriades D, Chahwan S, et al. Angiographic embolization for arrest of bleeding after penetrating trauma to the abdomen. *Am J Surg*. 1999;178(5):367-373.
344. Asensio JA, Forno W, Roldan G, et al. Abdominal vascular injuries: injuries to the aorta. *Surg Clin North Am*. 2001;81(6):1395-1416.
345. Asensio JA, Berne JD, Chahwan S, et al. Traumatic injury of the superior mesenteric artery. *Am J Surg*. 1999;178(3):235-239.
346. Asensio JA, Britt LD, Borzotta A, et al. Multiinstitutional experience with the management of superior mesentery artery injuries. *J Am Coll Surg*. 2001;193(4):354-365; discussion 365-366. Erratum in: *J Am Coll Surg* 2001;193(6):718.
347. Asensio JA, Petrone P, Kimbrell B, et al. Lessons learned in the management of thirteen celiac axis injuries [Review]. *South Med J*. 2005;98(4):462-466.
348. Asensio JA, Petrone P, Garcia-Nuñez L, et al. Superior mesenteric venous injuries: to ligate or to repair remains the question. *J Trauma*. 2007;62(3):668-675; discussion 675.
349. Asensio JA, Forno W, Roldán G, et al. Visceral vascular injuries [Review]. *Surg Clin North Am*. 2002;82(1):1-20, xix.
350. Tillou A, Romero J, Asensio JA, et al. Renal vascular injuries [Review]. *Surg Clin North Am*. 2001;81(6):1417-1430.
351. Asensio JA, Petrone P, Roldán G, et al. Analysis of 185 iliac vessel injuries: risk factors and prediction of outcome. *Arch Surg*. 2003;138(11):1187-1193; discussion 1193-1194.
352. Asensio JA, Demetriades D, Chahwan S, et al. Approach to the management of complex hepatic injuries. *J Trauma*. 2000;48(1):66-69.
353. Asensio JA, Roldán G, Petrone P, et al. Operative management and outcomes in 103 AAST-OIS grades IV and V complex hepatic injuries: trauma surgeons still need to operate, but angioembolization helps. *J Trauma*. 2003;54(4):647-653; discussion 653-654.
354. Asensio JA, Roldán G, Petrone P, et al. Operative management and outcomes in 103 AAST-OIS grades IV and V complex hepatic injuries: trauma surgeons still need to operate, but angioembolization helps. *J Trauma*. 2003;54(4):647-653; discussion 653-654.
355. Malbrain ML, Cheatham M, Kirkpatrick A, et al. Results from the international conference of experts on intra-abdominal hypertension and abdominal compartment syndrome. *Int Care Med*. 2006;32:1722-1732.
356. Cheatham ML, et al. Results from the International Conference of experts on intra-abdominal hypertension and abdominal compartment syndrome. II. Recommendations. *Intensive Care Med*. 2007;33:951-962.
357. Malbrain MLNG. Abdominal pressure in the critically ill: measurement and clinical relevance. *Int Care Med* 1999;25:1453-1458.
358. Deeren D, Dits H, Malbrain ML. Correlation between intraabdominal and intracranial pressure. *Int Care Med*. 2005;31:1577-1581.
359. Nick WV, Zollinger RW, Pace WG. Retroperitoneal hemorrhage after blunt abdominal trauma. *J Trauma*. 1967;7(5):652-659.
360. Goins WA, Rodriguez A, Lewis J, et al. Retroperitoneal hematoma after blunt trauma. *Surg Gynecol Obstet*. 1992;174(4):281-290.
361. Henao F, Aldrete JS. Retroperitoneal hematomas of traumatic origin. *Surg Gynecol Obstet*. 1985;161(2):106-116.
362. Evers BM, Cryer HM, Miller FB. Pelvic fracture hemorrhage: priorities in management. *Arch Surg*. 1989;124(4):422-424.
363. Kudsk KA, Sheldon GF. Retroperitoneal hematoma. In: Blaisdel FW, Trunkey DD, eds. *Abdominal Trauma*. New York, NY: Thieme-Stratton; 1982:398-413.
364. Estes WL, Bowman TL. Non-penetrating abdominal trauma: with special references to abdomen and pancreas. *Am J Surg*. 1952;83:432-452.
365. Flint LM, Broman A, Richardson JD, et al. Definite control for severe pelvic fracture. *Ann Surg*. 1979:189(6):709-715.
366. Trunkey DD, Chapman MW, Lim RC. Management of pelvic fractures in blunt trauma injury. *J Trauma*. 1974;16(11):912-923.

CHAPTER 29 ■ GENITOURINARY TRAUMA

BRADLEY A. ERICKSON AND JACK W. MCANINCH

RENAL TRAUMA

Epidemiology

Trauma patients suffer renal injury at rates of 1.4%-3.25% with proportionally higher rates seen in younger patients and in men (3:1 male to female).[1–3] Most renal trauma in the United States and Europe is blunt (95%-97%),[2,4] but there are major worldwide differences in the mechanism of renal injury (i.e., Turkey 31% blunt).[5,6] The most common blunt mechanism is motor vehicle accident and the most common penetrating injuries are from stab and gunshot wounds, with penetrating traumas having a proportionally higher rate of severe injury.[2] With the advent of sophisticated renal trauma imaging and grading systems, the majority of contemporary renal traumas can be managed nonoperatively.[7]

Pathophysiology

Blunt Renal Trauma. The kidneys are relatively protected organs, surrounded by the abdominal viscera anteriorly, the diaphragm and liver superiorly, and the back muscles and spine anteriormedially. This degree of protection means that only major blunt forces to the body lead to renal trauma, explaining the high rate of associated injuries to surrounding viscera (20%-94%).[8,9]

Motor vehicle accidents and falls are the most common mechanism for blunt renal trauma, with injuries coming both from direct impact of the abdominal wall and ribs with the kidney and from secondary impacts during the acute deceleration. The renal pedicle is especially prone to deceleration injuries. Because the renal vein and artery are the kidney's most secure attachments, they absorb the majority of the force during deceleration, leading to both tears and thrombosis of the renal vasculature. Parenchymal injuries of the kidney can result from both direct and secondary impacts with the surrounding musculature, the 11th and 12th ribs and the spinous processes[8,10] (Fig. 29.1).

Penetrating Renal Trauma. Penetrating trauma tends to be more severe and more unpredictable than blunt trauma. Gunshot injuries can damage the kidney from both direct impact of the bullet (permanent cavity) and from the bullets blast effect (temporary cavity), with high-velocity bullets leading to relatively more damage.[6] With stab wounds, the path of the injury can sometimes provide insight into the severity of injury. Wounds posterior to the anterior axillary line will more often lead to parenchymal injury only, most of which can be managed nonoperatively. Conversely, anterior renal injuries are more likely to injure the hilar strictures, which tend to be more life threatening in nature and require operative management, though use of these anatomical landmarks should never supplant appropriate imaging when possible.[11]

Initial Evaluation

Physical Exam. Historical and clinical findings suggestive of blunt renal trauma include hematuria, flank pain, flank ecchymoses, fractured ribs, and abdominal distention, with hematuria being the most common finding (80%-94%)[12] (Fig. 29.2).

Laboratory. An evaluation of the urine should be done in all trauma patients, including both gross evaluation and either dipstick or microscopic analysis. Hematuria should alert one to genitourinary injury, though the degree of hematuria does not always correlate well with the severity of renal injury, especially with penetrating and hilar injuries.[13] Serum creatinine at the time of trauma is rarely helpful as it generally reflects serum creatinine before injury. However, elevated creatinine may indicate preexisting renal pathology which has been cited as a risk factor for renal injury in the event of trauma.[14]

Imaging. The gold-standard imaging modality for genitourinary trauma in the hemodynamically stable patient is an IV contrast CT scan with both arterial and excretory phases (10 minutes after initial injection) (Fig. 29.3).[15] The excretory phase can be eliminated if no renal pathology is seen on the arterial phase, but is helpful in diagnosing the collecting system and ureteral injuries. Understanding which patients should undergo imaging is critical in the proper management of renal trauma and in general, all trauma patients with gross hematuria should be imaged with a CT scan. In blunt trauma patients with microscopic hematuria (>3RBCs/hpf) only, imaging can be reserved for adults who are unstable (systolic BP < 90) and in children with >50 RBCs/hpf, as major genitourinary injury has been found in only 0.2% and 2% of these patients, respectively.[16]

There are other less ideal imaging modalities including ultrasound, which in skilled hands can diagnose perinephric fluid collections but generally not the severity of renal injury.[17] Renal angiography is unnecessarily invasive to diagnose renal trauma in the era of CT scan, but can be used in conjunction with angioembolization when used to treat hemorrhage.[18] IVP can be especially useful in the setting of unstable patients, where renal injury is suspected, but imaging is not obtained prior to laparotomy. A single, on-table abdominal plain-film 10 minutes after a rapid bolus of contrast (2 mL/kg) can rule out most major renal injuries if found to be normal.[19]

Injury Classification. The American Association for the Surgery of Trauma (AAST) grading system for renal trauma, which has been recently modified (Table 29.1; Fig. 29.4), has been validated as a predictor of both injury severity and negative patient outcomes in large retrospective studies.[4,20] It relies on a properly performed CT scan for accurate grading and staging. Most grade I-III injuries can be managed conservatively. With the new grading modifications, many grade IV injuries can also be initially managed nonoperatively, whereas, nearly all grade V injuries will require intervention.[4,20,21]

Management

Conservative Renal Management. Directed conservative management is the mainstay of most contemporary renal trauma management algorithms (Algorithms. 29.1 and 29.2). While historically penetrating trauma to the kidney from

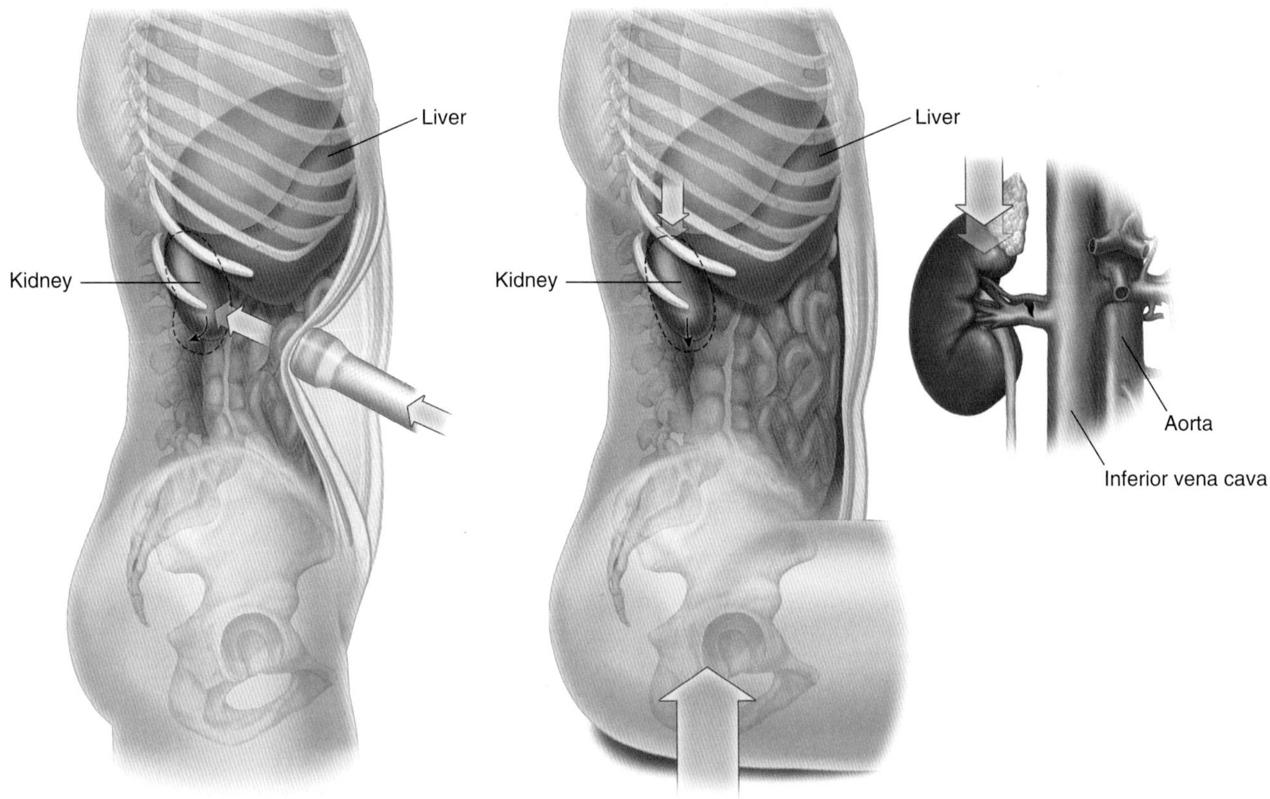

FIGURE 29.1. Mechanisms for blunt injury of the renal parenchyma.

gunshot and stab wounds resulted in renal exploration, it is no longer an absolute indicator for surgery with the advent of modern imaging techniques allowing for more accurate staging.[2] The protected retroperitoneal location of the kidney and its enveloping by Gerota's fascia will often be sufficient to tamponade renal bleeding.[8] Many conservative protocols include serial hematocrit concentration and bed rest for 24–48 hours, though these have never been rigorously validated.[16] Repeat imaging is also recommended for conservatively managed grade III-V injuries and for those patients with worsening clinical findings and/or Hct concentration as late bleeds can occur in up to 25% of patients.[22]

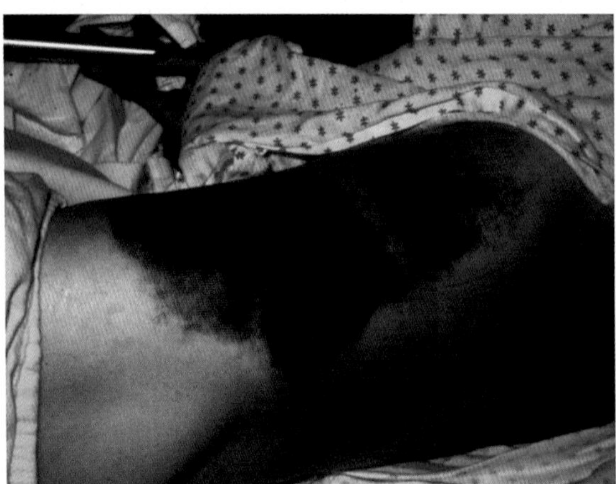

FIGURE 29.2. Typical physical exam findings in a patient that has suffered blunt renal trauma. (From Dr. Jack McAninch, with permission).

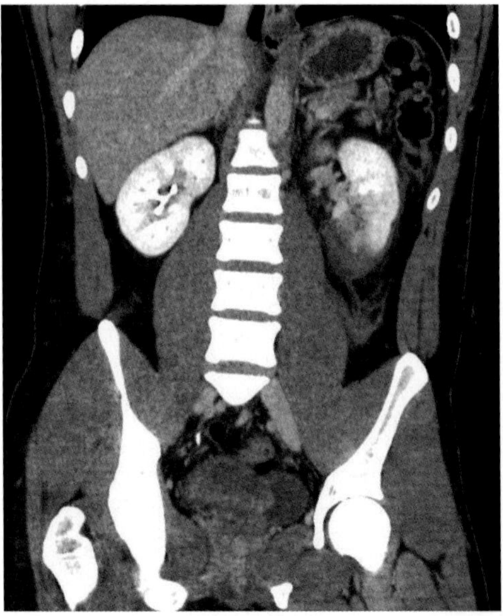

FIGURE 29.3. Grade IV renal trauma. (From Dr. Jack McAninch, with permission).

TABLE 29.1

AAST GRADING SYSTEM

GRADE	LOCATION	INJURY DEFINITION
I	Parenchyma Collecting system	Subcapsular hematoma and/or contusion No injury
II	Parenchyma Collecting system	Laceration <1 cm in depth and into cortex, small hematoma contained within Gerota's fascia No injury
III	Parenchyma Collecting system	Laceration >1 cm in depth and into medulla, hematoma contained within Gerota's fascia No injury
IV	Parenchyma Collecting system	Laceration through the parenchyma into the urinary collecting system Vascular segmental vein or artery injury Laceration, one or more into the collecting system with urinary extravasation Renal pelvis laceration and/or complete ureteral pelvic disruption
V	Vascular	Main renal artery or vein laceration or avulsion main renal artery or vein thrombosis

From Buckley JC, McAninch JW. Revision of current american association for the surgery of trauma renal injury grading system. *J Trauma* 2011;70(1):35–37.

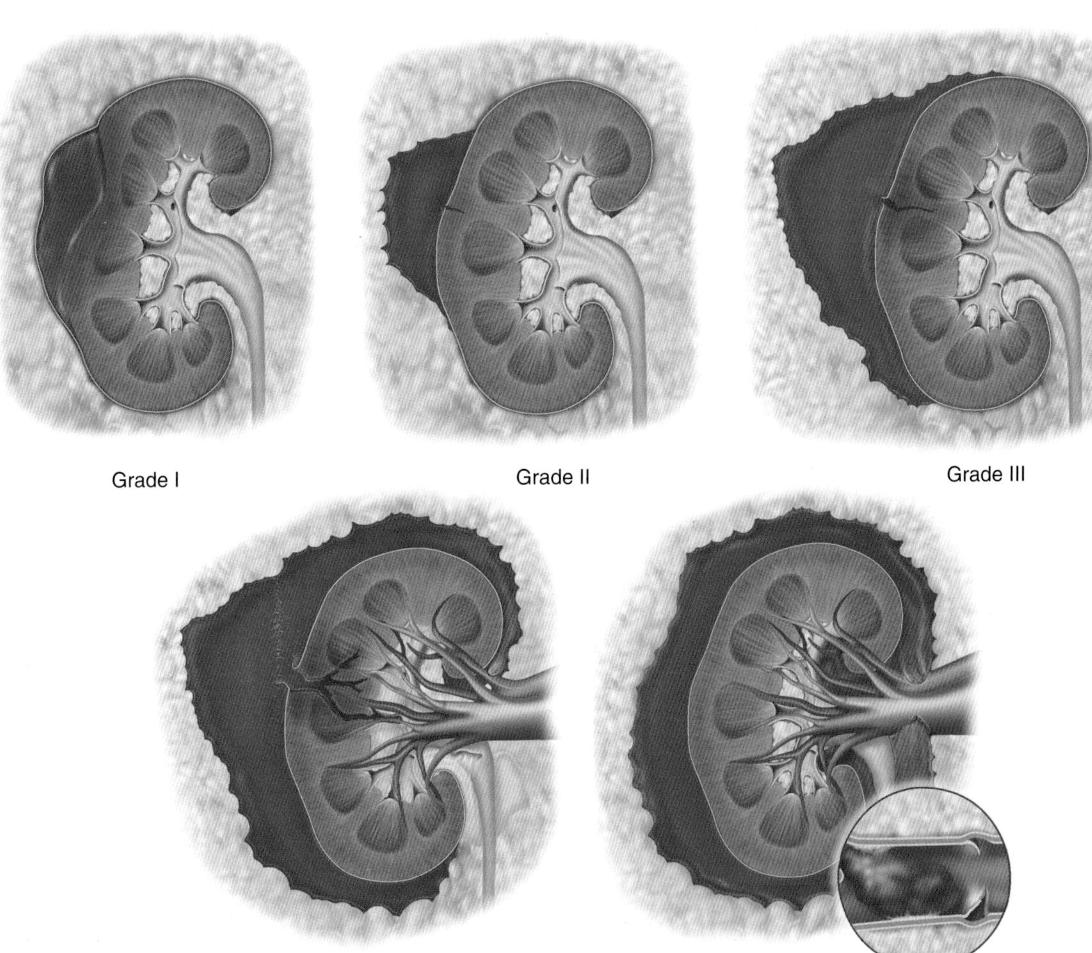

FIGURE 29.4. Modified AAST renal trauma grading system.

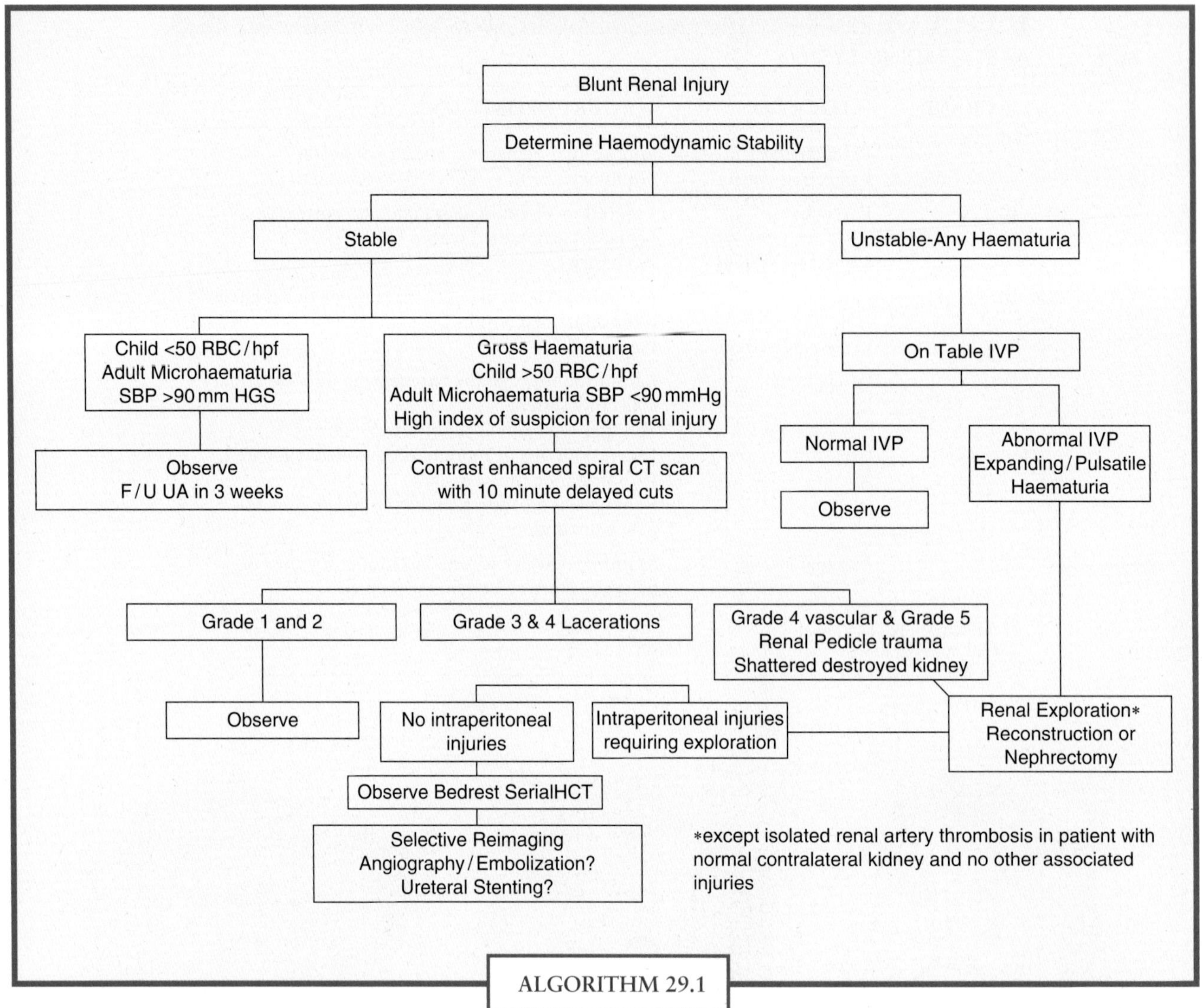

ALGORITHM 29.1 Blunt Renal Trauma Management algorithm. (From Santucci R, Wessels H, Bartsch G, et al. Evaluation and management of renal injuries: consensus statement of the renal trauma subcommittee. *BJU Int.* 2004;93(7):937–954.)

Surgical Management. Absolute indications for surgical management are few (Table 29.2), but prompt recognition is important as renal hemorrhage can be life threatening. The surgical approach to the damaged kidney is complicated and controversial. We have found that control of the renal vasculature prior to opening Gerota's fascia can decrease the likelihood of nephrectomy and make any subsequent renal surgery more controlled as bleeding can be managed prospectively, though others have disagreed with these findings.[2,23–25]

The initial surgical approach after laparotomy when vascular control is obtained, begins with identification of the aorta, where an incision of the posterior peritoneum is then made superior to the inferior mesenteric artery, gaining access to the retroperitoneum. Extension of the incision superiorly will lead to the left renal vein, which is the key anatomical landmark. The right renal artery can be found superior and medial to the left renal vein, often located with cephalad retraction of the vein and dissection between the aorta and inferior vena cava. The left renal artery lies just posterior and superior to the left renal vein. The right renal vein can be found on the opposite the left renal vein on the contralateral side of the IVC. Once the vessels are isolated, vessels loops are placed, but not occluded. The colon ipsilateral to the injury is then retracted medially and Gerota's fascia is opened. If uncontrollable bleeding is encountered, the vessels are then occluded by the vessel loops, starting with the respective renal artery and followed by the renal vein if necessary[23] (Fig. 29.5).

Renorrhaphy should be attempted for renal parenchymal injuries if possible (Fig. 29.6). All nonviable tissue should first be removed sharply. If greater than two-third of the kidney is nonviable, a nephrectomy should be strongly considered. Any bleeding parenchymal vessels should then be suture ligated with 4-0 chromic suture and any collecting system lacerations with a watertight running 4-0 chromic. Adequate collecting system closure can be confirmed by injection of methylene blue into the renal pelvis.[26]

Coverage of the repaired parenchymal bed is essential. If the renal capsule is still present, it can be used for coverage. Alternatively, coverage with off-the-shelf agents, such as Gelfoam, has been shown to assist with both parenchymal hemostasis and wound compression.[27,28] Bolsters made from these materials are secured to the remaining capsule with carefully placed 3-0 monofilament sutures. Additional coverage can be achieved with omentum, perinephric fat, and peritoneal flaps as needed.

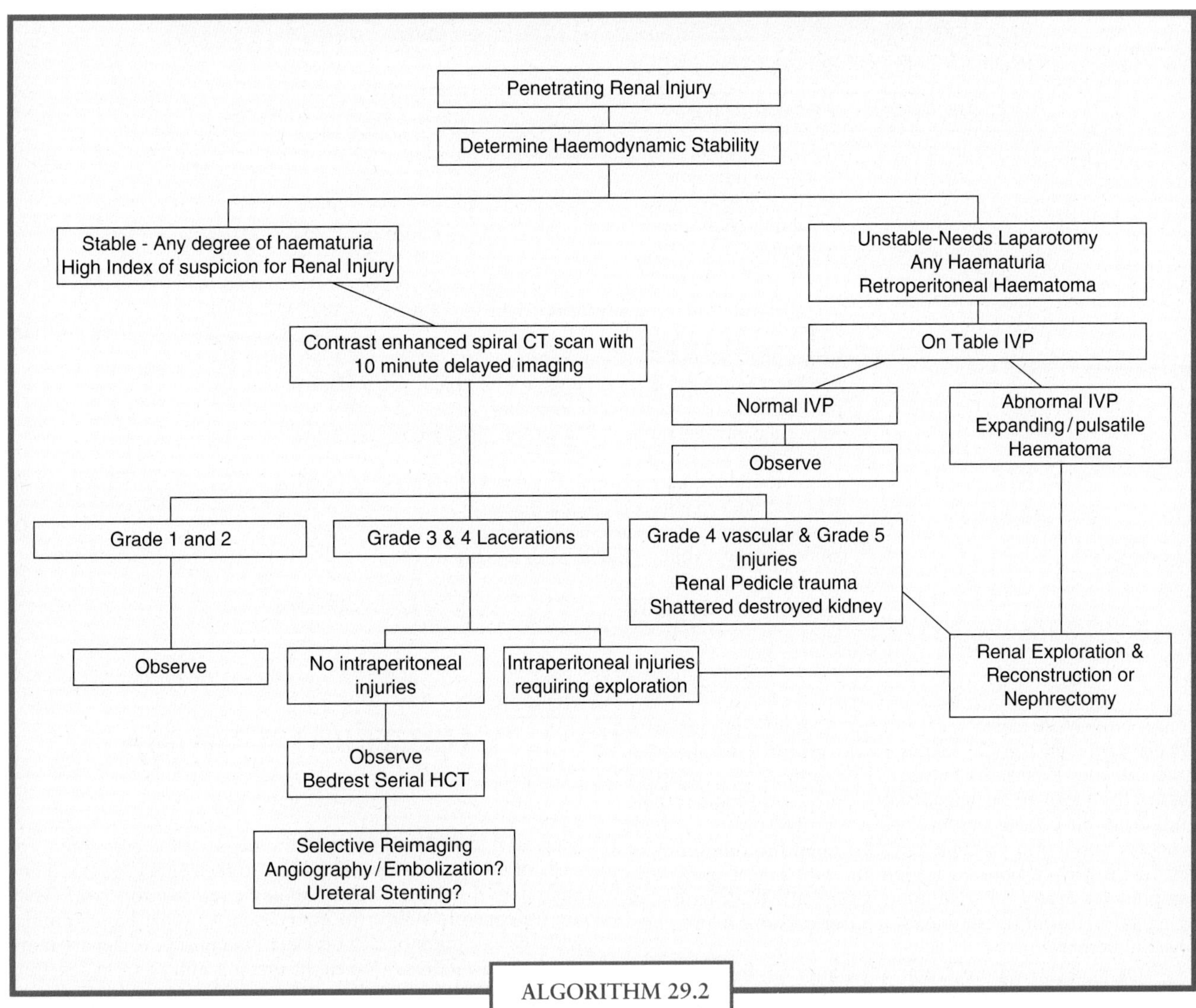

ALGORITHM 29.2 Penetrating Renal Trauma algorithm. (From Santucci R, Wessels H, Bartsch G, et al. Evaluation and management of renal injuries: consensus statement of the renal trauma subcommittee. *BJU Int.* 2004;93(7):937–954.)

Renal vascular injuries that require surgical intervention can be managed with the same initial operative approach. Incomplete renal arterial injuries can be repaired primarily with fine interrupted monofilament suture. Complete disruptions will often require nephrectomy, but if it's clinically necessary to attempt repair, arterial debridement and thrombectomy are usually required before the reanastomosis is attempted. In cases where a tension-free anastomosis is not possible, interposition with the hypogastric artery is preferred over the saphenous vein.[23,29]

Renal vein injuries are often more difficult to diagnose and to treat. Venous tears can be repaired primarily, but complete disruptions generally lead to nephrectomy. With left renal vein injuries near the IVC, ligation of the vein does not necessitate nephrectomy if collateral venous drainage provided by the adrenal, gonadal, and lumbar veins remains intact.[30]

Relative indications for surgical exploration of the kidney are shown in Table 29.2. If the retroperitoneum is incompletely staged and a large hematoma is noted at the time of surgery, an IVP should be obtained with abnormalities dictating exploration.[31] Repairing the kidney when concomitant abdominal visceral injuries are present can minimize complications such as postoperative infection and fistula.[32,33] With large devitalized segments present, exploration and removal of the segments may minimize postoperative abscesses, urinomas, and late hemorrhage.[34] Late or persistent bleeds may also require renal exploration, though angioembolization is being utilized at trauma centers more often with initial outcomes comparable to surgery.[18] Urinomas seen on CT scan will generally resolve spontaneously, but may require late percutaneous or endoscopic procedures, and rarely open surgery.[35]

Interventional Radiology. In patients with major renal injuries who are not undergoing laparotomy for other concomitant injuries, persistent renal bleeding that has failed conservative management (persistent bleeding requiring transfusion) may be managed with angioembolization of the kidney.[36] Early outcomes with this approach have been favorable, but failures do occur and open surgical management must always be considered if embolization fails to control bleeding.

Complications of Renal Injury and Management. Secondary hemorrhage and arteriovenous fistula formation in

TABLE 29.2

INDICATIONS FOR RENAL EXPLORATION

INDICATION	DESCRIPTION	TYPE
Absolute	Persistent, life-threatening hemorrhage believed to stem from renal injury	Acute
	Renal pedicle avulsion	Acute
	Expanding, pulsatile or uncontained retroperitoneal hematoma	Acute
Relative		
	A large laceration of renal pelvis or avulsion of the UPJ with major urinary leak	Acute/delayed
	Coexisting abdominal visceral injuries	Acute/delayed
	Persistent urinary leakage or abscess after failed percutaneous or endoscopic management	Delayed
	Abnormal intraoperative IVP in setting of suspected renal injury	Acute
	Large devitalized parenchymal segment with urinary leak after failed endoscopic management	Delayed
	Complete renal artery thrombosis of both kidneys, or of a solitary kidney with preserved renal perfusion	Acute
	Renovascular hypertension	Delayed

conservatively managed renal injuries is more common with deeper and higher-grade lesions, with rates of late bleeds in grade III and IV lesions between 13% and 25%.[37] Most of these bleeds can be managed successfully with angiographic embolization. Late bleeds have been reported up to 1 month after the initial injury which may correspond to the timing of retroperitoneal hematoma resolution, exposing a previously tamponaded artery.[38] Presentation is generally flank pain and/or hematuria or in the setting of an arteriovenous fistula, new onset hypertension.

Urinary extravasation from UPJ injury or from calyceal injury from a devitalized segment can successfully be managed with ureteral stent and/or percutaneous drain placement in >90% of cases, but may require open repair if a large devitalized renal segment is preventing healing or if leakage persists.[35] Abscesses associated with these leaks can be usually managed with percutaneous drainage alone.

New onset hypertension is noted in 5% of patients with conservatively managed renal trauma, with higher rates (40%-50%) in individuals with severe renal arterial injuries.[39] The mechanism is thought to be from renal ischemia and inappropriate renin release. Nephrectomy is the most common and most effective treatment. Renal insufficiency after conservative management has not been well studied, but angioembolization of renal hemorrhage leads to a 10% ipsilateral renal function and it is thought that some loss of function should be expected, especially with severe injury.[40]

Summary. With the advent of improved imaging techniques, outcomes data and grading criteria, the contemporary management of renal trauma has become mostly nonoperative. Grade V injuries and unstable patients will require surgery most often and in instances where the kidney must be explored, appropriate surgical techniques can lead to preservation of renal parenchyma in many cases. Prompt recognition of potential renal injuries followed by appropriate laboratory studies and imaging techniques can decrease renal trauma morbidity and mortality considerably.

URETERAL TRAUMA

Epidemiology

Ureteral injuries from external trauma are rare, accounting for <1% of urologic trauma, likely due to their small size, mobility, and relatively protected location in the retroperitoneum.[41] They are infrequently subject to injury from external blunt trauma, with the exception of UPJ deceleration injuries, which are more common in children.[42] When the ureter is injured from penetrating trauma, it is frequently associated with other abdominal injuries which can make them difficult to diagnose since the other injuries will often take diagnostic and management precedent.[43]

Most ureteral trauma experience comes from iatrogenic injury, usually encountered during difficult pelvic or ureteroscopic stone surgery, occurring at rates of 0.05%-30% depending on the type and difficulty of surgery being performed.[44] The most common types of iatrogenic injury are suture ligation, crush injury, and ureteral devascularization from aggressive ureteral skeletonization. Gynecologic surgery accounts for over half of injuries, with the remainder occurring during urologic, colorectal, general, and vascular surgery. Iatrogenic injuries can be prevented with good exposure and a thorough understanding of surgical anatomy. Preoperative imaging[45] and ureteral stenting have not been shown to decrease injury rate, but may make identification of the injury and subsequent repair easier.[46]

Diagnosis

Presentation. Early signs and symptoms of ureteral trauma are generally vague and nonspecific and include flank pain and hematuria. However, hematuria can be absent in up to 30% of cases and therefore, a high index of suspicion must be present whenever there is concern for a ureteral injury if an accurate diagnosis is to be made.[41] The surgical field/anatomy,

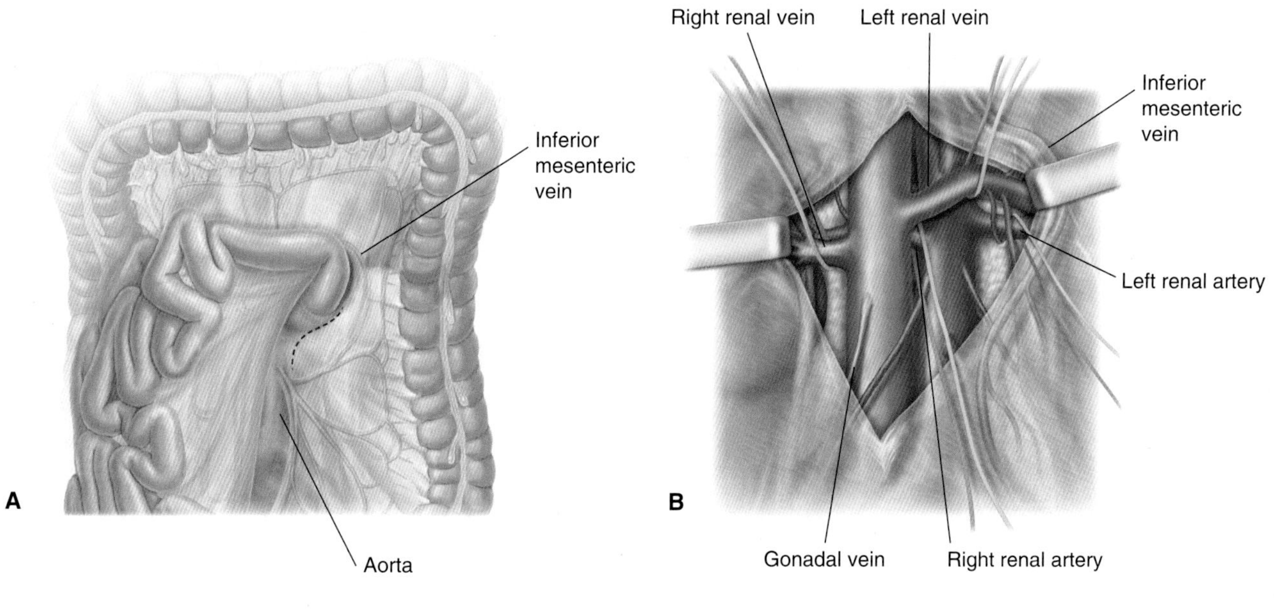

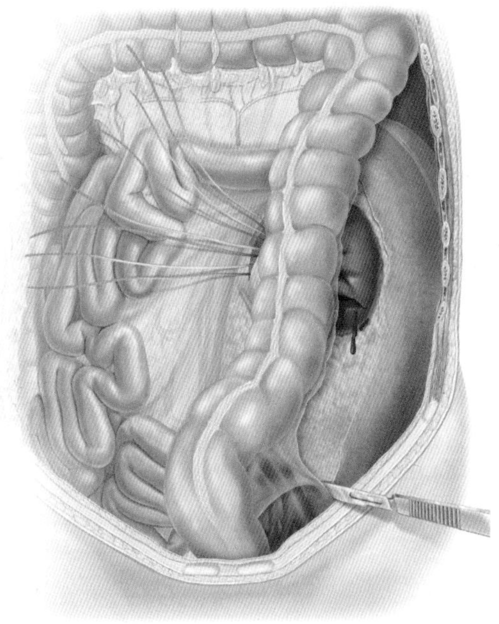

FIGURE 29.5. Surgical Approach to obtaining Hilar Control.

mechanism of injury, and path of the external trauma must be scrutinized with a low threshold to image and/or explore the ureter if injury is suspected.

Unfortunately, many ureteral injuries will present in a delayed fashion (65%-93%), often with symptoms such as prolonged ileus, low urine output, flank/abdominal pain, acute renal failure, or high drain output.[47] Morbidity from ureteral trauma is significantly higher when the diagnosis is delayed, resulting in higher rates of urinoma, infection, and renal unit loss.[48]

Imaging. With penetrating trauma, the best imaging modality to diagnose ureteral injury is a CT scan with delayed images obtained 10 minute after injection of IV contrast dye (Fig. 29.7). Delayed extravasation of contrast medial to the kidney is common for UPJ injuries and more distal extravasation for ureteral injuries. Ureteral injuries may also show hydronephrosis, delayed nephrograms, and contrast absent in the distal ureter. A complete IVP will also accurately diagnose most injuries, though this is rarely used anymore in the acute setting.[49] When a laparotomy is being performed without preoperative imaging and ureteral injury is suspected, a one-shot IVP can be utilized, which has high test specificity. However, the sensitivity is unacceptably low to rule out injury (20%-30%) and in these cases surgical exploration is probably the best way to diagnose injury, which can be improved by injection of intravenous methylene blue and inspection of the surgical field for dye extravasation. Retrograde pyelograms are both sensitive and specific but are logistically difficult to

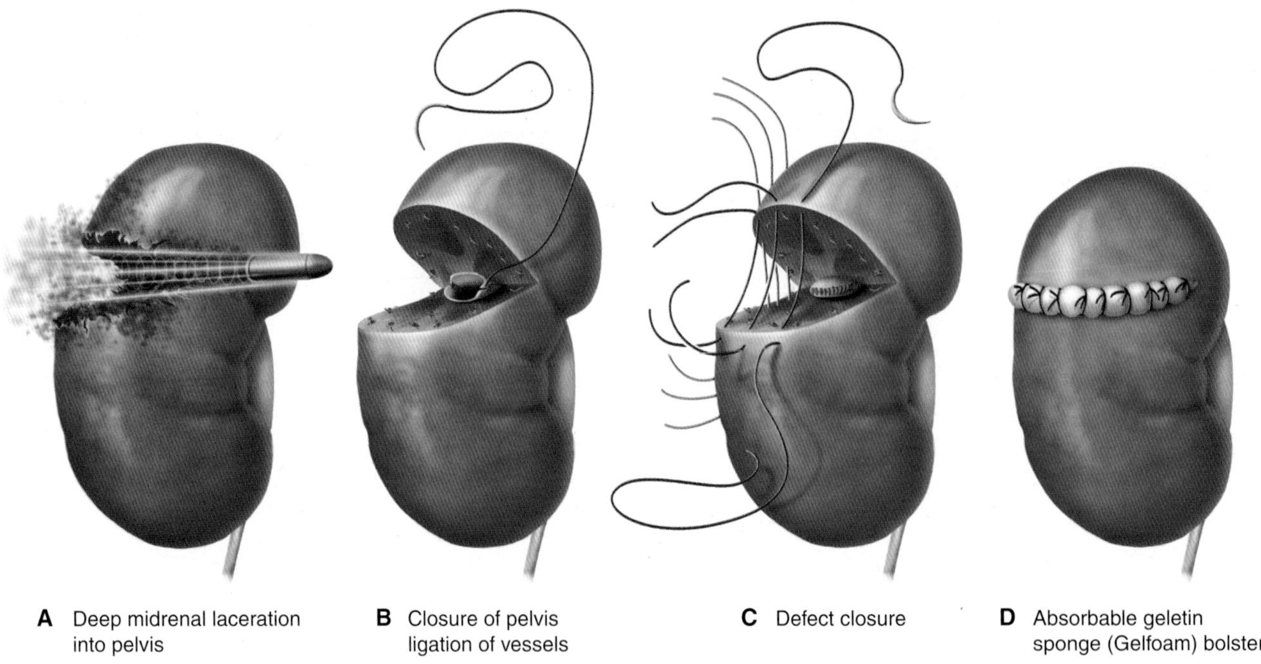

FIGURE 29.6. Renorrhaphy technique.

perform in the trauma setting and best used for diagnosing iatrogenic or delayed ureteral injuries or in the setting where IVP or CT scan results are equivocal.

Treatment (Algorithm. 29.3)

ENDOSCOPIC MANAGEMENT

Endoscopic management with a ureteral stent can be utilized in patients with incomplete injuries, including those in the UPJ, that are not otherwise undergoing surgical exploration. In patients with delayed presentation of iatrogenic injuries after surgery, placing a ureteral stent is a reasonable first option as these injuries are often caused by inadvertent stitch placement that may dissolve with time relieving the obstruction.[43] Outcomes of partial ureteral and UPJ injuries managed with stenting alone are excellent, with open intervention required rarely.

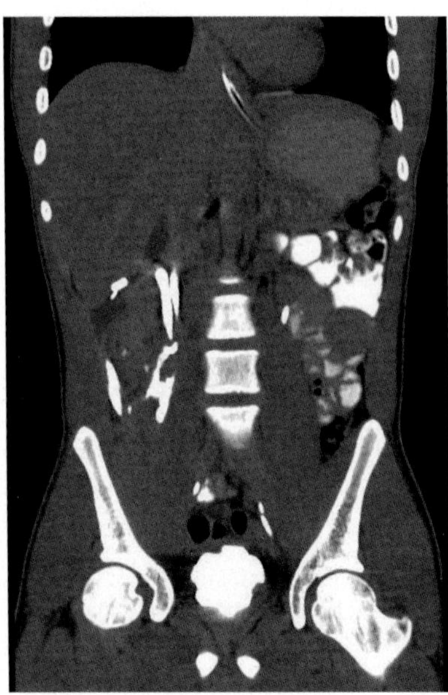

FIGURE 29.7. CT scan showing ureteral trauma on excretory images.

SURGICAL MANAGEMENT

Most penetrating injuries will be diagnosed during surgical exploration. Repair options are generally dictated by the patient's overall clinical picture, but in general, the ureter should be repaired in the same operative setting. The type of repair is dependent on both the mechanism and location of the injury. Gunshot injuries will often be associated with other abdominal injuries, but these should never preclude ureteral repair in the stable patient. Careful attention must be paid to the path of the bullet and any concern for injury to the ureter warrants exploration of the retroperitoneum with careful attention to the blast cavity. Any discoloration of the ureter may indicate devascularization injury and would warrant surgical repair as late leaks are common.[44]

Principles of a good ureteral repair are the same regardless of location and include careful mobilization of the ureter with adventia sparing so not to devascularize the segment, aggressive debridement of the damaged ureter until healthy, bleeding ends are encountered, and, finally, a stented, tension-free watertight anastomosis.

Proximal ureteral injuries are best managed with excision of the injured segment and reanastomosis with either the healthy proximal ureter (ipsilateral ureteroureterostomy, IUU) or the renal pelvis. Mid-ureteral injuries can be managed with an IUU if the distal segment is healthy. However, in cases where the distal segment is unreliable or damaged, the ureter can be anastomosed to the contralateral ureter (transureteroureterostomy) or a Boari flap (tabularized bladder flap) can be created. Distal ureteral injuries should be managed with reimplantation since the distal blood supply is less reliable after injury. If the distance from the injury to the bladder cannot be bridged without tension, a psoas hitch can be utilized. Additional options for longer-segment injuries include ileal interposition and autotransplantation, though these are seldom utilized in the acute traumatic setting. Outcomes for ureteral injuries of

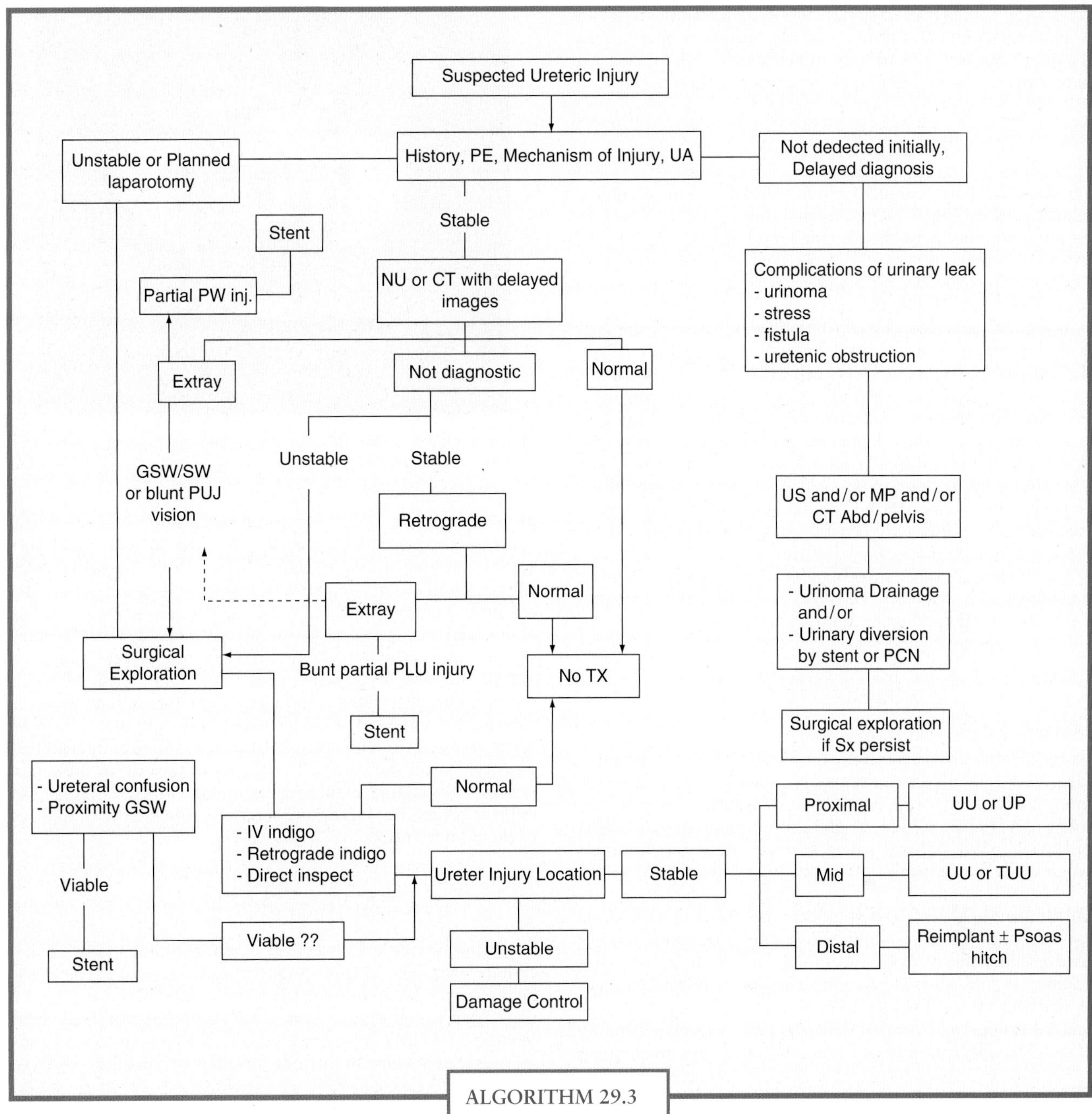

ALGORITHM 29.3 Ureteral Trauma algorithm. (From Brandes S, Chelsky M, Armenakas N, McAninch J. Diagnosis and management of ureteric injury: an evidence based analysis. *BJU Int.* 2004;94(3):277–289.)

all kinds are excellent if the above-mentioned principles are followed, though comparison outcomes studies are lacking.

With ureteral injuries in traumatic situations, a damage control approach to the injury should always be considered. Suture ligation of the ureter proximal to the injury with subsequent percutaneous nephrostomy tube is a reasonable option in the unstable patient and is much preferable to leaving the ureter drain into the surgical cavity. If the patient stabilizes, delayed repair can then be performed with improved outcomes.

Conclusion. Ureteral trauma is rare and will most often be encountered after iatrogenic injury. Early diagnosis is key to successful management, though this can often be difficult in a traumatic situation. Maintaining a high index of suspicion followed by appropriate imaging and intraoperative techniques can minimize morbidity from injury. Surgical repair of ureteral injuries is generally straightforward and often successful if proper repair principles are followed.

BLADDER TRAUMA

Epidemiology

Traumatic bladder injury is a result of blunt trauma 65%-85% of the time.[50] Nearly 2% of blunt abdominal trauma will injure the bladder, with 80% of these a result of pelvic fracture.[51] Of all pelvic fractures, 5%-10% will suffer a major bladder injury.[50,52]

Penetrating trauma is less common, with bladder injuries reported in 3.6% of abdominal gunshot wounds. Iatrogenic injury to the bladder occurs in 0.1%-10% of all pelvic cases, with increasing complexity of cases leading to higher rates of injury.[53]

Pathophysiology

The most common cause of blunt bladder trauma is motor vehicle accident (90%), either from a direct blow to the bladder, most commonly by the steering wheel or lap belt, or in the setting of a pelvic fracture.[53] Driving while intoxicated is an independent risk factor for bladder injury, as it predisposes to both MVAs and full bladders.[54]

When pelvic fractures lead to bladder injury, they are generally located at the fascial attachments of the bladder to pelvis, with pubic symphysis diastasis (RR 9.8) and obturator ring fractures (RR 3.2) being the most predictive fracture patterns for bladder injury.[55] Fractures in other locations can lead to bladder injury when fragments secondarily penetrate the bladder.[56] Bladder injuries from pelvic fracture are associated with urethral disruption in up to 15% of cases.[57] Direct blows to the bladder from external trauma lead to high intravesical pressures and ruptures are generally found at the dome of the bladder, generally the weakest location.

Penetrating trauma to the bladder is most often a result of gunshot or stab wounds. These will rarely be isolated injuries and will many times lead to multiple vesicotomies.[58]

Initial Evaluation

Physical Exam. The most common signs and symptoms of bladder trauma are hematuria (80%-100%) and abdominal pain (62%).[53] With direct trauma, bruising may be seen on the anterior abdominal wall, and urine extravasation may also be noted as perineal, scrotal, thigh, and abdominal wall edema and swelling.[58] In patients with a delayed diagnosis, symptoms may include low urine output or prolonged ileus.

Laboratory. A urinalysis should be obtained in all trauma patients, and hematuria should alert one to the possibility of genitourinary injury. Gross hematuria in the setting of pelvic fracture should always raise the suspicion of bladder and/or urethral injury. Bladder injuries that are recognized in a delayed fashion may present with elevated Cr levels secondary to systemic absorption of urine or prolonged ileus after injury.

Imaging. Correct imaging is the single most important factor in guiding appropriate management of bladder injury. If blood is seen at the urethral meatus, begin with a retrograde urethrogram to rule out concomitant urethral injury. A catheter should then be placed when appropriate and used to perform either a static or CT cystogram. If a CT scan is already being performed, CT cystogram is usually the most appropriate study. Distention of the bladder with contrast is important, and a minimum of 350 mL of contrast should be instilled to improve diagnostic sensitivity, which when performed appropriately, is over 95%.[59] Clamping the catheter during CT scan with IV contrast is not an appropriate alternative and if <350 mL is used, clot or peritoneal contents, which nearly always initially fill the cystotomy, may not be sufficiently displaced and injuries will be missed.[58] Static cystograms will always require AP, lateral and excretory images. CT cystograms will require only pelvic imaging after the bladder is filled, though excretory images may help delineate the location of injury.[60]

Injury Classification. Injuries are most commonly separated into extra- and intraperitoneal, with combined injuries present in up to 5%.[53] Extraperitoneal ruptures will show contrast extravasation generally confined to perivesical soft tissues, often in a "flare" pattern (Fig. 29.8). Intraperitoneal ruptures will show contrast extravasating into the cul-de-sac, outlining loops of bowel and if large enough, extend to other abdominal viscera such as the spleen (Fig. 29.9). Of blunt injuries, approximately 40% will be intraperitoneal and 60% extraperitoneal. Most penetrating injuries to the bladder will have an intraperitoneal component and concomitant abdominal visceral injuries.[61] Bladder neck injuries, which are most often associated with pelvic fractures and extraperitoneal injuries, should be carefully looked for as well as these can dramatically change management and outcomes.[62] Medial and inferior contrast extravasation is commonly seen with injuries of the bladder neck.

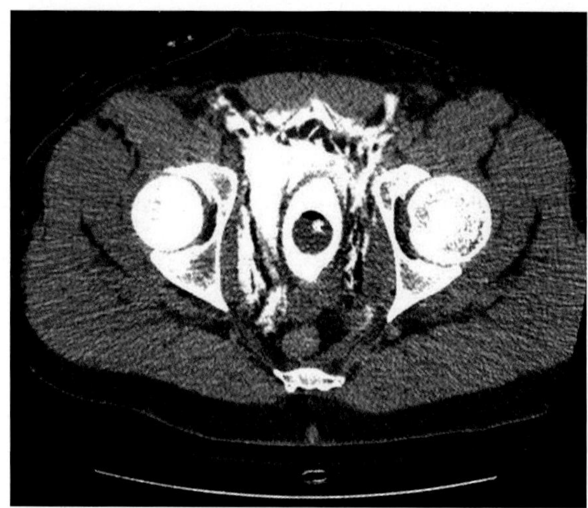

FIGURE 29.8. CT scan showing extraperitoneal bladder injury.

Management (Algorithm. 29.4)

Extraperitoneal. Conservative management with Foley catheter drainage is appropriate in most cases of extraperitoneal injury.[63] Foley drainage is usually maintained for 10–14 days after which time, a cystogram should be obtained demonstrating no leak before removal. Notable exceptions to conservative management include insufficient bladder drainage with the catheter, generally as a result of gross hematuria and clots, concomitant vaginal or rectal injury, bony fragments

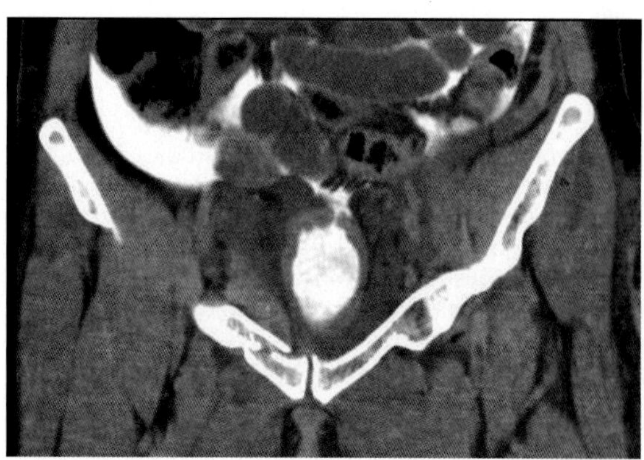

FIGURE 29.9. CT scan showing intraperitoneal bladder injury.

- No blood at the meatus AND
- Normal prostate on DRE

Gentle urethral catheterization

Gross haematuria

Stress Cystogram

Bladder Repture

Failed

Normal

Mlcrohaematuria

Normal

Extra-Peritoneal

Intra-Peritoneal

Urethrovesical Foley

Surgical Repair

Lower urinary tract management in the pelvic fracture patient

Retrograde urethrogram

Partial urethral repture

- Blood at the meatus OR
- Ascended or impalpable prostate on DRE

Total urethral repture

Suprapubic Cystostomy
(Consider stress cystogram if gross haematuriasuspicion of bladderinjury)

ALGORITHM 29.4

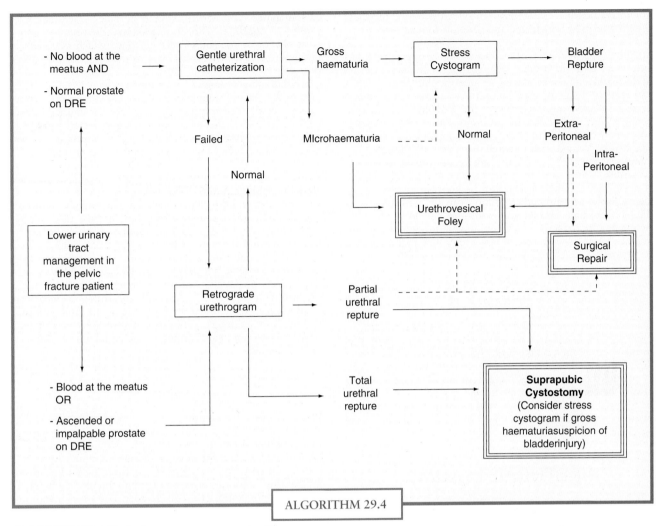

ALGORITHM 29.4 Urethral trauma management algorithm.

within the bladder, and bladder neck injury. Poor drainage from hematuria/clots or bony fragments can prevent coaptation of the bladder injury and impair healing. Concomitant vaginal and rectal injuries can lead to vagino- or rectovesical fistulas, which can be extremely difficult to manage and can be prevented with early bladder closure. Bladder neck injuries will generally not heal with catheter drainage alone since the injury involves sphincteric tissue, which will effectively hold the defect open, preventing healing and complicating catheter drainage. Additionally, if the patient is being explored surgically for other abdominal or orthopedic injuries, it is also generally felt that repair of the bladder should be performed concomitantly, since conservative management has a complication rate of up to 25%, including fistula formation, bladder calculi, delayed healing, and sepsis.[63]

Intraperitoneal. All intraperitoneal injuries should be repaired surgically, with the lone exception being small, iatrogenic injuries secondary to transurethral bladder tumor resection.[50] Most of these injuries will be a result of large external forces, which will often lead to large defects, most often at the dome, that are unlikely to heal spontaneously (Fig. 29.10). Given the extreme external force needed to rupture the bladder, concomitant injuries are common and overall mortality is high (20%-40%).[64] Gunshot and stab wounds will

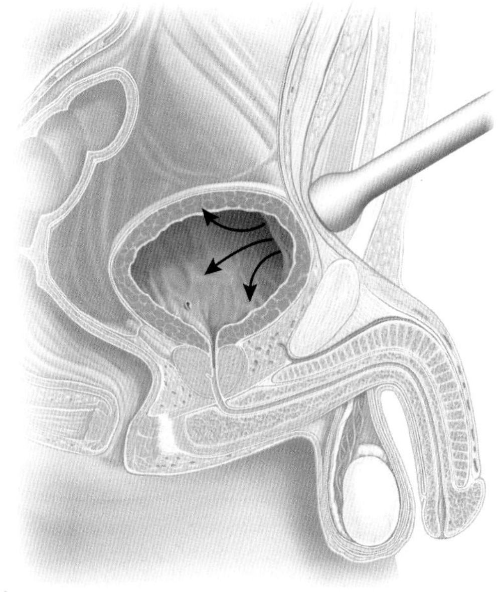

FIGURE 29.10. Mechanism of blunt bladder injuries.

often have multiple cystotomies (entry/exit wound), and these should always be anticipated and carefully looked for.

Surgical Technique. The bladder should be approached surgically in a uniform fashion, regardless of the size and location of the bladder injury, by making an anterior midline cystotomy, which allows for complete visualization of bladder mucosa and ureters.[50] Bladder injuries should be repaired intravesically with a single layer of 3-0 chromic suture to ensure the mucosa is adequately coapted. If the extravesical component of the injury can also be located with minimal dissection and difficulty, an additional muscle layer closure can be performed using Vicryl suture on the outside of the bladder. If ureteral integrity is questioned, methylene blue can be given intravenously, or alternatively, ureteral cathcterization can be performed with the bladder open. The surgical cystotomy should be closed in two layers, and a catheter and suprapubic tube should be left in place for at least 10 days, at which time a cystogram should be performed which will dictate catheter removal.[58]

Summary

Bladder injuries are rare and are most commonly secondary to blunt trauma associate with pelvic fractures. A properly performed cystogram has high diagnostic sensitivity and can help direct proper management. Most extraperitoneal injuries can be managed conservatively, but exceptions to this rule should always be considered. Intraperitoneal injuries should always be repaired surgically. Regardless of location or mechanism of bladder injury, with prompt injury recognition outcomes are excellent.

URETHRAL TRAUMA

Anatomy/Epidemiology

A thorough understanding of the urethral anatomy is important when discussing urethral trauma, since gender and age variations of the urethra as well as the specific trauma location will have important management implications. The male urethra is nearly 18–20 cm in length and is separated into two distinct anterior and posterior parts, both of which are relatively vulnerable to trauma, though from different mechanisms.[65] Conversely, the female urethra is only 4–6 cm in length, is well protected, and is rarely injured. The gender differences are especially evident when comparing posterior urethral injuries from pelvic fractures, which result in injury in up to 10% of male pelvic fractures but in only 1%-2% of similar fractures in females.[66] The anterior urethra, which is absent in females, is 14–16 cm in length in males and spans from the bulbar urethra to the urethral meatus, all of which is vulnerable to blunt injury.

Pathophysiology

Posterior Urethra. The majority (90%) of traumatic posterior urethral injuries in males will occur as a result of blunt trauma and pelvic fractures.[67] The prostatic and the membranous urethra have ligamentous attachments to the bony pelvis and shearing of these attachments from fractures can lead to tearing of urethral segments. Fracture patterns most predictive of urethral trauma include Malgaigne's fractures (anterior fracture through both rami of the symphysis pubis with posterior pelvic disruption either from facture of the sacrum or sacroiliac joint; OR 3.4), straddle fractures (fracture of all four pubic rami; OR 3.85), and straddle + sacroiliac fractures (OR 24.02).[67] The most common location for injury is at the prostatomembranous junction, which is relatively unsupported and therefore subject to the most shearing force (Fig. 29.11). Concomitant injury to the bladder (10%) and/or other abdominal organs (27%) is common, which can be attributed to the massive trauma generally required for a pelvic fracture to occur.[68] Penetrating trauma is rare but is usually from gunshot wounds. Other mechanisms of injury include iatrogenic injury from urethral instrumentation and from surgical removal of the prostate, both of which are usually ischemic injuries.

Anterior Urethra. Most injuries to the anterior urethra are a result of blunt trauma. The bulbar urethra is particularly vulnerable to straddle injury since it is relatively immobile and can be compressed by direct force against the underlying symphysis pubis (Fig. 29.12). Common culprits are bicycle handlebars and the tops of fences and not surprisingly, they are more common in younger males.[69] The penile urethra is much more mobile and less commonly injured. However, in nearly 20% of patients with penile fractures, a concomitant urethral injury will be noted, usually presenting as immediate detumescence with blood at the urethral meatus.[70] Gunshot wounds and stabbings more often involve the penile urethra with concomitant penile, testicular and rectal injuries happening frequently.[71]

Initial Evaluation

Presentation. Hematuria, and, more specifically, blood at the urethral meatus, is the most common sign of urethral injury, though it can be absent in up to 50% of posterior and 25% of anterior urethral injuries.[72] However, clinical suspicion should always dictate workup for urethral injury. For posterior urethral injuries, any type of pelvic fracture should alert one to the possibility of urethral injury. For anterior injuries, any type of straddle mechanism, especially when bruising is seen on physical exam, should alert one to injury. Frequently, patients will also present with painful urination or the inability to urinate. A high-riding prostate on digital rectal exam has often been implemented as a way to diagnose posterior

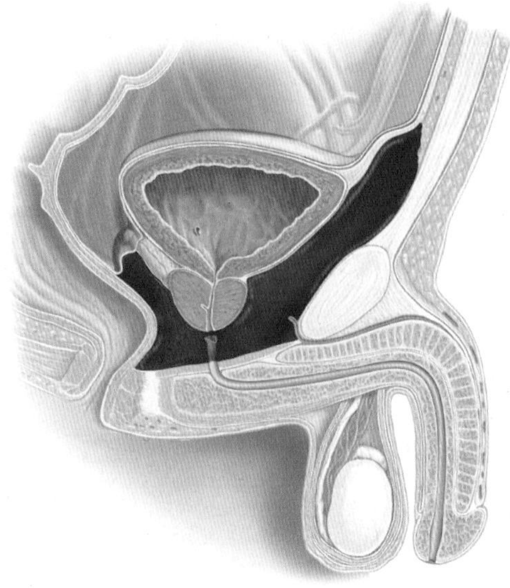

FIGURE 29.11. Posterior urethral disruption.

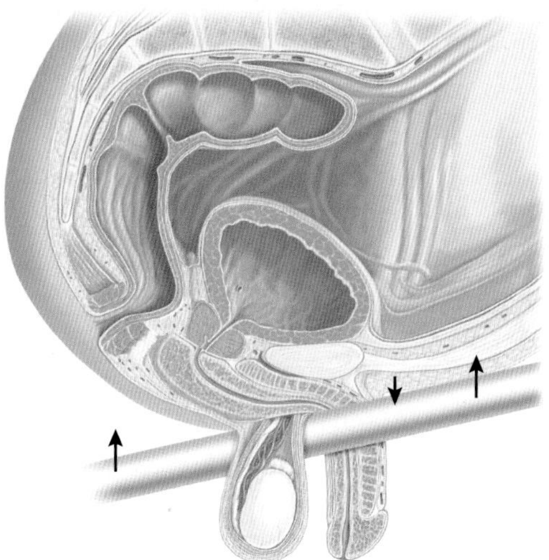

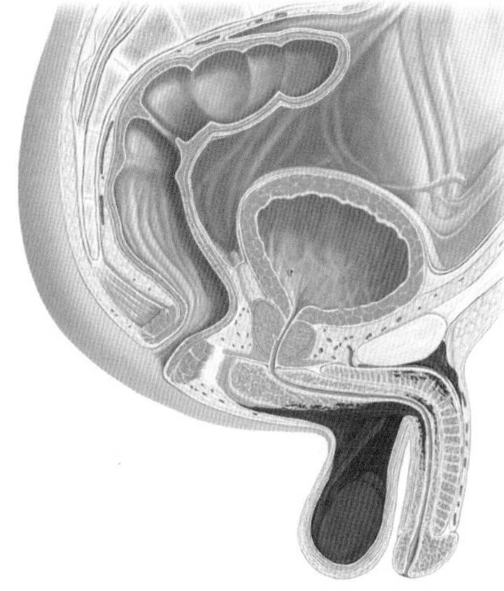

FIGURE 29.12. Anterior urethral trauma.

urethral injury, but has been shown to have both poor sensitivity and specificity, especially in young patients.[73]

Diagnosis. If blood is seen at the urethral meatus or if a urethral injury is suspected, a retrograde urethrogram should be performed before attempt at catheterization is made. These studies are best performed with the patient in a 30-degree oblique position, though this may not be possible in patients with a pelvic fracture. A 12–14F Foley catheter is then inserted into the tip of the penis and 1–2 mL is placed into the balloon to seed the catheter in the fossa navicularis. Retrograde injection through the catheter of full-strength contrast medium is then performed. This should be done under fluoroscopy if possible, but otherwise, radiographs should be obtained after at least 10 mL has been injected. Grading systems for urethral injuries vary, but in general, anterior injuries are classified as either partial or complete disruptions. In the posterior urethra, they are classified as partial, complete, or complex, with the latter pertaining to a complete injury that also involves the bladder neck.[65] Cystourethrography should not be used as a diagnostic tool for urethral injuries, except in females, but can later be utilized to help with catheter placement in certain injuries. Other imaging modalities such as ultrasound, CT, and MRI have little utility in the acute setting.

Management

Anterior Urethral Injury. With partial and complete disruptions from blunt trauma in males, injuries can be managed with either a Foley catheter or a suprapubic tube. A suprapubic tube has advantages over urethral catheterization in that it diverts the urine but also avoids urethral manipulation, which has been theorized to possibly worsen the injury and increase the need for subsequent complex urethral reconstruction.[74] Many penetrating injuries and all injuries that are the result of penile fractures should be explored in the acute setting. If a small segment is injured, it can be excised and the urethra can be repaired primarily. With larger injuries, the urethra should be marsupialized and delayed urethroplasty can be performed, usually at 3 months.[65]

Many traumas to the anterior urethra will result in urethral stricture disease. These injuries are best repaired at least 3 months after the initial trauma to allow for resolution of the hematoma and stabalization of the scar tissue. Repair technique is dependent on the length and location of stricture. Some strictures will be amenable to endoscopic stricture incision, but many perineal straddle injuries will be associated with important spongiofibrosis and will require open urethroplasty, many of which can be repaired with excision of the scar with primary anastomosis.[75]

Posterior Urethral Injury.

URINARY DIVERSION

Many posterior urethral injuries, especially those from with pelvic fractures, will be associated with other abdominal and orthopedic traumas that will often take management precedent to the urethral injury. Because of this, suprapubic tube placement is often the best initial management for posterior urethral injuries as it is a simple procedure that safely diverts the urine away from the injury. Suprapubic tubes be placed percutaneously or in an open fashion, often during abdominal exploration for other injury.[76]

IMMEDIATE PRIMARY REPAIR

Immediate repair of posterior urethral injuries has been associated with higher rates of impotence, incontinence, and stricture rates as compared with either delayed repair or primary endoscopic realignment and is not advised in most situations.[65] Exceptions to this rule include those injuries associated with bladder neck injuries, since the urine will preferentially drain through the bladder neck injury despite diversion, and rectal injuries, with the goal of preventing devastating rectoprostatic fistulas.[77]

IMMEDIATE PRIMARY REALIGNMENT

Primary realignment can be attempted in the stable patient either using purely endoscopic techniques or in an open fashion. Realignment differs from repair in that no attempt is made to secure the ends of the urethral segments to one another, and is simply to bring the transected ends in line with one another and achieve bladder drainage via a urethral catheter. Traction should not be placed on the catheter as bladder neck injury can ensue.[75] Aligning the urethral ends may decrease the need for subsequent urethroplasty versus suprapubic tube alone (62% vs. 100%) and likely makes delayed urethroplasty technically easier.[76]

DELAYED RECONSTRUCTION

Many posterior urethral injuries will result in subsequent stricture formation. Repair of these distraction injuries can be extremely challenging, with the difficulty directly correlating with the distance between the transected ends. Repair should be performed only by experienced surgeons, at least 3 months after the injury,[65] with restricture rates of <10%. Impotence (40%) and incontinence (5%) rates probably reflect damage done at the time of initial injury and are not from the surgery itself.

FEMALE URETHRAL INJURY

Injuries to the female urethra are rare. Distal injuries can be repaired primarily, generally through a vaginal approach. Proximal injuries are often associated with bladder injuries and are best repaired transvesically or retropubically. Long injuries with intact bladder necks may be best managed with initial suprapubic tube diversion with delayed repair to reduce the risk of urethral loss and incontinence.[78]

PEDIATRIC URETHRAL INJURY

The prostate is less developed in the pediatric male and the bladder neck becomes the most vulnerable segment of urethra to injury. If a bladder neck injury is suspected, immediate repair is advised. Injuries to more distal segments should follow management principles similar those of the adult male.[69]

Summary

Urethral injuries are rare and can often be challenging to manage in the acute trauma setting. In general, supraprostatic diversion is an acceptable option for the initial management of all injuries to the urethra. Delayed repair of any resulting urethral injury can then be performed by experienced hands after other injuries have been resolved and the patient is stable. However, no two urethral injuries are alike and each patient should be assessed and managed according to their initial clinical situations.

EXTERNAL GENITALIA TRAUMA

Epidemiology

Injuries to the male genitalia are rarely life threatening, but without prompt intervention, long-term sexual and psychological effects may result. Over one-third of all urologic trauma in the United States involves the genitalia.[79] In modern warfare, the genitalia are particularly vulnerable to injury, present in over 50% of unique urologic traumas.[80]

Scrotal/Testicular Trauma

Etiology. Nearly 85% of scrotal trauma is blunt, with the most common mechanisms being assault (33%), MVA (22%), and athletic activity (10%).[81] Penetrating trauma can be a result of knife, gunshot, bite, and blast injuries. Self-mutilation can also occur, usually during acute psychotic episodes.[82]

Diagnosis. Most scrotal injuries will be diagnosed by physical examination alone. However, when the integrity of the underlying testicular tissue is questioned, ultrasound is the imaging modality of choice. A high-frequency transducer (10 MHz) will give the best resolution of the testicular parenchyma, but may not always provide enough tissue penetration if a large scrotal hematoma is present, in which case lower frequencies (5 MHz) may be required. Change in the normal homogeneous pattern of the testicle is suggestive of injury (Fig. 29.13). Ultrasound is specific but not sensitive (<50%) for tunica albuginea ruptures, and ultrasound findings should never preclude surgical exploration if the suspicion is high for testicular rupture.[83]

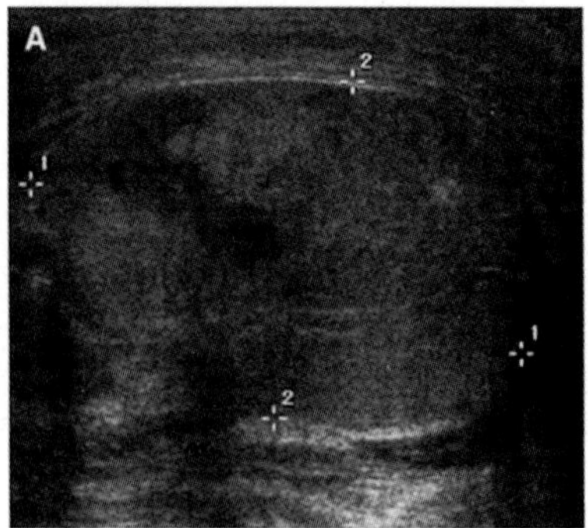

FIGURE 29.13. Ultrasound (10 MHz) imaging of testicle suggestive of injury.

Management. All testicular rupture injuries should be explored surgically, with prompt (<72 hours after injury) intervention leading to a decreased risk of testicular loss, infection, infertility, and pain.[81,84] Scrotal hematomas and hematoceles can be managed nonoperatively, but if testicular integrity is at all questioned, exploration is advised. A scrotal incision is made over the testicle, which is then delivered into the field. The hematoma is evacuated and the tunica vaginalis is opened, exposing the underlying tunica albuginea and testicle. All nonviable tissue should be excised and the tunical injury should then be repaired using absorbable sutures over all viable seminiferous tubules. In cases where tunica is unavailable or insufficient for coverage, use of autologous tunica vaginalis or Gore-Tex graft can be substituted.[85] A penrose drain is placed postoperatively.

Penile Trauma

Etiology. The majority of penile injuries will be penile fractures, or, more specifically, rupture of the fascial covering of the corpus cavernosum. These are nearly always the result of injury during sexual activity when an erect penis slips out of the vagina during intercourse and thrusts against the perineum or symphisis pubis. The relatively inelastic tunica albuginea will then absorb the majority of the bending force and subsequently tear. Nearly 10% of all penile fractures will also involve the urethra. Other mechanisms of injury include self-mutilation (including penile amputation), gunshot injury, and crush injury.

DIAGNOSIS

Diagnosing a penile injury is usually done by physical exam alone. When a tunical injury occurs, the patient will often hear a loud snapping noise, with resulting detumesence. Blood that had once filled the cavernosal bodies can now escape through the tunical injury, often quickly filling the space between the tunica albuginea and the skin. When Buck's fascia remains intact, the classic "eggplant" deformity ensues (Fig. 29.14). If Buck's fascia is compromised, the blood can also travel within the fascial planes to the scrotum and anterior abdominal wall. If blood is seen at the urethral meatus after injury or if the patient has hematuria, a concomitant urethral injury should be suspected. The tunical injuries are nearly always distal to the penile suspensory ligaments and unilateral,[86] ranging from 0.5 to 4 cm in length. The location of the injury can often be palpated and may cause point tenderness. If the diagnosis of

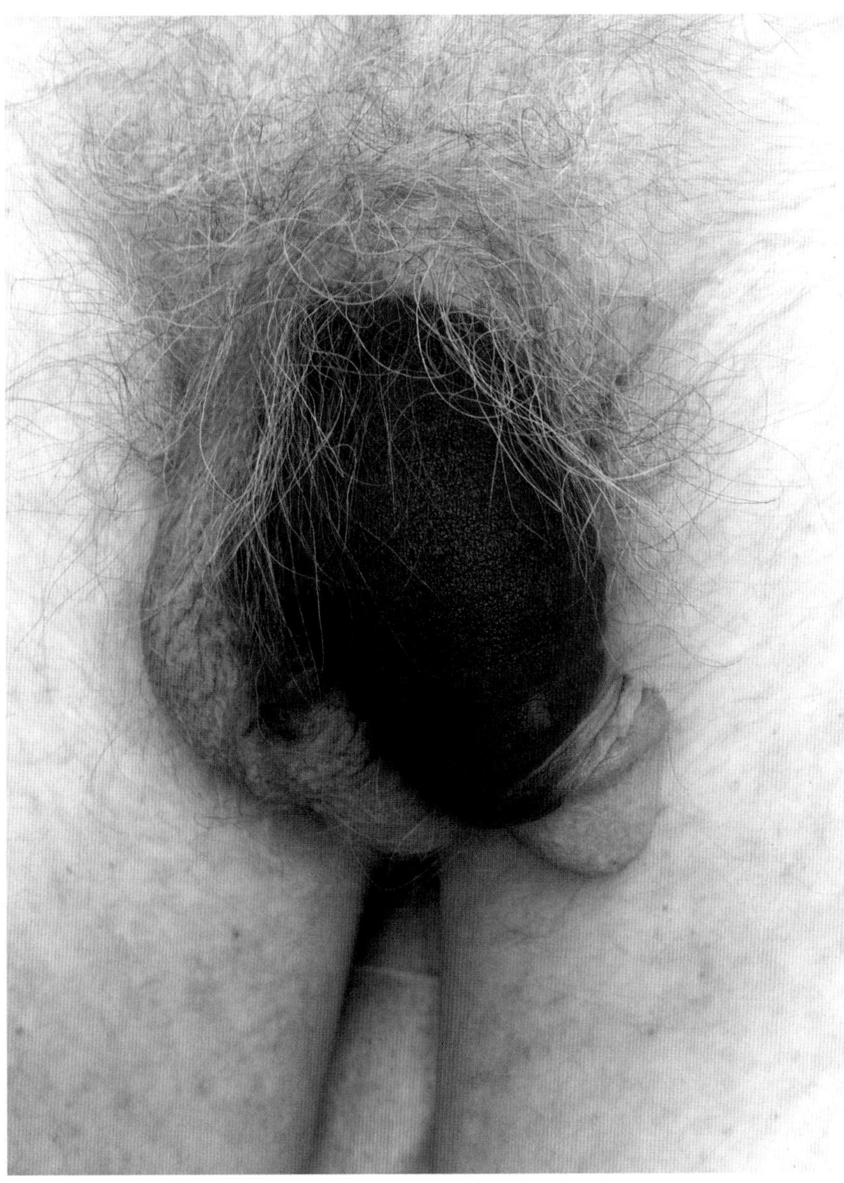

FIGURE 29.14. Penile fracture with classic "eggplant" deformity.

fracture is in question, ultrasound, cavernosometry, and MRI have been reported to be of some use.[86]

MANAGEMENT

All penile fractures should be explored surgically since reports comparing operative versus conservative nonoperative management show decreased rates of penile curvature, erectile dysfunction, and abscess formation in the surgical group.[87] Exploration is likely beneficial up to 1 week after the injury.[88] The penis can be explored either by degloving the penis via a circumcision incision or by a single linear incision over the injury if it can be easily localized. Any hematoma is evacuated and the tear is closed with interrupted 2-0 absorbable (polydioxanone) suture, with care to avoid the dorsal neurovascular bundles. The urethra should be thoroughly inspected through the same incision and repaired in a tension-free fashion over a urethral catheter if injured.

All deep-penetrating trauma to the penis and genitalia should be explored to assess the extent of damage with the goal of preserving reproductive organ function.[89] Penetrating injuries of the cavernosal bodies should be repaired as described above with the goal to preserve function and avoid penile curvature. When the spermatic cord is injured, ligation of vessels is often necessary but this does not mandate orchiectomy if collateral circulation from the cremasteric and/or vasal blood supply remains intact.[86] Vas deferens injuries should usually be ligated and then formally repaired using the microscope in a delayed fashion.

Penile amputation is a rare event and is usually the result of an acute psychotic episode or severe gender dysphoria.[90] Preservation of the penis can and should be sought whenever possible. The amputated penis should initially be wrapped in a saline-soaked gauze, put in a sealed sterile bag and then placed on ice, with care to avoid direct contact of the ice with the penis. The repair should begin with a spatulated urethral anastomosis over a catheter, followed by reattachment of the corporeal bodies with absorbable sutures. A microscopic reconstruction of the dorsal nerves, arteries, and veins should then ensue whenever possible, to improve penile sensation and decrease the risk of skin loss.[91] Erectile function can generally be preserved if the repair occurs <24 hours after amputation.

Genital Skin Loss

Etiology. The most common etiology for genital skin loss is infectious, usually the result of Fournier's gangrene (75%).[92] Traumatic avulsion of skin from accidents (farm machinery and motorcycle) and bite wounds can also occur. Avulsion injuries usually result when the genital skin becomes entangled in clothing that is traumatically ripped from the individual's body.

Management. Gangrenous skin should be immediately and aggressively excised. Secondary debridements are often necessary and should be planned in most cases. Reconstruction should take place only after the disease and the patient have fully stabilized.[93] A myriad of techniques are often necessary including primary closure, skin grafting, local tissue/thigh flaps, and combinations thereof. When the scrotal skin is involved and the testicles are left uncovered, scrotal pouches can be created or saline-soaked gauze can be used for protection in anticipation of eventual reconstruction.

Minor avulsion injuries can generally be repaired primarily after copious irrigation. Complete, circumferential avulsion injuries of the penis will usually require a more aggressive debridement because blood supply to the distal penile skin is often unrecoverable.[94] In these situations, observation after debridement followed by either primary repair (once skin integrity has declared itself) or skin grafting is recommended. Animal bite wounds can usually be closed primarily after irrigation and debridement.[95] Human bite wounds to the penis, which are more likely to present late and therefore, more likely to be grossly contaminated at presentation, should generally be left open and allowed to heal by secondary intention.[95] Most injuries to the scrotal skin can be repaired primarily if <70% of the skin has been lost.

CONCLUSION

Injuries to the external genitalia are rare, but can have lasting sexual and psychological sequelae if not managed in a timely and appropriate fashion. Goals of all management should be to first preserve sexual and urodynamic function, followed by cosmetic appearance if possible.

References

1. Baverstock R, Simons R, McLoughlin M. Severe blunt renal trauma: a 7-year retrospective review from a provincial trauma centre. *Can J Urol.* 2001;8(5):1372–1376.
2. Wessells H, Suh D, Porter JR, et al. Renal injury and operative management in the United States: results of a population-based study. *J Trauma.* 2003;54(3):423–430.
3. Krieger JN, Algood CB, Mason JT, et al. Urological trauma in the Pacific Northwest: etiology, distribution, management and outcome. *J Urol.* 1984;132(1):70–73.
4. Santucci RA, McAninch JW, Safir M, et al. Validation of the American Association for the Surgery of Trauma organ injury severity scale for the kidney. *J Trauma.* 2001;50(2):195–200.
5. Gray N. Renal trauma in a South African hospital: a two year study. *J R Army Med Corps.* 1985;131(1):19–20.
6. Ersay A, Akgun Y. Experience with renal gunshot injuries in a rural setting. *Urology.* 1999;54(6):972–975.
7. Broghammer JA, Fisher MB, Santucci RA. Conservative management of renal trauma: a review. *Urology.* 2007;70(4):623–629.
8. Schmidlin F, Farshad M, Bidaut L, et al. Biomechanical analysis and clinical treatment of blunt renal trauma. *Swiss Surg.* 1998(5):237–243.
9. McAninch JW, Carroll PR, Armenakas NA, et al. Renal gunshot wounds: methods of salvage and reconstruction. *J Trauma.* 1993;35(2):279–283; discussion 283–274.
10. Farshad M, Barbezat M, Flueler P, et al. Material characterization of the pig kidney in relation with the biomechanical analysis of renal trauma. *J Biomech.* 1999;32(4):417–425.
11. Bernath AS, Schutte H, Fernandez RR, et al. Stab wounds of the kidney: conservative management in flank penetration. *J Urol.* 1983;129(3):468–470.
12. Mendez R. Renal trauma. *J Urol.* 1977;118(5):698–703.
13. Carlin BI, Resnick MI. Indications and techniques for urologic evaluation of the trauma patient with suspected urologic injury. *Semin Urol.* 1995;13(1):9–24.
14. Brower P, Paul J, Brosman SA. Urinary tract abnormalities presenting as a result of blunt abdominal trauma. *J Trauma.* 1978;18(10):719–722.
15. Bretan PN Jr, McAninch JW, Federle MP, et al. Computerized tomographic staging of renal trauma: 85 consecutive cases. *J Urol.* 1986;136(3):561–565.
16. Santucci RA, Wessells H, Bartsch G, et al. Evaluation and management of renal injuries: consensus statement of the renal trauma subcommittee. *BJU Int.* 2004;93(7):937–954.
17. McGahan JP, Richards JR, Jones CD, et al. Use of ultrasonography in the patient with acute renal trauma. *J Ultrasound Med.* 1999;18(3):207–213; quiz 215–206.
18. Kantor A, Sclafani SJ, Scalea T, et al. The role of interventional radiology in the management of genitourinary trauma. *Urol Clin North Am.* 1989;16(2):255–265.
19. Eastham JA, Wilson TG, Ahlering TE. Urological evaluation and management of renal-proximity stab wounds. *J Urol.* 1993;150(6):1771–1773.
20. Buckley JC, McAninch JW. Revision of current american association for the surgery of trauma renal injury grading system. *J Trauma.* 2011;70(1):35–37.
21. Dugi DD III, Morey AF, Gupta A, et al. American Association for the Surgery of Trauma grade 4 renal injury substratification into grades 4a (low risk) and 4b (high risk). *J Urol.* 2010;183(2):592–597.
22. Blankenship JC, Gavant ML, Cox CE, et al. Importance of delayed imaging for blunt renal trauma. *World J Surg.* 2001;25(12):1561–1564.
23. Meng MV, Brandes SB, McAninch JW. Renal trauma: indications and techniques for surgical exploration. *World J Urol.* 1999;17(2):71–77.
24. Gonzalez RP, Falimirski M, Holevar MR, et al. Surgical management of renal trauma: is vascular control necessary? *J Trauma.* 1999;47(6):1039–1042; discussion 1042–1034.
25. Atala A, Miller FB, Richardson JD, et al. Preliminary vascular control for renal trauma. *Surg Gynecol Obstet.* 1991;172(5):386–390.
26. McAninch JW, Carroll PR, Klosterman PW, et al. Renal reconstruction after injury. *J Urol.* 1991;145(5):932–937.
27. Santucci RA, McAninch JW. Diagnosis and management of renal trauma: past, present, and future. *J Am Coll Surg.* 2000;191(4):443–451.
28. Pursifull NF, Morey AF. Tissue glues and nonsuturing techniques. *Curr Opin Urol.* 2007;17(6):396–401.
29. Haas CA, Dinchman KH, Nasrallah PF, et al. Traumatic renal artery occlusion: a 15-year review. *J Trauma.* 1998;45(3):557–561.
30. Turner WW Jr, Snyder WH III, Fry WJ. Mortality and renal salvage after renovascular trauma. A review of 94 patients treated in a 20 year period. *Am J Surg.* 1983;146(6):848–851.
31. Cass AS, Luxenberg M, Gleich P, et al. Management of perirenal hematoma found during laparotomy in patient with multiple injuries. *Urology.* 1985;26(6):546–549.
32. Safir MH, McAninch JW. Diagnosis and management of trauma to the kidney. *Curr Opin Urol.* 1999;9(3):227–231.
33. Rosen MA, McAninch JW. Management of combined renal and pancreatic trauma. *J Urol.* 1994;152(1):22–25.
34. Moudouni SM, Patard JJ, Manunta A, et al. A conservative approach to major blunt renal lacerations with urinary extravasation and devitalized renal segments. *BJU Int.* 2001;87(4):290–294.
35. Matthews LA, Smith EM, Spirnak JP. Nonoperative treatment of major blunt renal lacerations with urinary extravasation. *J Urol.* 1997;157(6):2056–2058.
36. Breyer BN, McAninch JW, Elliott SP, et al. Minimally invasive endovascular techniques to treat acute renal hemorrhage. *J Urol.* 2008;179(6):2248–2252; discussion 2253.
37. Heyns CF, de Klerk DP, de Kock ML. Stab wounds associated with hematuria—a review of 67 cases. *J Urol.* 1983;130(2):228–231.
38. Teigen CL, Venbrux AC, Quinlan DM, et al. Late massive hematuria as a complication of conservative management of blunt renal trauma in children. *J Urol.* 1992;147(5):1333–1336.
39. Watts RA, Hoffbrand BI. Hypertension following renal trauma. *J Hum Hypertens.* 1987;1(2):65–71.
40. Khan AB, Reid AW. Management of renal stab wounds by arteriographic embolisation. *Scand J Urol Nephrol.* 1994;28(1):109–110.
41. Brandes SB, Chelsky MJ, Buckman RF, et al. Ureteral injuries from penetrating trauma. *J Trauma.* 1994;36(6):766–769.
42. Morey AF, Bruce JE, McAninch JW. Efficacy of radiographic imaging in pediatric blunt renal trauma. *J Urol.* 1996;156(6):2014–2018.
43. Selzman AA, Spirnak JP. Iatrogenic ureteral injuries: a 20-year experience in treating 165 injuries. *J Urol.* 1996;155(3):878–881.
44. Palmer LS, Rosenbaum RR, Gershbaum MD, et al. Penetrating ureteral trauma at an urban trauma center: 10-year experience. *Urology.* 1999;54(1):34–36.
45. Mann WJ. Intentional and unintentional ureteral surgical treatment in gynecologic procedures. *Surg Gynecol Obstet.* 1991;172(6):453–456.

46. Sieben DM, Howerton L, Amin M, et al. The role of ureteral stenting in the management of surgical injury of the ureter. *J Urol.* 1978;119(3):330–331.
47. Brandes S, Coburn M, Armenakas N, et al. Diagnosis and management of ureteric injury: an evidence-based analysis. *BJU Int.* 2004;94(3):277–289.
48. Ghali AM, El Malik EM, Ibrahim AI, et al. Ureteric injuries: diagnosis, management, and outcome. *J Trauma.* 1999;46(1):150–158.
49. Mulligan JM, Cagiannos I, Collins JP, et al. Ureteropelvic junction disruption secondary to blunt trauma: excretory phase imaging (delayed films) should help prevent a missed diagnosis. *J Urol.* 1998;159(1):67–70.
50. Corriere JN Jr, Sandler CM. Management of the ruptured bladder: seven years of experience with 111 cases. *J Trauma.* 1986;26(9):830–833.
51. Udekwu PO, Gurkin B, Oller DW. The use of computed tomography in blunt abdominal injuries. *Am Surg.* 1996;62(1):56–59.
52. Palmer JK, Benson GS, Corriere JN Jr. Diagnosis and initial management of urological injuries associated with 200 consecutive pelvic fractures. *J Urol.* 1983;130(4):712–714.
53. Gomez RG, Ceballos L, Coburn M, et al. Consensus statement on bladder injuries. *BJU Int.* 2004;94(1):27–32.
54. Dreitlein DA, Suner S, Basler J. Genitourinary trauma. *Emerg Med Clin North Am.* 2001;19(3):569–590.
55. Avey G, Blackmore CC, Wessells H, et al. Radiographic and clinical predictors of bladder rupture in blunt trauma patients with pelvic fracture. *Acad Radiol.* 2006;13(5):573–579.
56. Cass AS. Diagnostic studies in bladder rupture. Indications and techniques. *Urol Clin North Am.* 1989;16(2):267–273.
57. Cass AS, Gleich P, Smith C. Simultaneous bladder and prostatomembranous urethral rupture from external trauma. *J Urol.* 1984;132(5):907–908.
58. Morey AF, Hernandez J, McAninch JW. Reconstructive surgery for trauma of the lower urinary tract. *Urol Clin North Am.* 1999;26(1):49–60, viii.
59. Quagliano PV, Delair SM, Malhotra AK. Diagnosis of blunt bladder injury: a prospective comparative study of computed tomography cystography and conventional retrograde cystography. *J Trauma.* 2006;61(2):410–421; discussion 421–412.
60. Horstman WG, McClennan BL, Heiken JP. Comparison of computed tomography and conventional cystography for detection of traumatic bladder rupture. *Urol Radiol.* 1991;12(4):188–193.
61. Petros FG, Santucci RA, Al-Saigh NK. The incidence, management, and outcome of penetrating bladder injuries in civilians resultant from armed conflict in Baghdad 2005–2006. *Adv Urol.* 2009:275634.
62. Mundy AR, Andrich DE. Pelvic fracture-related injuries of the bladder neck and prostate: their nature, cause and management. *BJU Int.* 2010;105(9):1302–1308.
63. Kotkin L, Koch MO. Morbidity associated with nonoperative management of extraperitoneal bladder injuries. *J Trauma.* 1995;38(6):895–898.
64. Thomae KR, Kilambi NK, Poole GV. Method of urinary diversion in nonurethral traumatic bladder injuries: retrospective analysis of 70 cases. *Am Surg.* 1998;64(1):77–80; discussion 80–71.
65. Chapple C, Barbagli G, Jordan G, et al. Consensus statement on urethral trauma. *BJU Int.* 2004;93(9):1195–1202.
66. Perry MO, Husmann DA. Urethral injuries in female subjects following pelvic fractures. *J Urol.* 1992;147(1):139–143.
67. Koraitim MM, Marzouk ME, Atta MA, et al. Risk factors and mechanism of urethral injury in pelvic fractures. *Br J Urol.* 1996;77(6):876–880.
68. Chapple CR, Png D. Contemporary management of urethral trauma and the post-traumatic stricture. *Curr Opin Urol.* 1999;9(3):253–260.
69. Koraitim MM. Posttraumatic posterior urethral strictures in children: a 20-year experience. *J Urol.* 1997;157(2):641–645.
70. Nicolaisen GS, Melamud A, Williams RD, et al. Rupture of the corpus cavernosum: surgical management. *J Urol.* 1983;130(5):917–919.
71. Gomez RG, Castanheira AC, McAninch JW. Gunshot wounds to the male external genitalia. *J Urol.* 1993;150(4):1147–1149.
72. Lim PH, Chng HC. Initial management of acute urethral injuries. *Br J Urol.* 1989;64(2):165–168.
73. Fallon B, Wendt JC, Hawtrey CE. Urological injury and assessment in patients with fractured pelvis. *J Urol.* 1984;131(4):712–714.
74. Park S, McAninch JW. Straddle injuries to the bulbar urethra: management and outcomes in 78 patients. *J Urol.* 2004;171(2 Pt 1):722–725.
75. Koraitim MM. Pelvic fracture urethral injuries: evaluation of various methods of management. *J Urol.* 1996;156(4):1288–1291.
76. Webster GD, Mathes GL, Selli C. Prostatomembranous urethral injuries: a review of the literature and a rational approach to their management. *J Urol.* 1983;130(5):898–902.
77. Mundy AR, Andrich DE. Pelvic fracture-related injuries of the bladder neck and prostate: their nature, cause and management. *BJU Int.*;105(9):1302–1308.
78. Koraitim MM. Pelvic fracture urethral injuries: the unresolved controversy. *J Urol.* 1999;161(5):1433–1441.
79. Brandes SB, Buckman RF, Chelsky MJ, et al. External genitalia gunshot wounds: a ten-year experience with fifty-six cases. *J Trauma.* 1995;39(2):266–271; discussion 271–262.
80. Serkin FB, Soderdahl DW, Hernandez J, et al. Combat urologic trauma in US military overseas contingency operations. *J Trauma.* 2010;69(Suppl 1):S175–S178.
81. Buckley JC, McAninch JW. Diagnosis and management of testicular ruptures. *Urol Clin North Am.* 2006;33(1):111–116, vii.
82. Aboseif S, Gomez R, McAninch JW. Genital self-mutilation. *J Urol.* 1993;150(4):1143–1146.
83. Jeffrey RB, Laing FC, Hricak H, et al. Sonography of testicular trauma. *AJR Am J Roentgenol.* 1983;141(5):993–995.
84. Kukadia AN, Ercole CJ, Gleich P, et al. Testicular trauma: potential impact on reproductive function. *J Urol.* 1996;156(5):1643–1646.
85. Sharma AC, Sam AD II, Lee LY, et al. Effect of NG-nitro-L-arginine methyl ester on testicular blood flow and serum steroid hormones during sepsis. *Shock.* 1998;9(6):416–421.
86. Morey AF, Metro MJ, Carney KJ, et al. Consensus on genitourinary trauma: external genitalia. *BJU Int.* 2004;94(4):507–515.
87. Tan LB, Chiang CP, Huang CH, et al. Traumatic rupture of the corpus cavernosum. *Br J Urol.* 1991;68(6):626–628.
88. Asgari MA, Hosseini SY, Safarinejad MR, et al. Penile fractures: evaluation, therapeutic approaches and long-term results. *J Urol.* 1996;155(1):148–149.
89. Cline KJ, Mata JA, Venable DD, et al. Penetrating trauma to the male external genitalia. *J Trauma.* 1998;44(3):492–494.
90. Jezior JR, Brady JD, Schlossberg SM. Management of penile amputation injuries. *World J Surg.* 2001;25(12):1602–1609.
91. Bhanganada K, Chayavatana T, Pongnumkul C, et al. Surgical management of an epidemic of penile amputations in Siam. *Am J Surg.* 1983;146(3):376–382.
92. Carroll PR, Cattolica EV, Turzan CW, et al. Necrotizing soft-tissue infections of the perineum and genitalia. Etiology and early reconstruction. *West J Med.* 1986;144(2):174–178.
93. Sorensen MD, Krieger JN, Rivara FP, et al. Fournier's gangrene: management and mortality predictors in a population based study. *J Urol.* 2009;182(6):2742–2747.
94. McAninch JW. Management of genital skin loss. *Urol Clin North Am.* 1989;16(2):387–397.
95. Wolf JS Jr, Turzan C, Cattolica EV, et al. Dog bites to the male genitalia: characteristics, management and comparison with human bites. *J Urol.* 1993;149(2):286–289.

CHAPTER 30 ■ ACUTE CARE SURGERY: SKELETAL AND SOFT-TISSUE INJURY

GUSTAVO X. CORDERO, GARY S. GRUEN, PETER A. SISKA, AND IVAN S. TARKIN

Expert care of musculoskeletal injury in the polytrauma patient will lead to optimized long-term clinical outcomes. After the initial assessment and stabilization of the patient, the orthopedic trauma surgeon has the responsibility of thoroughly evaluating the pelvis and extremities for both bone and soft-tissue injury during the secondary survey. A collaborative effort, however, between the general trauma surgeon and the orthopedic surgeon is required to coordinate care and promote safe and efficacious treatment of the multiply injured patient.[1]

GENERAL PRINCIPLES

The evaluation of the trauma patient with musculoskeletal injury includes a complete history and physical with an extensive neurologic and vascular examination. Specific fractures and dislocations will pose a greater risk to surrounding neurovascular structures, and the status of these structures should be noted (Table 30.1). The soft tissue surrounding the fracture site needs to be scrutinized for any defects to determine if the fracture is open or closed. Musculoskeletal emergencies such as compartment syndrome or vascular injury need to be promptly identified.

Further, a tertiary survey is of the utmost importance considering that 15–20% of musculoskeletal injuries are initially missed in the polytrauma patient.[2] This should be performed after the initial 24–48 hours. At this point of time in the patient's treatment course, distracting injuries would have been stabilized and the patient can sometimes assist with localizing further sites of musculoskeletal trauma.

Beyond physical examination, imaging is a critical aspect of the orthopedic workup. At least two orthogonal radiographs that include the proximal and distal joints of the injured extremity should be obtained. Further dedicated radiographs and imaging modalities (computed tomography and magnet resonance imaging) should be ordered by the consulting orthopedist.

Initial Care: Realignment and Reduction

After achieving the diagnosis of fracture or dislocation, prompt delivery of orthopedic care is essential to stop the cycle of injury. Prompt reduction/relocation and splinting protects the soft-tissue envelope, including nerves and vasculature from further traumatic insult. Reductions and relocations should be performed after completion of the secondary survey. Fractures can be immobilized with a well-padded, plaster splint spanning the joint proximal and distal to the fracture site.

Open Fractures

Open fractures in a trauma patient are a site for bacterial proliferation and need to be treated with debridement of debris and necrotic tissue followed by irrigation to decrease bacterial loads. The energy imparted to produce an open fracture causes major stripping of muscle and periosteum with considerable devascularization to the bone. Inadequate debridement increases the risk of developing osteomyelitis, nonunion, and potential loss of limb. Antibiotics are an adjunct treatment to a thorough debridement of an open wound and cannot be used independently.

The Gustilo and Anderson classification continues to be the most commonly used system to describe and guide treatment of open fractures.[3] The grade of the fracture is determined by the extent of soft-tissue disruption, degree of contamination of the wound, and severity of the fracture. In applying the classification system, the extent of soft-tissue disruption can only be determined after a thorough debridement has been performed. A grade I fracture is the result of low-energy trauma with a wound that is <1 cm that was caused by protrusion of the bone through the skin or a low-velocity bullet. A wound >1 cm with minimal devitalized soft tissue and contamination that was caused by moderate energy is classified as a grade II fracture. Grade III fractures are caused by high-energy trauma and have extensive soft-tissue injury, gross contamination, a laceration >10 cm, or a segmental fracture. High-power rifles and close-range shotgun blasts impact substantial soft-tissue injury and should be treated as grade III fractures. The presence of adequate soft-tissue coverage with intact periosteum, substantial soft-tissue loss with exposed bone that will require tissue transfer for coverage, and the presence of a vascular injury requiring repair for limb preservation subdivide grade III fractures into grade IIIa, IIIb, and IIIc, respectively.

The initial management of open fractures begins in the trauma resuscitation area. Gross contamination should be removed from the wound. Following the application of a dressing and fracture reduction, fractures should be splinted to decrease pain, reduce hemorrhage, and prevent further soft-tissue injury. Patients with open wounds need antibiotic prophylaxis with tetanus toxoid and a first-generation cephalosporin. Grade III fractures and contaminated wounds also receive an aminoglycoside to prevent gram-negative infection. Barnyard injuries warrant prophylaxis against anaerobes, such as clostridium, with penicillin. In the operating room, it is recommended to debride tissue that lacks contractility, consistency, and the ability to bleed.[4] Loose, devitalized bone should be removed regardless of whether or not it is crucial to stabilization. It has been shown that delays of up to 24 hours do not influence infection rates; however, it is recommended to not delay surgical care of open fractures in a stable patient and perform the initial debridement within 6 hours.[5] The combination of low-pressure irrigation with mechanical scrubbing is effective in reducing bacterial loads.[6] There is no consensus regarding the use of additives in the irrigation fluid. Bacitracin has been shown to not degrade in irrigation solutions; it interferes in the cell wall synthesis of microbes without the risk of cell necrosis and delayed wound healing seen with povidone–iodine and chlorhexidine.[7] Definitive fixation can be performed with an infection rate of <2% following debridement and irrigation in grade I fractures and grade II fractures with minimal soft-tissue loss.[3] Grade III fractures and wounds with severe soft-tissue damage are treated in a staged fashion with temporary immobilization with an external fixator.

TABLE 30.1

NEUROVASCULAR INJURIES ASSOCIATED WITH ORTHOPEDIC TRAUMA

ORTHOPEDIC INJURY	NEUROVASCULAR INJURY
Anterior shoulder dislocation	Axillary nerve injury, axillary artery injury
Humeral shaft fracture	Radial nerve injury
Supracondylar humeral fracture	Brachial artery
Distal radius fracture	Median nerve injury
Perilunate dislocation	Median nerve injury
Posterior hip dislocation	Sciatic nerve injury
Supracondylar femoral fracture/knee dislocation	Popliteal artery injury/ thrombosis
Proximal fibular fracture	Peroneal nerve injury
Mangled extremity/tibial fracture	All neurovascular structures of the lower leg

Following a thorough debridement, soft-tissue defects can be temporarily covered with an antibiotic bead pouch or a vacuum-assisted wound closure. High concentrations of antibiotics can be delivered to a wound through the use of antibiotic cement. Traditionally, tobramycin or vancomycin have been combined with one package of bone cement. The antibiotic cement can then be formed into beads on a stainless-steel wire and placed within a soft-tissue defect at an open fracture. If there is inadequate tissue to close the wound, a bead pouch can be formed by sealing the wound with an adhesive drape (i.e., Ioban and Tegaderm).[8] The use of vacuum-assisted wound closure (VAC) has gained popularity in the treatment of traumatic wounds. Vacuum-assisted wound dressing devices have been shown to dramatically increase the formation of granulation tissue, decrease the wound bacterial count, and decrease edema following fasciotomies.[9,10] The rate of deep infections following open tibial fractures has been shown to decrease fivefold when using VAC dressings rather than standard wound care.[11] External fixators can be used to span fracture sites and maintain immobilization while allowing for monitoring of soft tissues. By restoring limb length and alignment, improved circulation promotes healing, reduces inflammation, and increases revascularization of devitalized tissue.

Wounds should continue to be taken to the operating room for repeat irrigation and debridement every 48–72 hours. Debridements need to be thorough with early removal of nonviable tissue to allow for timely preparation of the wound for soft-tissue coverage. Decreased infection and flap complication rates occur when flap coverage is performed within 7 days of injury.[12] The early involvement of a plastic surgeon will aid in the planning of reconstructive options.

Compartment Syndrome

Compartment syndrome is a surgical emergency. The diagnosis of compartment syndrome can be challenging, especially in a trauma patient who is sedated or intubated. The devastating outcomes associated with a missed compartment syndrome stress the importance of early diagnosis and fasciotomies (Fig. 30.1A). Compartment syndrome is the result of an elevated pressure within a closed myofascial compartment that results in microcirculatory failure and tissue ischemia. Fifty percent of compartment syndromes are associated with a fracture and are caused by hemorrhage and edema in the injured soft tissue around the fracture. Other etiologies include vascular injuries with reperfusion injury and crush injuries. A constrictive dressing or splint can cause circumferential constriction of an extremity with resulting compartment syndrome that generally resolves with loosening of the dressings. The leg and the forearm are the most common sites for compartment syndrome secondary to tighter, more robust fascial boundaries. Compartment syndrome can also occur in the hand or foot, and rarely does it occur in the deltoid, arm, buttock, or thigh.[13] The presence of an open fracture does not exclude the possibility of a concurrent compartment syndrome. Compartment syndrome has been noted to be present in 9% of open tibial fractures.[14]

The diagnosis is based on clinical examination findings. Compartment pressure measurements are reserved for uncooperative, intoxicated, sedated, or obtunded patients. The classic signs of compartment syndrome are the five Ps: pressure, paresthesia, pain, paralysis, and pulselessness. The presence of tense, noncompressible compartments is generally the presenting sign that will initiate evaluation for compartment syndrome. Pain that is out of proportion to what would be expected for a particular injury and pain with passive stretch of muscles are key signs that confirm the diagnosis. Increasing demands for pain medication are also indicative of a developing compartment syndrome. Pulselessness, paralysis, and paresthesias are late signs that indicate a missed compartment syndrome. The presence of pulses and a normal neurologic examination should not be used to exclude a compartment syndrome.

Invasive compartment measurements can be used to assist in making the diagnosis when clinical findings are questionable. The delta *P* can be calculated by the difference between the diastolic blood pressure and compartment pressure. Values of <30 mm Hg are associated with inadequate oxygen delivery to tissues and require fasciotomies for treatment of compartment syndrome.[15] The use of continuous monitoring of compartment pressures has been advocated for the obtunded patient.[16] In general, compartment pressures of >20 mm Hg should raise suspicion for the development of a compartment syndrome. If suspicion of a compartment syndrome is high, it is better to perform a preemptive fasciotomy rather than miss a compartment syndrome and face potential limb loss.

The treatment of compartment syndrome is emergent decompressive fasciotomies. In compartment syndromes involving the leg, the anterior, lateral, and deep posterior compartments are the most frequently involved. The two-incision technique provides a reliable method for decompressing all four compartments. A lateral incision is made between the tibial crest and the fibula to release the anterior and lateral compartments. Longitudinal fasciotomies are made over both compartments until the muscles are soft (Figs. 30.1B and 30.2). Care should be taken to protect the superficial peroneal nerve as it courses posterior to the lateral intermuscular septum (Fig. 30.1C). A medial incision is then made 2 cm posterior to the posterior boarder of the tibia. The proximal aspect of the soleus is released from the tibia to allow access to the deep posterior compartment. Longitudinal fasciotomies are then made through the deep and superficial posterior compartments.

Compartment syndrome in the forearm also requires decompressive fasciotomies with two incisions. A curvilinear incision is made over the volar aspect of the forearm from the antecubital fossa to the palm (Figs. 30.3 and 30.4). The superficial fascia, deep intramuscular fascia, and carpal tunnel should be released. If the dorsal compartments remain tense

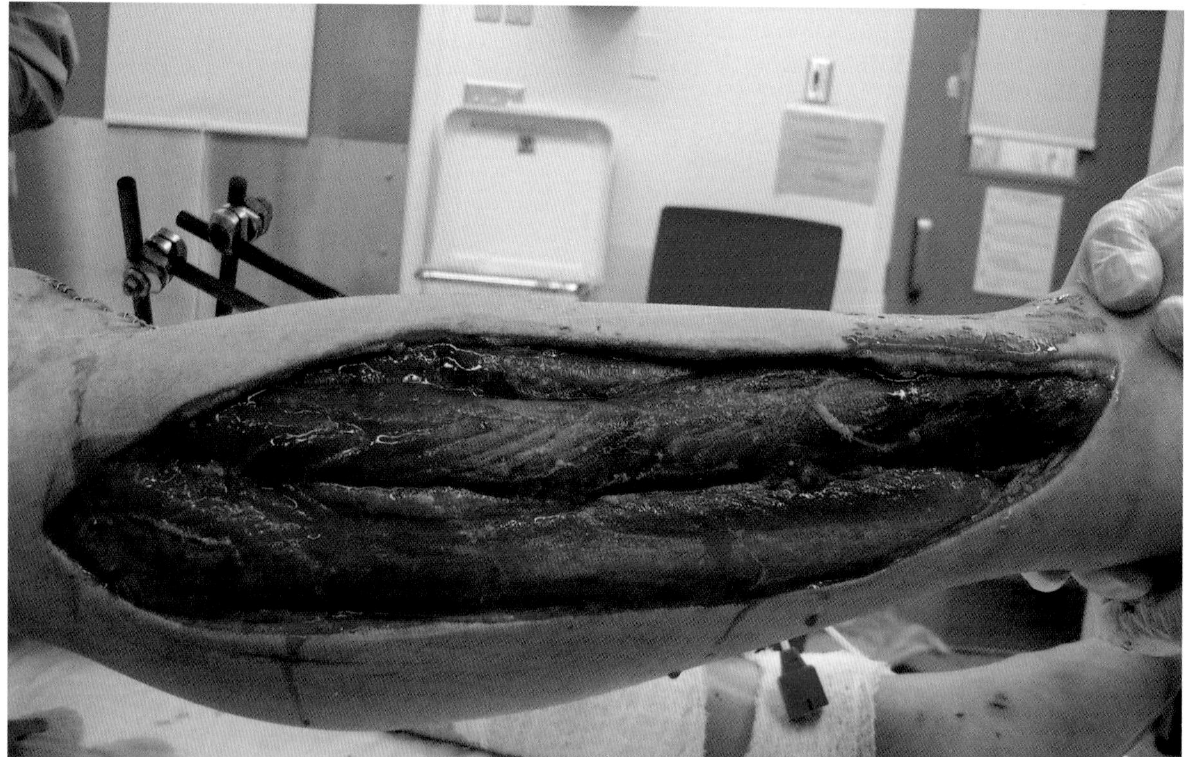

A

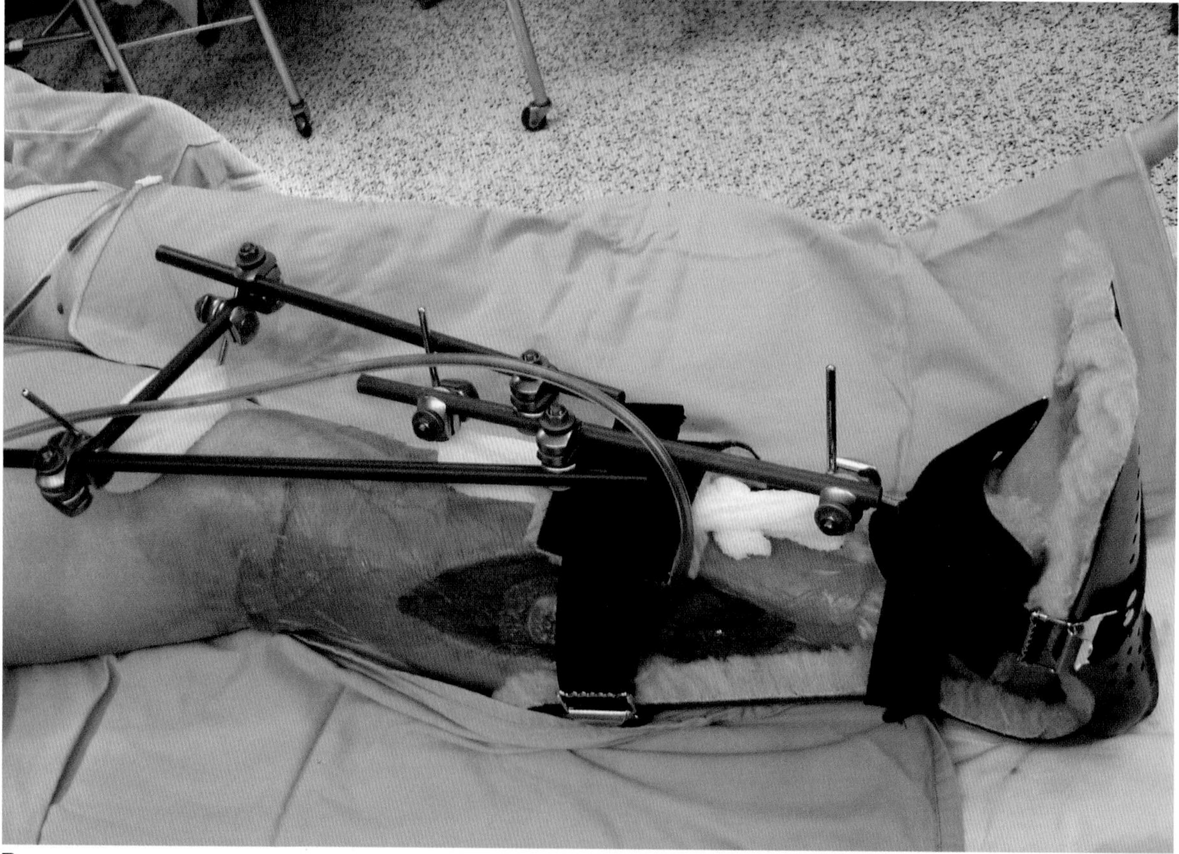

B

FIGURE 30.1. A: Necrotic muscle (anterior compartment) identified at the time of fasciotomy after delayed presentation of a compartment syndrome that resulted in permanent foot drop. B: Lateral-based longitudinal incision for release of both the anterior and lateral compartments of the leg in a patient with a segmental tibial shaft fracture. The fracture was provisionally stabilized with a spanning external fixation and a VAC was utilized to help decreased edema.

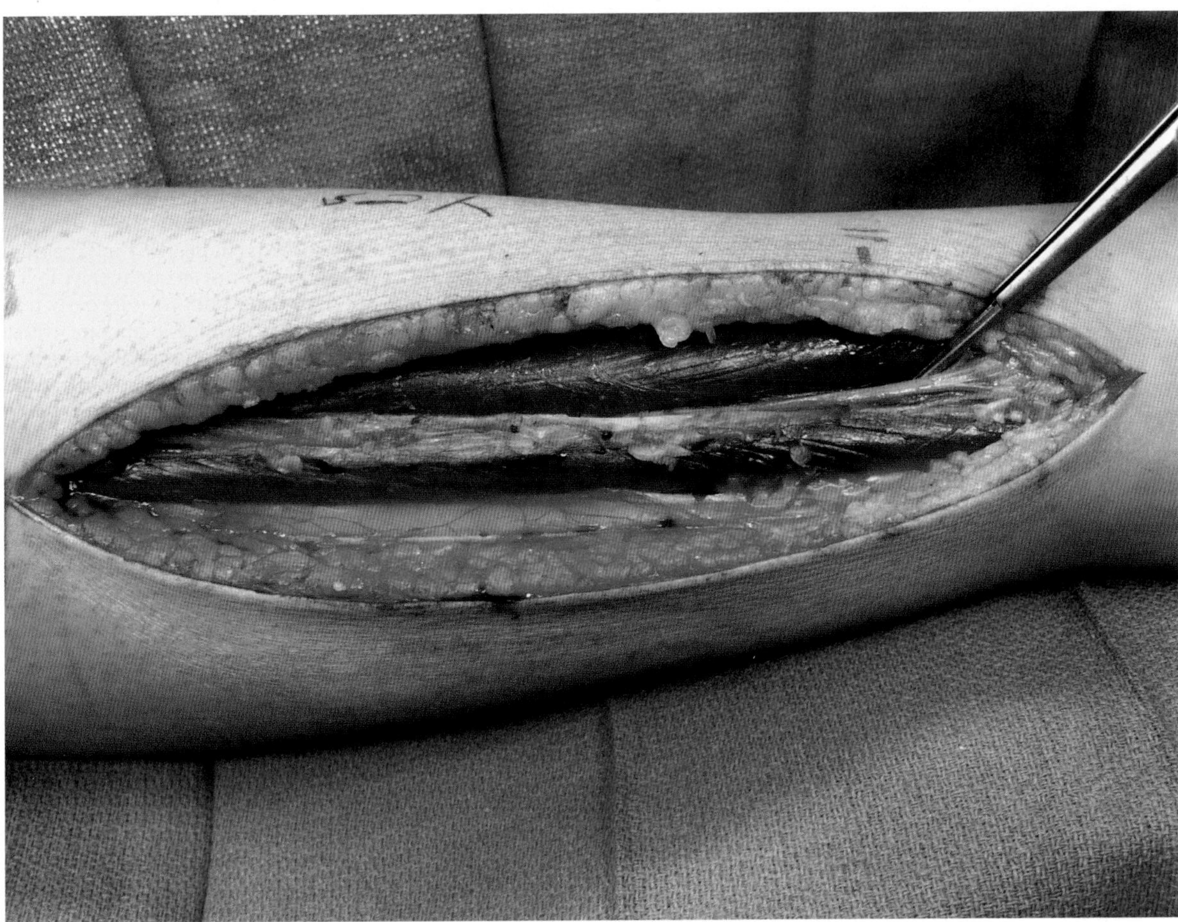

C

FIGURE 30.1. *(Continued)* C: The forceps marks the superficial peroneal nerve as it pierces through the fascia of the lateral compartment.

following volar fasciotomies, a longitudinal incision is made over the dorsal aspect of the forearm. Fasciotomies are then performed over the extensor compartment and mobile wad.

Vacuum-assisted dressing application following fasciotomies has been shown to significantly decrease the time to definitive wound closure (delayed primary closure or skin grafting) when compared to not using a VAC, 6.7 days and 16.1 days, respectively.[17] Irrigation and debridement of fasciotomy sites should be performed every 48–72 hours until delayed closure or skin grafting is performed.

Vascular Injury

A vascular consultation should be obtained if distal pulses are not equal to the contralateral extremity after reduction. In a patient in shock, pulses may be difficult to palpate and further evaluation with an ankle–brachial index (ABI) or an arteriogram can identify a vascular injury. If revascularization is deemed necessary, it should be emergently performed within 6 hours. Temporary or definitive fracture-dislocation stabilization needs to be performed prior to vascular repair to prevent reinjury or inappropriate tensioning of the vessel. An external fixator provides immediate, portable stabilization and can be applied quickly. The external fixator restores length and stability to facilitate vascular repair. Prophylactic fasciotomies should be performed to prevent reperfusion compartment syndromes.

Deep Vein Thrombosis and Pulmonary Embolism Prevention

The risk factors associated with the development of deep venous thrombosis (DVT) and pulmonary embolism (PE) are surgery, immobilization, fractures, and coagulopathy.[18] All of these risk factors are present in a multiply injured patient. The mortality rate for an untreated PE is 30%.[18] There continues to be controversy regarding the best prophylaxis for DVT. No significant decrease in the occurrence of DVT has been noted with the use of low-dose heparin, pneumatic compression devices, or arteriovenous foot pumps in the trauma patient.[19] Low-molecular-weight heparin has been indicated for DVT prevention in patients with pelvic fractures, complex lower extremity fractures that require surgical fixation, prolonged bed rest, and spinal cord injuries with complete or incomplete paralysis.[19] The use of vena cava filters has been recommended in patients who cannot receive anticoagulation secondary to ongoing bleeding or severe head injuries.[20]

MANAGEMENT OF INJURIES

Extremity Fractures

Fractures that involve the extremities can result in significant morbidity, decreased mobility, and post-traumatic arthritis.

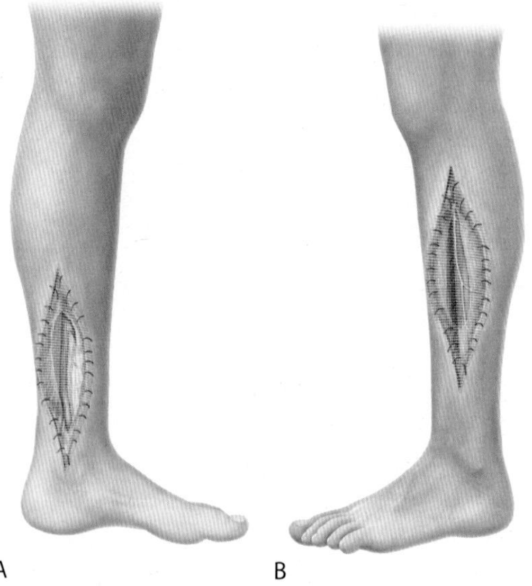

FIGURE 30.2. **A:** A lateral fasciotomy of the leg is performed by making a longitudinal incision from the proximal end of the fibula to the lateral malleolus and decompresses the anterior and lateral compartments. **B:** A medial incision situated between the anterior and posterior crests of the tibia provides a decompressive fasciotomy for the deep and superficial posterior compartments of the leg.

Extremity fractures can be seen in young patients who sustain high-energy trauma as well as elderly patients who sustain insufficiency fractures from low-energy mechanisms. The treatment modality and timing of surgical intervention for these injuries varies depending on the physiologic status of the multiply injured patient.

Damage Control Orthopedics

Early total care is the concept of stabilizing long-bone fractures acutely, especially for polytrauma patients. By stabilizing long-bone fractures, there is a subsequent decrease in fat emboli syndrome, mortality rate, and length of hospital stay. Over time, it was noted that some patients did not tolerate early total care and worsened with immediate definitive fracture treatments. This has led to the emergence of damage control orthopedics (DCO), with patients at risk of developing complications with acute fracture management being initially stabilized with provisional external fixation and less evasive procedures. However, it is still unclear what parameters can be used to identify at-risk patients who will benefit from DCO rather than early total care.

Patients with multiple trauma who survive the initial insult and the acute resuscitation period are subsequently faced with a 50% mortality rate from infection, acute respiratory distress syndrome (ARDS), and multiple organ failure.[21,22] Early total care is the preferred treatment in most polytrauma patients; however, an unfavorable immunologic response will be seen in a rare subset of these patients following acute definitive fracture fixation within the first 24 hours after injury.[23] The initial trauma has been referred to as the "first-hit" and the impact of the subsequent surgical burden as the "second-hit" phenomenon. To reduce the negative impact of the second hit, the principles of DCO were introduced.[24,25] The "second-hit" phenomenon may impact in particular those patients with more severe injury and initial physiologic derangement.[24] It appears the timing of secondary-hit phenomena may be most evident between days 3 and 5 following injury.[26]

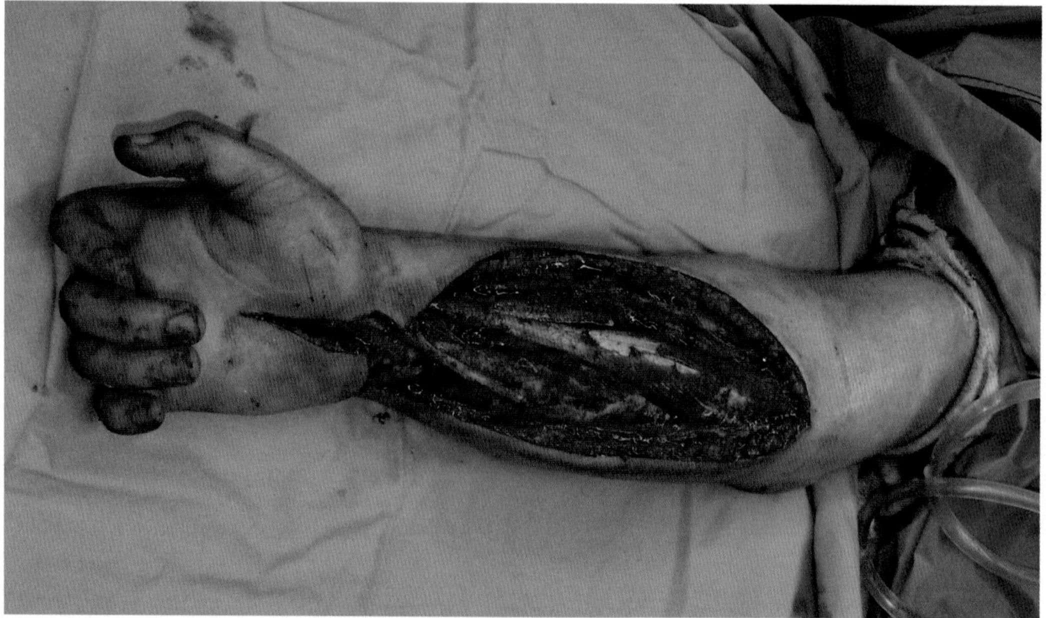

A

FIGURE 30.3. **A:** A patient with compartment syndrome of the forearm that was treated with complete release of the superficial fascia, deep intramuscular fascia, and carpal tunnel.

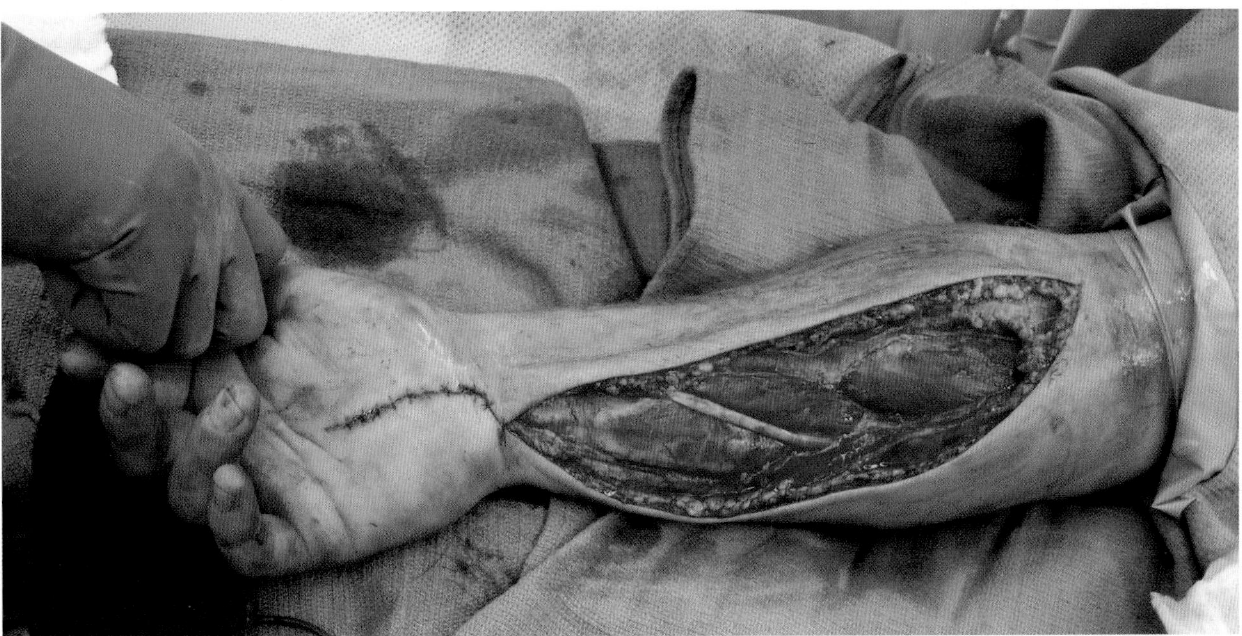

B

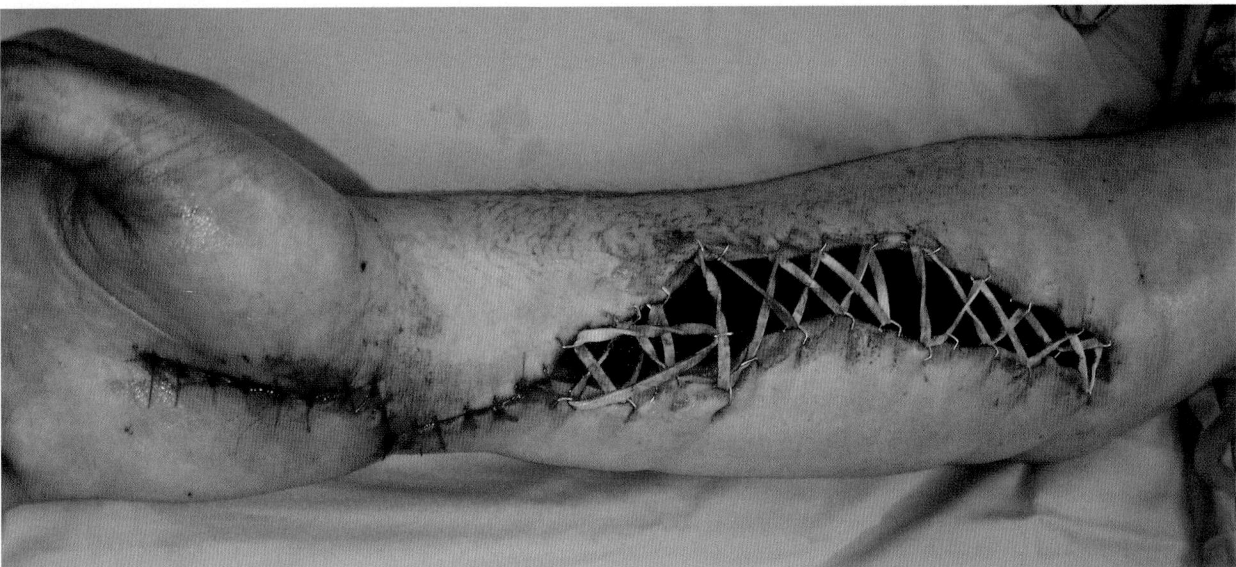

C

FIGURE 30.3. *(Continued)* B: Only the carpal tunnel portion could be reapproximated. C: A Jacob's ladder, utilizing vessel loop and staples, was used to approximate the tissues and minimize the area that would ultimately require a skin graft.

Diaphyseal Fractures

Diaphyseal fractures are frequently associated with high-energy traumas and many have associated injuries. Surgical goals are to restore limb length, alignment, and rotation while allowing for early mobilization of the patient. The use of provisional external fixation with delayed definitive treatment has been recommended to limit adverse surgical insult in unstable polytrauma patients. In the absence of pin-site infections, provisional fracture fixation with an external fixator for <2 weeks does not adversely affect definitive treatment with IMN.[27,28]

Initial imaging modalities of a grossly deformed lower extremity include orthogonal radiographs of the diaphysis and the proximal and distal joints. Fractures involving the articular margins are frequently seen with diaphyseal fractures. A computed tomography scan should be obtained prior to proceeding with surgical intervention if there is any concern for an articular fracture that would alter management. Femoral neck fractures are associated with 10% of femoral shaft fractures and approximately 30% are missed on initial evaluation.[29] A protocol with a dedicated internal rotation AP radiograph of the hip, fine-cut CT scan through the femoral neck, intraoperative fluoroscopic lateral radiograph of the hip, and postoperative AP and lateral radiographs of the proximal femur has been recommended to better detect and treat associated femoral neck fractures.[30]

Acute intramedullary nailing is the treatment choice for most diaphyseal fractures. Fat embolism syndrome occurs when marrow fat macroglobules are released from the intramedullary canal following a long-bone fracture, especially

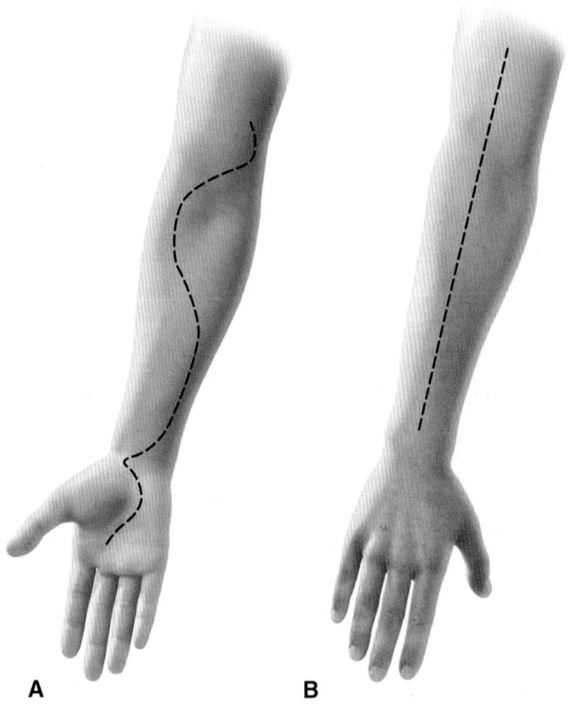

FIGURE 30.4. **A:** A curvilinear incision spanning over the volar aspect of the forearm from the antecubital fossa to the palm is used to decompress the superficial and deep compartments of the volar forearm. **B:** The dorsal compartments are released by performing a longitudinal incision over the dorsal aspect of the forearm.

in the femoral shaft. The lack of venous valves in the femur allows canal contents to drain into the bloodstream. After the fat emboli are released to the bloodstream, the emboli are surrounded by activated platelets that together cause an intense inflammatory response in the lung. The inflammatory response results in increased vasoconstriction and increased pulmonary artery pressures that can exacerbate pulmonary problems in a multiply injured patient.[31] Urgent stabilization of long-bone fractures has been recommended to decrease fat embolization, which is primarily accomplished with intramedullary nailing. The use of early external fixation followed by delayed intramedullary nailing has been shown to have decreased systemic inflammation when compared to early intramedullary nailing.[32] The degree of fat embolization has been shown to be greatest during nailing insertion with only minor differences during reaming.[27]

Open reduction and internal fixation (ORIF) with plates and screws is infrequently used to treat diaphyseal fractures since IMN minimizes soft-tissue stripping, devascularization of bone fragments, and infection rates. ORIF does have a role in the treatment of proximal and distal metadiaphyseal fractures with articular extension, ipsilateral femoral neck fracture, the presence of a total joint arthroplasty, extremely small intramedullary canals, and when there is a preexisting deformity that prevents the use of IMN.

Periarticular Fractures

The treatment of periarticular fractures varies from the management of diaphyseal fractures in that the articular surface must be anatomically reduced in addition to restoring alignment, length, and rotation. Inadequate restoration of the articular surface predisposes the patient to post-traumatic arthritis. Surgery must frequently be delayed to allow for soft-tissue swelling to decrease as well fracture blisters to resolve prior to definitive treatment. This is most evident in the treatment of tibial plateau and distal tibial pilon fractures.[33,34] The extensive surgical approaches that must be made to reduce and stabilize periarticular fractures may lead to further soft-tissue insult and failure to allow for the resolution of the initial swelling can result in postoperative wound complications. Patients must be closely monitored for signs of compartment syndrome and if fasciotomies are performed, the incisions must be placed to allow for subsequent surgical approaches to be made during definitive fixation.

A two-staged approach is frequently utilized in treating tibial plateau and pilon fractures when significant soft-tissue injury is present.[33] Initial management requires reduction of the fracture with realignment of the articular segment through ligamentotaxis. Acute application of a spanning external fixator allows for realignment of the joint, restoration of length, and immobilization to facilitate soft-tissue healing. In pilon fractures, the fibula can be acutely plated to assist in restoration of length and to maintain the talus reduced in the mortise if, soft tissues allow. Plain radiographs and CT scans are required to adequately visualize the fracture. CT scans should be obtained after the fracture has been reduced and length restored. CT scans allow for evaluation of intra-articular depression that must be addressed during definitive fixation.

When soft-tissue swelling has decreased, fracture blisters have reepithelialized, and skin wrinkles have returned definitive fixation can be performed. The surgical principles of ORIF of periarticular fractures are restoration of length, anatomic reduction of the articular surface, and bone grafting of metaphyseal defects. Nonsurgical management of periarticular fractures is generally reserved for patients that are nonambulatory, a poor surgical candidate secondary to comorbidities, or significant soft-tissue injury that precludes surgery.[35]

PELVIC FRACTURES

Incidence, Mechanism, and Associated Injuries

Pelvic fractures can result from low-energy trauma, such as a ground-level fall in the elderly, or from high-energy trauma, such as motor vehicle and motorcycles crashes, pedestrians struck by motor vehicles, and falls from heights. Stable fracture patterns generally result from low-energy trauma and can be managed nonoperatively. Surgery is generally required for the treatment of the unstable fractures that are caused by high-energy trauma.

Between 3% and 5% of traffic accidents are associated with pelvic injuries and account for 74% of unstable pelvic ring disruptions.[36,37] Among the unstable pelvic ring disruptions, more than 88% are associated with injuries to the head, chest, abdomen, spine, or long bones.[38] Urogenital injury (bladder disruption, urethra disruption, and vaginal tear), vascular injury, or bowel injury are the most commonly associated intrapelvic injury.[36] The mortality rate may be as high as 50% in complex pelvic ring disruptions.[39]

Clinical Evaluation

A trauma patient should be evaluated for a pelvic injury concurrently with resuscitation, especially in the setting of hypotension. The evaluation begins with obtaining a history and clinical examination. The involvement of the orthopedic team should occur as soon as a pelvic disruption is suspected. A communicative patient with a pelvic fracture may complain of pelvic pain and the inability to void if there is a urethral disruption.[37]

During the physical examination, it is critical to thoroughly examine the soft tissue around the pelvis for a laceration or degloving injury. While maintaining spine precautions, a patient can be logrolled to allow adequate evaluation of the posterior pelvis for lacerations or hematomas. The early identification of an open pelvic injury can facilitate an urgent exploratory laparotomy and a diverting colostomy. Approximately 4% of pelvic fractures are open and have a 50% mortality rate.[37],[40] Active bleeding through a soft-tissue defect in an open pelvic fracture poses a major challenge. The patient can rapidly exsanguinate since the fracture is no longer contained. Early blood transfusions, pressure tamponade of soft-tissue bleeding in the trauma room, urgent laparotomy for control of bleeding from extrapelvic sources, pelvic packing, and an arteriogram with embolization can assist with management of this problem.[40,41] Only 1% of pelvic fractures have a major vascular disruption; however, these disruptions result in a 75% mortality rate.[42]

In males, the scrotum should be examined for testicular displacement and the urethral meatus for blood. A urethral injury cannot be excluded by the absence of blood at the urethral meatus and can be further evaluated with a retrograde urethrogram or cystogram. The pubic symphysis should be palpated for diastasis and the rami for crepitus. A visual and bimanual pelvic examination should be conducted in females to evaluate for lacerations of the urethra, vagina, or rectum. Vaginal lacerations with healthy tissue should be irrigated and closed, whereas perineal lacerations are generally managed with serial debridements and delayed closure.

Urethral injuries should be evaluated with a rectal examination before inserting a Foley catheter. Urethral disruptions are more common in males and commonly occur below the urogenital diaphragm. A displaced prostate is indicative of a urethral disruption. The presence of blood with a digital rectal examination requires further evaluation with anoscopy and proctoscopy. A rectal tear with a pelvic fracture warrants irrigation of the wound and a diverting colostomy. Proctoscopy should also be considered for all patients with significantly displaced pelvic fractures, which can perforate the rectum.

Pelvic instability can be difficult to assess manually. Rotational stability can be evaluated with direct pelvic compression and vertical stability with the push–pull maneuver of the lower leg. Once pelvic instability has been identified, further stressing should be avoided to prevent excessive bleeding and patient discomfort. A detailed motor and sensory examination of the lower extremities should also be performed to assess for a neurologic injury.

Radiographic Evaluation

An anteroposterior pelvis radiograph should be obtained on all patients involved in a high-energy trauma and those with pelvic pain following a low-energy trauma. Pelvic inlet and outlet views should be obtained to evaluate anteroposterior and vertical displacement of the hemipelvis, respectively. It is important to remember that the displacement observed on radiographs is a static representation of a dynamic process that could have recoiled following the initial injury.

A computed tomography (CT) scan of the pelvis with 3 mm contiguous cuts should be obtained to evaluate the magnitude of the fracture or joint displacement and compression of the sacral foramina. Displacement of the posterior pelvic complex by >5 mm indicates significant posterior or vertical instability. The CT defines the pelvic injury in greater detail than radiographs and allows for more accurate preoperative planning.

Classification

There are various classification systems used to describe pelvic injuries; however, Tile's classification system based on the instability of the bony injury is the most commonly used (Table 30.2). The force vectors involved during injury correlate with the associated injuries seen with pelvic fractures.[44] Lateral compression fractures are associated with lung, spleen, liver, and closed head injuries, whereas anteroposterior compression fractures are associated with bladder, urethra, rectum, lower extremity, and chest injuries. Vertical shear fractures are associated with neurovascular injury, calcaneal fractures, and thoracolumbar fractures.

Type A fractures are stable, minimally displaced, and usually associated with low-energy trauma (Fig. 30.5A). They are further divided by the presence of pubic rami fractures, avulsion injuries, and transverse sacral or coccyx fractures. Type B fractures are characterized by rotational instability but maintain vertical stability (Fig. 30.5B). The pubic symphysis, rami, or both are involved anteriorly and the sacrum, sacroiliac joint, or both are involved posteriorly. Injuries can be ipsilateral and contralateral. Vertical instability characterizes type C fractures. Disruptions of the anterior and posterior pelvis result in vertical displacement of one or both hemipelvis (Fig. 30.5C).

Treatment

Patients with pelvic injuries can present hemodynamically unstable and require immediate pelvic immobilization during resuscitation (Algorithm. 30.1). Exposed fracture surfaces, venous plexus disruptions, and arterial tears can lead to pelvic hemorrhage. By closing down the potential space in the pelvis, blood loss can be decreased through tamponade. Circumferential pelvic antishock sheeting (CPAS), pelvic binder, C-clamp, military antishock trousers (MAST), or external fixation can be utilized to temporarily immobilize an unstable pelvis.

TABLE 30.2

TILE'S CLASSIFICATION SYSTEM FOR PELVIC RING INJURIES

TYPE	STABILITY	SUBTYPE
A	Stable	A1—Fractures of the pelvis not involving the ring A2—Stable, minimally displaced fractures of the ring
B	Rotationally unstable, vertically stable	B1—Open book B2—Lateral compression: ipsilateral B3—Lateral compression: contralateral (bucket handle)
C	Rotationally and vertically unstable	C1—Unilateral C2—Bilateral C3—Associated with an acetabular fracture

Ref. [43] (From Tile M. Pelvic ring fractures: should they be fixed? *J Bone Joint Surg.* 1988;70:1–12.)

TRAUMA

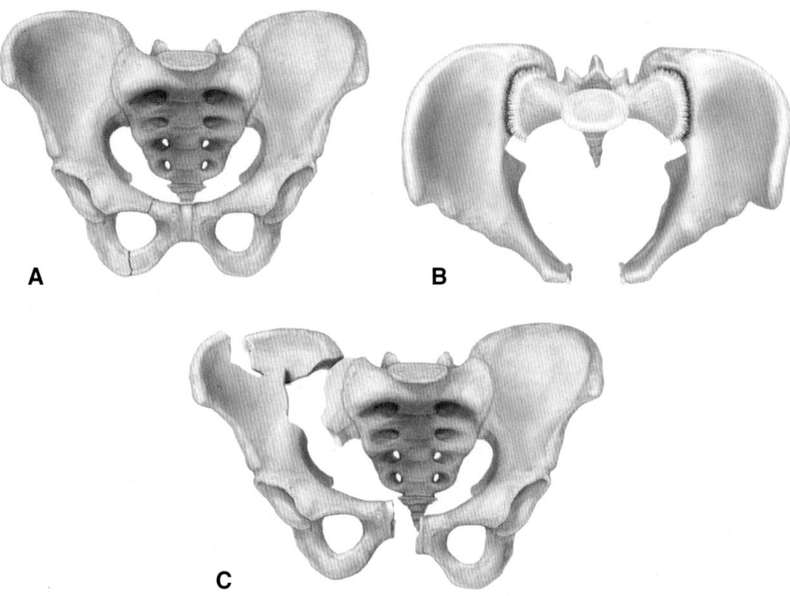

FIGURE 30.5. **A:** Stable, minimally displaced pelvic ring fracture. **B:** Rotationally unstable with pubic symphysis diastasis. **C:** Vertically and rotationally unstable pelvic fracture with disruption of both the anterior and posterior elements with vertical displacement of the hemipelvis.

CPAS has gained great acceptance since it is small, transportable, inexpensive, easily applied, provides satisfactory pelvic stability, and continues to allow access to the abdomen and lower extremities.[45] CPAS is applied by taking a sheet that has been folded lengthwise into widths of approximately 18 inches and placing it around the pelvis at the level of the pubic symphysis. The pelvis is then closed and stabilized as the sheet is tensioned and crossed anteriorly as a compressive force is applied on the lateral buttocks.

External fixators are commonly used to rapidly stabilize pelvic ring disruptions. There are both anterior and posterior systems available to treat specific injury patterns. Anterior pelvic external fixation provides stability by closing the pelvis anteriorly through the use of pins placed into the iliac crests or supra-acetabular area. In some patients, the posterior pelvic deformity may be increased with anterior pelvic stabilization and a pelvic C-clamp has been advocated.[39] The C-clamp compresses and stabilizes the posterior pelvic ring through two pins that are placed in the posterior ilium. The application of a C-clamp can be challenging especially in patients with posterior pelvic deformities and a too posterior position can result in insufficient stabilization. External fixation is the initial treatment of choice for open pelvic fractures.

Patients who continue to have hemodynamic instability despite adequate volume resuscitation, correction of coagulopathy, treatment of extrapelvic sources of bleeding, and temporary pelvic stabilization require angiographic evaluation and embolization [46]. Hemodynamic instability from the pelvis is defined as ongoing resuscitation of >6 units of packed red blood cells in a 4-hour time span. Superior gluteal artery injuries have been associated with displaced pelvic fractures through the sciatic notch.

Definitive treatment of a pelvic ring disruption is with open reduction and internal fixation in order to stabilize all disrupted elements (Algorithm. 30.1). Internal fixation should be delayed in the setting of an open fracture, and the use of an external fixator with serial debridements should continue until a clean wound is produced. The anterior pelvis can be stabilized acutely during a laparotomy in a hemodynamically unstable patient or on a delayed basis in a stable patient.[47] Incisions used for a laparotomy or placement of a suprapubic tube should be placed as cephalad and central as possible to prevent future compromise of surgical incisions used for anterior pelvic open reduction and internal fixation. Posterior pelvic fractures can be treated with either open reduction internal fixation or percutaneous placement of iliosacral screws under fluoroscopic guidance. A posterior approach with foraminal decompression may be required to treat displaced sacral fractures with nerve root impingement.

KNEE DISLOCATIONS

Knee dislocations are limb-threatening injuries that require evaluation for neurovascular disruptions. Many knee dislocations present spontaneously reduced; therefore, a knee with multiligamentous injuries should be considered a reduced knee dislocation. There can be significant stretching of the popliteal artery with a knee dislocation. The popliteal artery is tethered proximally at the adductor hiatus and distally deep to the soleus. During a knee dislocation, the popliteal artery is tethered at these two fibrous tunnels and a vascular injury can result. Knee dislocations are commonly described as the position of the tibia relative to the femur. Anterior knee dislocations are usually the result of a hyperextension injury and can injure the artery by traction with a resulting intimal tear 39% of the time.[48] A complete arterial transection can occur in up to 44% of posterior dislocations, which are the result of a posterior force applied to the anterior tibia.[48] The initial disruption may be a minor intimal tear and the vascular examination can remain normal.[49] Intimal tears are thrombogenic and a delayed thrombosis can occur many hours after injury. If the lower extremity is splinted to stabilize the knee dislocation, the thrombosis may not be recognized and significant damage can occur that results in subsequent limb loss.

The evaluation of a patient with a knee dislocation begins with a physical examination. The neurovascular status of the

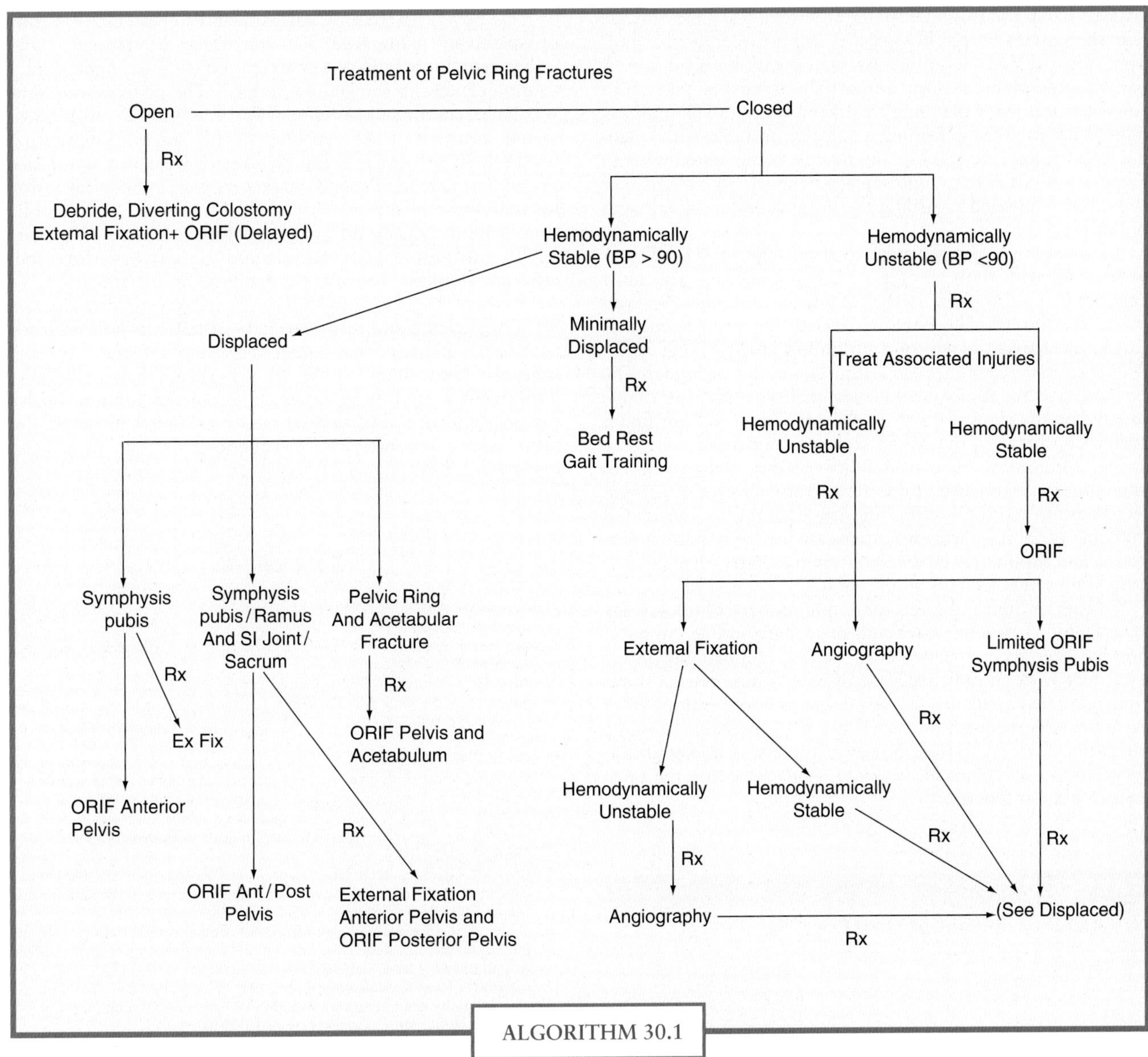

ALGORITHM 30.1 Algorithm for the treatment of polytrauma patients with pelvic ring fractures.

extremity should be noted and an immediate reduction of the dislocated knee should be performed. If pulses (dorsalis pedis and posterior tibial arteries) are absent prior to reduction and do not return following reduction, the patient should be taken immediately to the operating room for vascular exploration. Once a damaged segment is identified, it should be excised and reanastomosed with a reverse saphenous vein graft. A spanning knee external fixator should be considered prior to vascular repair to maintain the joint reduced, prevent damage to the neurovascular structures, and protect the articular surfaces.

If pulses are present before and after reduction, it is recommended to obtain an ankle–brachial index (ABI), especially if pulses are asymmetrical. A palpable pulse can remain despite vascular injury secondary to collateral blood flow.[50] An ABI of <0.9 has yielded sensitivities of 95%-100% in detecting clinically significant popliteal artery injury and warrants further evaluation with a duplex ultrasound.[50] Confirmation of arterial injury on the duplex ultrasound requires arteriography to further delineate the lesion and evaluate for possible vascular intervention.[51] ABIs of >0.9 have been associated with negative predictive values of 99% for major flow limiting arterial injury and should be followed with serial examinations every 4 hours for 48 hours.[52] Once vascular injuries have been addressed and the knee has been stabilized with an external fixator, surgical versus nonsurgical management can be discussed with the patient.

THE MANGLED LOWER EXTREMITY

The mangled lower extremity includes a wide spectrum of injuries with possible severe bony injury, soft-tissue disruption, vascular compromise, neurologic injury, and gross contamination. These injuries are difficult to manage and require the effort of many subspecialties, including general surgery, orthopedic surgery, vascular surgery, and plastic surgery. It is critical that prior to undertaking an attempt at limb salvage that the patient be physiologically able to tolerate the multiple surgeries and blood loss associated with limb salvage. A patient's underlying medical comorbidities must be taken into consideration when planning treatment options. The multiply injured patient that is hemodynamically unstable with ongoing hemorrhage or coagulopathy may be better suited with an amputation rather than limb salvage, whereas a stable patient should be counseled regarding the benefits and disadvantages of limb salvage.

Many scoring systems exist to determine the viability of proceeding with limb salvage versus amputation. The most commonly used system is the Mangled Extremity Severity Score (MESS).[53,54] The MESS is based on age, presence of shock, mechanism of injury, and limb ischemia (Table 30.3). Amputation is recommended with a score of 7 or higher. The Lower Extremity Assessment Project (LEAP) study was unable to validate the clinical utility of the MESS and did not find a correlation between the MESS score and functional outcome at 6 or 24 months.[55] The availability of subspecialty resources and surgeon experience at different treatment centers are not factored into scoring systems and can account for substantial outcome variability. Scoring systems are unable to predict outcomes and should not be the determining factor when considering limb salvage versus amputation.

Further recommendations for amputation over limb salvage have included ischemia time and neurologic injury. Amputation has been recommended in the setting of a mangled lower extremity with an ischemia time of over 6 hours or an unreconstructable vascular injury. An insensate foot resulting from a tibial nerve transection has historically been an absolute indication for amputation; however, there was no significant difference in outcomes in the LEAP study based on the presence of plantar sensation.[56]

TABLE 30.3

MANGLED EXTREMITY SEVERITY SCORE

AGE (Y)	POINTS
<30	0
30–50	1
>50	2
SHOCK	**POINTS**
Systolic blood pressure > 90 mm Hg	0
Transient hypotension	1
Persistent hypotension	2
EXTREMITY INJURY	**POINTS**
Low energy	1
Medium energy	2
High-energy crush	3
High-energy contamination	4
LIMB ISCHEMIA	**POINTS**
Normal perfusion	0
Pulseless, paresthesias	1
Cool, paralyzed	2

From Johansen K, Daines M, Howey T, et al. Objective criteria accurately predict amputation following lower extremity trauma. *J Trauma*. 1990;30(5):568–573.

The Lower Extremity Assessment Project (LEAP) study prospectively compared the outcomes of patients who underwent limb salvage versus amputation at eight level 1 trauma centers in the United States.[57] The primary outcome was based on the sickness impact profile (SIP), a multidimensional measure of self-reported health status. Amputation versus limb salvage and injury severity were not significant prognostic factors. Prognostic factors were rehospitalization for major complication, a low educational level (noncompletion of high school), poverty, nonwhite race, lack of private health insurance, poor social-support network, low self-efficacy, smoking history, or pending injury litigation.[58,59] At 7 years, both groups demonstrated severe disability in 40% of patients and just over 50% of patients had returned to work.[59] Patients that underwent limb salvage were significantly more likely to be rehospitalized than those who underwent amputation; however, projected lifetime health care costs were found to be three times higher in the amputation group secondary to prosthetic costs than those who underwent limb salvage.[60]

References

1. Agnew SG, Anglen JO. Delivery of orthopaedic trauma care. In: Baumgaertner MR, Tornetta III, eds. *Orthopaedic Knowledge Update Trauma 3*. 3rd ed. Rosemont, IL: American Academy of Orthopaedic Surgeons; 2005:11–20.
2. Pape HC, Giannoudis P, Rockwood C. The care of the multiply injured patients. In: Bucholz RB, Heckman JD, Brown CC, eds. *Rockwood and Green's Fractures in Adults*. 6th ed. Philadelphia, PA: Lippincott Williams & Wilkins; 2005.
3. Gustilo RB, Anderson JT. Prevention of infection in the treatment of one thousand and twenty-five open fractures of long bones: retrospective and prospective analyses. *J Bone Joint Surg Am*. 1976;58:453–458.
4. Scully RE, Artiz CP, Sako Y. An evaluation of the surgeon's criteria for determining the viability of muscle during debridement. *Arch Surg*. 1956;72:1031–1035.
5. Crowley DJ, Kanakaris NK, Giannoudis PV. Debridement and wound closure of open fractures: the impact of the time factor on infection rates. *Injury*. 2007;38:879–889.
6. Svoboda SJ, Bice TG, Gooden HA, et al. comparison of bulb syringe and pulsed lavage irrigation with use of a bioluminescent musculoskeletal wound model. *J Bone Join Surg Am*. 2006;88(10):2167–2174.
7. Petrisor B, Jeray K, Schemitsch E, et al. FLOW Investigators: fluid lavage in patients with open fracture wounds (FLOW): an international survey of 984 surgeons. *BMC Musculoskelet Disord*. 2008;9:7.
8. Henry SL, Ostermann PA, Seligson D. The antibiotic bead pouch technique. The management of severe compound fractures. *Clin Orthop Relat Res*. 1993;295:54–62.
9. Tarkin IS. The versatility of negative pressure wound therapy with reticulated open cell foam for soft tissue management after severe musculoskeletal trauma. *J Orthop Trauma*. 2008;22(10 suppl):S146–S151. Review.
10. Webb LX. New techniques in wound management: Vacuum-assisted wound closure. *J Am Acad Orthop Surg*. 2002;10(5):303–311.
11. Stannard JP, Volgas DA, Stewart R, et al. Negative pressure wound therapy after severe open fractures: A prospective randomized study. *J Orthop Trauma*. 2009;23(8):552–557.
12. Bhattacharyya T, Mehta P, Smith M, et al. Routine use of wound vacuum-assisted closure does not allow coverage delay for open tibia fractures. *Plast Reconstr Surg*. 2008;121(4):1263–1266.
13. Thorpe SW, Tarkin IS. Deltoid compartment syndrome is a surgical emergency. *J Shoulder Elbow Surg*. 2010;19(8):e11–e13.
14. Blick SS, Brumback RJ, Poka A, et al. Compartment syndrome in open tibial fractures. *J Bone Joint Surg Am*. 1986;68(9):1348–1353.
15. McQueen MM, Christie J, Court-Brown CM. Compartment pressure monitoring in tibia fractures. *J Bone Joint Surg Br*. 1996;78:99–104.
16. White TO, Howell GE, Will EM, et al. Elevated intramuscular compartment pressures do not influence outcome after tibial fracture. *J Trauma*. 2003;55(6):1133–1138.
17. Yang CC, Chang DS, Webb LX. Vacuum-assisted closure for fasciotomy wounds following compartment syndrome of the leg. *J surg Orthop Adv*. 2006;15(1):19–23.
18. Carson JL, Kelley MA, Duff A, et al. The clinical course of pulmonary embolism. *N Engl J Med*. 1992;326(19):1240–245.
19. Rogers FB, Cipolle MD, Velmahos G, et al. Practice management guidelines for the prevention of venous thromboembolism in trauma patients: the EAST practice management guidelines work group. *J Trauma*. 2002;53(1):142–164.

20. Velmahos GC, Kern J, Chan LS, et al. Prevention of venous thromboembolism after injury: an evidence-based report–part II: analysis of risk factors and evaluation of the role of vena caval filters. *J Trauma*. 2000;49(1):140–144.
21. Bone RC. Toward an epidemiology and natural history of SIRS (systemic inflammatory response syndrome). *JAMA* 1993;270(8):939.
22. Pfeifer R, Tarkin IS, Rocos B, et al. Patterns of mortality and causes of death in polytrauma patients: has anything changed? *Injury*. 2009;40(9):907–911.
23. Pape HC, Schmidt RE, Rice J, et al. Biochemical changes after trauma and skeletal surgery of the lower extremity: quantification of the operative burden. *Crit Care Med*. 2000;28(10):3441–3448.
24. Pape HC, Hildebrand F, Pertschy S. Changes in the management of femoral shaft fractures in polytrauma patients: from early total care to damage control orthopedic surgery. *J Trauma*. 2002;53(3):452–462.
25. Schreiber VM, Tarkin IS, Hildebrand F, et al. The timing of definitive fixation for major fractures in polytrauma: a matched-pair comparison between a US and European level 1 centres: analysis of current fracture management practice in polytrauma. *Injury*. 2010;42(7):650–654.
26. Brundage SI, McGhan R, Jurkovich GJ, et al. Timing of femur fracture fixation: effect on outcome in patients with thoracic and head injuries. *J Trauma*. 2002;52(2):299–307.
27. Bhandari M, Zlowodzki M, Tornetta P III, et al. Intramedullary nailing following external fixation in femoral and tibial shaft fractures. *J Orthop Trauma*. 2005;19(2):140–144.
28. Harwood PJ, Giannoudis PV, Probst C, et al. The risk of local infective complications after damage control procedures for femoral shaft fracture. *J Orthop Trauma*. 2006;20(3):181–189.
29. Watson JT, Moed BR. Ipsilateral femoral neck and shaft fractures: complications and their treatment. *Clin Orthop Relat Res*. 2002;399:78–86.
30. Tornetta P III, Kain MS, Creevy WR. Diagnosis of femoral neck fractures in patients with femoral shaft fracture: improvement with a standard protocol. *J bone Joint Surg Am*. 2007;89(1):39–43.
31. Pape HC, Rixen D, Morely J, et al. Impact of the method of initial stabilization for femoral shaft fractures in patients with multiple injuries at risk for complications (borderline patients). *Ann surg*. 2007;246(3):491–501.
32. Harwood PJ, Giannoudis PV, van Griensven M, et al. Alterations in the systemic inflammatory response after early total care and damage control procedures for femoral shaft fracture in severely injured patients. *J Trauma*. 2005;58(3):446–452.
33. Tarkin IS, Clare MP, Marcantonio A, et al. An update on the management of high-energy pilon fractures. *Injury* 2008;39:142–154.
34. Tarkin IS, Sop A, Pape HC. High-energy foot and ankle trauma: principles for formulating an individualized care plan. *Foot Ankle Clin*. 2008;13(4):705–723.
35. Kline AJ, Gruen GS, Pape HC, et al. Early complications following the operative treatment of pilon fractures with and without diabetes. *Foot Ankle Int*. 2009;30(11):1042–1047.
36. Gansslen A, Pohlemann T, Paul C, et al. Epidemiology of pelvic ring injuries. *Injury*. 1996;27(suppl 1):S-A13–A20.
37. Routt ML Jr, Nork SE, Mills WJ. High-energy pelvic ring disruptions. *Orthop Clin North Am*. 2002;33:59–72.
38. Flint L, Babikian G, Anders M, et al. Definitive control of mortality from severe pelvic fractures. *Ann Surg*. 1990;211:703–706.
39. Giannoudis PV, Pape HC. Damage control orthopaedics in unstable pelvic ring injuries. *Injury*. 2004;35:671–677.
40. Poole GV, Ward EF, Muakassa FF, et al. Pelvic fractures from major blunt trauma: outcome is determined by associated injuries. *Ann Surg*. 1991;213:532–538.
41. Riemer BL, Butterfield SL, Diamond DL, et al. Acute mortality associated with injuries to the pelvis: the role of early patient mobilization and external fixation. *J Trauma*. 1993;35:671–675.
42. Rothenberger D, Velasco R, Strate R, et al. Open pelvic fracture: a lethal injury. *J Trauma* 1978;18(3):184–187.
43. Tile M. Pelvic ring fractures: should they be fixed? *J Bone Joint Surg*. 1988;70:1–12.
44. Dalal SA, Burgess AR, Siegel JH, et al. Pelvic fracture in multiple trauma: classification by mechanism is key to pattern of organ injury, resuscitative requirements, and outcome. *J Trauma*. 1989;29(7):981–1002.
45. Routt ML Jr, Falicov A, Woodhouse E, et al. Circumferential pelvic antishock sheeting: a temporary resuscitation aid. *J Orthop Trauma*. 2002;16:45–48.
46. Panetta T, Scalfani SJ, Goldstein AS, et al. Percutaneous embolization for massive bleeding from pelvic fractures. *J Trauma* 1985;25:1021–1029.
47. Gruen GS, Leit ME, Gruen RJ, et al. The acute management of hemodynamically unstable multiple trauma patients with pelvic ring fractures. *J Trauma*. 1994;36:706–711.
48. Green NE, Allen BL. Vascular injuries associated with dislocation of the knee. *J Bone Joint Surg Am*. 1977;59:236–239.
49. Wagner WH, Clakins ER, Weaver FA, et al. Blunt popliteal artery trauma: one hundred consecutive injuries. *J Vasc Surg*. 1988;7:736.
50. Seroyer ST, Musahl V, Harner CD. Management of the acute knee dislocation: the Pittsburgh experience. *Injury*. 2008;39(7):710–718.
51. Mills WJ, Barei DP, McNair P. The value of the ankle-brachial index for diagnosing arterial injury after knee dislocation: a prospective study. *J Trauma*. 2004;56:1261–1265.
52. Johansen K, Lynch K, Paun M, Copass M. Non-invasive vascular tests reliably exclude occult arterial trauma in injured extremities. *J Trauma*. 1991;31:515–522.
53. Helfet DL, Howey T, Sanders R, et al. Limb salvage versus amputation: preliminary results of the Mangled Extremity Severity Score. *Clin Orthop*. 1990;256:80–86.
54. Johansen K, Daines M, Howey T, et al. Objective criteria accurately predict amputation following lower extremity trauma. *J Trauma*. 1990;30(5):568–573.
55. Ly TV, Travison TG, Castillo RC, et al. LEAP study group: ability of lower-extremity injury severity scores to predict functional outcome after limb salvage. *J bone Joint Surg Am*. 2008;90(8):1738–1743.
56. Bosse MJ, McCarthy ML, Jones AL, et al. Lower Extremity Assessment Project (LEAP) Study Group: The insensate foot following severe lower extremity trauma: an indication for amputation? *J Bone Joint Surg Am*. 2005;87(12):2601–2608.
57. MacKenzie EJ, Bosse MJ, Kellam JF, et al. Characterization of patients with high-energy lower extremity trauma. *J Orthop Trauma*. 2000;14(7):455–466.
58. Bosse MJ, MacKenzie EJ, Kellam JF, et al. An analysis of outcomes of reconstruction or amputation after leg-threatening injuries. *N Engl J Med*. 2002;347(24):1924–1931.
59. Cannada LK, Jones AL. Demographic, social and economic variables that affect lower extremity injury outcomes. *Injury*. 2006;37(12):1109–1116.
60. MacKenzie EJ, Jones AS, Bosse MJ, et al. Health-care costs associated with amputation or reconstruction of a limb-threatening injury. *Bone Joint Surg Am*. 2007;89(8):1685–1692.

CHAPTER 31 ■ EXTREMITY VASCULAR INJURIES

DAVID V. FELICIANO

HISTORY

Vascular injuries in the extremities have been reported since antiquity. Aulus Cornelius Celsus (25 BC-50 AD) first described that hemorrhage from such injuries could be treated by placing "ligatures... above and below the wounded part."[1] For the next 18 centuries, control of hemorrhage dominated all medical writings on extremity vascular injuries. Repair of an injured brachial artery was first performed in 1759 and reported by Hallowell in 1762.[2] The first repair of an injured artery in an extremity (the common femoral artery) in the United States was reported by John B. Murphy in Chicago in 1897.[3] Essentially all the modern suture techniques of vascular repair in the extremities were described by Charles C. Guthrie and Alexis Carrel during and after their collaboration in the Hull Physiological Laboratory at the University of Chicago from 1905 to 1906.[4,5]

Surgeons in military conflicts who made considerable contributions to the repair of vessels in the extremities over the past century have included the following: Sir George Henry Makins (1853–1933) in World War I; Michael E. DeBakey (1908–2008), Daniel C. Elkin (1883–1958), and Harris B. Shumacker, Jr. (1908–2009) in World War II; Frank C. Spencer (1925-) and Carl W. Hughes (1914-) in the Korean War; and Norman M. Rich (1934-) during the Vietnam War.[6] Recognizing that other forms of therapy are now used on occasion to treat vascular injuries in the extremities, the early laboratory description of stents/stent grafts was by the late Charles T. Dotter in 1969.[7]

EPIDEMIOLOGY

When considering all injuries admitted to military or civilian hospitals prior to the current conflicts in Iraq and Afghanistan, vascular injuries are uncommon. Frykberg and Schinco[8] noted that the incidence of vascular injuries in four military reports (1913; 1946; 1952; 1978) ranged from 0.4% to 2%, while two civilian reports (1991; 1992) had incidences ranging from 0.8% to 3.7%. Of interest, the distribution of vascular injuries varies widely in the United States. The incidence of vascular injuries in the extremities as a percentage of all vascular injuries has ranged from 38% to 50% in centers dealing with a significant number of gunshot wounds to >75% in centers dealing primarily with blunt trauma.[9]

TYPES OF INJURIES/ PATHOPHYSIOLOGY

There are seven recognized types of vascular injuries: (1) intimal injuries (flaps, defects, or subintimal hematomas); (2) partial wall defects (intima and media) presenting as traumatic "true" aneurysms; (3) complete wall defects presenting as traumatic "false" aneurysms or hemorrhage; (5) complete transections; (6) arteriovenous fistulas; and (7) spasm. Intimal injuries and partial wall defects continue to be most commonly associated with blunt trauma (i.e., blunt posterior dislocation of the knee joint with secondary thrombosis of the popliteal artery). In contrast, complete wall defects, near-complete or complete transections, and arteriovenous fistulas are most commonly associated with penetrating wounds. Arterial spasm can occur after either blunt or penetrating trauma to an extremity and is frequently noted distal to a proximal arterial injury that is occlusive.

PROGNOSTIC FACTORS

The age of the patient is a major factor in the success of peripheral arterial repair. With most peripheral arterial injuries occurring in patients under the age of 35 years, repairs are straightforward as vessels are soft, mobile, and without appreciable atherosclerosis. These characteristics allow for easy debridement and primary repair or end-to-anastomosis without the insertion of substitute vascular conduits in many patients. On the other hand, young patients do not have as many collateral vessels as might be seen in an older patient with slow atherosclerotic occlusion of the superficial femoral artery at Hunter's canal. For this reason, the superficial femoral artery, popliteal artery, and tibioperoneal trunk should be regarded as "end" arteries in which acute occlusion is a threat to the viability of the ipsilateral leg or foot.

Shock secondary to the injury to the extremity or to other injuries has many adverse effects on a subsequent arterial or venous repair. The "viscerocutaneous vasoconstriction" that is associated with hypovolemic shock decreases whatever arterial inflow that remains through an injured artery or any regional collaterals and increases distal ischemia. With decreased distal flow, in situ thrombosis of capillaries, arterioles, or even named arteries may occur in the lower leg. Finally, ischemia followed by restoration of arterial inflow is the classical sequence of the "ischemia-reperfusion" syndrome.[10] This syndrome increases edema of ischemic tissues distal to an arterial injury and may cause a compartment syndrome in the leg or forearm after arterial repair.[11]

The magnitude of a peripheral arterial or venous injury obviously impacts the success of a repair. When segmental resection of an injured vessel and insertion of an interposition graft, particularly a small Teflon one, are necessary, long-term patency is decreased.[12]

The impact of delay of an arterial repair on the success of salvaging an injured extremity is well known. The original description of the "6-hour window" to complete a major arterial repair in an injured extremity in dogs was described in 1949.[13] Of interest, the 6-hour window continues to be valid in humans with major arterial injuries in extremities based on the time of onset of neural necrosis and myonecrosis when "cold ischemia" (no collateral flow) is present.[14]

The presence of an associated venous injury has a major impact on outcome. The need to simultaneously clamp an injured major artery and vein in a lower extremity increases the likelihood that a postrepair distal compartment syndrome will occur.[11] In addition, ligation of a major vein in the lower extremity, such as the common femoral vein, had a significant adverse effect on femoral arterial inflow in one laboratory study.[15] Finally, the presence of multiple associated injuries to soft tissue, tendons, bones, and nerves in an extremity—the so-called "mangled extremity"—will result in amputation rates of 28%-78% when the major artery is occluded or transected.[16]

DIAGNOSIS

Physical Examination

A patient with "hard" signs of a peripheral arterial injury (external hemorrhage, pulsatile hematoma, decrease in or loss of pulse and distal ischemic signs or palpable thrill/audible bruit) should be moved to the operating room immediately with several exceptions.[17] It is appropriate to realign any displaced fracture with traction or a splint or to reduce any dislocated joint in the pulseless extremity to see if distal pulses return. In patients who are pulseless at the ankle or wrist and there is a shotgun wound to the extremity with wide dispersal of pellets or blunt trauma with fractures at several levels, some type of imaging study will be useful in localizing the site of injury. The final exception would include a patient with multiple injuries in whom there is a need to rule out life-threatening injuries to the brain, thorax, or abdomen using CT before moving the patient to the operating room.

Most patients present with "soft" signs of an arterial injury (history of arterial bleeding, proximity of extremity injury to a named artery, nonpulsatile hematoma, or injury to adjacent nerve).[18] These patients still have an arterial pulse at the ankle or wrist on physical examination or with use of the Doppler device. Depending on which soft sign or combination of soft signs is present, the incidence of arterial injuries in such patients ranges from 3% to 25%.[19–21] Most but not all, of these arterial injuries can be managed without surgery because they are small and, by definition, allow for continuing distal perfusion. In some centers, serial physical examinations alone are used to monitor distal pulses, and no CT—arteriogram or conventional arteriogram—is performed to document the magnitude of a possible arterial injury. This approach has been safe and accurate in asymptomatic patients with penetrating wounds to an extremity in proximity to a major artery.[20,22] Its accuracy is similar in higher kinetic energy injuries associated with blunt fractures or dislocations, particularly dislocations of the knee.[23] Observation is appropriate only with complete and continuing out-of-hospital follow-up.[19,20] When there is concern about a distal pulse deficit, inability to properly examine for distal arterial pulses, or a combination of soft signs of an arterial injury in an extremity, CT, conventional, or surgeon-performed arteriography or a duplex ultrasound should be performed.

Based on the discussion above, it is obvious that a comprehensive physical examination of the injured extremity is the prime diagnostic maneuver in patients with possible peripheral vascular injuries. Relying on physical examination, particularly in patients with "soft" signs of an arterial injury in an extremity, has decreased considerably the number of imaging studies performed in the past 20 years.

Arterial Pressure Index

An adjunct to the physical examination is the measurement of the arterial pressure index (API). The API is defined as the Doppler systolic pressure in the injured extremity divided by that in an uninjured extremity.[24–26] In a study by Lynch and Johansen[25] in which clinical outcome was the standard, an API lower than 0.90 had a sensitivity of 95%, specificity of 97.5%, and accuracy of 97% in predicting an arterial injury. An alternative when both lower extremities are injured is to use the ankle brachial index, which uses brachial artery pressure as the denominator.

When the patient has an API < 0.9, the current standard of care is to perform an imaging study on the injured extremity.[18,24–26]

Imaging Studies

Multidetector computed tomography arteriography (MDCTA) is rapidly replacing conventional radiology suite arteriography or surgeon-performed arteriography in the emergency center or operating room.[27,28] It can be performed rapidly with a reasonable amount of contrast and accuracy approaching conventional arteriography. When MDCTA is not available or the result is equivocal and the patient is hemodynamically stable, percutaneous intraarterial digital subtraction arteriography performed in a radiology suite by the interventional radiologist is the most commonly used invasive diagnostic technique. Of interest, this technique can now be performed in the trauma room with a mobile device.[29] Multiple sequential views of areas of suspected arterial injury can be obtained at differing intervals after injection of limited amounts of dye. The accuracy of this multiple-view technique has been demonstrated in many studies, although false-negative results have occurred. The disadvantages of the technique are the delays in diagnosis when on-call technicians must return to the hospital, the cost of modern equipment, and the distortion of images when metallic fragments are present (e.g., shotgun wound).[16]

When the patient is hemodynamically unstable or has multiple injuries, a rapid one- or two-shot surgeon-performed percutaneous arteriogram can be performed in the emergency center or operating room.[30,31] A thin-walled 18-gauge Cournand-style disposable needle is inserted either proximal to the area of suspected injury (e.g., in the common femoral artery for evaluation of the superficial femoral artery) or distal to it (e.g., in retrograde evaluation of axillary or subclavian arteries above a blood pressure cuff inflated to 300 mm Hg). Rapid hand injection of 35 mL of 60% diatrizoate meglumine dye is performed, and an anteroposterior radiographic view is taken or fluoroscopy is utilized. The timing for exposure of an x-ray film of the patient's extremity depends on which artery is to be evaluated. Proper evaluation of the tibial and peroneal arteries in the patient with a complex fracture of the tibia mandates that exposure not take place until 4–5 seconds after the injection of dye into the common femoral artery. The plane of the film is often changed before the second injection to examine the area in question more thoroughly. False-negative and false-positive results are rare when the technique is performed on a daily basis by experienced practitioners. If a patient has severe combined intracranial or truncal trauma and possible peripheral arterial lesions, life-threatening injuries should be treated first, followed by percutaneous intraoperative arteriography of the involved extremity.[16]

Duplex ultrasonography, a combination of real-time B-mode ultrasound imaging and pulsed Doppler flow detection, has been used extensively to evaluate patients with suspected peripheral vascular injuries. Accuracy has ranged from 96% to 100% in several studies.[32–34] The major disadvantage is the need for the study to be performed and interpreted by an experienced vascular surgeon or registered vascular technologist.

MANAGEMENT IN THE EMERGENCY CENTER

Hemorrhage resulting from a peripheral vascular injury is controlled by direct compression with a finger or compression dressing, compression at a "pressure point" or the application of a blood pressure cuff or tourniquet just proximal to the area of injury. Once hemorrhage is under temporary control in the patient with multisystem blunt trauma, a decision is made on which diagnostic imaging studies are necessary before transfer to the operating room.

When a peripheral arterial occlusion is associated with a delay in treatment or distal "cold ischemia" (inadequate or no collateral flow), the administration of intravenous heparin (100 U/kg) in the emergency center is appropriate. Contraindications include near-exsanguination from other injuries (coagulopathy may occur), a traumatic brain injury, a traumatic false aneurysm of the descending thoracic aorta or any other truncal artery, or CT documentation of an injury to a solid organ in the abdomen. Hemodynamically stable patients with isolated injuries to the extremities and "soft" signs undergo diagnostic evaluation and/or observation as described previously.

NONOPERATIVE MANAGEMENT/ STENTS/EMBOLIZATION

Nonoperative Management

Nonocclusive arterial injuries including intimal defects or flaps, subintimal or intramural hematomas, spasm, and small pseudoaneurysms that are nonobstructing are present on imaging in some patients with "soft" signs on presentation. On follow-up arteriograms, 87%-95% of these lesions have healed without any surgical or radiologic intervention.[35,36] Early arteriographic follow-up is necessary in patients who develop new symptoms while being observed. Careful follow-up of the injured patient and the extremity in an outpatient setting for a period of 2 months is mandatory.

Endovascular Stents

Currently, there is limited experience with the use of stents or stent grafts to treat peripheral arterial injuries.[37,38] This is a reflection of the excellent results obtained with operative management of these injuries for the past 60 years.[8,12,16] Therefore, the use of endovascular stents or stent grafts for peripheral vascular injuries should be limited to institutions in which there are approved protocols with plans for long-term follow-up of patients.[18]

Therapeutic Embolization by Interventional Radiology

Extravasation, a pseudoaneurysm, and arteriovenous fistula in the profunda femoris artery, one of the arteries in the leg or one of the branches of a major peripheral artery can be managed by embolization by an interventional radiologist. The ideal patient for such an intervention would be one with multisystem injuries, closed fractures, or late diagnosis of a traumatic aneurysm following orthopedic reconstruction.[36]

OPERATIVE MANAGEMENT

Preparation/Draping

Extensive preparation and draping of the skin is necessary. For a vascular repair in the upper extremity, this includes the chin to umbilicus and contralateral nipple to ipsilateral fingernails as well as one entire lower extremity to the toenails. In the lower extremity, preparation and draping would be from nipples to bilateral toenails. The hand or foot is then placed in a sterile plastic bag to allow for easy palpation of pulses after the arterial repair has been performed. Another option is to cover the entire extremity with an orthopaedic stockinette.

Preliminary or Concurrent Fasciotomy

Some patients have symptoms and signs of a compartment syndrome in the upper or lower extremity related to the peripheral vascular injury when first evaluated in the emergency center. For example, a patient with occlusion of the popliteal artery or a large hematoma in the anterior compartment of the leg might present with the following: (1) hypesthesia in the dorsal first web space; (2) weakness of toe extension and foot dorsiflexion; and (3) pain on passive toe flexion and foot plantar flexion.[11] A measurement of compartment pressure is appropriate when symptoms and signs are suggestive, but unclear, or when there does not appear to be excessive swelling of the compartment. If there is physical evidence or a compartment pressure documenting the presence of a compartment syndrome distal to an arterial injury, a preliminary or concurrent (with the arterial repair) fasciotomy is indicated.[39]

Incisions

A longitudinal incision is made over the area of the peripheral vascular injury. Examples would include the medial arm incision in the biceps–triceps groove to expose the brachial artery or the anteromedial thigh incision to expose the superficial femoral artery beyond its origin in the groin. When the area of injury is in proximity to a joint, a gently curved incision is made to prevent a postoperative scar contracture. Examples would include the following: (1) axillobrachial "S" over an injury to the distal axillary/proximal brachial vessels (Fig. 31.1); (2) medial-to-lateral "S" over the antecubital area of the upper extremity to expose the distal brachial artery and its bifurcation; and (3) obtuse incision over the medial knee joint to expose the entire popliteal artery.

Proximal and Distal Vascular Control

Once the skin incision is made, it is deepened proximally and distally around the area of the presumed vascular injury to allow for vascular control. In other words, the part of the incision over the area of the presumed vascular injury is only deepened when proximal and distal vascular control has been

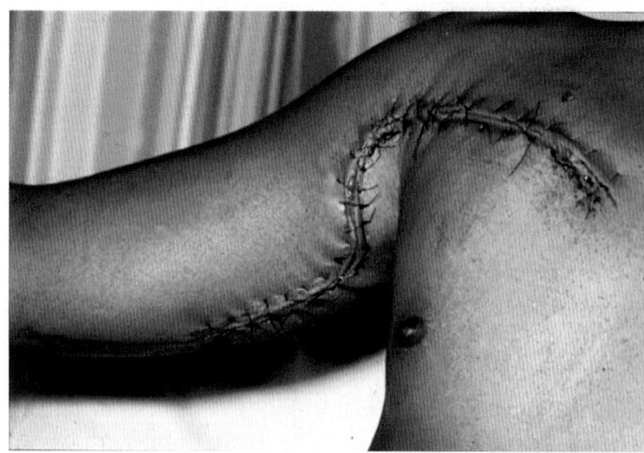

FIGURE 31.1. Standard incision for exposure of entire axillary and brachial arteries. (Reprinted from Feliciano DV. Peripheral vasculature. In: Britt LD, Trunkey DD, Feliciano DV, eds. *Acute Care Surgery. Principles and Practice*. New York: Springer;2007:661, with permission from Springer.)

attained with the use of small DeBakey vascular clamps, bulldog clamps, or vessel loops.

When hemorrhage cannot be controlled or a large hematoma is present, it is appropriate to enter the area of injury and rapidly apply vascular clamps directly around the perforation in the peripheral artery and/or vein. Adequate suction devices and appropriate retractors are mandatory to limit blood loss during this approach, but it allows for quicker vascular control in experienced hands.

Temporary Intraluminal Vascular Shunts

Once proximal and distal vascular control has been attained, there are two clinical scenarios in which insertion of a temporary intraluminal vascular shunt rather than repair or ligation is appropriate. The first is near-exsanguination with secondary hypothermia, a metabolic acidosis, or a coagulopathy likely to occur during resuscitation and operation. Rather than follow the classical dictum of "life over limb" and perform a ligation of an injured major artery of vein that may lead to an ultimate amputation, a shunt is inserted into the injured vessel. Once damage control resuscitation in the intensive care unit has reversed the "metabolic failure" of near-exsanguination, the patient is returned to the operating room for removal of the shunt and vascular repair.[40,41]

The second scenario is when a "mangled extremity" has resulted from a high kinetic injury impact (i.e., car bumper, motorcycle crash, penetrating wound from a military rifle) (Fig. 31.2). As previously noted, the combination of injuries to artery, bone, soft tissue, muscles/tendons, and peripheral nerves has resulted in ultimate amputation rates of 42%-78% in older series.[42,43] There are, however, patients without all the components of injury listed who will be candidates for limb salvage instead of amputation. These patients have an intact posterior tibial nerve in the lower extremity or a crush injury with a limited warm ischemia time (i.e., <6 hours) in the upper or lower extremity. If limb salvage is to be considered or if the patient and family object to an immediate amputation, a shunt is inserted into the injured vessel.

The technique for insertion of a temporary intraluminal shunt is quite simple. For peripheral arterial injuries, a No. 14-Fr. or smaller rigid carotid artery-type shunt is cut to a length approximating the distance between the two ends of the debrided vessel plus another 3–4 cm. A 2-0 silk tie is placed around the middle of the shunt as a marker, a hemostat is applied to the same location, and the shunt is inserted into the proximal arterial stump for 1.5–2.0 cm. Another 2-0 silk tie is placed around the end of the artery containing the short segment of shunt and tied tight to compress the artery down onto the shunt. Proximal arterial control is released, the hemostat around the middle of the shunt is removed, and flow through the shunt is verified. The hemostat is placed on the middle of the shunt again, and the distal end of the shunt is directed into the distal end of the artery for 1.5–2.0 cm. Another 2-0 silk tie is placed to compress the distal artery around the distal end of the shunt, and the hemostat on the shunt is removed. Arterial pulsations in the distal extremity are then verified by physical examination or use of a Doppler-device. When a large peripheral vein is to be shunted rather than ligated, thoracostomy tubes in the No. 16–24 Fr. size range are used rather than the smaller arterial shunts described above.

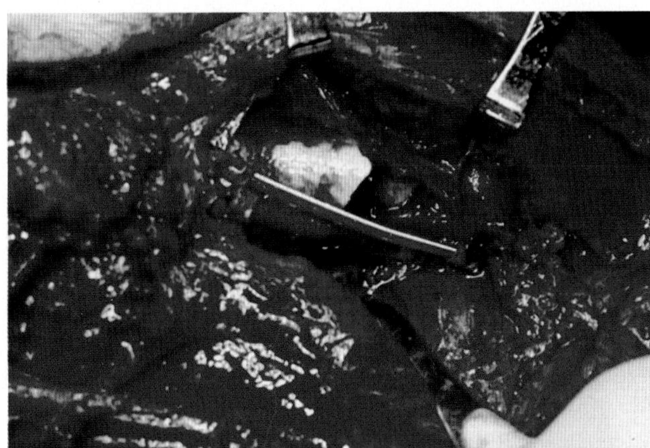

FIGURE 31.2. A 14-F "carotid artery" shunt in the popliteal artery and a 24-F thoracostomy tube shunt in the popliteal vein in a railroad worker with a crush injury to the distal thigh. (Reprinted from Feliciano DV. Peripheral vasculature. In: Britt LD, Trunkey DD, Feliciano DV, eds. *Acute Care Surgery. Principles and Practice*. New York, NY: Springer; 2007:670, with permission from Springer.)

The largest possible shunt that can be inserted in either a peripheral artery or vein is chosen. With use of a large shunt, postoperative anticoagulation is neither necessary nor appropriate in patients with multiple injuries or with substantial defects in soft tissues as might be seen with a mangled extremity. Thrombosis of an arterial shunt occurs when too small or too long a shunt is inserted, when a major adjacent vein is ligated rather than shunted, or when a delay in treatment has allowed for distal in situ thrombosis of multiple small arteries or veins in the leg or forearm. Thrombosis of an arterial shunt is an ominous predictor in that many such patients will eventually require amputation. This is particularly true when there is a delay in recognition of the thrombosis in the intensive care unit.

The longest dwell time for an arterial intraluminal shunt in a recent large civilian series was 52 hours,[41] but there is one report of a patient with a 10-day dwell time in the right axillary artery without anticoagulation.[44] Once the patient is stable or a decision has been reached that limb salvage is appropriate, the patient is returned to the operating room for removal of the shunt. The prior segmental resection of the injured vessel and the placement of crushing 2-0 silk ties on the remaining ends to hold the shunt in place mandate that an interposition graft will be inserted into the injured vessel. Therefore, an appropriate length of saphenous vein from the thigh or ankle of an uninjured lower extremity is removed in the usual fashion prior to removal of the arterial shunt. Should there be a large soft tissue defect over the arterial defect, a much longer segment of saphenous vein will have to be removed so that an extra-anatomic bypass (to be discussed) can be performed.[44,45] When a large peripheral vein such as the axillary, common femoral, or superficial femoral is to be repaired (to be discussed), no retrieval of the saphenous vein will be necessary unless the surgeon is committed to constructing a panel or spiral vein graft. In many centers, this type of complex reconstruction is avoided and a large ringed polytetrafluoroethylene (PTFE) graft is inserted.[12]

Arterial Repair—Upper Extremity

Injuries to the axillary, brachial, radial, or ulnar arteries account for approximately 45%-52% of peripheral arterial injuries treated in civilian trauma centers.[8,9] Because of its length and exposed position in the upper extremity, injuries to the brachial artery are 3–3.5 times more common than those to the axillary artery.

With suspected or documented injuries to the axillary artery, it is helpful to cover the entire upper extremity in an orthopedic stockinette and place it at the side of the patient if

TRAUMA

an injury to the first or second portion is suspected. This will allow for more room for the operating team as well as relax the muscles around the shoulder girdle as dissection proceeds. With a suspected injury to the third portion of the axillary artery, the upper extremity is abducted at 90° and placed on an armboard.

The axillary artery starts at the lateral border of the first rib and becomes the brachial artery at the lateral border of the teres major muscle. The operative approach varies depending on whether the arterial injury is located in the first portion (lateral border of the first rib to medial border of the pectoralis minor muscle), second portion (behind the pectoralis minor muscle), or third portion (lateral border of the pectoralis minor muscle to lateral border of teres major muscle). Injuries to the first or second portions that are not actively hemorrhaging are most commonly approached through an infraclavicular incision centered on the midclavicle.[46] After splitting the upper fibers of the pectoralis major muscle in a transverse fashion, the clavipectoral fascia is divided. Proximal arterial control is obtained by retracting the anteriorly positioned axillary vein in an inferior fashion and placing a vessel loop around the axillary artery just inferior to the clavicle. Distal control is obtained, as needed, by extending the infraclavicular incision into an incision in the deltopectoral groove. Should active hemorrhage from the second portion of the artery occur during dissection or the tamponaded injury is in the second portion, lateral retraction of the tendon of the pectoralis minor tendon is necessary. Persistent inadequate exposure of this arterial location mandates division of the tendon of the pectoralis minor muscle near the coracoid process to preserve the medial pectoral nerve. An injury in the third portion can be approached through the aforementioned incision in the deltopectoral groove. An alternate, but uncommonly utilized, approach involves a lateral pectoral incision along the edge of the pectoralis major muscle.

Injuries to the axillary artery, particularly those that are bleeding actively, are challenging because of the adjacent cords of the brachial plexus. The blind application of angled vascular clamps often entraps portions of the cords, leading to a partial brachial plexopathy for 12–24 months. Therefore, elevation of the injured artery proximally and distally with vessel loops is mandatory before vascular clamps are applied. The second problem in dealing with injuries at this location is the somewhat fragile nature of the axillary artery. This artery is rarely involved with substantial atherosclerosis and is extraordinarily soft with a consistency that sometimes approaches that of the subclavian artery. Lateral repairs performed with suture bites that are too thin or end-to-end repairs performed under tension will lead to sutures tearing through when vascular clamps are released.

The brachial artery starts at the lateral border of the teres major muscle, courses through the medial arm, and bifurcates at the radial tuberosity of the forearm. The operative approach in the arm has been described previously. When an injury occurs near the elbow, the standard S-shaped incision extending from the medial biceps–triceps groove is used. This incision crosses the antecubital fossa and then turns longitudinally beyond the midaspect of the volar side of the forearm. The fascia overlying the neurovascular bundle medially and the bicipital aponeurosis beneath the antecubital fossa are divided to allow for complete exposure of the brachial artery proximal to its bifurcation.

There is a logical sequence for performing a complex repair (end-to-end anastomosis or insertion of a graft) of the axillary or brachial artery after proximal and distal arterial control has been obtained with vessel loops (Fig. 31.3). When an end-to-end anastomosis is to be performed, a posterior knot is usually placed at 6 o'clock. If exposure is limited, as in an end-to-end anastomosis performed near the clavicle, it is helpful to

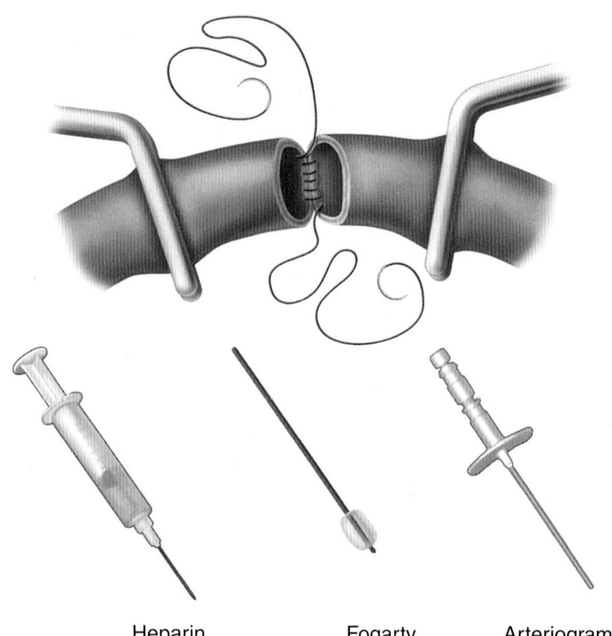

FIGURE 31.3. Fine points in peripheral arterial repair include use of small vascular clamps or Silastic vessel loops, open anastomosis technique, regional heparinization, passage of a Fogarty catheter proximally and distally, and arteriography on completion.

perform the first one-third of the posterior anastomosis in an open fashion (no posterior knot) in both directions to allow for complete visualization of all suture bites.[47] After this portion of the anastomosis is complete, the ends of the artery are pushed together as both sutures are pulled tight. Because both ends of the artery are now stabilized, a No. 5 or 6 Fogarty embolectomy catheter is passed proximally and distally to remove any thrombotic or embolic material. Approximately 10–15 mL of heparinized saline solution (50 U/mL of solution) is then injected into each end of the artery, and the vascular clamps are reapplied. The remaining two-thirds of the anastomosis is completed by running one end of the continuous suture along one side and the other end along the other side. The last few loops of suture, however, are left loose to allow for flushing before the anterior knot is tied. The proximal vascular clamp is removed for flushing and then reapplied. The distal vascular clamp is removed to allow for flushing as well. As air is evacuated by the distal flushing, the two suture ends are pulled up tight and tied. Once the first knot has been tied, the proximal arterial clamp is released. Bleeding from suture holes is controlled by the application of oxidized regenerated cellulose (Surgicel, Johnson & Johnson Medical, Inc., Arlington, TX) or Avitene (Med Chem Products, Inc., Woburn, MA). Because distal in situ thrombosis is very unusual during proximal arterial repairs in the upper extremity, the return of palpable pulses at the ipsilateral wrist obviates the need for a completion arteriogram. When distal pulsations are diminished or absent after removal of the vascular clamps, a completion arteriogram is mandatory.

When an interposition graft will be necessary to restore arterial continuity in the upper extremity, a reversed autogenous saphenous vein graft from the thigh of an uninjured lower extremity is the first choice. In the 15%-20% of young male patients with saphenous veins that are too small for replacement of a major vessel such as the axillary artery, a ringed PTFE synthetic graft is an acceptable alternative. The operative technique for each anastomosis may be as described above, or a more traditional approach may be used. The triangulation approach described by Carrel[48] involves placing stay sutures at 120 degree intervals on the circumference of the graft and on the recipient vessel. After these are tied and the ends of the graft and recipient vessel are in apposition, each 120 degree segment of the anastomosis may be readily approximated by a continuous suture technique. A related approach that is pertinent to the use of a rigid PTFE interposition graft is to place only two stay sutures 180 degree apart to appose the ends of the graft and recipient vessel. When an interposition graft has been inserted, the terminal flushing maneuvers and evacuation of air are performed as described previously as the second anastomosis is completed.

When an interposition graft has been inserted to complete an arterial repair in the upper extremity, it is the practice of the author to place all adult patients on an intravenous drip of 10% dextran 40 in 5% dextrose (10% Gentran 40, Baxter Healthcare Corp., Deerfield, IL) at a dose of 40 mL per hour × 3 days. This agent can prevent or reverse cellular aggregation and will prolong the bleeding time. In addition, adult patients are started on 81-mg aspirin tablets twice a day by rectal suppository or orally starting in the recovery room and maintained on this medication for the next 3 months.[49]

Venous Repair—Upper Extremity

Injuries to veins in the upper extremities are infrequently discussed. Diagnostic tests such as venograms are not employed to document the presence of a peripheral venous injury as the consequences of missing such an injury are so modest; that is, pressure dressings usually control venous hemorrhage from small injuries, and late venous pseudoaneurysms are extraordinarily rare. The only indications for operation are venous bleeding not controlled by a pressure dressing or the suspected or known presence of an associated arterial injury.

The incisions previously described for arterial injuries in the upper extremities are the same ones used for possible venous injuries. Proximal and distal control around a major venous injury, however, can be awkward because of multiple venous branches. As the venous system is characterized by low pressure, the use of small, medium, and large metal clips for ligation followed by division of venous branches is appropriate as exposure and control are obtained. Proximal and distal control around an area of injury can usually be maintained with use of vessel loops under tension rather than with angled vascular clamps.

Because of the presence of valves in the venous system, injection of heparinized saline toward the hand after distal venous control has been obtained is not performed. For the same reason, passage of a Fogarty balloon catheter toward the hand or toward the heart is inappropriate.

Essentially, all major injuries to the brachial or axillary venae comitantes or veins can be ligated as there are extensive venous collaterals throughout the upper extremity. On rare occasions in stable patients with an isolated major injury to the axillary vein, resection and an end-to-end anastomosis or insertion of a saphenous vein interposition graft has been performed. Lateral venorrhaphies for lesser injuries are performed with interrupted or continuous sutures of 7-0 polypropylene. With a meticulous suture technique, peripheral venous repairs (most studied in the lower extremities) have been documented to have short-term patencies exceeding 75% in several reports.[50,51]

Arterial Repair—Lower Extremity

Injuries to the femoral, popliteal, or shank arteries account for approximately 48%-55% of peripheral arterial injuries treated in civilian trauma centers. Because of its length and exposed position in the lower extremity, injuries to the common or superficial femoral artery are 2–2.5 times more common than those to the popliteal and shank arteries.

Injuries to the common femoral, proximal superficial femoral, or profunda femoris arteries are approached through the previously described longitudinal groin incision inferior to the inguinal ligament. An injury right at the inguinal ligament or the presence of a large pulsatile hematoma overlying the groin and inguinal ligament will mandate obtaining more proximal arterial control. An ipsilateral oblique incision is made in the lower quadrant 3 cm above the inguinal ligament. Successive muscle and aponeurotic layers including the transversus abdominis muscle and transversalis fascia laterally are divided. The peritoneum is pushed medially using spongesticks to enter the retroperitoneal space and expose the psoas muscle. After the ureter is elevated with the peritoneum, the external iliac artery is encircled with a vessel loop and clamped for proximal arterial control.

Once proximal and distal control has been obtained around arterial injuries in the groin, certain principles should be kept in mind. One is that the profunda femoris artery should not be sacrificed for reasons of exposure. Even if an end-to-end anastomosis or insertion of an interposition graft into the common femoral artery has been necessary, it is not difficult to reimplant the end of the profunda femoris artery into this reconstructed segment. This involves rotating the vascular clamps on the common femoral artery 90 degrees toward the midline. A small posterolateral arteriotomy in the common femoral artery or graft replacement will then allow for an end-to-side anastomosis to the profunda femoris artery using 6-0 polypropylene suture. Injuries to arteries below the groin are approached through longitudinal incisions as well. The superficial femoral artery in the proximal three-fourths of the thigh lies posterior to the inferior edge of the sartorius muscle. With anterior mobilization of this muscle and division of the surrounding sheath, the superficial femoral artery (and vein) is easily exposed. In the distal one-fourth of the thigh, exposure of the proximal popliteal artery involves mobilizing the sartorius muscle posteriorly and the vastus medialis muscle anteriorly. Occasionally, the adductor magnus tendon comprising the edge of the adductor hiatus may have to be divided, as well.[52] The entire popliteal artery system is exposed by extending the medial distal thigh incision into an incision 1 cm posterior to the edge of the tibia. The tendons of the sartorius, gracilis, and semitendinosus muscles will often require division 1–2 cm away from their insertions on the tibia for complete exposure. Each tendon should be divided between two colored sutures, with different colors used for each of the three tendons. This will allow for accurate reapproximation of the tendons following the arterial repair.

Exposure of the infrageniculate popliteal artery, proximal anterior tibial artery, tibioperoneal trunk, or proximal posterior tibial and peroneal arteries is obtained through a proximal medial incision in the leg. An 8-cm longitudinal incision beginning at the posterior edge of the condyle of the tibia is made in the medial infrapopliteal area, approximately 1 cm below the posterior edge of the tibia. It is imperative to avoid injury to the greater saphenous vein, which usually lies posterior to the incision described. After the fascia is incised posterior to the edge of the tibia and inferior to the overlying tendons of the sartorius, gracilis, and semitendinosus muscles, the medial head of the gastrocnemius muscle is retracted posteriorly. To obtain appropriate exposure in large patients, the electrocautery may be used to separate the medial attachments of the soleus muscle to the tibia as well. The deep dissection is somewhat tedious, especially if there is associated atherosclerosis at this location. Proper exposure of all vessels will usually involve careful ligation and division of the anterior tibial vein and separation of the posterior tibial and peroneal arteries from their associated veins.

One area in which the repair of arteries in the lower extremity differs from that in the upper extremity is in the management of extensive distal injuries. Although loss or ligation of the radial or ulnar artery will rarely result in loss of the hand, the loss of two shank arteries from an extensive blunt injury will often lead to a below- or above-knee amputation. Certain patients with these injuries have true mangled extremities and will be served best by an immediate amputation. Others will have disruption or thrombosis of the tibioperoneal trunk or of the anterior tibial artery and one of the branches of the tibioperoneal trunk. The combination of a crushing or shearing injury and loss of two main arteries will often leave one or more muscle compartments of the leg and/or the foot ischemic. In such patients, innovative bypasses originating in the distal popliteal artery and crossing over a fracture site may be necessary to restore adequate arterial flow to the leg and foot.

Venous Repair—Lower Extremity

As with venous injuries in the upper extremities, the only indications for operation are venous bleeding not controlled by a pressure dressing or the suspected or known presence of an arterial injury.

Venous injuries in the lower extremities are approached through the usual longitudinal incisions and managed as previously described. The one unique aspect of management is the much stronger emphasis on repair rather than ligation. The popliteal vein and superficial femoral vein inferior to its junction with the profunda femoris vein are true end veins draining the leg. Ligation of either of these veins has some theoretical disadvantages. There is always the concern that a below-knee compartment syndrome will develop in the early postoperative period, that there will be an acute adverse impact on arterial inflow into the shank, and that chronic edema of the leg will occur.[53–57] Several civilian series have documented, however, that venous ligation in the popliteal and superficial femoral veins is surprisingly well tolerated in young trauma patients.[53,54,56,57] This is particularly true if absolute bed rest and elevation of the injured lower extremity for the first 5–7 days after ligation are mandatory.[55] There is no clear-cut increase in the need for postligation fasciotomy, amputations are rare, and edema of the leg often resolves over time.[53,54,56,57] This is in marked contrast to the 50% edema reported after ligation of the popliteal vein during the Vietnam War.[58]

Nonetheless, in the absence of near exsanguination and sequelae of shock such as severe hypothermia, profound metabolic acidosis, and an intraoperative coagulopathy, the superficial femoral and popliteal veins should be repaired. Options for repair include lateral venorrhaphy with 6-0 polypropylene suture, vein patch venoplasty using the greater saphenous vein from the contralateral ankle, or insertion of an autogenous saphenous vein graft, or externally supported PTFE graft.[12,50,53,54,56,57,59] Because of the time needed to make spiral and panel vein grafts and the mixed patency rates reported, these are rarely performed in American trauma centers.[59,60]

After any type of complex venous repair in the lower extremity, it is the practice of the author to wrap the entire lower extremity with an elastic bandage at modest tension to avoid causing a compartment syndrome. The lower extremity is elevated on three to four pillows for 5–7 days, and strict bed rest is mandatory as previously described. Dextran 40 is administered intravenously at 40 mL per hour × 3 days, and an 81-mg aspirin tablet is administered twice a day by rectal suppository or orally starting in the recovery room and continuing for 3 months. Finally, a duplex venous study is performed before discharge.

Extra-anatomic Bypass

In the acute care setting, the indications for use of an extra-anatomic bypass include the following: (1) loss of soft tissue over injured artery or vein (Fig. 31.4); (2) postoperative wound infection with blowout of underlying arterial repair; and (3) simultaneous infections in soft tissue and underlying native artery secondary to injection of illicit drugs.[44,45] Injured patients in whom this technique has been used include those with shotgun wounds or with high kinetic energy blunt trauma to extremities.

The operative technique involves obtaining proximal and distal vascular control of the injured artery (and/or vein) through the open wound. Intraluminal shunts are inserted to maintain arterial inflow and venous outflow. Contused, necrotic, or infected soft tissue is then debrided rapidly, followed by debridement of the exposed artery to the edges of the defect in soft tissue. Longitudinal incisions are made over the course of the proximal and distal ends of the artery, which are mobilized so that they are no longer in contact with the defect in soft tissue. Following completion of the proximal anastomosis to a saphenous vein graft, the bypass graft is tunneled subcutaneously and, on occasion, intramuscularly around the defect in soft tissue. As has been noted in the use of extra-anatomic bypasses in patients with atherosclerotic disease, unusual courses of such grafts do not impair patency if kinks or twists are avoided (Fig. 31.4). After confirmation of pulsatile flow through the distal end of the graft, the graft is anastomosed in an end-to-end or end-to-side fashion to the distal end of the mobilized artery. Completion arteriography is mandatory to confirm a gentle curve without kinks in the extra-anatomic bypass graft and the absence of distal arterial thrombi or emboli. Because of the large size of the proximal veins of the extremities, it is appropriate to use an externally supported extra-anatomic PTFE graft for venous replacement. The incisions over the proximal and distal anastomoses to the graft then are closed, thereby placing the graft in a protected extra-anatomic subcutaneous tunnel.

In the postoperative period, packing of the defect in soft tissue can be performed as many times a day as the surgeon desires. Vigorous physical therapy is appropriate during the period of packing to avoid the formation of contractures in adjacent joints. Early coverage of the defect in soft tissue with

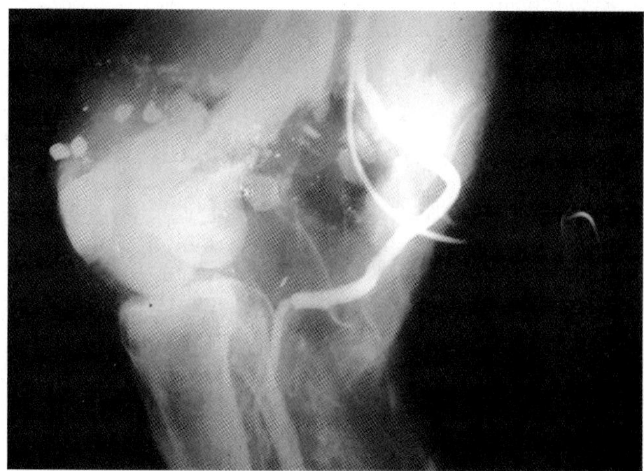

FIGURE 31.4. Extra-anatomic saphenous vein graft posterior to knee joint in patient with close-range shotgun wound to medial thigh, femur, and popliteal artery and vein. (Reprinted from Feliciano DV, et al. Extraanatomic bypass for peripheral arterial injuries. *Am J Surg*. 1989;58:506–509, with permission from Elsevier.)

a split-thickness skin graft and continuing physical therapy after healing occurs should minimize loss of function in the involved extremity. A baby aspirin tablet (81 mg) is administered every 12 hours to any patient without a history of gastrointestinal hemorrhage or known ulcers for 3 months to aid in patency of the grafts and in decreasing neointimal hyperplasia at the distal arterial suture line. If signs of aspirin toxicity, such as ringing in the ears, occur, the dose is decreased to 81 mg once a day.

Management of Wound in Soft Tissue

In patients with major peripheral vascular injuries and a transfusion-associated coagulopathy, extensive oozing often occurs in soft tissue as the operation is completed. In such patients, placement of closed suction drains into the blast cavity or area of dissection may be required for several hours postoperatively. The placement of drains prevents formation of a postoperative hematoma that could compress and possibly occlude the vascular repairs.

If a large blast cavity is present in soft tissue near the vascular repairs, some muscle or soft tissue should be sutured in a position that separates the two. A closed or open drain or open packing of the cavity exiting on the opposite side of the extremity from the skin incision and vascular repairs should then be inserted. This allows for drainage of the large blast cavity away from the vascular repairs and helps to avoid the problems of compression by hematoma and of cellulitis and late abscesses near a vascular repair.

Occasionally, primary wound closure is undesirable in patients with extensive muscle hematomas, soft tissue edema, or a severe coagulopathy after a peripheral vascular repair. In such patients, porcine xenografts (pigskin) are placed over the vascular repairs and the wound is packed open with antibiotic-soaked gauze.[61,62] After 24 hours of elevation of the injured extremity, the patient is returned to the operating room for delayed primary closure, or closure with a muscle rotation flap, or myocutaneous flap performed by the plastic surgery service.

The Mangled Extremity

As previously noted, a mangled extremity results from high-energy transfer or crushing trauma that causes some combination of injuries to artery, bone, soft tissue, tendon, and nerve. Approximately, two-thirds of such injuries are caused by motorcycle, motor vehicle, or vehicle–pedestrian accidents, reflecting the substantial transfer of energy that occurs during such incidents. Chapman[63] has emphasized that the kinetic energy dissipated in collision with an automobile bumper at 20 mph (100,000 ft-lb) is 50 times greater than that from a high-velocity gunshot (2,000 ft-lb).

When a patient with a mangled extremity arrives in the emergency center, the trauma team must work its way through the following series of decisions in patient care:

1. If the patient's life is in danger, should the mangled limb be amputated?
2. If the patient is stable, should an attempt be made to salvage the mangled limb?
3. If salvage is to be attempted, what is the sequence of repairs? (see previous section.)
4. If salvage fails, when should amputation be performed?

The most difficult decision is whether to attempt salvage of the limb. Since 1985, at least five separate scoring systems that describe the magnitude of injuries in a mangled extremity have been published.[24,64–67] All attempts to predict the need for amputation based on a total score were derived from the combination of injuries in the extremity and other factors. The applicability of any of these systems outside the institutions in which they originated has been questioned.[68,69]

Two major criteria are used most frequently in clinical decisions regarding immediate amputation versus attempted salvage. If either of the following factors is present, amputation is a better choice than prolonged attempts at salvage.

1. Loss of arterial inflow for longer than 6 hours, particularly in the presence of a crush injury that disrupts collateral vessels[13,70]
2. Disruption of the posterior tibial nerve[24,70,71]

Lange et al.[71] and Hansen[72] have described relative indications for immediate amputation in patients with Gustilo IIIC tibial fractures as well. These include serious associated polytrauma, severe ipsilateral foot trauma, anticipated protracted course to obtain soft tissue coverage, and tibial reconstruction. If two of these are present, immediate amputation is once again recommended.[71,72]

Compartment Syndromes and Fasciotomies

A compartment syndrome is defined as increased pressure within a closed fascial space that reduces capillary perfusion to a level less than that required for the viability of tissues.[73] Most compartment syndromes result from an increase in content of the compartment as caused by edema, hemorrhage, ischemic edema, reperfusion injury, or, on rare occasions, by chronic overexertion of muscles. Trauma and/or ischemia to the extremity remain the most common causes.

A history of a delay in presentation when ischemia in an extremity is present should make the attending physician suspicious that a compartment syndrome is present or is likely to develop. The patient will often complain of pain out of proportion to the extent of an injury. General findings on physical examination that increase the likelihood of a compartment syndrome occurring include systemic shock in combination with an ischemic extremity, evidence of a crush injury, and marked swelling of the extremity.[74,75] The presence of a tender or tight musculofascial compartment does not, however, precisely correlate with the presence of a compartment syndrome.

Rather, pain on passive stretch of muscles in the compartment is strongly suggestive. Other neurologic findings that often suggest the presence of an established compartment syndrome include hypesthesia in the sensory distribution of a nerve that courses through the compartment in question or weakness of the involved muscles. Finally, restoration of arterial inflow after more than a 4- to 6-hour delay, the need to clamp arterial inflow and venous outflow vessels at the time of vascular repair, and ligation of a major outflow vein are procedures at operation that make a compartment syndrome more likely to develop. Also, it is important to note that distal pulses in an extremity are often still palpable or audible by a Doppler device after a revascularization procedure even though a compartment syndrome is present.

One approach in vascular or trauma surgery services has been to perform a fasciotomy to relieve a suspected compartment syndrome whenever any of the historical, physical, or operative factors described earlier are present. An aggressive approach such as this will avoid missing a compartment syndrome, but will surely result in some unnecessary or "prophylactic" fasciotomies. Another approach is to measure the intracompartmental pressure (normal, 4–8 mm Hg) and only perform fasciotomy when a certain elevated pressure has been reached. A large number of techniques for measurement of intracompartmental pressure have been described including (1) needle injection, (2) wick catheter, (3) slit catheter, (4) arterial transducer, and (5) the STIC device (Solid-State Transducer IntraCompartmental Monitor System, Stryker Surgical, Kalamazoo, MI).[11,76] Unfortunately, there is little consensus in the literature about the absolute intracompartmental pressure that mandates a fasciotomy to avoid permanent muscular or neural damage. A rising pressure of more than 30 mm Hg, a pressure more than 45 mm Hg or a <20 mm, or a 30 mm Hg difference between diastolic blood pressure and the intracompartmental pressure have all been suggested over the past 25 years.[11] In a somewhat ecumenical approach, the American College of Surgeons Committee on Trauma poster entitled "Management of Peripheral Vascular Trauma" (2002) suggests that fasciotomy be performed for pressures ">30–35 mm Hg."[77]

Fasciotomies to relieve compartment syndromes in the upper extremities account for only 20% of all fasciotomies performed after trauma and even less after nontrauma vascular occlusions. Therefore, many surgeons are not familiar with the operative techniques that are utilized.

The forearm is divided into three musculofascial compartments, including volar, dorsal, and the "mobile wad."[78] Other authors describe superficial flexor, deep flexor, and extensor compartments.[76] The volar compartment (flexion, pronation, supination) is opened first using the "volar ulnar approach." The incision begins on the lateral (radial side) of the forearm distal to the antecubital fossa, proceeds transversely across the forearm parallel to the arm–forearm fold, and then makes a right angle turn down the ulnar volar aspect of the forearm (Fig. 31.5). At this right angle turn, the "mobile wad" can be decompressed by opening the underlying fascia. At the wrist, the ulnar incision curves toward the radial side until it crosses the carpal tunnel along the thenar crease of the palm. The fascia overlying the flexor digitorum sublimis and flexor carpi ulnaris muscles is divided from the aponeurosis of the elbow down to the carpal tunnel at the wrist (decompression of superficial flexor compartment). These two muscles are separated with retractors, the ulnar nerve and artery are identified overlying the flexor digitorum profundus, and the fascia overlying this muscle and the flexor pollicis longus is divided as well (decompression of deep flexor compartment). After complete decompression of the volar compartment, it is worthwhile to remeasure the intracompartmental pressure in the dorsal (extensor) compartment. Should its pressure still be elevated, the dorsal compartment is approached through a skin incision in the pronated forearm from the lateral epicondyle of the humerus to the midline of the wrist. The fasciotomy is performed in the interval between the extensor digitorum communis and extensor carpi radialis brevis muscles toward the radial side of the forearm. The role of the epimysiotomy of decompressed muscles is unclear, and a carpal tunnel release at the wrist is often added if the wrist and hand are swollen.

Any pale forearm muscle that still contracts with stimulation from the electrocautery device should be left in place at the first operation. The entire forearm is then covered with a bulky dressing and elevated by attaching a forearm stockinette to an intravenous pole. After 3–7 days of elevation in patients with obviously viable forearm muscles, the patient is returned to the operating room. Closure of the skin incision is best accomplished by undermining the subcutaneous tissues and placing multiple interrupted vertical mattress skin-only sutures of 2-0 nylon. When the tension is too great to complete the skin closure with sutures, a split-thickness skin graft harvested from the anterolateral thigh is applied.

Because the anterior compartment of the leg is prone to developing a compartment syndrome in high-risk patients, the pressure is always measured first in this compartment. If the pressures in this compartment and in the deep posterior compartment immediately posterior to the tibia are >30–35 mm Hg, a below-knee two-incision four-compartment fasciotomy is performed (Fig. 31.6). The leg is divided into four musculofascial compartments, including anterior, peroneal, superficial posterior, and deep posterior. The anterior and peroneal compartments are approached through a 25- to 30-cm longitudinal incision 2 cm anterior to the upper edge of the fibula. The subcutaneous tissue and skin of both flaps are mobilized using traction with rake retractors and manual pressure with a laparotomy pad over fingers. Perforating vessels are divided and ligated with 3-0 silk ties to eliminate postoperative oozing in coagulopathic patients. When the intermuscular septum is clearly visualized or palpated, separate longitudinal fasciotomies approximately 4–5 cm apart are made over the entire anterior and peroneal compartments. The superficial and deep posterior compartments are approached through a 25- to 30-cm longitudinal incision 2 cm posterior to the lower edge of the tibia. Care should be taken to avoid injury to the greater saphenous vein and nerve. The subcutaneous tissue and skin of both flaps are mobilized as above. The superficial posterior compartment is visualized by further traction on the posterior

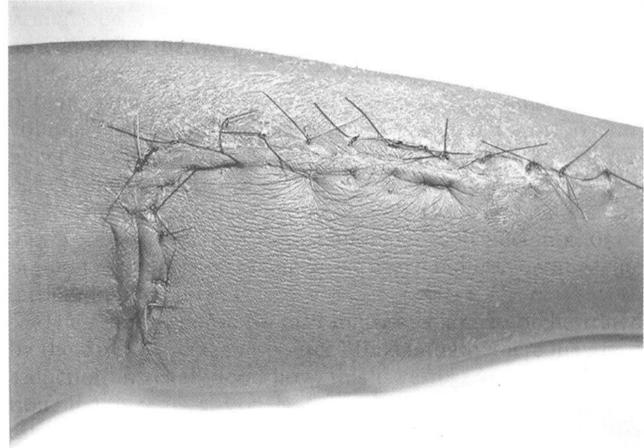

FIGURE 31.5. Proximal aspect of skin incision in volar-ulnar approach to decompress the volar and lateral ("mobile wad") compartments of the forearm. (Reprinted from Dente CJ, et al. Fasciotomy. *Curr Probl Surg*. 2009;46:769–840, with permission from Elsevier.)

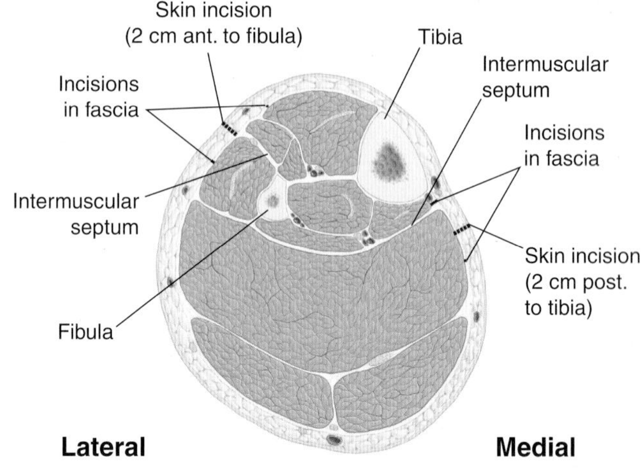

FIGURE 31.6. Two-skin incision four-compartment fasciotomy for decompression of compartments of the leg.

skin flap and opened over its entire length with a longitudinal incision. The deep posterior compartment may often be visualized in the distal aspect of the calf through the standard skin incision. Complete decompression of this musculofascial compartment posterior to the tibia and medial to the fibula will, however, require detachment of the soleus muscle from the back of the tibia.[76]

A compartment syndrome of the thigh in uncommon, but it has occurred in patients with severe pelvic fractures, ligation of the common or external iliac vein or common femoral vein, or, on rare occasions, with severe fractures of the femur. This entity will be present in many patients with the secondary extremity compartment syndrome following resuscitation from near exsanguination as well.[74,75] A compartment pressure >30–35 mm Hg in either the anterior or posterior compartment is an indication to perform a thigh two-incision three-compartment fasciotomy. The thigh is divided into three musculofascial compartments, including the quadriceps (anterior), hamstrings (posterior), and adductors (medial). The quadriceps compartment is approached through a 30-cm longitudinal anterolateral incision along the iliotibial tract from the intertrochanteric space to the lateral epicondyle of the distal femur. A longitudinal fasciotomy is made, and the fascia can be lifted off the rectus femoris muscle anteriorly as well. Access to the hamstrings compartment is obtained by mobilizing the vastus lateralis muscle anteriorly. The thick intermuscular septum medial to this muscle is then opened with a longitudinal incision to decompress the hamstrings compartment. If pressure in the adductor compartment is still elevated after the other two compartments of the thigh have been opened, the adductor compartment is approached through a 30-cm medial and longitudinal skin incision posterior to the sartorius muscle. After minimal mobilization of the skin and subcutaneous flaps, a longitudinal fasciotomy incision is made over the adductor muscles.

POSTOPERATIVE CARE

After the patient has been returned to the ward or intensive care unit, the injured extremity should be elevated and wrapped with elastic bandages if venous ligation was performed. Care must be taken to monitor intracompartmental pressure in such a situation, since the combination of venous hypertension and external compression may create an early compartment syndrome. Distal arterial pulses are monitored by palpation or with a portable Doppler unit. Intravenous antibiotics are continued for 24 hours if a primary repair or end-to-end anastomosis was performed. If a substitute vascular conduit was inserted, intravenous antibiotics are continued for 72 hours in some centers, much as in elective vascular surgery.

COMPLICATIONS

Early Occlusion of Arterial Repair

In-hospital occlusion of an arterial repair is always related to delayed presentation of the patient after injury, delayed diagnosis of the injury by a physician, a technical mishap in the operating room, or occlusion of venous outflow from the area of injury. In a patient with a delay in presentation or diagnosis, in situ distal arterial thrombosis may occur within 6 hours.[13] The passage of a Fogarty embolectomy catheter may not be helpful in such a situation, because it does not remove thrombi from arterial collateral vessels.

Technical mishaps at operation that lead to postoperative thrombosis of a repair include too much tension on an end-to-end anastomosis, failure to remove any thrombi or emboli in the distal arterial tree with a Fogarty embolectomy catheter, narrowing of a circumferential suture line, and failure to flush the proximal and distal arteries before final closure of the repair. Also, ligation or occlusion of a repair in the popliteal vein can lead to occlusion of an arterial repair at the same level.

If distal pulses disappear, the patient is returned immediately to the operating room for thrombectomy or embolectomy and revision of the repair as necessary. If there is no obvious reason for occlusion of the arterial repair at a reoperation, standard coagulation tests are performed immediately to screen for a thrombotic disorder. Examples include heparin-associated thrombocytopenia, antithrombin III deficiency, deficiency of protein C or S, and the antiphospholipid syndrome.

Delay in Diagnosis of an Arterial Injury

Occasionally, a patient has a traumatic false aneurysm or an arteriovenous fistula from a previous arterial injury that was not diagnosed.[79] The insertion of an endovascular stent with or without trans-stent angiographic embolization is possible for many of these lesions, and it can be accomplished readily by an experienced vascular surgeon or interventional radiologist.[80] If a major artery is involved, operative intervention using the principles described previously may be necessary.

Soft Tissue Infection over an Arterial Repair

A dreaded complication of combined orthopedic-vascular injuries, particularly in the lower extremity, is infection in the soft tissue overlying the arterial repair. If debridement of the soft tissue infection results in exposure of the arterial repair, one option is to attempt coverage of the arterial repair with a porcine xenograft and hope for the gradual growth of granulation tissue over the healthy artery. If the arterial repair starts to leak or suffers a blowout, the patient is returned to the operating room. The exposed portion of the artery is resected, and the aforementioned extra-anatomic saphenous vein bypass graft is placed around the area of soft tissue infection, making sure that both end-to-end anastomoses are covered by healthy soft tissue outside the wound.

Another option after debridement is for immediate coverage with a local muscle or myocutaneous rotation flap or for coverage with a free flap performed by the plastic surgery service.

Late Occlusion of Arterial Repair

Because saphenous vein grafts placed in peripheral arteries undergo the degenerative changes of atherosclerosis over time, late occlusions of some of these grafts can be expected. Management is the same as if the patient had occlusion of a primary artery—arteriography is performed based on symptoms, and bypass grafting is chosen if runoff is adequate to support another graft.

References

1. Zimmerman LM, Veith I. *Celsus and the Alexandrians (Chapter 3). Great Ideas in the History of Surgery*. Baltimore, MD: Williams & Wilkins; 1961:28-38.
2. Hallowell. Extract of a letter from Mr. Lambert, Surgeon at Newcastle upon Tyne, to Dr. Hunter, giving an account of new method of treating an aneurysm. *Med Obser Inq*. 1762;30:360. Cited by Rich NM. Historical and military aspects of vascular trauma. In: Rich NM, Mattox KL,

TRAUMA

Hirshberg A, eds. *Vascular Trauma*. 2nd ed. Philadelphia, PA: Elsevier; 2004:69.
3. Murphy JB. Resection of arteries and veins injured in continuity—end-to-end suture—experimental and clinical research. *Med Rec*. 1897;51:74-88.
4. Dente CJ, Feliciano DV. Alexis Carrel (1873–1944). Nobel Laureate, 1912. *Arch Surg*. 2005;140:609-610.
5. Stephenson HE Jr, Kimpton RS. *America's First Nobel Prize in Medicine or Physiology. The Story of Guthrie and Carrel*. Boston, MA: Midwestern Vascular Surgery Society; 2000.
6. Rich NM. Historical and military aspects of vascular trauma. In: Rich NM, Mattox KL, Hirshberg A, eds. *Vascular Trauma*. 2nd ed. Philadelphia, PA: Elsevier; 2004:3-72.
7. Dotter CT. Transluminally-placed coilspring endarterial tube grafts. Long-term patency in canine popliteal artery. *Invest Radiol*. 1969;4:329-332.
8. Frykberg ER, Schinco MA. Peripheral vascular injury. In: Feliciano DV, Mattox KL, Moore EE, eds. *Trauma*. 6th ed. New York, NY: McGraw-Hill; 2008:941-970.
9. Mattox KL, Feliciano DV, Burch J, et al. Five thousand seven hundred sixty cardiovascular injuries in 4,459 patients: epidemiological evolution 1958 to 1987. *Ann Surg*. 1989;209:698-707.
10. McCord JM. Oxygen-derived free radicals in postischemic tissue injury. *New Engl J Med*. 1985;312:159-163.
11. Dente CJ, Wyrzykowski AD, Feliciano DV. Fasciotomy. *Curr Probl Surg*. 2009;46:769-840.
12. Feliciano DV, Mattox KL, Graham JM, et al. Five-year experience with PTFE grafts in vascular wounds. *J Trauma*. 1985;25:71-82.
13. Miller HH, Welch CS. Quantitative studies on the time factor in arterial injuries. *Ann Surg*. 1949;130:428-438.
14. Heppenstall RB, Scott R, Sapega A, et al. A comparative study of the tolerance of skeletal muscle to ischemia. Tourniquet application compared with acute compartment syndrome. *J Bone Joint Surg Am*. 1986;68:820-828.
15. Hobson RW II, Howard EW, Wright CB, et al. Hemodynamics of canine femoral venous ligation: significance in combined arterial and venous injuries. *Surgery*. 1973;74:824-829.
16. Feliciano DV. Evaluation and treatment of vascular injuries. In: Browner BD, Jupiter JB, Levine AM, et al., eds. *Skeletal Trauma, Basic Science, Management, and Reconstruction*. 4th ed. Philadelphia, PA: Saunders Elsevier; 2009:323-340.
17. Snyder WH, Thal ER, Bridges RA. The validity of normal arteriography in penetrating trauma. *Arch Surg*. 1978;113:424-428.
18. Feliciano DV. Management of peripheral arterial injury. *Curr Opin Crit Care*. 2010;16:602-608.
19. Dennis JW, Frykberg ER, Crump JM, et al. New perspectives on the management of penetrating trauma in proximity to major limb arteries. *J Vasc Surg*. 1990;11:84-93.
20. Dennis JW, Frykberg ER, Veldenz HC, et al. Validation of nonoperative management of occult vascular injuries and accuracy of physical examination alone in penetrating extremity trauma. *J Trauma*. 1998;44:243-253.
21. Reid JDS, Weigelt JA, Thal ER, et al. Assessment of proximity of a wound to major vascular structures as an indication for arteriography. *Arch Surg*. 1988;123:942-946.
22. Frykberg ER, Dennis JW, Bishop K, et al. The reliability of physical examination in the evaluation of penetrating extremity trauma for vascular injury: results at one year. *J Trauma*. 1991;31:502-511.
23. Miranda FE, Dennis JW, Veldenz HC, et al. Confirmation of the safety and accuracy of physical examination in the evaluation of knee dislocation for popliteal artery injury: a prospective study. *J Trauma*. 2002;52:247-252.
24. Johansen K, Daines M, Howey T, et al. Objective criteria accurately predict amputation following lower extremity trauma. *J Trauma*. 1990;30:568-573.
25. Lynch K, Johansen K. Can Doppler pressure measurement replace "exclusion" ateriography in the diagnosis of occult extremity arterial trauma? *Ann Surg*. 1991;214:737-741.
26. Nassoura ZE, Ivatury RR, Simon RJ, et al. A reassessment of Doppler pressure indices in the detection of arterial lesions in proximity penetrating injuries of the extremities: a prospective study. *Am J Emerg Med*. 1996;14:151-156.
27. Seamon MJ, Smoger DM, Torres DM, et al. A prospective validation of a current practice: the detection of extremity vascular injury with CT angiography. *J Trauma*. 2009;67:238-244.
28. White PW, Gillespie DL, Feurstein I, et al. Sixty-four slice multidetector computed tomography angiography in the evaluation of vascular trauma. *J Trauma*. 2010;68:96-102.
29. Morozumi J, Ohta S, Homma H, et al. Introduction of mobile angiography into the trauma resuscitation room. *J Trauma*. 2009;67:245-251.
30. Itani KMF, Burch JM, Spjut-Patrinely V, et al. Emergency center arteriography. *J Trauma*. 1992;32:302-307.
31. O'Gorman RB, Feliciano DV. Arteriography performed in the emergency center. *Am J Surg*. 1986;152:323-325.
32. Bergstein JM, Blair JP, Edwards J, et al. Pitfalls in the use of color-flow duplex ultrasound for screening of suspected arterial injuries in penetrated extremities. *J Trauma*. 1992;33:395-402.
33. Gagne PJ, Cone JB, McFarland D, et al. Proximity penetrating extremity trauma: the role of duplex ultrasound in the detection of occult venous injuries. *J Trauma*. 1995;39:1157-1163.
34. Kuzniec S, Kauffman P, Molnar LJ, et al. Diagnosis of limb and neck arterial trauma using duplex ultrasonography. *Cardiovasc Surg*. 1998;6:358-366.
35. Frykberg ER, Vines FS, Alexander RH. The natural history of clinically occult arterial injuries: a prospective evaluation. *J Trauma*. 1989;29:577-583.
36. Stain SC, Yellin AE, Weaver FA, et al. Selective management of nonocclusive arterial injuries. *Arch Surg*. 1989;124:1136-1141.
37. Spirito R, Trabattoni P, Pompilio G, et al. Endovascular treatment of a post-traumatic tibial pseudoaneurysm and arteriovenous fistula: case report and review of the literature. *J Vasc Surg*. 2007;45:1076-1079.
38. White R, Krajcer Z, Johnson M, et al. Results of a multicenter trial for the treatment of traumatic vascular injury with a covered stent. *J Trauma*. 2006;60:1189-1196.
39. Feliciano DV, Moore EE, West MA, et al. Evaluation and management of peripheral vascular injury: part II. *J Trauma* (In press).
40. Cotton BA, Gunter OL, Isbell J, et al. Damage control hematology: the impact of a trauma exsanguination protocol on survival and blood product utilization. *J Trauma*. 2008;64:1177-1183.
41. Subramanian A, Vercruysse G, Dente C, et al. A decade's experience with temporary intravascular shunts at a civilian level I trauma center. *J Trauma*. 2008;65:316-326.
42. Caudle RJ, Stern RJ. Severe open fractures of the tibia. *J Bone Joint Surg Am*. 1987;69:801-807.
43. Gustilo RB, Mendoza RM, Williams DN. Problems in the management of type III (severe) open fractures: a new classification of type III open fractures. *J Trauma*. 1984;24:742-746.
44. Feliciano DV, Accola KD, Burch JM, et al. Extraanatomic bypass for peripheral arterial injuries. *Am J Surg*. 1989;158:506-510.
45. Feliciano DV. Heroic procedures in vascular injury management. The role of extra-anatomic bypass. *Surg Clin North Am*. 2002;82:115-124.
46. Graham JM, Mattox KL, Feliciano DV, et al. Vascular injuries of the axilla. *Ann Surg*. 1982;195:232-238.
47. Feliciano DV. Managing peripheral vascular trauma. *Infect Surg*. 1986;5:659-669, 682.
48. Carrell A. The surgery of blood vessels. *John Hopkins Hosp Bull*. 1907;18:18-28.
49. The Dutch Bypass Oral Anticoagulants or Aspirin Study Group. Efficacy of oral anticoagulants compared with aspirin after infrainguinal bypass surgery. The Dutch Bypass Oral Anticoagulants or Aspirin (BOA) Study: a randomized trial. *Lancet*. 2000;355:346-351.
50. Parry NG, Feliciano DV, Burke RM, et al. Management and short-term patency of lower extremity venous injuries with various repairs. *Am J Surg*. 2003;186:631-635.
51. Sharma PVP, Shah PM, Vinzons AT, et al. Meticulously restored lumina of injured veins remain patent. *Surgery*. 1992;112:928-932.
52. Wind GG, Valentine RJ. Axillary artery. In: Wind GG, Valentine RJ, eds. *Anatomic Exposures in Vascular Surgery*. Baltimore, MD: William & Wilkins; 1991:384-388.
53. Bermudez KM, Knudson MM, Nelken NA, et al. Long-term results of lower-extremity venous injuries. *Arch Surg*. 1997;132:963-968.
54. Feliciano DV, Herskowitz K, O'Gorman RB, et al. Management of vascular injuries in the lower extremities. *J Trauma*. 1988;28:319-328.
55. Mullins RJ, Lucas CE, Ledgerwood AM. The natural history following venous ligation for civilian injuries. *J Trauma*. 1980;20:737-743.
56. Timberlake GA, O'Connell RC, Kerstein MD. Venous injury: to repair or ligate—the dilemma. *J Vasc Surg*. 1986;4:553-558.
57. Yelon JA, Scalea TM. Venous injuries of the lower extremities and pelvis: repair versus ligation. *J Trauma*. 1992;33:532-536.
58. Rich NM, Hobson RW, Collins GJ Jr, et al. The effect of acute popliteal venous interruption. *Ann Surg*. 1976;183:365-368.
59. Pappas PJ, Haser PB, Teehan EP, et al. Outcome of complex venous reconstructions in patients with trauma. *J Vasc Surg*. 1997;25:398-404.
60. Zamir G, Berlatzky Y, Rivkind A, et al. Results of reconstruction in major pelvic and extremity venous injuries. *J Vasc Surg*. 1998;28:901-908.
61. Ledgerwood AM, Lucas CE. Split-thickness porcine graft in the treatment of close-range shotgun wounds to extremities with vascular injury. *Am J Surg*. 1973;125:690-695.
62. Ledgerwood AM, Lucas CE. Biological dressings for exposed vascular grafts: a reasonable alternative. *J Trauma*. 1975;15:567-574.
63. Chapman MW. Role of bone stability in open fractures. *Instr Course Lect*. 1982;31:75-87.
64. Gregory RT, Gould RJ, Peclet M, et al. The mangled extremity syndrome (M.E.S.): a severity grading system for multisystem injury of the extremity. *J Trauma*. 1985;25:1147-1150.
65. Howe HR Jr, Poole GV Jr, Hansen KJ, et al. Salvage of lower extremities following combined orthopedic and vascular trauma: a predictive salvage index. *Am Surg*. 1987;53:205-208.
66. Seiler JC III, Richardson JD. Amputation after extremity injury. *Am J Surg*. 1986;152:260-264.
67. Russell WL, Sailors DM, Whittle TB, et al. Limb salvage versus traumatic amputation: a decision based on a seven-part predictive index. *Ann Surg*. 1991;213:473-481.
68. Bonanni P, Rhodes M, Lucke JP. The futility of predictive scoring of mangled lower extremities. *J Trauma*. 1993;34:99-104.
69. Roessler MS, Wisner DH, Holcroft JW. The mangled extremity: when to amputate? *Arch Surg*. 1991;126:1243-1249.
70. Lange RH. Limb reconstruction versus amputation decision making in massive lower extremity trauma. *Clin Orthop Relat Res*. 1989;243: 92-99.

71. Lange RH, Bach AW, Hansen ST Jr, et al. Open tibial fractures with associated vascular injuries: prognosis for limb salvage. *J Trauma*. 1985;25:203-208.
72. Hansen ST Jr. The type IIIC tibial fracture: salvage or amputation? *J Bone Joint Surg Am*. 1987;69:799-800.
73. Matsen FA III. *Compartmental Syndromes*. New York, NY: Grune & Stratton; 1980.
74. Goaley TJ Jr, Wyrzykowski AD, MacLeod JBA, et al. Can secondary extremity compartment syndrome be diagnosed earlier? *Am J Surg*. 2007;194:724-727.
75. Tremblay LN, Feliciano DV, Rozycki GS. Secondary extremity compartment syndrome. *J Trauma*. 2002;53:833-837.
76. Twaddle BC, Amendola A. Compartment syndromes. In: Browner BD, Jupiter JB, Levine AM, et al., eds. *Skeletal Trauma, Basic Science, Management, and Reconstruction*. 4th ed. Philadelphia, PA: Saunders Elsevier; 2009:341-366.
77. Feliciano DV. *Management of Peripheral Vascular Trauma (Poster)*. American College of Surgeons Committee on Trauma/Subcommittee on Publications. Chicago, IL: American College of Surgeons; 2002.
78. Whitesides TE Jr, Heckman MM. Acute compartment syndrome: update on diagnosis and treatment. *J Am Acad Orthop Surg*. 1996;4:209-218.
79. Feliciano DV, Cruse PA, Burch JM, et al. Delayed diagnosis of arterial injuries. *Am J Surg*. 1987;154:579-584.
80. Stanton PE Jr, Rosenthal D, Clark M, et al. Percutaneous transcatheter embolization of injuries to the profunda femoris artery. *Angiology*. 1985;36:650-655.

CHAPTER 32 ■ BURNS*

BASIL A. PRUITT JR AND RICHARD L. GAMELLI

The organ system changes that occur following burn injury represent the stereotypic response to injury and make the burn patient the universal trauma model (Table 32.1). Those changes and the frequency of burn injury make burn patient management a challenge often presented to the trauma/acute care surgeon. The acute care surgery components of initial burn care include fluid resuscitation, and ventilatory support, as well as preservation and restoration of function of other organs and tissues. Following resuscitation, burn patient management is focused on wound care and provision of the necessary metabolic support. The involvement of the trauma/acute care surgeon in burn wound management is dependent upon the extent of the wound, depth of the wound, and site of care, that is, a general hospital in which a trauma/acute care surgeon might provide definitive wound care for a patient with burns of limited extent as opposed to a burn center where the wound care of a patient with extensive burns would be provided by a burn surgeon. The trauma/acute care surgeon must be able to identify those patients who are best cared for at a burn center and oversee their safe, prompt transfer.

EPIDEMIOLOGY

Only 21 states require the reporting of burn injury and in 9 of those states, only specific burns defined by etiology or extent must be reported. Consequently, an estimated total number of burns has been obtained only by extrapolation of the data collected in those states to the entire population. In 1996, 1.25 million was regarded as a realistic estimate of the annual incidence of burns in the United States.[1]

On the basis of data from federal surveys and the National Burn Registry, the American Burn Association estimates that in the United States, 450,000 burn injury patients receive medical treatment annually. The percentage of burn patients cared for at burn centers has increased steadily in recent years and of the 40,000 (~130 patients per million population) admitted to hospitals for treatment of their burn injury, two-thirds or 26,400 (~86 patients per million population) are cared for at the 125 hospitals with specialized burn centers of which 54 are verified by the American Burn Association.[2] That subset of patients defined by the American Burn Association (Table 32.2), as best cared for in a burn center[3] consists of 40 patients per million population with major burns and 46 patients per million population having lesser burns but a complicating cofactor. The geographic distribution of burn centers, which correlates closely with population density,[4] necessitates the use of aeromedical transfer by either fixed wing or rotary wing aircraft to transport burn patients to those facilities from remote areas.

There are identifiable populations at high risk for specific types of injuries that will require treatment by the trauma/acute care surgeon. Thermal burns outnumber scald burns by more than a factor of 2 in children of all ages treated in emergency departments for burns[5] even though scald burns are the most frequent form of burn injury overall.[6] The occurrence of tap water scalds can be minimized by adjusting the temperature settings on hot water heaters or by installing special faucet valves that prevent delivery of water at unsafe temperatures.

In adults, flames and the ignition of flammable liquids are the most common causes of burns. In patients of 80 or more years, scalds and flames each cause approximately 30% of burn injuries. Preexisting disease contributes to the injury event in approximately two-thirds of elderly patients and also contributes to their morbidity and mortality rates, which are higher than in younger patients.[7]

The vast majority of the burns treated at hospitals involve <20% of the total body surface area (TBSA) as reflected by the overall survival rate of 94.8%. The American Burn Association National Burn Registry Advisory Committee has estimated that there are only "4,000 fire and burn deaths each year with 75% of those occurring at the scene or during initial transport". Of patients admitted to burns centers, 63% are Caucasian and 70% are male. The cause of the burn injury in those patients was flame/fire 42%, scald 31%, hot object contact 9%, electric injury 4%, chemical injury 3%, and other 11%. Personal assault and self-inflicted injuries each accounted for approximately 2% of the burns. The home was the site of occurrence of the burn injury in two-thirds of the patients and, only 1 in 10 occurred at the work place.[2] However, one-fifth to one-quarter of all serious burns are employment related. Kitchen workers are at relatively high risk for scald injury, and roofers and paving workers are at greatest risk for burns due to hot tar.

In 1988, there were 236,200 patients treated in emergency rooms for chemical injuries.[8] Many chemical injuries are employment related. Strong acid injuries are of greatest incidence in those involved in plating processes and fertilizer manufacture and strong alkali injury is of greatest incidence in those involved in making soap. Injuries caused by phenol, hydrofluoric (HF) acid, anhydrous ammonia, cement, and petroleum distillates are also strongly associated with employment.

Injuries due to white phosphorus and mustard gas are most frequent in military personnel. Civilian recreational explosive devices, fireworks, are a seasonal cause of burn injury. The highest incidence of firework injuries occurs during the 4th of July holiday in the United States, and during religious celebrations in countries such as India.

Electric current causes approximately 1,000 deaths per year.[9] One-quarter of electric injuries occur on farms or industrial sites, and one-third occur in the home. Young children have the highest incidence of electric injury caused by household current as a consequence of inserting objects into an electrical receptacle or biting or sucking on electric cords and sockets. Adults at greatest risk of high voltage electric injury are the employees of utility companies, electricians, construction workers (particularly those manning cranes), farm workers moving irrigation pipes, oil field workers, truck drivers, and individuals installing antennae. National death certificate data document an average of 107 lightning deaths annually.[10] The vast majority (92%) of lightning-associated deaths occur during the summer months when thunderstorms are most common. Slightly more than one-half of patients killed by

*Some of the material in this chapter has been extracted, adapted, and revised from Pruitt BA Jr, Gamelli RL. "Chapter 9: Burns:" in Acute Care Surgery Principles and Practice (ed Britt LD, Trunkey DL, Feliciano DV) Springer, New York 2007, pg 125-160.

TABLE 32.1

ORGAN SYSTEM RESPONSE TO BURN INJURY

ORGAN SYSTEM	EARLY CHANGE	LATER RESPONSE
Cardiovascular	Hypovolemia	Hyperdynamic state
Pulmonary	Hypoventilation	Hyperventilation
Endocrine	Catabolism	Anabolism
Urinary	Oliguria	Diuresis
Gastrointestinal	Ileus	Hypermotility
Skin	Hypoperfusion	Hyperemia
Immunologic	Inflammation	Anergy
CNS	Agitation	Obtundation

lightning were engaged in outdoor activities such as golfing or fishing, and a quarter of patients who died from lightning injury were engaged in employment-related activities.[11]

Child abuse is a special form of burn injury, typically inflicted by parents but also perpetrated by siblings and child care personnel. The most common form of thermal injury abuse in children is caused by intentional application of a lighted cigarette. Burning the dorsum of a hand by application of a hot clothing iron is another common form of child abuse. The burns in abused children who require in-hospital care are most often caused by immersion in scalding water with the injury typically involving the feet, posterior legs, buttocks, and sometimes the hands (Fig. 32.1). It is important that the trauma/acute care surgeon identify and report child abuse because if it is undetected and the child is returned to the abusive environment, repeated abuse is associated with a high risk of fatality. In recent years, elder abuse has become more common and it too should be reported and the victim protected.

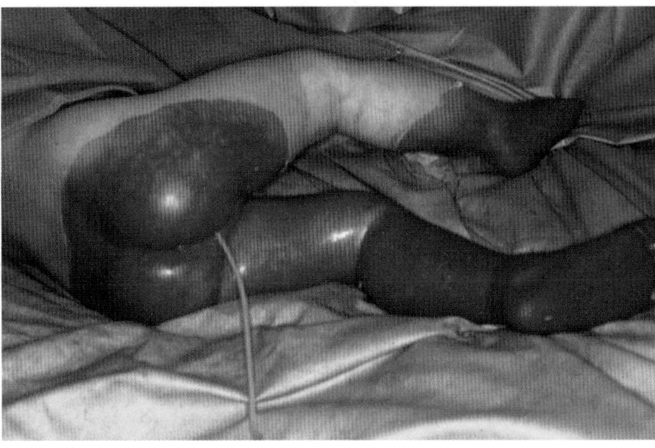

FIGURE 32.1. The distribution of the burns on this child (feet, legs, posterior thighs, buttocks, and perineum) is characteristic of abuse by intentional immersion scalding. The bright red moist burns of the buttocks and left posterior thigh were partial thickness burns, while the darker red, dry burns of the legs and feet, which darkened further with time, were full thickness injuries, which required grafting for closure.

TABLE 32.2

ABA BURN CENTER REFERRAL CRITERIA

I. Partial thickness burns of >10% TBSA.

II. Burns that involve the face, hands, feet, genitalia, perineum, or major joints

III. Third degree burns in any age group.

IV. Electrical burns including lightning injury.

V. Chemical burns.

VI. Inhalation injury.

VII. Burn injury in patients with preexisting medical disorders that could complicate management, prolong recovery, or affect mortality.

VIII. Any patient with burns and concomitant trauma (such as fractures) in which the burn injury poses the greatest risk of morbidity or mortality. In such cases, if the trauma poses the greater immediate risk, the patient's condition may be stabilized initially in a trauma center before transfer to a burn center. Physician judgment will be necessary in such situations and should be in concert with the regional medical control plan and triage protocols.

IX. Burned children in hospitals without qualified personnel or equipment for the care of children.

X. Burn injury in patients who will require special social, emotional, or rehabilitative intervention.

PATHOPHYSIOLOGY

Local Effects

The depth of burn injury produced, that is, partial thickness or full thickness, is related to the temperature of the energy source, the duration of the exposure, and the tissue surface involved. At temperatures <45°C, tissue damage is unlikely to occur in either adults or children even with an extended period of exposure. In the adult, exposure for 30 seconds when the temperature is 54°C will cause a burn injury.[12] In the child with relatively thinner skin, exposure to this same temperature for 10 seconds produces a substantial degree of tissue destruction. When the temperature is elevated to 60°C, a not uncommon setting for home water heaters, tissue destruction can occur in <5 seconds in children. At 71°C, a full thickness burn can occur in a near instantaneous manner. It is no surprise that when patients come in contact with boiling liquids, live flames, or are injured in industrial accidents where temperatures can exceed 1,000°C, substantial depths of injury occur. The systemic consequences of the injuries are proportional to the extent of the body surface area involved and may be modified by the patient's underlying physiological status and the presence of concomitant mechanical trauma. As the depth of the burn increases from partial to full thickness, the systemic response increases but to a lesser degree than that associated with increase in burn extent.

A burn injury causes three zones of damage (Fig. 32.2A). Centrally located is the zone of coagulation necrosis. Surrounding this is an area of lesser cell injury, the zone of stasis, and surrounding that an area of minimally damaged tissue, the zone of hyperemia, which abuts undamaged tissue. In a full thickness burn, the zone of coagulation involves all layers of the skin extending down through the dermis and into the subcutaneous tissue (Fig. 32.2B). In partial thickness injuries, this zone extends down only into the dermis and there are surviving epithelial elements capable of ultimately resurfacing

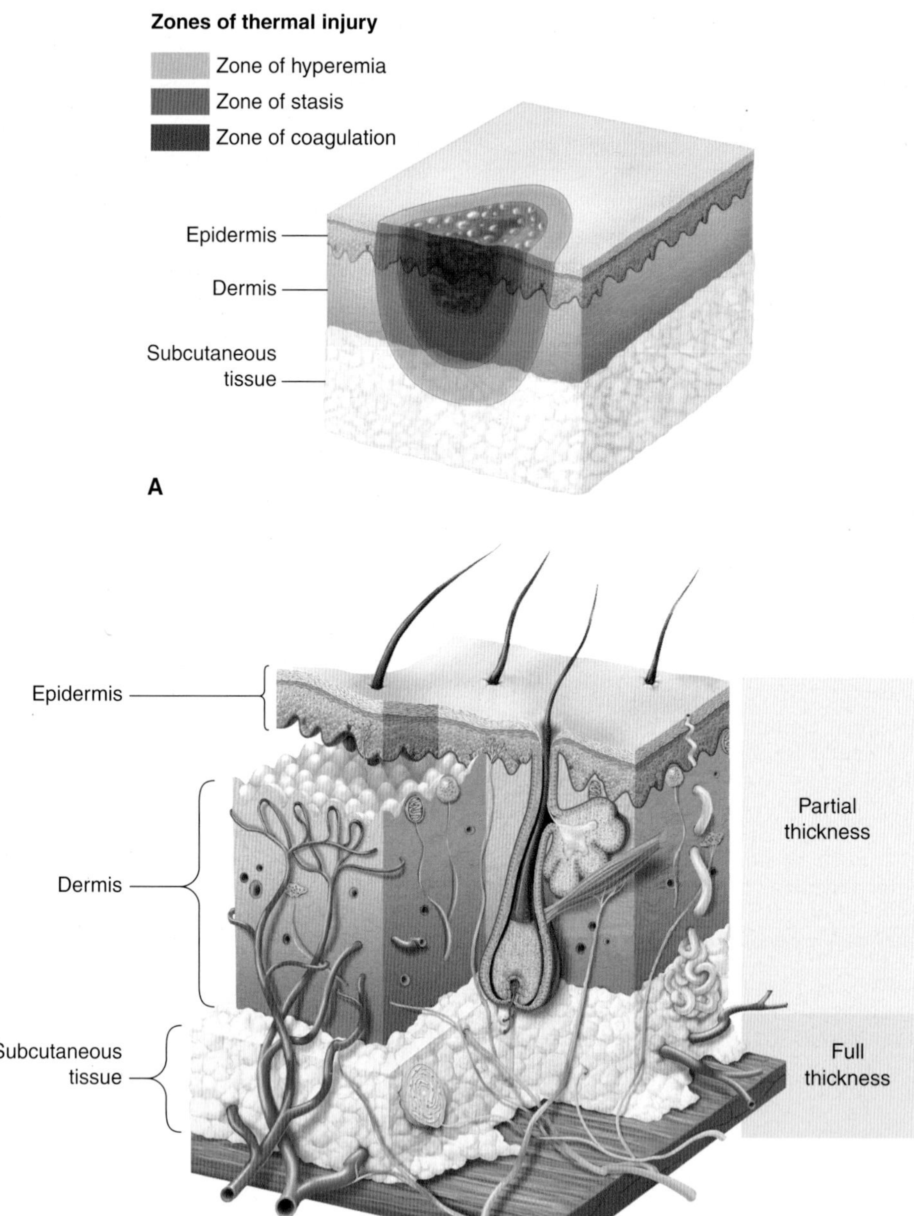

FIGURE 32.2. **A:** In any burn there are three identifiable concentric zones of injury. The most severe injury is in the zone of coagulation in which all tissue is nonviable. Surrounding that is the zone of stasis in which injured tissue with impaired blood flow can progress to necrosis if resuscitation is inadequate or be salvaged with adequate resuscitation. Surrounding the zone of stasis is the zone of hyperemia that contains the least injured tissue and is characterized by surface erythema and increased blood flow as manifestations of the inflammatory response. **B:** Diagram of the skin showing the levels of tissue injury defining second degree or partial thickness burns in which epithelial cells migrating from skin adnexa will resurface the wound and third degree or full thickness burns in which the dermis and adnexa are destroyed and must be closed by grafting.

the wound. In the zone of stasis, blood flow is altered but is restored with time as resuscitation proceeds. If thrombosis were to occur in a patient who is not adequately resuscitated, the zone of stasis can be converted to a zone of coagulation. The zone of hyperemia is best seen in patients with superficial partial thickness injuries as occur with severe sun exposure.

Along with the changes in wound blood supply there is considerable formation of edema in the burn-injured tissues. Release of local mediators from the burned tissue as well as from leukocytes causes alterations in local tissue homeostasis. Factors elaborated in the damaged tissues include histamine, serotonin, bradykinin, prostaglandins, leukotrienes, and interlukin-1. Complement is also activated, which can further modify transcapillary fluid flux. The changes in tissue water content have been ascribed to increased capillary filtration as well as changes in interstitial hydrostatic pressure.[13-16] The net effect of these various changes is appreciable movement of fluid into the extravascular fluid compartment. The ongoing development of edema fluid in the burn-injured tissue conceptually represents increased vascular permeability. Subsequent changes in lymph flow from burned tissue have been ascribed to changes in lymphatic vessel patency with obstruction occurring due to serum proteins that have transmigrated from the damaged capillaries.[17] Maximum accumulation of both water and protein in the burn wound occurs at 24 hours post injury.[18] This accumulation in tissues can remain beyond the first week post-burn. In addition to the changes in transcapillary fluid movement within the burn injured tissues, patients who have greater than a 20%-25% body surface burn have similar fluid movement in undamaged tissue beds including the gut and the lung. This may in part be related to the changes in transcapillary fluid flux and also be in response to the volume of resuscitation fluids administered.[19,20]

The appearance of the injuries is determined by the level of tissue destruction (Fig. 32.3A). When the wounds are superficial, they are associated with hyperemia, fine blistering, increased sensation, and intense pain upon palpation. The wounds are erythematous, warm, and readily blanch. These types of injuries represent first-degree burns or alternatively are termed superficial partial thickness injuries. With a second degree or deeper partial thickness burn, the wound presents with intact or ruptured blisters or is covered by a thin coagulum or crust. The key physical finding is preservation of sensation in the burned tissue although it is reduced (Table 32.3).

With proper care, superficial and even deeper partial thickness injuries are capable of healing. Even though burn blister fluid represents a near pure acellular filtrate of plasma, studies have revealed that this fluid may not necessarily promote wound healing.[21] Infection risk in deep partial thickness wounds is considerable and if an infection develops it can lead to greater tissue destruction and conversion to a full thickness injury. When the injury penetrates all layers of the skin or extends into the subcutaneous or deeper tissues, the wound will appear pale or waxy, be anesthetic, dry, and inelastic, and contain thrombosed vessels (Fig. 32.3B). Occasionally in children or young women, the wound may initially be cherry or brick red in appearance and be mistakenly considered to be partial thickness injury (Fig. 32.1). Such wounds typically have substantial edema, and are inelastic and insensate. Over the ensuing days, the wound darkens and becomes characteristic of a full thickness wound as the extravasated hemoglobin, which when fully oxygenated immediately post injury is responsible for the misleading wound color, undergoes reduction. Full thickness wounds are infection prone wounds, as they no longer provide any viable barrier to invading organisms and if left untreated are rapidly colonized and become a portal for invasive burn wound sepsis.

Systemic Response

The organ system response to a major burn injury results in some of the most profound physiologic changes that can occur. The magnitude of the response is proportional to the burn size and in some organ systems reaches a maximum at about a 50% body surface area burn. The duration of the changes is related to the persistence of the burn wound and the changes resolve with wound closure. The organ specific response follows the pattern that occurs with other forms of trauma with an initial level of hypofunction followed by the hyperdynamic flow phase. The changes in the cardiovascular response are some of the more critical ones and directly impact the initial care and management of the burn patient. Following burn injury, there is a transient period of decreased cardiac performance in association with elevated peripheral vascular resistance. This can be further compounded by failure to replace adequately the patient's intravascular volume loss leading to further impairments of cardiac filling, decreased cardiac output, and worsening organ hypoperfusion. Systemic hypoperfusion can result in further increases in systemic vascular resistance and reprioritization of regional blood flow. Whether the burn is responsible for causing a myocardial depressant to appear in the circulation or the impaired cardiac performance is simply a consequence of inadequate volume restoration remains an open question. What seems to be clear from experimental studies is that when there is a failure to resuscitate a burn patient adequately there is substantial impaired myocardial performance.[22] Conversely, the provision of adequate resuscitation volumes can preserve cardiac performance.[23]

Patients receiving appropriate volume restoration during the course of their resuscitation, develop normal cardiac performance values within 24 hours of injury and by the second

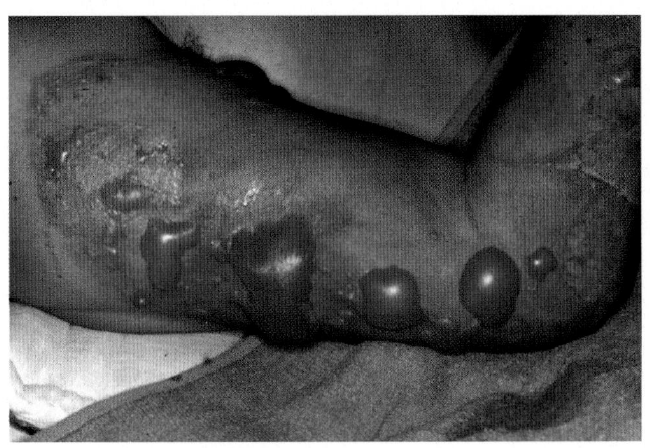

A

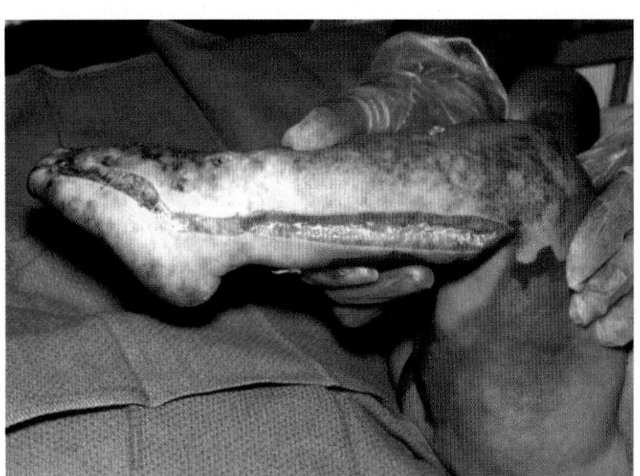

B

FIGURE 32.3. **A:** The partial thickness burns on this patient's arm display the characteristic blisters and areas of exfoliation of superficial epithelium revealing a pink moist wound shown just below the elbow. **B:** The full thickness burns on the left leg and foot of this child display the leathery, pallid, coagulated eschar characteristic of third degree burns. Edema beneath the circumferential eschar necessitated the escharotomy incision evident in the midlateral line of the burned leg and the lateral aspect of the foot. Note that the escharotomy was carried across the involved ankle joint.

TABLE 32.3

CLINICAL CHARACTERISTICS OF BURN INJURIES

	PARTIAL THICKNESS BURNS		FULL THICKNESS BURNS
	FIRST DEGREE	SECOND DEGREE	THIRD DEGREE
Cause	Sun or minor flash	Higher intensity or longer exposure to flash Relatively brief exposure to hot liquids, flames	Higher intensity or longer exposure to flash Longer exposure to flames or "hot" liquids Contact with steam or hot metal High voltage electricity Chemicals
Color	Bright red	Mottled red	Pearly white translucent and parchment-like Charred
Surface	Dry No bullae	Moist Bullae present	Dry, leathery, and stiff Remnants of burned skin present Liquefaction of tissue
Sensation	Hyperaesthetic	Pain to pin prick inversely proportional to depth of injury	Surface insensate Deep pressure sense retained
Healing	3–6 days	Time proportional to depth of burns—10–35 days	Requires grafting.

24 hours, those values further increase to supranormal levels. It is not uncommon to see adult patients with cardiac outputs in excess of 10 Liters per minute. In association with changes in cardiac output, there is a reduction in the systemic vascular resistance to 30%-40% of normal values. This hyperdynamic flow phase, part of the hypermetabolic response to the injury, will decrease toward normal levels with wound closure, but some degree of metabolic rate increase persists in major burn survivors for more than a year as the healed wounds fully mature.

Pulmonary changes following burn injury are the consequences of direct parenchymal damage as occurs with inhalation injury and the pathophysiologic effects of the burn per se. With isolated burn injury, neutrophil sequestration occurs in the lungs and may mediate lung injury. One mediator of this response appears to be the platelet-activating factor, which serves to prime neutrophils.[24] The changes in the pulmonary vascular response parallel those of the peripheral circulation though the increase may be to a greater degree and with a longer duration of change.[25] Capillary permeability in the lung appears to be mostly preserved following burn injury with the primary change being an increase in the lung lymph flow but no change in the lymph-to-plasma protein ratio.[26] Lung ventilation increases in proportion to the extent of burn with the patient having both an increase in respiratory rate and tidal volume. The increases are primarily related to the overall hypermetabolic response to the burn injury. Further perturbations in the patient's ventilatory status not related to the presence of an inhalation injury would indicate a supervening process such as sepsis, pneumonia, occult pneumothorax, pulmonary embolism, congestive heart failure, or an acute intraabdominal process.

The renal response to burn injuries is largely orchestrated by the cardiovascular response. While initially there may be a reduction in renal blood flow, this is restored with resuscitation. If the resuscitation is delayed or the fluid need underestimated, renal hypoperfusion will occur with early onset renal dysfunction secondary to renal ischemia. If the patient also experiences myoglobinuria or hemoglobinuria, which are capable of causing direct tubular damage, sequential injury can occur leading to further impairment of renal function. The changes in renal blood flow following burn injury require adjustment of the dosing schedule of a variety of medications such as aminoglycoside antibiotics to attain therapeutic levels. In patients who are receiving nutritional support, large doses of carbohydrates can cause glycosuria resulting in an inappropriate osmotic diuresis necessitating therapeutic intervention, that is, reduction of glucose load and/or administration of insulin. Daily urinary outputs in burn patients who are receiving protein loads greater than normal may be increased by the effects of the urinary urea load necessitating adjustment of fluid intake in order to excrete the increased solute load and avoid hypovolemia.

Burn-induced changes in gastrointestinal (GI) tract motility and a reduced capacity to tolerate early feedings had been previously thought to preclude the use of the GI tract as the primary route for nutritional support. With near immediate institution of enteral feedings via nasogastric or nasoduodenal tubes, GI motility can be preserved, mucosal integrity protected, and effective nutrient delivery achieved. It seems that delay in the initiation of enteral feeding is associated with the onset of ileus, which can also occur when the burn resuscitation has been complicated. Patients who are under-resuscitated will have alterations in GI tract motility and mucosal integrity as a consequence of intestinal hypoperfusion. Patients who have received massive resuscitation volumes will have considerable edema of the retroperitoneum, bowel mesentery, and bowel wall leading to a paralytic ileus. In patients who are intoxicated at the time of their burn injury, there may be further alterations in the GI tract with changes in the mucosal barrier function and alterations in local immunity.[27] In the past, the major GI complications following burn injuries were related to upper GI ulceration and bleeding. However, there has been a relative shift in the site of post-burn GI complications with the small bowel and colon now being more often affected.[28]

Burn injury results in an elevated hormonal and neurotransmitter response similar in magnitude to that of the "fight or flight" response.[29] The duration of the neurohumoral response is prolonged and it can be further increased with surgical stress. This can adversely impact the burn-induced metabolic changes and immune response. The increases in glucocorticoids and catecholamines correctly support the stress response of the injured patient except where this response becomes dysfunctional. In pathologic studies in humans as well as in animals, when there is an insufficient stress-hormone response, an otherwise survivable insult becomes fatal. Many of the multisystem changes occurring postburn can be related in part to the alterations in catecholamine secretion particularly the changes in resting metabolic expenditure, substrate utilization, and cardiac performance. As wound closure is accomplished, the altered neurohumoral response abates as the catabolic hormones recede and the anabolic hormones become predominant.

Burn injury results in the loss of balance in both leukocyte and erythrocyte production and function. Burns of >20% TBSA are associated with alterations in red cell production resulting in anemia.[30] Patients with major thermal injuries may lose up to 20% of their red cell mass in the first 24 hours due to thermal destruction of red cells in the cutaneous circulation. Such loss can be further compounded by frequent blood draws, blood loss related to surgical procedures, hemodilution with resuscitation and transient alterations in erythrocyte membrane integrity. Longer-term changes appear to be related to hyporesponsiveness of the erythroid progenitor cells in the bone marrow to erythropoietin.[31] Burn patients manifest increased circulating levels of erythropoietin following injury and attempts to augment those levels to improve red cell production have met with little success. During the early stages of resuscitation, reductions in platelet number, depressed fibrinogen levels, and alterations in coagulation factors return to normal or near normal values with appropriate resuscitation. Subsequent changes if they occur may be related to a septic process or in the case of platelets, heparin-induced platelet antibodies if heparin flushes are used as part of the maintenance protocol for intravascular devices. Changes in white cell number occur early with an increase in neutrophils due to demargination and accelerated bone marrow release. With uncomplicated burn injury, bone marrow myelopoiesis is relatively preserved.[32] With a septic complication, there appears, based on experimental evidence, to be a reduction in granulocyte formation and a relative shift to monocytopoiesis.[33] This defect appears not to be related to a lack of granulocyte colony stimulating factor but a growth arrest within the bone marrow of granulocyte precursor cells.[34,35]

In addition to the changes occurring in the bone marrow and the nonspecific aspects of the host defense mechanisms, there are substantial further depressions in the immune response. Burn injury causes a global impairment in host defense mechanisms. Alterations of the humoral immune response include reductions in IgG and IgM secretion, decreased fibronectin levels, and increases in complement activation. Cellular changes include alterations in T-cell responsiveness, changes in the T-cell subpopulations favoring the cytotoxic/suppressor T-cell, alterations in antigen processing and presentation, reductions in IL-2 release, and impairment of delayed type hypersensitivity reactions. In addition to the changes noted in granulocytes and monocytes and their release from the bone marrow, there are corresponding functional changes. Granulocytes have been noted to have impaired chemotaxis, decreased phagocytic activity, decreased antibody-dependent cell cytotoxicity, and a relative impairment in their capacity to respond to a second challenge.[36] The relative shift to monopoiesis is associated with an increase in secretion of PGE_2.[37] Dendritic cells, a critical component in the immune response, have also been found to be considerably altered following burn injury with infection.[38] Majetschak et al., who studied circulating proteasomes after burn injury identified elevation of 20 S proteasomes, which peaked on the day of injury, gradually declined during the ensuing 7 days, and had returned to baseline by postburn day 30. The proteasome levels did not discriminate for sepsis, multiple organ failure, or survival, but the circulating 20 S proteasomes were considered to be biomarkers of tissue damage and potentially useful in diagnosing inhalation injury.[39]

Recent studies of 242 pediatric patients with burns of more than 40% of the TBSA by Jeschke et al.[40] have documented the pervasiveness, intensity, and duration of the pathophysiologic response evoked by a major burn. Every patient was markedly hypermetabolic throughout their hospital stay and sustained substantial muscle protein loss and loss of lean body mass. Bone mineral density and bone mineral content decreased as well. Serum proteomic analysis revealed profound changes immediately after injury which, with variable changes across time, persisted throughout hospital stay. Cardiac function was compromised immediately after burn and was still abnormal at discharge. Insulin resistance was evident in the first week after injury and still present at discharge. Striking changes in IL-8, MCP-1, and IL-6 induced an inflammatory state and were associated with infections and sepsis. The clinical importance of these observations is that the burn patient is at significant risk for postburn infectious complications. This mandates the strictest adherence to aseptic technique in the management of the wounds and the insertion of intravascular devices, the judicious use of antimicrobial agents, aggressive nutritional support, and the achievement of rapid wound closure.

RESUCITATION

Priorities

In the immediate postburn period, the changes induced in the cardiovascular system by burn injury receive therapeutic priority. If the early postburn plasma volume loss is unreplaced, burn shock may occur accompanied by kidney and other organ failure and even death. In all patients with burns of more than 20% of the TBSA and those with lesser burns in whom physiologic indices indicate a need for fluid infusion, a large caliber intravenous cannula should be placed in an appropriately sized peripheral vein underlying unburned skin. If no such sites are available, a vein underlying the burn wound may be cannulated. If there are no peripheral veins available, the cannula can be placed in a femoral, subclavian, or jugular vein. Lactated Ringers solution should be infused at an initial rate of 1 Liter per hour in the adult and 20 mL/kg/h for children who weigh 50 kg or less. That infusion rate is adjusted following estimation of the fluid needed for the first 24 hours following the burn.

Fluid Administration

Resuscitation fluid needs are proportional to the extent of the burn (combined extent of partial and full thickness burns expressed as a percentage of TBSA) and are related to body size (most readily expressed as body weight) and age (the surface area per unit body mass is greater in children than in adults.) The patient should be weighed on admission and the extent of partial and full thickness burns estimated according to standard diagrams (Fig. 32.4) or, in the adult, by the use of the rule of nines that recognizes the fact that the surface area of various body parts represents 9% or a multiple thereof of the TBSA, that is, each upper limb and the head and neck 9%, each lower limb, posterior trunk and buttocks, and anterior trunk 18%, and the perineum and genitalia 1%. Those surface area relationships differ in children in whom the head and neck represent 21% of the TBSA and each lower limb, 14% at age one. The fraction of the TBSA represented by the head decreases progressively and that represented by the lower limbs increases progressively reaching adult proportions at age 16. The fact that the palmar surface of the patient's hand (palm and digits) represents 1% of his or her total body surface can be used to estimate the extent of irregularly distributed burns, that is, the number of the patient's "hands" needed to cover the patient's burn wounds.[41]

BURN ESTIMATE AND DIAGRAM

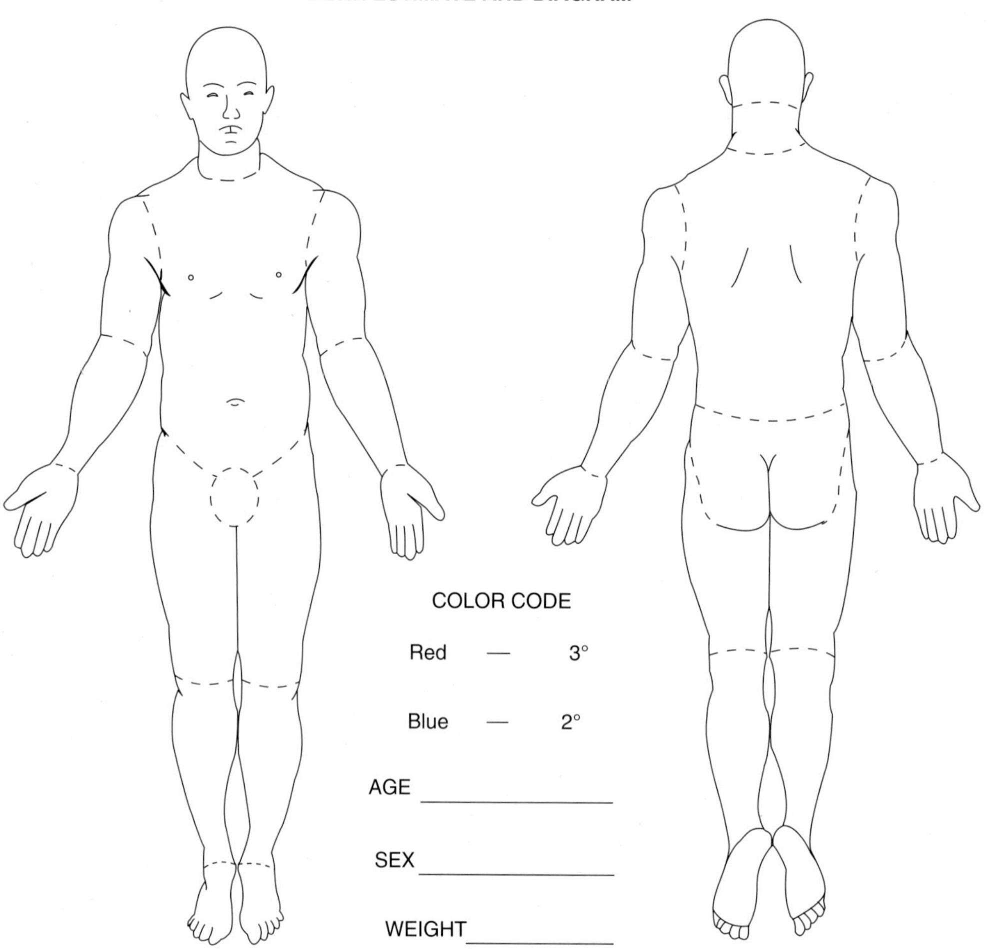

Area	Birth 1 yr	1 - 4 yr	5 - 9 yr	10 - 14 yr	18 yr	Adult	2°	3°	Total	Donar Area
Head	19	17	13	11	9	7				
Neck	2	2	2	2	2	2				
Ant. Trunk	13	13	13	13	13	13				
Post. Trunk	13	13	13	13	13	13				
R. Buttock	2 1/2	2 1/2	2 1/2	2 1/2	2 1/2	2 1/2				
L. Buttock	2 1/2	2 1/2	2 1/2	2 1/2	2 1/2	2 1/2				
Gentilia	1	1	1	1	1	1				
R.U. Arm	4	4	4	4	4	4				
L.U. Arm	4	4	4	4	4	4				
R.L. Arm	3	3	3	3	3	3				
L.L. Arm	3	3	3	3	3	3				
R. Hand	2 1/2	2 1/2	2 1/2	2 1/2	2 1/2	2 1/2				
L. Hand	2 1/2	2 1/2	2 1/2	2 1/2	2 1/2	2 1/2				
R. Thigh	5 1/2	6 1/2	8	8 1/2	9	9 1/2				
L. Thigh	5 1/2	6 1/2	8	8 1/2	9	9 1/2				
R. Leg	5	5	5 1/2	6	6 1/2	7				
L. Leg	5	5	5 1/2	6	6 1/2	7				
R. Foot	3 1/2	3 1/2	3 1/2	3 1/2	3 1/2	3 1/2				
L. Foot	3 1/2	3 1/2	3 1/2	3 1/2	3 1/2	3 1/2				

FIGURE 32.4. This diagram can be used to determine the extent of a patient's burn. Areas of the figures are colored with a blue pencil to indicate partial thickness burns and a red pencil to indicate full thickness burns. The columns with numbers, to the left below the figures, indicate how the percentage of body surface represented by various body parts changes with age.

In recent years, increased recognition of the association between resuscitation volume and compartment syndromes has focused interest on minimizing resuscitation fluid volume and increased use of those formulae estimating the fluid needed for the first 24 hours as 2.0 mL/kg body weight/percent of body surface burned as opposed to those formulae estimating first 24 hour fluid resuscitation needs as 4.0 mL/kg body weight/percent body surface area burned.[42-44]

In a study of 105 combat casualties with burns of more than 20% of the TBSA, the investigators reported that resuscitation guided by the modified Brooke Formula resulted in significantly lower first 24-hour fluid volume without any greater morbidity and mortality than in those for whom resuscitation was guided by the Parkland Formula. A greater percentage of those patients resuscitated with the Parkland Formula exceeded the Ivy index (250 mL of resuscitation fluid per kilogram body weight), which was associated with a high risk for abdominal compartment syndrome and was an independent predictor of death.[45]

In line with such reports, the American Burn Association's 2010 Advanced Burn Life Support (ABLS) manual has revised the recommendations for estimating the first 24-hour resuscitation fluid needs of burn patients.[46] One half of the estimated volume should be administered in the first 8 hours after the burn. If the initiation of fluid therapy is delayed, the initial half of the volume estimated for the first 24 hours should be administered in the hours remaining before the eighth postburn hour. The remaining half of the fluid is administered over the subsequent 16 hours. The infused volume is increased only as needed to achieve adequate resuscitation (Table 32.4).

The limited glycogen stores in a child may be rapidly exhausted by the marked stress hormone response to burn injury. Serum glucose levels in the burned child should be monitored and 5% dextrose in half normal saline administered if serum glucose decreases to hypoglycemic levels. In the case of small children with small burns, the resuscitation fluid volume as estimated on the basis of burn size may not meet normal daily metabolic requirements. In such patients, maintenance fluids should be added to the resuscitation regimen.

A "Rule of Ten" has recently been proposed as a simplified means of estimating the initial fluid infusion rate for adult burn patients and has been compared with existing formulae.

Rule of Ten.

1. Estimate burn extent to the nearest 10% of the TBSA
2. Extent of burns as estimated × 10 = initial infusion rate in mL per hour (for adults of 40–80 kg).
3. Increase rate by 100 mL per hour for each 10 kg body weight >80 kg.

In 100,000 simulations evaluated in silico, 88% of the initial infusion rates calculated by the Rule of Ten fell between those calculated by the Modified Brooke Formula (MB) and the Parkland (PL) Formula. The majority of the calculated rates clustered about the MB infusion rate.[47]

The infusion rate is adjusted according to the individual patient's response to the injury and the resuscitation regimen. The high circulating levels of catecholamines evoked by the burn and the progressive edema formation in burned and even unburned limbs commonly make measurements of pulse rate, pulse quality, and even blood pressure difficult and unreliable as indices of resuscitation adequacy. Since the hourly urinary output is a generally reliable and readily available index of resuscitation adequacy, an in-dwelling urethral catheter should be placed and the urinary output measured and recorded each hour. The fluid infusion rate is adjusted to obtain 30–50 mL of urine per hour in the adult and 1 ml per kg body weight per hour in children weighing <30 kg. To avoid excessive fluctuation of the infusion rate, the administration of fluid is increased or decreased only if the hourly urinary output is one-third or below or more 25% or more above the target level for 2 or 3 successive hours. If in either adults or children the resuscitation volume infused in the first 12 hours to achieve the desired urinary output or other indices of resuscitation adequacy exceeds estimated needs by more than twofold or will result in administration of six or more mL per percent body surface area burned per kg body weight in the first 24 hours, human albumin diluted to a physiologic concentration in normal saline should be infused and the volume of crystalloid solution reduced by a comparable amount. Inasmuch as functional capillary integrity is gradually restored during the first 24 hours postburn, such use of colloid-containing fluid is best reserved for the latter half of the first postburn day.

TABLE 32.4

ESTIMATION OF FIRST 24 HOUR FLUID RESUSCITATION NEEDS

I. Adult patients:
- A. Thermal and chemical burns: 2 mL lactated Ringers × body weight in kg × % TBSA[a] with second and third degree burns
- B. High voltage electric injury; 4 mL lactated Ringers × body weight in kg × % TBSA[a] with second and third degree burns

II. Pediatric patients (<14 years and <40 kg);
- A. Thermal and chemical burns; 3 mL[b] lactated Ringers × body weight in kg × % TBSA[a] with second and third degree burns
- B. High voltage electric injury; consult referral burn center immediately for guidance

[a]TBSA, total body surface area.
[b]The greater surface area per unit body mass in children necessitates a greater first 24' resuscitation fluid volume.

Restoration of functional capillary integrity and the establishment of a new transvascular equilibrium across the burn wound are manifested by the fact that both protein and water content of the burn-injured tissue reach maxima at or near 24 hours after injury.[18] Consequently, the volume of fluid needed for the second 24 hours postburn is less and colloid-containing fluids can be infused to reduce further volume and salt loading. Human albumin diluted to physiologic concentration in normal saline is the colloid-containing solution infused in a dosage of 0.3 mL per percent burn per kg body weight for patients with 30%-50% burns, 0.4 mL per percent burn per kg body weight for patients with 50%-70% burns, and 0.5 mL per percent burn per kg body weight for patients whose burns exceed 70% of the TBSA. Electrolyte-free, 5% glucose in water is also given in the amount necessary to maintain an adequate urinary output. The colloid-containing fluids for the second 24 hours for burned children are estimated according to the same formula, but half-normal saline is infused to maintain urinary output and avoid inducing physiologically substantive hyponatremia by infusion of large volumes of electrolyte-free fluid into the relatively small intravascular and interstitial volume of the child.

During the second 24 hours after injury, fluid infusion "weaning" should be initiated to minimize further volume loading. In a patient who is assessed to be adequately resuscitated, the volume of fluid infused per hour should be arbitrarily decreased by 25%-50%. If urinary output falls below target level, the prior infusion rate should be resumed. If urinary output remains adequate, the reduced infusion rate should be maintained over the next 3 hours at which time another similar fractional reduction of fluid infusion rate should be made. This decremental process will establish the minimum infusion rate that maintains resuscitation adequacy in the second postburn day.

Escharotomy

As resuscitation proceeds and edema forms beneath the inelastic eschar of encircling full thickness burns of a limb, blood flow to underlying and distal unburned tissue may be compromised. Circulatory compromise can occur in limbs with mixed depth partial thickness burns and on occasion in limbs with less than completely circumferential burns. Edema and coolness of distal unburned skin on a burned limb are normal accompaniments of the injury and are not indicative of circulatory compromise requiring surgical release. Cyanosis of distal unburned skin and progressive parasthesias, particularly unrelenting deep tissue pain, which are the most reliable clinical signs of impaired circulation, may become evident only after relatively long periods of relative or absolute ischemia. Those limitations can be overcome by scheduled (q1–2 h) monitoring of the pulse signal in the palmar arch vessels and the posterior tibial artery using an ultrasonic flowmeter. In an adequately resuscitated patient, absence of pulsatile flow or progressive diminution of the pulse signal on repetitive examinations is an indication for escharotomy.

Since the full thickness eschar is insensate, an escharotomy can be performed as a bedside procedure without anesthesia using a scalpel or an electrocautery device. On an extremity, the escharotomy incision, which is carried only through the eschar and the immediately subjacent superficial fascia, is placed in the midlateral line and must extend from the upper to the lower limit of the burn wound (Fig. 32.5). The circulatory status of the limb should then be reassessed. If that escharotomy has not restored distal flow, another escharotomy should be placed in the midmedial line of the involved limb. A fasciotomy may be needed when there has been a delay in restoring the patient's limb circulation and in particular if the patient is receiving a massive fluid load. Mistakes in the performance of escharotomies include injuries to extensor tendons and digital neurovascular bundles, insufficient depth and length of the incision, and delay in performing the escharotomy. Additionally, delayed bleeding from previously thrombosed vessels transected during the escharotomy should be promptly controlled. Continuous elevation and active exercise of a burned extremity for 5 minutes every hour limits edema formation and may eliminate the need for escharotomy.[48]

Edema formation beneath encircling full thickness truncal burns can restrict the respiratory excursion of the chest wall. If the limitation of chest wall motion is associated with hypoxia and progressive increase in the work of breathing, and peak inspiratory pressure as well, escharotomy is indicated to restore chest wall motion and improve ventilation. These escharotomy incisions are placed in the anterior axillary line bilaterally, and if the eschar extends onto the abdominal wall, the anterior axillary line incisions are joined by a costal margin escharotomy incision (Fig. 32.5). Rarely, encircling full thickness burns of the neck or penis will require release by placement of an escharotomy incision in the midlateral line(s) of the neck or the dorsum of the penis.

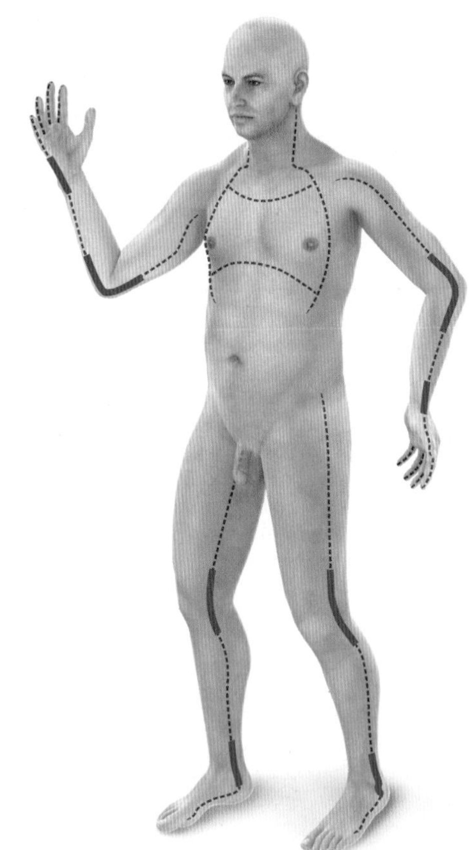

FIGURE 32.5. The *dashed lines* indicate the preferred sites of escharotomy of circumferential burns of the limbs, trunk, and other body parts. The thickened areas on those lines denote the importance of extending the escharotomy incisions across involved joints.

Post Resuscitation Fluid Therapy

Fluid management after the first 48 hours postburn should permit excretion of the retained fraction of the water and salt loads infused to achieve resuscitation, prevent dehydration and electrolyte abnormalities, and allow the patient to return to preburn weight by the 8th to 10th postburn day.[41] Infusion of the large volumes of lactated Ringers required for resuscitation commonly produces a weight gain of 20% or more and a reduction of serum sodium concentration to approximate that of lactated Ringers, that is, 130 mEq/L. Such patients do not need additional sodium and, in fact, have an elevated total body sodium mass in association with increased total body water. Correction of that relative hyponatremia is facilitated by the prodigious evaporative water loss from the surface of the burn wound, which is the major component of the markedly increased insensible water loss that is present following resuscitation. Insensible water loss, which must be taken into account in postresuscitation fluid management, can be estimated according to the formula:

Insensible water loss (mL per hour)
= (25 + % TBSAB) × TBSA in square meters

where TBSAB= Total Body Surface Area Burn, and TBSA= Total Body Surface Area.[49]

That water loss should be replaced only to the extent that will permit a daily loss of 2%-2.5% of the resuscitation-associated weight gain (as measured 48 hours after the burn) until preburn weight is attained. Inadequate replacement of insensible water loss makes hypernatremia the most commonly encountered electrolyte disturbance in the extensively burned patient following resuscitation. Such hypernatremia should be managed by provision of sufficient electrolyte-free water to allow excretion of the increased total body sodium mass and replace insensible water loss to the extent needed to prevent hypovolemia.

During resuscitation, hyperkalemia is the most frequently encountered electrolyte disturbance and is typically a laboratory sign of hemolysis and muscle destruction by high voltage electric injury or a particularly deep thermal burn. Hyperkalemia may also occur in association with acidosis in patients who are grossly underresuscitated. Hyperkalemia in the burn patient is treated as in any other surgical patient. In the case of patients with high voltage electric injury, emergency debridement of nonviable tissue and even amputation may be necessary to remove the source of the potassium. Hypokalemia may occur after the resuscitation period in association with alkalosis as a consequence of hyperventilation and may also accompany postresuscitation muscle wasting. Potassium losses are increased by the kaluretic effect of the mafenide acetate in Sulfamylon burn cream and, as noted below, by transeschar leaching in patients treated with 0.5% silver nitrate soaks.

Major depression of ionized calcium levels is uncommon, but total calcium levels may be depressed if calcium-binding proteins such as albumin decrease as may happen in patients receiving a high volume of resuscitation fluid. In extensively burned children, hypocalcemia has been associated with hypoparathyroidism and renal resistance to parathyroid hormone.[50] Symptomatic acute hypocalcemia should be treated with intravenous calcium (90–180 mg of calcium infused over 5–10 minutes) to control cardiac dysfunction and neuromuscular hyperactivity. Prolonged administration of parenteral nutrition and/or failure to supply sufficient phosphate to meet the needs of tissue anabolism following wound closure may cause hypophosphatemia. Administration of large volumes of antacids for stress ulcer prophylaxis is an infrequent cause of hypophosphatemia now that acid secretion inhibitors are used for that purpose. Hypophosphatemia can be prevented and treated by appropriate dietary phosphate supplementation.

The timely administration of adequate fluid as detailed above has essentially eliminated acute renal failure as a complication of inadequate resuscitation of burn patients. In a recent 10-year period, only 2 out of 2,132 burn patients treated at the U. S. Army Burn Center developed early renal failure, and those patients had established anuria when they were received in transfer from other institutions.[51] Far more common today are the complications of excessive resuscitation, that is, compartment syndromes and pulmonary compromise (Table 32.5). Compartment syndromes can be produced in the calvarium, muscle compartments beneath the investing fascia, and the abdominal cavity. Cerebral edema, which may efface the epidural space and compress the ventricular system, is most apt to occur in burned children and is manifested by obtundation and changes evident on computerized tomographic scans. Such changes should be addressed by maintaining cerebral perfusion pressure and minimizing further edema formation by reducing fluid infusion rate and inducing diuresis. Anterior ischemic optic neuropathy manifested by visual field defects and even blindness, is another manifestation of excessive fluid infusion. This complication has typically occurred in association with other compartment syndromes and anasarca in critically ill patients, particularly in those who are nursed in a prone position. Consequently, prone positioning should be avoided in severely injured, critically ill burn patients requiring large volumes of parenteral fluids. The occurrence of visual field defects should prompt alteration of fluid therapy and induction of a diuresis.[52]

Excessive fluid administration may also cause formation of enough ascitic fluid and edema of the abdominal contents to produce intra-abdominal hypertension. The abdominal compartment syndrome represents progression of intra-abdominal hypertension to the point of organ dysfunction, that is, typically oliguria, and/or altered pulmonary mechanics. Infusion of resuscitation fluid volumes in excess of 25% of body weight has been associated with a high incidence of abdominal compartment syndrome.[53] In all patients who have received that volume of resuscitation fluid, hourly monitoring of peak inspiratory pressure and intracystic pressure should be instituted.

TABLE 32.5

CONSEQUENCES OF EXCESS RESUSCITATION

I. Compartment syndrome
   A. Muscle compartments of unburned limbs
   B. Abdominal compartment syndrome
   C. Cerebral edema
   D. Anterior ischemic optic neuropathy

II. Pulmonary compromise
   A. Airway edema
   B. Pulmonary edema

Elevation of peak inspiratory pressure above 40 mm Hg and/or elevation of intracystic pressure above 25 mm of mercury, as measured through a urethral catheter, should prompt therapeutic intervention beginning with adequate sedation, reduction of fluid infusion rate, diuresis, and paracentesis. If organ failure becomes evident, a midline abdominal incision should be made to reduce the elevated intra-abdominal pressure. That incision can be temporarily closed with a polyethylene "bag," or a vacuum-assisted closure device. The abdomen can be definitively closed as soon as visceral edema resolves.

Compartment syndromes may also occur in the muscle compartments underlying the investing fascia of the limbs of burn patients, even in limbs that are unburned. To assess compartment pressure, the turgor of the muscle compartments should be assessed on a scheduled basis by simple palpation. A stony hard compartment is an ominous finding that should prompt further evaluation. The adequacy of arterial flow in all limbs of a burn patient should be monitored on a scheduled basis using the ultrasonic flowmeter. Ultrasonic detection of pulsatile flow is reassuring but the ultrasonic flow signals can be misleading since flow in large vessels may be maintained even though microcirculatory flow is severely compromised within a muscle compartment. Direct measurement of intracompartmental pressure using either a wick or needle catheter is much more reliable. A muscle compartment pressure of 25 mm of mercury or more necessitates performing a fasciotomy of the involved compartment in the operating room using general anesthesia.

Edema causing airway obstruction, in the absence of inhalation injury, has also been attributed to excessive resuscitation fluid. This complication, which necessitates endotracheal intubation, has been of particular concern in small children with extensive scald burns who have received in excess of 6 mL of lactated Ringers per percent body surface area burned per kilogram body weight. Pulmonary edema is rare during the initial 48-hour resuscitation period, but may occur in patients with extensive burns following resuscitation when the edema fluid is being resorbed and the protective early postburn pulmonary vascular changes have dissipated.

Mackie et al. have recently suggested that the application of mechanical ventilation alters postburn fluid dynamics and complicates fluid management by increasing net fluid balance independent of the presence of inhalation injury. Those investigators recorded a significantly greater cumulative fluid balance on the third and seventh postburn days in 186 patients with burns of more than 20% of the body surface who received mechanical ventilation as compared to that in patients who did not require mechanical ventilation.[54] Careful monitoring of intake and output in such patients is mandatory. The treatment of pulmonary edema in the burn patient is the same as for other patients.

A closed loop computerized system to adjust resuscitation fluid infusion rate on the basis of urinary output measured at a scheduled frequency, for example, each hour or as recently proposed every 10 minutes has also been evaluated as a means of reducing resuscitation volume and decreasing the incidence of compartment syndromes. When the system was employed in patients with massive burns, the investigators reported better maintenance of the urinary output target and that the prompt response to minute systemic changes resulted in a lower total infused volume and net fluid balance.[55]

Pathophysiologic studies have also identified pharmacologic agents and physiologic mechanisms that may reduce resuscitation fluid needs. In studies of a murine model of a 30% burn, a threefold increase in intestinal myosin light chain kinase (MLCK) was observed 4 hours after burn injury in association with a marked (fivefold) increase in intestinal permeability.[56] Postburn administration of pentoxifylline decreased the burn-induced phosphorylation of intracellular kinases and was associated with a decrease in histologic evidence of gut injury at 6 hours postburn and lung injury at 24 hours postburn.[57] The authors concluded that pentoxifylline attenuated the activation of the tight junction protein (MLCK) as a consequence of its reduction in tumor necrosis factor—alpha synthesis and nuclear factor kappaB activation after burn injury. Because of its anti-inflammatory effects, pentoxifylline has been proposed as an immunomodulatory additive of resuscitation fluid. Recently, that same group of investigators has identified a protective effect of vagal nerve stimulation on intestinal barrier integrity in a murine model of severe burn injury. Vagal stimulation was found to reduce the postinjury increase in intestinal permeability, decrease histologic changes in the intestinal mucosa, and prevent loss of occludin localization at points of intestinal epithelial cell-to-cell contact.[58]

VENTILATORY SUPPORT AND TREATMENT OF INHALATION INJURY

Pathophysiology

Patients suffering both inhalation injury and thermal burns have a considerably increased incidence of complications and probability of death. While an inhalation injury alone carries a mortality of 5%-8%, a combination of a thermal injury plus inhalation injury can easily result in a mortality 20% above that predicted on the basis of age and burn size.[59] Patients who have an otherwise survivable injury may succumb to their burn as a consequence of their inhalation injury and the complications that occur, particularly a gram negative pneumonia.[60] Injuries to the airway are most often due to direct damage by inhaled products of combustion or pyrolysis that cause inflammation and edema. Damage to the airway, while in part related to the heat content of the inhaled material in the oropharynx is, in the more distal airways, principally related to the particulate material contained within the smoke and the chemical composition of inhaled materials. Moist heat, which occurs with steam, has 4,000 times the heat-carrying capacity of dry smoke and is capable of causing more extensive thermal damage of the tracheobronchial tree.[61]

Presenting patient signs and symptoms are stridor, hypoxia, and respiratory distress.[62] The probability that a patient has suffered an inhalation injury is highly correlated with being burned in an enclosed space, having burns of the head and neck, and having elevated carbon monoxide levels. The extent and severity of the inhalation injury are directly related to the duration of exposure and the various toxins contained within the smoke. Injury due to heat is typically confined to the upper airway and supraglottic structures.[63] Particulate material within smoke is the vehicle by which the toxic materials are carried to the distal airway.

Particles of <5 μ in size can reach the terminal bronchi and the alveoli. Upper airway injuries involve the mucous membranes, nasopharynx, hypopharynx, epiglottis, glottis, and larynx. The lining mucous membranes as well as the cartilage of the glottis are easily damaged and can cause acute airway compromise.[63] Direct thermal injury to the lower airway is uncommon as rapid dissipation of heat occurs as the gases move through the upper airway. Injury to the tracheobronchial structures and pulmonary parenchyma is related to the toxins in the inhaled smoke and the ensuing host inflammatory response. Activation of the inflammatory cascade results in the recruitment of neutrophils and macrophages that propagate the injury.[64] Cellular damage is perpetuated by those cells that further the inflammatory response, which in turn leads to progressive pulmonary dysfunction.[65] Altered surfactant release causes obstruction and collapse of distal airway segments.[66] As part of the response to injury there is a marked and near immediate change in bronchial artery blood flow that can increase by up to twentyfold.[64] These changes in bronchial blood flow are also associated with marked alterations in vascular permeability within the lung and are thought to play an important role in the pathophysiologic response to inhalation injuries.[67] The net effect is that extensive destruction and inflammation reduce pulmonary compliance and impair gas exchange resulting in altered pulmonary blood flow patterns and ventilation perfusion mismatches.[68,69]

Asphyxiants

Carbon monoxide and cyanide gases are present in smoke and when inhaled are rapidly absorbed and cause systemic toxicity as well as impaired oxygen utilization and delivery. Carbon monoxide is an odorless, nonirritating gas that rapidly diffuses into the blood stream and rapidly binds to the iron moiety of the hemoglobin molecule. Carbon monoxide has a 240 times greater affinity for hemoglobin than does oxygen; thus it easily displaces oxygen. Carbon monoxide directly impairs the ability of hemoglobin to deliver oxygen to the tissues. Carbon monoxide also binds to enzymes within the mitochondria involved in intracellular oxygen utilization and cellular energetics.[70] Signs and symptoms of carbon monoxide poisoning are typically mild to none at all when carbon monoxide–hemoglobin (carboxyhemoglobin) levels are 10% or less. When carboxyhemoglobin levels are between 10% and 30%, symptoms are present and often manifested by headache and dizziness. Severe poisoning is seen in patients with carboxyhemoglobin levels of >50% that may be associated with syncope, seizures, and coma.

The diagnosis of carbon monoxide poisoning is made in a patient with burns on the basis of circumstances of injury, physical findings, and the measurement of blood carboxyhemoglobin level. It is important to note that pulse oximetry values do not differentiate between carboxyhemoglobin and oxyhemoglobin. Patients with appreciable carbon monoxide intoxication can have elevated oxygen saturations but will not have satisfactory blood oxygen contents. The primary treatment modality for carbon monoxide intoxication is provision of increased levels of inspired oxygen. The carbon monoxide "half-life" will decrease from 6 to 8 hours with room air to 40–80 minutes with 100% of FIO_2. Administration of oxygen in a hyperbaric chamber can further decrease the "half-life" to 15–30 minutes.[71] In a recently reported randomized trial, Weaver et al.[72] found that hyperbaric oxygen therapy significantly benefited patients with acute carbon monoxide poisoning. The utility of this in patients suffering major burns in association with carbon monoxide poisoning is yet to be demonstrated. It is an important practical question whether a patient can safely undergo treatment with hyperbaric oxygen therapy when there are other life-saving treatments that are needed. An approach that has worked well is to maintain the patient on 100% FIO_2 until carboxyhemoglobin levels are <15% and then to maintain this level of increased oxygen for an additional 6 hours at which time weaning of the FIO_2 can be initiated and conducted in accordance with standard criteria.

Cyanide poisoning, which has been considered uncommon except in combination with carbon monoxide intoxication, further disrupts normal cellular utilization of oxygen by binding to the cytochrome oxidase resulting in cellular lactic acid production and greater cellular dysfunction. Blood concentrations of cyanide >0.5 mg/L are toxic. Treatment of cyanide poisoning includes the administration of oxygen as well as decontaminating agents such as amyl and sodium nitrates. These compounds induce the formation of methemoglobin, which can act as a scavenger of cyanide.[73] Sodium thiosulphate, which can be administered intravenously, enhances the enzymatic detoxification of cyanide to thiocyanate but acts slowly. Hydroxycobalamin, which acts more rapidly and has few side effects, is the antidote of choice. The ready availability of cyanide antidote kits containing amyl nitrite pearls, 10% sodium nitrite, and 25% sodium thiosulfate or Cyanokits containing 5 g of hydroxycobalamin and their frequent use by emergency medical personnel must alert emergency department and burn physicians to the possibility that the patient has received such treatment in the field.[74]

Smoke may also contain a variety of toxic compounds that cause or initiate further damage to the airway (Table 32.6). The composition of each fire is different adding to the difficulty in caring for these patients. Such additional products in smoke include acrolein, hydrogen chloride, phosgene, ammonia, nitric oxide, and sulfur dioxide all of which are capable of causing substantial injury.

Airway Management

The most critical factor in the initial assessment of a burn patient is the patency of the airway and the ability of the patient to maintain and protect the airway. Standard criteria should be used to determine the need for mechanical stabilization of the airway also keeping in mind the systemic response to a major burn and the local response to an airway injury that may combine to cause progressive airway swelling and edema that will impair airflow. In an adult trachea of 14 mm, 1 mm of edema will result in a 25% reduction in cross sectional area. A similar degree of swelling in a 6 mm trachea of a child will result in greater than a 50% reduction in cross sectional area. Circumferential torso burns will further impair the ability of the patient to respire. Allowing airway compromise to proceed to a critical state before intubating the patient and stabilizing the airway is not appropriate care. The safest approach when there is concern about the airway, particularly in a patient needing transport for definitive care, is to perform early intubation.

Part of the initial management of the patient with inhalation injury should include a thorough evaluation of the airway including bronchoscopy. The clinical findings of an inhalation injury on bronchoscopy include airway edema, inflammation, increased bronchial secretions, presence of carbonaceous material that can diffusely carpet the airway, mucosal ulcerations and even endoluminal obliteration due to sloughing mucosa, mucous plugging, and cast formation (Fig. 32.6). Signs of gastric aspiration may also be evident. Bronchoscopy can be performed repeatedly for removal of debris and casts as well as surveillance for infection.

Direct airway treatment has been attempted with variable response. Desai et al. conducted an open label trial of the use of aerosolized heparin and *N*-acetylcysteine in children with inhalation injuries. The treated patients had an improved outcome (lesser incidence of atelectasis, decreased reintubation rate, and reduced mortality) compared to an untreated cohort.[75] A randomized prospective study has not yet been performed to confirm the utility of this approach particularly in adults. One noticeable effect with the empiric use of aerosolized heparin is the rapid clearing of particulate material and carbonaceous deposits from the airway. Laboratory studies have shown that the effectiveness of aerosolized heparin was increased when combined with intravenous administration of lisofylline. The synergistic effect of that antiinflammantory agent supports clinical evaluation of such combination therapy.[76] Inasmuch as the development of pneumonia in patients with inhalation injuries negatively impacts outcome, it is disappointing that prophylactic antibiotics have not been effective.[77] As a practical matter, it is best to culture these patients early to identify the organisms that have colonized their airways as a consequence of their injury and urgent airway manipulation. That information can guide therapy should the patient develop the signs and symptoms of early onset pneumonia. Steroids are not recommended in patients with inhalation injuries.[78]

Mechanical Ventilation

The critical feature in the management of patients suffering inhalation injuries is to minimize further damage to the airway and lung parenchyma while providing adequate gas exchange.[79] A major emphasis in the management of patients with inhalation injuries is to control airway pressures and thereby limit

TABLE 32.6

TOXIC AGENTS IN SMOKE

IRRITANT	CHARACTERISTICS	MECHANISM OF TOXICITY
Acrolein	Lipophilic	Direct epithelial damage
Hydrogen chloride	Water soluble	Forms free radicals
Phosgene	Low solubility	Causes the release of arachidonic acid metabolites
Ammonia	Water soluble	Forms hydroxyl ions and causes liquefactive necrosis
Nitric oxide	Lipid soluble	Causes lipid peroxidation
Sulfur dioxide	Water soluble	Causes lipid peroxidation

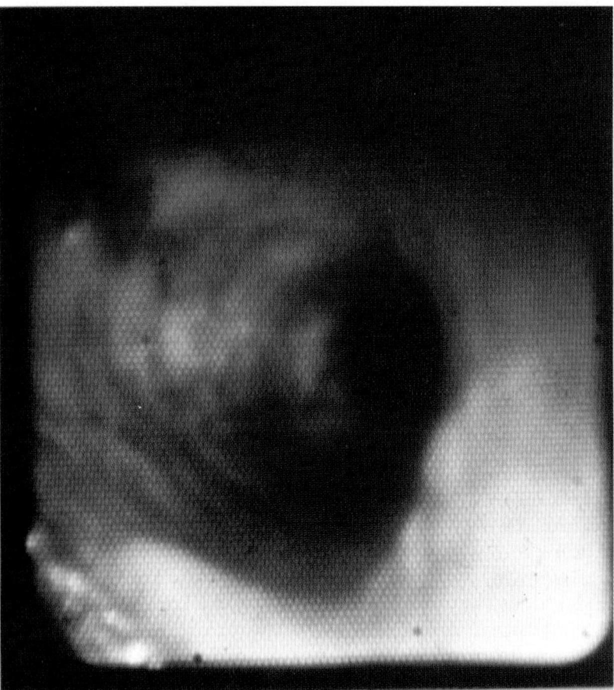

FIGURE 32.6. A bronchoscopic view of the airway in a patient with inhalation injury. Note the extensive deposition of carbonaceous material on the bronchial mucosa. Note also the erythematous areas of mucosal inflammation and pale focal areas of mucosal ulceration.

ventilation-induced barotraumas.[62] It is important to recognize that lung damage is not homogenous but patchy in distribution and requires that the level of positive end expiratory pressure (PEEP) used to maximize airway recruitment be limited to avoid ventilator-associated lung injury.[80,81] In states of severe lung injury, mechanical ventilation can lead to increases in sheer forces and changes in pulmonary blood flow. This in association with reductions in elasticity and alterations in lung compliance results in further lung injury and ventilation perfusion abnormalities.[82,83]

Using a standard volume mode of ventilation does not represent the best management of the damaged airway. Inverse ratio ventilation provides a strategy one can use in an attempt to counteract these changes and allow reductions in the level of PEEP and respiratory pressures to improve oxygenation.[84] Unfortunately, a clear advantage of inverse ratio ventilation over standard approaches has not been consistently shown.[85]

High-frequency ventilation is widely utilized at present in the form of high-frequency percussive ventilation (HFPV). High-frequency interrupted flow positive pressure ventilation delivers small tidal volumes (4 mL/kg) at flow rates of 250 liters per minutes with a frequency of 100 breaths per minute. In this mode, expiration is passive and thus there is an increased risk of air trapping and over distention. Allan et al.[86] recently reviewed and compared the use of HFPV using the VDR-4, (a volumetric diffusive respirator), high-frequency oscillatory ventilation, and high-frequency jet ventilation. Those investigators considered that HFPV in comparison to conventional ventilation improved oxygen and carbon dioxide tensions, attenuated lung inflammation and histologic lung injury, and improved static lung compliance, ventilation, oxygenation index, and the oxygen tension/fraction of inspired oxygen. That form of ventilation, which was also associated with a decrease in ventilator-associated pneumonia and an increase in survival of inhalation injury patients, was considered to have the unique capacity to exploit both high- and low-frequency ventilation to favorably influence gas exchange in a lung protective low tidal volume ventilation strategy.

There has been limited experience with the use of extracorporeal membrane oxygenation in the management of inhalation injuries in selected centers.[87] A carbon dioxide removal device has been developed to provide limited extracorporeal support to patients with chronic obstructive pulmonary disease. Investigators have reported that removal of carbon dioxide by that device permitted reduction in a patient's minute ventilation to one-third of baseline values.[88] The device has been proposed as a treatment modality for patients with pulmonary failure as a consequence of inhalation injury.

An approach that has worked well in many patients with inhalation injuries has been to identify promptly the presence of airway compromise and ensure that the patient is intubated with a properly sized endotracheal tube. Currently, it is our preference in the pediatric population to use a cuffed tube that may need to be inflated to achieve maximum ventilatory efficiency. In patients who have signs of inhalation injury on bronchoscopy, there is aggressive management of retained secretions with the use of bronchodilators and mucolytic agents along with aerosolized heparin. Meticulous control of airway pressure is practiced with the early performance of torso escharotomies and prompt treatment of an abdominal compartment syndrome particularly in the burned child. Mean airway pressures are maintained at <32–34 cm of water and ready use is made of chemical paralysis of the patient with a low threshold for conversion to pressure-controlled ventilation with titration of tidal volumes to lessen further the risk of ventilator-associated barotrauma. This may require the acceptance of smaller than usual tidal volumes and permissive hypercapnia, which is acceptable as long as arterial blood pH is above 7.26 and the patient is hemodynamically stable. These approaches along with a tightly controlled fluid resuscitation will in most circumstances avoid the need for alternative ventilator strategies in the care of these patients. Others including the senior author prefer to use HFPV prophylactically. In all patients with documented inhalation injury, HFPV is initiated on admission to minimize airway obstruction, maintain lung volume, and reduce the risk of pneumonia.

Early extubation and cessation of mechanical ventilation in patients with inhalation injury reduce the incidence of ventilator-associated pneumonia and limit barotrauma. The use of sedation "holidays" and spontaneous breathing trials enable one to assess pulmonary reserve and predict extubation success, but the results can be misleading. White and associates at the U.S. Army Burn Center evaluated interbreath interval complexity during spontaneous breathing trials as a means of predicting extubation success and reducing extubation failure.[89] Those investigators identified that lower interbreath interval complexity was associated with extubation failure. Analysis of wave form data identified lower sample entropy in the failure group with other nonlinear metrics moving in concert with entropy.

OTHER ORGAN SYSTEM SUPPORT

Pain Control

The pain experienced by patients suffering from acute thermal injuries is a complex integration of the objective neurologic input from the damaged tissue and the patient's fear and anxiety resulting from the traumatic event. The patient's pain is compounded further by wound care and the therapy required to maintain functional status. If the patient begins to perceive that there is no escape from this situation, fear and anxiety will be amplified and may be magnified further by the appearance and expression of concern by family and friends. Furthermore, as the burn begins to heal, there may be increased wound sensitivity during dressing changes and therapy sessions. This can further distress patients, as they perceive that instead of the pain improving with recovery it seems to be worsening. Pain is a fifth vital sign and it should be monitored, its level documented, and treatment be properly planned. Appropriate therapeutic options must be available to provide pain control to patients.

In patients who are hospitalized for ongoing care or require surgery, it is best to initiate long acting oral narcotic agents for background pain control and administer shorter acting narcotics either orally or parenterally, along with anxiolytic agents, for procedure related pain. For an acutely injured patient undergoing a procedure in the ICU or ward, intravenous morphine remains the main stay for analgesia along with oral compounds such as hydrocodone, which is preferable to oxycodone, which has a greater propensity for abuse. Clonidine can also be added to the pain regimen in patients who are having an initial poor response to narcotics and anxiolytic agents.[90] In patients who are intubated and are being maintained on mechanical ventilation, the two commonly used regimens are the continuous administration of intravenous morphine and diazepam or propofol and fentanyl to achieve pain control and sedation and prevent unplanned extubation. In the postoperative care of patients having skin graft procedures, the most painful wound is often not the burn wound but the donor site. Jellish et al.[91] have reported that the treatment of the skin graft harvest site with local anesthetic agents significantly improved the patient's pain score postoperatively. Patient-controlled analgesia is also a very effective strategy in patients who understand and can manipulate the delivery system. An important factor leading to effective pain control is to have established protocols that all members of the team understand and can use safely. There must be flexibility in the medication regimen and the patients must be fully informed that every attempt will be made to provide them the greatest comfort within the context of safe and compassionate care.

Neurological Deficits

Immediately following burn injury, the patient with an altered mental status needs to undergo a careful evaluation for injuries occurring during and prior to the time of the fire. Additionally, the patient's preinjury neurological status needs to be determined for any prior impairment. In patients who are obtunded, the primary concern is central nervous system (CNS) injury due to hypoxia and carbon monoxide poisoning. The use of alcohol or drugs in the time leading up to the burn injury can confound the assessment of the burn-injured victim. Testing for alcohol and drugs aids in the evaluation of such patients.[92] This is particularly important since the impact of alcohol appears to substantially modify the patient's chance for survival. The patient, particularly an elderly patient, should also be evaluated for a primary CNS event that might have precipitated their injury such as a seizure, stroke, or intracranial hemorrhage. The possibly of an assault must always be foremost in one's thoughts particularly in children when the history of the injury does not match the findings. It is not uncommon to find that a burn is a signal finding for child abuse.[93] This can also be the case in adults where the initial event was an assault and the burn is an attempt to disguise the physical attack.

Patients presenting with agitation must be rapidly evaluated for hypoxia and treated. The initial management of a patient who has a deteriorating mental status is a review of the medications and medication doses that have been administered to determine whether reversal agents should be given. In the treatment of children, the doses should be age and weight appropriate and carefully titrated to the patient's need. Later in the course of a burn patient's care, changes in mental status require a detailed review of medications for pain and sedation, measurement of serum electrolyte values particularly sodium, and evaluation for a septic process and the onset of renal or hepatic failure. Patients with impaired mental status either early or late must always be assessed for the status of their airway, their ability to maintain a patent airway, and the need for tracheal intubation.

Gastrointestinal Responses and Complications

Impaired GI motility and focal gastric mucosal ischemia occur in virtually all patients with burns involving more than 25% of the total body surface with the severity of change proportional to the extent of the burn.[94] The resulting ileus necessitates nasogastric intubation to prevent emesis and aspiration. If the mucosa is unprotected by instillation of antacid or treatment with an H_2 histamine receptor antagonist, ischemic erosions in the mucosa may progress to frank ulceration with associated bleeding or even perforation. Sufficient antacid (typically 30 mL but 60 mL may be needed) should be instilled each hour to maintain the pH of the gastric contents above 5. At the present, a histamine H_2 receptor antagonist (e.g., 400 mg of cimetadine given intravenously every 4 hours) or proton pump inhibitors are more commonly used for stress ulcer prophylaxis. When GI motility returns, enteral feeding should be initiated and the antacid therapy, for example, a 1,200–2,400 mg daily dose of cimetadine, can be added to enteral feeds. A randomized study comparing antacid prophylaxis and nonacid buffering sucralfate prophylaxis showed no difference in recovery of gram-negative organisms from the upper GI tract, and no difference in the occurrence of gram-negative pneumonia, but lesser gastric mucosal protection and a higher incidence of gram positive pneumonia in the sucralfate-treated group.[95]

WOUND CARE

Initial Wound Care

Initial wound care is focused on preventing further injury. Immediately upon removal of the burn victim from the site of injury, attention should be given to removal of burning clothing, disrupting contact with metal objects that may retain heat, and cooling of any molten materials adherent to the skin surface. Attempted cooling of burn wounds must be done with caution as local vasoconstriction can impair wound blood flow and extend the depth of the injury. The use of surface cooling of the burn is limited to patients with small burns typically not requiring hospitalization. Hypothermia can rapidly occur in children as well as adults particularly elderly patients if they are placed in cool or wet dressings. Patients being prepared for transport or admitted for definitive care should be placed in sterile or clean dry dressings and be kept warm. Prolonged exposure of the burn victim's wounds leads to cooling and further impairs the patient's response to their injury. Items of clothing or jewelry that may impair circulation should be removed prior to the onset of burn wound edema to prevent further compromise of the circulation. In cases of chemical injury, removal of contaminated clothing and copious water lavage of liquid chemicals and removal by brushing of powdered materials at the scene can limit the extent of the resultant burn injury. The ability to perform these maneuvers at the scene must be balanced against the patient's associated injuries that would mandate immediate transport for the care of life threatening injuries. No attempt should be made at chemical neutralization of the suspected chemical agent as such treatment would result in an exothermic reaction and cause additional tissue damage. The care provider must exercise extreme caution when working with victims of chemical injury to prevent self-contamination and personal injury. In all circumstances, those individuals caring for burn patients should wear personal protection devices. After admission to the hospital and as soon as resuscitative measures have been instituted, the patient should be bathed and the burn wounds cleansed with a detergent disinfectant. Chlorhexidine gluconate is a cleansing agent with an excellent antimicrobial spectrum.

During cleansing of the wound, the patient must not be allowed to become hypothermic. The treatment area and the cleansing fluids should be warm and the procedure should be done expeditiously. Materials that are densely adherent to the wound such as wax, tar, plastic, and metal should be gently removed or allowed to separate during the course of subsequent dressing changes. Sloughing skin, devitalized tissue, and ruptured blisters should be gently trimmed from the wound. No formal attempt is made to remove the burned tissue during these wound-dressing debridements. Patients may experience considerable pain and apprehension during these dressing changes and should receive adequate pain medication. In the patient on whom blisters are present, whether to remove them or allow them to remain is a matter of opinion. Blisters that are intact, particularly thick blisters on the palm of a hand maybe left intact.[96] Intact blisters must be closely monitored for signs of infection or rupture at which time they should be debrided and the wound treated. If a blister can be kept intact wound healing should be complete in <3 weeks. The notion that intact blisters are an effective biologic dressing has been called into question and some authors recommend removing all blisters and treating the burn as an open wound.[21] Careful wound cleansing should be done at each dressing change with serial debridement of devitalized tissue performed as necessary. The wound should be monitored for signs of infection and change in depth from the initial assessment. It is not uncommon for the initial wound depth to have been underestimated in children and young women. Additionally, the extent of body surface involvement should be recalculated to ensure that the initial burn size determination was accurate.

Topical Antimicrobial Therapy

The burn injury sets in progress a series of events leading to impaired local and systemic immunity. The damaged skin surface can serve as the portal for microbial invasion if it becomes progressively colonized. As microbial numbers increase within the wound to levels of 100,000 organisms per gram of tissue, an invasive wound infection and ultimately systemic sepsis may occur. Topically applied antimicrobial agents, which penetrate the burn eschar, are capable of achieving sufficient levels to control microbial proliferation within the wound. Systemic antibiotics do not achieve sufficiently high concentrations in the wound to achieve therapeutic levels, as the eschar is in large part avascular. These concepts form the basis for the use of topical antimicrobial agents in the prophylactic treatment of the burn wound and as a part of the management of burn wound infections.[97] Topical agents per se do not heal the wound but prevent local burn wound infection from destroying viable tissue in wounds capable of spontaneous healing. In burns that will require excision and grafting, control of the burn wound microbial density prevents the development of systemic sepsis secondary to invasive burn wound infection. The utility of topical agents is most clearly apparent in improving patient outcome in burns of >30% TBSA. The need for the use of topical antimicrobial compounds in the management of small burns has never been demonstrated and these injuries can be effectively managed with a petroleum-based dressing.[98-101] That being said, it has become common practice to apply topical antimicrobial agents to even small burn wounds despite the fact that there are no data to support this approach. Topical antimicrobial burn wound agents include cream, ointment, and liquid based products that require daily to twice daily dressing changes and reapplication. Also available are materials impregnated with antimicrobial compounds that typically are changed following a several day period of application.

Silver sulfadiazine, the most widely used agent, is available as a 1% suspension in a water-soluble micronized cream base. The cream is easily applied, causes little or no pain on application, and can be used open or as a closed dressing. As a closed dressing, the cream can be directly applied to the wound as a continuous layer, then covered over with a dressing or be impregnated into the dressing, which is then applied to the wound. At each dressing change, the cream should be totally removed and not allowed to form a caseous layer that will obscure the wound bed. When silver sulfadiazine is used in the management of superficial partial thickness burns, the dressing becomes discolored, the wound exudate appears infected, and the wound develops a yellow-gray pseudoeschar that is easily removed. The ability of silver sulfadiazine to penetrate an eschar and prevent wound infectious complication in burns >40%-50% TBSA is thought to be poor. However, wound cleansing with chlorhexidine as a part of the wound management along with silver sulfadiazine has proven to be a very effective combination in patients with larger burns. The most common toxic side effect of silver sulfadiazine is a transient leukopenia, which when it does occur in up to 15% of treated patients, resolves spontaneously without discontinuation of the drug.[102] The proposed mechanisms for this response have ranged from leukocyte margination in the wound (not drug related) to a direct cytotoxic effect of the drug on the bone marrow granulocyte and macrophage progenitor cells.[103] Silver sulfadiazine is active against a wide range of microbes including *Staphylococcus aureus*, *Escherichia coli*, *Klebsiella* species, many but not all *Pseudomonas aeruginosa*, *Proteus* species, and *Candida albicans*.

Mafenide acetate was one of the first effective topical agents introduced for the management of the burn wound. It was initially available as Sulfamylon burn cream (an 11.1% suspension in a vanishing cream base). It is commonly used on exposed wounds treated by the open technique though it is possible to use it under a light dressing. Mafenide acetate is highly effective against gram-positive and gram-negative organisms, but provides little antifungal activity.[104] Mafenide acetate readily diffuses into the eschar and is the agent of choice for major burns of the ears because it is also capable of penetrating cartilage. Drawbacks with the use of mafenide acetate include pain on application to partial thickness burns, and limited activity against methicillin-resistant S. *aureus*. Mafenide acetate also inhibits carbonic anhydrase, which increases urinary loss of bicarbonate, which may cause hyperchloremic acidosis and accentuate postburn hyperventilation. Fortunately, this affect is time limited because the kidney typically escapes from such inhibition in 8–10 days. Mafenide acetate has more recently become available as a 5% aqueous solution and is an excellent agent to use on freshly grafted wounds and is not associated with the problems found with the cream formulation.

Silver nitrate as a 0.5% solution has also been available since the 1960s and is effective against gram-positive and gram-negative organisms. The silver moiety is deposited on the burn wound and does not penetrate the eschar to any great extent. Silver nitrate soak solution leaches sodium, potassium, chloride, and calcium from the wound in association with trans-eschar water absorption, which can result in mineral deficits, alkalosis, and water loading. Those side effects can be minimized by giving sodium and other mineral supplements and modifying fluid therapy. These problems and the labor required to use silver nitrate effectively limit its routine use currently and most see silver sulfadiazine as a highly acceptable alternative.

Silver impregnated dressings consisting of a polyethylene mesh coated with a nanocyrstalline film of pure silver ions bonded to a flexible rayon-polyester sheet have recently become available for clinical use.[105] When the fabric base is in contact with wound fluids, the silver is released continuously to maintain a silver concentration of 50–100 mg/L on the wound for up to 48 hours. The treatment interval with such a composite may extend up to several days depending on the fabrication design with dressing changes needed only once or twice per week. On the basis of a multicenter randomized controlled trial it was concluded that Acticoat has better antimicrobial activity and fewer adverse effects than topical silver sulfadiazine, and reduces healing times.[106] The investigators considered the ease of application and low frequency of change to make Acticoat an ideal dressing for burn wounds. However, one must know that the wound has not become compromised during extended periods between reapplication. It is not advisable to use this approach in the care of perineal wounds particularly in small children with frequent bowel movements or wounds with excessive drainage or difficulty in maintaining contact between the dressing and the burn wound surface. The effectiveness of this membrane in treating extensive full thickness burns is unconfirmed and at present it is used to treat partial thickness burns.

In superficial partial thickness burns, the use of bacitracin ointment represents a satisfactory alternative particularly in patients with a known sulfa allergy. It may be used open especially with superficial facial burns or as a component of a closed dressing. Other topical agents include antibiotic combinations such as triple antibiotic ointment (neomycin, bacitracin zinc, and polymyxin B) and polysporin (bacitracin zinc and polymyxin B). In the case of methicillin-resistant staphylococci, mupirocin represents a useful agent.[107] These agents are also capable of being used with open or closed dressing techniques.

The application of topical antimicrobial agents to the burns of patients who will be transferred to a burn center may preclude the use of biological membrane dressings that will adhere to the wound surface to be effective. Additionally, upon admission to a burn center, any previously placed dressing will be removed to permit the burn team to make a precise assessment of the extent of the burn and the depth of injury. In addition to burn wound evaluation, the burned child must be inspected for any signs of abuse, which includes a detailed examination of the entire skin surface. Unless there will be an extended period of time before patient transfer to a burn center, placing the patient in a dry dressing, particularly if it is one with a nonadherent lining, and keeping the patient warm is the preferred initial management.

The sterile gloved hand is used to apply the burn cream of choice in a thickness sufficient to obscure the surface of the burn (Fig. 32.7). The wounds are then either left exposed or covered by a light occlusive dressing. Twelve hours later, the topical agent is reapplied to the entire burn wound. If a dressing is used over the topical agent, it is removed prior to reapplication of the topical agent following which a new dressing is applied. To optimize antimicrobial coverage and minimize side effects, one can alternate topical agents, that is, apply Sulfamylon burn cream after the morning cleansing and apply Silvadene burn cream in the evening.[108] If 0.5% silver nitrate soaks are used for topical wound care (as may be necessary in a patient allergic to sulfonamides), they should be changed two or three times a day and kept moist between changes by infusing additional soak solution every 2 hours. All environmental surfaces and equipment as well as the clothing and exposed skin of attending personnel must be protected from contact with the silver nitrate solution, which will cause dark brown discoloration of virtually anything with which it comes in contact.

Each day the topical agent is totally removed in the course of the daily cleansing and the entirety of the burn wound is examined to detect any signs of infection. If signs of infection are identified, a biopsy of the eschar and the underlying viable tissue should be obtained from the area of the wound suspected of harboring infection (Fig. 32.8). The biopsy sample is subjected to histologic examination and should also be cultured to determine predominant organisms. Histologic confirmation of invasive infection (the presence of bacteria or fungi in viable tissue underlying or adjacent to the burned tissue) necessitates a change to Sulfamylon burn cream topical therapy (mafenide acetate can diffuse into nonviable tissue to limit microbial proliferation), subeschar antibiotic infusion, physiologic fine tuning of the patient, and prompt surgical excision of the infected tissue.[109]

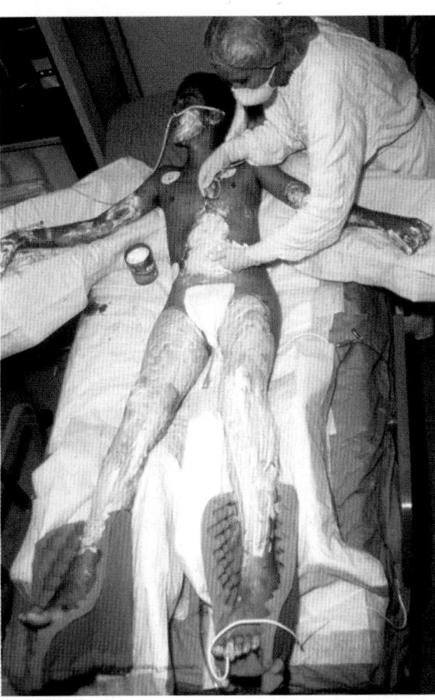

FIGURE 32.7. Following the initial cleansing and debridement, the burn wounds are covered with a topical antimicrobial burn cream as shown here. The topical agent is reapplied 12 hours later. The wounds are cleansed each day and thoroughly examined to identify signs of burn wound infection and if no such signs are evident the burn cream is reapplied.

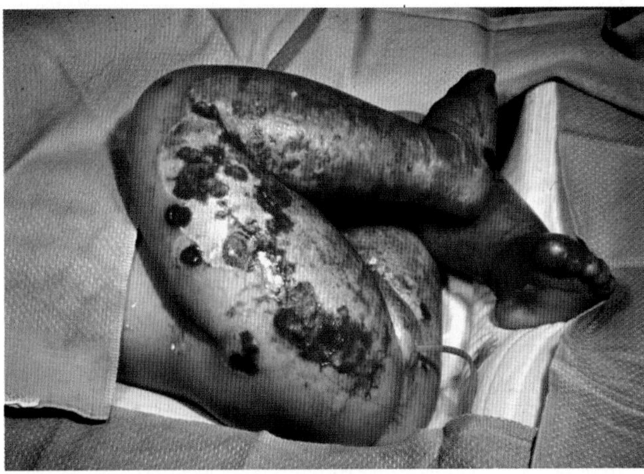

FIGURE 32.8. The dark brown areas in the leg burns of this child were sites of bacterial invasion. The smaller foci of black/red discoloration in unburned tissue at and near the periphery of the leg burns were ecthyma gangrenosa, which are pathognomonic of hematogenous spread of invasive Pseudomonas burn wound infection as confirmed by histologic examination of tissue biopsied from one of the lesions.

Burn Wound Excision and Grafting

Topical antimicrobial chemotherapy is typically employed to control microbial density on and in the burned tissue prior to excision with emphasis placed on early excision that is now considered to be optimum management of full thickness burns and those of mixed depth. If the patient is otherwise stable, burn wound excision can be carried out within a matter of hours postinjury. In the patient with a small burn, delay is often related to scheduling of the operating room and the surgical team. Timely excision for the patient with a small burn reduces the period of disability and the overall cost of the injury. In patients with a large burn wound, the timing and extent of the surgery is based on the patient's relative physiologic stability and his capacity to undergo a major operative procedure. Early burn wound excision and closure in patients with large wounds shortens the length of hospitalization, reduces cost, and favorably impacts overall burn mortality.[110,111] The presence of the burn wound is the primary stimulus for the ongoing problems facing the burn patient. Closure of the burn serves to ameliorate much of the postburn pathophysiology and is one of the most effective means by which to improve a burn patient's outcome. Wounds that are capable of spontaneous closure within two to three weeks postinjury can be managed expectantly provided the cosmetic and functional outcomes will be acceptable.

Wounds that are small in size or linear in shape can be managed by excision of the burn and primary wound closure. This is of use in burns of the upper inner arm in the elderly, localized burns of a pendulous breast, abdominal burns, buttock injuries, and thigh burns. Primary wound closure can also be achieved in some wounds with local tissue transfer techniques. This approach works quite well when these wounds are excised early before substantial microbial colonization of the wound occurs. In such cases, the burn is transformed into a healing surgical incision and creation of a skin graft donor site is avoided.

In selected cases, the injury may be of such a nature that amputation of the burned part is the most appropriate plan. In the patient with considerable multisystem trauma, the expeditious removal of the burn injury might be seen as the best option for the patient's overall survival. In a recent report, Santaniello et al.[112] found that the mortality in trauma victims with significant burn injuries and trauma was 28.3%, whereas in patients with burns only it was 9.8% and in patients with trauma only it was 4.3%. The management of these challenging patients requires a coordinated well-conceived plan of care that accounts for all of the patient's injuries and integrates the treatment needs of each injury to achieve an overall satisfactory outcome. A mangled extremity, which has also suffered a severe burn that is deemed nonsalvageable, should undergo early amputation. It is not necessary to extend the amputation to a level that allows closure with unburned tissue. If viable muscle is available to close the amputation site, that wound bed can be resurfaced with an autogenous skin graft. A grafted amputation site can, with a modern prosthesis, function as a durable stump. In a patient who is paraplegic and suffers an extensive deep lower extremity burn injury, amputation can be a viable alternative to excision and grafting.

A similar option may need to be considered for the patient in whom substantial preexisting peripheral vascular disease makes the likelihood of a healed and functional extremity highly unlikely. This unfortunately has become an all too frequent occurrence in the care of elderly burn patients who have progressive complications from long standing diabetes mellitus. The amputation level should be that which will maintain maximum function. This might be a transmetatarsal or Chopart-type amputation in patients with injuries of the distal foot. In patients confined to a wheel chair who have injuries to the leg, a through-knee amputation as opposed to an above-knee amputation provides a weight-bearing platform for sitting. In the patient in whom the initial insult represents a deep composite injury, repeated failed attempts at salvage are not in the patient's ultimate best interest. Such wounds often become infected and tissue that could have been preserved now must in the end be sacrificed with the functional end result less than that which would have occurred with early amputation.

Excision and grafting will be required for wounds not amenable to primary closure. The extent of the procedure that a patient can undergo is related to the patient's age, physiologic status, and skill of the operating team. A 17% surface area burn should be a universally survivable injury in 17-year-old patient while in patients in the eighth decade of life the mortality can easily be 50%. An otherwise healthy individual with available donor sites can well tolerate a 20%-25% total body burn excision and autografting in one procedure. Implicit in this approach is the use of experienced operating teams, an anesthesiologist who thoroughly understands the unique problems of the patient with a major body surface area burn, and an operating room fully equipped to treat such a patient, as well as ready availability of blood products and the capacity to care for the patient postoperatively. A patient having this extent of surgery in essence undergoes a doubling of the surface area of "injury"—the now excised and grafted wound along with the partial thickness wound produced by the donor site. In patients with wounds of a larger size (>30% TBSA) or those who cannot tolerate a single procedure to achieve closure, staged excision of burned tissue is performed and the resulting wounds are closed with available cutaneous autografts or a biologic dressing.[113]

The technique of burn wound excision is based on the depth of the wound and anatomic site to be excised. Excision of deep partial thickness wounds to the level of a uniformly viable bed of deep dermis, by the tangential technique pioneered by Janzekovic, and immediate coverage with cutaneous autograft results in rapid wound closure with a typically excellent result.[114] This can be done with an unguarded Weck knife, a Goulian/Weck guarded knife, a hand held dermatome or by using a powered dermatome set at 0.0016–0.0030 of an inch depending on the area to be excised and the age and gender of the patient. Optimally, the desired wound bed is achieved in one pass of the knife as evidenced by diffuse bleeding. If that end point is not realized another pass of the knife will be needed. A frequent error is attempting this technique in wounds of an inappropriate depth and assuming that punctate bleeding indicates a viable bed. Such wounds will heal with a poor take of the grafted skin as the bed contains marginally viable tissue incapable of supporting the cutaneous autograft. These wounds at the initial graft dressing change may appear to be doing well only to fail at 5–10 days postoperatively. Tangential excision as originally reported, was employed early in the first week postburn, however, it can be successfully applied any time to a wound that is not infected or heavily colonized. During the performance of this procedure, the amount of blood loss can be minimized with the use of a tourniquet on extremity burns or subeschar clysis containing epinephrine or ornithine vasopressin. The decision that the depth of the excision is satisfactory with these adjuncts will be based primarily on the appearance of the wound, an appreciation of which most experienced burn surgeons have had to learn to some degree through trial and error. High-pressure hydrosurgical devices are also available to excise burned tissue but are considered by some to be associated with greater blood loss and the sacrifice of more viable tissue.

A modification of tangential excision is wound excision via layered escharectomy. Using this technique, the wound is sequentially excised to a viable bed of subcutaneous tissue and elements of deep dermis particularly at the wound margin. This allows relative preservation of body part contour, a graft with ultimately more pliability, decreased limb edema, and a cosmetically more acceptable transition at the juncture of the grafted wound with the unburned skin of the wound margins.

An alternative to layered excision is to excise the wound with a scalpel or electrocautery. Using knife excision, the wound is excised to the muscle fascia or to viable deep subcutaneous tissue. As bleeding can be substantial with such procedures, the excision and control of bleeding must be done efficiently. The use of electrocautery to perform the dissection limits the blood loss without compromising the recipient graft site. Imperative with electrocautery excision into the deep fat is avoidance and limitation of thermal injury to the wound bed, which will compromise the "take" of the applied skin graft. The use of the cutting mode with rapid dissection is necessary. In cases where excision to fascia has been performed, the viability of the fascia should be assessed. The surgeon must determine if the fascia requires removal and the underlying muscle used as the graft bed. In the performance of fascial excisions, caution should be exercised during the dissection to avoid entrance into a joint or bursa and injury of extensor tendons in the hand or the Achilles' tendon at the ankle.

The blood loss occurring with burn wound excision is related to the time of excision postburn, the area to be excised, the presence of infection, and type of excision, that is, fascial or tangential. Donor sites can also represent a considerable portion of the blood loss. The use of the scalp or previously harvested donor sites is associated with increased bleeding. The quantity of blood loss has been estimated to range from 0.45 to 1.25-mL/cm^2 burn area excised.[115] Adjunctive measures that can be used to control blood loss include elevation of limbs undergoing excision, applications of topical thrombin and/or vasoconstrictive agents in solutions to the excised wound and donor site, clysis of skin graft harvest sites and/or the eschar prior to removal, and application of tourniquets. Spray application of fibrin sealant can also reduce bleeding from the excised wound after release of the tourniquet. Blood loss will be compounded if the patient has become coagulopathic, hypothermic or acidotic during the procedure. Perioperative cold stress, which may induce hypothermia, can be reduced by maintaining the temperature of the operating room between 30°C and 32°C and by using warmed fluids for wound irrigation. Oda et al.[116] have emphasized the importance of maintaining a warm operating room environment and limiting the duration of excision and other procedures to prevent hypothermia in patients with extensive burns. In 16 patients with extensive burns, pulmonary compromise characterized by a significant decrease in the PaO_2/FIO_2 ratio in association with an increase in neutrophils in bronchoalveolar lavage fluid occurred if body temperature decreased more than 1°C during the operation. The authors concluded that hypothermia during surgery showed little correlation with blood loss, transfusion, or duration of surgery alone but was significantly correlated with the development of acute lung injury.

The harvest, application, and postoperative care of split thickness skin grafts and skin graft donor sites are the same as for any other surgical patient. A silver containing hydrofiber gel sheet has recently been evaluated as a dressing for split thickness skin graft donor sites.[117] When applied to donor sites, either under a gauze dressing or a transparent film, the hydrofiber dressing was assessed to have the advantages of ease of application, management of drainage, and removal; reduction in donor site pain; and the ability to remain in place for up to 5 days. Grafting of the burn wound is usually done at the time of excision, but the surgeon must be aware of the patient's status throughout the surgical procedure and if necessary reassess the extent of the planned procedure. There will be instances where it will be best to perform the excision only and stage the timing of skin graft application. Additionally, if the wound bed is suspect as to its viability then only excision should be performed. The wound can be dressed with a 5% Sulfamylon solution dressing or covered with allograft skin or any of several biologic dressings and subsequently reevaluated. The use of cutaneous allografts is a very useful approach when excising facial burns where the goal is to preserve all possible elements and perform the definitive grafting procedure on a "tested" recipient bed. In cases where an infected wound is being excised, no attempt at placing autograft skin should be considered until the infection has been resolved following treatment with topical and systemic antimicrobial agents as determined by culture results and inspection of the wound.

The choice of the donor site in the performance of a cutaneous autograft will in some patients be limited to those skin sites that have not been injured with burns. When there is a choice of donor sites, the requirements of the recipient site and the potential for donor site morbidity should be factored into selecting the site of graft harvest. In the grafting of facial burns, color match is an important consideration and obtaining a graft from a site above the clavicles or the inner aspect of the thigh will provide the best result. In children, harvest of a graft from the scalp results in a donor site that is not particularly painful postoperatively and has no long-term cosmetic consequences. The harvest of grafts from posterior body surfaces provides, in general, a more acceptable wound for most patients. While the anterior thigh is an often-selected site, it can heal with considerable hypertrophic change and cause a patient more problems and distress than the grafted burn.

The use of sheets of autograft skin for resurfacing the burn represents the gold standard. This is the only acceptable approach for burns of the face and neck and the best choice in grafting of the hands and breast. Every attempt should be made to use such autografts in children, since they provide the best long-term results. It may not be possible to achieve these objectives in patients with extensive burns or those in whom the pattern and location of the injury limits donor site availability. The use of meshed cutaneous autografts allows the surgeon to increase the area covered. Skin graft meshing devices of various design and manufacture are available with expansion ratios from 1:1 to 1:9. The wider the mesh the greater the wound area covered, however, it will take the wound longer to close by ingrowth from the margins of the mesh reticulum to fill the open interstices during which time there is the very real potential for graft loss and wound infection to occur. Additionally, widely meshed autografts have a greater propensity to form hypertrophic burn scars, and may provide a skin surface with unsatisfactory mechanical stability, inadequate pliability, permanently poor cosmetic appearance, and restricted joint mobility. Despite these potential limitations, the use of meshed cutaneous autografts is an important strategy and potentially lifesaving approach in patients with extensive body surface area burns.

The technique of skin graft harvesting would seem a relatively simple procedure, yet it is often not done well. As noted above, the harvest site should be the one that will yield a graft with the desirable characteristics and the least donor site morbidity. Grafts should be of sufficient size to achieve wound closure with a minimum of intergraft seams. Powered dermatomes are available with up to 6 inch cutting widths that provide excellent sheets of skin for facial grafts or when meshed can cover a major burn area. Donor site preparation is essential to obtain a uniform graft. Powered clysis can rapidly be accomplished over an extensive harvest site using an air powered surgical wound irrigating system equipped with a 14 or 16 gauge needle attached to 3 L bags of normal saline. This provides a stable uniform surface for graft harvest and limits the difficulties encountered when harvesting over contoured surfaces or bony prominences. The thickness of the harvested graft should be related to the site to be grafted, whether the graft is to be meshed, the mesh ratio, and to some degree surgeon preference. The desired thickness of the graft also influences donor site selection, that is, a "thick" graft should be harvested from an area of "thick" skin. Harvest of a "thick" graft from an area of "thin" skin, that is, the inner arm, can produce a full thickness wound that will have to be grafted.

Skin grafts through which one can read printed material are primarily epithelial autografts with a minimal amount of dermis (0.004 0.006 inch) while those, which are more opaque contain a variably greater amount of dermis (0.008–0.012 inch). Thinner grafts yield a better donor site and function well on a dermal wound bed but may not do well when placed on a wound excised to fascia. In elderly patients, thin grafts that contain insufficient numbers of keratinocyte progenitor cells are considered the cause of melting graft syndrome and prolong the time of re-epithelization. Thicker grafts are more pliable, heal with less contraction, and will do better than thin grafts when meshed. The thicker grafts may result in donor site scarring and delay in donor site closure especially in the elderly patient.

The harvested graft should be placed on the prepared burn wound parallel to the major flexion creases and can be attached mechanically with staples or sutures or secured with tissue adhesives such as fibrin glue. A properly placed set of grafts on an extremity should at the end of the operation be able to remain in place as the extremity is put through a gentle range of motion. One of the most important aspects of a skin grafting procedure is the application of a proper dressing. A highly successful approach is to use multiple layers of a nonadherent linen dressing moistened with a 5% solution of mafenide acetate applied circumferentially to the excised and grafted wounds on an extremity. A bolster produced by using net dressings drawn tightly over the burn dressings and stapled to the skin is used to "fix" the grafts on torso wounds. Graft failure occurs as a result of inadequate excision, inadequate hemostasis, infection, subgraft seroma formation, mechanical sheering during postoperative care, or rarely, "upside down" application. The first dressing change is typically done 48–72 hours postoperatively. If a sheet graft is well intact at that time, a nonadherent dressing is reapplied to protect the wound. In the case of meshed autografts, the moist dressings of mafenide acetate solution, changed daily or more often as required, are continued until the mesh is closed.

To increase graft conformity to wound base, remove exudate, and to reduce shearing, topical negative pressure therapy is often used to cover and hold freshly applied split thickness skin grafts in place. Recently, investigators have reported that topical negative pressure dressings reduce shearing forces, restrict seroma and hematoma formation, simplify wound care, and improve patient tolerance.[118] Contrary to the speculation of others, those investigators could identify no major beneficial effects of topical negative pressure dressings on the rate of neovascularization of skin grafts.

Skin Substitutes

While split thickness cutaneous autografts are the usual method of wound closure there is often the need for a skin substitute. Alternative wound coverings are used to achieve wound closure when the available donor surface area is not sufficient, there is a need to test the wound bed, or for primary management of selected partial thickness wounds. The goal with a skin substitute is to obtain temporary physiologic wound closure and protect the wound from microbial invasion. Although a wide variety of skin substitutes have been developed and evaluated to replace the epidermis, the dermis, or the epidermis and dermis together, all currently available skin substitutes except for cultured autologous keratinocytes, must be considered temporary with autografting required for definitive wound closure.[119]

The two most commonly used naturally occurring biologic dressings are human cutaneous allograft and porcine cutaneous xenograft. Human allograft skin is commercially available as split-thickness grafts in either fresh viable or cryopreserved form. Both of these preparations are capable of becoming vascularized, however, this best occurs with fresh allograft skin. Allograft skin can provide wound coverage for 3–4 weeks before rejection.[120] Porcine xenograft tissue is available as reconstituted sheets of meshed porcine dermis or as fresh or frozen split-thickness skin. Porcine skin impregnated with silver ions to suppress wound colonization is also available. Xenograft skin can be used to cover partial thickness injuries or donor sites, which reepithelialize beneath the xenograft.[121] Using a murine model of burn injury, Wang et al. found that transgenic expression of cytotoxic T-lymphocyte—Associated Antigen4-immunoglobulin (CTLA4Ig) increased xenogeneic skin graft survival almost twofold without inducing systemic immunosuppression.[122] Such tissue may represent a readily available source of extended survival skin grafts for use in patients with massive burns. Similarly, nanofiber patches containing poly-n-acetyl glucosamine have been reported to accelerate closure of a murine model full thickness skin wound in association with an increase of cell proliferation and vascularity in granulation tissue.[123] This treatment was also credited with hemostatic action by virtue of platelet activation and vasoconstrictive properties all of which suggest usefulness in the treatment of complicated wounds.

Various synthetic membranes have been developed that provide wound protection and possess vapor and bacterial barrier properties. Biobrane (Dow-Hickham, Sugarland, Texas), is one such product that has been used in the management of partial thickness and donor site wounds.[124] This bilaminate membrane consists of a collagen gel adherent to a nylon mesh as the dermal analog to promote fibrovascular ingrowth and a thin outer silastic film as the epidermal analog to provide barrier properties. Biobrane has also been used as the scaffold for the growth of allogenic fibroblasts that secrete, while in culture, various growth factors along with other mediators. The fibroblasts are then removed by freezing to complete preparation of the membrane. These membranes are currently approved for use in fully excised wounds, donor sites, and superficial partial thickness burns.[125] Another collagen-based skin substitute is the dermal replacement developed by Burke and Yannas, presently in use as Integra (Integra LifeScience Corporation, Plainsboro, New Jersey). This membrane consists of an inner layer of collagen fibrils with added glycosaminoglycan and an outer barrier membrane of polysiloxane. It is placed over freshly excised full-thickness wounds and once fully vascularized, the epidermal analog is removed, and the vascularized "neodermis" is covered with a thin split thickness cutaneous autograft.[126]

StrataGraft skin tissue is another skin substitute that has a dermal equivalent populated with human dermal fibroblasts and a stratified biologically active epidermis derived from a pathogen free, long-lived, human keratinocyte progenitor near-diploid immortalized keratinocyte S (NIKS) cells. A comparison of StrataGraft® with cadaveric allograft applied to full thickness wounds for 1 week prior to autografting on 15 patients found there to be no differences in the number of T or B lymphocytes or Langerhans cells present in the grafts after 1 week. In the patients to whom the skin substitute was applied, no proliferation of peripheral blood mononuclear cells to NIKS, no enhancement of cell-mediated lysis of NIKS, *in vitro*, and no antibody generation targeted to NIKS were observed.[127] The authors concluded that StrataGraft "is well tolerated and not acutely immunogenic in patients..." and proposed it for use "in epidermal development, tissue engineering, and transplant studies" as well as facilitation of the healing of traumatic cutaneous wounds.

A permanent skin substitute represents a definitive means of wound closure for extensively burned patients. Presently, cultured epithelial autografts are commercially available but have been limited in use because of suboptimal graft take, fragility of the skin surface, and high cost.[128] Sood et al.[129] recently reported, on the basis of a retrospective review of the use of cultured epithelial autografts placed on an allodermis base, that take of the cultured autografts at 7 and 21 days was 72% and 67%, respectively. Those investigators concluded that when applied to an allodermis base, cultured epithelial autografts are useful in the treatment of extensive burn wounds.

New directions in the development of cultured epithelial autografts include the production of chimeric allogeneic-autologous cultured epithelium, the use of keratinocyte suspensions, and the application of low amperage direct current to allodermal/autoepidermal composite grafts as well as the development of culture-derived bilaminate membranes. Black et al have identified what they consider to be a neovascular network to form in a tissue-engineered skin equivalent in which keratinocytes, fibroblasts, and umbilical vein endothelial cells were cocultured in a collagen biopolymer.[130] Development of an autogenous vascular system in such a skin equivalent would permit inosculation to establish prompt vascularization by the host and achieve permanent adherence.

Sheng et al. have reported that bone marrow mesenchymal stem cells can be induced to acquire the phenotype of sweat gland cells. Implantation of such cells into anhydrotic areas of scars of healed, deep burn injury in five patients was reported to restore perspiration function in the transplanted areas. Histologic and biochemical studies confirmed that the transformed cells were involved in the recovery of functional sweat glands that produced sweat similar to that produced in areas of normal skin.[131] Confirmation of these findings offers the possibility of improved thermoregulation in patients who survive extensive thermal injury. Luo et al.[132] have assessed the ability of mesenchymal stem cells from human umbilical cord blood to promote cutaneous wound healing in an animal model of burn injury. Such cells differentiated into keratinocytes in the wound tissues and enhanced the healing of the burn wounds. The authors noted that mesenchymal stem cells can be isolated and proliferated but the need for human umbilical blood may limit subsequent clinical applicability.

Use of any biologic dressing requires that the excised wound and the dressing that has been applied be meticulously examined on at least a daily basis. Submembrane suppuration or the development of infection necessitates removal of the dressing, cleansing of the wound with a surgical detergent disinfectant solution, and even reexcision of the wound if residual nonviable or infected tissue is present. Following such wound care, a biologic dressing can again be applied and if it remains adherent and intact for 48–72 hours without suppuration, that biologic dressing can be removed and the wound closed definitively with cutaneous autografts.

The proper management of the patient's burn wounds is critical to achieve the optimum cosmetic and functional outcome and the timely return of the patient to full activity. In patients with major burns, the wound must be properly cared for and closure achieved expeditiously to lessen the level of physiologic disruption that accompanies a major burn. Failure to do so can result in invasive wound infection, chronic inflammation, erosion of lean body mass, scar formation, progressive functional deficits, and even death. As more patients with extensive burns survive, scar formation that impairs joint motion or limb function or causes disfigurement has become of greater concern. Recent studies of keloid scars have assessed the role of proteoglycans in the scaring process. Tissue from keloid scars was characterized by increased expression of syndecan-2 and fibroblast growth factor-2, and downregulation of decorin.[133] Decorin decreased extracellular matrix protein production and that action as well as its antifibrotic effect suggests therapeutic potential to ameliorate scaring.

Similarly, increased survival of extensively burned patients has focused attention on other outcomes such as the incidence of posttraumatic stress disorder (PTSD). A recent study has identified the fact that the incidence of PTSD is similar in military burn patients from the current conflicts in Iraq and Afghanistan and in civilian burn patients.[134] In both groups, the extent of burn and severity of injury but not age were significantly associated with PTSD. Earlier studies of burned children identifying an association between acute stress (ASD) and PTSD prompted a study to evaluate the effect of propranolol on the incidence of ASD.[135] A diagnosis of ASD was made in only 22 of 363 acutely burned children who had participated in a randomized trial of propranolol for control of postburn hypermetabolism. The incidence of ASD was found to be indifferent to propranolol, a result credited to "aggressive" treatment of anxiety and pain with opiates and benzodiazepines which appears to have decreased the incidence of ASD and reduced the incidence of the PTSD in burned children.

Effective topical antimicrobial therapy and early burn wound excision have considerably reduced the incidence of invasive bacterial infections. In a recent multiyear period, only 2.3% of patients treated at the U.S. Army Burn Center developed invasive burn wound infection but 72% of the 90 invasive infections that occurred in 3,876 patients were caused by opportunistic fungi (Fig. 32.9). Of the 90 patients who developed invasive burn wound infections, 55% or 61% expired. The most common nonbacterial opportunists recovered from burn patients are *Candida* species. Compared to the filamentous fungi, *Candida* sp. seldom invade but may be recovered from the blood of patients with multiple sites of colonization, extensive burns, prolonged hospital and ICU stay, multiple operative procedures, and receipt of total parenteral nutrition. A mortality of 15% has been attributed to candidemia

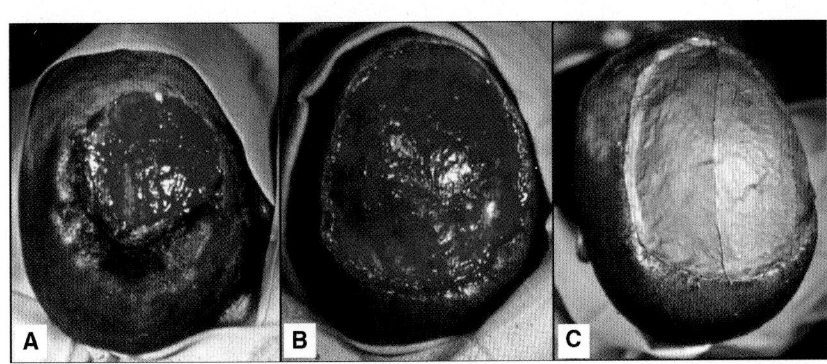

FIGURE 32.9. **A:** The rapid centrifugal spread of the necrosis in the scalp burn of this patient was caused by invasive mucormycosis. **B:** The extent of excision required to remove all the infected tissue encompassed the edematous tissue shown in "A" and produced a wound, which could be closed with split thickness skin grafts as shown in "C".

TRAUMA

with early empirical antifungal therapy recommended for burn patients with multiple site colonization.[136] A review of patients treated at the U.S. Army Burn Center who developed infections caused by filamentous fungi has identified a comorbid effect equal to that of an additional body surface area burn injury of 33%.[137]

The immunosuppression induced by burn injury also renders extensively burned patients susceptible to systemic viral infections typically caused by herpes simplex viruses and cytomegalovirus. A recent retrospective review of autopsy reports of 97 burn patients attributed death to bacterial infection in 27 and viral infection in 5.[138] In the patients in whom death was attributed to bacterial infection, the predominant organisms were *P. aeruginosa*, *E. coli*, *Klebsiella pneumoniae*, and *S. aureus*. The principal sites of infection were the blood stream in 50%, lungs in 44%, and the wound in only 6%. In two-thirds of those patients, the time of death was 21 or less days. The viral infections uniformly arose in the lower respiratory track and the time of death was often later ranging from 4 to 42 days. The herpes infections have typically been caused by HSV1 but recently a fulminant and fatal HSV-2 infection with pneumonitis and hepatitis has been reported in a patient with a 68% TBSA full thickness burn.[139]

TREATMENT OF SPECIAL THERMAL INJURIES

Electric Injury

The principal mechanism by which electricity damages tissue is by conversion to thermal energy. Currents of 1,000 V and above are classified as high voltage. Upon contact with such currents, the body acts as a volume conductor with small differences in conductivity among tissues of little consequence. At contact points where current density is greatest, tissue charring may limit current flow but at very high voltages current flow persists until the contact is interrupted. The electric current may induce cardiac and/or respiratory arrest necessitating cardiopulmonary resuscitation at the site of injury, on the way to the hospital, and in the emergency department. Arrhythmias may also occur after admission to the hospital necessitating electrocardiogram (EKG) monitoring for at least 24 hours after the last recorded episode of arrhythmia.

Two characteristics of high voltage electric injury increase the incidence of acute renal failure in patients with such injury. First, there may be only a small charred contact site evident with extensive inapparent subcutaneous tissue injury in a limb underlying unburned skin. The limited cutaneous injury may lead to gross underestimation of resuscitation fluid needs. Secondly, the mass of muscle injured by the electric current may liberate large amounts of hemochromogens that may damage the renal tubules. In addition to the electric injury, arcing of the current may ignite the patient's clothing to cause conventional thermal burns. Resuscitation fluids should be based on the extent of burn visible plus the estimated daily needs of the patient and adjusted according to the patient's response. If the urine contains hemochromogens (dark red pigments) fluid should be administered to obtain 75–100 mL of urine per hour with sodium bicarbonate added to the fluids to alkalinize the urine. If the hemochromogens do not clear promptly, or the patient remains oliguric, 25 g of mannitol should be given as a bolus and 12.5 g of mannitol added to each liter of lactated Ringers until the pigment clears. After administration of mannitol, urinary output is no longer an index of resuscitation adequacy and other indices of physiologic well being must be monitored to assess resuscitation status.

When the body functions as a volume conductor, current flow is proportional to the cross-sectional area of the body part involved. Consequently, severe tissue destruction may occur in a limb with relatively small cross section area and relatively little tissue damage occurs as current flows through the trunk. With cessation of current flow, body parts that acted as volume conductors now act as volume radiators with periosseous tissue deep in the limbs being exposed to elevated temperatures for longer periods of time.[140] Damage to the muscle in a limb is often associated with marked increase in the pressure within the compartment containing the damaged muscle which, if unrelieved, may cause further tissue necrosis. A limb muscle compartment that is stony hard to palpation should alert one to the need for surgical exploration. Evidence of extensive deep tissue necrosis, development of a compartment syndrome, and persistent or progressively severe hyperkalemia mandate operative intervention. At the time of exploration, the investing fascia is widely opened and the muscles of the involved limb thoroughly examined including the periosseous muscles of the limb, which can be necrotic yet overlain by more superficial viable muscle (Fig. 32.10). The extent of destruction may necessitate amputation at the time of exploration, particularly if the nonviable muscle is the source of persistent hyperkalemia. If the extent of muscle necrosis in a limb is indefinite, an arteriogram may be helpful. The identification of "pruning" of the intramuscular branches of the arterial tree identifies injured muscle and defines the level of amputation required to encompass the nonviable tissue.[141] Following debridement or amputation, the wound should be dressed open. The patient is returned to the operating room in 24–36 hours for reinspection and further debridement of nonviable tissue if necessary. When all tissue in the wound is viable, it may be closed definitively.

A detailed neurologic examination must be performed on all patients with high voltage electric injury at the time of admission and at scheduled 24–48 hour intervals thereafter. Signs of peripheral nerve and central nervous system impairment may be evident immediately after injury or may appear later. It is uncommon

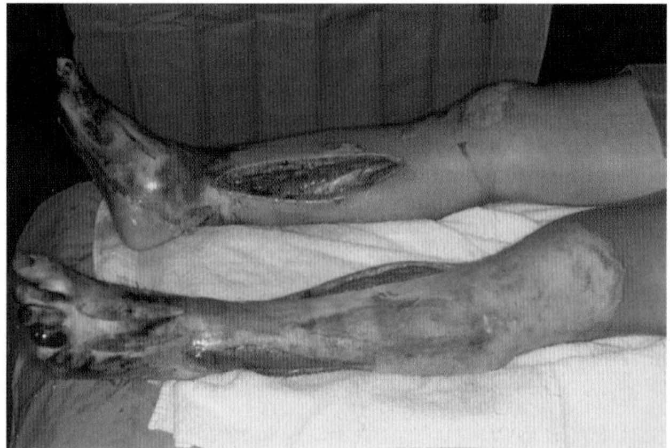

FIGURE 32.10. High Voltage electric injury caused desiccation and destruction of toes and the distal feet where cross-sectional tissue area was least. Thrombosed vessels are visible in the base of the linear incisions over the metatarsals of each foot. Edema of the pale damaged muscles which underlaid uninjured skin of the legs causes them to bulge above the edges of the fascia at the base of the fasciotomy incisions on the legs. The severity and extent of muscle damage necessitated bilateral below knee amputations.

for a nerve directly injured by electric current to regain function. The immediate functional impairment caused by nondestructive injury to which motor nerves are more sensitive than sensory nerves commonly resolves. Late occurring parasthesias and other polyneuritic symptoms causing deficits in the function of peripheral nerves remote from the sites of electric contact have been attributed to electroporation, the cellular effects of millivoltage electric fields.[142] Immediate neurologic impairments caused by direct nerve damage of the spinal cord more commonly resolve than do spinal cord deficits of later onset. Delayed onset spinal cord dysfunction can range from quadriplegia to localized nerve deficits with signs of ascending paralysis and even an amyotrophic lateral sclerosis-like syndrome.[143]

Remote organ injury is rare in patients with high voltage injury, but intestinal perforation, gall bladder necrosis, and direct liver injury have all been reported. Delayed hemorrhage from medium to large sized vessels has been attributed to electric injury-induced arteritis but inadequate debridement of injured tissue or transmural necrosis of the vessel wall as a consequence of exposure and desiccation appear to be more likely causes.

The formation of cataracts has also been associated with high voltage electric injury, particularly in those patients with a contact site on the head or neck. The patient should be informed that such cataracts may occur, commonly 3 or more years after the injury, but often much sooner. In patients with a head contact site, exfoliative debris may be evident in the anterior chamber of the eye immediately after injury. Such debris is slowly cleared and typically requires no specific treatment.

Tissue damage can also be caused by low voltage house current. Burns of the oral commissure occur in young children who bite electric cords or suck on the end of a live extension cord or an electric outlet. The lesion may have the characteristics of full thickness tissue damage but early surgical debridement may only accentuate the defect and should be avoided. These injuries will usually heal with minimal cosmetic sequelae, which can be addressed electively if needed. In the course of spontaneous healing, labial artery bleeding may occur. The parents should be warned that such bleeding, which can be impressive, may occur and instructed in how to apply manual pressure for temporary control until the vessel can be ligated.

Cardiopulmonary arrest is particularly common in patients struck by lightning and necessitates the immediate institution of cardiopulmonary resuscitation. Subsequent ECG abnormalities are uncommon and signs of acute myocardial damage, though rare, may become evident later. Coma immediately following injury is common, but typically transient. Keraunoparalysis (lightning paralysis) characterized by paresthesias and paralysis typically involving the lower limbs may develop over several days after lightning injury in association with vasomotor disorders.[144] This paralysis typically resolves without residual deficit. Lightning injury of the skin is generally superficial with a "splashed on" arborescent and spidery appearance.[145] The tip-toe sign refers to the small, circular full thickness burns on the tips of the toes that are common in patients with lightning injury. Prompt institution of cardiopulmonary resuscitation has increased the survival rate of patients struck by lightning to 70% and improved management of the systemic effects of lightning injury has reduced the incidence of acute renal failure and other complications.[11]

Chemical Injuries

A variety of chemical agents can cause tissue injury as a consequence of an exothermic chemical reaction, protein coagulation, desiccation, and delipidation. The severity of a chemical injury is related to the concentration and amount of chemical agent and the duration with which it is in contact with tissue.[146] Consequently, initial wound care to remove or dilute the offending agent takes priority in the management of patients with chemical injuries (Fig. 32.11). Immediate copious water lavage should be instituted while all clothing, including gloves, shoes, and underwear exposed to the chemical are being removed. The lavage is continued for at least 30 minutes or until dilution has lowered the concentration of the agent below that which will cause tissue damage or until testing the involved surface with litmus paper confirms that the agent has been removed. For patients in whom extensive surface injury has occurred, the irrigation fluid should be warmed to prevent the induction of hypothermia. Although seldom needed, if a patient with concentrated alkali injuries requires prolonged irrigation and is hemodynamically stable he can be cared for while sitting in a chair under a shower.

The appearance of skin damaged by chemical agents can be misleading. In the case of patients injured by strong acids, the involved skin surface may have a silky texture and a light brown appearance that may be mistaken for a suntan rather than the full thickness injury that it is. Skin injured by delipidation caused by petroleum distillates may be dry, show little if any inflammation, and appear to be undamaged but found to be a full thickness injury on histologic examination.

Variable degrees of pulmonary insufficiency may occur in patients with cutaneous injuries caused by volatile chemical agents that can also be inhaled, such as anhydrous ammonia, the ignition products of white phosphorus, mustard gas and chlorine, and even the vapors of strong acids. Additionally, pulmonary insufficiency may be caused by the inhalation of the gaseous products of petroleum distillates as may occur in patients who sustain delipidation injuries due to partial immersion in gasoline and other petroleum products.

In the case of patients with anhydrous ammonia injury, any powdery condensate adherent to the skin should be brushed off prior to irrigation. Irrigation is initiated at the scene and continued for the first 24 hours.[147] HF acid injury is most common in those involved in etching processes, the cleaning of air conditioning equipment, patio grills and other metallic objects with spray products containing HF, and petroleum refining. After contact with HF acid there is a characteristic pain-free interval of variable duration with subsequent appearance of focal pallor that progresses to penetrating necrosis, typically accompanied by severe pain. Immediately after injury, calcium gluconate gel should be applied topically, or prolonged irrigation with a solution of benzalkonium chloride instituted. The

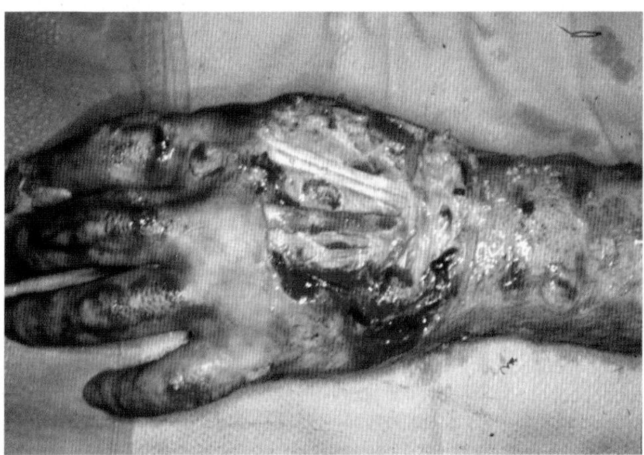

FIGURE 32.11. Failure to remove the glove into which concentrated lye had spilled and failure to start water lavage to remove the lye prior to arrival at the hospital resulted in the severe liquefaction necrosis of the skin, thrombosis of the vessels, and destruction of extensor tendons on the dorsum of the hand of this soap factory worker.

persistent severe pain that may occur in digits injured by HF acid can be relieved by injecting 10% calcium gluconate into the artery supplying that finger. Local tissue injection of calcium gluconate is an alternate route of delivery but may in itself compromise the blood supply of the involved digit. Persistent pain caused by subungual HF acid is best treated by removal of the nail under digital block anesthesia. The pain typically relents and the nail grows back with little or no deformity. If these measures fail to control pain, local excision and skin grafting will be needed to remove the damaged tissue and achieve pain relief.[148] Extensive HF acid injury may induce systemic hypocalcemia that is treated by intravenous infusion of calcium.

Burns caused by phenol should be treated with immediate water lavage to remove, by physical means, the liquid phenol on the cutaneous surface. Following that lavage, the involved area should be washed with a lipophilic solvent such as polyethylene glycol to remove any residual adherent phenol, which is only slightly soluble in water.[149] Intensive systemic support is required for patients with extensive phenol burns, in whom absorption of the agent can cause central nervous system depression, hypothermia, hypotension, intravascular hemolysis, and even death.

Injuries caused by white phosphorous are usually discussed with other chemical injuries but are actually conventional thermal burns caused by the ignition of the particulate phosphorus. These injuries are most commonly encountered in military personnel injured by explosive antipersonnel devices (grenades) that may cause mechanical tissue damage and drive fragments of white phosphorus into the soft tissues. All wounds containing white phosphorus particles should be covered with a wet dressing that is kept moist to prevent ignition of the particles by exposure to air. If the interval between injury and definitive wound care will be so long as to permit dessication of the wet dressings, the wounds can be briefly washed with a freshly mixed dilute 0.5%-1% solution of copper sulfate followed by copious rinsing. Such treatment generates a blue-gray cupric phosphide coating on the retained phosphorus particles that both impedes ignition and facilitates identification.[150] Whatever form of topical treatment is employed, the wound should be debrided and all retained phosphorus particles, which can be readily identified with an ultraviolet lamp, removed. The removed particles should be placed under water to prevent them from igniting and causing a fire in the operating room.

Strong acids and alkali can cause devastating ocular injuries and must be treated immediately, even before leaving the scene of the injury, by irrigation with water, saline, or phosphate buffer. In the hospital, eye irrigation must continue until the pH of the eye surface returns to normal. The rapid penetration of ocular tissue by strong alkalis necessitates prolonged irrigation (12–72 hours). Such irrigation is best carried out with a modified scleral contact lens with an irrigating side arm. The effects of iritis induced by chemical ocular injury are minimized by installation of a cycloplegic such as 1% atropine following irrigation. If irrigation and removal of the offending agent is delayed, the entire globe may be so damaged as to lose turgor and all visual function. Even with early irrigation, corneal damage can be severe and late complications of symblepharon and xerophthalmia may occur. An ophthalmologist should be involved in the care of such patients from the time of admission.

Bitumen Burns

Bitumen injuries are commonly caused by hot tar coming in contact with the skin. The injury that results is a thermal contact burn that is not associated with any important component of a chemically mediated injury. There is no appreciable absorption of materials unless the patient is in an explosion and has ingested or inhaled the material. The primary initial treatment is urgent cooling of the molten material with no attempt made to remove the tar. By cold application the transfer of heat can be limited and the degree of tissue damage minimized. There are various agents that have been advertised as being effective for the removal of tar and asphalt products. These have varied from mayonnaise to simple petroleum-based jellies and seem to be similar in terms of efficacy. Considering that the initial temperature of liquid tars and asphalts are typically in excess of 600°F, early concerns about infection would seem to be unfounded and offer no support for urgent removal with potential destructive consequences to underlying otherwise viable tissue. It is preferable to apply an emulsifying petroleum-based ointment and allow the tar to separate during the first day or two after admission.[146]

Cold Injuries

Injuries occurring secondary to environmental exposure can result in local injuries, frostbite, or systemic hypothermia. During the wintertime in urban environments, the most common mechanism of injury involves homeless persons or an elderly patient who has become disoriented and wandered from home. The pathophysiology of the local injuries consists essentially of crystal formation due to freezing of both extracellular and intracellular fluids. Consequently, the cells dehydrate and shrink and blood flow is altered to the exposed area resulting in tissue death. During the thawing of damaged tissues, micro emboli that have formed further occlude the microvascular circulation adding insult to injury.[151] It is important to note that the initial clinical presentation of the patient is not likely representative of the ultimate degree of tissue loss. Patients presenting with frostbite will have coldness of the injured body part with loss of sensation and proprioception. On initial exam, the limb may well appear pale, cyanotic or have a yellow white discoloration. During rapid rewarming for 15–30 minutes in water at 40–42°C, hyperemia will occur followed by pain, paresthesias, and sensory deficits. Over the subsequent 24 hours, edema and blistering will develop and it may be the better part of a week before one can determine the true depth and extent of the injury. In the initial management of the patient, rewarming is critical but it must be done only when there is no chance for an episode of refreezing. If blisters appear, whether they should be preserved or debrided has proponents on both sides of the answer. Some authors suggest that white blisters can be debrided while purplish blue blisters should be left intact. The injured extremity should be elevated in an attempt to control edema and padded to avoid pressure-induced ischemia as a secondary insult. Administration of pain medication is based on the patient's response. Frostbite wounds are tetanus prone wounds and therefore tetanus toxoid should be administered based on the patient's immunization status.

Before any definitive plans are made for surgical intervention, sufficient time should be allowed to pass so that a clear demarcation between viable and nonviable tissue is apparent (Fig. 32.12). If only minimal distal digital necrosis is evident and remains dry, spontaneous separation and healing with minimal soft tissue loss are commonly achieved. However, if extensive tissue loss is evident it is not in the patient's best interest to follow the adage of "freeze in January and amputate in June."[152] While it will take some time for definitive delineation of the depth of the injury, once the wounds have begun to mummify the thought that there will be tissue salvage seems more than naive. Patients suffering frostbite injuries should be evaluated for other potential trauma and treated for systemic hypothermia if it is present. The posthospitalization disposition of cold injury patients requires a clear understanding of their preexisting health status and the factors that predisposed them to injury such as dementia or major psychological disease.[153]

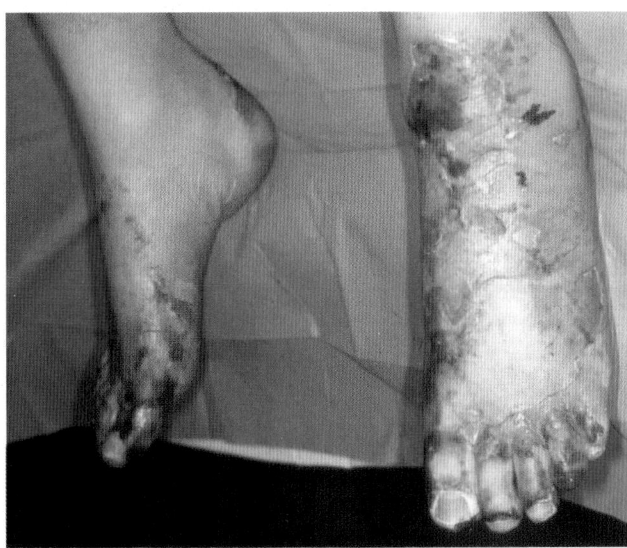

A

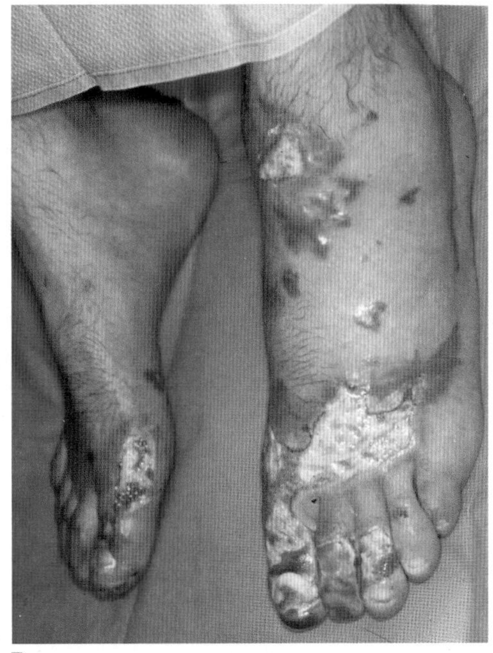

B

FIGURE 32.12. A: This photo taken 11 days after frostbite injury sustained during arctic maneuvers shows the extent of tissue damage, which was greatest on the great and second toes of the left foot. B: This photo shows the extent of healing that had occurred after 67 days of nonoperative management. Subsequent separation of the necrotic eschar from the left great and second toes revealed the wounds to be healed with minimal loss of distal digit soft tissue.

NON THERMAL CUTANEOUS INJURIES

Radiation Injury

Radiation exposure secondary to the detonation of a thermonuclear device is not as likely as is exposure from an industrial or medical accident, misuse of radiation materials, or acts of terrorism. The dispersal of radioactive substances can take several forms including accidents during storage and mishandling, accidents during transportation of radioactive materials, intentional dispersal either alone or in combination with other agents, and intentional dispersal through an explosive device. In both storage and transport accidents, the dispersal and subsequent exposure to radioactive materials is usually limited to the people immediately involved and is well contained geographically once the event is recognized. It is typically difficult to expose large numbers of individuals to substantial doses of radiation at any given time and the risks are limited to those involved in a given incident. Small-dose radiation exposure does not affect health for many years and is associated with few acute problems although it is still a major health risk. In the event of intentional radiation dispersal, the risk of exposure and injury as well as the source involved needs to be evaluated. The risk of trauma is related to the primary explosive device itself as well as trauma related to the secondary effects of the explosion such as shell fragments, structure collapse, or injury from debris. Psychological trauma due to either patients witnessing the primary event or the experience of living through the event with the associated physical manifestations may pose a further problem in the handling of a large number of injured victims.

Exposure risk is related to primary contamination from the particles released from the explosive device, secondary contamination from particles that have become mixed with debris, debris dust and fallout, and tertiary contamination from exposure to particles in contact with patients. Ionizing radiation is composed of two types: radiation that has mass and that which is energy only. Exposure to alpha particles, which are relatively large, slow moving, highly charged particles, and penetrate only a few microns into tissue can be effectively shielded with ordinary substances such as paper, cardboard, or clothing. Alpha particles can be a source of secondary and tertiary contamination. Beta particles made up of either positively or negatively charged species have greater energy and can penetrate more deeply into tissues and require shielding with material such as aluminum to prevent exposure. Both alpha and beta particles result from the decay of a radioactive source. Gamma and x-rays are produced by radioactive decay or an x-ray source; they have neither mass nor charge; however, they penetrate deeply and shielding requires the use of such materials as lead, steel, or thick cement. Following removal from the source of radiation no further exposure occurs and the patient poses no danger to those providing care. Radiation due to neutrons requires special consideration. Nuclear reactors are the major source of neutron emission and create radiation that penetrates deeply causing widespread damage to underlying tissues.

Radiation exposure of 2–4 gray (Gy) can cause nausea and vomiting, hair loss, and bone marrow injury leading to death from infection up to 2 months after exposure. Exposures of 6–10 Gy result in the destruction of the bone marrow, and injury to the GI tract with a mortality approaching 50% within 1 month. When the exposure is 10–20 Gy, there is severe injury to the GI tract and death may occur in as little as 2 weeks. When exposure is >30 Gy, cardiovascular and nervous system damage occur primarily as a result of hypotension and cerebral edema. There is almost immediate nausea, vomiting, prostration, hypotension, ataxia, and convulsion, and death can occur in a matter of hours. At present, there appears to be no effective treatment following radiation exposure. For treatment to be effective, it would need to be given prior to the exposure. In cases of accidental exposure, treating bone marrow suppression while successful has not prevented death, which usually occurs from radiation pneumonitis, GI tract injury, and hepatic and renal failure.[154,155]

The burn injuries resulting from radiation exposure are usually localized and represent a high radiation dose to the skin. They appear identical to a thermal burn and may present with erythema as with a first-degree burn that will heal following some sloughing of the skin. With higher dose exposures, blisters may occur as with a partial thickness burn and healing occurs in a similar manner. When the radiation exposure has been substantial such as 20 Gy, radionecrosis occurs. If the event leading to the radiation exposure causes surface contamination, decontamination needs to be done prior to dealing with the wound. This consists of saline irrigation of the wound and treatment with standard aseptic techniques. It is not necessary to excise the wound urgently unless it is contaminated with long-life radionuclides such as alpha emitting particles. Patients who have greater than a 1 Gy, whole body exposure should be considered for early wound closure so that the wound itself does not become the site of a lethal infection.[156]

To manage radiation-exposed victims effectively, a hospital must have a well-organized plan in place and the appropriate decontamination facility within the emergency room. The goals are to save the patients life and to prevent further injury. The decontamination must be done so that the personnel providing care to the patient do not become exposed. All contaminated materials must be carefully handled to prevent contamination of the hospital and its facilities and the public sewage system.

Toxic Epidermal Necrolysis (TEN)

TEN is a rare life threatening mucocutaneous form of exfoliative dermatitis that is often secondary to drug sensitivity. The incidence of TEN has been estimated at 0.4–1.2 cases per million population per year.[157] These patients may give a history of sore throat, burning eyes, fever, and malaise, and present with systemic toxicity. Physical findings can include rash, bullae, and diffuse exfoliation with the large areas of separation having the appearance of a partial thickness burn. When lateral stress is applied to the involved skin it separates at the dermal–epidermal junction, Nikolsky's sign. The resulting wounds give the appearance of a wet surface as seen in a second-degree burn. The mechanism of injury is thought to be keratinocyte apoptosis induced by interactions between the cell surface death receptor Fas and its receptor FasL or CD95L.[158] Lyle in 1956 was the first to describe two entities in the initial description of TEN consisting of staphylococcal-scalded skin syndrome (SSS) and what today is recognized as TEN.[159]

Staphylococcal-SSS is a generalized exfoliative dermatitis due to infections with staphylococcal organisms. In SSS, the lesion is at the intraepidermal layer with blister formation followed by desquamation of large sheets of skin with relatively rapid reeptheliazation over 7–10 days. The outcome in patients with SSS is significantly better than that in TEN patients. In TEN, there is necrosis of all layers of the skin and mortality between 30 and 40% while with SSS it is 3%-4%. Stevens Johnson Syndrome (SJS) is an entity in which there is also extensive epidermolysis often presenting with target shaped skin lesions with differentiation from TEN related to the extent of cutaneous involvement. One current delineation classifies patients with <10%-30% cutaneous involvement as SJS and those with >10%-30% as TEN particularly if it involves oral-genital and ocular mucosa.[160] Whether SJS and TEN represent the same process differing only in the extent of cutaneous involvement and sites affected or are pathologically distinct entities has not been answered with any degree of certainty.

Patients with TEN have wound care needs identical to those of patients with extensive second-degree wounds. They exhibit considerable fluid losses and have specialized nutritional needs. Care of these patients in a Burn Center by experienced surgeons has resulted in a substantial improvement in outcome.[161] General principles of management in these patients include the cessation of potential precipitating drugs, the discontinuance of systemic steroids if recently initiated, ophthalmologic evaluation, and skin biopsy confirmation of the diagnosis.[162] Additionally, systemic antibiotics should be reserved for those cases in which infection is highly likely. Replacement of fluid and electrolytes and provision of nutritional support and aggressive wound care are critical elements in the care of these patients. Wound care may consist of the application of a biologic dressing once all of the nonviable tissue is fully debrided or the use of silver-impregnated dressings (Fig. 32.13). The most frequent mistakes in the care and management of these patients are underestimating the extent of the cutaneous involvement, airway compromise, and not understanding how rapidly these patients can become critically ill. To date, the results of studies of various modalities that can be employed to control the degree of skin slough have been too inconsistent to recommend their general use.[163]

Mechanical Injury

The combination of burn injury and multisystem trauma occurs in up to 4%-5% of all burn patients.[164,165] Patients suffering combination injuries are typically male with their injuries having occurred from a flame ignition during an assault or motor vehicle crash. Victims suffering a combination of burns and trauma tend to have a higher incidence of inhalation injury, higher mortality, higher injury severity score (ISS), and longer length of stay despite no differences in TBSA burned when compared to patients with only burns. Trauma victims with burns with an inhalation injury have a near threefold increase in their mortality rate.[110] Those victims not surviving their injuries typically are considerably older, have a higher ISS, and a larger body surface area burn compared to trauma victims with burns who survive their injuries. The management priorities in patients suffering burns plus trauma must be as for patients with trauma. Understanding the mechanism of injury is vital in determining the probability of associated injuries and provides a guide in the work-up of the patient. A formal trauma evaluation should

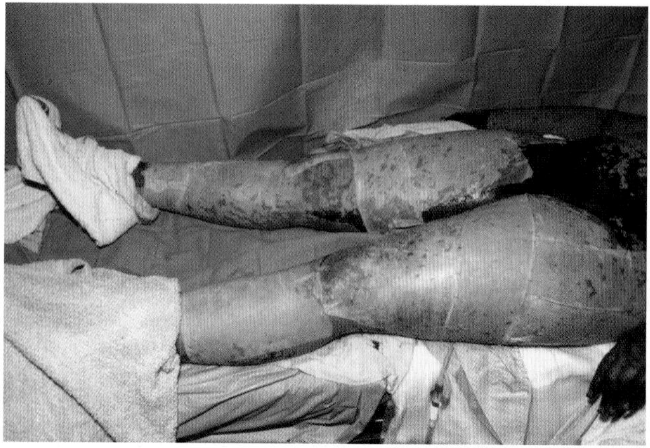

FIGURE 32.13. After the exfoliating epidermis was cleansed with sterile saline and gently debrided, the wounds on this patient with TEN were covered with a translucent collagen-based skin substitute (Biobrane) as shown here. The membrane decreases pain, prevents desiccation of the exposed dermis, and serves as a microbial barrier. If the membrane remains adherent to the wound, it can be left in place until the wound heals at which time the Biobrane will slough.

be performed on all burn victims when the history of the event points to the possibility of combined mechanisms of injury. In patients with major long bone injuries, early operative intervention with stabilization by use of an external fixator if necessary will facilitate the patient's overall management as well as that of the burn. In selected circumstances, early burn excision with skin graft wound closure may be the best approach to facilitate the operative management of the orthopedic injury.

The management of patients with substantial burn injuries in conjunction with mechanical trauma requires a highly coordinated plan of care. The patient must be continuously reassessed to avoid missing an injury and the surgeon vigilant to the development of trauma-related complications.

METABOLIC AND NUTRITIONAL SUPPORT

Estimation and Measurement of Metabolic Rate

Burn injury alters central and peripheral thermoregulatory mechanisms, the predominant route of heat loss, the distribution and utilization of nutrients, and metabolic rate. All of these postburn metabolic changes must be considered in planning the metabolic support and nutritional management of the hypermetabolic burn patient necessary to minimize loss of lean body mass, accelerate convalescence, and restore physical abilities. Metabolic support includes patient care procedures and environmental manipulations in addition to the provision of adequate nutrition.

The perceived temperature of comfort of burn patients (on average 30.4°C) is higher than that of unburned control patients and necessitates maintaining the ambient temperature at that level in the patient's room to prevent the imposition of added cold stress that would exaggerate an already elevated metabolic rate.[166] Physical therapy with active motion to the extent possible and passive motion to stretch muscles in the absence of spontaneous motion is instituted on admission to minimize muscle wasting secondary to disuse. Analgesic and anxiolytic agents should be used as needed to prevent pain- and anxiety-related increases in circulating catecholamine levels, which can further increase metabolic rate. Assiduous monitoring is necessary to facilitate early diagnosis and prompt treatment of infections and thereby reduce their metabolic impact. The importance of excision and grafting of the burn wound has been emphasized by recent studies showing that such treatment reduces resting energy expenditure in burn patients, even if the entire wound cannot be excised and grafted at a single sitting.

Even though metabolic rate can be reduced by pharmacologic means, studies indicating that the hypermetabolic response to burn injury is wound-directed speak for meeting caloric needs rather than reducing nutrient supply to the burn wound by pharmacologic intervention. One must determine the resting energy expenditure in order to calculate the nutrients required to meet the patient's needs. Bedside indirect calorimetry is the most accurate means of determining metabolic rate, but a bedside metabolic cart may not always be available. A number of formulas permit one to make close approximations of daily energy expenditure in a variety of surgical patients. A formula based on studies of extensively burned patients is useful in estimating burn patient calorie needs.[167]

$$\text{EER} = [\text{BMR} \times (0.89142 + 10.01335 \times \text{TBS})] \times m^2 \times 24 \times \text{AF}$$

where EER = estimated energy requirements, BMR = basal metabolic rate, TBS = total burn size, m^2 = total body surface area in square meters, and AF = activity factor of 1.25 for burns.

A rule of thumb estimate for nutritional needs of patients whose burns involve >30% of the body surface is 2,000–2,200 kilocalories and 12–18 g of nitrogen per square meter of body surface per day.[41]

Nutritional Support

Meeting the metabolic needs of the burn patient can be accomplished by providing nutritional support via the GI tract or by the intravenous route. After determining what the metabolic needs will be for an individual burn patient, the next question is will the patient be capable of meeting the needs by oral intake? In patients who can eat, it is not likely that a standard hospital diet will meet the calculated needs and it is often necessary to supplement the patient's intake with various nutritional supplements. A calorie count should be recorded to verify that the patient is capable of consistently meeting the daily nutrient intake goal. In the patient who is incapable of achieving the necessary nutrient intake or cannot eat, one must decide how to deliver the feedings. Total parenteral nutrition in the past provided a way by which patients could receive the majority or all of their calorie and protein needs but at present has largely been supplanted by the use of enteral nutritional support. As compared to total parenteral nutrition, enteral nutritional support is technically easier to accomplish, lower in cost, supports the health of the GI tract, and ameliorates the systemic inflammatory response syndrome.[168-172]

At the time of admission, a patient who will require specialized nutritional support should have either a nasogastric or nasoduodenal tube placed. Patients can safely and effectively be fed by either of these routes with appropriate precautions. It is not necessary that one use custom made feedings to meet the patient's nutrient needs. It is possible by using combinations of currently available commercial products to obtain the necessary blend of nutrients, feeding density, water, and protein requirements while avoiding the cost of compounding specialized enteral feedings. It is preferable to start enteral feedings soon after the patient is admitted. The patient should be fed with the head of the bed elevated to 30° with feeding residuals checked frequently to avoid gastric distention and possible aspiration. A potential advantage of early enteral feedings is modulation of the hypermetabolic response although the actual ability of early feedings to achieve this goal has been called into question.[173-175] When feedings are initiated early postinjury, the desired rate of administration can typically be reached within 24–48 hours of admission. There are multiple recommendations regarding the initial concentration, rate, incremental increase, and the frequency of the increases. Starting a tube feeding of standard concentration at 20–40 mL/hour and advancing the rate by a similar amount every 4 hours works well in most patients. The most important issues are that the nursing staff understands the goals, knows how to monitor for feeding intolerance, and appreciates the attention to detail necessary to achieve consistent delivery of the feedings.

If a patient is intolerant of gastric feedings and gastric aspirate volume exceeds the total of two hourly feedings, the administration of metaclopramide will often resolve the problem. If the patient fails to respond to metaclopramide, an attempt should be made to place either a nasoduodenal or nasojejunal feeding tube, which will minimize this feeding difficulty and lessen the risk of aspiration. Patients who become septic will often manifest changes in feeding tolerance along with new onset hyperglycemia or changes in insulin needs as early signs pointing to this problem. In patients receiving central vein alimentation, the risk of catheter sepsis must be evaluated as an etiology for the patient's septic process. In patients who become intolerant of enteral feedings or develop GI complications that prevent use of the GI tract, total parenteral nutrition will be required. However, with careful attention to detail and a well-designed, patient-specific enteral feeding protocol, this should rarely be needed in the care of a burn patient.

Blood is not part of the initial resuscitation for patients with only burn injuries but when there is multiple trauma, blood transfusions may be necessary in the early management of the patient. Often the presence of a major burn wound results in the patient being viewed as having only a burn and the standard assessment of a trauma patient is not done. Patients with impaired neurological status should undergo a computerized axial tomographic scan to rule out intracranial pathology along with evaluation for a spinal injury. This is particularly important if the patient jumped from a burning building to escape the fire, was injured in an industrial accident, or involved in a motor vehicle crash. Potential thoracic, abdominal, or pelvic injuries should be evaluated with chest, abdominal, and pelvic roentgenograms as well as with abdominal CT and Focused Assessment with Sonography for Trauma (FAST) examinations. Diagnostic peritoneal lavage may also be used in the unstable patient to verify the presence of an injury requiring exploratory laparotomy.

The nonoperative management of substantial injuries of the spleen or liver requires thoughtful consideration in patients with a major burn and it maybe prudent to opt for surgical management particularly if the abdominal wall is extensively burned.

Monitoring

The complications associated with the use of enteral or parenteral support in the burn patient are in large part similar. Burn injury induces insulin resistance that may lead to hyperglycemia. The maintenance of blood glucose values with aggressive insulin replacement has a favorable impact on the outcome of critically ill patients.[176] In critically ill patients, the preferable route of administration of insulin is intravenously with the goal of maintaining plasma glucose values between 80 and 110 mg/dl. There is a well-recognized limit to the carbohydrate calorie load that a critically ill patient can tolerate and for a 70-kg patient this is approximately 1,800 kilocalories per day from glucose.[177] Excessive amounts of glucose can result in respiratory quotient (RQ) values >1, which may cause hepatic steatosis and complicate ventilatory management. The effect of thermal injury on metabolic rate and insulin function has been further dissected by Duffy et al.[178] Those investigators identified elevation of circulating resistin levels in association with postburn elevation of insulin and glucose. "Insulin resistance" increased in concert with resistin expression. The marked increase in resistin transcript expression by the activated macrophages present in the soft tissues at the burn wound margins was considered to impair insulin function in the burn patients studied.

Sufficient protein to meet metabolic demands must be provided. To estimate protein needs 24-hour urine urea nitrogen is measured to which an additional 0.1–0.2 g of nitrogen per % TBSA burn remaining is added to account for wound exudate protein loss. These determinations can be done on a weekly basis unless there is a special need to perform them more frequently. Numerous studies have been done to determine precise protein needs and the optimum balance of protein and nonprotein calories. In adult patients, 1.5–2.0 g of protein per kg lean body mass per day is a reasonable goal and for children 3 g of protein per kg lean body mass. [179,180] A nonprotein calorie-to-nitrogen ratio of 100:1 provides the patient with sufficient calories to support protein synthesis in the face of ongoing protein breakdown and reduces net protein loss.[181,182] The provision of dietary protein at these levels has been shown to positively impact patient outcome.[183] An increasing blood urea nitrogen level must be evaluated in terms of nitrogen over feeding and the protein load recalculated to avoid uremia and an associated diuresis. Measurements of visceral proteins such as serum transferrin and albumin can be used to monitor the impact of the nitrogen content of the diet on the patient's nutritional status. Those proteins are simply markers that can be followed over time and are probably best utilized in a trend analysis based on weekly determinations since albumin has a half-life of 20 days and transferrin 8 days. Thyroid prealbumin with a half-life of 2 days and retinal binding protein with a 12-hour half-life can be used to track short-term responses in selected patients.

To prevent the development of essential fatty acid deficiencies, lipids must be included in the diet but should not exceed more than 40% of the total calorie load or more than 3 g/ kg BW/ day. Most enteral diets will contain adequate fat to prevent the development of essential fatty acid deficiency and parenteral diet formulations typically contain long chain fatty acids. The serum triglyceride concentration and the triene/tetraene ratio should be measured weekly to assess fatty acid status. If that ratio is >0.4 an essential fatty acid deficiency exists, which necessitates adjustment of the dietary fat content.[184] Supplemental medium chain triglycerides can be given enterally but are associated with increased ketone production and may cause diarrhea.[41]

Complications

Serum electrolytes must be monitored to make necessary adjustments in the amount of free water, sodium, chloride, potassium, phosphorus, calcium, magnesium, copper, and selenium provided to the patient. Laboratory values should be obtained at initiation of the feedings and daily during the stabilization phase and with each change in the patient's clinical status. During the first several days after admission, and with the initiation of nutritional support, there can be dramatic shifts in serum and plasma values of electrolytes and minerals. As noted above, hypernatremia can develop if free water replacement is insufficient to account for insensible water loss through the burn wound, which can be 2.0–3.1 mL/kg body weight/% burn/day.[185] Hypernatremia can also develop with persistent febrile episodes if free water replacement does not match the patient's needs. Hyponatremia may represent under replacement of sodium but typically is related to free water excess. Correction of hyponatremia should be attempted with restriction of free water intake. In adults, an increase in body weight of more than 400 g per day reflects water loading and should prompt a review of fluid intake and output records and adjustment of fluid administration.[12] Potassium and phosphorous must be given to meet the patient's needs, which often exceed initial estimates particularly when large loads of glucose are being given along with exogenous insulin. Recent reports have called attention to the effects of trace metal deficiency and the need for assiduous nutritional monitoring. Copper deficiency was implicated as a cause and copper then given to reverse indolent donor site healing in a pediatric burn patient receiving total parenteral nutrition.[186] A report of high urinary selenium excretion and low plasma selenium levels in association with an increased incidence of infection during the first 8 weeks in pediatric burn patients suggests that the recommended selenium intake for healthy children is insufficient for burned children and should be increased until the wound is healed.[187]

In the course of the patient's care, as the open wound area decreases and the hypermetabolic state slowly resolves, the nutrient load should be adjusted so that balance is maintained between metabolic needs and substrates delivered and the patient is not overfed. Alternatively, if a patient is found to have lost more than 10% of his or her admission weight, it is likely that caloric estimates are not being achieved or were underestimated. While most experienced clinicians possess the skill to assess patient needs accurately, the performance of bedside indirect calorimetry can provide objective information as to the patient's resting energy expenditure, respiratory quotient, oxygen consumption, and carbon dioxide production. The results may indicate the need to adjust the total calorie load if the resting energy expenditure has been underestimated or modify the fuel substrate load if the respiratory quotient is approaching or is >1.

The burn patient should receive increased amounts of vitamin C, at recommended doses of a gram per day in adults and 500 mg per day in children, which will aid in wound healing.[188] In patients with burns of >20% of the TBSA, zinc at doses of 220 mg per day will support wound healing as well as white cell function.[189] The routine provision of these nutrients avoids complications related to insufficient delivery and obviates the need to measure their levels in the patient.

In patients with prior surgery or preexisting medical conditions, special attention may be required to monitor for feeding intolerance and to insure that adequate amounts of iron, folate, and vitamin B_{12} are being effectively delivered. In patients who have received extended courses of broad-spectrum antibiotics, vitamin K replacement beyond standard recommendations may be required to avoid the development of nutritionally related coagulopathy. The preservation of lean body mass requires more than just the appropriate amounts and blend of nutrients. Physical activity is important in directing the nutrients to muscle and reducing truncal fat deposition and the risk of hepatic steatosis.

In addition to providing appropriate calorie, protein, and nutrient loads to burn patients, it is now possible to modulate the metabolic response. Administration of beta antagonists in children has been shown to be safe and to have an appreciable positive effect on outcome.[190] The administration of growth hormone, which is depressed following burn injury, has met with variable results. Herndon et al.[191] have reported a positive effect in burned children given growth hormone but a recent multicenter trial from Europe in critically ill patients showed an increased mortality in treated patients.[192] An alternative strategy that seems not to be associated with problems in adults and is efficacious in children is the use of the drug oxandrolone, although a recent study reported that the agent was associated with prolonged need for mechanical ventilation in trauma patients.[193-196] Additional strategies that might be utilized are the provision of selected nutrients in increased amounts. Glutamine, arginine, nucleotides, and omega-3 fatty acids have all been used in attempts to improve immune function above that seen with the optimal use of standard nutritional formulations.[197-201] The routine use of these measures requires a full understanding of the therapeutic benefits and the potential adverse consequences of each. Additionally, some studies have found such supplements to be ineffective.[202]

In patients who have established chronic renal failure or develop renal insufficiency during their course of care, changes in the nutritional formulation will have to be made to accommodate their altered clinical status. In patients who require dialysis, the frequency of dialysis should be adjusted so that the protein intake needed to meet metabolic needs can be given. In patients with substantial injuries who are receiving large amounts of feeding through the GI tract, the health of the GI tract itself must be continuously monitored. The development of major GI complications while not common can adversely impact the patient's outcome. Complications can include ischemic necrotic bowel disease, intestinal obstruction, the development of *Clostridium difficile* colitis and noninfectious diarrhea.[203-207] The patient's clinical status should be continuously monitored and any changes in abdominal findings on physical examination should be aggressively followed up with appropriate diagnostic radiographic studies, endoscopy, stool cultures, and abdominal exploration before the patient deteriorates and develops an irreversible condition.

TRANSPORTATION AND TRANSFER

Many important advances have been made in the care and management of burn-injured victims during the past 50 years. One of the more important advances has been the recognition of the benefits of a team approach in the care of critically injured burn patients. The American College of Surgeons and the American Burn Association have developed optimal standards for providing burn care and a burn center verification program that identifies those units that have undergone peer review of their performance and outcomes. Patients with burns and/or associated injuries and conditions listed in Table 32.2 should be referred to a burn center.

Once the decision has been made to transfer a patient to a Burn Center, there should be physician-to-physician communication regarding the patient's status and need for transfer.[208] Institutions should have preexisting interhospital transfer policies in place to facilitate communication and patient transfers. It is critical that the patient be properly stabilized in preparation for the transfer. The flight transfer team should have the capability of providing the care required for a critically injured, severely burned patient throughout the entire transfer procedure. A surgeon, a respiratory therapist, and a licensed practical nurse, all experienced in burn care comprise such a team for long distance, fixed wing aircraft transfers (Fig. 32.14). For short distance transport by rotary wing aircraft, inclusion of a burn physician in the flight team optimizes the safety and quality of care of extensively burned patients, but patients with lesser burns may be adequately cared for by nonphysician helicopter flight team members (a flight nurse and/or an advanced paramedic) who are in ready contact with medical control. A flight team roster should be maintained and published so the surgeons and other members of the team will be available when needed. Physicians and other team members should be assigned to the flight (transfer) team only after 6–12 months experience at a burn center, which will enable them to become familiar with the complications that occur in burn patients during resuscitation and develop competence in the prevention, treatment, and resolution of those problems.

During transport, the need to perform life-saving interventions such as endotracheal intubation or reestablishing vascular access may be very difficult to accomplish in the relatively unstable and limited space of a moving ambulance or a

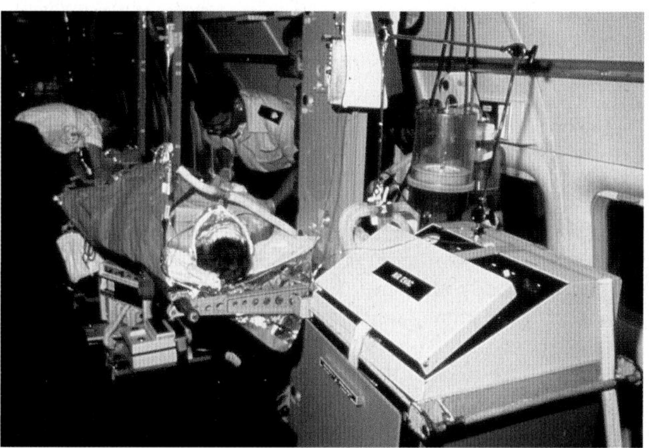

FIGURE 32.14. Long-distance transfer of severely burned critically ill patients is best carried out in fixed wing aircraft in which ICU capabilities can be provided including mechanical ventilation as well other supportive and monitoring equipment as shown here.

TRAUMA

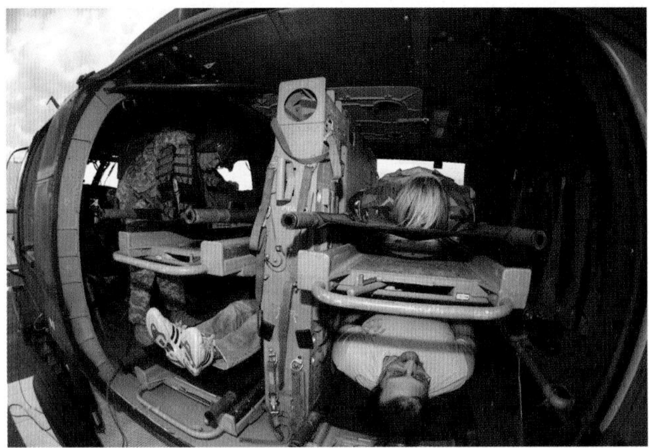

FIGURE 32.15. Patients are often transported to burn centers by helicopter. The noise, poor lighting, and vibration compromise monitoring. This photo of a U.S. Army UH-60 Blackhawk helicopter loaded with three simulated patients illustrates that space limitations and restricted patient access limit therapeutic interventions and necessitate preflight stabilization of patients being transferred.

TABLE 32.7

CHANGES IN BURN PATIENT MORTALITY AT U. S. ARMY BURN CENTER, 1945-2002

AGE GROUP–	PERCENTAGE OF BODY SURFACE BURN CAUSING 50% MORTALITY (LA_{50})	
	1945-1957	1992-2002
Children (0–14 y)	51	71[a]
Young adults (15–40 y)	43	75[b]
Another young adult		65[c]
Older adults	23	45[d]

[a]5 years.
[b]21 years.
[c]40 years.
[d]60 years.

helicopter in flight (Fig. 32.15). That difficulty makes it important to institute hemodynamic and pulmonary resuscitation and achieve "stability" prior to undertaking transfer by either aeromedical or ground transport. A secure large-bore intravenous cannula must be in place to permit continuous fluid resuscitation. Patients should be placed on 100% oxygen if there is any suspicion of carbon monoxide exposure. If there is any question about airway adequacy an endotracheal tube should be placed and mechanical ventilation instituted before transfer begins. Inflight mechanical ventilatory support can be provided by a transport ventilator with oxygen supplied from a lightweight kevlar tank transported in backpack fashion by the respiratory therapist. Patient safety during transport may necessitate chemical paralysis of the patient to prevent loss of the airway or vascular access. In-transit monitoring for helicopter transfer includes pulse rate, blood pressure, EKG, pulse oximetry, end tidal CO_2 levels, and respiratory rate. For long distance transfer, the same physiologic indices should be monitored. In addition, the ultrasonic flow meter should be used to assess the presence and quality of pulsatile flow in all four limbs on a scheduled basis and excursion of the chest wall should be monitored to identify a need for limb or chest escharotomy, respectively. The hourly urinary output should also be monitored with fluid infusion adjusted as necessary. All patients should be placed NPO (nothing by mouth) and those with a >20% body surface area burn require placement of a nasogastric tube. In essence, a mini ICU should be established for the duration of the long-distance flight.

The burn wound should be covered with a clean and/or sterile dry sheet. The application of topical antimicrobial agents is not necessary prior to transfer, since they will have to be removed on admission to the burn center. Maintenance of the patient's body temperature is vital. Wet dressings that can lead to hypothermia, particularly in small adults and children, should be avoided. The patient should be covered with a heat reflective space blanket to minimize heat loss. Pain medication is given in sufficient dosage to control the patient's pain during transport while avoiding respiratory depression, airway comprise or hypotension. Burn wounds, as tetanus prone wounds, mandate immunization in accordance with the recommendations of the American College of Surgeons. As in the case of the transfer of any trauma victim, documentation must be thorough, flow sheets should be clearly marked, and a listing of all medications, including IV fluids that have been given must be provided to the receiving physician. In the case of a patient suffering from substantial multisystem trauma and burn injuries, it may be necessary to treat the patient's life-threatening mechanical injury prior to transfer if the transport time will be of long duration or the patient is unstable. [113]

SURVIVAL DATA

During the course of the past half century, early postburn renal failure as a consequence of delayed and/or inadequate resuscitation has been eliminated and inhalation injury as a comorbid factor has been tamed. Invasive burn wound sepsis has been controlled and early excision with prompt skin grafting and general improvements in critical care have reduced the incidence of infection, eliminated many previously life threatening complications, and accelerated the convalescence of burn patients.[209] All of these improvements have considerably reduced the mortality of burn patients of all ages.

A simplified "Rule of Thumb" method of predicting mortality in burn patients has been the BAUX score, which consisted of adding the patient's age and extent of burn to estimate the percentage of mortality. That score has now been refined to account for the effect of inhalation injury and recent advances in burn care.[210] A single-term logistic regression model based on data from 39,888 patients in the National Burn Registry included inhalation injury to recalibrate the BAUX score. The authors identified a mortality effect of age and percent burn, which was virtually equal with inhalation injury adding the equivalent of 17 years or 17% burn. A recent report has suggested that pre-injury statin use reduces the odds of sepsis and death in elderly burn patients.[211] If that is confirmed by additional studies, further revision of mortality predictors may be necessary.

Revised BAUX Score (RBS) = age + persent burn + 17*

The revised BAUX score can be readily used at the bedside but the inverse logit transformation that requires the use of a calculator or nomogram provides more precise mortality predictions. The more complex thermal injury mortality model (TIMM) had better discrimination and calibration achieved by the use of nonlinear transformations of age and burn extent and two-way interactions among main effects.

*only if inhalation injury is present

A more detailed analysis has documented the improvement in burn patient survival over the past half century. At the midpoint of the last century, a burn of 43% of the total body surface would have caused the death of 50 of 100 young adult patients (15–40 years) with such burns. Since that time, the extent of burn causing such 50% mortality (the LA_{50}) in 21-year-old patients has increased to 75% of the total body surface and in 40-year-old patients to 65% of the total body surface. In children (0–14 years), the LA_{50} has increased from 51% of the total body surface in the 1950s to 71% today, and in the elderly (>40 years), the LA_{50} has increased from 23% of the TBSA to 45% (Table 32.7). Not only has survival improved, but the elimination of many life threatening complications and advances in wound care have improved the quality of life of even those patients who have survived extensive severe thermal injuries.

References

1. Brigham PA, McLaughlin E. Burn incidence and medical care use in the United States: estimates, trends, and data sources. *J Burn Care Rehabil.* 1996;17:95-107.
2. American Burn Association, 2011 National Burn Repository, Report of Data from 2001–2010. Version 7.0 All Rights Reserved Worldwide. www.ameriburn.org.
3. Stabilization, transfer, and transport, Chapter 9. In: *Advanced Life Burn Support Course Providers Manual.*Chicago, IL: American Burn Association; 2011:99-100.
4. *Burn Care Resources in North America.* Chicago, IL: American Burn Association; 2011:99-100.
5. *Burn Injury Fact Sheet, National Safe Kids Campaign (NSKC).* Washington DC: NSKC; 2004.
6. Graitcer PL, Sniezek JE: Hospitalizations Due to Tap Water Scalds, 1978–1985. *MMWR Morb Mortal Wkly Rep.* 1988; 37:35-38.
7. Cadier MA, Shakespeare PG. Burns in octogenarians. *Burns.* 1995;21:200-204.
8. Acute Chemical Hazards to Children and Adults. NEISS Data Highlights Vol. 12, Jan-Dec. 1988, *Washington DC Directorate for Epidemiology U. S. Consumer Product Safety Commission.*
9. Baker SP, O'Neill B, Karpf RS. *The Injury Fact Book.* Lexington, MA: Lexington Books; 1984:139-154.
10. Lopez RE, Holle RL. Demographics of lightning casualties. *Semin Neurol.* 1995;15:286-295.
11. Pruitt BA Jr, Goodwin CW, Mason AB Jr. Epidemiological, demographic, and outcome characteristics of burn injury. In: Herndon DN, ed. *Total Burn Care.* New York, NY: WB Saunders; 2002:16-30.
12. Pruitt BA Jr, Goodwin CW, Cioffi WG Jr. Thermal injuries. In: Davis JH, Sheldon GF. *Surgery A Problem-Solving Approach.* 2nd ed. St. Louis, MO: Mosby; 1995:642-720.
13. Arturson G, Mellander S. Acute changes in capillary filtration and diffusion in experimental burn injury. *Acta Physiol Scand.* 1964;62:457-463.
14. Lund T, Bert JL, Onarheim H, et al. Microvascular exchange during burn injury I: a review. *Circ Shock.* 1989;28:179-197.
15. Lund T, Wiig H, Reed RK, et al. A new mechanism for oedema generation: strongly negative interstitial fluid pressure causes rapid fluid flow into thermally injured skin. *Acta Physiol Scand.* 1987;129:433-436.
16. Arturson G, Soed AS. Changes in transcapillary leakage during healing of experimental burns. *Acta Chir Scand.* 1967;133:609-614.
17. Arturson G. Capillary permeability in burned and nonburned areas in dogs. *Acta Chir Scand.* 1961;274:55-103.
18. Brown WL, Bowler EG, Mason AD Jr. Studies of disturbances of protein turnover in burned troops: use of an animal model. In: *Annual Research Progress Report. U.S. Army Institute of Surgical Research, Fort Sam Houston, Texas*; 1981:233-259
19. Demling RH, Kramer GC, Gunther R, et al. Affect of nonprotein colloid on postburn edema formation in soft tissues and lungs. *Surgery.* 1984;95:593-602.
20. Mason AD Jr. The mathematics of resuscitation: 1980 Presidential Address, American Burn Association. *J Trauma.* 1980;20:1015-1020.
21. Nissen NN, Gamelli RL, Polverini PJ, et al. Differential angiogenic and proliferative activity of surgical and burn wound fluids. *J Trauma.* 2003;54:1205-1211.
22. DeMeules JE, Pigula FA, Mueller M, et al. Tumor necrosis factor and cardiac function. *J Trauma.* 1992;32:686-692.
23. Cioffi WG, DeMeules JE, Gamelli RL. The effects of burn injury and fluid resuscitation on cardiac function in-vitro. *J Trauma.* 1986;26:638-642.
24. Ayala A, Chaudry IH. Platelet activating factor and its role in trauma, shock, and sepsis. *New Horiz.* 1996;4:265-275.
25. Asch MJ, Fellman RJ, Walker HL, et al. Systemic and pulmonary hemodynamic changes accompanying thermal injury. *Ann Surg.* 1973;178:218-221.
26. Demling RH, Wong C, Jin LJ, et al. Early lung dysfunction after major burns: role of edema and vasoactive mediators. *J Trauma.* 1985;25:959-966.
27. Choudhry MA, Fazal N, Goto M, et al. Gut-associated lymphoid T-cell suppression enhances bacterial translocation in alcohol and burn injury. *Am J Physiol, Gastrointest Liver Physiol.* 2002;282:G937-947.
28. Kowal-Vern A, McGill V, Gamelli RL. Necrotic bowel is a complication in the thermally injured population. *Arch Surg.* 1997;132:440-443.
29. Murton SA, Tan ST, Prickett PC, et al. Hormone response to stress in patients with major burns. *Br J Plast Surg.* 1998;51:388-392.
30. Loebel DC, Baxter CR, Curreri PW. The mechanism of erythrocyte dysfunction in the early postburn period. *Ann Surg.* 1973;178:681-686.
31. Deitch EA, Sittig KM. A serial study of the erythropoietic response to thermal injury. *Ann Surg.* 1993;217:293-299.
32. Gamelli RL, Hebert JC, Foster RS Jr. Effect of burn injury on granulocyte and macrophage production. *J Trauma.* 1985;25:615-619.
33. McEuen DD, Ogawa M, Eurenius K. Myelopoiesis in the infected burn. *J Lab Clin Med.* 1997;89:540-543.
34. Gamelli RL, He LK, Liu H. Marrow granulocyte-macrophage progenitor response to burn injury as modified by endotoxin and endomethycin. *J Trauma.* 1994;37:339-346.
35. Santangello S, Gamelli RL, Shankar R. Myeloid commitment shifts toward monocytopoiesis after thermal injury and sepsis. *Ann Surg.* 2001;233:97-106.
36. Rico RM, Ripamonti R, Burns AL, et al. The effect of sepsis on wound healing. *J Surg Res.* 2002;102:193-197.
37. Hahn EL, Tai HH, He L-K, et al. Burn injury with infection alters prostaglandin E2 synthesis and metabolism. *J Trauma.* 1999;47:1051-1057.
38. Sen S, Muthu K, Jones S, et al. Thermal injury and sepsis deplete precursor dendritic cells and alter their function. *JACS.* 2003;197:539-540.
39. Majetschak M, Zedler S, Romero J, et al. Circulating proteasomes after burn injury. *J Burn Care Rest* 2010;31:243-250.
40. Jeschke MG, Chinkes DL, Finnerty CC, et al. The pathophysiologic response to severe burn injury. *Ann Surg* 2008;248:387-401.
41. Pruitt BA Jr, Goodwin CW Jr. Critical care management of the severely burned patient. In: Parrillo JE, Dellinger RP, eds. *Critical Care Medicine.* 2nd ed. St. Louis, MO: Mosby 2001;1475-1500.
42. Pruitt BA Jr. Protection from excessive resuscitation: "Pushing the Pendulum Back." *J Trauma.* 2000;49:567-568.
43. Klein MB, Hayden D, Elson C, et al. The association between fluid administration and outcome following major burn. A multicenter study. *Ann Surg.* 2007;245:622-628.
44. Gore DC, Hawkins HK, Chinkes DC, et al. Assessment of adverse events in the demise of pediatric burn patients. *J Trauma.* 2007;63:814-818.
45. Chung KK, Wolf SE, Cancio LC, et al. Resuscitation of severely burned military casualties: fluid begets more fluid. *J Trauma* 2009;67:231-237.
46. Shock and fluid resuscitation, Chapter 4. In: *Advanced Burn Life Support Course Provider Manual.* Chicago, IL: *American Burn Association* 2011;46-48.
47. Chung KK, Salinas J, Renz EM, et al. Simple derivation of the initial fluid rate for the resuscitation of severely burned adult combat casualties: In silico validation of the rule of 10. *J Trauma.* 2010;69:S49-S54.
48. Salisbury RE, Loveless S, Silverstein P, et al. Postburn edema of the upper extremity: evaluation of present treatment. *J Trauma.* 1973;13:857-862.
49. Warden GB, Wilmore DW, Rogers PW, et al. Hypernatremic state in hypermetabolic burn patients. *Arch Surg.* 1973;106:420-427.
50. Klein GL, Langman CV, Herndon DN. Persistent hypoparathyroidism following magnesium repletion in burn-injured children. *Pediatr Nephrol.* 2000;14:301-304.
51. Pruitt BA Jr. The development of the International Society for Burn Injuries and Progress in Burn Care: the whole is greater than the sum of its parts. *Burns* 1999;25:683-696.
52. Cullinane DC, Jenkins JM, Reddy S, et al. Anterior ischemic optic neuropathy: a complication after systemic inflammatory response syndrome. *J Trauma.* 2000;48:381-387.
53. Ivy ME, Atweh NA, Palmer J, et al. Intra-abdominal hypertension and abdominal compartment syndrome in burn patients. *J Trauma* 2000;49:387-391.
54. Mackie DP, Spoelder EJ, Paauw RJ, et al. Mechanical ventilation and fluid retention in burn patients. *J Trauma.* 2009;67:1233-1238.
55. Salinas J, Drew G, Gallagherj J, et al. Closed-loop and decision-assist resuscitation of burn patients. *J Trauma.* 2008;64:S321-S332.
56. Costantini TW, Peterson CY, Kroll L, et al. Pentoxifylline (PTX) modulates intestinal tight junction signaling after burn injury: effects on myosin light chain kinase. *J Trauma.* 2009;66:17-25.
57. Costantini TW, Peterson CY, Kroll L, et al. Burns, inflammation, and intentional injury: protective effects of an anti-inflammatory resuscitation strategy. *J Trauma.* 2009;67:1162-1168.
58. Costantini TW, Bansal V, Peterson CY, et al. Efferent vagal nerve stimulation attenuates gut barrier injury after burn: modulation of intestinal occludin expression. *J Trauma.* 2010;68:1349-1356.
59. Shirani KZ, Pruitt BA Jr, Mason AD Jr. The influence of inhalation injury and pneumonia on burn mortality. *Ann Surg. 1987*;205:82-87.
60. Tasaki O, Goodwin CW, Saitoh D, et al. Effects of burns on inhalation injury. *J Trauma.* 1997;43:603-607.
61. Balakrishnan C, Tijunelis AD, Gordon DM, et al. Burns and inhalation injury caused by steam. *Burns.* 1996;22:313-315.

62. Rabinowitz, PM, Siegel MB. Acute inhalation injury. *Clin Chest Med.* 2002;23:707-715.
63. Robinson M, Miller RH. Smoke inhalation injuries. *Am J Otolaryngol.* 1986;7:375-380.
64. Soejima K, Schmalstieg FC, Sakura H, et al. Pathophysiological analysis of combined burn and smoke inhalation injuries in sheep. *Am J Physiol Lung Cell Mol Physiol.* 2001;280:L1233-L1241.
65. Abraham E. Neutrophils in acute lung injury. *Crit Care Med.* 2003;31:S195-S199.
66. Chen CM, Fan CL, Chang CH. Surfactant and corticosteroid effects on lung function in a rat model of acute lung injury. *Crit Care Med.* 2001;29:2169-2175.
67. Suchner U, Katz DP, Furst P, et al. Impact of sepsis lung injury and the role of lipid infusion on circulating prostocyclin and thromboxane A2. *Intensive Care Med.* 2002;28:122-129.
68. Willey-Courand DB, Harris RS, Galletti GG, et al. Alterations in regional ventilation, perfusion, and shunt after smoke inhalation measured by PET. *J Appl Physiol.* 2002;93:1115-1122.
69. Shimazu T, Yukioka T, Ikeuchi H, et al. Ventilation-perfusion alterations after smoke inhalation injury in a ovine model. *J Appl Physiol.* 1996;81:2250-2259.
70. Ernst A, Zibrak JD. Carbon monoxide poisoning. *N Engl J Med.* 1998;339:1603-1608.
71. Weaver LK. Carbon monoxide poisoning. *Crit Care Clin.* 1999;15:297-317.
72. Weaver LK, Hopkins RO, Chan KJ, et al. Hyperbaric oxygen for acute carbon monoxide poisoning. *N Engl J Med.* 2002;347:1057-1067.
73. Mokhlesi B, Leikin JB, Murray P, et al. Adult toxicology in critical care: part II specific poisoning. *Chest.* 2003;123:897-922.
74. Barillo DJ. Diagnosis and treatment of cyanide toxicity. *J Burn Care Res.* 2009;30:148-152.
75. Desai MH, Mlcak R, Richardson J, et al. Reduction in mortality in pediatric patients with inhalation injury with aerosolized heparin/N-acetylcysteine therapy. *J Burn Care Rehab.* 1998;119:210-212.
76. Tasaki O, Mozingo DW, Dubick MA, et al. Effects of heparin and lisofylline on pulmonary function after smoke inhalation injury in an ovine model. *Crit Care Med.* 2002;30:637-643.
77. Combes A, Figliolini C, Trouillet JL, et al. Factors predicting ventilator-associated pneumonia recurrence. *Crit Care Med.* 2003;31:1102-1107.
78. Levine BA, Petroff PA, Slade Cl, Pruitt BA Jr. Prospective trials of dexamethazone and aerosolized gentamicin in the treatment of inhalation injury in the burned patient. *J Trauma.* 1978;18:188-193.
79. Brower RG, Fessler HE. Mechanical ventilation and acute lung injury and acute respiratory distress syndrome. *Clin Chest Med.* 2000;21:491-510.
80. Wang SH, Wei TS. The outcome of early pressure-controlled inverse rational ventilation on patients with severe acute respiratory distress syndrome in surgical intensive care unit. *Am J Surg.* 2002;183:151-155.
81. Gattinoni L, D'Andrea L, Pelosi P, et al. Regional effects and mechanism of positive end-expiratory pressure in early adult respiratory distress syndrome. *JAMA.* 1993;269:2122-2127.
82. Rouby JJ, Lu Q, Goldstein I. Selecting the right level of positive end-expiratory pressure in patients with acute expiratory distress syndrome. *Am J Respir Crit Care Med.* 2002;165:1182.1186.
83. Esteban A, Alia I, Gordo F, et al. Prospective randomized trial comparing pressure-controlled ventilation and volume-controlled ventilation in ARDS for the Spanish Lung Failure Collaborative Group. *Chest.* 2000;117:1690-1696.
84. Johnson B, Richard JC, Strauss C, et al. Pressure-volume curves and compliance in acute lung injury: evidence of recruitment above the lower inflection point. *Am J Respir Crit Care Med.* 1999;159:1172-1178.
85. Tripathi M, Pandy RK, Dwivedi S. Pressure controlled inverse ration ventilation in acute respiratory distress syndrome patients. *J Postgrad Med.* 2002;48:34-36.
86. Allan PF, Osborn EC, Chung KK, et al. High frequency percussive ventilation revisited. *J Burn Care Res.* 2010;31:510-520.
87. Kornberger E, Mair P, Oswald E, et al. Inhalation injury treated with extracorporeal CO_2 elimination. *Burns.* 1997;23:354-359.
88. Cardenas VJ Jr, Lynch JE, Ates R, et al. Venovenous carbon dioxide removal in chronic obstructive pulmonary disease: experience in one patient. ASOA IO. *J Trauma.* 2009;55:420-422.
89. White CE, Batchinsky AI, Necsoiu C, et al. Lower interbreath interval complexity is association with extubation failure in mechanically ventilated patients during spontaneous breathing trials. *J Trauma.* 2010;68:1310-1316.
90. Lyons B, Casey W, Doherty P, et al. Pain relief with low dosage intravenous clonidine in a child with severe burns. *Intensive Care Med.* 1996;22:249-251.
91. Jellish WS, Gamelli RL, Flurry P, et al. Effect of topical local anesthetic application to skin graft harvest site for pain management in burn patients undergoing skin grafting procedures. *Ann Surg.* 1999;229:115-120.
92. McGill V, Kowal-Vern A, Gisher SG, et al. The impact of substance use on mortality and morbidity from thermal injury. *J Trauma.* 1995;38:931-934.
93. Bennett B, Gamelli RL. Profile of an abused child. *J Burn Care Rehabil.* 1998;19:88-94.
94. Czaja AJ, McAlhany JC, Pruitt BA Jr. Acute gastro-duodenal disease following thermal injury: an endoscopic evaluation of incidence and natural history. *N Engl J Med.* 1974;291:925.
95. Cioffi WG, McManus AT, Rue LW III, et al. Comparison of acid neutralizing and non-acid neutralizing stress ulcer prophylaxis in thermally injured patients. *J Trauma.* 1994;36:541-547.
96. Swain, AH, Azadian BS, Wakeley CJ, et al. Management of blisters in minor burns. *Br Med J (Clin Res Ed).* 1987;295:181.
97. Hartford CE. The bequests of Moncrief and Moyer: an appraisal of topical therapy of burns-1981 American Burn Association presidential address. *J Trauma.* 1981;21:827-834.
98. Hunter GR, Chang FC. Outpatient burns: a prospective study. *J Trauma.* 1976;16:191-195.
99. Miller SF. Outpatient Management of Minor Burns. *Am Fam Physician.* 1977;16:167-172.
100. Nance FC, Lewis VL Jr, Hines JL, et al. Aggressive outpatient care of burns. *J Trauma.* 1972;12:144-146.
101. Heinrich JJ, Brand DA, Cuono CB. The role of topical treatment as a determinant of an infection in outpatient burns. *J Burn Care Rehabil.* 1988;9:253-257.
102. Smith-Choban P, Marshall WJ. Leukopenia secondary to silver sulfadiazine: frequency, characteristics, and clinical consequences. *Am Surg.* 1987;53:515-517.
103. Gamelli RL, Paxton TO, O'Reilly M. Bone marrow toxicity by silver sulfadiazine. *Surg Gyn Obstet.* 1993;177:115-120.
104. Lindberg RB, Moncrief JA, Mason AD. Control of experimental and clinical burn wound sepsis by topical application of sulfamylon compounds. *Ann NY Acad Sci.* 1968;150:950-972.
105. Yin HQ, Langford R, Burrell RE. Comparative evaluation of the antimicrobial activity of Acticoat™ antimicrobial barrier dressing. *J Burn Care Rehabil.* 1999;20:195-200.
106. Khundkar R, Malic C, Burge T. Use of Acticoat™ dressing in burns: what is the evidence? *Burns.* 2010;36:751-758.
107. Strock LL, Lee MM, Rutan RL, et al. Topical Bactroban® (Mupirocin) efficacy in treating burn wounds infected with methicillin-resistant staphylocci. *J Burn Care Rehabil.* 1990;11:454-460.
108. Pruitt BA Jr. Burn wound. In: Cameron JL, ed. *Current Surgical Therapy.* 5th ed. St. Louis, MO: Mosby; 1995:872-879.
109. Pruitt BA Jr, McManus AT, Kim JH, et al. Burn wound infections: current status. *World J Surg.* 1998;22:135-145.
110. Tompkins RG, Remensynder JP, Burke JF, et al. Significant reductions in mortality for children with burn injuries through the use of prompt eschar excision. *Ann Surg.* 1988;208:577-585.
111. Burke JF, Bondoc CC, Quinby WC. Primary burn excision and immediate grafting:a method of shortening illness. *J Trauma.* 1974;14:389-395.
112. Santaniello JM, Luchette FA, Esposito TJ, et al. Ten years experience of burn trauma and combined burn/trauma injuries comparing outcomes. *J Trauma.* 2004; 57:696-701.
113. McManus WF, Mason AD Jr, Pruitt BA Jr. Excision of the burn wound in patients with large burns. *Arch Surg.* 1989;124:718-720.
114. Janzekovic Z. A new concept in the early excision and immediate grafting of burns. *J Trauma.* 1970;10:1103-1108.
115. Desai MH, Herndon DN, Broemeling L, et al. Early burn wound excision significantly reduces blood loss. *Ann Surg.* 1990;211:753-759.
116. Oda J, Kasai K, Noborio M, et al. Hypothermia during burn surgery and post operative acute lung injury in extensively burned patients. *J Trauma.* 2009;66:1525-1530.
117. Blome-Eberwein S, Johnson RM, Miller SF, et al. Hydrofiber dressing with silver for the management of split-thickness donor cites: a randomized evaluation of two protocols of care. *Burns* 2010;36:665-672.
118. Moiemen NS, Yarrow J, Kamel D, et al. Topical negative pressure therapy: does it accelerate neovascularization within the dermal regeneration template, integra? A prospective histological in vivo study. *Burns.* 2010;36:764-768.
119. Brusselaers N, Pirayesh A, Hoeksema H, et al. Skin replacement in burn wounds. *J Trauma.* 2010;68:490-501.
120. Herndon DN. Perspectives in the use of Allograft™. *J Burn Care Rehabil.* 1997;18:S6.
121. Chatterjee DS. A controlled comparative study of the use of procine xenograft in the treatment of partial thickness skin loss in an occupational health center. *Curr Med Res Opin.* 1978;5:726-733.
122. Wang Y, Wei H, Ni Y, et al. Transgenic expression of cytotoxic T-lymphocyte-associated antigen 4-immunoglobulin (CTLA4Ig) prolongs xenogeneic skin graft survival without extensive immunosuppression in rat burn wounds. *J Trauma.* 2008;65:154-162.
123. Pietramaggiori G, Yang H-J, Scherer SS, et al.: Effects of poly-N-acetyl glucosamine (pGlcNAc) patch on wound healing in db/db mouse. *J Trauma.* 2008;64:803-808.
124. Demling RH. Burns. *N Engl J Med.* 1985;313:1389-1398.
125. Supple K, Halerz M, Aleem R, et al. Transcyte™ as an alternative dressing for use in the pediatric burn patient. *J Burn Care Rehabil.* 2003;24:5129.
126. Sheridan RL, Choucair RJ. Accellular allodermis in burn surgery: 1 year results of a pilot trial. *J burn Care Rehabi.l* 1998;19:528-530.
127. Centanni JM, Straseski JA, Wicks A, et al. StrataGraft© skin substitute is well-tolerated and is not acutely immunogenic in patients with traumatic wounds. *Ann Surg.* 2011;253:672-683.
128. Rue LW III, Cioffi WG, McManus WF, et al. Wound closure and outcome in extensively burned patients treated with cultured autologous keratinocytes. *J Trauma.* 1993;34:662-667.

129. Sood R, Roggy D, Zieger M, et al. Cultured epithelial autografts for coverage of large burn wounds in eighty-eight patients: The Indiana University experience. *J Burn Care Res*. 2010;31:559-568.
130. Black AF, Berhod F, L'heureaux N, et al. In vitro reconstruction of a human capillary-like network in a tissue-engineered skin equivalent. *FASEB J*. 1998;12:1331.
131. Sheng ZY, Fu X, Cai S, et al. Regeneration of functional sweat gland-like structures by transplanted differentiated bone marrow mesenchymal stem cells. *Wound Repair Reg*. 2009;17(3):427-435.
132. Luo G, Cheng W, He W, et al. Promotion of cutaneous wound healing by local application mesenchymal stem cells derived from human umbilical cord blood. *Wound Rep Reg*. 2010;18:506-513.
133. Mukhopadhyay A, Chan SY, Yi M, et al. Syndecan-2 and decorin: proteoglycans with a difference-implications in keloid pathogenesis. *J Trauma*. 2010;68:999-1008.
134. Mora, Alejandra G, Ritenour AE, et al. Posttraumatic stress disorder in combat casualties with burns sustain primary blast and concussive injuries. *J Trauma*. 2009;66: S178-S185.
135. Sharp S, Thomas C, Rosenberg L, et al. Propranolol does not reduce risk for acute stress disorder in pediatric burn trauma. *J Trauma*. 2010;68:193-197.
136. Moore EE, Padiglione AA, Wasiak J, et al. Canada in burns: risk factors and outcomes. *J Burn Care Res*. 2010;31:257-263.
137. Horvath EE, Murray CK, Vaughan GM, et al. Fungal wound infection (not colonization) is independently associated with mortality in burn patients. *Ann Surg*. 2007;245:978-985.
138. D'Avignon LC, Hogan BL, Murray CK, et al. Contribution of bacterial and viral infections to attributable mortality in patients with severe burns: an autopsy series. *Burns*. 2010;36:773-779.
139. Peppercorn A, Veit L, Sigel C, et al. Overwhelming disseminated herpes simplex virus type 2 infection in a patient with severe burn injury: case report and literature review. *J Burn Care Res*. 2010;31:492-498.
140. Hunt JL, Mason AD Jr, Masterson TS, et al. The pathophysiology of acute electric injuries. *J Trauma*. 1976;16:335-340.
141. Hunt JL, McManus WF, Haney WP, et al. Vascular lesions in acute electric injuries. *J Trauma*. 1974;14:461-473.
142. Lee RC, Gottlieb LJ, Krizek TJ. Pathophysiology and clinical manifestations of tissue injury in electrical trauma. *Adv Plastic Recon Surg*. 1992;8:1-29.
143. Levine MS, Atkins A, McKeel D, et al. Spinal cord injury following electrical accidents: case reports. *J Trauma*. 1975;15:459-463.
144. Fahmy FS, Brinsdon MD, Smith J, et al. Lightning: the multisystem group injuries. *J Trauma*. 1999;46:937-940.
145. Amy BW, McManus WF, Goodwin CW Jr, et al. Lightning injury with survival in five patients. *JAMA*. 1985;253:243-245.
146. Mozingo DW, Smith AA, McManus WF, et al. Chemical burns. *J Trauma*. 1988;28:642-647.
147. Amshel CE, Fealk MH, Phillips BJ, et al. Anhydrous ammonia burn case report and review of the literature. *Burns*. 200;26:493-497.
148. Kohnlein HE, Merkle P, Springorum HW. Hydrogen fluoride burns: experiments in treatment. *Surg Forum*. 1973;24:50.
149. Pardoe R, Minami RT, Sato RM, et al. Phenol burns. *Burns*. 1976;3:29-41.
150. Pruitt BA Jr. Management of burns in the multiple injury patient. *Surg Clin N Am*. 1970;50:1283-1299.
151. Bangs CC. Hypothermia and frostbite. *Emerg Med Clin North Am*. 1984;2:475-487.
152. Miller BJ, Chasmar LR. Frostbite in Saskatoon: a review of 10 winters. *Am J Surg*. 1980;23:423-426.
153. Britt LD, Dascombe WH, Rodriguez A. New horizons in management of hypothermia and frostbite injury. *Surg Clin North Am*. 1991;71:345-370.
154. *The Radiological Accident in Nesvizh*. Vienna, Austria: International Atomic Energy Agency; 1996.
155. Tsuii H, Akashi M, eds. The criticality accident in Tokaimura: medical aspects. *Proceedings of an International Conference, December 14 and 15. Chiba, Japan: National Institute of Radiological Sciences*, 2000 (NIRS-M-146).
156. Mettler, FA, Voelz GL. Major radiation exposure—what to expect and how to respond. *N Eng J Med*. 2002;346:1554-1561.
157. Roujeau JC, Kelly JP, Naldi L, et al. Medication use and the risk of Stevens Johnson Syndrome or toxic epidermal necrolysis syndrome. *N Engl J Med*. 1995;333:1600-1607.
158. Viard I, Wehrli P, Bullani R, et al. Inhibition of toxic epidermal necrolysis by clockade of CD95 with human intravenous immunoglobulin. *Science*. 1998;282:490-493.
159. Becker DS. Toxic epidermal necrolysis. *Lancet*. 1998;351:1417-1420.
160. Rasmussen JE. Erythema multiforme, Stevens-Johnson syndrome and toxic epidermal necrolysis. *Dermatol Nurs*. 1995;7:37-43.
161. Heimbach DM, Engrav LH, Marvin JA, et al. Toxic epidermal necrolysis a step forward in treatment. *JAMA*. 1987;2171-2175.
162. Speron S, Gamelli RL. Toxic epidermal necrolysis syndrome versus mycosis fungoides. *J Burn Care Rehabil*. 1997;18:421-423.
163. Brown KM, Silver GM, Halerz M, et al. Toxic epidermal necrolysis: does immunoglobulin make a difference? *J Burn Care Rehabil*. 2004;25:81-88.
164. Dougherty W, Waxman K. The complexities of managing severe burns with associated trauma. *Surg Clin North Am*. 1996;76:923-958.
165. Purdue GF, Hunt JL. Multiple trauma and the burn patient. *Am J Surg*. 1989;158:536-539.
166. Wilmore DW, Orcutt TW, Mason AD Jr, et al. Alterations in hypothalamic function following thermal injury. *J Trauma*. 1975;15:697-703.
167. Carlson DE, Cioffi WG Jr, Mason AD Jr, et al. Resting energy expenditure in patients with thermal injuries. *Surg Gynecol Obstet*. 1992;174:270-276.
168. Alverdy J, Aoys E, Moss GS. Total parenteral nutrition promotes bacterial translocation from the gut. *Surgery*. 1988;104:185-190.
169. Wilmore D, Long J, Mason A, et al. Catecholamines: mediators of the hypermetabolic response to thermal injury. *Ann Surg*. 1974;180:653-669.
170. Kudsk K, Brown R. Nutritional support. In: Mattox K, Feliciano D, Moore E, eds. *Trauma*. New York, NY: McGraw-Hill; 2000:1369-1405.
171. Demling RH, Seigne P. Metabolic management of patients with severe burns. *World J Surg*. 2000;24:673-680.
172. Bessey PQ, Jiang ZM, Johnson DT, et al. Posttraumatic skeletal muscle proteolysis: the role of the hormonal environment. *World J Surg*. 1989;13:465-470.
173. Mochizuki H, Trocki O, Dominion L, et al. Mechanism of prevention of postburn hypermetabolism and catabolism by early enteral feeding. *Ann Surg*. 1984;200:297-300.
174. Wood RH, Caldwell F Jr, Bowser-Wallace BH. The effect of early feeding on postburn hypermetabolism. *J Trauma*. 1988;28:177-183.
175. Chiarelli A, Enzi G, Casadei A, et al. Very early nutrition supplementation in burned patients. *Am J Clin Nutr*. 1990;51:1035-1039.
176. Van Den Berghe G, Wouters P, et al. Intensive insulin therapy in critically ill patients. *N Engl J Med*. 2001;345:1359-1367.
177. Askanazai J, Rosenbaum S, Hyman A, et al. Respiratory changes induced by the large glucose loads of total parenteral nutrition. *JAMA*. 1980;243:1444-1447.
178. Duffy SL, Lagrone L, Herdon DN, et al. resistin and postburn insulin dysfunction. *J Trauma*. 2009;66:250-254.
179. Peck M. Practice guidelines for burn care: nutritional support. *J Burn Care Rehabil*. 2001;12:59s-S-66S.
180. Waymack J, Herndon D. Nutritional support of the burned patient. *World J Surg*. 1992;16:80-86.
181. Wolf R, Goodenough R, Burke J, et al. Response of proteins and urea kinetics in burn patients to different levels of protein intake. *Ann Surg*. 1983;197:163-171.
182. Matsuda T, Kagan R, Hanumadass M, et al. The importance of burn wound size in determining the optimal calorie, nitrogen ratio. *Surgery*. 1983;94:562-568.
183. Alexander J, MacMillan B, Stinnet J, et al. Beneficial effects of aggressive protein feeding in severely burned children. *Ann Surg*. 1980:192:505-517.
184. O'Neill JA, Caldwell MD, Meng HC. Essential fatty acid deficiency in surgical patients. *Ann Surg*. 1977;185:535-542.
185. Harrison HN, Moncrief JA, Duckett JW Jr, et al. The relationship between energy metabolism and water loss from vaporization in severely burned patients. *Surgery*. 1964;56:203-211.
186. Liusuwan RA, Palmieri T, Warden G, et al. Impaired healing because of copper deficiency in a pediatric burn patient; a case report. *J Trauma*. 2008;65:464-466.
187. Dylewski ML, Bender JC, Smith AM, et al. The selenium status of pediatric patients with burn injuries. *J Trauma*. 2010:69:584-588.
188. Mayes T, Gottschlich M, Warden G. Clinical nutrition protocols for continuous quality improvement in the outcomes of patients with burns. *J Burn Care Rehabil*. 1997;18:365-368.
189. Selmanpakoglu ACC, Sayal A, Isimer A. Trace element (Al, Se Zn, Cu) levels in serum, urine and tissues of burn patients. *Burns*. 1994;20:99-103.
190. Herndon DN, Hart DW, Wolf SE, et al. Reversal of catabolism by betablockade after severe burns. *N Engl J Med*. 2001;345:1223-1229.
191. Herndon D, Barrow R, Kunkel K, et al. Effects of recombinant human growth hormone on donor site healing in severely burned children. *Ann Surg*. 1990;212:424-429.
192. Talala J, Ruokonen E, Webster N, et al. Increased mortality associated with growth hormone treatment in critically ill adults. *N Engl J Med*. 1999;341:785-792.
193. Demling R. Comparison of the anabolic effects and complications of human growth hormone and the testosterone analog, oxandrolone, after severe burn injury. *Burns*. 1999;25:215-221.
194. Demling R, Orgill D. The anticatabolic and wound healing effects of the testosterone analog oxandroline after severe burn injury. *J Crit Care*. 2000;15:12-17.
195. Demling R, DeSanti L. Oxandrolone, an anabolic steroid, significantly increases the rate of weight gain in the recovery phase after major burns. *J Trauma*. 1997;43:47-51.
196. Bulger EM, Jurkovich GJ, Farver CL, et al. Oxandrolone does not improve outcome of ventilator-dependent surgical patients. *Ann Surg*. 2004;240(3):472-480.
197. Saito H, Trocki O, Wang S, et al. Metabolic and immune effects of dietary arginine supplementation after burn. *Arch Surg*. 1987;122:784-789.
198. Souba W. Glutamine: a key substrate for the splanchnic bed. *Annu Rev Nutr*. 1991;11:285-308.
199. Alverdy JC. Effects of glutamine-supplemented diets on immunology of the gut. *JPEN*. 1990;14:109S-113S.
200. Ziegler T, Young L, Benfell K, et al. Clinical and metabolic efficacy of glutamine supplemented parenteral nutrition after bone marrow transplantation: a randomized double-blind controlled trial. *Ann Int Med*. 1992;116:821-830.

201. Alexander J, Saito H, Trocki O, et al. The importance of lipid type in the diet after burn injury. *Ann Surg*. 1986;204:1-8.
202. Saffle JR, Wiebke G, Jennings K, et al. Randomized trial of immune-enhancing enteral nutrition in burn patients. *J Trauma*. 1997;42: 793-802.
203. Kowal-Vern A, McGill V, Gamelli R. Ischemic necrotic bowel disease in thermal injury. *Arch Surg*. 1997;132:440-443.
204. Scaife C, Saffle J, Morris S. Intestinal obstruction secondary to enteral feedings in burn trauma patients. Proceedings of the Western Trauma Association, Crested Butte, CO, February 1999. *J Trauma;* 1991: 859-863.
205. Marvin R, McKinley B, McQuiggan M, et al. Nonocclusive bowel necrosis occurring in critically ill ttrauma patients receiving enteral nutrition manifests no reliable clinical signs for early detection. *Am J Surg*. 2000;179:7-12.
206. Grube B, Heimbach C, Marvin J. *Clostridium difficile* diarrhea in critically ill burned patients. *Arch Surg*. 1987;122:655-661.
207. Gottschlich M, Warden G, Havens P, et al. Diarrhea in tube-fed burn patients: incidence, etiology, nutritional impact and prevention. *JPEN* 1988;12:338-345.
208. Cioffe WG, Pruitt BA Jr. Aeromedical transport of the thermally injured patient. *Med Corp Int*. 1989;4:23-27.
209. Pruitt BA Jr. Centennial changes in surgical care and research. *Ann Surg*. 2000;233:287-301.
210. Osler T, Glance LG, Hosmer DW. Simplified estimates of the probability of death after burn injuries: extending and updating the Baux score. *J Trauma*. 2010;68:690-697.
211. Fogerty MD, Efron D, Morandi A, et al. Effect of preinjury statin use on mortality and septic shock in elderly burn patients. *J Trauma*. 2010;69:99-103.

CHAPTER 33 EVALUATION OF THE ACUTE ABDOMEN

GRETA L. PIPER, MATTHEW R. ROSENGART, ANDREW B. PEITZMAN, AND RAQUEL FORSYTHE

Abdominal pain is one of the most common conditions encountered, serving as the chief complaint in 5%-10% of emergency department visits.[1] Although this prevalence has not changed significantly over the last few decades, diagnostic accuracy has markedly improved. Hence, a more appropriate definition of an acute abdomen is the presence of abdominal pathology, which if left untreated (<72 hour history), will result in patient morbidity and mortality.

The goal of this chapter is to provide a guideline for the evaluation of the acute abdomen in the increasingly varied and complex populations of patients that has evolved with medical advancement and innovation. As risk factor analysis clearly identifies an association between time to diagnosis and therapy and outcome, a systematic approach is paramount.[2-6] *Pathophysiology*. Abdominal pathology can cause visceral, parietal, or referred pain.

Visceral pain originates from bilateral innervation of the autonomic and visceral afferent type C fibers. Pain is sensed secondary to stretch but also distension, contraction, traction, compression, and torsion. In addition, mucosal pain receptors respond to chemical stimuli including ischemia and inflammation. The pain perceived is usually dull, not well localized, midline, and corresponds to the embryologic origin of the affected organ. Epigastric pain generally indicates a foregut etiology, as visceral afferent nerves from the foregut travel with the celiac trunk. Periumbilical pain indicates a midgut etiology as these afferent nerves travel with superior mesenteric artery branches. Lower midline pain indicates hindgut or pelvic pathology as these fibers travel with the inferior mesenteric artery branches. Parietal pain results from irritation of the parietal peritoneum leading to somatic nerve activation (type C and A delta fibers).[6,7] Chemical peritonitis occurs from irritation by blood, urine, or gastrointestinal (GI) secretions. However, intraperitoneal blood alone causes little inflammation or pain. Secondary infection of blood or breakdown products of blood leads to chemical peritonitis.

In contrast to visceral pain, parietal pain is sharp and well-localized. Appendicitis demonstrates both visceral and parietal pain. The inflammation and distension of the appendix (part of the midgut) classically results in poorly localized, dull periumbilical pain. As the inflammation progresses and irritates the parietal peritoneum, pain becomes sharper and better localized to the right lower quadrant (RLQ).

Referred pain is pain that is sensed on the superficial surface but caused by a visceral process; common patterns associated with certain abdominal processes are shown in Figure 33.1.[8] Referred pain is the result of nerves carrying both autonomic and somatic innervation with both being activated. For example, the phrenic nerve and other afferents (derived from C3–C5 dermatomes) innervate the diaphragm and the associated peritoneum. Somatic C3–C5 dermatomes innervate the shoulder. Thus, the pain from intra-abdominal pathology irritating the underside of the diaphragm is referred to the shoulder via the common C3–C5 dermatome.[6]

Differential diagnosis is extensive for acute abdominal pain. Thus, it is a clinical challenge for the acute care surgeon. Etiologies of acute abdominal pain can be divided into GI, vascular, gynecologic, urologic, and nonabdominal causes (Table 33.1).[7]

HISTORY

A comprehensive *history of present illness (HPI)*, complete review of systems, and past medical history will rapidly narrow the differential diagnosis, and generally, yield an accurate diagnosis. A careful and detailed history is the most helpful factor in leading to a diagnosis. Ideally, the HPI would be the patient's own description of the onset and progression of abdominal pain including duration, quality, location, intensity, radiation, and any ameliorating or aggravating factors. Identification of the *location* of pain helps to narrow the differential (Fig. 33.2).[7,8] However, location of the pain can be deceptive. For example, in perforated peptic ulcer disease, the source is the stomach but pain may be perceived along the RLQ secondary to gastric and pancreatic/biliary fluid tracking down the right paracolic gutter.

Radiation of Pain. There are classic pain radiation patterns that strengthen a diagnosis (Fig. 33.1).

Periumbilical pain radiating to the back is associated with pancreatitis, perforated peptic ulcer disease, or aortic dissection. Subcostal left-sided abdominal pain with radiation to the shoulder may indicate an evolving myocardial infarction (MI), splenic pathology, or left subdiaphragmatic abscess. Right-sided abdominal pain may be seen with pleurisy or pneumonia. Pain from the flank radiating to the groin may indicate the presence of a ureteral stone.

Onset of Pain. Acute or abrupt onset of pain can be associated with a vascular etiology (acute mesenteric embolism, abdominal aortic aneurysm [AAA] rupture) or a perforated viscus. On the other hand, more gradual onset of pain is more characteristic of nonperforated peptic ulcer disease, cholecystitis, pancreatitis, diverticulitis, or appendicitis.

Character of Pain. Taken together with location, the character of pain gives further insight as to the abdominal process (Fig. 33.2). Cramping pain (colicky) is characteristic of bowel obstruction or gastroenteritis. Steadily increasing, constant pain indicates inflammatory and infectious etiologies, such as appendicitis, pancreatitis, cholecystitis, or diverticulitis.

Severity of Pain. Usually the greater the severity of the pain, the higher the likelihood of significant abdominal pathology.

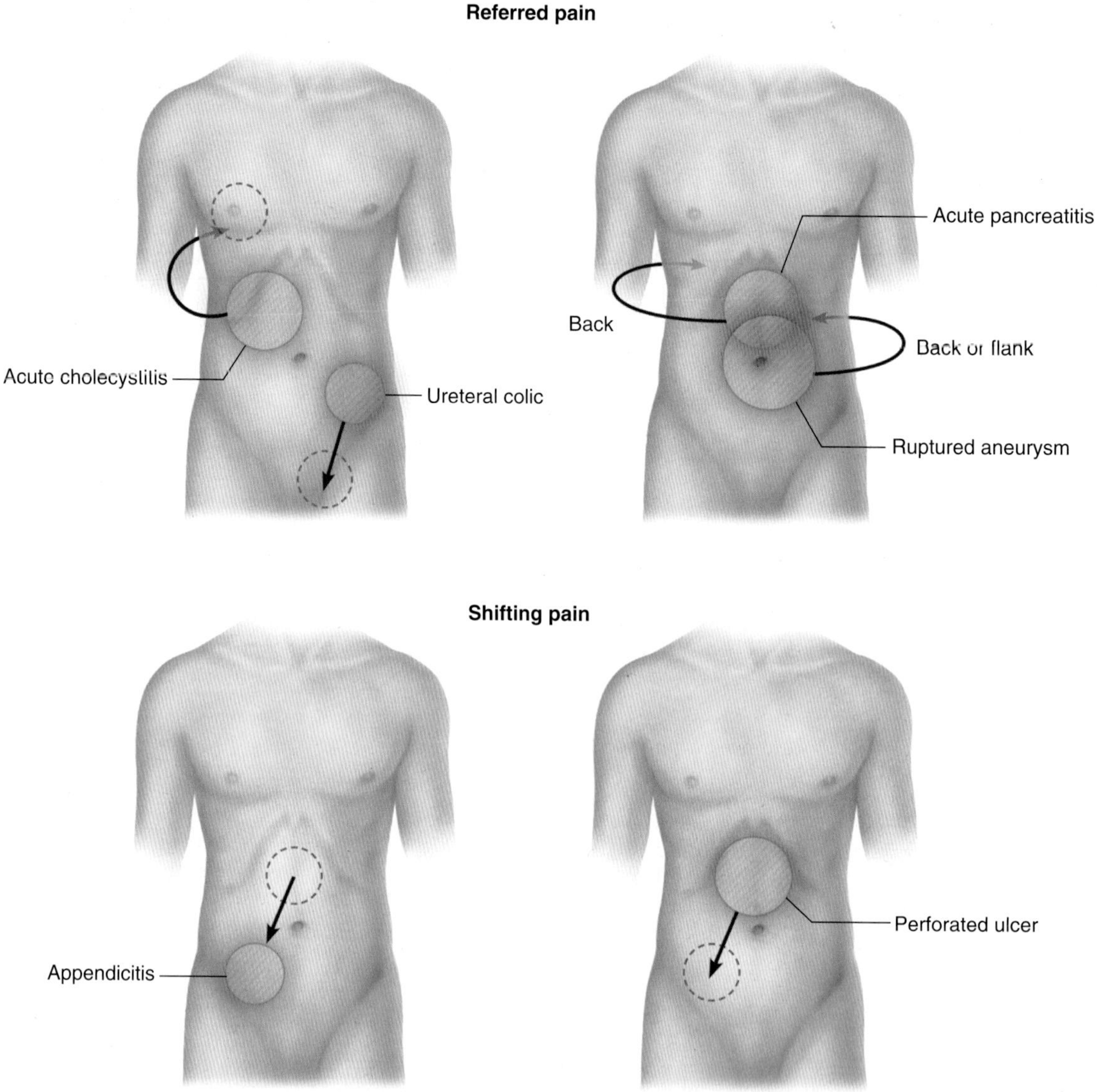

FIGURE 33.1. Referred pain and shifting pain in the acute abdomen. *Solid circles* indicate the site of maximum pain; dashed circles indicate sites of lesser pain. (Adapted from Doherty GM. The acute abdomen. In: Doherty GM, ed. *Current Surgical Diagnosis and Treatment.* 13th ed. New York, NY: McGraw-Hill/Lange; 2009: Figure 21.2, pg 453.)

On the other hand, patient characteristics, such as personality, medications, age, comorbidities, can influence the perceived pain. Serially following the severity of abdominal pain is important; this should be performed by the same examiner whenever possible to avoid interobserver variability. Pain scales can also help reduce this variability. Determination of *aggravating or alleviating factors* can be helpful in evaluation of the pain. Sitting up and leaning forward classically decreases pain in patients with pancreatitis. Any movement aggravates pain in patients with peritonitis; someone bumping the bed, hitting potholes on the ride to the hospital. *Associated symptoms* help narrow a differential diagnosis. For example, bloody diarrhea, fever, and abdominal pain may indicate acute mesenteric ischemia or inflammatory bowel disease. Nausea and vomiting with diarrhea prior to the onset of pain helps make the diagnosis of gastroenteritis. *Gynecologic/menstrual history* must be obtained in all women. Pain in the middle of the menstrual cycle may indicate ovulatory pain. Absence of menses when expected may indicate the possibility of an

TABLE 33.1

ETIOLOGIES OF ABDOMINAL PAIN

Gastrointestinal
Stomach/esophagus
Peptic ulcer disease
Gastritis/Esophagitis
Gastroesophageal reflux
Boerhaave's syndrome
Mallory-Weiss syndrome
Small bowel
Gastroenteritis
Mesenteric adenitis
Crohn's disease
Meckel's diverticulitis
Small bowel obstruction
Small bowel ischemia

TABLE 33.1

ETIOLOGIES OF ABDOMINAL PAIN *(Continued)*

Large bowel
Appendicitis
Large bowel obstruction/volvulus
Diverticulitis
Ulcerative colitis
Ischemic colon
Epiploic appendagitis
Other
Perforated viscus
Hernia
Cancer
Hepatobiliary/pancreatic
Cholecystitis
Pancreatitis
Cholangitis
Hepatitis
Hepatic abscess
Sphincter of Oddi dysfunction
Hepatic tumor
Acute liver swelling from right heart failure
Splenic
Splenic infarct
Splenic rupture
Urological
Kidney stone
Renal infarct
Urinary tract infection/acute cystitis
Acute pyelonephritis
Ruptured bladder
Acute epididymitis
Testicular torsion
Gynecological
Ovarian torsion
Ectopic pregnancy
Ovulation
Ovarian cyst
Pelvic inflammatory disease
Tubo-ovarian abscess
Endometriosis
Vascular
Abdominal aortic aneurysm
Acute mesenteric ischemia
Aortic dissection
Mesenteric venous thrombosis
Other
Pneumonia
Myocardial infarction
Diabetes mellitus
Porphyria
Sickle cell anemia
Henoch-Schonlein purpura
Muscular contusion/hematoma
Familial Mediterranean fever
Retroperitoneal hemorrhage

Adapted from Sahai RK, Forsythe RM. Evaluation of acute abdominal pain. In: Peitzman AB, Rhodes M, Schwab CW, et al., eds. *The Trauma Manual. Trauma and Acute Care Surgery*. Philadelphia, PA: Wolters Kluwer; 2008:574–584.

ectopic pregnancy. Previous pelvic infections or sexually transmitted diseases may raise suspicion of pelvic inflammatory disease. Monthly cyclical lower abdominal/pelvic pain may indicate endometriosis.

Past medical history paints a picture of the patient's overall health. In addition, known medical problems, prior operations and procedures (especially in our era of coronary stents and percutaneous angioplasty, and arterial stents), and current medications should be detailed. Comorbidities should be interpreted as potential sources of abdominal pathology (i.e., thromboembolic, mesenteric ischemia due to chronic atrial fibrillation). Diabetes or an immunosuppressed state may diminish perceived abdominal pain and minimize physical findings; the threshold for operative or other definitive intervention may be lower. Previous operations may suggest a postoperative complication or adhesions as a cause of bowel obstruction. A medication history is also important; certain diagnoses become more likely. For example, the use of nonsteroidal antiinflammatory drugs (NSAIDs) or corticosteroids would raise suspicion of a peptic ulcer or a perforated ulcer; digoxin use may raise the possibility of acute mesenteric ischemia; corticosteroids may mask significant underlying abdominal pathology. Allergies should be documented. A social history includes smoking, alcohol, and drug. Equally important are home, occupational, and travel exposures. For the unresponsive ICU patient, interview close family members, question the nursing staff, and review medical records.[7]

PHYSICAL EXAM

The general appearance of a patient helps with diagnosis and determination of the acuteness of treatment. Begin treatment of the acutely ill patient while working through the assessment and search for a diagnosis; treat the sick patient empirically, without a definitive diagnosis. A hypotensive patient with acute abdominal pain usually indicates concomitant septic shock, ruptured ectopic pregnancy, or rupture of a visceral or AAA. Other findings on examination may suggest the etiology of the abdominal pain. Patients with jaundice usually have a hepatobiliary source of their pain. A patient who is restless suggests renal colic as opposed to the patient with peritonitis who tries to lie motionless. Findings such as lethargy, sunken eyes, and poor skin turgor indicate dehydration, seen in cases of bowel obstruction, pancreatitis, and colitis with prolonged diarrhea.

Attention should then focus on the patient's vital signs, considering that the threshold for concern must be tailored to the information gleaned from the historical exam. For instance, elderly patients will not match the physiologic response of younger patients. Similar forme fruste presentations are encountered in immunosuppressed or immunocompromised patients, who comprise an increasing proportion of the general population.

The abdominal examination is performed with the patient supine. *Inspection* of the abdomen for signs of bruising, mottling, erythema, and prior surgical scars should be noted. A bulge in the groin or umbilicus may be secondary to an incarcerated hernia and also the cause of the patient's bowel obstruction. A flank hematoma (Grey-Turner's sign) or periumbilical hematoma (Cullen's sign) suggests severe hemorrhagic pancreatitis or ruptured AAA. *Auscultation* of the abdomen should document presence and character of bowel sounds. The presence of active, high-pitched bowel sounds indicates a mechanical small bowel obstruction. Absent or hypoactive bowel sounds suggest peritonitis or ileus. Bruits over the renal veins or visceral aneurysms may also be heard.

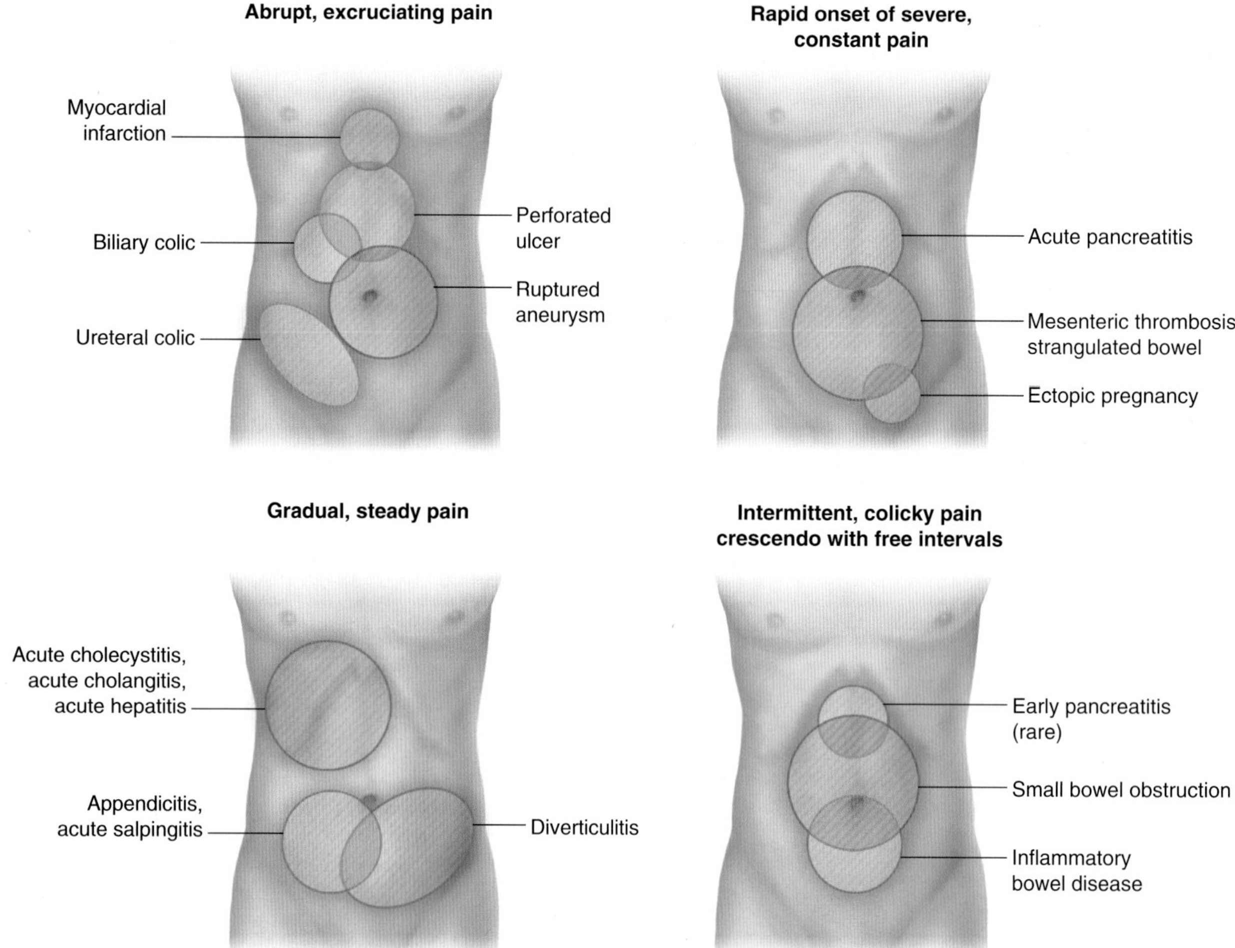

FIGURE 33.2. The location and character of pain are helpful in the differential diagnosis of the acute abdomen. Adapted from Doherty GM. The acute abdomen. In: Doherty GM, ed. *Current Surgical Diagnosis and Treatment*. 13th ed. New York, NY: McGraw-Hill/Lange; 2009: Figure 21.3, pg 454.)

If the patient is able, have him or her indicate with one finger the point of greatest pain. *Percussion* of the abdomen in all four quadrants may reveal tympany or dullness, and at times, peritonitis. Start with shallow *palpation* in the area of least pain and progress to the most painful area; this will help maintain a relaxed patient and enable a thorough exam. Involuntary guarding and rebound tenderness indicate peritonitis. A patient with rebound tenderness has exacerbation or onset of pain immediately after rapid removal of the examiner's hand pushing deeply into the abdomen. The presence of peritonitis should not be tested by this method because of the extreme pain it causes; you will lose your patient's trust. Instead, peritonitis can be assessed effectively by percussion, gentle palpation, rocking the patient's bed, or tapping the patient's heel. In a child, this can be assessed by having the child hop on one foot. Furthermore, the diffuseness of peritonitis dictates management. Diffuse peritonitis usually indicates an abdominal catastrophe and mandates surgical exploration. In a patient with altered mental status, grimacing, increased agitation, or purposeful attempts to move the hand of the examiner are "peritonitis equivalents," as are physiologic changes of tachycardia, tachypnea, and hypertension in response to palpation. The costovertebral areas should also be palpated or lightly tapped. Tenderness may indicate acute pyelonephritis. *Rovsing's sign* is more pain in the RLQ when pressure is applied to the left lower quadrant (seen with appendicitis). *Psoas sign* is pain with flexion or extension of the hip (seen in patients with psoas abscess or appendicitis, often retrocecal). The *obturator sign* is pain with internal/external rotation of the hip (appendicitis). *Murphy's sign* is an abrupt stop in inspiration during palpation over the right subcostal area (seen in patients with acute cholecystitis).

The rectal exam with stool guaiac is an important part of a complete physical exam. Tenderness along the right rectal vault supports the diagnosis of appendicitis or an abscess. A guaiac-positive study suggests colitis, GI bleeding (i.e., peptic ulcer or colitis), or cancer.

In women with abdominal pain, a pelvic exam is essential to differentiate gynecological from other abdominal causes of pain. Cervical discharge is consistent with pelvic infection and pelvic inflammatory disease. A bimanual exam should be performed and can help diagnose pelvic inflammatory disease, an ovarian mass, or a tubo-ovarian abscess (TOA). Right upper quadrant pain may be from Fitz-Hugh-Curtis disease, perihepatitis from pelvic inflammatory disease.

Palpation of an uninvolved region (i.e., thorax) can help distinguish pain of true abdominal pathology from a response to mere tactile stimulation. Serial exams can provide invaluable information in the patient without an obvious indication for operative intervention. Ideally, serial exams are performed by the same individual to allow more accurate comparison and avoid interrater variability. Analgesia is often withheld under the premise it obfuscates evaluation of the pain and its progression. A 2007 Cochrane Review by Manterola et al. identified six randomized control trials evaluating the use of narcotic analgesia in the evaluation of acute abdominal pain. The review demonstrated that administration of pain medication increases patient comfort without impact on the timing or accuracy of diagnosis.[3,4]

LABORATORY DATA

Laboratory data are adjunctive measures to support a diagnosis and should be tailored to the circumstances of the patient's history and physical (Table 33.2). The commonly encountered "shotgun" battery of biochemical testing does little other than consume valuable resources and potentially obscure the diagnosis with superfluous information.[5] However, in evaluation of a complex intensive care patient, in which time is of the essence, a broader approach is employed, which may incorporate an initial comprehensive set of biochemical and hematological studies. Nonetheless, these too should be customized to a differential obtained from the historical and physical examination. Test results should be evaluated not only as low, high, or normal, but also trended over time. Although the patient with an acute abdomen generally presents with an elevated white blood cell (WBC) count, an elevated WBC is not always seen in the acute abdomen. A "left shift" or "bandemia" can occur even if the total WBC is normal and is also indicative of an infection. The patient with dehydration (i.e., after excessive vomiting, third-spacing, or diarrhea) will present with hemoconcentration (elevated hemoglobin and hematocrit); an increased blood urea nitrogen/ creatinine (BUN/Cr) ratio (>20:1) is also indicative of dehydration. Hypochloremic, hypokalemic, metabolic alkalosis is often seen after prolonged vomiting. An anion gap metabolic acidosis (serum [Na]–serum [Cl]–serum [HCO_3] >= 12) indicates uremia, diabetic ketoacidosis, or lactic acidosis as concomitant processes. Creatinine determination is often needed prior to a contrast computed tomography (CT) scan to determine risk versus benefit.

Liver Function Tests. Transaminases (aspartate aminotransferase/alanine aminotransferase (AST, ALT)) may be elevated from numerous hepatobiliary disease states. Significant elevations indicate a hepatic process (i.e., viral hepatitis, abscess, ischemia, acetaminophen poisoning), usually with levels greater than three times normal. Lower levels can be nonspecific and due to a variety of causes including common bile duct stones, pancreatitis, steatohepatitis, and medications (i.e., statins). Alkaline phosphatase is produced by the cells lining the biliary tree. Elevation in its levels suggests a biliary process such as common bile duct stone, cholangitis, primary biliary sclerosis, or primary sclerosing cholangitis. However, alkaline phosphatase is produced by other organs including the gut, placenta, and bone. Therefore, a gamma-glutamyl transpeptidase GGTP level can be useful as it isolates the increased alkaline phosphatase as originating from the biliary tree.

The prothrombin time (PT) and albumin level indicate synthetic *function* of the liver. An elevated PT or decreased albumin level can indicate long-standing liver disease such as cirrhosis, important in the event a patient needs an operation. *Pancreatic Enzymes*. Amylase levels are elevated in pancreatitis with rise within 2–12 hours of symptoms and return to

TABLE 33.2

BIOCHEMICAL AND HEMATOLOGICAL LABORATORY ANALYSES

STUDY	COMPONENTS	INTERPRETATION/CAVEATS
Arterial blood gas (Acid–base status)	• Base deficit (BD) • Lactate	• Initial BD > 6 or lactate > 4, as well as, failure to correct these values within 24–48 hours are independent risk factors for increased mortality. • Elevated lactate levels may occur in the setting of accelerated production (i.e., catecholamine administration) or diminished metabolism (i.e. hepatic dysfunction).
Complete blood count	• WBC count and differential • Hemoglobin (Hgb) • Platelet count	• Normal WBC with bandemia is synonymous with leukocytosis. • Leukocytosis may be induced with corticosteroid use. • Acute anemia may indicate bleeding or dilutional effects of resuscitation. • Normal platelet count may not reflect normal platelet function (i.e., Aspirin, Clopidogrel)
Chemistry	• Electrolytes • BUN/creatinine • Glucose	• Consider GI losses, fluid resuscitation, diuretics, medications, and transcellular shifts due to acid-base disorders in the evaluation of electrolyte abnormalities. • BUN/creatinine ratio > 20 suggests hypovolemia (i.e., dehydration), but may also occur with upper GI hemorrhage • Hyperglycemia or hypoglycemia may occur with sepsis or corticosteroid use, in addition to diabetes. • Hypoglycemia due to hepatic insufficiency is indicative of severe hepatic dysfunction
Hepatobiliary tests	• Liver function tests (LFT) • Bilirubin • Amylase/lipase	• Elevated LFTs, in particular the transaminases, may be induced by severe shock due to hemorrhage or sepsis. • Elevated bilirubin, gamma-glutamyl transferase, and alkaline phosphatase are markers of biliary obstruction. • Hyperamylasemia typically occurs with pancreatitis, but may also be secondary to acute renal insufficiency or a perforated hollow viscus.
Coagulation studies	• Prothrombin time • INR	• Markers of hepatic synthetic function. • May be abnormally elevated from DIC, hepatic insufficiency, prior Coumadin use, or severe malnutrition.

normal over next 3–5 days. Peak levels occur within the first 48 hours of symptoms.[3,9] Because of pancreas "burn-out" in chronic pancreatitis, levels can be normal despite an episode of acute, often severe, pancreatitis. Thus, amylase levels do not correlate with etiology or severity of pancreatitis. In addition, hyperamylasemia is nonspecific and may be seen with inflammation of the GI tract, many gynecological diseases, renal failure, and salivary gland inflammation. Lipase levels are elevated in pancreatitis, will rise slightly later (4–8 hours), peak earlier (24 hours), and return to normal longer (8–14 days) than amylase.[3] Similar to amylase levels, lipase levels can be elevated in other intraabdominal pathology and renal insufficiency. Lipase levels are considered more specific than serum amylase for acute pancreatitis, especially in alcoholic pancreatitis.[3,9] However, levels *do not* correlate with etiology or severity.

Urinalysis (UA). Microscopic hematuria raises the possibility of a kidney stone or urological cancer. Pyuria, positive nitrite, and leukoesterase indicate acute pyelonephritis or cystitis. On the other hand, a "positive" urinalysis (i.e., with positive leukoesterase and few WBC's) may be secondary to an inflammatory process in the abdomen such as appendicitis rather than a urinary tract infection. A *pregnancy test* is mandatory in women of child-bearing age.

Erythrocyte sedimentation rate and C-reactive protein are nonspecific markers of inflammation and acute stress that are not useful in the acute abdomen but may be followed over time to trend a patient's response to treatment. Further study is needed to delineate the diagnostic utility in the acute abdomen of biomarkers such as procalcitonin.[10]

IMAGING

Improvements in abdominal imaging modalities have fostered a better appreciation of the advantages and limitations of each study in the evaluation of the acute abdomen.

X-ray. Plain radiographs of the abdomen and chest are inexpensive, portable, quickly performed tests, yet insensitive. They are a 'confluence of shadows,' dependent upon contrasting densities of apposed organs. Nonetheless, plain radiographs can reveal the dilated loops of a mechanical bowel obstruction, pneumoperitoneum of a perforated hollow viscus, or the thumbprinting indicative of pneumatosis. Portal venous gas may be seen in plain radiographs, related to intestinal ischemia or gas producing organisms. Calcifications may be seen in the pancreas, gallbladder, or aorta. Only 15% of gallstones are radiopaque, but 90% of kidney stones are opaque. The finding of a fecolith, occurring in 50% cases of appendicitis can be helpful.

Serial x-rays may be used to show the passage of previously administered oral contrast. However, if a CT scan is planned, no additional value is obtained from plain films in the evaluation of undifferentiated acute abdominal pain.[11-13]

Computed Tomography Scan. CT is a rapidly performed exam, although more expensive than plain films, which provides specific information about hollow and solid viscera, vasculature, muscles, and bones. However, the patient must be physiologically stable, as the CT suite is rarely equipped with resources to treat an unstable patient. Furthermore, the data would suggest that for moribund patients, the decision to operate should not be based on CT findings, and completion of the scan only delays surgical intervention.[14]

CT can be performed with or without intravenous or oral contrast. Patients with contrast allergies can be premedicated with a steroid and benadryl protocol. The administration of intravenous contrast provides an evaluation of organ perfusion, parenchymal injury, areas of differing perfusion (i.e., hematoma vs. parenchyma), and even thrombosis of vessels, but it has not been demonstrated to increase the rate of diagnosis.[15-17] Oral contrast requires time for intestinal passage. It is generally not necessary for the evaluation of small bowel obstruction or trauma patients and is relatively contraindicated in patients for whom an emergent scan is desired. A recent retrospective study of various combinations of intravenous, oral, and rectal contrast for CT of patients with an acute abdomen noted no difference in accuracy of diagnosis in enhanced compared to unenhanced scans.[16,17] In the acutely ill patient, an unenhanced scan eliminates the risks associated with contrast aspiration and renal injury. If contrast is used, extraluminal free fluid can be evaluated by Hounsfield units (HU) to help determine its source and significance. Typically, serous fluid is 0–20 HU, exudative or purulent fluid is 20–40 HU, and blood is 40 HU.[18] Although CT may be used to confirm the inflammatory changes of acute cholecystitis, remember that gallstones are commonly not seen (one-third) on CT.

Ultrasound. Ultrasound exams are noninvasive tests that can be performed at the patient's bedside. Focused abdominal sonography for trauma (FAST) is a rapid ultrasound exam used in trauma patients to evaluate the presence of fluid in four regions: the pericardium, the perihepatic region, the perisplenic area, and the pelvis. Right upper quadrant ultrasound can be used to evaluate liver parenchyma and the biliary system for ductal dilatation, stones, and surrounding fluid. Sensitivity is less than that of a CT scan in diagnosis of acute abdominal pathology (70% vs. 89%), but it is noninvasive and eliminates the risks of radiation.[19] Vaginal and RLQ ultrasound can be used to diagnose ovarian torsion and cysts and to confirm the diagnosis of appendicitis. Sonograms are routinely used in the pediatric population to evaluate abdominal pain. The primary limitations of ultrasonography include poor acoustic windows (i.e., obesity, clothing, or splints) and the study is operator-dependent.

Magnetic Resonance Imaging. MRI studies are less practical in the acute abdominal setting due to the time required to perform the test. An unstable patient does not belong in the MRI scanner; the closed environment is even less conducive to prompt treatment than CT. Also, patients with pacemakers or other metallic implants are not candidates for an MRI. MRI is often more useful in the investigation of chronic abdominal pain and abdominal masses. Magnetic resonance cholangiopancreatography is sensitive in the diagnosis of biliary and pancreatic pathology, associated with equal accuracy as endoscopic retrograde cholangiopancreatography (ERCP), but it is not a therapeutic option.[20] Unlike plain radiography and CT imaging, surgeons are less proficient at reading MRI than x-rays, ultrasound, and CT, and so a radiologist's interpretation is often necessary.

Angiography. Although the gold standard for vascular imaging and rapidly becoming the first line of intervention for vascular pathology, angiography has been supplanted by CT angiography as the diagnostic method of choice. There are circumstances, however, in which angiography is invaluable: type B aortic dissection, acute thromboembolism, chronic mesenteric ischemia, and rectus sheath or retroperitoneal hematomas. These are clinical situations in which angiographic therapies (i.e., stenting, embolization) may be the best treatment option.

DIAGNOSTIC ADJUNCTS

Once the differential diagnosis of acute abdominal pain has become more focused, specific invasive adjunctive tests can aid precise diagnosis, and may also be therapeutic.

Diagnostic Peritoneal Lavage (DPL). Introduced in 1965, diagnostic peritoneal lavage (DPL) had been primarily limited to the evaluation of the unstable trauma patient. Performance of a DPL involves the insertion of a catheter into the peritoneum, followed by lavage with warm saline. For trauma patients, frank blood, intestinal contents, or a cytologic assessment >500 WBCs per mm^3 or >100,000 RBCs per mm^3 is considered indicative of injury, necessitating either CT to evaluate solid injury in the hemodynamically stable patient or surgical exploration in the unstable patient. Recent studies have shown that DPL may be useful in the assessment of the nontraumatic acute abdomen to confirm or disprove the presence of intraabdominal pathology in the hypotensive, septic patient.[21,22] Equipoise persists regarding the WBC threshold for operative intervention. Cytology results of >200 WBCs per mm^3 is our generally accepted threshold for operative exploration in the nontrauma patient suspected of harboring acute abdominal pathology.

Endoscopy. Upper endoscopy allows evaluation of the esophagus, stomach, and first part of the small intestine. It can be performed in the patient's ICU room, provided that sedation can be administered, and adequate oxygenation and respiration can be maintained and monitored. Esophagitis, gastritis, and peptic ulcer disease can be diagnosed, biopsies can be taken, and if bleeding is noted, cautery, clipping, or injections of epinephrine may be therapeutic as well.

Colonoscopy/Sigmoidoscopy may be helpful in diagnosis or exclusion of certain pathology. Flexible sigmoidoscopy or colonoscopy is often used to diagnose colonic ischemia, especially in the setting of abdominal pain and diarrhea after abdominal aorta surgery. They can also be used in the evaluation of possible inflammatory bowel disease, infectious colitis (i.e. presence of pseudomembranes), and volvulus.

Laparoscopy. While exploration of the abdomen is one endpoint of the algorithm in evaluation of the patient with an acute abdomen, an unstable patient may not tolerate a nontherapeutic trip to the operating room. Diagnostic laparoscopy can be an extension of a DPL and can be performed under sterile conditions in the ICU if necessary. Walsh et al.[23] found bedside laparoscopy to be more accurate than DPL at prediction of need for laparotomy.

Hepatobiliary Imaging (HIDA). Nonfilling of the gallbladder 60 minutes after administration of intravenous biliary radiopharmaceutical can be used to diagnose cholecystitis with equivocal ultrasound results or in acalculous cholecystitis. The specificity can be increased by giving morphine. False positives do occur in critically ill, malnourished, or patients on total parental nutrition.

COMMON CAUSES OF THE ACUTE ABDOMEN

Acute appendicitis can occur in any patient (see chapter 37). A history of several hours of periumbilical or epigastric pain that eventually settles in the RLQ is classic. It is frequently associated with anorexia and nausea; emesis may also be present. No specific past medical history is predictive except the presence of an appendix. On exam, focal peritonitis at McBurney's point (one-third of the distance between the anterior superior iliac spine and the umbilicus) is the most common finding. A psoas sign, pain upon active flexion, or passive extension of the right hip, supports the diagnosis. With associated leukocytosis, no further studies or imaging are needed prior to operative intervention. In female patients, gynecologic etiologies must also be considered, including a ruptured ovarian cyst, ovarian torsion, TOA, and ectopic pregnancy. The differential diagnosis also includes terminal ileitis associated with inflammatory bowel diseases. Ultrasound or CT scan can be performed to confirm the diagnosis of appendicitis.[24-26] Alternatively, a laparoscopic approach to appendectomy allows intraoperative evaluation of the appendix, small bowel, and pelvic structures when the diagnosis is unclear.

Cholelithiasis/Cholecystitis. (See Chapter 39) Ultrasound is the study of choice for diagnosis. Gallstones can be detected in most (>95%) patients with cholelithiasis. CT is commonly used as a screening test in patients with abdominal pain; one-third of gallstones are not visualized on CT. The patient with postprandial right upper quadrant abdominal pain, gallstones, but no tenderness, leukocytosis, or fever has biliary colic. This patient can be scheduled for elective cholecystectomy. However, the patient with right upper quadrant tenderness, confirmed gallstones, and leukocytosis or fever has acute cholecystitis. Positive findings of cholecystitis on ultrasound or CT include gallbladder wall thickening (>3mm), pericholecystic fluid, and sonographic Murphy's sign, in addition to the presence of stones. Dilation of the common bile duct (CBD) (variable according to age but >7–8 mm) may indicate biliary obstruction secondary to a stone, stricture, or mass. The treatment for acute cholecystitis is intravenous antibiotics, bowel rest, and ideally laparoscopic cholecystectomy within 24 hours of admission.

Acute Pancreatitis. Acute pancreatitis is most commonly due to choledocholithiasis or alcohol ingestion. Acute pancreatitis is an inflammatory process diagnosed by the combination of epigastric abdominal pain, elevation of serum pancreatic enzymes (amylase or lipase), or CT evidence of pancreatic inflammation. In the majority of patients, pancreatitis is a self-limited process with mild abdominal pain and rapid resolution. If the etiology is choledocholithiasis and the patient improves clinically within several days as generally occurs (presumably with the stone passing through the common bile duct), laparoscopic cholecystectomy should be performed during the same hospital admission. The utility of intraoperative cholangiogram in this setting is still debated (see Chapter on Pancreatitis). However, in one-quarter of patients, acute pancreatitis is a severe, life-threatening condition. Thus, optimal treatment varies significantly, based on severity of the disease, underlying etiology and potential complications such as pseudocyst, necrosis, infection, or abdominal compartment syndrome (ACS) (see Chapter 38).

Acute Mesenteric Ischemia commonly presents as sudden onset of severe, diffuse abdominal pain frequently in the context of preexisting coronary artery disease, peripheral vascular disease, or atrial fibrillation. Prior AAA repair eliminates the inferior mesenteric artery, making more of the bowel dependent upon perfusion from the superior mesenteric artery. Vital sign abnormalities include tachycardia (if the patient is not receiving beta blockade), with or without hypotension, and tachypnea depending on the degree of ischemia and acidosis. The classic physical finding is pain which is out of proportion to examination; deep palpation may elicit a degree of tenderness less than anticipated. Aortic occlusion or a state of global low perfusion can also cause mottling of the skin of the lower abdomen and lower extremities. High doses of vasopressors can exacerbate this condition. Decreased or absent urine output is associated with mesenteric ischemia, and an elevated WBC count, lactate, and base deficit are generally seen. Abdominal x-rays may demonstrate a thumbprinted appearance of the intestine and Doppler ultrasound may reveal decreased or occluded mesenteric blood flow. CT tends to be more specific, showing thickened bowel wall, pneumatosis, free fluid, or occlusion of the aorta, celiac, or superior mesenteric artery.[27,28] Diagnosis is confirmed at the time of laparotomy. Eltarawy et al. showed that surgical consultation >24 hours after disease onset and operation >6 hours after the time of consult were associated with increased mortality.[14] Patients with delayed surgical consultation were more likely to have abdominal distension, elevated lactate concentration, acute renal failure, and vasopressor administration, and performing a CT scan further delayed definitive treatment.[14] Hence, the ideal approach is a good history and exam, combined with a low threshold of suspicion.

Bowel Obstruction. The history of illness includes abdominal pain and distension associated with nausea, emesis, obstipation or constipation, typically in a patient with prior abdominal surgery. Distension, with or without focal or diffuse tenderness, is typical. Abdominal scars and hernias should be carefully noted; an incarcerated hernia is especially concerning. Leukocytosis is not uncommon. X-rays may show air-fluid levels; a paucity of air in the distal colon and rectum indicates complete obstruction. CT can identify a specific transition point of obstruction. Bowel obstruction due to an internal hernia is seen as spiraling of the mesentery on CT imaging. CT may also provide evidence of impending or complete strangulation; thickened bowel wall, ascites, or lack of enhancement with IV contrast.[29] Oral contrast provides little benefit and poses the risks of emesis and aspiration pneumonitis.[17] Symptoms of a partial small bowel obstruction often improve with nasogastric decompression, while acute mesenteric ischemia continues to progress until treated.[14] Complete bowel obstruction or closed loop obstruction requires immediate laparotomy (see Chapter 36).

Clostridium difficile Colitis. The epidemiology of *Clostridium difficile* has changed significantly over the last two decades, although it remains the most common cause of antibiotic-associated colitis. *C. difficile* colitis is an increasing nosocomial problem in North America and Western Europe. Since 2002, the incidence has increased, relapses have become more frequent, and the fatality rate has increased.[30] The three major risk factors are the administration of antibiotics, age > 65 years, and prior hospitalization.[31] Even a single dose of antibiotics can induce the disease. Abdominal cramping, fever, and diarrhea are common symptoms at presentation. Diarrhea may be absent in up to 20% of patients. On exam, the patient is often distended and diffusely tender. The most notable change is a marked leukocytosis (WBC ≥ 30,000/mm^3).[32] Stool specimens should be evaluated for the presence of toxins A and B, although if suspicion is high, treatment should be initiated without delay. Radiographs are nonspecific. CT will show a thickened colon with or without associated ascites. On lower endoscopy, the patient will have pseudomembranes, although this is rarely performed in the acute setting. In a study by Dallal et al. the false negative rate of stool studies and endoscopy approached 15%, while the sensitivity of diagnosis by CT scan was 100%.[31] As the infection progresses, tachycardia, hypotension, and renal failure can develop quickly. A prompt response to metronidazole is consistent with this antibiotic-associated colitis, although with increasingly virulent and resistant strains, enteral vancomycin is now recognized as the first line treatment of severe *C. difficile* infection in the ICU setting.[30] When patients fail to respond to medical management, operative intervention is necessary. Traditionally, these patients underwent total abdominal colectomy and end ileostomy. A colon-sparing technique of laparoscopic loop ileostomy with subsequent serial vancomycin flushes through the colon is currently being evaluated at our institution with encouraging initial results (see chapter 35).

Peptic Ulcer Disease. Risk factors for peptic ulcer disease include NSAIDs, smoking, chronic illness, burns, steroid use, and a prior history of peptic ulcer disease (see chapter 35). Postprandial epigastric pain is a classic symptom, although with perforation, the pain becomes sharp and diffuse. It is not uncommon for the patient to report the exact time of symptom onset. The pain may be associated with nausea and vomiting, and peritonitis is frequent. The most common lab abnormality is leukocytosis, and hyperamylasemia may be seen. Upright chest x-ray will often show free air under the diaphragm. CT may show thickening, inflammation, and stranding around the stomach and duodenum as well as free air or free fluid. In the absence of perforation, upper endoscopy is highly accurate for peptic ulcer disease, and enables the acquisition of tissue for assessment of *Helicobator pylori*. Details regarding management are in chapter 35.

Ovarian/Uterine Pathology. Ovarian cysts or masses leading to ovarian torsion, TOA, or ectopic pregnancy usually present as unilateral lower abdominal pain, while pelvic inflammatory disease presents with more midline pelvic pain. The investigation of lower abdominal pain in a female patient must include a detailed gynecologic, obstetric, and social history. All females of childbearing age should undergo a pregnancy test. Women who have ovarian cysts may experience sharp pain around the time of ovulation and cyst rupture. Cysts or masses >5 cm in size are at risk for torsion, which is typically accompanied by severe, sharp, and continuous pain. The pain often resolves with spontaneous detorsion. Pain due to ectopic pregnancy lateralizes to one side of the abdomen soon after a missed period, and may be accompanied by vaginal spotting bleeding. Ectopic pregnancy can be life-threatening due to fallopian rupture and hemorrhage. Primary TOA develops in the majority of cases as a complication of pelvic inflammatory disease (PID), although they may develop after pelvic surgery.[33] Secondary TOAs result from bowel perforation (appendicitis, diverticulitis) with intraperitoneal spread of infection or in association with pelvic malignancy. Distinguishing between primary and secondary TOA is difficult. Primary TOA is the most common diagnosis in premenopausal women who are sexually active. However, in postmenopausal women, the presence of a gynecologic malignancy or other pelvic pathology causing secondary TOA must be excluded.[34] Pelvic ultrasound is the most frequently used method for characterization of ovarian pathology (see chapter 44).[35]

Intraabdominal Hypertension (IAH)/Abdominal Compartment Syndrome (ACS). The World Society of Abdominal Compartment Syndrome defines normal intraabdominal pressure (IAP) in critically ill adults as 5–7 mm Hg and abdominal hypertension as IAPs > 12 mm Hg. ACS is a sustained IAP > 20 mm Hg associated with new organ dysfunction. IAH and ACS occur in approximately 35% and 5% of ICU patients, respectively.[36] ACS is traditionally thought of as a traumatic or surgical entity, but it is being equally recognized in medical ICUs.

Patients at risk for IAH include critically ill patients, who have some element of decreased organ perfusion with a systemic inflammatory response that leads to capillary leakage. Aggressive fluid resuscitation leads to tissue edema, including the bowel wall and the mesentery, resulting in IAH.[37] This increased pressure compresses tissues and vessels leading to decreased perfusion and organ dysfunction. Conditions that predispose patients to the development of ACS include sepsis; ascites; intraperitoneal, retroperitoneal or abdominal wall bleeding; intraabdominal malignancy; laparotomy closed under tension; a positive intraoperative fluid balance >6 L; and polysystem traumatic or thermal injury.[36]

IAH leads to physiologic alterations that can result in falsely elevated central venous pressure and pulmonary artery wedge pressure. All patients at risk for ACS should have IAP measured and trended. Kirkpatrick et al. and Sugrue et al. compared IAP measurements to physical examination. Clinical judgment failed to detect significant IAH > 40% of the time.[38,39] IAP can be measured using gastric, bladder, or rectal manometry. Obeid et al.[40] found bladder pressure to be the most accurate and the most technically reliable method. Measurements are obtained by instilling 25–50 mL of saline into the bladder with the foley clamped, attaching IV pressure tubing to the foley, and transducing at the level of the bladder. Using volumes >50 mL may cause overestimation of IAP.[41]

The treatment of ACS is urgent surgical decompression. Interventions to manage IAH include the following: (1) decompression of intraluminal contents (stomach, bladder, colon), (2) evacuation of extraluminal contents (i.e., ascites), (3) increased abdominal wall compliance by neuromuscular blockade, (4) careful fluid and vasopressor management to maintain tissue perfusion, and (5) treatment of the underlying source of the inflammatory response.

UNIQUE POPULATIONS

Certain patient populations may present a more complicated picture of acute abdominal pain. Pregnant, immunosuppressed, and morbidly obese patients may present the same pathology with different signs and symptoms, obscuring the diagnosis. Consideration of etiologies specific to these populations and prompt diagnosis are important, as these patients may present late in the course of their disease, already with compromised physiology.

Pregnancy. The anatomic, physiologic, and biochemical changes associated with pregnancy must be taken into consideration in evaluation of the pregnant patient. As the gravid uterus increases in size, other structures including small and large intestine and appendix are displaced laterally and superiorly. Peritoneal signs are often absent because of the lifting and stretching of the anterior abdominal wall; the inflamed viscera are not apposed to the parietal peritoneum, thereby precluding any muscular response or guarding. GI motility is decreased due to elevated levels of progesterone, leading to constipation. Gallbladder function is impaired because of the hypotonia of the smooth muscle wall. Thus, emptying time is slowed and often incomplete, and bile stasis may lead to gallstone formation. There are no apparent morphologic changes in the liver during pregnancy, but there are functional alterations. Serum alkaline phosphatase activity may increase due to placental alkaline phosphatase isoenzymes. Plasma volume increases earlier and faster than red blood cell volume, until the end of the second trimester, when an increase in the red blood cells compensates. Hence, a mild anemia (e.g., Hct 33%) should be interpreted with caution. Total blood leukocyte count increases during pregnancy to as high as 16,000/mm^3 in later trimesters. Polymorphonuclear (PMN) leukocytes primarily contribute to this increase, as lymphocyte and monocyte numbers remain stable.[42-44]

The most useful diagnostic modalities in the pregnant patient are the history and serial exams. Laboratory values are unpredictable with the normal changes of pregnancy. Ultrasound is a useful noninvasive adjunct with no risk to the fetus. In general, maternal mortality is rare, but fetal mortality is higher when diagnosis is delayed. The most common reason for an acute abdomen in the pregnant patient is *acute appendicitis*. If the appendix progresses to perforation, fetal mortality may be as high as 36%; thus, suspicion must be high.[45] The appendix is displaced upward starting in the third month and progresses to the level of the iliac crest in the sixth month. Despite these changes, the most reliable symptom is still RLQ pain.[45] Symptoms of nausea and heartburn are nonspecific in the pregnant patient, as is leukocytosis.[46] Ultrasound is the diagnostic imaging method of choice with close to 100% sensitivity and 96% specificity, though the yield is user-dependent.[47] The risks of radiation (i.e., CT scan) are greatest during fetal organogenesis. The most sensitive time period for central nervous system teratogenesis is between 10 and 17 weeks of gestation. Of note, appendiceal rupture is twice as frequent during the third trimester.[48]

Cholecystitis affects 1/1,600–1/10,000 pregnancies.[43] Typical signs and symptoms occur, although Murphy's sign is uncommonly present. Laboratory data may demonstrate an elevated direct bilirubin and transaminases, although an elevated alkaline phosphatase is usually physiologic. Ultrasound is again the test of choice with 95% accuracy. The differential diagnosis includes MI, acute fatty liver of pregnancy, and HELLP syndrome. HELLP syndrome (hemolysis, increased liver function tests, and low platelets) carries a significant risk of both maternal and fetal mortality. It is easily confused with cholecystitis/cholelithiasis, as 65%-90% of patients with HELLP present with right upper quadrant pain.[49] HELLP must be excluded in all patients with preeclampsia, although it can present without hypertension.

Bowel obstruction occurs in 1/2,500- 1/3,500 pregnancies, usually during the third trimester.[43] Adhesions are the etiology in >60% of cases. Less common causes include volvulus, intussusception, hernia, and tumor. Patients complain of crampy abdominal pain, obstipation, and emesis. In small bowel obstruction, the pain tends to be diffuse, poorly localized upper abdominal pain that occurs in 5-minute intervals. Large bowel obstruction presents as lower abdomen or perineal pain that occurs in 15–20 minute intervals. Abdominal x-rays are generally the only imaging needed.[50] Morbidity is related to diagnostic and therapeutic delay. A common misdiagnosis is hyperemesis gravidarum, which also occurs late in pregnancy.

Pancreatitis, commonly associated with choledocholithiasis, most frequently occurs in the third trimester because of increased abdominal pressure on the biliary ducts.[43] Patients have sudden, severe epigastric pain that radiates to the back. Diagnosis is confirmed with elevated amylase and lipase levels, although these levels may be mildly elevated at baseline during the first and second trimesters. Ultrasound typically shows gallstones, ductal dilatation, or pseudocyst. *Adnexal torsion* is more common in the pregnant than in the nonpregnant patient. It presents as lateralized lower quadrant pain and is diagnosed with Doppler ultrasound to confirm decreased blood flow.

Immunosuppression. Circumstances of immunosuppression occur with organ transplantation, chemotherapy for malignancy, immunosuppressive therapy (i.e., Crohn's disease, idiopathic pulmonary fibrosis), and immunodeficiencies (i.e., HIV and AIDS). Causes of acute abdominal pain in this population can be categorized as (1) pathology closely associated with the immunocompromised state, or (2) illnesses that occur in any patient, independent of immune status.

Because recent and continuing medical advances have increased the life expectancies for this population, acute abdominal pain in immunosuppressed patients is more frequently encountered.[51,52] Classic clinical, laboratory, and radiographic evidence of intraabdominal pathology may be absent. As patients experience blunted symptoms, they tend to seek care later, often after the illness has progressed to a severe state.[53-55] The most common cause of the acute abdomen in the neutropenic patient is *neutropenic enterocolitis*, or typhilitis, with reported incidences of 0.8%-26%.[56] It has been described in other immunosuppressive states, and neutropenia is not requisite. The pathology involves mucosal injury often by cytotoxic drugs, profound neutropenia, and impaired host defense to invasion by microorganisms. Microbial infection leads to necrosis of various layers of the bowel wall.[57,58] The cecum is almost always affected because of its distensibility and decreased vascularization, compared to the rest of the colon.[59] The process often extends into the ascending colon and terminal ileum. Patients typically present with fever, RLQ pain, nausea with emesis, and watery or bloody diarrhea. CT demonstrates circumferential terminal ileum and cecal thickening with stranding of the mesentery.[60] Initial medical management is supportive; bowel rest, fluid resuscitation, total parenteral nutrition (TPN), and broad-spectrum antibiotics. Surgical intervention is reserved for cases with evidence of perforation, ischemia, persistent hemorrhage, or unresolving sepsis or peritonitis. Mortality rates are reported between 30% and 50%.[56-60]

Between 50% and 80% of the world's population is seropositive for cytomegalovirus (CMV), but primary *CMV infection* in the immunocompetent host typically is mild and clinically undetectable. Symptomatic reactivation occurs with immunocompromise or immunosuppression and may present as CMV enterocolitis. Mucosal ulcers can develop throughout the entire GI tract, although most commonly in the colon and esophagus.[61,62] These ulcers begin with bleeding and may progress to perforation. The diagnosis may be difficult. If endoscopic biopsies are negative for CMV, testing for the presence of CMV DNA in peripheral blood by polymerase chain reaction and for CMV antibodies may confirm the diagnosis. Gancyclovir is the initial medical treatment.

The incidence of *radiation enteritis* has increased with the current trend of combined chemotherapy and radiation.[63] Caused by a progressive occlusive vasculitis, it results in bowel lumen narrowing and mucosal damage that may lead to ulceration, obstruction, fistula, and perforation. Current treatment is mainly supportive.

Ascites associated with increased abdominal girth and nausea may cause abdominal pain. The diagnosis is made through biochemical and cytologic analysis of ascitic aspirate. These patients are also at risk for spontaneous bacterial peritonitis (SBP), particularly with low protein ascites that lacks complement factors. Bloody ascites may result from a traumatic tap or be secondary to malignancy. Dark brown ascitic fluid may indicate biliary perforation or leak. The upper limit of an absolute PMN leukocyte count in uncomplicated ascitic fluid is 250 per mm^3.[64] SBP is the most frequent cause of an increased ascitic WBC count with PMN predominance. A positive culture in conjunction confirms the diagnosis and is used to guide antibiotic therapy. Tuberculous peritonitis and peritoneal carcinomatosis give rise to an increased ascitic WBC count, but with lymphocyte predominance.

Posttransplant lymphoproliferative disorder (PTLD) refers to a group of B cell lymphomas occurring in immunosuppressed patients following organ transplant. The immunosuppression impairs T cell immunity and allows uncontrolled proliferation of Epstein-Barr virus (EBV)-infected B cells, resulting in monoclonal or polyclonal plasmacytic hyperplasia, B-cell hyperplasia, B-cell lymphoma, or immunoblastic lymphoma. PTLD can present as localized or disseminated disease. Clinical features may include fever, lymphadenopathy, pulmonary symptoms, central nervous system alterations, and weight loss. GI manifestations can result in an acute abdomen from bowel obstruction, ischemia, or perforation. The incidence varies with the type of allograft, occurring in 2%-3% of liver transplant recipients.[65] A higher risk is observed in children and recipients of heart and small bowel transplants. The diagnosis is based on a high index of suspicion. EBV titers should be noted, although this does not always correlate with the presence of disease.[66] Initial management of PTLD involves reduction or discontinuation of immunosuppressive agents. Several chemotherapy and radiation protocols are also available. EBV titer trends can be followed; a declining viral load suggests response to treatment. It is a difficult balance between eradication of the disease and preservation of graft function, but the diagnosis must be considered in all transplant patients with an acute abdomen.

The Obese Patient. The prevalence of obesity in the United States has been steadily increasing; overweight and obese adults constitute more than 60% of the population.[67] These patients are at greater risk of Type 2 diabetes mellitus, hypertension, hyperlipidemia, obstructive sleep apnea, cardiovascular disease, gallbladder disease, and gastroesophageal disease. The annual rate of bariatric surgical procedures performed to decrease these risks increased nearly sixfold between 1990 and 2000.[68] Obese patients with acute abdominal pain are a diagnostic challenge both before and after they have had weight loss surgery.

Physical examination can be more challenging in the overweight patient. Hernias and masses are difficult to palpate, and the degree of abdominal distension is difficult to ascertain. Radiologic imaging of the obese patient is difficult; imaging equipment and tables have size and weight limitations. Poor acoustic penetration and increased attenuation of the beam by dense subcutaneous and intraperitoneal fat yield low quality images. Low-frequency ultrasound provides the best opportunity for quality images.[69] CT can be used for a patient who does not exceed the diameter or weight limits of the machine.

Causes of the acute abdomen in this population include incisional and internal hernias, gastric outlet stenosis, marginal ulcers, band erosions, and gallstone disease. Any obese patient with epigastric pain should also be evaluated for acute cardiac pathology. Hernias from both open and laparoscopic bariatric and nonbariatric surgical procedures can lead to pain from obstructive symptoms. Increased abdominal wall laxity and difficulty performing adequate fascial closures at laparoscopic port sites contribute to the significant prevalence.[70] Internal hernias occur in up to 6% of all patients who have had gastric bypass surgery.[71] They typically occur at three locations: the transverse colon mesentery at the Roux limb hiatus, around the mesentery of the Roux limb, or at the mesenteric defect of the enteroenterostomy. CT findings may include a dilated gastric remnant, oral contrast that refluxes into the gastric remnant, or swirling of the mesenteric vessels. Persistent tachycardia despite fluid resuscitation, leukocytosis, and lactic acidemia are ominous signs of ischemia. Stenosis of the gastric outlet occurs in up to 12% of both gastric bypass and vertical banded gastroplasty patients.[72,73] The gastrojejunostomy may become inflamed and edematous or stricture due to marginal ulceration. Patients who have undergone gastric banding are at risk for band erosion into the stomach with an incidence of 0.3%-1.9%.[74-76] Pain, emesis immediately after eating, or hematemesis should prompt endoscopic evaluation.

Obese patients are more likely to have gallbladder disease than nonobese patients; however, routine cholecystectomy during bariatric surgery is not uniformly practiced. Right upper quadrant pain, nausea, and emesis after eating are common presenting symptoms. Liver function tests should be evaluated. It should be noted that after gastric bypass surgery, common bile duct stones cannot be removed via traditional ERCP. ERCP may be performed via open or laparoscopic approach through the gastric remnant at the time of cholecystectomy.[77,78]

CONCLUSION

While diagnostic and treatment innovations continue to evolve, the need for prompt diagnosis and intervention for the patient with acute abdominal pain persists. A thorough history and physical followed by specifically indicated labs and imaging provide the foundation for solving the diagnostic dilemma of the acute abdomen in increasingly complex patient populations.

References

1. Stone R. Acute abdominal pain. *Lippincotts Prim Care Pract.* 1998;2(4):341-357.
2. Powers RD, Guertler AT. Abdominal pain in the ED: stability and change over 20 years. *Am J Emerg Med.* 1995;13(3):301-303.
3. Thomas SH, Silen W, Cheema F, et al. Effects of morphine analgesia on diagnostic accuracy in emergency department patients with abdominal pain: a prospective, randomized trial. *J Am Coll Surg.* 2003;196:18-31.
4. Manterola C, Astudillo P, Laosada H, et al. Analgesia in patients with acute abdominal pain. *Cochrane Database Syst Rev.* 2007;18(3):CD005660.
5. Myakis S, Karamanof G, Liontos M, et al. Factors contributing to inappropriate ordering of tests in an academic medical department and the effect of an educational feedback strategy. *Postgrad Med J.* 2006;82(974):823-829.
6. Graff LG, Robinson D. Abdominal pain and emergency department evaluation. *Emerg Med Clin N Am.* 2001;19:123-136.
7. Sahai RK, Forsythe RM. Evaluation of acute abdominal pain. In: Peitzman AB, Rhodes M, Schwab CW, et al., eds. *The Trauma Manual. Trauma and Acute Care Surgery.* Philadelphia, PA: Wolters Kluwer; 2008:574-584.
8. Doherty GM, Boey JH. The acute abdomen. In: Way LW, Doherty GM. *Current Surgical Diagnosis and Treatment.* 11th ed. New York, NY: McGraw-Hill; 2003:505-506.

9. Smotkin J, Tenner S. Laboratory diagnostic tests in acute pancreatitis. *J Clin Gastroenterol.* 2002;34:459-462.
10. Becker KL, Snider R, Nylen ES. Procalcitonin assay in systemic inflammation, infection, and sepsis: clinical utility and limitations. *Crit Care Med.* 2008;36(3):941-952.
11. David V. Radiology of abdominal pain. *Lippincotts Prim Care Pract.* 1999;3:498-513.
12. Smith JE, Hall EJ. The use of plain abdominal x rays in the emergency department. *Emerg Med J.* 2009;26:160-163.
13. Ahn SH, Mayo-Smith WW, Murphy BL, et al. Acute nontraumatic abdominal pain in adult patients: abdominal radiography compared with CT evaluation. *Radiology.* 2002;225:159-164.
14. Eltarawy IG, Etman YM, Zenati M, et al. Acute mesenteric ischemia: the importance of early surgical consultation. *Am Surg.* 2009;75(3):212-219.
15. Meth MJ, Maibach HI. Current understanding of contrast media reactions and implications for clinical management. *Drug Saf.* 2006;29(2):133-141.
16. Basak S, Nazarian LN, Wechsler RJ, et al. Is unenhanced CT sufficient for evaluation of acute abdominal pain? *Clin Imaging.* 2002;26(6):405-407.
17. Hill BC, Johnson SC, Owens EK, et al. CT scan for suspected acute abdominal process: impact of combinations of IV, oral, and rectal contrast. *World J Surg.* 2010;34(4):699-703.
18. Rupanagudi VA, Sahni AK, Kanagarajan K, et al. Can pleural fluid density measured by Hounsfield units (HU) on chest CT be used to differentiate between transudate and exudates? *Chest.* 2005;128:361S.
19. Lameris W, van Randen A, van Es HW, et al. Imaging strategies for detection of urgent conditions in patients with acute abdominal pain: diagnostic accuracy study. *BMJ.* 2009;338:b2431.
20. Hekimoglu K, Ustundag Y, Dusak A, et al. MRCP vs. ERCP in the evaluation of biliary pathologies: review of current literature. *J Dig Dis.* 2008;9(3):162-169.
21. Hay JM, Peyrard P, Lautard M, et al. Closed peritoneal lavage in the diagnosis of non traumatic acute abdomen. *Ital J Surg Sci.* 1988;18(2):115-120.
22. Powell DC, Bivins BA, Bell RM. Diagnostic peritoneal lavage. *Surg Gynecol Obstet.* 1982;155(2):257-264.
23. Walsh RM, Popovich MJ, Hoadley J. Bedside diagnostic laparoscopy and peritoneal lavage in the intensive care unit. *Surg Endosc.* 1998;12(12):1405-1409.
24. Balthazar EJ, Birnbaum BA, Yee J, et al. Acute appendicitis: CT and ultrasound correlation in one hundred patients. *Radiology.* 1994;190:31-35.
25. Rao PM, Rhea JT, Novelline RA, et al. Helical CT technique for the diagnosis of appendicitis: prospective evaluation of a focused appendix CT examination. *Radiology.* 1997;202:139-144.
26. Terasawa T, Blackmore CC, Bent S, et al. Systematic review: computed tomography and ultrasonography to detect acute appendicitis in adults and adolescents. *Ann Int Med.* 2004;141:537-546.
27. Wolf EL, Sprayregen S, Bakal CW. Radiology in intestinal ischemia: plain film, contrast, and other imaging studies. *Surg Clin N Am.* 1992;72:107-124.
28. Taourel PG, Deneuville M, Pradel JA, et al. Acute mesenteric ischemia: diagnosis with contrast-enhanced CT. *Radiology.* 1996;199:632-636.
29. Maglinte DT, Balthazar EJ, Kelvin FM, et al. The role of radiography in diagnosis of SBO. *Am J Roentgenol.* 1997;168:1171-1180.
30. Leclair MA, Allard C, Lesur O, et al. *Clostridium difficile* infection in the intensive care unit. *J Intensive Care Med.* 2010;25(1):23-30.
31. Dallal RM, Harbrecht BG, Boujoukas AJ, et al. Fulminant *Clostridium difficile*: an underappreciated and increasing cause of death and complications. *Ann Surg.* 2002;235(3):363-372.
32. Wanahita A, Goldsmith EA, Musher DM. Conditions associated with leukocytosis in a tertiary care hospital, with particular attention to the role of infection caused by clostridium difficile. *Clin Infect Dis.* 2002;34(12):1585-1592.
33. Golde SH, Israel R, Ledger WJ. Unilateral tubo-ovarian abscess: a distinct entity. *Am J Obstet Gynecol.* 1977;127:807.
34. Protopapas AG, Diakomanolis ES, Milingos SD, et al. Tub-ovarian abscesses in postmenopausal women: gynecological malignancy until proven otherwise? *Eur J Obstet Gynecol Reprod Biol.* 2004;114:203.
35. Brown DL, Dudiak KM, Laing FC. Adnexal masses: US characterization and reporting. *Radiology.* 2010;254(2):342-354.
36. Malbrain ML, Cheatham ML, Kirkpatrick A, et al. Results from the international conference of experts on intra-abdominal hypertension and abdominal compartment syndromes. I. Definitions. *Intensive Care Med.* 2006;32(11):1722-1732.
37. Ball CG, Kirkpatrick AW. Intra-abdominal hypertension and the abdominal compartment syndrome. *Scand J Surg.* 2007;96:197-204.
38. Kirkpatrick AW, et al. Is clinical examination an accurate indicator of raised intra-abdominal pressure in critically injured patients? *Can J Surg.* 2000;43(3):207-211.
39. Sugrue M. et al. Clinical examination is an inaccurate predictor of intraabdominal pressure. *World J Surg.* 2002;26(12):1428-1431.
40. Obeid F, et al. Increases in intra-abdominal pressure affect pulmonary compliance. *Arch Surg.* 1995;130(5):544-547; discussion 547-548.
41. Malbrain ML, Deeren DH. Effect of bladder volume on measured intravesical pressure: a prospective cohort study. *Crit Care.* 2006;10:R98.
42. Hill CC, Pickinpaugh J. Physiologic changes in pregnancy. *Surg Clin North Am.* 2008;88(2):391-401.
43. Sharp HT. The acute abdomen during pregnancy. *Clin Obstet Gynecol.* 2002;45(2):405-413.
44. Amos JD, Schorr SJ, Norman PF, et al. Laparoscopic surgery during pregnancy. *Am J Surg.* 1997;174:222.
45. Hee P, Viktrup L. The diagnosis of appendicitis during pregnancy and maternal and fetal outcome after appendectomy. *Int J Gynaecol Obstet.* 1999;65:129-135.
46. Tamir IL, Bongard FS, Klein SR. Acute appendicitis in the pregnant patient. *Am J Surg.* 1990;160:571-576.
47. Lim HK, Bae SH, Seo GS. Diagnosis of acute appendicitis in pregnant women: value of sonography. *Am J Roentgenol.* 1992;159:539-542.
48. Tracey M, Fletcher HS. Appendicitis in pregnancy. *Am Surg.* 2000;66:555-559; discussion 559-560.
49. Sibai BM, Ramadan M, Usta I, et al. Maternal morbidity and mortality in 442 pregnancies with hemolysis, elevated liver enzymes, and low platelets (HELLP syndrome). *Am J Obstet Gynecol.* 1993;155:501-509.
50. Perdue PW, Johnson HW, Stafford PW. Intestinal obstruction complicating pregnancy. *Am J Surg.* 1992;164:384-388.
51. Hogg R, Lima V, Sterne JA, et al. Life expectancy of individuals on combination antiretroviral therapy in high income countries: a collaborative analysis of 14 cohort studies. *Lancet.* 2008;372(9635):293-299.
52. Chinen J and Buckley RH. Transplantation immunology: solid organ and bone marrow. *J Allergy Clin Immunol.* 2010;125(2 Suppl 2):S324-S335.
53. Steed DL, Brown B, Reilly JJ, et al. General surgical complications in heart and heart-lung transplantation. *Surgery.* 1985;98:739-745.
54. Mueller XM, Tevaearai HT, Stumpe F, et al. Gastrointestinal disease following heart transplantation. *World J Surg.* 1999;23:650-655; discussion 655-656.
55. Markogiannakis H, Konstadoulakis M, Tzertzemelis D, et al. Subclinical peritonitis due to perforated sigmoid diverticulitis 14 years after heart-lung transplantation. *World J Gastroenterol.* 2008;14(22):3583-3586.
56. Ullery BW, Pieracci FM, Rodney JR, et al. Neutropenic enterocolitis. *Surg Infect.* 2009;10(3):307-314.
57. Wade DS, Nava HR, Douglass HO Jr. Neutropenic enterocolitis: clinical diagnosis and treatment. *Cancer.* 1992;69:17-23.
58. Newbold KM. Neutropenic enterocolitis: clinical and pathological review. *Dig Dis.* 1989;7:281-287.
59. Alt B, Glass NR, Sollinger H. Neutropenic enterocolitis in adults: review of the literature and assessment of surgical intervention. *Am J Surg.* 1985;149:405-408.
60. Frick MP, Maile CW, Crass JR, et al. Computed tomography of neutropenic colitis. *Am J Roentgenol.* 1984;143:763-765.
61. Murray RN, Parker A, Kadakia SC, et al. Cytomegalovirus in upper gastrointestinal ulcers. *J Clin Gastroenterol.*1994;19:198-201.
62. Weber FH, Frierson HF, Myers B. Cytomegalovirus as a cause of isolated severe ileal bleeding. *J Clin Gastroenterol.* 1992;14:52-55.
63. Ooi BS, Tjandra JJ, Green MD. Morbidities of adjuvant chemotherapy and radiotherapy for resectable rectal cancer: an overview. *Dis Col Rectum.* 1999;42:403-418
64. Riggio O, Angeloni S. Ascitic fluid analysis for diagnosis and monitoring of spontaneous bacterial peritonitis. *World J Gastroenterol.* 2009;15(31):3845-3850.
65. Fung JJ, Jain A, Kwak EJ, et al. De novo malignancies after liver transplantation: a major cause of late death. *Liver Transplant.* 2001;7:S109-S118.
66. Nalesnik MA, Makowka L, Starzl TE. The diagnosis and treatment of post transplant lymphoproliferative disorders. *Curr Probl Surg.* 1988;25:367-472.
67. Flegal KM, Carroll MD, Ogden CL, et al. Prevalence and trends in obesity among US adults, 1999–2008. *JAMA.* 2010;303(3):235-241.
68. Trus TL, Pope GD, Finlayson SR. National trends in utilization and outcomes of bariatric surgery. *Surg Endosc.* 2005;19:616-620.
69. Uppot RN, Sahani DV, Hahn PF, et al. Impact of obesity on medical imaging and image-guided intervention. *Am J Roentgenol.* 2007;188(2):433-440.
70. Byrne TK. Complications of surgery for obesity. *Surg Clin North Am.* 2001;81:1181-1193; vii-viii.
71. Comeau E, Gagner M, Inabnet WB, et al. Symptomatic internal hernias after laparoscopic bariatric surgery. *Surg Endosc.* 2005;19:34-39.
72. Blachar A, Federle MP, Pealer KM, et al. Gastrointestinal complications of laparoscopic Roux-en-Y gastric bypass surgery: clinical and imaging findings. *Radiology.* 2002;223:625-632.
73. Sanyal AJ, Sugerman HJ, Kellum JM, et al. Stomal complications of gastric bypass: incidence and outcome of therapy. *Am J Gastroenterol.* 1992;87:1165-1169.
74. Cherian PT, Goussous G, Ashori F, et al. Band erosion after laparoscopic gastric banding: a retrospective analysis of 865 patients over 5 years. *Surg Endosc.* 2010;24(8):2031-2038.
75. Fielding GA, Ren CJ. Laparoscopic adjustable gastric band. *Surg Clin North Am.* 2005;85(1):129-140.
76. Carelli AM, Youn HA, Kurian MS, et al. Safety of the laparoscopic adjustable gastric band: 7-year data from a U.S. center of excellence. *Surg Endosc.* 2010;24(8):1819-1823.
77. Ceppa FA, Gagne DJ, Papasavas, et al. Laparoscopic transgastric endoscopy after Roux-en-Y gastric bypass. *Surg Obes Relat Dis.* 2007;3(1):21-24.
78. Patel JA, Patel NA, Shinde T, et al. Endoscopic retrograde cholangiopancreatography after laparoscopic Roux-en-Y gastric bypass: a case series and review of the literature. *Am Surg.* 2008;74(8):689-693; discussion 693-694.

CHAPTER 34 ■ ACUTE GASTROINTESTINAL HEMORRHAGE

CHRISTOPHER J. CARLSON AND GRANT E. O'KEEFE

GENERAL CONSIDERATIONS, DEFINITIONS, AND EPIDEMIOLOGY

Gastrointestinal (GI) hemorrhage is common and remains an important cause of morbidity and mortality. The differential diagnosis of acute GI hemorrhage includes a large number of conditions and lesions, which are listed in Tables 34.1 and 34.2. The implications for the surgeon vary and depend upon the cause, location, and severity of the hemorrhage. Bleeding may be the initial manifestation of an underlying condition that requires surgery in its own right (typically GI tract malignancy). In other cases, surgery may only be required to control hemorrhage and in increasingly rare situations, may be required to control active bleeding and also treat the underlying disease (recalcitrant peptic ulcer disease). This chapter will focus on bleeding of recent onset and duration that may result in hemodynamic instability and the need for blood transfusion.

Many lesions cease bleeding spontaneously and others are so effectively treated with endoscopic methods that they rarely require surgical therapy. That surgical therapy is not often needed for the majority of GI bleeding has likely led to a general lack of experience on the part of surgeons in their management. Given that when surgery is needed, it is often emergent and patients are often critically ill, there is little room for error. With this in mind, this chapter aims to address GI hemorrhage as it is encountered by surgeons and discusses important components of nonoperative and operative management in general and where important, for specific sources of bleeding.

Bleeding has historically been categorized as "upper" or "lower" depending upon its origin relative to the ligament of Treitz. However, recent diagnostic advances (double-balloon enteroscopy and capsule endoscopy) have lead to a reevaluation of this classification scheme, in part, because small intestinal sources can now be directly visualized, which allows them to be classified separately from colonic sources.[1,2] Upper GI hemorrhage (bleeding from the esophagus, stomach, or duodenum) accounts for 80% of cases of acute GI blood loss. Lower intestinal bleeding (colon and rectum) is responsible for 15%–20% of cases. Small intestinal lesions are responsible for <1% of cases in adults. Although difficult to estimate, approximately 100 hospital admissions per 100,000 persons in the United Kingdom were related to GI hemorrhage in 1989. The incidence of both upper and lower GI hemorrhage increases markedly with age.[3]

Patients with overt GI bleeding typically present to the hospital after an episode of hematemesis (the vomiting of blood), melena, or hematochezia. Melena is a black, tarry stool due to bacterial degradation of blood and can be evident after a 100 mL hemorrhage. Bleeding from the small intestine or right colon may also appear black. Hematochezia is the passage of bright red blood from the rectum and is usually indicative of a lower GI source. However, it may also be present in cases of massive upper GI hemorrhage. Patients with acute GI bleeding may present with the hemodynamic consequences of hemorrhage, including orthostatic syncope or near-syncope, complaints of dizziness, lightheadedness, and shortness of breath or palpitations.

History and physical examination can provide important clues to the cause and severity of bleeding. For example, melena after several days of worsening epigastric pain suggests peptic ulcer disease; whereas hematemesis or melena following vomiting or retching strongly suggests a Mallory-Weiss tear. Massive, painless upper GI hemorrhage in a patient with cirrhosis suggests bleeding from gastroesophageal varices, although other causes are responsible for bleeding in a significant number of patients with chronic liver disease.

A systematic physical examination is aimed at estimation of the magnitude of bleeding and the patient's ability to compensate. Signs and symptoms of hypovolemia include cool, clammy, mottled skin, tachycardia, tachypnea, collapsed jugular veins, oliguria, and perhaps hypotension. Advanced age, concomitant medical conditions, and their treatment (β-adrenergic blockade) can obscure these physical findings. Physical examination should also document evidence of cirrhosis and portal hypertension, and rectal examination is mandatory and may demonstrate bright red blood or melena.

INITIAL RESUSCITATION AND OVERALL DIAGNOSTIC APPROACH

Many patients will require intravenous fluid resuscitation. The need for two large-bore peripheral intravenous lines is determined by the estimated blood loss based upon history and physical examination. Most bleeding stops spontaneously and intravenous crystalloid resuscitation may be all that is required. However, in all cases, blood is drawn for type and crossmatch, complete blood count with platelet count, serum electrolyte, glucose, BUN and creatinine concentrations, liver function tests, and coagulation profile.

Patients presenting with hypotension or evidence of impaired end organ perfusion (oliguria, confusion, cardiac ischemia) should receive blood and blood products early. There are no data to support a target hemoglobin concentration, and the goal is to achieve hemodynamic stability and restore tissue perfusion and oxygen delivery rapidly. The observation that transfusion of stable critically ill patients only when hemoglobin concentration drops below 7 mg/dL is safe cannot be applied to patients with active GI hemorrhage who were excluded from the study.[4] In patients with active GI hemorrhage, a lower hemoglobin concentration was found to correlate with elevated troponin concentrations with several patients having chest pain to indicate ischemia.[5] In summary, blood transfusion should be used when there is evidence of hemodynamic compromise and not based upon predefined transfusion thresholds.

Recently, resuscitation strategies have focused on an earlier and more balanced use of red blood cells (RBCs), plasma and platelet transfusions, and a relatively more restricted use of crystalloids. This approach has been considered beneficial primarily in the context of traumatic hemorrhage requiring

TABLE 34.1

CAUSES OF ACUTE UGI HEMORRHAGE

Esophagus
Esophagitis
Reflux
Infectious (fungal, viral)
Esophageal varices
Neoplasms
Aortoesophageal fistula
Stomach
Gastric ulcer
Gastric varices
Gastric antral vascular ectasia (watermelon stomach)
Dieulafoy lesion
Arteriovenous malformation
GI stroma tumors
Lymphoma
Adenocarcinoma
Carcinoid tumors
Mallory-Weiss tear
Stress-related mucosal disease
Duodenum
Duodenal ulcer
Arteriovenous malformation
Neoplasms
Duodenal adenocarcinoma
Pancreatic adenocarcinoma
Carcinoid tumors
Dieulafoy lesion
Aortoduodenal fistula
Diverticula
Biliary and Pancreatic
Hemobilia
Pancreatitis-induced pseudoaneurysm (hemosuccus pancreaticus)

TABLE 34.2

CAUSES OF ACUTE MID AND LGIH

Small Intestine
NSAID-induced ulcers
Diverticula
Meckel's diverticula
Pseudodiverticula
Neoplasms
Lymphoma
GI stroma tumors (leiomyoma, leiomyosarcoma)
Adenocarcinoma
Carcinoid tumor
Inflammation
Crohn's disease
Radiation enteritis
Ischemic enteritis
Infectious enteritis
Arteriovenous malformations
Aortoenteric fistula
Colon and Rectum
Diverticulosis
Colitis
Crohn's disease
Ulcerative colitis
Radiation colitis
Infectious colitis
Ischemic colitis
Neoplasms
Adenocarcinoma
GI stromal tumors (leiomyoma, leiomyosarcoma)
Lymphoma
Carcinoid tumors
Arteriovenous malformation
Iatrogenic
Polypectomy sites
Benign rectal diseases
Hemorrhoids
Rectal ulcers

massive resuscitation, but seems applicable to patients with GI bleeding who also require multiple units of packed RBCs. It is particularly important to correct coagulopathy and thrombocytopenia with plasma and platelets. Platelet transfusion can also be considered in patients taking aspirin or other nonsteroidal anti-inflammatory agents who may have impaired platelet function. However, data to support this practice is limited and platelet transfusion is not routinely recommended.[6,7]

Careful hemodynamic monitoring is vital to successful management. Patients who are actively bleeding and those who have sustained substantial hemorrhage should be admitted to an intensive care unit for close hemodynamic monitoring. The presence of chronic comorbidities, such as cardiac, renal, hepatic, or pulmonary disease, increases the risk of death and requires close observation, ideally in an intensive care unit. Bladder catheterization to monitor urine output, continuous transcutaneous oxygen saturation monitoring, frequent measurement of heart rate and blood pressure and the assessment of mental status are required. Invasive monitoring (central venous pressure and oxygen saturation monitoring, pulmonary artery catheter, arterial catheter for continuous pressure and blood gas monitoring) may be helpful in certain situations. However, none have been clearly demonstrated to improve outcomes in patients with GI hemorrhage. An organized system for caring for patients with GI hemorrhage that includes observation in a dedicated intensive care unit and management by a multidisciplinary team has been shown to improve processes of care and, in some studies, to improve outcomes.[8,9]

Flexible endoscopy will identify the source of bleeding in the majority of cases and is the mainstay for the evaluation of acute GI hemorrhage. Upper endoscopy (esophagogastroduodenoscopy [EGD]) should also be considered as the initial test in patients presenting with hemodynamic instability and hematochezia, as 13% of patients presenting with maroon stools or bright red blood have an upper gastrointestinal (UGI) source.[10] Nasogastric saline lavage and aspiration with bloody return confirms an UGI source. However, a non-blood effluent does not reliably eliminate an UGI source nor does it confirm cessation of bleeding. Timely colonoscopy can identify the source of lower gastrointestinal hemorrhage (LGIH) in the majority of cases. Thorough cleansing of the colon facilitates visualization of mucosal lesions, and improves diagnostic accuracy. For this reason, colonoscopy is generally delayed to allow mechanical cleansing with a large volume polyethylene glycol-based solution.

Prognostic Factors and Scores

Several classification systems have been developed and tested for their ability to characterize a patient's risk for rebleeding and for death after GI hemorrhage. Prognostic systems for upper GI hemorrhage have been more widely adopted than those for bleeding from the lower GI tract. The Rockall score was developed to estimate the risk of death in patients with upper GI hemorrhage and is summarized in Table 34.3. A clinical or preendoscopic Rockall score can be assigned and is useful to identify patients at low risk who can be managed as outpatients, without early endoscopy.[11] The addition of endoscopic findings increases the accuracy of mortality predictions. The score can also be used, but is less predictive, to estimate the risk of recurrent bleeding. Based upon the original data, and including endoscopic findings, rebleeding and death were rare in patients with scores of 0–2.[12] A score of ≥ 5 was associated with a 10% risk of death and >25% risk of rebleeding. Other scores, based solely on clinical factors are less accurate than those that include endoscopic findings and have not been widely adopted. Three risk stratification scores have been developed for the assessment of lower gastrointestinal bleeding; however, none has garnered widespread use.[13]

NONSURGICAL DIAGNOSTIC MODALITIES AND INTERVENTIONS

The most useful diagnostic studies are also the primary therapeutic approaches in the majority of cases of GI hemorrhage. Most lesions that can be visualized endoscopically can be successfully treated with endoscopic methods. Diagnostic angiography with transcatheter embolization has demonstrated effectiveness as a second-line approach and may safely allow the patient to avoid operation, particularly in high-risk patients and situations. When endoscopy does not identify the source of bleeding, other tests may be helpful. These diagnostic and therapeutic tests are discussed in this section. Algorithm 34.1 highlights a suggested approach to management of GI bleeding.

Esophagogastroduodenoscopy

EGD is the procedure of choice in patients suspected of bleeding from the esophagus, stomach, or duodenum and will identify the site of bleeding in 95% of cases. There are advantages to performing EGD within 12–24 hours of presentation ("early upper endoscopy"). First, early endoscopy has been shown to reduce transfusion needs and hospital length of stay, in part, through more rapid control of bleeding.[14,15] Endoscopy can identify peptic ulcers at high risk of ongoing and recurrent bleeding (active bleeding, visible vessel, adherent clot) and allow patients without high-risk features to be discharged. Endoscopy will also identify non-peptic ulcer causes with a high risk of continued hemorrhage and mortality, (i.e., gastroesophageal varices) and distinguish them from lesions with a low risk, for example, Mallory-Weiss tears. Other causes of bleeding, such as Dieulafoy lesions, while often difficult to identify are typically treated successfully with endoscopic methods.[16] Effective endoscopic control of hemorrhage from a duodenal ulcer is shown in Figure 34.1. An example of perhaps the greatest benefit of upper endoscopy has been in the diagnosis and management of variceal hemorrhage secondary to portal hypertension; relegating surgery to a minimal role in the acute management. Because of its prominence in the differential diagnosis of acute upper GI hemorrhage and despite the rarity with which surgery is required to control bleeding, portal hypertension is discussed in detail in the section Four.

Colonoscopy

Colonoscopy is the diagnostic and sometimes the treatment modality of choice for most patients with lower GI bleeding.[1] The role of early or urgent colonoscopy in the evaluation of patients with acute lower GI bleeding is less clear than is the role for endoscopy in upper GI bleeding. While best suited for patients who are actively bleeding at the time of the study, massive colonic bleeding may obscure the bleeding site and lesion, limiting the utility of colonoscopy.

Stigmata of recent hemorrhage for lower GI bleeding are similar to those of upper GI lesions and include an actively bleeding site, a non-bleeding visible vessel, and an adherent clot. Although more difficult to discover in the colon, given the large surface area and potential issues with the preparation, these findings have been associated with continued hemorrhage and the need for urgent colectomy.[17] Not all studies have found colonoscopy to be accurate in the diagnosis of

TABLE 34.3

ROCKALL RISK SCORING SYSTEM

	SCORE			
VARIABLE	**0**	**1**	**2**	**3**
Age	<60 y	60–79 y	≥80 y	
Shock	"No shock" Systolic blood pressure ≥ 100 mmHg, heart rate <100/min	"Tachycardia" Systolic blood pressure ≥ 100 mmHg, heart rate ≥ 100/min	"Hypotension" Systolic blood pressure < 100 mmHg	
Comorbidity	None	None	Cardiac failure Ischemic heart disease Any major comorbidity	Renal Failure Liver failure Disseminated malignancy
Diagnosis	Mallory-Weiss tear No lesion identified No stigmata of recent hemorrhage	All other diagnosis	Malignancy of the upper GI tract	
Major stigmata of recent hemorrhage	None or dark spot only		Blood in upper GI tract Adherent clot Visible or spurting vessel	

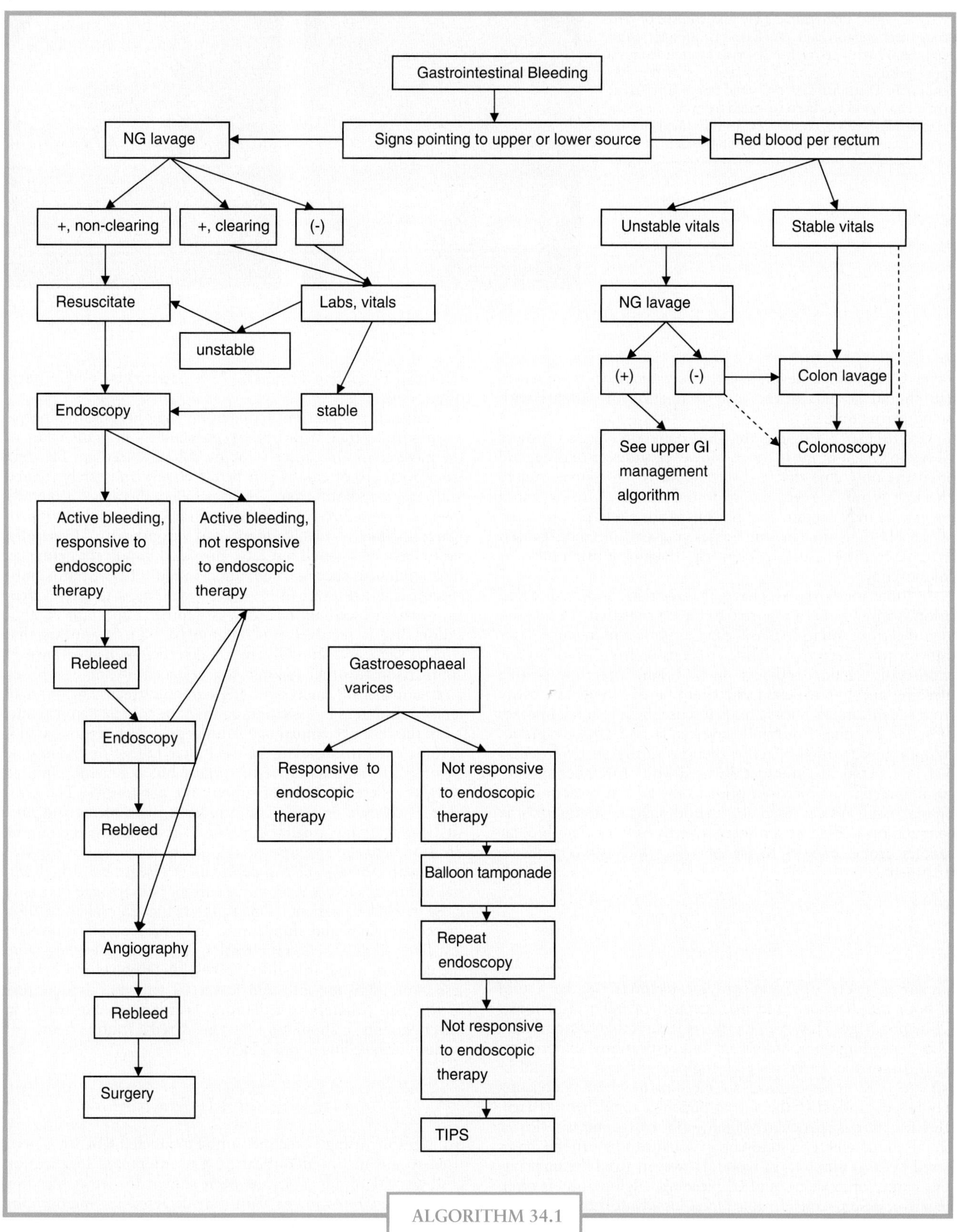

ALGORITHM 34.1 General diagnostic approach to gastrointestinal hemorrhage. The initial approach to any source of GI bleeding starts with resuscitation and stabilization of vital signs. Nasogastric lavage can help risk stratify and direct the initial endoscopic approach, but note that a negative nasogastric lavage does not rule out an UGI source of bleeding. In general, in UGI bleeding not responsive to up to two attempts at endoscopic therapy, surgery or alternative techniques (angiography) are considered. For lower gastrointestinal bleeding, colon lavage is not essential as blood can act as a cathartic, but is typically given when possible as visualization is usually much better.

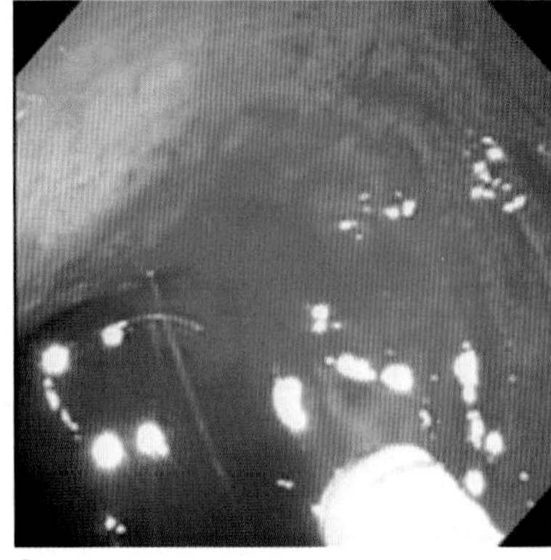

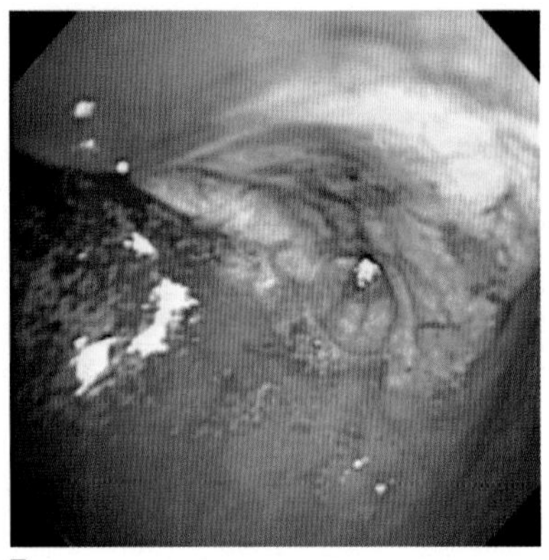

FIGURE 34.1. Endoscopic view and control of duodenal ulcer hemorrhage. **A:** Demonstrates intraduodenal blood with active hemorrhage evident from the upper posterior wall of the first portion of the duodenum. **B:** Demonstrates the same lesion after treatment. The blood has been irrigated from the duodenal lumen, and the ulcer crater is evident. Epinephrine has been injected adjacent to the bleeding vessel.

lower GI bleeding. Nevertheless, it is valuable in many cases and should be part of the early evaluation of patients with blood per rectum.

Diverticular bleeding is the most common source of lower GI hemorrhage in most series. However, indirect findings are often the only clue that a diverticulum is the source. Active bleeding is rarely seen, as are visible vessels. One or more diverticula may contain clot, but this is not a reliable indicator of the bleeding site. In some cases, massive bleeding caused by colonic diverticula can limit the diagnostic usefulness of colonoscopy.

Colonic angiodysplasia has a characteristic appearance and colonoscopy has been reported to have a sensitivity of 80% in identification. Angiodysplasia can be subtle and in some cases difficult to discern from subtle erosions or from traumatic or endoscopic suction artifacts. In addition, after appreciable bleeding and hypovolemia, the shunting of blood flow away from the intestinal mucosa may obscure these lesions. In cases of active bleeding from both diverticula and angiodysplasia, colonoscopy is often effective therapeutically. In diverticular bleeding, hemoclips are typically used with or without submucosal epinephrine injection; prior to the advent of hemoclips, bipolar cautery was used. In angiodysplasia, argon plasma coagulation is used as an alternative to cautery. The bipolar cautery probe can stick to the mucosa, which can complicate treatment.

Visceral Angiography and Transcatheter Treatment

Similar to endoscopy, angiographic methods can be a tool in both the diagnosis and management of upper and lower GI hemorrhage. However, its role is less established and may vary depending upon individual and institutional experience. As a diagnostic study, visceral angiography can be useful in patients with upper or lower GI bleeding in whom endoscopy has failed to identify the site of ongoing, rapid hemorrhage. This situation is particularly likely in the case of massive lower GI bleeding where colonoscopic visualization can be hampered by large amounts of blood. However, given the intermittent nature of most cases of GI bleeding, angiography is often negative, despite considerable blood loss. Unfortunately, there are no clinical features (e.g., shock, large amount or bright red appearance of blood) that correlate with positive angiographic findings.

Certain lesions often have characteristic angiographic findings that can assist in the diagnosis and guide treatment, whether angiographic, endoscopic, or surgical. Characteristic angiographic findings of angiodysplasia include a densely opacified and slowly emptying, dilated, tortuous vein (90% of patients), a vascular tuft (66%–75% of patients), and an early filling vein.

Transcatheter therapy, based upon angiographic findings, is an important treatment option, particularly in many cases of the most common causes of acute colonic bleeding. Bleeding from a variety of causes can be effectively and safely treated with angioembolization. Transcatheter therapies generally involve super-selective injection of one or a combination of materials (micro-coils, gelfoam, and vasopressin).[18] Generally, series have been small but have provided important guidance. First, technical success is common (often >90%), but clinical success is much lower (50%–65%), with most failure evident as recurrent bleeding. Ischemia is another important complication, but is relatively uncommon (< 5%). It appears that clinical success is most likely for diverticular hemorrhage in comparison to other colonic sources such as angiodysplasia and neoplasms.[19] Successful angiographic treatment of small intestinal sources is less common than for colonic hemorrhage.

In the case of hemorrhage from peptic ulcer disease, angiographic embolization can be used after failure of endoscopic treatment as an alternative to surgery but is generally limited to cases where the risks of surgery are prohibitive. The presence of chronic or acute comorbidities, such as morbid obesity and acute myocardial infarction should be weighed in the decision between attempts at angiographic control or surgical treatment. Angiography in peptic ulcer disease has a high initial technical success rate, but recurrent hemorrhage occurs in close to 50% of patients. Due to the rich collateral circulation of the stomach and duodenum, ischemic complications are less likely than when embolization is used for bleeding from the colon or small intestine. Successful embolization may be less likely than for mid and lower GI sources, also because of the rich collateral circulation. Therefore, while useful in select patients, it should not be considered a routine treatment option for bleeding peptic ulcers.

Radionuclide Scans

Scintigraphy using ^{99m}technetium (Tc)-labeled RBCs has been used to aid in the identification and attempted localization of lower GI bleeding. It has been shown to detect bleeding occurring at rates lower than that detected by angiography but lacks the spatial resolution and diagnostic precision of angiography and endoscopy. It may be useful in the detection of intermittently bleeding lesions or those with very low rates of hemorrhage. In the past, scintigraphy was often used in cases of obscure bleeding. However, in the case of rapid bleeding, angiography may be the better option when upper and lower endoscopy have not been diagnostic. The choice between angiography and scintigraphy has typically been guided by estimates of the rate and nature of bleeding. Angiography is considered able to detect bleeding rates of >0.5–1 mL/min (30–60 mL/h) and scintigraphy is able to detect slower (>0.1 mL/min [6 mL/h]) or intermittent bleeding. However, the clinical use of these thresholds is questionable and generally they are not relevant in the determination of the appropriate test. Active hemorrhage can be detected, localized and potentially treated with angiography. Therefore, the use of scintigraphy is limited and has typically been replaced by other studies.

One area where radionuclide scanning has a clear role is in the diagnosis of Meckel's diverticulum. ^{99}Tc-pertechnetate is secreted by ectopic gastric mucosa in Meckel's diverticula. This study should be considered early in the evaluation of children and young adults with lower GI bleeding.

Abdominal Computed Tomography Angiography

Standard computed tomography (CT) scanning has historically not been a reliable tool in the diagnosis of GI hemorrhage. However, technological advances allow for rapid acquisition and accurate timing of contrast administration with scanning to visualize vascular anatomy, abnormalities, and contrast extravasation.[20] Multi-detector CT angiography has a number of advantages over conventional angiography. CT angiography is possible in situations where conventional angiography may not be available. Movement artifact (from respiration and peristalsis) is essentially abolished with rapid acquisition times and the use of multi-planar images to remove overlying bowel loops. Cross-sectional imaging and multi-planar reconstruction facilitates accurate anatomical localization of the bleeding site and assessment of the underlying pathology.

Approaches to Obscure Gastrointestinal Hemorrhage

Obscure GI bleeding refers specifically to bleeding that persists or recurs without an obvious source after endoscopic evaluation.[2,21] Repeat endoscopy when the patient is better resuscitated may detect lesions such as ulcers or vascular ectasias that were obscured by blood or vasoconstriction at the time of initial examination. Generally, radiographic evaluation of the small bowel, including angiography or radionuclide scanning has failed to determine a source of bleeding. Most cases of obscure bleeding will eventually be found in the stomach, duodenum, or colon, and only 5% are eventually localized to the small intestine. The need for surgical evaluation is rare and is now almost entirely limited to treatment as newer diagnostic techniques have allowed lesions of the small bowel to be visualized. The techniques of balloon enteroscopy and wireless capsule enteroscopy have each facilitated the diagnosis of small intestinal sources that were previously impossible to visualize directly. Algorithm 34.2 illustrates a suggested diagnostic approach to patients with obscure GI hemorrhage.

Balloon Enteroscopy

Balloon endoscopy was developed as a technique to visualize the entire small intestine, in which the bowel is held apart by a balloon attached to the distal end of a soft overtube, through which a long enteroscope is passed. The technique has been reported to be useful for not only diagnosis but also endoscopic therapy. Single- and double-balloon techniques have been developed. Single-balloon enteroscopy is considered easier; however, double-balloon enteroscopy may have an edge in rate of complete enteroscopy and therapeutic yield. Both methods are labor intensive (require general anesthesia) and time-consuming and are performed in relatively few centers.[22,23] Enteroscopy may be primarily useful in situations where standard endoscopy, CT angiography, and angiography have failed to determine the source of obscure hemorrhage and bleeding is ongoing.[24,25]

Wireless Capsule Endoscopy

Imaging of the small intestine is also now possible with a wireless capsule endoscope consisting of a battery, light source, imaging-capturing system, and transmitter. The typical capsule endoscope is 11 mm x 26 mm and is moved solely by peristalsis. This system captures and sends up to two images per second for about 8 hours to an ultra-high frequency band radiotelemetry unit worn by the patient. The location of the capsule is suggested by the strength of the signal. Several studies have shown high diagnostic yields using this technique and found it to be superior to push enteroscopy in patients with obscure GI bleeding.[26] For an 8-hour study, approximately 57,000 images are generated. Although still considered tedious, with software advancements allowing up to four viewing frames at a time, the experienced reviewer can read an 8-hour study in <1 hour.

Intraoperative Endoscopy

Intraoperative enteroscopy using a combination of push enteroscopes per os and per rectum or via enterotomy can allow examination of the entire small bowel. While the endoscopist manipulates the scope, the surgeon manually advances the bowel over the endoscope. After the bowel is telescoped onto the endoscope, it is slowly withdrawn while the endoscopist examines the mucosal lumen and the surgeon watches the transilluminated bowel wall. With the advent of balloon enteroscopy and capsule endoscopy, interoperative endoscopy is rarely required.

SURGICAL CONSIDERATIONS AND PROCEDURES IN PATIENTS WITH GASTROINTESTINAL HEMORRHAGE

Surgery is generally reserved for patients with life-threatening hemorrhage who have failed previously discussed management options. Perhaps the greatest challenge is to identify patients requiring surgical therapy as early as possible in their course and avoid delays that may lead to increased instability and risk for complications while safely pursuing the nonsurgical approaches discussed in previous sections. Previously recommended indications for surgery, which have often reflected the severity of hemorrhage (shock, need for >4–6 units of RBCs), may no longer be appropriate. For example, in the case of bleeding from peptic ulcer disease, endoscopic retreatment after initial control of bleeding has been shown to decrease the need for surgery and results in fewer complications than surgical management, even in the presence of large-volume blood transfusion.[27] In the setting of colonic diverticular disease, an association between number of units of blood transfused and risk of rebleeding has been observed; however, no clear threshold exists for units of blood transfused and the need for operation.[28] In all cases, multiple factors including the source of hemorrhage, the appearance of the bleeding site at time of endoscopy, and patient comorbidities must be considered. Thus, the decision to proceed with surgery ultimately

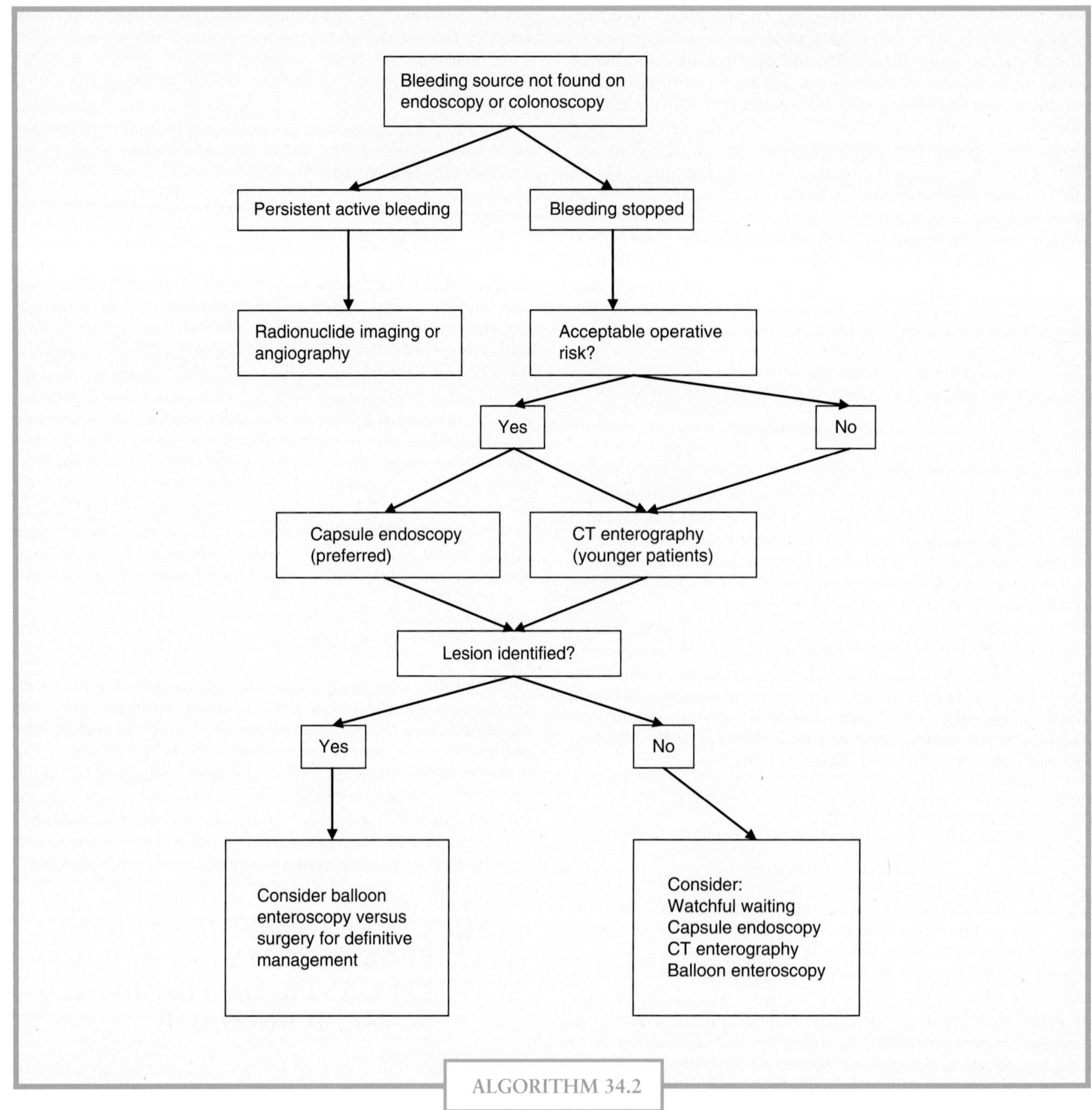

ALGORITHM 34.2 Approach to obscure gastrointestinal hemorrhage. In overt obscure bleeding that is active, radionuclide imaging and angiography may complement each other for the highest diagnostic and therapeutic yield. If bleeding has stopped, capsule endoscopy is preferred, although multiphase CT enterography should be considered in poor operative candidates (given the 1.4% rate of capsule retention), younger patients (where small bowel tumors are higher in the differential), and cases of suspected obstruction or neoplasm. Balloon enteroscopy may be considered to follow up on a positive preliminary study, or if bleeding persists and there is a high index of clinical suspicion for a small bowel lesion.

depends on clinical judgment rather than predefined, objective thresholds. In this section, the focus is on specific circumstances where operation is indicated and important aspects of specific procedures are detailed.

Peptic Ulcer Disease

Close collaboration between the endoscopist and surgeon is important when managing patients with high-risk peptic ulcers. Ideally, the surgeon should be available to view the endoscopy. This is particularly important in patients at high risk for needing surgical therapy (e.g., patients undergoing a repeat endoscopy for recurrent bleeding). This will facilitate surgical planning as the site of the bleeding lesion is rarely evident visually or by palpation without incision of the stomach or duodenum.

Even in cases of massive bleeding, patients can be stabilized with blood and blood product transfusion prior to induction of anesthesia. In most cases, access to the peritoneal cavity is via an upper midline incision. For proximal gastric ulcers, mobilization and retraction of the lateral segment of the left lobe of the liver is helpful for exposure and critical for the management of ulcers near the GE junction and for access to the esophagus if a truncal vagotomy is being considered.

For bleeding gastric ulcers, the operation of choice depends primarily on the location of the ulcer. Extensive gastric resections such as antrectomy, subtotal or total gastrectomy are generally not performed given that these patients are generally quite ill, at high risk of complications, and are best served by the quickest procedure that controls bleeding. Where possible, excision of the ulcer and closure of the resultant defect is ideal. This is generally applicable to ulcers of the gastric fundus, body and proximal antrum. Ulcers located near the GE junction pose a challenge, both in obtaining access and in determination of the appropriate method to control bleeding. Excision and primary closure should be done if possible without narrowing the GE junction. Alternatively, the ulcer can be oversewn after exposure through a high anterior gastrotomy.

Rarely, large ulcers on the posterior wall of the gastric antrum or body have eroded into the splenic artery or its branches, causing brisk hemorrhage. Resection is generally not possible and this circumstance is best treated by direct ligation, proximal and distal to the bleeding site, through the ulcer base. As with ulcers located near the GE junction, access to these posterior ulcers is obtained via an anterior longitudinal gastrotomy. The stomach should not be dissected from the pancreas to access the bleeding. When a gastric ulcer is left *in situ*, biopsy at the time of surgery is generally not necessary and instead follow-up endoscopy 6–8 weeks later is used to confirm healing or obtain tissue to exclude malignancy.

The typical duodenal ulcer that requires surgical therapy is located on the posterior–medial aspect of the first portion of the duodenum and has eroded into the gastroduodenal artery, often where it bifurcates into the superior pancreaticoduodenal and the right gastroepiploic arteries. Attention to the arterial anatomy is important to ensure successful control of bleeding. This rich anastomotic plexus often requires control of retrograde flow from these two branches in addition to suture ligation of the gastroduodenal artery. Access is obtained via a longitudinal duodenotomy and if additional exposure is needed, the incision is extended proximally across the pylorus. The ulcer and bleeding site are exposed, and active bleeding controlled with direct pressure. Ligation with 2.0 nonabsorbable suture must be done carefully as the common bile duct is typically located near and just to the right of the gastroduodenal artery. U-stitches must be placed in three quadrants to ensure control of the bleeding. Stitches are placed cephalad and caudally to the bleeding ulcer (12 o'clock and 6 o'clock) to directly control the gastroduodenal artery. A U-stitch must also be placed medially (3 o'clock) to control collateral flow from a transverse pancreatic artery. At times, the gastroduodenal artery may be additionally ligated at the superior border of the duodenum, as it dives behind the duodenum. The duodenum can then be closed longitudinally or transversely. However, if the pylorus is divided, a Heineke-Mikulicz pyloroplasty is generally indicated. The need for a vagotomy in this circumstance is debated and its reported use had been variable but definitively declining in recent years.[29,30] Postoperative treatment with proton-pump inhibitors and *Helicobacter pylori* infection can safely prevent recurrence in lieu of vagotomy.[31] Nevertheless, there may be circumstances, such as failure following *H. pylori* treatment, where control of gastric acid secretion by vagotomy is indicated. Vagotomy is contraindicated in the presence of hemodynamic instability, coagulopathy or acidosis. Cirrhosis, particularly when accompanied by portal hypertension, makes access to the esophagus hazardous and is a contraindication. A truncal rather than selective or highly selective vagotomy is indicated when vagotomy is performed.

Stress-Related Mucosal Disease (Gastritis and Ulceration)

Minor bleeding from gastric mucosal damage in critically ill patients is frequent, but clinically important hemorrhage is uncommon. Although surgery is rarely required, an organized management approach may reduce mortality associated with this condition.[32]

Coffee-ground or bloody emesis or nasogastric aspirate, coupled with hemodynamic instability, or the need for a blood transfusion mandates upper endoscopy to determine the source of bleeding. Endoscopic findings range from diffuse and superficial mucosal erosions to discrete, typically multiple, deeper ulcerations throughout the stomach.

A variety of techniques have been employed with variable success in arresting hemorrhage from stress gastropathy including endoscopic and embolization techniques and the selective catheterization of the left gastric artery with continuous infusion of vasopressin.

Surgical treatment options include gastrotomy with suture ligation of bleeding sites, hemigastrectomy, total gastrectomy, and gastric devascularization. Unfortunately, these critically ill patients poorly tolerate the more extensive procedures and lesser operations often fail to control hemorrhage. As with other causes of upper GI bleeding, endoscopic findings are important to guide surgical therapy. Regardless of the operation performed, mortality risk depends on the underlying illness, particularly in the presence of multiple organ failure. Mortality rates between 30% and 60% are commonly quoted, with as many as one-fourth of the deaths resulting from continued hemorrhage. Recurrent bleeding rates from 25% to 61% have been reported. The combination of vagotomy, hemigastrectomy, and oversewing of bleeding points has been touted as more successful in these patients. However, rebleeding rates of 11%–44% and operative mortality ranging from 33% to 63% have been associated with this procedure. More extensive operations such as near total gastrectomy or total gastrectomy are associated with significant mortality, although they successfully stop hemorrhage.

Gastroesophageal Varices

In developed countries, variceal hemorrhage is typically secondary to cirrhosis leading to portal hypertension. Generally, endoscopic therapies achieve effective immediate and longer-term control of hemorrhage and surgery is very rarely required. As a result, few surgeons have experience with emergent operative treatment of portal hypertension and variceal hemorrhage. This has further reduced the role of emergent surgery to specific and highly limited situations.

As with other sources of upper GI hemorrhage, early endoscopy is imperative for successful diagnosis and therapy in most situations. The identification of varices alone is not adequate to incriminate them as the source of the hemorrhage and it is helpful to visualize active bleeding or stigmata of recent hemorrhage. The entire esophagus, stomach, and duodenum must be adequately visualized to exclude alternate sources of hemorrhage, such as peptic ulcer disease and gastritis, which may coexist with portal hypertension and varices.

Endoscopic ligation (banding) is the most widely used modality for control of bleeding esophageal varices and is effective in up to 95% of cases. In general, a patient bleeding from esophageal varices should undergo urgent banding of the varices at the initial endoscopy.

In addition to endoscopic therapy, medical management is crucial to successful outcome. Avoiding excessive crystalloid resuscitation, which contributes to ascites formation, is important. Pharmacologic reduction in splanchnic blood flow can be helpful in reduction of variceal hemorrhage. Somatostatin or its synthetic analog, octreotide are the agents of choice and have replaced vasopressin for this indication. Meta-analyses have shown that the infusion of somatostatin is equally effective and safer than vasopressin in the pharmacologic control of variceal hemorrhage.[33] In the United States, the somatostatin analog octreotide is preferentially used because it is widely available. Octreotide is typically given as an initial injection of 50 μg, followed by a 50 μg/h continuous infusion for 2–5 days. Somatostatin and its analogs are an adjunct to established methods of controlling hemorrhage, as they have never been shown to reduce mortality and their effect is to reduce transfusion requirement by about one-half unit of packed RBCs per patient.[34]

The use of prophylactic antibiotics in cirrhotics with GI bleeding has been shown to decrease the rate of all infections, reduce the rate of variceal rebleeding, and decrease mortality.[35,36] This benefit applies to patients with and without ascites. Typically, a 3–7 day course of antibiotics, which covers gut organisms, is used, for example, ciprofloxacin 500 mg orally twice per day times seven days. Ceftriaxone is considered the preferred agent in centers with a high prevalence of quinolone-resistant organisms.[37]

In massively bleeding patients, balloon tamponade can be effective in temporary control of hemorrhage, and allows resuscitation, stabilization and attempts at endoscopic control when the patient is more stable. A Sengstaken-Blakemore tube consists of a single gastric lumen with proximal gastric and esophageal balloons. In a Minnesota tube, a second, proximal esophageal lumen allows the aspiration of secretions proximal to the balloons. Inflation of the gastric (and if required esophageal) balloon compresses the varices, and effectively controls hemorrhage in the majority of cases. However, hemorrhage recurs in 25%–50% of patients upon deflation, limiting this technique to a temporizing role, allowing time for resuscitation and stabilization in anticipation of definitive endoscopic treatment or as a bridge to TIPS.

These tubes can be associated with significant morbidity and mortality. Complications occur in 4%–9% of patients with the most frequent being aspiration pneumonitis. Measures to prevent pulmonary complications include endotracheal intubation before tube insertion and the placement of an esophageal tube to remove swallowed salivary secretions. Other important complications include esophageal rupture or necrosis and airway occlusion during the attempted removal of an incompletely deflated gastric balloon.

Typically, portal decompression has been recommended in the 10%–15% of cases where endoscopic and medical therapy has failed to control bleeding. Transjugular intrahepatic portosystemic shunting (TIPS) has replaced emergent surgical decompression in the acute management in these patients, but its use has typically been limited to manage recurrent hemorrhage.[9] Recently, earlier use of TIPS has been advocated and appears to be associated with both better control of bleeding and increased survival at 1 year.[38] Therefore, it may be reasonable to consider TIPS in patients whose bleeding has been controlled with endoscopic methods but who remain at high risk for recurrence (Child-Pugh Class C disease, or Class B with active bleeding at the time of endoscopy).

Hemorrhage from gastric varices in the context of cirrhosis and portal hypertension has been more resistant to standard endoscopic therapies.

Gastric Varices Secondary to Sinistral Portal Hypertension

This represents a unique variant of portal hypertension in which surgical therapy is primary and generally curative.[39] Splenic vein thrombosis leads to portal hypertension that is generally limited to the gastrosplenic circulation and manifest as gastric varices. Chronic pancreatitis is the most common factor leading to splenic vein thrombosis, which, in turn, leads to gastric varices. The natural history of asymptomatic splenic vein thrombosis and gastric varices is benign, with few patients apparently progressing to hemorrhage. Figure 34.2 demonstrates the appearance of gastric varices that have recently bled. Splenectomy is the procedure of choice in patients who have bled from gastric varices secondary to splenic vein thrombosis.

Aortoenteric Fistula

Most aortoenteric fistulae are secondary to prosthetic replacement or bypass of the infrarenal abdominal aorta. Erosion into the distal duodenum at the proximal anastomosis is the most frequent site. Less commonly, fistulae may involve an iliac limb of a bifurcated graft and the distal small intestine or sigmoid colon and present as hematochezia. It is postulated that erosion of the graft through the bowel wall results in perigraft infection, leading to dehiscence of the vascular anastomosis and eventually to GI hemorrhage. Primary aortoenteric fistulae (no aortic prosthetic graft) are a rare cause of GI hemorrhage, but should be considered in the differential diagnosis of obscure bleeding, particularly in patients with aneurismal disease.

Patients may initially experience a non-catastrophic episode of GI bleeding that is eventually followed by massive hemorrhage. This window of time may provide an opportunity for treatment if the diagnosis is entertained. Therefore, the diagnosis must be considered early in patients with GI hemorrhage and a history of aortic bypass grafting. Accompanying symptoms may include back or abdominal pain. Signs of infection, when present, are minimal.

The diagnosis can be made endoscopically (Figure 34.3) and every effort must be made to visualize the distal duodenum and proximal jejunum in patients who have bled and have a history of abdominal aortic grafting. However, even if endoscopy fails to demonstrate a fistula, the diagnosis must still be considered unless another convincing source of bleeding is

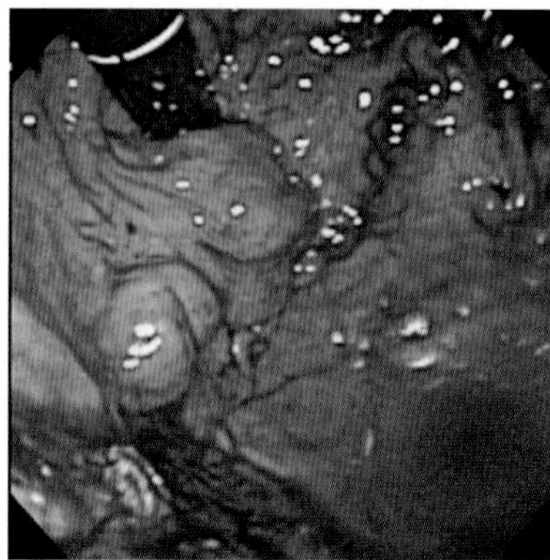

FIGURE 34.2. Endoscopic view of proximal gastric varices. This is a view of gastric fundal varices through the retroflexed gastroscope. In this case, the varices are evident as protuberances with intact, overlying mucosa, without active hemorrhage.

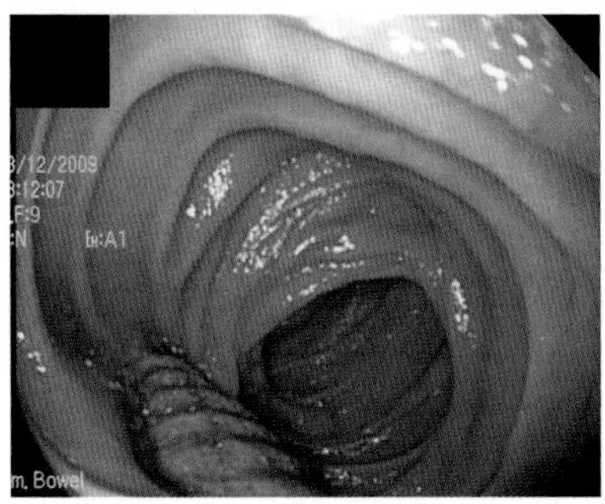

FIGURE 34.3. Endoscopic view of aortoenteric fistula. In some cases of hemorrhage from aortoenteric fistula, the graft, having eroded into the duodenum, may be visualized endoscopically. Here, the prosthetic aortic graft is seen in the proximal jejunum.

identified. If the patient is hemodynamically stable, CT is the next diagnostic test of choice.

In recent years, endovascular stent management has been employed, either as sole treatment in high-risk patients or in combination with open repair or resection of the fistula. The long-term outcome with endovascular repair is unknown and suspect if the original graft is left *in situ*.[40]

Other Causes of Gastric and Duodenal Bleeding

A *Mallory-Weiss tear* is a mucosal tear near the GE junction that leads to acute upper GI hemorrhage that occurs after retching or vomiting. While classically described as occurring in a patient who retches and vomits after a drinking binge, Mallory-Weiss tears may also be found following any bout of vigorous emesis. Initially, the emesis consists of gastric contents without blood and, subsequently, the patient develops hematemesis or melena. These lesions account for 5%–10% of cases of upper GI bleeding.

Most tears have stopped bleeding by the time endoscopy is performed and endoscopic treatment is typically effective when active bleeding is encountered. If surgery is required, treatment is simply oversewing the laceration. The main challenges are localization and access to the tear. The endoscopist can aid the surgeon by injecting tattoo ink, which can then be seen on the serosal surface and guide placement of the gastrotomy.

Dieulafoy lesions are an uncommon source, in which bleeding originates from an unusually large (1–3 mm diameter) artery running through the submucosa. Most are located in the stomach, but can be found in the duodenum, small bowel, and colon. They may therefore present as lower GI hemorrhage or may be the source of obscure GI bleeding. Erosion of the mucosa overlying the vessel results in necrosis of the arterial wall and brisk hemorrhage. The size of the mucosal defect is usually small (2–5 mm) and without evidence of chronic inflammation. Dieulafoy lesions of the stomach and duodenum can cause massive hemorrhage and, as discussed above, are usually successfully treated with endoscopic or angiographic methods. When surgery is required, treatment is generally oversewing the lesion via an appropriately placed enterotomy. Localization is the challenge and can be facilitated as described for Mallory-Weiss tears.

Uncommonly, the source of the GI bleeding may be a tumor. Metastatic or primary cancers may erode and induce GI bleeding anywhere in the GI tract. GIST, lymphoma, and vascular tumors account for a small percentage of GI bleeding. Treatment of these tumors is bowel resection.

Colonic Diverticular Disease

Colonic diverticula are common, but fewer than 5% hemorrhage. Classically, patients present with a sudden occurrence of mild lower abdominal discomfort, rectal urgency, and the subsequent passage of a large maroon stool. Despite considerable hemorrhage, often presenting with hypovolemic shock, bleeding typically ceases spontaneously but frequently recurs. Recurrent episodes also typically stop spontaneously or can be localized and treated angiographically. As a result, surgery is infrequently required.

However, when surgery is needed, the bleeding diverticulum is often not precisely localized preoperatively. For this reason, and to assure inclusion of the source of hemorrhage in the resection, segmental colectomy is the minimal procedure.

Subtotal colectomy for ongoing colonic hemorrhage that has not been successfully localized may occasionally be necessary. However, it is associated with greater perioperative morbidity than segmental resection and postoperative diarrhea may present a considerable problem to elderly patients. Nevertheless, operation may be necessary when a patient continues to bleed massively and preoperative localization has failed. In this circumstance, intraoperative colonoscopy has been suggested in an attempt to localize the bleeding and avoid subtotal colectomy. There are no data to support whether this approach is effective and its use is rare in most series of lower GI hemorrhage.[41] Intraoperative colonoscopy may prolong the operation, leading to increased complications.

Colonic Angiodysplasia

The approach to surgical therapy for bleeding from colonic angiodysplasia is similar to that described above for diverticular hemorrhage. In comparison to diverticular bleeding, hemorrhage from angiodysplasia is usually less severe, but somewhat more likely to recur. However, and as with diverticular bleeding, the majority of patients will stop bleeding spontaneously after the initial episode of hemorrhage.[42] The lesions are located most frequently in the cecum and ascending colon, although they may be found more distally in 20%–30% of cases. Multiple lesions may be present in as many as 40%–75% of all cases. The prevalence of colonic angiodysplasia in the general population appears to be <1%.

The rare patient acutely bleeding from angiodysplasia, in whom endoscopic or angiographic methods are unsuccessful or unavailable, can be treated with colectomy following preoperative localization of the bleeding site. The value of preoperative localization cannot be overstated as it will facilitate appropriate segmental colon resection.

Thus, the majority of cases of lower GI bleeding are related to diverticulosis or angiodysplasia. Although diverticula are more common in the left colon than right colon, substantial lower GI bleeding is generally from right-sided diverticulosis where there has been erosion through the vasa vasorum within the thin-walled diverticulum. Considering both diverticulosis and angiodysplasia, two-thirds of cases of massive lower GI bleeding are from the right colon. Thus, a blind right hemicolectomy results in rebleeding in one-third of patients. The alternative, a total abdominal colectomy, effectively eliminates the bleeding but adds morbidity.

Ischemic Colitis

Ischemic colitis is a common cause of lower GI hemorrhage, especially in the elderly. Bleeding is a common presentation occurring in approximately one-half to three-fourths of

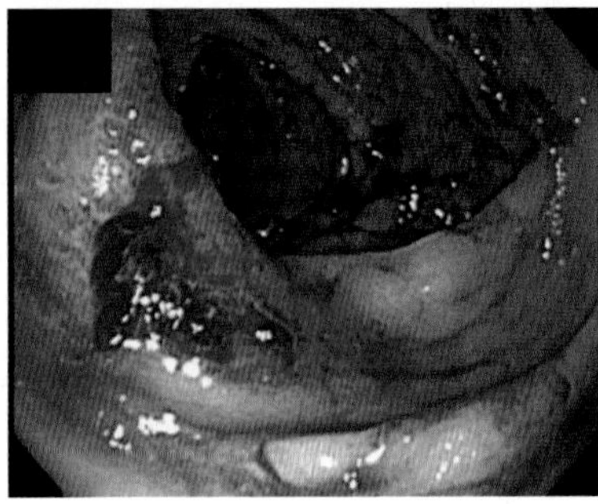

FIGURE 34.4. Endoscopic view of acute ischemic colitis. Pale, ischemic mucosa, in conjunction with mucosal ulceration and hemorrhage together are hallmarks of ischemic colitis. All are seen in this colonoscopic view.

patients, but is usually not massive. In most cases, it results from impaired local microvascular perfusion of the colonic wall. It occurs most commonly in the elderly who often have substantial medical comorbidities. Renal failure requiring hemodialysis, hypertension, cardiovascular disease, vasoactive medications, and a variety of other risk factors have been associated with ischemic colitis, but in many cases a specific initiating event cannot be identified. Any segment of the colon may be involved. Transmural necrosis can result in peritonitis and perforation. Mucosal ischemia may result in vague abdominal pain, diarrhea, and mild to moderate bleeding. Life-threatening hemorrhage is uncommon.

The endoscopic features of ischemic colitis are varied, but include erythema, granularity, friability, and sometimes erosions or ulcers, all of which may be patchy or confluent. Active hemorrhage is uncommon (Fig. 34.4). Once the diagnosis is made, treatment is generally observational as many patients will recover uneventfully with supportive care alone. Surgery may be indicated acutely for ongoing bleeding or for signs of full-thickness necrosis and peritonitis. There is no role for angiography in the acute management of these patients. If the patient recovers from the initial event, healing may be accompanied by fibrosis and clinical evidence of obstruction that may require resection weeks to months after the initial presentation.

Meckel's Diverticulum

Meckel's diverticula are present in approximately 2% of the population and the lifetime risk of a complication is low. Bleeding from a Meckel's diverticulum is rare, but is one of the most common causes of lower GI hemorrhage in children. It is an exceedingly rare cause of bleeding in adults, but must be considered in the differential diagnosis of obscure bleeding. The bleeding is due to ectopic gastric mucosa in the diverticulum with peptic ulceration of adjacent bowel mucosa. Abdominal scintigraphy following the intravenous injection of ^{99}technetium pertechnetate demonstrates the ectopic gastric mucosa within the diverticulum, suggesting the correct diagnosis. Treatment requires resection of the diverticulum with a cuff of adjacent bowel. Diverticulectomy alone will be associated with persistence of the ulcer and the possibility of recurrent hemorrhage.

References

1. Barnert J, Messmann H. Diagnosis and management of lower gastrointestinal bleeding. Nature reviews. *Gastroenterol Hepatol.* 2009;6(11):637-646.
2. Raju GS, et al.. American Gastroenterological Association (AGA) Institute technical review on obscure gastrointestinal bleeding. *Gastroenterology.* 2007;133(5):1697-1717.
3. Rockall TA, et al. Incidence of and mortality from acute upper gastrointestinal haemorrhage in the United Kingdom. Steering Committee and members of the National Audit of Acute Upper Gastrointestinal Haemorrhage. *BMJ.* 1995;311(6999):222-226.
4. Hebert PC, et al. A multicenter, randomized, controlled clinical trial of transfusion requirements in critical care. Transfusion Requirements in Critical Care Investigators, Canadian Critical Care Trials Group. *N Engl J Med* 1999;340(6):409-417.
5. Bellotto F, et al. Anemia and ischemia: myocardial injury in patients with gastrointestinal bleeding. *Am J Med* 2005;118(5):548-551.
6. Kwok A, Faigel DO. Management of anticoagulation before and after gastrointestinal endoscopy. *Am J Gastroenterol.* 2009;104(12):3085-3097; quiz 3098.
7. Anderson MA, et al. Management of antithrombotic agents for endoscopic procedures. *Gastrointest Endosc.* 2009;70(6): 1060-1070.
8. Baradarian R, et al. Early intensive resuscitation of patients with upper gastrointestinal bleeding decreases mortality. *Am J Gastroenterol.* 2004;99(4):619-622.
9. McAvoy NC, Hayes PC. The use of transjugular intrahepatic portosystemic stent shunt in the management of acute oesophageal variceal haemorrhage. *Eur J Gastroenterol Hepatol* 2006;18(11):1135-1141.
10. Wilcox CM, Alexander LN, Cotsonis G. A prospective characterization of upper gastrointestinal hemorrhage presenting with hematochezia. *Am J Gastroenterol.* 1997; 92(2):231-235.
11. Barkun AN, et al. International consensus recommendations on the management of patients with nonvariceal upper gastrointestinal bleeding. *Ann Intern Med.* 2010;152(2):101-113.
12. Rockall TA, et al. Risk assessment after acute upper gastrointestinal haemorrhage. *Gut.* 1996;38(3):316-321.
13. Strate LL, Naumann CR. The role of colonoscopy and radiological procedures in the management of acute lower intestinal bleeding. *Clin Gastroenterol Hepatol.* 2010;8(4):333-343; quiz e44.
14. Spiegel BM, Vakil NB, Ofman JJ. Endoscopy for acute nonvariceal upper gastrointestinal tract hemorrhage: is sooner better? A systematic review. *Arch Intern Med.* 2001;161(11):1393-1404.
15. Lin HJ, et al. Early or delayed endoscopy for patients with peptic ulcer bleeding. A prospective randomized study. *J Clin Gastroenterol.* 1996;22(4):267-271.
16. Lim W, et al. Endoscopic treatment of dieulafoy lesions and risk factors for rebleeding. *Korean J Intern Med* 2009;24(4): 318-322.
17. Jensen DM, et al. Urgent colonoscopy for the diagnosis and treatment of severe diverticular hemorrhage. *New Engl J Med* 2000;342(2):78-82.
18. Tan KK, Wong D, Sim R. Superselective embolization for lower gastrointestinal hemorrhage: an institutional review over 7 years. *World J Surg.* 2008;32(12): 2707-2715.
19. Khanna A, Ognibene SJ, Koniaris LG. Embolization as first-line therapy for diverticulosis-related massive lower gastrointestinal bleeding: evidence from a meta-analysis. *J Gastrointest Surg.* 2005;9(3):343-352.
20. Anthony S, Milburn S, Uberoi R. Multi-detector CT: review of its use in acute GI haemorrhage. Clin Radiol 2007;62(10):938-949.
21. Raju GS, et al. American Gastroenterological Association (AGA) Institute medical position statement on obscure gastrointestinal bleeding. *Gastroenterology.* 2007;133(5):1694-1696.
22. Domagk D, et al. Single- vs. double-balloon enteroscopy in small-bowel diagnostics: a randomized multicenter trial. *Endoscopy.* 2011;43(6): 472-476.
23. May A, et al. Prospective multicenter trial comparing push-and-pull enteroscopy with the single- and double-balloon techniques in patients with small-bowel disorders. *Am J Gastroenterol* 2010;105(3):575-581.
24. Monkemuller K, et al. A retrospective analysis of emergency double-balloon enteroscopy for small-bowel bleeding. *Endoscopy* 2009;41(8):715-717.
25. Katsinelos P, et al. Single-balloon enteroscopy in life-threatening small-intestine hemorrhage. *Endoscopy* 2010;42(1):88.
26. Triester SL, et al. A meta-analysis of the yield of capsule endoscopy compared to other diagnostic modalities in patients with obscure gastrointestinal bleeding. *Am J Gastroenterol.* 2005;100(11):2407-2418.
27. Lau JY, et al. Endoscopic retreatment compared with surgery in patients with recurrent bleeding after initial endoscopic control of bleeding ulcers. *N Engl J Med.* 1999;340(10):751-756.
28. McGuire HH Jr. Bleeding colonic diverticula. A reappraisal of natural history and management. *Ann Surg.* 1994;220(5):653-656.
29. Gilliam AD, et al. Current practice of emergency vagotomy and *Helicobacter pylori* eradication for complicated peptic ulcer in the United Kingdom. *Br J Surg.* 2003;90(1):88-90.
30. Reuben BC, et al. Trends and predictors for vagotomy when performing oversew of acute bleeding duodenal ulcer in the United States. *J Gastrointest Surg.* 2007;11(1): 22-28.
31. van Rensburg C., et al. Clinical trial: intravenous pantoprazole vs. ranitidine for the prevention of peptic ulcer rebleeding: a multicentre, multinational, randomized trial. *Aliment Pharmacol Ther.* 2009;29(5): 497-507.
32. Constantin VD, et al. Multimodal management of upper gastrointestinal bleeding caused by stress gastropathy. *J Gastrointest Liver Dis.* 2009;18(3): 279-284.
33. Imperiale TF, Teran JC, McCullough AJ. A meta-analysis of somatostatin versus vasopressin in the management of acute esophageal variceal hemorrhage. *Gastroenterology.* 1995;109(4):1289-1294.

34. Gotzsche PC, Hrobjartsson A. Somatostatin analogues for acute bleeding oesophageal varices. *Cochrane Database Syst Rev*. 2008(3):CD000193.
35. Chavez-Tapia NC, et al. Antibiotic prophylaxis for cirrhotic patients with upper gastrointestinal bleeding. *Cochrane Database Syst Rev*. 2010;9:CD002907.
36. Hou MC, et al. Antibiotic prophylaxis after endoscopic therapy prevents rebleeding in acute variceal hemorrhage: a randomized trial. *Hepatology*. 2004;39(3):746-753.
37. Garcia-Tsao G, et al. Prevention and management of gastroesophageal varices and variceal hemorrhage in cirrhosis. *Hepatology*. 2007;46(3): 922-938.
38. Garcia-Pagan JC, et al. Early use of TIPS in patients with cirrhosis and variceal bleeding. *N Engl J Med*. 2010;362(25):2370-2379.
39. Sakorafas GH, et al. The significance of sinistral portal hypertension complicating chronic pancreatitis. *Am J Surg*. 2000;179(2):129-133.
40. Lew WK, et al. Endovascular management of mycotic aortic aneurysms and associated aortoaerodigestive fistulas. *Ann Vasc Surg*. 2009;23(1):81-89.
41. Gayer C, et al. Acute lower gastrointestinal bleeding in 1,112 patients admitted to an urban emergency medical center. Surgery. 2009;146(4):600-606; discussion 606-607.
42. Foutch PG, Colonic angiodysplasia. *Gastroenterologist*. 1997;5(2):148-156.

CHAPTER 35 ■ INFLAMMATORY CONDITIONS OF THE GASTROINTESTINAL TRACT

MATTHEW SCHUCHERT, VAISHALI SCHUCHERT, AND BRIAN ZUCKERBRAUN

INFLAMMATORY EMERGENCIES OF THE ESOPHAGUS

Acute, inflammatory conditions of the esophagus requiring urgent treatment are associated with significant morbidity, and can result in the rapid progression of mediastinitis, sepsis and death.[1] Thoughtful and expeditious diagnostic testing and prompt operative intervention (when required) are critical in optimization of patient outcome. In this section, we review three severe inflammatory conditions of the esophagus: esophagitis, perforation, and caustic ingestion. Other esophageal emergencies related to obstruction, bleeding, trauma, and foreign bodies will be covered in the respective chapters devoted to these conditions.

Esophagitis

Acute inflammation of the esophagus can occur due to a variety of causes (Table 35.1). A careful History and Physical Examination can frequently reveal the probable etiology. Symptoms may include heartburn, chest pain, dysphagia, or odynophagia. Chest radiograph is frequently negative, but may reveal effusion or signs of aspiration. Barium esophagography may demonstrate irregular mucosal contour, ulceration, or stricture. Computed tomography (CT) can reveal esophageal thickening or distension. Esophagogastroduodenoscopy (EGD) is the most accurate diagnostic modality, providing both visual inspection and the opportunity for biopsy and pathologic confirmation of the underlying inflammatory process.

Gastroesophageal Reflux Disease. The most common cause of esophageal inflammation is gastroesophageal reflux disease (GERD). It is the most common benign condition affecting the esophagus encountered in the emergency room,[2] and accounts for up to 75% of patients with esophageal pathology.[3] Over 60 million Americans suffer from heartburn and indigestion (overall prevalence: 10%–20%).[4] The prevalence of GERD has been steadily increasing over the last two decades and may contribute to the rapid rise in the incidence of other complications of GERD (Barrett's esophagus, adenocarcinoma) along with the large societal costs associated with the treatment of reflux disease.[3]

Reflux esophagitis arises from repeated exposure of the distal esophagus to both acidic and bilious gastric contents secondary to an incompetent lower esophageal sphincter, hiatal hernia, or impaired gastric emptying. Symptoms are frequently episodic, and can be acute in nature. At endoscopy, the degree of mucosal damage can be assessed and graded based upon severity. The most widely-recognized grading systems are that of Savary and Miller[5] and the Los Angeles Classification[6] (Table 35.2). The degree of esophagitis can range from focal mucosal erythema to severe, circumferential hemorrhagic esophagitis. The optimal management for severe, reflux esophagitis is the institution of proton-pump inhibitor (PPI) therapy, which will resolve the inflammatory mucosal changes and patient symptoms in the majority of cases.[7] Other antacid therapy (calcium carbonate, H2-blockers, carafate) can be added to PPI therapy, as necessary. Acute surgical intervention is rarely required beyond endoscopy to secure the diagnosis. In patients with refractory end-organ damage and persistent symptoms despite maximal medical therapy, a definitive antireflux procedure (e.g., Nissen fundoplication) may be beneficial.[8]

Candida Esophagitis. Infectious causes of acute esophagitis are rare, and most commonly encountered in the immunocompromised host (e.g., HIV or posttransplantation setting), in cases of prolonged antibiotic use or in association with an underlying structural esophageal abnormality (e.g., stricture).[9] The most commonly encountered infectious pathogen within the esophagus is *Candida albicans*. The most common symptoms of *Candida esophagitis* are dysphagia and odynophagia. The diagnosis should be suspected if oral thrush is evident on physical examination, although the absence of thrush does not negate the possibility of esophageal candidiasis. The diagnosis is confirmed with EGD, which reveals characteristic white mucosal plaques and pseudomembranes (Fig. 35.1). For mild cases, the institution of fluconazole or ketoconazole, in addition to oral nystatin swish and swallow, is effective in eradication of the infection in conjunction with the withdrawal of any predisposing antibiotic or corticosteroid therapy. *C. esophagitis* can become severe, with circumferential, pseudomembranous exudative infiltrates. The infectious process can penetrate the esophageal wall, leading to the development of candidal sepsis or massive hemorrhage.[10] Patients manifesting signs of systemic illness are frequently treated with amphotericin B or caspofungin.

Viral Esophagitis. The most commonly encountered causes of viral esophagitis are cytomegalovirus (CMV) and herpes simplex virus (HSV). CMV is more common in the setting of AIDS, but each of these infections can occur in immunocompetent patients as well.[11] The most prominent presenting complaint is odynophagia. EGD reveals multiple shallow ulcerations or vesicles, in the case of HSV esophagitis. The degree of esophagitis can be severe, and patients can present with inability to swallow or gastrointestinal (GI) hemorrhage. Endoscopic biopsy confirms the diagnosis. Cytologic specimens reveal cytopathic effect restricted to the squamous epithelium and intranuclear eosinophilic inclusion bodies (Cowdry type A bodies). Severe HSV esophagitis generally responds to 2–4 weeks of acyclovir therapy.

CMV esophagitis is unusual in the normal host. CMV esophagitis can be associated with deep, longitudinal ulcers. The cytologic damage extends through the mucosa to involve underlying mesenchymal cells. Gancyclovir given over 2–4 weeks is the treatment of choice for CMV esophagitis. Long-term prophylaxis may be required in the transplant setting.

Bacterial Esophagitis. Bacterial etiologies of acute esophagitis are extremely rare. *Mycobacterium tuberculosis* has been associated with the development of esophagitis and ulceration.

TABLE 35.1

CAUSES OF ESOPHAGITIS

Gastroesophageal reflux disease
Infectious—*Candida*, Herpes, CMV, Bacterial
Iatrogenic—Nasogastric tube, EGD, Endoluminal Therapy
Drug-induced
Eosinophilic
Radiation
Caustic ingestion

This disease is believed to be more commonly the result of direct extension from infected nodal tissue.[12] Primary tuberculous infection can also present as an exophytic mass, or pseudotumor.[13] Patients typically present with dysphagia. EGD with biopsy typically will reveal the diagnosis. Standard antimycobacterial regimens are the treatment (e.g., isoniazid, rifampin, ethambutol).[14]

Radiation Esophagitis. Patients who have undergone prior radiation for intrathoracic malignancy (e.g., lung or esophageal cancer, lymphoma) can develop inflammatory changes within the esophagus that are proportional to the dose administered.[15] The esophageal mucosa becomes thickened and friable. Swallowing can become painful (odynophagia). Dysphagia can result from esophageal muscular fibrosis and stricture formation. Treatment is typically symptomatic (viscous lidocaine) until symptoms improve. Dilation or stenting of strictures may ultimately become necessary for recurrent, refractory dysphagia.[16]

Pill Esophagitis. The esophagus can become acutely inflamed from direct contact with ingested medications. Symptoms typically include chest pain and dysphagia within 4–6 hours of medication consumption. Common causes include antibiotics (esp. tetracycline), quinidine, potassium, and antiinflammatory medications. Treatment requires washing down the medication with water or physical removal of the pill by endoscopy in cases of underlying esophageal motor disorder or obstruction.[17]

Eosinophilic Esophagitis. Eosinophilic esophagitis is a unique disorder of the esophagus more commonly found in men. Patients present with dysphagia, heartburn, and recurrent food impaction. Symptoms typically will not respond to conservative measures or standard antisecretory therapy. EGD reveals multiple concentric rings in the proximal-mid esophagus. Mucosal biopsies reveal the presence of >20 eosinophils per high power field.[18] The etiology of this condition is not well understood, but is believed to represent an immunologic derangement in cytokine and T-cell function.[19] Symptomatic treatment with systemic or topical corticosteroids is recommended.

TABLE 35.2

ESOPHAGITIS GRADING SYSTEMS

Savary-Miller Stage I—Nonconfluent erythematous changes or erosions Stage II—Confluent, but not circumferential, erosions Stage III—Circumferential erosive and/or exudative lesions Stage IV—Chronic ulcer, stenosis or Barrett's esophagus
Los Angeles Classification Grade A—Mucosal break ≤ 5 mm in length Grade B—Mucosal break > 5 mm Grade C—Mucosal break continuous over > 2 mucosal folds Grade D—Mucosal break ≥75% of esophageal circumference

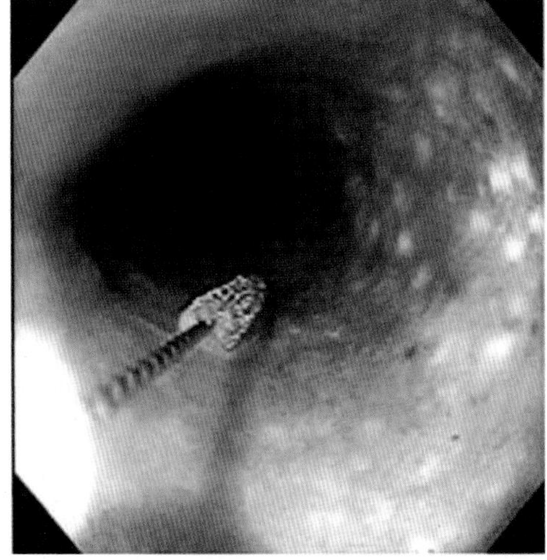

FIGURE 35.1. *C. esophagitis*. Severe inflammation of the esophagus is accompanied by the development of white plaques and pseudomembranes. (From Postma GN, Belafsky PC, Aviv JE. *Atlas of Transnasal Esophagoscopy*. Philadelphia, PA: Lippincott Williams & Wilkins. Figure 4.6.)

Iatrogenic Causes. Significant esophageal erosions can occur following long-term placement of nasogastric or feeding tubes. These erosions are typically an incidental finding of no clinical significance. Rarely, erosions can become severe resulting in esophagitis or bleeding. Treatment is removal of the offending foreign body to allow mucosal healing.[20] Esophageal inflammation can also occur following esophageal instrumentation (EGD), PEG tube placement, or following endoscopic esophageal interventions (photodynamic therapy, endoscopic mucosal resection).[21]. In select cases, patients may demonstrate an elevated white blood cell count and chest discomfort. Conservative management with intravenous antibiotics and hydration typically will lead to resolution of symptoms. Barium esophagography can be utilized to exclude full thickness perforation.

Uncommon Inflammatory Disorders. The esophagus can demonstrate involvement with primary dermatologic conditions, such as epidermolysis bullosa, pemphigus, erythema multiforme, or Behcet's disease. Sarcoidosis may present with nodularity and ulceration of the esophagus. Crohn's disease can occur anywhere from the mouth to the anus, but esophageal involvement is noted in only 1%–3% of cases.[22] Similar to ileocolic disease, Crohn's disease is characterized by aphthous ulceration, esophagitis, and long fibrotic strictures. In patients undergoing bone marrow transplantation, graft-versus-host disease may present with dysphagia, ulceration, and fibrosis. Protozoan infections (e.g., cryptosporidiosis and pneumocystis) in the setting of AIDS are rare, but have also been reported.[17]

Esophageal Perforation

Esophageal perforation is a life-threatening problem associated with high mortality rate (9%–36%).[23,24] Perforation can occur spontaneously in the setting of forceful retching/vomiting (Boerhaave's syndrome). More commonly perforation results from penetrating trauma or following esophageal instrumentation (EGD, dilation). Typical presenting symptoms include acute chest pain, shortness of breath and fever. Additional symptoms include dysphagia, odynophagia, epigastric pain, or productive cough. The clinical presentation may be fulminant, with signs of toxicity and shock. Chest x-ray reveals pneumomediastinum and subcutaneous emphysema, mediastinal air-fluid levels, and pleural effusions. Esophagography confirms and localizes the site of leak. CT is valuable in further definition of the site and extent of the leak, as well as the detection of undrained fluid collections, which is of particular value to plan the most appropriate surgical approach.[25]

The hallmarks of therapy include expeditious diagnosis, prompt institution of broad-spectrum antibiotics and early, aggressive surgical intervention directed at drainage, débridement, and control of the perforation site to prevent or treat sepsis.[26] Several surgical approaches can be employed in the management of spontaneous or iatrogenic esophageal perforation including débridement and primary closure, mediastinal drainage, placement of an esophageal T-tube, esophageal exclusion with proximal diversion, and esophagectomy. The selection of approach is influenced by the underlying cause and duration of the perforation, the degree of tissue injury and inflammation as well as the clinical condition of the patient. As expertise is gained in video-assisted esophageal surgery, minimally invasive surgical approaches to esophageal perforation and leak have been developed, and have become the preferred approach in many situations.[27] Given the lack of level 1 evidence to establish clear standards, a lack of consensus exists regarding various aspects of management of this complex and life-threatening problem.

The decision to operate is typically based upon the extent of mediastinal contamination and systemic sepsis rather than cause of perforation. The extent of perforation may be classified as contained or noncontained. A *noncontained* perforation is defined by free extravasation of contrast in the mediastinal or peritoneal cavities (Fig. 35.2). A *contained* perforation is defined as minimal extravasation of contrast at the perforation site, or the presence of pneumomediastinum or pneumoperitoneum without apparent extravasation of contrast (Fig. 35.3). The interval between the time of perforation and initiation of treatment is also considered in the management decision. The surgical tenets in management of esophageal perforation include: (1) identification and localization of the esophageal perforation, (2) débridement of all infected and necrotic tissue, (3) control of the leak (primary closure or T-tube placement), and (4) wide drainage of the mediastinum.[28]

Nonoperative management can be considered in patients with contained perforation and no clinical signs of sepsis. Patients are managed with no oral intake (NPO) for 24–72 hours, intravenous hydration, and antibiotics. Covered esophageal stents can be placed in select patients to occlude the perforation. The extent of contamination and signs of sepsis are the most important clinical variables in the outcome of esophageal perforation. The patient with a contained leak without signs of sepsis may generally be safely managed with a nonoperative approach.[29] Surgical intervention can subsequently be performed if clinical signs of sepsis arise.

In cases of noncontained perforation, esophageal repair represents the preferred surgical approach, when feasible. Primary repair is typically undertaken in patients with limited mediastinal contamination and necrosis, regardless of the time interval from perforation event to surgery.[30] During repair, it is critical to identify the full extent of injury. Devitalized esophageal and mediastinal tissues are first debrided. The full extent of mucosal injury is exposed, and the esophagus is closed in layers. Mobilization of a flap of vascularized tissue (e.g., intercostal muscle, pleura, pericardial fat, omentum) is recommended to buttress the repair. Multiple closed suction drains and chest tubes are inserted to achieve wide drainage of the mediastinum and pleura. Repair over a drain (e.g., T-tube) is a useful option when formal repair is not feasible. Repair can be performed by either minimally-invasive or open technique. The side chosen for thoracotomy or VATS is selected on the basis of known extravasation within the pleural space, taking into consideration extent of contamination and CT or endoscopic findings. Laparotomy or laparoscopy can be performed for the repair of gastroesophageal junction perforation into the peritoneal cavity. Gastrostomy and jejunostomy tubes are placed as adjuncts

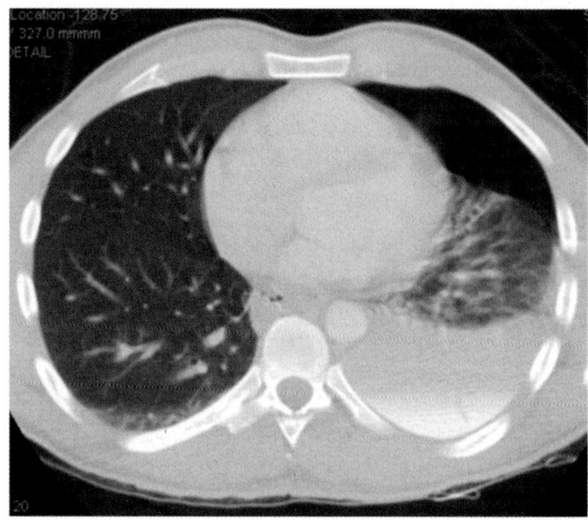

FIGURE 35.2. Esophageal perforation. Uncontained perforation with free flow of contrast material into the left pleural space. (Figure 1 from Abbas G, Schuchert MJ, Pettiford BL, et al. Contemporaneous management of esophageal perforation. *Surgery*. 2009;146(4):749–756.)

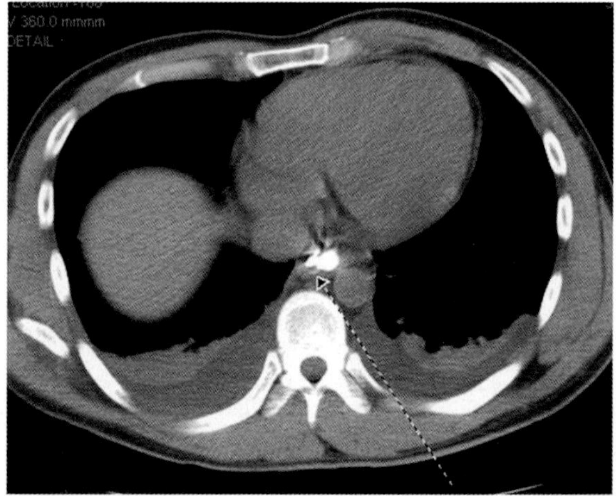

FIGURE 35.3. Esophageal perforation. Contained perforation of the distal esophagus. (Figure 2 from Abbas G, Schuchert MJ, Pettiford BL, et al. Contemporaneous management of esophageal perforation. *Surgery*. 2009;146(4):749–756.)

for drainage and enteral feeding access, respectively. Esophagectomy may be required in the setting of perforation and cancer or severe esophageal stricture. Esophageal exclusion is rarely performed, but can represent a life-saving option to the unstable patient with severe contamination.

Transcervical drainage is efficacious in the control of proximal esophageal perforation, usually secondary to trauma (gunshot wound, difficult intubation). This approach allows adequate exposure to control and repair perforations extending into the upper mediastinum down to the level of the carina. Transcervical drainage is also useful in the treatment of descending cervical mediastinitis, which may be odontogenic, peritonsillar, cervicofacial, or esophageal in origin.[31] Aided by gravity, as well as negative intrathoracic pressure, organisms and pus rapidly accumulate in the deep cervical and mediastinal fascial planes, with mortality rates as high as 30%–40%.[32] Esophageal leak after esophagectomy can be managed in most instances by opening the neck incision and packing the wound. Cervical exploration via this wound allows access to the upper mediastinum, facilitating assessment of the leak, the condition of the gastric tube, and esophagogastric anastomosis. It permits adequate exposure for débridement and drain placement.

Mid-distal esophageal perforation typically requires transthoracic drainage. Some authors advocate the routine use of thoracotomy to provide maximal exposure for thorough débridement, repair, and drainage. Increasingly, thoracoscopy is supplanting thoracotomy when conditions are appropriate.[33] The initial step is retraction of the lung and evacuation of fibrinous debris and purulent exudate. Intraoperative endoscopy is performed to assist in identification of the site of perforation. The suspected region can be submerged under irrigation during endoscopic insufflation to pinpoint the precise location of perforation. Once identified, the devitalized margins of the perforation are debrided, and the decision whether to attempt a primary closure, depending on the degree of surrounding tissue injury as well as the clinical condition of the patient, is made. If the defect is small (<1 cm), and surrounded by viable tissue, a primary closure can be performed with interrupted sutures. In the case of larger injury or perforation, surrounded by severely inflamed tissue, wide drainage is performed with placement of a T-tube to control the leak. Wide defects may allow direct placement of a T-tube through the perforation site. Jackson-Pratt drains as well as a 28–32 French chest tube are positioned strategically to provide wide drainage of the mediastinum and chest.

Special circumstances encountered during esophageal perforation provide opportunities for creative surgical approaches to this serious problem. Perforation involving an esophageal diverticulum can be managed by diverticulectomy (when possible) and drainage.[34] An important part of the surgical approach is to relieve distal obstruction with myotomy of either the cricopharyngeus (Zenker's diverticulum) or lower esophageal sphincter (epiphrenic diverticulum). Perforation of the distal esophagus after esophageal dilatation for achalasia occurs with a frequency of up to 15%. The location of the perforation is typically the left posterior esophagus. Full-thickness perforation tends to begin within a centimeter of the squamocolumnar junction, and extends proximally from a few millimeters to as much as 10 cm. These perforations can usually be repaired utilizing a thoracoscopic[35] or trans-abdominal[36] laparoscopic technique with suture closure of the perforation, contralateral Heller myotomy, and Toupet posterior fundoplication. A contralateral myotomy is performed extending 5 cm along the length of the esophagus and extending 1 cm onto the surface of the stomach, with care taken to spare the vagus nerves. A posterior fundoplication is then performed in the manner of Toupet, suturing the edges of the myotomy to the edges of the plicated stomach over a length of 4 cm.[37] This technique has the advantage of covering the closed esophageal perforation with a gastric serosal patch, at the same time treating the underlying motility disorder. A closed suction drain is placed into the mediastinum prior to closure.

Caustic Injury of the Esophagus

Caustic ingestion can result in significant injury to the esophagus and stomach. This condition is most commonly encountered with accidental ingestion in children, adults with underlying psychiatric conditions, or those with suicidal ideation. Caustic ingestion can involve both acidic and alkaline substances which produce severe esophagitis and gastritis. Full thickness esophageal and gastric injuries are not uncommon in this setting. Inciting agents include strong alkali products such as sodium or potassium hydroxide (lye), commonly utilized in drain/pipe cleaners. Strong acid compounds include hydrochloric, sulfuric, and phosphoric acid that are primary constituents of many household cleaners. Bleach ingestion (sodium hypochlorite) is commonly encountered in this setting but is rarely associated with significant esophageal injury.[38] The degree of damage depends upon the specific corrosive properties of the ingested agent, the amount, concentration, physical form (solid, liquid), and the duration of contact with the esophageal and gastric mucosa.

Acid burns result in coagulative necrosis. Given their reduced viscosity, these solutions typically pass quickly to the stomach resulting in a greater degree of gastric injury, and a lesser degree of esophageal damage. Outcome following acid injury has been reported to be worse than following alkaline injuries, with an associated higher rate of transmural injury and perforation.[39] In contrast to acid ingestion, alkaline injuries typically result in more extensive damage to both the esophagus and stomach. The degree of mucosal damage can be deep and penetrating (liquefaction necrosis); esophageal injury may be severe in this setting. The stomach itself may be partially preserved by neutralization by gastric acid. The affected mucosa is devitalized by direct contact with the alkaline agent. Severe concomitant inflammation ensues in viable tissues with vascular thrombosis, mucosal ulceration, and sloughing. Depending upon injury severity, progressive thinning of the esophageal wall may ultimately result in perforation and mediastinitis several days after the initial injury.

Patients will typically present with a known or suspected history of toxic substance ingestion reported by family members or EMS personnel. Symptoms commonly include severe nausea, vomiting, and hematemesis. The patient may complain of chest pain and severe abdominal pain. Inability to swallow and drooling may also result. The presence of fever, tachycardia, or hypotension portends a severe injury and a poor prognosis. Patients may have severe lip and oropharyngeal burns, associated with dysphonia and stridor. These findings should heighten suspicion of laryngeal and airway involvement, and early definitive control of the airway should be accomplished.[40] If there is evidence of significant laryngeal edema or stridor, tracheostomy should be performed urgently.

Initial therapeutic measures include prompt assessment and control of the airway, volume resuscitation, and institution of intravenous antibiotics. No attempt should be made to induce vomiting, as this may worsen the caustic injury. Nasogastric tubes should not be placed blindly as this may induce vomiting and may create a full thickness esophageal perforation. Radiographic evaluation with chest and abdominal x-rays is performed. Upper endoscopy is performed within the first 24 hours following ingestion. This permits assessment of the extent of esophageal and gastric damage and is critical in guiding therapy. The development of clinical manifestations of mediastinitis, peritonitis, and sepsis are indications for emergent surgery.

At endoscopy, mucosal injury can be categorized based upon the degree of injury. Grade 1 is associated with esophagitis and hyperemia. Grade 2 is denoted by esophageal mucosal ulcerations. Grade 3 is associated with necrosis extending into the wall of the esophagus, and may be focal or circumferential.[41] Superficial (grade 1) injuries typically resolve without chronic sequelae. Grade 2 injuries associated with significant or penetrating ulcers are associated with a significant risk of stricture formation. Grade 3 injuries typically result in mediastinitis and sepsis. Esophagectomy is commonly required in Grade 3 injuries, with delayed reconstruction following recovery from the initial presentation. The stomach is frequently unsuitable for reconstruction, and delayed re-construction with a colonic conduit is often required. Late sequelae of caustic injuries include the development of strictures and squamous cell carcinoma within the injured segment. Long-term endoscopic surveillance is recommended.[42]

INFLAMMATORY DISEASES OF THE STOMACH AND SMALL INTESTINE

When planning elective operations surgeons have the luxury of time to properly consider and execute an operation under optimal circumstances. Under emergent conditions, however, acute care surgeons and general surgeons must make rapid decisions both inside and outside the operating room. The decision of whether and if so, which operation should be performed, will usually determine surgical success. The patient's underlying medical condition and hemodynamic status should guide the type of operation and approach. This section focuses on inflammatory emergencies of the intestine that the acute care and general surgeons are likely to encounter in practice.

Gastroduodenal Perforation

Surgeons may encounter perforations of the stomach or duodenum secondary to trauma, neoplasm, foreign body ingestion, and iatrogenic perforations from diagnostic or therapeutic procedures. The most common cause of gastroduodenal perforation today remains ulcer disease with an incidence between 2% and 10% in patients with ulcers.[43,44]

Surgery is almost always indicated in the case of perforated peptic ulcer. Nonsurgical management can occasionally be considered in the carefully selected stable patient without evidence of a free leak. It is estimated that approximately half the perforations will seal spontaneously. Patients under the age of 70 without peritonitis or signs of sepsis and with the onset of symptoms of <24 hours may be candidates for a trial of nonoperative management. CT abdomen with oral contrast or gastroduodenography with water-soluble contrast should be performed. Free contrast extravasation mandates operation regardless of the patient's symptoms or clinical status.

The treatment plan for nonoperative management should include nasogastric tube decompression, fluid resuscitation, intravenous PPI, antimicrobial therapy, and close observation of hemodynamic status with serial abdominal exams. Any clinical deterioration warrants operation. Observation longer than 12 hours without improvement worsens the outcome and is not recommended. While favorable outcomes have been demonstrated in healthy patients, results in patients with major comorbidities are unknown.[44–46]

Most perforated peptic ulcers occur in the first portion of the duodenum (35%–65%); 25%–45% occur in the pylorus, and 5%–25% in the stomach. The pathophysiology of peptic ulcer has shifted from acid hypersecretion to *Helicobacter pylori* infection. Most patients with peptic ulcer disease will have evidence of *H. pylori* infection of the antral mucosa. The proportion of peptic ulcer caused by NSAID use is increasing, particularly in the elderly population. This is likely a significant contributing factor to the increasing frequency of complicated peptic ulcer disease requiring surgical intervention. Cigarette smoking and excessive alcohol consumption have traditionally been considered risk factors in the development of peptic ulcer but recent studies have not definitively confirmed their significance. Smoking does appear to increase the likelihood of requiring surgery for complications of peptic ulcer.[47–51]

In an emergency operation the surgeon must focus on the goals of the operation. Indeed, there is inherent danger in trying to accomplish more than what is necessary to achieve a good outcome for the patient. In the case of a gastroduodenal perforation, the primary goal is closure of the perforation, providing adequate drainage, and controlling abdominal sepsis. The patient's age, medical comorbidities, nutritional status, NSAID use, history of previous peptic ulcer disease, prior medical therapy for ulcer disease, and most importantly, hemodynamic status must be considered in plan and emergency operation for perforated peptic ulcer. Simple closure is associated with decreased morbidity and mortality in the acute setting, but with a higher rate of recurrence when compared with definitive resective procedures.[52] With the currently available highly effective acid suppression medications and *H. pylori* treatments, a definitive acid-reducing operation in the emergent setting is rarely indicated. Simple patch closure alone should be performed in patients with hemodynamic instability and with perforation of more than 24 hours' duration[53–56] (Fig. 35.4). In more stable patients, truncal vagotomy with pyloroplasty incorporating the ulcer has shown favorable results. Postoperative medical therapy with PPIs with or without therapy to eradicate *H. pylori* is indicated (Table 35.3). *H. pylori* infection can be demonstrated by tissue biopsy, serologic studies, or urea breath test. *H. pylori* eradication rates are similar between quadruple and triple therapy with comparable compliance. Prescribed therapy should be tailored to the individual patient.[57,58]

Formal gastric resection with reconstruction (Billroth I, Billroth II, Roux-en-Y) with or without vagotomy is rarely required today but should be considered for stable patients with recent (<12 hours) perforation and history of chronic or refractory ulcer disease.[44,59] The stable patient who is deemed unreliable or noncompliant may also be better served with a definitive ulcer operation. Any ulcer clearly associated with NSAID use may be managed with simple closure and discontinuation of the offending medication.

Unlike duodenal ulcers, gastric ulcers (GUs) are generally treated by excision. There are five types of GUs classified according to location and relationship to acid hypersecretion (Fig. 35.5). Type I GUs are the most common and are found at the incisura along the lesser curvature. There are two ulcers present in type II GUs—one in the body of the stomach and the other in the duodenum. Type III GUs are prepyloric. Type IV GUs are the least common and are found high on the lesser curve near the gastroesophageal junction. Type V GUs are caused by NSAIDs and respond to discontinuation of NSAID use.[52,60]

In elective or semielective surgery for intractable or recurrent ulcer, the operation of choice depends on the type of GU. Type II and Type III GUs are associated with acid hypersecretion and are typically treated with vagotomy and antrectomy including the GU. In an emergency operation for perforation, the surgeon must focus on the primary goals of the operation—to eliminate the defect, ensure adequate drainage, and treat abdominal sepsis. Perforated GUs tend to occur in elderly patients with multiple medical comorbidities and carry

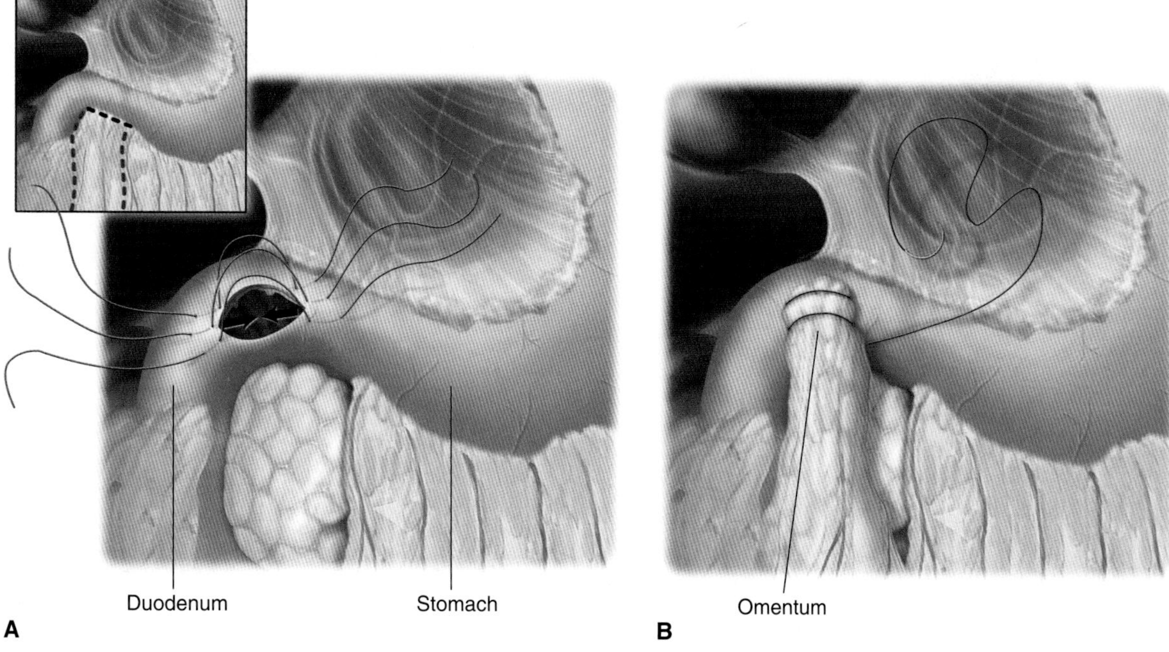

FIGURE 35.4. Omental patch closure of perforated ulcer. **A:** The right upper quadrant may be accessed through an upper midline incision. **B:** Adjacent omentum is placed over the perforation site.

an associated mortality rate as high as 40%.[61,62] Local wedge excision with or without truncal vagotomy and drainage are recommended for perforation (Figs. 35.6 and 35.7). In the stable patient with a history of chronic peptic ulcer disease or failed prior operation, distal gastrectomy is preferred with the addition of vagotomy in type II or III GUs. When excision or resection is not possible because of patient instability or prohibitive risk, eight to ten biopsies of the ulcer should be taken to evaluate for malignancy and *H. pylori* infection. Follow-up endoscopy should be performed in 6 weeks to ensure healing of the ulcer and eradication of *H. pylori*.[63] The operation performed for a given patient will depend on the patient's history, preexisting and current clinical status, as well as the type and location of the ulcer (Algorithm 35.1).

TABLE 35.3

MEDICAL TREATMENT FOR ERADICATION OF *H. PYLORI* (10–14 DAY REGIMEN)

Triple therapy	PPI[a] Amoxicillin 1 g bid Clarithromycin 500 mg bid
Penicillin allergy	PPI[a] Metronidazole 500 mg bid Clarithromycin 500 mg bid
Quadruple therapy (in cases of resistance or recent use of clarithromycin and/or metronidazole)	PPI[a] Bismuth 525 mg qid Metronidazole 250 mg qid Tetracycline 500 mg qid

[a]PPI (proton pump inhibitor) choices include: lansoprazole 30 mg bid, omeprazole 20 mg bid, pantoprazole 40 mg bid, rabeprazole 20 mg bid, and esomeprazole 40 mg qd.

Morbidity after perforation is common, ranging from 17% to 63%.[44,64] The Boey score is a useful scoring system to predict perioperative morbidity and mortality for a given patient[65–67] (Table 35.4). Pneumonia is the most common complication (up to 30%) followed by wound and intraabdominal infections. Fungal infection after perforation is common and associated with high mortality (up to 21%). Perioperative shock, renal failure, cirrhosis, advanced age, immunocompromise, and delayed operative intervention are identified risk factors for major morbidity and mortality. A history of diabetes mellitus or cardiopulmonary disease is associated with mortality up to 50%. Delay of more than 24 hours dramatically increases mortality. Morbidity and mortality is significantly higher with perforated GUs than with duodenal ulcers.[44,46,65,68]

The minimally invasive approach to perforated gastroduodenal perforation is increasingly utilized for select patients with good results.[69,70] As with many other minimally invasive operations, laparoscopic repair of perforated duodenal ulcer has been associated with decreased postoperative analgesia requirements, decreased incidence of wound infection, shorter hospital stay, and earlier return to work.[71] In a recent review of 56 papers, overall conversion rate from laparoscopic to open correction of perforated peptic ulcer was 12.4% (range 0%–28.5%). The main reason for conversion was diameter of the perforation. Generally, perforations larger than 1 cm should be converted to open repair. The next two most common reasons for conversion are inability to adequately localize the ulcer and technical difficulties in placing reliable sutures due to inflammation.[43] A Boey score of 2 or 3, age over 70 years, and symptoms >24 hours were associated with higher morbidity and mortality and should be considered relative contraindications to laparoscopic intervention,[64,72] although several authors have demonstrated good results with laparoscopic repair in patients with prolonged peritonitis.[43,73] A few papers have reported higher incidence of leakage with a laparoscopic approach, but the techniques used for repair were not necessarily comparable.[43,72] Shock is a contraindication to a laparoscopic approach.

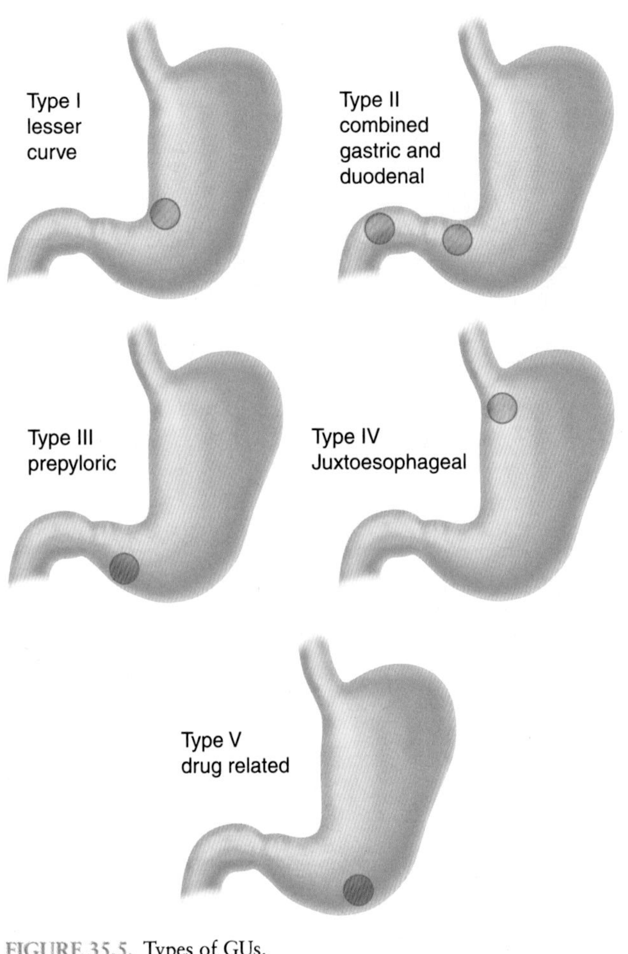

FIGURE 35.5. Types of GUs.

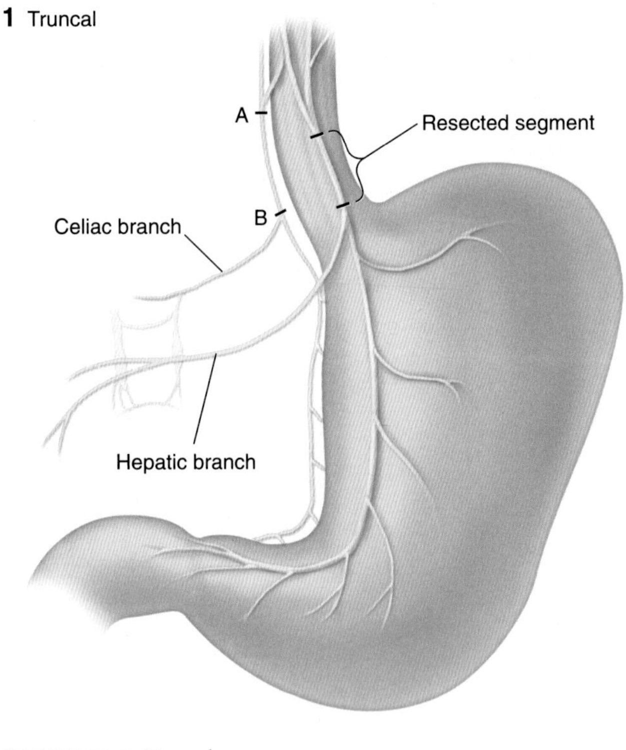

FIGURE 35.6. Truncal vagotomy.

Available data on recurrence rates should be considered in the context that most data predates the routine use of PPIs and eradication of *H. pylori*. Ulcer recurrence is <2% with vagotomy and antrectomy, 5%–15% with vagotomy and pyloroplasty, and 5%–20% with proximal gastric vagotomy.[50,52,60] Recent studies have shown patch closure of perforated duodenal ulcer followed by *H. pylori* eradication and a PPI to yield excellent results with low recurrence. This lends support to current practices of performing simple patch repair in the acute setting.[74,75] A careful history should be obtained from patients with recurrent ulcers with attention to potential contributing risk factors such as smoking, alcohol intake, and NSAID use. In patients who underwent resective procedures without identifiable etiology for ulcer recurrence, incomplete vagotomy, retained gastric antrum, or Zollinger-Ellison's syndrome should be considered. The diagnosis of Zollinger-Ellison's syndrome is confirmed by fasting hypergastrinemia while off PPIs and a secretin stimulation test. An increase in serum gastrin of 200 pg/mL (or possibly 120 pg/mL) or greater suggests the presence of a gastrinoma.[76]

Marginal Ulcer

A perforated marginal or perianastomotic ulcer presents a unique problem in a patient whose anatomy is already surgically altered from previous gastrojejunostomy or other gastric anastomosis. With increasing number of patients undergoing bariatric surgery, short- and long-term complications are better understood.[77] Elective surgery is occasionally performed for intractable ulcers, or ulcers not responding to maximal medical therapy after 3 months. Emergency surgery may be necessary in the case of perforated marginal ulcer and quite often it is the on-call general or acute care surgeon who finds himself/herself performing these challenging operations.

Roux-en-Y-gastric bypass (RYGB) remains the most commonly performed operation for obesity in the United States (Fig. 35.8). The reported incidence of marginal ulcers after RYGB varies widely, from <1% up to 16%.[78,79] A large single center study reported a 1% incidence of perforated marginal ulcer with the median time of presentation 18 months after RYGB.[78] A higher incidence of marginal ulcer may be associated with gastric partition without transection (commonly performed in open gastric bypass) than with transection of the stomach. Smoking, excessive alcohol intake, NSAID use, and steroids have been implicated as risk factors for the development of marginal ulcers, but results of studies have varied. The role of *H. pylori* is unclear although most authors recommend treatment if positive. Ulceration is more often on the jejunal side of the anastomosis, suggesting acid exposure from the stomach as an instigating factor. However, neither prophylactic acid suppression nor vagotomy has definitively been shown to reduce the rate of marginal ulcers after RYGB. Some studies suggest decreased incidence of marginal ulcer formation with retrocolic rather than antecolic gastrojejunal anastomosis.[78–83]

The goals of an emergency operation for perforated marginal ulcer are the same as in any upper GI perforation—close the defect, ensure adequate drainage, and manage sepsis. Establishment of alternate enteral access for nutritional support may be required. In the case of a prohibitively large ulcer or abscess, resection may be necessary. Creation of an anastomosis in the face of frank purulence or shock is not advisable and should be deferred until the patient has recovered physiologically and inflammation has subsided. Laparoscopic repair of perforated marginal ulcer has been described with favorable results in stable patients without abscess.

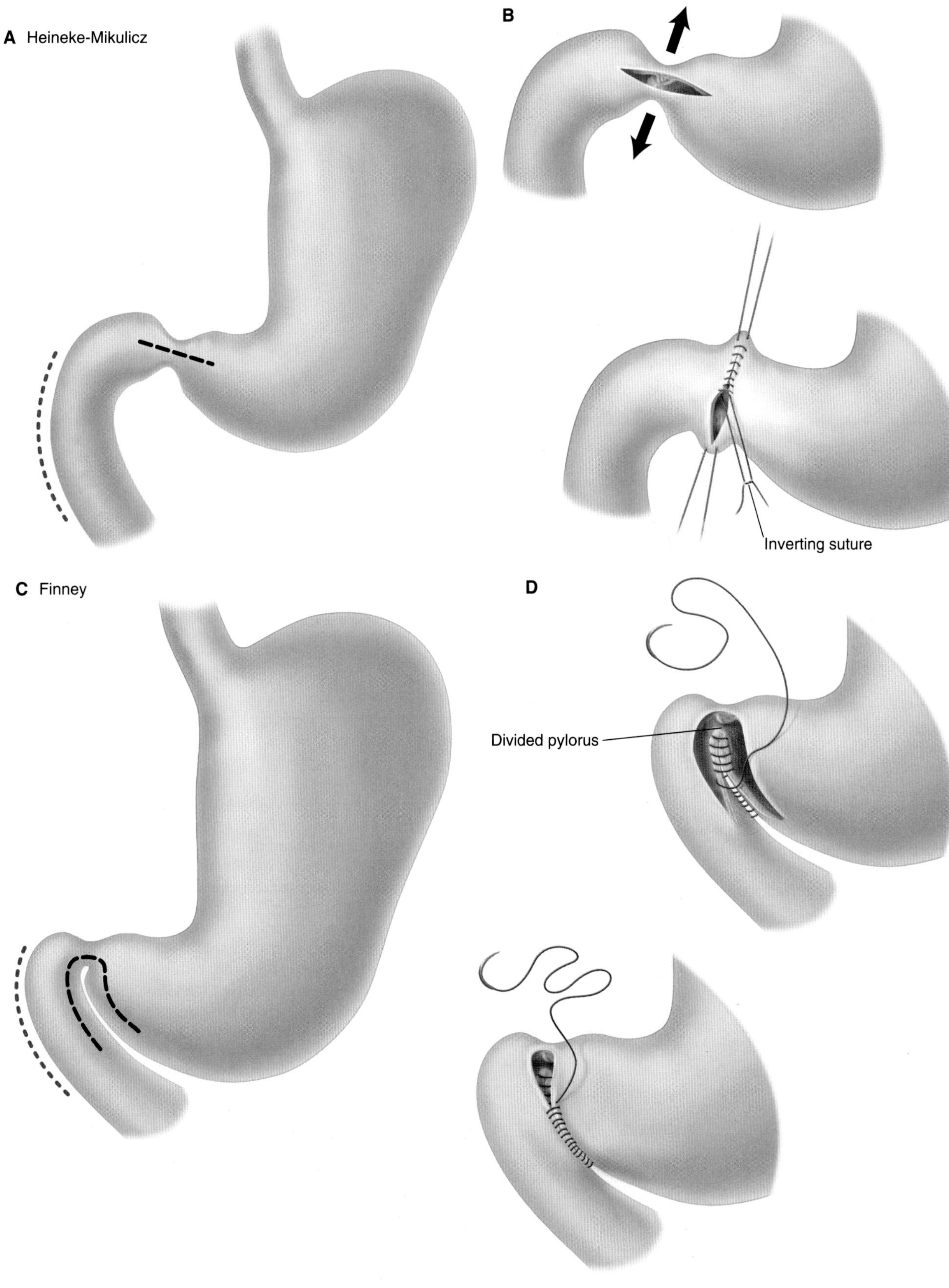

FIGURE 35.7. Pyloroplasty techniques.

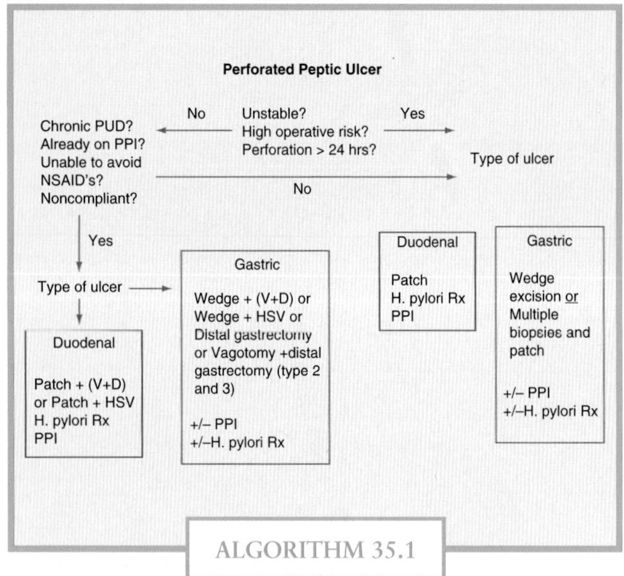

ALGORITHM 35.1. Algorithm for management of perforated peptic ulcers. (Adapted from Figure 26.44, p. 924 from Dempsey DT. Stomach. In: Brunicardi FC, ed. *Schwartz's Principles of Surgery*. 9th ed. The McGraw-Hill Companies, Inc.; 2010.)

Iatrogenic Perforation

Iatrogenic injury is an increasingly common cause of gastroduodenal perforation with more liberal use of esophagoduodenoscopy for diagnostic and therapeutic purposes. ERCP (endoscopic retrograde cholangiopancreatography) carries a risk of perforation between 0.5% and 2%.[84,85] Perforation has also been described as a complication following placement of inferior vena cava filters and biliary stents.[86,87] Microperforation, secondary to a wire or sphinchterotomy during ERCP may be managed conservatively in many cases. However, the standard therapy for free duodenal wall rupture has traditionally been surgical repair. Advances in endoscopic techniques now allow for possible closure of a duodenal perforation endoscopically if recognized immediately and the defect is not too large.[88,89] Intravenous antibiotics and close observation are mandated. If surgical repair of an iatrogenic gastric or duodenal perforation is indicated, the patient's hemodynamic status should guide surgical management.[90] Repair of the defect, peritoneal lavage, and placement of drains can be achieved laparoscopically as well as with laparotomy. The patient with frank peritonitis and in shock is better managed with laparotomy.[91] A repaired gastric defect may not require extraluminal drains, but a duodenal injury should be drained widely. Proximal decompression in either case is achieved adequately with a well-positioned nasogastric tube on sump suction. We do not recommend lateral duodenostomy, but rather favor placement of closed suction drains near the site of repair to provide an outlet for potential duodenal leak in the form of a controlled fistula. Surgical enteral access for postoperative nutritional support should be obtained. In cases of gross peritonitis or septic shock antifungal coverage should be included in the perioperative antimicrobial therapy.

TABLE 35.4

BOEY SCORE

RISK FACTORS	SCORE
Number of hours since perforation	
24 or less	0
More than 24	1
Preoperative systolic blood pressure (mm Hg)	
100 or greater	0
<100	1
Systemic illness: severe heart disease, severe pulmonary disease, renal failure, diabetes mellitus, liver failure	
Absent	0
Present	1

The predicted mortality is 0% with a score of 0, 10% with a score of 1, 45.5% with a score of 2, and 100% with a score of 3. (Adapted from Boey J, Choi SK, Poon A, et al. Risk stratification in perforated duodenal ulcers: A prospective validation of predictive factors. *Ann Surg*. 1987;205:22.)

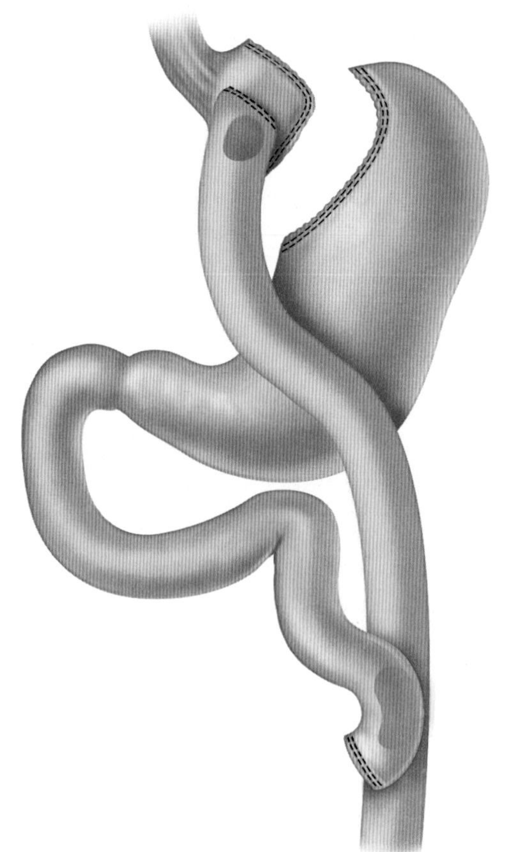

FIGURE 35.8. Roux-en-Y gastric bypass.

Crohn's Disease of the Small Bowel

Crohn's Disease is the most common primary surgical disease of the small intestine. It is an inflammatory process that can affect any portion of the alimentary tract from mouth to anus but most commonly affects the terminal ileum. Forty to fifty-five percent of patients with Crohn's disease have ileocolic disease, 30% have small bowel disease, and 15%–30% have disease involving only the colon or anorectum.[92,93] Grossly, the affected bowel is characterized by creeping fat and a thickened

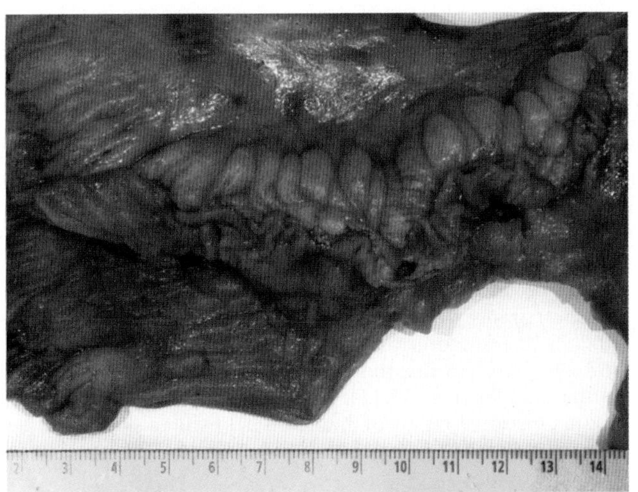
A

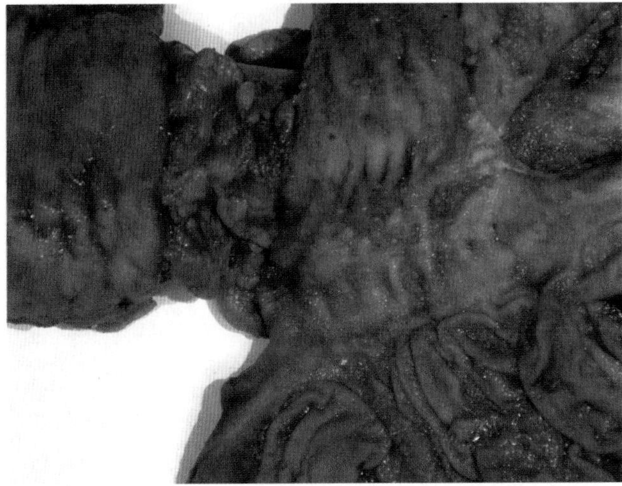
B

FIGURE 35.9. **A,B:** Crohn's disease of the small intestine.

bowel wall and mesentery (Fig. 35.9A). Cobblestoning of the mucosa is characteristic but is not pathognomonic of Crohn's disease (Fig. 35.9B). In contradistinction to ulcerative colitis, Crohn's disease is transmural and discontinuous (segmental) with rectal sparing. Crohn's disease is also associated with a greater degree of extraintestinal manifestations as compared to ulcerative colitis with up to 25% of patients having at least one extraintestinal manifestation of disease (Table 35.5). The incidence of Crohn's disease is highest in North America and Northern Europe. African Americans and Caucasian Americans are affected equally though certain ethnic groups, particularly Jews, have a greater incidence. Males and females appear to be affected equally. Risk is increased in smokers and in urban populations. Peak incidence is in the third decade of life with a smaller peak in the sixth decade of life. Genetic, immunologic, and infectious etiologies have been proposed and there appears to be a familial association but the cause of Crohn's disease remains elusive.[92,93]

TABLE 35.5

EXTRAINTESTINAL MANIFESTATIONS OF CROHN'S DISEASE

Eyes	Uveitis Iritis Episcleritis Conjunctivitis
Skin	Erythema nodosum Erythema multiforme Pyoderma gangrenosum
Blood	Deep venous thrombosis/pulmonary embolism Hemolytic anemia Thrombocytosis
Liver and pancreas	Sclerosing cholangitis Triaditis Pancreatitis
Joints and bones	Ankylosing spondylitis Arthritis Spondyloarthropathy Osteoporosis Clubbing
Kidney	Nephrotic syndrome Amyloidosis
Nervous system	Seizure Stroke Myopathy Peripheral neuropathy Headache

There is no cure for Crohn's disease. The goals of treatment are amelioration of symptoms and improvement in quality of life.[94] Symptoms and complications of Crohn's disease are treated medically with operation reserved for refractory cases or serious complications. Most patients (50%–70%) will require surgery at some point in their lives. Patients with Crohn's disease are optimally managed using a multidisciplinary team approach involving gastroenterologists and surgeons who specialize in inflammatory bowel disease, as well as radiologists, nutritionists, and stoma and wound care nursing specialists. Venous thromboembolism prophylaxis should be routine in hospitalized patients as inflammatory bowel disease is a risk factor for development of deep venous thrombosis.[95]

The three clinical patterns of Crohn's disease are *stricturing*, *perforating*, and *inflammatory*. Fibrosis and stenosis of discontinuous segments of bowel are the hallmark of the stricturing pattern. Repeated episodes eventually lead to strictures that no longer respond to medical therapies and patients ultimately require surgery. The perforating pattern is characterized by abscess or fistula formation. A combination of medical and surgical therapy is generally utilized. The inflammatory pattern is characterized by a more diffuse distribution along the alimentary tract and is treated medically with operation reserved for refractory cases.

Treatment of Inflammatory Crohn's Disease

The first line of therapy for mild symptoms is 5-ASA (Pentasa, Asacol). For a severe acute episode, or Crohn's flare, corticosteroids are the gold standard treatment to induce remission. Budesonide, a synthetic glucocorticoid, is often used to induce remission because of its reduced systemic absorption and more tolerable side effects when compared with prednisone. Antibiotics, typically metronidazole, may be used as adjunctive therapy. Infliximab, a monoclonal antibody against tumor necrosis factor-α (TNF-α), is used for the treatment of severe active Crohn's disease resistant to conventional therapy. Infliximab is effective as an induction agent with up to 70% patients responding within 1–2 weeks from a single infusion. Unfortunately infliximab use is associated with an increased risk of opportunistic infections such as tuberculosis, aspergillosis, and listeriosis. It is also generally necessary to administer immunosuppressants concomitantly with infliximab to prevent transfusion reactions due to the formation of antibodies to infliximab. Following successful induction therapy the goal of treatment becomes maintenance of remission. Steroids are ineffective as maintenance therapy. The two most common agents used for maintenance of remission are azathioprine and 6-mercaptopurine. Treatment with these agents is usually initiated during induction therapy because of their delayed onset of action. Patients must be monitored closely for complications such as bone marrow suppression, hepatotoxicity, and pancreatitis.[96]

Treatment of Perforating Crohn's Disease

The primary goal of treatment for abscess or fistula is control of sepsis. Image-guided drainage of an abdominal abscess with parenteral antibiotics is the mainstay of therapy (Fig. 35.10). Nutritional and metabolic support is essential. The three most important types of fistulae are enterocutaneous, enteroenteral, and enterovesical.

Enterocutaneous fistulae (ECF) occur in 4% of patients with Crohn's disease, either as a direct extension from the diseased bowel to the skin or from ongoing drainage via a percutaneous drainage site. They may also occur as a postoperative complication in patients who have recently undergone operation. Medical management should be initiated with antibiotics, nutritional support, and infliximab.[97] Infliximab has been associated with >60% response rate for closure of Crohn's related fistulae.[98,99] However, more recent studies have not demonstrated a positive impact of infliximab on operative rates for bowel resection or fistula repair.[100]

Enteroenteral fistulae in themselves also do not necessarily mandate operation. Surgery is indicated, however, if the fistulae are associated with an acute inflammatory exacerbation refractory to medical management, abdominal mass, hemorrhage, or uncorrectable malnutrition. Enterovesical fistula is characterized by chronic or recurrent urinary tract infections (88%), pneumaturia (88%), fecaluria (38%), and hematuria (63%).[92,93] CT of the abdomen and pelvis typically shows air in the bladder (Fig. 35.11). Diagnosis is confirmed by cystoscopy. Operative repair of enterovesical fistulae should be performed to prevent injury to the kidneys from recurrent urinary tract infections.

Surgical therapy in Crohn's disease is aimed at treatment of complications, relief of symptoms, and optimization of quality of life. Urgent operation may be necessary for free perforation (rare), acute hemorrhage, or uncontrolled sepsis from abscesses not amenable to percutaneous drainage. Less urgent operations are indicated for enterovesical fistula or acute Crohn's flare, obstruction, or fistula refractory to medical management.[101]

The preoperative workup for an elective operation for Crohn's disease should include a contrast radiographic study (small bowel follow through) to determine the length of bowel, location of disease, identify fistulae, and evaluate strictures. CT identifies masses, fluid collections, and bowel wall thickening. Colonoscopy and video capsule endoscopy may help establish

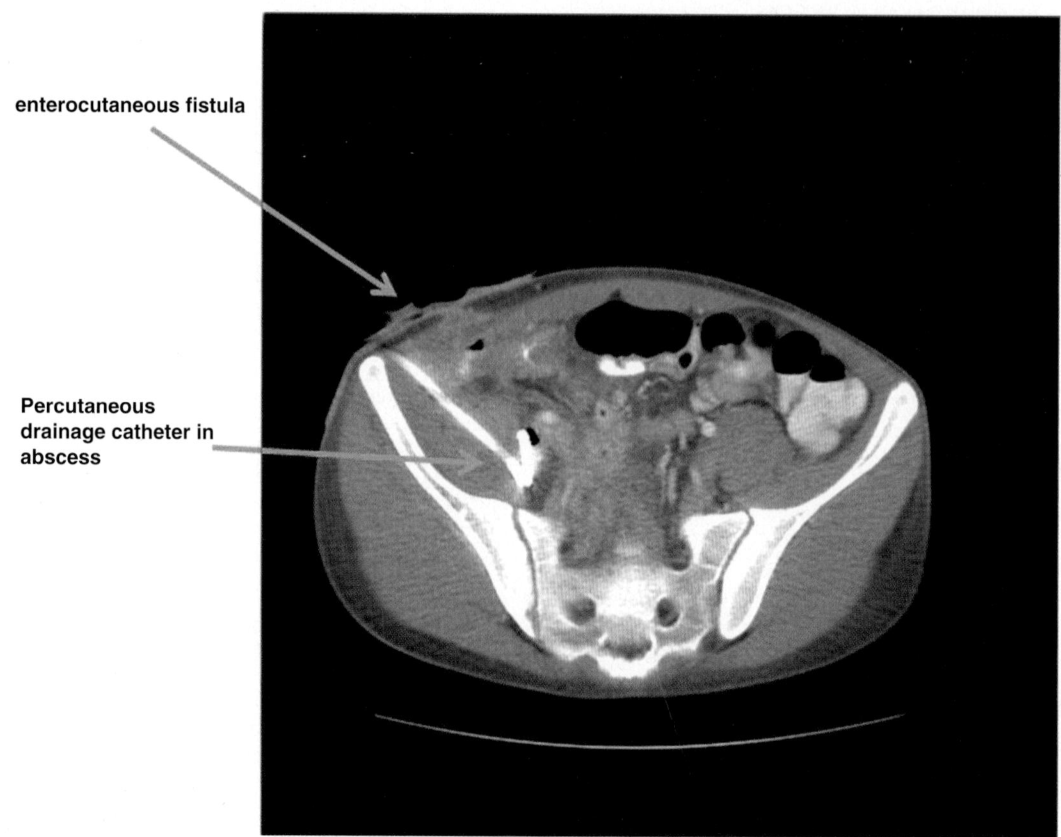

FIGURE 35.10. Abdominal abscess from Crohn's disease.

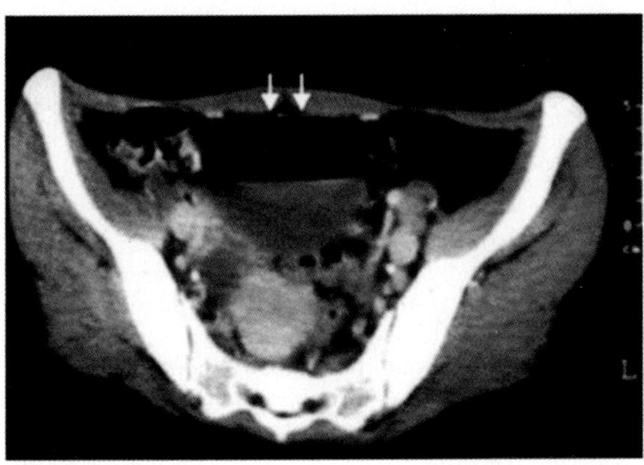

FIGURE 35.11. CT demonstrating air in the bladder. (From Chebli JM, Gaburri PD, Pinto JR. Enterovesical fistula in Crohn's disease. *Lancet*. 2004;364–368.)

the presence and extent of disease. The patient's nutritional status should ideally be optimized prior to surgery. Except in the case of high-grade obstruction, a standard mechanical and antimicrobial bowel prep should be performed. Consultation with the stoma care nursing team for preoperative counseling and marking for potential stoma sites is helpful to both the surgeon and to the patient. It is imperative that a history of any recent corticosteroid use be elicited to determine whether perioperative steroid replacement will be necessary. Other immunosuppressive medications may be safely discontinued preoperatively. Corticosteroid use in the perioperative period is associated with increased postoperative complications so a rapid taper postoperatively should be the goal when possible.[102]

In emergency operations for abdominal catastrophe with significant contamination or shock, a damage control approach may be prudent. The emergency "damage control" operation would consist of resection of the offending segment of bowel to grossly negative margins and peritoneal lavage with evacuation of any GI spillage or purulence. The surgeon must then determine whether to complete the operation with an assessment of the length of disease-free bowel, creation of an end ostomy (if applicable), and primary closure of the fascia, or to defer the second stage until hemodynamic stability has been achieved and gross peritonitis resolved. Primary anastomosis in the face of shock or gross contamination is associated with a high incidence of anastomotic leak and should be avoided if possible. Temporary closure may be achieved with either a running nonabsorbable suture closure of the skin or placement of a negative pressure vacuum dressing designated for the abdomen. The second, reconstructive operation 24–48 hours later consists of further lavage of the abdominal cavity, reestablishment of GI continuity with creation of an end ostomy or with primary anastomosis with or without protective loop ileostomy, and definitive closure of the abdomen. In the difficult case of duodenal disease, options include resection or bypass with gastrojejunostomy if resection is not feasible.

Operative management of fistulae involves identification of the inciting segment of bowel and the target structure. The abnormal connection is divided and the instigating segment of bowel resected. Resection of the target organ should only be performed if it is not amenable to simple repair. In cases of enterovesical fistula, division of the fistula is followed by primary repair of the bladder. Preoperative placement of ureteral stents may prove useful for identification of the ureters while navigating through the complex inflammatory mass. Foley catheter drainage of the bladder postoperatively is generally sufficient although an additional perivesical drain may be utilized in cases of severe inflammation or tenuous repair.

When dealing with obstruction due to stricture, viable alternatives to resection include balloon dilatation or stricturoplasty, particularly for short segment strictures (<4 cm). These alternatives may be more appropriate than resection when there is concern for short gut.[103–105] A Heinecke-Mikulicz-type stricturoplasty (longitudinal enterotomy with transverse repair) is typically used for strictures <10–12 cm in length. For longer strictures up to 25 cm in length a Finney-type strictureplasty is preferred. In the case of duodenal stricture, options include endoscopic balloon dilatation, stricturoplasty, bypass with gastrojejunostomy, or resection.[106] Leaving the diseased segment of bowel does however expose the patient to potential future complications such as hemorrhage or malignant degeneration.[107]

Recurrence rates after bowel resection and anastomosis have not been shown to have increased with microscopic involvement of resection margins.[108] The type of anastomosis, stapled or hand sewn, also does not seem to have impact on anastomotic recurrence rate, although patients with a side-to-side anastomosis may have a lower incidence of reoperation for anastomotic recurrence than those with end-to-end anastomosis.[109–111] We prefer a two-layer side-to-side hand sewn anastomosis when bowel is inflamed or edematous.

Selected patients are candidates for laparoscopic surgery for Crohn's disease.[112,113] Length of stay, morbidity, and overall cost in the first 3 postoperative months have been shown to be lower in patients who underwent a minimally invasive surgical approach. A laparoscopic approach also allows faster initiation of steroid therapy when needed and potentially reduces adhesion formation for future operations. Diagnostic laparoscopy is an excellent tool in the workup of patients in whom Crohn's disease is suspected but cannot be confirmed otherwise.[114,115] Contraindications to laparoscopic surgery in Crohn's disease include a known "frozen" abdomen and emergency surgery in an acutely ill patient with peritonitis, bleeding, or complete bowel obstruction. General medical contraindications to laparoscopy such as severe COPD, severe heart failure, and coagulopathy must be considered in planning the operative approach. The presence of dense adhesions is the most common reason for conversion from laparoscopic to open operation. Extensive inflammation, large inflammatory mass, and the inability to safely dissect a fistula are other cited reasons for conversion.[116] The number of prior abdominal operations has not been shown to be a predictor of conversion. When laparoscopy is utilized, resection may be performed externally or within the abdomen using the Ligasure device or ultrasonic scissors. A 5 cm periumbilical or suprapubic incision is used to deliver the specimen. Anastomosis is typically performed externally.

When Crohn's disease is first diagnosed during laparoscopy or laparotomy for suspected appendicitis or bowel obstruction, it may be advisable to treat the Crohn's disease medically rather than with resection. Intraoperative decision-making should take into account the patient's age, clinical status, and nature of the disease (inflammation, stricture). If the surgeon elects to treat surgically he/she should adhere to the basic principles of surgical management in Crohn's disease.

Whether elective or emergent, open or laparoscopic, certain basic principles apply to the surgical management of Crohn's disease. (1) Only the segment causing complications should be resected and only to grossly (not microscopically) negative margins. (2) Stricturoplasty may be the better choice when dealing with obstruction. (3) Bypass should be considered a last resort because of the risk of bleeding, perforation, and future malignancy in the bypassed portion, though it may be the only viable option with duodenal disease. (4) In high-risk patients (high dose steroids, profound malnutrition) end ostomy or protective loop ileostomy for a distal anastomosis is advisable. (5) Appendectomy should be performed when possible and safe to avoid future diagnostic dilemmas.

Crohn's Disease During Pregnancy

Active Crohn's disease during pregnancy is associated with increased risk of fetal loss, preterm delivery, low birth weight, and developmental defects.[93] Diagnosis and workup become challenging and may involve endoscopy, ultrasound, and magnetic resonance imaging in lieu of traditional studies associated with radiation exposure. Continued severe disease poses greater risk to both mother and fetus than does surgery. A frank, detailed discussion of risks, benefits, and alternatives is indicated preoperatively as is consultation with Maternal-Fetal Medicine. If surgical resection is required, ileostomy may be preferred to anastomosis to reduce the risk of postoperative complications.

Enterocutaneous Fistula

The management of ECF continues to challenge even seasoned surgeons. Fistulae are often complicated by sepsis, fluid and electrolyte abnormalities, malnutrition, and complex wound management issues. Mortality ranges from 10% to 20% depending upon coexisting conditions. ECF develop as a result of technical factors from a previous operation, factors related to healing and tissue integrity inherent to the patient, and factors related to specific disease processes.[117]

The vast majority of ECF occur as a complication of an abdominal operation. ECF may occur as a result of anastomotic leak, unrecognized enterotomy, incorporation of bowel in the fascial closure, and ischemia. Emergency abdominal procedures and contaminated operations are additional risk factors. Factors related to the patient's ability to heal include severe malnutrition, steroid use, radiation, and chemotherapy. A serum albumin <3.0 g/dL is a well-established risk factor for the development of ECF.[117] Enterocutaneous or enteroatmospheric fistulae are common among patients with an open abdomen related to multiple trauma or abdominal compartment syndrome. We recommend managing the open abdomen with vacuum negative pressure dressings specialized for the abdomen with a nonadherent plastic sheet placed over exposed bowel before the vacuum sponge is applied (Fig. 35.12A). While some studies have suggested increased risk of fistula formation with the use of negative pressure dressings, other studies have not been able to demonstrate this. When early fascial closure cannot be achieved after open abdomen we close the abdomen either with a skin-only closure with a heavy, running nonabsorbable suture (Fig. 35.12B), or with an absorbable mesh followed by skin grafting when a satisfactory bed of granulation tissue is present. The resulting ventral hernia can be repaired electively in 6–12 months.

An ECF classically presents as a wound infection following abdominal surgery. Drainage from the wound with the appearance and odor of enteric contents is diagnostic. The underlying fascial integrity should be evaluated as ongoing leakage of enteric contents may lead to fascial dehiscence and evisceration. Conversely, ECF should be in the differential diagnosis of a patient presenting with fascial dehiscence or evisceration.

An upper GI contrast study or CT with oral contrast may demonstrate an ECF. A chronic fistula tract can be injected with oral contrast to locate the site of communication with the intestinal tract (fistulogram). In general, the more proximal the fistula, the more pronounced the electrolyte abnormalities, fluid losses, and malnutrition. Distal fistulae may essentially function as an ileostomy or colostomy and may not be associated with any fluid, electrolyte, or nutritional abnormalities. More proximal fistulae may produce management problems with volume loss and electrolyte abnormalities.

The initial primary goal of treatment of an ECF is source control and control of sepsis. Correction of fluid and electrolyte imbalances, nutritional support, and skin care are essential adjuncts. Uncontrolled sepsis is the major cause of mortality in patients with ECF. Image-guided drainage of an abdominal abscess usually precludes the need for early operation which is associated with high morbidity and mortality. Early surgical intervention may be necessary in septic patients with uncontrolled leakage of enteric contents into the abdomen or abscesses not amenable to percutaneous drainage. If the patient is not septic despite having an intra-abdominal fluid collection, an attempt at nonoperative management can be made. A trial of medical management may eliminate the need for surgery in some patients altogether; in those patients who still require operation, the additional time allows the fistula tract to mature and inflammation to subside, creating a less hostile abdomen at the time of operation. Consultations should be held with the wound and ostomy care nursing team to assist with the complex wound management that most of these patients will have. Many surgeons champion the use of specially-fashioned abdominal negative pressure vacuum

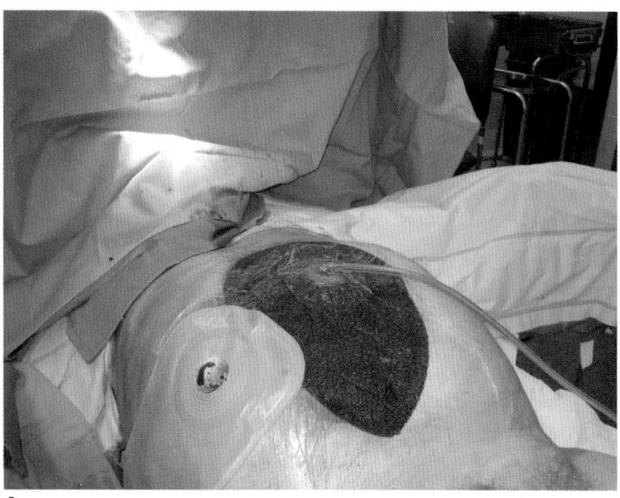
A

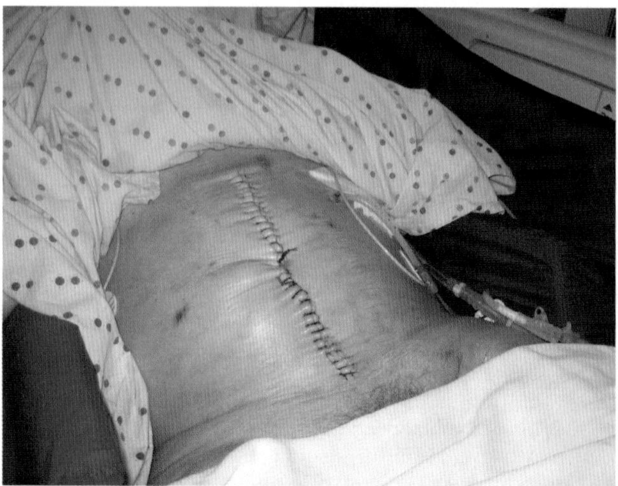
B

FIGURE 35.12. **A:** Abdominal VAC dressing. **B:** Running suture for skin-only closure of the abdomen.

dressings in the management of enteroatmospheric fistulae to promote healing. Creative skin grafting around the fistula may simplify wound care and provide patient comfort while the fistula matures or closes.

Adequate nutritional support is essential for spontaneous closure of an ECF. Patients with ECF are often profoundly catabolic and depleted in lean body mass, albumin, and prealbumin. Protein and caloric requirements may be double their baseline requirements. Enteral feeding, either by mouth or by a small-caliber nasogastric or nasoenteral tube, should be the first line of nutritional support in the absence of a contraindication.[118] Providing as little as 10%–20% of nutritional needs enterally is associated with maintenance of gut mucosal integrity and immunological function. Parenteral nutrition is associated with more infectious complications but may be the only means of providing nutrition to a patient with a high output fistula, obstruction, or short gut. Parenteral nutrition may sometimes be used to supplement enteral feeding for profoundly malnourished patients or patients who cannot tolerate full enteral feeds. If fistula output increases in response to enteral feeding it may be beneficial to provide nutritional support parenterally to try to allow for spontaneous closure of the fistula.[119]

The overall spontaneous closure rate of an ECF is 10%–40% with conservative management. The use of octreotide, an analogue of somatostatin, as adjunctive therapy may decrease fistula output, making a high-output fistula more manageable, but has not been shown to definitively impact spontaneous closure.[120,121] An ECF that persists 6–8 weeks after resolution of sepsis and correction of nutritional deficits is unlikely to close spontaneously, especially if the output is high (>500 mL/d). Up to 90% of ECF that are going to close spontaneously, close within 5 weeks after sepsis is controlled. Factors associated with failure of an ECF to close spontaneously include high output fistula, ongoing malnutrition, distal bowel obstruction, short fistula tract, abscess, and foreign body (including mesh). Malignancy, radiation, and steroids are also risk factors for nonclosure of ECF.

In planning an elective operation to repair an ECF preoperative imaging such as fistulogram and CT is obtained to identify the location of the fistula, evaluate for distal obstruction or potential foreign body, and to evaluate the abdominal wall in cases of loss of domain (large ventral defect) for possible abdominal wall reconstruction. A small but important subset of patients may benefit from earlier operation rather than delaying time to operation which exacerbates the catabolic state and leads to further debilitation and morbidity despite control of sepsis and aggressive nutritional support.

A mechanical and oral antimicrobial bowel prep should be performed when possible preoperatively. At laparotomy the bowel should be fully mobilized to allow proper identification of involved segments, ensure patency of the length of the bowel, and to perform segmental resection of the fistulae with tension-free anastomosis; fastidious technique is essential. Closure of the abdominal wall and distancing the repair from the incision should be routine. Surgical enteral access for postoperative nutritional support should be considered.

Infectious Enteritis

About 200–500 cases of typhoid fever and typhoid enteritis are reported annually in the United States. About 80% of cases occur in people with a history of recent travel to endemic areas. Typhoid enteritis is an acute systemic infection caused by ingestion of Salmonella typhi through contaminated food or water. Fever, abdominal pain, rash, and diarrhea (sometimes bloody) along with lymphadenopathy and hepatosplenomegaly are characteristic. Diagnosis is by positive blood or stool culture.[92] Because of high resistance to the original first-line therapy (ampicillin, chloramphenicol, trimethoprim-sulfamethoxazole) the recommended treatment for adults with typhoid fever and uncomplicated typhoid enteritis is now with fluoroquinolones or third generation cephalosporins. In areas of high fluoroquinolone resistance, azithromycin 1 g orally for 5 days is recommended.[122,123] Hemorrhage or perforation through an ulcerated Peyer's patch may necessitate operation. Perforation is usually solitary in the antimesenteric terminal ileum and managed with either simple closure or segmental resection. In the unusual event of multiple perforations resection with primary anastomosis or creation of end ileostomy may be required.[124]

Patients with AIDS or on immunosuppressive agents after organ transplantation are susceptible to GI infection by a host of pathogens. Protozoa (Cryptosporidium, Isospora, Microsporidium) are the most frequent class of pathogens causing diarrhea in patients with AIDS. The small bowel is the most common site of infection. Cryptosporidial transmission is by fecal–oral route. Public swimming pools have been implicated as a significant source of infection. Cryptosporidial enteritis generally resolves spontaneously in nonimmunocompromised hosts. In patients with AIDS, it is characterized by severe watery diarrhea (>10 L/d), cramps, nausea, and weight loss. Biliary involvement is common. Diagnosis is by isolation of oocysts in stool, bile, or tissue. Treatment is primarily HAART (highly active antiretroviral therapy) as raising the CD4 count to >100 cells/mm^3 usually leads to resolution of enteritis. Supportive care with oral or parenteral hydration and antidiarrheal agents may be life-saving and continues until there is resolution of diarrhea. A trial of nitazoxanide in conjunction with HAART may be considered.[125]

Enteric bacterial infection with *Salmonella*, *Shigella*, and *Campylobacter* are more common and more virulent in immunocompromised patients than healthy individuals. Affected patients present with abdominal pain, high fever, tenesmus, and hematochezia. Stool cultures will usually diagnose Salmonella and Shigella but may be falsely negative with *Campylobacter* infection. Treatment is parenteral antibiotics.

Mycobacterial infection in the immunocompromised patient may be due to either *M. tuberculosis* or the atypical *Mycobacterium avium* complex (MAC). Infection is characterized by fever, night sweats, abdominal pain, diarrhea, and weight loss. Routes of entry to the intestinal tract include the oral route (infected sputum or contaminated food or milk), hematogenous spread from pulmonary or military tuberculosis, or by contiguous spread. Intestinal tuberculosis involves the ileocecal region in 85%–90% of cases. Up to half of affected patients will have a palpable right lower quadrant mass and ascites is often present. Gross findings include ulcerations or tubercles covering the bowel surface and mesenteric lymphadenopathy. Strictures and fistula formation may be present. The diagnosis of mycobacterial infection is made by identification of the organism in tissue, either by acid-fast stain, by culture of the excised tissue, or by PCR. The treatment is similar for immunocompromised and immunocompetent hosts with multi-drug antimicrobial therapy. Most fistulae will respond to medical management.[126,127] Obstruction is the most common indication for surgery. Stricturoplasty may be an option for obstruction related to stricture as may be colonoscopic balloon dilatation.

The MAC organisms (*M. avium* and *M. intracellulare*) are ubiquitous in the environment and contracted by inhalation or ingestion.[128] Risk of infection is increased with CD4 count <50 cells/mm^3. Diagnosis is made with positive blood culture. MAC infection is characterized by massive thickening of the proximal small bowel. Perforation or other surgical emergencies are rare. Multi-drug therapy with clarithromycin or azithromycin and ethambutol is standard therapy. MAC infection in patients infected with HIV increases the risk of death independent of CD4 count.[125]

CMV is the most common viral cause of diarrhea in immunocompromised patients. Patients present with abdominal pain, fever, and weight loss. Diagnosis is made by demonstration of viral inclusions histologically or by serology. The treatment is usually ganciclovir or foscarnet.[129] Perforation of the distal small bowel or colon or massive hemorrhage may rarely necessitate urgent operation.

GI histoplasmosis occurs in association with disseminated histoplasmosis, a disease primarily of immunocompromised patients. Diagnosis is made by fungal smear and culture of infected tissue or blood. Treatment is most often amphotericin B.[130]

Small Bowel Diverticular Disease

Small bowel diverticulosis is a relatively rare entity and <4% of all small bowel diverticula will become symptomatic in a person's lifetime. Because the clinical presentation may be dramatic with bleeding, perforation, or acute inflammation, the acute care surgeon should be prepared to manage complications that may arise from these diverticula. There are two types of small bowel diverticula. False diverticula are acquired defects with herniation of mucosa and submucosa along the mesenteric side of the bowel where vessels penetrate the bowel wall. True diverticula are congenital anomalies arising in the antimesenteric side of the distal ileum (Meckel's diverticula).[131,132]

Duodenal Diverticula

A duodenal diverticulum typically presents during or after the fifth decade of life as a solitary outpouching along the mesenteric side of the duodenal wall. Duodenal diverticula are the most common small bowel diverticula, 45%–79% of all small bowel diverticula. Less than 1% require treatment.[133,134] Diagnosis is by EGD, ERCP, contrast radiography, or CT with oral contrast. They are reported to be found in 10%–20% of patients undergoing ERCP.[135]

The majority of duodenal diverticula (61%–75%) are located in the periampullary area, or within 2 cm of the ampulla of Vater. The inherent defects in the muscularis propria caused by the penetration of the pancreatic and biliary ducts predispose to the development of these false diverticula. Patients typically present with symptoms related to biliary or pancreatic ductal obstruction including cholangitis, jaundice, or pancreatitis. Patients with duodenal diverticula have a higher incidence of choledocholithiasis and pigment and bilirubinate stones. Duodenal diverticula should be considered in the differential diagnosis for patients with pancreatitis of unclear etiology.[135–138]

Asymptomatic or incidentally found duodenal diverticula should not be resected. The patient should be informed of the incidental finding and potential sequelae. Choledocholithiasis in association with a duodenal diverticulum should be managed conventionally as in patients without duodenal diverticula. Inflammation, perforation into the retroperitoneum or peritoneal cavity (Fig. 35.13), and hemorrhage occur less frequently but may necessitate intervention acutely.

Surgery for duodenal diverticula is associated with significant morbidity and mortality related to the patient's age, comorbidities, and technical challenges of the operation itself. The surgical approach begins with a complete Kocher maneuver and identification of the pancreaticobiliary structures and their relationship to the diverticulum. Cannulation of the ampulla of Vater with a metal probe or red rubber catheter helps to maintain orientation and avoid injury. Diverticulectomy with primary closure is the procedure of choice when the ductal structures are not involved and when there is no retroperitoneal contamination. For duodenal diverticula distal to the ampulla, options include diverticulectomy with jejunal serosal patch repair or segmental resection with end-to-end anastomosis. Roux-en-Y biliary bypass may be necessary when the ampulla is involved. In cases of retroperitoneal contamination secondary to a perforated duodenal diverticulum, options include antrectomy with Billroth II reconstruction or

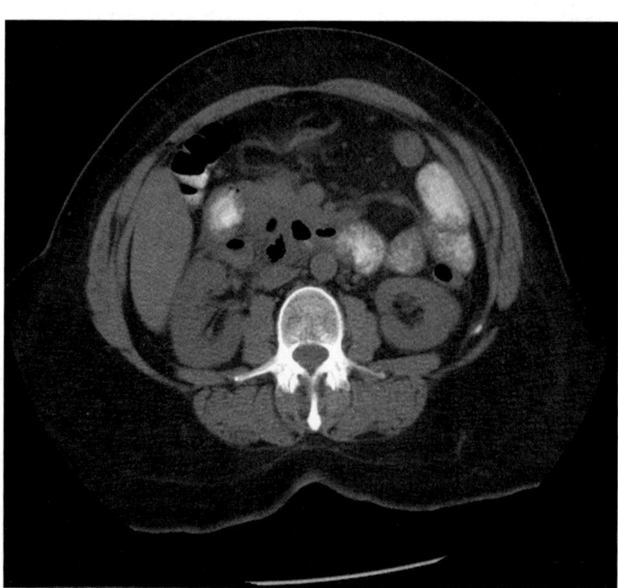

A

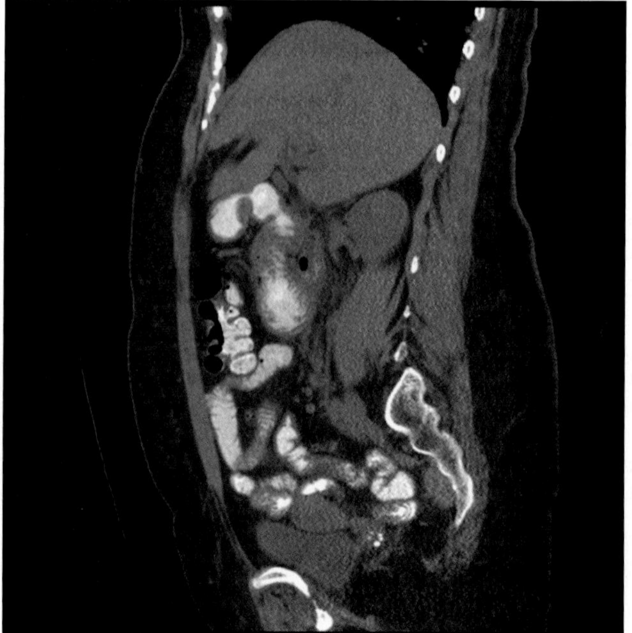

B

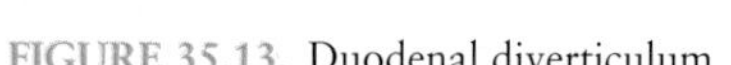

FIGURE 35.13. Duodenal diverticulum.

duodenal exclusion with placement of gastrostomy and jejunostomy tubes. To avoid biliary stasis and future diagnostic dilemmas, cholecystectomy should be performed in patients requiring surgery for duodenal diverticula.

Intraluminal or "windsock" diverticula are large, congenital, saccular diverticula in the second portion of the duodenum. They are associated with a myriad of other congenital anomalies including annular pancreas, choledochocele, malrotation, and superior mesenteric artery (SMA) compression syndrome. Cardiac and urogenital anomalies are also common. Obstruction is the most frequently encountered complication associated with an intraluminal diverticulum. The preferred treatment for symptomatic intraluminal diverticula is duodenotomy and excision.[139] Endoscopic excision has also been performed successfully.[140,141]

Jejunoileal Diverticula

Jejunoileal diverticula occur in 1%–3% of the general population and comprise only 25% of all small bowel diverticula, but are the most likely to be symptomatic.[142] They are often multiple, with 80% occurring in the jejunum, 15% in the ileum, and 5% along the full length. Patients typically present at age 50 or greater. Patients may present acutely with perforation, obstruction, hemorrhage, or inflammation causing peritonitis. More commonly, patients present with symptoms related to the intestinal dysmotility that is the underlying pathophysiology for the development of these acquired diverticula. Signs and symptoms related to stasis and malabsorption may include abdominal pain, steatorrhea, megaloblastic anemia, and neuropathy. Small bowel follow through establishes the diagnosis. CT with oral contrast has the added benefit of assessment of inflammation or subtle signs of perforation as well as the anatomic relationship of diverticula to surrounding structures. Diagnosis is often made at laparoscopy or laparotomy. In patients with symptoms related to malabsorption due to bacterial overgrowth, medical therapy with metronidazole and amoxicillin clavulanate, and nutritional support with vitamin supplementation is successful in 75% of cases. Surgical intervention may be indicated in patients in whom medical therapy fails. Segmental resection of the involved diverticula is the treatment of choice for symptomatic diverticula. Diverticula encountered incidentally during laparoscopy or laparotomy should not be excised.[142–144]

Meckel's Diverticulum

Meckel's diverticula, true diverticula on the antimesenteric side of the bowel, are the most common congenital anomaly of the small bowel and account for 25% of all small bowel diverticula (Fig. 35.14). Failure of the vitelline (omphalomesenteric) duct to obliterate may manifest as an ileoumbilical fistula, vitelline duct cyst, but most commonly as a Meckel's diverticulum. Its blood supply is derived from a persistent right vitelline artery from the SMA. The defining features of a Meckel's diverticulum are described by the "rule of two": 2% of the population, 2 inches long, within 2 feet of the ileocecal valve, and two types of heterotopic mucosa. It typically presents within the first 2 years of life but occasionally presents in adult patients. Half of Meckel's diverticula contain heterotopic mucosa with 75% being gastric mucosa and 15% pancreatic. It is the most common cause of lower GI bleeding in pediatric patients. Acid secretion from heterotopic mucosa within the diverticulum leads to ulcer formation on the opposite side of the bowel wall which may bleed. A "Meckel's scan," used to identify uptake of radioisotope by gastric mucosa, may be helpful in the workup of GI bleeding but plays no role in the workup of an acute abdomen. The most common presentation of a symptomatic Meckel's diverticulum in adults is bowel obstruction which may be secondary to intussusception, volvulus, or incarceration within an inguinal hernia (Littre's hernia).[145,146] Meckel's diverticulitis occurs in 25% of symptomatic patients and is often found at laparoscopy for what is initially thought to be appendicitis. In cases of obstruction or localized inflammation, stapled diverticulectomy or wedge excision with primary closure is adequate. With significant inflammation or with a wide-based diverticulum, segmental bowel resection is preferred. With hemorrhage, segmental resection is necessary to include the bleeding ulcer on the opposing bowel wall. Appendectomy should be performed to avoid future diagnostic dilemmas.

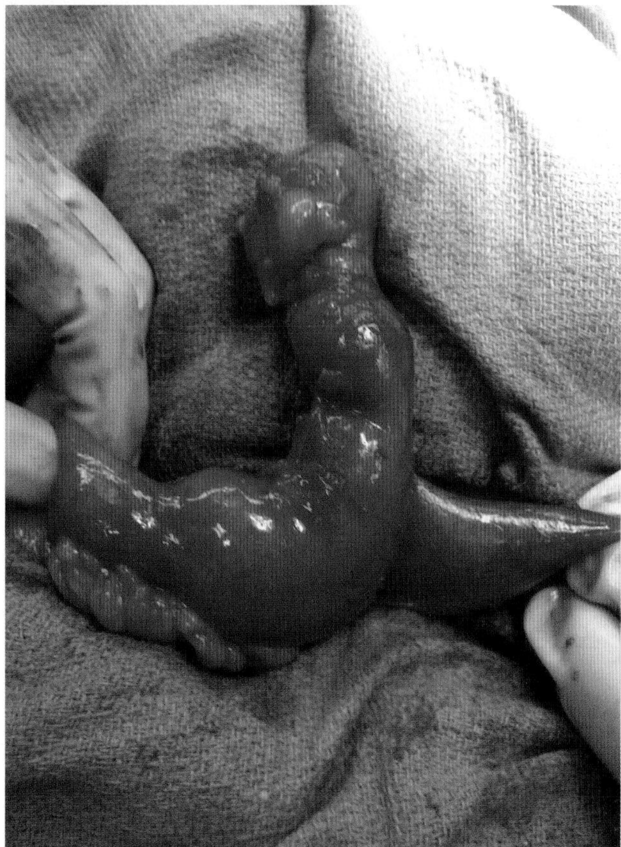

FIGURE 35.14. Meckel's diverticulum.

Incidentally found Meckel's diverticula in the pediatric population should be removed. Removal of an incidentally discovered Meckel's diverticulum in adults is controversial. Relative indications for removal include evidence of heterotopic tissue, signs of prior diverticulitis, or the presence of a mesodiverticular band. The initial indication for operation and implications for future planning should also be considered. Presently, most surgeons do not favor removing a Meckel's diverticulum found incidentally in an adult patient.[143,147]

INFLAMMATORY AND INFECTIOUS DISEASES OF THE COLON

An understanding of the management of inflammatory and infectious diseases of the colon is essential for the acute care surgeon. Multiple pathologies of the colon will prompt surgical consultation and consideration of operative management; these include colonic ischemia, bleeding, obstruction, diverticulitis, infectious colitides, and acute, severe manifestations of inflammatory bowel disease. This section will focus on inflammatory and infectious pathophysiology of the colon and will review current strategies of diagnosis and management. Under conditions of health, the complex microbiome of the colonic wall and lumen exists in symbiotic harmony. However, in the setting of the diseased colon, the colonic microbiome can result in life-threatening infection that may require source control, including surgical management.

Anatomy/Physiology

The colon extends from the end of the ileum to just above the peritoneal reflection at the junction of the sigmoid colon and rectum. Embryologically, the colon is derived from two origins.[149] The cecum, ascending, and proximal transverse colon are derived from the midgut and receive blood supply from the SMA, while the distal transverse colon and beyond are derived from the hindgut and receive blood supply from the inferior mesenteric artery (IMA) (Fig. 35.15). In general the venous and lymphatic drainage parallel the arteries. Grossly, the colon is 115–150 cm in length and ranges in diameter from 7.5 cm at the cecum to 2.5 cm at the rectosigmoid junction.[149] The colon rotates during development and attaches laterally on the right as the ascending colon and on the left as the descending colon. The mesentery at these locations most often fuses to the posterior peritoneum. The transverse and sigmoid colons have long, mobile peritoneum and allows significant variability in the location of these structures.

Histologically, the colon is divided into a mucosa, submucosa, muscularis propria, and serosa.[150] The mucosa is comprised of an epithelial layer, lamina propria and the muscularis mucosa. The epithelium is organized into crypts of nonbranching tubules. Various cell types include simple columnar cells, goblet cells, and undifferentiated amine precursor uptake and decarboxylation and enterochromaffin cells. The mucosa is in continuity with the lumen of the colon. The submucosa is a layer of connective tissues containing blood vessels, lymphatics, and nerves. The muscularis propria of the colon is an inner, continuous, circular muscle that is innervated by the myenteric plexus of Auerbach. The longitudinal muscle is organized into three cables of muscle, the tenia coli, which run from the cecum to the distal sigmoid, at which point these fibers disperse to form a circumferential layer over the rectum. The peritonealized surfaces of the colon are covered by a serosa throughout its length.

The major functions of the colon are absorption and digestion. Absorption of salts and water from the output of the small intestine is essential for normal physiological maintenance of fluids and electrolytes. Sodium is actively absorbed against concentration and electrical gradients and this drives the absorption of water. Chloride is also actively absorbed and exchanged for bicarbonate. Urea metabolizing bacteria in the colon form ammonia, which is also absorbed.[151] The colonic mucosa secretes mucus that contains high levels of potassium.

Colonic metabolism is interesting and depends at least in part on the symbiotic relationship with the colonic microflora. Colonic bacteria are predominately anaerobic, followed by gram negative aerobes.[152] Colonic bacteria ferment proteins, fibers, and carbohydrates. Bacteria ferment carbohydrates to short chain fatty acids (SCFA). These fatty acids are the preferred metabolic fuel of colonocytes and are readily absorbed. SCFA increase sodium, chloride, and water absorption and may also regulate proliferation, differentiation, motor, and immune functions in the colon.[149]

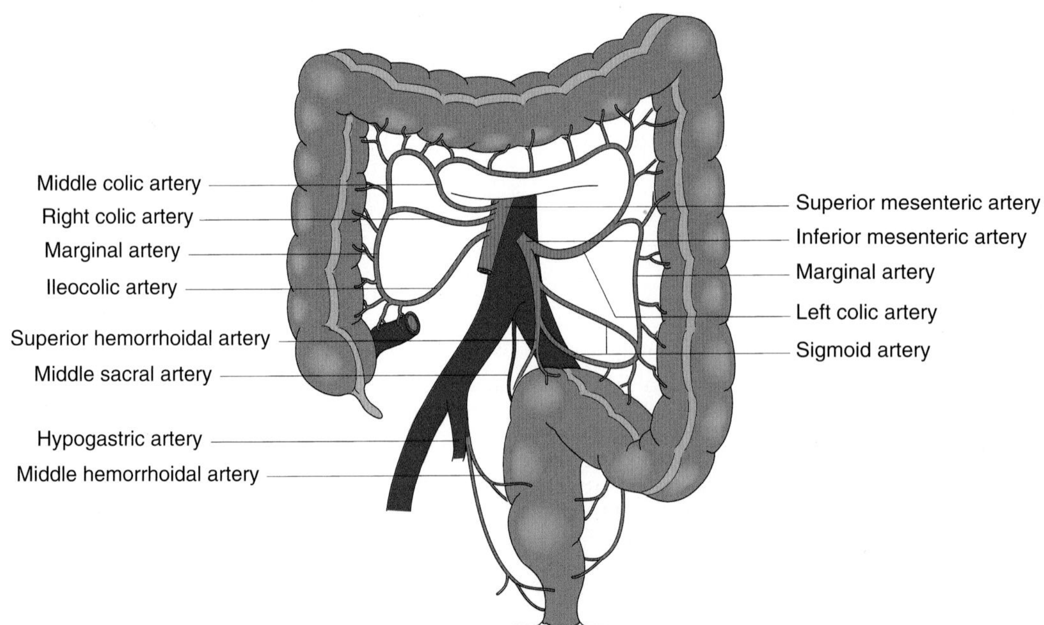

FIGURE 35.15. *Arterial anatomy of the colon.* The right colon and proximal transverse colon, which are embryologically derived from the midgut, have blood supply from the SMA, while the distal transverse, descending, and sigmoid colon, which are derived from the hindgut, have blood supply from the IMA. Rectal blood supply is from the IMA and the internal iliac arteries. (Reprinted from Greenfield LJ, Mulholland MW. *Greenfield's Surgery: Scientific Principles and Practice*. 4th ed. Philadelphia, PA: Wolters Kluwer Health/Lippincott Williams & Wilkins; 2006, with permission. Figure 65.3. Arterial blood supply of the colon.)

The motor function of the colon is complex and involves an interplay between propulsive and storage functions.[149,151] Contractions can be nonpropulsive, as well as both retrograde and antegrade propulsive movements. Grossly understated, segmental colonic motility matches functional properties of the colon. The right colon acts as a reservoir to mix and store, allowing the interplay of the complex microbiome and luminal nutrients, as well as absorption of salts and electrolytes. The left colon functions as a conduit, and the rectum and anus enable storage and continence.

An understanding of normal colon anatomy and physiology is essential to understand pathophysiology and disease, as well as to guide management of both acute and chronic colonic disease.

INFLAMMATORY AND INFECTIOUS EMERGENCIES OF THE COLON

The risk with most inflammatory processes of the colon is associated with compromise of the integrity of the colonic mucosa or perforation, both of which can result in life-threatening infection and sepsis. It is imperative as a surgeon to understand the natural history of these disease processes, appreciate the role of medical and surgical therapies, and to achieve timely source control if necessary. For most of these disease processes, delayed operative management in the setting of colonic necrosis or perforation significantly increases mortality. This section will focus on the most common inflammatory/infectious disease processes relevant to acute care surgery including diverticulitis, ischemic colitis, inflammatory bowel disease, and *Clostridium difficile* associated disease (CDAD).

Diverticulitis

Colonic diverticulosis refers to the presence of diverticulum in the colon in the absence of inflammation, while diverticulitis refers to the presence of inflammation and infection associated with a diverticulum.[153,154] The clinical spectrum of diverticulitis can range from relatively mild abdominal pain to sepsis. The term "diverticular disease" refers to all pathophysiological processes associated with colonic diverticulosis, including diverticulitis and diverticular bleeding. The diverticula in diverticulosis are pulsion or "false" diverticula, containing mucosa that essentially herniated through the muscular layers of the colon. Diverticula are typically 0.5–1 cm saccular outpouchings of the colon.[153]

Colonic diverticulosis is common in Western population and the incidence increases with age.[155] Diverticulosis is rarely seen in individuals younger than age 30. However, in Western society, the prevalence increases to 40% by the age of 60 years and 60%–80% by 80 years of age.[155–157] In most cases, diverticula involve the sigmoid and left colon. With increasing age, there is an increased prevalence of diverticulosis that extends more proximally in the colon. Interestingly, diverticulosis in Asian countries occurs more commonly as isolated diverticulosis of the right colon.

It is estimated that 10%–25% of patients with diverticulosis develop diverticulitis.[158–160] Although it is difficult to determine, the number, size, or extent of diverticula, it does not seem to correlate with the risk of developing diverticulitis. Studies suggest that the incidence of diverticulitis has been increasing over the past several decades in the U.S. population, but this may be in part secondary to the increased availability and use of CT.

Pathophysiology. As previously stated most colonic diverticula are pulsion diverticula. The formation is thought to be associated, in part, to increased intraluminal pressure.[153] The diverticula typically "herniate" or penetrate the colonic wall where the nutrient vessels (vasa recta) penetrate the circular muscle layer. Diverticula typically occur along either side of the mesenteric tenia or on the mesenteric border of the two antimesenteric tenias. Several hypotheses to explain the development of diverticulosis include generation of high intracolonic pressures secondary to disordered motility and the role of dietary fiber.[161–165] An alternative hypothesis has focused on collagen deposition in the colon wall and decreased colonic elasticity. This is referred to as tenia specific elastosis.[166] Additional risk factors for the development of diverticulosis include increasing age, geographic factors, cigarette smoking, nonsteroidal antiinflammatory use, obesity, decreased physical activity, and caffeine ingestion.[157]

The etiology of acute diverticulitis is thought to be similar to the development of acute appendicitis, in which obstruction of the diverticulum can lead to bacterial overgrowth, distention, and tissue ischemia. This results in localized inflammation, and possibly contained perforation with the formation of a peridiverticular abscess or free intraperitoneal perforation with peritonitis.[154,155] It is also possible for the inflammatory process to fistulize into adjacent structures, most commonly the bladder. The most commonly cultured isolates from abscesses or perforations associated with diverticulitis are anaerobic bacteria (*Bacteroides, Clostridium, Peptostreptococcus,* and *Fusobacterium*) followed by gram negative aerobes (*Escherichia coli*). *Enterococcus* is the most common gram positive aerobe.[167,168]

Symptoms/Clinical Manifestations. Approximately 10%–25% of patients with diverticulosis develop diverticulitis. The symptoms of diverticulitis range from mild abdominal pain to peritonitis and sepsis. Although the extent of symptoms often varies with the extent of inflammation, the degree of symptomatology likely depends on a number of other features including location of inflammation, extent of muscular dysfunction, and varying visceral sensitivity. The most common symptom complex during acute diverticulitis involves left lower quadrant pain and fever. Depending upon the location of inflammation and the redundancy of the sigmoid colon, pain may be also midline or in the right lower quadrant. Patients often describe a change in bowel habits with mild diarrhea. Bleeding per rectum is usually not associated with diverticulitis and would suggest other etiologies of colitis, including inflammatory bowel disease or ischemia. Nausea or vomiting may be present secondary to an associated ileus, a small bowel or large bowel obstruction secondary to phlegmon formation or inflammatory stricture. Physical examination most often reveals tenderness, at times with an associated mass. Laboratory evaluation often demonstrates leukocytosis.

Most often symptoms resolve after treatment with antibiotics. However, some patients will have "smoldering" disease that only partially improves and is marked by continued symptoms of left sided abdominal pain and low grade fevers.[169] Patients will often have crampy pain associated with a partial obstruction secondary to a continued phlegmon or stricture. Other patients with smoldering disease have more elusive symptoms of pain without fever or leukocytosis or imaging findings and this may be difficult to differentiate from irritable bowel syndrome.

When diverticulitis is associated with a colovesicular fistula, the infection or abscess is essentially drained by decompression into the urinary bladder and symptoms are marked by cystitis, pneumaturia, pyuria, or fecaluria.[170] Laboratory evaluation often reveals an abnormal urinalysis and polymicrobial urine culture. Similarly, colovaginal or uterine fistulae may present with vaginal discharge, passage of air or stool per vagina.

Differential Diagnosis. The differential diagnosis for patients with diverticulitis includes appendicitis, colorectal cancer, bowel obstruction, inflammatory bowel diseases, ischemic colitis, gynecological disease, and irritable bowel syndrome. Other diagnoses may include pyelonephritis, ureteral calculi, endometriosis, stercoral ulcer, or colonic volvulus. The use of CT as a diagnostic adjunct to history and physical can often confirm the diagnosis of diverticulitis or distinguish among the other potential diagnoses. Following the initial presentation of diverticulitis, the importance of endoscopy to exclude an underlying malignancy must be underscored; this is critical. Colonoscopy or sigmoidoscopy is most often performed at least 6 weeks after the episode of diverticulitis due to concerns of exacerbating microperforations secondary to intraluminal insufflation associated with performing these procedures.

Diagnostic Imaging. Although multiple imaging modalities are of potential use to diagnose suspected diverticulitis, none are as useful as CT.[171–173] Plain films are of limited value in confirmation of the diagnosis of diverticulitis, but may identify free intraperitoneal air as a nonspecific finding. Contrast enemas may be of utility to diagnose diverticulosis or strictures/mucosal abnormalities associated with diverticulitis. Water-soluble contrast should be used if an urgent operation or perforation is suspected, whereas barium should be avoided in this setting. Additionally, water soluble contrast may be of use in relieving partial obstruction secondary to the "slippery" nature of these agents and because high osmolarity may decrease tissue edema. It has been shown that ultrasound can demonstrate wall thickening, extraluminal air, and abscesses. However, ultrasound has not played a major role in the clinical diagnosis of diverticulitis in the United States.[174]

CT is both widely available and accurate. CT can accurately determine the diagnosis of diverticulitis, its complications, as well as other diagnoses (Fig. 35.16). Furthermore, severity-staging systems based upon CT findings in diverticulitis have been developed and are useful for determination of the morbidity and mortality, as well as the clinical course.[173,175] Moreover, CT severity scoring also correlated with recurrence in patients who were managed nonoperatively.[176] The scoring system that has gained the most wide spread acceptance is the Hinchey classification system (Fig. 35.17).

Management. Uncomplicated diverticulitis is treated with antibiotic therapy.[157,168] Based upon the common culture

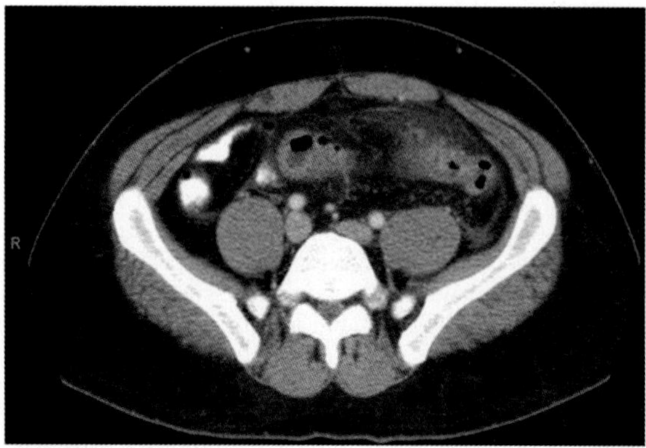

FIGURE 35.16. CT scans of the colon revealing changes of acute diverticulitis.

results in patients with diverticular abscesses or perforations, most isolates are polymicrobial. The most common aerobic gram negative is *Escherichia coli*, aerobic gram positive is *Enterococcus*, and anaerobic is *Bacteroides fragilis*. Antibiotic regimens for the treatment of diverticulitis should have: (1) activity against these common bacteria, (2) good tissue penetration, (3) minimal toxicity, and (4) clinical efficacy.[168] There are a number of single or combination regimens that will satisfy at least the first three of these criteria (Table 35.6). Recommendations have been put forth by multiple societies including the American Society of Colon and Rectal Surgeons and the American College of Gastroenterology.[159,177] Additionally, the Surgical Infection Society and the Infectious Disease Society of America have also put forth applicable antibiotic regimens for complicated intraabdominal infections. However, these guidelines also involve source control (drainage procedures or surgical resection) and may not be as applicable to patients with uncomplicated diverticulitis who are treated with antibiotics alone.[168] The ideal regimen(s) has not been determined. Piperacillin/tazobactam or carbapenems are often used in hospitalized or higher risk patients based upon their broad spectrum of activity. Fluoroquinolones plus metronidazole are often used in uncomplicated diverticulitis based upon the ability to convert to oral therapy without need to change the antibiotic. Oral regimens include amoxicillin/clavulanic acid, moxifloxacin, ciprofloxacin and metronidazole, or trimethoprim/sulfamethoxazole and metronidazole. The ideal duration of antibiotic therapy in uncomplicated or complicated diverticulitis is not defined.

Patients with minimal symptoms and mild clinical findings on exam are often treated as outpatients on oral regimens for 7–14 days. Patients who present with more severe tenderness, fever, systemic symptoms, or inability to tolerate oral intake are most often hospitalized. These patients most often will undergo laboratory evaluations as well as CT. Patients with uncomplicated disease (Hinchey stages 0 or I) are generally treated with bowel rest and a parenteral regimen and then transitioned to an oral regimen following clinical improvement.

Some studies have demonstrated a benefit of immunomodulatory agents in the treatment of diverticulitis that does not require source control.[168,178–180] These have included 5-ASA products and mesalamine. Because of the inflammation involved in diverticulitis, these agents may prove to have a role in treating diverticulitis, particularly to decrease future recurrences. Additional therapies under investigation include rifaximin or probiotics.[181]

Diverticular abscesses are present in approximately 15% of patients with diverticulitis who have undergone CT. These abscesses can be mesocolic or pericolic (Hinchey stage I) or pelvic or retroperitoneal (Hinchey stage II). Patients with diverticular abscesses that are larger and have a radiologic window (accessible) are treated with percutaneous drainage as a means of source control, in addition to antibiotic therapy.[182] "Large" is a subjective term and usually is an abscess larger than 4 cm.[183] Percutaneous drainage may be more successful in patients with simple, nonloculated abscesses, or patients with mesocolic or pericolic abscesses. Transabdominal drainage is generally preferable, however, transgluteal, transperineal, transvaginal, or transrectal drainage are alternatives.

The ideal therapy for patients with diverticular abscess is actively debated. In general, percutaneous drainage is added as an adjunctive therapy in patients with larger abscesses that have a radiologic window.[183–186] The decision for operation in these patients is made on a case-by-case basis. Clinical response is followed. If the patient fails to improve or the clinical condition worsens, repeat CT to evaluate for recurrent or persistent abscesses is often performed or operation is recommended. Although the role and timing for elective surgical resection is also debated, patients with Hinchey stage 0, I, and

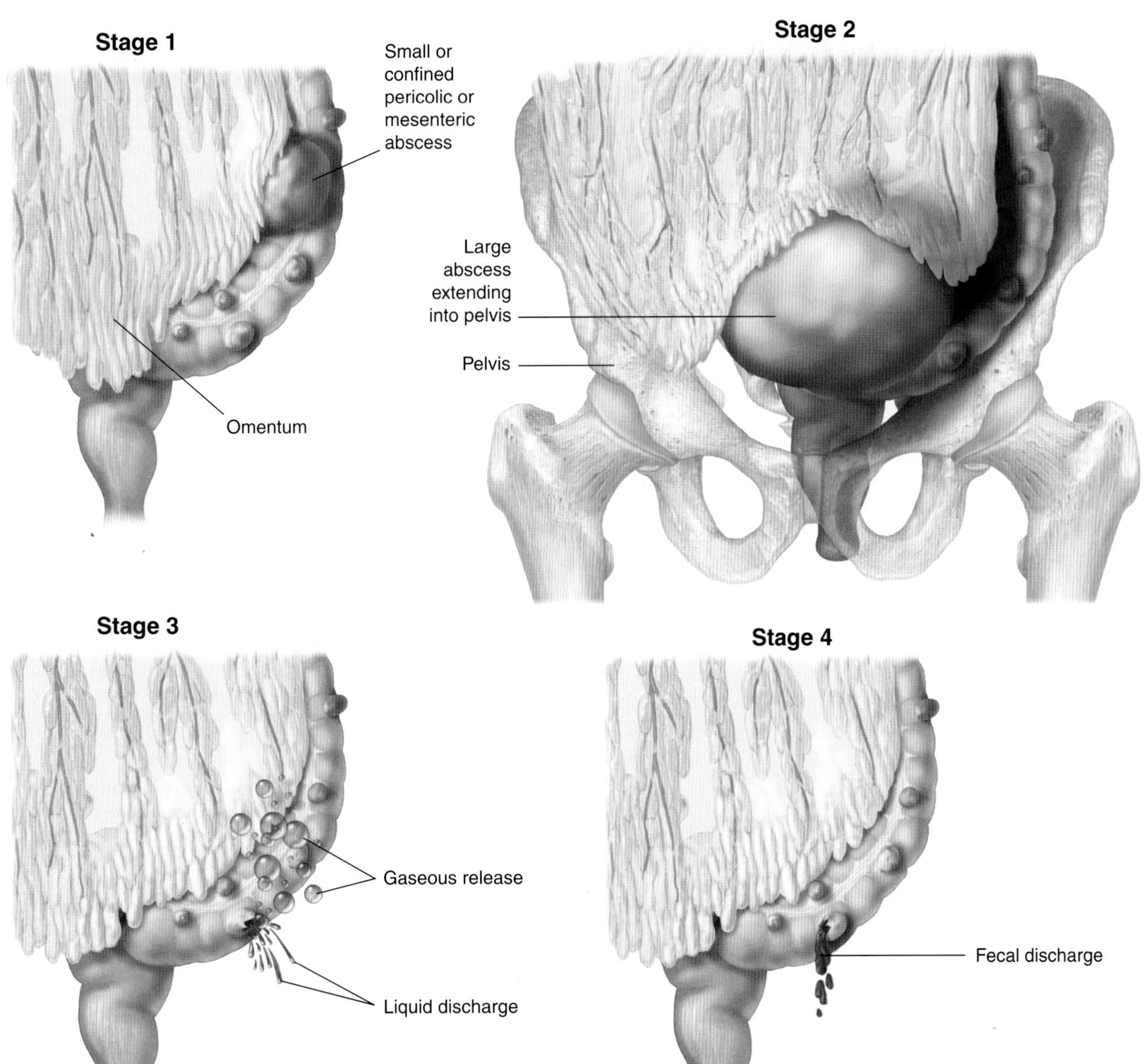

FIGURE 35.17. Representative Hinchey staging of diverticulitis. Stage 0 (not depicted) is mild diverticulitis without abscess formation. Stage I disease consists of small, pericolic of mesenteric abscesses, whereas stage II disease has abscesses that are either pelvic or distant intra-abdominal sites. Stage III consists of purulent peritonitis, while stage IV represents fecal peritonitis.

II ideally can be treated with antibiotics with or without percutaneous drainage and elective surgical resection offered in the future if indicated. As suggested, patients with complicated diverticulitis should undergo elective laparoscopic sigmoid resection after resolution of the acute episode.

When and if to operate on the patient with repeated bouts of uncomplicated diverticulitis is far more controversial. Traditional teaching until recently was that colon resection was offered for patients with two or more bouts of uncomplicated diverticulitis (inflammation limited to the colon) or any patient under age 50 with an episode of diverticulitis. The rationale was that these patients had high risk of recurrent disease, with concern for perforation. More recent data have disproven this assumption. In fact, 70% of patients with free perforation from diverticulitis have no prior episode of symptomatic disease. The 2006 recommendation by the Society of Colorectal Surgeons states, "the decision to recommend elective sigmoid colectomy after recovery from acute diverticulitis (uncomplicated) should be made on a case by case basis as the number of attacks is not necessarily the overriding factor in defining the appropriateness of surgery."[159] On the other hand, diverticulitis in immunosuppressed patients, specifically transplant patients, does seem to be more virulent. Elective sigmoid resection should be considered after the first episode of diverticulitis.

Patients with free perforation and purulent peritonitis or feculent peritonitis (Hinchey stage III or IV) should be treated with surgical management. Only 1% of patients will develop

TABLE 35.6

ANTIMICROBIAL THERAPY OPTIONS FOR ACUTE DIVERTICULITIS

Single agent regimens
Cephalosporin
Cefoxitin[a]
Penicillin/beta-lactamase inhibitor combinations
Ampicillin/sulbactam[c]; Ticaricillin/clavulinic acid;
Piperacillin/tazobactam
Carbapenem
Imipenem/cilastatin; Meropenem; Doripenem; Ertapenem
Glycylcycline
Tigecycline
Fluoroquinolone
Moxifloxacin
Combination regimens
Aminoglycoside[c] + an antianaerobic agent[d]
Tobramycin; Gentamicin
Cephalosporin + an antianaerobic agent[d]
Cefotaxime; Ceftriaxone; Ceftazidime; Cefepime
Monobactam + an antianaerobic agent
Aztreonam
Trimethoprim/sulfamethoxazole[e] + an antianaerobic agent[d]
Fluoroquinolone + an antianaerobic agent
Ciprofloxacin
Levofloxacin
Oral regimens
Moxifloxacin
Amoxicillin/clavulanic acid
Ciprofloxacin + metronidazole
Trimethoprim/sulfamethoxazole + metronidazole

[a]Not recommended because of increased resistance of *B. fragilis*.
[b]Not recommended as first line therapy because of increased resistance of *E. coli*.
[c]Not recommended as first line therapy because of toxicity concerns.
[d]Metronidazole or clindamycin have been used; however the utility of clindamycin is questioned because of increased resistance of *B. fragilis* and the association with *Clostridium* difficile colitis.
[e]Not FDA approved for intra-abdominal infections.

free perforation, and this is most often the initial attack of diverticulitis. Historically, surgical therapy was performed as a three stage operation (upstream diversion, followed by resection and colorectal anastomosis, and finally restoration of continuity). The mainstay of surgical treatment for perforated diverticulitis or complicated diverticulitis requiring urgent operation has been the Hartmann procedure. This involves resection of the involved disease segment, end colostomy and a blind pouch at the rectum. This procedure eliminates the septic focus, but has the disadvantage of requiring a second major operation. Studies have demonstrated that a high number of patients (up to 35%), particularly those of advanced age or with severe comorbidity never undergo reversal of their end colostomy.[187,188] Retrospective review has illustrated that Hartmann's procedures were associated with an 18.8% mortality, a wound infection rate of 24.2%, and stoma complications in 10.3%.[189] For this procedure, resect the minimal amount of colon necessary for source control, with limited pelvic mobilization or mobilization of the splenic flexure, essentially performing a "perforectomy" with margins only as extensive to allow creation of an ostomy and closure of the Hartmann stump. This approach makes the subsequent operation less difficult and facilitates dissection of the rectal stump and mobilization of the splenic flexure for anastomosis. A wide mesenteric resection is not necessary. Identification of the ureter is preferred. It should be noted that additional resection of the distal sigmoid colon down to the site of splaying of the tenia coli is advocated at the time of second operation, that is, do not leave the sigmoid colon distally. Proximal resection is usually still limited to soft pliable colon without diverticula at the site of anastomosis. If proximal colon contains diverticula and the colon is otherwise grossly normal, this is left in place.

There is increased interest in alternative surgical treatment other than the Hartmann procedure. Several studies have suggested that in select patients with Hinchey stages III or IV diverticulitis, resection with primary anastomosis is superior to Hartmann resection.[190–192] In these studies, there is a selection bias in patients who underwent resection with primary anastomosis. Several clinical and patient-related issues should be considered as contraindications to this approach, including hemodynamic instability, diffuse peritonitis, significant bowel wall edema, ischemia, immunocompromised state, and ischemia.

An additional alternative that is being utilized for the acute presentation is laparoscopic exploration with peritoneal lavage.[193–199] Laparoscopic exploration is performed; if feculent peritonitis is found, the patient is converted to a laparotomy and a resection is performed. However, if the finding is purulent peritonitis, the patient's sigmoid colon is not mobilized or resected and the peritoneum is lavaged laparoscopically and a drain is left. Early studies demonstrate this approach to be promising. In a review of 213 patients from 8 studies with a 38-month follow up, 3% of cases were converted to an open procedure.[193] Ten percent of patients had complications and thirty-one percent of patients went on to have an elective resection with primary anastomosis.

Colovesical fistulae often require surgical treatment, however an urgent operation is rarely required, as the fistula usually serves to "drain" or decompress the infection.[170,200]. If a patient is highly symptomatic with symptoms of cystitis, then suppressive antibiotics are utilized. Management of a colovesical fistula at the time of operative exploration infrequently requires resection of the bladder. The fistula is usually "pinched off" the colon and the fistulous tract often may not be identified. A suture repair is necessary in few cases. We advocate an indwelling foley catheter with a cystogram prior to removal of the catheter, usually after 7–10 days postoperatively. When managed electively, as in all cases of diverticulitis, colonoscopy or sigmoidoscopy should be performed preoperatively to exclude a malignancy, in addition to cystoscopy to exclude primary bladder neoplasm.

Diverticular strictures can result in partial or complete bowel obstruction. Most often this is associated with repeated attacks of diverticulitis. The management of obstruction is covered in more detail in Chapter XX).

Infectious Colitides

There are a number of infections which can result in colitis. These include *C. difficile*, *Campylobacter*, *Salmonella*, *Yersinia*, *Shigella*, and *E. coli*. Additionally, CMV can result in colitis, particularly in immunosuppressed patients. Additional infections include amebic colitis from *Entamoeba histolytica* and toxic megacolon in Chagas disease from *Trypanosoma cruzi*. This chapter will focus on CDAD as this bacterium is now considered the leading nosocomial infection.

C. Difficile Associated Disease

C. difficile is a gram positive, spore forming anaerobe. *CDAD* affects over 3 million patients annually, causing 15%–35% of antibiotic-associated diarrhea, and 70% of cases of antibiotic-associated colitis.[201] *C. difficile* colitis was initially identified in the 1970s and has since gained increasing notoriety due to its associated high morbidity (30%–80%) and mortality (4%–10%).[202] The reported incidence of "fulminant" or "severe, complicated" *CDAD*, defined as the most severe manifestation of *CDAD* with concomitant systemic toxicity and organ dysfunction is increasing. Additionally, recurrence is common, occurring in approximately 25% of patients.[203]

Pathophysiology. *CDAD* is acquired through the oral ingestion of *C. difficile* spores, which are resistant to gastric acidity and thus able to germinate into the vegetative form in the small intestine. Kyne et al. demonstrated that 31% of patients who received antibiotics in the hospital were colonized with *C. difficile*, and 56% of these patients developed symptomatic disease.[204] With colonization and depletion of competitive flora the *C. difficile* is free to overgrow and produce exotoxins (principally toxins A and B), which induce mucosal death and inflammatory changes. Essentially, this is a disease of colonic bacterial overgrowth. Most often, the consequences of toxin production are limited to the colon, resulting in the stereotypical diarrhea associated with this infection. In that small subset of patients with severe and fulminant disease, the consequences of the toxemia become systemic.[203]

Why only a subset of patients exposed to antibiotics become colonized, why only a fraction of these patients develop symptomatic disease, and why some patients suffer more severe disease compared to others is largely unknown. Some authors suggest that differing humoral antibody responses to the toxins are largely responsible for both the development of infection/colitis and the varying severity of disease.[205–207] Major risk factors for the development of *CDAD* are antibiotic exposure, hospitalization and advanced age (Table 35.7).

Symptoms/Clinical Manifestation. The severity of symptoms from *CDAD* ranges from mild diarrhea to sepsis. The most common clinical presentation is diarrhea associated with history of antibiotic use (either a few days after the antibiotic is started up to 12 weeks after the termination of antibiotics). Patients with diarrhea may have cramps, fever, and fecal leukocytes. Bowel movements are usually watery, with a characteristic foul smell. Fever, high leukocytosis, and abdominal pain usually localized to the lower quadrants accompany the diarrhea. Hypoalbuminemia often occurs as a result of large protein losses and is a sign of severe disease. For most mild cases, diarrhea is usually the only symptom. However, there are rare occasions, especially in toxic patients with ileus, during which diarrhea may be absent.

TABLE 35.7

RISK FACTORS FOR THE DEVELOPMENT OF CDAD

Antibiotics
Hospitalization
Long-term care facilities
Immunosuppression
Advanced age
Postoperative
Proton pump inhibitors
Elemental diets
Inflammatory bowel disease

Diagnosis. Having an index of suspicion is the most important component to making the diagnosis of *CDAD*. The diagnosis of *CDAD* is based on a combination of clinical and laboratory findings: symptoms, almost always diarrhea, plus a stool test positive for *C. difficile* toxins or toxigenic *C. difficile*. Visual or pathologic evidence of pseudomembranous colitis is also diagnostic. A careful history will usually confirm exposure to antibiotics; abatement of diarrhea in response to medical therapy supports the diagnosis. There are multiple laboratory tests available, however, the clinically most useful test with greatest sensitivity and specificity is cell cytotoxicity assay, which relies on the cytotoxic effects of toxin from stool samples on cells in culture.[208–210]

CT, with or without contrast, is a useful adjunct for evaluation of the colon in a patient with suspected *CDAD*. It is far less sensitive than stool toxin assays, and the changes seen are rarely diagnostic. The sensitivity and specificity of CT to identify colonic abnormalities in these patients is 52%–85% and 48%–93%, respectively.[211] In cases in which surgical consultation is desired, fulminant colitis characteristically features colonic-thickening, pericolonic-stranding, and the "accordion sign" (oral contrast material with high attenuation in the colonic lumen alternating with an inflamed mucosa with low attenuation). A "double-halo sign"/"target sign" is often seen with IV contrast representing varying degrees of attenuation of the mucosa secondary to hyperemia and submucosal inflammation). Most severe *CDAD* will show changes throughout the entire colon (pancolitis) and moderate quantities of ascitic fluid (Fig. 35.18). In one series, CT predicted the operative findings in 94% of cases.[212]

Management. In all cases, standard hospital isolation precautions must be instituted to reduce the spread of the disease. If possible, the antibiotics previously employed for the treatment of systemic infections should be discontinued, a goal which cannot always be accomplished because of persistent systemic infections. The recommended oral medications (metronidazole or vancomycin) must be given into the digestive tract so that the highest concentrations reach the colon. The two drugs are equally effective for mild or moderate disease, but metronidazole is less expensive.[213–215] Mild or moderate disease in adults usually responds to oral metronidazole 500 mg three times per day or 250 mg four times per day for 10–14 days. Severe disease, most often characterized by fever, leukocytosis [15–20,000 cells/mm^3], cramps, and diarrhea but without hypotension, ileus, or megacolon is better treated with vancomycin 125 mg four times per day for 10–14 days.[203]. First recurrences can be successfully retreated with either drug regimen but second and subsequent recurrences require a course of vancomycin with a taper of therapy over time. Patients who cannot tolerate oral antibiotics may be treated with intravenous metronidazole 500 mg IV every 8 hours. Parenteral metronidazole achieves therapeutic concentrations in the colon via biliary secretion but only in patients with diarrhea. It is important to remember that neither oral nor parenteral metronidazole reaches therapeutic concentrations in normal stool; thus continuing its administration more than 14 days in patients whose diarrhea resolves has no therapeutic value. Oral vancomycin, on the other hand, achieves effective concentrations in both normal and unformed stool so that recurrences are best treated with oral vancomycin. Vancomycin by the intravenous route is totally ineffective against *CDAD* because it does not reach the intestinal lumen.

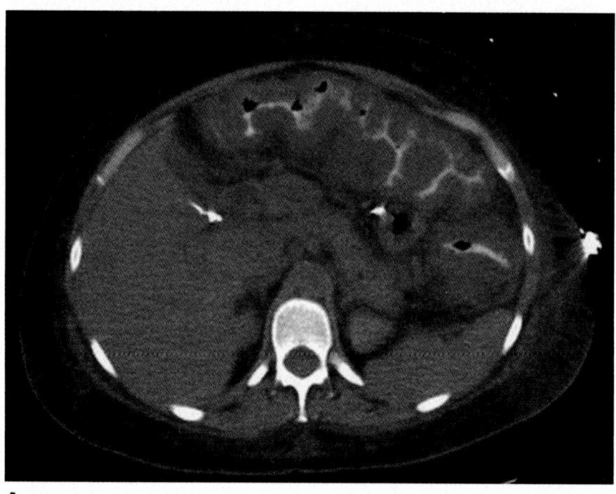

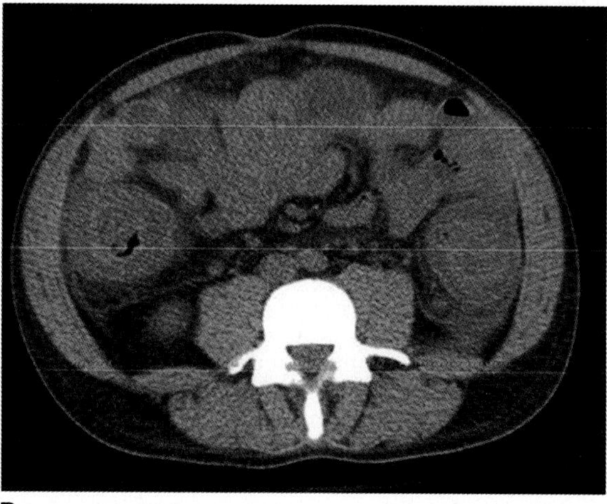

FIGURE 35.18. CT scans showing colitis in CDAD. CT scan findings of CDAD include colonic wall thickening, often involving the entire colon (pancolitis), pericolonic edema and mesenteric fat stranding, and ascites.

These therapeutic guidelines require amplification when patients do not respond or deteriorate during treatment. In any patient with severe disease, whether presenting initially with fever and leukocytosis complicating the diarrhea or these findings develop during medical treatment, early surgical consultation is required so that concurrent medical/surgical treatment planning can proceed for the unusual case in which operative intervention will be required. Surgical treatment has been demonstrated to improve outcomes in severe complicated *CDAD*, that is, in patients admitted to intensive care units with organ failure, or the need for vasoactive agents or ventilatory assistance. Although successful in many patients, the timing of operative intervention is difficult. Total abdominal colectomy, for example, the standard treatment of severe complicated disease, often referred to as "fulminant" *CDAD*, carries considerable morbidity and mortality (35%–85%).[203,216] The fear of these complications of treatment can lead to excessive deferral of surgical consultation, and an even less favorable outcome.

Early experiences from our group suggest that severe, complicated CDAD can be treated operatively (avoiding colon resection) with creation of a loop ileostomy and intraoperative colonic lavage, followed by antegrade vancomycin flushes of the colon via the ileostomy (in print). Using this approach, mortality has significantly decreased at our institution. Ileostomy can be reversed 3 months after the initial operation if the patient's clinical condition allows. This approach has the hypothetical advantages of improved short-term and long-term outcomes and avoidance of colectomy. However, it remains to be validated as an alternative to colectomy for the treatment of severe, complicated CDAD. Algorithm 35.2 highlights a recommended treatment strategy for patients with CDAD.

Bacterial Enterocolitides

A number of bacterial infections can cause enterocolitis. These include *E. coli, Campylobacter*, *Salmonella*, *Yersinia*, and *Shigella*. The most common symptom from these infections is diarrhea. The care is mainly supportive from a fluid and electrolyte standpoint. Additionally, treatment with antibiotics can hasten recovery. Typically, fluoroquinolones are first line antibiotics. The nonabsorbable rifamycin-based antibiotic rifaximin can be used for noninvasive *E. coli* infections. Although these infections can be quite serious, they typically do not require surgical consultation or treatment.

Cytomegalovirus Colitis

CMV is a double stranded DNA herpes virus. Although 50%–80% of the world's population is seropositive for CMV, generally, only immunocompromised patients develop invasive CMV infection. In an immunocompetent host, the CMV virus stays in a chronic latent state in the host's cells and viral proliferation is prevented by host cell-mediated immunity.[217] Although, there are reports of CMV causing colitis in older patients without obvious immunodeficiency, it is generally limited to patients with immunodeficiency.[218] CMV colitis is seen in 2%–16% of patients with solid organ transplants and 3%–5% of patients with HIV/AIDS.[219,220] Another population prone to CMV colitis is the group of patients with ulcerative colitis. CMV colitis has been reported in 27.3% of patients with steroid refractory colitis and 9.1% of patients with nonrefractory colitis.[221] Symptoms usually involve watery diarrhea, fever, and weight loss. However, there may be little diarrhea and blood per rectum in up to 30% of patients.

CMV colitis may be difficult to discern from other forms of colitis. When the colon becomes affected by tissue-invasive CMV, ulcerative changes can be seen. As ulcers increase in depth, erosion into blood vessels can cause profuse bloody diarrhea. Over time, inflammatory polyps may develop, which, rarely, may obstruct the colon. Colonoscopy and biopsy should diagnose CMV infection. Histological findings include giant cells (25–35 μm) with cytomegaly and large ovoid or pleomorphic nuclei containing basophilic inclusions (owl's eyes, halo rim). Culture for CMV may be positive, but testing for viral antigens using immunofluoresecent antibodies increases the sensitivity for detection of CMV.[222] CMV infection of the colon causes a vasculitis that may cause severe pain. Initially, because of the severe pain and peritonitis that can be found on exam, exploratory laparotomy and surgical resection

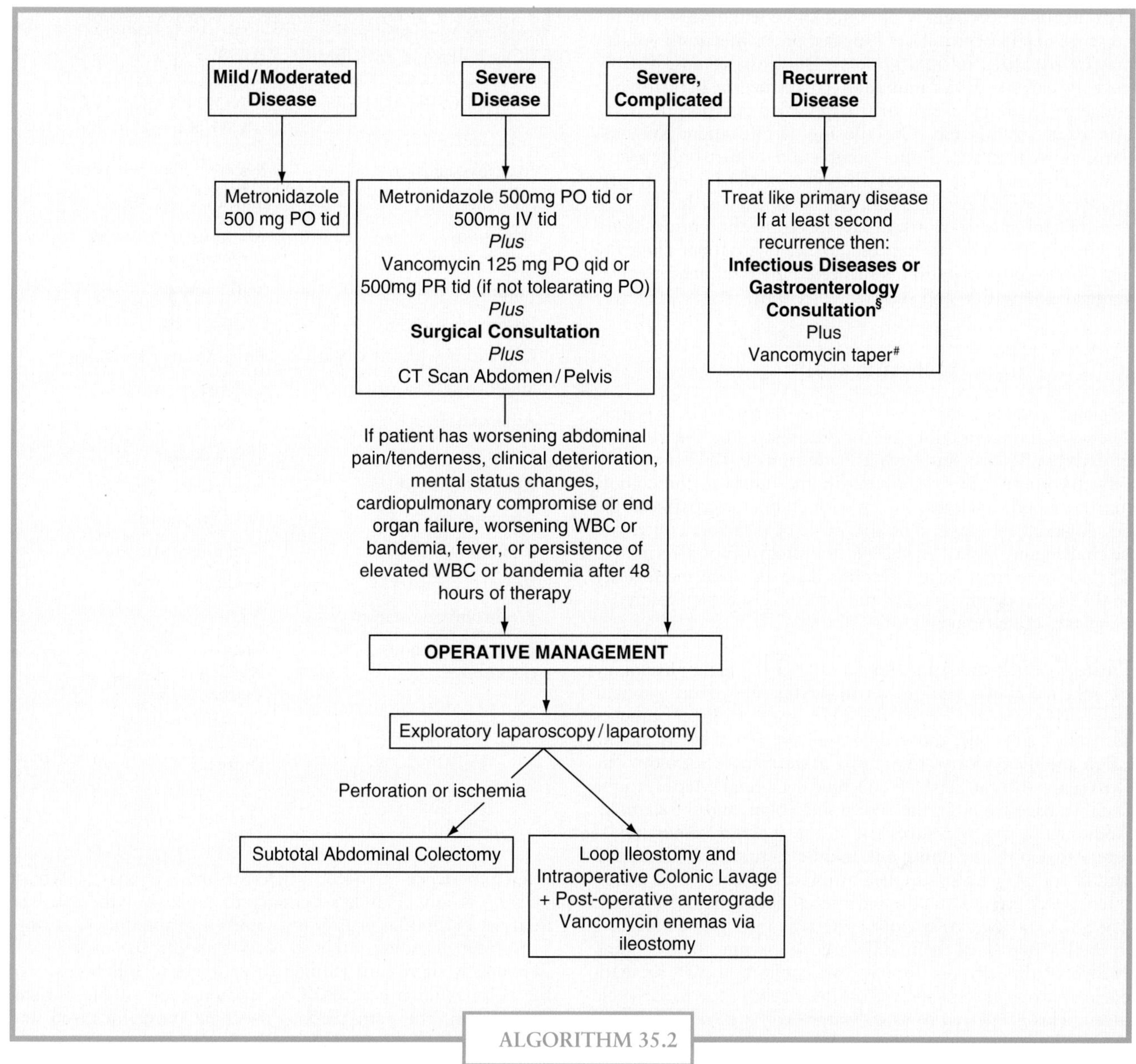

ALGORITHM 35.2 Treatment algorithm for *CDAD*. This protocol lowers what has been the standard threshold for operative therapy when compared to typical strategies that utilize operative management as a salvage type of procedure. Severe and severe complicated CDAD as defined by Society for Healthcare Epidemiology of America (SHEA) and the Infectious Diseases Society of America (IDSA). (Cohen SH, Gerding DN, Johnson S, et al. Clinical practice guidelines for Clostridium difficile infection in adults: 2010 update by the society for healthcare epidemiology of America (SHEA) and the infectious diseases society of America (IDSA). *Infect Control Hosp Epidemiol.* 2010:31(5):431–455.) §For second or more recurrent episodes we recommend consultation and management in conjunction with either the Infectious Diseases or Gastroenterology Divisions, depending on local practices. #Second recurrences are most often treated with a vancomycin course in which the frequency of dosing is decreased over multiple weeks.

was common. Additionally, if left untreated the severe inflammation and vasculitis may lead to ischemia and transmural necrosis of the bowel, resulting in perforation and peritonitis. With increased awareness of CMV infection in immunocompromised patients and treatment with antivirals, the need for operation is now rare. However, a continued challenge exists in patients with ulcerative colitis, where CMV colitis is also prevalent and can result in toxic megacolon. Antiviral therapy may resolve this condition, but if the diagnosis is not considered in patients with ulcerative colitis and therapy is initiated late in the course, colectomy may be necessary. First line antiviral therapy is ganciclovir, with foscarnet used as a second line therapy in most cases.[223]

Amebic Colitis

Amebic colitis, also known as amebiasis, is caused by invasion of the intestine by the protozoan parasite, *E. histolytica*. Although primarily a disease found in underdeveloped countries, this condition may exist in patients who have recently traveled outside the United States.[224,225] An accurate history, including travel and sexual history, is crucial to make the diagnosis. *E. histolytica* is found worldwide, but is most prevalent in Africa, Central and South America, and Asia. Symptoms usually include fever, crampy abdominal pain and diarrhea that may be bloody. Physical exam is not specific.

Fecal examination usually does not show leukocytes, and the presence of leukocytes should suggest other infections. Ameba may be visualized in stool samples. Diagnosis is most reliably made by enzyme-linked immunoassay testing for *E. histolytica* antigens. Treatment is primarily supportive care plus the addition of metronidazole. Oral dosing of the aminoglycoside paromomycin is added after completion of metronidazole if symptoms resolve to destroy the cysts in the lumen. Loperamide is avoided in the treatment of amebiasis. In the case of fulminant amebic colitis, broad-spectrum antibiotics should be given in addition to metronidazole. If a patient clinically deteriorates or perforation is suspected the treatment involves surgical exploration and subtotal colectomy.

Ischemic Colitis

Ischemic colitis is the most common form of GI ischemia. There are numerous etiologies for ischemic colitis, but all result in decreased blood supply that is injurious to the colon.[226–228] Ischemic colitis can range from limited injury to the colonic mucosa to full thickness injury with colonic necrosis and the development of sepsis. The diagnosis of ischemic colitis can be challenging, and often the exact etiology is not determined. The outcome from ischemic colitis depends upon the severity of the injury, the duration of the ischemia, and the rapidity of diagnosis and treatment.

Pathophysiology. An understanding of the pathophysiology of ischemic colitis requires an understanding of the vascular supply (Fig. 35.15).[151,229–231] The SMA gives off direct branches (ileocolic, right colic, and middle colic arteries) to the ascending colon and the proximal two thirds of the transverse colon. The IMA gives off branches (left colic and sigmoidal arteries) to the distal transverse colon, the descending colon, and the sigmoid. Additionally, the IMA gives rise to the superior hemorrhoidal artery to supply the upper and middle rectum. The lower and middle rectum are also supplied by direct branches of the paired internal iliac arteries (middle and inferior hemorrhoidal arteries). The SMA and IMA collateralize primarily through a connection in the left branch of the middle colic artery and the ascending branch of the left colic artery. This connection may be inadequate leaving the splenic flexure relatively prone to ischemic insult. This is referred to as a "watershed" area or "Griffiths" point'.[232] Another region that may be prone to ischemic insult is the area of the colon between that supplied by the distal sigmoid branches and the superior hemorrhoidal artery.[229,231]

Blood flow to the colon can be decreased secondary to changes in perfusion that affect the systemic vasculature or local changes in blood flow in the mesenteric vasculature. The etiologies are often classified as occlusive or nonocclusive (Table 35.8).[233] Examples of *occlusive* include embolic phenomena, thrombosis, atherosclerosis, or small vessel disease. Examples of *nonocclusive* include shock states, medication effects, or colonic obstructions. Nonocclusive ischemia results in a low flow state to the colon or mesenteric vasoconstriction. Interestingly, systemic low flow states often affect the right colon, whereas localized nonocclusive ischemia tends to affect watershed areas. Specific clinical situations that can precipitate ischemic colitis include aortic surgery that compromises flow to the IMA, as well as angiographic embolization to treat GI bleeding.[234–236]

TABLE 35.8

ETIOLOGIES OF ISCHEMIC COLITIS

OCCLUSIVE CAUSES	NON-OCCLUSIVE CAUSES
Arterial occlusion	Systemic hypoperfusion
Embolus	Shock
Thrombosis	Major cardiovascular surgery/bypass
Trauma	Snake venom
Postaortic surgery	Anaphylaxis
Colectomy with IMA ligation	Long-distance running
Small vessel disease	Colonic obstruction
Atherosclerosis	Volvulus
Vasculitis	Colon cancer
Rheumatoid arthritis	Strangulated hernia
Amyloidosis	Fecal impaction
Radiation injury	Pseudo-obstruction
Venous occlusion	Medications
Prothrombotic states	Digoxin
Mesenteric venous thrombosis	Cocaine NSAIDs Vasopressors Pseudoephedrine Interferon-ribavirin Diuretics

Symptoms/Clinical Manifestation. Although there are varied etiologies, the clinical presentation of ischemic colitis is quite uniform. Often, the onset is sudden, crampy abdominal pain that is poorly localized. Pain from ischemia of the left sided colon often is appreciated vaguely in the left lower quadrant or flank, and that of right sided ischemia is appreciated centrally. After the onset of abdominal pain, patients will often experience the need to defecate and will pass bloody or maroon stools. This is secondary to mucosal ischemia. The quantity of blood is usually not significant, and if there is more substantial bleeding, other etiologies should be suspected. If ischemia is significant enough to progress to full necrosis of the colon, which can result in inflammation of the parietal peritoneum, the pain tends to become more localized and significant.

Physical examination generally reveals mild tenderness that may be more pronounced over the ischemic segment. Peritonitis is present when there is transmural necrosis. Depending upon the etiology of the ischemic colitis, the patient may have hemodynamic instability. The majority of patients who develop ischemic colitis in nonhospitalized settings present with normal hemodynamics and mild tenderness as the only findings.

Laboratory evaluations are nonspecific. Patients with more substantial ischemia may have an elevated white blood cell count. Electrolytes may be abnormal if a patient is dehydrated. If there is more significant ischemia, patients may have a metabolic acidosis, an elevated base deficit on arterial blood gases, as well as an elevated lactate; all are nonspecific. D-Lactate may be a more useful value to follow, as D-Lactate is produced by bacterial fermentation in the colon.[237] In the setting of mucosal ischemia, D-Lactate levels can increase in the systemic circulation secondary to increased mucosal permeability to this stereoisomer. D-Lactate levels have a sensitivity of 82%–90% and a specificity of 77%–87% in prediction of early colonic ischemia.[237,238]

Diagnosis. Diagnosis of ischemic colitis is made by history and physical examination in combination with radiologic studies and colonoscopic inspection. Plain films of the abdomen are of limited utility and not sensitive, but may demonstrate thickened colon wall, thumbprinting on the colon wall, and rarely pneumatosis coli. Some advocate air contrast enemas, which may enhance visualization of thumbprinting.[239,240] Contrast enemas are generally avoided in the acute setting of ischemic colitis as they do not offer much information and can worsen ischemia if the colon is over distended. These studies may have a role in the follow up on the consequences of ischemia such as stricture.

CT with intravenous contrast is useful to assess acute mesenteric ischemia, as well as other pathology. Intravenous contrast allows visualization of the mesenteric arteries as well as the mesenteric venous system. CT angiography or conventional angiography may be indicated if mesenteric ischemia is suspected. Findings of ischemic colitis on CT scan are nonspecific, including colon thickening and ascites.[241] Ultrasound and Doppler flow studies are not reliable to consistently make a diagnosis.[242]

Colonoscopy is the most sensitive and specific diagnostic test. Early ischemia is visualized as changes in the mucosa. It will appear pale and edematous, and there may be hyperemic appearing patches. Advancing ischemia can be visualized as blackish nodules protruding into the lumen. These occur as a result of submucosal hemorrhage. If there are areas of mucosa that are gray-green or black, this suggests more advanced ischemia and should raise concern for transmural ischemia. Colonoscopy also allows biopsy to help differentiate inflammatory, ischemic, and infectious causes of colitis if these are in the differential diagnosis. Colonoscopy should be performed with caution as to not over distend the colon, which may exacerbate ischemia or precipitate perforation.

Management. In the absence of signs of colonic gangrene or perforation, ischemic colitis is managed nonoperatively.[243] Most patients with colonic ischemia have mucosal limited disease and fall into this category. Intravenous fluids are started and patients are resuscitated if there is evidence of volume depletion. Patients are placed on bowel rest and should not eat or drink. If patients have significant ileus or bowel distension then a nasogastric tube is placed for suction. Cardiac function is optimized and drugs which can impair mesenteric blood flow are limited if possible. Although there is little data to support this practice, most patients are placed on broad spectrum antibiotics to cover the usual colonic anaerobic and aerobic bacteria. Other pharmacologics that can improve mesenteric blood flow such as glucagon and papaverine have not been studied rigorously enough to support their use. Bowel preps or enemas are typically avoided as this may worsen ischemia. Patients are monitored for signs of deterioration, including fever, tachycardia, worsening exam, leukocytosis, or sepsis.

If transmural colonic necrosis, infarction, or perforation is suspected, prompt operative exploration is indicated. The ischemic colon is resected. Margins of resection should be based upon any evidence of ischemia and most would advocate resection to points with normal mucosa. This may be difficult to assess by inspection of the serosal surface of the colon and may be aided by direct mucosal inspection, either by colonoscopy or opening the resected specimen to evaluate mucosa at the margins for variability. Exploratory laparotomy allows assessment of colonic blood flow via visible inspection and palpation of pulses. If ischemia involves multiple segments or is more advanced, a subtotal colectomy may be performed. The decision to perform an end colostomy or ileostomy depends upon the etiology of the ischemic colitis. Anastomosis is usually avoided in patients with hemodynamic instability or immunocompromised patients. If the ischemic segment is focal, the bowel margins are clearly viable and healthy, and there is no ongoing pathology to precipitate further ischemia, anastomosis can be performed. The adjunct of intraoperative colonic lavage or the addition of upstream fecal diversion, usually with a diverting loop ileostomy should be contemplated when an anastomosis is being performed.

The prognosis of patients with ischemic colitis is generally good if disease is limited to the mucosa, as in most patients.[233,244] Long-term consequences may be ulcerating segmental colitis or stricture formation. Strictures are seen in 10% of patients who recover and may require an elective segmental resection.[245] If the patient develops a segmental colitis, which can manifest as persistent diarrhea and rectal bleeding, this too may be treated with elective resection. Patients who require urgent exploration and operation for more substantial ischemia have a worse prognosis, with mortalities approaching 40%. This may be secondary to associated comorbidities in this patient population.

Acute Presentation of Inflammatory Bowel Disease

Severe acute ulcerative colitis can be defined as >6 bowel movements per day plus one of the following: (1) Temperature >37.8°C, (2) large amounts of rectal bleeding, (3) heart rate >90 beats per minute, (4) hemoglobin <10.5 g/dL, or (5) an erythrocyte sedimentation rate >30 mm/h.[246–248] Historically, untreated severe ulcerative colitis was associated with a mortality of 24%, but this has decreased to <1% using a combination of corticosteroids and immunomodulatory drugs and timely surgical intervention. The approach should be multidisciplinary and surgical therapy reserved as a salvage therapy. Toxic megacolon is a general term for an acute form of colonic distension associated with significant inflammation and colonic failure, and can lead to sepsis. Toxic megacolon can develop from inflammatory bowel disease and is an emergency that requires surgical therapy. Although approximately 10% of patients will satisfy criteria for severe colitis upon initial presentation for ulcerative colitis, most often patients who present with severe colitis from inflammatory bowel disease will already have a diagnosis or have sought medical care prior to the acute presentation. Therefore, we will not focus on the pathophysiology and initial diagnostic workup of inflammatory bowel disease, but rather the management of patients with acute severe colitis.

Diagnosis. Patients with criteria for severe colitis should be admitted to the hospital. It is important in patients who do not have an established diagnosis of inflammatory bowel disease to consider alternative diagnoses including infectious and ischemic colitis. In patients with a diagnosis of inflammatory bowel disease, it is also important to specifically consider CMV infection, as well as *C. difficile* infection.[249–252]

Sigmoidoscopy or colonoscopy is useful to evaluate the severity of an attack of colitis.[246,253,254] The extent of mucosal inflammation and ulceration can be determined. Biopsy can also be performed to diagnose CMV. Biopsy and inspection may also help diagnose ischemic colitis or Crohn's colitis. It should be noted that differentiation of inflammatory disease limited to the colon as Crohn's disease or ulcerative colitis may be difficult; in addition, 15% of patients will be given a diagnosis of indeterminate colitis. However, the management in acute severe colitis for each of these entities is similar. Inspection of the mucosa and stool samples can also be collected for analysis or culture to evaluate for *C. difficile* or other infections, including, *Campylobacter*, *Salmonella*, *Yersinia*, *Shigella*, *E. histolytica*, and *E. coli*.

Plain films can evaluate for perforation, disease extent, or toxic megacolon. Modern day availability of CT makes this a diagnostic adjunct which can more accurately determine all of these features. However, it is not as easy to perform, is more costly, and exposes patients to more radiation compared to plain films. Plain films can be performed daily and used as an adjunct to clinical exam to help guide management. Physical exam findings may be masked by steroids and other immunomodulatory treatments.

Laboratory examination for leukocytosis, blood counts, electrolytes, and inflammatory markers should be followed. Patients with severe colitis are prone to dehydration and electrolyte abnormalities, specifically hypokalemia. This may be exacerbated by corticosteroids.

Management. One of the most important facets of management is the multidisciplinary approach of gastroenterologist and surgeon. Patients should receive supportive care with intravenous fluids. Patients with severe colitis may be prone to venous thromboembolic disease secondary to protein losses and should receive prophylaxis against venous thrombosis even in the presence of bloody diarrhea. An algorithm for the treatment of severe colitis is highlighted in Algorithm 35.3.

The mainstay of treatment for acute severe colitis is corticosteroids.[247,248] Treatment is usually for 5 days but may extend up to 10 days. If a patient's clinical status improves, they are typically started on oral steroids, which are then tapered over time. Approximately 60% of patients do not respond completely to steroids.[246,247,255,256] There are multiple prognostic indices that can predict the outcome of patients with severe colitis and failure to respond to steroid therapy. If treatment failure seems likely, then additional "rescue" therapies should be considered earlier in the course. If the patient deteriorates, operation should be considered immediately. This underscores the importance of surgical consultation early in the hospitalization.

Cyclosporine is a calcineurin inhibitor that prevents T-cell activation and proliferation. It is used in an attempt to avoid surgery when corticosteroids fail.[256–258] Cyclosporine is often started on day 3 when steroids are failing, and converted to oral dosing once symptoms improve. Importantly, cyclosporine does not seem to increase the risk of perioperative complications in patients who do not respond and undergo surgery.

Infliximab is a monoclonal antibody that binds to TNFα. The use of infliximab was first established in Crohn's disease. Several smaller trials have supported the use of this antibody for the treatment of steroid refractory severe colitis.[259–262] The use of this agent is in evolution, but will likely prove to be of benefit. Infliximab has a good short term safety profile. However, the perioperative risks in patients who progress to

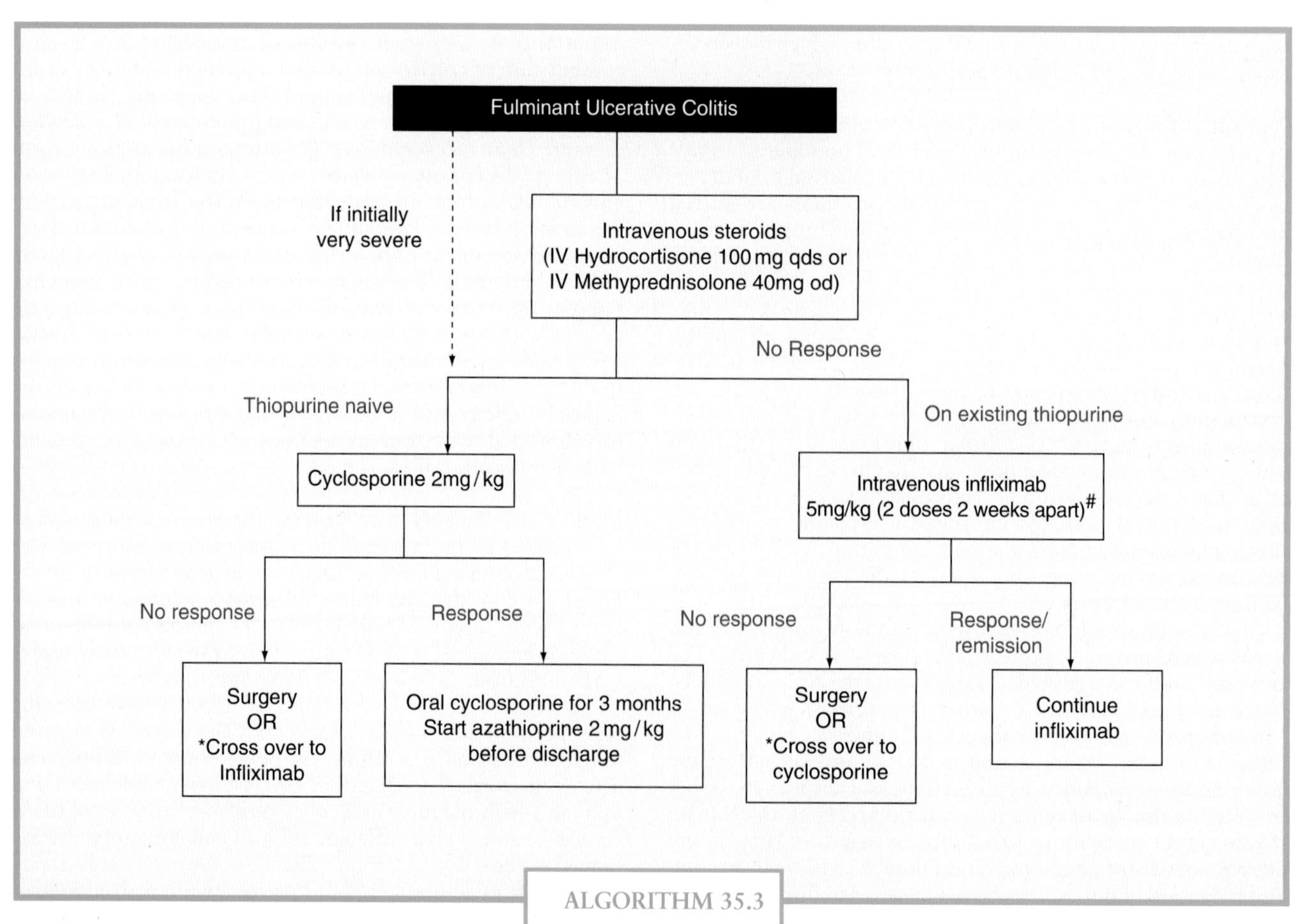

ALGORITHM 35.3 Clinical management strategy for severe/fulminant ulcerative colitis. #Infliximab has been associated with increased risk of infections. (Reprinted from Ng SC, Kamm MA. Therapeutic strategies for the management of ulcerative colitis. *Inflamm Bowel Dis*. 2009;15(6):935–950, with permission. Figure 4 p. 946.)

surgery may be more substantial, specifically for infectious complications. This remains to be determined.

Trials comparing infliximab to cyclosporine are underway.[263] Additional immunomodulatory agents are being investigated and show promise. These include immunoglobulin G2 against CD3 epsilon chains on T-cells, the calcineurin inhibitor tacrolimus, and leucocytapheresis to selectively remove populations of white blood cells.[264–268]

Surgery is still the definitive treatment. Failure of medical therapy in the acute setting, clinical deterioration, perforation, or toxic megacolon are indications for operation. In the setting of severe colitis, patients will generally undergo a subtotal abdominal colectomy, end ileostomy, and creation of a Hartmann's pouch. If the distal colon and rectum are severely inflamed and creation of a Hartmann's pouch does not seem possible, a mucous fistula can be created. Alternatively, the distal colon and rectum can be left as a Hartmann's pouch and the end can be secured above the fascia at the inferior extent of the midline wound. The fascia is not closed at this point. If the stump breaks down, it will manifest as a controlled mucous fistula. With either management, total proctocolectomy is usually avoided in this acute setting if a restorative procedure is contemplated in the management of the patient in the future. Not extending the resection down to the peritoneal reflection, thus leaving a longer Hartmann's pouch, will facilitate future dissection and creation of an ileal pouch with anal anastomosis in the future, if the patient is a candidate. Again, early surgical involvement and consultation with a stoma therapist will help guide management, as well as enhance patient understanding and acceptance of surgical management.

Colectomy is an effective treatment to manage this disease acutely. It can improve quality of life, and in the long term can decrease the need for immunomodulatory drugs and the risk of cancer. In patients who undergo a restorative procedure, complications from surgery are high, including anastomotic leak, stricture, small bowel obstruction, and pouchitis. This needs to be balanced with the long-term morbidity or mortality of medical therapy, which is still to be defined.

MISCELLANEOUS CAUSES OF COLONIC INFLAMMATION

Epiploic Appendagitis

Colonic epiploic appendages are fatty appendages on the peritoneal surface of the colon along its entire length. Torsion or spontaneous venous thrombosis of these appendages are rare, but diagnosed more commonly secondary to increased use of CT (Fig. 35.19). Symptoms manifest as localized abdominal pain. It most commonly occurs in the sigmoid or cecum, thus mimicking diverticulitis or appendicitis.[269,270] Laboratory findings are nonspecific. CT can diagnose this pathologic entity, although depending on the location, it can be difficult to discern epiploic appendagitis from early diverticulitis.[271–274] Ultrasound may aid in the diagnosis as well.[275,276] The disease is thought of as self limiting and treatment generally involves pain control and nonsteroidal anti-inflammatory medications. Some reports have demonstrated recurrence and would advocate, either in the primary setting or following recurrence, exploration (preferably laparoscopic if possible) with ligation and excision of the inflamed appendage.[277]

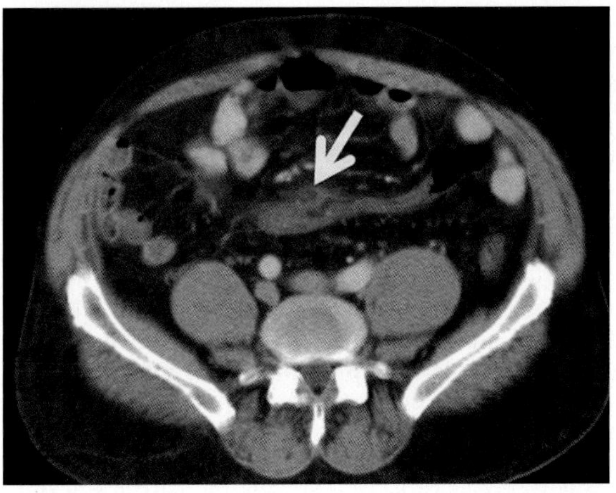

FIGURE 35.19. CT scan showing appendagitis. Appendagitis may appear as an abnormality of the fat adjacent to the colon, with or without pericolonic fat stranding. White arrow points out a change in fat density of the colonic appendage adjacent to the sigmoid colon.

Neutropenic Enterocolitis

Neutropenic enterocolitis (also known as typhlitis) is a syndrome in neutropenic patients characterized most typically by fever and right lower quadrant pain. Patients may have distension, diarrhea, or lower GI bleeding. It can occur in patients with hematologic malignancies, myelodysplastic syndromes, AIDS, or in the setting of immunosuppressive therapies.[278–282] The etiology is uncertain but may occur as a result of mucosal injury from cytotoxic drugs and impaired host defense. Other diagnoses must be considered, such as appendicitis, ischemic colitis, CDAD, and other infectious colitis. CT can be useful to exclude other diagnoses. CT may demonstrate a dilated cecum, right lower quadrant inflammation, or pericecal inflammation or ascites. Treatment is usually supportive with intravenous fluids, bowel rest, and antibiotics. Immunosuppressive therapy should be stopped and consideration should be given to correct neutropenia using recombinant therapies, such as granulocyte colony-stimulating factor.[283] Operation is considered for patients with continued bleeding despite aggressive correction of hematologic abnormalities, perforation, or clinical deterioration. In this immunosuppressed population, most surgeons would advocate resection of the affected region (ileocecectomy versus right hemicolectomy) with end ileostomy and mucous fistula.

Radiation Proctitis

Radiation proctitis is characterized by injury to the distal colon or rectum following radiation therapy. Acute proctitis occurs within 6 weeks of therapy and is characterized by diarrhea, urgency, and rectal bleeding. These symptoms usually resolve spontaneously over time and therapy is aimed at prevention of perianal skin irritation and breakdown. Chronic radiation proctitis is delayed in onset and usually occurs at least 1 year after radiation therapy. It occurs as a result of radiation-induced obliterative endarteritis that results in mucosal ischemia.[284] This results in stricture formation and bleeding. The diagnosis is made by a history of radiation and endoscopic evaluation demonstrating mucosal edema, erythema, telangiectasias, ulcers, and strictures. Treatment should be based on the symptom complex. Sucralfate enemas have a low side effect profile and may be successful.[285,286] Ablative therapies, including argon plasma coagulation, lasers, and electrocautery can successfully treat bleeding.[287] Argon plasma coagulation has the advantage of being widely available, cheap, and having a minimal depth of penetration.[288–290] Some reports suggest that SCFA enemas or formaldehyde enemas can stop bleeding.[291,292] Surgery is reserved for recalcitrant bleeding, significant strictures, or pain.[293]

SUMMARY

Acute inflammatory processes of the intestinal tract may require urgent operation. The acute care surgeon must apply critical decision making to the management of patients presenting with inflammatory emergencies in an expeditious and well-thought-out manner. Surgeons must resist the temptation to do too much in the operating room during an emergency operation. The primary goals of the operation must remain the focus and a damage control approach may better serve some critically ill patients. Allowing the patient's health and hemodynamic status to guide decision making will generally lead to better outcome.

References

1. Duncan M, Wong RKH. Esophageal emergencies: things that will wake you from a sound sleep. *Gastroenterol Clin North Am*. 2003;32:1035–1052.
2. Meyer GW, Castell DO. Evaluation and management of diseases of the esophagus. *Am J Otolaryngol*. 1981;2:336–344.
3. DeMeester TR, Stein HJ. Surgical treatment of gastroesophageal reflux disease. In: *The Esophagus*. Boston, MA: Little-Brown; 1992:579.
4. El-Serag HB. Time trends of gastroesophageal reflux disease: a systematic review. *Clin Gastroenterol Hepatol*. 2007;5(1):17–26.
5. Miller G, Savary M, Monnier P. Notwendige diagnostic: endoskopie. In: Blum AL, Siewert JR, eds. *Reflux-therapie*. Berlin, Germany: Springer-Verlag; 1981:336.
6. Lundell L, Dent J, Bennett J, et al. Endoscopic assessment of esophagitis: clinical and functional correlates and further validation of Los Angeles Classification. *Gut*. 1999;45:172–180.
7. Leedham S, Jankowski J. The evidence base of proton pump inhibitor chemoprotective agents in Barrett's esophagus—the good, the bad and the flawed. *Am J Gastroenterol*. 2007;102:21–23.
8. DeVault KR, Castell DO. Updated guidelines for the diagnosis and treatment of gastroesophageal reflux disease. *Am J Gastroenterol*. 2005;100:190–200.
9. Baehr PH, McDonald GB. Esophageal infections: risk factors, presentation, diagnosis and treatment. *Gastroenterology*. 1994;106:509–532.
10. Kumar A. Massive gastrointestinal bleeding due to *Candida esophagitis*. *Southern Med J*. 1994;87(6):669–671.
11. Ramanathan J, Rammouni M, Baran J Jr, et al. Herpes simplex esophagitis in the immunocompetent host: an overview. *Am J Gastroenterol*. 2000;95(9):2171–2176.
12. Jain SK, Jain S, Jain M, Yaduvanshi A. Esophageal tuberculosis: is it so rare? Report of 12 cases and review of literature. *Am J Gastroenterol*. 2002;97: 293–296.
13. Fujiwara Y, Osugi H, Takada N, et al. Esophageal tuberculosis presenting with an appearance similar to that of carcinoma of the esophagus. *J Gastroenterol*. 2003;38:477–481.
14. Welzel TM, Kawan T, Bohle W, et al. An unusual case of dysphagia: esophageal tuberculosis. *J Gastrointest Liver Dis*. 2010;19(3):321–324.
15. Werner-Wasik M, Yorke E, Deasy J, et al. Radiation dose-volume effects in the esophagus. *Int J Radiat Oncol Biol Phys*. 2010;76 (3 suppl):S86–S93.
16. Davila M, Bresalier RS. Gastrointestinal complications of oncologic therapy. *Nat Clin Pract Gastroenterol Hepatol*. 2008;5(12):682–696.
17. Swann LA, Munter DW. Esophageal emergencies. *Emerg Med Clin N Am*. 1996;14(3):557–570.
18. Alexander JA, Kratzka DA. Therapeutic options for eosinophilic esophagitis. *Gastroenterol Hepatol*. 2011;7(1):59–61.
19. Mishra A, Hogan SP, Brandt EB, et al. An etiological role for aeroallergens and eosinophils in experimental esophagitis. *J Clin Invest*. 2001;107(1):83–90.
20. Metheny NA, Meert KL, Clouse RE. Complications related to feeding tube placement. *Curr Opin Gastroenterol*. 2007;23(2): 178–182.
21. Litle VR, Luketich JD, Christie NA, et al. Photodynamic therapy as palliation for esophageal cancer: experience in 215 patients. *Ann Thorac Surg*. 2003;76(5):1687–1692.
22. Geboes K, Jannsens J, Rutgeerts P, et al. Crohn's disease of the esophagus. *J Clin Gastroenterol*. 1986;8(1):31–37.
23. Skinner DB, Lttle AG, DeMeester TR. Management of esophageal perforation. *Am J Surg*. 1988;139:760–764.
24. Bufkin BL, Miller Jr JI, Mansour KA. Esophageal perforation: emphasis on management. *Ann Thorac Surg*. 1996;61:1447–1451
25. Young CA, Menias CO, Bhalla S, et al. CT features of esophageal emergencies. *Radiographics*. 2008;28:1541–1553.
26. Port JL, Kent MS, Korst RJ, et al. Thoracic esophageal perforations: a decade of experience. *Ann Thorac Surg*. 2003;75:1071–1074.
27. Collins C, Arumugasamy M, Larkin J, et al. Thoracoscopic repair of instrumental perforation of the oesophagus: first report. *Ir J Med Sci*. 2002;171(2):68–70.
28. Nguyen NT, Follette DM, Roberts PF, et al. Thoracoscopic management of postoperative esophageal leak. *J Thorac Cardiovasc Surg*. 2001;121(2):391–392.
29. Vogel Sb, Rout WR, Martin TD, et al. Esophageal perforation in adults: aggressive, conservative treatment lowers morbidity and mortality. *Ann Surg*. 2005;241:1016–1023.
30. Abbas G, Schuchert MJ, Pettiford BL, et al. Contemporaneous management of esophageal perforation. *Surgery*. 2009;146:749–756.
31. Kiernan PD, Hernandez A, Byrne WD, et al. Descending cervical mediastinitis. *Ann Thorac Surg*. 1998;65:1483–1488.
32. Wheatley MJ, Stirling MC, Kirsh MM, et al. Descending necrotizing mediastinitis: transcervical drainage is not enough. *Ann Thorac Surg*. 1990;49:780–784.
33. Chung DA, Ritchie AJ. Videothoracoscopic drainage of mediastinal abscess: an alternative to thoracostomy. *Ann Thorac Surg*. 2000;69:1573–1574.
34. Tinoco RC, Tinoco AC, El-Kadre L. Perforated epiphrenic diverticulum treated by video laparoscopy. *Surg Endosc*. 1999;13(3):270–272.
35. Nathanson LK, Gotley D, Smithers M, et al. Videothoracoscopic primary repair of early distal oesophageal perforation. *Aust N Z J Surg*. 1993;63:399–403.
36. Bell RC. Laparoscopic closure of esophageal perforation following pneumatic dilation for achalasia: report of two cases. *Surg Endosc*. 1997;11(5):476–478.
37. Swanstrom LL, Pennings J. Laparoscopic esophagomyotomy for achalasia. *Surg Endosc*. 1995;9(3): 286–290.
38. Wasserman RL, Ginsburg CM. Caustic substance injuries. *J Pediatr*. 1985;107(2):169–174.
39. Poley JW, Steyerberg EW, Kuipers EJ, et al. Ingestion of acid and alkaline agents: outcome and prognostic value of early upper endoscopy. *Gastrointest Endosc*. 2004;60(3): 372–377.
40. Kikendall J. Caustic ingestion injuries. *Gastroenterol Clin North Am*. 1991;220:847–857.
41. Zargar SA, Kochhar R, Mehta S, et al. The role of fiberoptic endoscopy in the management of corrosive ingestion and modified endoscopic classification of burns. *Gastrointest Endosc*. 1991;37(2):165–169.
42. Zhou JH, Jiang YG, Wang RW, et al. Management of corrosive esophageal burns in 149 cases. *J Thorac Cardiovasc Surg*. 2005;130:449–455.
43. Bertleff MJO, Lange JF. Laparoscopic correction of perforated peptic ulcer: first choice? A review of literature. *Surg Endosc*. 2010;24:1231.
44. Lui FY, Davis KA. Gastroduodenal perforation: maximal or minimal intervention? *Scand J Surg*. 2010;99:73.
45. Crofts TJ, Park KG, Steele RJ, et al. A randomized trial of nonoperative treatment for perforated peptic ulcer. *N Engl J Med*. 1989;320:970.
46. Hermansson M, von Holstein CS, Zilling T. Surgical approach and prognostic factors after peptic ulcer perforation. *Eur J Surg*. 1999;165:566.
47. Gisbert J, Legido J, Garcia-Sanz I, et al. *Helicobacter pylori* and perforated peptic ulcer: prevalence of the infection and role of nonsteroidal anti-inflammatory drugs. *Dig Liver Dis*. 2004;36:116–120.
48. Kurata JH, Nogawa AN. Meta-analysis of risk factors for peptic ulcer: nonsteroidal anti-inflammatory drugs, *Helicobacter pylori*, and smoking. *J Clin Gastroenterol*. 1997;24:2.
49. Lee SW, Chang CS, Lee TY, et al. Risk factors and therapeutic response in Chinese patients with peptic ulcer disease. *World J Gastroenterol*. 2010;16:2017–22.
50. Mulholland, MW. Gastroduodenal ulceration. In: Mulholland MW, Lillemoe KD, Doherty GM, et al. *Greenfield's Surgery: Scientific Principles and Practice*. 4th ed. Lippincott Williams and Wilkins; 2006.
51. Talamini G, Tommasi M, Amadei V, et al. Risk factors of peptic ulcer in 4943 inpatients. *J Clin Gastroenterol*. 2008;42:373–80.
52. Dempsey DT. Stomach. In: Brunicardi FC, Andersen DK, Billiar TR, et al., eds. *Schwartz's Principles of Surgery*. 9th ed. McGraw Hill Co., Inc.; 2010.
53. Kate V, Ananthakrishnan N, Badrinath S. Effect of *Helicobacter pylori* eradication on the ulcer recurrence rate after simple closure of perforated duodenal ulcer: retrospective and prospective randomized controlled studies. *Br J Surg*. 2001;88:1054.
54. Lau WY, Leow CK. History of perforated duodenal and gastric ulcers. *World J Surg*. 1997;21:890.
55. Ng EK, Larn YH, Sung JJ, et al. Eradication of *Helicobacter pylori* prevents recurrence of ulcer after simple closure of duodenal ulcer perforation: randomized controlled trial. *Ann Surg*. 2000: 231:153.
56. Stabile BE. Redefining the role of surgery for perforated duodenal ulcer in the *Helicobacter pylori* era. *Ann Surg*. 2000;231:159.
57. Graham DY, Fischbach L. *Helicobacter pylori* treatment in the era of increasing antibiotic resistance. *Gut*. 2010;59:1143–1153.
58. Luther J, Higgins PD, Schoenfield PS, et al. Empiric quadruple versus triple therapy for primary treatment of *Helicobacter pylori* infection: systematic review and meta-analysis of efficacy and tolerability. *Am J Gastroenterol*. 2010;105:65–73.
59. Jordan PH, Morrow C. Perforated peptic ulcer. *Surg Clin North Am*. 1988;68:315–329.

60. Newman NA, Mufeed S, Makary MA. The stomach: benign gastric ulcers. In: Cameron JL, Cameron AM, eds. *Current Surgical Therapy*. 10th ed. Churchill Livingstone; 2010.
61. Bulut OB, Rasmussen C, Fischer A. Acute surgical treatment of complicated peptic ulcer with special reference to the elderly. *World J Surg*. 1996;20:574–577.
62. Herrington JL Jr, Sawyers JL. Gastric ulcer. *Curr Probl Surg*. 1987;24:759.
63. Hodnett RM, Gonzalez F, Lee WC, et al. The need for definitive therapy in the management of perforated gastric ulcers. Review of 202 cases *Ann Surg*. 1989;209:36.
64. Lunevicius R, Morkevicius M. Systematic review comparing laparoscopic and open repair for perforated peptic ulcer. *Br J Surg*. 2005;92:1195.
65. Boey J, Choi SK, Poon A, et al. Risk stratification in perforated duodenal ulcers: a prospective validation of predictive factors. *Ann Surg*. 1987;205:22.
66. Boey J, Wong J, Ong GB. A prospective study of operative risk factors in perforated duodenal ulcers. *Ann Surg*. 1982;195:265.
67. Lohsiriwat, V, Prapasrivorakul, S, Lohsiriwat, D. Perforated peptic ulcer: clinical presentation, surgical outcomes, and the accuracy of the Boey scoring system in predicting postoperative morbidity and mortality. *World J Surg*. 2009;33:80.
68. Svanes C, Salvesen H, Stangeland L, et al. Perforated peptic ulcer over 56 years. Time trends in patients and disease characteristics. *Gut*. 1993;34:1666–1671.
69. Karamanakos SN, Sdralis E, Panagiotopoulos S, et al. Laparoscopy in the emergency setting: a retrospective review of 540 patients with acute abdominal pain. *Surg Laparosc Endosc Percutan Tech*. 2010;20:119.
70. Memon MA, Fitzgibbons RJ Jr. The role for minimal access surgery in the acute abdomen. *Surg Clin North Am*. 1997;77:1333.
71. Siu W, Leong H, Law B, et al. Laparoscopic repair for perforated peptic ulcer: a randomized controlled trial. *Ann Surg*. 2002;235:313.
72. Lee FY, Leung KL, Lai BS, et al. Predicting mortality and morbidity of patients operated on for perforated peptic ulcers. *Arch Surg*. 2001;136:90.
73. Vaidya BB, Garg CP, Shah JB. Laparoscopic repair of perforated peptic ulcer with delayed presentation. *J Laparoendosc Adv Surg Tech*. 2009;19:153
74. Blomgren LGM. Perforated peptic ulcer: long-term results of simple closure in the elderly. *World J Surg*. 1997;21:412–415.
75. Yetkin G, Uludag M, Akgun I, et al. Late results of a simple closure technique and *Helicobacter pylori* eradication in duodenal ulcer perforation. *Acta Chir Belg*. 2010;110:537–542.
76. Ellison EC. Zollinger Ellison syndrome. In: Cameron JL, Cameron AM, eds. *Cameron: Current Surgical Therapy*. 10th ed. Churchill-Livingstone; 2010.
77. Ali MR, Fuller WD, Choi, MP, et al. Bariatric surgical outcomes. *Surg Clin North Am*. 2005;4:835.
78. Felix EL, Kettelle J, Mobley E, et al. Perforated marginal ulcers after laparoscopic gastric bypass. *Surg Endosc*. 2008;22:2128.
79. Patel RA, Brolin RE, Gandhi A. Revisional operations for marginal ulcer after Roux-en-Y gastric bypass. *Surg Obes Relat Dis*. 2009;5:317.
80. Ben-Meir A, Sonpal I, Patterson L, et al. Cigarette smoking, but not NSAIDs or alcohol use or comorbidities, is associated with anastomotic ulcers in Roux-en-Y gastric bypass (RYGB) patiets. *Surg Obes Relat Dis*. 2005;1:263.
81. Lublin M, McCoy M, Waldrep J. Perforating marginal ulcers after laparoscopic gastric bypass. *Surg Endosc*. 2006;20:51.
82. Pope GD, Goodney PP, Burchard KW. Peptic ulcer/stricture after gastric bypass: a comparison of technique and acid suppression variables. *Obes Surg*. 2002;12:30.
83. Rasmussen JJ, Fuller W, Ali MR. Marginal ulceration after laparoscopic gastric bypass: an alalysis of predisposinjg factors in 260 patients. *Surg Endosc*. 2007;21:1090.
84. Jalihal A, Chong VH. Duodenal perforations and haematoma: complications of endoscopic therapy. *ANZ J Surg*. 2009;79:767–768.
85. Mao Z, Zhu Q, Wu W, et al. Duodenal perforations after endoscopic retrograde cholangiopancreatography: experience and management. *J Laparoendosc Adv Surg Tech*. 2008;18:691–695.
86. Freezor RJ, Huber TS, Welborn MB 3rd, et al. Duodenal perforation with an inferior vena cava filter: an unusual cause of abdominal pain. *J Vasc Surg*. 2002;35(5):1010–1012.
87. Zeb F, Kevans D, Muir K, et al. Duodenal impaction/perforation of a biliary stent-a rare complication in the management of choledocholithiasis. *J Gastrointestin Liver Dis*. 2009;18:391–392.
88. Charabaty-Pishvaian A, Al-Kawas F. Endoscopic treatment of duodenal perforation using a clipping device: case report and review of the literature. *Southern Med J*. 2004;97:190–193.
89. Mangiavillano B, Viaggi P, Masci E. Endoscopic closure of acute iatrogenic perforations during diagnostic and therapeutic endoscopy in the gastrointestinal tract using metallic clips: a literature review. *J Digest Dis*. 2010;11:12–18.
90. Stapfer M, Selby RR, Stain SC, et al. Management of duodenal perforation after endoscopic retrograde cholangiopancreatography and sphinchterotomy. *Ann Surg*. 2000;232:191–8.
91. Palanivelu C, Jategaonkar PA, Rangarajan M, et al. Laparoscopic management of a retroperitoneal duodenal perforation following ERCP for periampullary cancer. *JSLS*. 2008;12:399–402.
92. Evers BM. Small intestine. In: Townsend CM Jr, ed. *Sabiston Textbook of Surgery: The Biological Basis of Modern Surgical Practice*. 18th ed. Saunders 2007.
93. Stein SL, Michelassi F. Small bowel: Crohn's disease of the small bowel. In: Cameron JL, Cameron AM, eds. *Cameron: Current Surgical Therapy*. 10th ed. Churchill Livingstone; 2010.
94. Delaney CP, Kiran RP, Senagore AJ, et al. Quality of life improves within 30 days of surgery for Crohn's disease. *J Am Coll Surg*. 2003;196:714.
95. Novacek G, Weltermann A, Sobala A, et al. Inflammatory bowel disease is a risk factor for recurrent venous thromboembolism. *Gastroenterol*. 2010;139:779.
96. Lichtenstein GR, Hanauer SB, Sandborn WJ; Practice Parameters Committee of the American College of Gastroenterologists. Management of Crohn's disease in adults. *Am J Gastroenterol*. 2009;104:465–83.
97. Felly C, Vader JP, Juillerat P, et al. Appropriate therapy for fistulizing and fibrostenotic Crohn's disease: results of a multidisciplinary expert panel-EPACT II. *J Crohns Colitis*. 2009;3:250–256.
98. Present DH, Rutgeerts P, Targan S, et al. Infliximab for the treatment of fistulas in patients with Crohn's disease. *N Engl J Med*. 1999;340:398.
99. Sands BE, Anderson FH, Bernstein CN, et al. Infliximab maintenance therapy for fistulizing Crohn's disease. *N Engl J Med*. 2004;350:876–85.
100. Jones DW, Finlayson SR. Trends in surgery in Crohn's disease in the era of infliximab. *Ann Surg*. 2010;252:307.
101. Fichera A, Michelassi F. Surgical treatment of Crohn's disease. *J Gastrointest Surg*. 2007;11:791.
102. Aberra FN, Lewis HD, Hass D, et al. Corticosteroids and immunomodulators: postoperative infectious complication risk in inflammatory bowel disease patients. *Gastroenterology*. 2003;125:320.
103. Dietz DW, Laureti S, Strong SA, et al. Safety and longterm efficacy of strictureplasty in 314 patients with obstructing small bowel Crohn's disease. *J Am Coll Surg*. 2001;192:330.
104. Fearnhead NS, Chowdhury R, Box B, et al. Long-term follow-up of strictureplasty for Crohn's disease. *Br J Surg*. 2006;93:475.
105. Hassan C, Zullo A, De Francesco V, et al. Systematic review: endoscopic dilatation in Crohn's disease. *Aliment Pharmacol Ther*. 2007;26:1457.
106. Worsey MJ, Hull T, Ryland L, et al. Strictureplasty is an effective option in the operative management of duodenal Crohn's disease. *Dis Colon Rectum*. 1999;42:596.
107. Menon AM, Mirza AH, Moolla S, et al. Adenocarcinoma of the small bowel arising from a previous strictureplasty for Crohn's disease: report of a case. *Dis Colon Rectum*. 2007;50:257.
108. Fazio VW, Marchetti F, Church M, et al. Effect of resection margins on the recurrence of Crohn's disease in the small bowel. A randomized controlled trial. *Ann Surg*. 1996;224:563.
109. McLeod RS, Wolff BG, Ross S, et al. Recurrence of Crohn's disease after ileocolic resection is not affected by anastomotic type: results of a multicenter, randomized, controlled trial. *Dis Colon Rectum*. 2009;52:919.
110. Scarpa M, Angriman I, Barollo M, et al. Role of staped and hand-sewn anastomoses in recurrence of Crohn's disease. *Hepato Gastroenterol*. 2004;561:1053.
111. Simillis C, Purkayastha S, Yamamoto T, et al. A meta-analysis comparing conventional end-to-end anastomosis vs. other anastomotic configurations after resection in Crohn's disease. *Dis Colon Rectum*. 2007;50:1674.
112. Hasegawa H, Watanabe M, Nishibori H, et al. Laparoscopic surgery for recurrent Crohn's disease. *Br J Surg*. 2003;90:970.
113. Moorthy K, Shaul T, Foley RJE. The laparoscopic management of benign bowel fistulas. *J Soc Laparoendosc Surg*. 2004;8:356.
114. Tan JJ, Tjandra JJ. Laparoscopic surgery for Crohn's disease: a meta-analysis. *Dis Colon Rectum*. 2007;50:576.
115. Young-Fadok TM, HallLong K, McConnell EJ, et al. Advantages of laparoscopic resection for ileocolic Crohn's disease. Improved outcomes and reduced costs. *Surg Endosc*. 2001;15:450.
116. Alves A, Panis Y, Bouhnik Y, et al. Factors that predict conversion in 69 consecutive patients undergoing laparoscopic ileocecal resection for Crohn's disease: a prospective study. *Dis Colon Rectum*. 2005;48:2302.
117. Visschers RG, Olde Damink SW, Winkens B, et al. Treatment strategies in 135 consecutive patients with enterocutaneous fistulas. *World J Surg*. 2008;32:445–53.
118. Martindale RG, McClave SA, Vanek VW, et al. Guidelines for the provision and assessment of nutrition support therapy in the adult critically ill patient: Society of Critical Care Medicine and American Society for Parenteral and Enteral Nutrition: Executive Summary. *Crit Care Med*. 2009;37:1757–1761.
119. Sepehripour S, Papagrigoriadis S. A systematic review of the benefit of the total parenteral nutrition in the management of enterocutaneous fistulas. *Minerva Chir*. 2010;65:577–85.
120. Alivizatos V, Felekis D, Zorbalas A. Evaluation of the effectiveness of octreotide in the conservative treatment of postoperative enterocutaneous fistulas. *Hepatogastroenterol*. 2002;49:1010–1012.
121. Makhdoom ZA, Komar MJ, Still CD. Nutrition and enterocutaneous fistulas. *J Clin Gastroenterol*. 2000;31:195–204.
122. Lynch MF, Blanton EM, Bulens S, et al. Typhoid fever in the United States 1999–2006. *JAMA*. 2009;302:859.
123. Parry CM, Hien TT, Dougan G, et al. Typhoid fever. *N Engl J Med*. 2002;347:1770.

124. Ameh EA, Dogo PM, Attah MM, et al. Comparison of three operations for typhoid perforation. *Br J Surg*. 1997;84:558.
125. Grinsztejn B, Fandinho FC, Veloso VG, et al. Mycobacteremia in patients with the acquired immunodeficiency syndrome. *Arch Int Med*. 1997;157:2359.
126. Horvath KD, Whelan RL. Intestinal tuberculosis: return of an old disease. *Am J Gastroenterol*. 1998;93:692.
127. Marshall JB. Tuberculosis of the gastrointestinal tract and peritoneum. *Am J Gastroenterol*. 1993;88:989.
128. Reed C, von Reyn CF, Chamblee S, et al. Environmental risk factors for infection with *Mycobacterium avium* complex. *Am J Epidem*. 2006;164:32.
129. Blanshard C, Benhamou Y, Dohin E, et al. Treatment of AIDS-associated gastrointestinal cytomegalovirus infection with foscarnet and ganciclovir: a randomized comparison. *J Infec Dis*. 1995;172:622.
130. Kahi CJ, Wheat LJ, Allen SD, et al. Gastrointest histoplasmosis. *Am J Gastroenterol*. 2005;100:1896.
131. Gallagher SF, Fabri PJ. Management of diverticulosis of the small bowel. In: Cameron JL, Cameron AM, eds. *Cameron: Current Surgical Therapy*. 10th ed. Churchill Livingstone; 2010.
132. Tavakkolizadeh A, Whang EE, Ashley SW, et al. Small intestine. In: Brunicardi FC, Andersen DK, Billiar TR, et al. eds. *Schwartz's Principles of Surgery*. 9th ed. McGraw Hill Co., Inc.; 2010.
133. Akhrass R, Yaffe MB, Fischer C. Small-bowel diverticulosis: perceptions and reality. *J Am Coll Surg*. 1997;184:383.
134. Psathakis D, Utschakowski A, Muller G, et al. Clinical significance of duodenal diverticula. *J Amer Coll Surg*. 1994;178:257.
135. Egawa, N, Anjiki, H, Takuma K, et al. Juxtapapillary duodenal diverticula and pancreaticobiliary disease. Dig Surg 2010;27:105.
136. Lotveit T, Osnes M, Larsen S. Recurrent biliary calculi: duodenal diverticula as a predisposing factor. *Ann Surg*. 1982;196:30.
137. Uomo G, Manes G, Ragozzino A, et al. Periampullary extraluminal duodenal diverticula and acute pancreatitis: an underestimated etiological association. *Am J Gastroenterol*. 1996;91:1186.
138. Zoepf T, Zoepf DS, Arnold JC, et al. The relationship between juxtapapillary duodenal diverticula and disorders of the biliopancreatic system: analysis of 350 patients. *Gastrointest Endosc*. 2001;54:56.
139. D'Alessio MJ, Rana A, Martin JA, et al. Surgical management of intraluminal duodenal diverticulum and coexisting anomalies. *J Am Coll Surg*. 2005;201:143–148.
140. Badaoui A, Piessevaux H. A new endoscopic therapy for an intraluminal diverticulum of the duodenum. *Endoscopy*. 2007;39(suppl 1):E99–E100.
141. Lee SH, Park SH, Lee JH, et al. Endoscopic diverticulotomy with an isolated-tip papillotome (Iso-Tome) in a patient with intraluminal duodenal diverticulum. *Gastrointest Endosc*. 2005;62:817–19.
142. Chow DC, Babaian M, Taubin HL. Jejunoileal diverticula. *Gastroenterologist*. 1997;5:78–84.
143. Longo WE, Vernava AM III. Clinical implications of jejunoileal diverticular disease. *Dis Colon Rectum*. 1992;35:381.
144. Tsiotos GG, Farnell MB, Ilstrup DM. Nonmeckelian jejunal or ileal diverticulosis: an analysis of 112 cases. *Surgery*. 1994;116:726–731.
145. Skandalakis PN, Zoras O, Skandalakis JE, et al. Littre hernia: surgical anatomy, embryology, and techniques of repair. *Am Surg*. 2006;72:238–43.
146. Yahchouchy EK, Marano AF, Etienne JCF, et al. Meckel's diverticulum. *J Am Coll Surg*. 2001;192:658–62.
147. Zani A, Eaton S, Rees CM, et al. Incidentally detected Meckel's diverticulum: to resect or not to resect? *Ann Surg*. 2008;247:276–281.
148. Guidelines for prevention and treatment of opportunistic infections in HIV-infected adults and adolescents: Recommendations of the National Institutes of Health (NIH), the Centers for Disease Control and Prevention (CDC), and the HIV Medical Association of the Infectious Diseases Society of America (HIVMA/IDSA), 2008.
149. Shackelford RT, Yeo CJ, Peters JH. *Shackelford's Surgery of the Alimentary Tract*. 6th ed. Philadelphia, PA: Saunders; 2007.
150. Ross MH, Pawlina W, Barnash TA. *Atlas of Descriptive Histology*. Sunderland, MA: Sinauer Associates; 2009.
151. Mulholland MW. *Greenfield's Surgery: Scientific Principles and Practice*. 4th ed. Philadelphia, PA: Lippincott Williams & Wilkins; 2006.
152. Hebuterne X. Gut changes attriuted to aging: effects on intestinal microflora. *Curr Opin Clin Nutr Metab Care*. 2003;6(1):49–54.
153. Slack WW. The anatomy, pathology, and some clinical features of diverticulitis of the colon. *Br J Surg*. 1962;50:185–190.
154. West AB. The pathology of diverticulitis. *J Clin Gastroenterol*. 2008;42(10):1137–1138.
155. Jacobs DO. Clinical practice. Diverticulitis. *N Engl J Med*. 2007;357(20):2057–2066.
156. Almy TP, Howell DA. Medical progress. Diverticular disease of the colon. *N Engl J Med*. 1980, 302(6):324–331.
157. Hall J, Hammerich K, Roberts P. New paradigms in the management of diverticular disease. *Curr Probl Surg*. 2010;47(9):680–735.
158. Stollman N, Raskin JB. Diverticular disease of the colon. *Lancet*. 2004;363(9409):631–639.
159. Rafferty J, Shellito P, Hyman NH, et al. Practice parameters for sigmoid diverticulitis. *Dis Colon Rectum*. 2006;49(7):939–944.
160. Janes S, Meagher A, Frizelle FA. Elective surgery after acute diverticulitis. *Br J Surg*. 2005, 92(2):133–142.
161. Painter NS. The cause of diverticular disease of the colon, its symptoms and its complications. Review and hypothesis. *J R Coll Surg Edinb*. 1985;30(2):118–122.
162. Heise CP. Epidemiology and pathogenesis of diverticular disease. *J Gastrointest Surg*. 2008;12(8):1309–1311.
163. Commane DM, Arasaradnam RP, Mills S, et al. Diet, ageing and genetic factors in the pathogenesis of diverticular disease. *World J Gastroenterol*. 2009;15(20):2479–2488.
164. Fisher N, Berry CS, Fearn T, et al. Cereal dietary fiber consumption and diverticular disease: a lifespan study in rats. *Am J Clin Nutr*. 1985;42(5):788–804.
165. Strate LL, Liu YL, Syngal S, et al. Nut, corn, and popcorn consumption and the incidence of diverticular disease. *JAMA*. 2008;300(8):907–914.
166. Whiteway J, Morson BC. Elastosis in diverticular disease of the sigmoid colon. *Gut*. 1985;26(3):258–266.
167. Brook I, Frazier EH. Aerobic and anaerobic microbiology in intraabdominal infections associated with diverticulitis. *J Med Microbiol*. 2000;49(9):827–830.
168. Byrnes MC, Mazuski JE. Antimicrobial therapy for acute colonic diverticulitis. *Surg Infect (Larchmt)*. 2009;10(2):143–154.
169. Horgan AF, McConnell EJ, Wolff BG, et al. Atypical diverticular disease: surgical results. *Dis Colon Rectum*. 2001;44(9):1315–1318.
170. Woods RJ, Lavery IC, Fazio VW, et al. Internal fistulas in diverticular disease. *Dis Colon Rectum*. 1988;31(8):591–596.
171. Rosen MP, Sands DZ, Longmaid HE 3rd, et al. Impact of abdominal CT on the management of patients presenting to the emergency department with acute abdominal pain. *AJR Am J Roentgenol*. 2000;174(5):1391–1396.
172. Halligan S, Saunders B. Imaging diverticular disease. *Best Pract Res Clin Gastroenterol*. 2002;16(4):595–610.
173. Ambrosetti P, Becker C, Terrier F. Colonic diverticulitis: impact of imaging on surgical management—a prospective study of 542 patients. *Eur Radiol*. 2002;12(5):1145–1149.
174. Schwerk WB, Schwarz S, Rothmund M. Sonography in acute colonic diverticulitis. A prospective study. *Dis Colon Rectum*. 1992;35(11):1077–1084.
175. Baker ME. Imaging and interventional techniques in acute left-sided diverticulitis. *J Gastrointest Surg*. 2008;12(8):1314–1317.
176. Poletti PA, Platon A, Rutschmann O, et al. Acute left colonic diverticulitis: can CT findings be used to predict recurrence? *AJR Am J Roentgenol*. 2004;182(5):1159–1165.
177. Stollman NH, Raskin JB. Diagnosis and management of diverticular disease of the colon in adults. Ad Hoc Practice Parameters Committee of the American College of Gastroenterology. *Am J Gastroenterol*. 1999;94(11):3110–3121.
178. Tursi A. Mesalazine for diverticular disease of the colon—a new role for an old drug. *Expert Opin Pharmacother*. 2005;6(1):69–74.
179. Tursi A, Papagrigoriadis S. Review article: the current and evolving treatment of colonic diverticular disease. *Aliment Pharmacol Ther*. 2009;30(6):532–546.
180. Trivedi CD, Das KM. Emerging therapies for diverticular disease of the colon. *J Clin Gastroenterol*. 2008;42(10):1145–1151.
181. Tursi A, Brandimarte G, Daffina R. Long-term treatment with mesalazine and rifaximin versus rifaximin alone for patients with recurrent attacks of acute diverticulitis of colon. *Dig Liver Dis*. 2002;34(7):510–515.
182. Saini S, Mueller PR, Wittenberg J, et al. Percutaneous drainage of diverticular abscess. An adjunct to surgical therapy. *Arch Surg*. 1986;121(4):475–478.
183. Siewert B, Tye G, Kruskal J, et al. Impact of CT-guided drainage in the treatment of diverticular abscesses: size matters. *AJR Am J Roentgenol*. 2006;186(3):680–686.
184. Brandt D, Gervaz P, Durmishi Y, et al. Percutaneous CT scan-guided drainage vs. antibiotherapy alone for Hinchey II diverticulitis: a case-control study. *Dis Colon Rectum*. 2006;49(10):1533–1538.
185. Kumar RR, Kim JT, Haukoos JS, et al. Factors affecting the successful management of intra-abdominal abscesses with antibiotics and the need for percutaneous drainage. *Dis Colon Rectum*. 2006;49(2):183–189.
186. Soumian S, Thomas S, Mohan PP, et al. Management of Hinchey II diverticulitis. *World J Gastroenterol*. 2008;14(47):7163–7169.
187. Salem L, Anaya DA, Roberts KE, et al. Hartmann's colectomy and reversal in diverticulitis: a population-level assessment. *Dis Colon Rectum*. 2005;48(5):988–995.
188. Maggard MA, Zingmond D, O'Connell JB, et al. What proportion of patients with an ostomy (for diverticulitis) get reversed? *Am Surg*. 2004;70(10):928–931.
189. Krukowski ZH, Matheson NA. Emergency surgery for diverticular disease complicated by generalized and faecal peritonitis: a review. *Br J Surg*. 1984;71(12):921–927.
190. Constantinides VA, Heriot A, Remzi F, et al. Operative strategies for diverticular peritonitis: a decision analysis between primary resection and anastomosis versus Hartmann's procedures. *Ann Surg*. 2007;245(1):94–103.
191. Constantinides VA, Tekkis PP, Athanasiou T, et al. Primary resection with anastomosis vs. Hartmann's procedure in nonelective surgery for acute colonic diverticulitis: a systematic review. *Dis Colon Rectum*. 2006;49(7):966–981.
192. Aydin HN, Tekkis PP, Remzi FH, et al. Evaluation of the risk of a nonrestorative resection for the treatment of diverticular disease: the

Cleveland Clinic diverticular disease propensity score. *Dis Colon Rectum.* 2006;49(5):629–639.
193. Alamili M, Gogenur I, Rosenberg J. Acute complicated diverticulitis managed by laparoscopic lavage. *Dis Colon Rectum.* 2009;52(7):1345–1349.
194. Lam HD, Tinton N, Cambier E, et al. Laparoscopic treatment in acute complicated diverticulitis: a review of 11 cases. *Acta Chir Belg.* 2009;109(1):56–60.
195. Mutch MG. Complicated diverticulitis: are there indications for laparoscopic lavage and drainage? *Dis Colon Rectum.* 2010;53(11):1465–1466.
196. Myers E, Hurley M, O'Sullivan GC, et al. Laparoscopic peritoneal lavage for generalized peritonitis due to perforated diverticulitis. *Br J Surg.* 2008;95(1):97–101.
197. Swank HA, Vermeulen J, Lange JF, et al. The ladies trial: laparoscopic peritoneal lavage or resection for purulent peritonitisA and Hartmann's procedure or resection with primary anastomosis for purulent or faecal peritonitisB in perforated diverticulitis (NTR2037). *BMC Surg.* 2010;10:29.
198. Taylor CJ, Layani L, Ghusn MA, et al. Perforated diverticulitis managed by laparoscopic lavage. *ANZ J Surg.* 2006;76(11):962–965.
199. White SI, Frenkiel B, Martin PJ. A ten-year audit of perforated sigmoid diverticulitis: highlighting the outcomes of laparoscopic lavage. *Dis Colon Rectum.* 2010;53(11):1537–1541.
200. Moss RL, Ryan JA Jr. Management of enterovesical fistulas. *Am J Surg.* 1990;159(5):514–517.
201. Gravel D, Miller M, Simor A, et al. Health care-associated *Clostridium difficile* infection in adults admitted to acute care hospitals in Canada: a Canadian Nosocomial Infection Surveillance Program Study. *Clin Infect Dis.* 2009;48(5):568–576.
202. Gujja D, Friedenberg FK. Predictors of serious complications due to *Clostridium difficile* infection. *Aliment Pharmacol Ther.* 2009;29(6):635–642.
203. Cohen SH, Gerding DN, Johnson S, et al. Clinical practice guidelines for *Clostridium difficile* infection in adults: 2010 update by the society for healthcare epidemiology of America (SHEA) and the infectious diseases society of America (IDSA). *Infect Control Hosp Epidemiol.* 2010;31(5):431–455.
204. Kyne L, Hamel MB, Polavaram R, et al. Health care costs and mortality associated with nosocomial diarrhea due to *Clostridium difficile. Clin Infect Dis.* 2002;34(3):346–353.
205. Drudy D, Calabi E, Kyne L, et al. Human antibody response to surface layer proteins in *Clostridium difficile* infection. *FEMS Immunol Med Microbiol.* 2004;41(3):237–242.
206. Katchar K, Taylor CP, Tummala S, et al. Association between IgG2 and IgG3 subclass responses to toxin A and recurrent *Clostridium difficile*-associated disease. *Clin Gastroenterol Hepatol.* 2007;5(6):707–713.
207. Dawson AE, Shumak SL, Redelmeier DA. Treatment with monoclonal antibodies against *Clostridium difficile* toxins. *N Engl J Med.* 2010;362(15):1445; author reply 1445–1446.
208. Curry S. *Clostridium difficile. Clin Lab Med.* 2010;30(1):329–342.
209. Wren M. *Clostridium difficile* isolation and culture techniques. *Methods Mol Biol.* 2010;646:39–52.
210. Wren MW, Sivapalan M, Kinson R, et al. Laboratory diagnosis of *clostridium difficile* infection. An evaluation of tests for faecal toxin, glutamate dehydrogenase, lactoferrin and toxigenic culture in the diagnostic laboratory. *Br J Biomed Sci.* 2009;66(1):1–5.
211. Kirkpatrick ID, Greenberg HM. Evaluating the CT diagnosis of *Clostridium difficile* colitis: should CT guide therapy? *AJR Am J Roentgenol.* 2001;176(3):635–639.
212. Sailhamer EA, Carson K, Chang Y, et al. Fulminant *Clostridium difficile* colitis: patterns of care and predictors of mortality. *Arch Surg.* 2009;144(5):433–439; discussion 439–440.
213. Wenisch C, Parschalk B, Hasenhundl M, et al. Comparison of vancomycin, teicoplanin, metronidazole, and fusidic acid for the treatment of *Clostridium difficile*-associated diarrhea. *Clin Infect Dis.* 1996;22(5):813–818.
214. Teasley DG, Gerding DN, Olson MM, et al. Prospective randomised trial of metronidazole versus vancomycin for Clostridium-difficile-associated diarrhoea and colitis. *Lancet.* 1983;2(8358):1043–1046.
215. Zar FA, Bakkanagari SR, Moorthi KM, et al. A comparison of vancomycin and metronidazole for the treatment of *Clostridium difficile*-associated diarrhea, stratified by disease severity. *Clin Infect Dis.* 2007;45(3):302–307.
216. Dallal RM, Harbrecht BG, Boujoukas AJ, et al. Fulminant *Clostridium difficile*: an underappreciated and increasing cause of death and complications. *Ann Surg.* 2002;235(3):363–372.
217. Taylor GH. Cytomegalovirus. *Am Fam Physician.* 2003;67(3):519–524.
218. Rafailidis PI, Mourtzoukou EG, Varbobitis IC, et al. Severe cytomegalovirus infection in apparently immunocompetent patients: a systematic review. *Virol J.* 2008;5:47.
219. Whitley RJ, Jacobson MA, Friedberg DN, et al. Guidelines for the treatment of cytomegalovirus diseases in patients with AIDS in the era of potent antiretroviral therapy: recommendations of an international panel. International AIDS Society-USA. *Arch Intern Med.* 1998;158(9):957–969.
220. Slifkin M, Tempesti P, Poutsiaka DD, et al. Late and atypical cytomegalovirus disease in solid-organ transplant recipients. *Clin Infect Dis.* 2001;33(7):E62–E68.
221. Maconi G, Colombo E, Zerbi P, et al. Prevalence, detection rate and outcome of cytomegalovirus infection in ulcerative colitis patients requiring colonic resection. *Dig Liver Dis.* 2005;37(6):418–423.
222. Kandiel A, Lashner B. Cytomegalovirus colitis complicating inflammatory bowel disease. *Am J Gastroenterol.* 2006;101(12):2857–2865.
223. Lawlor G, Moss AC. Cytomegalovirus in inflammatory bowel disease: pathogen or innocent bystander? *Inflamm Bowel Dis.* 2010;16(9):1620–1627.
224. Huston CD. Parasite and host contributions to the pathogenesis of amebic colitis. *Trends Parasitol.* 2004;20(1):23–26.
225. Stanley SL Jr. Amoebiasis. *Lancet.* 2003;361(9362):1025–1034.
226. Brandt LJ, Boley SJ. Colonic ischemia. *Surg Clin North Am.* 1992;72(1):203–229.
227. Brandt LJ, Boley SJ. AGA technical review on intestinal ischemia. American Gastrointestinal Association. *Gastroenterology.* 2000;118(5):954–968.
228. Marston A, Pheils MT, Thomas ML, et al. Ischaemic colitis. *Gut.* 1966;7(1):1–15.
229. Michels NA, Siddharth P, Kornblith PL, et al. The variant blood supply to the descending colon, rectosigmoid and rectum based on 400 dissections. Its importance in regional resections: a review of medical literature. *Dis Colon Rectum.* 1965;8:251–278.
230. Griffiths JD. Extramural and intramural blood-supply of colon. *Br Med J.* 1961;1(5222):323–326.
231. Griffiths JD. Surgical anatomy of the blood supply of the distal colon. *Ann R Coll Surg Engl.* 1956;19(4):241–256.
232. Meyers MA. Griffiths' point: critical anastomosis at the splenic flexure. Significance in ischemia of the colon. *AJR Am J Roentgenol.* 1976;126(1):77–94.
233. MacDonald PH. Ischaemic colitis. *Best Pract Res Clin Gastroenterol.* 2002;16(1):51–61.
234. Kuo WT, Lee DE, Saad WE, et al. Superselective microcoil embolization for the treatment of lower gastrointestinal hemorrhage. *J Vasc Interv Radiol.* 2003;14(12):1503–1509.
235. Zelenock GB, Strodel WE, Knol JA, et al. A prospective study of clinically and endoscopically documented colonic ischemia in 100 patients undergoing aortic reconstructive surgery with aggressive colonic and direct pelvic revascularization, compared with historic controls. *Surgery.* 1989;106(4):771–779; discussion 779–780.
236. Brewster DC, Franklin DP, Cambria RP, et al. Intestinal ischemia complicating abdominal aortic surgery. *Surgery.* 1991;109(4):447–454.
237. Poeze M, Froon AH, Greve JW, et al. D-lactate as an early marker of intestinal ischaemia after ruptured abdominal aortic aneurysm repair. *Br J Surg.* 1998;85(9):1221–1224.
238. Murray MJ, Gonze MD, Nowak LR, et al. Serum D(-)-lactate levels as an aid to diagnosing acute intestinal ischemia. *Am J Surg.* 1994;167(6):575–578.
239. Wolf EL, Sprayregen S, Bakal CW. Radiology in intestinal ischemia. Plain film, contrast, and other imaging studies. *Surg Clin North Am.* 1992;72(1):107–124.
240. Bower TC. Ischemic colitis. *Surg Clin North Am.* 1993;73(5): 1037–1053.
241. Balthazar EJ, Yen BC, Gordon RB. Ischemic colitis: CT evaluation of 54 cases. *Radiology.* 1999;211(2):381–388.
242. Teefey SA, Roarke MC, Brink JA, et al. Bowel wall thickening: differentiation of inflammation from ischemia with color Doppler and duplex US. *Radiology.* 1996;198(2):547–551.
243. Scharff JR, Longo WE, Vartanian SM, et al. Ischemic colitis: spectrum of disease and outcome. *Surgery.* 2003;134(4):624–629; discussion 629–630.
244. Longo WE, Ballantyne GH, Gusberg RJ. Ischemic colitis: patterns and prognosis. *Dis Colon Rectum.* 1992;35(8):726–730.
245. Paterno F, McGillicuddy EA, Schuster KM, et al. Ischemic colitis: risk factors for eventual surgery. *Am J Surg.* 2010;200(5):646–650.
246. Travis SP, Farrant JM, Ricketts C, et al. Predicting outcome in severe ulcerative colitis. *Gut.* 1996;38(6):905–910.
247. Truelove SC, Jewell DP. Intensive intravenous regimen for severe attacks of ulcerative colitis. *Lancet.* 1974;1(7866):1067–1070.
248. Truelove SC, Witts LJ. Cortisone in ulcerative colitis; final report on a therapeutic trial. *Br Med J.* 1955;2(4947):1041–1048.
249. Criscuoli V, Casa A, Orlando A, et al.Severe acute colitis associated with CMV: a prevalence study. *Dig Liver Dis.* 2004;36(12):818–820.
250. Bossuyt P, Verhaegen J, Van Assche G, et al. Increasing incidence of *Clostridium difficile*-associated diarrhea in inflammatory bowel disease. *J Crohns Colitis.* 2009;3(1):4–7.
251. Clayton EM, Rea MC, Shanahan F, et al. The vexed relationship between *Clostridium difficile* and inflammatory bowel disease: an assessment of carriage in an outpatient setting among patients in remission. *Am J Gastroenterol.* 2009;104(5):1162–1169.
252. Cottone M, Pietrosi G, Martorana G, et al. Prevalence of cytomegalovirus infection in severe refractory ulcerative and Crohn's colitis. *Am J Gastroenterol.* 2001;96(3):773–775.
253. Daperno M, Sostegni R, Pera A, et al. The role of endoscopic assessment in ulcerative colitis in the era of infliximab. *Dig Liver Dis* 2008;40(suppl 2):S220–S224.
254. Carbonnel F, Lavergne A, Lemann M, et al. Colonoscopy of acute colitis. A safe and reliable tool for assessment of severity. *Dig Dis Sci.* 1994;39(7):1550–1557.
255. Jarnerot G, Rolny P, Sandberg-Gertzen H. Intensive intravenous treatment of ulcerative colitis. *Gastroenterology.* 1985;89(5):1005–1013.

256. Van Assche G, D'Haens G, Noman M, et al. Randomized, double-blind comparison of 4 mg/kg versus 2 mg/kg intravenous cyclosporine in severe ulcerative colitis. *Gastroenterology*. 2003;125(4):1025–1031.
257. Kornbluth A, Present DH, Lichtiger S, et al. Cyclosporin for severe ulcerative colitis: a user's guide. *Am J Gastroenterol.* 1997;92(9): 1424–1428.
258. Lichtiger S, Present DH, Kornbluth A, et al. Cyclosporine in severe ulcerative colitis refractory to steroid therapy. *N Engl J Med.* 1994;330(26):1841–1845.
259. Chey WY. Infliximab for patients with refractory ulcerative colitis. *Inflamm Bowel Dis.* 2001;7(suppl 1):S30–S33.
260. Chey WY, Shah A. Infliximab for ulcerative colitis. *J Clin Gastroenterol.* 2005;39(10):920; author reply 920.
261. Jarnerot G, Hertervig E, Friis-Liby I, et al. Infliximab as rescue therapy in severe to moderately severe ulcerative colitis: a randomized, placebo-controlled study. *Gastroenterology*. 2005;128(7):1805–1811.
262. Rutgeerts P, Sandborn WJ, Feagan BG, et al. Infliximab for induction and maintenance therapy for ulcerative colitis. *N Engl J Med.* 2005;353(23):2462–2476.
263. Hanauer SB. Infliximab or cyclosporine for severe ulcerative colitis. *Gastroenterology*. 2005;129(4):1358–1359;author reply 1359.
264. Baumgart DC, Pintoffl JP, Sturm A, et al. Tacrolimus is safe and effective in patients with severe steroid-refractory or steroid-dependent inflammatory bowel disease—a long-term follow-up. *Am J Gastroenterol.* 2006;101(5):1048–1056.
265. Baumgart DC, Wiedenmann B, Dignass AU. Rescue therapy with tacrolimus is effective in patients with severe and refractory inflammatory bowel disease. *Aliment Pharmacol Ther.* 2003;17(10):1273–1281.
266. Fellermann K, Tanko Z, Herrlinger KR, et al. Response of refractory colitis to intravenous or oral tacrolimus (FK506). *Inflamm Bowel Dis.* 2002;8(5):317–324.
267. Hanai H, Iida T, Takeuchi K, et al. Intensive granulocyte and monocyte adsorption versus intravenous prednisolone in patients with severe ulcerative colitis: an unblinded randomised multi-centre controlled study. *Dig Liver Dis.* 2008;40(6):433–440.
268. Hanai H, Watanabe F, Takeuchi K, et al. Leukocyte adsorptive apheresis for the treatment of active ulcerative colitis: a prospective, uncontrolled, pilot study. *Clin Gastroenterol Hepatol.* 2003;1(1):28–35.
269. Schnedl WJ, Krause R, Tafeit E, et al. Insights into epiploic appendagitis. *Nat Rev Gastroenterol Hepatol.* 2011;8(1):45–49.
270. Sorser SA, Maas LC, Yousif E, et al. Epiploic appendagitis: the great mimicker. *South Med J.* 2009;102(12):1214–1217.
271. Sandrasegaran K, Maglinte DD, Rajesh A, et al. Primary epiploic appendagitis: CT diagnosis. *Emerg Radiol.* 2004;11(1):9–14.
272. Singh AK, Gervais DA, Hahn PF, et al. CT appearance of acute appendagitis. *AJR Am J Roentgenol.* 2004;183(5):1303–1307.
273. Sirvanci M, Tekelioglu MH, Duran C, et al. Primary epiploic appendagitis: CT manifestations. *Clin Imaging.* 2000;24(6):357–361.
274. Uslu Tutar N, Ozgul E, Oguz D, et al. An uncommon cause of acute abdomen—epiploic appendagitis: CT findings. *Turk J Gastroenterol.* 2007;18(2):107–110.
275. Seitz K. Sonographic diagnosis of diverticulitis: the burdensome way to acceptance. *Ultraschall Med.* 2004;25(5):335–336.
276. van Breda Vriesman AC, Puylaert JB. Old and new infarction of an epiploic appendage: ultrasound mimicry of appendicitis. *Abdom Imaging.* 1999;24(2):129–131.
277. Sand M, Gelos M, Bechara FG, et al. Epiploic appendagitis—clinical characteristics of an uncommon surgical diagnosis. *BMC Surg.* 2007;7:11.
278. Davila ML. Neutropenic enterocolitis. *Curr Opin Gastroenterol.* 2006;22(1):44–47.
279. Katz JA, Wagner ML, Gresik MV, et al. Typhlitis. An 18-year experience and postmortem review. *Cancer.* 1990;65(4):1041–1047.
280. Monkemuller KE, Wilcox CM. Diagnosis and treatment of colonic disease in AIDS. *Gastrointest Endosc Clin N Am.* 1998;8(4):889–911.
281. Sloas MM, Flynn PM, Kaste SC, et al. Typhlitis in children with cancer: a 30-year experience. *Clin Infect Dis.* 1993;17(3):484–490.
282. Urbach DR, Rotstein OD. Typhlitis. *Can J Surg.* 1999;42(6):415–419.
283. Wade DS, Nava HR, Douglass HO Jr. Neutropenic enterocolitis. Clinical diagnosis and treatment. *Cancer.* 1992;69(1):17–23.
284. Babb RR. Radiation proctitis: a review. *Am J Gastroenterol.* 1996;91(7):1309–1311.
285. Sasai T, Hiraishi H, Suzuki Y, et al. Treatment of chronic post-radiation proctitis with oral administration of sucralfate. *Am J Gastroenterol.* 1998;93(9):1593–1595.
286. Stockdale AD, Biswas A. Long-term control of radiation proctitis following treatment with sucralfate enemas. *Br J Surg.* 1997;84(3):379.
287. Leiper K, Morris AI. Treatment of radiation proctitis. *Clin Oncol (R Coll Radiol).* 2007;19(9):724–729.
288. Dees J, Meijssen MA, Kuipers EJ. Argon plasma coagulation for radiation proctitis. *Scand J Gastroenterol Suppl.* 2006(243):175–178.
289. Taieb S, Rolachon A, Cenni JC, et al. Effective use of argon plasma coagulation in the treatment of severe radiation proctitis. *Dis Colon Rectum.* 2001;44(12):1766–1771.
290. Tjandra JJ, Sengupta S. Argon plasma coagulation is an effective treatment for refractory hemorrhagic radiation proctitis. *Dis Colon Rectum.* 2001;44(12):1759–1765;discussion 1771.
291. al-Sabbagh R, Sinicrope FA, Sellin JH, et al. Evaluation of short-chain fatty acid enemas: treatment of radiation proctitis. *Am J Gastroenterol.* 1996;91(9):1814–1816.
292. Biswal BM, Lal P, Rath GK, et al. Intrarectal formalin application, an effective treatment for grade III haemorrhagic radiation proctitis. *Radiother Oncol.* 1995;35(3):212–215.
293. Lucarotti ME, Mountford RA, Bartolo DC. Surgical management of intestinal radiation injury. *Dis Colon Rectum.* 1991;34(10):865–869.
294. Ng SC, Kamm MA. Therapeutic strategies for the management of ulcerative colitis. *Inflamm Bowel Dis.* 2009;15(6):935–950.

CHAPTER 36 ■ INTESTINAL OBSTRUCTION AND DYSMOTILITY SYNDROMES

LOUIS H. ALARCON

Few clinical conditions are as common yet potentially perplexing as intestinal obstruction. Intestinal obstruction is a frequent presenting problem and accounts for a large percentage of surgical consults for acute abdominal pain. As many as 15% of surgical admissions are for mechanical small bowel obstruction.[1]

Intestinal obstruction develops when gas and succus are prevented from passing distally through the gastrointestinal tract as a result of either intrinsic or extrinsic compression (i.e., mechanical obstruction) or gastrointestinal paralysis (i.e., nonmechanical obstruction, either ileus or pseudo-obstruction). Many different etiologies may account for this pathology. Ileus is the most common form of dysmotility, although not an obstruction *per se*. It frequently develops after abdominal surgery or in association with intra-abdominal or extra-abdominal inflammatory conditions.[2] Mechanical small bowel obstruction is slightly less common. Postoperative intra-abdominal adhesions account for the majority of mechanical small-bowel obstructions. Cancer and hernia account for the majority of the remaining cases of small-bowel obstruction. Mechanical colonic obstruction is less frequent than small-bowel obstruction, and accounts for 10%–15% of cases of mechanical bowel obstruction. The most common causes of mechanical large-bowel obstruction include obstructing carcinoma, diverticulitis, or volvulus. Acute colonic pseudo-obstruction occurs most often in elderly patients, in response to acute medical illness, or in the postoperative period.

PATHOPHYSIOLOGY OF INTESTINAL OBSTRUCTION

Mechanical small-bowel obstruction develops as gastrointestinal secretions and gas accumulate in the distended intestine proximal to an obstructed segment. As the distension progresses, the intraluminal hydrostatic pressure compresses the intestinal mucosal villus lymphatics, causing lymphedema of the bowel wall. With increasing intraluminal pressures, the hydrostatic pressure at the venous end of the postcapillary venules causes a shift in the Starling dynamics across the capillary bed, leading to the net filtration of fluids, electrolytes, and proteins into the bowel wall and lumen. This so-called "third spacing" can lead to the loss of massive amounts of intravascular volume, causing dehydration, hypovolemia, and end-organ hypoperfusion if untreated. Venous hypertension may also lead to arterial hypoperfusion and bowel ischemia in some cases, but, more often, direct arterial occlusion occurs due to the mechanical forces associated with a segment of bowel, which has twisted upon its mesentery (volvulus) or due to strangulation in an incarcerated hernia. If the bowel ischemia is not treated in a timely fashion, intestinal necrosis, perforation, and peritonitis ensue. Furthermore, the normal intestinal mucosal barriers are disrupted, theoretically allowing gut bacteria to translocate into the systemic circulation.[3,4] Enteric bacteria have been isolated in the mesenteric lymph nodes of approximately 60% of patients undergoing laparotomy for simple bowel obstruction (without strangulated intestine) compared to only 4% of patients undergoing laparotomy for conditions other than bowel obstruction.[5]

DIAGNOSIS AND EVALUATION

Patients with mechanical bowel obstruction or ileus often present with abdominal pain and distension, nausea, vomiting, and obstipation.[6] Several clinical features may help distinguish mechanical obstruction from ileus or pseudo-obstruction. The pain associated with mechanical obstruction is typically moderate to severe and crampy in nature, while patients with ileus tend to have less pain and in some cases no pain.

A detailed past surgical history must be obtained in all patients. Prior abdominal surgery places the patient at risk for the development of adhesive small-bowel obstruction. The lack of prior abdominal surgery or inflammatory conditions makes adhesive disease unlikely as the etiology of the patient's obstruction. Any prior history of malignancy must be taken into account, as recurrent cancer must be in the differential diagnosis.

PHYSICAL EXAMINATION AND INITIAL MANAGEMENT

The patient with bowel obstruction often requires simultaneous evaluation and initial resuscitation. It is important to rapidly assess the degree of physiologic impairment, and address it expeditiously. Common physiologic abnormalities include hypovolemia, electrolyte abnormalities, and prerenal azotemia. Establishment of intravenous access and fluid resuscitation are important parts of the initial management of these patients. Careful monitoring of urinary output with an indwelling Foley catheter may serve as an important endpoint of resuscitation. Nasogastric decompression may be necessary to reduce the incidence of vomiting and aspiration. The character of the nasogastric tube output may be useful as far as diagnosis is concerned. A nonbilious output implies a gastric outlet obstruction. Bilious but nonfeculent aspirate is usually seen in proximal small-bowel obstructions or colonic obstruction with a competent ileocecal valve. Distal small-bowel obstruction often presents with feculent nasogastric output.

It is also important to exclude other medical conditions, which may be associated with nausea, vomiting, and abdominal distention such as an acute coronary syndrome or pneumonia.

Examination of the abdomen proceeds in an orderly fashion: inspection, auscultation, palpation, and percussion. With the patient in the supine position, general inspection of the abdomen is performed. The degree of abdominal distension may vary with the level of the obstruction: proximal small-bowel obstruction may be associated with minimal abdominal distension. Surgical scars from prior abdominal surgery should be noted. Visible peristaltic waves are often associated with mechanical small-bowel obstruction.

Auscultation with a stethoscope should be performed for at least 5 minutes to determine the presence and quality of bowel sounds. The typical bowel sounds in a patient with a mechanical small-bowel obstruction are high-pitched and hyperactive. Patients with ileus often have a silent abdomen. However, patients with long-standing intestinal obstruction or perforation associated with peritonitis may have a silent abdomen.

Palpation of the abdomen should start gently and become progressively deeper as the patient's pain is assessed. If the patient complains of pain in one discrete region area, it is useful to begin the palpation on the opposite side of the abdomen. Most patients with bowel obstruction have diffuse abdominal tenderness, but less than half will have mild tenderness, guarding, or rigidity.[6] Traditionally, many surgeons believe that the findings of localized tenderness, guarding, or rebound are indicative of underlying bowel strangulation and mandate operation. However, these findings are neither sensitive nor specific for the detection of underlying bowel ischemia[7] or obstruction.[6] Furthermore, patients with ileus may also have abdominal tenderness and may be difficult to distinguish from mechanical bowel obstruction in this regard. Gentle percussion should be performed to assess for tympany associated with underlying distended, gas-filled intestine; dullness, indicative of an underlying mass; or peritoneal irritation associated with ischemic bowel or peritonitis secondary to perforation.

A comprehensive evaluation for abdominal wall herniae must be performed in all patients. This includes careful inspection for inguinal, femoral, umbilical, incisional, and other abdominal wall herniae. Herniae should be assessed for the presence of incarcerated intestine. If local signs of infarcted intestine are present such as erythema or cellulitis, the patient should undergo immediate operation without attempt at reduction. Otherwise, careful reduction should be attempted, but care taken to avoid further injury to the intestine during this maneuver, or of reducing already ischemic bowel. Some herniae, such as obturator hernia or internal hernia, may not be readily detectable on physical exam and require imaging to detect. Digital rectal examination is performed to evaluate for masses, fecal impaction, and occult blood. Similarly, digital examination of any existing stoma is important to assess obstruction at a colostomy or ileostomy site.

DIAGNOSTIC STUDIES

Plain Radiographs

While abdominal radiographs should be obtained routinely on all patients suspected of having a bowel obstruction, plain films may be diagnostic in only half of such patients.[8,9] Plain films are more sensitive in the detection of high-grade obstruction but less sensitive to detect low-grade obstruction. A chest x-ray helps to exclude an acute pulmonary process such as pneumonia, as well as detect subdiaphragmatic air, indicative of hollow viscus perforation. Plain abdominal x-rays (upright, lateral decubitus, and supine) can distinguish between mechanical bowel obstruction and ileus in many cases and may establish the location of the obstruction (small vs. large intestine). Except for inguinal hernia or gallstone ileus, the cause of the obstruction is often not discernable on plain radiographs. It is helpful to distinguish between gas-filled loops of small and large intestine. The small intestine contains valvulae conniventes or plicae circulares, which

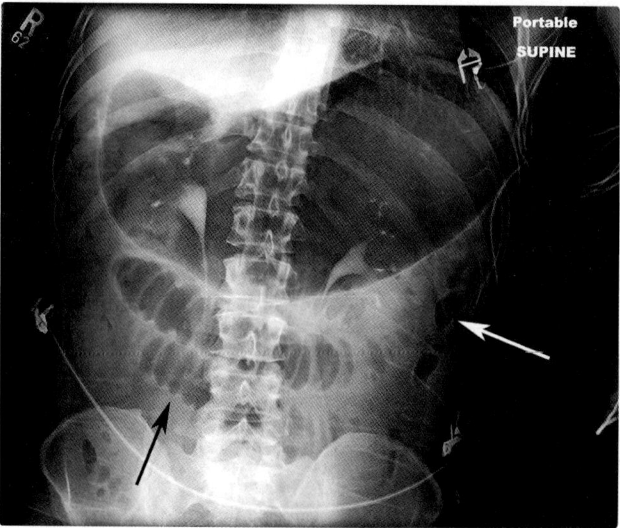

FIGURE 36.1. Abdominal radiograph of a supine patient with small-bowel obstruction. The stomach is markedly distended. There are several dilated small-bowel loops, which demonstrate prominent valvulae conniventes with bowel wall edema (*black arrow*). Scant gas is seen within the decompressed colon (*white arrow*).

encompass the entire lumen of the bowel. Colon, which contains gas demonstrates colonic haustral markings, which cross only part of the bowel lumen (Fig. 36.1). Normally, the small intestine does not contain visible gas, so the finding of substantial gas in the small intestine is abnormal. The presence of air–fluid levels is also indicative of either mechanical obstruction or ileus. Gas throughout the small intestine and colon is usually associated with ileus, but can also be seen in cases of distal (rectal) obstruction. The presence of distended, air–fluid-filled loops of small intestine with absent colonic gas suggests high-grade small-bowel obstruction. However, in the early stages of small-bowel obstruction or in cases of partial obstruction, some gas may remain within the colon. Patients with closed-loop obstruction or very proximal small-bowel obstruction may have few or no dilated loops of intestine. Massive distension of the colon is seen in cases of pseudo-obstruction or colonic volvulus. Thickened intestinal walls with mucosal thumbprinting occurs when the intestine is edematous or ischemic (Fig. 36.1). Also, pneumatosis of the intestinal wall and portal venous gas result from advanced cases of intestinal ischemia. Free intraperitoneal air indicates perforation of a hollow viscus.

Laboratory Studies

Patients with mechanical bowel obstruction often have fluid and electrolyte disturbances that should be corrected during the resuscitation phase and prior to surgical intervention. Likewise, patients with ileus often have an associated metabolic or infectious etiology that should be sought as part of the diagnosis and treatment of the condition. Serum electrolytes, creatinine, hemoglobin, and coagulation parameters should be checked routinely. Serum lactate may be elevated in cases of bowel ischemia. Patients with considerable physiologic impairment may need assessment of acid–base status with arterial blood gas. For patients with ileus, additional studies that should be obtained include serum magnesium, phosphate, ionized calcium, urinalysis, pancreatic enzymes, and a search for potential infectious sources.

ADJUNCTIVE TESTS

Computed Tomography

Many clinicians rely on computed tomography (CT) to determine the etiology and location of intestinal obstruction,[10–14] and CT has become the radiographic modality of choice for the diagnosis of intestinal obstruction.[9] The diagnosis of small-bowel obstruction on CT involves the identification of dilated loops of intestine proximally with normal or collapsed loops distally. A small-bowel caliber > 2.5 cm is considered dilated. If a transition point is identified, the diagnosis of obstruction is more certain. The transition point often resembles a bird's beak (Figs. 36.2 and 36.3), and this "beak sign" is present in 60% of cases of small-bowel obstruction.[9] The small-bowel feces sign, the presence of small-bowel particulate material in a dilated segment (Fig 36.4), is present in 56% of cases of small-bowel obstruction.[15] CT has a sensitivity of 81%–94% and specificity of 96% for diagnosis of high-grade bowel obstruction.[9] The accuracy of CT scan is reduced in cases of partial intestinal obstruction, although recent advances in CT technology are improving its accuracy in these cases. CT has several advantages over other imaging modalities: it can accurately determine the level, etiology, and degree of the obstruction and can readily indentify closed-loop obstruction and bowel ischemia. CT can detect extrinsic mass lesions or inflammatory processes not visible on plain radiographs.[16] CT is the most sensitive modality to detect intraperitoneal free air and pneumatosis intestinalis (Fig. 36.4C). CT is also the preferred modality to distinguish mechanical colonic obstruction from pseudo-obstruction.[17] Administration of oral contrast may not be tolerated by acutely ill and obstructed patients and is usually not essential for the CT identification of obstruction; luminal fluid and air can easily be distinguished within the bowel lumen. However, enteral contrast may be useful in discriminating partial from complete obstruction and the level of the obstruction. The use of intravenous contrast during CT is recommended so the bowel wall can be visualized in contrast to its luminal contents.[18–20] The most important information that CT can provide is whether strangulation (bowel ischemia) is present. The sensitivity of contrast-enhanced CT for diagnosis of intestinal ischemia is as high as 90%.[9] Signs of intestinal ischemia on contrast-enhanced CT include thickened bowel wall, ascites, the target sign (trilaminar appearance of bowel wall from enhanced mucosa and muscularis with edematous submucosa in between), lack of contrast enhancement of bowel wall, pneumatosis intestinalis, gas in mesenteric or portal veins, and the "whirl sign" (twisting of mesenteric vessels in volvulus).

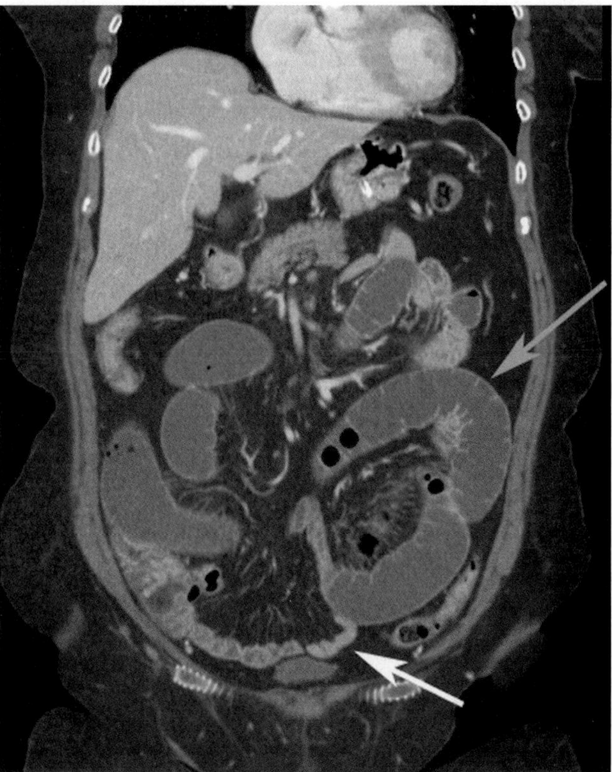

FIGURE 36.3. Coronal CT scan demonstrating small-bowel obstruction with dilated proximal small intestine (*gray arrow*) and decompressed distal small intestine (*white arrow*) beyond the level of the obstruction.

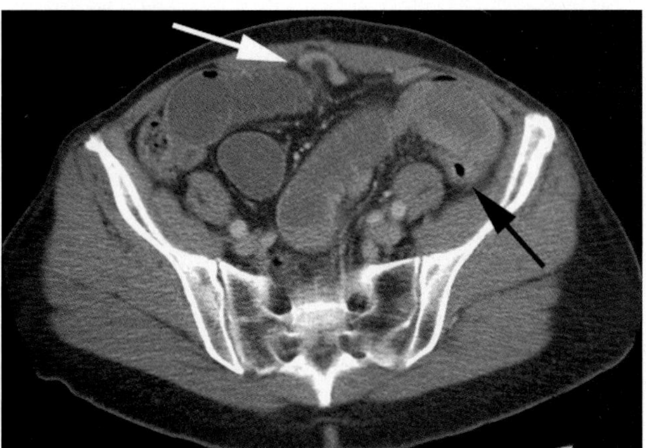

FIGURE 36.2. CT demonstrating high-grade small-bowel obstruction with a transition point or "bird's beak" (*white arrow*) between distended and decompressed loops of small intestine. The decompressed descending colon is also seen (*black arrow*).

Other Radiographic Modalities

Given the limitations of plain abdominal radiographs described above, other adjunctive radiographic modalities have been advocated. Clearly, CT is the modality of choice given its availability and accuracy. However, in some instances, ultrasonography and magnetic resonance imaging (MRI) have been proposed. Both modalities are highly sensitive and specific for intestinal obstruction when performed and interpreted by experienced clinicians. Two prospective trials found that ultrasonography was as sensitive as and more specific than plain radiographs in the diagnosis of intestinal obstruction.[21,22] The accuracy of ultrasonography is operator dependent, and most surgeons are not yet comfortable in the interpretation of sonographic images for the diagnosis of intestinal obstruction. These reasons, plus the accuracy and widespread availability of CT, limit the clinical utility of ultrasonography in this setting. However, for patients who are hemodynamically unstable and not suitable candidates for transport to CT, bedside ultrasonography may be a useful modality.[21]

There is evidence suggesting that MRI is more sensitive and specific than contrast-enhanced CT in determining the etiology and location of bowel obstruction.[23] However, continuing evolution and technological advances in CT imaging, such as

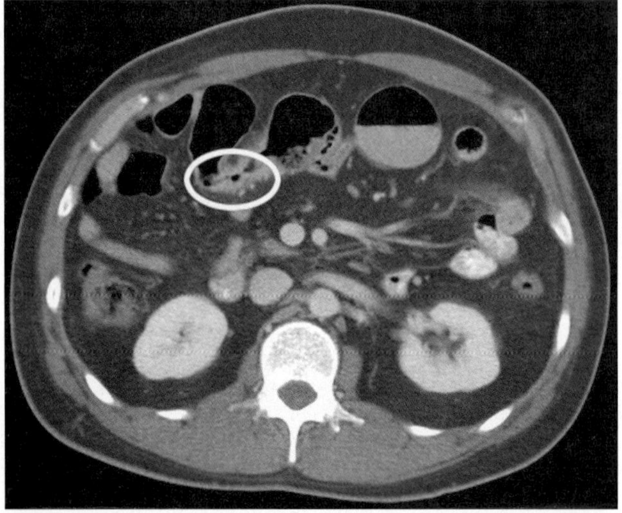

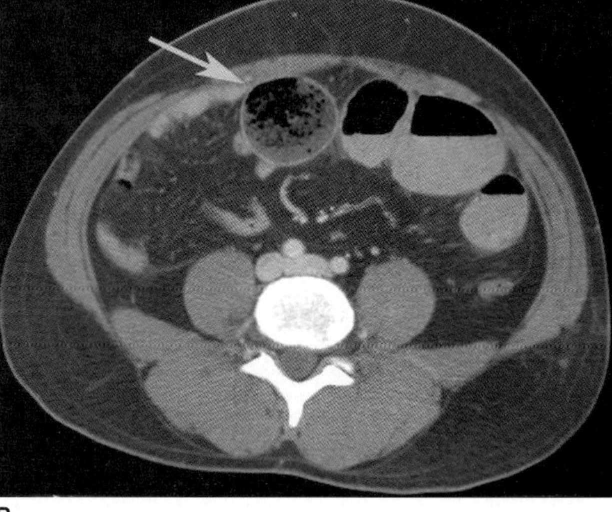

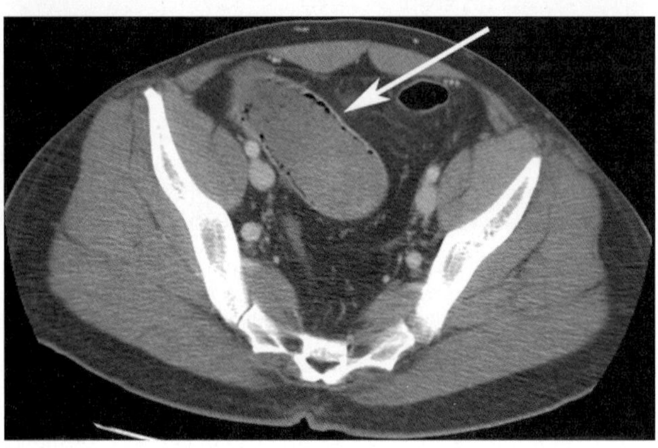

FIGURE 36.4. A: CT scan showing small-bowel obstruction with transition point at a focal area of wall thickening (*white ellipse*). B: proximal to the obstruction, there is marked dilation of the small bowel with small-bowel feces sign (*gray arrow*). C: pneumatosis intestinalis of a segment of ischemic, obstructed small intestine (*white arrow*).

multiphasic scanning, faster scanners, and 3D reconstruction, have increased the accuracy of this modality, further reducing the utility of ultrasonography and MRI.

Gastrointestinal contrast studies may be useful diagnostic modalities in some instances, but best used in the subacute or chronic setting. Oral contrast studies such as small-bowel follow-through can offer information about the location and degree of the obstruction and the bowel transit time. Limitations of the small-bowel follow-through include logistics, the length of time required to complete the study, the dilution of contrast as it travels distally, and the risk of contrast aspiration. Enteroclysis allows nondistensible segments of intestine to be more readily identified. Enteroclysis is performed by placing a catheter in the small intestine and infusion of contrast material. Enteroclysis is accurate at detection of low-grade and intermittent obstruction and can serve as an adjunct to CT in these cases; it has no advantage over CT in the diagnosis of high-grade obstruction.[9] The administration of contrast enemas may be useful in cases of colonic distension to evaluate for mechanical obstruction, for example, due to mass lesions or stricture.

Sigmoidoscopy

For patients with distal colon or rectal obstruction, sigmoid volvulus, or colonic pseudo-obstruction with massive colonic distension, flexible or rigid sigmoidoscopy may be both diagnostic and therapeutic. When the radiographs demonstrate distended colon with gas extending to the sigmoid or rectum, sigmoidoscopy will readily exclude a distal colon or rectal mass as the etiology of the obstruction. Care must be exercised to avoid instillation of a large amount of air during the sigmoidoscopy; this will increase the chances of iatrogenic perforation of the colon.

DETERMINATION OF THE NEED FOR SURGERY

For patients with suspected bowel obstruction, the decision to operate and the timing of surgery can be determined based on the history, physical exam, laboratory data, plain radiographs, and CT. It is important to distinguish mechanical obstruction from ileus. Patients with nonmechanical obstruction usually do not require immediate surgery. Early identification of patients with obstruction and bowel ischemia is critical. Also, in patients with mechanical obstruction, determination of whether the obstruction is complete (which requires immediate operation) vs. partial (which does not) is important. Similarly, determination of the level and etiology of the obstruction has important therapeutic implications. Patients with complete or partial bowel obstruction generally should be admitted to a surgical service as admission to nonsurgical service is associated with increased patient morbidity and mortality.[24,25] In one series of 166 cases of small-bowel obstruction, 20 patients underwent immediate surgery due to concern for bowel ischemia and 45% of these proved to have ischemic bowel at laparotomy. Among those selected for conservative management, about two-thirds resolved without surgery, but 6% had strangulated bowel and 2% died.[26]

MECHANICAL OBSTRUCTION

There are many potential causes of bowel obstruction (see Tables 36.1 and 36.2). Patients with mechanical, complete bowel obstruction should undergo immediate surgery after expeditious correction of hypovolemia and fluid and electrolyte disorders. Nonoperative management of complete intestinal obstruction is associated with increased morbidity and mortality due to delayed recognition and treatment of strangulated bowel.[7] Immediate operation is also indicated for patients with bowel obstruction in the presence of peritonitis or signs of systemic toxicity, incarcerated or strangulated herniae, pneumatosis intestinalis, cecal volvulus, or sigmoid volvulus with systemic toxicity. CT will help identify the presence of these conditions in equivocal cases. Exceptions to this rule for immediate operation for these conditions include patients with terminal illness whose goals of care are palliation of symptoms, or those who have cardiopulmonary instability, which requires resuscitation prior to surgery.

ADHESIVE SMALL-BOWEL OBSTRUCTION

Postoperative adhesions are the most common cause of intestinal obstruction and account for 60% of cases of small-bowel obstruction.[29] Adhesive intestinal obstruction usually occurs in the small intestine. In the setting of colonic obstruction, an alternative etiology should be sought as adhesions rarely cause colonic obstruction. Intestinal obstruction resulting from adhesions may occur as early as days to as late as many years after surgery.[30] Adhesive small-bowel obstruction most frequently occurs after prior appendectomy, colorectal surgery, gynecologic procedures, or upper gastrointestinal surgery. One-fourth of patients with mechanical small-bowel obstruction had multiple prior laparotomies.[29] Laparoscopic surgery is associated with a lower incidence of postoperative bowel obstruction compared to comparable open surgery.[31] Initial treatment of adhesive small-bowel obstruction includes bowel rest, nasogastric decompression, intravenous fluids, correction of metabolic and electrolyte abnormalities, and analgesia.

TABLE 36.1

ETIOLOGY AND INCIDENCE OF SMALL-BOWEL OBSTRUCTION

ETIOLOGY	RELATIVE INCIDENCE (%)
Adhesions	60
Neoplasm	20
Hernia	10
Inflammatory bowel disease	5
Volvulus	3
Others	2

From Hayanga AJ, Bass-Wilkins K, Bulkley GB. Current management of small-bowel obstruction. *Adv Surg.* 2005;39:1–33.

TABLE 36.2

ETIOLOGY AND INCIDENCE OF LARGE-BOWEL OBSTRUCTION

ETIOLOGY	RELATIVE INCIDENCE (%)
Neoplasm (malignant or benign)	86
Volvulus	5
Hernia	3
Diverticular disease	2
Ischemic colitis	1
Others	3

From Biondo S, Pares D, Frago R, et al. Large-bowel obstruction: predictive factors for postoperative mortality. *Dis Colon Rectum.* 2004;47:1889–1897.

In this setting, nonoperative management is associated with resolution of symptoms in approximately 90% of patients.[32–34] However, as many as half of these patients will experience recurrent obstruction.[34–36]

Some studies suggest that the probability of resolution of the bowel obstruction with conservative management can be predicted based on the nature of the prior abdominal surgery.[37–39] Procedures associated with a higher failure rate for conservative management of adhesive small-bowel obstruction include those which were performed through a midline laparotomy, those involving the aorta, colon, rectum, appendix or pelvic adnexa, and those done to alleviate previous obstruction due to carcinomatosis. In these cases, a shorter duration of observation during conservative management should be considered.

For patients with partial bowel obstruction due to adhesions, there is no clear consensus on how long such patients should be treated conservatively. However, beyond 48 hours of observation, the risks of complications increase substantially and the probability of nonoperative resolution decreases considerably.[40] In general, patients who are likely to resolve with conservative management begin to show clinical improvement in the first 12 hours. Consideration for surgical intervention should be made for patients who fail to show signs of improvement or who deteriorate in this time frame. Patients selected for conservative management must be examined serially and frequently, preferably by the same clinician. The degree of abdominal distension, amount and character of the nasogastric output (e.g., feculent output correlates with complete obstruction, necessitating surgery), the passage of flatus or bowel movement, and the development of new or worsening abdominal tenderness should be carefully assessed at frequent intervals. Follow-up plain radiographs may be useful to demonstrate persistence or resolution of the radiographic abnormality.

It should be possible to determine with a high degree of accuracy which patients will require surgery to address adhesive small-bowel obstruction within 24–48 hours of admission. Using CT, patients with complete bowel obstruction or closed-loop obstruction, that is, those who require urgent operation, can be readily identified and treated appropriately.[11–13] For those with partial obstruction, close clinical observation will identify those who are failing to progress and warrant surgical intervention. In addition, the success or failure of nonoperative management can be predicted by the time it takes for orally administered contrast to reach the right colon. Arrival of contrast within 8–24 hours predicts success of conservative management with >95% sensitivity and specificity.[41–43]

SURGICAL ADHESIOLYSIS

Laparotomy with surgical adhesiolysis is the traditional surgical modality to treat patients with adhesive bowel obstruction who require operative intervention. The principles of this technique involve midline laparotomy with careful entry into the peritoneal cavity to avoid iatrogenic bowel injury, identification and sharp lysis of the adhesions that contribute to the obstruction, careful inspection of the intestine to identify injury or ischemia, repair or resection of perforated intestine, and resection of ischemic or gangrenous segments. When operative adhesiolysis is required for small-bowel obstruction, the mortality ranges from <5% for uncomplicated obstruction, to as high as 30% in cases where bowel resection is required for intestinal strangulation or gangrene.[30]

Laparoscopic lysis of adhesions relieves obstruction in the majority of patients and compares favorably to open surgery.[44–49] To reduce the chance of bowel injury during trocar placement, the first port should be placed using open technique under direct visualization and in an area away from prior surgical incisions.[50,51] In retrospective, case-control matched series, about half of patients treated with laparoscopic adhesiolysis required conversion to open surgery due to inability to complete the procedure laparoscopically or to manage complications.[49] Patients with two or more prior laparotomies had a considerably higher rate of intraoperative complication during laparoscopy. Despite the high conversion rate, the group of patients who underwent laparoscopic adhesiolysis experienced an overall reduction in postoperative complications. Other studies have also shown that patients explored laparoscopically who required conversion to open laparotomy did not fair worse than those initially treated with laparotomy.[52]

One potential advantage of laparoscopic surgery for adhesive bowel obstruction over open surgery is that it results in a reduced risk of causing additional intra-abdominal adhesions, which may lead to subsequent adhesive bowl obstruction.[53,54] However, patients who undergo laparoscopic surgery for adhesive bowel obstruction may be at increased risk for early unplanned reoperation due to complications or incomplete relief of obstruction.[44] Another problem is that iatrogenic bowel perforation during laparoscopic adhesiolysis may not be detected during the initial surgery.[50] Thus, a low threshold to convert to open surgery is advocated when laparoscopic adhesiolysis fails to identify and treat an obvious point of obstruction or when the adhesiolysis is difficult or unsafe. Preemptive conversion to open laparotomy when there is poor visualization or dense adhesions is preferable to reactive conversion after an iatrogenic injury has occurred.[55] In addition, careful patient selection is also important; the laparoscopic approach may best be suited for patients who have undergone one or two prior abdominal operations, especially if they have undergone appendectomy only, and in whom the etiology of the obstruction is felt to be adhesive bands.[56] Patient selection for laparoscopic adhesiolysis is important. Indications for laparoscopic exploration include proximal obstruction, partial obstruction, anticipated single band, localized radiographic distension, and mild abdominal distension. Contraindications to laparoscopy for bowel obstruction include coagulopathy, inability to tolerate general anesthesia, severe abdominal distension, massively dilated loops of intestine, peritonitis, sepsis, hemodynamic instability, and dense adhesions with fused loops of intestine or multiple prior laparotomies. The surgeon's experience and advanced laparoscopic skills may also be an important factor in determining the safety and efficacy of laparoscopic adhesiolysis for bowel obstruction.[57,58]

INTESTINAL OBSTRUCTION IN THE EARLY POSTOPERATIVE PERIOD

A common surgical dilemma is the patient who develops abdominal distension, obstipation, nausea, vomiting, and pain early after abdominal surgery. It may be difficult to differentiate postoperative ileus from mechanical small-bowel obstruction in this patient population. As many as 10% of postoperative patients develop mechanical small-bowel obstruction,[59] and in 90% of these cases, the etiology is adhesive disease.[60,61] In most cases, plain abdominal radiographs will help differentiate between ileus and mechanical bowel obstruction in this patient population.[60]

Furthermore, it is imperative to exclude technical complication as the etiology of the patient's postoperative ileus or obstruction. Complications such as anastomotic leak, abscess, internal hernia, perforation, anastomotic stricture, or stomal obstruction must be identified and treated appropriately. These conditions are unlikely to resolve with nasogastric decompression and bowel rest. When plain abdominal radiographs are unrevealing, CT is the appropriate study in this situation.

In most patients without peritoneal irritation or systemic toxicity, intestinal obstruction in the early postoperative period can be managed safely with bowel rest, intravenous fluids, and nasogastric decompression.[59,60] Because the risk of intestinal strangulation in patients with early postoperative adhesive obstruction is lower (<1%)[60,62] than those who present with obstruction in a delayed fashion, these patients are usually managed conservatively for longer periods of time. Close to 90% of patients resolve spontaneously after 2 weeks of conservative management. Approximately 70% of those who will resolve with nonoperative management do so in the first week, with another 25% responding by the second week. Beyond 2 weeks, patients with persistent obstruction are unlikely to resolve spontaneously and should undergo operation to manage the obstruction.[60,61] Parenteral nutritional support should be initiated in patients who will be treated conservatively and with bowel rest and no enteral nutrition for >7–10 days.[63] In the past, long intestinal tubes were advocated to manage postoperative bowel obstruction.[33] However, a randomized trial of long intestinal tubes versus standard nasogastric tubes found no difference in time to resolution of obstruction, the need for operation, or the duration of postoperative ileus.[64]

BOWEL OBSTRUCTION IN PATIENTS WITHOUT PRIOR ABDOMINAL SURGERY

While adhesive disease is the etiology of intestinal obstruction in most patients with prior abdominal surgery, patients who have never undergone surgery and who develop intestinal obstruction should be carefully evaluated for an underlying etiology that requires surgical intervention. Such patients who have partial obstruction can be appropriately admitted for conservative management during this evaluation. These patients often have an external or internal hernia, tumor, malrotation, volvulus, or intussusception. Malignant tumors account for 20% of small-bowel obstructions, and is the most common cause of small-bowel obstruction after postoperative adhesions.[65] The most commonly utilized first-line test is CT, which will identify the etiology in the majority of cases. Once the obstruction resolves and if CT is unrevealing, a small-bowel follow-through may provide a diagnosis. In some cases, elective exploratory laparoscopy or laparatomy may be necessary to diagnose and treat the underlying etiology.

STRANGULATION AND CLOSED-LOOP OBSTRUCTION

The type, location, and etiology of intestinal obstruction will impact the likelihood of resolution without surgery as well as the morbidity and mortality. Strangulation occurs when blood supply to a segment of intestine is compromised, usually due to a loop of intestine trapped in an abdominal wall or internal hernia, a volvulus or intussusception. Venous flow is usually affected first, leading to bowel wall edema, which first affects the mucosa and submucosal layers. Decreased arterial flow and pressure to the affected segment follows. These factors contribute to reduced blood flow to the segment of intestine and increased permeability and edema of the involved bowel. Substantial fluid sequestration and systemic hypovolemia can result. As the local process progresses, inadequate blood flow leads to release of inflammatory mediators, the potential for bacterial translocation, intestinal gangrene, and perforation with peritonitis.

Strangulation occurs in approximately 10% of patients with mechanical small intestinal obstruction. While the mortality associated with uncomplicated intestinal obstruction is <5%, when strangulation develops, mortality increases to 10%–37%.[7,40,66] The goal of surgical intervention is to relieve the obstruction prior to the development of intestinal strangulation to reduce the associated morbidity and mortality. Patients at highest risk for strangulation are those who present with an incarcerated hernia, volvulus, closed-loop or complete intestinal obstruction. Early identification of these processes by careful physical exam and radiographs (plain abdominal radiographs or CT) is paramount to timely surgical management and are indications for immediate surgery. Unfortunately, physical exam alone has a poor sensitivity to detect early signs of obstruction with strangulation,[7] prompting many clinicians to recommend routine use of CT for patients with mechanical bowel obstruction admitted for a trial of conservative management. Contrast-enhanced CT can demonstrate compromised blood supply and intestinal wall edema in early cases of intestinal strangulation.[14,67,68] Radiographic evidence of pneumatosis intestinalis and free intraperitoneal air are late findings of gangrene and perforation, and indications for immediate operation; but the goal should be to intervene prior to the development of these findings.

Closed-loop obstruction is a specific type of obstruction in which two points along the course of the bowel are obstructed at a single location, thus forming a closed loop. Usually this is due to adhesions, volvulus, or internal herniation. Closed-loop obstruction is more likely to cause intestinal ischemia than obstruction due to simple adhesive disease, but may also be more difficult to diagnose on plain radiographs. CT often demonstrates a "whirl sign."[69]

INTESTINAL OBSTRUCTION DUE TO HERNIA

Hernia is the etiology of 10% of cases of small-bowel obstruction, and is more likely to be associated with strangulation than obstruction due to adhesions.[7,70] For patients without a history of prior abdominal surgery, hernia is the second leading cause of intestinal obstruction after neoplasm. Any hernia that is incarcerated, tender to palpation, is associated with skin changes such as erythema or induration, is an indication for immediate surgery. Ultrasonography and CT are appropriate diagnostic modalities in cases where the hernia is difficult to detect on physical examination.

Paraduodenal hernia, which is a congenital abnormality resulting from intestinal malrotation, has been recognized as an important cause of closed-loop obstruction in adults.[71,72] It may account for as many as half of internal herniae. Patients present with a spectrum of symptoms ranging from mild abdominal discomfort and nausea to catastrophic closed-loop obstruction with intestinal gangrene and perforation. The diagnosis is readily made by CT or upper gastrointestinal contrast study, and operation should be performed expeditiously to prevent strangulation and peritonitis.[71]

VOLVULUS

Intestinal volvulus is a closed-loop obstruction caused by twisting of the intestine on its mesentery, leading to obstruction and impaired blood supply to the segment of intestine. Patients present with acute colicky abdominal pain, nausea, vomiting, and distension. Small-bowel volvulus may not be readily apparent on abdominal radiographs because the closed-loop fills with fluid and air–fluid levels may be absent, but the fluid-filled loop is usually apparent on CT. The finding of small-bowel volvulus mandates surgical intervention.

Colonic volvulus can occur anywhere in the large intestine, but is most common in the sigmoid (Fig. 36.5) followed by the cecum. Plain abdominal radiographs are often diagnostic, usually making CT unnecessary. Patients with colonic volvulus who have signs of systemic toxicity, signs of peritoneal inflammation on physical examination, or bloody rectal output require immediate operation. For patients with sigmoid volvulus, in the absence of these indications for immediate surgery, endoscopic decompression is the most appropriate first-line treatment and is effective in approximately 95% of patients.[73] During sigmoidoscopy, careful navigation of the sigmoidoscope with minimal air insufflation should be performed to reduce the risk of perforation. The finding of mucosal gangrene during sigmoidoscopy is an indication to abort the procedure and proceed immediately for surgery. Plain abdominal radiographs should be obtained after the endoscopic decompression to exclude the possibility of perforation. After successful endoscopic decompression, the patient should be evaluated and prepared for definitive surgical therapy during the same hospital admission since the likelihood of recurrent volvulus is high; sigmoidectomy with primary anastomosis is the preferred operation in suitable candidates. Patients with colonic volvulus proximal to the sigmoid colon usually require surgical intervention; endoscopic decompression is usually unsuccessful and associated with a considerably higher rate of complications.

INFLAMMATORY CONDITIONS

Partial bowel obstruction secondary to inflammatory conditions such as inflammatory bowel disease, radiation enteritis, or diverticulitis usually resolve with conservative management: nasogastric decompression, bowel rest, intravenous fluids. Crohn's disease accounts for approximately 5% of all cases of small-bowel obstruction.[74] For patients with intestinal obstruction due to an exacerbation of Crohn's disease, the addition of antiinflammatory agents may reduce the duration of obstruction and the need for surgery.[75] Surgery may become necessary in some of cases of Crohn's disease if the patient has persistent obstruction, fails to improve with medical management, or develops peritonitis. Stricturoplasty and other non-resectional therapies are preferable to removal of segments of bowel in these patients due to the risk of short gut syndrome. Similarly, surgery is a last resort effort in patients with obstruction due to radiation enteritis. Radiation strictures with obstruction that does not resolve after a prudent course of conservative management may require operation. Resection to grossly normal sections of bowel may become necessary.

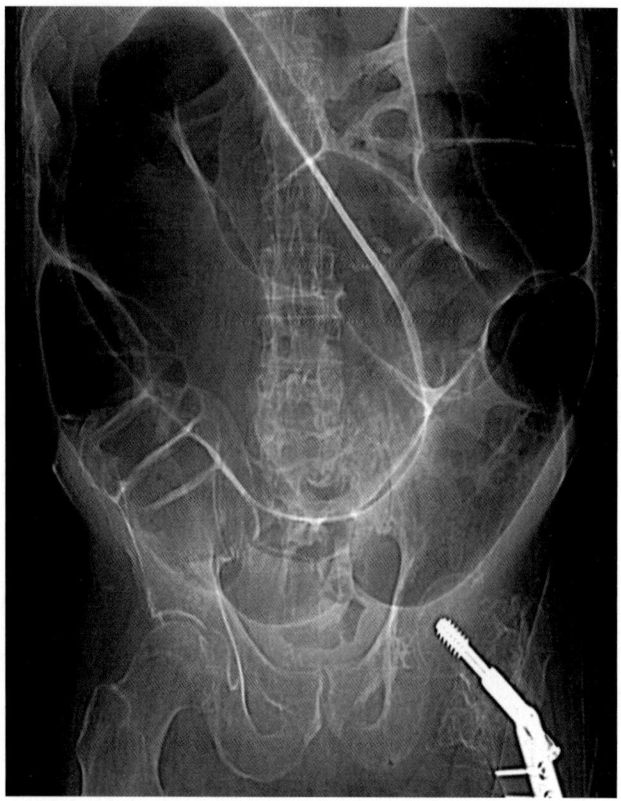

A

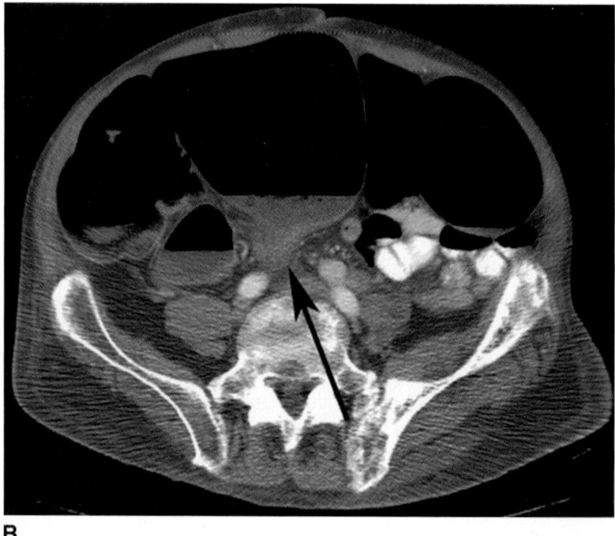

B

FIGURE 36.5. A: Abdominal radiograph of a patient with sigmoid volvulus, demonstrating massively distended sigmoid colon, which extends from the left lower quadrant to the right upper quadrant. B: CT scan of the same patient demonstrates a "beak sign" (*black arrow*) where the sigmoid colon twists upon itself, resulting in complete obstruction.

Patients with acute diverticulitis may also present with partial colonic obstruction in 20% of cases. CT should be obtained in most cases of diverticulitis which require hospital admission to detect complications such as an associated abscess, which may need percutaneous drainage or free perforation requiring laparotomy.[76] Partial colonic obstruction usually resolves with conservative management and intravenous antibiotics directed at the underlying diverticulitis. Surgery is indicated if the patient develops peritonitis, if the obstruction does not resolve after an appropriate period of observation, or if chronic diverticular stricture develops, causing recurrent obstruction. Full colonic evaluation to exclude colorectal neoplasm is indicated in cases where elective resection is contemplated.

PARTIAL COLONIC OBSTRUCTION

Common etiologies of partial colonic obstruction include cancer, diverticulitis, and strictures; adhesive disease is a rare cause of colonic obstruction. In the evaluation of patients with colonic obstruction, digital rectal examination and sigmoidoscopy are done to assess any rectal mass, fecal impaction, sigmoid volvulus, or stricture. If these tests are unrevealing, contrast enema should be performed to evaluate the more proximal colon. Failure to find an obstructing lesion in the patient with distension of the entire colon is usually associated with colonic pseudo-obstruction.

Patients with partial colonic obstruction should initially be treated conservatively, since the morbidity, mortality, and need for colostomy are all increased in the setting of emergency colonic resection for obstruction. Patients with distal sigmoid and rectal tumors causing partial obstruction may benefit from endoluminal colonic stenting. Approximately 90% of such patients will improve clinically within 96 hours of colonic stenting,[77] allowing patient preparation for one-staged open[77,78] or laparoscopic[79] colonic resection.

MALIGNANT BOWEL OBSTRUCTION

Bowel obstruction due to malignant disease may complicate the course of patients with abdominal and pelvic tumors, and occurs in 5%–43% of patients with advanced primary or metastatic intra-abdominal malignancy.[80] Some of these patients will have advanced, unresectable disease, and the goal of care is palliation of symptoms. The etiology of malignant bowel obstruction may be multifactorial, and can involve extrinsic compression of the bowel by tumor, infiltration of the mesentery, luminal obstruction by tumor, as well as impaired intestinal motility due to opioids, electrolyte disorders, certain medications, and adrenal insufficiency.[81] The rate of benign intestinal obstruction in patients with known malignancy ranges between 3% and 48%,[80] so a benign etiology must be considered in these patients. Regardless of the etiology of the obstruction, it may be desirable to avoid surgery in this population of patients. Bowel rest and early pharmacologic therapy with analgesics, antiemetics, and antisecretory drugs are the mainstays of treatment and have been shown to be effective at controlling gastrointestinal symptoms.[82] Octreotide has been shown to reduce the severity of abdominal pain and vomiting, and the duration of nasogastric decompression needed in patients with inoperable malignant bowel obstruction in randomized controlled trials.[83–85] Intraluminal stents may be deployed endoscopically in patients with malignant bowel obstruction and are associated with improved quality of life and avoidance of laparotomy and colostomy in patients with inoperable malignant colorectal obstruction.[86–89] Palliative percutaneous endoscopic gastrostomy may be effective for long-term gastric decompression in terminally ill patients with gastric or proximal small-bowel obstruction.[90]

INTESTINAL DYSMOTILITY DISORDERS

Ileus

Ileus is a hypomotility state defined as the disruption of normal gastrointestinal propulsive activity in the absence of mechanical bowel obstruction. Implicit in this definition is that mechanical obstruction has been excluded. Ileus is fairly common immediately after abdominal surgery; however, it can also occur in association with a number of metabolic, inflammatory, or infectious processes in the abdomen, chest, or systemically. A common clinical mistake is failure to identify and treat the underlying etiology. The pathophysiology of ileus is complex and poorly understood, but involves the following factors: spinal–intestinal neural reflexes, local and systemic inflammatory mediators, sympathetic hyperactivity, and other exacerbating factors such as endogenous and exogenous opioids, intraperitoneal surgery and bowel manipulation, electrolyte and metabolic abnormalities.[91,92]

Postoperative ileus usually occurs after major abdominal surgery and manifests as atony of the stomach, small and large intestines. Under normal circumstances, intestinal motility returns at about 24 hours in the small intestine, followed subsequently by the stomach and colon. Perhaps contrary to traditional teaching, the duration of postoperative ileus can be shortened by the early removal of nasogastric tubes,[93,94] early initiation of enteral nutrition,[95–97] use of multi-modality pain prevention techniques, including: minimization of opioids, use of nonsteroidal anti-inflammatory agents[98] and regional blocks,[99] and the chewing of gum.[100,101] A comprehensive protocol of controlled rehabilitation with early ambulation and diet shortens the duration of postoperative ileus and reduces hospital length of stay after laparotomy with bowel resection.[102] The theory in support of early feeding is that it stimulates gastrointestinal hormones, elicits gut propulsive activity, and thus coordinated gut motility. Concern over an increased incidence of anastomotic leak with early feeding is unfounded.[103] In addition, studies have shown that laparoscopic surgery is associated with a shortened duration of postoperative ileus compared to open surgery.[104–106]

Treatment of persistent postoperative ileus must include a search for potentially contributing etiologies such as electrolyte disturbances (hypokalemia, hyponatremia, hypocalcemia, hypomagnesemia), offending medications (opioids, anticholinergics, calcium channel blockers, certain antiemetics), and other medical conditions such as infection (urinary tract infection, pneumonia, bacteremia, intra-abdominal abscess, peritonitis), uremia, pancreatitis, hypothyroidism, and low cardiac output state (myocardial infarction). Failure to identify and treat these underlying etiologies will result in increased morbidity and length of stay. Patients with established postoperative ileus may require nasogastric decompression, intravenous fluids, and bowel rest until the underlying etiology has been addressed and peristalsis returns. Diagnostic evaluation usually involves CT, which can help distinguish between ileus and mechanical obstruction in most patients, and identify the underlying etiology in some cases. A randomized, controlled trial demonstrated the efficacy of a peripherally acting μ-opioid receptor antagonist, alvimopan, in reducing the duration of postoperative ileus after laparotomy with bowel resection without compromising pain control in these patients.[107]

Pseudo-obstruction

Intestinal pseudo-obstruction is a motility disorder similar to ileus, which may develop in the small or large intestine, but is most common in the colon, where it carries the eponym of Ogilvie's syndrome. Acute colonic pseudo-obstruction develops classically in elderly hospitalized or institutionalized patients, and has many of the same risk factors as ileus. Patients usually present with abdominal distension, discomfort, nausea, vomiting, and obstipation.[108] It is important to exclude mechanical bowel obstruction, as the etiology and treatment of these entities is very different. Radiographs usually demonstrate dilated colon with no clear transition point. Usually, the cecum is the most distended portion of the colon, and is most at risk for perforation. Despite frequent assertions to the contrary, there is no clear linear relationship between cecal diameter and perforation. Some patients have recovered after reaching a cecal diameter of 25 cm,[109] while others have perforated at <10 cm.[110] The risk of perforation may also be associated with the duration of colonic distension.[111] The risk of spontaneous perforation is between 3% and 15% and is associated with a mortality of 50%.[110]

Treatment of acute colonic pseudo-obstruction is directed at the underlying etiology. Patients with signs of peritonitis or systemic toxicity require operation, and may need total abdominal colectomy. Otherwise, a trial of bowel rest, decompression, management of fluid, electrolyte and metabolic disturbances should be initiated. These measures alone will result in resolution of symptoms in 33%–100% of patients, with a mean response time of 3 days.[109] Colon decompression with rectal tube or sigmoidoscopy may be therapeutic and help identify underlying colonic ischemia. Colonoscopic decompression is effective in 70% of patients, with a 40% recurrence rate, 3% complication rate, and 1% mortality rate.[112] More recently, pharmacologic management has replaced endoscopic decompression in appropriate candidates. The potent parasympathomimetic agent, neostigmine, has been shown to be effective and safe in a randomized controlled trial of patients with acute colonic pseudo-obstruction. Neostigmine administration leads to prompt colonic evacuation and resolution of symptoms in most patients within minutes, with a low rate of recurrence (11%).[113,114] Contraindications to neostigmine include mechanical bowel obstruction, colonic ischemia or perforation, bradycardia, reactive airway disease, recent coronary occlusion, vagotonia, hyperthyroidism, and cardiac arrhythmias. Neostigmine should be used with caution in elderly patients with coronary artery disease, and should be administered in a cardiac monitored setting. Colonoscopic decompression or operation should be reserved for patients with a contraindication to, or who fail to respond to, neostigmine.

References

1. Irvin TT. Abdominal pain: a surgical audit of 1190 emergency admissions. *Br J Surg*. 1989;76:1121-1125.
2. Luckey A, Livingston E, Tache Y. Mechanisms and treatment of postoperative ileus. *Arch Surg*. 2003;138:206-214.
3. Berg RD, Garlington AW. Translocation of certain indigenous bacteria from the gastrointestinal tract to the mesenteric lymph nodes and other organs in a gnotobiotic mouse model. *Infect Immun*. 1979;23:403-411.

4. Reed LL, Martin M, Manglano R, et al. Bacterial translocation following abdominal trauma in humans. *Circ Shock*. 1994;42:1-6.
5. Deitch EA. Simple intestinal obstruction causes bacterial translocation in man. *Arch Surg*. 1989;124:699-701.
6. Eskelinen M, Ikonen J, Lipponen P. Contributions of history-taking, physical examination, and computer assistance to diagnosis of acute small-bowel obstruction. A prospective study of 1333 patients with acute abdominal pain. *Scand J Gastroenterol*. 1994;29:715-721.
7. Sarr MG, Bulkley GB, Zuidema GD. Preoperative recognition of intestinal strangulation obstruction. Prospective evaluation of diagnostic capability. *Am J Surg*. 1983;145:176-182.
8. Maglinte DD, Reyes BL, Harmon BH, et al. Reliability and role of plain film radiography and CT in the diagnosis of small-bowel obstruction. *AJR Am J Roentgenol*. 1996;167:1451-1455.
9. Nicolaou S, Kai B, Ho S, et al. Imaging of acute small-bowel obstruction. *AJR Am J Roentgenol*. 2005;185:1036-1044.
10. Balthazar EJ. For suspected small-bowel obstruction and an equivocal plain film, should we perform CT or a small-bowel series? *AJR Am J Roentgenol*. 1994;163:1260-1261.
11. Daneshmand S, Hedley CG, Stain SC. The utility and reliability of computed tomography scan in the diagnosis of small bowel obstruction. *Am Surg*. 1999;65:922-926.
12. Donckier V, Closset J, Van Gansbeke D, et al. Contribution of computed tomography to decision making in the management of adhesive small bowel obstruction. *Br J Surg*. 1998;85:1071-1074.
13. Peck JJ, Milleson T, Phelan J. The role of computed tomography with contrast and small bowel follow-through in management of small bowel obstruction. *Am J Surg*. 1999;177:375-378.
14. Zalcman M, Sy M, Donckier V, et al. Helical CT signs in the diagnosis of intestinal ischemia in small-bowel obstruction. *AJR Am J Roentgenol*. 2000;175:1601-1607.
15. Lazarus DE, Slywotsky C, Bennett GL, et al. Frequency and relevance of the "small-bowel feces" sign on CT in patients with small-bowel obstruction. *AJR Am J Roentgenol*. 2004;183:1361-1366.
16. Balthazar EJ. George W. Holmes Lecture. CT of small-bowel obstruction. *AJR Am J Roentgenol*. 1994;162:255-261.
17. Frager D, Rovno HD, Baer JW, et al. Prospective evaluation of colonic obstruction with computed tomography. *Abdom Imaging*. 1998;23:141-146.
18. Joyce WP, Delaney PV, Gorey TF, et al. The value of water-soluble contrast radiology in the management of acute small bowel obstruction. *Ann R Coll Surg Engl*. 1992;74:422-425.
19. Sandikcioglu TG, Torp-Madsen S, Pedersen IK, et al. Contrast radiography in small bowel obstruction. A randomized trial of barium sulfate and a nonionic low-osmolar contrast medium. *Acta Radiol*. 1994;35:62-64.
20. Stordahl A, Laerum F. Water-soluble contrast media compared with barium in enteric follow-through. Urinary excretion and radiographic efficacy in rats with intestinal ischemia. *Invest Radiol*. 1988;23:471-477.
21. Ogata M, Mateer JR, Condon RE. Prospective evaluation of abdominal sonography for the diagnosis of bowel obstruction. *Ann Surg*. 1996;223:237-241.
22. Grunshaw ND, Renwick IG, Scarisbrick G, et al. Prospective evaluation of ultrasound in distal ileal and colonic obstruction. *Clin Radiol*. 2000;55:356-362.
23. Beall DP, Fortman BJ, Lawler BC, et al. Imaging bowel obstruction: A comparison between fast magnetic resonance imaging and helical computed tomography. *Clin Radiol*. 2002;57:719-724.
24. Schwab DP, Blackhurst DW, Sticca RP. Operative acute small bowel obstruction: admitting service impacts outcome. *Am Surg*. 2001;67:1034-1038; discussion 1038-1040.
25. Oyasiji T, Angelo S, Kyriakides TC, et al. Small bowel obstruction: outcome and cost implications of admitting service. *Am Surg*. 2010;76:687-691.
26. Fevang BT, Jensen D, Svanes K, et al. Early operation or conservative management of patients with small bowel obstruction? *Eur J Surg*. 2002;168:475-481.
27. Hayanga AJ, Bass-Wilkins K, Bulkley GB. Current management of small-bowel obstruction. *Adv Surg*. 2005;39:1-33.
28. Biondo S, Pares D, Frago R, et al. Large bowel obstruction: predictive factors for postoperative mortality. *Dis Colon Rectum*. 2004;47:1889-1897.
29. Cox MR, Gunn IF, Eastman MC, et al. The operative aetiology and types of adhesions causing small bowel obstruction. *Aust N Z J Surg*. 1993;63:848-852.
30. Ellis H. The clinical significance of adhesions: focus on intestinal obstruction. *Eur J Surg Suppl*. 1997:5-9.
31. Duepree HJ, Senagore AJ, Delaney CP, et al. Does means of access affect the incidence of small bowel obstruction and ventral hernia after bowel resection? Laparoscopy versus laparotomy. *J Am Coll Surg*. 2003;197:177-181.
32. Bizer LS, Liebling RW, Delany HM, et al. Small bowel obstruction: the role of nonoperative treatment in simple intestinal obstruction and predictive criteria for strangulation obstruction. *Surgery*. 1981;89:407-413.
33. Gowen GF. Long tube decompression is successful in 90% of patients with adhesive small bowel obstruction. *Am J Surg*. 2003;185:512-515.
34. Williams SB, Greenspon J, Young HA, et al. Small bowel obstruction: Conservative vs. surgical management. *Dis Colon Rectum* 2005;48:1140-1146.
35. Barkan H, Webster S, Ozeran S. Factors Predicting the Recurrence of Adhesive Small-Bowel Obstruction. *Am J Surge*. 1995;170:361-365.
36. Landercasper J, Cogbill TH, Merry WH, et al. Long-term outcome after hospitalization for small-bowel obstruction. *Arch Surg*. 1993;128:765-770; discussion 770-761.
37. Ellis H, Moran BJ, Thompson JN, et al. Adhesion-related hospital readmissions after abdominal and pelvic surgery: a retrospective cohort study. *Lancet*. 1999;353:1476-1480.
38. Miller G, Boman J, Shrier I, et al. Natural history of patients with adhesive small bowel obstruction. *Br J Surg*. 2000;87:1240-1247.
39. Parker MC, Ellis H, Moran BJ, et al. Postoperative adhesions: ten-year follow-up of 12,584 patients undergoing lower abdominal surgery. *Dis Colon Rectum*. 2001;44:822-829; discussion 829-830.
40. Sosa J, Gardner B. Management of Patients Diagnosed as Acute Intestinal-Obstruction Secondary to Adhesions. *Am Surg*. 1993;59:125-128.
41. Blackmon S, Lucius C, Wilson JP, et al. The use of water-soluble contrast in evaluating clinically equivocal small bowel obstruction. *Am Surg*. 2000;66:238-242; discussion 242-234.
42. Chen SC, Lin FY, Lee PH, et al. Water-soluble contrast study predicts the need for early surgery in adhesive small bowel obstruction. *Br J Surg*. 1998;85:1692-1694.
43. Abbas SM, Bissett IP, Party BR. Meta-analysis of oral water-soluble contrast agent in the management of adhesive small bowel obstruction. *Br J Surg*. 2007;94:404-411.
44. Bailey IS, Rhodes M, O'Rourke N, et al. Laparoscopic management of acute small bowel obstruction. *Br J Surg*. 1998;85:84-87.
45. Fischer CP, Doherty D. Laparoscopic approach to small bowel obstruction. *Semin Laparosc Surg*. 2002;9:40-45.
46. Metzger A, LuquedeLeon E, Tsiotos GG, et al. Laparoscopic management of SBO (small bowel obstruction): Indications and outcome. *Gastroenterology*. 1997;112:A1459-A1459.
47. Strickland P, Lourie DJ, Suddleson EA, et al. Is laparoscopy safe and effective for treatment of acute small-bowel obstruction? *Surg Endosc Ultrasound Interven Tech*. 1999;13:695-698.
48. Suter M, Zermatten P, Halkic N, et al. Laparoscopic management of mechanical small bowel obstruction: are there predictors of success or failure? *Surg Endosc*. 2000;14:478-483.
49. Wullstein C, Gross E. Laparoscopic compared with conventional treatment of acute adhesive small bowel obstruction. *Br J Surg*. 2003;90:1147-1151.
50. Chapron C, Pierre F, Harchaoui Y, et al. Gastrointestinal injuries during gynaecological laparoscopy. *Hum Reprod*. 1999;14:333-337.
51. Vrijland WW, Jeekel J, van Geldorp HJ, et al. Abdominal adhesions: intestinal obstruction, pain, and infertility. *Surg Endosc*. 2003;17:1017-1022.
52. Chopra R, McVay C, Phillips E, et al. Laparoscopic lysis of adhesions. *Am Surg*. 2003;69:966-968.
53. Garrard CL, Clements RH, Nanney L, et al. Adhesion formation is reduced after laparoscopic surgery. *Surg Endosc Other Interven Tech*. 1999;13:10-13.
54. Tittel A, Treutner KH, Titkova S, et al. Comparison of adhesion reformation after laparoscopic and conventional adhesiolysis in an animal model. *Langenbecks Arch Surg*. 2001;386:141-145.
55. Reissman P, Spira RM. Laparoscopy for adhesions. *Semin Laparosc Surg*. 2003;10:185-190.
56. Levard H, Boudet MJ, Msika S, et al. Laparoscopic treatment of acute small bowel obstruction: A multicentre retrospective study. *Anz J Surg*. 2001;71:641-646.
57. Kirshtein B, Roy-Shapira A, Lantsberg L, et al. Laparoscopic management of acute small bowel obstruction. *Surg Endosc*. 2005;19:464-467.
58. Franklin ME Jr, Gonzalez JJ, Jr., Miter DB, et al. Laparoscopic diagnosis and treatment of intestinal obstruction. *Surg Endosc*. 2004;18:26-30.
59. Ellozy SH, Harris MT, Bauer JJ, et al. Early postoperative small-bowel obstruction—a prospective evaluation in 242 consecutive abdominal operations. *Dis Colon Rectum*. 2002;45:1214-1217.
60. Pickleman J, Lee RM. The management of patients with suspected early postoperative small bowel obstruction. *Ann Surg*. 1989;210:216-219.
61. Stewart RM, Page CP, Brender J, et al. The incidence and risk of early postoperative small bowel obstruction. A cohort study. *Am J Surg*. 1987;154:643-647.
62. Spears H, Petrelli NJ, Herrera L, et al. Treatment of Bowel Obstruction after Operation for Colorectal-Carcinoma. *Am J Surg*. 1988;155:383-386.
63. Braga M, Ljungqvist O, Soeters P, et al. ESPEN Guidelines on Parenteral Nutrition: surgery. *Clin Nutr*. 2009;28:378-386.
64. Fleshner PR, Siegman MG, Slater GI, et al. A prospective, randomized trial of short versus long tubes in adhesive small-bowel obstruction. *Am J Surg*. 1995;170:366-370.
65. Mucha P, Jr. Small intestinal obstruction. *Surg Clin North Am*. 1987;67:597-620.
66. Brolin RE. Partial small bowel obstruction. *Surgery*. 1984;95:145-149.
67. Ha HK. CT in the early detection of strangulation in intestinal obstruction. *Semin Ultrasound CT MR*. 1995;16:141-150.
68. Kim JH, Ha HK, Kim JK, et al. Usefulness of known computed tomography and clinical criteria for diagnosing strangulation in small-bowel obstruction: analysis of true and false interpretation groups in computed tomography. *World J Surg*. 2004;28:63-68.
69. Balthazar EJ, Birnbaum BA, Megibow AJ, et al. Closed-loop and strangulating intestinal obstruction: CT signs. *Radiology*. 1992;185:769-775.

70. Shatila AH, Chamberlain BE, Webb WR. Current status of diagnosis and management of strangulation obstruction of the small bowel. *Am J Surg*. 1976;132:299-303.
71. Yoo HY, Mergelas J, Seibert DG. Paraduodenal hernia—A treatable cause of upper gastrointestinal tract symptoms. *J Clin Gastroenterol*. 2000;31:226-229.
72. Mathieu D, Luciani A. Internal abdominal herniations. *AJR Am J Roentgenol*. 2004;183:397-404.
73. Mangiante EC, Croce MA, Fabian TC, et al. Sigmoid volvulus. A four-decade experience. *Am Surg*. 1989;55:41-44.
74. Miller G, Boman J, Shrier I, et al. Etiology of small bowel obstruction. *Am J Surg*. 2000;180:33-36.
75. Pelletier AL, Kalisazan B, Wienckiewicz J, et al. Infliximab treatment for symptomatic Crohn's disease strictures. *Aliment Pharmacol Ther*. 2009;29:279-285.
76. Hulnick DH, Megibow AJ, Balthazar EJ, et al. Computed tomography in the evaluation of diverticulitis. *Radiology*. 1984;152:491-495.
77. Binkert CA, Ledermann H, Jost R, et al. Acute colonic obstruction: clinical aspects and cost-effectiveness of preoperative and palliative treatment with self-expanding metallic stents–a preliminary report. *Radiology*. 1998;206:199-204.
78. Mainar A, Ariza MAD, Tejero E, et al. Acute colorectal obstruction: Treatment with self-expandable metallic stents before scheduled surgery—results of a multicenter study. *Radiology*. 1999;210:65-69.
79. Dulucq JL, Wintringer P, Beyssac R, et al. One-stage laparoscopic colorectal resection after placement of self-expanding metallic stents for colorectal obstruction—a prospective study. *Digest Dis Sci*. 2006;51:2365-2371.
80. Krouse RS. Surgical management of malignant bowel obstruction. *Surg Oncol Clin N Am*. 2004;13:479-490.
81. Poon D, Cheung YB, Tay MH, et al. Adrenal insufficiency in intestinal obstruction from carcinomatosis peritonei—a factor of potential importance in symptom palliation. *J Pain Symptom Manage*. 2005;29:411-418.
82. Mercadante S, Ferrera P, Villari P, et al. Aggressive pharmacological treatment for reversing malignant bowel obstruction. *J Pain Symptom Manage*. 2004;28:412-416.
83. Mercadante S, Ripamonti C, Casuccio A, et al. Comparison of octreotide and hyoscine butylbromide in controlling gastrointestinal symptoms due to malignant inoperable bowel obstruction. *Support Care Cancer*. 2000;8:188-191.
84. Mystakidou K, Tsilika E, Kalaidopoulou O, et al. Comparison of octreotide administration vs conservative treatment in the management of inoperable bowel obstruction in patients with far advanced cancer: a randomized, double- blind, controlled clinical trial. *Anticancer Res*. 2002;22:1187-1192.
85. Ripamonti C, Mercadante S, Groff L, et al. Role of octreotide, scopolamine butylbromide, and hydration in symptom control of patients with inoperable bowel obstruction and nasogastric tubes: a prospective randomized trial. *J Pain Symptom Manage*. 2000;19:23-34.
86. Hosono S, Ohtani H, Arimoto Y, et al. Endoscopic stenting versus surgical gastroenterostomy for palliation of malignant gastroduodenal obstruction: a meta-analysis. *J Gastroenterol*. 2007;42:283-290.
87. Masci E, Viale E, Mangiavillano B, et al. Enteral self-expandable metal stent for malignant luminal obstruction of the upper and lower gastro-intestinal tract: a prospective multicentric study. *J Clin Gastroenterol*. 2008;42:389-394.
88. Trompetas V. Emergency management of malignant acute left-sided colonic obstruction. *Ann R Coll Surg Engl*. 2008;90:181-186.
89. Xinopoulos D, Dimitroulopoulos D, Theodosopoulos T, et al. Stenting or stoma creation for patients with inoperable malignant colonic obstructions? Results of a study and cost-effectiveness analysis. *Surg Endosc*. 2004;18:421-426.
90. Scheidbach H, Horbach T, Groitl H, et al. Percutaneous endoscopic gastrostomy/jejunostomy (PEG/PEJ) for decompression in the upper gastrointestinal tract. Initial experience with palliative treatment of gastrointestinal obstruction in terminally ill patients with advanced carcinomas. *Surg Endosc*. 1999;13:1103-1105.
91. Nezami BG, Srinivasan S. Enteric nervous system in the small intestine: pathophysiology and clinical implications. *Curr Gastroenterol Rep*. 2010;12:358-365.
92. Behm B, Stollman N. Postoperative ileus: etiologies and interventions. *Clin Gastroenterol Hepatol*. 2003;1:71-80.
93. Cheatham ML, Chapman WC, Key SP, et al. A meta-analysis of selective versus routine nasogastric decompression after elective laparotomy. *Ann Surg*. 1995;221:469-476; discussion 476-468.
94. Nelson R, Edwards S, Tse B. Prophylactic nasogastric decompression after abdominal surgery. *Cochrane Database Syst Rev*. 2007;(3):CD004929.
95. Choi J, O'Connell TX. Safe and effective early postoperative feeding and hospital discharge after open colon resection. *Am Surg*. 1996;62:853-856.
96. Stewart BT, Woods RJ, Collopy BT, et al. Early feeding after elective open colorectal resections: a prospective randomized trial. *Aust N Z J Surg*. 1998;68:125-128.
97. Velez JP, Lince LF, Restrepo JI. Early enteral nutrition in gastrointestinal surgery: a pilot study. *Nutrition*. 1997;13:442-445.
98. Sim R, Cheong DM, Wong KS, et al. Prospective randomized, double-blind, placebo-controlled study of pre- and postoperative administration of a COX-2-specific inhibitor as opioid-sparing analgesia in major colorectal surgery. *Colorectal Dis*. 2007;9:52-60.
99. Jorgensen H, Wetterslev J, Moiniche S, et al. Epidural local anaesthetics versus opioid-based analgesic regimens on postoperative gastrointestinal paralysis, PONV and pain after abdominal surgery. *Cochrane Database Syst Rev*. 2000;CD001893.
100. Asao T, Kuwano H, Nakamura J, et al. Gum chewing enhances early recovery from postoperative ileus after laparoscopic colectomy. *J Am Coll Surg*. 2002;195:30-32.
101. Schuster R, Grewal N, Greaney GC, et al. Gum chewing reduces ileus after elective open sigmoid colectomy. *Arch Surg*. 2006;141:174-176.
102. Delaney CP, Zutshi M, Senagore AJ, et al. Prospective, randomized, controlled trial between a pathway of controlled rehabilitation with early ambulation and diet and traditional postoperative care after laparotomy and intestinal resection. *Dis Colon Rectum*. 2003;46:851-859.
103. Correia MI, da Silva RG. The impact of early nutrition on metabolic response and postoperative ileus. *Curr Opin Clin Nutr Metab Care*. 2004;7:577-583.
104. Basse L, Madsen JL, Billesbolle P, et al. Gastrointestinal transit after laparoscopic versus open colonic resection. *Surg Endosc*. 2003;17:1919-1922.
105. Lacy AM, Garcia-Valdecasas JC, Pique JM, et al. Short-term outcome analysis of a randomized study comparing laparoscopic vs open colectomy for colon cancer. *Surg Endosc*. 1995;9:1101-1105.
106. Milsom JW, Bohm B, Hammerhofer KA, et al. A prospective, randomized trial comparing laparoscopic versus conventional techniques in colorectal cancer surgery: a preliminary report. *J Am Coll Surg*. 1998;187:46-54; discussion 54-45.
107. Wolff BG, Michelassi F, Gerkin TM, et al. Alvimopan, a novel, peripherally acting mu opioid antagonist: results of a multicenter, randomized, double-blind, placebo-controlled, phase III trial of major abdominal surgery and postoperative ileus. *Ann Surg*. 2004;240:728-734; discussion 734-725.
108. Vanek VW, Al-Salti M. Acute pseudo-obstruction of the colon (Ogilvie's syndrome). An analysis of 400 cases. *Dis Colon Rectum*. 1986;29:203-210.
109. Sloyer AF, Panella VS, Demas BE, et al. Ogilvie's syndrome. Successful management without colonoscopy. *Dig Dis Sci*. 1988;33:1391-1396.
110. Rex DK. Colonoscopy and acute colonic pseudo-obstruction. *Gastrointest Endosc Clin N Am*, 1997;7:499-508.
111. Johnson CD, Rice RP, Kelvin FM, et al. The radiologic evaluation of gross cecal distension: emphasis on cecal ileus. *AJR Am J Roentgenol*. 1985;145:1211-1217.
112. Kahi CJ, Rex DK. Bowel obstruction and pseudo-obstruction. *Gastroenterol Clin North Am*. 2003;32:1229-1247.
113. Hutchinson R, Griffiths C. Acute colonic pseudo-obstruction: a pharmacological approach. *Ann R Coll Surg Engl*. 1992;74:364-367.
114. Ponec RJ, Saunders MD, Kimmey MB. Neostigmine for the treatment of acute colonic pseudo-obstruction. *N Engl J Med*. 1999;341:137-141.

CHAPTER 37 ■ APPENDICITIS

D. PATRICK BRYANT AND HEIDI FRANKEL

In the time of Leonardo da Vinci, the appendix was ascribed a function as an organ capable of expanding and contracting, to deal with excessive wind and prevent perforation of the cecum. Over the ensuing years, others have recognized that the appendix served an immune function as well, namely, in the lymphocyte response. This is particularly true in ruminators.[1] Bollinger et al.[2] theorize that the appendix is responsible for maintaining homogeneity in the flora of the colon.

EMBRYOLOGY

The appendix is an organ derived from the midgut. It begins as a outpouching of the embryonic cecum and then lines up at the confluence of the taeniae. The vermiform appendix becomes visible in the eighth week of gestation (when fetal length is 10–12 cm), and the first accumulations of lymphatic tissue develop during the 14th and 15th weeks directly below the epithelium. Some lymphocytes penetrate into the epithelial layer of the vermiform appendix that distinctly contains fewer goblet cells than the other colic mucosa. The vermiform appendix, tonsils, and Peyer's patches possess no draining lymphatic vessels.

ANATOMY

The appendix varies in size, but on average it is generally 6–9 cm in length and may be in a retrocecal, pelvic, retroileal, or right pericolic position, and at times within the wall of the cecum. The blood supply is from the appendiceal artery; the terminal branch of the ileocolic artery. It is an end artery and the ischemia that is part of the process in acute appendicitis is the result of no collateralized flow. Occasionally, the artery itself becomes thrombosed as part of the inflammatory process, resulting in a gangrenous appendix with perforation.

HISTORY

Perityphlitis was a diagnosis without a known causative factor until Dr. Reginald Fitz published his work in 1886 demonstrating that perityphlitis and perforated appendicitis were one and the same disease. In 1889, Dr. Charles McBurney presented his report on the early surgical intervention of appendicitis to the New York Surgical Society. In 1894, he presented his paper on the muscle splitting incision that bears his name. The procedure for appendectomy was largely unchanged for almost a century.

The first laparoscopic appendectomy was performed by Dr. Kurt Semm in May of 1980.[3] Currently, well over half of the approximately 250,000 appendectomies performed annually in the United States are laparoscopically done. In addition to laparoscopy, the major advances in the care of appendicitis included the introduction of broad spectrum antibiotics, the improvement in preoperative diagnostic testing, and the use of interventional radiology to perform drainage procedures for periappendiceal abscesses.

EPIDEMIOLOGY

The incidence of appendicitis peaks in the mid to late teens with a slight male predominance (~1.3: 1). The incidence of 84 per 100,000 patients has remained stable over time.[4] The overall mortality of appendicitis is 0.5%, 1.7% in cases with perforation, and over 20% in patients over the age of 70.[5]

PATHOPHYSIOLOGY

Acute appendicitis is the most common surgical emergency treated in the acute care setting. Its classic presentation remains relatively unchanged over time; present in about 80% of those who present with lower abdominal pain. The standard presentation in a relatively young person is a result of luminal obstruction of the appendix. This obstruction may be related to hyperplasia of the germinal follicles or from a fecalith impacted in the appendiceal orifice. The capacity of the appendix is about 0.5 mL. With the orifice obstructed, the pressure in the lumen quickly rises above 60 mm Hg and ischemia results. The ensuing distension stimulates the visceral afferent nerves, leading to the nausea and emesis, as well as the periumbilical pain, which is emblematic of early disease. As the inflammatory process continues, the pain localizes to McBurney's point when the inflamed appendix comes in contact with the peritoneum and the somatic afferent nerves are stimulated. As the pressure increases, vascular compromise develops and along with it, bacterial overgrowth, after which, perforation can be expected.

Perforation is clearly more of a problem in the pediatric population. Nearly one-half of young pediatric patients with acute appendicitis present to care after perforation.[5,6] Perforation is associated with vomiting, prolonged illness, and higher body temperatures. Perforation is also an important factor in morbidity and mortality, including prolongation of the hospital stay, development of a secondary abscess (pelvic, psoas, hepatic, tubo-ovarian), urinary retention, hematuria, and subacute and delayed bowel obstruction. Alternatively, patients with acute appendicitis who perforate may develop a "contained" abscess.

The entity of chronic appendicitis describes a disease process with symptoms over 7 or more days. The pathology tends to show more lymphocytic or eosinophilic infiltration. These patients have a greater diversity of abdominal complaints as well; pelvic, back, and bilateral lower abdominal pain, which makes diagnosis more difficult.

DIAGNOSIS

The "classic" history for appendicitis involves the patient presenting with periumbilical pain, which subsequently localizes to the right lower quadrant. At this point, the pain character changes from a dull ache or vague discomfort to a sharp "finger point" pain. This change is due to the change in the neurologic pathway involved. Periumbilical pain is due to the distenson of the appendix sending nociceptive signals via the celiac pathway through visceral afferents. Localized right lower quadrant pain develops from the irritation of the parietal peritoneum that corresponds to the dermatomal distribution of the somatic afferent nerve roots at McBurney's point. Patients generally have a low-grade fever; it is rare for them to have a very high fever. They will invariably have malaise and lethargy. After the pain starts, patients often have some degree of nausea and emesis. These symptoms transpire over a 12–24 hours period; however, that can be variable as well.

On physical exam, the patient will often delineate the area of maximal tenderness (McBurney's point). Rovsing's sign is a peritoneal sign elicited by pressing on the left lower quadrant with resultant pain in the right lower quadrant. The psoas sign pertains to irritation of the psoas muscle that is described as pain in the pelvis after the patient extends his/her right thigh while lying on the left side. The obturator sign is demonstrated with the patient in the supine position and rotating a flexed right lower extremity medially.

A child with acute retrocecal or retroileal appendicitis (appendix deep to distal ileal bowel loops) may walk with exaggerated lumbar lordosis and have a slightly flexed right hip as a result of right psoas muscle spasm. Pain with extension of the right hip with the patient in left lateral decubitus position (psoas sign) and with internal rotation of the thigh (obturator sign) may be found with retrocecal appendicitis. If present, this indicates peritonitis.

Symptoms are contingent on the location of the appendix. For those patients with a retrocecal appendix, the pain is often posterior radiating to the groin, simulating the pain of renal colic. The patient may have associated microscopic hematuria. The anterior abdominal findings of tenderness and localized rebound are often less impressive in the patient with a retrocecal appendix. Those patients with an appendix lying in the pelvis can have pelvic pain with urinary symptoms.

LABORATORY DATA

The most diagnostic laboratory value for most patients with acute appendicitis is an elevated white blood count. This finding is most reliable in young persons, but less so in the elderly. If the WBC is normal without left shift, then the diagnosis of acute appendicitis should be reconsidered, although a normal WBC occurs in up to 30% of those with appendicitis. Of course, a markedly elevated WBC should raise the possibility of perforation. Urinalysis should be obtained to exclude nephrolithiasis. The presence of microhematuria may be caused by ureteral or bladder irritation from the adjacent appendicitis. In females of child-bearing age, a serum pregnancy test should be obtained. Additionally, a liver panel with amylase and lipase levels can be useful; pancreatitis should be considered in the differential diagnosis. Another marker that may be helpful is the C-reactive protein level. A normal C-reactive protein level has been associated with the absence of acute appendicitis.[6]

RADIOLOGY

An abdominal x-ray series (flat and upright) is a mainstay of the workup for abdominal pain, but generally will be unrevealing in appendicitis, with the rare exception of the radio-opaque fecalith. The other benefit of the plain radiograph is when it suggests bowel obstruction in a patient without a hernia or previous surgery. This can be the sign of a perforated appendicitis in someone with an atypical presentation.

The accuracy **of ultrasound** (US) depends upon the skill level of the sonographer. US findings suggestive of acute appendicitis include a noncompressible appendix of at least 6 mm in diameter. US has become a mainstay of diagnosis in the pediatric population. US does have its limitations, and while the ranges of reported specificity (88%–99%) and accuracy (82%–99%) for US have been acceptable, sensitivity (50%–100%) has varied considerably. Furthermore, US is relatively inexpensive and safe. Its biggest drawback is that negative findings do not exclude appendicitis with a high degree of confidence unless a normal appendix is visualized. However, appendiceal visualization rates in normal individuals without appendicitis vary widely in the published literature, from a high of 98%,[7] to a low of 22%.[8] A meta-analysis of three United States and three European studies with varied prevalence of acute appendicitis indicated that US was inferior to **computed tomography** (CT) in all instances.[9]

CT has become the diagnostic test of choice in many emergency departments and primary care facilities. CT findings of acute appendicitis include a visualized appendix >6 mm in size with periappendiceal stranding or wall thickening. A fecalith can be visualized in one quarter of cases of acute appendicitis. A contrast-filled appendiceal lumen without other abnormalities on CT essentially eliminates the diagnosis of acute appendicitis. If the appendix cannot be visualized on CT, the diagnosis cannot be excluded. Current generation high-resolution scanners produce sensitivity rates of 91%–97% and specificity rates of 91%–93%[10] (Fig. 37.1). Particularly in centers where OR access is at a premium, utilization of CT to eliminate the negative appendectomy appears prudent. Further, a recent review suggests that a noncontrast CT compared to CT with contrast may provide equivalent diagnostic accuracy, expediting the workup.[11] Mere introduction of CT into a care algorithm in and of itself does not lower the published 10%–20% negative appendectomy rate. However, integrating its use into a management strategy that uses senior surgeon consultation early in the workup can dramatically lower this rate as reported by Antevil et al.[12] Clearly, the best use of this technology is in the premenopausal female, where Wagner and colleagues have demonstrated a nearly two-thirds reduction in the negative appendectomy rate.[13] On the other hand, liberal use of CT does not appear to affect the rate of perforation. As a general rule, however, with a reliable history and physical exam, there is little reason for an adjunctive CT scan.[14] The benefit of CT is

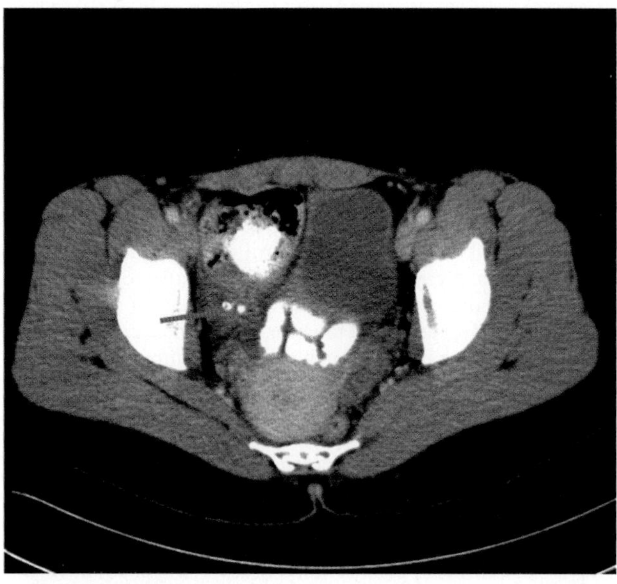

FIGURE 37.1. Pelvic CT with 16-slice scanner showing the obstructing fecalith at the base of the appendix.

in the patient with an unreliable exam or the inconsistent story. In addition, in elderly populations where other surgical conditions are common (ischemic colitis, *Clostridium difficile* colitis, colon cancer), CT may provide essential information. There is certainly concern for exposing the pediatric population to unnecessary radiation. This must be balanced with the morbidity of delaying the diagnosis in this population, one with a high perforation rate—20% in recent study.[15]

SPECIAL SITUATIONS

Approximately 5% of patients with appendicitis present in a delayed fashion, well after rupture. Patients with *perforated appendicitis* and a contained abscess can undergo percutaneous drainage and subsequent interval appendectomy after 8–12 weeks. There are some who question whether this delayed appendectomy is necessary.[16] The risk for recurrence appears higher in the presence of an appendicolith[17] and, certainly, an interval appendectomy can address the issue of an incidental finding, albeit rare. Invariably, the procedure can be performed laparoscopically when done in a staged fashion, even as an outpatient.[18]

Of course, if the perforation is encountered in the process of the initial operation, then the procedure should carry forward; understanding the risk of postoperative abscess formation is increased. It may be prudent to place a drain and abort further surgery if dense adhesions are present and the anatomy is unclear.[19] Although acute or gangrenous appendicitis without perforation may be treated with 24 hours or less of antibiotics, perioperatively, those with perforation and abscess formation warrant longer therapy. Regimens should cover common aerobic and anaerobic enteric flora without concern for enterococcus. Both single agent and combination intravenous therapy are appropriate and may be completed with an oral regimen of either ciprofloxacin/metronidazole or amoxicillin/clavulanic acid in those able to tolerate an oral diet.[20]

In patients with a history of *inflammatory bowel disease*, it is incumbent on the treatment team to exclude an active flair prior to surgical intervention. However, in a new presentation for Crohn's disease, the diagnosis process should proceed as is prudent. If the diagnosis of Crohn's is made at the time of surgery, if the patient is not obstructed, perforated or bleeding, then the operation should end and medical treatment begun. Many favor appendectomy at this operation, if the cecum at the base of the appendix is normal.

In *female patients*, the differential diagnosis includes many other entities (ovarian cyst, torsion, tubo-ovarian abscess, pelvic inflammatory disease, endometriosis, ectopic pregnancy, and Mittelschmerz), that CT would be reasonable, provided that the pelvic exam, ultrasound, and lab results were equivocal. In **pregnancy**, the application of the CT exam becomes more problematic, although still useful, and in this scenario the addition of MRI becomes helpful. The diagnosis of acute appendicitis is always difficult during pregnancy due to blunting of signs and symptoms, and the change in the relative position of the appendix. However, the correct diagnosis and prompt treatment in pregnancy is of great importance. Delay in intervention with perforation or unnecessary intervention increases mortality and morbidity for both the fetus and the mother. The rate of perforation has been reported as 25%–40% during pregnancy and increases the rates of spontaneous abortion, preterm labor, perinatal morbidity, and mortality. Mortality (combined miscarriage and infant mortality) increases from 7% to 20% with appendiceal perforation.[21,22] The laparoscopic approach may be safe in most; however, there is a lack of high-grade evidence to unequivocally support this approach. In the most recent large series, the rate of fetal loss is doubled (from 3.1% to 5.6%) with the laparoscopic technique; however, the rate of preterm delivery (2.1% vs. 8.1%) is substantially lower.[23]

The accurate diagnosis of appendicitis in *children* is often difficult, particularly with reluctance to utilize CT with the attendant risks of ionizing radiation. In children with abdominal pain, either the presence of a fever or of rebound tenderness triples the likelihood of appendicitis.[24] Symptoms and signs are most useful in combination, especially for identification of patients who require no further evaluation or intervention, and have been incorporated into several scoring systems.[25,26] The antibiotic management of both simple and complicated appendicitis in children should be similar to that in adult patients.[27]

In the *elderly*, the need for CT might only be limited by the comorbidities of the patient, especially, renal failure or use of certain medications. The elderly are another group where increased utilization of CT due to unreliability of exam or history may be appropriate (Algorithm. 37.1).

Immunosuppressed patients, particularly children, may develop acute appendicitis. The diagnosis may be difficult and CT may be warranted. The distinction between appendicitis and typhlitis is challenging and CT may not be definitive. The disease usually presents in complicated form and outcome is poor in the face of neutropenia.[28] Acute appendicitis may occur at a higher incidence in HIV-infected patients than in the general population, particularly in those with a high viral load or on a medication regimen that does not include highly active antiretroviral therapy. Presentation is often complicated as well.[29]

The incidence of *carcinoid* in the appendix at the time of appendectomy is 0.3%.[16] Currently, appendectomy for carcinoids <2 cm is adequate. Carcinoids over 2 cm in size require a right hemicolectomy for definitive management, with dissection to the root of the mesentery for lymphatic control. There is some recent literature to support the adequacy of a simple appendectomy for some carcinoids over 2 cm.[30]

For *appendiceal adenocarcinoid* (goblet cell carcinoma), the current management also includes right hemicolectomy for tumors over 1 cm in diameter.[31] Appendiceal adenocarcinoma is also a rare finding, with an incidence of 1 per 10 million cases. Those with stage I or II disease are treated with a simple appendectomy, whereas a right hemicolectomy should be performed for those with advanced disease.[32]

Another pathology that may be seen in the appendiceal specimen is a **mucocele or mucinous cystadenoma.** These are generally benign but should be removed early when found. If the base is uninvolved, then they can be removed via a standard appendectomy. For those that involve the cecum, a right hemicolectomy is indicated. The possibility to remove them laparoscopically is also available as long as the involved segment of the appendix is not grasped, to avoid the risk of perforation and spillage of epithelial tissue. Spillage could lead to the devastating condition of pseudomyxoma peritonei.[33,34] Pseudomyxoma can lead to chronic and acute bowel obstruction that often leads to mortality.

OPERATIVE PROCEDURE

As previously mentioned, the procedure for removal of the appendix had not changed substantially for 100 years, until the advent of laparoscopy. Currently, the debate continues as to which is the better modality. The most recent review shows that although laparoscopic appendectomy is becoming more prevalent, it is more costly and has unique complications. Laparoscopic appendectomy does have a slight advantage in earlier hospital discharge, decreased postoperative wound infection rate, and earlier return to activities. However, there is some question as to whether these benefits outweigh the initial increase in cost.[35]

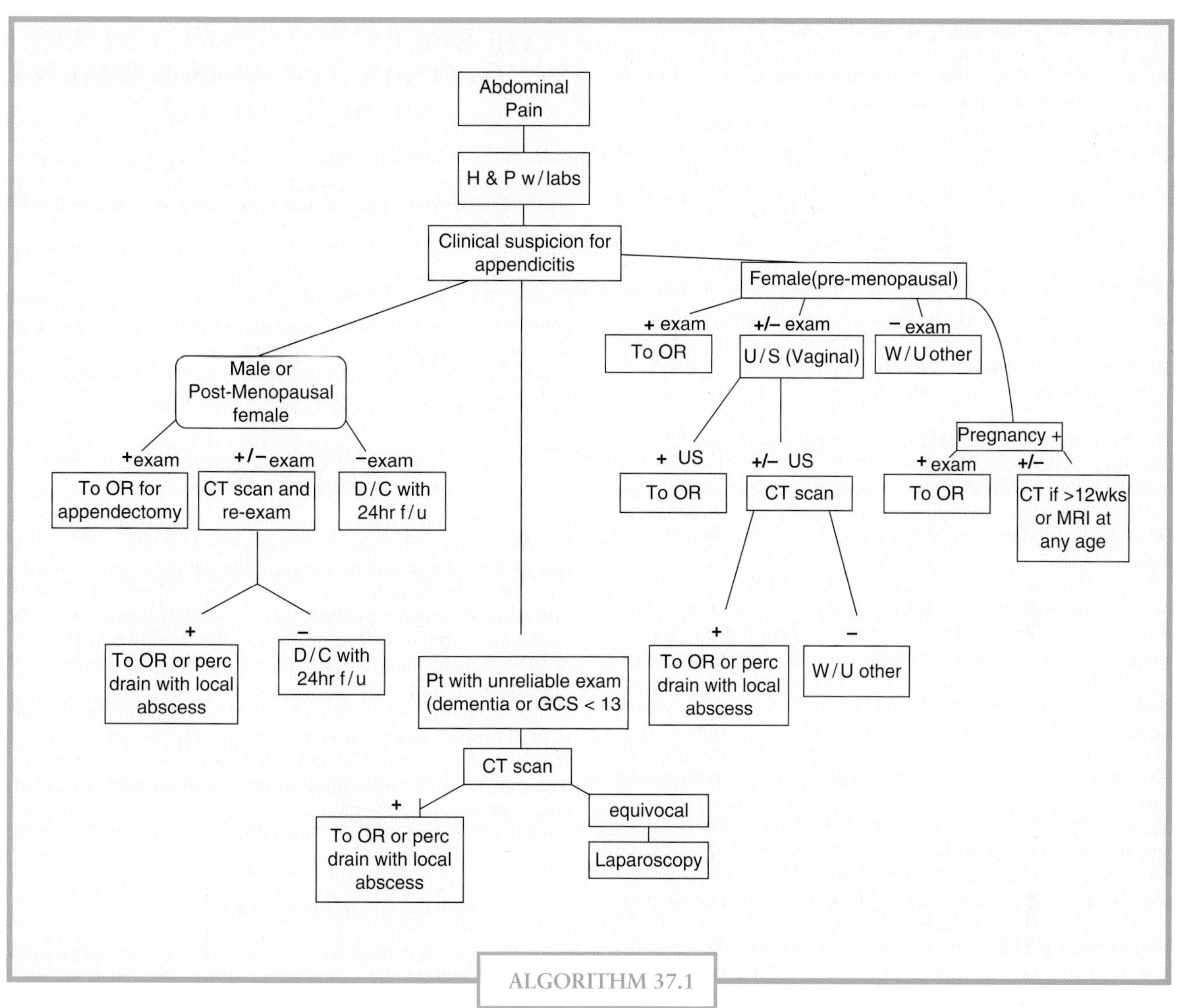

ALGORITHM 37.1 Algorithm for the diagnosis of acute appendicitis.

There is also discussion about laparoscopy being advantageous in the ability to view the whole abdomen when the appendix seems normal, as well as the ability to irrigate and aspirate into the pelvis to prevent postoperative abscess.

Regardless, the procedure itself starts with a patient who has been evaluated with a decision to proceed to the operating room. Depending upon the duration of illness or suspicion of perforation, preoperative resuscitation should occur, with early use of antibiotics. Informed consent should address the appropriate risks involved and also be clear in regard to the risk of more extensive surgery, including the possibility of an ileocecectomy or right hemicolectomy. There should also be a clear communication about the post-op risks of abscess, urinary retention, bleeding, wound infection, bowel obstruction, and potential hernia.

There is some debate as to whether surgery for a patient with a known diagnosis of acute appendicitis can "wait until the morning" if this diagnosis is established at nighttime. The practice does appear reasonable provided the delay is <6 hours.[36,37] The abdominal landmarks are noted and having established the point of maximal tenderness prior to induction, the choice of incision is determined. The use of a transverse Rocky-Davis incision versus an oblique McBurney incision is surgeon preference. The skin incision is carried down to the external oblique and continues in the direction of its fibers. Muscle splitting through the internal oblique and the transversus abdominis muscles in the direction of their fibers is accomplished until the peritoneum is reached. The peritoneum is opened and the use of self-retaining retractors is considered. The cecum is identified and followed to the confluence of the taeniae so that the base of the appendix can be identified. Depending upon the level of inflammation, the appendix is delivered into the wound. The amount of fibrinous attachment will dictate how easy or difficult this may be.

There is no benefit from routinely culturing peritoneal fluid as >10 organisms are typically identified.[38] The most commonly isolated bacteria include *Escherichia coli, Bacteroides fragilis*, streptococcus species, and *Pseudomonas*. These are generally well treated with any third-generation cephalosporin or fluoroquinolone, with the addition of metronidazole or clindamycin for anaerobic coverage.

As the appendix is brought up into the wound, the decision to approach the mesoappendix versus the appendix first is addressed. If the mesoappendix is manageable, then serial ligation between clamps is ideal. This should be ligated with minimum of 2-0 absorbable suture. The base of the appendix is clamped and a heavy absorbable suture is used to tie off the base. A clamp is placed distal to the sutures and the appendix is transected above the ties and removed from the patient. The protruding mucosa is fulgurated to prevent mucocele. Alternatively, the stump may be invaginated with a purse-string or Z-stitch as per surgeon preference. There is no evidence to support the invagination of the appendiceal stump. The area is copiously irrigated and the attempt to include the pelvis in the irrigation is made. The wound is closed in layers and the skin may be closed if the appendix was not perforated. Antibiotic therapy is then based on the guidelines. Non-perforated appendicitis requires only 24 hours of IV antibiotic therapy, whereas perforated appendicitis requires therapy until there are no clinical signs of infection.[27]

Those patients who have diffuse peritonitis after free spillage after a perforated appendix may be best served with a lower midline incision to deal with the diffuse contamination and prepare for the possibility of doing an ileocecectomy or right hemicolectomy should the cecum be considerably inflamed.

The laparoscopic approach is also adequate and is used often preferentially due to the potential benefit of shorter hospital stay and improved pain control. Additionally, it may be the procedure of choice for obese patients. The laparoscopic approach begins with the same previous initial resuscitation and antibiotic administration. The camera port is placed first; we prefer an open technique with the placement of a Hassan trocar. The 5 mm port for grasping the appendix can be in the suprapubic position or the right upper quadrant. The dissection port can be a 12 mm left lower quadrant port, as is our preference, or a 5 mm left lower quadrant port. The dissection of the window between the mesoappendix and the appendix is usually performed with the Maryland dissector. The mesoappendix can then be controlled with the harmonic scalpel, the LigaSure device, or a division with the GIA stapler with a vascular load, which requires a larger port. The appendix may then be divided at its base with the same stapler, or with an endoloop. The appendix is then removed in an endocatch bag and the area and pelvis irrigated with saline. After final inspection of the appendiceal stump and mesoappendix, the trocars are removed under direct inspection and the fascial defects closed with a figure eight fascial stitch. The skin closure is by subcuticular suture. The recent Cochrane analysis suggests that laparoscopic surgery for suspected appendicitis has diagnostic and therapeutic advantages compared to conventional "open" surgery. However, due to small differences, it does not advocate one therapy over the other. The advantages noted in the analysis of 67 studies were reduced pain, wound infection, and hospital length of stay.[39] Another recent meta-analysis of laparoscopic versus open appendectomy for complicated appendicitis suggests that the former has a reduced incidence of surgical site infection but no difference with regard to intra-abdominal abscess occurrence.[40]

For both the open and the laparoscopic approach, the patient is kept on IV fluids until a diet is tolerated. Treatment with antibiotics is as described above. Diet is started by postoperative day one and patients prepared for discharge.

Finally, because some patients may recover from an episode of acute appendicitis without operative intervention, there has been some interest in nonoperative management of this disease. However, a high readmission rate ranging from 14% to 35% was associated with antibiotic therapy alone.[41] Certainly, this strategy is fraught with danger in children and elderly patients and not the approach that we advocate.

THE ROLE OF THE ACUTE CARE SURGEON IN THE MANAGEMENT OF APPENDICITIS

Two studies address the role of the in-house acute care surgeon (ACS), also covering trauma patients, in caring for patients with appendicitis. They reach conflicting conclusions. The group from the University of Pennsylvania note that after adoption of an ACS model, the time to the operating room was shortened by 4 hours, the complication and rupture rate decreased by 10%, and length of stay was lessened by a day[42] compared to a traditional staffing model. The group from Wright State reports an identical time to the operating room and perforation rate, but a greater usage of the laparoscopic technique (that may be a function of evolution).[43]

SUMMARY

Acute appendicitis is the most common surgical emergency for the ACS. With advanced imaging and early intervention, the risk of mortality today is related to the patient's comorbidities. Current best practices lead to early surgery and treatment of abscess with surgery or drainage, given the presentation. The use of percutaneous drainage is a major advance in the care of these patients and allows a staged approach to complicated appendicitis.[44] Laparoscopy has added an important diagnostic and therapeutic tool for the management of appendicitis; particularly in females of childbearing age. The use of antibiotics should follow established practice guidelines. A problem yet to be solved is the substantial difference in the early diagnosis and treatment of the youngest of the population, who often are already perforated prior to the intervention of the medical staff.

References

1. Craig SW, Cebra JJ, Rabbit Peyer's patches, Appendix, and popliteal lymph node B lymphocytes: a comparative analysis of their membrane immunoglobulin components and plasma cell precursor potential. *J Immunol.* 1975;114(1 pt 2):492-502.
2. Bollinger R, Barbas AS, Bush EL, et al. Biofilms in the large bowel suggest an apparent function of the human vermiform appendix. *J Theoretic Biol.* 2007;249(4):826-831.
3. Bhattacharya K. Kurt Semm: a laparoscopic crusader. *J Min Access Surg.* 2007;3:35-36.
4. Körner H, Söreide JA, Pedersen EJ, et al. Stability in incidence of acute appendicitis. *Digest Surg.* 2001;18:61-66.
5. Nelson DS, Bateman B, Blote, RG. Appendiceal perforation in children diagnosed in a pediatric emergency department. *Pediatric Emerg Care.* 2000;16(4):233-237.
6. Asfar A, Safar H, Khoursheed M, et al. Would measurement of C-reactive protein reduce the rate of negative exploration for acute appendicitis? *J R Coll Surg Edinburgh.* 2000;45(1):21-24.
7. Lowe LH, Perez R, Scheker LE, et al. Appendicitis and alternate diagnoses in children: findings on unenhanced limited helical CT. *Pediatr Radiol.* 2001;31:569-577.
8. Karakas SP, Guelfguat M, Leonidas JC, et al. Acute appendicitis in children: comparison of clinical diagnosis with ultrasound and CT imaging, *Pediatr Radiol.* 2000;30:94-98.
9. van Randen A, Bipa S, Zwinderman AH, et al. Acute appendicitis: meta-analysis of diagnostic performance of CT and graded compression US related to prevalence of disease. *Radiology.* 2008;249:97-106.
10. Kim YJ, Kim JE, Kim HS and Hwang HY. MDCT with coronal reconstruction: clinical benefit in evaluation of suspected acute appendicitis in pediatric patients. *Am J Roentgenol.* 2009;192(1):150-152.
11. Hlibczuk V, Dattaro JA, Zin Z, et al. Diagnostic accuracy of noncontrast computed tomography for appendicitis in adults: a systematic review. *Ann Em Med.* 2010;55:51-59.
12. Antevil JL, Rivera L, Langenberg BJ, et al. Computed tomography-based clinical diagnostic pathway for acute appendicitis: prospective validation. *J Am Coll Surg.* 2006;203(6):849-856.
13. Wagner PL, Eachempati SR, Soe K, et al. Defining the current negative appendectomy rate: for whom is preoperative computed tomography making an impact? *Surgery.* 2008;144(2):276-282.

14. Lin KH, Leung WS, Wang CP, et al. Cost analysis of management in acute appendicitis with CT scanning under a hospital global budgeting scheme. *Emerg Med J*. 2008;25(3):149-152.
15. Colvin JM, Bachur R, Kharbanda A. The presentation of appendicitis in preadolescent children. *Pediatr Emerg Care*. 2007;23(12):849-855.
16. Kaminski A, Liu IL, Applebaum H, et al. Routine interval appendectomy is not justified after initial nonoperative treatment of acute appendicitis. *Arch Surg*. 2005;140:897-892.
17. Tsai HM, Shan YS, Shey JC, et al. Clinical analysis of the predictive factors for recurrent appendicitis after initial nonoperative treatment for perforated appendicitis. *Am J Surg*. 2006;192:311-315.
18. Whyte C, Tran E, Lopez ME, et al. Outpatient interval appendectomy after perforated appendicitis. *J Pediatr Surg* 2008;43:1970-1973.
19. Petrowsky H, Demartines N, Rousson V, et al. Evidence-based value of prophylactic drainage in gastrointestinal surgery: a systematic review and meta-analyses. *Ann Surg*. 2004;240(6):1074-1084.
20. Mazuski JE, Sawyer RG, Nathens AB, et al. The Surgical Infection Society Guidelines on antimicrobial therapy for intra-abdominal infections: evidence for the recommendations. *Surg Infections*. 2002;3:175-233.
21. Bailey LE, Finley RK Jr, Miller SF, et al. Acute appendicitis during pregnancy. *Am Surg*. 1986;52:218-221.
22. Yilmaz HG, Akgun Y, Bac B, et al. Acute appendicitis in pregnancy-risk factors associated with principal outcomes: a case control study. *Int J Surg*. 2007;5:192-197.
23. Walsh CA, Tang T, Walsh SR. Laparoscopic versus open appendicectomy in pregnancy: a systematic review. *Int J Surg*. 2008;6:339-344.
24. Bundy DG, Byerley JS, Liles EA, et al. Does this child have appendicitis. *JAMA*. 2007;298:438-451.
25. Alvarado A. A practical score for the early diagnosis of acute appendicitis. *Ann Em Med*. 1986;15:557-564.
26. Samuel M. Pediatric appendicitis score. *J Pediatr Surg*. 2002;37:877-881.
27. Nadler EP, Gaines BA. The Surgical Infection Society guidelines on antimicrobial therapy for children with appendicitis. *Surg Infections*. 2008;9:75-83.
28. Chui CH, Chan MY, Tan AH et al. Appendicitis in immunosuppressed children: still a diagnostic and therapeutic dilemma? *Ped Blood Cancer*. 2008;50:1282-1283.
29. Crun-Cianflone N, Weekes J, Bavaro M. Appendicitis in HIV-infected patients during the era of highly active antiretroviral therapy. *HIV Med*. 2008;9:421-426.
30. Moertel CG, Dockery MB, Judd ES. Carcinoid tumors of the vermiform appendix. *Cancer*. 1968;21:270-278.
31. Bamboat ZM, Berger DL. Is right hemicolectomy for 2.0-cm appendiceal carcinoids justified? *Arch Surg*. 2006;141(4):349-352.
32. Geode AC, Caplin ME, Winslet MC. Carcinoid tumour of the appendix. *Br J Surg*. 2003;90(11):1317-1322.
33. Walters KC, Paton BL, Schmelzer TS, et al. Treatment of appendiceal adenocarcinoma in the United States: penetration and outcomes of current guidelines. *Am Surg*. 2008;74(11):1066-1068.
34. Chiu CC, Wei PL, Huang MT, et al. Laparoscopic resection of appendiceal mucinous cystadenoma. *J Laparoendosc Adv Surg Tech*. 2005;15(3):325-328.
35. Sporn E, Petroski GF, Mancini GJ, et al. Laparoscopic appendectomy—is it worth the cost? Trend analysis in the US from 2000 to 2005. *J Am Coll Surg*. 2009;208(2):179-185.
36. Ditillo MF, Dziura JD, Rabinovici R. Is it safe to delay appendectomy in adults with acute appendicitis? *Ann Surg*. 2006;1244:656-660.
37. Surana R, Quinn F, Puri P. Is it necessary to perform appendectomy in the middle of the night for children? *Br Med J*. 199;306(6886):1168.
38. Foo FJ, Beckingham IJ, Ahmed I. Intra-operative culture swabs in acute appendicitis: a waste of resources. *Surg J R Coll Surg Edinburgh Ireland*. 2008;6(5):278-281.
39. Sauerland S, Jaschinksi T, Neugebauer EAM. Laparoscopic versus open surgery for suspected appendicitis. *Cochrane Database Syst Rev*. 2010;(10):CD001546.
40. Markides G, Subar D, Riyad K. Laparoscopic versus open appendectomy in adults with complicated appendicitis: systematic review and meta-analysis. *World J Surg*. 2010;34: 2026-2040.
41. Humes DJ, Simpson J. Acute appendicitis. *Br Med J*. 2006;333(7567): 530-534.
42. Earley AS, Pryor JP, Kim PK, et al. An acute care surgery model improves outcomes in patients with appendicitis. *Ann Surg*. 2006;244:498-504.
43. Ekeh AP, Monson B, Wozniak CJ, et al. Management of acute appendicitis by an acute care surgery service: is operative intervention timely? *J Amer Coll Surg*. 2008;207:43-48.
44. Brown CV, Abrishami M, Muller M, et al.Appendiceal abscess: immediate operation or percutaneous drainage? *Am Surg*. 2003;69(10):829-832.

CHAPTER 38 ■ ACUTE PANCREATITIS

PATRICIO POLANCO AND STEVEN J. HUGHES

Acute pancreatitis (AP) is an inflammatory process readily diagnosed by the combination of epigastric abdominal pain, abnormal elevation of pancreatic enzymes (amylase or lipase) in the serum, or computed tomography evidence of pancreatic inflammation.[1] In 75% of affected patients, AP is a self-limited process presenting as mild pain with rapid, spontaneous resolution. However, AP is a severe, life-threatening condition in the remaining quartile of patients, characterized by a systemic inflammatory response syndrome (SIRS) associated with the potential of multiple organ system failure (MOSF) and other complications including death. Thus, optimal treatment varies considerably, driven by accurate assessment of the severity of the disease, determination of the underlying etiology, and identification of potential complications such as pseudocyst, necrosis, infection, hemorrhage, and abdominal compartment syndrome (ACS).

EPIDEMIOLOGY

The annual incidence of AP varies among populations, ranging between 4.9 and 35 per 100,000 persons per year.[2] Russo et al[3]. reported 218,188 patients admitted in the United States for AP, with an overall mortality rate of 1.8% in the year 2000. In fact, the incidence of AP is increasing in western countries, resulting in an increasing rate of outpatient visits and admissions for acute and chronic pancreatitis (Fig. 38.1) in the United States. This is attributed to increasing alcohol consumption, and an increased incidence of gallbladder disease and obesity in this population.[4] AP can occur at any age, but the mean age for the first attack is the sixth decade.

ETIOLOGY AND PATHOGENESIS

Calculus biliary tract disease is the most common cause of AP and when combined with ethanol alcohol abuse as the second most common causative factor, these etiologies account for over 80% of the cases. The other etiologies of AP are rare and can be difficult to definitively diagnose. Table 38.1 summarizes these various etiologies.

Mechanical

The most common cause of AP is the passage of biliary tract precipitates in the form of crystalline sludge or frank gallstones from the gallbladder into the common bile duct, leading to temporary or persistent obstruction of the pancreatic duct at the level of the ampulla of Vater. Data are inconclusive as to whether the ensuing AP is due to a chemical injury from reflux of bile or enteric contents or an increase in hydrostatic pressure. Biliary AP is more common in females.

The second most common mechanical etiology of AP is endoscopic retrograde cholangiopancreatography (ERCP). Asymptomatic hyperamylasemia is observed following ERCP in 35%-70% of patients. However, clinical symptoms consistent with pancreatitis occur in fewer than 5% of the cases,[5,6] and the current frequency of pancreatitis following ERCP is considerably lower through efforts to avoid pancreatic duct injection when unnecessary and avoidance of vigorous injection of contrast when the duct does need to be visualized.

Anatomical abnormalities of the pancreas can also lead to mechanical causes of AP. Periampullary neoplasms or diverticuli, and duodenal duplication cysts may rarely lead to AP. *Pancreas divisum* is a relatively common anatomic variant of the pancreas seen in 5%-7% of the healthy population and is due to failure of the dorsal and ventral ducts to fuse during embryogenesis. This abnormality is thought to result in a relative stenosis of the lesser ampulla, resulting in ductal hypertension and subsequent AP. Annular pancreas is often associated with aberrant ductal anatomy, but rarely presents with pancreatitis.

Finally, AP occurs in 5% of patients with blunt abdominal trauma; hyperamylasemia without frank AP is present in a substantial percentage of other blunt trauma patients. Penetrating trauma involving the pancreas also causes AP; the energy distribution of a firearm missile places this mechanism at considerably higher risk for pancreatitis than that of relatively low-energy stab injuries.[7]

Toxic

Alcohol-induced pancreatitis is more common among men and is the second most common cause of AP, but only a small percentage of alcoholic subjects develop pancreatitis. This disparity is thought to be due to a combination of environmental and genetic factors which are poorly understand. Alcohol-induced pancreatitis may present as AP or as chronic pancreatitis. Not all alcoholic pancreatitis patients progress to chronic pancreatitis; even with continued alcohol abuse, some patients have nonprogressive, repetitive AP.[8]

Pharmacologic

Certain pharmacologic agents cause AP in idiosyncratic fashion due to poorly understood pharmacogenetic factors (e.g., aminosalicylates, 6-mercaptopurine) or direct, dose-related toxic effects (e.g., diuretics, sulfonamides). Table 38.1 lists the most common agents associated with drug-induced AP. The estimated incidence of drug-induced pancreatitis is 0.1%-2%. Balani et al.[9] described certain subpopulations who may be at higher risk such as children, women, the elderly, and patients with advanced HIV infection or inflammatory bowel disease. Most cases of drug-induced pancreatitis are mild and self-limiting, and the diagnosis of the etiology is usually implied rather than proven.

Metabolic

Hypertriglyceridemia and hypercalcemia are the two most common metabolic disorders associated with AP, but account for fewer than 3% of AP cases. Serum triglyceride concentrations must be markedly elevated, above 1,000 mg/dL to provoke AP. Thus, this etiology of AP is usually associated with

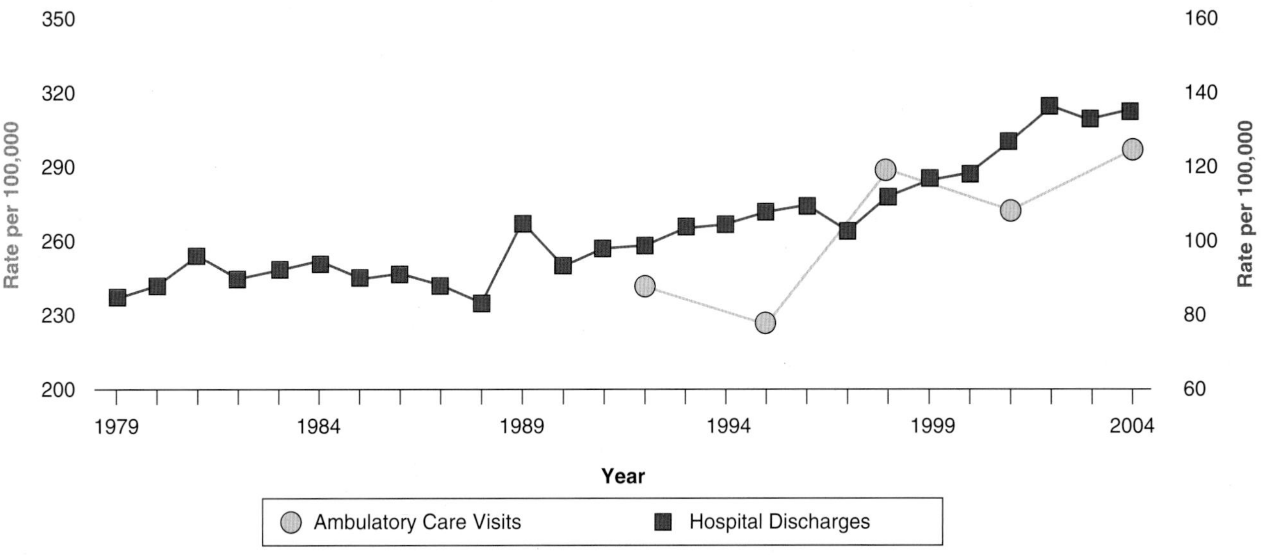

FIGURE 38.1 Age-adjusted rates of ambulatory care visits and hospital discharges with Pancreatitis in the United States of America 1979–2004. Source: National Ambulatory Medical Care Survey and National Hospital Ambulatory Medical Care and National Hospital Discharge Survey. With permission from Everhart JE et al., *Gastroenterology,* 2009;**136**:1134–1144.

type I, II, and V hyperlipidemia, but elevated triglycerides secondary to obesity, diabetes, estrogen or tamoxifen therapy, or nephrotic syndrome can also provoke AP. Triglyceride concentrations need to be measured at admission; after fluid resuscitation, the serum values may reduce considerably and thus prove misleading. Hypercalcemia of any etiology can occasionally cause AP, representing <1% of cases, and not clearly correlating with the degree of hypercalcemia. This disorder is usually a manifestation of hyperparathyroidism, but can also be seen in patients with excessive doses of vitamin D, familial hypocalciuric hypercalcemia, metastatic cancer, and total parenteral nutrition (TPN).

Infectious

Although several infectious agents can cause AP, this etiology accounts for <1% cases of AP.[10] The viruses, Mumps, Coxsackievirus, Hepatitis B, Cytomegalovirus, Varicella-Zoster and Herpes simplex can induce AP. More recently, HIV infection has been related to AP. Although it is hypothesized that AP can be caused by HIV itself, most commonly it is associated with opportunistic infections or medications (e.g., didanosine). Bacterial infections including Mycoplasma, Legionella, Leptospira and Salmonella, and fungal infections (Aspergillus) and parasites (Toxoplasma, Cryptosporidium, and Ascaris) have been reported as agents causing AP.

Hereditary Pancreatitis

Some genetic mutations are associated with AP, most notably mutations of the *serine protease 1* (*prss*1) and *serine protease inhibitor Kazal 1* (*spink*1) genes. SPINK1 is described as disease modifier and can promote AP in combination with alcohol abuse. Also, at least one mutant variant of the *cystic fibrosis transmembrane conductance regulator* (*cftr*) gene has been identified in some patients with idiopathic chronic and acute recurrent pancreatitis. These possible inherited forms of AP should be suspected when the following criteria are present: Idiopathic recurrent pancreatitis, relatives with pancreatitis-associated mutations or family history of recurrent pancreatitis, idiopathic chronic pancreatitis, or pancreatitis in childhood.[11] Genetic testing and counseling are recommended for this group of patients.

Autoimmune

Autoimmune pancreatitis is poorly understood, but is often associated with elevations in serum IgG4 concentrations, and resection specimens stain strongly for IgG4 expression. The process can be localized, or involve the entire gland. These patients typically present with a constellation of symptoms and findings consistent with pancreatic cancer including pancreatic and biliary strictures and low-attenuation masses by CT, rather than AP.

Vascular

AP secondary to ischemia is a very rare event but it has been described as a complication of lupus and other etiologies of vasculitis, atheroembolic events, intraoperative hypotension, and hemorrhagic shock. This etiology of AP needs to be particularly considered in patients that develop AP following cardiopulmonary bypass status.

PATHOGENESIS

The inflammatory processes that occur with AP are extraordinarily similar regardless of the etiology, and include both structural and biochemical changes. Early events are characterized by changes in secretion, intracellular activation of enzymes, and generation of inflammatory mediators. Intra-acinar activation of trypsinogen, uncontrolled by endogenous antagonists such as SPINK 1, alpha-1 antitrypsin, and alpha-2-macroglobulin, leads to activation of other enzymes such as

TABLE 38.1

ETIOLOGIC FACTORS OF ACUTE PANCREATITIS

ETIOLOGIC CATEGORY	SPECIFIC ITEM
Mechanical	Gallstones or biliary sludge Neoplastic process Periampullary diverticulum Sphincter of Oddi dysfunction Blunt or penetrating trauma Post ERCP
Toxic	Alcohol Scorpion toxin
Drugs	Azathioprine Sulfonamides Thiazides Furosemide Pentamidine Didanosine Methyldopa Tetracycline Estrogens Valproic acid Sulindac 5-aminosalicylic acid 6-mercaptopurine L-Asparaginase
Metabolic	Hypertriglyceridemia Hypercalcemia Hyperuricemia
Infectious	Viral Parasites Mycoplasm
Vascular	Circulatory shock Ischemia–reperfusion Embolic Hypothermia Malignant hyperthermia Autoimmune vasculitis
Hereditary	Serine protease 1 (*prss1*) mutation Serine protease inhibitor Kazal 1 (*spink1*) mutation Cystic fibrosis transmembrane conductance regulator (*ctfr*) mutation
Autoimmune	IgG4

proelastase, procarboxypeptidase, prophospholipase A2 and other cascades including kallikrein–kinin, complement components, and fibrinolysis. Pancreatic digestion characterized by necrosis, apoptosis, and autophagy ensues. Microcirculatory injury and leukocyte chemoattraction with release of cytokines further mediate these processes.

The release into the circulation of activated pancreatic enzymes and cytokines (phospholipase, elastase, TNF, IL-2, platelet-activated factor—PAF, complement, etc.) mediate the SIRS seen in patients with severe pancreatitis. In these patients, these mediators affect distant organs, leading to increased vascular permeability, vasodilation, liver injury, pulmonary injury, myocardial depression, and acute kidney injury. Thus, severe AP can lead to MOSF.[12] Why a subset of individuals develop severe AP with SIRS is poorly understood and is an area of intense investigation.

CLINICAL FINDINGS

The most consistent symptom of AP is severe epigastric pain, often extending through or with band-like radiation to the back. Anorexia, nausea, and vomiting are also reported by the majority of patients. Systemic findings such as fever, tachycardia, dehydration, and in severe cases, shock and coma subsequently may be present. The typical, temporal history of biliary pancreatitis is onset of pain within 2 hours of a large meal, usually high in fat content. The onset of symptoms from alcohol-induced AP typically ensues 1–3 days after a drinking binge.

Importantly, findings on the initial physical exam are rarely indicative of the severity of the disease. Hemodynamic changes or signs of pulmonary, hepatic, or renal injury should not be expected at presentation, nor should their absence suggest the patient is likely to follow a self-limited clinical course. Epigastric tenderness is a constant finding. Guarding, abdominal distension, decreased bowel sounds, and even rebound tenderness may be present. The mucous membranes may appear dry and the urine typically appears concentrated.

Later in the disease course, if the AP process is caused by choledocholithiasis or liver injury leading to cholestasis has occurred, jaundice or scleral icterus may be noted. Similarly, physical findings of pulmonary injury will develop in severe AP including rales and decreased breath sounds, usually in left base associated with a pleural effusion. Without adequate volume replacement or in the setting of severe renal injury, oliguria or anuria may be observed. Although classically described, Grey-Turner sign (ecchymotic discoloration of flank) and Cullen sign (ecchymotic discoloration of periumbilical region) are seen in only 1%-2% of patients and indicate severe AP with retroperitoneal hemorrhage dissecting into these areas. These findings have been associated with a mortality rate of 37%.[13]

DIAGNOSIS OF AP: BIOCHEMICAL MARKERS AND IMAGING

The diagnosis of AP is first suspected clinically then confirmed by biochemical or radiologic evidence. According to guidelines published by the American College of Gastroenterology, the diagnosis of AP requires two of the following three features: (1) abdominal pain characteristic of AP, (2) serum amylase or lipase ≥3 times the upper limit of normal, and (3) characteristic findings of AP on CT scan.[14]

Biochemical Markers

Amylase and lipase are the most accepted confirmatory biomarkers in AP. Serum amylase concentrations rise within 6–12 hours of the onset of pain and with a half-life of approximately 10 hours. Serum lipase concentrations more slowly elevate, typically peaking 24 hours after the onset of pain, and then normalize over 2–3 weeks. In episodes of mild and uncomplicated pancreatitis, serum amylase should normalize within 3–5 days. Elevated serum amylase is considered a sensitive but nonspecific test for AP. Hyperamylasemia can be found in diseases that affect other organs, which produce amylase, such as salivary glands (e.g., parotiditis, trauma, calculi) and fallopian tubes (ectopic pregnancy and salpingitis). Hyperamylasemia can be observed in chronic renal failure patients or found in almost any peripancreatic inflammatory process including intestinal ischemia or a perforated viscus. In contrast, elevated serum lipase is both sensitive (85%-100%) and specific for the diagnosis of AP. Thus, it is ultimately a superior diagnostic tool except early in the clinical course;

additional, later sampling may be necessary.[15] Importantly, the level of pancreatic enzyme elevation does not correlate with severity of disease and has no value in the assessment of clinical progress or prognosis; therefore, daily measurement of amylase and lipase is not recommended.

Several other biochemical tests or biomarkers have been forwarded as having merit in the diagnosis of AP, but for a variety of reasons, none have been routinely employed. Urine amylase and clearance of amylase can be diagnostic tools for AP, but are only used to diagnose macroamylasemia (in which urine amylase is normal). The serum elevation of other pancreatic enzymes (phospholipase A, trypsin, carboxipeptidase A, colipase, and carboxylester lipase) currently lacks clinical utility. Pancreatitis-associated protein, Trypsinogen activation peptide (TAP), and Trypsinogen-2 are nonenzymatic pancreatic peptides that are elevated in AP. Serum concentrations of TAP have been described as a predictor of disease severity.[16]

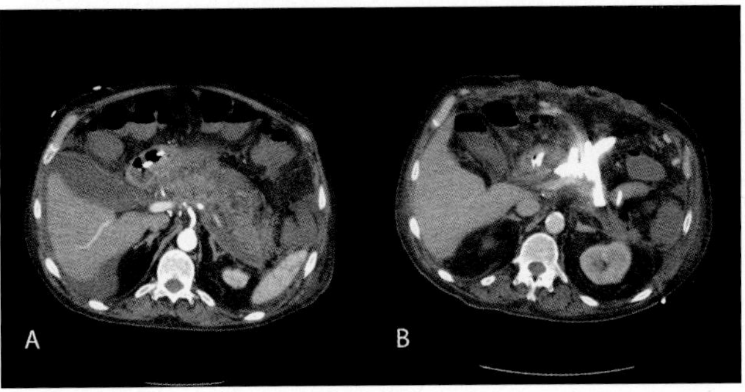

FIGURE 38.2 Computed tomography of pancreatic necrosis. **A:** Arterial phase image of the pancreas from a dynamic, contrast-enhanced CT shows lack of enhancement of nearly the entire pancreas, suggesting necrosis of more than 80% of the Gland. **B:** CT of the same patient after open debridement and external drainage demonstrating control of peripancreatic fluid collections.

IMAGING

Recent advances in imaging have led to significant progress in the diagnosis, assessment, prognostication, and treatment of AP and associated complications. Of historical interest, a series of abdominal roentograms was once the only option for imaging patients with abdominal pain and suspicion of AP. Classically, the findings of AP are localized or may be only a segmental ileus called the "sentinel loop sign" and the "colon cut-off sign." In severe cases, a generalized ileus can be observed.

Contrast-enhanced Computed Tomography (CT) is currently the preferred imaging tool for the diagnosis of AP and assessment of severity. CT at the initial evaluation of a patient with abdominal pain can exclude pancreatitis and many other acute intra-abdominal processes. However, CT is not necessary to implement appropriate initial treatment for a patient with even severe AP, and CT is not cost-effective when patients present with clear clinical and biochemical features of mild AP. If CT is obtained in a patient with self-limited AP, the findings range from a normal appearing pancreas without peripancreatic abnormalities to diffuse enlargement of the gland with heterogeneous attenuation of the parenchyma and stranding of the peripancreatic fat.[17] Focal involvement of the gland can be seen in up to 18% of patients and this pattern is commonly seen in patients with chronic alcohol abuse.[18]

If a patient presents with clinical features predictive of a severe episode or the patient's clinical condition deteriorates despite adequate initial medical management, a dynamic, contrast-enhanced CT should be obtained. In severe AP, all the findings described above can be observed, but the true value of dynamic contrast administration is the potential identification of regions of the gland that lack arterial enhancement representing an area(s) of necrosis. Beger *et al.* showed an overall accuracy of 87% for detection of necrosis (confirmed by surgical intervention) with 100% sensitivity for the detection of extended pancreatic necrosis, but only 50% sensitivity for the detection of minor necrotic areas identified at surgery; the specificity of CT for necrosis was 100% in this series.

The normal pancreatic parenchyma attenuates x-rays to 40–50 Hounsfield units (HU) on unenhanced CT images; this increases to 100–150 HU during the arterial phase of contrast administration. Typically, delineation of necrosis by dynamic, contrast-enhanced CT becomes identifiable 24–48 hours after the initiation of symptoms (Fig. 38.2). Thus, early CT (within 12–24 hours of initial presentation) may be equivocal or may underestimate the amount of necrosis and severity of disease, and more informative results are obtained with a dynamic, contrast-enhanced CT 48–72 hours after the onset of an acute attack of pancreatitis.[19] This timing also allows intravascular resuscitation prior to the administration of intravenous contrast, thus reducing the risk of contrast-induced renal injury. If contrast cannot be given due to severe allergy or tenuous renal function, the criterion of pancreatic parenchyma displaying attenuation <30 HU correlates to regions of ischemia, and the development of necrosis has been described.[19]

CT also plays an essential role in the identification and management of AP complications, such as focal fluid collections, abscess, and pseudocyst. Throughout the course of severe AP, repeated CT studies may be needed according to clinical evolution or anticipation of complications. However, routine serial CT scan is not recommended unless there has been a change in the patient's clinical condition.

Ultrasound (US) evaluation is appropriately obtained in patients with AP when cholelithiasis is a possible etiology. A diffusely enlarged pancreas with hypoechoic areas are distinctive ultrasonographic findings of AP. However, in almost a third of the patients, the interposition of bowel gas obscures the pancreas. For this reason, US has a limited role in diagnosis and assessment of the severity of AP.[20] US is helpful in the assessment of the intra- and extrahepatic biliary tree. A dilated common bile duct may suggest impaction rather than spontaneous passage of the biliary and pancreatic duct obstruction, and should prompt evaluation for the appropriateness of ERCP.

Magnetic Resonance Imaging (MRI)/Magnetic Resonance Cholangiopancreatography (MRCP) is similar in accuracy to contrast-enhanced CT in diagnosis and staging the severity of AP. MRI/MRCP is not the standard imaging technique for AP and its use will depend on availability, local expertise, and institutional algorithms. MRI is a good alternative when intravenous contrast cannot be administered and necrosis is suspected. Purported advantages of MRI include no radiation exposure, lack of nephrotoxicity of gadolinium, superior tissue characterization, and potential ability to detect pancreatic duct disruptions.[21] Disadvantages include patient intolerance or ineligibility, significantly longer durations of image acquisition, and variability in technique and access. MRCP is the only noninvasive method to assess the pancreatic duct and is appropriate when delineation of biliary and pancreatic duct anatomy is important or to identify the potential etiology of AP such as biliary calculi and pancreas divisum, or there is clinical need to assess the pancreatic duct for evidence of disruption or stricture (Fig. 38.3). If pancreatic stricture is suspected, the sensitivity of the technique is dependent upon imaging before and after the administration of secretin.

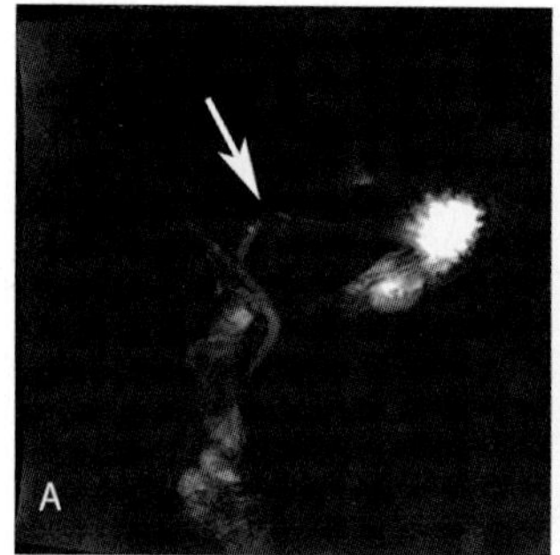

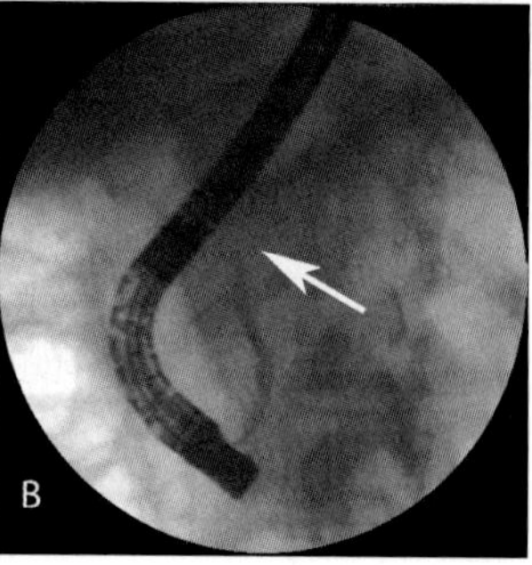

FIGURE 38.3 Disrupted pancreatic duct. Pancreatitis can result in disruption and/or stricture of the main pancreatic duct, complicating care. **A:** MRCP suggests a stricture or disruption of the pancreatic duct near the neck of the gland. **B:** Subsequent ERCP confirms disruption with an abrupt termination of filling and inability to visualize the proximal duct with contrast injection.

Endoscopic Ultrasound (EUS) is an increasingly important imaging tool in evaluation of the pancreas and biliary tree. However, knowledge of the value of EUS in AP is in evolution and access to this modality is currently limited for the most part to academic institutions. EUS may prove valuable in minimally invasive approaches to management of AP complications, including drainage or debridement of peripancreatic fluid collections, pseudocysts, and focal necrosis. Although not commonly used in AP, it could be useful in patients with recurrent pancreatitis with uncertain etiology since it has a high sensitivity for calculi, small pancreatic duct tumors, and duct abnormalities.[18] EUS criteria for chronic pancreatitis have been defined, but remain controversial versus traditional approaches of secretin stimulation and ERCP.

CLASSIFICATION AND PROGNOSIS OF ACUTE PANCREATITIS

Once the diagnosis of AP has been made, it is essential to determine the probable severity of the disease. Based upon the Atlanta Criteria established during a consensus conference in 1992, AP can be categorized in mild and severe cases. Mild AP is associated with minimal organ dysfunction and an uneventful recovery, and occurs in more than 75% of the patients. These patients usually experience rapid normalization of symptoms and laboratory values in response to the conservative measures of bowel rest, pain management, and crystalloid administration. Failure to improve within 48–72 hours should prompt investigation for complications or another diagnosis. In contrast, severe AP is associated with organ dysfunction or local complications, such as necrosis, abscess, or pseudocyst. Severe AP can be anticipated upon initial presentation by the identification of three or more Ranson's criteria, an APACHE II score >7, or Glasgow prognostic criteria (Table 38.2).

The Ranson's prognostic criteria, initially described in 1974, include 11 parameters, five of which are evaluated at admission, and six which are assessed after 48 hours. In the original report, the sensitivity of three or more criteria to predict severe disease was 65% with a specificity of 99%, yielding a positive predictive value (PPV) of 95% and a negative predictive value (NPV) of 86%. More recently, a meta-analysis that included 1,307 patients revealed an overall sensitivity for predicting severe AP of 75%, specificity of 77%, a PPV of 49%, and an NPV of 91%. These data reveal the fact that there is a high false-positive rate of Ranson's criteria and many patients with a score more than 3 will not develop clinically severe pancreatitis.[22] Preferentially used in the United Kingdom, the Glasgow's prognostic criteria examine eight factors.

The acute physiology and chronic health evaluation (APACHE), initially developed in 1981, included 34 factors, thus complicating its use. It was subsequently simplified to 12 factors in APACHE II (1985). This assessment is widely used and accepted today for critically ill patients. The APACHE II score produces comparable accuracy to Ranson's criteria in distinguishing mild from severe pancreatitis, with an accuracy of about 70%-80%. Later modifications of the score, APACHE III (1991) and APACHE O-Obesity (1996), have been proposed but are not broadly used.

CT can predict the severity of AP. Balthazar et al[23]. described a grading system based upon findings of unenhanced CT (Table 38.3). This initial grading system described five distinct groups based on pancreatic and peripancreatic inflammation with presence of fluid collections and/or free air. This was subsequently modified to include findings of contrast-enhanced CT that included the amount of necrosis (<30%, 30%-50%, and >50%) to create a CT severity index (CTSI).[24] Several studies have shown that the amount of necrosis strongly correlates with organ failure and mortality. A recent series of 276 patients

TABLE 38.2

SEVERITY SCORING SYSTEMS FOR ACUTE PANCREATITIS

RANSON'S CRITERIA		GLASGOW'S CRITERIA	APACHE (0–4 POINTS EACH)
On admission	*Within 48 h*	Age >55 y	Temperature
Age >55 y	Hemoglobin ↓ below 10 mg/dL	White cell count > 15 × 10^9/L	Mean arterial pressure
WBC >16,000/mm^3	Blood urea Nitrogen ↑ >5 mg/dL	PaO_2 <60 mmHg (8 kPa)	Heart rate
LDH >350 U/L	Calcium ↓ <8 mg/dL	LDH >600 U/L	Respiratory Rate
AST >250 U/L	PaO_2 <60 mmHg (8 kPa)	AST >200 U/L	Oxygenation
Glucose >200 mg/dL	Base deficit >4 mEq/L Fluid sequestration >6 L	Albumin <32 g/L Ca <2 mmol/L Glucose >10 mmol/L Urea >16 mmol/L	Arterial pH HCO_3^- Na^+ K^+ Creatinine Hematocrit White blood count Glasgow Coma Scale

TABLE 38.3

COMPUTED TOMOGRAPHY SEVERITY INDEX

GRADE	CT FINDING	POINTS	NECROSIS PERCENTAGE	ADDITIONAL POINTS
A	Normal pancreas	0	0	0
B	Pancreatic enlargement	1	0	0
C	Pancreatic inflammation and/or peripancreatic fat	2	<30	2
D	Single peripancreatic fluid collection	3	30–50	4
E	Two or more fluid collections and/or retroperitoneal air	4	>50	6

reported that organ failure occurred in 5%, 20%, and 50% of the patients with <30% necrosis, 30%-50% of necrosis, and >50% of necrosis, respectively.[25] Furthermore, a statistically significant correlation between the incidence of morbidity and mortality and the CTSI score has been established. Patients scoring 0–1 point had no morbidity or mortality, while those with a score of 2 have a morbidity of 4% without mortality. In the group of patients with CTSI scores of 7–10, mortality was 17% and 92% had complications.[26] Thus, the CTSI score has been validated as one of the most reliable prognostic factors of severity, morbidity, and mortality.

Finally, other immunologic markers of inflammation including C-reactive protein, IL-6, IL-8, IL-10, TNF, procalcitonin, and PMN elastase can be assayed from the serum and have been forwarded as predictors of AP severity. C-reactive protein is an acute-phase reactant, largely studied as a marker of inflammation and severity in AP. Concentrations of C-reactive protein above 150 mg/dL at 48 hours discriminate mild from severe AP.[20] Procalcitonin is another acute-phase reactant that has not only been described as a marker of severe AP with organ failure (when concentration >0.5 ng/mL at 24 hours after admission),[27] but also as a discriminator of infected pancreatic necrosis (when concentration >1.8 ng/mL).[28] Although the utility of these immunologic biomarkers has been reported, a positive impact on the clinical management of patients with AP remains unproven, and as such, few clinicians utilize them.

MANAGEMENT

Mild Acute Pancreatitis

The majority of the AP cases (>75%) can be classified as mild according to the Atlanta criteria. These patients usually recover in 3–5 days and only require conservative, supportive medical management. This consists of bowel rest, fluid resuscitation, pain control, and correction of electrolytes and metabolic disorders. Vigilance must be maintained to identify early signs of SIRS and organ dysfunction. Even in mild cases, considerable redistribution and subsequent loss of intravascular volume can occur. In addition to exacerbating potential renal injury, inadequate resuscitation can result in further pancreatic injury and pancreatic necrosis.[29] Thus, aggressive fluid resuscitation with close monitoring of hydration status, urine output, and vital signs is recommended for all patients with AP. Typical electrolyte abnormalities include hypokalemia, hypocalcemia, hypomagnesemia, and hyperglycemia. These electrolytes should be evaluated daily and corrected as indicated.

In mild AP, there is no role for antibiotics. Analgesia is essential and should be administered parenterally to ensure adequate delivery. Opioids, typically via patient-controlled analgesia, are appropriate. Hydromorphone is the pharmacologic agent of choice. While morphine and meperidine have historically been used, morphine increases the sphincter of Oddi pressure, a theoretically undesired effect. However, there is no clinical evidence that morphine can worsen or exacerbate AP.[30] Meperidine has fallen out of favor due to its known potential to induce neuromuscular irritation and seizures due to accumulation of a neurotoxic metabolite (normeperidine).

Since the inflammation in mild AP subsides within a week, nutrition is not usually a concern. Bowel rest should be prescribed until the pain has resolved and the patient has return of appetite. Initial intake is restricted to water or clear liquids with advancement to a low-fat diet as tolerated. If symptoms recur, CT evaluation of potential complications is warranted. If complications are absent, in addition to the resolution of pain, delaying a second challenge to oral intake until there has been normalization of serum pancreatic enzymes is reasonable.

Cholecystectomy for Biliary Pancreatitis

If biliary pancreatitis is confirmed by US, laparoscopic cholecystectomy during the same hospitalization is safe and cost-effective. Even a 2-week delay in operative intervention is associated with a 13% rate of recurrent pancreatitis.[31] Furthermore, two prospective studies showed that laparoscopic cholecystectomy can be done safely in mild AP, even before normalization of amylase and lipase, and resolution of pain.[32,33] A recent randomized trial in mild AP compared this approach versus delaying intervention until serum enzymes normalized and abdominal pain had resolved. This study showed shorter length of stay in the early group without an increase in perioperative morbidity or technical difficulty.[34]

Inherent to the diagnosis of biliary pancreatitis is that particulate matter has been and may remain within the common bile duct. There is consensus that ERCP should not be performed prior to cholecystectomy in cases of mild, biliary pancreatitis unless data such as an elevated conjugated bilirubin or dilated common bile duct suggests persistent occlusion. Even then, some authors argue that intraoperative cholangiography is safer and more cost-effective than ERCP, noting that it has been shown that recent cholecystectomy does not increase the risks of ERCP. However, debate continues as to the appropriateness of routine intraoperative cholangiography. The incidence of retained stones is approximately 9%, but the incidence of subsequent symptoms in patients who do not undergo cholangiography is only 1%.[35] Once a retained stone is identified, it should be addressed. Thus, routine intraoperative cholangiography in the setting of AP will result in a significant number of common bile duct explorations or ERCPs that do not provide clinical benefit.

Other Causes of Acute Pancreatitis

Patients with alcohol-induced pancreatitis should receive assessment for alcoholism and other addictions, and referral to therapy if appropriate. It is most cost-effective to make the assumption of essential nutrient deficiency, and thiamine and folate should be administered. These patients should be carefully monitored for signs of acute withdrawal from alcohol, and prophylaxis against seizure using benzodiazepines implemented immediately if such symptoms arise.

Management of hypercalcemia or hypertriglyceridemia etiologies should be addressed prior to discharge from the hospital. If the AP is drug-induced, the causative agent should be permanently withdrawn and listed as an allergy. Evaluation and management of other etiologies can be pursued after discharge in the outpatient setting.

Severe Acute Pancreatitis

The natural history of severe AP follows two distinct phases. The first phase is characterized by SIRS and varying organ dysfunction or failure with subsequent clinical stabilization or improvement, and the second phase occurs in patients who develop infectious complications, most typically occurring 3–6 weeks from the onset of symptoms.

Early Phase Interventions. When severe AP is probable (Ranson's criteria > 3, APACHE > 7), the patient should be admitted and monitored in an intensive care unit for aggressive fluid resuscitation with continuous surveillance of vital signs and pulmonary, renal, and other organ functions in preparation for the probable need to subsequently support failing organs systems. If SIRS does ensue, central venous and arterial pressure monitoring is warranted. This monitoring is critical in the setting of a severe capillary leak to minimize the risk of inadequate crystalloid replacement leading to inadequate tissue perfusion, shock, altered mental status, acute tubular necrosis and acute renal failure, and worsening pancreatic necrosis, or conversely, excessive resuscitation, exacerbating pulmonary edema, worsening ARDS, or intra-abdominal hypertension and subsequent ACS.

Abdominal Compartment Syndrome

ACS is a severe complication of AP that requires emergent surgical intervention. The etiology of ACS in severe AP is due to retroperitoneal and peripancreatic inflammation that results in large fluid shifts, leading to visceral and abdominal wall edema in addition to ascites, and the ileus that often accompanies severe pancreatitis. Spontaneous hemorrhage can also increase retroperitoneal and intra-abdominal contents. ACS can be a devastating complication of AP, and the related mortality is estimated to be between 50% and 75%.[36,37] Treatment for ACS is emergent, decompressive laparotomy to relieve intra-abdominal hypertension. ACS occurs early in AP, most often within the first week and potentially within the first 24 hours of presentation. Urgent decompressive laparotomy results in immediate improvement in hemodynamics and ventilator requirements, and can save a subset of these patients. Importantly, decompression does not mandate future pancreatic debridement in all patients; exploration of the pancreas during release of an ACS is unwarranted, thus this procedure can be performed in the ICU to avoid transfer of these critically ill patients.

Nutrition in Severe AP

Patients with severe AP should be anticipated to be at high risk for the development of malnourishment during their illness. Enteral nutrition (EN) via nasojejunal feeding access is superior to TPN for patients with severe AP. Several randomized controlled trials and subsequent meta-analysis have consistently showed that EN significantly reduces infections, surgical interventions, and mortality in patients with severe AP.[38-40] The use of EN instead of TPN has the notable advantages of prevention of catheter-related infections and preservation of the intestinal barrier, preventing bacterial translocation from the intestines, likely the major source of bacteria that lead to infected necrosis. When elemental or semi-elemental supplements versus complex polymeric formulas are delivered distal to the ligament of Treitz, the stimulation of the pancreas is reduced by 50%. Importantly, the presence of gastric ileus, peripancreatic fluid collections, necrosis or elevated pancreatic enzymes are not contraindications for enteral feeding.

Antibiotic prophylaxis in Severe AP

Infection is the leading cause of morbidity and mortality in severe AP and complicates the disease in 20%-40% of patients with necrotizing pancreatitis.[41,42] The extent of necrosis is predictive of the subsequent risk of infection. This complication usually occurs 3–6 weeks after the onset of symptoms. The risk of mortality increases to 40% if initially sterile pancreatic necrosis becomes infected. The majority of cases represent monomicrobial infections with *Escherichia coli, Pseudomona, Klebsiella, Enterococcus,* and *Bacteriodes* species. With the increasing use of antibiotic prophylaxis, polymicrobial infections and other organisms including *Staphylococcus* and *Candida* species have been increasingly observed.

Based on controlled and uncontrolled trials, the use of antibiotic prophylaxis was suggested as part of the conservative medical management of necrotizing pancreatitis. Initial meta-analyses further suggested that mortality and morbidity can be reduced through the administration of prophylactic, broad-spectrum antibiotics.[43] Imipenem–cilastatin, meropenem and the combination of ciprofloxacin and metronidazol (in penicillin-allergic patients) were the antibiotics recommended due to their better penetration into the necrotic material. Subsequently, superiorly designed and controlled studies failed to demonstrate such a benefit.[42,44-46] The most recent Cochrane Database Review (2010)[47] of seven randomized, controlled trials that compared antibiotics versus placebo in CT-proven pancreatic necrosis failed to demonstrate a statistically significant difference between the two groups with respect to mortality, rates of infected pancreatic necrosis, need for surgical intervention, fungal infection, and nonpancreatic infection. Despite these data, antibiotic prophylaxis in necrotizing pancreatitis is an unsettled topic of discussion and some guidelines and experts still recommend this practice.

ERCP and Sphincterotomy in Severe Biliary Pancreatitis

Initial studies of the potential benefit of ERCP in patients with severe AP provided disparate results, with some suggesting ERCP actually worsened the disease. In fact, the most recent meta-analysis by Petrov et al.[48] that included three trials encompassing 405 patients showed that early ERCP in patients with either mild or severe acute biliary pancreatitis without concomitant acute cholangitis did not lead to a substantial reduction in the risk of overall complications and mortality.[48] However, approximately 10% of patients with severe biliary pancreatitis present with persistent occlusion of the ductal systems. Multiple studies and meta-analyses suggest that early ERCP and papillotomy benefits the course of the disease in this setting, leading to a substantial reduction in complications.[49,50] When there is high suspicion of persistent bile duct stones (i.e., jaundice, dilated bile duct) or evident choledocholithiasis on noninvasive imaging (US, CT, MRCP), ERCP should be performed within 72 hours. If a patient presents with concomitant cholangitis, ERCP should be performed within 24 hours.

Medical Approaches to Modulate the Severity of Acute Pancreatitis

Multiple agents have been investigated in hope they can prevent the development of severe AP. A noninclusive list includes probiotics, somatostatin analogs, antiproteases, drotrecogin alfa (Xigris), and lexipafant. Many of these agents modulate the severity of AP in animal models that typically administer the agent prior to the pancreatic insult; a timing scheme that cannot be duplicated clinically. However, clinical trials of these agents have failed to demonstrate benefit to placebo. In fact, lexipafant did not reduce ERCP-induced pancreatitis even when given prior to the procedure, and the use of probiotics has recently been found to be associated with worse outcomes. Thus, there are no current proven strategies/agents that prevent or reduce severe AP.

Late-Phase Interventions

Late-phase interventions are required when complications of AP occur, including infected pancreatic necrosis, hemorrhage, and pseudocyst or other fluid collection. Disruption of the pancreatic duct and persistent pancreatic fistula may also occur and are briefly addressed.

Infected Pancreatic Necrosis. Infectious complications of pancreatic necrosis usually occur 3–6 weeks after the onset of symptoms, and the mortality without surgical intervention can reach 100%. The reported mortality of infected necrosis with surgical management ranges between 15 and 28%.[51] The diagnosis of infected pancreatic necrosis is suspected by worsening abdominal pain, fever, and leukocytosis. The presence of gas within the pancreas by CT is considered highly suggestive of infected necrosis. Alternatively, infected necrosis can be confirmed by CT-guided fine needle aspiration.

Open surgical debridement and external drainage was once the predominant surgical approach to management of pancreatic necrosis in the United States. This typically included serial laparotomies to facilitate further debridement of evolving peripancreatic necrotic tissues. Unfortunately, this approach is associated with an approximately 20% enteric fistula rate and near-universal abdominal wall hernia. Given that several other less invasive techniques have been reported to successfully drain the infected pancreatic bed including percutaneous, laparoscopic, or retroperitoneal approaches with or without continuous lavage, many large-volume centers have abandoned this approach for an incremental treatment ladder, or step approach. This approach tries to delay or even avoid surgical intervention.

Delayed intervention has proven to reduce mortality to 27% [52] from 65% compared to early surgical intervention.[53] One of the advantages of delayed intervention is that the demarcation of necrotic tissues and subsequent liquefaction facilitates the use of nonsurgical approaches such as percutaneous or endoscopic drainage that can temporize or even prevent the need for surgery. In fact, endoscopic techniques of pancreatic drainage via transgastric or transduodenal approaches that eliminate the risk of persistent pancreaticocutaneous fistula are becoming increasingly common in carefully selected patients. Percutaneous necrosectomy has also been described in small series of patients in this setting with good clinical success, but typically require repeated drainage or procedures to upsize the catheters.[54,55] Reported failure rates for this approach are highly variable (31%-87%). Nonetheless, should these approaches fail, they do not typically complicate subsequent surgical intervention.

Minimally invasive pancreatic debridement and external drainage have been reported with encouraging results. A retroperitoneal approach to debridement and drainage of infected pancreatic necrosis was initially described by Gambiez *et al.* in a series of 20 patients with clinical success in 75% of patients, but a transperitoneal laparoscopic approach mimicking the traditional open procedure with either retrocolic or antecolic access of the lesser sac is the most commonly reported. A combined approach of percutaneous drainage followed by use of these catheters to guide laparoscopic trochars into the cavity and then perform an intracavitary, laparoscopic debridement has been successfully employed at our institution. Other authors have described various alternatives and combined percutaneous techniques with retroperitoneal approaches. Thus, there are multiple approaches to the management of infected pancreatic necrosis, but no studies have prospectively compared them. The favored approach continues to be driven by institutional experience and expertise.

Pancreatic Pseudocyst and Peripancreatic Fluid Collections. Extravasation of pancreatic secretions from ductal structures into the parenchyma or surrounding structures resulting in pseudocyst or persistent peripancreatic fluid collection(s) complicates approximately one-third of severe AP cases. Such collections of either pancreatic juice or transudate range dramatically in size, location, and clinical significance. In half of these patients, multiple collections are present. Pseudocysts typically expand over the first week following the onset of symptoms, and then evolve over the ensuing 4–12 weeks, although this process can be further prolonged in some patients (Fig. 38.4). Once contained by anatomic planes, the ensuing inflammatory response eventually produces a fibrous capsule that lacks an epithelial lining. As above, the evolution of these collections over time also includes liquefaction of particulate and necrotic material. Intervention should be delayed until this process has matured. The likelihood of spontaneous resolution is related to the size, but not strongly enough to produce a clinically reliable rule relating size, location, and symptoms to the need for intervention. When present, these collections pose the risk of becoming infected, and often produce mass effect that leads to symptoms of pain, early satiety, nausea, or biliary obstruction.

Surgical management is reserved for the relief of symptoms or infection. The potential for pancreatic duct stricture or disruption must be considered as these conditions alter the

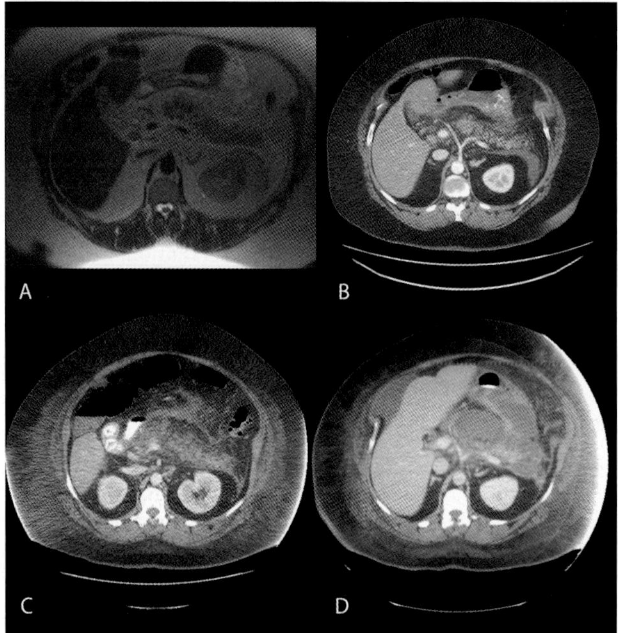

FIGURE 38.4 Evolution of pancreatitis. **A:** MRI of patient with acute pancreatitis 24 hours after the onset of symptoms demonstrates pancreatic edema without signs of necrosis. Gallstones and sludge were also identified, confirming the etiology. **B:** CT of the same patient obtained at 48 hours. **C:** CT of the same patient 1 week after presentation demonstrates areas of necrosis. **D:** CT of the same patient 3 weeks after presentation demonstrates the development of peripancreatic fluid collections.

surgical procedure of choice. MRCP is preferred over ERCP given the potential of infecting a previously sterile collection with ERCP. If a pancreatic duct stricture or disruption is identified, distal pancreatectomy rather than enteric drainage is typically indicated. However, in select circumstances, ERCP and placement of a pancreatic stent may subsequently be appropriate, but must be performed as part of a collaborative plan that is prepared to address subsequent infection or treatment failure.

In the majority of cases, enteric drainage is the surgical treatment of choice. The size, location, and complexity of the pseudocyst determine whether cyst gastrostomy or cyst Roux-En-Y is performed. Minimally invasive and endoscopic approaches for both of these procedures have been reported with similar success compared to open techniques. Biopsy of the pseudocyst wall is indicated for intraoperative assessment of an epithelial lining suggestive of a neoplastic rather than inflammatory process. Even with removal of debris and septations, and creation of a large communication between the collection and the intestine, most series report about a 20% failure rate with persistent fluid collection following the surgical procedure.

Hemorrhage

AP-associate hemorrhage is a rare but lethal complication. If pancreatic secretions are exposed to retroperitoneal structures due to necrosis or peripancreatic fluid collections, the potential for life-threatening hemorrhage exists. The hemorrhage can be retroperitoneal, intraperitoneal, or hemosuccus pancreaticus. When hemorrhage occurs, the splenic artery is the most frequently involved named vessel, followed by the gastroduodenal artery. Diagnostic and treatment modalities include endoscopy, angiography including embolization, and surgical exploration and ligation, and are dependent upon clinical scenario, expertise, and availability. Operative approaches include opening the causative fluid collection with control and ligation of the involved artery, packing if control cannot be obtained because the source is diffuse or venous, or distal pancreatectomy if warranted and technically feasible. The potential for hemorrhage is particularly significant when fluid is identified by CT to be tracking into the splenic hilum and under the capsule of the spleen, and most experts agree this is an indication for urgent surgical intervention of splenectomy, debridement, and external drainage.

References

1. Bradley EL III. A clinically based classification system for acute pancreatitis. Summary of the International Symposium on Acute Pancreatitis, Atlanta, GA, September 11 through 13, 1992. *Arch Surg*. 1993;128(5):586-590.
2. Vege SS. *GI Epidemiology*. Malden, MA: Blackwell Publishing; 2007.
3. Russo MW, Wei JT, Thiny MT, et al. Digestive and liver diseases statistics, 2004. *Gastroenterology*. 2004;126(5):1448-1453.
4. Everhart JE, Ruhl CE. Burden of digestive diseases in the United States Part III: liver, biliary tract, and pancreas. *Gastroenterology*. 2009;136(4):1134-1144.
5. Aliperti G. Complications related to diagnostic and therapeutic endoscopic retrograde cholangiopancreatography. *Gastrointest Endosc Clin N Am*. 1996;6(2):379-407.
6. Wang P, Li ZS, Liu F, et al. Risk factors for ERCP-related complications: a prospective multicenter study. *Am J Gastroenterol*. 2009;104(1):31-40.
7. Cappell MS. Acute pancreatitis: etiology, clinical presentation, diagnosis, and therapy. *Med Clin North Am*. 2008;92(4):889-923.
8. Hanck C, Singer MV. Does acute alcoholic pancreatitis exist without preexisting chronic pancreatitis? *Scand J Gastroenterol*. 1997;32(7):625-626.
9. Balani AR, Grendell JH. Drug-induced pancreatitis: incidence, management and prevention. *Drug Saf*. 2008;31(10):823-837.
10. Parenti DM, Steinberg W, Kang P. Infectious causes of acute pancreatitis. *Pancreas*. 1996;13(4):356-371.
11. Fink EN, Kant JA, Whitcomb DC. Genetic counseling for nonsyndromic pancreatitis. *Gastroenterol Clin North Am*. 2007;36(2):325-33, ix.
12. Waldthaler A, Schutte K, Malfertheiner P. Causes and mechanisms in acute pancreatitis. *Dig Dis*. 2010; 28(2):364-372.
13. Dickson AP, Imrie CW. The incidence and prognosis of body wall ecchymosis in acute pancreatitis. *Surg Gynecol Obstet*. 1984;159(4):343-347.
14. Banks PA, Freeman ML. Practice guidelines in acute pancreatitis. *Am J Gastroenterol*. 2006;101(10):2379-2400.
15. Agarwal N, Pitchumoni CS, Sivaprasad AV. Evaluating tests for acute pancreatitis. *Am J Gastroenterol* 1990;85(4):356-366.
16. Tenner S, Fernandez-del CC, Warshaw A, et al. Urinary trypsinogen activation peptide (TAP) predicts severity in patients with acute pancreatitis. *Int J Pancreatol*. 1997;21(2):105-110.
17. Maher MM, Lucey BC, Gervais DA, et al. Acute pancreatitis: the role of imaging and interventional radiology. *Cardiovasc Intervent Radiol*. 2004;27(3):208-225.
18. Koo BC, Chinogureyi A, Shaw AS. Imaging acute pancreatitis. *Br J Radiol*. 2010;83(986):104-112.
19. Balthazar EJ. Acute pancreatitis: assessment of severity with clinical and CT evaluation. *Radiology*. 2002;223(3):603-613.
20. Dervenis C, Johnson CD, Bassi C, et al. Diagnosis, objective assessment of severity, and management of acute pancreatitis. Santorini consensus conference. *Int J Pancreatol*. 1999;25(3):195-210.
21. Arvanitakis M, Koustiani G, Gantzarou A, et al.Staging of severity and prognosis of acute pancreatitis by computed tomography and magnetic resonance imaging-a comparative study. *Dig Liver Dis*. 2007;39(5):473-482.
22. Larvin M. Acute pancreatitis assesment of clinical ceverity and prognosis. In: *The Pancreas*. Oxford: Blackwell Science; 1998.
23. Balthazar EJ, Ranson JH, Naidich DP, et al. Acute pancreatitis: prognostic value of CT. *Radiology*. 1985;156(3):767-772.
24. Balthazar EJ, Robinson DL, Megibow AJ, et al. Acute pancreatitis: value of CT in establishing prognosis. *Radiology*. 1990;174(2):331-336.
25. Garg PK, Madan K, Pande GK, et al. Association of extent and infection of pancreatic necrosis with organ failure and death in acute necrotizing pancreatitis. *Clin Gastroenterol Hepatol*. 2005;3(2):159-166.
26. Balthazar EJ, Freeny PC, vanSonnenberg E. Imaging and intervention in acute pancreatitis. *Radiology*. 1994;193(2):297-306.
27. Mofidi R, Suttie SA, Patil PV, et al. The value of procalcitonin at predicting the severity of acute pancreatitis and development of infected pancreatic necrosis: systematic review. *Surgery*. 2009;146(1):72-81.
28. Olah A, Belagyi T, Issekutz A, et al. Value of procalcitonin quick test in the differentiation between sterile and infected forms of acute pancreatitis. *Hepatogastroenterology*. 2005;52(61):243-245.

29. Brown A, Baillargeon JD, Hughes MD, et al. Can fluid resuscitation prevent pancreatic necrosis in severe acute pancreatitis? *Pancreatology*. 2002;2(2):104-107.
30. Thompson DR. Narcotic analgesic effects on the sphincter of Oddi: a review of the data and therapeutic implications in treating pancreatitis. *Am J Gastroenterol*. 2001;96(4):1266-1272.
31. Ito K, Ito H, Whang EE. Timing of cholecystectomy for biliary pancreatitis: do the data support current guidelines? *J Gastrointest Surg*. 2008;12(12):2164-2170.
32. Taylor E, Wong C. The optimal timing of laparoscopic cholecystectomy in mild gallstone pancreatitis. *Am Surg*. 2004;70(11):971-975.
33. Rosing DK, De VC, Yaghoubian A, et al. Early cholecystectomy for mild to moderate gallstone pancreatitis shortens hospital stay. *J Am Coll Surg*. 2007;205(6):762-766.
34. Aboulian A, Chan T, Yaghoubian A, et al. Early cholecystectomy safely decreases hospital stay in patients with mild gallstone pancreatitis: a randomized prospective study. *Ann Surg*. 2010;251(4):615-619.
35. No Authors Listed. NIH state-of-the-science statement on endoscopic retrograde cholangiopancreatography (ERCP) for diagnosis and therapy. NIH state-of-the-science statements 19[1], 1-26. 1–14–2002. 1–14–2002.
36. Chen H, Li F, Sun JB, et al. Abdominal compartment syndrome in patients with severe acute pancreatitis in early stage. *World J Gastroenterol*. 2008;14(22):3541-3548.
37. Al-Bahrani AZ, Abid GH, Holt A, et al. Clinical relevance of intra-abdominal hypertension in patients with severe acute pancreatitis. *Pancreas*. 2008;36(1):39-43.
38. McClave SA, Chang WK, Dhaliwal R, et al. Nutrition support in acute pancreatitis: a systematic review of the literature. *J Parenter Enteral Nutr*. 2006;30(2):143-156.
39. Marik PE, Zaloga GP. Meta-analysis of parenteral nutrition versus enteral nutrition in patients with acute pancreatitis. *BMJ*. 2004; 328(7453):1407.
40. Petrov MS, Pylypchuk RD, Emelyanov NV. Systematic review: nutritional support in acute pancreatitis. *Aliment Pharmacol Ther*. 2008;28(6):704-712.
41. Villatoro E, Bassi C, Larvin M. Antibiotic therapy for prophylaxis against infection of pancreatic necrosis in acute pancreatitis. *Cochrane Database Syst Rev*. 2006;(4):CD002941.
42. Isenmann R, Runzi M, Kron M, et al. Prophylactic antibiotic treatment in patients with predicted severe acute pancreatitis: a placebo-controlled, double-blind trial. *Gastroenterology*. 2004;126(4):997-1004.
43. Sharma VK, Howden CW. Prophylactic antibiotic administration reduces sepsis and mortality in acute necrotizing pancreatitis: a meta-analysis. *Pancreas*. 2001;22(1):28-31.
44. Dellinger EP, Tellado JM, Soto NE, et al. Early antibiotic treatment for severe acute necrotizing pancreatitis: a randomized, double-blind, placebo-controlled study. *Ann Surg*. 2007;245(5):674-683.
45. Xue P, Deng LH, Zhang ZD, et al. Effect of antibiotic prophylaxis on acute necrotizing pancreatitis: results of a randomized controlled trial. *J Gastroenterol Hepatol*. 2009;24(5):736-742.
46. Garcia-Barrasa A, Borobia FG, Pallares R, et al. A double-blind, placebo-controlled trial of ciprofloxacin prophylaxis in patients with acute necrotizing pancreatitis. *J Gastrointest Surg*. 2009;13(4):768-774.
47. Villatoro E, Mulla M, Larvin M. Antibiotic therapy for prophylaxis against infection of pancreatic necrosis in acute pancreatitis. *Cochrane Database Syst Rev*. 2010;(5):CD002941.
48. Petrov MS, van Santvoort HC, Besselink MG, et al. Early endoscopic retrograde cholangiopancreatography versus conservative management in acute biliary pancreatitis without cholangitis: a meta-analysis of randomized trials. *Ann Surg*. 2008;247(2):250-257.
49. Ayub K, Imada R, Slavin J. Endoscopic retrograde cholangiopancreatography in gallstone-associated acute pancreatitis. *Cochrane Database Syst Rev*. 2004;(4):CD003630.
50. Heinrich S, Schafer M, Rousson V, et al. Evidence-based treatment of acute pancreatitis: a look at established paradigms. *Ann Surg*. 2006; 243(2):154-168.
51. Tonsi AF, Bacchion M, Crippa S, et al. Acute pancreatitis at the beginning of the 21st century: the state of the art. *World J Gastroenterol*. 2009;15(24):2945-2959.
52. Mier J, Leon EL, Castillo A, et al. Early versus late necrosectomy in severe necrotizing pancreatitis. *Am J Surg*. 1997;173(2):71-75.
53. Kivilaakso E, Fraki O, Nikki P, et al. Resection of the pancreas for acute fulminant pancreatitis. *Surg Gynecol Obstet*. 1981;152(4):493-498.
54. Echenique AM, Sleeman D, Yrizarry J, et al. Percutaneous catheter-directed debridement of infected pancreatic necrosis: results in 20 patients. *J Vasc Interv Radiol*. 1998;9(4):565-571.
55. Gmeinwieser J, Holstege A, Zirngibl H, et al. Successful percutaneous treatment of infected necrosis of the body of the pancreas associated with segmental disruption of the main pancreatic duct. *Gastrointest Endosc*. 2000;52(3):413-415.

CHAPTER 39 ■ CHOLECYSTITIS, CHOLANGITIS, AND JAUNDICE

UMUT SARPEL AND H. LEON PACHTER

Disorders of the biliary tract often demand the attention of the acute care surgeon. These disorders can run the gamut from the benign attack of biliary colic, to the rapidly fatal entity—suppurative cholangitis. However, attention to key features in the history and physical exam, when coupled with the appropriate labs and imaging tests, allows an accurate diagnosis and treatment plan in most instances.

ANATOMY

Simplistically, the biliary system can be thought of as the plumbing of the liver, providing drainage of bile into the intestines. Most surgical disorders of the biliary tract are secondary to an obstruction along this drainage tract. As such, the diagnosis and treatment of biliary disorders requires a thorough understanding of biliary anatomy.

Biliary Anatomy

The intrahepatic bile ducts course alongside their arterial and portal venous counterparts to form the portal triads of the liver parenchyma. These ducts coalesce into the right and left hepatic ducts. The caudate lobe has its own system of small ducts which drain directly into both the right and left main ducts. As the right and left hepatic ducts exit the liver, they remain sheathed in Glisson's capsule, hiding them from direct view. The right duct has a short course outside the liver, whereas the left duct has a long extrahepatic course as it travels along the undersurface of the left lobe to the hilum. The point of biliary convergence into the main hepatic duct is variable; in some individuals the bifurcation is well outside the liver, while in others it is practically intraparenchymal.

The gallbladder is nestled along the undersurface of the liver at the junction of the right and left lobes. It is separated from the liver parenchyma by the cystic plate, which is a continuation of Glisson's capsule. A common mistake during cholecystectomy is to dissect the gallbladder en bloc with the cystic plate off the liver bed, which leads to unnecessary bleeding. The true plane for cholecystectomy is found close to gallbladder wall, leaving the whitish cystic plate intact on the liver.

The cystic duct empties into the common hepatic duct, forming the common bile duct (CBD). The length of the cystic duct may be short, or it may run along the hepatic duct for some distance before joining it. This anatomical variability is of paramount significance during cholecystectomy when extreme care should be taken to avoid inadvertent injury to the CBD while ligating the cystic duct.

The main bile duct runs vertically in the hilum, anterior to the portal vein and lateral to the hepatic artery. The normal diameter of the CBD is approximately 5 mm, although it can be slightly wider in the elderly.[1] A useful rule of thumb is that the diameter of the bile duct increases 1 mm for every decade of life. While an 8 mm CBD could be a normal finding in an 80-year-old, it should be considered dilated in an otherwise healthy 30-year-old. The cystic duct usually measures 3 mm in diameter. Thus, any difficulty in ligation of the cystic duct with a 5-mm clip applier should be a red flag to the surgeon that the structure in question may in fact be the CBD.

When dealing with the biliary tree, anatomical variations are common and unpredictable. If appropriate vigilance is not exercised, an elective cholecystectomy can become a disaster with injury to the bile ducts, arteries or both. It cannot be stressed enough that the possibility of anomalies in biliary anatomy must be foremost in the mind of any surgeon performing a hepatobiliary procedure. Moreover, awareness of these variations is essential for the proper interpretation of an intraoperative cholangiogram.

A relatively common and potentially critical variation is the low-inserting posterior sectoral duct. In most individuals, this duct, which drains segments VI and VII of the liver, joins the anterior sectoral duct to form the right hepatic duct. However, in some individuals, this duct travels independently to enter the common hepatic duct, the cystic duct, or even the CBD as a separate structure. This low-inserting posterior duct may be injured during cholecystectomy leading to a persistent bile leak or atrophy of intrahepatic liver segments.

Arterial Anatomy

In most instances, the hepatic artery arises from the celiac trunk. However, the right hepatic artery (or even the entire hepatic) may originate from the superior mesenteric artery. In these cases, the hepatic artery will lie posterior to the CBD for its entire length. As a result, the cystic artery's position within Calot's triangle will be altered, which may lead to confusion during cholecystectomy.

Another common variant is the accessory left hepatic artery. Instead of arising from the common hepatic artery, this vessel arises from the left gastric artery. In most cases, this is actually an accessory artery which supplies segments II and III, while a smaller branch off the common hepatic still supplies segment IV.

After the hepatic artery bifurcates, the right hepatic artery dives behind the CBD where is becomes vulnerable to injury during cholecystectomy. The right hepatic artery sometimes curves near the cystic duct in its course towards the liver; this has been termed "Moynihans' hump."[2,3] In these cases, the cystic artery is short, and attention must be paid to avoid either injury to the right hepatic artery or ligation when mistaken for the cystic artery. Anterior and posterior branches of the cystic artery are often identifiable; these can originate from the main cystic artery or may arise independently from the right hepatic artery.

When an injury to the CBD occurs in the course of a cholecystectomy, it is often a paired injury; that is, the common duct is mistaken for the cystic duct and as part of the illusion and the right hepatic artery is mistaken for the cystic artery. Therefore, in all cases of iatrogenic bile duct injury, it is important to investigate the patency of the right hepatic artery.[4,5]

Venous Anatomy

The venous drainage from the gallbladder is directly into the liver parenchyma. Variations in hepatic venous and portal venous anatomy are common, but rarely clinically relevant to the acute care surgeon. However, special mention of the anatomy of the middle hepatic vein is warranted. The course of the middle hepatic vein within the hepatic parenchyma becomes quite superficial as it nears the gallbladder fossa. The vein can be injured during cholecystectomy if the surgeon veers off the correct plane and violates the liver parenchyma. Dark venous blood quickly fills the field, and can turn an ambulatory case into one with major blood loss. Direct pressure applied to the liver bed usually allows temporary hemostasis while assistance is en route. Depending upon the degree of injury, definitive control can be obtained with either argon beam coagulation, clipping, or with a parenchymal suture.

PHYSIOLOGY

Hepatocytes import unconjugated bilirubin from the plasma and conjugate it with glucuronic acid to make it water soluble. Conjugated bilirubin is then excreted into the bile canaliculi, and is eventually emptied into the duodenum. Through this process, approximately 1 L of bile is produced per day.[6] The function of bile is (1) to deliver bile salts to the intestines to aid in digestion of fats, (2) to excrete bilirubin, which is an oxidative product of heme, resulting from the destruction of senescent red blood cells, and (3) to excrete toxins.

Jaundice is the physical manifestation of hyperbilirubinemia, and usually becomes noticeable when the bilirubin level exceeds 3 mg/dL. Jaundice can result from an aberration anywhere along the process from bile production through excretion. The etiology of jaundice can be determined by whether the hyperbilirubinemia is predominantly unconjugated or conjugated. Unconjugated hyperbilirubinemia is seen with overproduction of bilirubin, impaired uptake of bilirubin, or impaired conjugation of bilirubin. Conjugated hyperbilirubinemia is seen with impaired excretion or obstruction of the biliary tree.

A conjugated hyperbilirubinemia can also be seen in cholestasis. In this clinical scenario, the ratio of total to direct bilirubins will mimic an obstructive pattern, although no downstream obstruction is present and biliary dilatation will accordingly be absent. Any systemic inflammatory process can affect bile secretion and result in cholestatic jaundice. This is often the case in the chronically ill or septic intensive care unit (ICU) patient whose labs demonstrate direct hyperbilirubinemia and otherwise unimpressive liver function studies. This cholestatic jaundice may be profound and will not resolve until the underlying process is controlled.

Surgical emergencies of the biliary system are usually due to acute obstruction of the biliary tree. Obstructive jaundice has several physiologic consequences which have relevance to surgeons, including aberrations in cardiac output, coagulation, renal function, wound healing, and the immune system. These issues should be considered for any jaundiced patient on the surgical service.

Cardiac Physiology

Obstruction of the biliary system can cause hemodynamic disturbances including decreased peripheral vascular resistance and depressed cardiac contractility.[7,8] Jaundiced patients display more labile blood pressure and are more susceptible to shock. Obstructed patients who undergo biliary decompression can become acutely hypotensive. It is unclear if this is due to cardiac lability, or secondary to instrumentation-induced bacteremia.

Coagulation

In patients with obstructive jaundice, impaired vitamin K absorption from the gut occurs due to a lack of intestinal bile, and is evidenced by a prolonged prothrombin time.[9] The effect is reversible with parenteral administration of vitamin K. There is little risk to vitamin K administration, therefore any jaundiced patient undergoing an operation should receive preoperative supplementation.

Renal

The decreased cardiac function associated with jaundice leads to renal hypoperfusion and acute renal failure. Hepatorenal syndrome is well-known in advanced cirrhotics, but renal insufficiency can also occur in patients with obstructive jaundice. When undergoing surgery, special attention needs to be paid to maintenance of intravascular volume. The mortality rate of patients with obstructive jaundice who develop renal failure is close to 70%.[10]

Wound Healing

Delayed wound healing and a high incidence of wound dehiscence have been reported in patients undergoing surgery to relieve obstructive jaundice. This may be related to decreased activity of the enzyme prolyl hyrdoxylase, which is required for normal collagen synthesis, in the skin of jaundiced patients. Levels of this enzyme return to normal following relief of the obstruction.[11] Accordingly, meticulous wound closure technique must be used in this group of patients.

Immune System

Jaundiced patients have numerous defects in cellular immunity which make them prone to infection; including impaired T-cell proliferation, decreased neutrophil chemotaxis, and defective phagocytosis.[12–14] In addition, bacterial translocation from the gut is increased when bile is absent the intestinal lumen. Jaundiced patients should be considered immunocompromised.

IMAGING OF THE BILIARY TREE

Ultrasound

Ultrasound is inexpensive, fast, and noninvasive making it the ideal method for visualization of the gallbladder and intrahepatic bile ducts. Views of the more distal CBD are usually obscured by overlying bowel gas and cannot be adequately examined by ultrasound. In addition, it is of limited use in obese patients and in cirrhotics because of the poor image quality caused by these conditions. Lastly, it is important to keep in mind that sonography is highly user-dependent, and thus only as reliable as the skill of the user.

Stones and sludge in the gallbladder are hyperechoic and cast an acoustic shadow. The sensitivity of ultrasound in the detection of stones is high, and the lack of stones on an ultrasound should bring into question the diagnosis of biliary colic or cholecystitis in an otherwise healthy patient.

Sonographic findings suggestive of acute cholecystitis are: (1) the presence of stones or sludge, (2) gallbladder wall thickening >4 mm, (3) pericholecystic fluid, and (4) a sonographic Murphy's sign, or tenderness elicited when the sonographer presses the ultrasound probe onto the visualized gallbladder.

When making a diagnosis of cholecystitis, it is important to note that bilirubin levels should be normal and on imaging the CBD should be of normal size. If jaundice or a dilated CBD is seen in a patient with abdominal pain, cholangitis must be suspected instead. Rarely, a markedly edematous gallbladder or a large stone impacted within the gallbladder can cause external compression of the CBD; a process known as Mirizzi's syndrome. In this case, intrahepatic biliary dilatation may be seen on ultrasound; however the CBD distal to the gallbladder (downstream from the obstruction) should not be dilated.

Computed Tomography

Computed tomography (CT) is not the initial test of choice for evaluation of the biliary system since approximately one-third of stones are not dense enough to be seen on CT.[15] In addition, the cost and radiation exposure make CT undesirable as first-line imaging. Nevertheless, in reality, CT is often the first test performed on patients with abdominal pain.

In acute cholecystitis, CT will demonstrate a thickened gallbladder; streaking and edema may be present in the pericholecystic fat. However, the CT appearance of the gallbladder can be misleading: the gallbladder may become slightly thick-walled due to other intraabdominal processes (e.g., ascites) which can mislead the clinician. Alternatively, the CT appearance of the gallbladder may be underwhelming even in genuine cases of acute cholecystitis. The absence of stones on CT scan should never be used in clinical decision making, since stones may be missed on CT.

Despite its limitations in stone-related disease, CT is well-suited to identify tumors and other non-stone sources of obstruction of the biliary tree. CT is also useful in patients with postoperative complications, since it can demonstrate the presence of a bile collection (biloma), hematoma, or vascular injury. When present, pneumobilia is easily seen with CT. While this is a normal finding following biliary enteric bypass or sphincterotomy, in patients who have not been instrumented, pneumobilia may indicate the presence of a biliary enteric fistula or may be a manifestation of suppurative cholangitis.

Scintigraphy

Hepatobiliary scintigraphy involves the intravenous injection of a radiopharmaceutical tracer (e.g., technetium-iminodiacetic acid compound) which is taken up by the liver and excreted into the bile. Sequential images show activity in the liver, then in the bile ducts and gallbladder, and eventually in the small bowel. The gallbladder is seen within 30 minutes, and the intestines within 60 minutes in most subjects. Nonvisualization of the gallbladder implies obstruction of the cystic duct and, in the appropriate clinical setting, confirms the presence of cholecystitis. Scintigraphy is the most accurate test for acute cholecystitis and sensitivity rates exceed 95%.[16] Specificity rates are also high, but false positives can be seen during prolonged fasting, and when acute pancreatitis hypoalbuminemia is present. Scintigraphy can be a useful tool for the confirmation of biliary tract pathology in patients where the clinical picture is unclear. It is particularly useful to confirm *acalculous cholecystitis*, where ultrasound findings may be equivocal.

Cholangiography

Direct cholangiography can be obtained by injection of contrast (1) percutaneously through the liver, (2) retrograde via the ampulla during endoscopic retrograde cholangiopancreatography (ERCP), or (3) directly into the biliary tree during surgery. Cholangiography provides the highest resolution imaging of biliary anatomy. The technique of intraoperative cholangiography is discussed later. Noninvasive imaging of the biliary tree can be obtained by magnetic resonance cholangiopancreatography (MRCP). However, unlike ERCP, MRCP does not provide the opportunity for a concomitant therapeutic component.

DISORDERS OF THE GALLBLADDER

Surgical pathology of the biliary tree usually results from physical obstruction of bile drainage; most often due to stones. Treatment depends upon the site of obstruction and whether there is concomitant infection.

Asymptomatic Cholelithiasis

Bile is maintained in a liquid state by the delicate balance of bile salts, lecithin, and cholesterol. Cholelithiasis results when these factors become unbalanced. The vast majority of gallstones are cholesterol stones which form in the gallbladder. Pigment stones, which form secondary to hemolysis, are fairly unusual. Results from autopsy studies and ultrasound screening studies suggest that cholelithiasis is present in 10%-20% of the population. Surveillance of individuals with known gallstones suggests that only 15% of patients ever develop symptoms.[17,18] Gallstones are often detected incidentally on an ultrasound or CT obtained for other reasons. These asymptomatic stones do not require any surveillance or surgical follow-up.

Biliary Colic

Gallstones may intermittently obstruct the cystic duct, causing pain known as biliary colic. This term is actually a misnomer, since within each attack the pain is constant, not colicky. When the cystic duct is obstructed, the patient usually experiences right upper-quadrant or epigastric pain that typically lasts for 4–6 hours. The pain may radiate to the back, shoulder or the subscapular area. Nausea is usually present, and vomiting may occur, but is not the dominant symptom. Classically, the pain starts after a fatty meal, due to cholecystokinin release. The resulting contraction of the gallbladder against an obstructed cystic duct causes intense pain. The pain often subsides without treatment when the offending stone slips back into the gallbladder, thereby resolving the obstruction.

Some patients with biliary colic will develop intractable pain with a crescendo of symptoms. These patients may experience symptoms with nearly every meal and often present with documented weight loss or dehydration. Cholecystectomy should be performed expeditiously in these cases.

It is important to note that in biliary colic, while obstruction of the cystic duct is present, infection is not. Accordingly, the treatment is does not require antibiotics, only bowel rest with IV hydration, pain control, and elective cholecystectomy. Once infection develops, right upper-quadrant tenderness, leukocytosis and fever invariably follow. With these findings, biliary colic has now evolved into acute cholecystitis. Careful physical examination and the use of ultrasonography will usually distinguish between these two entities.

Acute Cholecystitis

Acute cholecystitis occurs when obstruction of the cystic duct is accompanied by infection of the bile and gallbladder. These patients will present with complaints of pain and nausea similar to biliary colic; however the pain of cholecystitis will persist for 1–2 days if left untreated. On physical examination, right upper quadrant tenderness will be present due to inflammation of the gallbladder. A classic Murphy's sign describes the focal gallbladder tenderness that is elicited when, upon taking a deep breath, the patient abruptly halts inspiration due to the sudden pain that occurs when the descending gallbladder hits the examiner's hand, which is pressed into the right subcostal margin. Fever and mild leukocytosis are typically present, consistent with infection. Liver function tests should be normal, except in rare cases of Mirizzi's syndrome described below.

The treatment of acute cholecystitis generally consists of antibiotics, bowel rest with IV hydration, pain control, and cholecystectomy. Common biliary pathogens are the enteric gram-negative organisms including *Escherichia coli* and *Klebsiella*.[19] Bile is normally sterile; the sphincter of Oddi prevents enteric bacteria from entering the biliary system, and the flow of bile helps prevent infection with its mechanical flushing action. However, when cystic duct obstruction occurs, as in cholecystitis, stasis of bile within the gallbladder allows bacterial proliferation and infection.

The definitive treatment of cholecystitis is cholecystectomy. In the past, delayed cholecystectomy was advocated as safer than cholecystectomy performed during the acute inflammatory phase. However, a meta-analysis of 12 prospective, randomized trials showed that prompt cholecystectomy does not result in higher rates of CBD injury, and actually results in substantially lower length of stay and decreased hospital costs.[20,21] Therefore, unless there are medical contraindications, early cholecystectomy should be performed.

Variations of Cholecystitis

Routine cholecystitis is relatively straightforward in its diagnosis and treatment. However, certain types of cholecystitis can be more challenging to identify and manage.

Mirizzi's Syndrome

Mirizzi's syndrome, occurs when an inflamed gallbladder causes external compression of the CBD, thereby leading to obstructive jaundice (Fig. 39.1).[22] The compression may be due to an enlarged and inflamed gallbladder, or from a large stone impacted in the gallbladder neck. Mirizzi's syndrome is rare, one study states that it occurs in approximately 0.1% of patients with gallstone disease[23]; therefore, Mirizzi's syndrome is diagnosis of exclusion. Direct hyperbilirubinemia should never be attributed to Mirizzi's syndrome unless other causes of obstructive jaundice have been excluded, since the consequences of a missed cholangitis can be severe.

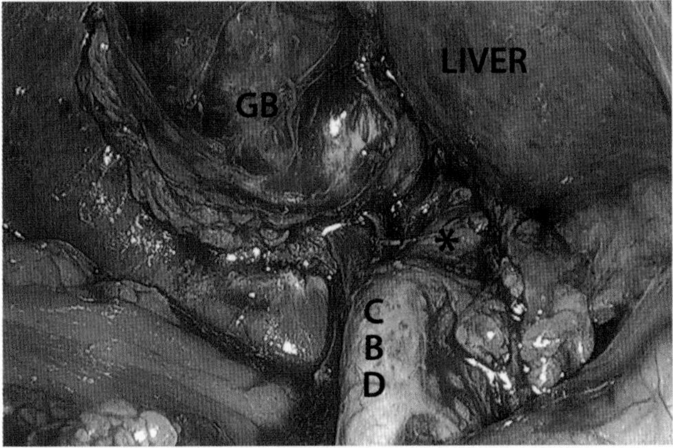

FIGURE 39.1. Mirizzi's syndrome. *Asterisk* marks area of CBD compression by the infundibulum of the gallbladder.

Acalculous Cholecystitis

Acalculous cholecystitis occurs almost exclusively in patients with severe comorbidities, and is classically seen in hospitalized patients who are septic, receiving parenteral nutrition, on vasopressors, or who have suffered major trauma or burns. The precise etiology of this entity is unknown, but theories include gallbladder ischemia and presence of inspissated bile.[24,25] Since the cystic artery is a small terminal vessel, global hypoperfusion is thought to result in gallbladder wall ischemia and eventually necrosis. The diagnosis of acalculous cholecystitis is challenging because, by definition, it occurs in patients who are ill, have confounding histories, and are usually unable to verbalize their symptoms. Acalculous cholecystitis is often found as the result of a CT done for fever of unknown origin in a patient in the ICU. Gangrene and perforation occur commonly, due to the frequent delay in diagnosis.

Often, ultrasound or CT show only a distended, mildly thickened gallbladder. Diagnosis can be difficult since gallbladder distension may simply be due to a prolonged NPO status with total parenteral nutrition, and not cholecystitis. Nuclear scintigraphy (e.g., HIDA scan) can be useful in unclear cases of acalculous cholecystitis. Since many patients with acalculous cholecystitis are quite ill, often immediate cholecystectomy is not possible or prudent. In this setting, imaging-guided percutaneous drainage of the gallbladder allows drainage of bile and release of the infection. This treatment is sufficient in most cases, less commonly a cholecystectomy may be required if tissue necrosis has set in. If the patient resolves the episode of acalculous cholecystitis with percutaneous cholecystostomy, cholecystectomy is seldom necessary at a later time.

Gangrenous Cholecystitis

Gangrenous cholecystitis occurs when infection and inflammation cause thrombosis of the cystic artery; this leads to ischemia and gangrene of the gallbladder wall, eventually resulting in liquefaction necrosis and perf oration of the gallbladder. Gangrene occurs first at fundus of the gallbladder because this is the most distant site from the blood supply of the cystic artery. In patients with free perforation, bile stained ascites may be present. Gangrenous cholecystitis is more common in diabetics due to their underlying small vessel disease.[26] Once gangrene has developed, a cholecystostomy tube will most likely be insufficient to halt the process. The problem that arises is ascertaining which patients can be managed with a tube cholecystostomy and which cannot. If the patient with acute or gangrenous cholecystitis has not improved within 24 hours of placement of the tube, it is possible that tissue necrosis is present, for which the patient should undergo urgent cholecystectomy. Other causes for the lack of response to cholecystostomy include malposition or dislodgement of the catheter or incorrect diagnosis of cholecystitis.

Emphysematous Cholecystitis

The imaging appearance of gas within the gallbladder wall is pathognomonic of emphysematous cholecystitis and indicates the presence of gas-forming bacteria such as clostridia species, *E. coli*, or *Klebsiella*.[27] The infection progresses in stages from the presence of gas in the gallbladder lumen, to within the gallbladder wall, and ultimately into pericholecystic tissues.[28] The presence of gas can obscure ultrasound imaging of the gallbladder, however the diagnosis is easily made with CT (Fig. 39.2). Emphysematous cholecystitis occurs more commonly in elderly or diabetic males, and is more frequently associated with acalculous cholecystitis.[29] Expeditious cholecystectomy is warranted if the patient will tolerate the operation.

Hydrops of the Gallbladder

The normal physiologic function of the gallbladder is to take up and store the bile excreted from the liver. In long-standing cases of cystic duct obstruction the bile within the gallbladder is slowly resorbed. Continuing secretion from the mucosa of the gallbladder results in its filling with a clear mucoid fluid termed "white bile". This is known as *hydrops* or a mucocele of the gallbladder. Typically, these patients have a distended gallbladder that cannot be grasped during laparoscopic cholecystectomy. The diagnosis is usually made when the surgeon aspirates the gallbladder to decompress it and clear mucous is returned.

Cholecystitis During Pregnancy

Cholecystitis is the second most common nongynecologic process to complicate pregnancy, following appendicitis.[30] Estrogen through its negative effect on smooth muscle activity is thought to be responsible for the increased rate of cholecystitis in women, and in pregnancy in particular. Although the pathophysiology of cholecystitis is the same as in the nonpregnant state, the natural hesitancy of clinicians to image and treat a pregnant patient can lead to a delay in diagnosis and intervention (see Chapter 44). This delay can be more harmful to the mother and fetus than cholecystitis itself. While straightforward attacks can be treated with antibiotics, recurrent cholecystitis can lead to maternal dehydration and malnutrition, with obvious deleterious effects to the fetus. In these cases, cholecystectomy may be necessary during pregnancy. If possible, the procedure should be performed during the second trimester; surgery during the first trimester is associated with increased fetal loss, and surgery during the third trimester may induce premature contractions. As a general rule, all attempts should be undertaken, if possible, to bring the patient to term and then perform an elective cholecystectomy. The approach is similar for biliary pancreatitis in pregnancy.

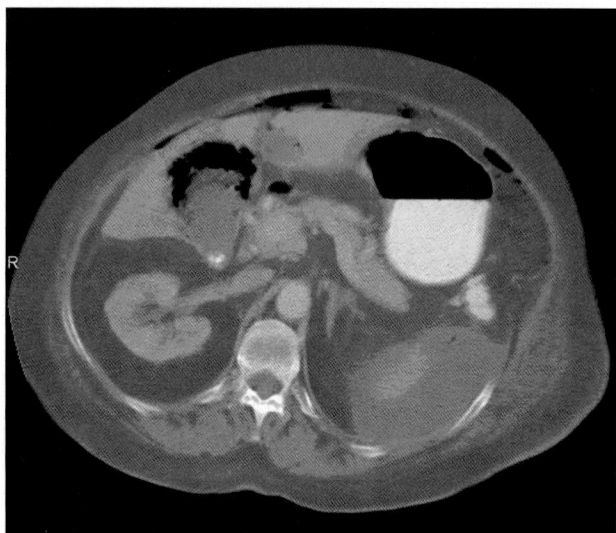

FIGURE 39.2. Emphysematous cholecystitis on CT.

Gallstone Ileus

Gallstone ileus is another misnomer of medical terminology. Whereas ileus implies the absence of mechanical obstruction, in gallstone ileus there is a physical obstruction of the GI tract by a gallstone. Long-standing, recurrent attacks of cholecystitis eventually lead to erosion of a gallstone through the gallbladder wall into a neighboring loop of bowel. Cholecystoduodenal fistulization is most common, but cholecystocolic fistulae may also develop. The fistula itself is asymptomatic; gallstone ileus occurs when the offending stone occludes the bowel lumen leading to obstruction. Classically, the gallstone erodes into the duodenum and travels to the narrowest point in the GI tract, the ileocecal valve, where it causes small bowel obstruction in the terminal ileum. An abdominal x-ray showing dilated loops of small bowel along with a pneumogram of the biliary tree is pathognomonic for gallstone ileus. At operation, an enterotomy is performed to remove the obstructing stone (Fig. 39.3). If possible, the stone should be milked proximally so that the enterotomy can be performed through normal, nondilated bowel, rather than at the site of obstruction which is typically edematous. A full examination of the small bowel is necessary to detect additional nonobstructing stones which may be present.[31] Once the patient recovers from surgery, elective cholecystectomy and the division of the cholecystoenteric fistula may be considered, but is usually unnecessary. Cholecystectomy should absolutely not be attempted during the acute presentation since the right upper quadrant is hostile due to the inflammation caused by the recent fistulization.[32,33] If later cholecystectomy is contemplated an open approach should be undertaken to minimize inadvertent injury to the CBD and to have maximal exposure for repair of the bowel fistula.

DISORDERS OF THE COMMON BILE DUCT

Choledocholithiasis

In studies where routine intraoperative cholangiography is performed, approximately 6% of asymptomatic patients are found to have incidental CBD stones.[34] However, unlike asymptomatic cholelithiasis, the discovery of asymptomatic choledocholithiasis should prompt intervention due to the potentially severe consequences of jaundice, gallstone pancreatitis, or cholangitis.

The presence of stones in the CBD should be suspected in any patient with:

- direct hyperbilirubinemia
- intrahepatic biliary dilatation seen on preoperative imaging
- dilated CBD seen on imaging or by intraoperative visualization
- history of gallstone pancreatitis, or with elevated amylase or lipase levels

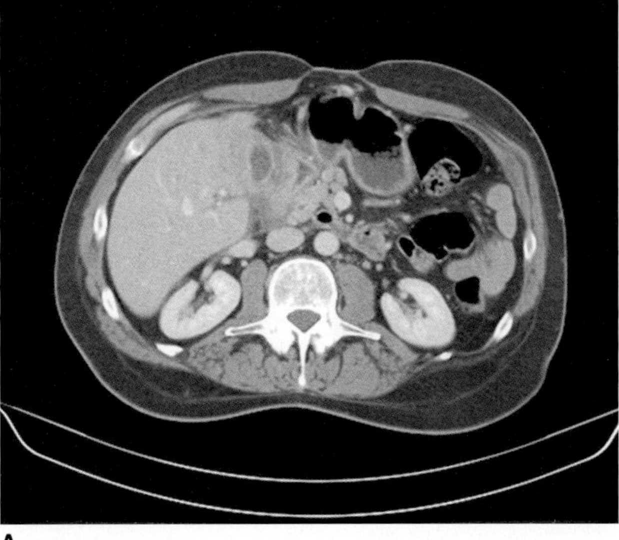

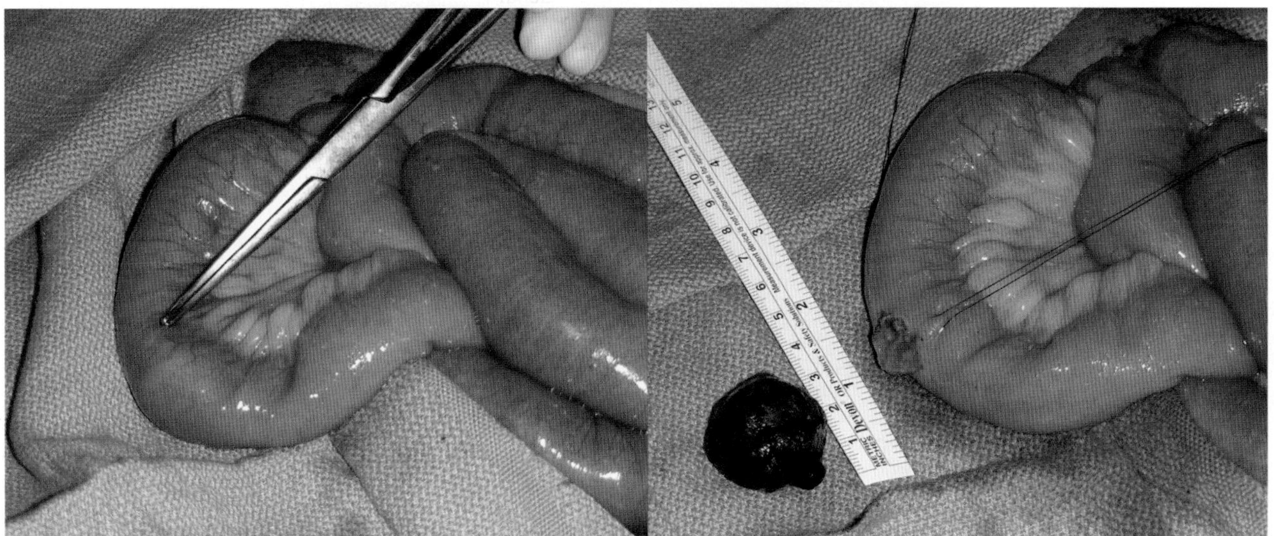

FIGURE 39.3. Gallstone ileus. **A:** CT showing Inflammation of the gallbladder and duodenum. **B:** Gallstone obstructing distal small bowel, after enterotomy with extraction of gallstone.

In these patients, the CBD must be imaged by either preoperative MRCP, ERCP, or by intraoperative cholangiography. at the time of cholecystectomy Preoperative ERCP is usually the method of choice, since it is therapeutic as well as diagnostic. In addition, if a preoperative ERCP is unsuccessful, a CBD exploration can then be performed at the time of cholecystectomy.

Cholangitis

Cholangitis occurs when the flow of bile from the liver is obstructed and the static column of bile proximal to the obstruction becomes infected. Cholangitis rarely ensues when the biliary obstruction occurs gradually over a period of time, as with tumors or strictures. Choledocholithiasis or the sudden clogging of a biliary stent is the usual etiology.

The presentation of cholangitis is described by *Charcot's Triad*: fever, jaundice, and right upper-quadrant pain. On examination, the liver is diffusely tender, as opposed to the focal gallbladder tenderness seen with cholecystitis. This finding can be elicited by palpation in the epigastrium where the liver is not shielded by the rib cage. *Reynaud's Pentad*, the addition of hypotension and mental status changes, heralds the onset of septic shock. Laboratory values demonstrate marked leukocytosis and direct hyperbilirubinemia, often accompanied by mildly elevated transaminases; which reflect the hepatotoxic effect of the infection. The predominance of conjugated bilirubin points to obstruction as the cause of the jaundice, as opposed to acute hepatitis.

Ultrasonography will typically reveal intrahepatic biliary dilatation and a dilated CBD due to downstream obstruction. However, due to the presence of overlying gas in the duodenum, the offending stone itself, which is lodged at the ampulla, will not be seen on sonography. The ultrasound can determine if there are stones in the gallbladder; if gallstones are present, the clinician can reasonably assume that the cause of the cholangitis is stones; although it is possible to have had a single gallstone, which traveled into the CBD, which then left the gallbladder empty, this is decidedly unusual.

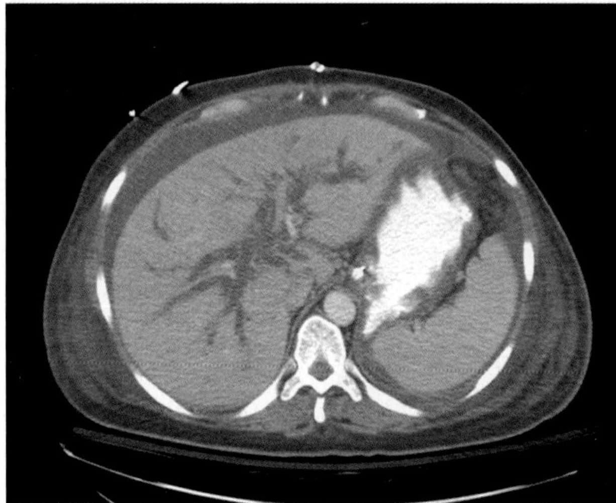

FIGURE 39.4. Intrahepatic biliary dilatation.

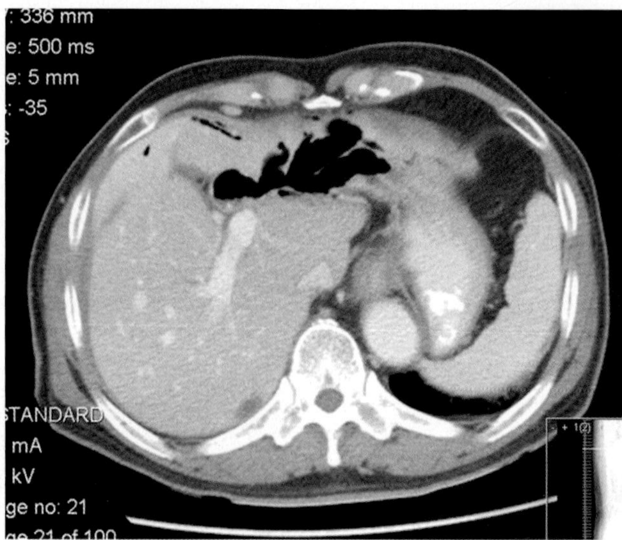

FIGURE 39.5. Recurrent pyogenic cholangitis due to chronic intrahepatic stone formation. Note the biliary dilatation, pneumobilia, and parenchymal atrophy of the left lobe, while the right hepatic lobe is spared. The left lobe is thought to be more commonly affected due to the sharper angle of insertion of the left duct into the CBD.

CT will also demonstrate biliary dilatation (Fig. 39.4), although ultrasound is the first imaging that should be obtained since many gallstones are not apparent on CT. It is important to point out that the CBD diameter may be normal during the early stages of cholangitis this finding can mislead the clinician. In the setting of sudden obstruction, it may take 24–48 hours for appreciable biliary dilatation to develop. Therefore, the absence of biliary dilatation on initial imaging studies should not exclude the diagnosis of obstructive cholangitis. If uncertainty exists, an MRI/MRCP can both identify the presence and location of stones, or reveal if a tumor or other process is responsible. Scintigraphy will demonstrate lack of bile flow into the small bowel, although the poor image resolution and logistic difficulties with arranging a HIDA scan make it less commonly used in the setting of cholangitis.

Bile in its natural state is golden-brown in color and does not contain bacteria. In contrast, infected bile becomes bright green secondary to bacterial metabolism of bilirubin. As the infection progresses further, the obstructed bile becomes purulent, and is known as suppurative cholangitis. The most common isolated pathogens are *E. coli*, *Klebsiella*, *Enterobacter*, and *Enterococci*; anaerobes are also present in a minority of cases.[19] Intravenous antibiotic therapy for cholangitis must provide excellent gram-negative coverage. Patients with long-standing biliary obstruction may also have *Pseudomonas* and *Candida* in their systems.

Antibiotic treatment for cholangitis is necessary but not sufficient for its treatment. It is critical to underscore that the urgently needed treatment for cholangitis is decompression.[35] This is especially true for suppurative cholangitis, where the mortality is 100% if not promptly drained. Similar to lancing an abscess, drainage is absolutely necessary; antibiotics alone are insufficient to treat the infection. Patients with an obstructed duct may develop post-decompression shock following CBD instrumentation.[36] It is not unusual for patients to become transiently bacteremic with fevers and rigors following decompression. A short duration of vasopressor support may be required in these cases. Once the acute cholangitis has resolved, cholecystectomy is indicated during the same admission to prevent further attacks.

Recurrent Pyogenic Cholangitis

This entity is characterized by repeated bouts of cholangitis as a result of stones and strictures in the intrahepatic bile ducts. The exact etiology of this disease is still unknown, although a causal relationship with *Chlonorchis sinensis* infection has been implicated.[39] While biliary strictures and intrahepatic stones are at the root of the disease, it remains unclear which is the initial event. Strictures lead to biliary stasis and stone formation, and alternately stones cause biliary strictures, thus resulting in a vicious cycle. Over the years, these patients develop progressively severe biliary dilatation and eventually atrophy of the involved hepatic segments. The left hepatic lobe is more commonly affected than the right lobe, perhaps due to the angle of insertion of the left duct into the CBD.[38] Over time, the involved liver atrophies into a thin, fibrotic parenchyma containing dilated bile cisterns packed with columns of stones (Fig. 39.5). In addition, years of irritation of the bile ducts can lead to malignant degeneration, resulting in cholangiocarcinoma.

Patients usually report multiple previous attacks of abdominal pain and frequently have already undergone cholecystectomy. However, since these stones form within the intrahepatic bile ducts, cholecystectomy is not curative, and the cholangitic attacks continue. ERCP is typically unsuccessful at biliary decompression since the affected bile ducts are usually packed with large stones. Percutaneous transhepatic biliary drainage is necessary if antibiotics are unsuccessful in treating the infection.

Once the acute cholangitis resolves, the patient needs to be evaluated for definitive treatment. Simple stone extraction or destruction with laser lithotripsy is not effective. Since the ducts themselves are abnormal and strictured, new stone formation and infection invariably occur. If anatomically feasible, the most definitive therapy is resection of the affected liver. Bile duct resection and hepaticojejunostomy are commonly required in complex cases.

LAPAROSCOPIC CHOLECYSTECTOMY

Identification of Anatomy

Laparoscopic cholecystectomy, when uncomplicated, results in little physiologic insult to the patient, and allows outpatient surgery or discharge home within 24 hours. The guiding principle of safe cholecystectomy is the clear identification of the gallbladder-cystic duct junction. The use of laparoscopic cholecystectomy allows much faster patient recovery, but has resulted in a higher rate of injury to the CBD (compared to open cholecystectomy) ranging from 0.3% to 0.6%.[39] The lower rate of injury in open surgery is likely due to the anterograde, or fundus-down, approach which allows definitive identification of the CBD before any structures are ligated. However, in laparoscopic cholecystectomy, initial dissection in the hepatocystic triangle can create visual ambiguity, leading to confusion of the CBD for the cystic duct.[40]

One method to assure correct anatomy is to always obtain the *critical view* before ligation of any structure. In this approach, the fat in the hepatocystic triangle is dissected away until the liver bed can be seen with only two structures traversing it; by definition these structures can only be the cystic duct and cystic artery (Fig. 39.6).[39]

Universal intraoperative cholangiography is another method to confirm correct anatomy. Advocates of universal intraoperative cholangiography point out that this method can also identify unsuspected CBD stones. Opponents state that the discovery of small asymptomatic stones, which would probably pass on their own, leads to transcystic duct exploration or the necessity of a postoperative ERCP, which have their own inherent risks and complications.

The Difficult Cholecystectomy

In patients with chronic cholecystitis, repeated attacks lead to fibrosis of the gallbladder and bile ducts, making identification of anatomy challenging. Interestingly, difficult cholecystectomy occurs more often in males than females,[41] perhaps because cholecystitis is less often suspected as the diagnosis in men. It is important for the general surgeon to have several different approaches to cholecystectomy in his/her armamentarium.

The "dome-down" anterograde technique of open surgery, whereby the gallbladder is taken off the liver bed from the fundus downward, can be used in laparoscopic surgery as well. This approach allows the surgeon to dissect down to the vital structures before ligating them. However, this method can be challenging since the liver retraction normally provided by the gallbladder is lost.

In severe cases of inflammation, when the cystohepatic triangle cannot be recognized or dissected, a subtotal or partial

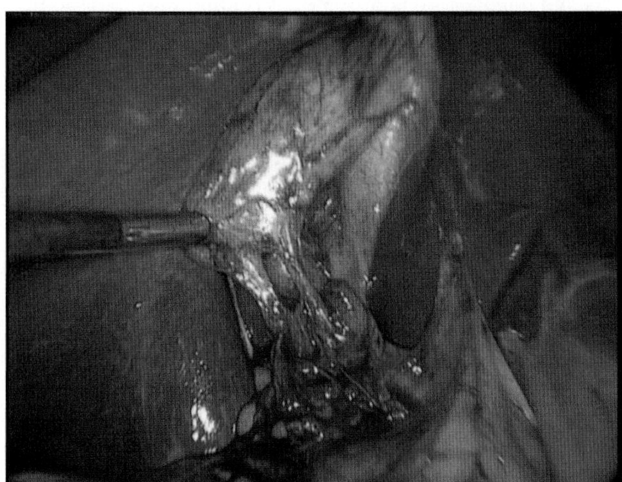

FIGURE 39.6. The critical view of safety for laparoscopic cholecystectomy. Note that only 2 structures are seen traversing the liver bed: the cystic duct and the cystic artery.

cholecystectomy may be the most prudent course of action. In this technique, the gallbladder is filleted open to the level of Hartmann's pouch and the anterior wall is excised. Any stones are removed, including any impacted in the neck of the gallbladder. The posterior wall of the gallbladder is left *in situ* and the mucosa is cauterized; a drain is left behind in the liver bed. Closure of the cystic duct is not needed and should not be attempted, since inadvertent injury to the CBD may result.

Spillage of stones is not uncommon during laparoscopic cholecystectomy. However, every reasonable attempt should be made to retrieve them since several long-term complications have been reported from retained stones. Frequently the stone acts as a nidus for infection, leading to the formation of an intraperitoneal abscess.[42] Less commonly, gallstones have been reported to fistulize into the bronchial tree, the bladder, and through the skin.[43,44]

Conversion from laparoscopic to open cholecystectomy is indicated in the setting of a difficult cholecystectomy. However, an open approach does not guarantee an easier operation. Clear identification of anatomy and strict adherence to surgical principles is necessary to avoid injury to the biliary tree.

For patients with severe comorbidity or those who are hemodynamically unstable, an ultrasound-guided, percutaneous cholecystostomy tube can be used to decompress an infected gallbladder.[45] Percutaneous cholecystostomy is especially useful in severely ill patients who develop acalculous cholecystitis. Once the acute infection has resolved, cholecystectomy can be performed. Alternatively, in patients who are poor operative candidates if contrast injected into the cholecystostomy tube shows flow into the CBD and duodenum, the cholecystostomy tube may be removed with no further intervention.

Intraoperative Cholangiography

Various techniques can be used to perform intraoperative cholangiography. Typically a clip is first applied high on the cystic duct at the level of the gallbladder. The anterolateral wall of the cystic duct is incised to create a small "ductotomy." The cystic duct can be gently milked to deliver any stones within. A cholangiography catheter is then introduced either percutaneously across the abdominal wall or via a cholangiography clamp, and is then guided into the ductotomy and secured in place. The smooth insertion of the catheter may be impeded by stones impacted in the cystic duct, or by the valves of Heister, the spiral mucosal folds of the cystic duct. Great care should be taken not to force the catheter into position; this can lead to an unrecognized injury to the back wall of the cystic duct, resulting in a bile leak postoperatively.

To be complete, cholangiography must demonstrate filling of bilateral hepatic ducts, the full length of the CBD, and flow into the duodenum. If the hepatic ducts do not fill, placing the patient in Trendelenburg position and administering morphine may be effective. Gentle compression of the CBD may also be needed in patients with dilated, compliant ducts to force dye to fill the proximal system. On the other hand, if the duodenum does not fill, the administration of glucagon to relax the sphincter of Oddi can be attempted. A filling defect may represent a stone, or may be a bubble of air inadvertently introduced into the tubing. Bubbles will tend to float into a different position if the table is tilted.

Common Bile Duct Exploration

The natural history of stones in the CBD is not certain, and has not been studied prospectively. Incidentally discovered small stones will likely pass into the duodenum without clinical impact. However, since cholangitis and gallstone pancreatitis are potentially lethal, it is generally advisable to remove CBD stones upon discovery. If suspected preoperatively, ERCP is the method of choice for clearing the CBD. However, if CBD stones are discovered during the course of cholecystectomy, the surgeon has the choice of an immediate laparoscopic CBD exploration or a postoperative ERCP.

Laparoscopic CBD exploration is a technically challenging procedure, particularly if the duct is normal sized. The surgical team and nursing staff need to be well-versed in the use of the choledochoscope and various methods of stone extraction. Open CBD exploration is now rarely necessary; however, it is a vital technique for all general surgeons to possess. A wide Kocher maneuver is necessary to be able to palpate the distal, retroduodenal CBD. A longitudinal, choledochotomy is made in the distal portion of the CBD, keeping in mind that the blood supply of the CBD is at 3 o'clock and 9 o'clock. The duct is held open with stay sutures on either side, and can then be atraumatically swept with a Fogarty's balloon or stone clamp.

Following laparoscopic or open CBD exploration, a T tube is left within the common duct. This allows egress of bile during the immediate postoperative period when distal ampullary edema or spasm may occur. In addition, the T tube allows access for postoperative cholangiography to assess for retained stones or bile leak. Stone extraction can be performed by interventional radiology via a 14 French T tube if the stones are ≤5 mm in size.[46]

Following CBD exploration, a biliary-enteric anastomosis may be needed, such as in patients with retained intrahepatic stones, or in those with a stone impacted at the ampulla. Patients in whom a large number of stones are retrieved should be presumed to have a retained stone even if none is seen, and bypass should be considered. Finally, any patient with multiple large should undergo biliary-enteric bypass, since ERCP can generally only retrieve stones < 1 cm in size. A side-to-side choledochoduodenostomy is the easiest type of bypass to perform, since the duodenum has already been mobilized and can usually be easily rolled upwards to meet the CBD.

Complications of Biliary Surgery

Complications from biliary surgery generally result from either bleeding from the hepatic parenchyma or injury to the biliary tree.

Hemorrhage

Bleeding during cholecystectomy can occur from (1) injury to the cystic or hepatic artery, (2) oozing from the hepatic parenchyma, or (3) laceration of the middle hepatic vein.

During laparoscopic dissection of the hepatocystic triangle, the cystic artery may be damaged or inadvertently transected before control is obtained. Typically, a fine-tipped instrument can be used to grasp the bleeding stump and a clip can be applied under direct vision. Under no circumstances should clips be placed blindly in this region. Although the brisk, pulsatile bleeding from the cystic artery stump can be visually impressive, gentle pressure will usually allow temporary hemostasis until the camera is cleaned and the instruments are prepared. It is important to ascertain whether the injured vessel is indeed the cystic artery. Injury to the right hepatic artery is not uncommon, and if suspected should prompt conversion to open surgery for close inspection and repair. Ligation of the hepatic artery generally does not cause any immediate ramifications since the hepatic parenchyma will continue to receive blood supply from the portal vein. However, since the bile ducts are fed predominantly by the hepatic artery, biliary strictures may occur over time.

During cholecystectomy, oozing from the liver bed commonly occurs from dissection in the wrong plane. When removing the gallbladder, the cystic plate, a whitish extension of Glisson's capsule, should be left intact on the liver bed. The correct plane is usually closer to the gallbladder than initially suspected; visualization of the yellow-brown hepatic parenchyma indicates that the dissection has gone too deep. A useful method to control bleeding from the liver bed is argon beam coagulation. Alternatively, electrocautery on a high setting can be used to paint the bleeding liver surface for hemostasis. Although not immediately hemodynamically significant, if this oozing is not controlled a hematoma in the liver bed can result. Postoperatively, this hematoma may become infected or cause compression of the bile duct.

Sudden, massive, dark-colored hemorrhage from the liver bed indicates laceration of the middle hepatic vein. This major vessel lies just below the bed of the gallbladder, and is vulnerable to injury during cholecystectomy.[47] Fortunately, the hepatic veins are a low pressure system, and direct compression of the site will tamponade the bleeding. Depending upon the degree of injury, definitive control can be obtained with either argon beam coagulation, clipping, or a parenchymal suture.

Bile Leak

Bile leak following cholecystectomy is discovered when bile is seen in a drain either left at surgery, or in one placed by interventional radiology upon discovery of a fluid collection. The source of the bile may be from (1) the liver bed, (2) the cystic duct stump, (3) the CBD, (4) a posterior sectoral duct, or (5) a duct of Luschka. The most important first step in the treatment of a bile leak is to ascertain whether the leak is controlled. The following step is to determine whether there is downstream obstruction; either from a retained stone or from iatrogenic injury.

Most cases of bile leak are from the cystic duct stump; these are typically low volume and well controlled by a drain. Patients with an uncontrolled bile leak despite drainage likely have a severe injury or transection of the CBD. Bile is extremely irritating to the peritoneum, and if the leak is uncontrolled, biliary peritonitis will result. Patients with an uncontrolled bile leak will have marked abdominal tenderness and manifest signs of sepsis. It is important to note, that even patients with severe bile leaks may have normal bilirubin levels since there is no obstruction to the flow of bile out of the liver. Once the sepsis is controlled, these patients must be reexplored by an experienced hepatobiliary surgeon. The irritation of the peritoneum caused by bile can make reexploration challenging, particularly if the bile leak was initially unrecognized and drainage delayed.

On the other hand, if the bile leak is well-controlled by a drain, the patient will be asymptomatic with normal hemodynamic parameters. A minor bile leak from the gallbladder bed will result in trace amounts of bile within the drain which resolves within 1–2 days without intervention. However, the patient with more substantial amounts of bile in the drain, or with abdominal pain, should be evaluated with ERCP. The most common site of bile leak is from the cystic duct stump,[48] either due to a dislodged clip or due to increased pressure caused by a retained stone downstream. Injection of contrast during ERCP can demonstrate the source of the bile leak, confirm that extravasation is controlled by the drain, and exclude distal obstruction as the cause of the leak. In addition, sphincterotomy and insertion of a biliary stent can be performed to change the pressure gradient, allowing flow of bile out of the ampulla rather than through the site of injury. Typically, the bile leak will resolve immediately following ERCP and the patient can be safely discharged.

While a bile leak which originates from the cystic duct or the CBD will be clearly seen on ERCP, other sources of leak may not be visualized. For example, if the leak is from a transected posterior sectoral duct, the liver side may continue to leak bile and no leak of contrast will be apparent from the biliary stump. In this case however, close inspection of the cholangiogram will reveal failure of the posterior right sector to fill with contrast, indicating the true diagnosis. Similarly, a duct of Luschka may not retain a connection to the main biliary tree, and therefore may not be seen on ERCP.[48] These etiologies should be suspected when there is bile in the drain, but the ERCP is nondiagnostic. Minor bile leaks will resolve over time, although several weeks of drainage may be required. However, a leak from transected posterior sectoral duct may persist and reoperation may be necessary.

Injury to the Common Bile Duct

While injury to the CBD is a serious complication, the sequelae of the injury can be greatly diminished if the injury is recognized at the time of surgery. During cholecystectomy, the surgeon must always be attentive to possible anatomical variations, and should maintain a degree of suspicion even in apparently straight-forward cases. Unclear anatomy can create an optical illusion where the surgeon mistakes one structure for another.

During cholecystectomy, the cystic duct and the cystic artery must be clearly identified before any structure is ligated. If there is any doubt as to the anatomy at hand, a cholangiogram should be performed, or the case should be converted to open. If bile is seen leaking into the operative field, the anatomy must be reexamined and a cholangiogram performed. If an unexpected ductal structure is encountered while taking the gallbladder off the liver bed, this should alert the surgeon that a biliary injury may have already occurred, as often the second structure is the cystic duct and the initially ligated structure is the CBD. In short, every attempt should be made to ascertain the correct anatomy, and any level of doubt should lead to an investigation.

If a CBD injury is recognized at the time of surgery, it is wise to recruit the assistance of a hepatobiliary surgeon to aid in the reconstruction. A limited, sharp injury to the CBD may be possible to repair over a T tube. However, most laparoscopic bile duct injuries result in complete discontinuity of the biliary tree and require Roux-en-Y hepaticojejunostomy. Cautery and crush injuries should categorically not be repaired primarily since the area of damage extends beyond what is immediately apparent.

Most instances of injury to the biliary tree are not recognized at the time of operation.[49] Postoperative manifestations of injury are bile leak, biliary obstruction, or both. The most important initial step in management is to determine the exact anatomy of the injury and to ascertain whether a bile leak is controlled. A detailed classification of biliary injuries by Strasberg et al.[5] and Bismuth[50] outline the varieties of biliary tree injuries that occur during cholecystectomy.

Any patient who develops abdominal pain, fever, or jaundice following cholecystectomy has a biliary injury until proven otherwise. Imaging is the first step in the evaluation of these patients. A CT of the abdomen may reveal the presence of intrahepatic biliary dilatation or a fluid collection in the liver bed. While a small hematoma can be managed expectantly, a biloma should be drained percutaneously by interventional radiology. If a biliary leak is present it should be managed with a drain and ERCP as detailed in the previous section.

Biliary obstruction following cholecystectomy is either due to a retained stone, or inadvertent ligation of the CBD. ERCP is necessary to delineate the etiology. Occasionally, a hematoma compressing the CBD causes biliary obstruction, and a biliary stent is sufficient treatment until the hematoma resorbs. When CBD injury has occurred, reconstruction with Roux-en-Y hepaticojejunostomy is necessary to restore biliary-enteric continuity. Over 90% of these patients will do well,[51] but some may suffer from anastomotic stricture and bouts of cholangitis over their lifetime.

Late Stricture of the Common Bile Duct

The development of a biliary stricture following cholecystectomy is usually the result of iatrogenic injury to the CBD. This may be the result of direct compression of the bile duct by a surgical clip which was placed too close to the CBD. Another common mechanism of injury results from or overly aggressive dissection near the junction of the cystic duct with the CBD, leading to a delayed ischemic stricture. Similarly, the use of cautery too close to the CBD can result in a thermal injury with delayed stricture. Lastly inadvertent ligation of the right hepatic artery can result in delayed biliary stricture formation from ischemic insult. ERCP with balloon dilation and stent can be attempted for stricture of the CBD; however the stricture usually recurs over time. Roux-en-Y hepaticojejunostomy may be necessary for long-term relief.

CONCLUSION

Diseases of the biliary tree are seen frequently by the acute care surgeon, and cholecystectomy is one of the most commonly performed operations, therefore a thorough understanding of the pathology and treatment of these disorders is vital. While cholecystectomy is relatively straightforward in some patients, in others the surgery can be fraught with danger. Major hemorrhage from injury to the hepatic artery or the middle hepatic vein can occur; severe biliary injury may result from misinterpretation of the anatomy or ischemic injury to the CBD. In addition, variations in anatomy are relatively common and further increase the complexity of surgery on the biliary tract.

References

1. Liu TH, Consorti ET, Kawashima A, et al. Patient evaluation and management with selective use of magnetic resonance cholangiography and endoscopic retrograde cholangiopancreatography before laparoscopic cholecystectomy. *Ann Surg*. 2001;234(1):33–40.
2. Adams DB. The importance of extrahepatic biliary anatomy in preventing complications at laparoscopic cholecystectomy. *Surg Clin N Am*. 1993;73:861–871.
3. Nagral S. Anatomy relevant to cholecystectomy. *J Min Access Surg*. 2005;1:53–58.
4. Davidoff AM, Pappas TN, Murray EA, et al. Mechanisms of major biliary injury during laparoscopic cholecystectomy. *Ann Surg*. 1992;215(3):196–202.
5. Strasberg SM, Hertl M, Soper NJ. An analysis of the problem of biliary injury during laparoscopic cholecystectomy. *J Am Coll Surg*. 1995;180:101–125.
6. Ong ES, Espat NJ. Bile secretion. In: Blumgart LH, ed. *Surgery of the Liver, Biliary Tract and Pancreas*. 4th ed. Philadelphia, PA: Elsevier Health Sciences; 2006:72–78.
7. Melzer E, et al. Recovery of pressor response to norepinephrine following relief of the obstructed common bile duct in the rat. *Res Exp Med*. 1993;193:163–167.
8. Padillo J, Puente J, Gómez M, et al. Improved cardiac function in patients with obstructive jaundice after internal biliary drainage: hemodynamic and hormonal assessment. *Ann Surg*. 2001;234:652–656.
9. Nakeeb A, Pitt HA. Pathophysiology of biliary tract obstruction. In: Blumgart LH, ed. *Surgery of the Liver, Biliary Tract and Pancreas*. 4th ed. Philadelphia, PA: Elsevier Health Sciences; 2006:79–86.
10. Fogarty BJ, Parks RW, Rowlands BJ, et al. Renal dysfunction in obstructive jaundice. *Br J Surg*. 1995;82:877–884.

11. Grande L, Garcia-Valdecasas JC, Fuster J, et al. Obstructive jaundice and wound healing. *Br J Surg*. 1990;77:440–442.
12. Thompson RL, Hoper M, Diamond T, et al. Development and reversibility of T lymphocyte dysfunction in experimental obstructive jaundice. *Br J Surg*. 1990;77:1229–1232.
13. Andy OJ Jr, Grogan JB, Griswold JA, et al. Peritoneal neutrophil chemotaxis is impaired in biliary obstruction. *Am Surg*. 1992;58:28–31.
14. Scott-Conner CE, Grogan JB, Scher KS, et al. Impaired bacterial killing in early obstructive jaundice. *Am J Surg*. 1993;166:308–310.
15. Barakos JA, Ralls PW, Lapin SA, et al. Cholelithiasis: evaluation with CT. *Radiology*. 1987;162:415–418.
16. Velasco J, Singh J, Ramanujam P, et al. Hepatobiliary scanning in cholecystitis. *Eur J Nucl Med*. 1982;7:11–13.
17. Attili AF, Carulli N, Roda E, et al. Epidemiology of gallstone disease in Italy: prevalence data of the Multicenter Italian Study on Cholelithiasis. *Am J Epidemiol*. 1995;141:158–165.
18. Muhrbeck O, Ahlberg J. Prevalence of gallstones in a Swedish population. *Scand J Gastroenerol*. 1995;30:1125–1128.
19. Thompson JE Jr, Pitt HA, Doty JE, et al. Broad spectrum penicillin as an adequate therapy for acute cholangitis. *Surg Gynecol Obstet*. 1990;171:275–282.
20. Johansson M, Thune A, Blomquist A, et al. Management of acute cholecystitis in the laparoscopic era; results of a prospective randomized clinical trial. *J Gastrointest Surg*. 2003;7:642–645.
21. Papi C, Catarci M, D'Ambrosio L, et al. Timing of cholecystectomy for acute calculous cholecystitis: a meta-analysis. *Am J Gastroenterol*. 2004;99:147–155.
22. Lai EC, Lau WY. Mirizzi syndrome: history, present and future development. *ANZ J Surg*. 2006;76(4)251–257.
23. Hazzan D, Golijanin D, Reissman P, et al. Combined endoscopic and surgical management of Mirizzi syndrome. *Surg Endosc*. 1999;13(6): 618–620.
24. Warren BL. Small vessel occlusion in acute acalculous cholecystitis. *Surgery*. 1992;111:163–168.
25. Hakala T, Nuutinen PJ, Ruokonen ET, et al. Micoangiopathy in acute acalculous cholecystitis. *Br J Surg*. 1997;84:1249–1252.
26. Fagan SP, Awad SS, Rahwan K, et al. Prognostic factors for the development of gangrenous cholecystitis. *Am J Surg*. 2003;186:481–485.
27. Sakai Y. Images in clinical medicine. Emphysematous cholecystitis. *N Engl J Med*. 2003;348:2329.
28. Gill KS, Chapman AH, Weston MJ. The changing face of emphysematous cholecystitis. *Br J Radiol*. 1997;70(838):986–991.
29. Chiu HH, Chen CM, Mo LR. Emphysematous cholecystitis. *Am J Surg*. 2004;188(3):325–326.
30. Date RS, Kaushal M, Ramesh A. A review of the management of gallstone disease and its complications in pregnancy. *Am J Surg*. 2008;196(4):599–608.
31. Doogue MP, Choong CK, Frizelle FA. Recurrent gallstone ileus: underestimated. *Aust N Z J Surg*. 1998;68(11):755–756.
32. Lobo DN, Jobling JC, Balfour TW. Gallstone ileus: diagnostic pitfalls and therapeutic successes. *J Clin Gastroenterol*. 2000;30:72–76.
33. Reisner BM, Cohen JR. Gallstone ileus: a review of 1001 reported cases. *Am Surg*. 1994;60:441–446.
34. Majeed AW, Ross B, Johnson AG, et al. Common duct diameter as an independent predictor of choledocholithiasis: is it useful? *Clin Radiol*. 1999;54:170–172.
35. Kinney TP. Management of ascending cholangitis. *Gastrointest Endosc Clin N Am*. 2007;17(2):289–306.
36. Tamakuma S, et al. Relationship between hepatic hemodynamics and biliary pressure in dogs: its significance in clinical shock following biliary decompression. *Jpn J Surg*. 1975;5:255–268.
37. Choi BI, et al. Clonorchiasis and cholangiocarcinoma: etiological relationship and imaging diagnosis. *Clin Microbiol Rev*. 2004;17:540–552.
38. Fan ST, Wong J. Recurrent pyogenic cholangitis. In: Blumgart LH, ed. *Surgery of the Liver, Biliary Tract and Pancreas*. 4th ed. Philadelphia, PA: Elsevier Health Sciences; 2006:971–988.
39. Strasberg SM. Avoidance of biliary injury during laparoscopic cholecystectomy. *J Hepatobiliary Pancreat Surg*. 2002;9(5):543–547.
40. Way LW, Stewart L, Gantert W, et al. Causes and prevention of laparoscopic bile duct injuries: analysis of 252 cases from a human factors and cognitive psychology perspective. *Ann Surg*. 2003;237(4):460–469.
41. Kanaan SA, et al. Risk factors for conversion of laparoscopic to open cholecystectomy. *J Surg Res*. 2002;106:20–24.
42. Memon MA, et al. The outcome of unretrieved gallstones in the peritoneal cavity during laparoscopic cholecystectomy. *Surg Endosc*. 1999;13:848–857.
43. Downie GH, et al. Cholelithoptysis: a complication following laparoscopic cholecystectomy. *Chest*. 1993;103:616–617.
44. Chia JKS, et al. Gallstones exiting the urinary bladder: a complication of laparoscopic cholecystectomy. *Arch Surg*. 1995;130:677.
45. Byrne MF, Suhocki P, Mitchell RM, et al. Percutaneous cholecystostomy in patients with acute cholecystitis: experience of 45 patients at a US referral center. *J Am Coll Surg*. 2003;197:206–211.
46. Blumgart LH. Stones in the common bile duct—clinical features and open surgical approaches and techniques. In: Blumgart LH, ed. *Surgery of the Liver, Biliary Tract and Pancreas*. 4th ed. Philadelphia, PA: Elsevier Health Sciences; 2006:528–547.
47. Ball CG, MacLean AR, Kirkpatrick AW, et al. Hepatic vein injury during laparoscopic cholecystectomy: the unappreciated proximity of the middle hepatic vein to the gallbladder bed. *J Gastrointest Surg*. 2006;10(8):1151–1155.
48. Massoumi H, Kiyici N, Hertan H. Bile leak after laparoscopic cholecystectomy. *J Clin Gastroenterol*. 2007;41(3):301–305.
49. Lillemoe KD, Martin SA, Cameron JL, et al. Major bile duct injuries during laparoscopic cholecystectomy. Follow-up after combined surgical and radiologic management. *Ann Surg*. 1997;225:459–468.
50. Bismuth H. Postoperative strictures of the bile duct. In: Blumgart LH, ed. *The Biliary Tract: Clinical Surgery International*. Edinburgh, UK: Churchill Livingstone; 1982:209–218.
51. Lillemoe KD, Melton GB, Cameron JL, et al. Postoperative bile duct strictures: management and outcome in the 1990s. *Ann Surg*. 2000;232:430–441.

CHAPTER 40 ■ GASTROINTESTINAL TRACT FOREIGN BODIES

ROBERT A. IZENBERG, ROBERT C. MACKERSIE

The ingestion or insertion of foreign bodies (FBs) into the gastrointestinal (GI) tract, whether accidentally or deliberately, represents a common problem for emergency medicine physicians and gastroenterologists, and a less common problem for general and acute care surgeons. The earliest reports of an ingested GI FBs date back to 1692 when a young (age 5) Frederick William I, the future King of Prussia, swallowed a shoe buckle. The buckle passed uneventfully several days later, aided by the oral administration of several grains of rhubarb. So celebrated was this event that the actual buckle was displayed in Berlin for many years afterwards.

Similar to King Frederick's shoe buckle, 80%-90% of ingested food boluses and FBs will pass spontaneously.[1] Studies have suggested that 10%-20% of patients will require nonoperative (generally endoscopic) removal, and approximately 1% will require surgical intervention.[2] The true incidence of FB obstruction is unknown, but a recent study by Longstreth, reported an estimated annual incidence rate of food impaction at 13 episodes per 100,000 in a Health Maintenance Organization (HMO) population with a 1.7:1 male to female ratio.[3] This same study ranked it as the third most common nonbiliary endoscopic emergency, ranking only behind acute upper GI hemorrhage and acute lower GI hemorrhage in its frequency. Although deaths from FB ingestions and insertions are rare, a recent review noted an estimated 1,500–1,600 deaths annually in the United States from FB ingestion/insertion.[4]

The following discussion of GI FBs will review general considerations in the surgical treatment of GI ingestions and insertions, followed by a more specific review of the management options for FB ingestions (upper GI) and insertions (colorectal).

GENERAL CONSIDERATIONS

The GI tract has a remarkable ability to pass indigestible material to which is attributed the (relatively) low incidence of problems created by FB ingestions. The tendency for peristaltic flow to be centered axially and to slow down as a result of irritating (FB) stimuli may facilitate the passage of foreign material. This same smooth muscle activity may also contribute to pushing the more easily passed blunt or smooth end of an object forward ahead of the less easily passed sharp or rough end.

With respect to impedance to forward motion, the GI tract is not created uniformly and several areas may create additional obstacles. The cricopharyngeal sphincter, for example, is anatomically the narrowest point in the GI tract, and the cervical esophagus has been the most common site of FB impaction in some series. Those objects which remain in the pharynx are usually sharp or slender such as fish or chicken bones, tacks, pins or toothpicks. These sharp objects can become trapped in the faucial or lingual tonsil, the tonsillar fossa, or lateral pharyngeal wall behind the posterior pillar. Occasionally, they are impaled between the base of the tongue and the surface of the epiglottis. Open safety pins can be caught in the hypopharynx with one end engaged in the piriform sinus.[5]

Other areas of anatomic esophageal narrowing are the lower esophageal sphincter (LES), and the levels of the aortic arch and left mainstem bronchus,[6] with the LES a more common point of obstruction. Areas where ingested FBs may be entrapped further downstream are the pyloric muscle, the duodenal sweep/ligament of Treitz and the ileocecal valve. In addition to these normal areas of FB impedance, pathologic changes to the GI tract may produce sufficient narrowing to entrap even smaller ingested material. Peptic stricture of the lower esophagus or duodenum, anastomotic stricture from previous GI surgery, fundoplication of the lower esophagus, Schatzki rings, scleroderma, Crohns strictures, and even achalasia may contribute to FB entrapment.

Two obvious factors to be considered with all upper GI ingestions or rectal insertions are size and contour of the FB (sharp/pointed/rough vs. blunt/smooth). In regard to size, while no precise cutoff can be used to absolutely determine which ingested objects will pass and which will not, as a general rule an object length of over 5 cm (~3 cm in children) and a diameter over 2 cm will typically be trapped at either the pylorus or ileocecal valve. The distinction between sharp/pointed and blunt/smooth ingested FB is important due to the increased risk (estimated at 15%-35%) of perforation with the former.[1,7]

Although seemingly straightforward, one of the more difficult challenges in the management of FB ingestions and insertions can sometimes be simply making the diagnosis. The majority of FB ingestions occur in young children who may or may not be able (or refuse) to give a reliable history and present with seemingly unrelated symptoms. Patients with recognized psychiatric illness may intentionally or unintentionally ingest FBs and present with a nonexistent or misleading history. Findings on physical examination, in the absence of complications, may be limited, and a high degree of suspicion is often needed leading to imaging studies and the correct diagnosis.

Surgical intervention for ingested or inserted FBs is generally reserved for either complications (perforation, obstruction, major hemorrhage, local/systemic toxicity), or intractability (failure to pass an otherwise benign FB). Given the enormous variety of ingested objects, (buttons, coins, beads, toothpicks, toothbrushes, pens, pins, hair, jewelry, hardware, fishhooks, razorblades, paperclips, silverware, toys, keys, crayons, rocks, dentures, batteries, drugs, bones, etc.), the diagnostic challenges, and the profile of the "at-risk" patient populations, management is often highly individualized. Well coordinated multidisciplinary management involving radiology and gastroenterology services can help minimize both the incidence of surgical intervention and complications.

FOREIGN BODY INGESTION (per os)

There are only two ways a FB can end up in the GI tract: ingested via the mouth (os), or inserted via the rectum. While there is some epidemiologic crossover, these two mechanisms

"The views expressed in this article are those of the author and do not necessarily reflect the official policy or position of the Department of the Navy, Department of Defense, nor the U.S. Government."

generally are associated with different patient populations, different foreign objects, and a different approach to the diagnosis and management. As such, the following discussion distinguishes between the two.

Patients who have ingested FBs present in several ways: (1) Without symptoms following a recognized ingestion, in order to be "evaluated," (2) With symptoms referable to a recognized ingestion, (3) With symptoms, but following an unrecognized, unwitnessed, or unacknowledged ingestion. These patterns maybe associated with distinct demographic groups. Group 1 includes the "worried well," the legitimately concerned, and sometimes prisoners who deliberately swallow objects for secondary gain. Group 3 is comprised mostly of young children, psychiatric patients, and very elderly adults.

Approximately 80% of the patients with ingested FBs are under 15 years of age[6] with the peak incidence occurring between the ages of 3 months and 3 years.[8] Adults are also at risk, especially those with preexisting anatomic or motility disorders in the case of unintentional food bolus ingestion, and those with psychiatric and behavioral disorders or dementia in cases of intentional or accidental ingestions of objects other than food. Edentulous adults are at particular risk of FB ingestion whether it is a food bolus or swallowing of dentures. The wearing of dentures decreases the normal oral tactile sensitivity making it difficult to sense the size of a food bolus or the presence of bones. Prisoners may also purposefully ingest/insert FBs into the GI tract, seeking secondary gain by movement from their place of incarceration to a medical facility for treatment. Purposeful ingestion of FBs to facilitate drug trafficking also occurs, and FB impactions have also been reported as part of hazing rituals in the past and also in college students playing the game of "quarters."[9]

Elements of a careful history include the object ingested (if known), past episodes of dysphagia, food impaction, previous abdominal operations, gastroesophageal reflux disease, known structural esophageal disease, and the contents of any associated meal. Symptomatic patients will often report sudden onset of dysphagia during the meal, which may be accompanied by chest pain, or odynophagia and an inability to tolerate secretions. In children and adults unable to give a history, any sudden refusal to eat, drooling, or respiratory symptoms such as a cough or wheezing due to aspiration are reasons to suspect FB ingestion. Often the patient's localization of the pain is unreliable as a means of identifying the location of the retained FB. As a general rule, pain/discomfort symptoms are referred more proximally in the esophagus and pharynx than the actual site of retention/impaction.[10]

Physical examination, to assess the patient's stability and to assess any complications of the impaction, is often unrevealing. Airway compromise, ventilation, and the risk of aspiration should first be assessed. The inability to handle secretions and drooling suggests a complete or near-complete obstruction of the esophagus by the object. Subcutaneous crepitus, swelling of the neck or chest, or peritoneal signs is suggestive of perforation and should trigger rapid diagnostic measures to confirm and localize the site of perforation or, in the case of frank peritonitis, immediate operation.

The use of radiographic imaging is mildly controversial, particularly for esophageal FBs. In patients symptomatic for an esophageal FB who are likely to be referred for endoscopic evaluation and FB extraction regardless of imaging results, plain imaging or computed tomography (CT) imaging may only add to the cost and delay definitive management. For those patients deemed to be candidates for imaging studies, plain film radiographs of the neck, chest and abdomen are the fastest and simplest means of detecting radio-opaque objects such as metal or larger bones. Most fish bones, chicken bones, plastic, and small pieces of glass however cannot be easily visualized on plain radiographs. Contrast studies using Gastrografin or thin barium will usually allow visualization (with or without the addition of cotton fiber), but the contrast agents themselves may create problems. Barium hinders visualization during any subsequent endoscopy and should not be used in the setting of suspected esophageal perforation. Gastrografin can cause pulmonary edema and severe pneumonitis if aspirated.

CT of the neck, chest and abdomen may be helpful if perforation abscess or fistula is suspected, or to visualize an object not seen with other modalities. In a 1999 study by Eliashar et al.,[11] helical CT was found to have sensitivity and specificity of 100% and 93.7%, respectively, for detecting esophageal bone impactions. CT imaging of the abdomen may also be used to characterize the location and extent of bowel obstruction for larger and more distal FB.

Flexible esophagogastroduodenoscopy is often both diagnostic (of the type and location of the impacted FB) as well as therapeutic (removal). Upper GI endoscopy has the additional advantage of diagnosis of the underlying pathology (e.g., web or stricture) which led to the impaction and to assess the degree of associated mucosal damage.

Clinical Management of Upper GI Foreign Bodies

Recognizing that the management of many cases of FB ingestion needs to be individualized, a general proposed management scheme is outlined in Algorithm 40.1. The discussion that follows roughly corresponds to the sequence outlined in the Algorithm 40.1.

Regardless of symptoms, there are two categories of FB ingestion that mandate early endoscopic retrieval: sharp or pointed objects in any accessible location (oropharynx, esophagus, stomach, duodenum), and small batteries often ingested by young children. As previously noted, the incidence of GI perforation with sharp/pointed objects is sufficiently high to justify pre-emptive retrieval.

In the case of battery ingestions, multiple mechanisms of injury are involved including electrical discharge and mucosal burns (that may occur very quickly), pressure necrosis with larger batteries, mercuric oxide toxicity, and caustic injury from leakage in a moist saline-rich environment. Most significant battery-related injuries occur in younger (age < 4 years) children ingesting cylindrical or larger (>18 mm) lithium type batteries. Liquefaction necrosis and perforation may occur rapidly (<2 hours) after the ingestion of these devices when they become lodged in the esophagus. Following radiologic confirmation of location and of battery versus coin ingestion, the former should be immediately removed via endoscopy to avoid serious or even fatal complications. If the battery cannot be extracted from the esophagus, an alternative is to push it into the stomach where it can be retrieved with a basket more easily. Batteries that have passed beyond the esophagus at presentation usually do not require removal unless the patient exhibits signs and symptoms of injury to the GI tract or a large diameter battery (those larger than 2 cm in size) remains in the stomach for greater than 48 hours as determined by repeat radiographs.[8]

In patients completely devoid of symptoms in whom a FB ingestion is known or suspected, plain radiographs may be obtained to verify ingestion, size, and location of radio-opaque objects. For non-radio-opaque objects, CT is usually necessary for visualization. Most patients with FB lodged in the esophagus will be symptomatic and will require endoscopic extraction. For those asymptomatic patients with gastric or duodenal FB, the decision to perform endoscopic extraction may be made on the basis of length (>5 cm for adults, 3–4 cm for children) or diameter (>2 cm). Asymptomatic patients ingesting smaller (nonsharp, nonpointed) objects may be managed expectantly and observed for the development of any symptoms.

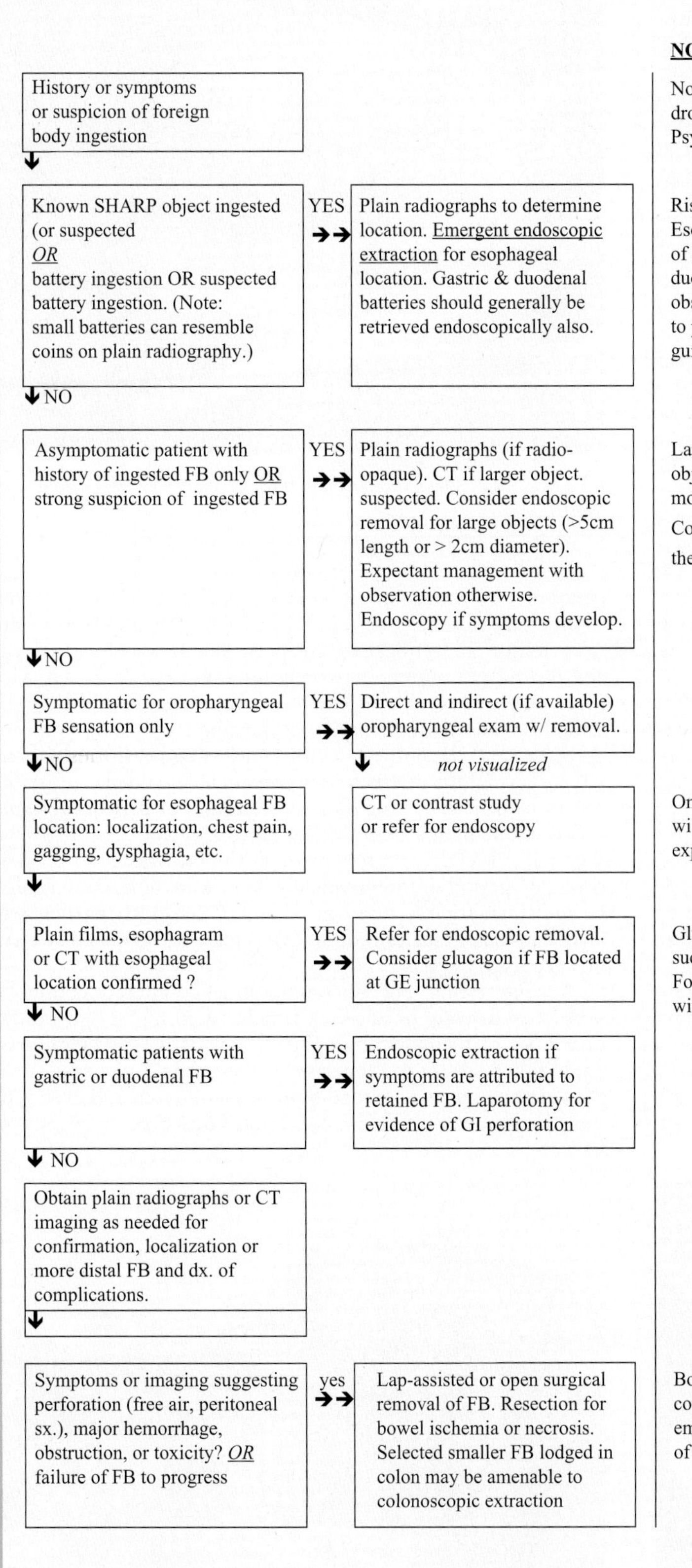

NOTES

Non-spcific complaints in children such as malaise, refusal of food, drooling or wheezing should raise the suspicion of FB ingestion. Psych patients should be similarly suspect.

Risk factors are size (>12 mm), younger age, and lithium type batteries. Esophageal damage may occur rapidly (<2 hours). Selected cases of smaller (< 12mm) button batteries found in the stomach or duodenum of older (>12 yrs) patients may be managed with observation for 24-48 hours with endoscopic extraction for failure to progress. Call the National Battery ingestion hotline for detailed guidance: 202-625-3333

Larger esophageal objects will generally create symptoms. Smaller objects in the stomach (or more distal) will pass spontaneously more than 90% of the time.

Confirmation of passage is most directly accomplished by straining the stool or (for radio-opaque objects), by repeat plain films.

Only a minority of patients with oropharyngeal FB sensation will have retained material. Selected patients may be managed expectantly if imaging studies are negative.

Glucagon relaxes the lower esophageal sphincter and has a variable success rate (10-50%). Nausea & vomiting may be a accompaniment. Foley catheter removal may be considered for cooperative patients with smooth impacted FBs.

Body "packers" and "stuffers" who ingest large quantities of contraband opiates may present with opiate toxicity and require emergency (open) operation for the expedient removal of intraluminal drugs.

ALGORITHM 40.1

ALGORITHM 40.1 Suggested Management for FB ingestion (upper GI).

Patients symptomatic for FB sensation only in the oropharynx should undergo direct and indirect (if available) examination with extraction of any identified objects. For patients with a negative exam, imaging studies may be obtained (contrast swallow or CT) to stratify patients in need of endoscopic evaluation and extraction. As only a minority (<25%-30%) of these patients will have a retained FB, some authors advocate expectant management for those patients with negative examination and negative imaging studies of the oropharynx.

Retained esophageal FB typically produces symptoms including dysphagia, odynophagia, gagging, excessive salivation, chest pain or heartburn, and patients usually seek early medical attention. While the majority of these patients will require endoscopic FB retrieval, there are less invasive techniques that may obviate this approach. Glucagon has been administered in this setting in an effort to relax the esophageal smooth muscle and promote passage of smaller FB or food boluses. Glucagon is known to relax GI tract smooth muscle and has been reported to relax the LES (lower esophageal sphincter) by 60% in normal subjects after IV administration.[12] Despite its promise, results with glucagon have been mixed with its success rate being reported at anywhere from 12% to 50%.[12] Some authors have attributed this to the inability of glucagon to relax the fixed stenosis of esophageal strictures. Contraindications to the use of Glucagon include insulinoma, pheocromocytoma, Zollinger-Ellison syndrome, and known hypersensitivity to the drug.

Foley catheter extraction is another technique used in the emergency departments (EDs) with success reported at over 85%. It requires a cooperative patient, <72 hours since ingestion, and the absence of respiratory symptoms or underlying esophageal disease. Contrast esophagography is first performed to confirm location, size, and "smoothness" of the FB and to exclude significant esophageal disease or the presence of multiple ingested objects. The Foley catheter is passed through the nose past the FB and the FB is then displaced up into the mouth using a (distally inflated) balloon much like an embolectomy catheter removes a clot.

At this point in the management scheme, asymptomatic patients and those with more proximal impactions have already been managed, leaving symptomatic patients with ingested objects located in the stomach, duodenum, or more distally. As previously mentioned, larger objects (>5 cm length or >2 cm diameter) and sharp or pointed objects should generally be extracted if endoscopically accessible in the esophagus, stomach, or duodenum. Past the duodenum, the next major anatomical obstacle is the ileocecal valve, but sharp or larger objects may hang up anywhere in the GI tract (Figs. 40.1–40.3). Management at this stage should be individualized based on the nature of the ingested object, symptom complex, and patient risk factors (including previous abdominal surgery). Indications for surgery include evidence of perforation such as free air on diagnostic studies or peritoneal signs, obstruction, major hemorrhage (rare), or the failure of the ingested object to progress through the GI tract after a "reasonable" period of time (typically 2–3 days). Surgery may also be indicated for the removal of higher risk FBs (particularly large or sharp) that cannot be extracted endoscopically or are not expected to pass.

An interesting but uncommonly encountered condition occurs exclusively in younger females who ingest substantial quantities of their own hair. These hair balls (trichobezoars), are highly resistant to GI peristalsis and usually accumulate in the stomach but may extend into the duodenum and even into the jejunum, constituting a condition known as the Rapunzel

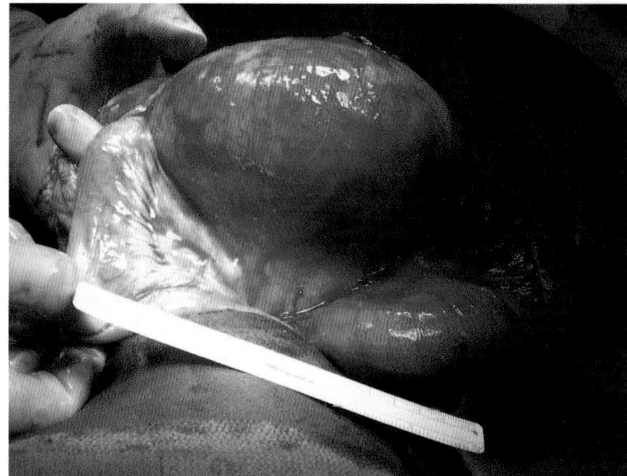

FIGURE 40.2. Obstructed small bowel. (Courtesy of Dr. Michael West.)

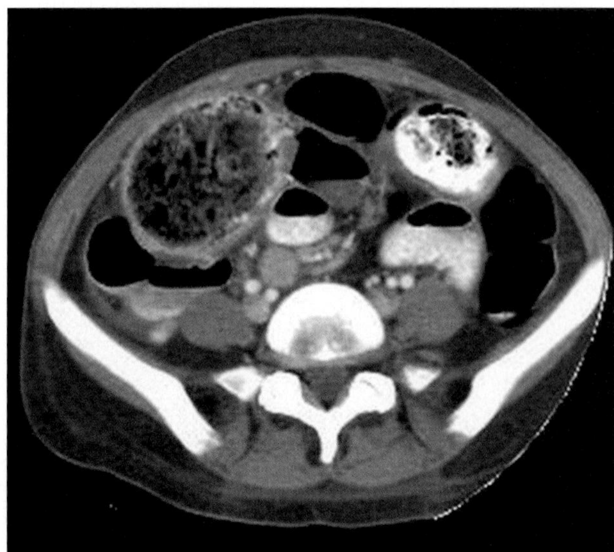

FIGURE 40.1. CT of small bowel bezoar. (Courtesy of Dr. Michael West.)

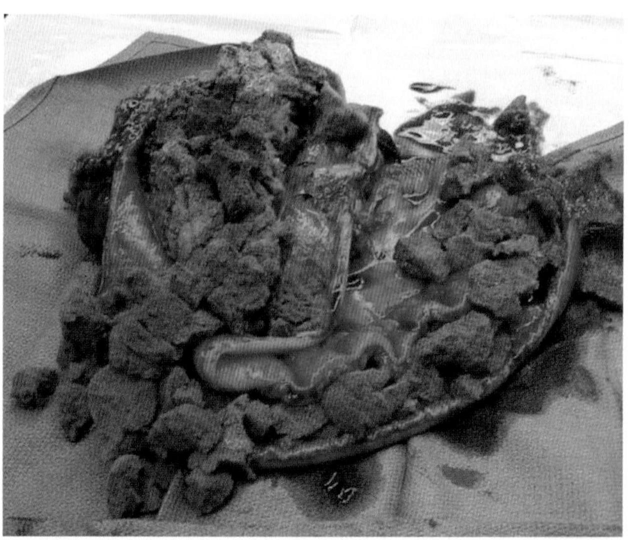

FIGURE 40.3. Bezoar containing furniture foam. (Courtesy of Dr. Michael West.)

syndrome. Most patients have associated psychiatric or eating disorders including trichotillomania (pulling out one's own hair), trichophagia (eating same), anorexia neverosa, depression, or pica. Complete endoscopic removal of large trichobezoars has proven difficult and most patients will require open surgical intervention for complete extraction.

The surgical procedures performed in the setting of complicated FB ingestions vary with regard to the level of the lesion and the severity of damage to the adjacent bowel. The variability of entrapped ingested objects and the limited number of cases requiring surgery do not allow any meaningful guidelines to be developed. In most cases the surgical approach is an extrapolation from management techniques applicable to other diseases or conditions.

As a general rule, larger FBs lodged in the GI tract may be identified and removed using laparoscopic assist techniques. Surgical options include simple enterotomy and extraction and repair or extraction and oversew of a small perforation with abdominal washout. Segmental ischemia or severe inflammation may require primary resection with anastomosis. More severe ileocecal lesions may require cecectomy or limited right colectomy. In most cases, a primary ileocolic anastomosis may be safely performed. Large, severely inflamed duodenal perforations, often more distal, may be the most troublesome, requiring complex or augmented repair (using small bowel loop or Roux-Y) with or without duodenal diversion. The morbidity of operation after perforation from a FB has been reported as high as 57% with mortality as high as 6%.[13]

One unique indication for surgical intervention pertains to the removal of wrapped packets of drugs, typically heroin, cocaine, or other opiates, that are swallowed and do not pass on their own causing obstruction or leak with systemic toxicity. This may occur with "body stuffers" or "body packers." These street slang terms denote users who more abruptly ingest quickly prepared packets of drugs to conceal them to avoid arrest and prosecution ("stuffers") and drug traffickers ("mules") who ingest more carefully wrapped packets of drugs for purposes of concealed transport. In addition to obstruction, these packets of drugs may leak or rupture, leading to GI absorption and overdose toxicity.

Risk factors for complications arising from ingested drug packets include: 1) a large number (>50) of packets, 2) large size packets, 3) signs of systemic toxicity, 4) bowel obstruction, 5) passage of disrupted packaging. Asymptomatic "stuffers" or "packers" may be managed expectantly with careful monitoring for laboratory of clinical evidence of drug absorption. Extraction of drug packets is indicated for obstruction, failure to pass, or evidence of systemic toxicity. Due to the greater likelihood of tearing the drug packets during retrieval, endoscopic removal is usually avoided. The preferred approach has been (open) laparotomy for both its speed and the lesser likelihood of inadvertent packet rupture.

FOREIGN BODY INSERTION (PER RECTUM)

Colorectal and lower GI tract FBs are approached and managed differently from those of the upper GI tract. Although one of the earliest case reports was published in 1919,[14] and Haft and Benjamin[15] referred to a case as long ago as the 16th century, retained rectal FBs were thought to be an uncommon occurrence in the past and more of a curiosity or a source of humor than a medical problem.[16]

Today, rectal FBs are no longer viewed as a medical oddity and have been reported with greater frequency in recent years. The vast majority of FBs ingested from above that are capable of making it past the esophagus, pylorus, duodenum, and ileocecal valve will rarely become lodged in the colon or rectum. As a result, the great preponderance of rectal FB encountered by physicians are inserted from below.

The transanal introduction of FBs has been observed in penitentiary prisoners, psychiatric patients, in association with homicide and suicide attempts, as an accompaniment to various erotic acts including sadomasochistic practices, in cases of sexual aggression or rape, in people under the effects of drugs or alcohol, and in drug "mules."[17] Objects can be inserted for diagnostic or therapeutic purposes, or self treatment of anorectal disease, by criminal assault, by accident, or most commonly for sexual purposes. One recent systemic review found that 48.7% of cases were reportedly for sexual stimulation followed by personal care or self treatment of constipation, hemorrhoids or pruritis ani (25%), assaults (11.8%), and accidents (9.2%).[19] While there appears to be more reports of retained rectal FBs in the western literature, it occurs worldwide, with a consistent male predominance.[19] A very strong male predominance is supported by reports from Kurer et al., who observed a male: female ratio of 37:1 in their review of the literature in 2009,[16] and by Busch and Starling,[20] who reported it to be 28:1.

A wide variety of retained rectal FBs have been reported, ranging from glass bottles to household tools, dildos, vibrators, vegetables and fruits, and many more[20,21] (Fig. 40.4). Kurer et al.,[16] found that the most commonly retained FBs in their review were household objects (42.2%) and that they were generally bottles of various shapes and sizes and drinking glasses.

While a detailed history should of course, be taken, it is often the case that the patient will present to the ED only after multiple prior attempts have been made to remove the object. The circumstances and even timing of the FB insertion may change due to general embarrassment on the part of the patient. The presenting complaint may be rectal bleeding, diarrhea, constipation, or obscure abdominal pain[22] in the majority of patients, with the denial of the rectal insertion of a FB.[16] The history should include the size and character of the device and the time lapse between insertion of the object and presentation to the hospital. Symptoms such as nausea, vomiting and abdominal pain are very significant and may point to complete obstruction or perforation, especially if coupled with fever, tenderness or peritoneal signs on abdominal examination.

Despite the fact that most rectal FBs are inserted knowingly or with consent, the potential for assaultive mechanisms, including rape and domestic violence (DV) must be considered. Suspicious cases are best managed in conjunction with appropriate investigative process and with the involvement of sensitive rape or DV counseling. In some cases, patients may not be aware of the presence of a retained rectal FB and present with other complaints.

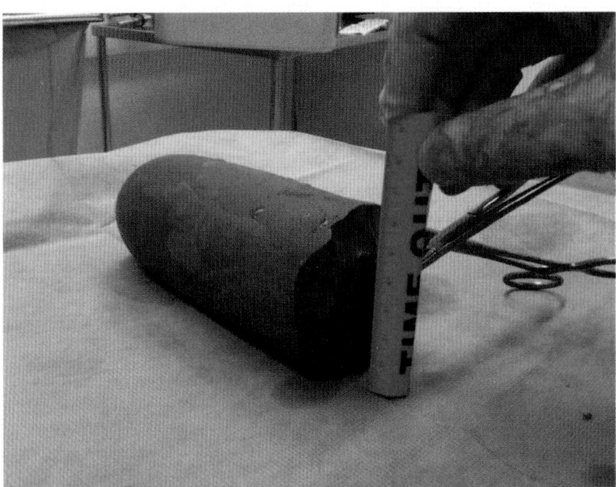

FIGURE 40.4. Rectal FB. (Courtesy of Dr. Michael West.

Clinical Management of Rectal Foreign Bodies

As with upper GI FBs, cases of retained rectal FB are highly individualized, and a considerable degree of flexibility and even creativity may be useful in successful extraction and management. A general scheme for the management of rectal FB is presented in Algorithm 40.2.

General, acute care, and colorectal surgeons are the specialists most commonly consulted when a patient presents with a retained rectal FB as many of these patients will require FB extraction in the operating room, with some patients requiring more extensive colorectal procedures. The major initial

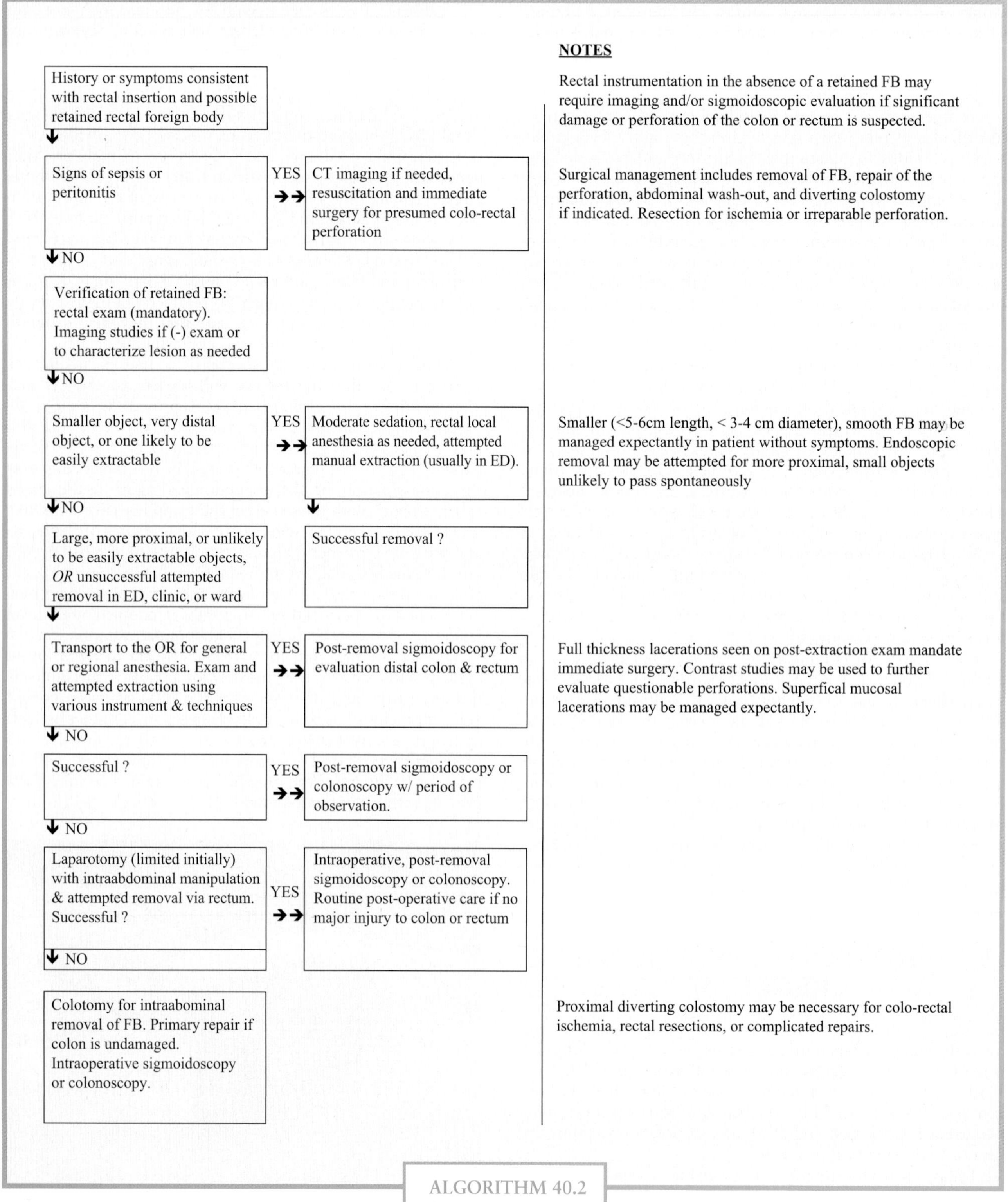

ALGORITHM 40.2 Suggested management for retained rectal FBs.

decision to be made is whether a given patient is best managed in the operating room or can potentially be managed in the ED or other treatment area. Evidence of colo-rectal perforation based on physical examination (peritonitis) or imaging (free air, rectal contrast extravasation, bowel ischemia, etc.) mandates operative exploration with or without a retained rectal FB. Other relative indications for using the OR as the venue for attempted FB extraction include large, sharp, pointed, or more proximal FBs, or those of a nature likely to make simple manual extraction difficult.

A digital rectal examination will often identify the presence of an object in the distal rectum. However, an object lodged at or above the rectosigmoid junction will not be palpable. Huang described these objects lying above the rectosigmoid junction (>10 cm above the dentate line in average sized adults) as high lying FBs, and reported that in his series, 33% of patients presented in this fashion.[18] Occasionally, objects will be palpable on abdominal examination either in the right or left lower quadrants.

Special attention should be paid to the condition of the anal sphincters on rectal exam. This is particularly important in patients who present without a previous history of FB placement or in those who are victims of assault. Many patients with retained rectal FBs will have lax anal sphincters from repeated anal penetration, however in patients without sphincter injury, the sphincters may have increased rectal tone secondary to muscle spasm. The examination and documentation of anal resting and squeeze tone along with perianal sensation is an integral part of the rectal evaluation.

Laboratory studies including white blood count can be used to assess the potential for occult perforation. Other lab values include an arterial blood gas or serum lactate suggestive of occult injury such as mucosal ischemia from pressure necrosis, or an extraperitoneal perforation which may not be immediately obvious on examination.[23]

Radiographic studies, specifically plain films of the abdomen (flat plate to include the kidneys, ureter and bladder, upright abdomen, and chest x-ray) will often demonstrate the size, shape and position of the object in the colon or rectum. Small air bubbles seen along the psoas muscle suggest a retroperitoneal rectal perforation but this sign is subtle and may not be appreciated. An upright chest radiograph may be obtained looking for free air under the diaphragm signifying an intraperitoneal perforation of the colon or rectum.[21]

In a stable or asymptomatic patient, an abdominal and pelvic CT scan will provide more detailed information regarding the size, character and location of the rectal FB as well as increasing the sensitivity for detection of extraperitoneal colorectal perforation. Rectal wall thickening, mesorectal air, fluid collections, and fat stranding all indicate a full-thickness injury and should be taken as evidence of perforation until proven otherwise.[23]

In the absence of colorectal perforation and for rectal FBs more likely to be extractable without general anesthesia, an attempt at transanal extraction of the FB in the ED or other treatment area may be undertaken. Some authors have further limited the patient population eligible for ED extraction to those whose FBs are narrow and made of either wood or latex rubber,[21] presumably because the ability to gain a purchase on the object with a tenaculum or Kocher clamp is easier when dealing with these substances.

Transanal Removal

If extraction in the ED is attempted, positioning and relaxation must be optimized. The patient may be positioned either in lithotomy on a pelvic exam table, in high lithotomy using candy cane stirrups, or in left lateral Sims position with the knees flexed to the chest making sure the buttocks are well off the bed. For relaxation and analgesia, a rectal field block may be administered subcutaneously, intersphincterically, and submucosally using either 0.5% or 1% Lidocaine (Xylocaine) mixed 50:50 with 0.5% Bupivicaine (Marcaine) both with epinephrine. A pudendal nerve block may also be used, infiltrating deeper tissues approximately 1 cm medial to the ischial tuberosities in the posterolateral location bilaterally.[23] Moderate sedation, typically with fentanyl and versed is usually necessary in addition to local anesthesia to ensure the patient's comfort during the procedure. Only after the patient has been sufficiently relaxed should attempts be made to remove the object.

If the object can be palpated lower in the rectum, the anal canal should be gently dilated to accommodate three fingers.[23] Attempts can then be made to deliver the object using any number of clamps or devices to extract the object. As previously mentioned, if the object cannot be palpated, or if aggressive actions are necessary to deliver the object, then the patient should be transferred to the operating room where more definitive anesthetic care can be delivered (deeper relaxation general or spinal anesthesia) before attempting to remove the object.

Lake et al.[24] noted that approximately one-third of the patients with rectal FBs had had an attempt at removal by the emergency medical service prior to the surgical service being summoned. This lead to successful removal of the object, in 16% of those patients, but in additional delay to treatment in the remaining 84%.

Whether the extraction is performed in the ED or the operating room, a rigid sigmoidoscopy should then be performed to evaluate the rectal mucosa, to ensure that there are no further objects within the colon, that there is no active bleeding and also to make sure there is no full-thickness injury to the bowel mucosa.

Extraction Methods

Multiple techniques have been proposed for removal of the myriad of objects that may be found as retained rectal FB, and a high degree of inventiveness is often helpful in devising "object-based" solutions.[25] For blunt or solid objects, most authors favor trying to manually remove the object and if that fails to use a Kocher clamp or ring forceps as graspers. The ability to use the surgeon's hand will depend on the laxity of the anal sphincters and also the density of the anal block (and the size of the hand). Patients treated under local or conscious sedation, may be asked to perform a Valsalva maneuver, to assist in the delivery of the object. Smooth objects such as bottles, jars, fruits and vegetables, dildos and vibrators often cannot be easily grasped, and care must be taken not to fragment the object *in vivo*. For glass objects this may lead to disaster, however, in the case of fruits and vegetables, fragmentation may actually assist in removal of the object, or in allowing the object to pass spontaneously. Schecter and Albo report using plaster of Paris powder mixed with water and inserted into the open end of the jar. As the plaster begins to harden, a ring forceps is introduced into the soft plaster and allowed to harden in place. The forceps can then be used to apply traction to extract the jar.[21]

Some smooth objects create a vacuum seal with the rectum making their removal more difficult. Several authors have reported the use of a Foley catheter, which is passed proximal to the object and followed by inflating the balloon. The inflation of the balloon and subsequent insufflation of the bowel proximal to the object can assist in breaking the vacuum, and the catheter can then be used as a handle to deliver the object thus manipulating it from both above and below. Other authors have reported using a Sengstaken-Blakemore or Minnesota tube in a similar manner to remove impacted jars.[23]

EMERGENCY SURGERY

Obstetrical forceps and obstetrical vacuum devices have also been employed to break the vacuum seal, widen the canal and extract foreign objects. Graspers however, should not be used to extract drug packets found in body packers (see previous section). Instead, these patients should be admitted, hydrated and observed for spontaneous passage. If the patient remains stable without signs of perforation, then the packets will invariably descend to a level where they can be manually extracted. If signs of perforation or systemic toxicity occur the patient should be taken to the operating room and the packets should be rapidly removed via the rectum or through laparotomy with colotomy.

More recently, flexible endoscopy has been advocated as an adjunct to the extraction process. This approach has been reserved for those objects which are in the proximal rectum or in the distal colon.[24] Of patients presenting with retained FBs, 55% of those within the sigmoid required laparotomy versus only 24% of those in the rectum.[24] Endoscopy has been advocated as a possible way to avoid open surgery, by extracting the object using a polypectomy snare or by using the scope to break the vacuum seal of objects further in the anorectal canal and distal colon thereby removing objects that would otherwise not be amenable to transanal extraction.[23]

Surgical Management

As stated previously, there are several occasions where surgery for a retained rectal FB is necessary. The first is the failure of transanal extraction in the ED using moderate sedation, whether from inadequate relaxation or from position or composition of the object. If the patient requires deeper anesthesia, further transanal extraction attempts may be made in the operating room using the same or similar techniques employed in the ED. In addition, abdominal pressure applied to the left lower quadrant may help to propel an object caudally to allow for transanal extraction[22]—a maneuver usually too painful to be performed in a sedated patient in the ED.

The complete failure of all efforts at transanal extraction generally mandates a laparotomy to remove the obstructing object. Once inside the abdomen, manual "milking" of the object into the distal rectum may aid in the extraction transanally. If this is not successful, then a colotomy may be made and the object removed from the colon. In the absence of any significant colon or rectal damage, the colotomy may be repaired primarily. Fecal diversion is generally not necessary in these patients.

Patients presenting initially with sepsis and peritoneal signs, as previously mentioned, require aggressive resuscitation, broad spectrum antibiotics, placement of appropriate monitors, and emergent abdominal exploration. The decision as to what specific procedure to perform on this group of patients is dependent on the location of the perforation, the duration of the perforation and the delay to presentation, the degree of surrounding tissue injury, the amount of fecal contamination in the area, and the patient's physiologic condition. As a general rule, patients with established peritonitis, fecal contamination, and hemodynamic instability should be treated as any other unstable perforated colorectal patient with washout, FB removal, closure or resection of the site of perforation, and a "damage control" laparotomy with temporary abdominal closure and staged proximal diversion.

Management Post Removal and Potential Complications

Major complications following the extraction of rectal FBs are rare but can be life threatening if missed. All patients are observed for some period of time to assess their clinical stability prior to discharge. The length of this period of observation depends on the clinical stability of the patient, the length of delay to presentation, as well as how difficult the extraction was and whether it was transanal or via laparotomy. Patients undergoing transanal FB removal should undergo post extraction endoscopy, and serial abdominal examinations with follow-up radiograph as needed.[24,26] Bleeding from laceration of the rectal mucosa is usually self-limiting; however, on occasion these patients may require repeat examination under anesthesia and suture ligation of the bleeding vessel. Delayed perforation from occult colorectal injury following FB extraction is a more serious problem that can require emergent laparotomy and possible colostomy. Sphincter problems may also be encountered post extraction especially if the FB was the result of an assault. Repair of these injuries should be delayed until adequate evaluation of the symptoms and defects can be performed. Referral to a colorectal surgeon experienced in complex rectal sphincteric reconstruction is sometimes necessary.

SUMMARY

FBs of the GI tract continue to present a challenge to physicians and surgeons. Although the vast majority of ingested FBs will pass spontaneously, those >2 cm in size, or 5 cm in length are at increased risk of impaction. Button batteries and narcotic packets pose additional risks because of their potentially fatal consequences. Endoscopy is the preferred method of retrieval for most impacted, orally ingested objects. Surgical intervention is reserved for complications of upper GI FBs and for objects requiring removal beyond the duodenal sweep.

With regard to rectal FBs, an attempt at transanal extraction either under local, sedation or general anesthesia will often be successful. Patients require sigmoidoscopic or colonoscopic examination of the involved colon or rectum and observation for delayed complications. Failed transanal extraction mandates open surgical intervention for either augmented transanal or direct (colotomy) FB extraction.

References

1. Webb WA. Management of foreign bodies of the upper gastrointestinal tract: update. *Gastrointest Endosc.* 1995;41(1):39-51.
2. Telford JJ. Management of ingested foreign bodies. *Can J Gastroenterol.* 2005;19(10):599-601.
3. Longstreth GF, Longstreth KJ, Yao JF. Esophageal food impaction: epidemiology and therapy. A retrospective, observational study. *Gastrointest Endosc.* 2001;53(2):193-198.
4. Eisen GM, Baron TH, Dominitz JA, et.al. Guideline for the management of ingested foreign bodies from the American Society for Gastrointestinal Endoscopy. *Gastrointest Endosc.* 2002;55(7):802-806.
5. Barnes WA. Management of foreign bodies in the alimentary tract. *Am J Surg.* 1964;107:422-428.
6. Smith MT, Wong RK. Foreign bodies. *Gastrointest Endosc Clin N Am.* 2007;17(2):361-382, vii.
7. Vizcarrondo FJ, Brady PG, Nord HJ. Foreign bodies of the upper gastrointestinal tract. *Gastrointest Endosc.* 1983;29(3):208-210.
8. Guideline for the management of ingested foreign bodies. American Society for gastrointestinal endoscopy. *Gastrointest Endosc.* 1995;42(6):622-625.
9. Conway WC, Sugawa C, Ono H, et al. Upper GI foreign body: an adult urban emergency hospital experience. *Surg Endosc.* 2007;21(3):455-460.
10. Wilcox CM, Alexander LN, Clark WS. Localization of an obstructing esophageal lesion. Is the patient accurate? *Dig Dis Sci.* 1995;40(10):2192-2196.
11. Eliashar R, Dano I, Dangoor E, et al. Computed tomography diagnosis of esophageal bone impaction: prospective study. *Ann Otol Rhinol Laryngol.* 1999;108(7 pt1):708-710.
12. Ko HH, Enns R. Review of food bolus management. *Can J Gastroenterol.* 2008;22(10):805-808.
13. Rodriguez-Hermosa JI, Codina-Cazador A, Sirvent JM, et al. Surgically treated perforations of the gastrointestinal tract caused by ingested foreign bodies. *Colorectal Dis.* 2008;10(7):701-707.
14. Smiley O. A glass tumbler in the rectum. *JAMA.* 1919;72:1285.
15. Haft JS, Benjamin HB. Foreign bodies in the rectum: some psychosexual aspects. *Med Asp Hum Sexual.* 1973;7:74-95
16. Kurer MA, Davey C, Khan S, et al. Colorectal foreign bodies: a systematic review. *Colorectal Dis.* 2010;12:851-861.

17. Pavlidis TE, Marakis GN, Triantafyllou A, et al. Management of ingested foreign bodies. How justifiable is a waiting policy? *Surg Laparosc Endosc Percutan Tech*. 2008;18(3):286-287.
18. Huang WC, Jiang JK, Wang HS, et al. Retained rectal foreign bodies. *J Chin Med Assoc*. 2003;66(10):607-612.
19. Hunter TB, Taljanovic MS. Foreign bodies. *Radiographics*. 2003;23(3):731-757.
20. Busch DB, Starling JR. Rectal foreign bodies: case reports and a comprehensive review of the world's literature. *Surgery*. 1986;100(3):512-519.
21. Schecter WP, Albo RJ. "*Removal of Rectal Foreign Bodies" Mastery of Surgery*. 4th ed. 2001.
22. Boon-Swee O, Yik-Hong H, Kong-Weng E, et al. Management of anorectal foreign bodies: a cause of obscure anal pain. *Aust N Z J Surg*. 1998;68(12):852.
23. Goldberg JE, Steele SR. Rectal foreign bodies. *Surg Clin North Am*. 2010;90(1):173-184.
24. Lake JP, Essani R, Petrone P, et al. Management of retained colorectal foreign bodies: predictors of operative intervention. *Dis Colon Rectum*. 2004;47(10):1694-1698.
25. Cohen JS, Sackier JM. Management of colorectal foreign bodies. *J R Coll Surg Edinb*. 1996;41(5):312-315.
26. Rodriguez-Hermosa JI, Codina-Cazador A, Ruiz B, et al. Management of foreign bodies in the rectum. *Colorectal Dis*. 2007;9(6):543-548.
27. Clarke DL, Buccimazza I, Anderson FA, et al. Colorectal foreign bodies. *Colorectal Dis*. 2005;7(1):98-103.
28. Colon V, Grade A, Pulliam G, et al. Effect of doses of glucagon used to treat food impaction on esophageal motor function of normal subjects. *Dysphagia*. 1999;14(1):27-30.
29. Digoy GP. Diagnosis and management of upper aerodigestive tract foreign bodies. *Otolaryngol Clin North Am*. 2008;41(3):485-496, vii-viii.
30. Fraser I. Foreign Bodies. *Br Med J*. 1939;1(4088):967-971.
31. Henderson C, Engel J, Schlesinger P. Foreign body ingestion: review and suggested guidelines for management. Endoscopy. *Gastroenterology*. 1987;19:68-71.
32. Koornstra JJ, Weersma RK. Management of rectal foreign bodies: description of a new technique and clinical practice guidelines. *World J Gastroenterol*. 2008;14(27):4403-4406.
33. McPherson RC, Karlan M, Williams RD. Foreign body perforation of the intestinal tract. *Am J Surg*. 1957;94(4):564-566.
34. Nandi P, Ong GB. Foreign body in the oesophagus: review of 2394 cases. *Br J Surg*. 1978;65(1):5-9.
35. Syrakos T, Zacharakis E, Antonitsis P, et al. Surgical intervention for gastrointestinal foreign bodies in adults: a case series. *Med Princ Pract*. 2008;17(4):276-279.
36. Webb WA. Management of foreign bodies of the upper gastrointestinal tract. *Gastroenterology*. 1988;94(1):204-216.
37. Weiland ST, Schurr MJ. Conservative management of ingested foreign bodies. *J Gastrointest Surg*. 2002;6(3):496-500.

CHAPTER 41 ■ ANORECTAL ABSCESS AND INFLAMMATORY PROCESSES

HERAND ABCARIAN

ANORECTAL ABSCESS

Anorectal abscess is by far the most common colorectal disease requiring acute care and surgery. The overwhelming majority of anorectal abscesses originate from infection in anal glands, which drain into the crypts of Morgagni at the dentate line. Occlusion of the draining channel in bacteria-rich environment produces an abscess in the intersphincteric space before spreading to adjacent spaces (Fig. 41.1).

Other causes of anorectal abscess include Crohn's disease, rare specific infections such as tuberculosis, actinomycosis, and pinworm infestation in children. Trauma with external (penetrating) injuries or internal perforation of anorectum (from ingested sharp objects such as toothpicks, fish or chicken bones) may cause an abscess, which can also appear acutely or as a smoldering infection, often difficult to diagnose.

The presenting symptoms of anorectal abscess vary depending upon the extension of infection in perianal or perirectal spaces and whether the abscess is located proximal or distal to the anorectal ring (Fig. 41.2). *Low abscesses*, that is, those located distal to the anorectal ring, include intersphincteric, perianal or ischiorectal, depending on the anatomic site of the purulent collection between the sphincters, at the anal verge or in the ischiorectal fossa. These abscesses are associated with intense localized symptoms such as pain, swelling, erythema, cellulitis, tenderness, and fluctuation later in the disease process. In intersphincteric abscesses, the pain is aggravated with Valsalva maneuver (coughing, sneezing, laughing) On the other hand, the patient may have little or no systemic symptoms of fever, chills, and malaise, probably because of earlier diagnosis and intervention. The *low abscesses* are easier to diagnose, with the exception of posterior midline intersphincteric abscesses in male patients where the infection is sequestered in the intersphincteric or deep postanal space. The only way to reliably make the diagnosis is a careful bidigital examination, which may need to be done under anesthesia if the patient is in too much pain to tolerate examination otherwise. With the index finger, gently pushing posteriorly and the thumb pressing between the coccyx and the anus, the warm, tender swelling and induration can be easily palpated. The more superficial perianal or ischiorectal abscess can be drained urgently in the office, clinic, or emergency department with liberal use of local infiltration anesthesia.

High abscesses, that is, those located proximal to the anorectal ring (e.g., high intermuscular/submucosal or supralevator), often present with minimal local symptoms such as pelvic or rectal pressure on sitting or defecation. However, they may be associated with more systemic symptoms of fever, chills and malaise, and ketoacidosis in diabetics. These patients often identified as having "fever of unknown origin" are subjected to unnecessary laboratory and imaging studies and ineffective nonoperative treatment with oral or intravenous antibiotics. A high index of suspicion and a careful gentle rectal examination is all that is needed to arrive at the correct diagnosis. If the patient does not tolerate the examination in the outpatient setting, then he/she should be examined under anesthesia where proper and expeditious surgical procedure can be performed at the same time.[1]

The principle of surgical therapy of anorectal abscess is early, adequate, and dependent drainage. Small superficial abscesses may be drained under local infiltration anesthesia. A cruciate incision is preferable to a simple incision because its edges retract and the corners can be excised with a scalpel or iris scissors to create a small opening and prevent premature sealing of the incision with the thick proteinaceous pus. The incision should be made on the prominent point of the abscess and it must be placed as close to the anus as possible to shorten the length of a subsequent fistula should one develop postoperatively. Packing or placement of mushroom drains is usually unnecessary and may cause undue pain at insertion and removal.

Larger abscesses must be drained in the operating room under regional or general anesthesia. This allows exploration of adjacent spaces to drain the abscess thoroughly and also to probe and identify an associated fistula tract. If the abscess is very large, multiple openings (unroofing) is preferable to a long anteroposterior incision. Smaller (1–2 cm) openings can be connected with Penrose drains looped around the intact skin bridges and sutured to itself to maintain postoperative drainage as long as necessary. These openings heal within 4–6 weeks of removal of Penrose drains while a long anteroposterior, circumanal incision undergoes a step-off deformity (due to retraction of sphincter mechanism medially) and may take months to heal, leaving significant postoperative scarring.[2] Contrary to popular belief, there is no septation in an abscess cavity to be broken up. Exploration of cavity is only indicated to exclude extension to adjacent spaces.

If infection spreads bilaterally (horseshoe abscess), the patient should be taken to the operating room for adequate drainage. A horseshoe abscess always originates from an infection in the deep postanal space. If the surgeon is adequately trained to deal with the primary source, a midline sphincterotomy should be done. Otherwise, bilateral abscesses should be drained to deal urgently with sepsis and leave the fistula to be dealt with subsequently and in more experienced hands if necessary.

High abscesses need to be drained in the operating room under anesthesia for good exposure. If the submucosal or high intermuscular abscess bulges into the rectal lumen, it should be drained into the rectum. A small (1 × 1 cm) window overlying the abscess should be excised for biopsy as well as for prolonging drainage and to delay premature healing of the incision. A supralevator abscess pointing into the rectum may be drained in a similar fashion. But if it has tracked caudad into the ischiorectal fossa, as it often does, it should be drained through ischiorectal space, providing it with dependent drainage. A supralevator abscess should never be drained both through the rectum as well as externally as this will result in an extrasphincteric fistula, which is extremely difficult if not impossible to cure later on.[3]

The natural history of anorectal abscesses after early drainage is as follows: (a) It may heal and never recur; (b) It may heal and recur at the same area, months or years later; or (c) It may never heal and remain as a persistent draining sinus. The latter two scenarios signify the presence of a fistula. Therefore,

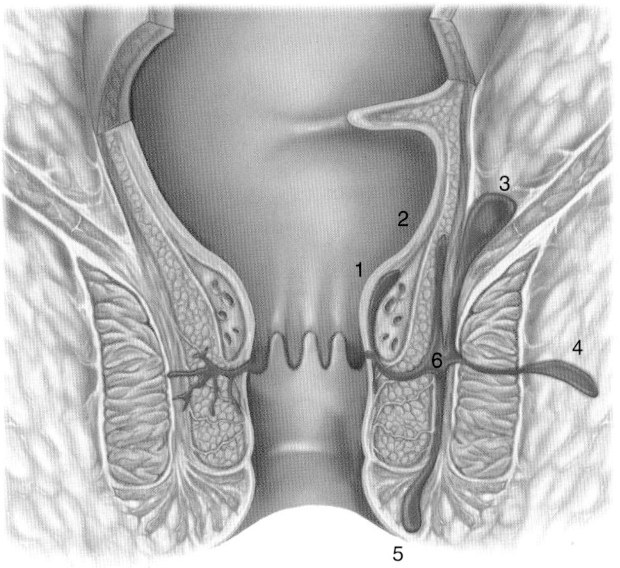

FIGURE 41.1. Left: Anal glands opening in anal crypts. Right: Extension of abscess to adjacent spaces: *1*. Submucosal; *2*. High intermuscular; *3*. Supralevator; *4*. Ischiorectal; *5*. Perianal; 6. Intersphincteric.

in select cases when a fistula is identified at the time of abscess drainage and the portion of the sphincter mechanism overlying the fistula tract is very small, the surgeon may elect to perform a primary fistulotomy. This will treat the fistulous abscess definitively, shorten sick days, minimize morbidity, and prevent recurrences.[4] However, primary fistulotomy in inexperienced hands may result in unintended extensive sphincterotomy and subsequent fecal incontinence. Therefore, when a fistula is identified but the surgeon is uncertain about its extent and complexity, it is best to place a nonabsorbable braided suture (No. 1 or 2 silk) or silastic (vessel) loop into the tract, tying it loosely as a draining Seton. This will provide long-term drainage, prevent recurrence of abscess, and allow the definitive treatment of the fistula to be postponed to a later date or referral to a more experienced surgeon.[5,6]

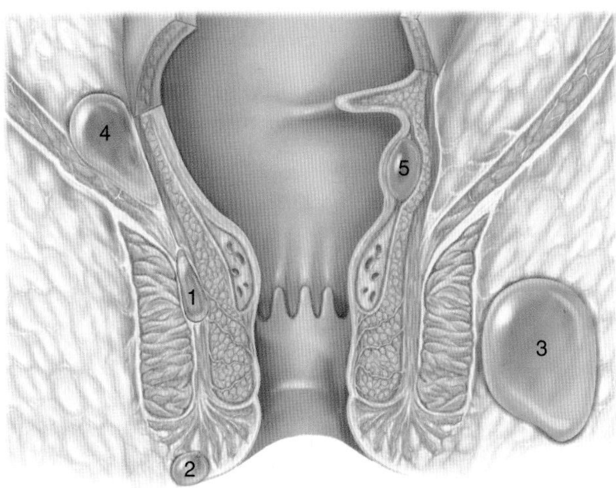

FIGURE 41.2. High abscesses: *1*. Intersphincteric; *2*. Perianal; *3*. Ischiorectal; *4*. Supralevator; *5*. Submucosal/intermuscular.

FOURNIER'S GANGRENE

Fournier's gangrene or synergistic perianal or scrotal gangrene was first described in 1883. The symptoms and tissue necrosis may evolve rapidly, within a few hours in young men, or follow a more insidious course lasting 2–3 days in the elderly. Enriquez et al.,[7] in a retrospective comparison of Fournier's gangrene, found that those secondary to GI causes had slower onset than those related to GU causes.

The illness typically begins with perianal, scrotal or penile pain, swelling, fevers, chills, and urinary retention. Symptoms may be present for a few days but the patient may present with septic shock without anorectal or urogenital complaints. A careful history must be taken to elicit presence of comorbidities, especially instrumentation, unusual sexual practices, HIV, and most importantly, diabetes mellitus which is present in over 50% of the patients.

Physical examination reveals gross swelling of perineum, penis, scrotum, and gluteal regions (Fig. 41.3). Overlying skin may show purpura, necrosis (black spots), and is often associated with crepitus. In extreme cases, these signs may extend to thighs, groins, lower abdominal wall, and anterior or posterior chest wall. The area may be exquisitely tender but necrotic skin is often anesthetic. Spontaneous drainage from watery brown liquid to frank pus may occur and is associated with characteristic feculent odor. Signs and symptoms of systemic toxicity such as fever, tachycardia, hypotension, or altered mental status may be present.

In a compilation of 164 cases of Fournier's gangrene from the literature, Cataldo found 41% to be of GI and 30% from GU sources. In 36% of patients, the cause was not identified.[8] Given the frequency of GI causes, that is, abscess–fistulas, it is easy to picture the spread of infection penetrating Colles fascia, leading to scrotal gangrene. On the other hand, if Fournier's gangrene is a result of subclinical urinary extravasation (e.g., instrumentation), the infected urine spreads to corpus cavernosum and penetrates tunica albuginea, leading to involvement of Buck's fascia. Once Buck's fascia is transgressed, involvement of Dartos fascia follows. Dartos fascia is an extension of Colles fascia, which itself is an extension of Scarpa's fascia of the abdominal wall. Thus, infection may easily spread to the buttocks, thighs, groins, and along the abdominal wall.[9]

In cases of GI origin, gram-negative bacteria and Bacteroides species predominate; whereas in cases due to GU origin, *Escherichia coli* and Streptococcus species are most common.

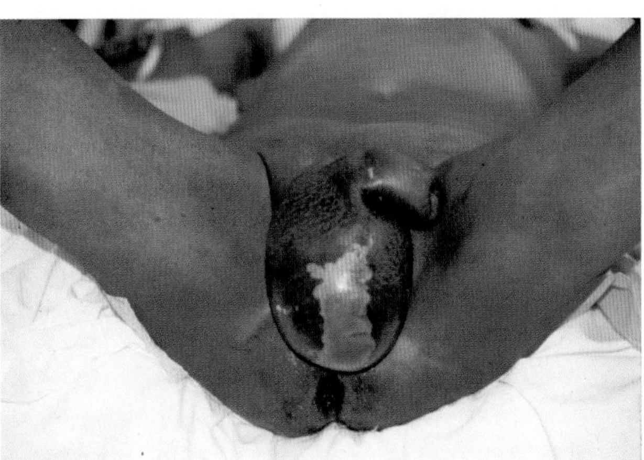

FIGURE 41.3. Fournier's gangrene involving bilateral ischiorectal fossa and scrotum.

In trauma-related cases, Staphylococcus and Streptococcus predominate. Irrespective of the source, bacterial synergism results in recovery of multiple types of organisms in over 80% of the cases, which includes Clostridial species as well. Pseudomonas is the most common pathogen found in gangrene associated with hematologic malignancies.[10,11] Just as there is no need for imaging studies to diagnose Fournier's gangrene, detailed, time-consuming bacterial cultures are often unnecessary as long as the treatment plan includes broad antibiotic coverage.

Treatment of Fournier's gangrene includes systemic resuscitation and support, broad-spectrum antibiotics, wide surgical excision, and debridement with delayed wound closure. Hyperbaric oxygen (HBO) therapy can be used as an adjunct but not in lieu of the above measures.

Systemic support includes administration of fluids and electrolytes, glucose control, and, in cases of septic shock, placement of central lines and pressors, as indicated. Broad-spectrum antibiotics to provide coverage for gram-negative rods, anaerobes, and clostridial species are essential. Surgical therapy includes debridement and excision of all necrotic areas. Lithotomy position allows access to perianal, perineal, external genital regions, as well as both groins and thighs. Debridement should be carried out to bleeding tissue. Anal sphincters and testicles are usually spared and need not be excised (Fig. 41.4).

In general, it is good policy to return to the OR in 24 hours to explore for further necrotic tissue left behind especially in questionable areas. If the patient remains febrile with elevated WBC, ESR, or CRP, a reexploration in 24–48 hours is mandatory. Suprapubic cystostomy is indicated for gross urinary leak (e.g., ureteral rupture 2° dilation of a stricture). Diverting colostomy should be reserved for patients in whom fecal contamination is a major problem. After initial aggressive debridement, the patient should be maintained on broad-spectrum antibiotics. Nutritional support is essential to aggressively combat the catabolic state.

HBO therapy has been used in the management of Fournier's gangrene. Even though the use of HBO is logically justified, no prospective randomized trials have been performed to study the efficacy of HBO. Published reports have dealt with small patient groups. HBO may be beneficial as bactericidal by increasing subcutaneous neovascularity, enhancing phagocytosis, inhibiting the production of Clostridial alphatoxins, bacteriostatic effect on many anaerobes (Bacteroids, Peptococcus, Peptostreptococcus) and actual bactericidal effect on Clostridium spores.

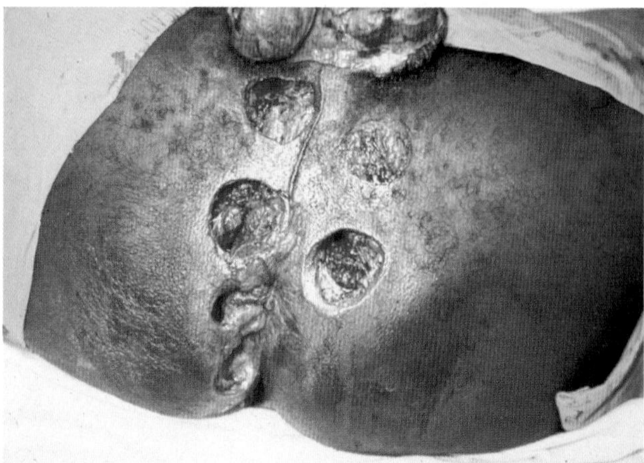

FIGURE 41.4. Same patient after third surgical intervention. Note scrotal debridement and multiple ischiorectal fossa counterincisions.

Fournier's gangrene remains a potentially lethal disease. Presence of advanced age, diabetes, alcoholism, and malignancy are associated with higher mortality.[12] Higher mortality in Fournier's gangrene of GI origin (28%) versus those secondary to GU disease (10%) has been reported.[6] Therefore, every effort must be made to control the spread of infection through wide debridement, supported with broad-spectrum antibiotics, nutritional support, and HBO. The survivors may undergo plastic and reconstructive operations, often in multiple stages, to provide skin coverage and preserve function.

ANAL FISSURE

The role of acute care and surgery in anal fissure is usually in two separate and distinct phases of the disease.

1. Acute anal fissure causes severe pain, which may last for hours following bowel movement and can be quite disabling. Gentle eversion of the anal canal by lateral traction on the buttocks generally helps in the diagnosis of midline anal fissure. In its acute stage, the base of this fissure is quite pink (corrugator ani muscle). Digital rectal examination is very painful, totally unnecessary, and must be avoided. Acute anal fissure will respond to bowel management (softening the stool), warm sitz baths, and use of "chemical sphincterotomy," a term used often to describe use of nitroglycerine, calcium channel blockers, and botulinum toxin in reducing the spasm and contracture of the internal sphincter which is the source of prolonged pain after defecation. 2% Diltiazem gel, 0.3% Nifedipine ointment, and 0.2% nitroglycerine ointment applied on anal surface two to three times daily often provides rapid pain relief. The main problem with all medications used to lower internal sphincter pressure is that even though temporarily effective, none is durable and the symptoms of fissure will recur in over 50% of the cases, necessitating surgical management.[13,14]
2. Chronic anal fissure can be just as painful as acute anal fissure. Gentle examination reveals that the midline fissure is lined with white fibers of the internal sphincter. It is unlikely for the medical management to succeed in such cases and elective lateral internal sphincterotomy is often necessary. Long-standing anal fissures may be associated with low intersphincteric abscess caused by infection undermining the posterior midline internal sphincter. Swelling, erythema, purulent drainage, or fluctuations are signs that mandate urgent surgical intervention. A minimal posterior midline internal sphincterotomy is all that is needed to unroof the abscess and lower the internal sphincter pressure permanently, allowing the fissure to heal. "Conservative" care using antibiotics, sitz baths, and analgesics are usually ineffective and delay the inevitable surgical procedure needed for permanent cure. There is minimal risk of fecal incontinence in conservative posterior midline fissurotomy and intersphincteric fistulectomy.

HEMORRHOIDS

Pelvic sepsis following rubber band ligation of hemorrhoids is a serious and potentially lethal complication if not diagnosed early and treated aggressively. Russell and Donahue originally described this complication in four patients. The warning signs of incipient pelvic sepsis are increasing pain after banding and dysuria or urinary retention. Spread of infection in perirectal tissues and pelvis is usually followed by septic shock and death.[15] If a patient complains of increasing pain after rubber band ligation of internal hemorrhoids, which is usually a painless procedure, he/she needs to be immediately examined, especially if worsening pain is associated with dysuria. Examination under anesthesia shows the necrotic hemorrhoid often with the rubber band still in place, surrounded by an irregular grayish area, which is the spreading submucosal infection. The band must be removed, the necrotic tissue debrided to bleeding tissue at depth and periphery, leaving the wound open to heal by secondary intention. Intravenous broad-spectrum antibiotics should be administered and the patient monitored for signs and symptoms of sepsis.[16] Colostomy is unnecessary but repeat debridement is indicated if the patient remains septic. In the absence of aggressive therapy, death from septic shock may result.

Uncomplicated hemorrhoids generally do not cause infectious complications except when there is circumferential, prolapsed internal and thrombosed external hemorrhoids. These set of findings have been coined "acute hemorrhoidal disease" by Salvati.[17] This can be seen after severe traveler's diarrhea or in women who had undergone a prolonged, difficult vaginal delivery with instrumentation. Erosion of thrombosed hemorrhoids or pressure necrosis of the skin from large thrombosis may lead to a superficial abscess. The abscess must be drained but the remainder of circumferential hemorrhoids need not be excised acutely to avoid excessive excision of anoderm and postoperative anal stricture. It is best to inject the edematous hemorrhoids with a mixture of lidocaine, epinephrine, and hyaluronidase. The latter chemical breaks down tissue barriers and causes immediate spread and dissipation of the edema with resolution of symptoms.[17]

PILONDIAL CYST/ABSCESS

Is an acquired condition unrelated to the anorectum. However, when acutely infected, it required expeditious incision and drainage to prevent spread of infection. Waiting for the abscess to "point," results in the infection spreading through normal uninvolved skin. Large pilonidal abscesses should be drained and not excised primarily because there is a tendency to excise the edematous area of cellulitis, leaving wounds two to three times larger than if the same cyst is excised when quiescent. Infected cysts, especially in cases of hirsute patients, recurrent infections, free drainage of pus, and lateral extension of the abscess must be treated with only excision and not subjected to a variety of plastic surgical closures due to high failure of wound closures.[18]

References

1. Abcarian H. Acute suppuratious of anorectum. *Surg Ann.* 1975;8:305-333.
2. Abcarian H, Eftaiha M. Floating free-standing anus: a complication of massive anorectal infection. *Dis Colon Rectum.* 1983;25:516-521.
3. Prasad ML, Abcarian H, Read DR. Supralevator abscess. Diagnosis and treatment. *Dis Colon Rectum.* 1981;24:456-462.
4. McElwain JW, McLean MD, Alexander RM, et al. Experience with primary fistulotomy for anorectal abscess. a report of 1000 cases. *Dis Colon Rectum.* 1975;18:646-649.
5. Ramanujam PS, Prasad ML, Abcarian H, et al. Perianal abscess and fistula. a study of 1023 patients. *Dis Colon Rectum.* 1984;7:593-597.
6. Ramanujam PS, Prasad ML, Abcarian H. The role of seton in fistulotomy of the anus. *Surg Gynec Obstet.* 1983;157:419-423.
7. Enriquez JM, Moreno S, DeVasa M. Fournier's syndrome of urogenital and anorectal origin. *Dis Colon Rectum.* 1987;33:33-37.
8. Cataldo PA. Fournier's Gangrene. In Surgery of the Anus, Rectum and Colon: Mazier, Levien, Luchtefeld and Senagore editors. W.B. Saunders Company, Philadelphia, PA, 1995. pp.986-993.
9. Spirnak JP, Resnick MI, Hampel N. Fournier's gangrene: report of 20 patients. *J Urol.* 1984;31:289-291.
10. Mackowiak PA. Microbial synergism in human infection. *N Eng J Med.* 1978;298:83.
11. Roberts DS. Synergic mechanisms in certain mixed infections. *J Infect Dis.* 1969;120:720.
12. Drake SG, King AM, Stack WK. Gas gangrene and related infection: classification, clinical features and aetiology, management and mortality. a report of 88 cases. *Br J Surg.* 1977;64:104-112.
13. Nelson RL. Systemic review of medical therapy for anal fissure. *Dis Colon Rectum.* 2004;47:422-431.
14. Richard CS, Gregoire R, Plewes EA, et al. Internal sphincterotomy is superior to topical nitroglycerin in the treatment of chronic anal fissure: results of a randomized, controlled trial by the Canadian Colorectal Surgical Trials Group. *Dis Colon Rectum.* 2000;43:1048-1057.
15. Russell TR, Donahue JH. Hemorrhoid banding. A warning. *Dis Colon Rectum.* 1985;28:291-293.
16. Quevedo-Bonilla G, Farkas AM, Abcarian H, et al. Septic complications of hemorrhoidal banding. *Arch Surg.* 1988;123:650-651.
17. Eisenstat T, Salvati EP, Rubin RJ. The outpatient management of acute hemorrhoidal disease. *Dis Colon Rectum.* 1979;22:351-357.
18. Eftaiha M, Abcarian H. The surgical treatment of pilonidal disease. *Dis Colon Rectum.* 1977;20:279-286.

CHAPTER 42 ABDOMINAL WALL HERNIAS: EMERGENCIES AND RECONSTRUCTION

TIMOTHY C. FABIAN AND MARTIN A. CROCE

INTRODUCTION

There are few conditions that test the combination of a surgeon's critical care skills, technical ability, and judgment more than a patient with an open abdomen. Successful management depends on appropriate initial operative intervention, temporary abdominal wall coverage (depending upon the etiology for open abdomen), delivery of surgical critical care, management of complications, and definitive abdominal wall reconstruction (AWR). The current chapter will address these issues. We will discuss acute abdominal wall coverage as it relates to the etiology of the defect and methods for temporary closure. Different options for definitive abdominal wall management will be presented, including technical points for reconstruction. Finally, data regarding outcomes for AWR will be presented.

Acute Coverage: Etiology

Abbreviated Laparotomy for Trauma. The concept of abbreviated laparotomy for critically injured patients was described by Stone et al.[1] in 1983. They described the concept of addressing life threatening hemorrhage quickly followed by immediate closure of the abdomen without definitive management of the hollow organ or other abdominal injuries. Ligation of injured bowel segments to control contamination was recommended. Gauze packing of major hepatic injury or other areas of the abdomen with "nonsurgical bleeding" was used to control hemorrhage. Patients later returned to the operating room when hemodynamically stable for definitive management—bowel resection and anastomoses, ostomy creation, omental packing of hepatic wounds, etc. These investigators demonstrated improved survival in patients who had laparotomy terminated as rapidly as possible to avoid further hemorrhage and its sequelae—particularly coagulopathy. The concept of traumatic coagulopathy was subsequently expanded upon by Moore[2] who referred to the "bloody vicious cycle" of metabolic acidosis, hypothermia, and progressive coagulopathy. Subsequently, the term "damage control" was introduced by Rotondo et al.[3] to describe the abbreviated laparotomy as initially reported by Stone.

While the concept of abbreviated laparotomy undoubtedly has saved numerous lives, it was not without its own problems; we have in some sense traded morbidity for decreased mortality. Some patients had temporary abdominal closure with prosthetic material. Usually, this material was polypropylene mesh. Contact with the underlying bowel sometimes led to fistula formation, especially if the mesh was left long enough to allow ingrowth of granulation tissue.[4] If the skin was simply closed over the mesh, the mesh frequently became infected.[5-7] Other patients still underwent attempts at abdominal closure, with the hope that abdominal closure would allow the gauze packing to effectively tamponade exsanguinating hemorrhage. The packing was effective, but the increased abdominal pressure led to a series of physiologic perturbations. Profound respiratory failure, renal failure, and subsequent cardiovascular collapse were observed, leading to the recognition of the entity "abdominal compartment syndrome" (ACS).

Abdominal Compartment Syndrome. While compartment syndrome may occur anywhere in the body, it is more likely to develop in anatomic compartments with low compliance.[8] Common anatomic sites are extremities, the intracranial vault, and the abdomen. Regardless of location, the most likely final common pathway is an ischemia/reperfusion injury (Algorithm 42.1). Endothelial damage from ischemia/injury initiates a series of inflammatory cascades resulting in the loss of endothelial cell tight junctions and subsequent interstitial edema and cellular swelling. Continued ischemia further exacerbates the hyperinflammatory response, resulting in continued ischemia. Reperfusion, with its attendant neutrophil activation and oxygen-free radical production, further accelerates the cellular damage and interstitial edema. This causes dramatic increase in interstitial edema, resulting in alterations in microvascular blood flow. Typically, pressures around 25 mm Hg are necessary for reduction in microvascular flow. Left untreated, this cascade of events usually leads to cellular death in the compartment. It is important to realize that the detrimental edema and microvascular flow alterations require reperfusion; that is, resuscitation from shock. This phenomenon is most evident following revascularization of the lower extremity following vascular injury. If four compartment fasciotomies are performed prior to vascular repair, minimal swelling of the muscle is seen. However, when fasciotomies follow vascular repair, the muscle typically will bulge.

The pathophysiology of the ACS is similar. ACS may be viewed as a global ischemia/reperfusion injury, resulting in significant visceral edema. The three characteristics of ACS are respiratory insufficiency, decreased splanchnic flow, and diminished renal function. In a series of experiments in dogs, Richardson and Trinkle[9] created a model of progressive intra-abdominal hypertension (IAH). This linear pressure increase resulted in a dramatic increase in peak inspiratory pressures, decreased cardiac output, and venous hypertension in both the inferior vena cava and renal veins; all at an abdominal pressure of 25 mm Hg. These findings were confirmed in a porcine model by Diebel et al.[10] They demonstrated that increased abdominal pressures reduced cardiac output (without alterations in pulmonary artery occlusion pressures), decreased superior mesenteric arterial flow, and decreased mucosal pH.

The three types of ACS are primary, secondary, and recurrent. *Primary ACS* typically follows injury, shock and resuscitation, and laparotomy (either abbreviated with or without gauze packing); this type is most commonly seen. *Secondary ACS* is typically seen in patients who receive massive fluid resuscitation following severe injury,[11] burns, or resuscitation from sepsis.[12] Secondary ACS was originally described by Maxwell et al.[11] in seven patients who developed ACS without previous laparotomy. All patients had dramatic improvement

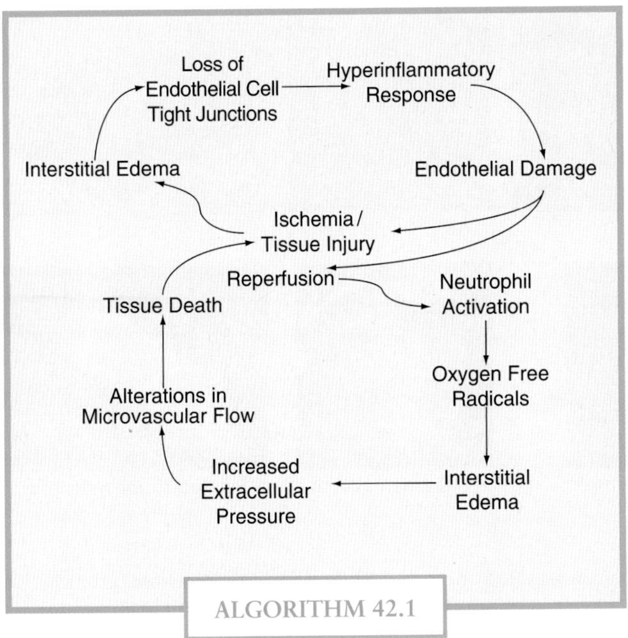

ALGORITHM 42.1 Ischemia/reperfusion injury.

following abdominal decompression. *Recurrent ACS* (formerly called tertiary ACS) is ACS, which recurs after initial treatment; likely due either to inadequate initial treatment or ongoing tissue ischemia.

In suspected cases with the clinical scenario of ACS, the diagnosis may be confirmed by measurement of the bladder pressure, which reflects abdominal pressure. There are many ways to measure bladder pressure,[13-16] and there are currently commercially available kits that allow continuous measurements. The World Society of the Abdominal Compartment Syndrome (www.wsacs.org) has offered standard definitions of IAH based on the intra-abdominal pressure (IAP) and standard methods of pressure measurement.[17] There are four proposed grades of IAH:

Grade I:	IAP 12–15 mm Hg
Grade II:	IAP 16–20 mm Hg
Grade III:	IAP 21–25 mm Hg
Grade IV:	IAP >25 mm Hg

Abdominal perfusion pressure (APP), which is analogous to cerebral perfusion pressure, may also be calculated:

$$\text{APP} = \text{mean arterial pressure} - \text{IAP}$$

Some have suggested that the APP is an accurate predictor of abdominal visceral perfusion.[18,19] A target APP of at least 60 mm Hg is associated with improved survival in patients with IAH and ACS.[18] ACS may be defined as sustained IAP > 20 mm Hg (with or without an APP < 60 mm Hg) that is associated with new organ dysfunction.[17] The management of patients with ACS is the same as for patients with compartment syndrome of any other body area; decompression. This, of course, results in a patient with an open abdomen. In less severe cases, nonoperative therapy may be beneficial.[20,21]

Severe Intra-abdominal Infection. There are instances when adequate source control may not be possible with a single laparotomy. Diseases such as perforated diverticulitis and necrotizing pancreatitis may result in diffuse suppurative peritonitis. Leaving the abdomen open in such instances allows easier access for repeat laparotomy for irrigation, debridement of nonviable tissue, and ultimately, source control. This practice of repeat laparotomy has not been shown to improve patient outcome in controlled trials.[22,23] Nonetheless, it has its proponents and may be performed in the operating room or at the bedside in the ICU in selected cases.[24-26] More importantly, repeat laparotomy is frequently required to obtain effective source control, and the open abdomen can avoid the development of ACS in these critically ill septic patients.

Mesenteric Ischemia. The management of patients with acute mesenteric ischemia is facilitated by use of the open abdomen. The "second look" procedure allows assessment of bowel viability and resection of ischemic or necrotic segments, if necessary.[27] Ward et al.[28] demonstrated improved outcome in patients with delayed bowel anastomosis and repeat laparotomy. Park et al. demonstrated improved survival with bowel resection at either the first or second look procedure.[29] By leaving the abdomen open, even in the patient deemed low risk for development of ACS, the fascial edges are spared repeat fascial closures and necrotic fascial edges.

Abdominal Wall Loss. Necrotizing soft tissue infections of the abdominal wall are devastating disease processes. Adequate source control requires prompt diagnosis and operative intervention, which may necessitate debridement of large portions of the abdominal wall.[30,31] Interestingly, this problem has decreased in frequency with more liberal uses of the open abdomen. Leaving the abdomen open avoids tight fascial closure. This tight closure may result in strangulation of the fascia, which can serve as a nidus for infection in contaminated wounds.

Other causes of abdominal wall loss include shotgun blasts and high-velocity gunshot wounds. It is imperative to adequately debride these wounds. In the case of shotgun injuries, the shell and wadding are frequently imbedded in the tissue and must be removed. In the case of high velocity injuries, the missile tract should be debrided of nonviable tissue. The kinetic energy imparted to the tissue will cause more extensive injury, and these wounds frequently result in significant tissue loss. These wounds should be reexamined frequently, because they often will require further debridement.

Acute Coverage: Options. The primary goal of acute, temporary coverage of the open abdomen is protection of the underlying viscera. This should be accomplished without compromising the fascia in anticipation of subsequent abdominal closure or reconstruction. Effective temporary closure allows control of fluid losses and helps reduce the catabolism associated with large wounds. To these ends, there are a number of options for temporary closure. The primary options are plastic, absorbable mesh, a vacuum device, skin, and nonabsorbable mesh (Fig. 42.1).

Plastic Closure. One of the easiest devices to use for temporary abdominal closure is a sterile 2-L IV infusion bag. Surgeons in Colombia described its use years ago for temporary abdominal closure; hence the term "Bogotá bag." Another plastic device for acute coverage is the x-ray cassette cover. These are inexpensive, readily available, and can cover a large area if necessary. Plastic temporary closure is a short-term method for coverage since it is not particularly durable. The plastic is typically sewn to the skin edges allowing for a fairly rapid closure. Another advantage to using plastic for acute coverage is it allows the underlying viscera to be visually inspected. Plastic closure is generally during the first 48–72 hours postinjury as ongoing resuscitation is necessary. If the patient survives this initial phase after injury, a more durable method of temporary abdominal closure will be necessary.

Absorbable Mesh. The use of absorbable mesh for acute coverage affords more durability for temporary closure than

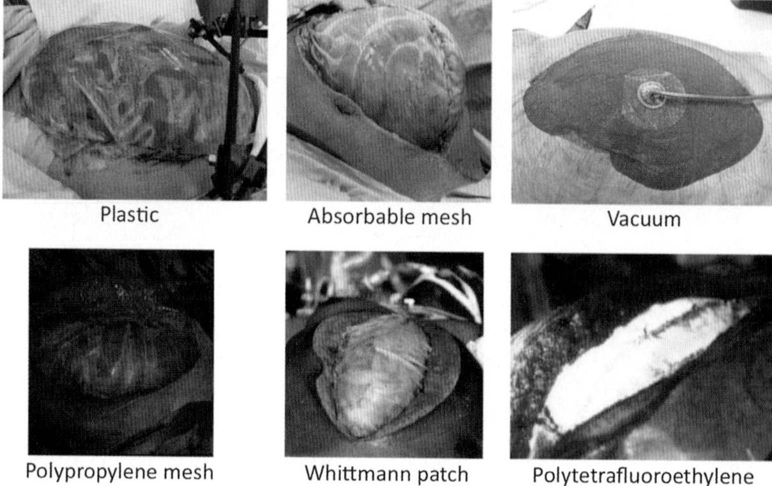

FIGURE 42.1. Six different methods of temporary abdominal closure.

does plastic. These meshes, polyglycolic acid (Dexon), and polyglactin 910 (Vicryl) may be sewn to the fascia and will prevent the progressive loss of abdominal domain that may be seen when the closure material is sewn to the skin. The authors' choice is woven polyglactin 910. It is not as elastic as polyglycolic acid or knitted polyglactin 910, but is similarly pliable. Since it does not stretch, it allows sequential pleating that can facilitate delayed fascial closure. It is important to note that pleating the mesh should be performed frequently to avoid adhesions between the viscera and abdominal wall. If the mesh is placed and no attempts are made to cinch and pleat it, adhesions will form, and the patient is destined for a planned ventral hernia. When the mesh is ready to be removed, it simply peels off the underlying viscera and early granulation tissue since there is a thin suppurative layer that forms under the mesh. In a small number of patients, there is rapid ingrowth of granulation tissue through the mesh. In these patients, skin graft may successfully be performed without attempts at mesh removal.

Vacuum Closure. Use of vacuum-assisted temporary abdominal closure is gaining in popularity due to its rapid placement and simplicity. There are also commercially available kits for vacuum-assisted closure of the abdomen. Since its original description by Brock et al.[32] in 1995, it has become one of the standards for acute coverage of the open abdomen. Whether the "homemade" vacuum device[32] or the commercial device is used, there are a number of real and theoretic advantages. Perhaps, the most important component is the sheet of plastic that is placed beneath the abdominal wall and superficial to the viscera. This sheet precludes adherence between the viscera and abdominal wall that may facilitate delayed fascial closure. Indeed, several investigators have reported high-delayed fascial closure rates for patients with vacuum-assisted acute coverage ranging from 65% to 100%.[33-35] However, only one prospective randomized study has been performed comparing vacuum with absorbable mesh for acute coverage of the open abdomen. Bee et al.[36] randomized 51 patients to either vacuum-assisted or polyglactin 910 coverage for patients with open abdomens.[36] There was no difference in delayed fascial closure rates (31% for vacuum and 26% for mesh). The lower delayed fascial closure rates occurred despite strict protocols with aggressive mesh pleating and repeated attempts at closure. It appears that the best predictor for delayed fascial closure is patient selection. It is unlikely that patients with massive visceral edema and hemorrhagic shock will undergo delayed fascial closure. On the other hand, patients without massive edema, or those left open for "second look" procedures, are excellent candidates for delayed closure. Regardless, careful attention to the abdomen with repeated attempts at closure is required to optimize delayed facial closure rates.

Nonabsorbable Mesh. Early materials for temporary abdominal coverage included polypropylene mesh. This mesh was sewn to the fascia, preventing loss of domain. It was either removed when granulation tissue began to grow through the interstices or left in place. If removed, a split-thickness skin graft was placed over the wound. If left in place, full-thickness skin and subcutaneous tissue were typically mobilized and reapproximated. This method had the advantage of eliminating a large ventral hernia. There were two problems with this management; fistula formation and mesh extrusion. Fistula rates around 20% were reported, with progressive mesh extrusion even higher over time.[4,5,37] Since there are better alternatives available, there is little need for polypropylene mesh for acute coverage of the abdomen. Another nonabsorbable option is use of the plastic artificial burr (Wittmann patch). Velcro-type sheets are sutured to the fascial edges and allowed stepwise reapproximation of the fascia. Investigators have reported high-delayed fascial closure rates.[38] A modification described by Fantus involves placement of a plastic sheet beneath the abdominal wall, similar to the vacuum device, to prevent adhesions and facilitate closure.[39]

Skin Closure. In patients with relatively small fascial defects where delayed fascial closure cannot be accomplished, there are basically three options: allow the wound to granulate, place a split-thickness skin graft, or mobilize skin and subcutaneous tissue for approximation. The latter allows a better cosmetic result, but does not change the need for ultimate ventral hernia repair. Split-thickness skin grafting provides optimal coverage for large defects and is a key component in the staged management of AWR as described later. A subset of patients may benefit from immediate skin reapproximation with a series of towel clips or suture. This closure can be beneficial in patients without significant visceral edema and are at low risk for the development of ACS. For example, patients with acute mesenteric ischemia and a "second look" procedure may be ideal candidates for initial towel clip closure.

Complications. Given the fact that patients managed with an open abdomen are critically ill and injured, it is not surprising that complications are not uncommon. Most are related to the wound. Patients who have acute coverage material sewn to the skin may develop skin edge necrosis, a relatively minor problem. For those patients with the material sewn to the fascial edge, development of fascial necrosis may be a more serious issue. Both require debridement back to healthy, viable tissue.

Some patients have a persistent systemic inflammatory state, which precludes adequate mobilization of fluids. This results in persistent visceral edema along with an edematous, nonpliable abdominal wall. Regardless of the method of temporary abdominal closure, these patients will not undergo delayed fascial closure. Adhesions will develop between the viscera and abdominal wall, creating a "frozen abdomen." When this occurs, it is imperative to obtain biologic coverage of the open, granulating viscera. This is best accomplished with split-thickness skin grafting. Wound coverage will reduce the catabolic demand of the open abdomen[40] and reduce the incidence of formation of enteroatmospheric fistula.

An enterocutaneous fistula is an epithelialized communication between the gastrointestinal tract and the skin. An enteroatmospheric fistula is a hole in the bowel that is exposed in an open abdomen. Should such a fistula occur before the open abdomen has granulated, the management is resection; this is a rare occurrence and is usually the result of a technical failure. The new anastomosis should be buried beneath viable tissue (loops of bowel or the abdominal wall) so that none of the suture line is exposed. Unfortunately, most of the enteroatmospheric fistulae occur in patients with a frozen abdomen, making reoperation precarious at best.

In a prospective study on temporary abdominal closure, Bee et al.[36] noted an increased rate of fistulae in patients managed with vacuum closure. Further analysis identified the subgroup more prone to fistula development; patients with tube jejunostomies, placed either for nutrition or for management of duodenal injury. These fistulae were likely due to the plastic drape, which is effective in preventing adhesion formation. While adhesion prevention is advantageous when trying to gradually close an abdomen, adhesion formation between viscera and the abdominal wall is beneficial when patients have tube enterostomies. It is our current practice to avoid vacuum temporary closure in patients with tube enterostomies.

Prevention, of course, is the best course of action. The longer the granulating abdomen is left open, the greater chance for a fistula.[40,41] Jernigan et al.[40] demonstrated a significant association between a prolonged open granulating abdomen and fistula formation. In their series of 274 patients initially managed with an open abdomen, 129 patients either survived with an open abdomen or had fascial closure. Ten of these patients developed a fistula and had skin grafting almost 10 days later than those without a fistula. Thus, early grafting is important for fistula prevention.

Fischer et al.[42] evaluated 2,224 patients who had laparotomy for trauma and found 43 patients with fistulae (1.9%). The fistula rate for the 380 patients with an open abdomen was 8.4%; nearly 70% occurred prior to skin grafting. Of note, 37% of the fistulae closed spontaneously. Management of these patients is difficult; control of the enteric output and support of nutrition are paramount. Control may be obtained by various tubes placed in the fistula, but this is rarely completely successful and often enlarges the size of the enterostomy (Fig. 42.2).

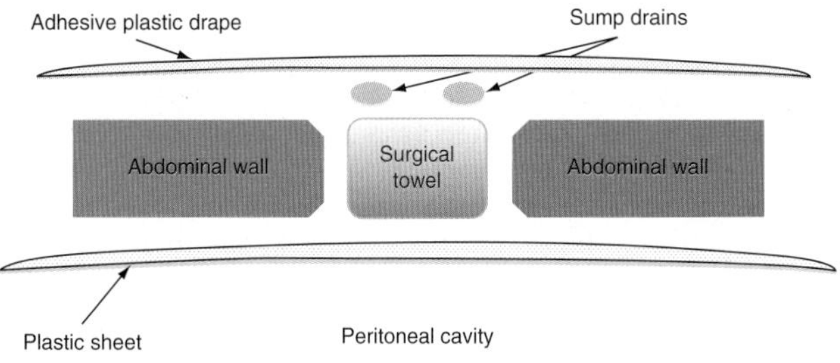

FIGURE 42.2. Vacuum dressing for management of open abdominal wound.

The bowel is protected, and the sponge is cut around the fistula; this allows output control. Skin grafting may be possible around the fistula so that an ostomy bag may be placed. As long as nutrition can be maintained, these patients can then undergo fistula resection at the time of AWR.

DEFINITIVE ABDOMINAL WALL RECONSTRUCTION

There are several issues to consider in determination of the proper time for AWR following damage control operations. Ideally, secondary fascial closure can be undertaken during the initial hospitalization. Secondary closure eliminates the need for rehospitalization for reconstruction and its attendant morbidity and costs. Gradual pleating of the prosthetic bridge will permit secondary fascial closure in some patients. When negative pressure therapy has been used, secondary closure rates up to 90% have been reported.[33] Others have experienced much lower success, approximating 25%.[36] While all of the reasons for such disparity are not entirely clear, it is likely in part related to institutional biases for performing temporary abdominal closure. Those institutions that have liberal indications will perform temporary closure in less severely injured patients than in those centers with more conservative criteria. Less severely injured patients will develop less intestinal edema and will consequently have high-fascial closure rates following the index laparotomy. Other contributing factors might include fluid resuscitation protocols, and the degree of aggressiveness applied to fascial reapproximation.

Another approach to achieve abdominal closure during the initial hospitalization for those patients, in whom fascial reapproximation is not possible, is hernia repair with prosthesis prior to discharge. Since the wounds are heavily contaminated with ICU pathogens, the use of synthetic meshes is prohibited. Biologic meshes have been utilized for these reconstructions since they have been shown to be more resistant to infection than synthetics. Guy et al.[43] reported one of the initial experiences with that technique in 10 patients. Early results provided enthusiasm for that approach. Others series with limited numbers of patients and short follow-up have been reported.[44,45] While that technique has the appeal of eliminating future AWR, there are several drawbacks. Most of these patients are very early in their recovery from massive insults and hernia repair at that time adds further insult. They are relatively immunocompromised, and their healing ability is likely impaired. It would be anticipated that hernia repair failure rate will be high when long-term follow-up is achieved.

When the open abdominal wound cannot be closed during the hospitalization for injury, the patient becomes a candidate for delayed AWR. The intestinal contents are covered with skin during convalescence. Occasionally, full-thickness skin and subcutaneous fat are mobile enough to cover the open wound; more commonly, STSG is required. The length of the interval from hospital discharge to AWR must be carefully timed. Reconstruction should be delayed until the patients have recovered from their injuries and have resumed an anabolic state. If operation is done prior to resolution of dense adhesions and inflammation, results are significantly compromised and morbidity increased. Enterotomies are predictable and lead to infectious wound complications and failure of reconstruction. On the other hand, when reconstruction is excessively deferred, loss of abdominal domain progresses. Loss of domain puts more tension on the repair and increases hernia recurrence rates. AWR should generally be undertaken 6–12 months following initial wound coverage. It takes that time for dense adhesions and inflammation to resolve with the development of predominantly filmy adhesions. This process can be easily followed by examination of the wound when a STSG has been used. During the early stages, the abdominal contents can be determined by palpation to be primarily an indurated sheet with minimal ability to separate thickened bowel loops. As time passes, resolution of the induration can be appreciated on examination. Eventually, the STSG can be pinched between the examiner's fingers and loosed adhesions appreciated along with the separation of nonindurated small bowel loops. Those findings signal the correct time for AWR.

METHODS OF RECONSTRUCTION

Two basic types of procedures are employed for delayed reconstruction. AWR can be accomplished by either prosthetic hernia repair or autologous tissue transfer. Autologous repair of these defects is usually by a component separation technique. The majority of reconstructions in North American are done with prostheses. A major advantage of this approach is the relative simplicity of repair and the ready availability of material for fascial replacement. Significant disadvantages include prosthetic infection, gastrointestinal fistulae, and repair failure with hernia recurrence. Mesh infection and fistula formation essentially always require mesh removal, a generally unpleasant task. The subsequent, tertiary reconstruction adds another layer of difficulty and even higher failure rates. While there is less experience with components separation reconstruction, advantages of autologous tissue transfer include avoidance of implantation of foreign material with the potential for fewer septic complications and a lower fistula rate. However, autologous tissue procedures are more complex and have the potential for wound complications including skin necrosis, wound infection, and repair failure.

Prosthetic Reconstruction

A wide variety of techniques described for prosthetic hernia repair and a vast number of prosthetic materials are available. Prosthetic use has become routine over the past two decades. Prior to that, direct suture of the fascial edges resulted in a 54% failure rate for ventral herniorrhaphy.[46] Failure occurred primarily due to closure under tension. Nearly all hernias larger than 3 cm are now repaired with prostheses. In the early years of prosthetic utilization, ventral hernia repairs were most commonly done by a fascial "bridging" or "inlay" technique. Following mobilization of skin flaps and dissection and excision of the hernia sac, healthy fascial edges were defined circumferentially. The edges of the prosthetic material are sewn to the edges of the fascia with either running or interrupted suture technique. Reports with long-term follow-up revealed high recurrence rates. Failures occurred where the prostheses pulled away from the fascial edge. Those poor results paved the way for the investigation of other surgical techniques.

Initial advances were made by overlapping the prostheses 3–5 cm beyond the fascial edge. Stoppa and Rives[47,48] led the way in this innovation. They described extraperitoneal mesh placement between the rectus muscle and posterior fascia with the wide overlap. Mesh placement in such fashion leads to tension-free attachment with a large surface area for tissue incorporation. It has been subsequently demonstrated that polypropylene meshes contract up to 30% over time,[49] providing a rationale for the overlap and perhaps explaining the higher recurrence rate with bridging techniques. The Rives-Stoppa technique of overlapping mesh 3–5 cm or more beyond normal fascial edges has been deemed the "gold standard" for prosthetic repair by the American Hernia Society.[50] Intraperitoneal foreign material carries the small but real risk of gastrointestinal erosion. Novitsky et al. have supported placement between the peritoneum and posterior fascia.[9] Placement of mesh in the retrorectus position is commonly referred to as an "underlay" technique. Using Stoppa's basic premise, others began placing mesh as an "onlay" anterior to the rectus fascia. Hence, the different techniques have been variously accompanied with peritoneal or posterior fascial closure to avoid direct bowel contact. A group from the Netherlands, led by de Vries Reilingh, has made many important contributions to the field of complex ventral hernia repair. They compared onlay, inlay, and underlay techniques (Fig. 42.3).[51] The underlay technique was associated with the lowest recurrence rate, 12% compared with 44% for inlay ($p = 0.03$) 23% for onlay (NS). The onlay technique had significantly higher wound complications compared with both of the others. The underlay technique has the greatest support at this time. Up to this point, only the basic components of mesh repair have been considered. A more confusing and controversial area is the type of mesh chosen for repair.

Mesh Types

A large array of mesh products are available for AWR. The surgeon is challenged to sort out the pros and cons of the varied materials. Unfortunately, there is little follow-up available to make truly informed decisions regarding mesh selection. Be that as it may, a general classification will follow in an attempt to highlight properties that merit consideration when considering mesh products for AWR.

Traditionally, the ideal fascial substitute was considered to possess the characteristics of strength, infection resistance, and being noncarcinogenic, and biologically inert. However, as we now know, the characteristic of being biologically inert has instead become a desirable feature that has attracted much attention and investment. There are currently three broad mesh categories: synthetic absorbable, synthetic nonabsorbable, and biologic. An excellent review of the available products was recently published.[52]

Absorbable meshes (glycolic acid and polyglycolic acid) are an important instrument in the toolbox of the acute care surgeon. They are a serviceable adjunct for temporary abdominal closure (discussed earlier in this chapter) and for coverage of defects associated with major abdominal wall loss from trauma or infection. However, they are not appropriate for definitive AWR since they will be totally absorbed between 3 and 6 months, and result in a 100% hernia recurrence rate.

Synthetics meshes have a long and interesting surgical history. While an in-depth historical discussion is beyond the scope of this chapter, a brief synopsis will aid in appreciation of the evolution of these products. A timeline for various materials is demonstrated in Figure 42.4. Prostheses for hernia repair were introduced in the late 19th century. The earliest materials were silver.[53,54] Silver is bactericidal and was associated with low recurrence; but the material fragmented over time and that deterioration was associated with fluid accumulations and sinus tracts. Nonetheless, it was the primary material used for half of a century. The chemical element tantalum (Ta) was introduced next.[55] Tantalum is a hard, corrosion resistant, inert material. Not surprisingly, it was associated with fistulae, and its use was relatively short-lived. Polyethylene terephthalate, a polyester fiber (Dacron), enjoyed another relatively short life for hernia repair,[56] but it has had a successful run as a vascular conduit since its introduction for that purpose by Michael DeBakey.[57] Polypropylene mesh was introduced in the late 1950s as Marlex. After a run similar to silver of

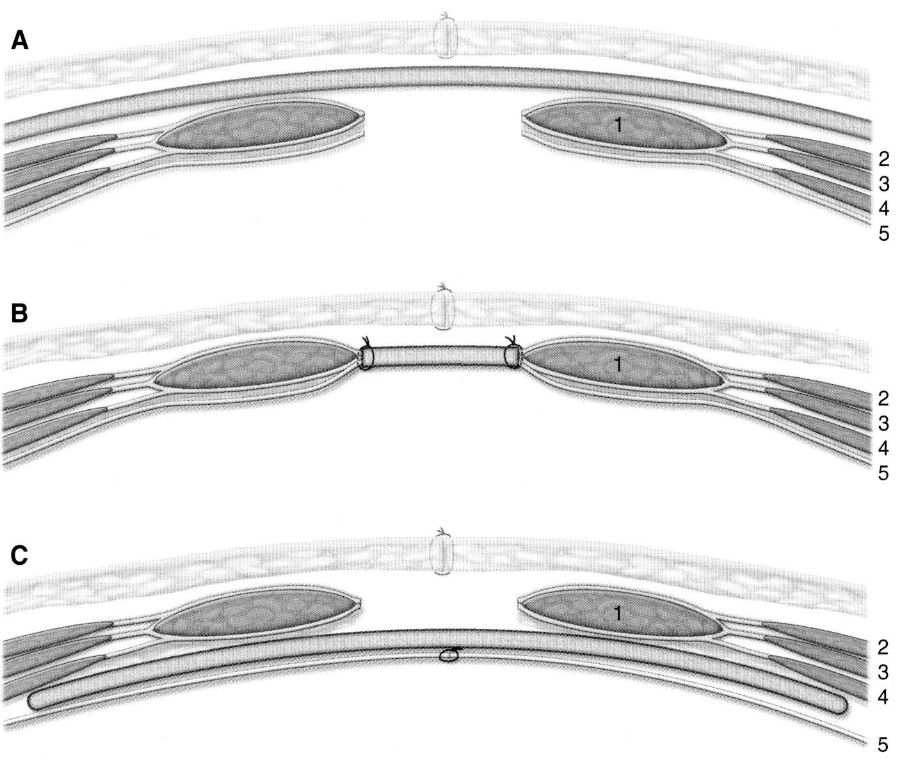

FIGURE 42.3. Reconstruction of a large incisional hernia using the (**A**) onlay, (**B**) inlay, and (**C**) underlay technique. PPM, polypropylene mesh; *1*, rectus abdominis muscle; *2*, the external oblique muscle; *3*, the internal oblique muscle; *4*, transverse muscle; *5*, peritoneum.

another half century, polypropylene has continued supremacy as the most common material used for ventral hernia repair today.[52] Polytetrafluoroethylene (PTFE) was introduced for hernia repair in 1970 and has remained the only real challenger to polypropylene as a synthetic prosthesis for hernia repairs. PTFE is a fluorocarbon that is extremely nonreactive and durable.

Polypropylene was first introduced in its heavyweight form (Marlex and Prolene) and is now also available as a lightweight mesh (Vypro). The heavyweight meshes have a tensile strength six times that of the abdominal wall, while the lightweight has strength similar to the abdominal wall.[58] Heavyweight meshes have been associated with chronic pain more frequently than those with lightweight mesh repair.[59] Data derived from implantation in animals suggest that there may be less inflammation associated with the lightweight materials and have less shrinkage and contraction over time.[60,61] However, there

Timeline of Mesh Introduction

Silver 1900
Tantalum 1948
Dacron 1956
Polypropylene 1963
PTFE 1970
ePTFE 1987

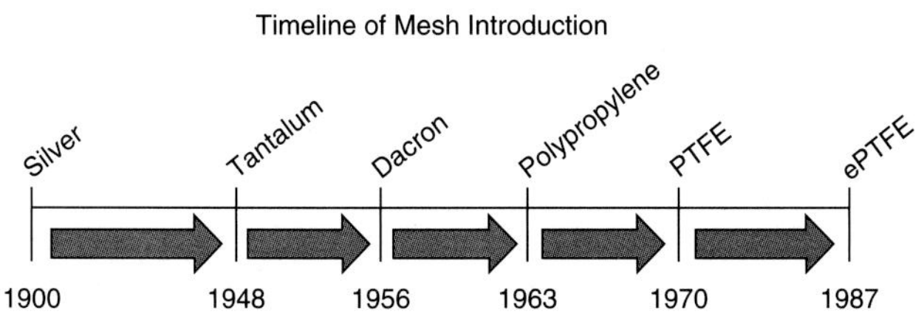

FIGURE 42.4. Timeline of mesh introduction.

is no clinical data that demonstrates clear superiority of any particular polypropylene product. It is widely accepted that polypropylene should not be placed in direct contact with the abdominal viscera.

Expanded polytetrafluoroethylene (ePTFE) provides the advantage of being biologically inert. This provides an appealing characteristic for intraperitoneal insertion. But that nonreactivity creates somewhat of a double-edged sword. ePTFE becomes incorporated to a lesser degree than polypropylene with less connective tissue ingrowth, contributing to higher recurrence rates at the mesh-fascial interface. Wound seromas are more commonly associated with ePTFE. For abdominal wall repairs, ePTFE is currently most commonly used in laparoscopic repairs or as a composite.

There are problems with both polypropylene and ePTFE meshes when used for AWR. A major drawback of polypropylene is when it is placed in the intraperitoneal surface and has potential contact with the gastrointestinal tract, there is a substantial risk for fistula to develop; fistula rates as high as 28% have been reported.[62] A disadvantage of PTFE is a tendency to not become incorporated well into the tissue. That may lead to hernia recurrences and to wound seromas. To surmount both of these shortcomings, products have been developed with coupled surfaces. The polypropylene surface is intended for use in contact with the abdominal wall fascia or muscles while the smooth PTFE side is intended for apposition to the bowel. While polypropylene is used in the major of these composite products, the undersurface has also been coated with various polymers including cellulose polymers instead of the PTFE. Another product, DualMesh, is a double-sided ePTFE prosthesis with differing surface properties on each side to allow for tissue incorporation on one and a smooth surface to avoid bowel erosion on the intra-abdominal surface. Most reports on these composites are in animal models, with the majority supporting the dual concepts of increased incorporation and decreased risk for erosion. However, there is minimal data from clinical trials to prove their superiority.

Biologic meshes were clinically introduced 20 years ago. Initial applications were for the treatment of third-degree burns, breast reconstruction, bladder slings, and an assortment of occasional reconstructive applications. They are derived from human, bovine, and porcine sources. The tissues are chemically decellularized, which leaves a lattice of collagen, elastin, and laminin for neovascularization and tissue regeneration. The primary products that are available at this time are human acellular dermal matrix (HADM), porcine acellular dermal matrix (PADM), and porcine small intestinal submucosa (PSIS). As previously noted, HADM has been used for one-stage AWR following damage control laparotomy in a small number of patients. When used for primary hernia repair, HADM has resulted in high eventration rate related to stretching of the material and 20% hernia recurrence rate when used as a reinforcement of fascial repair.[63] Eventration has not been less problematic with the other biologic meshes. HADM is harvested from cadavers, and it might be anticipated that there would be substantial variability among sections as opposed to the uniformity of synthetic materials. The PADM would seem likely to have more uniformity than HADM, but there has been minimal clinical study. Laboratory studies demonstrated that biologic prostheses placed intraperitoneally resulted in neovascularization and attained tensile strength greater than the surrounding tissues.[64] Currently, the greatest advantage for the biologic meshes is their use in contaminated fields. They resist infection to much higher degrees than synthetics; HADM may be more resistant than PSIS.[65,66] When surgical site infections develop, wounds with exposed biologic meshes can usually be managed with negative pressure dressings and mesh salvage. After a period of several weeks, neovascularization produces granulation tissue, which will be a satisfactory bed for STSG. That cannot be accomplished with synthetic meshes; the wound may clean up and even allow for skin closure. But they always become reinfected, sometimes in a few days, sometimes in a few weeks. Infected synthetic mesh requires excision.

It is important for surgeons to understand financial impacts of our management strategies. The most expensive prosthesis is HADM averaging \$26.00 per cm^2; bovine and porcine-based material cost between \$8.60 and \$22.00 per cm^2; absorbable mesh such as Vicryl and polypropylene cost \$.20 per cm^2 and \$1.00 per cm^2, respectively. A cost comparison of the different meshes demonstrated wide variation. The average size of defects resulting from temporary abdominal closure techniques that cannot be closed at the initial hospitalization has been reported from 600 to 960 cm.[36,41,67] Closure of those defects with biologic prostheses as inlays or fascial bridges would result in expenses of \$15,600-\$24,960.

Components Separation

Mesh reconstruction of the large abdominal wall defects resulting from damage control procedures is plagued by prosthetic infection and hernia recurrence. Intestinal contamination predisposes to those complications. Intestinal stomas and fistulas are common antecedents in these patients, and enterotomies during dissection at the time of AWR occur in 30%.[69] In 1990, Ramirez et al. first described the components separation technique for AWR.[30] This method of reconstruction relies on autologous tissues with local myofascial tissue advancement rather than mesh. The concept is simple and based on "relaxing incisions."

Incision of the external oblique component of the anterior rectus fascia is done bilaterally. Incision is begun in the midabdomen approximately 1–2 cm lateral to the rectus sheath. The incisions are extended superiorly over the costal margin and inferiorly to the area of the pubis. The plane between the external oblique and internal oblique muscles is then bluntly dissected laterally to the region of the anterior axillary line. The posterior rectus fascia is mobilized from the rectus abdominus muscles. This completes mobilization of the anterior rectus fascia and rectus muscle. The anterior fascia and muscle are approximated in the midline. This procedure provides advancement of approximately 10, 20, and 6 cm in the upper, mid, and lower thirds of the abdominal wound.[69] This procedure works well for moderate size hernias, but the majority of defects resulting from damage control laparotomy cannot be closed in a tension-free manner and require mesh supplement for repair. To accomplish closure of these very large defects with a minimal need for adjunctive mesh, we developed a modification of the Ramirez technique.[70]

Modified Components Separation will be described as a series of steps (Fig. 42.5).

Step 1. STSG Removal. This begins in an area that has loose adherence of graft to viscera, usually in the midabdomen. The graft is sharply incised and with a combination of blunt and sharp dissection the graft is freed from bowel, omentum, and liver. Adhesions are usually filmy, but are dense in some locations. Small areas of intact skin may be left without sequelae. There are usually dense adhesions of the skin to the liver, and caution should be taken to avoid disruption of Glisson's capsule in order to avoid troublesome bleeding. Dense adhesions are also encountered at the musculofascial junction. The STSG is excised from the abdominal wall to preserve the skin edges. Following graft excision, lysis of adhesions of viscera to the anterior abdominal wall is performed laterally to expose the posterior fascia for tissue advancement, generally to the region of the anterior axillary line. Step 1 usually takes 45–60 minutes; if adhesions are dense, this may take hours. Be prepared for a long operation and proceed with patience. Ostomy reversal is done at this time.

Step 2. Full-thickness Skin Flaps. Dissection is begun in the anatomic plane just superficial to the fascia. This is avascular except for musculocutaneous perforators. These should be preserved whenever possible to avoid wound problems associated with skin necrosis, which is rare. The flaps are raised to the area between the anterior and midaxillary lines to gain mobilization for midline closure. Meticulous hemostasis should be established to minimize infection and seroma formation.

Step3. Release of External Oblique Component of Anterior Rectus Fascia. The lateral edge of the rectus muscle is easily identified and confirmed by placing a hand in the abdomen with the palmar surface in contact with the posterior rectus sheath and the thumb on the anterior rectus sheath. In this manner, rubbing the fingers and thumb easily identifies the lateral border of the rectus muscle. A nick is made 1–2 cm lateral to that, which incises the external oblique component of the anterior rectus sheath, leaving the

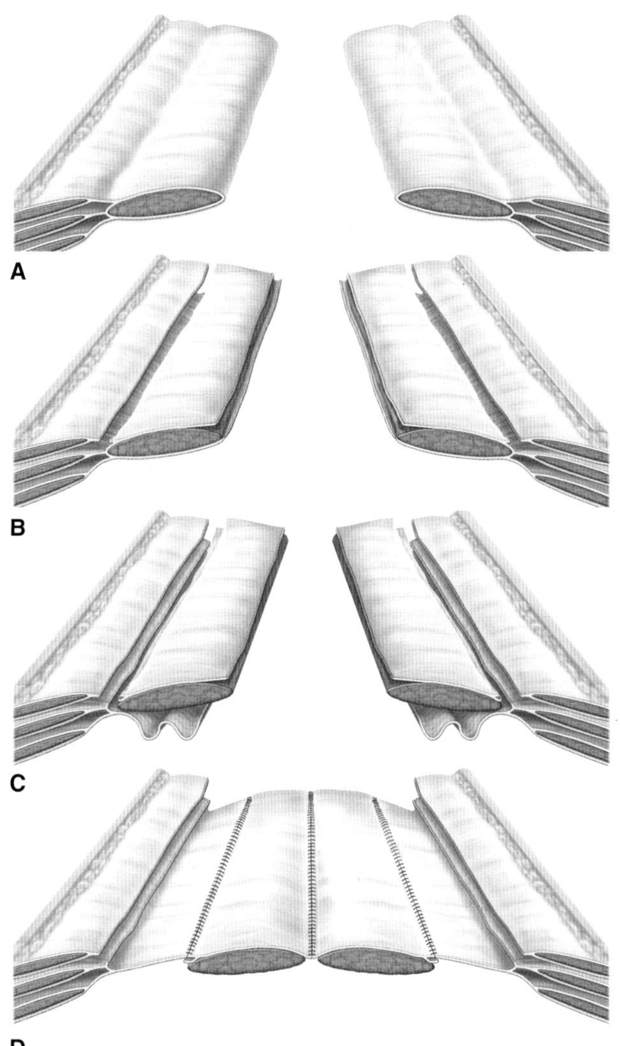

FIGURE 42.5. Modified components separation technique for AWR. (**A**) Normal anatomy above the arcuate line. (**B**) The posterior rectus sheath is mobilized from the rectus muscle, and the external oblique fascia is divided. (**C**) The internal oblique component of the anterior rectus sheath is divided down to the arcuate line. (**D**) Completed repair, suturing the medial border of the posterior sheath to the lateral border of the anterior sheath, with approximation of the medial portion of the anterior sheath in the midline.

interior oblique component intact. A hemostat is inserted, and the external oblique fascia is incised superiorly over the costal margin 5–7 cm, which results in division of some lower fibers of the serratus anterior muscle attachment. The external oblique fascia is incised inferiorly to the level of the pubis. The loose areolar tissue between the external and internal oblique muscles is then bluntly dissected to maximize medial mobilization.

Step 4. Dissection of the Posterior Rectus Sheath. The medial edge of the rectus sheath is incised for the entire length of the muscle. There is dense scar on the medial aspect that requires excision. This exposes the anterior and posterior fascia and muscle as three separate layers. The posterior sheath is freed from the muscle, the length of the muscle. Just below the umbilicus, the arcuate line can be seen, below which there is peritoneum but no posterior fascial component. The inferior epigastric vessels enter around the arcuate line, and care is necessary to avoid injury since they provide the great component of the blood supply to the rectus mechanism. Steps 1–4 comprise the Ramirez components separation, and if the wound can be closed without tension, the procedure is complete. The remaining steps make up the Memphis modification for wounds under tension.

Step 5. Release of Internal Oblique Component of the Anterior Rectus Fascia. Following release of the posterior sheath, a hand is placed between the rectus muscle and posterior sheath. With the hand cupping the muscle, the index finer should be at the most superior portion of the sheath. The anterior fascia is sharply incised over the index finger. This opens the anterior portion of the internal oblique fascia, while protecting the posterior sheath. A finger can then be seen through this incision. Using electrocautery, an incision is made through the interior oblique component of the anterior rectus fascia, stopping at the arcuate line. Further division inferiorly would create a lateral hernia defect since there is no posterior rectus fascia below this point. The rectus muscle with the adherent anterior sheath will be free medially and laterally.

Step 6. Translocation of the Anterior Fascia and Muscle. After release of the internal oblique fascia, the rectus muscle and anterior fascia will be attached only at the most superior and inferior portions. The posterior sheath remains in continuity with the native abdominal wall laterally. The rectus muscle and anterior fascia can be pulled medially, and this provides the additional mobilization gained by the modification. The medial aspect of the posterior sheath is sutured to the lateral aspect of the anterior sheath.

Step 7. Wound Closure. The anterior sheath is sutured in the midline. This results in three separate suture lines. The most difficult portion to gain adequate length is in the epigastric area. If closure cannot be accomplished without undue tension, mesh adjuncts will be required. This is necessary in 10%-20% of cases and is currently done with biologic mesh placed as an underlay. Four closed suction drains are placed and the skin closed. Abdominal binders are used in the postoperative period.

Aggressive pulmonary toilet and early mobilization are necessary postoperatively. Heavy lifting should be avoided for several months. Wound infection and necrosis of the medial skin edges are the major complications. Patients with thin body habitus are at greatest risk for skin necrosis. When major wound complications result in an open wound, negative pressure dressings are employed.

In evaluation of any surgical procedure, and especially when evaluating the success and failure rates of ventral hernia repair and AWR, careful consideration must be given to follow-up. We recently evaluated our AWR results from a 15-year experience.[71] Figure 42.6 clearly demonstrates that patients will continue to develop hernia recurrences for up to 4 years, and recurrences appear to cease at that time. Few ventral hernia studies report that duration of follow-up, and it is nonexistent for AWR following damage control procedures. This same principle applies to those patients who have secondary fascial approximation during the same hospitalization as the temporary abdominal closure, or when biologic mesh repair is done during the initial hospitalization. It could be

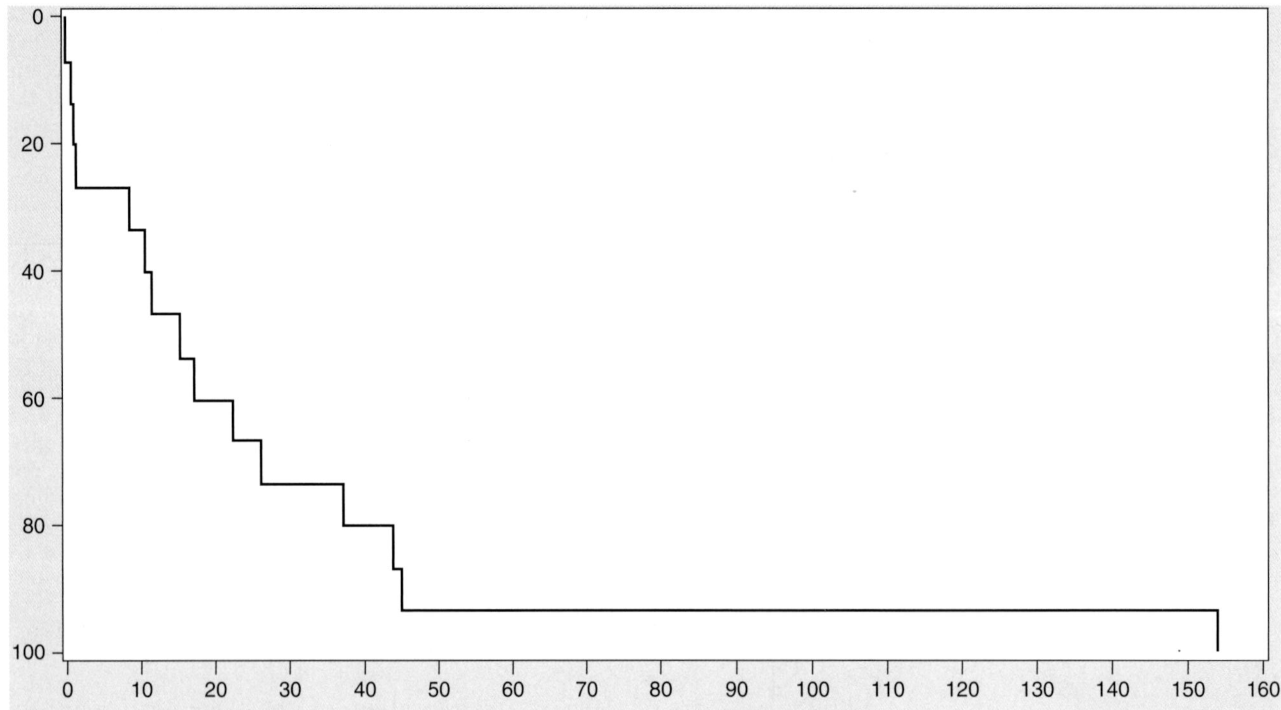

FIGURE 42.6. Time (months; horizontal axis) to hernia recurrence (14% rate) from 114 AWRs. The percentage of recurrence is represented on the vertical axis with the majority occurring within 48 months. From DiCocco JM, Magnotti LJ, Emmett KP, et al. Long-term follow-up of AWR after planned ventral hernia: a 15-year experience. *J Am Coll Surg* 2010;210:686–698.

expected that there will be a high-ventral hernia recurrence rate in those patients.

Over the past 15 years, most of the reconstructive techniques for AWR detailed in this chapter have been employed at our institution.[71] The hernia recurrence rate from this experience compares very favorably with other reports (Table 42.1). With one of the largest series reported, and with the longest follow-up (mean 5.6 years), our recurrence has proven to be one of the lowest (14%). The modified component separation technique has evolved into the workhorse for AWR at our institution. With long-term follow-up, the hernia recurrence rate for this procedure has been 5%.[71]

TABLE 42.1

HERNIA RECURRENCE RATE AFTER AWR

FIRST AUTHOR	N	FOLLOW-UP (MO)	RECURRENCE (%)	DEFECT SIZE (CM²)	BMI	METHODS USED
De Vries[74]	43	15.6	28	234	27.3	CS
Lowe[68]	30	9.5	10	240	33.2	CS + P
Jernigan[41]	73	24	6	600	n/a	MCS + P
De Vries[51]	37	36	57	400	28	CS vs. ePTFE
Rodriguez[67]	23	7	9	960	27.6	CS + P
DeMoya[72]	6	12	100	425	n/a	Human acellular dermis
Diaz[75]	165	10.4	25	201	30.7	CS + P vs. P only
Ko[73]	200	10.3	22	n/a	31.7	CS vs. P underlay
DiCocco[71]	114	63.6	14	621	27.3	CS, MCS, P

CS, components separation; P, prosthetic; MCS, modified components separation; ePTFE, expanded polytetrafluoroethylene.
From DiCocco JM, Magnotti LJ, Emmett KP, et al. Long-term follow-up of abdominal wall reconstruction after planned ventral hernia: a 15-year experience. *J Am Coll Surg*. 2010;210:686–698.

References

1. Stone HH, Strom PR, Mullins RJ. Management of the major coagulapathy with onset during laparotomy. *Ann Surg*. 1983;197:532-535.
2. Moore EE. Staged laparotomy for the hypothermia, acidosis, and coagulopathy syndrome. *Am J Surg*. 1996;172:405-410.
3. Rotondo MF, Schwab CW, McGonigal MD, et al. 'Damage control': an approach for improved survival in exsanguinating penetrating abdominal injury. *J Trauma*. 1993;35(3):375-383.
4. Stone HH, Fabian TC, Turkleson ML, et al. Management of acute full-thickness losses of the abdominal wall. *Ann Surg*. 1981;193(5):612-617.
5. Jones JW, Jurkovich GJ. Polypropylene mesh closure of infected abdominal wounds. *Am Surg*. 1989;1:73-76.
6. Nagy KK, Fildes JJ, Mahr C, et al. Experience with three prosthetic materials in temporary abdominal wall closure. *Am Surg*. 1996;62:331-335.
7. Voyles CR, Richardson JD, Bland KI, et al. Emergency abdominal wall reconstruction with polypropylene mesh: short-term benefits versus long-term complications. *Ann Surg*. 1981;194:219-223.
8. Fabian TC. Damage control in trauma: laparotomy wound management acute to chronic. *Surg Clin North Am*. 2007;87(1):73-93.
9. Richardson JD, Trinkle JK. Hemodynamic and respiratory alterations with increased intra-abdominal pressure. *J Surg Res*. 1976;20(5):401-404.
10. Diebel LN, Dulchavsky SA, Wilson RF. Effect of increased intra-abdominal pressure on mesenteric arterial and intestinal mucosal blood flow. *J Trauma*. 1992;33(1):45-49.
11. Maxwell RA, Fabian TC, Croce MA, et al. Secondary abdominal compartment syndrome: an underappreciated manifestation of severe hemorrhagic shock. *J Trauma*. 1999;47:995-999.
12. Rivers E, Mguyen B, Havstad S, et al. Early goal-directed therapy in the treatment of severe sepsis and septic shock. *N Engl J Med*. 2001;345:1368-1377.
13. Malbrain ML. Different techniques to measure intra-abdominal pressure (IAP): time for a critical reappraisal. *Intensive Care Med*. 2004;30:357-371.
14. Cheatham ML, Safcsak K. Intra-abdominal pressure: a revised method for measurement. *J Am Coll Surg*. 1998;186:594-595.
15. Sugrue M, Bauman A, Jones F, et al. Clinical examination is an inaccurate predictor of intra-abdominal pressure. *World J Surg*. 2002;26:1428-1431.
16. Balogh Z, Jones F, D'Amours S, et al. Continuous intra-abdominal pressure measurement technique. *Am J Surg*. 2004;188:679-684.
17. Malbrain MLNG, Cheatham ML, Kirkpatrick A, et al. Results from the international conference of experts on intra-abdominal hypertension and abdominal compartment syndrome. I. Definitions. *Intensive Care Med*. 2006;32:1722-1732.
18. Cheatham ML, White MW, Sagraves SG, et al. Abdominal perfusion pressure: a superior parameter in the assessment of intra-abdominal hypertension. *J Trauma*. 2000;49:621-626.
19. Deeren D, Dits H, Malbrain MLNG. Correlation between intra-abdominal and intracranial pressure in nontraumatic brain injury. *Intensive Care Med*. 2005;31:1577-1581.
20. Britt RC, Gannon T, Collins JN, et al. Secondary abdominal compartment syndrome: risk factors and outcomes. *Am Surg*. 2005;71(11):982-985.
21. Reed SF, Britt RC, Collins J, et al. Aggressive surveillance and early catheter-directed therapy in the management of intra-abdominal hypertension. *J Trauma*. 2006;61:1359-1363.
22. Christou NV, Barie PS, Dellinger EP, et al. Surgical Infection Society intra-abdominal infection study. Prospective evaluation of management techniques and outcome. *Arch Surg*. 1993;128:193-198.
23. Adkins, AL, Robbins J, Villalba M, et al. Open abdomen management of intra-abdominal sepsis. *Am Surg*. 2004;70:137-140.
24. Wittmann DH, Aprahamian C, Bergstein JM. Etappenlavage: advanced diffuse peritonitis managed by planned multiple laparotomies utilizing zippers, slide fastener, and Velcro analogue for temporary abdominal closure. *World J Surg*. 1990;14:218-222.
25. Ivatury RR, Nallathambi M, Rao PM, et al. Open management of the septic abdomen: therapeutic and prognostic considerations based on APACHE II. *Crit Care Med*. 1989;17:511-517.
26. Ivatury RR, Nallathambi M, Rohman PM, et al. Open management of the post-traumatic septic abdomen. *Am Surg*. 1990;56:548-552.
27. Park WM, Gloviczki P, Cherry KJ Jr, et al. Contemporary management of acute mesenteric ischemia: factors associated with survival. *J Vasc Surg*. 2002;35:445-452.
28. Ward D, Vernava AM, Kamiski DL. Improved outcome by identification of high-risk nonocclusive mesenteric ischemia, aggressive re-exploration, and delayed anastomosis. *Am J Surg*. 1995;170:577-581.
29. Park WM, Gloviczki P, Cherry KJ Jr, et al. Contemporary management of acute mesenteric ischemia: Factors associated with survival. *J Vasc Surg* 2002;35(3):445-452.
30. Bertram P, Treutner KH, Stumpf M, et al. Postoperative necrotizing soft-tissue infections of the abdominal wall. *Langenbeck's Arch Surg*. 2000;385:39-41.
31. Levy E, Palmer DL, Frileux P, et al. Septic necrosis of the midline wound in postoperative peritonitis. Successful management by debridement, myocutaneous advancement and primary skin closure. *Ann Surg*. 1988;207:470-479.
32. Brock WB, Barker DE, Burns RP. Temporary closure of open abdominal wounds: the vacuum pack. *Am Surg*. 1995;6(1):30-35.
33. Miller PR, Meredith JW, Johnson JC, et al. Prospective evaluation of vacuum-assisted fascial closure after open abdomen: planned ventral hernia rate is substantially reduced. *Ann Surg*. 2004;239(5):608-616.
34. Cothren CC, Moore EE, Johnson JL, et al. One hundred percent fascial approximation with sequential abdominal closure of the open abdomen. *Am J Surg*. 2006;192:238-242.
35. Scott BG, Feanny MA, Hirschberg A. Early definitive closure of the open abdomen: a quiet revolution. *Scand J Surg*. 2005;94:9-14.
36. Bee TK, Croce MA, Magnotti LJ, et al. Temporary abdominal closure techniques: a prospective randomized trial comparing polyglactin 910 mesh and vacuum-assisted closure. *J Trauma*. 2008;65(2):337-344.
37. Voyles CR, Richardson JD, Bland KI, et al. Emergency abdominal wall reconstruction with polypropylene mesh: short-term benefits versus long-term complications. *Ann Surg*. 1981;194:219-223.
38. Weinberg JA, George RL, Griffin RL, et al. Closing the open abdomen: improved success with Wittmann Patch staged abdominal closure. *J Trauma*. 2008;65(2):345-348.
39. Fantus RJ, Mellett MM, Kirby JP. Use of controlled fascial tension and an adhesion preventing barrier to achieve delayed primary fascial closure in patients managed with an open abdomen. *Am J Surg*. 2006;192: 243-247.
40. Schecter WP, Ivatury RR, Rotondo MF, et al. Open abdomen after trauma and abdominal sepsis: a strategy for management. *J Am Coll Surg*. 2006;203(3):390-396.
41. Jernigan TW, Fabian TC, Croce MA, et al. Staged management of giant abdominal wall defects: acute and long-term results. *Ann Surg*. 2003;238:349-357.
42. Fischer PE, Fabian TC, Magnotti LJ, et al. A ten-year review of enterocutaneous fistulas after laparotomy for trauma. *J Trauma*. 2009;67(5): 924-928.
43. Guy JS, Miller R, Morris JA, et al. Early one-stage closure in patients with abdominal compartment syndrome: fascial replacement with human acellular dermis and bipedicled flaps. *Am Surg*. 2003;69:1025-1029.
44. Lee EI, Chike-Obi CJ, Gonzalez P, et al. Abdominal wall repair using human acellular dermal matrix: a follow-up study. *Am J Surg*. 2009;198: 650-657.
45. Kim H, Bruen K, Vargo D. Acellular dermal matrix in the management of high-risk abdominal wall defects. *Am J Surg*. 2006;192:705-709.
46. Paul A, Korenkov M, Peters S, et al. Unacceptable results of the Mayo procedure for repair of abdominal incisional hernias. *Eur J Surg*. 1998;164:361-367.
47. Stoppa RE. The treatment of complicate groin and incisional hernias. *World J Surg*. 1989;13:545-554.
48. Rives J, Pire JC, Flament JB, et al. Treatment of large eventrations. New therapeutic indications apropos of 322 cases. *Chirurgie*. 1985;111:215-225.
49. Matthews BD, Pratt BL, Pollinger HS, et al. Assessment of adhesion formation to intra-abdominal polypropylene mesh and polytetrafluoroethylene mesh. *J Surg Res*. 2003;114:126-132.
50. Novitsky YW, Porter JR, Rusho ZC, et al. Open preperitoneal retrofascial mesh repair for multiply recurrent ventral incisional hernias. *J Am Coll Surg*. 2006;203:283-289.
51. de Vries Reilingh TS, van Geldere D, Langenhorst BLAM, et al. Repair of large midline incisional hernias with polypropylene mesh: comparison of three operative techniques. *Hernia*. 2004;8:56-59.
52. Shankaran V, Weber DJ, Reed RL II, et al. A review of available prosthetics for ventral hernia repair. *Ann Surg*. 2011;253(1):16-26.
53. Goepel R. Ueber die verschliessung von bruchpforten durch einheilung geflochtener, Fertiger Silberdrahtnetze (silberdrahtperlotten). *Verh Dsch Ges Chir*. 1900;19:174-179.
54. Witzel O. Uber den verschluss von bauchwunden und bruchpforten durch versenkte silverdrahtnetze (einheilung von filigranpelotten). *Centralb Chir*. 1900; 27:257-259.
55. Bothra R. Tantalum gauze in the repair of large postoperative ventral hernias: late onset small bowel fistula due to tantalum mesh. *Arch Surg*. 1973;125:649-650.
56. Wolstenholme JT. Use of commercial Dacron fabric in the repair of inguinal hernias and abdominal wall defects. *AMA Arch Surg*. 1956;73:1004-1008.
57. DeBakey ME, Cooley DA, Crawwford ES, et al. Clinical application of a new flexible knitted Dacron arterial substitute. *Am Surg*. 1958;24:862-869.
58. Klinge U, Klosterhalfen B, Conze J, et al. Modified mesh for hernia repair that is adapted to the physiology of the abdominal wall. *Eur J Surg*. 1998;164:951-960.
59. Schmidbauer S, Ladurner R, Hallfeldt KK, et al. Heavy-weight versus low-weight polypropylene meshes for open sublay mesh repair of incisional hernia. *Eur J Med Res*. 2005;10:247-253.
60. Matthews BD, Pratt BL, Pollinger HS, et al. Assessment of adhesion formation to intra-abdominal polypropylene mesh and polytetrafluoroethylene mesh. *J Surg Res*. 2003;114:126-132.
61. Costello CR, Bachman SL, Grant SA, et al. Characterization of heavyweight and lightweight polypropylene prosthetic mesh explants from a single patient. *Surg Innov*. 2007;14:168-176.
62. Jones JW, Jurkovich GJ. Polypropylene mesh closure of infected abdominal wounds. *Am Surg* 1989;55(1):73-76.
63. Butler CE, Langstein HN, Kronowitz SJ. Pelvic, abdominal, and chest wall reconstruction with AlloDerm in patients at increased risk for mesh-related complications. *Plast Reconstr Surg*. 2005;116:1263-1277.

64. Badylak S, Kokini K, Tullius B, et al. Strength over time of a resorbable bioscaffold for body wall repair in a dog model. *J Surg Res.* 2001;99:282-287.
65. Patton JH Jr., Berry S, Kralovich KA. Use of human acellular dermal matrix in complex and contaminated abdominal wall reconstructions. *Am J Surg.* 2007;193:360-363.
66. Helton WS, Fisichella PM, Berger R, et al. Short-term outcomes with small intestinal submucosa for ventral abdominal hernia. *Arch Surg.* 2005;140:549-562.
67. Rodriguez ED, Bluebond-Langner R, Silverman RP, et al. Abdominal wall reconstruction following severe loss of domain: the R. Adams Cowley Shock Trauma Center algorithm. *Plast Reconstr Surg.* 207;120:669-680.
68. Lowe JB, Lowe JB, Baty JD, et al. Risks associated with "components separation" for closure of complex abdominal wall defects. *Plast Reconstr Surg.* 2003;111:1276-1283.
69. Ramirez OM, Ruas E, Dellon AL. "Components separation" method for closure of abdominal wall defects: an anatomic and clinical study. *Plast Reconstr Surg.* 1990;86:519-526.
70. DiCocco JM, Fabian TC, Emmett KP, et al. Components separation for abdominal wall reconstruction: the Memphis modification. *Surgery.* 2012;151(1):118-25.
71. DiCocco JM, Magnotti LJ, Emmett KP, et al. Long-term follow-up of abdominal wall reconstruction after planned ventral hernia: a 15-year experience. *J Am Coll Surg.* 2010;210:686-698.
72. DeMoya MA, Dunham M, Inaba K, et al. Long-term outcome of acellular dermal matrix when used for large traumatic open abdomen. *J Trauma.* 2008;65:349-353.
73. Ko JH, Wang EC, Salvay DM, et al. Abdominal wall reconstruction, lessons learned from 200 "components separation" procedures. *Arch Surg.* 2009;144:1047-1055.
74. De Vries Reilingh TS, Van Goor H, Rosman C, et al. "Components separation technique" for the repair of large abdominal wall hernias. *J Am Coll Surg.* 2003;196:32-37.
75. Diaz JJ, Conquest AM, Ferzoco SJ, et al. Multi-institutional experience using human acellular dermal matrix for ventral hernia repair in a compromised surgical field. *Arch Surg.* 2009;144:209-215.

CHAPTER 43 ■ SURGICAL INFECTIONS OF SKIN AND SOFT TISSUE

VANESSA P. HO, SOUMITRA R. EACHEMPATI, AND PHILIP S. BARIE

Infections of skin and soft tissue (SSTI) encompass a diverse set of conditions and are a common cause of hospitalization and morbidity. For the purposes of clinical trials, the U.S. Food and Drug Administration (FDA) uses the term skin and skin structure infections (SSSI), further divided into "uncomplicated" and "complicated" subgroups.[1] Necrotizing tissue soft tissue infections (NSTIs) are studied separately and are therefore excluded from studies of complicated SSTI (cSSTI), although certainly not from the practices of acute care surgeons. The term "skin and soft tissue infections" is preferred and used herein as inclusive of the infections that may necessitate surgeon involvement.

New terminology has been proposed by the FDA for the study of antimicrobial therapy of SSTIs: "acute bacterial skin and skin structure infections (ABSSSI)."[2] This terminology, not in clinical use, describes infections of lesser severity that do not require surgical drainage or debridement, owing to the perceived difficulty of parsing whether it is the surgery or the antibiotic that is most important to achieve cure. For the purposes of this discussion of surgical therapy of SSSIs, the definition is irrelevant, and the question of efficacy is moot.

SSTI vary widely in severity; whereas some SSTIs can be treated non-operatively, others are life threatening and require radical surgical debridement in addition to broad-spectrum antibiotic therapy. Practice guidelines for treatment of SSTIs have been published by both the Infectious Diseases Society of America (Table 43.1)[1] and the Surgical Infection Society (Table 43.2).[3]

Uncomplicated SSTIs are superficial or self-limited. They may require only incision and drainage (without antibiotics) or oral antibiotics (without drainage) and rarely require hospitalization. Uncomplicated infections have historically been excluded from trials of antibiotic therapy for complicated SSTIs and vice versa, but may be included henceforth under the ABSSSI paradigm.

By contrast, cSSTIs involve deeper tissues or require major surgical intervention. An infection is also considered complicated if the patient has specific medical comorbidities, including chronic kidney disease, diabetes mellitus, or peripheral arterial disease. Examples of cSSTI include major abscesses, deep (organ/space) surgical site infections (SSIs), diabetic foot infections (DFIs), incisional SSIs with systemic signs of infection, infected decubitus ulcers, and NSTIs. Because clinical trials of drug therapy for cSSTI exclude NSTI, limited prospective data have been collected for their treatment.

UNCOMPLICATED SSTI

Uncomplicated infections include simple abscess, impetigo, furuncles, and nonnecrotizing cellulitis. Nonnecrotizing cellulitis is a diffuse, spreading skin infection without a suppurative focus, usually presenting as a complication from a breach of skin integrity.[4] The differential diagnosis of cellulitis includes both infectious and noninfectious entities, and serious underlying sources of infection should be ruled out. Cellulitis may be a sign of a deeper infection (e.g., spread of subjacent osteomyelitis, thigh cellulitis following colon perforation into the retroperitoneum). Clinicians must be aware that early NSTIs can be confused for cellulitis if initial symptoms are modest.

Cellulitis is caused most commonly by gram-positive cocci, either streptococci (usually *Streptococcus pyogenes*) or *Staphylococcus aureus*.[5] In cases where patients are immunocompromised, causative agents can also include *Haemophilus influenzae* and *S. pneumoniae*.[3] Predisposing factors include alterations of skin integrity or venous or lymphatic drainage or alterations in host defenses, such as diabetes mellitus. The diagnosis of cellulitis is made clinically, based on history and the appearance of the lesion; neither imaging studies nor cultures of the lesion have a high diagnostic yield. Needle aspiration or punch biopsy also has low yield; an organism is isolated 5%–40% of the time.[6–8]

Simple cutaneous abscesses are well-circumscribed collections of purulent material within the dermis and subcutis. These lesions are usually painful, tender, and fluctuant, with a central pustule and surrounding erythema and edema. These infections are typically polymicrobial, with *S. aureus* isolated in only one-quarter of cases. Treatment of cutaneous abscesses is incision and drainage, with mechanical destruction of intracavitary loculations (Table 43.1).[1] Gram stain, culture, or systemic antibiotics are rarely necessary unless a patient has systemic signs or severe immune compromise. Antibiotic coverage is usually unnecessary unless the patient has surrounding cellulitis.

In cases where antibiotic treatment is warranted for uncomplicated SSTI, oral therapy is appropriate unless the patient has systemic signs (e.g., fever, chills), medical comorbidity, or a rapidly spreading lesion. Appropriate oral agents include dicloxacillin, cephalexin, cephradine, or cefadroxil. For moderate-to-severe infections, parenteral penicillins are the treatment of choice; however, treatment failures may occur in severe cases. Other possible regimens for initial empiric parenteral therapy of severe nonnecrotizing cellulitis are antistaphylococcal penicillins such as nafcillin or cephalosporins such as cefazolin or ceftriaxone (Table 43.1). If methicillin-resistant *S. aureus* (MRSA) is suspected or the patient is highly allergic to penicillin (i.e., anaphylactoid reaction), vancomycin, telavancin, tigecycline, or linezolid may be chosen. A new "fifth-generation" cephalosporin with activity against MRSA, ceftaroline (see below), has also been approved, specifically for ABSSSI. Minocycline or linezolid may be appropriate for oral therapy of hospital-acquired MRSA.

MRSA IN SSTI

MRSA in SSTI requires particular mention. Approximately 60% of hospital isolates of *S. aureus* are MRSA[9]; hospitalized or recently hospitalized patients who develop a SSTI must be considered for empiric therapy against hospital-acquired strains of MRSA. Community-acquired MRSA (CA-MRSA) SSTIs are being observed increasingly among patients with

TABLE 43.1

SUMMARY OF RECOMMENDATIONS FROM PRACTICE GUIDELINE FOR DIAGNOSIS AND TREATMENT OF SKIN AND SOFT TISSUE INFECTIONS (SSTI)-INFECTIOUS DISEASES SOCIETY OF AMERICA

Level I	
Impetigo:	Mupirocin is the best topical agent and is equivalent to oral systemic antimicrobials when lesions are limited in number. Patients with numerous lesions or who do not respond to topical therapy should receive an oral antimicrobial agent. PCN or penicillinase-resistant PCN are TOCs for nonbullous lesions. PCN or 1-G cephalosporin is recommended for bullous lesions.
Erysipelas:	PCN is TOC for streptococcal infection. Penicillinase-resistant PCN or 1-G cephalosporin is recommended if staphylococci are suspected.
Cellulitis:	Penicillinase-resistant PCN or 1-G cephalosporin is the TOCs, unless resistant organisms are common in the community. Use clindamycin or vancomycin for PCN-allergic patients.
Cutaneous abscess:	Incision and drainage is the TOC.
Furunculosis:	Recurrent furunculosis may be treated with mupirocin to the anterior nares (for chronic staphylococcal carriers) or clindamycin 150 mg/d for 3 mos.
MRSA:	Linezolid, daptomycin, and vancomycin have excellent efficacy in SSTI in general and in particular those caused by MRSA.
NSTI:	Surgical intervention is the major therapeutic modality.
Type I NSTI:	Ampicillin–sulbactam plus ciprofloxacin plus clindamycin is TOC for community-acquired infection.
Type II NSTI:	Clindamycin/PCN combination therapy is TOC.
Level II	
Furunculosis:	Attempt to eradicate the staphylococcal carrier state among colonized persons.
Type I NSTI:	A variety of antimicrobials directed against aerobic gram-positive and -negative bacteria and anaerobes may be used in mixed necrotizing infection.
Type II NSTI:	Consider intravenous gamma globulin (IVIG) therapy. PCN/clindamycin combination therapy is the TOC for infections caused by *Clostridium perfringens*.
Animal bites:	Oral amoxicillin–clavulanic acid or intravenous ampicillin–sulbactam or ertapenem should be administered to non–PCN-allergic patients because of suitable activity against *Pasteurella multocida*. Acceptable alternative regimens include piperacillin–tazobactam, imipenem–cilastatin, and meropenem.
Level III	
Cutaneous abscess:	Gram stain, culture, and systemic antibiotics are rarely necessary.
Furunculosis:	Systemic antibiotics are usually unnecessary, absent fever, or extensive surrounding cellulitis.
Animal bites:	1-G cephalosporins, penicillinase-resistant PCN, macrolides, and clindamycin should be avoided as therapy because of poor activity against *P. multocida*.
Human bites:	Intravenous ampicillin–sulbactam or cefoxitin are the TOCs for non–PCN-allergic patients. A hand surgeon should evaluate clenched-fist injuries for penetration into synovium, joint capsule, or bone.

Suspicion of possible surgical site infection does not justify use of antibiotics without a definitive diagnosis and the initiation of other therapies, such as opening the incision. All infected surgical incisions should be opened.

1-G, first-generation cephalosporin; MRSA, methicillin-resistant *Staphylococcus aureus*; NSTI, necrotizing soft tissue infection; PCN, penicillin; SSI, surgical site infection; TOC, treatment of choice.

From Stevens DL, Bisno AL, Chambers HF, et al. Practice guidelines for the diagnosis and management of skin and soft-tissue infections. *Clin Infect Dis*. 2005;41:1373–1406

no prior contact with the health care system.[10] Molecular epidemiologic studies indicate that CA-MRSA is a genetically unique pathogen that has a distinct susceptibility pattern. The CA-MRSA clone likely arose from antibiotic selection pressure upon a commensal, saprophytic *Staphylococcus* sp. that is part of normal skin flora.[11] About 75% of CA-MRSA infections are SSTI, but this pathogen may cause pneumonia as well; either manifestation may be associated with tissue necrosis.[12] In many areas of the United States, CA-MRSA is now the predominant cause of SSTIs that present to emergency departments and should be considered when choosing empiric therapy.[13]

The antimicrobial susceptibilities of CA-MRSA differ from the hospital clones. CA-MRSA is similarly susceptible to vancomycin and linezolid, but CA-MRSA may also be susceptible *in vitro* to macrolides, clindamycin, and co-trimoxazole. Whereas the latter drug is most reliable for oral therapy,[14] severe infections usually require intravenous antibiotics.[15,16] Macrolide-inducible clindamycin resistance has been associated with treatment failures; therefore, caution is advised with clindamycin therapy,[17] especially in the presence of macrolide resistance.

Outbreaks of CA-MRSA have been associated with groups of people in close contact, including prison inmates, amateur and professional sports teams, military recruits, and clients of day-care centers.[18–21] Direct contact with skin is a definite risk factor, as are shared personal hygiene items (e.g., towels, bars of soap). Also at risk are young children and people of lower socioeconomic status. SSTI infections caused by CA-MRSA have a characteristic appearance that may aid in diagnosis. The lesions are usually superficial and well-demarcated, often with central necrosis. If uncomplicated, incision and drainage alone or topical mupirocin ointment or chlorhexidine solution may be sufficient therapy. If antibiotic therapy is required, oral co-trimoxazole should be considered, but severe infections are at risk of treatment failure with this regimen and should be treated with a parenteral glycopeptide or linezolid.

TABLE 43.2

SUMMARY OF RECOMMENDATIONS FROM GUIDELINES FOR TREATMENT OF COMPLICATED SKIN AND SOFT TISSUE INFECTIONS FROM THE SURGICAL INFECTION SOCIETY

Non-necrotizing Cellulitis
- Most frequent causative agent is β-hemolytic streptococci; other agents are *Haemophilus influenzae* and pneumococcus
- Parenteral penicillin is TOC; treatment failures may occur in severe cases
- Protein synthesis-inhibitory agents alone or in combination with cell wall-active agents should be given in severe cases, but macrolide resistance is increasing
- Other regimens may include antistaphylococcal penicillins, cefazolin, or ceftriaxone

Complicated Skin and Soft Tissue Infections
- Involve a broad variety of pathogens; frequently polymicrobial
- *Staphylococcus aureus* is most common isolate; CA-MRSA increasingly common
- Simple abscesses may respond to incision and drainage alone
- Complex abscesses and abscesses with cellulitis require adjuvant antibiotics
- Empiric antibiotic therapy should be directed toward the most likely pathogens, including CA-MRSA in most settings
- Suspected polymicrobial infections should be managed with coverage of enteric gram-negative and anaerobic pathogens

Necrotizing Soft Tissue Infections
- Delays in diagnosis increase morbidity and mortality
- Presence of gas in soft tissue is specific for necrotizing infections
- CT and MRI improve the detection of soft tissue gas, but radiographic findings of tissue fluid and edema are not sensitive or specific
- Clinical features suggestive of NSTI are:
  - Pain disproportionate to findings at physical exam
  - Tense edema
  - Bullae
  - Skin ecchymosis/necrosis
  - Cutaneous anesthesia
  - Systemic toxicity
  - Progression despite antibiotic therapy
- Predictive laboratory values are:
  - White blood cell count >14 × 10^9/L
  - Serum [sodium] <135 mmol/L
  - [Blood urea nitrogen] >15 mg/dL
- Early antibiotic coverage of likely pathogens is indicated; this depends on the clinical setting, inciting pathophysiology, and previous exposure to antibiotics
- Timely and adequate surgical debridement of involved tissue improves outcome
- Frequent reevaluation or return to the operating room within 24 hours should be undertaken to ensure adequacy of debridement and lack of progression
- Necrotizing infections are more frequently polymicrobial; they may involve anaerobic and aerobic gram-positive and gram-negative pathogens
- Possible single-agent regimens include imipenem/cilastatin, meropenem, ertapenem, piperacillin/tazobactam, ticarcillin/clavulanic acid, or tigecycline

Diabetic Foot Infections
- May involve a wide variety of pathogens; separating colonizing bacteria from pathogens may be difficult
- Monomicrobial infections caused by gram-positive cocci are most common, but gram-negative bacilli and anaerobes may be involved. Chronic wounds may have resistant pathogens.
- Empiric therapy should take local sensitivity patterns, previous antibiotic exposure, and previous pathogens into consideration.
- Adequate tissue cultures should be obtained. Superficial surface swabs are not recommended.
- Possible antibiotic regimens include cefazolin, ceftriaxone, cefoxitin, ampicillin/sulbactam, piperacillin/clindamycin, piperacillin/tazobactam, imipenem/cilastatin, and ertapenem; daptomycin and linezolid can be used with the addition of gram-negative coverage
- For MRSA infections, vancomycin, daptomycin, and linezolid can be considered[a]

Adjunctive Therapies
- Data are insufficient for extracorporeal plasma treatment, HBO, and intravenous immunoglobulin.

[a]Note that telavancin is FDA-approved for the treatment of SSTI caused by MRSA, but was approved subsequent to publication of this guideline

CA-MRSA, community acquired methicillin-resistant *Staphylococcus aureus*; CT, computed tomography, FDA, U.S. Food and Drug Administration; HBO, hyperbaric oxygen therapy; MRI, magnetic resonance imaging; MRSA, methicillin-resistant *Staphylococcus aureus*; NSTI, necrotizing soft tissue infection; SSTI, skin and soft tissue infections, TOC, treatment of choice.

From May AK, Stafford RE, Bulger EM, et al. Treatment of complicated skin and soft tissue infections. *Surg Infect (Larchmt)*. 2009;10:467–499.

COMPLICATED SSTI

Complicated SSTIs involve deeper tissues or require major surgical intervention. Infection in the presence of chronic kidney disease, diabetes mellitus, or peripheral arterial disease also defines a cSSTI. Examples of cSSTIs include major abscesses, organ/space SSIs, some incisional SSIs (those with systemic signs of infection), DFIs, infected decubitus ulcers, and NSTIs. Clinical trials of drug therapy for cSSTI exclude NSTIs because of high mortality rates and the crucial contribution of timely surgical debridement to outcome. An evidence-based summary of recent clinical trials of antibiotic therapy is shown in Table 43.3.[1,15,22–34] Most trials are designed to demonstrate "non-inferiority" of the tested regimen against the comparator regimen, and so numerous regimens appear comparable despite widely divergent spectra of activity. Notably, comparable outcomes are achieved by agents that treat only gram-positive cocci (e.g., vancomycin, linezolid, daptomycin, telavancin), but the many options available to investigators (e.g., choice of comparator in "standard therapy" regimens, addition of aztreonam) make the literature a challenge to interpret.

Three meta-analyses have been published recently to assess the literature comparing linezolid with vancomycin for cSSTI (n = 2)[35,36] and daptomycin versus comparator agents (either vancomycin or semisynthetic penicillins[37]; Table 43.4). Despite considering different trials for inclusion, the two meta-analyses of linezolid versus vancomycin each concluded that resolution of cSSTI is more likely after linezolid therapy, albeit with more nausea, diarrhea, and myelosuppression (nephrotoxicity is more common with vancomycin). Differences in cure rates of infection were not observed for daptomycin versus comparators.

Diabetic Foot Infection

Patients with diabetes mellitus are at risk for considerable morbidity as a result of chronic foot ulceration and foot infection, including limb loss.[38,39] DIFs are usually a consequence of skin ulceration, either from ischemia or trauma to an insensate, neuropathic foot. One-third of patients presenting with a DFI have had a chronic foot lesion for more than 1 month beforehand. Two-thirds of patients with DFI present with peripheral arterial disease, and the prevalence of sensory neuropathy is about 80%. Although most DFIs remain superficial, as many as 25% spread contiguously to involve subcutaneous tissue or bone (osteomyelitis). The compartmentalized anatomy of the foot, with its various spaces, tendon sheaths, and neurovascular bundles, allows ischemic necrosis to affect tissues within a compartment or spread along anatomic planes. Recurrent infections are common, and 10%-30% of affected patients eventually require amputation.[40]

Diabetic patients are predisposed to DFIs not only because of the portal of entry and poor perfusion, but also because of defective innate immunity, including impaired neutrophil and monocyte/macrophage function, which appear to correlate with the adequacy of glycemic control.[41,42] Adaptive immunity may be impaired as well. Diabetic patients also have a higher prevalence of nasal carriage of *S. aureus*, which predisposes patients to SSTIs.

Infections affect the forefoot most commonly, especially the toes and the metatarsal heads on the plantar surface. Infection must be diagnosed clinically because, as with all skin wounds, polymicrobial flora is present, many of which are nonpathogenic. Systemic signs (e.g., fever, chills), purulent drainage, or at least two local signs of inflammation (e.g., calor [warmth], rubor [redness], dolor [pain, or tenderness], and tumor [induration]) are suggestive. Deep infections may have few surface signs. Chronic wounds may manifest discoloration, friability, delayed healing, or be malodorous. Signs of systemic toxicity are uncommon in DFI, even with limb-threatening infection, but metabolic abnormalities (e.g., hyperglycemia, ketoacidosis, hyperosmolar state) imply severe disease. Many patients do not complain of pain, and more than one-half of patients have neither fever, nor leukocytosis, nor an elevated erythrocyte sedimentation rate. Whenever the diagnosis of DFI is considered, aggressive management is indicated because these infections may progress rapidly.

Several severity scores have been proposed for DFI,[43] but none has universal acceptance. Severity may be determined clinically by assessment of the depth of the wound and tissue perfusion. Local wound exploration with a sterile surgical instrument is important to identify necrotic tissue or the presence of a foreign body (e.g., a needle that the patient stepped on, but did not feel at the time) or osteomyelitis.[44,45] Assessment of severity is essential for antibiotic selection (including route of administration) and to determine the need for hospitalization and the necessity and timing of surgical debridement or level of amputation. Systemic signs should raise suspicion of a deep infection. Indications for hospitalization include correction of hypovolemia or metabolic abnormalities, parenteral antibiotic therapy, or the need for surgery. Other reasons to hospitalize a DFI patient include an inability or unwillingness of the patient to provide local wound care or to maintain non–weight-bearing status or likely noncompliance with outpatient oral antibiotic therapy. Antibiotic therapy alone cannot overcome suboptimal wound care and inadequate glycemic control.

Acute DFIs are usually caused by gram-positive cocci; *S. aureus* is the most important pathogen in DFI. Whereas *S. aureus* is often present as a monomicrobial infection[42,46] (Table 43.5), it is also usually an important pathogen in polymicrobial infections. Chronic wounds, recurrent infections, and infections of hospitalized patients are more likely to harbor complex flora, including aerobes and anaerobes.[47] Among gram-negative bacilli, bacteria of the family Enterobacteriaceae are common. *Pseudomonas aeruginosa* may be isolated from wounds that have been treated with hydrotherapy or wet dressings. Enterococci may be recovered from patients treated previously with a cephalosporin. Anaerobic bacteria seldom cause DFIs as the sole pathogen, but they may be isolated from deep infections or necrotic tissue.[47] Antibiotic-resistant bacteria, especially MRSA, may be isolated from patients who have received antibiotics previously or who have been hospitalized or reside in long-term care facilities.

Antibiotic Therapy. Forty to sixty percent of diabetic patients who are treated for a foot ulcer receive antibiotics, but antibiotic therapy does not improve the outcome of uninfected foot lesions in diabetic patients.[39,48] Successful antibiotic therapy requires a therapeutic concentration of antibiotic at the site of infection. Intravenous antibiotics are indicated for patients with systemic illness, severe infection, intolerance of oral antibiotics, or pathogens that are not susceptible to oral agents. After the patient stabilizes and shows signs of improvement, a switch to oral antibiotic therapy may be appropriate. Slower delivery of antibiotic after an initial oral dose is inconsequential for non–critically ill patients, and so the main consideration is the bioavailability of the chosen agent. Among the potential choices of oral antibiotics for DFIs, clindamycin, linezolid, and fluoroquinolones have good oral bioavailability. Even parenteral antibiotics may not penetrate tissue adequately in the presence of peripheral arterial disease, even when serum concentrations are adequate.[49]

Initial empiric therapy should be directed at common pathogens (Table 43.5).[46,48–51] Mild infections may be treated more narrowly because disease progression is unlikely to

TABLE 43.3

RECENT PROSPECTIVE TRIALS OF ANTIBIOTIC THERAPY FOR COMPLICATED SKIN AND SKIN STRUCTURE INFECTIONS

STUDY	DRUG	COMPARATOR	RESULT	NOTES
Stevens, 2002[23]	Linezolid 600 mg IV QD	Vancomycin 1 g IV Q12H	73% vs. 73% Cure, E population 95% CI (−16.6, 16.8)	MRSA only Open-label 7 days of therapy Underpowered
Seltzer, 2003[30]	Dalbavancin 1 g IV day 1 and 500 mg day 8	Standard therapy	94% vs. 76% E population Only result fortwo doses of dalbavancin shown	Open-label Dose-ranging phase 2 trial
Arbeit, 2004[22]	Daptomycin 4 mg/kg IV QD	Standard therapy or vancomycin 1 g IV Q12H, oral switch to synthetic penicillin OK if MSSA	83% vs. 84% cure, E population 95% CI (−4.0, 5.6)	Combined report of two phase 3 trials Non-inferior treatment for 7-14 d
Wilcox, 2004[24]	Linezolid 600 mg IV/PO Q12H	Teicoplanin dose determined by investigator	96% vs. 88% cure, ITT population 95% CI (2.5, 13.2)	Linezolid superior to teicoplanin, but dose of teicoplanin questionable
Giordano, 2005[25]	Moxifloxacin 400 mg IV/PO QD	Piperacillin–tazobactam 3.375 g IV Q6H, amoxicillin–clavulanate 800 mg PO Q12H	79% vs. 82% cure, E population 95% CI (−12.04, 3.29)	Non-inferior Treatment for 7-14 d
Ellis-Grosse, 2005[26]	Tigecycline 100 mg load then 50 mg IV Q12H	Vancomycin 1 g Q12H plus aztreonam 2 g IV Q12H	80% vs. 82% cure, mITT population 95% CI (−7,1, 2.8)	Combined report of two phase 3 trials Non-inferior
Jauregui, 2005[27]	Dalbavancin 1 g day 1, 500 mg day 8	Linezolid 600 mg IV/PO Q12H	89% vs. 91% E population 97.5% CI calculated, only lower limit of −7.28 reported	Randomized D:L 2:1 Treatment for 14 d
Weigelt, 2005[28]	Linezolid 600 mg Q12H IV/PO, aztreonam permitted	Vancomycin 1 g IV Q12H, switch to semisynthetic penicillin if MSSA, aztreonam permitted	92% vs. 89% cure, ITT population 95% CI (−0.11, 7.47)	Open-label Phase 4 Treatment up to 14 d Linezolid superior in MRSA subset 95% CI (6.08–25.70
Stryjewski, 2006[31]	Telavancin 10 mg/kg IV q24h	Standard therapy Antistaphylococcal penicillin or vancomycin 1g IV q12h	96% vs. 90% cure, in MRSA cases 92% vs. 78% ($p = 0.07$)	Randomized double-blind active-control phase 2
Fabian, 2005[29]	Meropenem 500 mg IV q8h	Imipenem–cilastatin 500 mg IV q8h	73% vs. 75% cure in mITT population 95% CI (−8.4, 4.7)	Randomized double-blind; imipemem–cilastatin underdosed?
Cenizal, 2007[15]	TMP-SMX 180/600 mg PO q12h for 7 days	Doxycycline 100 mg PO q12h for 7 days	79% vs. 100% cure ($p = 0.283$)	Randomized; underpowered
Stryjewski, 2008[32]	Telavancin 10 mg/kg IV q24h	Vancomycin 1 g IV q12h	88% vs. 87% cure 95% CI (−2.1, 4.6)	Pre-specified pooled analysis of two randomized double-blind trials
Corey, 2010[33]	Ceftaroline 10 mg/kg IV q24h	Vancomycin 1g IV q12h plus aztreonam	86% vs. 86% cure, mITT population	Randomized double-blind Phase 3
Itani, 2010[34]	Linezolid 600 mg IV q12h	Vancomycin 15 mg/kg IV q12h	81% vs. 74% cure, mITT population	Open-label randomized trial of patients with MRSA. Aztreonam and metronidazole permissible in either arm

"Standard therapy" means that selection of the comparator agent was at the discretion of the investigator. Non-inferiority is defined statistically when the lower limit of the 95% confidence interval is >−15, and the confidence interval contains zero. A trial with a relatively narrow confidence interval is likely to have greater statistical power (or more homogeneous results) than one with a wider interval.

CI, confidence interval; E, evaluable patient group; ITT, Intention-to-treat patient group; IV, intravenous; mITT, modified intention-to-treat patient group; PO, oral administration; TMP-SMX, trimethoprim-sulfamethoxazole.

TABLE 43.4

RESULTS OF META-ANALYSES OF LINEZOLD AND DAPTOMYCIN THERAPY FOR CSSTI

Bounthavong, 2010[35]	Linezolid vs. vancomycin	5 studies, 2,652 patients with MRSA
	Resolution of infection, CE patients	OR 1.41, 95% CI: 1.03–1.95
	mITT patients	OR 1.91, 95% CI: 1.33–2.76
	Mortality	OR 1.17, 95% CI: 0.85–1.62
Beibei, 2010[36]	Linezolid vs. vancomycin	9 studies, 2,489 patients
	Resolution of infection, CE patients	OR 1.40, 95% CI: 1.01–1.95
	Mortality not reported	
Bilziotis, 2010[37]	Daptomycin vs. comparators Clinical success (3 RCTs), CE patients OR 0.89; 95% CI 0.63–1.25	4 trials (3 randomized), 1,557 patients

CE, clinically evaluable; CI, confidence interval; cSSTI, complicated skin and soft tissue infections; mITT, modified intent-to-treat population; MRSA, methicillin-resistant *Staphylococcus aureus*; OR, odds ratios, RCT, randomized controlled trial.

prevent modification of the regimen when microbiology data become available. For severe infections, regimens should utilize broad-spectrum intravenous antibiotics. Any regimen must account for allergy, renal function, recent antibiotic therapy, local susceptibility patterns, and the possibility of antibiotic-resistant pathogens. Empiric coverage for gram-positive bacteria (staphylococci and streptococci) is almost always required, and so the usual question is whether to broaden the regimen to cover gram-negative bacteria (Table 43.5).[46,50,51] Anaerobic coverage should be considered for necrotic or malodorous wounds. If the patient responds to empiric therapy, the regimen may be narrowed according to microbiology susceptibility testing. The possibility of fastidious organisms missed by culture should be considered among nonresponders, or surgery may be needed.

Agents with demonstrated efficacy in clinical trials of therapy for DFIs include cephalosporins, β-lactamase inhibitor combination antibiotics, fluoroquinolones, clindamycin, carbapenems, glycopeptides, and linezolid (Table 43.6). The optimal duration of therapy for DFI has not been determined; common practice is to treat mild infections for 1 week, whereas serious infections that do not involve bone may require therapy for 2 weeks. Adequate debridement, resection, or amputation can shorten the necessary duration of therapy. Blood stream infection is a rare complication, for which many experts recommend a minimum of 2 weeks of therapy. Therapy may be discontinued when all signs and symptoms of infection have resolved; incomplete wound healing is not an indication to prolong antibiotic therapy.

TABLE 43.5

PATHOGENS ISOLATED IN A CLINICAL TRIAL OF ANTIBIOTIC THERAPY OF DIABETIC FOOT INFECTION

ORGANISMS	ISOLATES
Staphylococci	
Staphylococcus aureus (total)	158
Methicillin-sensitive *S. aureus*	127
Methicillin-resistant *S. aureus*	31
Coagulase-negative staphylococci	65
Streptococci	
Streptococcus agalactiae	52
β-Hemolytic streptococci	6
Streptococcus species	14
Enterococci	60
Pseudomonas species	27
Enterobacteriaceae	88

(50% of cases had only gram-positive cocci isolated).
Data from Lipsky BA, Itani K, Norden C, et al. Treating foot infections in diabetic patients: a randomized, multicenter, open-label trial of linezolid versus ampicillin-sulbactam/amoxicillin-clavulanate. *Clin Infect Dis*. 2004;38:17–24.

Adjuncts to Antibiotic Therapy. Hyperbaric oxygen (HBO) may improve wound healing and decrease the rate of amputation of DFI according to one double-blind, randomized trial.[52] However, most evidence of HBO effect in DFI is anecdotal[53] and difficult to interpret because of patient comorbidities that are poorly controlled for small sample sizes, and scant documentation of wound size and severity. Potential candidates for HBO therapy include patients at high risk for amputation (deep infections unresponsive to therapy). Objectively, HBO may be most beneficial when the transcutaneous oxygen tension is <40 mm Hg before therapy and increases to >200 mm Hg after therapy.[53]

Surgical revascularization may also be considered.[54] Improving blood flow to the ischemic, infected foot may be a crucial determinant of outcome. Initial debridement is undertaken in the presence of infection; revascularization is generally postponed until sepsis is controlled, but should not be postponed more than a few days lest there be additional tissue loss in the meanwhile. Successful revascularization of an ischemic, infected foot can result in 3-year limb salvage rates of up to 98%.[55]

A good outcome may be expected in 80%–90% of mild cases treated appropriately and 50%–60% for more advanced DFIs. Aggressive surgical debridement is often needed for infections of deep tissue or bone. Partial amputations (e.g., toe amputation, "ray" amputation of a metatarsal) may be foot-sparing and lead to effective control of infection in >80% of cases. Healing is facilitated when there is no exposed bone, absent tissue edema, a palpable popliteal pulse, ankle systolic blood pressure >80 mm Hg, and a white blood cell count <12,000 per mm^3. Infection recurs in 20%–30% of cases and should increase the suspicion of underlying osteomyelitis.

TABLE 43.6

RECENT PROSPECTIVE TRIALS OF ANTIBIOTIC THERAPY FOR COMPLICATED SKIN AND SKIN STRUCTURE INFECTIONS OF THE FOOT IN PATIENTS WITH DIABETES MELLITUS

STUDY	DRUG	COMPARATOR	RESULT	NOTES
Lipsky, 2004[46]	Linezolid (L) 600 mg IV/PO q12h	Ampicillin–sulbactam (A-S) 3 g IV q6h then amoxicillin–clavulanate 875 mg q 12 h	Clinical cure 81% vs. 71% (p = NS) Linezolid superior in post-hoc foot ulcer and nonosteo-myelitis groups	Open label randomized L:A-S 2:1 Treatment for 7–28 d
Harkless, 2005[50]	Piperacillin–tazobactam 4.5 g q8h IV	Ampicillin–sulbactam 3 g IV q6h	Clinical cure 81% vs. 83% Confidence interval not reported	Open label vancomycin 1 g IV q12h optional for both groups
Lipsky, 2005[51]	Ertapenem 1 g QD	Piperacillin–tazobactam 3.375 g Q6H for 5 d Amoxicillin–clavulanate 1 g PO Q12h for up to 23 d	94% vs. 92% cure, E Population 95% CI (-2,9, 6.9)	Non-inferior Treatment for up to 28 d

Osteomyelitis. Osteomyelitis is a feared complication of DFI (incidence, 50%–60% in serious DFIs; 10%–20% in mild infections).[39] However, because diabetic patients may have destructive bone lesions caused by peripheral neuropathy (e.g., Charcot joint), distinguishing between neuropathic and infectious destruction of bone can be difficult. The likelihood of osteomyelitis is increased with foot ulcers that are chronic (>4 weeks), large (>2 cm diameter), deep (>3 mm), or associated with a marked elevation of ESR (>70 mm/h).[39] Wound exploration that "probes to bone" has a positive predictive value of >90% for the diagnosis of osteomyelitis.

The initial diagnostic test should be plain radiographs of the foot. Radiographic changes may take 2 weeks to become manifest, and so repeating an initially negative study of a stable patient may be a better tactic than proceeding immediately to more sophisticated and expensive imaging. If clinical and plain radiographic findings are nondiagnostic, technetium 99m bone scans are 85% sensitive, but only 45% specific. Leukocyte scans (e.g., ^{111}In) have similar sensitivity, but higher specificity (~75%). Magnetic resonance imaging (MRI) is usually the diagnostic test of choice because of high sensitivity (>90%) and specificity (>80%), but is expensive. A definitive diagnosis of osteomyelitis requires a bone biopsy for culture and histology. Bone biopsy must be obtained through a clean surgical incision that does not traverse an open wound to avoid contamination by colonizing organisms. Biopsy is indicated if the diagnosis remains doubtful after imaging studies, or if the etiologic agent(s) cannot be ascertained because of previous antibiotic therapy or confusing culture results. Most cases of osteomyelitis are polymicrobial; *S. aureus* is isolated most commonly (~40%), but *S. epidermidis*, streptococci, and Enterobacteriaceae are also common isolates.

Antibiotic therapy of osteomyelitis should be based on results of bone culture, because soft tissue culture results do not predict bone pathogens accurately.[39] Empiric therapy should always cover *S. aureus*; broader coverage should be administered based on history or results of cultures. Most antibiotics penetrate bone poorly, and leukocyte function is impaired in these patients, and so long-term (at least 6 weeks) parenteral (at least initially) therapy is required. Osteomyelitis complicating DFI can be arrested by antibiotic therapy alone in about two-thirds of cases, and so resection of infected bone is not always necessary. Oral antibiotics with good bioavailability (e.g., fluoroquinolones, clindamycin) may be useful for most of the therapeutic course. If all infected bone is removed, a shorter course of therapy (e.g., 2 weeks) may be appropriate. Clinical resolution may be documented by a decrease to normal of the ESR or loss of increased uptake on a leukocyte scan.

SURGICAL SITE INFECTION

Infections of surgical incisions are now referred to as SSIs,[56] a common surgical complication that occurs after about 3% of all surgical procedures.[57] Potential complications of SSIs include tissue destruction, failure or prolongation of wound healing, incisional hernias, and occasionally blood stream infection. Recurrent pain and disfiguring scars may also result. Surgical site infections result in substantial morbidity, prolonged hospital stays, and increased direct patient costs, creating a huge economic burden on healthcare systems.[58]

Infection may occur within the surgical site at any depth, from the skin to the intracavitary operative field. Superficial incisional SSI involves tissues down to the fascia (Fig. 43.1), whereas deep incisional SSI extends into fascia and muscle, but not intracavitary. Organ/space infections are intracavitary, but, if related directly to an operation, are considered to be SSIs.

Epidemiology

Numerous factors determine whether a patient will develop a SSI, including factors contributed by the patient, the environment, and the treatment (Table 43.7).[59] As described by the National Nosocomial Infections Surveillance System (NNIS)[59–61] of the U.S. Centers for Disease Control and Prevention (CDC) (Table 43.8), the most recognized risk factors for SSI are the wound classification (contaminated or dirty—see below and Table 43.9), American Society of Anesthesiologists (ASA) class ≥ 3 (chronic active medical illness; Table 43.10),

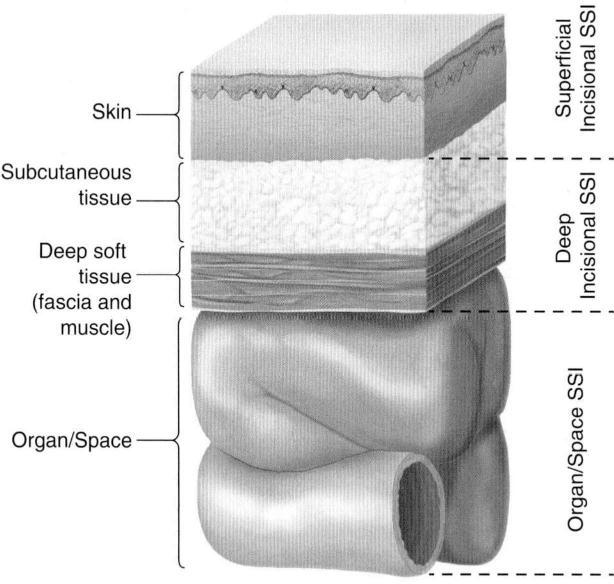

FIGURE 43.1. Cross-section of the abdominal wall depicting U.S. Centers for Disease Control and Prevention (CDC) classifications of surgical site infection.

TABLE 43.7

RISK FACTORS FOR THE DEVELOPMENT OF SURGICAL SITE INFECTIONS

Patient Factors
Ascites
Chronic inflammation
Corticosteroid therapy (controversial)
Obesity
Diabetes
Extremes of age
Hypocholsterolemia
Hypoxemia
Peripheral vascular disease (especially for lower extremity surgery)
Postoperative anemia
Prior site irradiation
Recent operation
Remote infection
Skin carriage of staphylococci
Skin disease in the area of infection (e.g., psoriasis)
Undernutrition

Environmental Factors
Contaminated medications
Inadequate disinfection/sterilization
Inadequate skin antisepsis
Inadequate ventilation

Treatment Factors
Drains
Emergency procedure
Hypothermia
Inadequate antibiotic prophylaxis
Oxygenation (controversial)
Prolonged preoperative hospitalization
Prolonged operative time

Adapted from Barie PS. Surgical site infections: epidemiology and prevention. *Surg Infect (Larchmt)* 2002;(3 suppl 1):S9–S21.

TABLE 43.8

NATIONAL NNIS RISK INDEX FOR SURGICAL SITE INFECTIONS

TRADITIONAL CLASS	0	1	2	3	ALL
Clean	1.0%	2.3%	5.4%	NA	2.1%
Clean/contaminated	2.1%	4.9%	9.5%	NA	3.3%
Contaminated	NA	3.4%	6.6%	13.2%	6.4%
Dirty	NA	3.1%	8.1%	12.8%	7.1%
All	1.5%	2.9%	6.8%	13.0%	2.8%

Adapted from National Nosocomial Infections Surveillance (NNIS) System Report, Data Summary from January 1992–June 2001, issued August 2001. *Am J Infect Control.* 2001;29:404–421.

and prolonged operative time, where time is longer than the 75th percentile for each such procedure. Clean surgical procedures (class I incisions; Table 43.9) involve only integumentary and musculoskeletal soft tissues (e.g., groin hernia, breast, thyroid). Clean-contaminated procedures (class II) open a hollow viscus (e.g., alimentary, biliary, genitourinary, respiratory tract) under controlled circumstances (e.g., elective colon surgery). Contaminated procedures (class III) involve extensive introduction of bacteria into a normally sterile body cavity, but too briefly to allow infection to become established (e.g., penetrating abdominal trauma, enterotomy during adhesiolysis for mechanical bowel obstruction). Dirty procedures (class IV) are those where the surgery is performed to control established infection (e.g., colon resection for complicated diverticulitis).

According to the NNIS classification, the risk of SSI increases with an increasing number of risk factors present, irrespective of the wound class and almost without regard for the type of operation (Table 43.11).[62] Laparoscopic abdominal surgery is associated with a decreased incidence of SSI under certain circumstances, which has required a modification of the NNIS risk classification.[61] For laparoscopic biliary, gastric, and colon surgery, one risk factor point is subtracted if the operation is performed via the laparoscope, so that the NNIS risk classification system grades risk from –1 to 3. Laparoscopy decreases the risk of SSI for several reasons, including decreased wound size, limited use of cautery, and a diminished stress response to tissue injury. Laparoscopic appendectomy, on the other hand, is a unique circumstance in that the risk of SSI is reduced by laparoscopy only if no risk factors are present (i.e., the patient is otherwise healthy, the appendix is not perforated, and the operation does not take more than 1 hour).

Outpatient surgery and early discharge protocols pose problems for surveillance of SSI.[63] Although many SSIs will develop in the first 5–10 days after surgery, a SSI may develop up to 30 days after surgery (1 year, if a prosthetic device was inserted); thus, SSIs do occur in the postdischarge setting. Therefore, estimates of the incidence of SSI after ambulatory surgery depend upon inherently unreliable voluntary self-reporting by surgeons. Therefore, the incidence of SSI reported by NNIS is almost certainly underestimated. Unfortunately, data reported by the NNIS also do not identify cases as incisional or organ/space SSIs.

Host-derived factors are important contributors to the risk of SSI that the ASA score may not capture. Increased age,[64] obesity, malnutrition, diabetes mellitus,[65,66] hypocholesterolemia,[67] previous radiation therapy, and other factors are

TABLE 43.9

SURGICAL SITE INFECTION WOUND CLASSIFICATION AND APPROXIMATE RATES OF INFECTION

CLASS	DEFINITION	EXAMPLES	RATE (%)
I: Clean	Atraumatic wound No inflammation No break in aseptic technique No entry of biliary, respiratory, GI, or GU tracts If drained, by closed drainage	Herniorrhaphy Excision of skin lesion Thyroidectomy	1–5
ID: Clean; prosthetic material implanted	Same as I, Clean	Vascular surgery with graft Cardiac valve replacement	1–5
II: Clean-contaminated	Atraumatic wound No inflammation Minor break in aseptic technique Biliary, respiratory, GI, or GU tract entered under controlled conditions with minimal contamination	Appendectomy without perforation Elective colectomy after bowel preparation Cholecystectomy	2–9
III: Contaminated	Traumatic wound with delay in therapy or exogenous contamination Acute non-purulent inflammation Major break in aseptic technique Entry of biliary, respiratory, GI, or GU tract with gross spillage of contents	Penetrating abdominal with hollow viscus injury Inadvertent enterotomy during adhesiolysis for mechanical small intestinal obstruction	3–13

GI, gastrointestinal; GU, genitourinary.

TABLE 43.10

AMERICAN SOCIETY OF ANESTHESIOLOGISTS (ASA) PHYSICAL STATUS SCORE

ASA 1 A normal healthy patient.
ASA 2 A patient with mild-to-moderate systemic disturbance that results in no functional limitations. Examples: hypertension, diabetes mellitus, chronic bronchitis, morbid obesity, and extremes of age.
ASA 3 A patient with severe systemic disturbance that results in functional limitations. Examples: poorly controlled hypertension, diabetes mellitus with vascular complications, angina pectoris, prior myocardial infarction, and pulmonary disease that limits activity.
ASA 4 A patient with a severe systemic disturbance that is life threatening with or without the planned procedure. Examples: congestive heart failure, unstable angina pectoris, advanced pulmonary, renal or hepatic dysfunction.
ASA 5 A morbid patient not expected to survive with or without the operative procedure. Examples: ruptured abdominal aortic aneurysm, pulmonary embolism, and traumatic brain injury with increased intracranial pressure.
ASA 6 Any patient in whom the procedure is an emergency. Example: ASA 4E.

not accounted for specifically by NNIS. In a study of 2,345 patients undergoing cardiac surgery, the incidence of SSI was 8.5% (199/2,345).[68] The relative risk (RR) of SSI among diabetic patients was 2.29 (95% confidence interval [CI] 1.15–4.54), and the RR among obese patients (body mass index >30) was 1.78 (95% CI, 1.24–2.55). Malone et al. found an incidence of SSI of 3.2% among 5,031 noncardiac surgery patients at a Veterans Affairs hospital. Independent risk factors for the development of SSI included ascites, diabetes mellitus, postoperative anemia, and recent weight loss, but not chronic obstructive pulmonary disease, tobacco use, or corticosteroid use.[69] Other studies have linked low-serum albumin concentration and increased serum creatinine concentration to an increased risk of SSI.[70]

Microbiology

Inoculation of the surgical site occurs during surgery, either inward from the skin or outward from the tissues being operated on. The microbiology of SSI depends on the type of operation, with an increased likelihood of gram-negative bacilli after gastrointestinal surgery or infrainguinal vascular surgery. However, most SSIs are caused by gram-positive cocci that are commensal skin flora (Table 43.12),[70] including *S. aureus*, coagulase-negative staphylococci (usually *S. epidermidis*), and *Enterococcus* spp. Head and neck surgery (if pharyngoesophageal structures are entered) and intestinal surgery may be associated with SSI caused by enteric facultative (e.g., *Escherichia coli*) and anaerobic (e.g. *Bacteroides fragilis*) bacteria. Properly administered antibiotic prophylaxis is an essential part of an ensemble of tactics to prevent surgical site infection and is discussed elsewhere (see Chapter 13).

TABLE 43.11

SURGICAL SITE INFECTION RATES AFTER COMMON OPERATIVE PROCEDURES BY RISK CATEGORY

PROCEDURE	NUMBER OF RISK FACTORS			
	0	1	2	3
Appendectomy	1.15	1.15	3.47	3.47
Bile duct, liver, or pancreatic surgery	8.07		13.65	
Breast surgery	0.95	2.95	6.36	6.36
Colon surgery	3.99	5.59	7.06	9.47
Gastric surgery	1.72		4.23	
Herniorrhaphy (inpatient)	0.74	2.42	5.25	
Peripheral vascular bypass surgery	2.93	6.98		
Small bowel surgery	3.44	6.75		

Adapted from Edwards JR, Peterson KD, Mu Y, et al. National Healthcare Safety Network (NHSN) report: Data summary for 2006 through 2008, issued December 2009. *Am J Infect Control.* 2009;37:783–805.

Preoperative Preparation

The patient should be assessed prior to elective surgery for modifiable risk factors. Open skin lesions should heal beforehand if possible. The patient should be free of bacterial infections of any kind and should preferably quit smoking at least 1 month prior to surgery. The patient must not be shaved the night before, considering that the risk of SSI is increased by bacteria that colonize the inevitable small cuts and abrasions.[70] Particular attention should be paid to the patient's nutritional status. Obese patients should lose as much weight as is safely possible. Malnourished patients can reduce the risk of SSI significantly with as few as 5 days of enteral nutritional support.[71,72]

TABLE 43.12

INCIDENCE OF PATHOGEN ISOLATION IN SURGICAL SITE INFECTION (COLLECTED SERIES)

ORGANISM	PERCENTAGE
Staphylococcus aureus	20
Coagulase-negative staphylococci	14
Enterococci	12
Pseudomonas aeruginosa	8
Escherichia coli	8
Enterobacter spp.	7
Proteus mirabilis	3
Streptococcus spp.	3
Klebsiella pneumoniae	3
Candida albicans	2

Diagnosis and Treatment

Specific criteria have been established by the CDC for the diagnosis of SSI (Table 43.13). Adherence to these diagnostic guidelines is important, because SSI can be misdiagnosed otherwise. Proper surveillance requires the prospective involvement of trained personnel, adhering to the aforementioned criteria, who inspect incisions directly and in prospect. Retrospective studies of SSI are plagued by diagnostic inaccuracy and therefore are inherently dubious. Likewise, voluntary self-reporting by surgeons produces notoriously underestimated incidence rates, because reporting does not occur; SSIs that become apparent in the outpatient setting escape hospital-based surveillance programs. Therefore, published data from NNIS (Table 43.8) probably are at or near the lower end of the confidence interval.

TABLE 43.13

CRITERIA FOR DIAGNOSIS OF INCISIONAL AND ORGAN/SPACE SURGICAL SITE INFECTIONS (SSIs) WITHIN 30 DAYS OF ALL PROCEDURES (1 YEAR IF PROSTHETIC MATERIAL IS IMPLANTED)

INCISIONAL SSI

Superficial—infection involves skin or subcutaneous tissue of the incision *and* at least one of the following:

1. Purulent drainage from the superficial incision
2. Organisms isolated from an aseptically obtained culture from the superficial incision
3. One or more of the following: pain, localized swelling, erythema, or heat, and incision is opened deliberately by surgeon, unless incision is culture negative.
4. Diagnosis of superficial incisional SSI by surgeon

Deep—infection involves fascial or muscle layer of the incision *and* at least one of the following:

1. Purulent drainage from the deep incision, excluding organ/space[a]
2. Incision that dehisces spontaneously or is opened deliberately by a surgeon in the presence of fever (>38°C), or pain, unless site is culture negative
3. Evidence of infection is found on direct examination, during repeat surgery, or by histopathologic or radiologic examination[b]
4. Diagnosis of deep incisional SSI by surgeon

ORGAN/SPACE SSI

Infection of any part of the anatomy (e.g., organs or surgically created spaces) opened or manipulated during an operation *and* at least one of the following:

1. Purulent drainage from a drain that is placed into the organ/space
2. Organisms isolated from an aseptically obtained culture from the organ/space
3. Evidence of infection is found on direct examination, during repeat surgery, or by histopathologic or radiologic examination[b]
4. Diagnosis of an organ/space SSI by surgeon

For all classifications, infection is defined as occurring within 30 d after the operation if no implant is placed or within 1 year if an implant is in place and the infection is related to the incision

[a]Report infection that involves both superficial and deep incision sites as a deep incisional SSI

[b]Report an organ/space SSI that drains spontaneously through the incision as a deep incisional SSI

Adapted from Mangram AJ, Horan TC, Pearson ML, et al. Guideline for prevention of surgical site infection, 1999. Hospital Infection Control Practices Advisory Committee. *Infect Control Hosp Epidemiol.* 1999;20:250–278.

Not all draining or erythematous incisions are infected. A superficial swab culture will likely become contaminated during specimen collection and be overinterpreted. Once a diagnosis of SSI is established, there is only one constant in the management: incise and drain the incision. Often, opening the incision and applying basic wound care (e.g., topical saline-soaked wet-to-dry cotton gauze dressings) is sufficient, provided that the incision is opened sufficiently to facilitate wound care and the diagnosis of associated conditions. An incision that is too small may fail to control the infection. Most nostrums other than physiologic saline applied to gauze dressings (e.g., modified Dakin solution, 0.25% acetic acid solution) actually suppress fibroblast proliferation and may delay secondary wound healing.

Opening the incision adequately is essential because it affords not only control of the infection but also an opportunity to diagnose and treat associated conditions such as skin, subcutaneous tissue, or fascial necrosis that requires debridement; fascial dehiscence or evisceration that requires formal abdominal wall reconstruction; or subfascial drainage that could signal an organ/space infection or an enteric fistula. Without control of complicating factors, a SSI will be difficult or impossible to control.

Antibiotic therapy is not required for uncomplicated superficial SSIs that are opened and drained adequately and that receive appropriate local wound care. If antibiotic therapy is unwarranted, then culture and susceptibility testing of wound drainage are of no value. In fact, routine swabs of drainage are not recommended because the risk of contamination by commensal skin flora is high. Rather, tissue specimens or an aliquot of pus collected aseptically and anaerobically into a syringe are recommended for analysis.

Antibiotics may be indicated if there is systemic evidence of toxicity (e.g., fever, leukocytosis) or cellulitis that extends more than 2 cm beyond the incision. Antibiotics are also indicated as adjunctive management of several of the complications mentioned earlier. The choice of antibiotic is defined by the operation performed through the incision and the likely infecting organism. Coverage against gram-positive cocci is indicated in most circumstances.

Wound closure by secondary intention can be protracted and disfiguring. Reports of vacuum-assisted wound closure (VAC) are proliferating. Putative benefits of VAC dressings include reduced inflammation, increased fibroblast activity, improved wound hygiene (fluid is aspirated continuously from the field), and more rapid wound contraction and closure.[73] However, these benefits remain conjectural in the absence of definitive class I data.

NECROTIZING SOFT TISSUE INFECTION

Necrotizing soft tissue infections (NSTIs) are dangerous because of rapid progression and much systemic toxicity, but fortunately also uncommon.[74] Bacterial proteases cleave tissue planes, facilitating rapid spread. Host defenses are overwhelmed, leading to hemodynamic instability and hypoperfusion. Ischemic tissue in turn is susceptible to progression of the infection, and organ dysfunction may result. Because NSTIs are uncommon and their initial manifestations are protean and can be subtle, clinicians must have a high index of suspicion in order to prevent diagnostic delay. Although most presentations are obvious, a NSTI must always be considered whenever a patient presents with severe pain, particularly of the perineum or an extremity, which is disproportionate to any physical findings. There may be no obvious portal. The presence of gas in the soft tissues (crepitus) on examination or by imaging study is helpful, but unreliable if absent.

Delayed definitive therapy (i.e., surgical debridement) is the major risk factor for mortality in cases of NSTI; therefore, familiarity is crucial for anyone (e.g., surgeon, emergency physician, primary care physician) who might encounter an early presentation. True NSTIs cannot be treated successfully with antibiotics alone (although broad-spectrum antibiotics are an essential adjunct to surgery), and so timely surgical consultation is mandatory.[75] Even with optimal therapy, mortality is approximately 25%–30%, and hospitalization is protracted, complicated, and expensive regardless of outcome.[75–77]

Although many names have been applied to these serious infections, such as synergistic gangrene and the eponymous Fournier gangrene (of the scrotum), it is most useful to characterize NSTIs based on the deepest tissue layer involved by necrosis. Involvement of the skin and subcutaneous tissue only is *necrotizing cellulitis*, whereas involvement of the fascia (most common) is referred to as *necrotizing fasciitis*, and involvement of underlying muscle is referred to as *necrotizing myositis* or sometimes myonecrosis. Some experts classify NSTIs further by the causative pathogen (e.g., clostridial myositis) or whether the infection is polymicrobial (type I) or caused by a single organism (type II). It is important to distinguish NSTI from nonnecrotizing SSTIs, because the latter may be treated effectively with intravenous antibiotics alone. However, only operative debridement can classify accurately the anatomic extent of NSTI; therefore, attempts to classify NSTIs preoperatively can only engender dangerous, even life-threatening delay.

Etiology

Necrotizing STIs can be primary or secondary events. Primary, or idiopathic, infections are less common and lack a portal of entry. Whether the source of bacteria in primary NSTIs is the blood stream or from epithelial disruptions too small to be apparent is debated; either mechanism is possible. One well-known example, the halophilic marine bacteria of the genus *Vibrio* (especially *V. vulnificus*),[78] can cause NSTIs after ingestion of raw seafood or skin trauma while wading in seawater. Another example is NSTI caused by *Clostridium septicum*, which is specifically associated with occult carcinoma of the colon and likely arises after a bacteremia.[79]

Much more common than primary infections are secondary infections, which may arise after burns or trauma, in recent surgical incisions, or as a consequence of unrecognized, neglected, or inadequately treated SSTIs. Other potential portals of entry include human, animal, or insect bites, and parenteral drug abuse.[80] Secondary NSTIs often have associated conditions that can predispose to tissue necrosis or impede containment by local host defenses. Inadequate treatment of SSTIs, such as decubitus ulcers,[81] ischemic leg ulcers, Bartholin cyst abscess, or perirectal or ischiorectal abscess, poses a high risk of progression to NSTI. However, for reasons that are unclear, SSTIs of the face, neck, or chest[82–85] progress less often to NSTI than infections of the perineum and lower extremity.

Microbiology

Necrotizing STIs are divided into two categories: polymicrobial (type I, 80%) and monomicrobial (type II, 20%). Monomicrobial NSTIs are caused most commonly by *S. pyogenes*, but *S. aureus* and *C. perfringens* can also be causative. Rare causes of monomicrobial NSTI include *V. vulnificus*, community-associated MRSA,[11] and *Bacillus cereus*.[86] *Pseudomonas aeruginosa* rarely is a pathogen of NSTI; rarer still are the infections caused by *C. septicum*. Phycomycotic NSTI (mucormycosis) caused by *Rhizopus*, *Mucor*, or *Absidia* spp. may occur in profoundly immunosuppressed patients or after accidental burial by a landslide. Much more common are the polymicrobial NSTIs, which account for approximately 80% of cases. Aerobic gram-positive and -negative bacteria and anaerobes are usually all present, and the bacteria may act synergistically to promote dissemination and increase toxicity. *Escherichia coli* and *B. fragilis* are the most common aerobic and anaerobic isolates, respectively.[87] The most likely gram-positive coccus to be isolated depends on the clinical context. For example, enterococci are more likely to be isolated when the NSTI complicates a recent abdominal incision.

Pathogenesis. After inoculation of susceptible tissue, several factors determine the extent of infection, including the size of the inoculum, the invasiveness of the organism,[88,89] the presence of a foreign body or ischemic tissue, and impaired host responses. Inoculation can occur from delayed or inadequate treatment of an initially localized process, inappropriate closure of a contaminated surgical incision that should have been left open, or in the presence of an enterostomy or retention sutures. Inoculation may also be occult; for example, NSTI of the thigh can be the initial manifestation of a colon perforation into the retroperitoneum.

The hallmark of NSTI is rapid progression and a fulminant clinical course. Both monomicrobial and polymicrobial NSTIs are true emergencies that require rapid diagnosis and definitive treatment. Several bacterial enzymes cause tissue damage and promote bacterial invasiveness, including hemolysin, fibrinolysin, hyaluronidase, and streptokinase elaborated by *S. pyogenes*; collagenase elaborated by *P. aeruginosa*; and lecithinase elaborated by *C. perfringens*. Polymicrobial NSTIs are characterized by synergistic interactions of facultative aerobes and anaerobes. Tissue hypoxia and impaired neutrophil function create conditions favorable for the proliferation of facultative bacteria, which consume oxygen in the microenvironment and lower the tissue redox state, thereby creating conditions favorable for the growth of anaerobes.

Extensive tissue necrosis develops from direct tissue injury caused by bacterial toxins, inflammation and tissue edema, and vascular thrombosis. The subcutaneous fat and fascia are more likely than the overlying skin to develop necrosis. Thus, there may be little or no early cutaneous evidence of underlying infection, but the patient will complain of severe pain. As the infection progresses, thrombosis of the cutaneous microcirculation leads to the characteristic erythema, edema, bullae, and overt gangrene of advanced NSTI.

Soft tissue gas may or may not be present, depending on the pathogens involved, but develops as a result of anaerobic wound conditions that allow gas-forming organisms to proliferate, including *C. perfringens*, *B. fragilis*, *E. coli*, *K. pneumoniae*, *P. aeruginosa*, and *Proteus* spp. These bacteria produce insoluble gases such as hydrogen, nitrogen, and methane, which remain in the tissue to a variable degree. Gas in the tissue tends to be a late finding in nonclostridial polymicrobial infections and to be absent in NSTI caused by *S. pyogenes*.

Diagnosis

The diagnosis of NSTI is based primarily on the history and physical examination. One notable early characteristic is a complaint of severe pain that is disproportionate to local physical findings. Inspection of the overlying skin may yield few early clues as cutaneous stigmata may be subtle. Clinicians should consider NSTI for all soft tissue manifestations of inflammation signs and symptoms such as pain, swelling, rubor, increased temperature, and loss of function. Characteristic features to elicit include edema and tenderness that extend beyond the margin of erythema, skin vesicles or bullae, crepitus, and the absence of lymphangitis and lymphadenitis. Erythema limits should be marked with a pen and should be reexamined frequently; failure to improve with appropriate antibiotics should prompt further investigation. Crepitus is a specific indicator but not commonly present in early NSTIs. As infection progresses, cutaneous anesthesia and necrosis develop along with clinical manifestations of sepsis (fever, tachycardia, hypotension, and encephalopathy). Occasionally, patients with clostridial sepsis will present with anemia and jaundice secondary to hemolysis, and patients with myonecrosis will present with myoglobinuria, rhabdomyolysis, and acute renal failure.

Some common laboratory tests may point the clinician toward the diagnosis of NSTI in the appropriate clinical context. Wall et al.[90,91] showed that hyponatremia ($[Na]_{serum} < 135$ mEq/dL) and leukocytosis (white blood cell count $>14 \times 10^9$/L) have good diagnostic accuracy (Table 43.14). Wong et al.[92] described the Laboratory Risk Indicator for Necrotizing Fasciitis (LRINEC) score (Table 43.15), which may be even more accurate. Although these observations have not been subjected to independent validation, they may be valuable to the extent that it *heightens* the suspicion of a clinician confronted with a possible NSTI.

If the diagnosis is not obvious by physical examination and laboratory testing, radiographic studies may be obtained, provided surgical exploration, which is the definitive diagnostic test as well as therapeutic intervention, is not unduly delayed. Plain radiographs can demonstrate gas in the soft tissues even in the absence of crepitus, but the absence of gas does not exclude the presence of NSTI. Computed tomography is sensitive for the presence of soft tissue gas, and it may also demonstrate asymmetric edema of tissue planes (a nonspecific finding). A CT scan may be helpful in the evaluation of the obese patient with a deep-seated infection, a circumstance where the physical examination can be unreliable. However, to the extent that obtaining any imaging study will delay the operative management of the patient, they should be avoided. Wheareas fine needle aspiration and incisional biopsy of questionably affected tissues may add information, these should only be used in the setting of operative debridement. Gram stain of the biopsy material can demonstrate causative organisms and an inflammatory cell infiltrate; frozen section demonstration of necrosis, thrombosis, or pathogens in tissue are diagnostic. The use of imaging or biopsy as "confirmatory" tests cannot be condoned. Clinical diagnosis alone is sufficient to begin broad-spectrum antimicrobial therapy and undertake surgical exploration and debridement.

Treatment

The management of NSTI is a true emergency. The elapsed time between the onset of symptoms and the initial operative treatment is the single most important factor influencing morbidity and mortality. Delay in diagnosis must be avoided at all costs, as the success of management depends on prompt recognition and operative debridement.[93–95] Once the diagnosis of NSTI is made, tissue salvage and patient survival can only be achieved by prompt, widespread debridement in the operating room. Operative debridement should not be delayed for resuscitation, as this may be performed in the operating room, and the patient may not respond to resuscitation until

TABLE 43.14

OBJECTIVE CRITERIA TO DISTINGUISH NECROTIZING SOFT TISSUE INFECTIONS FROM NON-NECROTIZING INFECTIONS

A. DIAGNOSTIC ACCURACY

	SENSITIVITY (%)	SPECIFICITY (%)	POSITIVE PREDICTIVE VALUE (%)	NEGATIVE PREDICTIVE VALUE (%)
Tense edema	38	100	100	62
Gas on x-ray	39	95	88	62
Bullae	24	100	100	57
WBC > 14 × 10^9/L	81	76	77	80
Sodium <135 mg/dL	75	100	100	77
Chloride <95 mg/dL	30	100	100	55
BUN > 15 mg/dL	70	88	88	71

B. INCIDENCE OF POSITIVE LABORATORY PARAMETERS (UNIVARIATE ANALYSIS)

	NECROTIZING FASCIITIS	OTHER INFECTION	*P* VALUE
WBC > 14 × 10^9/L	17/21 (81%)	5/21 (24%)	0.0002
Sodium <135 mEq/L	15/20 (75%)	0/17 (0%)	0.0001
Chloride <95 mEq/L	6/20 (30%)	0/17 (0%)	
BUN > 15 mg/dL	14/20 (70%)	2/17 (12%)	0.0007

BUN, blood urea nitrogen WBC, white blood cell Data from Wall DB, de Virgilio C, Black S, et al. Objective criteria may assist in distinguishing necrotizing fasciitis from nonnecrotizing soft tissue infection. *Am J Surg*. 2000;179:17–21; Wall DB, Klein SR, Black S, et al. A simple model to help distinguish necrotizing fasciitis from nonnecrotizing soft tissue infection. *J Am Coll Surg*. 2000;191:227–231.

the infected tissue is removed. Identification of the causative organism(s) and underlying pathology can wait. Antibiotics are a necessary adjunct and must be started immediately, but they are only an adjunct; the mortality of true NSTI managed nonoperatively is 100%.

The patient should have blood products available in the operating room and should have adequate IV access for resuscitation. The first surgical objective is a thorough wound exploration to confirm the presence and extent of NSTI. Debridement of all infected, devitalized tissue must be aggressive. The underlying tissue necrosis usually extends far beyond the boundary of the skin involvement; therefore, exposure must be wide and dissection must extend beyond the boundary of tissue viability. Considering that these infections spread rapidly, resection of a margin of viable tissue is prudent even at the cost of additional deformity or disability; certainly, all non-viable tissue should be removed at the initial operation. When the margin of viability is indistinct, frozen section examination of the limits of resection can occasionally be helpful. NSTIs are characterized by gray-brown fluid drainage, gray fascia, easy separation of subcutaneous fat from fascia, or dead muscle. Wound drainage must be submitted for comprehensive microbiologic testing. Fasciotomies should be performed if compartment syndrome is suspected or is a likely sequela of impending resuscitation. A temporary prosthesis may be necessary to reconstruct the abdominal wall to prevent evisceration in some cases. All open wounds are irrigated before loose packing with saline-moistened gauze.

Routine reexploration in the operating room is necessary at 24 hours to ensure that all necrotic tissue has been debrided. Patients with NSTIs are often unstable, so ICU management must also be aggressive with mechanical ventilation, fluids, blood and blood products, and hemodynamic support as appropriate so that the crucial return trip to the operating room can occur on schedule. End-organ dysfunction such as acute kidney injury and coagulopathy should be treated supportively and aggressively so that return trips to the operating room are not delayed. Operative debridement is continued daily until the infection is controlled. Extremity amputation or colostomy may be necessary to manage severe infections of the extremity or perineum, respectively.

Empiric antibiotics must be effective against a broad range of potential pathogens (gram-positive cocci, gram-negative bacilli including *Pseudomonas*, and anaerobes), because the infecting organism usually cannot be discerned from inspection alone. Empiric antifungal therapy is unnecessary in most cases of NSTI. Antibacterial monotherapy can be achieved with a carbapenem or piperacillin–tazobactam. Current guidelines recommend ampicillin–sulbactam, but activity may be inadequate against *E. coli* and *K. pneumoniae*. Clindamycin in high dosage may be preferable to penicillin G for streptococcal infections, because of *in vitro* evidence that clindamycin inhibits toxin production. Clindamycin is also effective against MSSA. Metronidazole can be substituted for clindamycin for therapy for type I infections if better anaerobic coverage is needed. Gentamicin is best avoided because of the additive risk of acute kidney injury in patients who may be hypovolemic or hypotensive. However, gentamicin is an efficient microbicide when given in adequate dosage; single-daily dose administration provides an adequate peak serum concentration while also minimizing toxicity. Combination therapy that includes vancomycin is now popular, especially considering that nearly 60% of *S. aureus* strains are now MRSA. Vancomycin or other

TABLE 43.15

LABORATORY RISK INDICATOR FOR NECROTIZING FASCIITIS (LRINEC) SCORE

PARAMETER	POINT VALUE
C-reactive protein, mg/L	
<150	0
≥150	4
White blood cell count, mm^3	
<15	0
15–25	1
>25	2
Hemoglobin, g/dL	
>13.5	0
11–13.5	1
<11	2
Sodium, mEq/L	
>135	0
≤135	2
Creatinine, mg/dL	
≤1.6	0
>1.6	2
Glucose, mg/dL	
≤180	0
>180	1

The maximum LRINEC score is 13 points. A score of ≥6 points should raise the suspicion of a necrotizing soft tissue infection, whereas a score of ≥8 points is strongly predictive. The model was constructed retrospectively but has a positive predictive value of 92% at a cutoff score of 6 points, and a negative predictive value of 96%.

Adapted from Wong CH, Khin LW, Heng KS, et al. The LRINEC (Laboratory Risk Indicator for Necrotizing Fasciitis) score: a tool for distinguishing necrotizing fasciitis from other soft tissue infections. *Crit Care Med.* 2004;32:1535–1541.

agents that are active against MRSA can be added to piperacillin–tazobactam or a carbapenem if appropriate.

All identified pathogens should be treated. The duration of therapy must be individualized, but most NSTIs will require a minimum of 10 days of therapy. Once culture and sensitivity data are available, the empiric antibiotic regimen should be adjusted accordingly. Adjustment can be challenging when multiple pathogens are isolated from a polymicrobial infection, but an attempt must be made to narrow the antibiotic spectrum as appropriate in order to decrease the chance of superinfection by multidrug-resistant pathogens. Clostridial infections are best treated with penicillin alone, but many clinicians prefer high-dose clindamycin to penicillin for NSTIs caused by *S. pyogenes* because of its antitoxin properties. Anaerobic infections of the head, neck, and upper extremity tend to be caused by penicillin-susceptible anaerobes, whereas those of the trunk and lower extremity tend to include *B. fragilis*, against which penicillin is ineffective. Rare phycomycotic infections may require amphotericin B; fluconazole is ineffective.

Patients with traumatic wounds should receive tetanus toxoid or immune globulin, depending on their immunization status. Other therapy is supportive, including early nutritional support and prophylaxis against venous thromboembolic disease. HBO therapy has been advocated, especially for clostridial infections.[92–94] Among the putative benefits of hyperbaric oxygen are inhibition of exotoxin production, increased tissue oxygen tension, and improved neutrophil function. However, there are no randomized trials of HBO therapy of NSTI. A "dive" is time-consuming, and patients may be too unstable for this setting; priority should always be timely diagnosis and rapid transfer to the operating room for wide debridement.

References

1. Stevens DL, Bisno AL, Chambers HF, et al. Practice guidelines for the diagnosis and management of skin and soft-tissue infections. *Clin Infect Dis.* 2005;41:1373–1406.
2. Draft guidance for industry: acute bacterial skin and soft tissue infections: developing drugs for treatment. www.fda.gov/downloads/drugs/.../guidances/ucm071185.pdf. Accessed March 20, 2011.
3. May AK, Stafford RE, Bulger EM, et al. Treatment of complicated skin and soft tissue infections. *Surg Infect (Larchmt).* 2009;10:467–499.
4. Swartz MN. Clinical practice. Cellulitis. *N Engl J Med.* 2004;350:904–912.
5. Brook I, Frazier EH. Aerobic and anaerobic bacteriology of wounds and cutaneous abscesses. *Arch Surg.* 1990;125:1445–1451.
6. Hook EW III, Hooton TM, Horton CA, et al. Microbiologic evaluation of cutaneous cellulitis in adults. *Arch Intern Med.* 1986;146:295–297.
7. Kielhofner MA, Brown B, Dall L. Influence of underlying disease process on the utility of cellulitis needle aspirates. *Arch Intern Med.* 1988;148:2451–2452.
8. Lebre C, Girard-Pipau F, Roujeau JC, et al. Value of fine-needle aspiration in infectious cellulitis. *Arch Dermatol.* 1996;132:842–843.
9. National Nosocomial Infections Surveillance (NNIS) System Report, data summary from January 1992 through June 2004, issued October 2004. *Am J Infect Control.* 2004;32:470–485.
10. Fridkin SK, Hageman JC, Morrison M, et al. Methicillin-resistant *Staphylococcus aureus* disease in three communities. *N Engl J Med.* 2005;352:1436–1444.
11. Charlebois ED, Perdreau-Remington F, Kreiswirth B, et al. Origins of community strains of methicillin-resistant *Staphylococcus aureus. Clin Infect Dis.* 2004;39:47–54.
12. Miller LG, Perdreau-Remington F, Rieg G, et al. Necrotizing fasciitis caused by community-associated methicillin-resistant *Staphylococcus aureus* in Los Angeles. *N Engl J Med.* 2005;352:1445–1453.
13. Frazee BW, Lynn J, Charlebois ED, et al. High prevalence of methicillin-resistant *Staphylococcus aureus* in emergency department skin and soft tissue infections. *Ann Emerg Med.* 2005;45:311–320.
14. Szumowski JD, Cohen DE, Kanaya F, et al. Treatment and outcomes of infections by methicillin-resistant *Staphylococcus aureus* at an ambulatory clinic. *Antimicrob Agents Chemother.* 2007;51:423–428.
15. Cenizal MJ, Skiest D, Luber S, et al. Prospective randomized trial of empiric therapy with trimethoprim-sulfamethoxazole or doxycycline for outpatient skin and soft tissue infections in an area of high prevalence of methicillin-resistant *Staphylococcus aureus. Antimicrob Agents Chemother.* 2007;51:2628–2630.
16. Markowitz N, Quinn EL, Saravolatz LD. Trimethoprim-sulfamethoxazole compared with vancomycin for the treatment of *Staphylococcus aureus* infection. *Ann Intern Med.* 1992;117:390–398.
17. Lewis JS II, Jorgensen JH. Inducible clindamycin resistance in staphylococci: should clinicians and microbiologists be concerned? *Clin Infect Dis.* 2005;40:280–285.
18. Barrett TW, Moran GJ. Update on emerging infections:news from the Centers for Disease Control and Prevention. Methicillin-resistant *Staphylococcus aureus* infections among competitive sports participants—Colorado, Indiana, Pennsylvania, and Los Angeles County, 2000–2003. *Ann Emerg Med.* 2004;43:43–45.
19. Herold BC, Immergluck LC, Maranan MC, et al. Community-acquired methicillin-resistant *Staphylococcus aureus* in children with no identified predisposing risk. *JAMA.* 1998;279:593–598.
20. David MZ, Mennella C, Mansour M, et al. Predominance of methicillin-resistant *Staphylococcus aureus* among pathogens causing skin and soft tissue infections in a large urban jail: Risk factors and recurrence rates. *J Clin Microbiol.* 2008;46:3222–3227.
21. Main CL, Jayaratne P, Haley A, et al. Outbreaks of infection caused by community-acquired methicillin-resistant *Staphylococcus aureus* in a Canadian correctional facility. *Can J Infect Dis Med Microbiol.* 2005;16:343–348.
22. Arbeit RD, Maki D, Tally FP, et al. The safety and efficacy of daptomycin for the treatment of complicated skin and skin-structure infections. *Clin Infect Dis.* 2004;38:1673–1681.
23. Stevens DL, Herr D, Lampiris H, et al. Linezolid versus vancomycin for the treatment of methicillin-resistant Staphylococcus aureus infections. *Clin Infect Dis.* 2002;34:1481–1490.
24. Wilcox M, Nathwani D, Dryden M. Linezolid compared with teicoplanin for the treatment of suspected or proven Gram-positive infections. *J Antimicrob Chemother.* 2004;53:335–344.
25. Giordano P, Song J, Pertel P, et al. Sequential intravenous/oral moxifloxacin versus intravenous piperacillin-tazobactam followed by oral amoxicillin-clavulanate for the treatment of complicated skin and skin structure infection. *Int J Antimicrob Agents.* 2005;26:357–365.
26. Ellis-Grosse EJ, Babinchak T, Dartois N, et al. The efficacy and safety of tigecycline in the treatment of skin and skin-structure infections: results of 2

double-blind phase 3 comparison studies with vancomycin-aztreonam. *Clin Infect Dis*. 2005;41(suppl 5S):341–353.

27. Jauregui LE, Babazadeh S, Seltzer E, et al. Randomized, double-blind comparison of once-weekly dalbavancin versus twice-daily linezolid therapy for the treatment of complicated skin and skin structure infections. *Clin Infect Dis*. 2005;41:1407–1415.
28. Weigelt J, Itani K, Stevens D, et al. Linezolid versus vancomycin in treatment of complicated skin and soft tissue infections. *Antimicrob Agents Chemother*. 2005;49:2260–2266.
29. Fabian TC, File TM, Embil JM, et al. Meropenem versus imipenem-cilastatin for the treatment of hospitalized patients with complicated skin and skin structure infections: Results of a multicenter, randomized, double-blind comparative study. *Surg Infect (Larchmt)*. 2005;6:269–282.
30. Seltzer E, Dorr MB, Goldstein BP, et al. Once-weekly dalbavancin versus standard-of-care antimicrobial regimens for treatment of skin and soft-tissue infections. *Clin Infect Dis*. 2003;37:1298–1303.
31. Stryjewski ME, Chu VH, O'Riordan WD, et al. Telavancin versus standard therapy for treatment of complicated skin and skin structure infections caused by gram-positive bacteria: FAST 2 study. *Antimicrob Agents Chemother*. 2006;50:862–867.
32. Stryjewski ME, Graham DR, Wilson SE, et al.; Assessment of Telavancin in Complicated Skin and Skin-Structure Infections Study. Telavancin versus vancomycin for the treatment of complicated skin and skin-structure infections caused by gram-positive organisms. *Clin Infect Dis*. 2008;46:1683–1693.
33. Corey GR, Wilcox M, Talbot GH, et al. Integrated analysis of CANVAS 1 and 2: Phase 3, multicenter, randomized, double-blind studies to evaluate the safety and efficacy of ceftaroline versus vancomycin plus aztreonam in complicated skin and skin-structure infection. *Clin Infect Dis*. 2010;51:641–650.
34. Itani KM, Dryden MS, Bhattacharyya H, et al. Efficacy and safety of linezolid versus vancomycin for the treatment of complicated skin and soft-tissue infections proven to be caused by methicillin-resistant *Staphylococcus aureus*. *Am J Surg*. 2010;199:804–816.
35. Bounthavong M, Hsu DI. Efficacy and safety of linezolid in methicillin-resistant *Staphylococcus aureus* (MRSA) complicated skin and soft tissue infection (cSSTI): a meta-analysis. *Curr Med Res Opin*. 2010;26:407–421.
36. Beibei L, Yun C, Mengli C, Nan B, et al. Linezolid versus vancomycin for the treatment of gram-positive bacterial infections: Meta-analysis of randomised controlled trials. *Int J Antimicrob Agents*. 2010;35:3–12.
37. Bliziotis IA, Plessa E, Peppas G, et al. Daptomycin versus other antimicrobial agents for the treatment of skin and soft tissue infections: a meta-analysis. *Ann Pharmacother*. 2010;44:97–106.
38. Lipsky BA. Medical treatment of diabetic foot infections. *Clin Infect Dis*. 2004;39(suppl 2S):104–114.
39. Lipsky BA, Berendt AR, Deery HG, et al. Diagnosis and treatment of diabetic foot infections. *Clin Infect Dis*. 2004;39:885–910.
40. Reiber GE, Pecoraro RE, Koepsell TD. Risk factors for amputation in patients with diabetes mellitus. A case-control study. *Ann Intern Med*. 1992;117:97–105.
41. Wilson RM. Neutrophil function in diabetes. *Diabet Med*. 1986;3:509–512.
42. Wheat LJ, Allen SD, Henry M, et al. Diabetic foot infections. Bacteriologic analysis. *Arch Intern Med*. 1986;146:1935–1940.
43. Armstrong DG, Lavery LA, Harkless LB. Validation of a diabetic wound classification system. The contribution of depth, infection, and ischemia to risk of amputation. *Diabetes Care*. 1998;21:855–859.
44. Jeffcoate WJ, Lipsky BA. Controversies in diagnosing and managing osteomyelitis of the foot in diabetes. *Clin Infect Dis*. 2004; 9(suppl 2):S115–S122.
45. Lipsky BA. Osteomyelitis of the foot in diabetic patients. *Clin Infect Dis*. 1997;25:1318–1326.
46. Lipsky BA, Itani K, Norden C, et al. Treating foot infections in diabetic patients: a randomized, multicenter, open-label trial of linezolid versus ampicillin-sulbactam/amoxicillin-clavulanate. *Clin Infect Dis*. 2004;38:17–24.
47. Gerding DN. Foot infections in diabetic patients: the role of anaerobes. *Clin Infect Dis*. 1995;20(suppl 2):S283–S288.
48. Lipsky BA. Evidence-based antibiotic therapy of diabetic foot infections. *FEMS Immunol Med Microbiol*. 1999;26:267–276.
49. Raymakers JT, Houben AJ, van der Heyden JJ, et al. The effect of diabetes and severe ischaemia on the penetration of ceftazidime into tissues of the limb. *Diabet Med*. 2001;18:229–234.
50. Harkless L, Boghossian J, Pollak R, et al. An open-label, randomized study comparing efficacy and safety of intravenous piperacillin/tazobactam and ampicillin/sulbactam for infected diabetic foot ulcers. *Surg Infect (Larchmt)*. 2005;6:27–40.
51. Lipsky BA, Armstrong DG, Citron DM, et al. Ertapenem versus piperacillin/tazobactam for diabetic foot infections (SIDESTEP): prospective, randomised, controlled, double-blinded, multicentre trial. *Lancet*. 2005;366:1695–1703.
52. Stone J, Cianci P. The adjunctive role of hyperbaric oxygen therapy in the treatment of lower extremity wounds in patients with diabetes. *Diabetes Spectrum*. 1997; 10:118–123.
53. Wunderlich RP, Peters EJ, Lavery LA. Systemic hyperbaric oxygen therapy: lower-extremity wound healing and the diabetic foot. *Diabetes Care*. 2000;23:1551–1555.
54. Estes JM, Pomposelli FB Jr. Lower extremity arterial reconstruction in patients with diabetes mellitus. *Diabet Med*. 1996;13(suppl 1):S43–S47.
55. Tannenbaum GA, Pomposelli FB Jr, Marcaccio EJ, et al. Safety of vein bypass grafting to the dorsal pedal artery in diabetic patients with foot infections. *J Vasc Surg*. 1992;15:982–988.
56. Horan TC, Gaynes RP, Martone WJ, et al. CDC definitions of nosocomial surgical site infections, 1992: a modification of CDC definitions of surgical wound infections. *Infect Control Hosp Epidemiol*. 1992;13:606–608.
57. Barie PS. Surgical site infections: epidemiology and prevention. *Surg Infect (Larchmt)*. 2002;3(suppl 1):S9–S21.
58. Fry DE. The economic costs of surgical site infection. *Surg Infect (Larchmt)*. 2002;3(suppl 1):S37–S43.
59. National Nosocomial Infections Surveillance (NNIS) System Report, Data Summary from January 1992–June 2001, issued August 2001. *Am J Infect Control*. 2001;29:404–421.
60. Dellinger EP, Hausmann SM, Bratzler DW, et al. Hospitals collaborate to decrease surgical site infections. *Am J Surg*. 2005;190:9–15.
61. Garibaldi RA, Cushing D, Lerer T. Risk factors for postoperative infection. *Am J Med*. 1991;91(3B):58S–163S.
62. Edwards JR, Peterson KD, Mu Y, et al. National Healthcare Safety Network (NHSN) report: data summary for 2006 through 2008, issued December 2009. *Am J Infect Control*. 2009;37:783–805.
63. Emori TG, Gaynes RP. An overview of nosocomial infections, including the role of the microbiology laboratory. *Clin Microbiol Rev*. 1993;6:428–442.
64. Raymond DP, Pelletier SJ, Crabtree TD, et al. Surgical infection and the aging population. *Am Surg*. 2001;67:827–832.
65. Latham R, Lancaster AD, Covington JF, et al. The association of diabetes and glucose control with surgical-site infections among cardiothoracic surgery patients. *Infect Control Hosp Epidemiol*. 2001;22:607–612.
66. Pomposelli JJ, Baxter JK III, Babineau TJ, et al. Early postoperative glucose control predicts nosocomial infection rate in diabetic patients. *JPEN J Parenter Enteral Nutr*. 1998;22:77–81.
67. Delgado-Rodriguez M, Medina-Cuadros M, Martinez-Gallego G, et al. Total cholesterol, HDL-cholesterol, and risk of nosocomial infection: a prospective study in surgical patients. *Infect Control Hosp Epidemiol*. 1997;18:9–18.
68. Malone DL, Genuit T, Tracy JK, et al. Surgical site infections: reanalysis of risk factors. *J Surg Res*. 2002;103:89–95.
69. Scott JD, Forrest A, Feuerstein S, et al. Factors associated with postoperative infection. *Infect Control Hosp Epidemiol*. 2001;22:347–351.
70. Mangram AJ, Horan TC, Pearson ML, et al. Guideline for prevention of surgical site infection, 1999. Hospital Infection Control Practices Advisory Committee. *Infect Control Hosp Epidemiol*. 1999;20:250–278.
71. Gianotti L, Braga M, Nespoli L, et al. A randomized controlled trial of preoperative oral supplementation with a specialized diet in patients with gastrointestinal cancer. *Gastroenterology*. 2002;122:1763–1770.
72. Tepaske R, Velthuis H, Oudemans-van Straaten HM, et al. Effect of preoperative oral immune-enhancing nutritional supplement on patients at high risk of infection after cardiac surgery: a randomised placebo-controlled trial. *Lancet*. 2001;358:696–701.
73. Fuchs U, Zittermann A, Stuettgen B, et al. Clinical outcome of patients with deep sternal wound infection managed by vacuum-assisted closure compared to conventional therapy with open packing: a retrospective analysis. *Ann Thorac Surg*. 2005;79:526–531.
74. File TM. Necrotizing soft tissue jnfections. *Curr Infect Dis Rep*. 2003;5:407–415.
75. Ahrenholz DH. Necrotizing soft-tissue infections. *Surg Clin North Am*. 1988;68:199–214.
76. Malangoni MA. Necrotizing soft tissue infections: are we making any progress? *Surg Infect (Larchmt)*. 2001;2:145–150.
77. McHenry CR, Piotrowski JJ, Petrinic D, et al. Determinants of mortality for necrotizing soft-tissue infections. *Ann Surg*. 1995;221:558–563.
78. Oliver JD. Wound infections caused by *Vibrio vulnificus* and other marine bacteria. *Epidemiol Infect*. 2005;133:383–391.
79. Kudsk KA. Occult gastrointestinal malignancies producing metastatic *Clostridium septicum* infections in diabetic patients. *Surgery*. 1992;112:765–770.
80. Ebright JR, Pieper B. Skin and soft tissue infections in injection drug users. *Infect Dis Clin North Am*. 2002;16:697–712.
81. Cunningham SC, Napolitano LM. Necrotizing soft tissue infection from decubitus ulcer after spinal cord injury. *Spine*. 2004;29:E172–E174.
82. Hohlweg-Majert B, Weyer N, Metzger MC, et al. Cervicofacial necrotizing fasciitis. *Diabetes Res Clin Pract*. 2006;72:206–208.
83. Praba-Egge AD, Lanning D, Broderick TJ, et al. Necrotizing fasciitis of the chest and abdominal wall arising from an empyema. *J Trauma*. 2004;56:1356–1361.
84. Skitarelic N, Mladina R, Morovic M. Cervical necrotizing fasciitis: Sources and outcomes. *Infection*. 2003;31:39–44.
85. Toran KC, Nath S, Shrestha S, et al. Odontogenic origin of necrotizing fasciitis of head and neck-a case report. *Kathmandu Univ Med J*. 2004;2:361–363.
86. Darbar A, Harris IA, Gosbell IB. Necrotizing infection due to *Bacillus cereus* mimicking gas gangrene following penetrating trauma. *J Orthop Trauma*. 2005;19:353–355.
87. Elliott D, Kufera JA, Myers RA. The microbiology of necrotizing soft tissue infections. *Am J Surg*. 2000;179:361–366.
88. Gillespie SH. New tricks from an old dog: Streptococcal necrotising soft-tissue infections. *Lancet*. 2004;363:672–673.

89. Chhatwal GS, McMillan DJ. Uncovering the mysteries of invasive streptococcal diseases. *Trends Mol Med.* 2005;11:152–155.
90. Wall DB, de Virgilio C, Black S, et al. Objective criteria may assist in distinguishing necrotizing fasciitis from nonnecrotizing soft tissue infection. *Am J Surg.* 2000;179:17–21.
91. Wall DB, Klein SR, Black S, et al. A simple model to help distinguish necrotizing fasciitis from nonnecrotizing soft tissue infection. *J Am Coll Surg.* 2000;191:227–231.
92. Wong CH, Khin LW, Heng KS, et al. The LRINEC (Laboratory Risk Indicator for Necrotizing Fasciitis) score: a tool for distinguishing necrotizing fasciitis from other soft tissue infections. *Crit Care Med.* 2004;32:1535–1541.
93. Voros D, Pissiotis C, Georgantas D, et al. Role of early and extensive surgery in the treatment of severe necrotizing soft tissue infection. *Br J Surg.* 1993;80:1190–1191.
94. Bilton BD, Zibari GB, McMillan RW, et al. Aggressive surgical management of necrotizing fasciitis serves to decrease mortality: a retrospective study. *Am Surg.* 1998;64:397–400.
95. Anaya DA, McMahon K, Nathens AB, et al. Predictors of mortality and limb loss in necrotizing soft tissue infections. *Arch Surg.* 2005;140:151–157.
96. Clark LA, Moon RE. Hyperbaric oxygen in the treatment of life-threatening soft-tissue infections. *Respir Care Clin N Am.* 1999;5:203–219.
97. Wilkinson D, Doolette D. Hyperbaric oxygen treatment and survival from necrotizing soft tissue infection. *Arch Surg.* 2004;139:1339–1345.
98. Riseman JA, Zamboni WA, Curtis A, et al. Hyperbaric oxygen therapy for necrotizing fasciitis reduces mortality and the need for debridements. *Surgery.* 1990;108:847–850.

CHAPTER 44 ■ OBSTETRIC AND GYNECOLOGIC EMERGENCIES

DAVID STREITMAN AND W. ALLEN HOGGE

ACUTE SURGICAL CARE CONSIDERATIONS IN THE PREGNANT PATIENT

Pregnant patients who require nonobstetrical surgical intervention pose unique challenges due to altered anatomy and physiology, as well as the impact of the surgical pathophysiology and its treatment upon the fetal environment. Disease processes amenable to surgical intervention are altered in their presentation, by both objective changes in maternal physiology and alteration of symptom perception by the gravid patient. Add to this the reluctance of providers to pursue a surgical therapeutic course for fear of complicating the pregnancy, and the delay of definitive treatment may become a major determinant of outcome. Furthermore, hesitancy to utilize certain diagnostic modalities can delay needed surgical intervention. Acute care surgeons should understand physiologic changes in pregnancy and abnormal presentations of common general surgical problems, since 0.5%-1% of pregnant patients will require nonobstetrical surgical intervention during pregnancy.[1]

To address these concerns, this section will review pertinent maternal physiology and typical diseases that require surgical therapy in pregnancy, provide normal laboratory values in the gravid patient, and give guidance on diagnostic modalities in pregnancy. If a gravid patient presents with signs and symptoms of disease requiring acute surgical intervention, two rules generally apply: treatment that supports or restores normal maternal physiology will help the fetus (*to help the fetus, treat the mother first*), and consultation with an obstetrician, if readily available, is advisable.

MATERNAL PHYSIOLOGY

Acid/Base

Respiratory changes during pregnancy produce a mild alkalosis via hyperventilation while maintaining normoxia. There is a concomitant, although smaller, increase in urinary excretion of bicarbonate. The result is a mild increase in pH with a lower pCO_2 and lower serum bicarbonate. These changes are reflected in the blood gas values typical of pregnancy as seen in the table of normal lab values in pregnancy (Table 44.1).[2]

Cardiovascular

Cardiac output increases in response to an increase in basal metabolic rate along with blood volume expansion that begins at 8 weeks, reaches 15% by 12 weeks, and peaks at 40%-45% increase in blood volume.[3] Reduction in systemic vascular resistance and an increase in resting heart rate of 10 beats per minute help achieve a cardiac output of 6–7 L/min in the third trimester, to 8–9 L/min in labor and in the immediate postpartum period. Maternal position can have a profound effect on cardiac output, with an increase of 1.2 L/min, about 20%, from a supine to left lateral decubitus position.[4] Uterine blood flow at term is 600 mL/min but decreases by as much as one-third in the supine position.[5] This uterine perfusion decline from supine positioning can alter fetal oxygen saturation by 10%[6] and create persistent fetal heart rate decelerations, which may result in fetal distress.

Respiratory

An increase in minute ventilation is produced by 21% increase in tidal volume, whereas respiratory rate remains stable. The diaphragm elevates 4 cm and thoracic diameter increases by 2 cm resulting in a chest circumference increase of 6 cm. However, the sum of these changes is a decrease in total lung capacity of about 200 mL. Expiratory reserve volume and residual volume (and their sum, functional residual capacity) decrease due to diaphragmatic elevation and increase in tidal volume. Inspiratory reserve volume and vital capacity are preserved. Peak expiratory flow decreases by 0.5 L/min/wk of gestation across pregnancy, translating to a loss of 10% in a woman of average height.[7] The total of these pulmonary changes is a diminished capacity of the gravida for tolerating respiratory insult, or exacerbation of underlying pulmonary disease, such as asthma.

Renal

Changes in renal function in pregnancy result in a temporarily hyperfunctioning organ. Both renal perfusion and glomerular filtration rate (GFR) increase early and rapidly. By 2 weeks postconception, GFR increases 25% over nonpregnant status; by the second trimester (13 weeks after the last menstrual period) GFR is up 50%. Renal perfusion increases to a greater degree, until late third trimester when renal perfusion declines slightly more than GFR. The increased urine production results in urinary frequency. Due to anatomic compression of the ureters and dextrorotation of the uterus, hydronephrosis and hydroureter occur, greater on the right than the left. High levels of progesterone from the placenta act as a smooth muscle relaxant, slowing ureteral peristalsis. The result is a higher risk for lower urinary tract infection, and pyelonephritis. Enhanced urine production results in a lower average serum creatinine of 0.5 mg/dL, with levels above 0.8 mg/dL considered abnormal in pregnancy. Hyperfunction allows greater excretion of bicarbonate, with a resulting decrease of serum bicarbonate by 4–5 mEq/dL, helping to balance the hyperventilation in the pulmonary system, and compensating partially for the respiratory alkalosis of pregnancy. Serum osmolarity is reduced by 10 mOsm/L, serum sodium is reduced by about 5 mEq/L, and amino acids and water-soluble vitamins are lost at a greater rate during urine production.

Metabolism

Pregnancy requires 10%-20% more caloric intake or approximately 300 kcal/d.[8] Growth of the fetus and placenta, maternal blood volume expansion, and uterine muscle hypertrophy

TABLE 44.1

NORMAL REFERENCE RANGES IN PREGNANT WOMEN

	NONPREGNANT ADULT	FIRST TRIMESTER	SECOND TRIMESTER	THIRD TRIMESTER
Hematology				
Erythropoietin (U/L)[a]	4–27	12–25	8–67	14–222
Ferritin (ng/mL)[a]	10–150[b]	6–130	2–230	0–116
Folate, red blood cell (ng/mL)	150–450	137–589	94–828	109–663
Folate, serum (ng/mL)	5.4–18.0	2.6–15.0	0.8–24.0	1.4–20.7
Hemoglobin (g/dL)[a]	12–15.8[b]	11.6–13.9	9.7–14.8	9.5–15.0
Hematocrit (%)[a]	35.4–44.4	31.0–41.0	30.0–39.0	28.0–40.0
Iron, total binding capacity (μg/dL)[a]	251–406	278–403	Not reported	359–609
Iron, serum (μg/dL)[a]	41–141	72–143	44–178	30–193
Mean corpuscular hemoglobin (pg/cell)	27–32	30–32	30–33	29–32
Mean corpuscular volume (μm^3)	79–93	81–96	82–97	81–99
Platelet (×10^9/L)	165–415	174–391	155–409	146–429
Mean platelet volume (μm^3)	6.4–11.0	7.7–10.3	7.8–10.2	8.2–10.4
Red blood cell count (×10^6/mm^3)	4.00–5.20[b]	3.42–4.55	2.81–4.49	2.71–4.43
Red cell distribution width (%)	<14.5	12.5–14.1	13.4–13.6	12.7–15.3
White blood cell count (×10^3/mm^3)	3.5–9.1	5.7–13.6	5.6–14.8	5.9–16.9
Neutrophils (×10^3/mm^3)	1.4–4.6	3.6–10.1	3.8–12.3	3.9–13.1
Lymphocytes (×10^3/mm^3)	0.7–4.6	1.1–3.6	0.9–3.9	1.0–3.6
Monocytes (×10^3/mm^3)	0.1–0.7	0.1–1.1	0.1–1.1	0.1–1.4
Eosinophils (×10^3/mm^3)	0–0.6	0–0.6	0–0.6	0–0.6
Basophils (×10^3/mm^3)	0–0.2	0–0.1	0–0.1	0–0.1
Transferrin (mg/dL)	200–400	254–344	220–441	288–530
Transferrin, saturation without iron (%)	22–46[a]	Not reported	10–44	5–37
Transferrin, saturation with iron (%)	22–46[a]	Not reported	18–92	9–98
Coagulation				
Antithrombin III, functional (%)	70–130	89–114	88–112	82–116
D-dimer (μg/mL)	0.22–0.74	0.05–0.95	0.32–1.29	0.13–1.7
Factor V (%)	50–150	75–95	72–96	60–88
Factor VII (%)	50–150	100–146	95–153	149–211
Factor VIII (%)	50–150	90–210	97–312	143–353
Factor IX (%)	50–150	103–172	154–217	164–235
Factor XI (%)	50–150	80–127	82–144	65–123
Factor XII (%)	50–150	78–124	90–151	129–194
Fibrinogen (mg/dL)	233–496	244–510	291–538	373–619
Homocysteine (μmol/L)	4.4–10.8	3.34–11	2.0–26.9	3.2–21.4
International Normalized Ratio	0.9–1.04	0.89–1.05	0.85–0.97	0.80–0.94
Partial thromboplastin time, activated (s)	26.3–39.4	24.3–38.9	24.2–38.1	24.7–35.0
Prothrombin time (s)	12.7–15.4	9.7–13.5	9.5–13.4	9.6–12.9
Protein C, functional (%)	70–130	78–121	83–133	67–135
Protein S, total (%)	70–140	39–105	27–101	33–101
Protein S, free (%)	70–140	34–133	19–113	20–65
Protein S, functional activity (%)	65–140	57–95	42–68	16–42
Tissue plasminogen activator (ng/mL)	1.6–13	1.8–6.0	2.4–6.6	3.3–9.2
Tissue plasminogen activator inhibitor-1 (ng/mL)	4–43	16–33	36–55	67–92
von Willebrand factor (%)	75–125	Not reported	Not reported	121–260
Blood chemical constituents				
Alanine transaminase (U/L)	7–41	3–30	2–33	2–25
Albumin (g/dL)	4.1–5.3[b]	3.1–5.1	2.6–4.5	2.3–4.2
Alkaline phosphatase (U/L)	33–96	17–88	25–126	38–229
Alpha-1 antitrypsin (mg/dL)	100–200	225–323	273–391	327–487
Amylase (U/L)	20–96	24–83	16–73	15–81
Anion gap (mmol/L)	7–16	13–17	12–16	12–16
Aspartate transaminase (U/L)	12–38	3–23	3–33	4–32
Bicarbonate (mmol/L)	22–30	20–24	20–24	20–24
Bilirubin, total (mg/dL)	0.3–1.3	0.1–0.4	0.1–0.8	0.1–1.1
Bilirubin, unconjugated (mg/dL)	0.2–0.9	0.1–0.5	0.1–0.4	0.1–0.5
Bilirubin, conjugated (mg/dL)	0.1–0.4	0–0.1	0–0.1	0–0.1
Bile acids (μmol/L)	0.3–4.8	0–4.9	0–9.1	0–11.3
Calcium, ionized (mg/dL)	4.5–5.3	4.5–5.1	4.4–5.0	4.4–5.3
Calcium, total (mg/dL)	8.7–10.2	8.8–10.6	8.2–9.0	8.2–9.7

TABLE 44.1

NORMAL REFERENCE RANGES IN PREGNANT WOMEN (*Continued*)

Ceruloplasmin (mg/dL)	25–63	30–49	40–53	43–78
Chloride (mEq/L)	102–109	101–105	97–109	97–109
Creatinine (mg/dL)	0.5–0.9[b]	0.4–0.7	0.4–0.8	0.4–0.9
Gamma-glutamyl transpeptidase (U/L)	9–58	2–23	4–22	3–26
Lactate dehydrogenase (U/L)	115–221	78–433	80–447	82–524
Lipase (U/L)	3–43	21–76	26–100	41–112
Magnesium (mg/dL)	1.5–2.3	1.6–2.2	1.5–2.2	1.1–2.2
Osmolality (mOsm/kg H_2O)	275–295	275–280	276–289	278–280
Phosphate (mg/dL)	2.5–4.3	3.1–4.6	2.5–4.6	2.8–4.6
Potassium (mEq/L)	3.5–5.0	3.6–5.0	3.3–5.0	3.3–5.1
Prealbumin (mg/dL)	17–34	15–27	20–27	14–23
Protein, total (g/dL)	6.7–8.6	6.2–7.6	5.7–6.9	5.6–6.7
Sodium (mEq/L)	136–146	133–148	129–148	130–148
Urea nitrogen (mg/dL)	7–20	7–12	3–13	3–11
Uric acid (mg/dL)	2.5–5.6[b]	2.0–4.2	2.4–4.9	3.1–6.3
Metabolic and endocrine tests				
Aldosterone (ng/dL)	2–9	6–104	9–104	15–101
Angiotensin converting enzyme (U/L)	9–67	1–38	1–36	1–39
Cortisol (μg/dL)	0–25	7–19	10–42	12–50
Hemoglobin A_{1C} (%)	4–6	4–6	4–6	4–7
Parathyroid hormone (pg/mL)	8–51	10–15	18–25	9–26
Parathyroid hormone-related protein (pmol/L)	<1.3	0.7–0.9	1.8–2.2	2.5–2.8
Renin, plasma activity (ng/mL/h)	0.3–9.0	Not reported	7.5–54.0	5.9–58.8
Thyroid-stimulating hormone (μIU/mL)	0.34–4.25	0.60–3.40	0.37–3.60	0.38–4.04
Thyroxine-binding globulin (mg/dL)	1.3–3.0	1.8–3.2	2.8–4.0	2.6–4.2
Thyroxine, free (ng/dL)	0.8–1.7	0.8–1.2	0.6–1.0	0.5–0.8
Thyroxine, total (μg/dL)	5.4–11.7	6.5–10.1	7.5–10.3	6.3–9.7
Triiodothyronine, free (pg/mL)	2.4–4.2	4.1–4.4	4.0–4.2	Not reported
Triiodothyronine, total (ng/dL)	77–135	97–149	117–169	123–162
Vitamins and minerals				
Copper (μg/dL)	70–140	112–199	165–221	130–240
Selenium (μg/L)	63–160	116–146	75–145	71–133
Vitamin A (retinol) (μg/dL)	20–100	32–47	35–44	29–42
Vitamin B_{12} (pg/mL)	279–966	118–438	130–656	99–526
Vitamin C (ascorbic acid) (mg/dL)	0.4–1.0	Not reported	Not reported	0.9–1.3
Vitamin D, 1,25-dihydroxy (pg/mL)	25–45	20–65	72–160	60–119
Vitamin D, 24,25-dihydroxy (ng/mL)	0.5–5.0	1.2–1.8	1.1–1.5	0.7–0.9
Vitamin D, 25-hydroxy (ng/mL)	14–80	18–27	10–22	10–18
Vitamin E (α-tocopherol) (μg/mL)	5–18	7–13	10–16	13–23
Zinc (μg/dL)	75–120	57–88	51–80	50–77
Autoimmune and inflammatory mediators				
C3 complement (mg/dL)	83–177	62–98	73–103	77–111
C4 complement (mg/dL)	16–47	18–36	18–34	22–32
C-reactive protein (mg/L)	0.2–3.0	Not reported	0.4–20.3	0.4–8.1
Erythrocyte sedimentation rate (mm/h)	0–20[b]	4–57	7–47	13–70
Immunoglobulin A (mg/dL)	70–350	95–243	99–237	112–250
Immunoglobulin G (mg/dL)	700–1,700	981–1,267	813–1,131	678–990
Immunoglobulin M (mg/dL)	50–300	78–232	74–218	85–269
Sex hormones				
Dehydroepiandrosterone sulfate (μmol/L)	1.3–6.8[c]	2.0–16.5	0.9–7.8	0.8–6.5
Estradiol (pg/mL)	<20–443[b,c]	188–2,497	1,278–7,192	6,137–3,460
Progesterone (ng/mL)	<1–20[b]	8–48	99–342	13, 52
Prolactin (ng/mL)	0–20	36–213	110–330	137–372
Sex hormone binding globulin (nmol/L)	18–114[b]	39–131	214–717	216–724
Testosterone (ng/dL)	6–86[b]	26–211	34–243	63–309
17-hydroxyprogesterone (nmol/L)	0.6–10.6[b]	5.2–28.5	5.2–28.5	15.5–84
Lipids				
Cholesterol, total (mg/dL)	<200	141–210	176–299	219–349
High-density lipoprotein cholesterol (mg/dL)	40–60	40–78	52–87	48–87
Low-density lipoprotein cholesterol (mg/dL)	<100	60–153	77–184	101–224

(*Continued*)

TABLE 44.1

NORMAL REFERENCE RANGES IN PREGNANT WOMEN (*Continued*)

Very-low-density lipoprotein cholesterol (mg/Dl)	6–40	10–18	13–23	21–36
Triglycerides (mg/dL)	<150	40–159	75–382	131–453
Apolipoprotein A-I (mg/dL)	119–240	111–150	142–253	145–262
Apolipoprotein B (mg/dL)	52–163	58–81	66–188	85–238
Cardiac				
Atrial natriuretic peptide (pg/mL)	Not reported	Not reported	28.1–70.1	Not reported
B-type natriuretic peptide (pg/mL)	<167 (age-and gender-specific)	Not reported	13.5–29.5	Not reported
Creatine kinase (U/L)	39–238[b]	27–83	25–75	13–101
Creatine kinase-MB (U/L)	<6	Not reported	Not reported	1.8–2.4
Troponin I (ng/mL)	0–0.08	Not reported	Not reported	0–0.064 (intrapartum)
Blood gas				
pH	7.38–7.42 (arterial)	7.36–7.52 (venous)	7.40–7.52 (venous)	7.41–7.53 (venous) 7.39–7.45 (arterial)
PO_2 (mm Hg)	90–100	93–100	90–98	92–107
PCO_2 (mm Hg)	38–42	Not reported	Not reported	25–33
Bicarbonate (HCO_3^-) (mEq/L)	22–26	Not reported	Not reported	16–22
Renal function tests				
Effective renal plasma flow (mL/min)	492–696[b]	696–985	612–1,170	595–945
Glomerular filtration rate (GFR) (mL/min)	106–132[b]	131–166	135–170	117–182
Filtration fraction (%)	16.9–24.7	14.7–21.6	14.3–21.9	17.1–25.1
Osmolarity, urine (mOsm/kg)	500–800	326–975	278–1,066	238–1,034
24-h albumin excretion (mg/24 h)	<30	5–15	4–18	3–22
24-h calcium excretion (mmol/24 h)	<7.5	1.6–5.2	0.3–6.9	0.8–4.2
24-h creatinine clearance (mL/min)	91–130	69–140	55–136	50–166
24-h creatinine excretion (mmol/24 h)	8.8–14	10.6–11.6	10.3–11.5	10.2–11.4
24-h potassium excretion (mmol/24 h)	25–100	17–33	10–38	11–35
24-h protein excretion (mg/24 h)	<150	19–141	47–186	46–185
24-h sodium excretion (mmol/24 h)	100–260	53–215	34–213	37–149

The references used to construct this table are listed in the UpToDate topic: Normal reference ranges for laboratory values in pregnancy.
[a]Range from references with and without iron supplementation.
[b]Normal reference range is specific range for females.
[c]Range is for premenopausal females and varies by menstrual cycle phase.
Reproduced with permission from: Abbassi-Ghanavati M, Greer LG. *Reference table of normal laboratory values in uncomplicated pregnancies.* In: Cunningham FG, Leveno KJ, Bloom S, et al., eds. *Williams Obstetrics*, 23rd ed. New York: McGraw-Hill; 2010.

occur via addition of 1,000 g of protein. Nitrogen balance is positive due to more efficient use of dietary protein. Urinary amino acid metabolites suggest that maternal muscle is not broken down to obtain the amino acids that the placenta concentrates in the fetus. Medication metabolism is altered with many of the CYP enzymes elevated substantially throughout pregnancy, but others are reduced.[9] Along with increased maternal plasma volume and weight, drug bioavailability and metabolism may be altered in difficult-to-predict patterns.

ANESTHESIA

General endotracheal anesthesia carries greater risk for the pregnant patient, primarily due to increased risk of aspiration and vascular congestion of the airway. Gastric emptying and pH are not altered in pregnancy, but progesterone relaxes the gastroesophageal sphincter, creating the equivalent of a full stomach. Laryngeal edema, soft tissue increases in the upper chest and neck, and the chest wall diameter increase in pregnancy may complicate airway management via face mask, laryngeal mask, or endotracheal tube. In addition, anesthetic agents, although known not to increase malformation risks for the fetus, are capable of hampering physiologic compensation for supine positioning and aortocaval compression in the second and third trimesters.

FETUS

Gestational age plays a key role in determining the approach to operative treatment in pregnancy. At term (>37 weeks gestation), delivery concomitant with surgical therapy may be an appropriate approach, though cesarean delivery is not uniformly indicated. Preterm birth occurs in about 5% of gravidas undergoing abdominal surgery before 37 weeks. Operative treatment for disease with a prominent infectious or inflammatory component is more likely to result in labor. Due to the increased risk of preterm birth, antenatal steroids (betamethasone 12 mg parenterally, 2 doses 24 hours apart) to accelerate fetal lung maturation should be considered between 24 and 34 weeks gestation, if the surgical condition is not adversely affected. Fetal lung surfactant production stimulated by betamethasone commences within hours and peaks by 48 hours after the first dose. However, operative intervention should not be postponed for that goal unless it is safe to do so. If maternal status allows, transfer to a tertiary care center should be made in case preterm delivery ensues. If transfer is not possible and delivery seems likely, then transport of the neonate needs to be arranged.

SURGICAL AND OBSTETRIC EMERGENCIES

Trauma

Trauma is a leading cause of maternal mortality, with homicide, accidents, and suicide being the most likely sources of trauma. Fetal death can occur, particularly after 12 weeks' gestation when the uterus becomes an abdominal organ. Severe motor vehicle crashes can result in maternal shock or death, or placental abruption, contributing to fetal loss rate of 8%.[10] Low birth weight and delivery within 48 hours are more common for unrestrained gravidas. If possible, a pregnant woman involved in a vehicular crash should be transported to a center with obstetric and intensive neonatal care capabilities. She should be placed in left lateral tilt position if injuries allow, to optimize cardiopulmonary function. The trauma survey should proceed normally, with attention to maintenance of adequate intravascular volume. Routine laboratory studies are obtained as are any imaging studies necessary for evaluating the injuries. If the mother is Rh negative, RhoGAM should be given after obtaining a type and screen and Kleihauer-Betke test to estimate the volume of any fetomaternal hemorrhage from blunt abdominal trauma. If known or thought to be 24 weeks or greater in gestation, assessment of fetal heart rate by ultrasound, or preferably, continuous external Doppler monitoring of the type used in labor and delivery, should be routine. An obstetric provider familiar with interpretation of fetal heart rate tracings (obstetrician, family practitioner, certified nurse-midwife or labor and delivery nurse) should assess fetal stability as early in the care as possible. If between 24 and 34 weeks' gestation, administration of betamethasone to accelerate fetal lung maturity should be considered, if not contraindicated.

When the pregnant patient presents with trauma, symptoms such as vaginal bleeding and abdominal pain, and signs, such as tachycardia and hypertension, can overlap with several potential pregnancy complications. With blunt trauma, separation of the placenta from deformation of the uterine wall as a result of direct impact or sudden deceleration can result in *placental abruption*. Blood loss of 1–2 L can be sequestered in the gravid uterus, resulting in severe abdominal pain or labor, and can lead to rapid onset DIC. This places the mother and fetus at grave risk, with need for immediate delivery to prevent fetal death. A large-volume transfusion protocol should be employed early in the management of abruption of this degree. In addition, a drug screen should be obtained. Illicit drug use is a common problem in obstetrical emergencies. Nearly half of trauma in pregnancy is associated with substance abuse. Heroin and methamphetamines are the most commonly abused drugs in pregnancy.

Penetrating abdominal trauma is likely to affect the uterus in the second and especially third trimesters, with the risk for fetal injury or death increasing as gestational age increases. Diagnostic peritoneal lavage can be used in the gravid patient safely, although the location for incision may be altered. Amniocentesis may be helpful to determine whether the uterus has been penetrated or the fetus directly injured. Amniotic fluid, obtained by ultrasound-guided needle aspiration, can also be sent for fetal lung maturity studies in late preterm fetuses (>30 weeks) to aid in decisions regarding delivery. Depending upon the degree of prematurity as estimated by gestational age and neonatal care capabilities of the facility, immediate delivery of a fetus injured by penetrating trauma may be indicated.

Nontraumatic Obstetric Hemorrhage

The uterus grows in weight from 70 g nonpregnant to 1,100 g near term. Enlargement is accomplished by myocyte hypertrophy and addition of fibrous and elastic tissue. Perfusion of the uterus increases to a peak of 450–650 mL/min at term[11] through uterine arteries that double their diameter by 20 weeks' gestation, resulting in flow velocity that is eightfold greater than nonpregnant. Venous dilation to accommodate this increased blood flow is accomplished through decreased elastin and reduced adrenergic innervation in response to various placental hormones. Cessation of blood loss from placental implantation site after delivery is accomplished primarily via contraction of myocytes interlaced with the uterine vasculature. In addition, there are substantial increases in several of the coagulation proteins during pregnancy, and platelet concentration is decreased only slightly at term despite a large increase in circulating volume.

However, there are several conditions that can precipitate hemorrhage before or during labor, or after delivery. Acute obstetric hemorrhage is usually evident as vaginal bleeding, but may be sequestered within the uterus. Rarely, hemorrhage can occur intraabdominally. The mother's complaints can range from painless vaginal bleeding to uterine contractions or even tetany; she may even present with signs of peritoneal irritation. Disseminated intravascular coagulation may occur with fetal death, massive placental abruption, or amniotic fluid embolism.

Abdominal Pain

Abdominal pain is a common complaint in normal pregnancy and frequently provokes acute visits to the obstetrician. Etiologies for abdominal pain may relate directly to pregnancy; "round ligament" pain, contractions, placental abruption, adnexal mass, ovarian torsion, or degenerating uterine fibroids. Other etiologies such as urinary tract infection, constipation, bowel gas, renal calculi, and gallstones are influenced by an enlarging gravid uterus and increasing levels of placental hormones. Some sources of abdominal pain are common, but unrelated to pregnancy *per se*, such as appendicitis, abdominal adhesions, bowel obstruction or intussception, and inflammatory bowel disease.

The most common diagnoses associated with abdominal pain that require surgical intervention are adnexal mass, appendicitis, and cholelithiasis/cholecystitis. Depending upon gestational age, these may be handled laparoscopically. Several series on third trimester laparoscopic operations appear to provide similar outcomes with the advantages of minimally invasive surgery. An altered approach to laparoscopic entry to the peritoneal cavity may be necessary depending upon the size of the gravid uterus. The greatest danger for appendicitis in pregnancy is delay in diagnosis, with a 50% negative appendectomy rate acceptable, given the high maternal morbidity and mortality as well as preterm birth risk of undiagnosed, ruptured appendicitis. Cholelithiasis can be treated conservatively with some success, although recurrent or prolonged symptoms may mandate cholecystectomy during pregnancy. The greatest danger is progression to cholecystitis, with a likely increase in preterm birth risk. Risk of untreated ovarian torsion is loss of the affected ovary and ovarian vein thrombus formation.

Surgery Outside the Abdomen

In general, surgery outside the abdomen is less likely to result in preterm birth. There is less opportunity for direct stimulation of the uterus, either by the disease or the surgical procedure. However, involvement of an obstetrician is advisable, and elective surgery should still await delivery of the pregnancy at term.

For orthopedic procedures prompted by trauma, the mechanism of trauma and any concomitant abdominal trauma are factors most likely to determine impact upon pregnancy. If prolonged immobilization is anticipated, thromboprophylaxis may be indicated, possibly for longer than is routine from the orthopedic perspective. Head and neck surgery may be impacted by anatomical alterations involving the airway secondary to vascular congestion as well as soft tissue accumulation in the upper chest and neck. Neurosurgical conditions may impact maternal cardiovascular and pulmonary physiology sufficiently to endanger maternal support of the fetus. At essentially all gestational ages, if management of neurosurgical disease mandates controlled hypotension to preserve maternal life or brain function, it should be used, knowing that the fetus is intolerant of prolonged maternal hypotension and may succumb. Thoracic surgical procedures may have the largest impact on preterm birth risk or pregnancy loss rate outside of abdominal nonobstetric surgery due to the severity of disease that mandates this approach. Cases of cardiopulmonary bypass have been reported with some fetal survival.[12]

The need for fetal monitoring may be driven by the pathophysiology requiring surgical treatment. For nonemergent surgery, recording fetal heart tones prior to and after surgery will be sufficient in most cases. If there is concern for fetal compromise from obstetric disease, fetal monitoring during surgery may be indicated. If need for fetal delivery during nonemergent, nonobstetric surgery is felt to be likely, then appropriate planning for the obstetric and pediatric teams needs to be included.

PREOPERATIVE WORKUP

Preoperative workup involving laboratory testing and imaging warrants special consideration in pregnancy. The table of normal laboratory values in pregnancy (Table 44.1) can aid in understanding expression of pathophysiology. There are some limits on imaging techniques in pregnancy due to fetal concerns. Ultrasound has been used for diagnostic imaging in pregnancy for several decades with a good safety profile and is typically the modality used first in evaluation of abdominal pathology during pregnancy. Ultrasound energy emission when the unit is set for obstetric imaging is half that of routine abdominal ultrasound. However, routine abdominal settings can still be used to image abdominal organs during pregnancy, as energy transfer to the fetus is minimal in most circumstances. Ionizing radiation from x-ray, computed tomography (CT), and fluoroscopy should be minimized or avoided if possible. If used, shielding of the uterus with a lead apron should occur if feasible. However, CT and x-ray imaging protocols that minimize the amount of radiation used in pregnant patients have been developed, and if critical, timely imaging information is required, they should not be withheld. For counseling purposes, the dose of ionizing radiation that reaches the uterus, and thus the increase in risk of childhood cancer for the fetus, can be estimated; the increase in risk is generally quite low. Magnetic resonance imaging (MRI) does not involve ionizing radiation and is thought to be safe for the fetus by most authorities. The use of MRI in pregnancy has expanded over the last 10 years, and more data are available on its diagnostic accuracy, particularly for nonobstetric abdominal pathology in pregnancy. Diagnostic accuracy for appendicitis in pregnancy approaches 95% with MRI.[13] Use of gadolinium in pregnant animals has raised a concern for fetal renal impact, and use in human pregnancy has been studied on a limited basis. Given our current understanding, gadolinium should only be used if the benefit outweighs the risk. Endoscopic and endoultrasonic techniques for gastrointestinal, pulmonary, and cardiac conditions can be done safely in pregnancy. Sedation can be used. However, involvement of an anesthesia provider familiar with anesthesia management in pregnancy may be prudent.

POSTOPERATIVE MANAGEMENT

Postoperative management for a pregnant surgical patient is altered little in most cases. The same postoperative goals of adequate pain control, early ambulation, and judicious advancement of diet should be pursued. Prolonged bladder drainage via catheter should be avoided if possible, as pyelonephritis from ascending infection is more likely in pregnancy. Wound healing is altered for laparotomy incisions, in that the growing uterus will place the incision under constant tension and it may result in a wider cicatrix.

Medications

There are several medications that should be avoided or judiciously used in pregnancy. Antibiotics that should be avoided include fluoroquinolones and tetracycline. Aminoglycosides should be used in the lowest effective dose for the shortest duration to avoid auditory nerve toxicity in the fetus. Narcotic analgesics are the drug class of choice for postoperative pain in a pregnant surgical patient. The lowest dose and shortest duration of narcotic that achieves analgesia adequate to allow ambulation should be used. Such dosing is unlikely to create fetal or maternal dependence for most surgical cases. If prolonged narcotic use is anticipated, then discussion of possible fetal dependence should involve the obstetric and pediatric teams. Nonsteroidal anti-inflammatory medications have limited fetal impact if used for <72 hours below 32 weeks' gestation, but are generally avoided in favor of oral narcotic analgesics because of their effect on the fetal ductus arteriosus. Thromboprophylaxis should be considered perioperatively, with use of compressive devices advisable in all cases where feasible. If surgical treatment is expected to result in prolonged immobilization, such as lower extremity orthopedic procedures, pharmacologic thromboprophylaxis may be warranted. A hematologist or maternal–fetal medicine specialist should be consulted for appropriate dosing and duration.

GYNECOLOGIC EMERGENCIES

Gynecological emergencies can best be classified into two categories: pregnancy related, and non–pregnancy related. For some conditions that are not directly related to pregnancy, the presence of a positive pregnancy test may make that condition more, or less, likely to be the etiology of the patient's presenting complaints. Likewise, management decisions may be altered by the presence of a concomitant pregnancy.

PREGNANCY-RELATED EMERGENCIES

Ectopic Pregnancy

An ectopic pregnancy is the implantation of a fertilized ovum outside the endometrial cavity of the uterus. Approximately 95% of these abnormal implantations are in the fallopian tubes. It is the number one cause of death in the first trimester of pregnancy, and accounts for 1 in 10 pregnancy-associated deaths.[14] It is a commonly misdiagnosed condition with emergency department (ED) physicians failing to make the diagnosis on an initial visit nearly 50% of the time.[15]

Table 44.2 lists the risk factors for ectopic pregnancy. The two main categories are conditions that result in tubal damage, and a history of infertility or infertility treatments.

In the modern era of highly sensitive home pregnancy testing kits, many ectopic pregnancies are diagnosed before the onset of symptoms. For purposes of these discussions, we will concentrate on the symptomatic patient. The classic presentation is a history of a missed menstrual period, abdominal pain, and vaginal bleeding or spotting. However, ectopic pregnancy should be considered in the differential diagnosis of any patient of reproductive age who presents with lower abdominal pain.

Unless there has been rupture of the tubal pregnancy, the physical findings may be minimal. There may be mild tenderness in the lower abdomen on deep palpation. Only 50% of patients will have adnexal tenderness, and about half will have cervical motion tenderness.[16] In contrast, the patient with a ruptured ectopic pregnancy presents with shock, severe abdominal pain, and peritoneal signs.

The key diagnostic tests in the evaluation of a possible ectopic pregnancy are a quantitative beta subunit of human chorionic gonadotrophin (β-hCG), and transvaginal ultrasound. While a single value of β-hCG alone is not useful in differentiation between a normal intrauterine pregnancy, an abnormal intrauterine pregnancy, or an ectopic pregnancy, it may be useful in association with transvaginal ultrasound. In the absence of previous gestational dating, many institutions have established a discriminatory zone for β-hCG, the level above which an intrauterine pregnancy should be visualized by transvaginal ultrasound. A commonly accepted cutoff is 1,500–2,500 IU/L. However, multiple gestations may have much higher levels of β-hCG for any given gestational age, and hCG levels should be interpreted with caution in patients undergoing infertility treatments.

The differential diagnosis for the patient presenting with abdominal pain and a positive pregnancy test includes rupture of the corpus luteum cyst of pregnancy, ovarian torsion, appendicitis, and in rare situations, acute salpingitis. It is possible to have both an ectopic pregnancy and an intrauterine pregnancy simultaneously (heterotopic pregnancy), and, thus, an ultrasound indicating a normal intrauterine pregnancy does not completely exclude an ectopic pregnancy. However, these pregnancies are quite rare, except in patients undergoing infertility treatments.

TABLE 44.2

RISK FACTORS FOR ECTOPIC PREGNANCY

- Prior ectopic pregnancy
- History of pelvic inflammatory disease (PID)
- History of tubal surgery
- Current IUD use
- History of infertility for ≥ 2 y
- Current infertility treatment
- Smoking
- Older maternal age

Management of the patient with a suspected ectopic pregnancy depends entirely on the patient's hemodynamic situation. In the patient with a surgical abdomen, appropriate fluid and blood resuscitation should be followed by laparotomy to remove the affected tube and establish hemostasis. The laparoscopic approach is favored in most cases except in the setting of hemodynamic instability. If possible, the ectopic pregnancy is removed through an incision in the fallopian tube (salpingostomy). The quantitative serum hCG should be followed after salpingostomy to insure complete removal of the pregnancy. If salpingostomy is not possible, the entire affected fallopian tube is removed (salpingectomy). In the hemodynamically stable patient without abdominal findings on examination; that is, the nonruptured ectopic pregnancy, gynecologic consultation is appropriate to determine whether surgical or medical management (special circumstances in the compliant patient) of the unruptured ectopic pregnancy is appropriate.

Spontaneous Abortion

Vaginal bleeding in the first trimester of pregnancy should prompt first the question of whether the pregnancy is intrauterine, or represents an ectopic pregnancy. Once the diagnosis of an intrauterine pregnancy is confirmed, an evaluation to determine the cause and implications of the bleeding can be undertaken. It is important to note, however, in the setting of potentially life-threatening hemorrhage, the priority is hemodynamic stabilization before proceeding with any evaluation.

Loss, or the potential loss, of the pregnancy prior to 20 weeks' gestation is termed an abortion, and abortion is generally subdivided into five categories (*threatened*, *inevitable*, *missed*, *incomplete*, *complete*); each is briefly discussed below. *Threatened abortion* is the most common diagnosis, and is given to any woman who presents with vaginal bleeding, a closed cervix, and an apparently normal intrauterine pregnancy by transvaginal ultrasound. Some of these patients will ultimately lose the pregnancy, but the majority will result in a normal outcome. Management of these patients is conservative, and should be done in consultation with the patient's gynecologist.

Missed abortion is the patient presenting with vaginal bleeding, a closed cervix, but an ultrasound revealing a nonviable fetus (embryonic demise) or an empty gestational sac (anembryonic demise). Rarely is vaginal bleeding excessive in this situation, and the patient can be referred to her gynecologist for either surgical or medical evacuation of the uterine contents.

The two situations most likely to present with severe vaginal hemorrhage are an *inevitable abortion*, and an *incomplete abortion*. In the circumstance of an inevitable abortion, the patient will be noted by speculum examination to have a dilated cervix, often with products of conception protruding through the open cervix. As the term implies, there is no therapy to maintain the pregnancy once the cervix has dilated, and suction curettage should be performed to remove the products of conception. Incomplete abortion is diagnosed when a portion of the products of conception have been passed, but vaginal bleeding persists and ultrasound indicates retained products of conception. Incomplete abortion is the most likely diagnosis when a patient presents with severe, or life-threatening vaginal hemorrhage in the first trimester. Once the patient has been stabilized, suction curettage should be performed to remove the remaining products of conception.

Complete abortion refers to the clinical circumstance where the patient has had intense bleeding and cramping that has resolved on presentation. Ultrasound will confirm that the uterus is "empty" and that pregnancy has been completely expelled. Once the patient is hemodynamically stable, she can be referred to her gynecologist for postabortion care.

NON–PREGNANCY-RELATED CONDITIONS

Ovarian Cysts

Ovarian cysts commonly cause pelvic pain, and are classified as either functional (arising as a result of the normal menstrual cycle) or neoplastic (a true cyst arising from the epithelium). The patient presents with pain from rupture, hemorrhage, or torsion. Diagnosis is made by history and physical examination; pelvic examination will confirm the diagnosis and define the type of cyst. Management is supportive, including appropriate pain therapy. Nonsteroidal agents are first-line choices, with opioids used for more severe discomfort (although more pain suggests ovarian torsion). Hemorrhagic cysts may require surgical management if there is ongoing hemorrhage.

Torsion of the Ovary

Ovarian torsion is caused by rotation of the ovary or the entire adnexa about the ovarian pedicle, resulting in arterial, venous, or lymphatic obstruction. It accounts for a small percentage of surgical emergencies in women but requires immediate surgical intervention when a presumptive diagnosis is made.

The symptoms of ovarian torsion classically are sudden onset of unilateral pelvic pain with radiation to the flank, associated with nausea and vomiting. In some cases, the patient will present with a history of dull aching pain, but with sharp exacerbations. A low-grade fever is often seen, and laboratory evaluation shows a moderate leukocytosis. Abdominal examination is characterized by rigidity, spasm, and tenderness with unilateral pain on deep palpation.

Huchon et al.[17] have recently published a scoring system to assist in the diagnosis of adnexal torsion. The five criteria most associated with torsion are the absence of vaginal bleeding or discharge, an ovarian cyst of >5 cm seen on ultrasonography, unilateral lumbar or abdominal pain, pain lasting <8 hours, and vomiting. However, the authors admit that their scoring system does not perform better than good clinical judgment. A patient with a documented ovarian mass by ultrasound, presenting with pain and vomiting, must be assumed to have adnexal torsion, and immediate surgical intervention is indicated. The early diagnosis and treatment of adnexal torsion may allow preservation of the affected adnexal structure.

Ruptured Tuboovarian Abscess

The life-threatening complication of pelvic inflammatory disease (PID), is rupture of a tuboovarian abscess. Rupture of a tuboovarian abscess is associated with septic shock, and a mortality rate that approaches 15%.[18] Key features in the history are previous diagnosis of a sexually transmitted infection, previous treatment of acute salpingitis, or the presence of an IUD. Physical findings are consistent with an acute surgical abdomen.

Immediate management involves aggressive fluid resuscitation, broad-spectrum antibiotics, and intravenous sympathomimetics, if necessary. Once the patient is stabilized, she should undergo exploratory laparotomy to remove the abscess, and irrigate the peritoneal cavity. The extent of the surgery will depend upon operative findings, and the patient's desires regarding future childbearing.

Endomyometritis is an infection of the endometrium with extension to the myometrium, commonly diagnosed following a therapeutic termination of pregnancy, with an incidence of 1 per 100 procedures. Pathogens include group B beta streptococcus, *Staphylococcus aureus*, *Bacteroides* species, *Neisseria gonorrhea*, and *Chlamydia trachomatis*. The patient commonly presents within 5 days of procedure or delivery with abdominopelvic pain, fever, and a foul-smelling discharge. Physical examination reveals uterine tenderness. Management requires admission to the hospital and broad-spectrum parenteral antibiotics. Ultrasound to detect retained products of conception is important in patients not responding to antibiotic therapy. Dilation and curettage is necessary in patients with endometritis and retained products of conception.

Endometriosis is a common condition, present in up to 15% of premenopausal women. The condition is the result of hormonally responsive implants of endometrial tissue in the abdominopelvic cavity on areas such as the peritoneum, bladder, and bowel.

The etiology of endometriosis is uncertain but may be related to retrograde menstruation through the fallopian tube. The most common complaint is cyclic abdominal pain and painful menses (dysmenorrhea). Physical examination reveals abdominal or pelvic tenderness. An ovarian or pelvic mass may be palpated and may represent an endometrioma. Rectovaginal examination may reveal nodularity in the rectovaginal septum or uterosacral ligaments. Similar to simple ovarian cysts, acute management centers on pain control. Patients with endometriosis will need outpatient gynecologic management to determine what medical or surgical treatment plan is most appropriate. Endometrial implants may also be found in incisions for obstetric or gynecologic procedures.

Pelvic Inflammatory Disease is an inflammatory condition of the upper genital tract thought to be caused by ascension of microorganisms from the lower genital tract. This disease may include infection of the endometrium (endometritis), fallopian tubes (salpingitis), or peritoneal cavity. The disease may progress to tuboovarian abscess, as mentioned above. Prompt diagnosis and treatment of PID is important to prevent both short- and long-term morbidity in women with the diagnosis. The consequences of PID include infertility, increased risk of ectopic pregnancy, and chronic pelvic pain.

The CDC estimates that there are approximately 780,000 new cases of PID being diagnosed annually in the United States. Risk factors for development of PID include young age, multiple sex partners, young age of sexual debut, and lack of use of barrier contraception. Cases caused by *N. gonorrhea* is 43%, 10% is by *C. trachomatis* alone, and 12% is caused by coinfection with both organisms; the remaining 30% of PID is caused by infection with anaerobic bacteria, *Mycoplasma*, and *Ureaplasma*.

Diagnosis is often difficult and inaccurate secondary to wide variation in severity of symptoms. The gold standard for diagnosis remains laparoscopy with directed biopsy and culture, although this is not practical or necessary for most patients. The CDC criteria for the diagnosis of PID require the presence of uterine or adnexal tenderness AND cervical motion tenderness. The patient may also have one or more of the following: temperature of >101°F, a mucopurulent cervical discharge, white blood cells on wet mount, elevated sedimentation rate, elevated C-reactive protein, or positive testing for *N. gonorrhea* or *C. trachomatis*.

The goals of management are treatment of the immediate symptoms of abdominal pain and pelvic pain, and prevention of later consequences: infertility, ectopic pregnancy, and chronic pelvic pain.

Vaginal Bleeding

Profuse vaginal blood loss to the extent to compromise hemodynamic status can either be pregnancy related or not. Regardless of the etiology, if the vital signs point to an acute and profound process, the patient should be managed as a trauma patient with fluid resuscitation and rapid transfusion. Vaginal examination should be performed to confirm the source of bleeding, search for vaginal trauma or cervical neoplasm, or ensure whether the source is intrauterine. Bimanual examination is helpful to assess for uterine size or adnexal pathology that might explain the etiology of the blood loss. The two key laboratory tests are complete blood count and a quantitative β-hCG. Once pregnancy is excluded, the first-line treatment for excessive intensive bleeding is high-dose estrogen, or combination of estrogen/progestin, therapy to control the bleeding. Once the bleeding has been controlled, the patient can be evaluated as an outpatient. In the rare circumstance where the bleeding does not respond to medical therapy, alternative therapies include endometrial ablation or uterine artery embolization.

Sexual Assault is a common problem in the United States, with increasing prevalence. Although most sexual assaults go unreported, many victims present for care following an assault. The true incidence is unknown, although in some studies, up to 24% of women report that they have been the victim of a completed rape, with another 20% reporting that they have been the victim of an attempted rape. Women between the ages of 17 and 25 are the most common victims of rape, and nearly three quarters of women know the assailant. One-third of rapes involve oral and/or anal penetration.

MANAGEMENT

Victims should be immediately taken to a private room in the ED. With the permission of the victims, and not to impede evaluation and treatment of medical conditions or injury, law enforcement personnel should be contacted early to aid with the combined medical–legal needs. If available, a sexual assault team, or an experienced clinician, is preferred to provide the best possible evaluation and care. Many EDs have a "rape kit" with guided evaluation to thoroughly obtain and protect evidence. A thorough history should be taken detailing all of the specifics of the assault that the patient can remember. Clothes should be gathered and labeled with the patient's name, date, and time of collection. Evidence should never be left unattended to maintain the chain of evidence of clinician to law enforcement. Physical examination should include a complete body examination. Any moist or dried secretions, stains, hair, or foreign material should be collected. A Wood's lamp may ease collection. A complete pelvic examination should be performed, with attention to the presence of any secretions, stains, hair, or foreign material. The pubic hair must be combed and the material collected sent with the comb to the laboratory. A speculum examination should be performed, with careful attention to trauma to the vaginal walls. Also, vaginal fluid should be collected, to be examined for the presence of sperm. Swabs should be obtained, to examine for gonorrhea, chlamydia, and Trichomonas. A bimanual examination should be performed, to assess for pelvic trauma. Rectal examination should be included as necessary, with the collection of appropriate specimens. Finally, blood should be obtained to test for HIV, hepatitis B, and syphilis. In select cases, directed toxicology screening may be needed. Emergency contraception should be offered to all victims of sexual assault. Immediate counseling should be available, along with structured follow-up for medical and psychologic assessment after the initial evaluation. Depending upon state and local regulations, other specimens may be collected such as blood, saliva, and fingernail debris.

References

1. Parangi S, Levine D, Henry A, et al. Surgical gastrointestinal disorders during pregnancy. *Am J Surg*. 2007;193:223-232.
2. Cunningham FG, Leveno KJ, Bloom S, et al. *Williams Obstetrics*. 23rd ed. New York: McGraw-Hill; 2009, Appendix.
3. Bernstein IM, Ziegler W, Badger GJ. Plasma volume expansion in early pregnancy. *Obstet Gynecol*. 2001;97:669.
4. Bamber JH, Dresner M. Aortocaval compression in pregnancy: the effect of changing the degree and direction of lateral tilt on maternal cardiac output. *Anesth Analg*. 2003;97:256.
5. Jeffreys RM, Stepanchak W, Lopez B, et al. Uterine blood flow during supine rest and exercise after 28 weeks of gestation. *Br J Obstet Gynecol*. 2006;113:1239.
6. Simpson KR, James DC. Efficacy of intrauterine resuscitation techniques in improving fetal oxygen status during labor. *Obstet Gynecol*. 2005;105:1362.
7. Harirah HM, Donia SE, Nasrallah FK, et al. Effect of gestational age and position on peak expiratory flow rate: a longitudinal study. *Obstet Gynecol*. 2005;105:372-376.
8. Hytten FE, Chamberlain G, ed. *Clinical Physiology in Obstetrics*. Oxford, UK: Blackwell Scientific; 1991:152.
9. Tracy TS, Venkataramanan R, Glover DD, et al. Temporal changes in drug metabolism (CYP1A2, CYP2D6 and CYP3A Activity) during pregnancy. *Am J Obstet Gynecol*. 2005;192:633-639.
10. Crosby WM. Trauma during pregnancy: maternal and fetal injury. *Obstet Gynecol Survey*. 1974;29:683-699.
11. Kauppila A, Koskinen M, Puolakka J, et al. Decreased intervillous and unchanged myometrial blood flow in supine recumbency. *Obstet Gynecol*. 1980;55:203.
12. Chambers CE, Clark SL. Cardiac surgery during pregnancy. *Clin Obstet Gynecol*. 1994;37:316-323.
13. Oto A, Ernst RD, Ghulmiyyah LM, et al. MR imaging in the triage of pregnant patients with acute abdominal and pelvic pain. *Abdom Imaging*. 2009;34:243-250.
14. Current trends ectopic pregnancy—United States, 1990–92, *MMWR Morb Mortal Wkly Rep*. 1995;44:46-48.
15. Abbott J, Emmans LS, Lowenstein SR. Ectopic pregnancy: ten common pitfalls in diagnosis. *Am J Emerg Med*. 1990;8:515-522.
16. Lipscomb GF, Stovall TG, Ling FW. Nonsurgical treatment of ectopic pregnancy. *N Engl J Med*. 2000;343:1325-1329.
17. Huchon C, Staraci S, Fauconnier A. Adnexal torsion: a predictive score for pre-operative diagnosis. *Hum Reprod*. 2010;25:2276-2280.
18. Benrubi GI, ed. *Handbook of Obstetrics and Gynecologic Emergencies*. Philadelphia, PA: Lippincott Williams and Wilkins; 2010:263.

CHAPTER 45 ■ NONTRAUMATIC VASCULAR EMERGENCIES

BRIAN L. CHEN, JARROD D. DAY, BABATUNDE H. ALMAROOF, SADAF S. AHANCHI, AND JEAN M. PANNETON

Nontraumatic vascular emergencies span the entirety of the body as would be expected given the life-essential nature of the vascular system. The diverse presentations reflect the specifics of each affected tissue bed. However, common themes unite the management of these conditions. First, thorough physical examination is essential as many of the vascular beds can be interrogated directly by examination or its extension, Doppler ultrasound. Second, imaging modalities, including color duplex ultrasound, computed tomographic angiography, and angiography, complement the evaluation of a vascular patient, helping to determine the optimal treatment. Finally, technologic advances in transcatheter intervention now present the surgeon with attractive alternatives to traditional open surgery. Some endovascular interventions complement rather than replace surgery, so multidisciplinary vascular skill sets are becoming essential. Given the rapid evolution of vascular surgery, continuing medical education is essential in caring for these conditions.

In this chapter, the breadth of both arterial and venous conditions most commonly presenting in the emergency room is addressed. For the arterial system, rupture and ischemia in multiple anatomic territories and acute aortic dissection are discussed. For the venous system, the management of venous thrombosis in multiple organ systems is reviewed.

ARTERIAL EMERGENCIES AND ARTERIAL RUPTURE

Abdominal Aortic Rupture. Approximately, 15,000 deaths per year due to ruptured abdominal aortic aneurysms (rAAAs) occur in the United States, making it the 13th leading cause of death.[1] These deaths represent a small fraction of the estimated 1.7 million patients with abdominal aortic aneurysm (AAA) in the United States, with 190,000 new cases discovered each year.[1]

To date, the cause of AAA in the majority of patients is unknown. Although atherosclerosis, hypertension, smoking (8:1), and male gender (4:1) have been found to be associated with AAA, no specific mechanism accounts for the development of AAA.[2] In a minority of patients, AAA is known to be related to underlying connective tissue disorders, such as Marfan's syndrome or Ehlers-Danlos syndrome, aortitis due to syphilis or other aggressive microorganisms, or degeneration of wall integrity with aortic dissection and cystic medial necrosis.

The classical presentation of rAAA is hypotension, abdominal or back pain, and a pulsatile abdominal mass. However, rAAA can present insidiously even while the rupture is contained by the retroperitoneum or if only a small leak has developed. Inevitably, acute decompensation with loss of tamponade occurs within 24 hours leading to hemorrhagic shock. The rupture frequently occurs through the left posterolateral aortic wall into the retroperitoneum (Fig. 45.1). Rupture into the gastrointestinal tract or inferior vena cava (IVC) (aortocaval fistula) have been reported. Patients with aortocaval fistula may also have an audible abdominal bruit and venous hypertension resulting in swollen cyanotic legs, lower gastrointestinal bleeding, and hematuria. Rarely, contained rAAA presents with radicular symptoms due to nerve root compression and bowel obstruction due to compression. Additionally, fever and leukocytosis in the presence of rAAA symptoms merit consideration of infected AAA, as these patients are at high risk for rupture.[3]

The classic presentation of rAAA remains an indication for proceeding directly to the operating room (OR). However, for patients who present with stable hemodynamics, the diagnostic algorithm has evolved over the last decade. With the increased availability of spiral computed tomography (CT), patients can be screened for rAAA within minutes. The anatomical information provided by a CT angiogram (CTA) helps determine suitability for an endovascular aortic repair (EVAR).

Controversy exists with regard to the optimal technique for repair of rAAA. However, multiple studies have been published demonstrating decreased mortality for EVAR compared to open repair. In a recent meta-analysis, a 38% reduction in mortality was reported in patients treated with EVAR versus open repair for rAAA.[4] However, the substantial institutional, material, and manpower commitments necessary to execute an emergent EVAR for rAAA must be emphasized.

Mehta published the Albany Vascular Group's standardized protocol for endovascular aneurysm repair of rAAA (Algorithm 45.1).[5] Hemodynamically unstable patients (systolic blood pressure <80 mm Hg) proceed directly to the OR. Permissive hypotension is utilized in these patients to limit further hemorrhage. Stable patients undergo emergent CTA to evaluate for EVAR anatomic suitability and then proceed to the OR. While in the OR, a femoral artery cutdown is completed to allow placement of a long 12–14 French arterial sheath, which is advanced over a guidewire into the juxtarenal aortic position, allowing both performance of an angiogram via the sheath and support of an aortic occlusion balloon. If a patient remains hemodynamically unstable, an aortic occlusion balloon is advanced over the wire into the supraceliac position. Inflation of the occlusion balloon replaces the traditional supraceliac aortic clamp, allowing the anesthesia team to resuscitate the patient with free rupture from the aorta thus controlled. An angiogram is performed to evaluate the neck of the aneurysm to determine if an EVAR is feasible. A detailed discussion of the technique of EVAR is beyond the scope of this chapter, but in short, the technique involves placement of a covered stent graft inside the aorta to cover the rupture and exclude the aneurysm. Current commercially available endografts require a 10–15 mm proximal neck and a 20 mm iliac landing zone to complete an EVAR successfully.

If the patient's anatomy is not compatible with EVAR, an open repair is necessary. First, an abdominal incision is made, either midline or wide transverse for a transperitoneal approach or a left flank lazy S incision for a retroperitoneal approach. If the retroperitoneal hematoma extends to the pararenal aorta or root of the mesentery, the supraceliac aorta is exposed by dividing the left triangular ligament of the liver and opening the lesser omentum. If the hematoma is

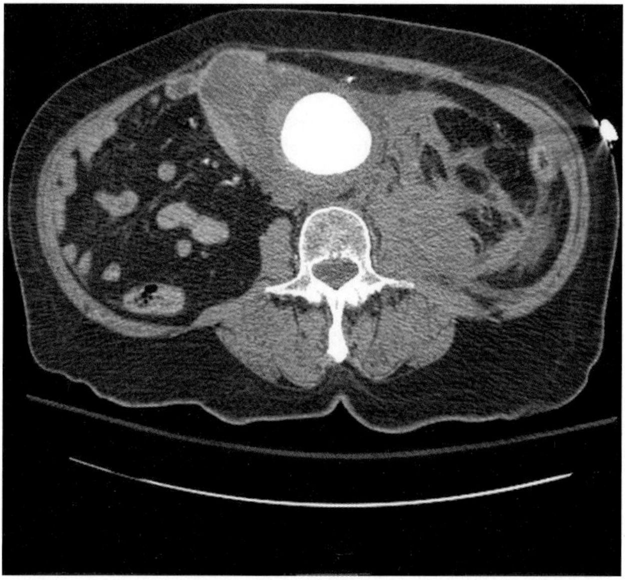

FIGURE 45.1. Abdominal aortic aneurysm ruptured with left posterolateral retroperitoneal hematoma.

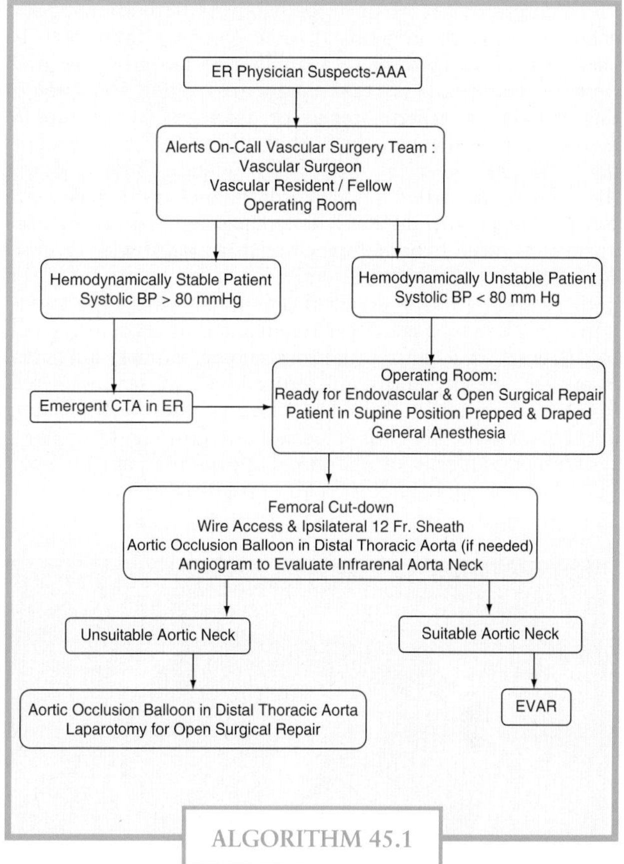

ALGORITHM 45.1 Albany vascular group ruptured AAA protocol. (Reproduced from Mehta M, et al. Establishing a protocol for endovascular treatment of ruptured abdominal aortic aneurysm: outcomes of a prospective analysis. *J Vasc Surg*. 2006;44:1–8, with permission.)

more contained, then direct exposure of the infrarenal aorta can be accomplished, taking care to avoid injury to the crossing left renal vein. Also, remember that the left renal vein is posterior to the abdominal aorta in 5% of patients. Once the supraceliac aorta is exposed, the occlusion balloon can be exchanged for a supraceliac clamp, if necessary. The distal extent of the aneurysm is determined with dissection of the distal aorta. Depending upon the status of the iliac arteries and aortic bifurcation, a bifurcated or tube graft replacement of the aorta is performed. Based on the clinical status of the patient, systemic heparinization may be used. The aorta is controlled proximally and distally with clamps and the aneurysm sac is opened longitudinally. The thrombus is removed from the aneurysm sac and lumbar arteries are suture ligated from within the aorta. If heavy back bleeding is present from the inferior mesenteric artery, its orifice is also suture ligated. A synthetic Dacron graft is sewn into place with permanent synthetic monofilament sutures. The sac should be reapproximated over the graft and the retroperitoneum is closed if possible. If not, a tongue of omentum is rotated into the retroperitoneum to cover the aortic repair in order to prevent aortoenteric fistula formation. Not infrequently, abdominal compartment syndrome develops in rAAA due to the fluid shifts associated with aggressive resuscitation, bowel edema, and accumulation of large intraperitoneal or retroperitoneal hematomas.[6] Thus, consideration of delayed fascia closure or temporary mesh closure may be necessary.

Thoracic Aortic Rupture. Similar to abdominal aortic rupture, ruptured thoracic aortic aneurysms (rTAAs) comprise the majority of the nontraumatic thoracic aortic ruptures. The literature documents an annual incidence of rTAA of 5 per 100,000.[7] The majority of rTAAs are localized to the ascending aorta and arch, with only 30% in the descending aorta.[7] These patients have a mortality rate as high as 97%, with the majority of patients dying before reaching the hospital.[7] In a recent meta-analysis, a male predominance of 70% was reported with an average age of 70 ± 5.6 years old.[8]

Thoracic aortic aneurysms (TAAs) most commonly result from age-related atherosclerotic medial degenerative disease (70%-93%) or aortic dissection (4%-30%).[9] Connective tissue disorders such as Marfan's syndrome (1.6%-10.9%) or Ehlers-Danlos syndrome (1.1%-4.2%), aortitis due to syphilis or granulomatous disease, aortitis such as Takayasu's disease (0.9%-2.1%), and trauma (0.1%-1.8%) have been reported as causes for development of TAA.[9]

Ruptured TAA frequently presents with a mixture of aneurysm and rupture symptoms. Pain is commonly cited: ascending aortic involvement presenting with anterior chest pain, aortic arch involvement leading to neck pain, descending aortic involvement presenting with back pain localized between the scapulae, and diaphragmatic level aortic involvement causing midback and epigastric pain. Interestingly, TAA tend to be more symptomatic (48%) and more likely to rupture than AAA.[9] Ascending aortic aneurysms can cause superior vena cava (SVC) obstruction, aortic valvular insufficiency, and heart failure. Arch aneurysms can cause hoarseness due to recurrent laryngeal nerve compression. Descending thoracic aneurysms can compress adjacent structures, causing dyspnea or stridor with compression of the trachea or a major bronchus, or dysphagia with compression of the esophagus. Thrombus from TAA can embolize to the anterior spinal artery, causing paraparesis or paraplegia, and also to distal tissue beds, resulting in a variety of symptoms dependent on the specific organ or limb affected. Rupture of the ascending aorta may result in pericardial tamponade, dissection of the aortic valve leading to aortic insufficiency, or dissection of the coronary arteries leading to a myocardial infarction. Rupture of a TAA into an adjacent structure can result in hemoptysis, hematemesis, gastrointestinal bleeding, and progressive dyspnea from parenchymal lung compression from intrapleural hemorrhage.

To date, surgical repair in the hands of cardiothoracic surgeons (or vascular surgeons at some centers) continues to be used in the management of ascending aorta and aortic arch rupture. The details of such repairs are beyond the scope of this chapter. In general, repair of ascending aortic rupture involves replacement of the aorta with a Dacron supracoronary tube graft from the sinotubular junction to the origin of the innominate artery under cardiopulmonary bypass with possible aortic valvuloplasty or replacement. For aortic arch aneurysms, deep hypothermic circulatory arrest with cerebral perfusion is used with replacement of the arch with a Dacron graft extending to the descending thoracic aorta. The supra-aortic trunk vessels are either reimplanted or sewn as a patch to the graft. If a concomitant descending thoracic aneurysm is present, an elephant trunk procedure may be completed, in which the graft is allowed to telescope into the descending aorta beyond the arch repair's distal anastomotic suture line.

With the advent of thoracic endovascular aortic repair (TEVAR), the paradigm for repair of ruptured descending TAA has evolved, although the rarity of rTAA limits the availability of class I evidence. TEVAR technology, in short, involves intravascular deployment of a covered stent, which covers the rupture and excludes blood flow from the aneurysm sac, (Fig. 45.2). TEVAR requires proximal and distal landing zones of 20 mm and a commercially available device large enough to exclude blood flow from the aneurysm at these seal zones. Other adjunctive procedures, such as common carotid to common carotid bypass, common carotid to subclavian bypass, or visceral debranching procedures may also be necessary. A recent meta-analysis for ruptured descending TAA demonstrated a lower 30-day mortality in patients treated with TEVAR compared to open repair, 18.9% versus 33.3%.[8] Additionally, myocardial infarction was less common, 3.5% versus 11.1%, and a trend toward improved stroke and permanent paraplegia rates was demonstrated.[10] Other retrospective series support the benefits of this paradigm shift in management.[10,11]

If the patient's anatomy is unfavorable for endovascular repair, surgical repair of the ruptured descending TAA is

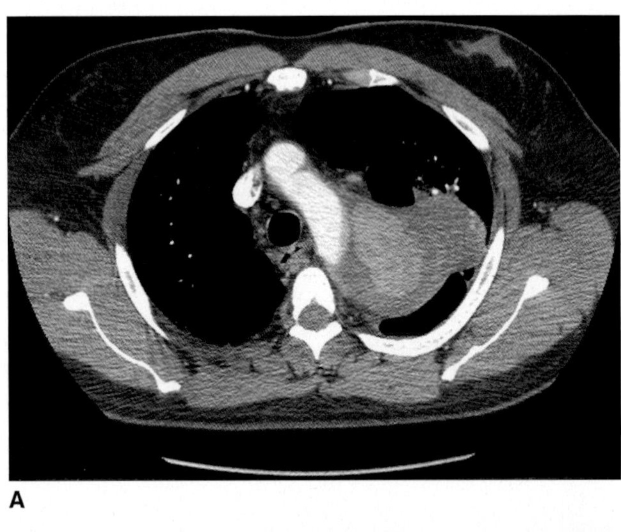

A

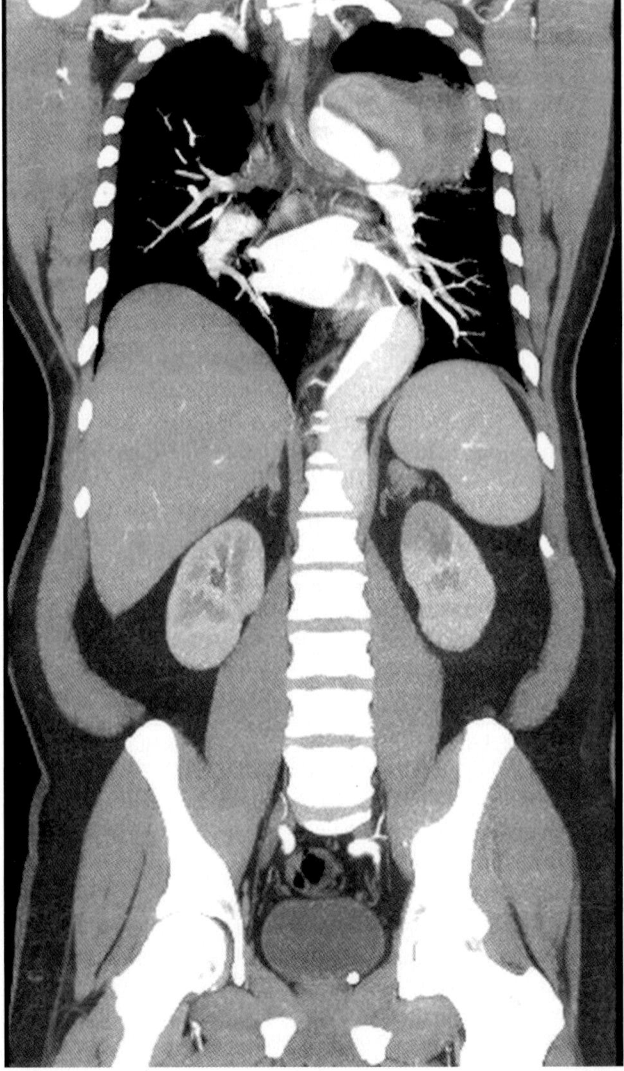

B

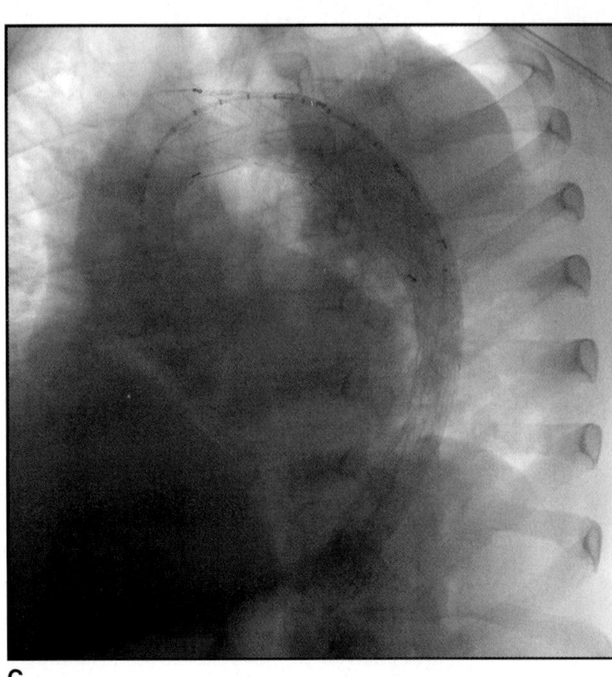

C

FIGURE 45.2. Ruptured thoracic aneurysm from chronic aortic dissection. A,B: Transverse and coronal section. C: After repair with TEVAR with left subclavian artery fenestration and stenting.

necessary. A detailed discussion of such surgical technique is beyond the scope of this chapter. Simplified, the surgical technique involves a left posterolateral thoracotomy or thoracoabdominal incision and clamping the aortic arch either distal to the left subclavian artery or between the left common carotid and left subclavian artery. At the surgeon's judgment, atrio-femoral bypass may be utilized to provide retrograde perfusion to the spinal cord, viscera, and kidneys. Finally, a segmental aortic clamp and sew technique is utilized to minimize segmental spinal ischemia, reimplanting large intercostals arteries as deemed necessary. If mesenteric and renal arteries are compromised by the aortic repair, they should be reimplanted either separately or via a Carrell patch including the compromised arteries.

Iliac Artery Rupture. Similar to rAAA, iliac artery rupture presents in the setting of preexisting iliac artery aneurysms (IAAs). Due to their location in the pelvis, IAAs frequently are not discovered until they are larger than the currently recommended repair size of 3.5 cm. The average mortality for emergent repair of ruptured arteries is 28% versus 5% for elective repair, emphasizing the importance of early detection.[12]

Isolated IAAs are rare with a prevalence of only 0.4%-1.9% of all aneurysms.[12] IAAs are more commonly found with AAAs, being prevalent in 10%-20% of cases of AAA.[12] The primary iliac artery segments involved are: common iliac artery (CIA) (70%), internal iliac artery (IIA) (20%), multiple segments (10%), and external iliac artery (rare).[12] Also, one-third of patients with an IAA will have an aneurysm in the contralateral iliac artery. Etiologies for these aneurysms are unknown, but thought to be similar to the etiologies observed for AAA, with medial degeneration from atherosclerosis being the most common cause.

Ruptured iliac arteries frequently present with sudden abdominal, groin, or thigh pain with a pulsatile mass in the affected groin. Prior to rupture, 50% of IAA will be symptomatic due to compression or erosion into surrounding structures: compression of ureters leading to pyelonephritis and sepsis, compression of the rectum leading to pain with defecation, and compression of pelvic nerves leading to paraesthesias of the lower extremities. Rarely, IAA present with thromboembolic symptoms or cardiac overload due to erosion into an iliac vein.

Open operative repair of IAA remains the gold standard. In short, CIA aneurysms are repaired with interposition graft and IIA aneurysms are repaired by ligation with or without interposition graft placement.[12,13] With the advent of endovascular interventions, multiple series now document endovascular treatment of IAA. IAA in the setting of AAA is now treated by exclusion with endograft iliac limbs as part of EVAR.[12,13] Additionally, embolization of the IIA, consisting of placement of coils in the main IIA trunk if nonaneurysmal and additional coiling of the anterior and posterior divisions of the IIA if aneurysmal, may be a necessary adjunct to prevent a type II endoleak in these cases. In the setting of isolated CIA aneurysm, an endograft iliac limb is deployed if the proximal CIA landing zone is ≥ 20 mm; otherwise, a bifurcated EVAR is completed with iliac limb coverage of the IIA.[12,13] If an isolated IIA aneurysm is present, the IIA is embolized as described above with or without coverage with an iliac endograft limb.[12,13]

Peripheral Artery Rupture. Nontraumatic rupture of peripheral arteries, consisting of arteries distal to and including the subclavian artery and distal to and including the femoral artery, is rare. This is in part due to the rarity of bland aneurysms of these arteries and their tendency to present with thromboembolic symptoms rather than rupture.

In contrast, mycotic aneurysms of peripheral arteries usually rupture. The root cause is infection with bacteria or fungi that lodge in vessels and cause transmural necrosis, leading to aneurysm formation. The clinical presentation of these aneurysms ranges from overwhelming sepsis to more insidious symptoms of fever, malaise, chills, night sweats, and pain. Often on examination, the skin demonstrates erythema, tenderness, and a palpable pulsatile mass.

The high rate of rupture of mycotic peripheral aneurysms justifies intervention in all cases, as antibiotics are inadequate to treat the compromised arterial wall. Debridement of necrotic tissue is essential in all cases. For subclavian and axillary arteries, a discussion of surgical approaches to repairing these arteries is beyond the scope of this chapter, as exposure of these arteries depends on location of involved segment, ranging from median sternotomy or left posterolateral thoracotomy to simple supraclavicular or axillary incisions. In short, if injury to the subclavian vein and brachial plexus can be avoided, treatment involves excision and reconstruction of artery with vein interposition graft.[14] If adjacent structures are likely to be injured, arterial ligation with incision and drainage of the aneurysm has been reported. Forearm and hand mycotic aneurysms usually require only excision and ligation.[15] Finally, femoral and popliteal artery mycotic aneurysms require aneurysm excision and arterial reconstruction with saphenous or femoral vein conduit.[14] Adjuncts such as a sartorius flap may be needed to help cover the arterial reconstruction, allowing then use of aggressive local wound care including negative pressure dressings.

Visceral Artery Rupture. Ruptured visceral arteries are rare yet lethal entities, with 20%-70% presenting as emergencies and 8.5%-75% of patients dying from their ruptured visceral artery.[16] In most cases, rupture is the result of unrecognized preexisting aneurysms, which themselves are rare with a 0.01%-0.2% incidence during autopsy.[17] More than 3,000 visceral artery aneurysms have been reported in the literature, with variable rupture rates depending on the tissue bed involved (Table 45.1). In decreasing order of prevalence in the general population, the most commonly involved visceral arteries include the splenic, hepatic, superior mesenteric, and celiac arteries.[18,19] In reported series, there is a male predominance for visceral artery aneurysms, except for splenic artery aneurysms where there is a 4:1 female predominance. Reported rupture rates are summarized in Table 45.1.[20,21]

In most series, atherosclerosis is cited as the most common etiology for ruptured visceral arteries.[16-19,22] Other etiologies include fibrodysplasia, mycotic aneurysms, blunt trauma, connective tissues disorders such as Marfan's syndrome and Ehlers-Danlos syndrome, vasculitides such as giant cell arteritis and

TABLE 45.1

COMPILATION OF REPORTED VISCERAL ARTERY ANEURYSM RUPTURE RATES AND ASSOCIATED MORTALITY

VISCERAL ARTERY INVOLVED	RUPTURE RATE	MORTALITY FROM RUPTURE
Splenic artery	2%	25%
Hepatic artery	<20%	21%-35%
Superior Mesenteric Artery	38%-50%	30%
Celiac artery	13%	50%

polyarteritis nodosa, and gastrointestinal conditions such as pancreatitis and chronic peptic ulcer disease.[16–19,22] Pregnancy merits special mention as the hormonal-mediated changes in vessel wall structure and increased splanchnic and splenic arterial flow result in an increased incidence of rupture with a maternal and fetal mortality rate of 64%-75% and 72.5%-95%, respectively.[23]

Clinical presentation of visceral artery rupture is dependent on the pattern of rupture, with free peritoneal rupture acutely presenting as hemorrhagic shock and retroperitoneal rupture possibly presenting delayed symptoms due to initial tamponade. Most commonly cited presentations are hypotension, abdominal and back pain, and gastrointestinal bleeding, including hemobilia in cases of hepatic artery rupture.[16,18,19] Splenic aneurysm rupture not infrequently presents with minimal symptoms followed by acute decompensation.

Traditional treatment of visceral artery rupture has been open surgical approach consisting of ligation and bypass or possible reconstruction of the vessel as tolerated by the patient. For splenic artery aneurysm rupture, splenic artery ligation as part of splenectomy has historically been the treatment of choice. However, with the recognition of the importance of the spleen in immune function, more attempts at splenic salvage, consisting of splenic artery aneurysmectomy or exclusion, have occurred. Of special note, because of the exceedingly high maternal and fetal mortality rates from ruptured splenic artery aneurysms, elective surgical management of splenic aneurysms in females of childbearing age should be recommended when the splenic artery aneurysm is ≥2 cm.[23] In fact, some experts recommend surgical intervention on all splenic artery aneurysms during pregnancy regardless of size, ideally after the first trimester.[23] Hepatic arterial rupture can be managed with aneurysmectomy or aneurysmal exclusion as long as gastroduodenal and gastroepiploic collaterals are patent. Superior mesenteric artery (SMA) rupture frequently requires aneurysmorrhaphy and simple ligation, assuming adequate collateral blood flow through the inferior pancreaticoduodenal and middle colic arteries. Given the importance of the SMA to intestinal perfusion, attempts at repair of the SMA in the hemodynamically stable patient with aneurysmorrhaphy or interposition graft have been reported. Celiac artery rupture has been treated with aneurysmectomy and primary reanastomosis or interposition graft.

With the advent of endovascular technology, multiple case series have been published on endovascular embolization with coils and glues and exclusion of visceral artery aneurysms with covered stent grafts. However, the numbers of endovascular interventions for ruptured visceral arteries are limited in these series and no long-term follow-up on these interventions is available. Common complications from endovascular interventions include inadequate embolization, end tissue infarction from embolization, abscess formation from infarcted tissue, and embolization of glue or coils from initial delivery site.[16,19,23–26]

Arterial Ischemia

The bulk of emergency vascular interventions can be attributed to arterial ischemia. This seemingly diverse group of disease processes shares a common mechanism—compromised arterial blood flow whether due to embolism, thrombosis, dissection or poor cardiac function (Table 45.2). Symptoms and long-term outcomes are partially dependent on the ischemic tolerance of the affected tissue bed, for example, 6 hours for lower extremities and 5 minutes for the brain. Even after successful revascularization, risk of reperfusion injury and development of a compartment syndrome or systemic inflammatory response syndrome plagues these patients. This section

TABLE 45.2

ETIOLOGIES OF ARTERIAL ISCHEMIA

EMBOLISM	THROMBOSIS	TRAUMA	OUTFLOW VENOUS OCCLUSION	LOW-FLOW STATES
Heart Atherosclerotic Acute MI Arrhythmia Valvular disease Rheumatic Bacterial Prosthetic Dysrhythmia Atrial fibrillation	Low-flow states CHF Hypovolemia Hypotension	Penetrating Direct vessel injury Indirect injury Missile emboli Proximity	Compartment syndrome	Cardiogenic
Artery-to-artery Aneurysm Atherosclerotic plaque	Atherosclerosis	Blunt Intimal flap Spasm	Phlegmasia	Hypovolemia
Idiopathic	Hypercoagulable states	Drug abuse Cocaine inhalation Drug toxicity		Drug effect
Paradoxical embolus	Vascular grafts Progression of disease Intimal hyperplasia Mechanical	Iatrogenic Intimal flap Dissection External compression		

will review arterial ischemia according to the limb or organ affected.

Lower Limb Ischemia. The incidence of acute leg ischemia (ALI) has been reported to be 9–14 per 100,000 with a peak incidence of 180 per 100,000 in patients older than 90 years.[27,28] The most common causes of lower limb ischemia are thrombosis and embolism. Most emboli to the lower extremities originate from the heart (80%-90%), and 60%-70% of these patients have an underlying cardiac condition.[27,29] These cardiogenic emboli lodge at branch points due to changes in laminar blood flow caused by vessel divisions and sequential reduction in diameter of branch arteries with each division. In decreasing order of relative frequency: the femoral bifurcation, the aortic bifurcation, the popliteal trifurcation. Aggressive medical management of atrial fibrillation with anticoagulation and rheumatic heart disease with antibiotics has shifted the incidence toward thrombosis.

The Trans-Atlantic Inter-Society Consensus (TASC II) Working Group in 2007 redefined acute limb ischemia as "any sudden decrease in limb perfusion causing a potential threat to limb viability."[30] As no reliable biochemical or radiologic indices of limb viability exists, a high index of clinical suspicion is required for rapid diagnosis and management. The clinical severity and presentation of ALI depends not only on the etiology, but on the location, proportion of luminal obstruction, and the capability of existing collateral circulation to transport blood around the obstruction. ALI due to emboli is more likely to present with sudden, severe limb-threatening ischemia. In contrast, patients with chronic arterial occlusive disease may also develop acute thrombosis, but their chronically diseased vascular beds develop collateral circulation, partially mitigating ischemia.

Acute limb ischemia is essentially a clinical diagnosis with a range of symptoms classically described as the 6 P's: pain, paresthesia, paralysis, pallor, pulselessness, and poikilothermia. Pain in the toes and feet is usually the first presenting symptom of ALI. As ischemia continues, paraesthesia develops as large sensory nerves transmitting pain, temperature, and light touch become malperfused. Finally, in the most severe ischemic conditions, paralysis ensues with loss of toe flexion and extension. This is followed by an absence of foot dorsiflexion and plantarflexion due to ischemic myopathy of the calf muscles. As the muscles infarct, the leg swells and becomes more tender, and eventually the foot loses passive movement. After 6–8 hours, muscles become rigid and contracted and the limb is unsalvageable. Amputation is necessary at this point to prevent renal failure from rhabdomyolysis.

The clinical findings of pallor include a white, waxy extremity with absent capillary refill. With thrombosis, as the collateral circulation dilates to restore flow, there may be gradual improvement in capillary refill. If there is still refill after blanching, the limb is still salvageable. However, with fixed mottling or cyanosis the capillaries have thrombosed or ruptured and limb recovery is unlikely. Pulselessness is the sine qua non of acute limb ischemia. Palpable pulses in the contralateral extremity suggest embolism as the cause. With thrombosis, there are usually signs of chronic limb ischemia such as thickened toe nails, loss of hair, reduced or absent contralateral pulses. Finally, poikilothermia, or perishing cold, is the finding of decreasing skin temperature from the proximal unaffected limb to the distal ischemic limb.

With the advent of endovascular therapy, the range of management options for acute limb ischemia has expanded. These options include open surgical revascularization, endovascular revascularization, or anticoagulation with observation. First, a determination of ischemia severity is completed using the clinical classification of acute limb ischemia listed in Table 45.3.[31] In this initial step, the degree of motor and sensory dysfunction is determined and the presence of arterial and venous flow verified with a handheld continuous Doppler unit. If no contraindication exists, the patient is started on systemic anticoagulation with heparin to prevent further clot propagation. Patients with level I ischemia should be treated with heparinization and close observation for symptom deterioration, especially older sedentary patients with substantial comorbidities who may become completely asymptomatic with aggressive management of associated comorbidities. In the younger, more active patient with level I ischemia, a more aggressive approach of proceeding directly to endovascular intervention, using catheter-directed thrombolysis or thrombectomy, or surgery is more prudent since the earlier the thrombus is removed, the better the outcome. This same strategy is employed for level IIA and IIB ischemia, but revascularization must be done expeditiously and four compartments calf fasciotomy much more likely to be needed to treat compartment syndrome. Most patients with level III ischemia should receive primary amputation only with treatment of comorbidities due to the potential consequences of reperfusion injury.

EMERGENCY SURGERY

TABLE 45.3

RUTHERFORD'S CLASSIFICATION OF ACUTE LIMB ISCHEMIA

CATEGORY	DESCRIPTION	PROGNOSIS	SENSORY LOSS	MOTOR DEFICIT	ARTERIAL DOPPLER	VENOUS DOPPLER
I	Viable	No immediate threat	None	None	Audible	Audible
IIA	Marginally threatened	Salvageable if promptly treated	Minimal (toes) or none	None	Inaudible	Audible
IIB	Immediately threatened	Salvageable if immediately revascularized	More than toes, rest pain	Mild/Moderate	Inaudible	Audible
III	Irreversible	Major tissue loss, permanent nerve damage inevitable	Profound, anesthetic	Profound, paralysis (rigor)	Inaudible	Inaudible

Modified from Rutherford RB, et al. Recommended standards for reports dealing with lower extremity ischemia: revised version. *J Vasc Surg.* 1997;26:517–538.

After addressing the embolus or thrombus with either endovascular or open surgical intervention, underlying atherosclerotic lesions are frequently revealed. For endovascular intervention, angioplasty and stenting may be utilized as indicated by the angiographic findings. For open surgical intervention, endarterectomy and patch angioplasty is often utilized. For more diffuse disease, surgical bypass is often preferred. However, endovascular methods have developed to provide transcatheter alternatives, which may be less morbid in a high risk patient.[32]

Popliteal Artery Aneurysm. Though popliteal artery aneurysms (PAAs) are the most common peripheral arterial aneurysm, they have only a reported prevalence of <1.0%.[33] Rupture of these aneurysms is so rare, that the exact prevalence is unknown. Rather than rupture, acute limb ischemia from thrombosis of PAA and subsequent embolization to the pedal arteries is the most common mode of presentation and has been reported in 17%-46% of cases.[33] These patients may present with a history of recent claudication consistent with compromise of the popliteal or tibial arteries. With progression of distal embolization, these patients usually develop the signs of acute limb ischemia discussed in the above section.

If Rutherford class IIB and III acute ischemia is present, immediate intervention in the OR is necessary to salvage the limb as catheter-directed thrombolysis frequently requires 24 hours. An above the knee medial exposure of the distal superficial femoral artery and below the knee exposure of the popliteal artery, trifurcation, and tibial arteries are necessary for proximal and distal ligation of the PAA to prevent further embolization and to allow direct thromboembolectomy of the tibial arteries. Intraoperative thrombolytic infusion can be used to facilitate thrombus clearance of the tibial arteries. Intraoperative angiogram is used to confirm tibial artery recanalization. Once this is verified, a bypass, preferably with saphenous vein conduit, is completed from the superficial femoral artery down to the distal popliteal artery or to the tibial artery with direct inline flow to the foot. If no tibial arteries are visualized and there is no obvious target for revascularization, prolonged catheter-directed thrombolytic infusion may be warranted to obtain limb salvage. In some situation when the runoff vessels are absent and the leg no longer deemed salvageable, the patient is placed on systemic Heparin to allow the limb to demarcate to minimize future amputation level. However, if substantial leg muscle ischemia is present, an urgent high level amputation, such as an above knee or through knee amputation may become necessary. If the patient presents with acute limb ischemia but without neurologic symptoms, a preoperative angiogram can be completed to identify any open tibial arteries and optimize the outflow with catheter-directed thrombolysis of thrombosed tibial arteries. If the patient's condition deteriorates or fails to improve, surgical revascularization as discussed above is recommended. To date, while complete endovascular treatment of thrombosed PAA has been reported, inadequate numbers and follow-up are available in the literature to recommend such therapy.[33,34]

Upper Extremity Ischemia. Acute arm ischemia is relatively uncommon and is usually not immediately limb-threatening due to the robust collateral circulation of the upper extremity. Studies report an incidence of acute arm ischemia of 1.2-3.5 per 100,000 population with a female predominance (2:1).[28] Unlike lower limb ischemia, embolus, due to atrial fibrillation most commonly, is the cause of 90% of acute arm ischemia. Other sources of emboli include recent myocardial infarction, ventricular aneurysms, atrial myxomas, and paradoxical emboli. Thrombosis comprises 5% of acute arm ischemia with atherosclerotic narrowing as the most common predisposing condition. Thoracic outlet syndrome, aneurysm, and arteritis are other thrombotic causes that deserve mention. Less common sources are hypercoagulable states, malignancy (Trousseau's syndrome), and radiation injury. Trauma and iatrogenic injuries make up the remainder of acute arm ischemia cases.

Patients with upper extremity ischemia present with acute pain and coolness of the extremity, the exact location depending on the level of obstruction. In most instances, emboli lodge in the brachial artery (60%) or axillary artery (26%). A slightly increased occurrence of embolic ischemia occurs in the right arm due to the brachiocephalic artery's proximity to the heart and larger ostium. The extremity appears pale with poor capillary refill compared to the contralateral unaffected arm. The hand may be weaker and numb, but muscle function is normally preserved. Examination often reveals the level of obstruction by the level of loss of pulse. With heparinization, some capillary refill may return to the distal extremity with improvement in neurologic function. Hand mottling is rarely observed in embolic disease, rather more often in the setting of shock where inotropes are used to support systemic blood pressure. The impact of underlying arterial stenosis is accentuated in this setting, as the blood pressure is inadequate to exceed the resistance caused by the stenosis. Also, inotropes used to augment cardiac function may cause peripheral vasoconstriction, further aggravating a difficult situation.

Nonoperative management consists of anticoagulation with heparin and treatment of contributing comorbidities such as cardiac failure or dysrhythmia. Most natural history studies demonstrate some degree of compromised arm function with nonoperative management and thus justify a more aggressive approach.[35,36] Thromboembolectomy is the most frequently performed procedure in this setting. Optimization of the patient's comorbidities is also essential to long-term success, as untreated comorbidities can cause recurrence. Thromboembolectomy of the brachial, radial, and ulnar arteries can be performed under local anesthesia through an antecubital fossa incision. Exposure of the brachial artery at its bifurcation allows proximal and distal embolectomy through a single incision. Long-term anticoagulation, unless contraindicated, should be routinely prescribed to reduce recurrence risk and postoperative mortality.[37] When the source of emboli is a proximal artery lesion, definitive surgery or angioplasty may be required after thromboembolectomy. After thromboembolectomy, atherosclerotic lesions of the subclavian or axillary arteries are increasingly managed with percutaneous angioplasty with selective stenting, falling back to surgical bypass if endovascular therapy fails.

Cerebrovascular Ischemia

Great Vessels. Conditions involving the great vessels for example, the subclavian, common carotid, and brachiocephalic arteries may cause low-flow states or embolization leading to stroke, transient ischemic attacks (TIAs) or arm ischemia. Atherosclerotic occlusive disease is the most common etiology, reported in 69%-100% of cases.[38] Takayasu's arteritis is the second most common cause, followed by radiation arteritis. Peak occurrence has been reported in the age range of 50–61 years old with slight female predominance of disease (53%). Also, cigarette smoking is an important risk factor for the development of atherosclerotic disease in this distribution, often with multiple vessel involvement.

Most patients are symptomatic (80%) with the mean interval between symptoms and revascularization of 15 years. Generally, atherosclerotic lesions cause thromboembolic events, in contrast to the smooth tapering lesions of Takayasu's aortitis that normally cause low-flow symptoms.[39] The Mayo Clinic series demonstrated that 63% of patients with an atherosclerotic lesion in the great vessels presented with embolic events: cerebrovascular (53%), upper extremity (10%) and mixed (5%).[38]

The presence of symptomatic disease is an indication for intervention. Direct surgical reconstruction via a transsternal approach has been the gold standard for patients with multiple branch involvement. Alternatively, ministernotomy to the third intercostal space can be performed with transection of the sternum. Cervical reconstruction through a transverse supraclavicular incision is the preferred option for isolated disease of the common carotid and proximal subclavian arteries. With subclavian lesions proximal to the vertebral origin, subclavian–carotid transposition is preferable to bypass due to the superior patency rates.[40] Synthetic conduits are preferred over vein grafts for surgical reconstruction of the great vessels. Endovascular management has been successfully performed for a variety of supra-aortic trunk diseases. Percutaneous angioplasty of lesions of varying lengths has been reported with high technical success. However, total occlusion has higher failure rates (65% vs. 100%) and worse patency rates when compared to stenoses.[41] Due to the inferior patency of endovascular management of subclavian occlusions, some advocate endovascular management for subclavian stenoses only, and surgery (subclavian–carotid transposition) for subclavian artery occlusions.[42]

Carotid Artery. Stroke is the third leading cause of death in the United States, and the most common cause of death as a result of a neurologic disease. The overall incidence of new stroke is approximately 160 per 100,000 population per year. Based on more recent data in a population-based study, the cerebral infarction rate approaches 632 per 100,000 population in the 65–74-year age group, and the older than 75-year age group had a stroke rate of 1,786 per 100,000 population per year.[43] The rates in men are approximately 1.5 times that of women of the same age. The primary pathologic process is atherosclerosis, responsible for 90% of lesions of the extracranial system. The remaining 10% of cases is due to fibromuscular dysplasia, kinking from arterial elongation and tortuosity, migraine vasospasm, spontaneous nontraumatic intimal dissection, inflammatory angiopathies, or radiation injury. Atherosclerotic plaques typically occur at branches or bifurcations. The most commonly affected sites include the bifurcation of the common carotid artery, the carotid siphon, and the origins of the middle and anterior cerebral arteries. The ratio of extracranial to intracranial lesions is over 2:1 in the Western world.

Many clinical syndromes are associated with carotid artery disease. These are classified as either a TIA or stroke. TIA is defined as a sudden focal neurologic deficit that completely resolves within 24 hours. Stroke is due to cerebral infarction as a result of hypoperfusion, embolization, or hemorrhage. Any of these mechanisms can result in speech deficits consisting of dysarthria, dysphasia, or aphasia. Motor deficits range from loss of fine motor skills to hemiplegia contralateral to the affected carotid disease. There may also be numbness or paresthesia. Transient visual disturbances consisting of monocular blindness or visual field defects, termed amaurosis fugax, can also arise. Occasionally, there may be global cerebral hypoperfusion causing decreased mentation, presyncope, or even vertebrobasilar symptoms.

The goal of therapy for carotid artery disease is prevention of cerebral infarction. Patients with symptomatic 70%-99% internal carotid artery (ICA) stenosis derive the greatest benefit from carotid endarterectomy (CEA) compared to best medical therapy (BMT). The North American Symptomatic Carotid Endarterectomy Trial (NASCET) demonstrated a reduction of ipsilateral stroke from 26% over 2 years with BMT alone to 9% with the addition of CEA.[44] In patients with symptomatic moderate grade (50%-69%) ICA stenosis, there is some benefit of CEA compared to BMT with a stroke risk reduction from 22% to 15%.[45] In this particular group of patients, subgroup analysis identified cohorts that benefitted the most from CEA: males, patients with stroke rather than TIAs, and patients with hemispheric stroke symptoms rather than retinal symptoms.

With the increased acceptance of carotid artery stenting (CAS), controversy remains regarding the optimal management of symptomatic patients with ICA stenosis. The Stenting and Angioplasty with Protection in Patients at High Risk for Endarterectomy (SAPPHIRE) trial showed noninferiority of CAS with distal embolic protection (DEP) compared to CEA in high-risk patients. Some surgeons use this data as a reason to offer CAS with DEP to patients who are considered at high-risk due to anatomic (prior neck irradiation, recurrent stenosis after CEA) or medical (severe cardiac or pulmonary disease) conditions.[46]

Regardless of the method selected to treat a symptomatic carotid stenosis (CEA vs. CAS), it is essential to rapidly start antiplatelet therapy with acetylsalicylic acid (ASA) or clopidogrel when a patient becomes symptomatic. Prior to initiating anticoagulation therapy, a hemorrhagic stroke needs to be ruled out by a head CT.

Visceral Ischemia

Mesenteric Ischemia. Acute mesenteric ischemia (AMI) is a vascular emergency with a mortality of 70%-90% that has not improved over the past 70 years.[47] Most patients with AMI present in the sixth to seventh decade with multiple comorbidities. In a Swedish autopsy study, the overall incidence rate was 12.9 per 100,000 person-years.[48] After normalizing for the increased longevity of females, the distribution is roughly equal between men and women.

The four well recognized clinical patterns of AMI include arterial embolism, arterial thrombosis, mesenteric vein thrombosis (MVT), and nonocclusive mesenteric ischemia (NOMI). MVT will be addressed in the venous emergency section. The two primary arterial causes of AMI are embolism and thrombosis. Arterial emboli are responsible for 40%-50% of cases and usually originate from a cardiogenic source such as a recent myocardial infarction, tachyarrhythmia, cardiomyopathy, or valvular disease. Emboli primarily lodge in the SMA and branches due to the oblique takeoff from the aorta. Most emboli (50%) lodge distal to the middle colic artery branch rather than at the origin (15%). Mesenteric arterial thrombosis occurs in 25%-30% of AMI cases and usually in the setting of chronic atherosclerotic SMA stenosis. The insidious nature of atherosclerosis allows collaterals to form; however, this capacity eventually is exceeded. Due to the pervasive nature of mesenteric arterial thrombosis, 70%-100% mortality rates have been reported. It remains unclear which particular patients with considerable mesenteric artery stenosis will ultimately develop thrombosis. Finally, NOMI is primarily a cardiogenic disease. Frequently, the mesenteric vessels are patent yet the heart fails to adequately perfuse the intestines. NOMI is frequently seen in the setting of critically ill patients in which the mesenteric blood flow is further constricted by inotropic drugs utilized to augment cardiac function.

Due to the rich collateral blood flow between the celiac, superior mesenteric, and inferior mesenteric arteries, compromise of at least two of these arteries is necessary to cause ischemic symptoms. Many of the signs and symptoms of AMI are similar to other acute abdominal pathologies (i.e. pancreatitis, small bowel obstruction) and depend on the underlying cause. With SMA embolism, there is an acute onset of unrelenting abdominal pain associated with immediate bowel evacuation. Classically, the pain is described as out of proportion to the physical examination. There is also nausea and vomiting, along with excessive third spacing, leading to dehydration and tachycardia, mental confusion, and sometimes respiratory collapse. Laboratory findings include hemoconcentration, leukocytosis, elevated lactate level, and metabolic acidosis with an increased anion gap. This should be contrasted against patients with chronic mesenteric ischemia who not infrequently have a prior history of postprandial abdominal pain with unintentional weight loss. As expected, chronic mesenteric ischemia patients can also present emergently with acute occlusion in the setting of chronically diseased mesenteric arteries. Regardless of the etiology, once bowel infarction occurs, the patient develops peritonitis and hemodynamic instability with multiorgan system failure if bowel resection is not performed expeditiously and the remaining viable bowel reperfused promptly.

In any patient older than 60 years with a history of atrial fibrillation, recent myocardial infarction, or any history of prior postprandial pain and weight loss, a high index of suspicion for AMI should be maintained. If the diagnosis is made in the first 24 hours, the survival rate is 50%, dropping to 30% with delay.[49] Older planar abdominal CT has poor sensitivity and specificity for the diagnosis of AMI; however, newer dynamic contrast-enhanced, multislice CT demonstrates greater sensitivity in detecting bowel ischemia. The gold standard for diagnosis continues to be angiography; however, this modality does not evaluate bowel viability. If an acute abdomen is present on exam, exploratory laparotomy is indicated regardless of availability of a mesenteric angiogram. Also with a high index of suspicion and contrast-enhanced CT findings suggestive of AMI, most vascular surgeons would proceed directly to exploratory laparotomy.

Once the diagnosis is made, treatment should begin immediately with aggressive fluid resuscitation, correction of metabolic abnormalities and optimization of any medical conditions. Broad-spectrum antibiotics should be started as early as possible. Efforts to reduce thrombus propagation should be initiated with systemic anticoagulation unless there is a contraindication. With peritoneal signs, bowel infarction is likely and emergency laparotomy is indicated. Even without peritonitis, surgical revascularization is indicated once the diagnosis is made. After laparotomy, visceral revascularization should proceed prior to bowel resection. For embolism, a standard embolectomy is performed through a transverse arteriotomy in the proximal SMA. If the etiology is unknown, a proximal SMA longitudinal arteriotomy can be completed instead to facilitate an aortomesenteric bypass. If embolectomy returns pulsatile back-bleeding, then the arteriotomy is closed with a patch angioplasty, preferably with vein. If an aortomesenteric bypass is needed, often the case with arterial thrombosis, inflow is obtained from either the infrarenal or supraceliac aorta. Vein is preferably used as the conduit in this setting, due to the presence of ischemic or necrotic bowel. After revascularization, the bowel is evaluated and frankly necrotic bowel is resected. Intraoperative assessment of bowel viability is often inaccurate and second-look laparotomy is the rule.

Another revascularization option in the setting of AMI is retrograde open mesenteric stenting (ROMS).[50] After the initial bowel exploration, the intestines are packed away to limit contamination. An infracolic exposure is obtained, which facilitates dissection of the SMA or a large SMA branch. The artery is cannulated with a micropuncture needle and a microwire is placed into the SMA in a retrograde fashion. A sheath is placed in the usual fashion and using a Glidewire and catheter, re-entry into the aorta is obtained. A limited aortogram is performed from this catheter, allowing identification of the length of the stenosis or obstruction. The catheter is exchanged for an appropriately sized angioplasty balloon that is inflated to profile to predilate the SMA, then a balloon expandable stent is placed to limit luminal recoil in the SMA. A completion angiogram is performed to document successful revascularization of the SMA. The puncture hole in the SMA or branch is repaired with a 6–0 nylon. The advantages of ROMS is greater speed, less physiologic stress as aortic clamping is avoided, and avoidance of any synthetic material in a potentially contaminated field.[50]

Due to the rarity of NOMI, with an incidence of only 2 per 100,000 person-years, guidelines for treatment of NOMI derive from reported case series.[48] Currently, authors recommend intra-arterial administration of vasodilators, including papaverin, nitroglycerin, or glucagon.[51] Antibiotics are also frequently administrated to treat bacterial translocation caused by the compromised mucosal integrity observed in NOMI.[51] Optimization of underlying cardiac function accompanies these interventions.

Renovascular Ischemia. Acute ischemic events involving the renal vasculature include embolism, thrombosis, renal artery dissection, trauma, and renal vein thrombosis (RVT). The first two will be discussed in this section and further discussion on RVT deferred to the venous emergency section. Embolic or thrombotic renal occlusion is a rare occurrence, reported as 1.4% of a series of 14,411 autopsies.[52] Emboli typically originate from the heart from conditions such as atrial fibrillation, mitral valvular disease, and acute myocardial infarction. Up to 30% of renal emboli from cardiogenic sequelae are bilateral. Proximal aortic aneurysms and aortic plaques can also be a source, especially after manipulation with percutaneous catheters. Concomitant embolism to other aortic branches is also common. Renal artery thrombosis occurs with advanced atherosclerotic disease of the aorta and can progress into the proximal renal artery. This condition is generally clinically silent due to the collateralization with ureteral, lumbar, adrenal or capsular arteries. As expected, this subset of patients is at highest risk of iatrogenic thromboembolism with catheter-based interventions.

The clinical presentation of acute renal ischemia is variable and vague, thus this diagnosis is rarely considered. Common symptoms are flank, back or abdominal pain, hematuria, or hypertensive crisis. Bilateral renal artery occlusion may present with pyrexia, acute renal failure, and anuria. On urinalysis, leukocytosis, erythrocytosis, and proteinuria are frequently found. Any patient with these symptoms and history of dysrhythmia, recent myocardial infarction, or malignancy should have renal artery occlusion in their differential diagnosis.

Due to its vague symptoms, renal artery compromise often is diagnosed only by radiographic studies. Contrast-enhanced CT scan demonstrates filling defects indicating abnormal perfusion. Angiography not only confirms the diagnosis but also the degree of atherosclerotic disease and the pattern of collateral blood flow to the distal renal artery, which helps in differentiating renal artery embolism from thrombosis.

Previous studies suggest that open surgical treatment is less effective than anticoagulation alone, especially when the duration of symptoms is >12 hours.[53] However, percutaneous thrombolysis is a viable option even for individuals with chronic symptoms.[53] For embolism, early open surgical embolectomy, percutaneous thrombolysis, or pharmacomechanical thrombectomy should be offered. Surgical intervention should especially be considered in otherwise healthy patients with partial renal occlusion, bilateral renal emboli, or an embolus to a solitary kidney. Mortality is considerably reduced if preoperative correction of metabolic abnormalities is initiated prior to embolectomy. Thrombolysis typically reveals the underlying atherosclerotic process which can then be treated with balloon angioplasty with or without stent placement.

Unlike renal artery embolism, arterial thrombosis less often requires urgent operative intervention. Surgical revascularization proceeds after resuscitation and correction of metabolic disturbances. Surgical options include aortorenal bypass with saphenous vein or synthetic grafts. With severe aortic atherosclerotic disease, extra-anatomic bypass including hepatorenal, splenorenal, or iliorenal bypasses may be necessary. Percutaneous thrombolysis has been performed in this group of patients with primary stenting and offers an alternative approach with good outcomes.[53]

ACUTE AORTIC DISSECTION

Aortic dissection is well recognized as a lethal aortic pathology, with most deaths resulting from malperfusion or rupture of the aorta. It involves an intimal tear that allows pressured systemic blood flow to hydrostatically dissect the aortic media. Eventually the pressure dissects back into the true lumen, in this process creating a false lumen. Early recognition of this entity is essential as acute ascending aortic dissection and descending aortic dissection with malperfusion require immediate intervention. In recent years, development of thoracic endograft technology has reshaped the management of aortic dissection.

Aortic dissection affects 3–4 per 100,000 people annually.[54] An early mortality rate as high as 1% per hour if untreated has been reported, and 21% of aortic dissection patients die before receiving treatment in the hospital.[55] The classic clinical profile for an aortic dissection patient is an elderly male with hypertension. Peak incidence has been reported for the 40- to 70-year old age groups, and males have two to five times increased incidence of aortic dissection.[56]

Chronic hypertension is the most commonly cited risk factor for aortic dissection, followed by increased age and male gender. Connective tissue disorders, such as Ehlers-Danlos syndrome, Loeys-Dietz syndrome, or Turner's syndrome, and aortic vasculitidies which destroy aortic medial layers, predispose patients to dissection. Bicuspid aortic valve has been linked to dissection, though the exact mechanism is unknown. Finally, pregnancy is a major risk factor, as one-half of aortic dissections in women younger than 40 years old occur during pregnancy.

According to the International Registry of Acute Aortic Dissection, most patients with aortic dissection present with an abrupt onset of pain, described as a sharp or tearing pain.[57] Interestingly, most patients present between 6 AM and noon with the highest rate of dissection occurring during winter. Stanford type A dissections (involving the ascending aorta) more frequently present with anterior chest pain, while Stanford type B dissections (originating distal to the origin of the left subclavian artery) frequently present with back pain radiating to the interscapular region. Other symptoms in type A are dependent on retrograde dissection into the aortic root leading to development of pericardial tamponade, aortic valvular regurgitation, or myocardial infarction. For type B, depending on visceral or lower extremity malperfusion, abdominal or leg pain with possible neurologic compromise may be present. Also, dissection in the aortic arch can lead to compromised blood flow in the great vessels, causing upper extremity and cerebrovascular ischemia.

Rapid diagnosis allows identification of appropriate therapy for these patients. CTA is considered the gold standard for identification of aortic dissection due to its speed and general availability. The limited availability and speed of magnetic resonance angiography make it a second tier imaging study, better suited for evaluation of chronic aortic dissection. Transesophageal echocardiogram can detect ascending aortic dissection and the presence of aortic root compromise and pericardial effusion.

The data for type A dissection continues to support open surgical interventions. 91% percent of patients with type A dissection die within 1 week without surgery. Even with ascending aortic replacement with aortic root valvuloplasty or replacement, a mortality rate of 13%-33% has been cited.[58]

In contrast, uncomplicated type B dissection is preferentially treated with maximal medical management consisting of antihypertensive and antiimpulse medications. The first line agents are beta blockers, followed by calcium channel blockers, angiotensin-converting enzyme inhibitors, and vasodilators such as nipride.[59] Even without medical therapy, 40% of these patients will survive to 1 year. However, with optimal medical management, a mortality rate of 7%-11% can be achieved, compared to 17%-19% with surgical intervention.[59] Complicated type B dissection, however, requires intervention for pain or hypertension recalcitrant to maximal medical therapy, rapidly increasing aortic diameter, imminent or verified aortic rupture, or evidence of visceral or limb malperfusion.[59,60]

Open surgical intervention on type B dissection consists of either a segmental aortic graft replacement or an open fenestration technique in which the dissection flap is excised to restore visceral flow.[61] An endovascular fenestration technique consists of endovascular perforation of the dissection septum and widening the perforation with an angioplasty balloon, usually at the level of the compromised visceral vessels. Similarly, aortic branch compromise from the aortic dissection can be managed through endovascular techniques with direct stenting of visceral, renal, or iliac arteries to restore flow.[60]

Since the advent of thoracic endografting, multiple thoracic centers are adopting TEVAR as their intervention of choice for complicated type B dissection. The operative goal of TEVAR for acute aortic dissection is to cover the proximal entry tear and reexpand the true lumen to help restore distal aortic perfusion (Fig. 45.2). Understand that most thoracic centers treating type B dissection are extrapolating TEVAR for aneurysmal disease into TEVAR for aortic dissection. However, no commercially available thoracic endograft has a Federal Drug Administration approved indication for aortic dissection. Additionally, the one randomized clinical trial for TEVAR use in aortic dissection (INSTEAD) focused on simple chronic dissection, not acute or complicated dissection.[62] Thus, the intervention offered to a complicated type B dissection patient will vary with the expertise of the local treatment center.

VENOUS EMERGENCIES

While arterial emergencies are often more dramatic clinically, venous disease is more pervasive than arterial disease, with an estimated two-thirds of the general population having varying degrees of venous disease. Venous emergencies can be as dramatic as phlegmasia cerulea dolens, with impending gangrene of the affected lower extremity, or as subtle as the insidious onset of renal vein thrombosis. These conditions are frequently discovered in the setting of other systemic diseases.

Lower Extremity

Superficial Vein Thrombosis. The majority of lower extremity superficial vein thrombosis (SVT) affects branches of the greater saphenous vein in patients with varicose veins. This is treated with rest and nonsteroidal anti-inflammatory drugs. Complications such as recurrent SVT, thrombus propagation, and pulmonary embolism (PE) occur in 5%-10% of patients. Patients with greater saphenous vein thrombus are at particular risk for thrombus propagation, mandating a follow-up duplex scan. If thrombus propagates to within 5 cm of the saphenofemoral junction, ligation should be performed as the thrombus often extends 5–10 cm beyond the imaged location.[63] If the junction itself is involved, the patient should receive anticoagulation therapy for at least 3 months.[63] Recent evidence suggests that patients with acute initial idiopathic greater saphenous vein thrombosis may benefit from a short course of fondaparinux.[64]

Lower Extremity Deep Vein Thrombosis. The incidence of lower extremity deep venous thrombosis (DVT) ranges from 56 to 160 per 100,000 annually. Stasis is the predominant factor causing DVT, especially in postoperative or trauma patients. DVT symptoms are nonspecific and include leg swelling, pain, fever, erythema or cyanosis. Venous duplex ultrasound is the initial diagnostic study of choice, demonstrating vein incompressibility, absence of phasic flow, and possibly hypoechoic appearance, which differentiates between acute and chronic thrombus. While D-dimer assay has an excellent negative predictive value for DVT, it is not specific during the postoperative period.

Treatment should be started promptly to prevent clot propagation and reduce the risk of PE and postthrombotic syndrome. Low molecular weight heparin or unfractionated heparin is used for initial treatment before conversion to Warfarin. Patients should be monitored for Heparin-induced thrombocytopenia while on heparin drip. If there are no contraindications, thrombolysis and thrombectomy may be beneficial in patients with venous gangrene or extensive iliofemoral thrombus. Prevention is the key to avoid DVT and its complications. Hallmarks of prevention are ambulation, application of graduated compression stockings or intermittent pneumatic compression, and pharmacologic prophylaxis with subcutaneous heparin, whether fractionated or unfractionated.

Phlegmasia Alba/Cerulea Dolens. The two clinical syndromes associated with extensive iliofemoral venous thrombosis are phlegmasia alba dolens and the more severe phlegmasia cerulea dolens. In phlegmasia alba dolens, the common iliac vein or external iliac vein is occluded but the internal iliac and collateral veins remain patent. The patient has moderate to severe swelling, leg tenderness, pallor but no ischemia. Management is either anticoagulation, catheter-directed lysis, or pharmacomechanical thrombectomy in good-risk patients.

Phlegmasia cerulea dolens occurs in patients with extensive thrombosis of the iliofemoral venous system with loss of collateral circulation. Half of these patients will progress to venous gangrene, with more than 90% of patients having an underlying malignancy. Patients typically present with pain, poikilothermia, and severe swelling of the affected limb but often have palpable pulses initially, then progress to loss of arterial inflow due to elevated compartment pressures caused by occlusion of the iliofemoral venous system. Management is systemic anticoagulation, intravenous fluid, and leg elevation. Also, both catheter-directed thrombolysis and pharmacomechanical thrombectomy have emerged as effective acute interventions. Surgical thrombectomy has been relegated to recalcitrant cases not responsive to other interventions. Palliative care is appropriate for those patients with disseminated malignancy.

Upper Extremity

Septic Phlebitis. Septic thrombophlebitis is characterized by venous thrombosis, inflammation, and bacteremia.[65] The clinical course and severity of septic thrombophlebitis is variable. Placement of an intravascular catheter is the main causative factor in the development of phlebitis and superficial septic thrombophlebitis. Many cases present as benign localized venous cords that resolve completely with removal of peripheral catheters. Some cases present as severe systemic infections culminating in profound shock that is refractory to management. These cases should be managed aggressively with surgical resection of the vein, broad-spectrum antibiotics, and intensive care. Any associated abscesses should be incised and drained.

Upper Extremity Deep Vein Thrombosis. Central venous catheters are the most common cause of upper extremity deep vein thrombosis. In young patients with spontaneous subclavian and axillary vein thromboses, Paget-Schroetter syndrome must be considered. Treated with anticoagulation alone, these patients are often left with chronic pain and swelling of the arm. Aggressive management with catheter-directed thrombolysis followed by delayed thoracic-outlet decompression and first-rib resection provides excellent functional results. Patients without evidence of Paget-Schroetter syndrome can be treated with heparin and warfarin, although consideration should be given to thrombolysis in good-risk patients.

Infected Internal Jugular Vein Thrombosis. Thrombus in the internal jugular veins is usually due to catheter insertion. Intravenous drug abuse is also a risk factor. A feared complication is secondary infection of the thrombus by a local oropharyngeal infection (Lemierre's syndrome), usually by anaerobes or methicillin-resistant *Staphylococcus aureus*. Other reported sources of secondary infection of internal jugular thrombus include pneumonia and liver abscess. Management of internal jugular vein thrombosis caused by catheters is catheter removal followed by anticoagulation. Septic complications are managed by intravenous antibiotics. Rarely, surgical excision of all the infected tissue may be necessary.[66]

Visceral Venous Thrombosis

Portal Vein Thrombosis. The exact frequency of portal vein thrombosis (PVT) is unknown, but segmental or complete PVT occurs in as many as 30% of patients with hepatocellular carcinoma. The incidence of PVT in patients with cirrhosis and portal hypertension is approximately 5%. Reduced portal blood flow caused by hepatic parenchymal disease, abdominal sepsis, and hypercoagulable syndromes are potential causes. PVT is often not discovered until gastrointestinal hemorrhage develops, unless the thrombosis is discovered during routine surveillance for a known underlying pathologic condition. In most patients, PVT occurs slowly and silently. The signs and symptoms of PVT can be subtle or nonspecific, and often are overshadowed by underlying diseases. The exceptions are patients with thrombophilia and portal and mesenteric venous thromboses who present with moderate or severe abdominal pain after acute or subacute development of PVT. The development of PVT can precipitate the need for emergency endoscopy for sclerotherapy of gastroesophageal varices, transjugular intrahepatic portosystemic shunt placement, surgical portocaval shunt creation, transjugular or transhepatic portomesenteric thrombolysis and thrombectomy, or even resection of ischemic bowel or liver transplantation.[67]

Mesenteric Vein Thrombosis. MVT accounts for 5%-10% of cases of AMI. As the venous end-branches of the SMV and inferior mesenteric vein are frequently also thrombosed, thromboembolectomy of the mesenteric veins is often inadequate. Treatment of the end-branches requires catheter-directed SMA delivery of a thrombolytic agent, assuming adequate exchange of the thrombolytic agent to the venous drainage of the intestines. As a survival advantage to aggressive therapy has not been demonstrated, the treatment of MVT is generally systemic anticoagulation therapy.[68]

Similar to patients with mesenteric ischemia secondary to nonocclusive mesenteric ischemia, close observation for signs of worsening bowel ischemia, peritonitis, and systemic inflammation are essential; up to one-third of patients with MVT require exploration for necrotic bowel. These patients should undergo second-look laparotomy to assess viability of marginally perfused bowel. In addition, patients with MVT should undergo a hypercoagulable workup to identify any underlying etiology that would necessitate lifelong anticoagulation therapy.[67]

Renal Vein Thrombosis. Occlusion due to thrombus in the major renal veins or tributaries is rare, as often these patients are asymptomatic or their symptoms are ascribed to other diseases. The renal veins, particularly on the left side, have a generous collateral network both inside and outside the kidney, reducing symptoms. Cases of spontaneous recanalization or resolution of RVT have been documented. RVT in both adults and children is associated with renal diseases and nephrotic syndrome.[69] The kidney's response to venous occlusion is determined by the acuteness of the disease, extent and timely development of collateral circulation, involvement of one or both kidneys, and origin of the underlying disease.[69] In renal vein occlusion, anticoagulation is the primary option, and catheter-directed pharmacomechanical thrombectomy with or without thrombolysis can be applied in selected cases.[70] The role of surgery in the treatment of RVT is limited because of high risk of rethrombosis. Nephrectomy may be indicated in rare cases of hemorrhagic infarction of the kidney with rupture and bleeding.

Central venous obstruction

Superior Vena Cava Obstruction. Superior vena cava syndrome (SVCS) is caused by obstruction of flow in the SVC because of either extraluminal compression or intraluminal obstruction of the SVC. The majority of cases of SVCS are caused by neoplastic progression into the venous wall with resultant compression of the tumor mass against the relatively fixed thin-walled SVC. Alternatively, SVC obstruction can also occur as a result of intravascular thrombosis caused by neoplastic involvement.

SVCS usually has an indolent course related to progression of the underlying malignancy. Clinical progression of SVCS usually takes place over the course of several weeks often with facial and upper extremity edema, distended neck veins, and visible chest wall venous collaterals. With an acute onset of SVCS, venous collaterals may not have sufficient time to develop and patients may exhibit more rapid worsening of clinical symptoms. Other symptoms include dyspnea, facial plethora, cough, headaches, dizziness, and stridor. In severe conditions, SVC obstruction can give rise to venous congestion resulting in cerebral edema, leading to altered mental status and even coma.[71]

The traditional treatment of SVCS associated with thoracic malignancy has been radiotherapy, chemotherapy, or both. Patients with nonmalignant SVCS traditionally underwent surgical reconstruction of the SVC, enabling future dialysis access or placement of a pacemaker.[72] Currently, the first line treatment of SVCS is catheter-based percutaneous interventions such as balloon angioplasty, stenting, and directed thrombolysis.[72] These interventions expedite the establishment of luminal patency and provide rapid symptom relief. In patients whose SVC obstruction is caused by intraluminal thrombosis, thrombolytic therapy is an effective means of dissolving the SVC thrombus. The only contraindication to endovascular therapy is a contraindication to thrombolytic therapy or anticoagulation. Patients who fail to respond or who are not candidates for endovascular therapy should be evaluated for surgical reconstruction or palliative care.

Inferior Vena Cava Obstruction. IVC occlusion is a rare condition associated with iliofemoral thrombus extension, congenital IVC anomalies, malignancy, hypercoagulable disorders, trauma, radiation, inflammation, pregnancy, or external compression by adjacent pathologies, IVC filter placement, or liver transplant. Clinical findings in these patients range from moderate bilateral lower extremity swelling to limb pain, discoloration, and venous stasis ulcerations. The symptoms are exacerbated by the presence of associated venous reflux. The patients may be asymptomatic if the occlusion is chronic and adequate venous collateralization has developed. When compared with patients with lower extremity DVT alone, these patients have a higher incidence of PE.[73] Diagnosis can be made with venous duplex ultrasound or with venography. Venous phase CT is another noninvasive means of making a rapid diagnosis. Severely symptomatic patients will usually require intervention in addition to anticoagulation. Front line of management is endovascular intervention with pharmacomechanical thrombectomy, catheter-directed thrombolysis, and balloon angioplasty and stenting of any stenotic lesions. Failure of endovascular treatment is an indication for surgical management in the form of an ilio-caval or cavo-atrial bypass.[74]

Pulmonary Embolism. In the United States, PE resulting from lower extremity DVT in 90% of patients, remains a significant cause of mortality, resulting in 300,000 deaths annually.[75] Symptomatic manifestation of PE depends not only on the burden of thrombosis within the pulmonary circulation, but also on the patient's underlying cardiopulmonary reserve. Clinical features of PE include chest pain, dyspnea, hypoxia, cough, and hemoptysis. Massive PE can present with hypotension or even full cardiac arrest. A CT pulmonary angiography is the diagnostic test of choice but a ventilation–perfusion scan may be a viable alternative in patients with renal failure or contrast allergy. Pulmonary angiography is reserved for cases where therapeutic interventions are considered. In severe cases, right heart dysfunction will be seen on echocardiogram or electrocardiogram.

Prompt anticoagulation with heparin is started once there is a high clinical suspicion for PE, even before confirmatory tests have been completed. Catheter-directed or systemic thrombolysis has been used in patients with severe cardiopulmonary collapse as it decreases clot burden and pulmonary hypertension. Pulmonary artery embolectomy is reserved for patients with massive PE who have contraindications to thrombolysis or respond poorly to them. This can be performed surgically or percutaneously with catheter-directed embolectomy devices but the mortality rate can be up to 50%.

Oral anticoagulation can be started once diagnosis is confirmed and the patient is fully heparinized. The duration of treatment is at least 3–6 months but also depends on the etiology of the PE. Inhaled nitric oxide can help improve cardiac output and oxygenation in patients with massive PE. IVC filters are recommended for patients who have recurrent PE despite adequate anticoagulation or have contraindications to anticoagulation. IVC filters can also be placed prophylactically in patients with documented proximal lower extremity DVT and contraindication to anticoagulation.

EMERGENCY SURGERY

References

1. Goldstone J. Aneurysms of the aorta and iliac arteries. In: Moore WS, ed. *Vascular and Endovascular Surgery: A Comprehensive Review*. 7th ed. Philadelphia, PA: Saunders Elsevier; 2006:488-510.
2. Taylor LM, Porter JM. Basic data related to clinical decision-making in abdominal aortic aneurysms. *Ann Vasc Surg*. 1987;1:502-504.
3. Oderich GS, Panneton JM, Bower TC, et al. Infected aortic aneurysms: aggressive presentation, complicated early outcome, but durable results. *J Vasc Surg*. 2001;34:900-908.

4. Sadat U, Boyle JR, Walsh SR, et al. Endovascular vs open repair of acute abdominal aortic aneurysms—a systematic review and meta-analysis. *J Vasc Surg*. 2008;48:227-236.
5. Mehta M, Taggert J, Darling RC 3rd, et al. Establishing a protocol for endovascular treatment of ruptured abdominal aortic aneurysm: outcomes of a prospective analysis. *J Vasc Surg*. 2006;44:1-8.
6. Rasmussen TE, Hallett JW Jr, Noel AA, et al. Early abdominal closure with mesh reduces multiple organ failure after ruptured abdominal aortic aneurysm repair: guidelines from a 10-year case control study. *J Vasc Surg*. 2002;35:246-253.
7. Johansson G, Markström U, Swedenborg J. Ruptured thoracic aortic aneurysm: a study of incidence and mortality rates. *J Vasc Surg*. 1995;21:958-958.
8. Jonker FH, Trimarchi S, Verhagen HJ, et al. Meta-analysis of open versus endovascular repair for ruptured descending thoracic aortic aneurysm. *J Vasc Surg*. 2010;51:1026-1032.
9. Panneton JM, Hollier LH. Nondissecting thoracoabdominal aortic aneurysms: part I. *Ann Vasc Surg*. 1995;9:503-514.
10. Jonker FH, Verhagen HJ, Lin PH, et al. Outcomes of endovascular repair of ruptured descending thoracic aortic aneurysms. *Circulation*. 2010;121:2718-2723.
11. Patel HJ, Williams DM, Upchurch GR Jr, et al. A comparative analysis of open and endovascular repair for the ruptured descending thoracic aorta. *J Vasc Surg*. 2009;50:1265-1270.
12. Sandhu RS, Pipinos II. Isolated iliac artery aneurysms. *Semin Vasc Surg*. 2005;18:209-215.
13. Patel NV, Long GW, Cheema ZF, et al. Open vs endovascular repair of isolated iliac artery aneurysms: A 12-year experience. *J Vasc Surg*. 2009;49:1147-1153.
14. Flanigan DP. Aneurysms of the peripheral arteries. In: Moore WS, ed. *Vascular and Endovascular Surgery: A Comprehensive Review*. 7th ed. Philadelphia, PA: Saunders Elsevier; 2006:512-521.
15. Leon LR, Psalms SB, Labropoulos N, et al. Infected upper extremity aneurysms: a review. *Eur J Vasc Endovasc Surg*. 2007;35:320-331.
16. Grotenmeyer D, Duran M, Park EJ, et al. Visceral artery aneurysms—follow-up of 23 patients with 31 aneurysm after surgical or interventional therapy. *Langenbecks Arch Surg*. 2009;394:1093-1100.
17. Røkke O, Søndenaa K, Amundsen S, et al. The diagnosis and management of splanchnic artery aneurysms. *Scan J Gastroenterol*. 1995;31:737-743.
18. Carr SC, Mahvi DM, Hoch JR, et al. Visceral artery aneurysm rupture. *J Vasc Surg*. 2001;33:806-811.
19. Pulli R, Dorigo W, Troisi N, et al. Surgical treatment of visceral artery aneurysms: a 25-year experience. *J Vasc Surg*. 2008;48:344-342.
20. Rectenwald JE, Stanley JC, Upchurch GR Jr. Splanchnic artery aneurysms. In: Hallett JW Jr, Mills JL Sr, Earnshaw JJ, Reekers JA, Rooke TW, eds. *Comprehensive Vascular and Endovascular Surgery*. 2nd ed. Philadelphia, PA: Mosby Elsevier, 2009;358-372.
21. Stanley JC, Messina LM, Zelenock GB. Splanchnic and renal artery aneurysms. In: Moore WS, ed. *Vascular and Endovascular Surgery: A Comprehensive Review*. 7th ed. Philadelphia, PA: Saunders Elsevier, 2006;523-536.
22. Oderich GS, Panneton JM, Bower TC, et al. The spectrum, management and clinical outcome of Ehlers-Danlos syndrome type IV: a 30-year experience. *J Vasc Surg*. 2005;42:98-106.
23. Ha JF, Phillips M, Faulkner K. Splenic artery aneurysm rupture in pregnancy. *Eur J Obstet Gynecol Reprod Biol*. 2009;146:133-137.
24. Berceli SA. Hepatic and splenic artery aneurysm. *Semin Vasc Surg*. 2005;18:196-201.
25. Hashim A, Allaqaband S, Bajwa T. Leaking hepatic artery aneurysm successfully treated with covered stent. *Catheter Cardiovasc Interv*. 2009;74:500-505.
26. Ruiz-Tovar J, Martínez-Molina E, Morales V, et al. Evolution of the therapeutic approach of visceral artery aneurysms. *Scand J Surg*. 2007;96:308-313.
27. Abbott WM, Maloney RD, McCabe CC, et al. Arterial embolism: a 44-year perspective. *Am J Surg*. 1982;143:460-464.
28. Dryjski M, Swedenborg J. Acute ischemia of the extremities in a metropolitan area during one year. *J Cardiovasc Surg (Torino)*. 1984;25:518-522.
29. Sheiner NM, Zeltzer J, MacIntosh E. Arterial embolectomy in the modern era. *Can J Surg*. 1982;25:373-375.
30. Norgren L, Hiatt W, Dormandy J, et al. Inter-society Consensus for the Management of Peripheral Arterial Disease (TASC II). *J Vasc Surg*. 2007;45(suppl):S5-S67.
31. Rutherford RB, Baker JD, Ernst C, et al. Recommended standards for reports dealing with lower extremity ischemia: revised version. *J Vasc Surg*. 1997;26:517-538.
32. Schwarzwalder U, Zeller T. Below-the-knee revascularization. Advanced techniques. *J Cardiovasc Surg (Torino)*. 2009;50:627-634.
33. Robinson WP, Belkin M. Acute limb ischemia due to popliteal artery aneurysm: a continuing surgical challenge. *Semin Vasc Surg*. 2009;22:17-24.
34. Kropman RHJ, Schrijver AM, Kelder JC, et al. Clinical outcome of acute leg ischaemia due to thrombosed popliteal artery aneurysm: systematic review of 895 cases. *Eur J Vasc Endovasc Surg*. 2010:39:452-457.
35. Fogarty TJ, Cranley JJ, Krause RJ, et al. A method for extraction of arterial emboli and thrombi. *Surg Gynecol Obstet*. 1963;116:241-244.
36. Savelyev VS, Zatevakhin II, Stepanov NV. Artery embolism of the upper limbs. *Surgery*. 1977;81:367-375.
37. Eyers P, Earnshaw JJ. Acute non-traumatic arm ischaemia. *Br J Surg*. 1998;85:1340-1346.
38. Rhodes JM, Cherry KJ Jr, Clark RC, Panneton JM, Bower TC, Gloviczki P, Hallett JW Jr, Pairolero PC. Aortic-origin reconstruction of the great vessels: risk factors for early and late complications. *J Vasc Surg*. 2000;31:260-269.
39. Fields CE, Bower TC, Cooper LT, et al. Takayasu's arteritis: operative results and influence of disease activity. *J Vasc Surg*. 2006;43:64-71.
40. Cinà CS, Safar HA, Lagana A, et al. Subclavian carotid transposition and bypass grafting: consecutive cohort study and systematic review. *J Vasc Surg*. 2002;35:422-429.
41. Düber C, Klose KJ, Kopp H, et al. Percutaneous transluminal angioplasty for occlusion of the subclavian artery: short and long-term results. *Cardiovasc Intervent Radiol*. 1992;15:205-210.
42. Linni K, Ugurluoglu A, Mader N, et al. Endovascular management versus surgery for proximal subclavian artery lesions. *Ann Vasc Surg*. 2008;22:769-775.
43. Matsumoto N, Whisnant JP, Kurland LT, et al. Natural history of stroke in Rochester, Minnesota, 1955 through 1969: an extension of a previous study, 1945 through 1954. *Stroke*. 1973;4:20-29.
44. Collaborators of NASCET. Beneficial effect of carotid endarterectomy in symptomatic patients with high-grade carotid stenosis. *N Engl J Med*. 1991;325:445-453.
45. Barnett HJ, Taylor DW, Eliasziw M, et al. Benefit of carotid endarterectomy in patients with symptomatic moderate or severe stenosis. *N Engl J Med*. 1998;339:1415-1425.
46. Yadav JS, Wholey MH, Kuntz RE, et al. Protected carotid-artery stenting versus endarterectomy in high-risk patients. *N Eng J Med*. 2004;351:1493-1501.
47. Wyers NC. Acute mesenteric ischemia: diagnostic approach and surgical treatment. *Semin Vasc Surg*. 2010;23:9-20.
48. Acosta S. Epidemiology of mesenteric vascular disease: clinical implications. *Semin Vasc Surg*. 2010;23:4-8.
49. Oldenburg WA, Lau LL, Rodenberg TJ, et al. Acute mesenteric ischemia: a clinical review. *Arch Intern Med*. 2004;164:1054-1062.
50. Stout CL, Messerschmidt CA, Leake AE, et al. Retrograde open mesenteric stenting for acute mesenteric ischemia is a viable alternative for emergent revascularization. *Vasc Endovascular Surg*. 2010;44:368-371.
51. Björck M, Wanhainen A. Nonocclusive mesenteric hypoperfusion syndromes: recognition and treatment. *Semin Vasc Surg*. 2010;23:54-64.
52. Hoxie HJ, Coggin CB. Renal infarction: Statistical study of two hundred five cases and detailed report of an unusual case. *Arch Intern Med*. 1940;65:587.
53. Robinson S, Nichols D, MacLeod A, et al. Acute renal artery embolism: a case report and brief literature review. *Ann Vasc Surg*. 2008;22:145-147.
54. Karthikesalingam A, Holt PJ, Hinchliffe RG, et al. The diagnosis and management of aortic dissection. *Vasc Endovascular Surg*. 2010;44:165-169.
55. Moon MR. Approach to the treatment of aortic dissection. *Surg Clin N Am*. 2009;89:869-893.
56. Patel PD, Arora RR. Pathophysiology, diagnosis, and management of aortic dissection. *Ther Adv Cardiovasc Dis*. 2008;2:439-468.
57. Suzuki T, Mehta RH, Ince H, et al. Clinical profiles and outcomes of acute type B aortic dissection in the current era: lessons from the International Registry of Aortic Dissection (IRAD). *Circulation*. 2003;108(suppl):II-312-II-317.
58. Subramanian S, Roselli EE. Thoracic aortic dissection: long-term results of endovascular and open repair. *Semin Vasc Surg*. 2009;22:61-68.
59. Moon MC, Morales JP, Greenberg RK. Complicated acute type B dissection and endovascular repair: indications and pitfalls. *Perspect Vasc Surg Endovasc Ther*. 2007;19:146-159.
60. Oderich GS, Panneton JM, Bower TC, et al. Aortic dissection with aortic side branch compromise: impact of malperfusion on patient outcome. *Perspect Vasc Surg Endovasc Ther*. 2008;20:190-200.
61. Panneton JM, Teh SH, Cherry KJ Jr, et al. Aortic fenestration for acute or chronic aortic dissection: an uncommon but effective procedure. *J Vasc Surg*. 2000;32:711-721.
62. Nienaber CA, Rousseau H, Eggebrecht G, et al. Randomized comparison of strategies for type B aortic dissection: the Investigation of STEnt Grafts in Aortic Dissection (INSTEAD) trial. *Circulation*. 2009;120:2519-2528.
63. Leon L, Giannoukas AD, Dodd D, et al. Clinical significance of superficial vein thrombosis. *Eur J Vasc Endovasc Surg*. 2005;29:10-17.
64. Decousus H, Prandoni P, Mismetti P, et al. CALISTO Study Group. Fondaparinux for the treatment of superficial-vein thrombosis in the legs. *N Engl J Med*. 2010;363:1222-1232.
65. Mermel LA, Allon M, Bouza E, et al. Clinical practice guidelines for the diagnosis and management of intravascular catheter-related infection: 2009 Update by the Infectious Diseases Society of America. *Clin Infect Dis*. 2009;49:1-45.
66. Strinden WD, Helgerson RB, Maki DG. Candida septic thrombosis of the great central veins associated with central catheters. Clinical features and management. *Ann Surg*. 1985;202:653-658.
67. Condat B, Pessione F, Hillaire S, et al. Current outcome of portal vein thrombosis in adults: risk and benefit of anticoagulant therapy. *Gastroenterology*. 2001;120:490-497.
68. Rhee RY, Gloviczki P, Mendonca CT, et al. Mesenteric venous thrombosis: still a lethal disease in the 1990s. *J Vasc Surg*. 1994;20:688-697.
69. Asghar M, Ahmed K, Shah SS, et al. Renal vein thrombosis. *Eur J Vasc Endovasc Surg*. 2007;34:217-223.

70. Day JD, Chen BL, Panneton JM. Bilateral renal vein thrombosis treated with percutaneous thrombolysis and mechanical thrombectomy. *J Vasc Surg*. 2009;50:1541.
71. Nieto AF, Doty DB. Superior vena cava obstruction: clinical syndrome, etiology, and treatment. *Curr Probl Cancer*. 1986;10:441-484.
72. Kalra M, Gloviczki P, Andrews JC, et al. Open surgical and endovascular treatment of superior vena cava syndrome caused by nonmalignant disease. *J Vasc Surg*. 2003;38:215-223.
73. Linnemann B, Schmidt H, Schindewolf M, et al. Etiology and VTE risk factor in distribution in patients with IVC thrombosis. *Thromb Res*. 2008;123:72-78.
74. Alimi YS, Hartung O. Ilio-caval venous obstruction: surgical treatment. In: Cronenwett JL, Johnston W, eds. *Rutherford's Vascular Surgery*. 7th ed. Philadelphia, PA: Saunders Elsevier; 2010:932-935.
75. Raskob GE, Silverstein R, Bratzler DW, et al. Surveillance for deep vein thrombosis and pulmonary embolism: recommendations from a national workshop. *Am J Prev Med*. 2010;38(suppl):S502-S509.

CHAPTER 46 ■ INTENSIVE CARE UNIT: THE ESSENTIALS—INCLUDING ASSESSMENT OF SEVERITY OF CRITICAL ILLNESS

MAYUR B. PATEL AND ADDISON K. MAY

Patients managed by acute care surgeons frequently present with organ system dysfunction or are at high risk to develop organ system dysfunction, increasing their risk of adverse outcome and death. The presence of infection, tissue injury, large volume transfusions, or ischemia/reperfusion in this patient population may contribute to the development of a systemic inflammatory response or subsequent immunosuppression contributing to altered tissue healing, infectious complications, organ injury, and organ failure.[1-6] Thus, critically ill or injured acute care surgery patients frequently require critical care management to provide timely and appropriate therapeutic interventions, achieve adequate endpoints of resuscitation, appropriately assess the risk and presence of complications, mitigate the risk of organ dysfunction, and treat organ dysfunction and failure. In this chapter, the contribution of intensive care unit (ICU) and critical care management for the acute care surgical patient is reviewed as (1) timely, targeted, and appropriate application of therapeutic interventions; (2) assessment and recognition of risk; and (3) prevention of complications and minimization of the propagation of organ injury.

THE CRITICAL CARE TEAM AND SYSTEM OF CARE

The concept of critical care has evolved dramatically since the first three-bed ICU was established by Walter Dandy at the Johns Hopkins Hospital in 1926.[7] ICUs were originally developed to provide increased nurse staffing ratios, increased monitoring, and ventilator management. As our understanding of the pathophysiology of critical illness and its treatment has progressed and as patient acuity has increased over time, the concept of critical care has evolved into one of a multidisciplinary team providing a system of care to deliver timely and targeted interventions to address the underlying pathologic condition and the global and organ-specific dysfunction. This is achieved while limiting the risk of complications and iatrogenic organ injury. Critical care may be defined as the process of high-intensity physiologic monitoring coupled with short response pharmacologic, hemodynamic, ventilatory, and procedural interventions. These efforts are designed to reestablish normal homeostasis and minimize primary, secondary, and iatrogenic injury. Importantly, the mitigation of risk of complications and further exacerbation of organ injury may be the most significant contribution of critical care systems. Critical care is generally the most expensive, technologically advanced, and resource intensive component of medical care. Despite the high incremental cost of providing intensivist-directed critical care management, numerous studies have demonstrated considerable incremental benefits of intensivist-directed critical care on mortality, morbidity, and overall cost.[8-15]

Considerable heterogeneity exists across ICUs relative to physician responsibility, physician staffing and availability, provision of ancillary services, and organization of teams and processes. This heterogeneity complicates the ability to assess the contribution of individual components of critical care to the outcome. In Table 46.1, various descriptions of physician staffing models are provided.[16] In general, closed unit staffing models provide reductions in mortality when compared to open unit models[9-13] and the inclusion of multidisciplinary teams appears to provide incrementally greater reductions in mortality when combined with closed unit models.[17]

TIMELY, TARGETED, AND APPROPRIATE APPLICATION OF THERAPEUTIC INTERVENTIONS

Regardless of the structural organization of individual ICUs, the provision of timely, targeted, and appropriate therapeutic interventions improves the outcome of critically ill and injured patients. These concepts are discussed in detail in Chapters 4, 7, 12, and 13 and in chapters in Section IV. Mainstays of therapy for the critically ill acute care surgery population include (1) goal-directed resuscitation and appropriate inotropic support, (2) appropriate and timely antibiotic therapy, and (3) timely and effective source control of infectious, hemorrhagic, or ischemic insults.

While early resuscitation has long been accepted to improve outcomes in the critically ill acute care surgery population, debate continues regarding strategies and appropriate endpoints.[4,18-23] Measures of tissue hypoxia such as base deficit, elevated lactate, and decreased mixed venous saturation correlate with the development of organ system dysfunction and mortality following the onset of

TABLE 46.1

TERMINOLOGIES TO DESCRIBE ICU PHYSICIAN STAFFING MODELS

Closed	Intensivist responsible for day-to-day management of patients, including all admissions and discharges, orders, and clinical management
Open	Primary physician responsible for day-to-day management decisions. ICU admission and discharge policies exist, but the primary physician is the ultimate decision maker. There may be no full-time intensivist or may be involved at the discretion of the primary physicians
High intensity and closed	Intensivist responsible for all patient care in a closed ICU
High intensity and open	The ICU is open but it is mandatory to consult the intensivist
Low intensity and open	The ICU is open and consulting the intensivist is optional
Low intensity	No intensivist available
High intensity	>80% of patients managed by intensivist
Intermediate intensity	>0 but <80% of patients managed by intensivist
No intensivist	No intensivist available
Choice	The ICU is open and consulting the intensivist is optional
No choice and closed	Closed ICU or mandatory ICU consultation
No choice and no intensivist	No intensivist available

Gajic O, Afessa B. Physician staffing models and patient safety in the ICU. *Chest*. 2009;135:1038–1044.

hemorrhage and sepsis and early correction (likely within 6 hours in at-risk groups) of these abnormalities is associated with improved outcomes.[4,18-21,23-29] Resuscitation strategies that target adequate tissue oxygenation as endpoints, and that both respond to the alteration in physiology and limit excessive fluids, appear to have better outcomes than those that do not employ these measures. However, no perfect set of markers has been identified to guide resuscitation in all settings.

For patients with both community and hospital-acquired infections, the time to appropriate antibiotic therapy has been shown to significantly alter outcomes. Thus, establishment of the likelihood of the presence of infection, the source of infection if present, likely pathogens, and potential resistance of pathogens involved, all factor into timing and selection of antibiotic therapy. Inadequate empiric antimicrobial therapy is associated with twice the mortality in studies of mixed hospital-acquired infections,[30] ventilator-associated pneumonia,[31-33] hospital-acquired bloodstream infections,[34,35] and peritonitis.[36,37] Prior antibiotic exposure was associated with inadequate empiric therapy in many of these studies with selection of more resistant pathogens.[30,34,36] As the severity of illness increases, the timing of antibiotic initiation appears to assume increasing importance in septic patients. In a study of 335 surgical ICU patients with infections, using logistic regression analysis, Barie et al.[38] demonstrated that each 30-minute delay in initiation of antibiotic therapy from the onset of fever was associated with a 2% increase in mortality. For patients with septic shock, the influence of antibiotic timing appears to be even greater. In a study of 2,731 patients with septic shock from 14 ICUs in the United States and Canada, Kumar et al.[39] demonstrated that each 1-hour delay in antibiotic therapy from the onset of hypotension was associated with a 12% increase in mortality. The increased risk of death was consistent across subcategories including intra-abdominal, skin and soft tissue, respiratory, blood stream, community, and nosocomial infections; only 50% of patients received therapy within 6 hours of the onset of hypotension. These studies highlight the importance of systems that enable the early identification of infectious processes and the administration of early empiric antibiotic therapy appropriate for the clinical setting.

A significant portion of critically ill patients managed by acute care surgeons require source control as part of therapeutic interventions, most commonly patients with intra-abdominal processes or skin and soft tissue infections. Severely septic patients may require rapid resuscitation and stabilization in an ICU setting prior to operative intervention for source control. For patients with necrotizing skin and soft tissue infections, the time to effective source control is associated with outcome and these patients may require multiple operative interventions before source control is achieved.[40,41] Critical care support may be required during this period for the treatment of sepsis and septic shock, to support and minimize organ system dysfunction, and to assist with wound management. Critically ill patients with peritonitis present the acute care surgeon with unique challenges. In general, critically ill patients with peritonitis are at higher risk for failure of primary source control and the development of secondary complications such as abdominal compartment syndrome, recurrent intra-abdominal infection (abscess and tertiary peritonitis), and fistula formation than patients with peritonitis who are not critically ill.

One clear demonstration of compliance with timely, targeted, appropriate interventions in critically ill patients is provided through the efforts of the Surviving Sepsis Campaign (SSC).[43] The SSC established evidence-based management guidelines and implemented a broad educational program to facilitate integration of these guidelines in clinical practice in North America, South America, and Europe. Elements of the guidelines were grouped or bundled into two sets of targets to be completed within either 6 hours or within 24 hours of admission. Numerous studies have demonstrated an associated benefit of compliance with the SSC.[45] A before and after analysis of participating sites was conducted on data submitted from January 2005 through March 2008. Compliance with elements in the bundle increased linearly throughout the period and resulted in a 5.4% adjusted absolute decline in mortality over the 2-year period.[46]

ASSESSMENT AND RECOGNITION OF RISK: ASSESSMENT OF PATIENTS WITH PERITONITIS

Patients with severe sepsis (organ dysfunction and criteria of systemic inflammatory response syndrome) secondary to peritonitis, while representing a small portion of all patients with peritonitis, are at higher risk of mortality.[47] Patients more likely to develop severe sepsis from peritonitis include those with more advanced age, those with diffuse peritonitis, and those with preexisting organ dysfunction.[47] Not surprisingly, factors that predict development of severe sepsis are similar to those that predict failure of treatment and mortality from peritonitis as well. Multivariate analysis in numerous studies has identified advanced age, low serum albumin, poor nutrition, preexisting organ dysfunction, and high Acute Physiology and Chronic Health Evaluation (APACHE) II scores as associated with failure of source control and death.[48-54] In an analysis of 217 patients entered into a randomized trial of complicated intra-abdominal infections, 14% of patients had APACHE II scores of 15 or greater with failure rates in these patients >40%. If APACHE II scores were >20, failure rate exceeded 50%.[55] Each of these risk factors is a measure of the degree of variance from the host's normal physiologic state. In addition to these physiologic risk factors, the degree of inflammation and bacterial burden within the peritoneum also predicts the risk of failure of source control. Diffuse peritonitis, moderate or extensive residual contamination at the completion of the source control procedure, or inability to achieve adequate source control also predicts failure.[54,56-58] Risk factors for failure of source control from intra-abdominal infections are summarized in Table 46.2. Knowledge of these risk factors should be utilized to estimate the postoperative clinical course, to help determine the level of support and monitoring, and predict the likelihood of postoperative intra-abdominal infectious complications. The assessment of risk of failure is important as delays to definitive therapy in patients who fail source control are associated with increased mortality.[62]

TABLE 46.2

CLINICAL FACTORS THAT PREDICT FAILURE OF SOURCE CONTROL FOR INTRA-ABDOMINAL INFECTIONS[55,59-61]

Delay in the initial intervention (>24 h)
High severity of illness (APACHE II ≥ 15)
Advanced age
Comorbidity and degree of organ dysfunction
Low albumin
Poor nutritional status
Degree of peritoneal involvement/diffuse peritonitis (Peritonitis severity score, Mannheim Peritonitis index)
Inability to achieve adequate debridement or control of drainage
Presence of malignancy

ASSESSMENT AND RECOGNITION OF RISK: MODELING SEVERITY OF ILLNESS IN THE ICU

Scoring systems for severity of illness can broadly be divided into those that are targeted for a specific disease process or organ system (e.g., the Model for End-Stage Liver Disease (MELD) score in liver disease, the Mannheim Peritonitis Index for intra-abdominal infection, and the Glasgow Coma Score for brain injury) and those that are generic for all ICU patients. This section focuses on these generic scores that can be divided into those that assess disease severity on admission and those that assess the degree of organ system derangement or injury at variable time points in any given patient. Scoring systems for severity of illness utilize a variety of demographic, clinical, physiological, and laboratory variables. The most common scoring systems that assess disease severity upon admission include the APACHE, the Simplified Acute Physiology Score (SAPS), and the Mortality Probability Model (MPM), all of which were developed to predict likelihood of survival.[63] Common scoring systems used to assess the presence and severity of organ dysfunction on admission and during the ICU stay include the Multiple Organ Dysfunction Score and the Sequential Organ Failure Assessment.[63]

Each of the three scoring systems used to assess disease severity upon admission and predict outcome (i.e., APACHE, SAPS, MPM) uses variables obtained within a 24-hour period of admission, typically the worst value recorded. Each has had multiple generations, with the most recent version undergoing adjustment of the prediction model based upon new datasets, equations for which are proprietary. Prediction equations for older, nonproprietary versions are no longer being adjusted. Versions of these scores are frequently used to stratify patient severity within studies or to control for variation in severity within a defined population when assessing performance.[63] They may also be used to determine eligibility for inclusion in clinical trials, for therapeutic interventions,[42,43] or to assess the likelihood of therapeutic failure.[55] Generally, these systems perform well when comparing outcome within specific critically ill patient populations, but not across varying populations of critically ill patients.

Measures of organ injury and dysfunction may be used to assess organ dysfunction at admission but may also be used as outcome variables. Thus, they are dynamic, varying among individuals and within a given individual over time and thus can be used to assess and quantitate change in organ function over time. However, outcome prediction and organ dysfunction scores are not mutually exclusive and provide different types of information, which together can complement the clinician's subjective evaluation of a patient's status. These scores may be employed to provide a quantitative response to therapy and direct subsequent therapeutic interventions.[64,65]

More recently, a new system for analysis of sepsis has been developed, the predisposition, insult, response, organ dysfunction (PIRO) system. The PIRO system was created so that a clinically useful staging system, similar to cancer staging, could stratify patients based on their baseline risk for an adverse outcome and their potential to respond to therapy across the very heterogenous patient population defined as septic.[66] While further studies are needed, performance for the prediction of outcome in sepsis is very promising.[67]

PREVENTION OF COMPLICATIONS AND MINIMIZATION OF THE PROPAGATION OF ORGAN INJURY

While relatively few interventions have been shown in randomized, controlled trials to consistently impact outcome in the ICU, outcome of critically ill patients is improving.[38] The improvement in outcome is likely related to both the introduction of specific therapeutic strategies that limit the development and progression of organ dysfunction as well as the complex systems of delivery required to provide highly specific and targeted therapies. Several therapeutic strategies that impact the outcome of patients include those involving respiratory management, sedation and delirium management, cardiovascular risk management, renal management, transfusion practices, endocrine support, infection control, nutritional provision, prevention of airway loss, skin breakdown, deep vein thrombosis, and stress ulcers, as well as the safe performance of invasive, bedside procedures. Each of these areas has a large body of literature that continues to support the advancement of care for the critically ill and injured patient. A full discussion of these topics is beyond the scope of a single chapter, although they will be discussed briefly below. Evidence-based guidelines may assist with the appropriate application of many of these areas listed. However, maintaining high level compliance with both simple and complex components of care within each is difficult and is aided by multidisciplinary teams and informatics support.

Respiratory Management

Appropriate respiratory management of mechanically ventilated, critically ill patients impacts the outcome considerably. Strategies directed toward liberation from ventilatory management, prevention of lung and remote organ injury through low volume ventilatory strategies (i.e., ARDS Net), and strategies to limit the development of ventilator-associated pneumonia have important implications for patient outcome.[43] Clear support for systems and teams that continuously evaluate the appropriateness and ability to wean patients from ventilator support have been shown to reduce the number of ventilator days and improve outcome.[43] Application of weaning protocols, avoidance of weaning of intermittent mandatory ventilation rate, daily spontaneous breathing trials, targeted sedation and daily cessation of sedation, and appropriate use of tracheostomies reduce ventilator days and improve outcomes in certain patient populations. Use of a low-volume ventilation strategy also limits the progression and severity of acute lung injury and acute respiratory distress syndrome, as well as measures of systemic inflammation. However, despite clear data from randomized studies, application of this strategy has been slow to be widely adopted in practice.[68] The need for mechanical ventilation and the presence of an endotracheal tube greatly increases the risk of the development of pneumonia. However, the application of several interventions has been shown to limit the risk of pneumonia in randomized studies.[69,70] These include spontaneous breathing trials, targeted sedation, head of bed elevation, dental and oral care, and hypopharyngeal suctioning. However, high level compliance with each of these may be difficult to achieve and systems to monitor and enhance compliance may improve their application.[71]

Sedation and Delirium Management

The complex interrelationships between sedation, pain management, sleep, delirium, cognitive dysfunction, and outcome are increasingly recognized but are incompletely understood. While the prevention of pain and anxiety remains an important goal in the management of critically ill patients, oversedation has been recognized to contribute to prolonged mechanical ventilation, altered sleep patterns, and increased delirium.[72-75] Targeted sedation and pain control and daily cessation of sedation have been shown to substantially decrease the time of mechanical ventilation, ICU and hospital length of stay, and outcome.[73,74] Delirium occurs in up to 80% of ICU patients but is frequently underrecognized.[76] The presence and severity of delirium correlates with both cognitive deficits post discharge and overall outcome.[76-78] Both the depth of sedation and agents used to provide sedation contribute to the severity of delirium. At present, inadequate data regarding pharmacologic therapy to limit the development of delirium exists to make recommendations.[73] For the treatment of agitated delirium, few randomized trials exist and the use of antipsychotics, either conventional (Haldol) or less common agents, may be considered. A summation of recommendations for nonpharmacologic efforts to limit delirium and approach to ICU sedation is provided in Table 46.3.

Cardiovascular Risk Management

Surgery is a physiologically stressful event and may precipitate myocardial infarction (MI) in high risk patients any time during the perioperative period. While several studies have shown a significant reduction in perioperative MI and death from cardiac causes with the institution of perioperative beta blockade in high risk patients, all cause mortality with beta blockade may be higher in lower risk patients.[73,79-81] Patients with

TABLE 46.3

RECOMMENDATIONS FOR DELIRIUM AND SEDATION MANAGEMENT IN THE ICU

Nonpharmacologic to limit delirium:

Systematic programs to enhance orientation and cognition sleep quality, and mobilization

- Noise reduction
- Light management to facilitate day/night cycles
- Minimization of sleep interruptions
- Introduction of therapeutic activities
- Early mobilization and physical and occupational therapy

Approach to ICU sedation:

1. Provide adequate analgesia first and monitor adequacy with validated assessment tool
2. Employ targeted sedation protocols with validated assessment tools
3. Consider daily cessation of sedation in conjunction with spontaneous breathing trials in ventilated patients.
4. Avoid the adverse effects commonly associated with standard sedative regimens
   - Propofol and dexmedetomidine may be beneficial when compared with benzodiazepines, particularly with short-term needs
   - Avoid midazolam accumulation with targeted sedation to the lightest appropriate target and daily cessation
   - Avoid continuous infusion lorazepam if possible to limit propylene glycol toxicity and monitor serum anion gap if dose exceeds 1 mg/kg.
   - Avoid prolonged or high dose (70 mg/kg/h) of propofol to limit the risk of propofol infusion syndrome.

preoperative history of beta blockade and those at high risk of cardiovascular events should undergo institution therapy with appropriate targets. However, appropriate limitation of hypotension and bradycardia should be achieved to minimize complications.

Renal Management

Acute kidney injury (AKI) is common in the critically ill population, occurring in one-third to two-thirds of patients, and is associated with a substantial increase in morbidity and mortality.[82] The mortality associated with AKI increases proportionally with the severity of injury and is >50% in those requiring renal replacement therapy. Serum creatinine, the most commonly used parameter to assess renal function, lacks both sensitivity and specificity. In addition, increases in serum creatinine lag considerably behind the decline in glomerular filtration rate. Thus, early decline in renal function may go unnoticed. The etiology of AKI in critically ill patients is commonly multifactorial and often difficult to assign to single insults. However, recognition of risk with avoidance of repeated insults is the mainstay of prevention. The most common cause of renal failure in the general ICU population is sepsis. Other causes/risk factors include hypovolemia, hypoperfusion, rhabdomyolysis, obstruction, abdominal syndrome, and nephrotoxic agents. Common nephrotoxic agents include nonsteroidal anti-inflammatory drugs, aminoglycosides, amphotericin, penicillins, acyclovir, and radio-contrast agents. Maintenance of adequate renal perfusion and renal perfusion pressure in the setting of sepsis and ischemia/reperfusion syndrome requires assurance of adequate volume resuscitation and inotropic and vasopressor therapy. Adequate data supports the use of prevention strategies for contrast-induced nephropathy including; hydration with either sodium chloride or sodium bicarbonate, the use of *N*-acetyl cysteine (NAC), and the use of low-volume nonionic, low-osmolar or iso-osmolar contrast. The choice of sodium chloride versus sodium bicarbonate remains controversial but the weight of the current evidence suggests that bicarbonate may be superior. Meta-analysis of the use of NAC provides conflicting results, although none have demonstrated harm.

Transfusion Practice

While transfusions are common in critically ill patients and may be lifesaving in severely anemic patients (Hgb < 5 g/dL) and actively hemorrhaging patients, transfusion of blood carries a significant risk of transfusion reactions, transmission of infectious agents, transfusion-related acute lung injury, and immunomodulation.[83-85] Hebert's landmark study published in 1999 compared a restrictive versus liberal transfusion strategy in critically ill patients. The authors demonstrated that patients restricted to a transfusion trigger of 7.0 g/dL Hgb with a target of 7.0–9.0 g/dL Hgb fared better than patients transfused at 10.0 g/dL Hgb and maintained at 10.0–12.0 g/dL.[86] The deleterious effect of severe postoperative anemia on mortality was shown in a study of 300 patients with a postoperative hemoglobin concentration <8.0 g/dL who refused blood transfusion for religious reasons with significant increases in mortality occurring when hemoglobin concentrations fell to <5 g/dL.[83] Patients with a recent history of acute MI or unstable angina may benefit from a higher transfusion threshold (trigger of 10 g/dL Hgb).[84,87] The benefit of transfusion in sepsis and in those with inadequate oxygen consumption remains to be established.[84] No single criterion should be used as an indication for red cell component therapy. Multiple factors related to the patient's clinical status and oxygen delivery needs should be considered. Accordingly, the decision to transfuse erythrocytes must be based upon an assessment of the risks of anemia versus the risks of transfusion.

Endocrine Support

Endocrine dysfunction has gained attention in critical care in the last decade. The most prominent areas of endocrine dysfunction include the development of stress-induced insulin resistance and resulting hyperglycemia, acute adrenal insufficiency in sepsis, and thyroid dysfunction in critical illness. Stress-related hyperglycemia occurs commonly following surgery, trauma, and sepsis. The magnitude of hyperglycemia is strongly associated with poor outcome in both the noncritically ill and the critically ill population, particularly in the nondiabetic patients.[88-90] The development of hyperglycemia, while multifactorial, is significantly related to stress-induced insulin resistance. Following the landmark Leuven study published in 2001,[91] glycemic control in the form of intensive insulin therapy (IIT) in the ICU has received much attention in a variety of critically ill populations. While the interpretation of data on this topic is confounded by variation in patient populations, incidence of hypoglycemia, variation of IIT protocols, and variation in nutritional provision, several conclusions can be drawn from the existing literature and are summarized:

- Hyperglycemia should be controlled in the critically ill surgical population[92]
- Intravenous insulin should be used to achieve this, but efforts to measure and limit hypoglycemia are essential[92-94]
- Periods of glycemic analysis longer than 2 hours result in poorer control and increased hypoglycemia[94,95]

Important areas of uncertainty exist regarding glycemic control that include

- The optimal target for glycemic control
- The optimal early nutritional provision and its influence on glycemic control

Adrenal insufficiency and relative adrenal insufficiency in critical illness and sepsis has also received considerable attention in the past decade. Following the publication by Annane et al.[96] with treatment of patients with refractory septic shock with low dose hydrocortisone, considerable debate has occurred over the appropriate indications. Current recommendations supported by meta-analysis of studies in sepsis include[43,97]:

- Consideration of intravenous hydrocortisone in doses of ≤300 mg/d for patients in septic shock when hypotension responds poorly to fluid resuscitation and vasopressors.
- Steroid therapy may be discontinued once vasopressors are no longer required.

Nutritional Provision

Critical illness is associated with a strongly catabolic state, the severity of which coincides with the severity of the systemic inflammatory response. The provision of nutritional support to critically ill patients is paramount and may preserve lean body mass, immune function, and reduce metabolic complications. Specific, targeted nutritional therapy may modulate the stress response in various settings and have a favorable impact on outcome.[98] Despite significant advances in our understanding of optimal nutritional provision, much remains unknown and this area has been inadequately studied. Enteral nutrition is strongly preferred over parenteral and can safely be delivered in the majority of patients within 48 hours of surgery or completion of resuscitation and achievement of hemodynamic stability. The role of early nutritional provision (<48 hours) via the parenteral route has been inadequately studied at this point and American and European organizations differ in their recommendations. Recommendations of the Society of Critical Care Medicine and the American Society for Parenteral and Enteral Nutrition have recently been published.[98,99]

Antibiotic Stewardship Programs

Critically ill patients are at high risk of health care-acquired infections that prolong ICU and hospital stay and increase morbidity and mortality. While antibiotics are paramount for prophylaxis and treatment, antibiotic exposure is associated with an increased risk of subsequent infection in critically ill patients and strongly associated with the acquisition of resistant pathogens.[30,100-104] Antibiotic stewardship programs have been shown to reduce antibiotic use, hospital-acquired infections, and antibiotic resistance in hospital-acquired pathogens.[105,106] Stewardship should assure appropriate empiric coverage with antibiotics, an organized diagnostic approach to identification of therapy, deescalation of antibiotics to known or highly suspected pathogens, limitation of antibiotic therapy to evidence-based treatment courses, and appropriate dosing regimens.

References

1. Dewar D, Moore FA, Moore EE, et al. Postinjury multiple organ failure. *Injury*. 2009;40:912-918.
2. Kohl BA, Deutschman CS. The inflammatory response to surgery and trauma. *Curr Opin Crit Care*. 2006;12:325-332.
3. Lenz A, Franklin GA, Cheadle WG. Systemic inflammation after trauma. *Injury*. 2007;38:1336-1345.
4. Rivers EP, Coba V, Whitmill M. Early goal-directed therapy in severe sepsis and septic shock: a contemporary review of the literature. *Curr Opin Anaesthesiol*. 2008;21:128-140.
5. Sihler KC, Napolitano LM. Complications of massive transfusion. *Chest*. 2010;137:209-220.
6. Talmor M, Hydo L, Barie PS. Relationship of systemic inflammatory response syndrome to organ dysfunction, length of stay, and mortality in critical surgical illness: effect of intensive care unit resuscitation. *Arch Surg*. 1999;134:81-87.
7. Bleck TP. Historical aspects of critical care and the nervous system. *Crit Care Clin*. 2009;25:153-164, ix.
8. Dimick JB, Pronovost PJ, Heitmiller RF, et al. Intensive care unit physician staffing is associated with decreased length of stay, hospital cost, and complications after esophageal resection. *Crit Care Med*. 2001;29:753-758.
9. Ghorra S, Reinert SE, Cioffi W, et al. Analysis of the effect of conversion from open to closed surgical intensive care unit. *Ann Surg*. 1999;229:163-171.
10. Hanson CW III, Deutschman CS, Anderson HL III, et al. Effects of an organized critical care service on outcomes and resource utilization: a cohort study. *Crit Care Med*. 1999;27:270-274.
11. Nathens AB, Rivara FP, MacKenzie EJ, et al. The impact of an intensivist-model ICU on trauma-related mortality. *Ann Surg*. 2006;244:545-554.
12. Pronovost PJ, Angus DC, Dorman T, et al. Physician staffing patterns and clinical outcomes in critically ill patients: a systematic review. *JAMA*. 2002;288:2151-2162.
13. Pronovost PJ, Jenckes MW, Dorman T, et al. Organizational characteristics of intensive care units related to outcomes of abdominal aortic surgery. *JAMA*. 1999;281:1310-1317.
14. Pronovost PJ, Needham DM, Waters H, et al. Intensive care unit physician staffing: financial modeling of the Leapfrog standard. *Crit Care Med*. 2004;32:1247-1253.
15. Pronovost PJ, Rinke ML, Emery K, et al. Interventions to reduce mortality among patients treated in intensive care units. *J Crit Care*. 2004;19:158-164.
16. Gajic O, Afessa B. Physician staffing models and patient safety in the ICU. *Chest*. 2009;135:1038-1044.
17. Kim MM, Barnato AE, Angus DC, et al. The effect of multidisciplinary care teams on intensive care unit mortality. *Arch Intern Med*. 2010;170:369-376.
18. Blow O, Magliore L, Claridge JA, et al. The golden hour and the silver day: detection and correction of occult hypoperfusion within 24 hours improves outcome from major trauma. *J Trauma*. 1999;47:964-969.
19. Englehart MS, Schreiber MA. Measurement of acid-base resuscitation endpoints: lactate, base deficit, bicarbonate or what? *Curr Opin Crit Care*. 2006;12:569-574.
20. Jansen TC, van Bommel J, Woodward R, et al. Association between blood lactate levels, Sequential Organ Failure Assessment subscores, and 28-day mortality during early and late intensive care unit stay: a retrospective observational study. *Crit Care Med*. 2009;37:2369-2374.
21. Moore FA, McKinley BA, Moore EE. The next generation in shock resuscitation. *Lancet*. 2004;363:1988-1996.
22. Rivers E, Nguyen B, Havstad S et al. Early goal-directed therapy in the treatment of severe sepsis and septic shock. *N Engl J Med*. 2001;345:1368-1377.
23. Rivers EP, Coba V, Visbal A, et al. Management of sepsis: early resuscitation. *Clin Chest Med*. 2008;29:689-704, ix-x.
24. Davis JW, Kaups KL, Parks SN. Base deficit is superior to pH in evaluating clearance of acidosis after traumatic shock. *J Trauma*. 1998;44:114-118.
25. Kincaid EH, Miller PR, Meredith JW, et al. Elevated arterial base deficit in trauma patients: a marker of impaired oxygen utilization. *J Am Coll Surg*. 1998;187:384-392.
26. Mikulaschek A, Henry SM, Donovan R, et al. Serum lactate is not predicted by anion gap or base excess after trauma resuscitation. *J Trauma*. 1996;40:218-224.
27. Moomey CB Jr, Melton SM, Croce MA, et al. Prognostic value of blood lactate, base deficit, and oxygen-derived variables in an LD50 model of penetrating trauma. *Crit Care Med*. 1999;27:154-161.
28. Scalea TM, Maltz S, Yelon J, et al. Resuscitation of multiple trauma and head injury: role of crystalloid fluids and inotropes. *Crit Care Med*. 1994;22:1610-1615.
29. Scalea TM, Simon HM, Duncan AO, et al. Geriatric blunt multiple trauma: improved survival with early invasive monitoring. *J Trauma*. 1990;30:129-134.
30. Kollef MH, Sherman G, Ward S, et al. Inadequate antimicrobial treatment of infections: a risk factor for hospital mortality among critically ill patients. *Chest*. 1999;115:462-474.
31. Alvarez-Lerma F. Modification of empiric antibiotic treatment in patients with pneumonia acquired in the intensive care unit. ICU-Acquired Pneumonia Study Group. *Intensive Care Med*. 1996;22:387-394.
32. Luna CM, Vujacich P, Niederman MS, et al. Impact of BAL data on the therapy and outcome of ventilator-associated pneumonia. *Chest*. 1997;111:676-685.
33. REllo J, Gallego M, Mariscal D, et al. The value of routine microbial investigation in ventilator-associated pneumonia. *Am J Respir Crit Care Med*. 1997;156:196-200.
34. Ibrahim EH, Sherman G, Ward S, et al. The influence of inadequate antimicrobial treatment of bloodstream infections on patient outcomes in the ICU setting. *Chest*. 2000;118:146-155.
35. Leibovici L, Shraga I, Drucker M, et al. The benefit of appropriate empirical antibiotic treatment in patients with bloodstream infection. *J Intern Med*. 1998;244:379-386.
36. Montravers P, Gauzit R, Muller C, et al. Emergence of antibiotic-resistant bacteria in cases of peritonitis after intraabdominal surgery affects the efficacy of empirical antimicrobial therapy. *Clin Infect Dis*. 1996;23:486-494.
37. Mosdell DM, Morris DM, Voltura A, et al. Antibiotic treatment for surgical peritonitis. *Ann Surg*. 1991;214:543-549.
38. Barie PS, Hydo LJ, Shou J, et al. Decreasing magnitude of multiple organ dysfunction syndrome despite increasingly severe critical surgical illness: a 17-year longitudinal study. *J Trauma*. 2008;65:1227-1235.
39. Kumar A, Roberts D, Wood KE, et al. Duration of hypotension before initiation of effective antimicrobial therapy is the critical determinant of survival in human septic shock. *Crit Care Med*. 2006;34:1589-1596.
40. May AK. Skin and soft tissue infections. *Surg Clin North Am*. 2009;89:403-420, viii.
41. May AK, Stafford RE, Bulger EM, et al. Treatment of complicated skin and soft tissue infections. *Surg Infect (Larchmt)*. 2009;10:467-499.
42. Bernard GR, Vincent JL, Laterre PF, et al. Efficacy and safety of recombinant human activated protein C for severe sepsis. *N Engl J Med*. 2001;344:699-709.
43. Dellinger RP, Levy MM, Carlet JM, et al. Surviving Sepsis Campaign: international guidelines for management of severe sepsis and septic shock: 2008. *Crit Care Med*. 2008;36:296-327.
44. Vincent JL, Bernard GR, Beale R, et al. Drotrecogin alfa (activated) treatment in severe sepsis from the global open-label trial ENHANCE: further evidence for survival and safety and implications for early treatment. *Crit Care Med*. 2005;33:2266-2277.
45. Townsend SR, Schorr C, Levy MM, et al. Reducing mortality in severe sepsis: the Surviving Sepsis Campaign. *Clin Chest Med*. 2008;29:721-733, x.
46. Levy MM, Dellinger RP, Townsend SR, et al. The Surviving Sepsis Campaign: results of an international guideline-based performance improvement program targeting severe sepsis. *Intensive Care Med*. 2010;36:222-231.
47. Anaya DA, Nathens AB. Risk factors for severe sepsis in secondary peritonitis. *Surg Infect (Larchmt)*. 2003;4:355-362.
48. Bohnen JM, Mustard RA, Oxholm SE, et al. APACHE II score and abdominal sepsis. A prospective study. *Arch Surg*. 1988;123:225-229.
49. Bohnen JM, Mustard RA, Schouten BD. Steroids, APACHE II score, and the outcome of abdominal infection. *Arch Surg*. 1994;129:33-37.
50. Christou NV, Barie PS, Dellinger EP, et al. Surgical Infection Society intra-abdominal infection study. Prospective evaluation of management techniques and outcome. *Arch Surg*. 1993;128:193-198.
51. Dellinger EP, Wertz MJ, Meakins JL, et al. Surgical infection stratification system for intra-abdominal infection. Multicenter trial. *Arch Surg*. 1985;120:21-29.

52. Ohmann C, Wittmann DH, Wacha H. Prospective evaluation of prognostic scoring systems in peritonitis. Peritonitis Study Group. *Eur J Surg.* 1993;159:267-274.
53. Pacelli F, Doglietto GB, Alfieri S, et al. Prognosis in intra-abdominal infections. Multivariate analysis on 604 patients. *Arch Surg.* 1996;131:641-645.
54. Wacha H, Hau T, Dittmer R, et al. Risk factors associated with intraabdominal infections: a prospective multicenter study. Peritonitis Study Group. *Langenbecks Arch Surg.* 1999;384:24-32.
55. Barie PS, Vogel SB, Dellinger EP, et al. A randomized, double-blind clinical trial comparing cefepime plus metronidazole with imipenem-cilastatin in the treatment of complicated intra-abdominal infections. Cefepime Intra-abdominal Infection Study Group. *Arch Surg.* 1997;132:1294-1302.
56. Grunau G, Heemken R, Hau T. Predictors of outcome in patients with postoperative intra-abdominal infection. *Eur J Surg.* 1996;162:619-625.
57. Hopkins JA, Lee JC, Wilson SE. Susceptibility of intra-abdominal isolates at operation: a predictor of postoperative infection. *Am Surg.* 1993;59:791-796.
58. Solomkin JS, Dellinger EP, Christou NV, et al. Results of a multicenter trial comparing imipenem/cilastatin to tobramycin/clindamycin for intra-abdominal infections. *Ann Surg.* 1990;212:581-591.
59. Biondo S, Ramos E, Fraccalvieri D, et al. Comparative study of left colonic Peritonitis Severity Score and Mannheim Peritonitis Index. *Br J Surg.* 2006;93:616-622.
60. Bosscha K, Reijnders K, Hulstaert PF, et al. Prognostic scoring systems to predict outcome in peritonitis and intra-abdominal sepsis. *Br J Surg.* 1997;84:1532-1534.
61. Seiler CA, Brugger L, Forssmann U, et al. Conservative surgical treatment of diffuse peritonitis. *Surgery.* 2000;127:178-184.
62. Koperna T, Schulz F. Relaparotomy in peritonitis: prognosis and treatment of patients with persisting intraabdominal infection. *World J Surg.* 2000;24:32-37.
63. Vincent JL, Moreno R. Clinical review: scoring systems in the critically ill. *Crit Care.* 2010;14:207.
64. van Ruler O, Lamme B, Gouma DJ, et al. Variables associated with positive findings at relaparotomy in patients with secondary peritonitis. *Crit Care Med.* 2007;35:468-476.
65. van Ruler O, Mahler CW, Boer KR, et al. Comparison of on-demand vs planned relaparotomy strategy in patients with severe peritonitis: a randomized trial. *JAMA.* 2007;298:865-872.
66. Dellinger RP, Carlet JM, Masur H, et al. Surviving Sepsis Campaign guidelines for management of severe sepsis and septic shock. *Crit Care Med.* 2004;32:858-873.
67. Rubulotta F, Marshall JC, Ramsay G, et al. Predisposition, insult/infection, response, and organ dysfunction: A new model for staging severe sepsis. *Crit Care Med.* 2009;37:1329-1335.
68. Kalhan R, Mikkelsen M, Dedhiya P, et al. Underuse of lung protective ventilation: analysis of potential factors to explain physician behavior. *Crit Care Med.* 2006;34:300-306.
69. Tablan OC, Anderson LJ, Besser R, et al. Guidelines for preventing health-care—associated pneumonia, 2003: recommendations of CDC and the Healthcare Infection Control Practices Advisory Committee. *MMWR Recomm Rep.* 2004;53:1-36.
70. Tolentino-DelosReyes AF, Ruppert SD, Shiao SY. Evidence-based practice: use of the ventilator bundle to prevent ventilator-associated pneumonia. *Am J Crit Care.* 2007;16:20-27.
71. Zaydfudim V, Dossett LA, Starmer JM, et al. Implementation of a real-time compliance dashboard to help reduce SICU ventilator-associated pneumonia with the ventilator bundle. *Arch Surg.* 2009;144:656-662.
72. Hooper MH, Girard TD. Sedation and weaning from mechanical ventilation: linking spontaneous awakening trials and spontaneous breathing trials to improve patient outcomes. *Crit Care Clin.* 2009;25:515-525, viii.
73. Riker RR, Fraser GL. Altering intensive care sedation paradigms to improve patient outcomes. *Crit Care Clin.* 2009;25:527-538, viii-ix.
74. Sessler CN, Pedram S. Protocolized and target-based sedation and analgesia in the ICU. *Crit Care Clin.* 2009;25:489-513, viii.
75. Skrobik Y. Delirium prevention and treatment. *Crit Care Clin.* 2009;25:585-91, x.
76. Pandharipande P, Jackson J, Ely EW. Delirium: acute cognitive dysfunction in the critically ill. *Curr Opin Crit Care.* 2005;11:360-368.
77. Girard TD, Jackson JC, Pandharipande PP, et al. Delirium as a predictor of long-term cognitive impairment in survivors of critical illness. *Crit Care Med.* 2010;38:1513-1520.
78. Griffiths RD, Jones C. Delirium, cognitive dysfunction and posttraumatic stress disorder. *Curr Opin Anaesthesiol.* 2007;20:124-129.
79. Angeli F, Verdecchia P, Karthikeyan G, et al. Beta-blockers and risk of all-cause mortality in non-cardiac surgery. *Ther Adv Cardiovasc Dis.* 2010;4:109-118.
80. London MJ, Zaugg M, Schaub MC, et al. Perioperative beta-adrenergic receptor blockade: physiologic foundations and clinical controversies. *Anesthesiology.* 2004;100:170-175.
81. White CM, Talati R, Phung OJ, et al. Benefits and risks associated with beta-blocker prophylaxis in noncardiac surgery. *Am J Health Syst Pharm.* 2010;67:523-530.
82. Dennen P, Douglas IS, Anderson R. Acute kidney injury in the intensive care unit: an update and primer for the intensivist. *Crit Care Med.* 2010;38:261-275.
83. Carson JL. Morbidity risk assessment in the surgically anemic patient. *Am J Surg.* 1995;170:32S-36S.
84. Napolitano LM, Kurek S, Luchette FA, et al. Clinical practice guideline: red blood cell transfusion in adult trauma and critical care. *Crit Care Med.* 2009;37:3124-3157.
85. Taylor RW, Manganaro L, O'Brien J, et al. Impact of allogenic packed red blood cell transfusion on nosocomial infection rates in the critically ill patient. *Crit Care Med.* 2002;30:2249-2254.
86. Hebert PC, Wells G, Blajchman MA, et al. A Multicenter, Randomized, Controlled Clinical Trial of Transfusion Requirements in Critical Care. *N Engl J Med.* 1999;340:409-417.
87. Hebert PC, Yetisir E, Martin C, et al. Is a low transfusion threshold safe in critically ill patients with cardiovascular diseases? *Crit Care Med.* 2001;29:227-234.
88. Dungan KM, Braithwaite SS, Preiser JC. Stress hyperglycaemia. *Lancet.* 2009;373:1798-1807.
89. Egi M, Bellomo R, Stachowski E, et al. Variability of blood glucose concentration and short-term mortality in critically ill patients. *Anesthesiology.* 2006;105:244-252.
90. Umpierrez GE, Isaacs SD, Bazargan N, et al. Hyperglycemia: an independent marker of in-hospital mortality in patients with undiagnosed diabetes. *J Clin Endocrinol Metab.* 2002;87:978-982.
91. Van den BG, Wouters P, Weekers F, et al. Intensive insulin therapy in the critically ill patients. *N Engl J Med.* 2001;345:1359-1367.
92. Griesdale DE, de Souza RJ, van Dam RM, et al. Intensive insulin therapy and mortality among critically ill patients: a meta-analysis including NICE-SUGAR study data. *CMAJ.* 2009;180:821-827.
93. Dortch MJ, Mowery NT, Ozdas A, et al. A computerized insulin infusion titration protocol improves glucose control with less hypoglycemia compared to a manual titration protocol in a trauma intensive care unit. *JPEN J Parenter Enteral Nutr.* 2008;32:18-27.
94. Dossett LA, Collier B, Donahue R, et al. Intensive insulin therapy in practice: can we do it? *JPEN J Parenter Enteral Nutr.* 2009;33:14-20.
95. Holzinger U, Warszawska J, Kitzberger R, et al. Real-time continuous glucose monitoring in critically ill patients: a prospective randomized trial. *Diabetes Care.* 2010;33:467-472.
96. Annane D, Sebille V, Charpentier C, et al. Effect of treatment with low doses of hydrocortisone and fludrocortisone on mortality in patients with septic shock. *JAMA.* 2002;288:862-871.
97. Minneci PC, Deans KJ, Eichacker PQ, et al. The effects of steroids during sepsis depend on dose and severity of illness: an updated meta-analysis. *Clin Microbiol Infect.* 2009;15:308-318.
98. McClave SA, Martindale RG, Vanek VW, et al. Guidelines for the Provision and Assessment of Nutrition Support Therapy in the Adult Critically Ill Patient: Society of Critical Care Medicine (SCCM) and American Society for Parenteral and Enteral Nutrition (A.S.P.E.N.). *JPEN J Parenter Enteral Nutr.* 2009;33:277-316.
99. Martindale RG, McClave SA, Vanek VW, et al. Guidelines for the provision and assessment of nutrition support therapy in the adult critically ill patient: Society of Critical Care Medicine and American Society for Parenteral and Enteral Nutrition: Executive Summary. *Crit Care Med.* 2009;37:1757-1761.
100. Fabian TC, Croce MA, Payne LW, et al. Duration of antibiotic therapy for penetrating abdominal trauma: a prospective trial. *Surgery.* 1992;112:788-794.
101. Kollef MH. Ventilator-associated pneumonia. A multivariate analysis. *JAMA.* 1993;270:1965-1970.
102. May AK, Fleming SB, Carpenter RO, et al. Influence of broad-spectrum antibiotic prophylaxis on intracranial pressure monitor infections and subsequent infectious complications in head-injured patients. *Surg Infect (Larchmt).* 2006;7:409-417.
103. Namias N, Harvill S, Ball S, et al. Cost and morbidity associated with antibiotic prophylaxis in the ICU. *J Am Coll Surg.* 1999;188:225-230.
104. Trouillet JL, Chastre J, Vuagnat A, et al. Ventilator-associated pneumonia caused by potentially drug-resistant bacteria. *Am J Respir Crit Care Med.* 1998;157:531-539.
105. Dellit TH, Owens RC, McGowan JE Jr, et al. Infectious Diseases Society of America and the Society for Healthcare Epidemiology of America guidelines for developing an institutional program to enhance antimicrobial stewardship. *Clin Infect Dis.* 2007;44:159-177.
106. Dortch M, Fleming S, Kauffmann R, et al. infection reduction strategies including antibiotic stewardship protocols in surgical and trauma intensive care units are associated with reduced resistant gram-negative healthcare-associated infections. *Surg Infect (Larchmt).* 2011;12:15-25.

CHAPTER 47 ■ ACUTE RESPIRATORY DYSFUNCTION

GIANA HYSTAD DAVIDSON AND EILEEN BULGER

The primary functions of the respiratory system are to adequately deliver oxygen from the external environment to meet the metabolic demands of tissues and eliminate the buildup of carbon dioxide. The acute care surgeon is faced with a number of injuries and acute illnesses that impair pulmonary function. This chapter focuses on acute respiratory dysfunction and the common conditions and treatment strategies important for the acute care surgeon.

PHYSIOLOGY OF RESPIRATION

The two main functions of the respiratory system are ventilation to eliminate carbon dioxide and oxygenation to deliver oxygen to the tissues. Efficiency of ventilation is achieved by matching ventilation to perfusion in the gas-exchange regions of the lung. Minute ventilation is calculated by multiplying the tidal volume by the respiratory rate and can be directly measured by collecting exhaled gas over a measured time. Higher minute ventilation represents greater carbon dioxide release. Normal minute ventilation volume is 5–8 L/minute for a 70 kg man. Increased cellular metabolism in response to injury results in increased CO_2 production, which must be matched by increased release from the lungs. Normally, a resting adult must eliminate 200 mL/kg/minute of CO_2. In the hypermetabolic state, CO_2 production increases to the range of 425 mL/kg/minute.[1] The minute ventilation required to maintain eucapnia rises concurrently from approximately 5 L/minute (resting rate) to 10 L/minute. This represents a 100% increase in the work of breathing required to meet metabolic demands under these circumstances.

Oxygenation is primarily dependent on binding to hemoglobin (Hb). Hb is composed of four polypeptide chains including two alpha and two beta chains totaling 146 amino acids. Each polypeptide contains an iron atom on the heme group that is capable of binding oxygen. For each gram of Hb, 1.39 mL of O_2 can be stored. Arterial O_2 content (CaO_2) is related to Hb concentration and Hb saturation (SaO_2) by the following equation[2]:

$$CaO_2 = [Hb] \times 1.36\ (mL\ O_2/gO_2) \times SaO_2 + 0.003\ mL \times PaO_2$$

The oxygen dissociation curve seen (Fig. 47.1) shows the percent saturation of Hb at various partial pressures of oxygen. As erythrocytes travel to areas with low oxygen saturation, the partial pressure of oxygen decreases leading to delivery of oxygen to tissue. Temperature, organic phosphates such as DPG and pH directly affect Hb affinity for oxygen and oxygen delivery.

Obstructive airway disease such as chronic obstructive pulmonary disease (COPD), asthma, chronic bronchitis, and emphysema decrease gas flow and therefore gas exchange. As a consequence, arterial partial pressure of O_2 drops (hypoxemia) and arterial partial pressure of CO_2 increases (hypercapnia). Interventions to improve the match between ventilation and pulmonary perfusion may be required. In the setting of acute respiratory failure secondary to acute respiratory distress syndrome (ARDS), pulmonary contusion, or severe pneumonia, hypoxia is the primary factor due to consolidation of the pulmonary parenchyma. In the setting of acute pulmonary embolism (PE), ventilation/perfusion (V/Q) mismatch is also enhanced secondary to disruption of perfusion to segments of lung tissue.

Basic features of respiratory dysfunction include dyspnea, hypoxia, and hypercarbia. There are a variety of medicine conditions leading to respiratory dysfunction, which is defined as a drop in PO_2 <60 mm Hg or a rise in PCO_2 >50 mm Hg. Table 47.1 is an overview of the four main mechanisms of respiratory dysfunction.

Hypoxemia

The rate and severity of hypoxia and hypercarbia affect the clinical and neurologic presentation of the patient. Patients may experience mild confusion and headache to loss of consciousness. Hypoxemia should always be considered a cause of altered mental status. Prolonged central nervous system hypoxia has the potential to lead to hypoxic–ischemic encephalopathy through neuronal death. Hypoxia may be secondary to airflow obstruction in conditions such as asthma or airspace flooding as seen in pneumonia, aspiration, or hemorrhage. Acute airflow obstruction can cause hypoxemia that is typically treatable with supplemental oxygen. However, conditions that result in airspace flooding typically require adjuvant therapies and are not reversible by additional oxygen alone. Pulmonary shunting occurs when the alveoli of the lung is perfused normally; however, there is ventilation failure to the perfused regions leading a change in the ventilation/perfusion ratio. In a healthy individual, the physiologic shunt is rarely over 4%.[3] Shunting is minimized by the reflexive constriction of pulmonary vasculature to hypoxia. In conditions such as pulmonary contusion, the shunt increases considerably and mechanical ventilation may be required. Therapy should always focus on treatment for the underlying cause of hypoxemia.

Ventilatory Failure

The etiology of hypocapnia and hypoxia are frequently different. With neurologic depression, the decrease in the drive to breathe reduces minute ventilation leading to increase $PaCO_2$. In patients who require a high minute ventilation to maintain a normal $PaCO_2$, there is often elevated CO_2, increased dead space, or a high degree of ventilated but poorly perfused alveoli.[4] This is a common etiology in our trauma and perioperative patients in combination with neurologic impairment.

Perioperative and Neurologic Impairment

The perioperative period is high risk for progression of respiratory dysfunction. Patients have a significant risk for atelectasis, which is the primary mechanism of perioperative respiratory

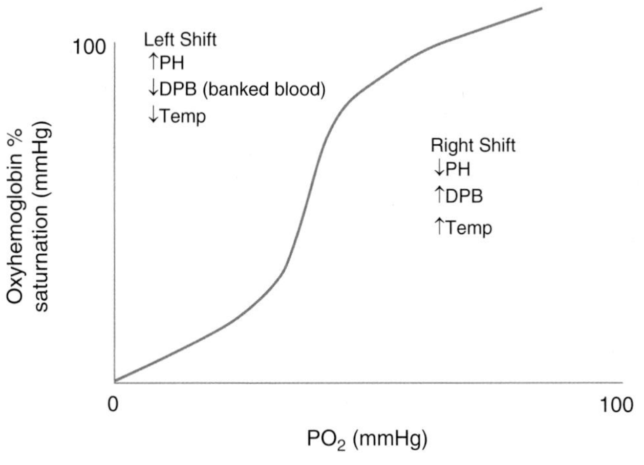

FIGURE 47.1. Oxygen dissociation curve.

dysfunction. Abnormal abdominal mechanics reduce the end-expired lung volume leading to progressive lung collapse in the dependent portions of the lung. The addition of narcotics or benzodiazepines can lead to a combination of ventilatory dysfunction leading to respiratory failure. Treatment of patients in the perioperative patients should focus on excellent bronchopulmonary hygiene to minimize atelectasis and clear secretions. This includes incentive spirometry, early ambulation, maintenance of euvolemia, and patient positioning. Attention to abdominal/thoracic pain and incisional pain is necessary and epidural anesthesia or transcutaneous electrical nerve stimulation should be considered for those individuals at high risk for pulmonary dysfunction including the obese, elderly, and patients with thoracic trauma. Lung collapse can be detected radiographically and on routine exam and should be treated aggressively with techniques for lung recruitment.

Shock

Patients with hypotension secondary to cardiogenic, hypovolemic, or septic shock often present with respiratory dysfunction. While there is no primary pulmonary mechanism, mechanical ventilation is often necessary. This allows for stabilization of gas exchange and minimizes cardiac steal until the underlying cause is identified and treated.

The mainstay of treating acute respiratory dysfunction is mechanical ventilatory support. Identification and treatment of the underlying cause is paramount. Prompt initiation of supportive ventilation during this time is key to preserving neurologic function and preventing permanent sequelae.

SPECIAL POPULATIONS

Children

The unique anatomy of children is important for both diagnosis and treatment of acute respiratory dysfunction. Children have a large head and tongue in proportion to the size of the oral cavity as well as prominent tonsils and adenoid tissue. Increased neck flexion from the prominent occipital bulge can lead to airway obstruction. Focus on proper head positioning including chin-lift and jaw-thrust is especially important in this population.[5] Equipment sizing is also imperative. Broselow tape and equipment of various sizes should be immediately available.

Neonates and infants are obligate nose breathers. Nasal obstruction can cause both increased work of breathing and

TABLE 47.1

MECHANISM OF RESPIRATORY DYSFUNCTION

	HYPOXEMIA	VENTILATORY FAILURE	PERIOPERATIVE	SHOCK
Mechanism	Intrapulmonary shunting	Alveolar hypoventilation	Atelectasis	Hypoperfusion
Etiology	Airspace obstruction	CNS depression, loss of neuromuscular coupling, Increased work of breathing/dead-space	Collapse of dependent portions of the lung	Cardiogenic shock Hypovolemic shock Sepsis
Clinical presentation	Hypoxemia often refractory to O_2 therapy	Hypercapnia with hypoxemia. Often corrects with O_2 therapy.	Hypoxemia, frequently tachypnea, May respond to O_2 therapy, maneuvers to improve lung collapse	Hypoxemia, hypotension, frequently tachypnea
Common manifestation	ARDS, cardiopulmonary edema, pneumonia, alveolar hemorrhage	Narcotic/benzodiazepine overdose, asthma, COPD, pulmonary fibrosis	Obesity, ascities, pain, anesthesia, fluid overload, smoking history, Secretions	MI, pulmonary hypertension, hemorrhage, tamponade, bacteremia
Treatment: mechanical ventilation if indicated.	Treat pneumonia, drain pleural effusions, minimize dead-space	Oxygen therapy, reverse sedation, bronchodilation, positioning and suctioning to clear secretions, chest tube, Pain control,	Positioning, suctioning secretions, 45 degree upright, pain control, drain ascities, re-expand atelectasis, stop smoking 6 wks preoperatively, maintain euvolemia	Correct underlying cause, treat sepsis, maintain euvolemia, appropriate management of electrolytes

respiratory distress. Nasal suctioning can help to improve respiratory status in these patients.[6] The larynx is well protected behind the mandibular arch and due to the relatively short neck; only a small portion of the trachea is unprotected above the manubrium. There is increased elasticity of the tracheobronchial tree. Laryngeal injuries are rare but often present with vague symptoms including hoarseness and subcutaneous emphysema, whereas tracheobronchial injuries often present with pneumothorax with or without a persistent airleak.[7]

Due to the increased plasticity of the chest wall in children, blunt injury to the chest is transmitted to deeper structures. Thirty-four percent of pediatric patients with pulmonary contusions do not show radiographic evidence of rib fractures.[8] Injuries such as pulmonary contusion, pneumothorax, hemothorax, blunt cardiac injury, and great vessel trauma can be found without rib fractures and a high index of suspicion is required for quick diagnosis.[6]

Elderly

A broad range of physiologic changes compromise the anatomic and functional integrity of the respiratory system in the elderly. This includes impaired elastic recoil of the lung and decreased dynamic compliance, both which increase airflow resistance leading to progressive airflow trapping. Decreased size and number of muscle fibers impairs the strength of intercostal and diaphram contraction. Individual response to hypoxemia and hypercapnia also wanes with age.[9–11] Reduced plasticity of the chest wall also increases the risk of the elderly for rib fractures and the associated complications.

Obesity

Excess adipose tissue in obese individuals reduces chest wall compliance, increases airway and pulmonary resistence, and increases work of breathing.[12] Obesity-hypoventilation syndrome (pickwickian syndrome) is found in one-third of individuals with a BMI of >35 (morbidly obese).[13] Nearly all have obstructive sleep apnea and >50% develop pulmonary hypertension.[14] Care must be taken to maintain adequate oxygen saturation (of >88%), especially in the setting of narcotics and/or benzodiazepines in trauma or postoperative patients. Continuous airway monitoring should be considered as diminished neuromuscular response to hypercapnia may quickly lead to hypoventilation, hypercapnia, acidemia, and respiratory distress.[14,15] The risk and rate of deterioration will be accelerated by intoxication, rib fractures, spine immobilization, and limited mobility in all patients, but perhaps to a greater degree in the obese and elderly population.

While the management of respriatory distress of obese patients is similar to normal weight individuals, bilevel positive airway pressure (BIPAP) should be considered in stable patients. However, BIPAP should never delay or be used instead of endotracheal intubation.[14]

Pregnancy

One of the principal causes of morbidity and mortality among pregnant women is acute respiratory dysfunction. Studies suggest that up to 30% of maternal deaths results from acute respiratory failure. Predominent causes include adult respiratory distress syndrome, thromboembolism, venous air embolism, beta-adrenergic tocolytic therapy, and amniotic fluid embolism.[16] The etiology of respiratory failure is similar in nonpregnant patients but the physiologic changes of pregnancy complicate standard management. In pregnancy, minute ventilation increases by 50% due to increased respiratory rate and tidal volume required to compensate for changes in maternal, fetal, and placental oxygen requirements and CO_2 production. There is a mild respiratory alkalosis in pregnancy with a reduction in $PaCO_2$ to 27–34 mm Hg (normal 35–45 mm Hg) and a compensatory reduction in bicarbonate to 18–21 mL/Eq/L (normal 22–30 mL/Eq/L) to maintain arterial blood pH of 7.4–7.45.[17,18] Oxygen consumption increases by up to 20%–30% in the third trimester and maternal cardiac output increases by 50% during the first two trimesters due to both an increased stroke volume and heart rate and a decrease in systemic vascular resistance. Fetal oxygenation depends on maternal cardiac output. Therefore, diuresis, positive end-expiratory pressure (PEEP), and vasopressor treatments, which may change the maternal blood flow and shunt blood away from the uterus, may put the fetus at risk.[19] As long as the maternal PaO_2 is maintained above 60 mm Hg and both cardiac output and fetal blood flow remains stable, the fetus will not be affected adversely.[17]

Standard treatment for respiratory dysfunction includes ventilatory, hemodynamic, and nutritional support. However, in pregnancy, maternal–fetal physiology and drug safety require additional consideration. Respiratory dysfunction in pregnancy results from hypoxic and hypercapnic–hypoxic physiologic causes. Hypoxic respiratory dysfunction is the predominant cause of pregnancy-related respiratory failure that includes ARDS, PE, venous air embolism and amniotic fluid embolism pneumonia, cardiogenic pulmonary edema, and pneumothorax. Hypercapnic–hypoxic respiratory dysfunction results from narcotics or sedatives, asthma, myasthenia gravis, and Guillain Barre.[17]

ARDS is a common final pathway of pulmonary injury and has a similar presentation and mortality rate for both gravid and nongravid patients. Outcomes are related to comorbidities, age, injury, and etiology and range in the literature from 30% to 70%.[16,20] Causes of ARDS unique to pregnancy include tocolytic-induced pulmonary edema, eclampsia, aspiration chorioamnionitis, amniotic fluid embolism, trophoblastic embolism, placental abruption, obstetric hemorrhage, endometritis, retained placental products, and septic abortion.[17] Pregnancy brings the additional challenge of evaluating for the presence and etiology of pulmonary edema and fetal monitoring. The use of a pulmonary artery catheter may aid in diagnosis and tailoring therapeutic decisions.[16] Fetal assessment is best with continuous fetal heart monitoring and sonographic biophysical profile done in consultation with obstetrics colleagues.[21] Hypovolemia of pregnancy, particularly during the 30th to 32nd week gestation, may also contribute to progression and poor outcomes of ARDS in this population.[16]

The mainstay of therapy in respiratory failure in the pregnant patient is maternal stabilization, fetal monitoring, treatment of underlying cause, prevention of aspiration, and low-tidal lung protective mechanical ventilation with the application of PEEP when indicated. As PEEP exceeds 10 cm H_2O, there is decreased venous return, decreased cardiac output, which worsens fetal oxygen delivery. The effect of hypercapnia on fetal blood flow is unknown.[17] Fluid restriction in pregnancy is controversial. While it improves oxygenation, fluid restriction worsens cardiac output and organ perfusion.[17]

COMMON CAUSES OF ACUTE RESPIRATORY DYSFUNCTION

Acute Respiratory Distress Syndrome

ARDS is characterized by dysfunction in respiratory mechanics and gas exchange. The mortality rate ranges from 40% to 50%.[22] The incidence in the United States is approximately

190,000 cases per year affecting a wide distribution of both medical and surgical patients and is associated with >74,000 deaths per year.[23] In 1994, the American-European Consensus Committee recommended seperating patients with lung disease into two groups, those with acute lung injury (ALI) and those with more severe hypoxia, ARDS. Criteria include: acute onset, bilateral infiltrates on chest radiograph, pulmonary artery wedge pressure <18 mm Hg or the absence of left atrial hypertension. ALI is considered to be present if the PaO_2:FiO_2 ratio is <300, whereas ARDS requires a PaO_2:FiO_2 ratio to be <200.[24]

Several studies have sought to improve outcome following ARDS. The only study that has demonstrated a major improvement in outcome utilized a lung-protective ventilation strategy with lower than usual tidal volumes.[20] The pathogenesis of ALI and ARDS in surgical patients is variable. These most commonly include sepsis, trauma, aspiration, near drowning, blood transfusion, pulmonary contusion, and inhalation injury.[25] Typically, an initial inflammatory stage with neutrophil infiltration and massive capillary leak is then followed by a fibroproliferative phase, drastically changing the elasticity of the lung.[24,25]

The clinical course of ARDS is variable with patients recovering within weeks to months of prolonged ventilation. Rather than respiratory failure itself, it is prolonged ventilation with superimposed infection and multisystem organ failure that ultimately leads to death. Treatment strategies include ventilatory support to minimize iatrogenic injury with a goal to avoid progression of pulmonary damage and modulation of inflammatory response through pharmocologic options.[25] Studies of treatment options have only shown a mortality benefit for patients with ARDS with low-tidal ventilation.[26] The Acute Respiratory Distress Syndrome network (ARDSnet) trial randomized patients to receive ventilatory support with 6 mL/kg versus 12 mL/kg based on predicted body weight. Allowing for hypercapnia, there is a goal plateau pressure of <30 cm H_2O. The low tidal volume group (6 mL/kg) had a significantly lower mortality rate (31% vs. 40%), and increased number of ventilator-free days.[20]

Pneumothoraces

A breach in the parietal or visceral pleural can result in air in the pleural space (pneumothorax). Diagnosis of small pneumothoraces is most commonly made by chest radiograph; however, the presence of a tension pneumothorax should be evident on physical exam. A small separation of space may translate into a large pneumothorax, particularly depending on the position of the patient during chest radiograph. A tension pneumothorax is created when a large amount of intrapleural air causes a shift in the mediastinum toward the contralateral lung. Stab or gunshot wounds may create a sucking chest wound. Ventilation and venous return of blood to the heart may be compromised resulting in hypotension that can lead to cardiovascular collapse. Open and tension pneumothoraces should be diagnosed clinically based on physical exam including decreased breath sounds and hypotension and treated as a surgical emergency.

Pneumothoraces are classically classified as spontaneous or acquired. Typically, spontaneous pneumothoraces are secondary to rupture of small blebs due to increased transpulmonary pressure. In addition to connective tissue disorders, common causes of spontaneous pneumothorax are rupture of subpleural blebs after coughing, blunt chest trauma, rapid fall in atmospheric pressure, rapid decompression (seen in scuba diving), and high altitude with flying. Presentation ranges from asymptomatic to pleuritic chest pain, decreased breath sounds, and dyspnea, and may progress to hypotension, tachycardia, diaphoresis, and cyanosis, and deviation of trachea if a pneumothorax progresses to a tension pneumothorax.[27]

Pneumothoraces are the most common intrathoracic blunt chest injury.[28] Delay in diagnosis or missed pneumothorax is a significant cause of preventable death.[29] The energency department use of CT scanning and ultrasound along with supine chest radiographs may contribute to the delay in diagnosis of occult pneumothoraces. The incidence of the occult pneumothorax varies in the literature. In children with blunt trauma, the incidence of undiagnosed pneumothorax is 3.7% on abdominal CT.[30] Intubated trauma patients with an average injury severity score (ISS) of 30 had an incidence of missed initial pneumothorax as high as 64%.[31] Ball et al.[32] demonstrated that at one trauma center, 15% of patients with an ISS of >11 had an occult pneumothorax on abdominal CT with 55% not detected by initial chest radiograph. There is no general consensus for treatment of the occult pneumothorax as progression is not well understood. Generally, in asymptomatic patients without mechanical ventilation, observation and monitoring for increasing size is safe and effective. Patients with positive-pressure ventilation have a higher likelihood for development of a tension pneumothorax and chest tube placement should be considered as these patients often have a low cardiopulmonary reserve.[33]

Hemothorax

Blood in the pleural space is typically secondary to trauma, iatrogenic injury, neoplasms, pulmonary infarction, or infections.[27] One-third of all thoracic traumas requires tube thoracostomy for hemothorax.[28] Effective drainage can frequently be done with a large (36 French) chest tube. Early evacuation of retained hemothorax has been shown to improve clinical outcomes.[34] A small number of patients will require thoracotomy for complete evacuation. The pleura is able to resorb a significant amount of fluid, however, it is unclear what quantity may be assumed to resolve spontaneously in adults. Retained clot is the primary predisposing risk factor in the development of posttraumatic empyema. Furthermore, in trauma patients there is significant upregulation of inflammatory cytokines causing recruitment of neutrophils to the site of injury and thickening of the pleura. This pleura thickening reduces the likelihood of resolution of the hemothorax.[35] The parietal peel may lead to chronic lung entrapement and recurrent pneumonia. If significant thrombus has formed following trauma, the patient is at risk for retained hemothorax and development of secondary infection may lead to empyema. Additionally, host immune system may be impaired by hypotension and blood transfusions. The reported prevalence of posttraumatic empyema is 5%–10%.[36] Penetrating chest injuries are often clean wounds. However, secondary contamination of the pleura from injuries to the gastrointestinal tract, devitalized tissue from chest wall trauma, unsterile chest tube placement or other foreign body, trapped lung or underlying pneumonia may lead to empyema. *Staphylococcus aureus* is the primary causative organism in posttraumatic empyema.[37,38]

Chest Wall Trauma

Blunt chest trauma at a regional trauma center has a reported incidence of 10% among all trauma patients.[39] Pulmonary contusion is reported in 25% of patients with blunt chest trauma.[40] Pathophysiology of blunt chest trauma includes increased alveolocapillary permeability, increased intrapulmonary shunting, pulmonary edema, ventilation–perfusion mismatching, and loss of compliance.[41] Clinically, presentation depends on degree of involvement, additional injuries, and comorbid conditions. Symptoms range from increased work of breathing to acute respiratory decompensation.[41] Complications following injury, including respiratory failure, ARDS, and pneumonia, are common and lead to a reported mortality rate between 9% and 50%, depending on associated injuries.[42,43] Flail chest and pulmonary contusion are associated with a mortality rate of nearly double either alone.[42]

Imaging modalities to evaluate blunt chest trauma include chest radiography and thoracic CT. In evaluating pediatric patients with a pulmonary contusion, Wylie et al. found that 15% of patients had an initial chest x-ray (CXR) that did not identify the lung contusion.[44] These results were similar to adult studies that show progression of radiographic findings over time. Thoracic CT has been found to be more sensitive for pulmonary contusion than CXR alone.[45] Typically, chest CT has been the gold standard for detection of pulmonary contusion with 100% sensitivity. Chest radiography sensitivity for pulmonary contusion on initial exam is typically reported at approximately 40%.[46] Despite decreased sensitivity, CXR is still the primary modality for initial evaluation in the unstable patient.

There is an inconsistent correlation between contused lung volume and severity of clinical disease. In 2009, Hamrick et al. attempted to quantify lung volume involved in pulmonary contusions using computerized topography. They found that patients with >20% of total contused lung volume frequently required mechanical ventilation within 48 hours of injury.[47] Rib fractures, patient age, inflammation, aspiration, sepsis, and possibly surfactant dysfunction all affect progression and severity of pulmonary dysfuntion with lung contusion.[48]

There is controversy surrounding fluid management in the treatment of patients with pulmonary contusions. Excessive crystalloid resuscitation has been associated with worsening hypoxia. However, prospective studies have failed prove causation.[49,50] Euvolemia is recommended with crystalloids and blood products as indicated for other injuries. The use of steroids has been shown to be of no benefit and may impair bacterial clearance within the pulmonary tissue.[49,51]

Associated injuries are largely predictive of morbidity and mortality in patients with blunt chest trauma. Rib fractures are clinically important as a marker for serious intrathoracic and abdominal injury. They are a source of significant pain and an independent predictor for respiratory failure, particularly in the elderly. The presence of three or more rib fractures is associated with increased intensive care and hospital stay and increased mortality.[52] In a retrospective study of patients over 65 years old with rib fractures, 31% of patients with rib fractures develop nosocomal pneumonia and 22% died.[53,54] Adequate analgesia and pulmonary hygiene are the mainstays of therapy for patients with multiple rib fractures. The pain associated with rib fractures impairs ventilatory function leading to poor outcomes. Bulger et al. demonstarted that when epidural anesthesia was used in adult patients with greater than three rib fractues, there was a sixfold decrease in the risk of pneumonia and twofold decrease in time on a ventilator. There was no difference demonstrated in mortality in this study.[54]

Blunt chest trauma affects a substantial portion of trauma patients and can result in considerable morbidity. Elderly patients are at hightened risk for decompensation and may require close monitoring. Mainstays of therapy include mechanical ventilation when indicated, pain control, and aggressive pulmonary toilet.

Laryngotracheal Trauma

Laryngotracheal trauma occurs in <1% of all trauma patients but has a mortality rate of 20%–40%.[55–57] The most commonly reported mechanism is blunt force trauma to the cervical region. This mechanism may also lead to damage to the esophogus, cervical spine, closed head and vascular injuries. The most immediate and fundamental treatment is securing the airway. Schaefer recommended tracheostomy with local anesthesia to avoid endotracheal intubation.[58] However, others argue that endotracheal intubation can be done safely with experienced personnel under direct visualization with a small endotracheal tube.[54,59] After securing the airway, a high index of suspicion should be maintained to rule out additional injuries. Larrngoscopy may be helpful in identifying edema, hematoma, laceration to thyroid cartilage, or laynx.[57] CT scan may be helpful in identifying additional injuries including fractures. After initial exam and radiography, consideration should be given to contrast swallow studies and esophagogastroduodenoscopy to rule out esophageal injury.[58]

Pulmonary Embolism

An estimated 250,000 deaths from PE occur in the United States per year.[60] Mortality is typically secondary to right ventricular failure.[61] The risk for thrombosis in surgical patients is greatest at the time of injury and during the perioperative phase.[62–64] In patients without prophylaxis against venous thromboembolic disease (VTE), deep vein thrombosis is reported in as many as 30% with a fatality rate of 1%.[59] Due to the significant mortality rate as well as the risk of respiratory compromise from PE, prevention of VTE is the mainstay of therapy.[65] We will focus on clinical presentation of respiratory dysfunction associated with PE as Chapter 57 provides more details on thromboembolic disease.

Diagnosis of PE requires suspicion based on risk factors, nonspecific signs and symptoms. The lack of specificity of clinical presentation leads to additional testing for confirmatory diagnosis. PE should be considered for any unexplained dyspnea or hypoxia. Common symptoms of PE include anxiety and pleuritic chest pain. Tachypnea and tachycardia are the most common clinical signs of PE.[60] Electrocardiographic (ECG) abnormalities include T-wave changes, ST segment abnormalities, and/or axis deviation, and have been demonstrated in 87% of patients with a diagnosed PE without underlying cardiac disease.[66] The low specificity of ECG change was confirmed in the prospective investigation of pulmonary embolism diagnosis (PIOPED) study.[67] Young patients with good functional pulmonary reserve may have a normal PaO_2. However, especially in the elderly, hypoxemia is commonly present. In patients over age 40, the PaO_2 has been found to be >80 mm Hg in 3% of patients while in those younger than age 40, 29% of patients with proven PE had a PaO_2 over 80 mm Hg.[68] The alveolar–arterial oxygen tension difference was >20 mm Hg in 86% of patients with diagnosed PE in the PIOPED study.[66] While helpful in developing the clinical picture, PaO_2 remains nonspecific and can be normal in a patient with normal cardiopulmonary reserve.

Chest radiography is often the appropriate first step in the work up for acute respiratory dysfunction. In the setting of acute respiratory dysfunction, a normal chest radiograph is strongly suggestive of PE. The most common radiograph findings for PE are both nonspecific and common in postoperative and trauma patients including atelectasis, pleural effusion, elevated hemidiaphragm, and pulmonary infiltrates.[69] Spiral CT remains the most common method for diagnosis of PE. Limitations include poor peripheral visualization and false positive results due to pulmonary lymph nodes.[60] Reliability of CT for diagnosis varies in the literature. Using pulmonary angiography as the gold standard gave a positive predictive value range of 60%–89% and negative predictive value of approximately 80% for spiral CT.[70] This indicates that interpretation by the radiologist plays a large role in diagnostic accuracy. Other studies have shown a 95% sensitivity and specificity of spiral CT scan for diagnosis of PE.[71,72] In patients with documented PE, >80% have right ventricular size or function abnormalities on echocardiography suggesting PE.[73,74] These are nonspecific findings and can be found in other causes of right heart dysfunction including COPD exacerbations.

If the patient has a low bleeding risk and suspicion is high, it is reasonable to start anticoagulation therapy during diagnostic testing. Patients presenting with hemodynamic compromise secondary to PE may be candidates for thrombolytic therapy. Indications include arterial hypotension (systolic blood pressure (SBP) <90 mm Hg or a decrease of >40 mm Hg), cardiogenic shock, circulatory collapse, right ventricular dilation or pulmonary hypertension, arterial–alveolar O_2 gradient of >50 mm Hg.[60] Systemic thrombolytic therapy is frequently contraindicated in postsurgical and trauma patients.

It is important to consider prevention of subsequent PE in the patient who has a history of PE. Inferior vena cava (IVC) filters are a therapeutic option in patients with VTE. Indications IVC filter placement include patients who have deep venous thrombosis (DVT) and contraindications to anticoagulation or in patients who have the risk of hemorrhage while anticoagulated.[75] In addition, the use of prophylactic IVC filters in high-risk patients has been evaluated in small studies. Thirty-nine patients at two institutions undergoing major spinal reconstruction had permanent IVC filters placed preoperatively. There were no PEs diagnosed in patients who had IVC filter placed compared to 12% of patients who developed PE in a matched cohort control group at the same institutions.[76] Trauma patients with injuries or comorbidities indicating high risk for DVT and PE may be candidates for prophylactic IVC filter placement. Those at highest risk include: severe head injury, spinal cord injuries with neurologic deficit, pelvic, and long bone fractures.[77] Prophylactic IVC filters have been increasingly placed in the trauma population over the past decade with minimal complications.[74] In evaluating placement of permanent filters placed for blunt trauma injuries, Wojcik et al. reported a series (N = 105) of patients who were treated with permanent IVC filters for DVT diagnosis and prophylaxis with a mean follow up of 29 months. They found no PEs in the patients with filters placed and no clinically identifiable complications related to insertion of the vena cava filters. In follow-up, they reported minimal migration one filter, one vena cava occlusion, 11 patients experienced lower extremity edema following discharge, and 28 of the 64 patients with prophylactic IVC filters developed a DVT following placement.[78] In an additional study using Greenfield filters placed within 48 hours of trauma, PE-related mortality decreased from 17% to 2.5%, with only 2 of 40 patients developing substantial venous stasis of the lower extremities.[79] Additional studies support prophylactic IVC filter placement in trauma patients at high risk for DVT and PE. However, above-mentioned studies are small and additional studies are needed to further elucidate clear populations that will benefit from prophylactic filter placement, long-term complications, and adequacy of filter removal. Modern IVC filters are frequently removable once the period of high thrombotic risk has passed; however, a recent study reported that poor follow-up of injured patients can lead to low retrieval rates.[80]

Fat Embolism

Fat embolism is associated most commonly with trauma and orthopedic fractures, particularity long bone fractures. Fat embolism is defined as the presence of fat droplets within the peripheral and lung microcirculation.[81] Fat embolism syndrome (FES) is a manifestation of fat embolism that occurs in the presence of fat in the pulmonary vasculature. FES presents with clinical signs typically 12–72 hours following trauma with symptoms of progressive respiratory failure with hypoxemia, petechial rash, and altered mental status variably present.[82] Additional clinical features include tachycardia, fever, retinal changes, jaundice, renal involvement (anuria or oliguria), fat in the urine or sputum, unexplained drop in Hb or platelets, and fat macroglobulinemia.[80] FES has a heterogeneous pattern of presentation. There is no confirmatory test and there is ongoing debate on the precise diagnostic criteria making diagnosis and accurate incidence rates difficult. FES is a diagnosis of exclusion based on clinical characteristics and risk factors. A 10-year review at a level-one trauma center identified 27 patients with clinically apparent FES from 1985 to 1995. This was 0.9% of all long-bone fractures treated during this time. These patients had a mean ISS of 9.5 and 44% required mechanical ventilation.[83] Treatment is primarily supportive and alternative causes for respiratory dysfunction should be excluded. Chest radiograph in patients with FES often have abnormalities. Classically, these include diffuse, bilateral interstitial and alveolar densities. However, findings are nonspecific and there is a lag time related to the clinical symptoms.[81] Intraoperative pulmonary fat embolism can be identified using transesophogeal echocardiography with a sensitivity of 80% and a specificity of 100% in patients with pulmonary fat embolism large enough to produce hemodynamic instability.[84] Treatment for FES is supportive.[83] Prophylactic strategies including early stabilization of fractures involving the pelvis or long bones have been shown to result in a decrease in the incidence of FES.[85] Early rigid fixation of fractures decreases the recurrent bouts of fat embolism.[81]

Inhalation Injuries

Inhalation injuries from smoke affect between 5% and 35% of hospitalized burn patients and lead to increased morbidity and mortality.[86] The incidence of respiratory dysfunction is high following inhalation injury. Furthermore, complications including pneumonia, hypoxemia, and prolonged ventilation are common.[84,87] Mortality increases by 20% in burn patients with inhalation injury compared to those without an inhalation component and complications such as pneumonia increase mortality by 60%.[88] There are various unreliable clinical signs of inhalation injury.[89,90] Bronchoscopy may diagnose mucosal erythema, airway edema, erosions, necrosis, and soot. Elevated carboxyhemoglobin (COHb) concentration is a poor marker of inhalation injury because the half-life of COHb with 100% oxygen therapy is 30–40 minutes. Smokers and urban residents exposed to significant pollution will have a COHb concentration elevated to 10% and COHb concentrations are not an accurate predictor of mortality.[91–93] A PaO_2/FIO_2 ratio of <300 after resuscitation in children with inhalation injury is considered predictive of mortality in children.[89] The PaO_2/FIO_2 ratio was lower in patients who received more fluids.[91] The goal of fluid resuscitation should be to achieve euvolemia.

THORACOSTOMY TUBE PLACEMENT

Potential complications of chest tube placement can be avoided by vigilant monitoring and strict adherence to sterility. Morbidity from chest tube placement includes vascular injury, improper positioning of the tube leading to both injury and poor function, inadvertent tube removal, increased length of hospital stay, undrained pneumothorax and/or hemothorax, empyema, and pneumonia. Complications are reported in up to 21% of cases. The risk of complication varies greatly by training of provider placing the thoracostomy tube. These complication rates from one level-one trauma center included 6% by surgeon, 13% by emergency physician, and 38% prior to transfer to the trauma center.[94]

Most patients with significant pneumothoraces (>30%) require placement of a closed-chest catheter for acceptable pulmonary re-expansion. This catheter then can be placed either to underwater suction drainage or to a Heimlich (one-way) valve. If a Heimlich valve fails to re-expand the lung fully or if the patient has additional injuries, admission to hospital and chest tube suction drainage is recommended. Unless contraindication exists, chest tubes should be placed in the midaxillary line at the level of the fifth intercostal space (nipple line). In women, the breast tissue should be retracted medially and avoided in the dissection to the chest wall. Placement of the thoracostomy tube with the use of blunt clamp dissection avoids the dangers of trocar insertion. Following resolution of any air leak and pneumothorax on upright chest radiograph, the tube may be taken off suction (water seal) and removed if the lung remains fully inflated.

The routine administration of systemic antibiotics for chest tube placement has remained controversial in the trauma literature. The risk of infectious complications, most commonly pneumonia and empyema, is reported between 2% and 25%.[95,96] When antibiotics are given prophylactically, they should be directed toward the most common organisms including gram-positive cocci and *Haemophilus*. There are a number of studies that show favorable effects of prophylactic antibiotics on empyema and pneumonia prevention and several that show no benefit. The Eastern Association for the Surgery of Trauma (EAST) Practice Management Guidelines Work Group concluded that there was insufficient data available to recommend routine use of presumptive antibiotics in the management of tube thoracostomy for traumatic hemopneumothorax.[97]

SUMMARY

Acute respiratory dysfunction has a broad etiology and clinical manifestations. However, treatment is straightforward with initial management always including airway management and consideration of mechanical ventilation. The etiology should then be elucidated and treated appropriately. Prevention of progression of respiratory dysfunction to respiratory failure is paramount in the care of the surgical patient.

- Trauma patients are at significant risk for infectious complications and development of ARDS.
- Goal of fluid management is euvolemia.
- Evidence shows that incomplete drainage of hemothorax is an important risk factor in empyema development. Prophylactic antibiotic therapy remains controversial.
- Low tidal ventilation with permissive hypercapnia is recommended for patients with ALI/ARDS.
- All staff should have training on pulmonary hygiene including suctioning, elevation of the head of bed, incentive spirometry, and early ambulation.
- DVT prophylaxis, IVC filters, and early fracture fixations are important for decreasing the incidence of PE.

References

1. Uehara M, Plank LD, Hill GL. Components of energy expenditure in patients with severe sepsis and major trauma: a basis for clinic care. *Crit Care Med.* 1999;7:1295-1302.
2. Hlastala MP, Berger A. *Physiology of Respiration.* New York, NY: Oxford University Press, Inc; 2001.
3. Garay S, Kamelar D. Pathophysiology of trauma-associated respiratory failure. In: Hood RM, Boyd AD, Culliford AT, eds. *Thoracic Trauma.* Philadelphia, PA: Saunders; 1989:328-332.
4. Wood L. The pathophysiology and differential diagnosis of acute respiratory failure. In: Schmidt G, Hall JB, eds. *Principles of Critical Care.* 3rd ed. New York, NY: McGraw-Hill; 2005:465-479.
5. Holm-Knudsen RJ, Rasmussen L. Paediatric airway management: basic aspects. *Acta Anaesthesiol Scand.* 2009;53(1):1-9.
6. Atkinson C, Bowman A. Pediatric airway differences. *J Trauma Nurs.* 2003;10:118-122.
7. Granholm T, Farmer DL. The surgical airway. *Respir Care Clin N Am.* 2001;7(1):13-23.
8. Roux P, Fisher R. Chest injuries in children: an analysis of 100 cases of blunt chest trauma from motor vehicle accidents. *J Pediatr Surg.* 1992;27:551-555.
9. Chan ED, Welsh C. Geriatric respiratory medicine. *Chest.* 1998;114:1704-1733.
10. Janssens JP, Pache JC, Nicod JP. Physiological changes in respiratory function associated with ageing. *Eur Respir J.* 1999;13:197-205.
11. Britto RR, Zampa CC, Oliveira TA, et al. Effects of the aging process on respiratory function. *Gerontology.* 2009;55:505-510.
12. Jensen D, Ofir D, O'Donnell D. Effects of pregnancy, obesity and aging on the intensity of perceived breathlessness during exercise in healthy humans. *Respir Physiol Neurobiol.* 2009;167:87-100.
13. Nowbar S, Burkart K. Obesity-associated hypoventilation in hospitalized patients: prevalence, effects, and outcome. *Am J Med.* 2004;116:1-7.
14. Nelson JA, Loredo JS, Acosta JA. The obesity-hypoventilation syndrome and respiratory failure in the acute trauma patient. *J Emerg Med.* 2011;40:e67-e69.
15. Redolfi S, Corda L, La Piana G, et al. Long-term non-invasive ventilation increases chemosensitivity and leptin in obesity-hypoventilation syndrome. *Respir Med.* 2007;101:1191-1195.
16. Deblieux P, Summer W. Acute respiratory failure in pregnancy. *Clin Obstet Gynecol.* 1996;39:143-152.
17. Bandi VD, Munnur U, Matthay MA. Acute lung injury and acute respiratory distress syndrome in pregnancy. *Crit Care Clin.* 2004;20:557-607.
18. Crapo R. Normal cardiopulmonary physiology during pregnancy. *Clin Obstet Gynecol.* 1996;39:3-16.
19. Eisenach JC. Uteroplacental blood flow. In: Chestnut DH, ed. *Obstetric Anesthesia: Principles and Practice.* St. Louis, MO: Mosby-Year Book, Inc; 1994:43-56.
20. Ventilation with lower tidal volumes as compared with traditional tidal volumes for acute lung injury and the acute respiratory distress syndrome. The Acute Respiratory Distress Syndrome Network. *N Engl J Med.* 2000;342(18):1301-1308.
21. Manning F. Fetal biophysical profile: a critical appraisal. *Clin Obstet Gynecol.* 2002;45(4):975-985.
22. Doyle RL, Szaflarski NK. Identification of patients with acute lung injury: predictors of mortality. *Am J Respir Crit Care Med.* 1995;152:1818-1824.
23. Rubenfeld GD, Caldwell E, Peabody E, et al. Incidence and outcomes of acute lung injury. *N Engl J Med.* 2005;353(16):1685-1693.
24. Bernard GR, Artigas1 A, Brigham1 KL, et al. Report of the American-European consensus conference on ARDS: definitions, mechanisms, relevant outcomes and clinical trial coordination.The Consensus Committee. *Intensive Care Med.* 1994;20:225-232.
25. Bulger EM, Jurkovich GJ, Gentilello LM, et al. Current clinical options for the treatment and management of acute respiratory distress syndrome. *J Trauma Inj Infect Crit Care.* 2000;48:562-572.
26. Tsushima K, King LS, Aggarwal NR, et al. Acute lung injury review. *Intern Med.* 2009;48:621-630.
27. Theodore PR,Jablons DM. Thoracic wall, pleura, mediastinum, & lung. In: Doherty GM, ed. *CURRENT Diagnosis & Treatment: Surgery.* 13th ed. New York, NY: The McGraw-Hill Companies, Inc. 2010.
28. Richardson J, Miller F, Carrillo E, et al. Complex thoracic injuries. *Surg Clin North Am.* 1996;76:725-748.
29. Di Bartolomeo S, Sanson G, et al. A population-based study on pneumothorax in severely traumatized patients. *J Trauma.* 2001;51:677-682.
30. Holmes JF, Brant W, Bogren H, et al. Prevalence and importance of pneumothoraces visualized on abdominal computed tomographic scan in children with blunt trauma. *J Trauma.* 2001;50:516-520.
31. Guerrero-Lopez F, Vázquez-Mata G, Alcázar-Romero PP, et al. Evaluation of the utility of computed tomography in the initial assessment of the critical care patient with chest trauma. *Crit Care Med.* 2000;28:1370-1375.
32. Ball CB, Kirkpatrick A, Laupland KB, et al. Incidence, risk factors, and outcomes for occult pneumothoraces in victims of major trauma. *J Trauma.* 2005;59:917-925.
33. Kollef MH. Risk factors for the misdiagnosis of pneumothorax in the intensive care unit. *Crit Care Med.* 1991;19:906-910.
34. Morrison CA, Lee T, Wall M. Use of a trauma service clinical pathway to improve patient outcomes for retained traumatic hemothorax. *World J Surg.* 2009;33:1851-1856.
35. Livingston DH, Hauser C. Chest wall and lung. In: Mattox K, Feliciano DV, eds. *Trauma.* 6th ed. New York: McGraw-Hill; 2008:525-552.
36. Coselli JS, Mattox KL, Beall AC. Reevaluation of early evacuation of clotted hemothorax. *Am J Surg.* 1984;148(6):786-790.
37. Caplan ES, Hoyt N. Empyema occurring in the multiply traumatized patient. *J Trauma.* 1984;24:785-789.

38. Hoth JJ, Burch P, et al. Pathogenesis of posttraumatic empyema: the impact of pneumonia on pleural space infections. *Surg Infect.* 2003;4:29-35.
39. Ziegler DW, Agarwal N. The morbidity and mortality of rib fractures. *J Trauma.* 1994;37:975-979.
40. LoCicero J III, Mattox K. Epidemiology of chest trauma. *Surg Clin North Am.* 1998;69:15-19.
41. Cohn SM, Zieg P. Experimental pulmonary contusion: review of the literature and description of a new porcine model. *J Trauma.* 1996;41:565-571.
42. Clark GC, Schecter WP, Trunkey DD. Variables affecting outcome in blunt chesl trauma: flail chest vs pulmonary contusion. *J Trauma.* 1988;28:298-304.
43. Demirhana R, et al. Comprehensive analysis of 4205 patients with chest trauma: a 10-year experience. *Interact CardioVasc Thorac Surg.* 2009;9: 450-453.
44. Wylie J, Morrison G, et al. Lung contusion in children—early computed tomography versus radiography. *Pediatr Crit Care Med.* 2009;10(6): 643-647.
45. Schild HH, Strunk H, et al. Pulmonary contusion: CT vs plain radiographs. *J Comput Assist Tomogr.* 1989;13:417-420.
46. McGonigal MD, Schwab CW, Kauder DR, et al. Supplemental emergent chest computed tomography in the management of blunt torso trauma. *J Trauma.* 1990;30:1431-1434.
47. Hamrick MC, Duhn R, et al. Critical evaluation of pulmonary contusion in the early post-traumatic period: risk of assisted ventilation. *Am Surg.* 2009;75:1054-1058.
48. Raghavendran K, Notter R, et al. Lung contusion: inflammatory mechanisms and interaction with other injuries. *Shock.* 2009;32:122-130.
49. Bongard FS, Lewis F. Crystalloid resuscitation of patients with pulmonary contusion. *Am J Surg.* 1984;148(1):145-151.
50. Johnson JA, Cogbill T, Winga E. Determinants of outcome after pulmonary contusion. *J Trauma.* 1986;26(8):695-697.
51. Wanek S, Mayberry J. Blunt thoracic trauma: flail chest, pulmonary contusion, and blast injury. *Crit Care Clin.* 2004;20:71-81.
52. Lee RB, Bass S, et al. Three or more rib fractures as an indicator for transfer to a Level I trauma center: a population-based study. *J Trauma.* 1990;30:689-694.
53. Bulger EM, Arneson MA, Mock CN, et al. Rib fractures in the elderly. *J Trauma.* 2000;48:1040-1046.
54. Bulger EM, Edwards T, et al. Epidural analgesia improves outcome after multiple rib fractures. *Surgery.* 2004;136:426-430.
55. Gussack GS, Jurkovich G, Luterman A. Laryngotracheal trauma: a protocol approach to a rare injury. *Laryngoscope.* 1986;96:660-665.
56. Edwards WH Jr, Morris J, et al. Airway injuries. The first priority in trauma. *Am Surg.* 1987;53:192-197.
57. Lambert GE Jr, McMurry G. Laryngotracheal trauma: recognition and management. *JACEP.* 1976;5:883-887.
58. Schaefer S. The acute management of external laryngeal trauma. A 27-year experience. *Arch Otolaryngol Head Neck Surg.* 1992;l18:598-604.
59. Bhojani RA, Rosenbaum D, et al. Contemporary assessment of laryngotracheal trauma. *J Thorac Cardiovasc Surg.* 2005;130:426-432.
60. Qadan M, Tyson M, et al. Venous thromboembolism in elective operations: balancing the choices. *Surgery.* 2008;144:654-661.
61. Tapson VF, Carroll BA, Davidson BL, et al. The diagnostic approach to acute venous thromboembolism: clinical practice guideline. *Am J Respir Crit Care Med.* 1999;160:1043-1066.
62. Hitos K, Cannon M, et al. Effect of leg exercises on popliteal venous blood flow during prolonged immobility of seated subjects: implications for prevention of travel-related deep vein thrombosis. *J Thromb Haemost.* 2007;5(9):1890-1895.
63. Bajzar L, Chan A, et al. Thrombosis in children with malignancy. *Curr Opin Pediatr.* 2006;18:1-9.
64. Barrett J, Hamilton W. Malignancy and deep vein thrombosis. *Br J Gen Pract.* 2006;56:886.
65. Eppsteiner RW, Shin JJ, Johnson J, et al.Mechanical compression versus subcutaneous heparin therapy in postoperative and posttrauma patients: a systematic review and meta-analysis. *World J Surg.* 2010;34(1):10-9.
66. The urokinase pulmonary embolism trial: a national cooperative study. *Circulation.* 1973;47(2 suppl):II1-108.
67. Investigators P. Value of the ventilation-perfusion scan in acute pulmonary embolism: results of the Prospective Investigation of Pulmonary Embolism Diagnosis (PIOPED). 1990;263(20):2753-2759.
68. Green R, Meyer T, Dunn M, et al. Pulmonary embolism in younger adults. *Chest.* 1992;101:1507-1511.
69. Stein PD, Terrin ML, et al. Clinical, laboratory, roentgenographic, and electrocardiographic findings in patients with acute pulmonary embolism and no pre-existing cardiac or pulmonary disease. *Chest.* 1991;100(3):598-603.
70. Drucker EA, Rivitz SM, et al. Acute pulmonary embolism: assessment of helical CT for diagnosis. *Radiology.* 1998;209:235-241.
71. Remy-Jardin M, Remy J, Wattinne L, et al. Central PE: diagnosis with spiral volumetric CT with single-breath-hold technique: comparison with pulmonary angiography. *Radiology.* 1992;185:381-387.
72. Van Rossum AB, Treurniet FE, Kieft GJ, et al. Role of spiral volumetric computed tomographic scanning in the assessment of patients with clinical suspicion of pulmonary embolism and an abnormal ventilation perfusion scan. *Thorax.* 1996;51(1):23-28.
73. Kasper W, Meinertz T, et al. Echocardiography in assessing acute pulmonary hypertension due to pulmonary embolism. *Am J Cardiol.* 1980;45:567-572.
74. Come P. Echocardiographic evaluation of pulmonary embolism and its response to therapeutic interventions. *Chest.* 1992;101:151S-162S.
75. Rectenwald J. Vena cava filters: uses and abuses. *Semin Vasc Surg.* 2005;18:166-175.
76. Rosner MK, Kuklo TR, et al. Prophylactic placement of an inferior vena cava filter in high-risk patients undergoing spinal reconstruction. *Neurosurg Focus.* 2004;17(4):E6.
77. Rogers FB, Shackford SR, et al. Prophylactic vena cava filter insertion in severely injured trauma patients: indications and preliminary results. *J Trauma.* 1993;35(4):637-641.
78. Wojcik R, Cipolle MD, et al. Long-term follow-up of trauma patients with a vena caval filter. *J Trauma.* 2000;49:839-843.
79. Rodriguez JL, Lopez JM, et al. Early placement of prophylactic vena caval filters in injured patients at high risk for pulmonary embolism. *J Trauma.* 1996;40:797-802.
80. Karmy-Jones R, Jurkovich GJ, et al. Practice patterns and outcomes of retrievable vena cava filters in trauma patients. An AAST multicenter study. *J Trauma Inj Infect Crit Care.* 2007;62:17-25.
81. Akhar S. Fat embolism. *Anesthesiol Clin.* 2009;27:533-550.
82. Levy D. The fat embolism syndrome. A review. *Clin Orthop Relat Res.* 1990;(261):281-286.
83. Bulger EM, Smith DG, Maier RV, et al. Fat embolism syndrome. A 10-year review. *Arch Surg.* 1997;132(4):435-439.
84. Pruszczyk P, Torbicki A, et al. Noninvasive diagnosis of suspected severe pulmonary embolism: transesophageal echocardiography vs spiral CT. *Chest.* 1997;112:722-728.
85. Svenninsen S, Nesse O, Finsen V, et al. Prevention of fat embolism syndrome in patients with femoral fractures—immediate or delayed operative fixation? *Ann Chir Gynaecol.* 1987;76:163-166.
86. Clark WR Jr. Smoke inhalation: diagnosis and treatment. *World J Surg.* 1992;16: 24-29.
87. Stephenson SF, Esrig BC, Polk Jr HC, et al. The pathophysiology of smoke inhalation injury. *Ann Surg.* 1975;182:652-660.
88. Shirani KZ, Pruitt Jr BA, Mason Jr AD. The influence of inhalation injury and pneumonia on burn mortality. *Ann Surg.* 1987;205(1):82-87.
89. Clark Jr WR, Nieman GF. Smoke inhalation. *Burns Incl Therm Inj.* 1988;14:473-494.
90. Clark WR, Bonaventura M, Myers W. Smoke inhalation and airway management at a regional burn unit: 1974–1983 part I: diagnosis and consequences of smoke inhalation. *J Burn Care Rehabil.* 1989;1:52-56.
91. Brown DL, Archer SB, et al. Inhalation injury severity scoring system: a quantitative method. *J Burn Care Rehabil.* 1996;16:552-557.
92. Smith DL, Cairns BA, et al. Effect of inhalation injury, burn size, age on mortality: a study of 1447 consecutive burn patients. *J Trauma.* 1994;37:655-659.
93. Hassan Z, Wong JK, Bush J, et al. Assessing the severity of inhalation injuries in adults. *J Int Soc Burn Injuries.* 2009. n.p. <http://www.biomedsearch.com/nih/Assessing-severity-inhalation-injuries-in/20006445.html>.
94. Etoch SW, Bar-Natan MF, et al. Tube thoracostomy: factors related to complications. *Arch Surg.* 1995;130(5):521-526.
95. Eddy AC, Luna G, Copass M. Empyema thoracis in patients undergoing emergent closed tube thoracostomy for thoracic trauma. *Am J Surg.* 1989;157:494-497.
96. Love NM, Smith JW, et al. Thoracostomy thoracic injurie preventive antibiotic usage in traumatic. *Chest.* 1994;106:1493-1498.
97. Luchette FA, Barrie PS, et al. Practice management guidelines for prophylactic antibiotic use in tube thoracostomy for traumatic hemopneumothorax: the EAST Practice Management Guidelines Work Group. *J Trauma.* 2000;48(4):758-757.

CHAPTER 48 ■ MULTIPLE ORGAN DYSFUNCTION SYNDROME

PHILIP S. BARIE AND FREDRIC M. PIERACCI

Multiple organ dysfunction syndrome (MODS) is a potentially progressive syndrome of reversible dysfunction of two or more organ systems as a consequence of acute, life-threatening, pathologic interactions among host defenses, the inflammasome, and the coagulation system that, once deranged, disrupt systemic homeostasis. Nearly 40 years since the initial description,[1] MODS is unquestionably the leading cause of death among critically ill surgical patients, and the leading cause of late deaths (not related to exsanguination or overwhelming central nervous system [CNS] injury) following trauma.[2] Moreover, the financial burden to both individual hospitals and the health care system as a result of the acute care of patients with MODS is astronomical, and the long-term needs of survivors are substantial.[3]

Currently, the MODS is believed to represent a severe manifestation of dysregulated or uncontrolled systemic inflammation.[4,5] Despite a sophisticated understanding of the pathogenesis of MODS, effective therapies have remained elusive; therefore prevention or early mitigation becomes crucial if lives are to be saved. This is likely because of the heterogeneous manifestations of MODS; organ dysfunction may follow a vast array of physiologic or metabolic insults, and may affect variable numbers of organ systems to varying degrees at different times. The development of targeted therapeutics has been hampered by the redundancy and interrelationships of the dysregulated immune response, or because such therapies have been targeted too narrowly, if not mistargeted altogether.[6] Better understanding of these interrelationships is crucial if patient care is to improve or new therapies are to be found.

HISTORICAL PERSPECTIVES

Multiple organ failure (MOF) following a severe physiologic insult was recognized first during the late 1960s as the unwanted consequence of advancements in the management of shock. Successful resuscitation of shock was followed by death from hitherto unidentified disease manifestations characterized by progressive, irreversible failure of several organs. In 1975, Baue coalesced early case reports of organ failure following severe injury[7,8] into the concept of MOF as a distinct entity, which he described as "the progressive failure of many or all systems after an overwhelming injury or operation."[9] In doing so, Baue gleaned two concepts fundamental to mortality during critical illness: First, that mortality in the intensive care unit (ICU) was the consequence of the interaction of multiple failing organs; and second, that individual organ systems were interrelated; injury to one organ system could cause dysfunction of another. For example, pulmonary failure was found more often than not to occur along with dysfunction of at least one other organ system.[10] Moreover, mortality from acute respiratory failure is usually determined by the magnitude of nonpulmonary organ dysfunction; the combination of respiratory and hepatic dysfunction is especially deleterious.[10,11] Furthermore, improvements in the treatment of the acute respiratory distress syndrome (ARDS), such as ventilation at low tidal volumes, also decreased the likelihood of additional, subsequent organ failure.[12,13] Soon after Baue's initial description of MOF, Fry et al.[14] reported a linear relationship between the number of failed organs and mortality during critical illness; whereas mortality following failure of a single organ was 30%, mortality following failure of four or more organs was 100%.

The etiology of MOF was believed initially to be always infection.[15] However, clinical, pathologic, and experimental findings have discredited this theory. Autopsies of patients with MOF did not always demonstrate a focus of infection; either infection was never present, or organ dysfunction progressed despite successful anti-infective therapy.[16,17] Trauma patients with organ failure were sometimes never infected.[18] When infection did occur during critical illness, it sometimes followed organ failure, rather than preceding it.[19] Under experimental conditions, characteristic hemodynamic and inflammatory derangements could be replicated absent any infection.[20,21]

This discrepancy was reconciled by observations that an occult reservoir of pathogens (e.g., the gastrointestinal [GI] tract) could initiate or perpetuate sepsis and organ dysfunction without any overt infection.[22,23] According to this "gut-motor" hypothesis, bacterial overgrowth during critical illness (secondary to gastric acid suppressive therapy, impaired intestinal immunity, or both) caused organ dysfunction. However, selective gut decontamination (topical oral antibiotics and enteral antibiotics by gavage, with or without systemic antibiotic prophylaxis) although effective in reducing the incidence of nosocomial infection, neither attenuated MODS nor improved mortality, calling the gut-motor hypothesis into question.[21,24] Even if ultimately correct, it may be that mediators (elaborated in intestinal lymph as a result of intestinal ischemia-reperfusion (I-R) injury, thence becoming systemic) are more important than the intestinal flora.

That infection was sufficient, but unnecessary to cause organ damage stimulated the reevaluation of the pathophysiology of MOF. Goris et al.[18] suggested "massive activation of inflammatory mediators by severe tissue trauma or intra-abdominal sepsis" as the etiology of MOF. Marshall and Sweeney[25] reinforced this theory by observing that the degree of the inflammatory response to infection predicted ICU mortality, rather than the type or extent of infection itself. Eventually, the hypothesis developed that a hypodynamic, excessive, or otherwise dysfunctional immune response was the principal cause of organ damage, rather than the cytotoxic effects of invading microorganisms *per se*.[4] This theory synthesized myriad, seemingly unrelated causes of organ failure into a unifying hypothesis, and was consistent with extant clinical and experimental observations. In recognition, and in an attempt at standardization, an American College of Chest Physicians/Society of Critical Care Medicine consensus statement defined diagnostic criteria for what was termed the *systemic inflammatory response syndrome* (SIRS) in 1992.[26] The diagnosis of SIRS was fulfilled by the presence of at least two of the host-response criteria: (1) Core body temperature >38°C or <36°C, (2) heart rate >90 beats/min, (3) respiratory rate >20 breaths/min (not ventilated) or $PaCO_2$ < 32 mm Hg (ventilated), and

TABLE 48.1

HISTORIC SYNONYMS FOR WHAT IS REFERRED TO CURRENTLY AS THE MODS

Sequential organ failure
Progressive systems failure
Remote organ failure
Multiple organ failure
Multiple organ failure syndrome
Multiple systems organ failure
Postinjury multiple organ failure

MODS, multiple organ dysfunction syndrome.

(4) WBC > 12,000, <4,000 or >10% immature forms (bands) absent any other cause, such as antineoplastic chemotherapy. *Sepsis* is the characterization of the host response to the insult and thus has a specific definition: SIRS caused by infection. *Severe sepsis* is sepsis complicated by dysfunction of at least one organ, whereas *septic shock* is severe sepsis with hypotension (cardiac dysfunction) that is refractory to fluid administration (see Chapter 14). Organ dysfunction is also recognized as a common consequence of SIRS, and the term MODS signifies the presence of altered organ function in critically ill patients such that homeostasis cannot not be achieved without intervention. But which intervention (see below)? Specifically, SIRS correlates with both the incidence and magnitude of MODS, and ultimately mortality.[27]

Currently, MODS remains the acronym used most commonly to describe organ dysfunction during critical illness. However, several other terms have been used, and may remain in use (Table 48.1).[28–31] No scoring system is "right or "wrong"; indeed, scores such as the MOD score[28] (Table 48.2) and the Sequential Organ Failure Assessment (SOFA) score[30] quantify largely the same pathophysiology and behave similarly.[32–35] However, the absence of a validated score that is recognized universally leads to conflicting reports of the incidence, time course, and mortality of MODS, hampering both research and clinical understanding.[36] Consensus is needed urgently.

EPIDEMIOLOGY

The MODS is the leading cause of death among nontrauma ICU patients.[37–40]. As many as 19% of ICU patients will develop MODS,[35,37–40] and MODS is responsible for approximately 50%[41,42] to 80%-94%[38,43,44] of ICU mortality. Patients who develop MODS experience a 25-fold increase in mortality[43] and a doubled length of stay compared to critically ill patients who do not develop organ dysfunction.[45] MODS is the most common ICU diagnosis in patients associated with prolonged stay (>21 days) in the ICU;[46] even modest degrees of MODS[47] prolong hospitalization.

Any biologic stress that activates systemic inflammation may precipitate SIRS, thus placing the patient at risk of MODS. Known precipitants of MODS are listed in Table 48.3; hypoperfusion/I-R injury without shock was the most common etiologic insult responsible for MODS in one study, followed by sepsis without shock, and shock regardless of etiology.[45] In another prospective study of elderly patients with ARDS, I-R injury was the leading cause.[48] Moreover, Sauaia et al.[49] found that an Injury Severity Score (ISS) of ≥25 points combined with a transfusion requirement of ≥ 6 units of red blood cell concentrates was associated with a 46% likelihood of developing MODS. Cryer et al.[50] further defined these risk factors, reporting a 66% incidence of MODS in patients with an ISS ≥ 25, regardless of transfusion requirement. For any given mechanism, both increased age[39] and number of comorbidities[39,51] increase the likelihood of MODS. Population data indicate that black persons may have higher case rates of infection, severe sepsis, acute organ dysfunction, and mortality.[52] Critically ill children may also develop MODS.[53,54] The pathophysiology appears to be similar[53] (see below), and neonates and younger children appear to be at higher risk than older children.[54]

Furthermore, certain individuals may harbor a genetic predisposition to MODS in the form of an exaggerated innate

TABLE 48.2

THE MULTIPLE ORGAN DYSFUNCTION SCORE

ORGAN SYSTEM	SCORE				
	0	1	2	3	4
Respiratory (PaO_2:FiO_2)[a]	>300	226–300	151–225	76–150	≤75
Renal (serum [creatinine])[b]	≤100	101–200	201–350	351–500	>500
Hepatic (serum [bilirubin])[c]	≤20	21–60	61–120	121–240	>240
Cardiovascular (PAR)[d]	≤10	10.1–15.0	15.1–20.0	20.1–30.0	>30.0
Hematologic (platelet count)[d]	>120	81–120	51–80	21–50	≤20
Neurologic (GCS)	15	13–14	10–12	7–9	≤6

[a]PaO_2:FiO_2 is calculated without reference to the use or mode of mechanical ventilation, and without reference to the use or level of positive end-expiratory pressure.
[b]The serum creatinine concentration is measured in mmol/L, without reference to the use of dialysis.
[c]The serum bilirubin concentration is measured in mmol/L.
[d]The platelet count is measured in platelets/mL × 10^{-3}; PAR, pressure adjusted heart rate; GCS, Glasgow Coma Scale score. To convert the serum creatinine concentration from mmol/L to mg/dL, divide by 88.4. To convert the serum bilirubin concentration from mmol/L to mg/dL, divide by 17.1.
Reproduced from Marshall JC, Cook DJ, Christou NV, et al. Multiple Organ Dysfunction Score: a reliable descriptor of a complex clinical outcome. *Crit Care Med.* 1995;23:1638–1652.

TABLE 48.3

CAUSES OF THE MODS

Sepsis
Multiple trauma
Burns
Pancreatitis
Gastric aspiration
Massive hemorrhage
Massive transfusion
Ischemia-reperfusion
Ischemic necrosis
Microvascular thrombosis
Interleukin-2 therapy ("cytokine-release syndrome")
Salicylate intoxication
Multiple sequential physiologic insults

TABLE 48.4

SNPs IDENTIFIED IN THE PATHOGENESIS OF TRAUMA, SEPSIS, AND MODS

Pattern and signal transduction receptors
Angiopoietin 2 gene (ANGPT2)
Calcitonin gene (CALCA1)
Heat shock protein A1B (HSPA1B)
Heat shock protein A1L (HSPA1L)
Interleukin-1 receptor–associated kinase-1 (IRAK-1)
Interleukin-1 receptor–associated kinase-4 (IRAK-4)
Lipopolysaccharide binding protein (LBP)
Mannose-binding lectin (MBL)
Mitochondrial ND1 gene (ND1)
Monocyte differentiation antigen CD14 (CD14)
Myelin and lymphocyte protein (MAL)
Myeloid differentiation 2 gene (MD-2)
Myosin light polypeptide kinase (MYLK)
Toll-interleukin 1 receptor (TIR) domain–containing adapter protein (TIRAP)
Toll-like receptor-1 (TLR_1)
Toll-like receptor-2 (TLR_2)
Toll-like receptor-4 (TLR_4)
Cytokines
I kappa beta
Interferon-gamma
Interleukin-1 alpha
Interleukin-1 beta
Interleukin-1 receptor antagonist
Interleukin-6
Interleukin-10
Macrophage inhibitory factor
Tumor necrosis factor-alpha
Tumor necrosis factor-beta
Coagulation proteins
Factor V
Fibrinogen
Plasminogen activator inhibitor-1
Thrombin-activatable fibrinolysis inhibitor

MODS, multiple organ dysfunction syndrome.

immunity/inflammatory response to illness.[55–58] Single nucleotide polymorphisms (SNPs) have now been identified for a number of genes and peptides related to pattern recognition receptors (PRRs), signal transduction molecules, effector cytokines, and coagulation proteins (Table 48.4), but owing to their multiplicity (with more likely to be identified), it is unlikely that causality will be established for a single SNP or combination. However, their assay does hold promise as a biomarker of risk, predisposition, or the development of MODS.

PATHOPHYSIOLOGY

Several phenotypes have been proposed to describe the onset of MODS[59] (Algorithm 48.1). According to the *one-hit model*, organ dysfunction develops as the direct result of a massive initial insult (e.g., burn or multiple injuries, severe pancreatitis), which itself is sufficient to cause MODS. By contrast, the *two-hit model* describes sequential insults, usually isolated temporally. According to the two-hit model, a "priming" insult (e.g., burn) is followed by a subsequent insult (e.g., central line–associated blood stream infection). The inflammatory response, "primed" by the first insult to react in an exaggerated manner to the second, induces further immune dysfunction and MODS. According to the *sustained-hit model*, a continuous, smoldering insult, such as ventilator-associated pneumonia caused by a difficult-to-treat, multi-drug-resistant bacterium, at once causes and sustains organ dysfunction. In reality, any of these mechanisms, alone or in combination, may result in MODS.

Organ failure may manifest in several organ systems (Table 48.5), and is no longer believed to follow a particular temporal sequence. Cardiovascular instability is often the first manifestation of dysfunctional homeostasis, resulting in I-R injury after resuscitation. The splanchnic and renal circulations are particularly susceptible to I-R injury. Pulmonary failure is equally common and is usually an early manifestation, whereas hepatic, hematologic, and GI dysfunctions and acute kidney injury usually are later manifestations, if they occur at all.[9,14,43,60] In particular, hepatic dysfunction may not be recognized promptly because the liver has redundant metabolic capacity; substantial hepatic dysfunction may precede elevation of the serum bilirubin concentration. Furthermore, certain combinations of organ failure have been shown to be especially deleterious (e.g., hepatic and pulmonary, or renal and pulmonary).[10,11]

Two distinct periods of altered immune function characterize MODS. The first is dominated by upregulated innate immunity (Table 48.6), uncontrolled inflammation, increased endothelial permeability, microvascular thrombosis, apoptosis (programmed cell death), and disruption of parenchymal cellular integrity.[61–63] The second involves a predominance of anti-inflammatory cytokines, downregulated adaptive immunity (Table 48.6), immunosuppression,[64] and an increased risk of infection. This general disruption of the normal regulation of the immune system during MODS has been termed *immunologic dissonance*.[65]

Inflammation and Tissue Injury

Organ damage following severe injury is believed to occur secondary to uncontrolled activation of the inflammatory response caused by tissue hypoxia. Following tissue injury,

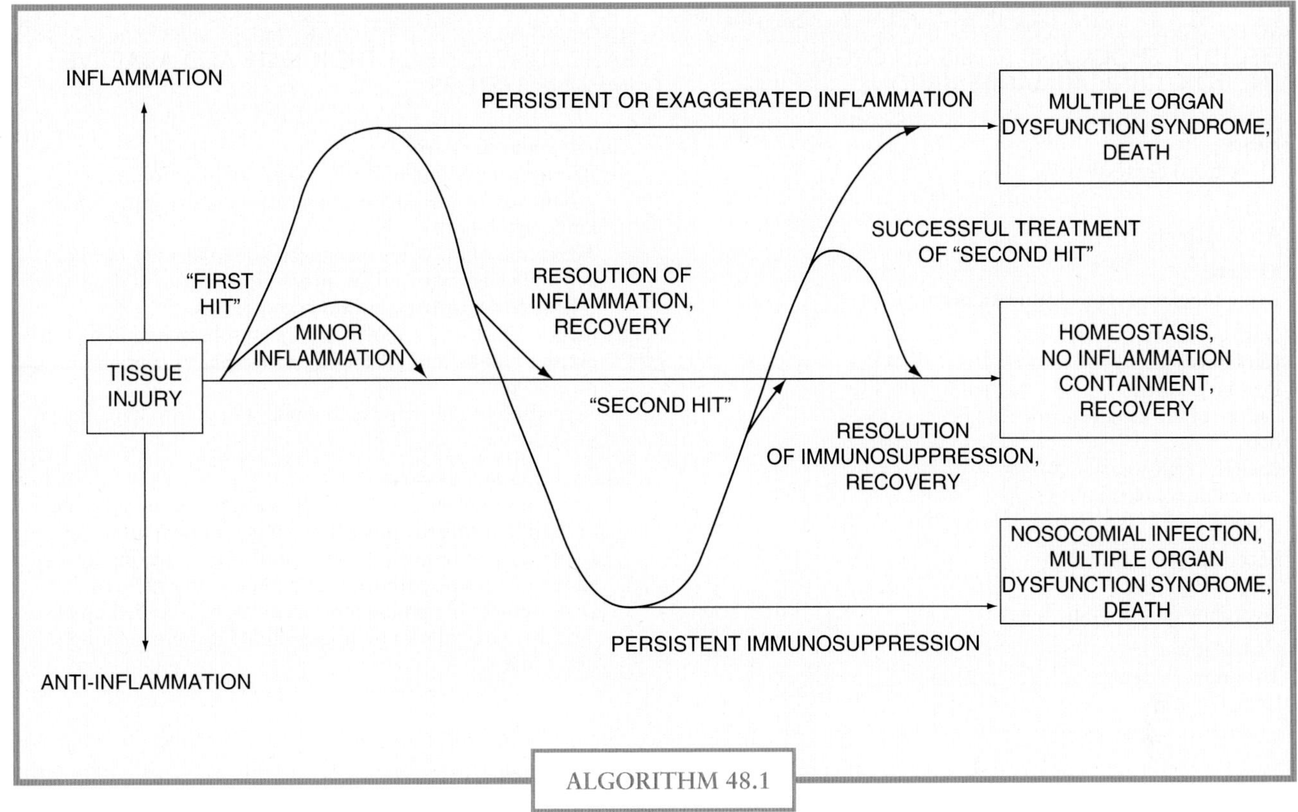

ALGORITHM 48.1 Ebb and flow of pro- and anti-inflammatory responses to tissue injury, resulting in recovery, organ dysfunction, nosocomial infection, or death.

the early stage of the inflammatory response is characterized by macrophage activation as well as secretion of inflammatory cytotoxins and cytokines. Cytotoxins are released primarily by cluster of differentiation 8 (CD8)+ cells (e.g., cytotoxic T cells, dendritic cells), a cell surface co-receptor for major histocompatibility Class II (MHC Class II); these cells act locally by causing damage to cell walls and tight junctions.[66] By contrast, cytokines mediate primarily the CD4+ (a cell surface co-receptor for MHC Class I) response, and may be secreted by a variety of cell types (e.g., platelets, endothelial cells) in addition to those of the immune system (e.g., T helper [Th] cells, regulatory T cells, monocytes, macrophages, and dendritic cells). Cytokines may act both locally and systemically. Although they may be classified broadly into groups by function (Table 48.7), the cytokine-mediated inflammatory response is redundant; each cytokine has multiple activities on different cell types, some of which are salutary. The balance of pro and anti-inflammatory responses is not always self-regulatory and balanced; predominance of either influence may be deleterious. As such, the inflammatory response has been challenging to manipulate for therapeutic effect.

Recruitment of polymorphonuclear (PMN) leukocytes into tissue represents a second prominent feature of MODS. Postmortem examination of patients with ARDS has demonstrated massive PMN leukocyte infiltration into lung parenchyma.[67] Neutrophil activation (respiratory burst) generates large amounts of reactive oxygen species and lipid mediators (e.g., prostaglandins, leukotrienes) that are autodestructive. Furthermore, depletion[68] or inhibition[69–71] of PMN leukocytes decreases the severity of lung injury in animal models of ARDS. Infiltration of PMN leukocytes is accompanied by upregulation of hepatic inflammatory proteins (e.g., C-reactive protein) and the complement system,[72] increased capillary permeability, and the formation of reactive oxygen and nitrogen species (Table 48.8). The clinical manifestation of increased capillary permeability is tissue edema, whether of connective tissue, lung, or brain.

Innate immune cells have evolved to sense microbial pathogens through PRRs, which interact with conserved pathogen-associated molecular patterns (PAMPs) to convey microbial information into immune cell signaling and activation events.[73] PRRs also recognize endogenous damage-associated molecular patterns (DAMPs) (also called alarmins or endokines) released during microbial invasion, mediated in part by Toll-like receptors (TLRs). The DAMP molecules, including high mobility group box-1 protein (HMGB1), heat-shock proteins (HSPs), uric acid, altered matrix proteins, and S100 proteins, represent important danger signals that mediate inflammatory responses through the receptor for advanced glycation end-products (RAGE) and TLRs, after release from activated or necrotic cells. The HMGB1 protein is released actively after stimulation of the innate immune system by PAMPs and is released passively by sterile ischemia or cell injury.[74–77] The RAGE is a multiligand MHC Class III receptor of the immunoglobulin gene superfamily. Infection is associated with the release of HMGB1 and S100A12. Engagement of RAGE by its diverse ligands, which include HMGB1, results in receptor-dependent signaling and activation of nuclear factor-kappa beta (NF-kB). Furthermore, RAGE acts as an endothelial adhesion receptor for leukocyte integrins and promotes leukocyte recruitment. Inhibition of RAGE signaling reduces inflammatory responses in several noninfectious and infection models of inflammation.

TABLE 48.5

EFFECTS OF SHOCK AND SEPSIS ON ORGAN FUNCTION: CLINICAL MANIFESTATIONS

Heart: Myocardial depression
Lungs: Acute respiratory distress syndrome
Kidneys: Acute tubular necrosis (acute kidney injury)
Gut: Cholestasis Erosive gastritis Failure of the hepatosplenic RE system Ileus Bacterial translocation (?) Acalculous cholecystitis (?)
CNS: Encephalopathy Polyneuropathy Neuromuscular dysfunction
Coagulation: Thrombocytopenia Coagulopathy

TABLE 48.6

BASIC FUNCTIONS OF THE INNATE AND ADAPTIVE IMMUNE SYSTEMS

Innate immune system:
- Recruitment of immune cells to sites of infection, via production of specialized chemical mediators (e.g., chemokines, cytokines).
- Activation of the complement cascade to identify bacteria, activate phagocytes, and to promote clearance of dead cells (efferocytosis) or antibody complexes.
- Identification and removal of foreign substances present in organs, tissues, and the blood and lymph, by specialized phagocytes.
- Activation of the adaptive immune system through antigen presentation.

Adaptive immune system:
- Recognition of specific "nonself" antigens in the presence of "self", during the process of antigen presentation.
- Generation of responses that are tailored to maximally eliminate specific pathogens or pathogen-infected cells.
- Development of immunologic memory, to be called upon quickly to eliminate a pathogen should a subsequent infection occur.

A key question concerns how sterile injury activates innate immunity to mediate damaging inflammation in the absence of invasion by pathogens. That HMGB1, a ubiquitous nuclear protein, mediates the activation of innate immune responses, led to the understanding that HMGB1 plays a crucial role at the intersection of the host inflammatory response to sterile and infectious threat through TLR4 signaling pathways that mediate cytokine release and tissue damage. The RAGE-HMGB1 complex also regulates *autophagy* (programmed cell survival) and *apoptosis* (programmed cell death), sustaining the former and inhibiting the latter.

Apoptosis is deranged in MODS. Markers of apoptosis such as the Fas receptor (also known as tumor necrosis factor [TNF] receptor superfamily member 6 and CD 95)[78] (a cell-surface protein receptor expressed on essentially all cells of the body that when bound to its ligand [FasL] is internalized and signals an initiator caspase cascade [caspase-8, -10], ultimately resulting in apoptosis), and nuclear matrix proteins[79] have been identified in patients with MODS. Interestingly, whereas some cell types (e.g., splenocytes and hepatocytes) demonstrate accelerated apoptosis, other cell types, such as circulating neutrophils, exhibit inhibited apoptosis. Still other tissues, such as the kidney and lung, show only minimal changes in rates of cellular death.[80–82]

There are two major pathways of apoptosis: The *death-receptor pathway*, which is mediated by activation of death receptors and the B-cell leukemia/lymphoma 2 (Bcl2)-regulated *mitochondrial pathway*, which is mediated by stimuli that ultimately lead to mitochondrial injury.[83] Ligation of death receptors recruits the adaptor protein, Fas-associated death domain, which in turn recruits caspase-8. This latter ultimately activates caspase-3, the key "executioner" caspase. In the mitochondrial pathway, proapoptotic Bcl homology (BH)-3 proteins are activated by noxious stimuli, which interact with and inhibit antiapoptotic Bcl2 or Bcl-extra large (BCL-XL) proteins. Thus, Bcl2-associated X protein (BAX, a proapoptotic antagonist of Bcl2) and BAK (Bcl-2 homologous antagonist/killer) act unopposed to alter transmembrane potential and induce mitochondrial permeability with release of cytochrome c, which ultimately results in the activation of caspase-9 through the apoptosome. Caspase-9 then activates caspase-3.

The uncontrolled inflammation characteristic of MODS is accompanied by microvascular thrombosis.[84,85] Indeed, the inflammatory and coagulation systems are related intimately,[85] manifesting as failure of the microcirculation. Several proinflammatory cytokines (e.g., TNF-α) may activate tissue factor and initiate the coagulation cascade.[86] In turn, the thrombin receptor activates nuclear factor kappa beta (NF-κB), which causes increased transcription of proinflammatory gene products.[87] Microvascular thrombosis results in tissue hypoxia, thus perpetuating the inflammatory response. Early coagulopathy increases the risk of developing MODS.[87]

Anti-inflammatory Response

Whereas the initial phase of MODS is characterized by a disruption of homeostatic mechanisms to favor inflammation, a second, distinct later period is characterized by impaired adaptive immunity and increased susceptibility to infection.[88] This phenomenon has been called the compensatory anti-inflammatory response system, and the result referred to as *immunoparalysis*.[65] During this later period, increased elaboration of anti-inflammatory cytokines such as IL-10 and -13 and transforming growth factor (TGF)-β, impaired antibody synthesis, and anergy of T lymphocytes are characteristic.[89–91]

In many cases of sepsis, failure of the immune system to eradicate pathogens presages a prolonged phase of immune suppression, characterized not only by failure to eradicate the primary infection but also by development of secondary nosocomial infections.[88] The immune suppression is mediated by multiple mechanisms, including massive apoptosis-induced depletion of lymphocytes and dendritic cells, decreased

TABLE 48.7

MAJOR CLASSES OF INFLAMMATORY CYTOKINES, REPRESENTATIVE MEMBERS, AND THEIR MAIN ACTION(S)

CYTOKINE	PRODUCER CELL	MAIN ACTIONS
Hematopoietins		
IL-1	Macrophages, epithelial cells	Fever, T-cell activation, macrophage activation
IL-2		T-cell proliferation
IL-6	T cells T cells, macrophages, astrocytes	T- and B-cell growth and differentiation, acute phase protein production
IL-7	Bone marrow stroma	Growth and differentiation of immature T cells and B cells, prevents apoptosis
IL-15	Mononuclear phagocytes	Increases production of natural killer cells, prevents apoptosis
Chemokines		
IL-8[a]	Macrophages, others	Chemotactic for neutrophils, T cells
MCP-1 (now CCL2)[b]	Macrophages, others	Chemotactic for monocytes
Modulators of immune response		
TNF-α	Macrophage, NK cells	Local inflammation, endothelial activation
TNF-β	T cells, B cells	Killing, endothelial activation
IL-4	Th2 cells, mast cells, macrophages	B- and T-cell proliferation, IgE and IgG synthesis
IL-6	T cells, macrophages, astrocytes	General upregulator of inflammation
IL-12	B cells, macrophages	NK cell activation, T-cell differentiation
IL-16	Lymphocytes, epithelial cells, CD8+	CD4+ chemoattractant
IL-17	T cells	Upregulates production of chemokines and antibacterial peptides. Antagonizes anti-inflammatory effects of T regulatory cells
IL-18	T helper 17 (Th17) cells	Induces IFN-γ production, natural killer cell activity
IFN-γ	Macrophages, T cells, natural killer cells	Macrophage activation, increased MHC production
Anti-inflammatory		
IL-10	T cells, macrophages	Inhibition macrophage function
IL-13	T cells	Inhibition of macrophage cytokine production
TGF-β	Monocytes, T cells	Inhibition of cell growth, anti-inflammatory

IL, interleukin; MCP, macrophage chemoattractant protein; TNF, tumor necrosis factor; NK, natural killer; IFN, interferon; MHC, major histocompatibility complex; TGF, transforming growth factor.
[a]Seventeen CXC chemokines (so named because one amino acid separates two cysteine molecules) have been identified in this subgroup of the chemokine family, of which IL-8 is one, along with seven G protein–coupled receptors.
[b]Twenty-seven CC chemokines (so named because of the adjacency of two cysteine molecules) have been identified in this subgroup of the chemokine family. CCL2: CC ligand 2.

expression of the HLA-DR cell-surface antigen-presenting complex, and increased expression of the negative costimulatory molecules programmed death 1, cytotoxic T-lymphocyte–associated antigen 4, and B- and T-lymphocyte attenuator and their corresponding ligands. Numbers of regulatory T cells and myeloid-derived suppressor cells are increased, and there is a phenotypic shift from inflammatory type 1 helper T (Th1) cells to an anti-inflammatory phenotype of type 2 helper T (Th2) cells that is associated with the production of IL-10. The innate and adaptive immune systems are both compromised severely with poorly functional "exhausted" CD8+ and anergic CD4+ T cells.

An alternative, systems biology-derived theory describes the pathogenesis of MODS as a disruption of interorgan or intercellular communication.[92] Accordingly, each organ system is viewed as a stochastic (random) biologic oscillator, whose activity varies periodically with time. The dynamic behavior of any one organ necessarily reflects the state of the organism as a whole. During normal homeostasis, variability within each oscillator is preserved through mechanical, neural, hormonal, and immune (e.g., cytokine and prostaglandin) inputs. As a result of massive physiologic insult, interoscillator communication becomes uncoupled, resulting in a regularization of normally variable organ outputs.

The majority of research in the area of biologic oscillators has been conducted using loss of normal heart rate variability as a marker of uncoupling. Clinical investigations have reported increased cardiac regularity after administration of endotoxin to healthy volunteers,[93] as well as in emergency department patients with sepsis.[94] Furthermore, low heart rate variability correlates with both ICU mortality[95,96] and mortality from MODS.[97,98] As a result, measurement of heart rate variability has emerged as a noninvasive, accurate, and validated tool to predict outcomes during critical illness.[99]

The uncoupling of stochastic biologic oscillators offers an intriguing alternative theory for the pathogenesis of MODS, and has been used to explain the failure of antimediator trials aimed at attenuating the inflammatory response in these patients (discussed below).[100] However, substantial additional research, as well as a fundamental shift in the current conceptualization of MODS, will be required to provide tangible options for the treatment of patient with MODS. One such

TABLE 48.8

OXIDANTS AND TISSUE INJURY

OXIDANT	DESCRIPTION
•O_2^-, superoxide anion	Formed in many auto-oxidation reactions and by the electron transport chain. Relatively unreactive but can release Fe^{2+} from iron–sulfur proteins and ferritin. Undergoes dismutation to form H_2O_2 spontaneously or by enzymatic catalysis, and is a precursor for metal-catalyzed •OH formation H_2O_2, hydrogen peroxide formed by dismutation of •O_2^- or by direct reduction of O_2. Lipid-soluble, and thus able to diffuse across membranes
•OH, hydroxyl radical	Formed by Fenton reaction and decomposition of peroxynitrite. Extremely reactive
RO• and ROO•, peroxy	Oxygen-centered organic radicals that participate in lipid peroxidation reactions
HOCl, hypochlorous acid	Formed from H_2O_2 by myeloperoxidase. Lipid-soluble and highly reactive. Oxidizes protein constituents, including thiol groups and amino groups
ONOO-, peroxynitrite	Formed in a reaction between •O_2^- and •NO. Lipid soluble and similar in reactivity to HOCl. Protonation forms peroxynitrous acid, which undergoes cleavage to form •OH and nitrogen dioxide (NO_2)

Production of oxidizing species plays a central role in killing of pathogens, with activated phagocytes producing both reactive oxygen and nitrogen species. These include superoxide (•$O2^-$), nitric oxide (•NO) and their particularly reactive product, peroxynitrite ($ONOO^-$). This effect is non-specific; almost every part of the target cell is damaged, preventing a pathogen from escaping destruction by mutation of a single molecular target, but damage to host tissues is problematic.

example suggested by Buchman involves a shift from traditional random or scheduled sampling of physiologic parameters to continuous sampling strategies in order to better capture loss of organ variability.[97] The feasibility of "physiologically dense data capture" has been demonstrated,[101] but outcomes have not been improved demonstrably.

ORGAN SYSTEM MANIFESTATIONS

Although uncontrolled inflammation exerts distinct, predictable effects on each organ system, organ dysfunction rarely occurs in isolation. Moreover, it is important to note that organ dysfunction in critical illness is usually multifactorial. For example, acute kidney injury is often iatrogenic, resulting from hypovolemia or nephrotoxic drugs such as radiocontrast media. Listed below are the known consequences of systemic inflammation on individual organ systems (Table 48.5).

Although cardiovascular failure manifested as shock is often the cause of SIRS and ultimately MODS, inflammation also results in impaired cardiac function.[102] TNF and reactive oxygen and nitrogen species inhibit cardiac contractility.[103] Inflammation also causes increased endothelial permeability and vasodilation, decreasing blood volume and systemic vascular resistance, respectively. Thus, each component of blood pressure is affected (preload, contractility, and afterload), resulting in hypotension that may be refractory to volume replacement, thus necessitating vasopressor therapy.

Lung inflammation results in impaired gas exchange that is manifested primarily as hypoxia rather than hypercarbia. The most severe pulmonary manifestation of MODS is ARDS, characterized by PaO_2:FIO_2 < 200 and diffuse, bilateral pulmonary infiltrates on chest radiography in the presence of a pulmonary wedge pressure <18 mm Hg. The ARDS is a relatively common complication of SIRS, its pathophysiology and management have been described in detail,[104,105] and it is discussed elsewhere in this volume (see Chapter 47). The interplay of coagulation and inflammation is a crucial determinant of acute lung inflammation in ARDS.[106]

In addition to alterations in leukocyte function, both thrombopoiesis and erythropoiesis are inhibited during MODS. Thrombocytopenia is a well-recognized sequela of both SIRS and sepsis and results not only from bone marrow suppression, but also from increased consumption and sequestration within the reticuloendothelial (RE) system.[85] Furthermore, IL-1, TNF-α, and TGF-β inhibit erythropoietin synthesis and action.[107–110] Recombinant TNF-α induces anemia and hypoferremia associated with decreased iron release from the RE system and incorporation into red blood cells.[111,112] Interleukin-1 and TNF-α also induce ferritin production as part of the *acute-phase reaction*, sequestering iron that would otherwise be available for erythropoiesis.[113] Both generalized inflammation and microvascular thrombosis lead to consumption of clotting factors, which may cause disseminated intravascular coagulation.

Manifestations of GI injury are protean in MODS. Patients may have gastric, small bowel, or colonic ileus (e.g., acute colonic pseudo-obstruction, or Ogilvie's syndrome) after GI surgery; an estimated 50% of patients have delayed gastric emptying during mechanical ventilation, and up to 80% with increased intracranial pressure after traumatic brain injury.[114] Furthermore, ileus, malabsorption, and diarrhea are common sequelae of mucosal inflammation. Potential causes of GI dysmotility during critical illness are numerous and common, including impaired innervation, inflammation, I-R injury, medications, electrolyte disturbances, and sepsis; it is likely that many cases are multifactorial, as interplay among inflammation, immunity, and neuronal pathways has been demonstrated.[115] The gut is innervated by intrinsic enteric nerves and extrinsic autonomic pathways (predominantly parasympathetic, via the vagus nerve). Vagal pathways mediate both a cholinergic anti-inflammatory pathway and act indirectly to modulate inflammatory processes via postganglionic neuromodulation of immune cells in organs such as the spleen. Manifestations of I-R injury range from stress-related gastric mucosal hemorrhage ("stress gastritis") to acute acalculous cholecystitis.[116] Disruption of intestinal mucosal integrity as a result of splanchnic I-R injury or due to the actions of inflammatory cytokines may facilitate the translocation of invading microorganisms and cause both bacteremia and infection (i.e., "gut-motor" hypothesis, see above).[22,117] Increased intestinal permeability has been associated with the subsequent development of both SIRS and MODS.[118] Unfortunately, most conventional tests for gut dysmotility are cumbersome in the ICU; measurement of the non-protein amino acid citrulline (which is derived almost entirely from enterocytes) as a marker of decreased enterocyte mass has been suggested as a way to quantify small bowel function in critical illness.[119]

Hepatic dysfunction in patients with MODS is characterized by cholestatic jaundice.[120] Leakage of bilirubin from the hepatic canalicula into the intracellular and eventually intravascular space results from disruption of tight junctions by cytotoxic inflammation.[66] Hepatic synthetic function during inflammation is characterized by early upregulation of positive acute-phase proteins (e.g., C-reactive protein and ferritin), and downregulation of negative acute-phase proteins (e.g., albumin and transferrin). This initial period is followed by generalized impairment, including decreased synthesis of coagulation factors manifest as hypoprothrombinemia that is not correctable by vitamin K administration. However, the liver has substantial redundant metabolic capacity, and up to 80% of hepatic synthetic function may be lost before the serum bilirubin concentration increases. Measurement of metabolites of drugs metabolized by the liver may provide an earlier and more sensitive quantitative assessment of hepatic dysfunction.[121]

The traditional assessment of neurologic dysfunction in MODS has been the calculation of the Glasgow Coma Scale (GCS) score, for which purpose it was not designed. Application of the GCS is complicated in critical illness due to the fact that many patients are intubated endotracheally (such that the verbal component cannot be assessed), and sedated, if not anesthetized recently. Nonetheless, and despite having to give patients substantial benefit of the doubt in calculation of the GCS, it remains a powerful predictor of outcome in MODS. Nonetheless, alternatives are sought. Hypoperfusion, microvascular thrombosis, and cerebral edema combine to cause encephalopathy in MODS, but neurologic manifestations may include neuropathies and myopathies.[122] Furthermore, the *critical illness polyneuropathy syndrome*, characterized by debility, muscle weakness, and eventual atrophy, has been associated with the development of MODS.[123] Risk factors for development of ICU-acquired weakness include bed rest, sepsis, and corticosteroid therapy. A strong association exists between weakness and long-term ventilator dependence, and may be present for months after recovery, if not indefinitely. Alterations of autonomic tone manifested as loss of normal heart rate variability, baroreflex sensitivity, and chemoreflex sensitivity are common in patients with MODS, and the degree of autonomic dysfunction correlates with mortality.[95,96] Critical illness polyneuropathy may prove to be a better indicator of neurologic dysfunction than encephalopathy, in that it may be quantified by electrophysiologic testing and is not affected by sedatives, analgesics, or anesthetics.

Hypoxic/ischemic insults to the kidney are the most common cause of acute kidney injury, characterized by oliguria, azotemia, fluid overload, and accumulation of nitrogenous waste (see Chapter 52). Other common causes of acute kidney injury include rhabdomyolysis and drug toxicity (e.g., iodinated radiocontrast media, antibiotics). Electrolyte abnormalities are not prominent unless caused by rhabdomyolysis (hyperkalemia and hyperphosphatemia), likely because they are monitored and corrected readily by the clinician. Although renal dysfunction usually becomes apparent (i.e., elevated serum creatinine concentration) later in the course of MODS, hypoxic injury likely occurs at the time of the initial insult. Even mild degrees of renal impairment (well short of the need for renal replacement therapy) translate into substantial morbidity and mortality. Proinflammatory cytokines such as TNF-α may also activate the renin–angiotensin–aldosterone axis.[45] Interleukin-1, TNF-α, and TGF-β inhibit erythropoietin synthesis and function,[111–113] which essentially cease below a glomerular filtration rate < 25 mL/min.

Diagnosis

Early characterizations depicted organ failure as an "all-or-nothing" response. Organ failure was described as a dichotomous event for each organ. Moreover, failure of each organ was accorded the same weight, regardless of severity. Organ failure was considered present if an iatrogenic intervention to support organ function was necessary (e.g., renal replacement therapy). Prognosis was related solely to the number of failed organs, rather than the severity and the timing of failure. The former observation remains true, but more subtle gradations of organ dysfunction are now recognized.

The current conceptualization of MODS is more nuanced: MODS is not an "all-or-nothing" phenomenon, not every organ "fails" even when dysfunction develops, and not every organ becomes dysfunctional to the same extent.[124] Rather, organ dysfunction is recognized to occur in a continuum of altered physiology. In response to this conceptualization, several scoring systems have been developed to quantify the extent of organ dysfunction associated with MODS.[28–32]

Organ systems typically considered in the scoring of MODS are: (1) Respiratory, (2) cardiovascular, (3) renal, (4) hepatic, (5) hematologic, and (6) CNS. Notably absent from this list are both the GI and endocrine systems, owing to a lack of objective descriptors of organ failure. Five scoring systems are currently employed with frequency.[28–32] Central to each is a gradation of organ dysfunction based on mostly objective measurements of altered physiologic function.

One such scoring system, the multiple organ dysfunction (MOD) score, is shown in Table 48.2.[28] The MOD score was developed from a MEDLINE review of clinical studies involving patients with MODS between 1969 and 1993. Five organ systems were evaluated using available physiologic markers: (1) Respiratory (PaO_2:FiO_2), (2) renal (serum creatinine concentration), (3) hepatic (serum bilirubin concentration), (4) hematologic (platelet count), and (5) CNS (GCS score—the most subjective of the measurements). Cardiovascular dysfunction is quantified by the pressure-adjusted heart rate, which is defined as the product of the heart rate and the ratio of central venous pressure to mean arterial pressure. Each organ system is graded on a scale from 0 to 4 points for a maximum total score of 24. A MOD score of 0 for any organ system corresponds to a mortality of <5%, whereas a score of 4 correlates with a mortality of >50%. The aggregate MOD score for survivors is calculated using the worst value for each organ system for each day, or can be scored on a cumulative basis for the episode of care.

Other scoring systems follow similar patterns and include the now-obsolete Brussels score,[29] the sepsis-related organ failure assessment (SOFA),[30] the logistic organ dysfunction system,[31] and the Denver MOF score.[32] These scoring systems have been validated similarly using cohorts of critically ill patients.

Data obtained using scoring systems is useful for prognostication. Initial, aggregate, and mean scores have all been correlated with mortality. For example, the total MOD score correlates in a linear fashion with ICU mortality both when calculated on ICU day one and when the maximum score is compared to the score on day 1.[28,44] Similarly, calculations of the initial, highest, and mean SOFA score all correlate with mortality.[124] Because daily scores may fluctuate, cumulative or aggregate scores possess the greatest prognostic utility.[44]

Because patients may demonstrate altered physiology in the immediate postoperative period related to anesthesia and recovery or transient, stereotypical surgical stress, some authors have criticized both SIRS and MODS scoring systems as being oversensitive during this time period. Furthermore, some scoring systems have traditionally omitted data obtained during the first 48 hours. However, evidence suggests that both SIRS and MODS scores calculated as early as 24 hours after injury can predict mortality from MODS.[27] These results have called into question the traditional pathophysiologic framework that depicts MODS as an occurrence relatively late in the ICU course (i.e., the two-hit model), and suggest that substantial organ dysfunction occurs much earlier. For these reasons, early resuscitation to avoid or minimize the consequences of I-R injury is of paramount importance.[125] Indeed, markers of organ dysfunction observed as early as post-injury day 1 are perhaps better viewed as outcome measures rather than risk factors.

Much interest has been afforded the use of biomarkers for the diagnosis of inflammatory states and infection and to guide therapy, but results have been modest. Disease processes are inherently heterogeneous, the appearance of biomarkers may be transitory, relevant biomarkers may not circulate in blood, or assay may be timed for an irrelevant period. Using pancreatitis as an example, nearly 40 putative biomarkers have been evaluated in at least three clinical reports,[126] but methodologic quality is poor and uneven, and little useful information has translated into clinical practice. Early clearance of lactate as a surrogate for resuscitation-related resolution of global tissue hypoxia after injury and during severe sepsis is validated as a marker of favorable outcome, and has been correlated with decreased concentrations of several biomarkers and decreased risk of MODS.[127] Among trauma and burns patients, increased plasma concentrations of IL-6 have been correlated with increased risk of organ dysfunction, but not invariably nosocomial infection or death.[128] Multiplexed cytokine assays of multiple candidate biomarkers have established associations between elevated concentrations of circulating cytokines in trauma patients[129,130] and patients with sepsis,[131] but other than for IL-6, the studies have little in common, and assay of IL-6 is not available routinely from clinical laboratories in the United States.

Procalcitonin has been studied extensively as a biomarker for infectious and inflammatory conditions, and as a guide to therapy. Some evidence suggests that procalcitonin has diagnostic and prognostic utility for diagnosis of MODS and outcomes thereof and from injury.[132–134] However, data are few, studies are heterogeneous, and correlations are modest. Further study is needed.

MANAGEMENT

Management of MODS may be classified broadly as either prophylaxis or treatment, which in turn is either supportive care or attenuation of the proinflammatory response. Supportive care involves early recognition, resuscitation, and artificial maintenance of organ function. Evidence-based strategies include ventilation with lower tidal volumes for ARDS,[12] renal replacement therapy for acute kidney injury,[135] and intensive insulin therapy (serum glucose concentration < 140 mg/dL).[136–138]

Of note, although tissue and cellular hypoxia play an important role in the initial pathophysiology of MODS, resuscitation to supranormal levels of tissue oxygenation to prevent or attenuate MODS using high FiO_2, inotropes (e.g., dobutamine), or blood transfusion has not improved outcomes, and may in fact worsen the severity of organ dysfunction during MODS.[139–142] Exacerbation of tissue damage following the introduction of supranormal levels of oxygen may be explained by increased substrate for the generation of cytotoxic reactive oxygen species.

Transfusion of blood and blood products must be parsimonious. Oxygen transport is not improved acutely by blood transfusion because the "storage lesion" characteristic of banked blood depletes erythrocyte high-energy phosphates, leading to two deleterious consequences. First, 2,3-diphosphoglycerate is depleted within 48 hours of storage, leading to a "left shift" of the oxyhemoglobin dissociation curve, inhibiting oxygen offloading. Second, loss of cell membrane adenosine triphosphate after about 2 weeks of storage leads to membrane fragility and deformation such that the erythrocyte cannot deform to transit the microcirculation, preventing oxygen offloading. Large-volume transfusion, transfusion of increasing quantities of blood stored more than 14 days, and administration of fresh frozen plasma have all to be associated with the development of ARDS and MODS,[143–146] but the observation regarding fresh frozen plasma remains controversial.[147]

Early, appropriate antibiotic therapy remains a cornerstone of successful therapy for severe sepsis and septic shock. Although dosing recommendations for renal insufficiency are plentiful (see Chapter 13), few data exist to guide antibiotic dosing in MODS.[148] The two pharmacokinetic factors likely to vary most in patients with MODS are volume of distribution and clearance (see Chapter 13). Disease- and resuscitation-driven increases in volume of distribution may lead to lower-than-expected plasma drug concentrations, at least for the first day of therapy. Thereafter, organ dysfunction may decrease drug clearance, leading to potential toxicity. Maintenance dosing must be guided by drug clearance and adjusted to the degree of MODS.

Anti-mediator Therapy

Efforts to manipulate the dysregulated immune response characteristic of MODS have constituted a substantial portion of experimental research in the field of critical care for two decades. Early attempts sought to achieve generalized immune suppression. However, treatment with nonspecific inhibitors of inflammation such as non-steroidal anti-inflammatory drugs, corticosteroids, and dietary fish oil did not improve outcomes. Indeed, non-steroidal anti-inflammatory agents may worsen organ dysfunction, particularly by decreasing renal perfusion and disrupting gastric mucosal integrity.

As understanding grew of the role of individual cytokines in the inflammatory response, attention turned towards targeted, mediator-directed therapy for MODS. Nearly 100 such clinical trials have been conducted to date, including anti-mediator monoclonal antibodies (e.g., anti-TNF, anti-endotoxin) and receptor antagonists or inhibitors (e.g., IL-1 receptor antagonist, tissue factor pathway inhibitor, TLR-4 antagonist). However, targeted interventions aimed at cytokine neutralization have been largely disappointing.[149,150] A recent, combined analysis of clinical trials of mediator-directed therapy in patients with SIRS reported only a modest (3%) overall reduction in 28-day mortality,[151] and no mediator-directed treatment has been licensed specifically for use in patients with established MODS in the United States.

The failure of mediator-directed therapy is likely multifactorial. Measurement of elevated serum concentrations of inflammatory cytokines during MODS does not confirm causality. Expression of mediators may vary over time, and is regulated by a variety of complementary mediators, each of which has several targets. Furthermore, measurement of serum concentrations may not reflect tissue activity. Finally, regional variations in ICU practice may explain partially the discrepancy between efficacy and effectiveness observed when comparing clinical trials.

Drotrecogin alfa (activated) (drotAA, or recombinant human activated protein C [rhAPC], an endogenous coagulation factor with anti-inflammatory, anticoagulant, and fibrinolytic properties), was approved from 2001–2011 for the treatment of severe sepsis associated with a high risk of death,[152] but has now been withdrawn from the market.[153] The development of drotAA galvanized appreciation of the interrelationship between inflammation and coagulation in the pathophysiology of both SIRS and MODS. Although the primary outcome variable reported following therapy with drotrecogin alfa (activated) was a reduction in 28-day mortality (19.4% relative risk reduction in death compared with placebo [$p = 0.005$]),[152] a subsequent analysis also revealed a substantial improvement in mean SOFA scores at 28 days in patients treated with drotrecogin alfa (activated) versus placebo[154] Additional therapies for the management of sepsis, distinct from mediator-based efforts, have been organized into "bundles" (see Chapter 12), with favorable effects upon mortality.[155,156]

OUTCOMES OF MULTIPLE ORGAN DYSFUNCTION SYNDROME

Both the heterogeneous patient population and lack of standardized scoring systems limit the tracking of progress in the management of MODS. Furthermore, both temporal and spatial comparisons are hindered by variations in severity of illness and thus likelihood of developing MODS. An earlier report of mortality following MODS reported no difference in either the incidence of (14%) or mortality from (60%) MODS when comparing patients admitted from 1979 to 1982 to those admitted from 1988 to 1990.[39] However, a substantial decrease in mortality was noted in those patients with what was considered severe organ failure (≥3 organs failed on day 4 or later). A later study (March-December 1997) found that mortality from MODS, defined as a MOD score of ≥2 for two organ systems and the necessity of an active ICU intervention, was 53%.[46] A still more recent prospective study (2005), reported a 17% incidence of MODS and 45% mortality in over 7,000 patients from 79 ICUs.[35] Barie et al.[44] showed that the severity-adjusted risk of mortality from MODS decreased steadily over a 17-year period of observation. Thus, mortality from MODS is decreasing over time. However, future studies using both standardized, incremental scoring systems and similar subject populations to compare outcomes in patients with organ failure are warranted.

Survival and Long-term Outcomes

Fewer than one-half of survivors of severe sepsis are alive 1 year later[157]; even less is known about survivors of MODS. Mortality is increased compared with life-table norms for several years thereafter. Risk factors for decreased long-term survival that are identifiable before hospital discharge have not been reported.

In one study, 56% of end-stage renal disease patients who required critical care for an episode of MODS survived their ICU stay.[158] Fifty-six percent of the survivors (31% of the total) were alive 2 years later; the mortality rate was higher for medical ICU patients as compared with surgical ICU patients. Survivors died at a faster rate than end-stage renal disease (ESRD) patients who did not require critical care, but this difference was abolished when deaths within 30 days of ICU discharge were discounted.

Ulvik et al.[159] examined long-term outcomes after trauma in a cohort of patients who developed MODS. Among 322 patients, 47% had MODS as assessed by the SOFA score, and 28% had single organ failure. The patients were contacted by telephone 2–7 years after discharge. At follow-up, 75% were still alive, and 52% had enjoyed a complete recovery. Long-term survival and functional status did not differ between survivors with no or single organ failure, whereas survivors of MODS had a six-fold increased risk of death, and a 3.9-fold increased risk of requiring assistance with activities of daily living.

THE FUTURE?

Understanding that sepsis and MODS are complex, chaotic systems and that taking a systems biology approach to their characterization is in its infancy, the future holds promise.[6] Genomic profiling may allow more useful characterizations of risk and outcomes.[160,161] Mathematical modeling (*translational systems biology*) aims to harness the power of computational simulation to streamline design of devices or drugs, identify therapeutic targets, simulate clinical trials, and predict the effects of drugs on individuals.[162–164]

The emerging field of metobolomics, a science of systems biology, is the global assessment of endogenous metabolites within a biologic system.[165] Detection of metabolites, whether in cells, tissues, or fluids, is conducted either by nuclear magnetic resonance spectroscopy or mass spectroscopy, with the data input into sophisticated multivariable analyses. Metobolomics could advance understanding of complex biologic systems such as ARDS and MODS, or aid in biomarker of drug target identification, it being reasonable to assume that a profile or pattern of indices is more likely to elucidate disease severity and progression than any one parameter (i.e., biomarker).

With new knowledge will come new approaches to therapy, likely in the realm of immunotherapy.[166] As sepsis-induced immunosuppression has come to be recognized as the overriding immune dysfunction in MODS, therapies may be directed in the future at enhancing immune responsiveness, as the opposite tactic (i.e., suppressing inflammation) clearly has not been successful. The prevention of sepsis-induced immune suppression, or its treatment if it occurs, is a research priority.[166] Although immunostimulatory therapy with agents such as IFN-γ and granulocyte-colony stimulating factor (G-CSF) has not been successful so far, IL- and IL-15 may be useful in the future. IL-7 (already in clinical trials to treat cancer and hepatitis C virus and human immunodeficiency virus infections) and IL-15 are anti-apoptotic, immunostimulatory cytokines that diminish the immunosuppressive effects on phagocytes by relieving them of the burden of clearing large numbers of apoptotic cells. IL-7 also improves the effector function of lymphocytes and their migration. Personalized medicine, for example, to use flow cytometry to identify patients with high levels of expression of negative co-stimulatory molecules on leukocytes, could be used to support the decision to use immunostimulatory therapy. Candidates for such therapy could be those patients with infections caused by opportunistic pathogens (e.g., *Stenotrophomonas*, *Acinetobacter*).

Ultimately, Cobb[167] has speculated that therapy of sepsis and MODS may evolve through several phases. Macrosystems engineering is possible now, in that performance improvement is a fixture of every ICU. Henceforth, advances in tissue engineering will allow the deployment of bioartificial organs for replacement. Ultimately, a new science of molecular engineering may permit the reprogramming of dysfunctional somatic cells by the manipulated overexpression of a few DNA transcription factors known to be central to the fate of embryonic stem cells. The reprogramming of the dysfunctional somatic cells to a more robust phenotype, referred to as *induced pluripotent stem cells*, has already been hailed as a scientific breakthrough.[168] These stem cells could be administered as cellular therapy to reprogram aged or dysfunctional organs to a state of renewed health, although many questions remain to be answered before these techniques are ready for the clinic.

References

1. Ashbaugh DG, Bigelow DB, Petty TL, et al. Acute respiratory distress in adults. *Lancet*. 1967;2:319-323.
2. Dutton RP, Stansbury LG, Leone S, et al. trauma mortality in mature trauma systems: Are we doing better? An analysis of trauma mortality patterns, 1997–2008. *J Trauma*. 2010;69:620-626.
3. Yende S, Angus DC. Long-term outcomes from sepsis. *Curr Infect Dis Rep*. 2007;9:382-386.
4. Gustot T. Multiple organ failure in sepsis: prognosis and role of systemic inflammatory response. *Curr Opin Crit Care*. 2011;17:153-169.
5. Singh S, Singh P, Singh G. Systemic inflammatory response syndrome outcome in surgical patients. *Indian J Surg*. 2009;71:206-209.
6. Papathanassoglou EDE, Bozas E, Giannakopoulou MD. Multiple organ dysfunction syndrome pathogenesis and care: a complex systems' theory perspective. *Nurs Crit Care*. 2008;13:247-259.
7. Skillman JJ, Goldman H, Silen W. Respiratory failure, hypotension, sepsis and jaundice. *Am J Surg*. 1969;117:523-530.
8. Tilney NL, Morgan AP. Sequential system failure after rupture of abdominal aortic aneurysms: an unsolved problem in postoperative care. *Ann Surg*. 1969;178:117-122.
9. Baue AE. Multiple, progressive, or sequential systems failure: a syndrome of the 1970s. *Arch Surg*. 1975;110:779-781.
10. Schwartz DB, Bone RC, Balk RA, et al. Hepatic dysfunction in the adult respiratory distress syndrome. *Chest*. 1989;95:871-875.
11. Barie PS, Hydo LJ, Eachempati SR. Nonpulmonary organ dysfunction and mortality with acute respiratory failure. *Chest*. 2008;134:467.
12. Brower RG, Matthay MA, Morris A, et al. Ventilation with lower tidal volumes as compared with traditional tidal volumes for acute lung injury and the acute respiratory distress syndrome. *N Engl J Med*. 2000;342:1301-1308.
13. Del Sorbo L, Slutsky AS. Acute respiratory distress syndrome and multiple organ failure. *Curr Opin Crit Care*. 2011;17:1-6.
14. Fry DE, Fulton RL, Polk HC Jr. Multiple system organ failure: The role of uncontrolled infection. *Arch Surg*. 1980;115:136-140.
15. Fry DE. Multiple organ dysfunction syndrome: past, present and future. *Surg Infect*. 2000;1:155-161.
16. Rowlands BJ, Soong CV, Gardiner KR. The gastrointestinal tract as a barrier in sepsis. *Br Med Bull*. 1999;55:196-211.
17. Sinanan M, Maier RV, Carrico CJ. Laparotomy for intra-abdominal sepsis in patients in an intensive care unit. *Arch Surg*. 1984;1:652-658.
18. Goris RJA, te Boekhorsh TPA, Nuytinic JKS, et al. Multiple organ failure: generalized autodestructive inflammation? *Arch Surg*. 1985;120:1109-1115.
19. Marshall JC, Christou NV, Horn R, et al. The microbiology of multiple organ failure: The proximal gastrointestinal tract as an occult reservoir of pathogens. *Arch Surg*. 1988;123:309-313.
20. Goris RJA, Boekholtz WKF, van Bebbler IPT, et al. Multiple organ failure and sepsis without bacteria: an experimental model. *Arch Surg*. 1986;121:897-901.
21. Goris RJA, van Bebber IP, Mollen RM, et al. Does selective decontamination of the gastrointestinal tract prevent multiple organ failure? An experimental study. *Arch Surg*. 1991;126:561-565.
22. Carrico CJ, Meakins JL, Marshall JC, et al. Multiple-organ failure syndrome: the gastrointestinal tract: the motor of MOF? *Arch Surg*. 1986;121:197-201.
23. Marshall JC, Christou NV, Horn R, et al. The microbiology of multiple organ failure. *Arch Surg*. 1988;123:309-315.
24. Cerra FB, Maddaus MA, Dunn DL, et al. Selective gut decontamination reduces nosocomial infections and length of stay but not mortality or organ failure in surgical intensive care unit patients. *Arch Surg*. 1992;127:163-169.
25. Marshall JC, Sweeney D. Microbial infection and the septic response in critical surgical illness: Sepsis, not infection, determines outcome. *Arch Surg*. 1990;125:17-23.
26. American College of Chest Physicians/Society of Critical Care Medicine Consensus Conference. Definitions for sepsis and organ failure, and guidelines for the use of innovative therapies in sepsis. *Crit Care Med*. 1992;20:864-874.
27. Talmor M, Hydo L, Barie PS. Relationship of systemic inflammatory response syndrome to organ dysfunction, length of stay, and mortality in critical surgical illness: effect of intensive care unit resuscitation. *Arch Surg*. 1999;134:81-87.
28. Marshall JC, Cook DJ, Christou NV, et al. Multiple Organ Dysfunction Score: a reliable descriptor of a complex clinical outcome. *Crit Care Med*. 1995;23:1638-1652.
29. Bernard G. The Brussels score. *Sepsis*. 1997;1:43-44.
30. Vincent JL, Moreno R, Takala J, et al. The SOFA (Sepsis-related Organ Failure Assessment) score to describe organ dysfunction/failure. On behalf of the Working Group of Sepsis-Related Problems of the European Society of Intensive Care Medicine. *Intensive Care Med*. 1996;22:707-710.
31. Le Gall JR, Klar J, Lemeshow S, et al. The logistic organ dysfunction system. A new way to assess organ dysfunction in the intensive care unit. *JAMA*. 1996;276:802-810.
32. Sauaia A, Moore EE, Johnson JL, et al. Validation of postinjury multiple organ failure scores. *Shock*. 2009;31:438-447.
33. Hanisch E, Brause R, Paetz J, et al. Review of a large clinical series: Predicting death for patients with abdominal septic shock. *J Intensive Care Med*. 2011;26:27-33.
34. Wang H, Ye L, Yu L, et al. Performance of sequential organ failure assessment, logistic orhan dysfunction, and multiple organ dysfunction score in severe sepsis within Chinese intensive care units. *Anaesth Intensive Care*. 2011;39:55-60.
35. Cabre L, Mancebo J, Solsona JF, et al. Multicenter study of the multiple organ dysfunction syndrome in intensive care units: the usefulness of Sequential Organ Failure Assessment scores in decision making. *Intensive Care Med*. 2005;31:927-933.
36. Dewar DC, Balogh ZJ. The epidemiology of multiple-organ failure: a definition controversy. *Acta Anesthesiol Scand*. 2011;55:248-249.
37. Heard SO, Fink MP. Multiple organ system failure syndrome—part I: epidemiology, prognosis, and pathophysiology. *J Intensive Care Med*. 1991;6:279-294.
38. Deitch EA. Multiple organ failure: pathophysiology and potential future therapy. *Ann Surg*. 1992;216:117-134.
39. Zimmerman JE, Knaus WA, Wagner DP, et al. A comparison of risks and outcomes for patients with organ system failure. *Crit Care Med*. 1996;24:1633-1641.
40. Wheeler AP, Bernard G. Treating patients with severe sepsis. *N Engl J Med*. 1999;340:207-214.
41. Tran DD, Groeneveld ABJ, van der Meulen J, et al. Age, chronic disease, sepsis, organ system failure, and mortality in a medical intensive care unit. *Crit Care Med*. 1990;18:474-479.
42. Tran DD, Cuesta MA, van Leeuwen PA, et al. Risk factors for multiple organ system failure and death in critically injured patients. *Surgery*. 1993;114:21-30.
43. Barie PS, Hydo LJ, Pieracci FM, et al. Multiple organ dysfunction syndrome in critical surgical illness. *Surg Infect* (*Larchmt*) 2009;10:369-377.
44. Barie PS, Hydo LJ, Shou J, et al. Decreasing magnitude of multiple organ dysfunction syndrome despite increasingly severe critical surgical illness: a 17-year longitudinal study. *J Trauma*. 2008;65:1227-1235.
45. Barie PS, Hydo LJ. Epidemiology of multiple organ dysfunction syndrome in critical surgical illness. *Surg Infect*. 2000;1:173-183.
46. Martin CM, Hill AD, Burns K, et al. Characteristics and outcomes for critically ill patients with prolonged intensive care unit stays. *Crit Care Med*. 2005;33:1922-1927.
47. Barie PS, Hydo LJ. Influence of multiple organ dysfunction syndrome on duration of critical illness and hospitalization. *Arch Surg*. 1996;131:1318-1323;
48. Eachempati SR, Hydo LJ, Shou J, et al. Outcomes of acute respiratory distress syndrome (ARDS) in elderly patients. *J Trauma*. 2007;63:344-350.
49. Sauaia A, Moore FA, Moore EE, et al. Early predictors of postinjury multiple organ failure. *Arch Surg*. 1994;129:39-45.
50. Cryer HG, Leong K, McArthur DL, et al. Multiple organ failure: by the time you predict it, it's already there. *J Trauma*. 1999;46:597-604.
51. Perl TM, Dvorak L, Hwang T, et al. Long-term survival and function after suspected gram-negative sepsis. *JAMA*. 1995;274:338-345.
52. Mayr FB, Yende S, Linde-Zwirble WT, et al. infection rate and acute organ dysfunction risk as explanations for racial differences in severe sepsis. *JAMA*. 2010;303:2495-2503.
53. Proulx F, Joyal JS, Mariscalco MM, et al. The pediatric multiple organ dysfunction syndrome. *Pediatr Crit Care Med*. 2009;10:12-22.
54. Bestati N, Leteurtre S, Duhamel A, et al. Differences in organ dysfunctions between neonates and older children: a prospective, observational, multicenter study. *Crit Care*. 2010;14:R202.
55. Knight JC. Kwiatkowski D. Inherited variability of tumor necrosis factor production and susceptibility to infectious disease. *Proc Assoc Am Physicians*. 1999;111:290-298.
56. Gu W, Jiang J. Genetic polymorphisms and posttraumatic complications. *Comp Funct Genomics* 2010:814086.
57. Hildebrand F, Mommsen P, Frink M, et al. Genetic predisposition for development of complications in multiple trauma patients. *Shock*. 2011;35:440-448.
58. Humphries SE, Luong LA, Montgomery HE, et al. Gene-environment interaction in the determination of levels of plasma fibrinogen. *Thromb Haemost*. 1999;82:818-825.
59. Moore FA, Moore EE. Evolving concepts in the pathogenesis of postinjury multiple organ failure. *Surg Clin North Am*. 1995;75:257-277.
60. Cryer HG. Advances in the understanding of multiple organ failure. *Surg Infect*. 2000;1:165-170.

61. Mevorach D, Trahtemberg U, Krispin A, et al. what do we mean when we write "senescence," "apoptosis," "necrosis," or "clearance of dying cells?" *Ann N Y Acad Sci.* 2010:1209:1-9.
62. Hattori Y, Takano K, Teramae H, et al. Insights into sepsis therapeutic design based on the apoptotic death pathway. *J Pharmacol Sci.* 2010;114:354-365.
63. Vanhorebeek I, Gunst J, Derde S, et al. Insufficient activation of autophagy allows cellular damage to accumulate in critically ill patients. *J Clin Endocrinol Metab.* 2011;96:E633-E645.
64. Kimura F, Shimizu H, Yoshidome H, et al. Immunosuppression following surgical and traumatic injury. *Surg Today.* 2010;40:793-808.
65. Bone RC. Immunologic dissonance: a continuing evolution in our understanding of the systemic inflammatory response syndrome (SIRS) and multiple organ dysfunction syndrome (MODS). *Ann Intern Med.* 1996;125:680-687.
66. Fink MP, Delude RL. Epithelial barrier dysfunction: A unifying theme to explain the pathogenesis of multiple organ dysfunction at the cellular level. *Crit Care Clin.* 2005;21:177-196.
67. Sessler CN, Bloomfield GL, Fowler AA. Current concepts of sepsis and acute lung injury. *Clin Chest Med.* 1996;17:213-235.
68. Stephens KE, Ishizaka A, Wu ZH, et al. Granulocyte depletion prevents TNF-mediated acute lung injury in guinea pigs. *Am Rev Respir Dis.* 1988;138:1300-1307.
69. Nathens AB, Marshall JC, Watson RWG, et al. Diethylmaleate ameriorates endotoxin-induced acute lung injury. *Surgery.* 1996;120:360-366.
70. Barie PS, Malik AB. Role of intravascular coagulation and granulocytes in lung vascular injury after bone marrow embolism. *Circ Res.* 1982;50:830-838.
71. Barie PS, Tahamont MV, Malik AB. Prevention of increased pulmonary vascular permeability after pancreatitis by granulocyte depletion in sheep. *Am Rev Respir Dis.* 1982;126:904-908.
72. Roumen RM, Redl H, Schlag G, et al. Inflammatory mediators in relation to the development of multiple organ failure in patients after severe blunt trauma. *Crit Care Med.* 1995;23:474-480.
73. Davicino RC, Eliçabe RJ, Di Genaro MS, et al. Coupling pathogen recognition to innate immunity through glycan-dependent mechanisms. *Int Immunopharmacol.* 2011;11:1457-1463.
74. Zoelen MA, Achouiti A, van der Poll T. RAGE during infectious diseases. *Front Biosci (Schol Ed).* 2011;3:1119-1132.
75. Andersson U, Tracey KJ. HMGB1 is a therapeutic target for sterile inflammation and infection. *Annu Rev Immunol.* 2011;29:139-162.
76. Huang W, Tang Y, Li L. HMGB1, a potent proinflammatory cytokine in sepsis. *Cytokine.* 201051:119-126.
77. Bopp C, Bierhaus A, Hofer S, et al. Bench-to-bedside review: The inflammation-perpetuating pattern-recognition receptor RAGE as a therapeutic target in sepsis. *Crit Care.* 2008;12:201.
78. Papathanassoglou ED, Moynihan JA, Vermillion DL, et al. Soluble Fas levels correlate with multiple organ dysfunction severity, survival, and nitrate levels, but not with cellular apoptotic markers in critically ill patients. *Shock.* 2000;14:107-112.
79. Yamada Y, Endo S, Nakae H, et al. Nuclear matrix protein levels in burn patients with multiple organ dysfunction syndrome. *Burns.* 1999;25:705-708.
80. Hotchkiss RS, Schmieg RE Jr, Swanson PE, et al. Rapid onset of intestinal epithelial and lymphocyte apoptotic cell death in patients with trauma and shock. *Crit Care Med.* 2000;28:3207-3217.
81. Jimenez MF, Watson RWG, Parodo J, et al. Dysregulated expression of neutrophil apoptosis in the systemic inflammatory response syndrome (SIRS). *Arch Surg.* 1997;132:1263-1270.
82. Hotchkiss RS, Swanson PE, Freeman BD, et al. Apoptotic cell death in patients with sepsis, shock, and multiple organ dysfunction. *Crit Care Med.* 1999;27:1230-1251.
83. Hotchkiss RS, Strasser A, McDunn JE, et al. Cell death. *N Engl J Med.* 2009;361:1570-1583.
84. Dorinsky PM, Gadek JE. Mechanisms of multiple nonpulmonary organ failure in ARDS. *Chest.* 1989; 96:885-892.
85. van der Poll T, Daan de Boer J, et al. The effect of inflammation on coagulation and vice versa. *Curr Opin Infect Dis.* 2011;24:273-278.
86. Ryu J, Pyo H, Jou I, et al. Thrombin induces NO release from cultured rat microglia via protein kinase C, mitogen-activated protein kinase and NF-kB. *J Biol Chem.* 2000;275:29955-2999.
87. Gando S, Nanzaki S, Kemmotsu O. Disseminated intravascular coagulation and sustained systemic inflammatory response syndrome predict organ dysfunctions after trauma: application of clinical decision analysis. *Ann Surg.* 1999;229:121-127.
88. Hotchkiss RS, Karl IE. The pathophysiology and treatment of sepsis. *N Engl J Med.* 2003;348:138-150.
89. Marchant A, Alegre ML, Hakim A, et al. Clinical and biological significance of interleukin-10 plasma levels in patients with septic shock. *J Clin Immunol.* 1995;15:266-273.
90. Miller-Graziano CL, Szabo G, Griffey K, et al. Role of elevated monocyte transforming growth factor β (TGF-β) production in posttrauma immunosuppression. *J Clin Immunol.* 1991;11:95-102.
91. Volk RP, Döcke WD. Immunostimulation with cytokines in patients with 'immunoparalysis.' In: Marshall JC, Cohen J, eds. *Immune Response in the Critically Ill.* Berlin, Germany: Springer-Verlag; 1999:393-404.
92. Godin PJ, Buchman TG. Uncoupling of biologic oscillators: a complementary hypothesis concerning the pathogenesis of multiple organ dysfunction syndrome. *Crit Care Med.* 1996;24:1107-1116.
93. Godin PJ, Fleisher LA, Eidsath A, et al. Experimental human endotoxemia increases cardiac regularity: results from a prospective, randomized, crossover trial. *Crit Care Med.* 1996;24:1117-1124.
94. Barnaby D, Ferrick K, Kaplan D, et al. Heart rate variability in emergency department patient with sepsis. *Acad Emerg Med.* 2002;9:661-670.
95. Winchell RJ, Hoyt DB. Spectral analysis of heart rate variability in the ICU: a measure of autonomic function. *J Surg Res.* 1996;63:11-16.
96. Winchell RJ, Hoyt DB. Analysis of heart-rate variability: a pnoninvasive predictor of death and poor outcome in patients with severe head injury. *J Trauma.* 1997;43:927-933.
97. Buchman TG. Nonlinear dynamics, complex systems, and the pathobiology of critical illness. *Curr Opin Crit Care.* 2004;10:378-382.
98. Schmidt H, Muller-Werdan US, Hoffman T, et al. Autonomic dysfunction predicts mortality in patients with multiple organ dysfunction syndrome of different age groups. *Crit Care Med.* 2005;33:1994-2004.
99. Buchman TG, Stein PK, Goldstein B. Heart rate variability in critical illness and critical care. *Curr Opin Crit Care.* 2002;8:311-315.
100. Seely AJ, Christou NV. Multiple organ dysfunction syndrome: exploring the paradigm of complex nonlinear systems. *Crit Care Med.* 2000;28:2193-2200.
101. Norris PR, Canter JA, Jenkins JM, et al. Personalized medicine: genetic variation and loss of physiologic complexity are associated with mortality in 644 trauma patients. *Ann Surg.* 2009;250:524-530.
102. Balija TM, Lowry SF. Lipopolysaccharide and sepsis-induced myocardial dysfunction. *Curr Opin Infect Dis.* 2011;24:248-253.
103. Ungureanu-Longrois D, Balligand J, Kelly RA, et al. Myocardial contractile dysfunction in the systemic inflammatory response syndrome: a cytokine-inducible nitric oxide synthase in cardiac myocytes. *J Mol Cell Cardiol.* 1995;27:155-167.
104. Del Sorbo L, Slutsky AS. Acute respiratory distress syndrome and multiple organ failure. *Curr Opin Crit Care.* 2011;17:1-6.
105. Burns KE, Adhikari NK, Slutsky AS, et al. Pressure and volume limited ventilation for the ventilatory management of patients with acute lung injury: A systematic review and meta-analysis. *PLoS One.* 2011;6(1):e14623.
106. Sebag SC, Bastarache JA, Ware LB. Therapeutic modulation of coagulation and fibrinolysis in acute lung injury and the acute respiratory distress syndrome. *Curr Pharm Biotechnol.* 2011 Mar 14 [Epub ahead of print].
107. Jelkmann W, Pagel H, Wolff M, et al. Monokines inhibiting erythropoietin production in human hepatoma cultures and in isolated perfused rat kidneys. *Life Sci.* 1992;50:301-308.
108. Jelkmann W. Proinflammatory cytokines lowering erythropoietin production. *J Interferon Cytokine Res.* 1998;18:555-559.
109. Faquin WC, Schneider TJ, Goldberg MA. Effect of inflammatory cytokines on hypoxia-induced erythropoietin production. *Blood.* 1992;79:1987-1994.
110. Frede S, Fandrey J, Pagel H, et al. Erythropoietin gene expression is suppressed after lipopolysaccharide or interleukin-1 beta injections in rats. *Am J Physiol.* 1997;273:R1067-R1071.
111. Moldawer LL, Marano MA, Wei H, et al. Cachectin/tumor necrosis factor alters red blood cell kinetics and induces anemia in vivo. *FASEB J.* 1989;3:1637-1643.
112. Alvarez-Hernandez X, Liceaga J, McKay IC, et al. Induction of hypoferremia and modulation of macrophage iron metabolism by tumor necrosis factor. *Lab Invest.* 1989;61:319-322.
113. Rogers JT, Bridges KR, Durmowicz GP, et al. Translational control during the acute phase response. Ferritin synthesis in response to interleukin-1. *J Biol Chem.* 1990;265:14572-14578.
114. Ukleja A. Altered GI motility in critically ill patients: current understanding of pathophysiology, clinical impact, and diagnostic approach. *Nutr Clin Pract.* 2010;25:16-25.
115. De Winter BY, De Man JG. Interplay between inflammation, immune system, and neuronal pathways: effect on gastrointestinal motility. *World J Gastroenterol.* 2010;16:5523-5525.
116. Barie PS, Eachempati SR. Acute acalculous cholecystitis. *Gastroenterol Clin North Am.* 2010;39:343-357.
117. Davis MG, Hagen PO. Systemic inflammatory response syndrome. *Br J Surg.* 1997;84:920-935.
118. Faries PL, Simon RJ, Martella AT, et al. Intestinal permeability correlates with severity of injury in trauma patients. *J Trauma.* 1998;44:1031-1036.
119. Peters JH, Beishuizen A, Keur MB, et al. Assessment of small bowel function in critical illness: Potential role of citrulline metabolism. *J Intensive Care Med.* 2011;26:105-110.
120. Franson TR, LaBrecque DR, Buggy BP, et al. Serial bilirubin determinations as a prognostic marker in clinical infections. *Am J Med Sci.* 1989;297:149-152.
121. Maynard ND, Bihari DJ, Dalton RN, et al. Liver function and splanchnic ischemia in critically ill patients. *Chest.* 1997;111:180-187.
122. Griffiths RD, Hall JB. Intensive care unit-acquired weakness. *Crit Care Med.* 2010;38:779-787.
123. Leijten FS, Harineck-de Werd JE, Poortvliet DC, et al. The role of polyneuropathy in motor convalescence after prolonged mechanical ventilation. *JAMA.* 1991;274:1221-1225.
124. Ferreira FL, Peres Bota D, Bross A, et al. Serial evaluation of the SOFA score to predict outcome in critically ill patients. *JAMA.* 2001;86:1754-1758.

125. Rivers E, Nguyen B, Navstad S, et al. Early goal-directed therapy in the treatment of severe sepsis and septic shock. *N Engl J Med.* 2001;345:1368-1377.
126. Sigounas DE, Tatsioni A, christoudoulou DK, et al. New prognostic markers for outcome of acute pancreatitis, overview of reporting in 184 studies. *Pancreas.* 2011;40:522-532.
127. Nguyen HB, Loomba M, Yang JJ, et al. early lactate clearance is associated with biomarkers of inflammation, coagulation, apoptosis, organ dysfunction, and mortality in severe sepsis and septic shock. *J Inflamm (Lond).* 2010;7:6.
128. Cuschieri J, Bulger E, Schaeffer V, et al. Inflammation and the Host Response to Injury Collaborative Research Project. Early elevation in random plasma IL-6 after injury is associated with development of organ failure. *Shock.* 2010;34:346-351.
129. Sun T, Wang X, Liu Z, et al. Plasma concentrations of pro- and anti-inflammatory cytokines and outcome prediction in elderly hip fracture patients. *Injury.* 2011;42:707-713.
130. Jastrow KM, Gonzalez EA, McGuire MF, et al. early cytokine production risk stratifies trauma patients for multiple organ failure. *J Am Coll Surg.* 2009;209:320-331.
131. Mera S, Tatulescu D, Cismaru C, et al. Multiplex cytokine profiling in patients with sepsis. *APMIS.* 2011;119:155-163.
132. Haasper C, Kalmbach M, Dikos GD, et al. Prognostic value of procalcitonin (PCT) and/or interleukin-6 (IL-6) plasma levels after multiple trauma for the development of multi organ dysfunction syndrome (MODS) or sepsis. *Technol Health Care.* 2010;18:89-100.
133. Castelli GP, Pognani C, Cita M, et al. Procalcitonin as a prognostic and diagnostic tool for septic complications after major trauma. *Crit Care Med.* 2009;37:1845-1849.
134. Ge QG, Yin CH, Wen Y, et al. [Clinical study of relationship between serum procalcitonin and severity of multiple organ dysfunction syndrome] (Chinese). *Zhongguo Wei Zhong Bing Ji Jiu Yi Xue.* 2005;17:729-731.
135. Latour-Perez J, Palencia-Herejon E, Gomez-Tello V, et al. Intensity of continuous renal replacement therapies in patients with severe sepsis and septic shock: a systematic review and meta-analysis. *Anaesth Intensive Care.* 2011;39:373-383.
136. Van den Berghe G, Wouters P, Weekers F, et al. Intensive insulin therapy in critically ill patients. *N Engl J Med.* 2001;345:1359-1367.
137. Bocchichio GV, Bocchichio KM, Joshi M, et al. Acute glucose elevation is highly preductive of infection and outcome in critically injured trauma patients. *Ann Surg.* 2010;252:597-602.
138. Griesdale DE, deSouza RJ, van Dam RM, et al. Intensive insulin therapy and mortality among critically ill patients: A meta-analysis including NICE-SUGAR study data. *CMAJ.* 2009;180:821-827.
139. Hayes MA, Timmins AC, Yau EF, et al. Elevation of systemic oxygen delivery in the treatment of critically ill patients. *N Engl J Med.* 1994;330:1717-1722.
140. Gattinoni L, Brazzi L, Pelosi P, et al. A trial of goal-oriented hemodynamic therapy in critically ill patients. *N Engl J Med.* 1995;333:1025-1032.
141. Herbert PC, Wells G, Blajchman MA, et al. A multicenter, randomized, controlled clinical trial of transfusion requirements in critical care: Transfusion Requirements in Critical Care Trials Group. *N Engl J Med.* 1999;340:409-417
142. Alia I, Esteban A, Gordo F, et al. A randomized and controlled trial of the effect of treatment aimed at maximizing oxygen delivery in patients with severe sepsis or septic shock. *Chest.* 1999;115:453-461.
143. Moore FA, Moore EE, Sauaia A. Blood transfusion. An independent risk factor for postinjury multiple organ failure. *Arch Surg.* 1997;132:620-624.
144. Watson GA, Sperry JL, Rosengart MR, et al. Inflammation and Host Response to Injury Investigators. Fresh frozen plasma is independently associated with a higher risk of multiple organ failure and acute respiratory distress syndrome. *J Trauma.* 2009;67:221-227.
145. Karam O, Tucci M, Bateman ST, et al. Association between length of storage of red blood cell units and outcome of critically ill children: a prospective observational study. *Crit Care.* 2010;14:R57.
146. Johnson JJ, Moore EE, Kashuk JL, et al. Effect of blood products transfusion on the development of postinjury multiple organ failure. *Arch Surg.* 2010;145:973-977.
147. Murad MH, Stubbs JR, Gandhi MJ, et al. The effect of plasma transfusion on morbidity and mortality: a systematic review and meta-analysis. *Transfusion.* 2010;50:1370-1383.
148. Ulldemolins M, Roberts JA, Lipman J, et al. Antibiotic dosing in multiple organ dysfunction syndrome. *Chest.* 2011;139:1210-1220.
149. Marshall JC. Clinical trials of mediator-directed therapy in sepsis: what have we learned? *Intensive Care Med.* 2000;26:S75-S83.
150. Spruijt NE, Visser T, Leenen LPH. A systematic review of randomized controlled trials exploring the effect of immunomodulative interventions on infection, organ failure, and mortality in trauma patients. *Crit Care.* 2010;14:R150.
151. Zeni F, Freeman B, Natanson C. Anti-inflammatory therapies to treat sepsis and septic shock. A reassessment. *Crit Care Med.* 1997;25:1095-1100.
152. Bernard GR, Vincent J, Laterre P, et al. Efficacy and safety of recombinant human activated protein C for severe sepsis. *N Engl J Med.* 2001;344:699-709.
153. Barie PS. Current role of activated protein C therapy for severe sepsis and septic shock. *Curr Infect Dis Rep.* 2008;10:368-376.
154. Vincent JL, Angus DC, Artigas A, et al. Effects of drotrecogin alfa (activated) on organ dysfunction in the PROWESS trial. *Crit Care Med.* 2003;31:834-40.
155. Dellinger RP, Levy MM, Carlet JM, et al., International Surviving Sepsis Campaign Guidelines Committee; American Association of Critical-Care Nurses; American College of Chest Physicians; American College of Emergency Physicians; Canadian Critical Care Society; European Society of Clinical Microbiology and Infectious Diseases; European Society of Intensive Care Medicine; European Respiratory Society; International Sepsis Forum; Japanese Association for Acute Medicine; Japanese Society of Intensive Care Medicine; Society of Critical Care Medicine; Society of Hospital Medicine; Surgical Infection Society; World Federation of Societies of Intensive and Critical Care Medicine. Surviving Sepsis Campaign: International guidelines for management of severe sepsis and septic shock: 2008. *Crit Care Med.* 2008;36:296-327. Erratum in: *Crit Care Med.* 2008;36:1394-1396.
156. Levy MM, Dellinger RP, Townsend SR, et al.; Surviving Sepsis Campaign. The Surviving Sepsis Campaign: results of an international guideline-based performance improvement program targeting severe sepsis. *Crit Care Med.* 2010;38:367-374.
157. Yende S, Angus DC. Long-term outcomes from sepsis. *Curr Infect Dis Rep.* 2007;9:382-386.
158. Chapman RJ, Templeton M, Ashworth S, et al. Long-term survival of chronic dialysis patients following survival from an episode of multiple-organ failure. *Crit Care.* 2009;13:R65.
159. Ulvik A, Kvale R, Wentzel-Larsen T, et al. Multiple organ failure after trauma affects even long-term survival and functional status. *Crit Care.* 2007;11:R95.
160. Warren HS, Elson CM, Hayden DL, et al. A genomic score prognostic of outcome in trauma patients. *Mol Med.* 2009;15:220-227.
161. Rajicic N, Cuschieri J, Finkelstein DM, et al.; Inflammation and the Host Response to Injury Large Scale Collaborative Research Group. Identification and interpretation of longitudinal gene expression changes in trauma. *PLoS One.* 2010;5:e14380.
162. An G, Mi Q, Dutta-Moscato J, Vodovotz Y. Agent-based models in translational systems biology. *Wiley Interdisp Rev Syst Biol Med.* 2009;1:159-171.
163. Luan D, Szlam F, Tanaka KA, et al. Ensembles of uncertain mathematical models can identify network response to therapeutic interventions. *Mol Biosyst.* 2010;6:2272-2286.
164. Luan D, Zai M, Varner JD. Computationally derived points of fragility of a human cascade are consistent with current therapeutic strategies. *PLoS Comput Biol.* 2007;3:e142.
165. Serkova NJ, Standiford TJ, Stringer KA. The emerging field of quantitative blood metobolomics for biomarker discovery in critical illnesses. *Am Rev Respir Crit Care Med.* 2011;184:647-655.
166. Hotchkiss RS, Opal S. Immunotherapy for sepsis-A new approach against an ancient foe. *N Engl J Med.* 2010;363:87-89.
167. Cobb JP. MORE for multiple organ dysfunction syndrome: Multiple Organ REanimation, REgeneration, and REprogramming. *Crit Care Med.* 2010;38:2242-2246.
168. Vogel G. Breakthrough of the year: reprogramming cells. *Science.* 2008;322:1766-1767.

CHAPTER 49 ■ MECHANICAL VENTILATOR SUPPORT

MARC J. SHAPIRO AND BRIAN M. HALL

The respiratory system is responsible for both oxygenation and ventilation. Oxygenation is the ability to provide oxygen to the tissues. Ventilation is the removal of carbon dioxide via the lungs to maintain a neutral pH. When the ability to breathe is compromised, whether it is secondary to hypoxia, acidosis, injury, oversedation, somnolence, muscle fatigue, or other issues, supplemental and artificial modes must be employed in order to provide adequate oxygenation and ventilation; these methods will be discussed.

NONINVASIVE VENTILATION

As part of the evaluation and treatment of patients, there are a number of adjuncts that can be utilized in an attempt to preclude the need for intubation with an artificial airway and mechanical ventilation.[1] To address hypoxemia, supplemental oxygen should be initiated.

The basic form of oxygen supplementation is via a nasal cannula. Oxygen is delivered through prongs that are inserted into the nares and can be regulated between a low flow (1–2 L/minute) and a high flow concentration (10 L/minute), although the higher flow rates can be uncomfortable for a patient. Flows up to 20 L/min with humidification have also been used to create a continuous positive airway pressure (CPAP) effect as well. This oxygen supply is either from a wall source via a regulator or from an oxygen tank. Caution must be exercised in patients with end-stage or chronic pulmonary disease as many of these patients rely on hypoxia to provide their respiratory drive. Providing too high an arterial oxygen saturation can abolish this drive.

If a nasal cannula is inefficient in oxygen delivery, that is, delivery of oxygen to a mouth breather, other modalities may be employed. Oxygen delivery via a face mask is a simple means to improve oxygenation in a patient. Oxygen flow from a wall circuit or a specialized tank can increase the concentration of oxygen in inspired air to approximately 55%. Openings on the side of the mask allow removal of CO_2 without effort. However, if an individual's tidal volume (TV) is high, room air may be entrained into the mask, thus diminishing the enriched oxygen concentration. To diminish this latter effect, the patient may be switched to a venturi mask. This apparatus is similar in appearance to a face mask, but has one way valves replacing the openings on the side of the mask. This allows an increase in enriched oxygen concentrations up to 80% at the tertiary bronchioles, as well as CO_2 removal. Another less frequently used noninvasive oxygen delivery system is a face tent. This fits below the chin and oxygen flow is directed into the oral and nasal passages without the mask actually touching the face. This is particularly useful in patients with burns, macerated facial skin, etc. and can provide up to 50% oxygen concentration levels.

Higher concentrated levels of oxygen can be provided by CPAP or bilevel positive airway pressure mask. This is a mask that is firmly secured over the nose and/or mouth, and delivers concentrated oxygen under positive pressure. Prior to initiation of this treatment, the patient should be awake, able to cough and may require gastric decompression via a nasogastric tube. This is done to avoid gastric distension and aspiration resulting from the aerophagia generated from the provided pressure.

MECHANICAL VENTILATION

Ventilation using mechanical means has seen changes from a century ago when the use of negative pressure ventilation and the so called "iron lung" was utilized during the polio epidemic. This has progressed to the current usage of positive pressure ventilation with digital rather than analogue technology. Advanced computer technology incorporating patient data and operator data, coupled with pharmacomanipulation and ancillary assistance described below has also led to the improvement of mechanical ventilation.[2–6]

Ventilation–perfusion ratio (V/Q) looks at oxygen consumption and CO_2 production. It assumes that there is a near linear relationship between CO_2 and PCO_2. Alveolar–capillary gas transport can be expressed as $DO_2I = (SaO_2 \times Hb \times 1.34) + (0.0031 \times PaO_2) \times CI \times 10$ where DO_2I is oxygen delivery index and normal values are 500–600 mL O_2/min/m^2. Oxygen consumption is generally 25% of oxygen delivery and together give rise to the extraction ratio or A-VO_2 difference, with normal being 5 mL O_2/dL of blood. In times of high O_2 demands, the normal tissues can extract 50% or more O_2 from the blood. In various conditions however, such as SIRS, the extraction is less.

Ventilation

The ventilator circuit is approximately 60 inches of corrugated plastic tubing connecting the ventilator to the artificial patient airway, for example, an endotracheal (ET) or tracheostomy tube. The circuit may contain filters, humidifiers, water traps, heated wires, artificial noses, closed suction catheters, and devices for aerosol administration or capnography and is directly connected to the ventilator.

To determine acceptable placement of the ET tube, a colorimetric CO_2 detector may be used. This device has a pH-sensitive chemical bonded to a specialized paper element that changes color with ventilation in the presence of CO_2. During CPR this detector is of limited value. The cardiac output, and thus the pulmonary blood flow, may both be diminished and CO_2 may not be exchanged, let alone exhaled. Another device available to verify ET tube placement into the trachea is the esophageal detection device. Negative pressure applied at the end of the artificial airway allows the bulb to inflate if the ET tube is in the trachea on inspiration. This relies on the fact that with inspiration the lungs are distended and the esophagus is collapsed and thus the bulb will not fill if the ET tube is in the esophagus, unless the patient has had a large amount of gas insufflated into the esophagus such as from manual ventilation.

Aside from the traditional ET tube, tubes impregnated with silver and tubes with a supraglottic suction port to prevent secretions from contaminating the respiratory tree, have been used. Both adjuncts add considerable cost to the tubes with little proven benefit.

The cycle of respiration using mechanical ventilation consists of the following steps:

1. A trigger either by the patient or the machine to initiate a breath may be in the form of a set time, pressure, or volume.
2. The volume or pressure goal, if set, is reached and may also be influenced by flow sensitivity.
3. Then based on whether volume cycled, time cycled, flow cycled, or pressure cycled, the inspiratory phase is completed and there may be a pause.
4. The exhalation phase then begins, which in most cases is passive and dependent in part on pulmonary compliance and airway and equipment resistance, the product of which is called the time constant (Tc).

Terms Utilized for Mechanical Ventilation

1. TV is the amount of air the patient inspires or is delivered by the ventilator during an inspiration (mL).
2. Respiratory rate or frequency is the number of breaths per minute and may include the patient's breaths, the ventilator breaths or both.
3. Minute volume ventilation (MVV) is the product of the TV and the frequency (L/minute).
4. Peak airway pressure (Paw) is the pressure required to deliver the set TV to the patient (cm H_2O).
5. Plateau pressure (Pplat) is the pressure necessary to distend the lung at end inspiration (cm H_2O).
6. Mean airway pressure (Maw) is the average pressure delivered (cm H_2O).
7. Inspiratory time (IT) is the number of seconds required to deliver a set TV.
8. Peak inspiratory flow is the highest flow during the inspiratory phase used to deliver the set TV (L/min).
9. FiO_2 is the fraction of inspired oxygen or the concentration of inspired oxygen gas with 0.21 (21%) being room air and 1.0 (100%) being the maximum short of using a hyperbaric chamber.
10. Compliance is the change in volume divided by the change in transthoracic pressure.
11. Elastance is the change in transthoracic pressure divided by the change in volume.
12. Resistance is the ratio of change in pressure to change in volume.
13. Static compliance is the ability of the alveoli to expand with increasing volume or pressure and is measured in a no-flow condition. It is expressed as the ratio of the change in volume over the change in alveolar pressure. Dynamic compliance is the same ratio while flow is occurring. The opposite of compliance is elastance.

Modes of Mechanical Ventilation

Mechanical ventilators operate via one of two modes: pressure control or volume control (Table 49.1). Pressure control is a mode of ventilation where the pressure delivered with each breath is constant.[7] Volume control ventilation is a mode where the volume of each breath delivered remains constant. Dual control implies that breaths are a combination of volume and pressure control. There are wide ranges of other modes of mechanical ventilation, which are detailed below (Table 49.2):

CMV is continuous mandatory ventilation in which all breaths are delivered by the ventilator at a minimum preset frequency to a preset volume (Table 49.1). It is rarely used today as it is considered an unnatural form of ventilation, and thus should only be considered in patients who are chemically paralyzed.

ACV is assist–control ventilation in which a set volume is delivered at a set minimum frequency. In addition, the patient can trigger the ventilator to deliver an additional breath at the preset volume or pressure above the preset frequency.

IMV is intermittent mandatory ventilation in which the machine breaths are delivered at a set frequency, volume, and pressure.[8] Any additional breaths are spontaneous with patient generated volumes or pressure. This form of ventilation is primarily utilized in the NICU.

SIMV is synchronized intermittent mandatory ventilation where the ventilator delivered breath is presented within a preset time, preferably in concert with the patient's inspiratory effort. If there is little or no spontaneous breathing, a time triggered breath is delivered in the absence of a patient generated breath. Patients can be weaned from this mode of ventilation.

PSV is pressure support ventilation in which the patient's inspiratory effort is assisted by the ventilator to a preset pressure. This mode of ventilation is patient triggered, pressure limited, and flow cycled, allowing patients to set their own frequency, IT, and volume. Patients can be weaned from this mode of ventilation (Algorithm 49.1).

CPAP is continuous positive airway pressure where a constant level of positive pressure is set while the patient is breathing spontaneously. This mode can be used prior to extubation or decannulation of a mechanically ventilated patient.

APRV is airway pressure release ventilation that allows spontaneous breathing. The patient ventilates with a high pressure (*Phi*) level, which is essentially CPAP, and during the inspiratory phase the *Phi* is released at a set low pressure level (*Plo*). The time spent at each level of ventilation is the T*hi* or the IT and T*lo*, which is the expiratory time. The spontaneous breaths are pressure controlled, pressure triggered, pressure limited, and pressure cycled. APRV allows spontaneous breaths during the inflation period. This mode is attractive in that it may limit acute lung injury (ALI) by decreasing maximal pressures and increasing mean pressures, thus improving oxygenation.[9–11]

PCIRV is pressure controlled inverse ratio ventilation and is a time triggered, pressure limited, and time cycled mode of ventilation in which all breaths are mandatory.[7] This mode generally has inspiration times longer than exhalation. When spontaneous breathing is absent this is similar to APRV.

PRVC is pressure-regulated volume control where the TV is set and the inspiratory pressure is adjusted by the ventilator to assure the preset volume delivery.

TABLE 49.1

CONTROLLED MANDATORY VENTILATION VS. PRESSURE CONTROLLED VENTILATION

	CMV	PCV
Tidal volume	Constant	Variable
Peak inspiratory pressure	Variable	Constant
Inspiratory time	Set directly or indirectly	Constant
Inspiratory flow	Set directly or indirectly	Variable
Inspiratory flow waveform	Constant	Variable

TABLE 49.2

BASIC MODES OF MECHANICAL VENTILATION

	TIDAL VOLUME (TV)	ADVANTAGE	DISADVANTAGE
Volume Assist Control (VAC)	Volume triggered	MVV set	Plateau pressure varies
Pressure Assist Control (PAC)	Pressure triggered	Comfortable for patient Pressure limited	Variable V_T
Pressure Support (PS)	Patient triggered Pressure target	Comfortable for patient Good synchrony	Requires patient respiratory drive
Synchronous Intermittent Mechanical Ventilation (SIMV)	Preset, synchronized TV	More natural form of ventilation	Increases work of breathing

HFOV is high-frequency oscillatory ventilation with low TVs and small airway fluctuations. The goal of this mode is to decrease mean airway pressures, while avoiding stacking of breaths. The frequencies may vary between 100 and 900 breaths per minute with gas transport via nonconvective mechanisms.[12] The most successful use for HFOV has been in the treatment of respiratory failure in premature infants.

PAV is proportional assist ventilation, which is an interactive ventilatory mode to improve synchrony between patient ventilatory demand and ventilator support.[13] The ventilator provides dynamic inspiratory pressure assistance in linear proportion to patient inspiratory effort. For PAV to work the patient must be spontaneously breathing. If the patient tires, PAV will not provide the ventilatory support for a targeted pressure or volume.

Permissive hypercapnia is a modality of ventilation utilized to remove carbon dioxide from the blood when more conventional methods, that is, increasing the rate and decreasing TV, are unsuccessful. The manipulation of the ventilator to allow the PCO_2 to rise upwards to 50–80 mm Hg or higher, while not jeopardizing arterial pH, is the goal of this therapy. This form of ventilation is another mode of lung-protective ventilation, and may be required in patients with a PaO_2:FiO_2 ratio below 300.

PEEP is positive end-expiratory pressure and occurs at the end of exhalation and prevents the deflation and collapse of an alveolus opened during inspiration. The primary role of PEEP is alveoli recruitment. Under normal circumstances, the alveolar and airway pressures are equal with complete lung emptying. Intrinsic PEEP occurs when lung emptying is not complete and the airway pressure rises to equal that of the elevated alveolar pressure. In this circumstance, if PEEP continues to rise, barotrauma to the lungs can lead to a pneumothorax.

Independent lung ventilation is a form of ventilation that commonly uses a dual lumen ET tube to allow individual lung ventilation. This may also be accomplished using two small ET tubes, one ending in each mainstem bronchus. This form of therapy is used during a thoracotomy or thoracoscopy, so the surgical side can be preferentially deflated and TV lowered to facilitate exposure for operation. Other indications for use in the operating room or the intensive care unit (ICU) include massive hemoptysis, pulmonary alveolar proteinosis, unilateral lung injury, single-lung transplantation, or bronchopleural fistula. A single or dual ventilator can be used and even set to different modes of ventilation for use with independent lung ventilation.

ACUTE LUNG INJURY

Mechanical ventilation is used to treat hypoxemia, acidosis, and other life-threatening conditions. Although lifesaving, it may incite ventilator-induced lung injury. This may occur by barotrauma manifesting as extra-alveolar air, volutrauma from mechanical stretch, atelectrauma from alveolar mechanical stress, and biotrauma from systemic inflammatory mediators.

A pneumothorax is extra-alveolar, intraplueral air and occurs in 4%–15% of patients mechanically ventilated over 24 hours. Patients most prone are those with asthma, chronic obstructive pulmonary disease (COPD), ALI, and the adult respiratory distress syndrome (ARDS). Due to the observation that this may be precipitated by right mainstem intubation, alveolar overdistension may play a major role in its pathogenesis.[14]

In 2000, the NIH-sponsored ARDS Network phase III study looked at two groups of patients with respiratory failure and divided them based on TV calculated from the predicted body weight.[15–17] These variables were 6 and 12 mL/kg, respectively. In the 6 mL/kg group, the plateau pressure goal of <30 cm H_2O was achieved by decreasing the TV to a minimum of 4 mL/kg predicted body weight. The study was terminated early due to the statistical superiority of diminished mortality in the low TV group and substantial decrease in ventilator free days. Parsons also found that these low TV patients had a substantial decrease in inflammatory mediators such as IL-6, 8, and 10.

PHARMACOLOGIC APPROACH TO MECHANICAL VENTILATION

Up to 71% of SICU and seriously ill patients experience considerable pain. If untreated pain can lead to increases in sympathomimetics, catecholamines, and cytokines.

Elevated cytokines such as TNF-alpha, IL-1, IL-6, IL-8, as well as a decrease in IL-2, can adversely affect the T cell mediated immune response. The hyperglycemia that pain and stress induce may decrease chemotaxis and phagocytosis by neutrophils, leading to an increase in the infection rate, specifically ventilator-associated pneumonias (VAPs). Increased fibrinogen concentrations, increased plasminogen activator inhibitor, and increased platelet reactivity from stress can lead to a hypercoagulable state and thrombosis. In addition, stress increases

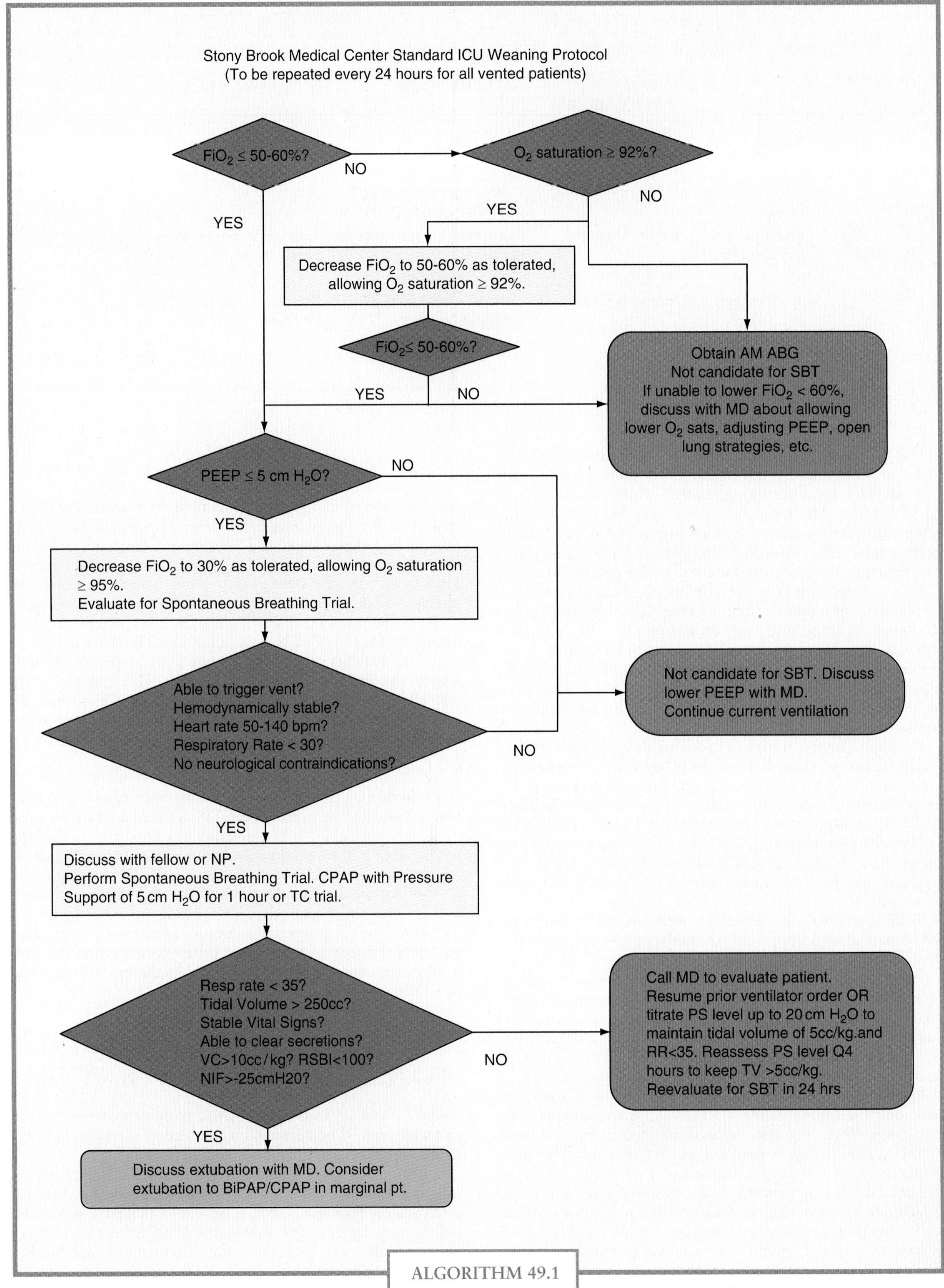
Stony Brook Medical Center Standard ICU Weaning Protocol
(To be repeated every 24 hours for all vented patients)
FiO2 ≤ 50-60%?
NO
O2 saturation ≥ 92%?
NO
YES
YES
Decrease FiO2 to 50-60% as tolerated, allowing O2 saturation ≥ 92%.
FiO2≤ 50-60%?
YES
NO
Obtain AM ABG
Not candidate for SBT
If unable to lower FiO2 < 60%, discuss with MD about allowing lower O2 sats, adjusting PEEP, open lung strategies, etc.
PEEP ≤ 5 cm H2O?
NO
YES
Decrease FiO2 to 30% as tolerated, allowing O2 saturation ≥ 95%.
Evaluate for Spontaneous Breathing Trial.
Able to trigger vent?
Hemodynamically stable?
Heart rate 50-140 bpm?
Respiratory Rate < 30?
No neurological contraindications?
NO
Not candidate for SBT. Discuss lower PEEP with MD.
Continue current ventilation
YES
Discuss with fellow or NP.
Perform Spontaneous Breathing Trial. CPAP with Pressure Support of 5 cm H2O for 1 hour or TC trial.
Resp rate < 35?
Tidal Volume > 250cc?
Stable Vital Signs?
Able to clear secretions?
VC>10cc/kg? RSBI<100?
NIF>-25cmH20?
NO
Call MD to evaluate patient.
Resume prior ventilator order OR titrate PS level up to 20 cm H2O to maintain tidal volume of 5cc/kg.and RR<35. Reassess PS level Q4 hours to keep TV >5cc/kg.
Reevaluate for SBT in 24 hrs
YES
Discuss extubation with MD. Consider extubation to BiPAP/CPAP in marginal pt.
ALGORITHM 49.1

ALGORITHM 49.1 Stony Brook Medical Center Standard ICU Weaning Protocol. To be repeated every 24 hours for all vented patients.

myocardial oxygen consumption, placing more stress on the heart. Thus, control of pain is important in controlling and weaning patients from mechanical ventilation. Attenuation or removal of painful and noxious stimuli is a crucial goal in oxygenation, ventilation, and weaning of these patients. Simple maneuvers such as proper positioning, using an appropriate type of bed, stabilization of fractures, and removing any physical irritants can also help decrease pain medication requirements.

Pharmacologic adjuncts are helpful, and include opioids, nonsteroidal anti-inflammatory drugs (NSAIDs), acetaminophen, and neural blockade. Opioids are the most common medications used for analgesia in the SICU (Table 49.3). They act centrally and peripherally via both mu and kappa receptors. Administration occurs by many avenues and includes oral, patch-transdermal, sublingual, epidural, intramuscular, or intravenous such as with a patient controlled analgesia device. There are a number of potential side effects of opioid use, the most important of which include respiratory depression, hypotension, altered mental status, constipation, and urinary retention. Naloxone is a narcotic antagonist that assists in reversal of unwanted opioid side effects.

IV ketamine, a nonopioid analgesic, may cause tachycardia, hypertension, hallucinations, and elevation in intracranial pressure, even at subanesthetic doses. Therefore, ketamine is generally avoided in the traumatic brain injured patient. Acetaminophen is used primarily for treatment of pyrexia, mild analgesic relief, and as an adjunct with narcotics. Hepatotoxicity may occur, especially in patients with depleted glutathione stores. NSAIDS can be used for analgesia; however their role is limited in ICU patients due to their side effects of gastric irritability and bleeding.

Epidural catheters are effective in control of more diffuse pain that may occur with multiple rib fractures or a laparotomy incision. Side effects include hypotension and respiratory depression. With the placement and removal of these catheters, be aware of recent anticoagulant or platelet inhibitor administration, due to the concern of developing an epidural hematoma.

Delirium

Delirium is an acute, potentially reversible impairment of consciousness and cognitive function that may occur in up to 80% of elderly ICU patients. There are a number of tools that can be used to identify and grade the degree of delirium in the ICU. The CAM-ICU confusion assessment method is based on the acute onset of mental status changes, inattention, disorganized thinking, and an altered level of consciousness. This tool has a high sensitivity and specificity.

Delirium is generally treated with neuroleptic drugs that antagonize basal ganglia dopamine. Intermittent IV boluses of haloperidol in dosages of 2–5 mg repeated every 15–20 minutes until agitation abates, up to a daily dose of 300 mg, may be used. However, with higher dosages the incidence of Torsades de pointes increases due to dose-dependent QT-interval prolongation. Cardiac monitoring, repletion of electrolytes, and extra caution in patients with a cardiac history are warranted. Neuroleptic agents can also lead to extrapyramidal side effects such as tremors and neuroleptic malignant syndrome. When possible, modification of behavior and environment should also be undertaken, such as limiting interruptions and noise. Other agents such as seroquel, which is only available via the oral route, can be beneficial.

Sedation and Anxiety

Anxiety or a state of apprehension in response to new or perceived threats is not uncommon in the ICU. It is an unfamiliar environment with bells and whistles leading to multiple types and forms of distractions. As with delirium, there are a number of scales available to assess the level of sedation, such as the Richmond Agitation-Sedation Scale, the Ramsay Scale, and the Motor Activity Assessment Scale.

There are many different classes of medications that are used for sedation. The use of benzodiazepines may actually assist in lowering the dosages of opioids required. If necessary, benzodiazepines can be reversed with flumazenil. These commonly used agents differ in their duration of action and rapidity of onset, as shown in Table 49.4. Propofol causes antegrade amnesia and sedation, and is only available in an intravenous formulation. It has also been used as an anticonvulsant. Propofol is a favored benzodiazepine in the ICU setting because of its rapid onset of action and quick metabolic elimination. Drawbacks of propofol are its increased cost as compared to other benzodiazepines, and the increased risk of hypertriglyceridemia and pancreatitis. Dexmedetomidine, another frequently used sedative, has the advantage of analgesic and sympatholytic properties with little respiratory suppression.

NEUROMUSCULAR BLOCKADE

With the increase in the variability of the different modes of mechanical ventilation, manipulations with flow rate and I:E ratio, and the availability of different sedative/analgesic agents, paralytics have seen a marked decrease in utilization in the ICU. Intensivists place patients on sedation vacations to assess ability to wean/extubate, to decrease the incidence of VAPs, and to decrease other conditions such as neuromuscular

TABLE 49.3

COMMONLY USED OPIOIDS IN THE ICU

DRUG	BOLUS DOSE	INFUSION RATE	HALF-LIFE	ELIMINATION	COMMENTS
Morphine sulfate	2.5–5.0 mg	5–35 mg/h or 0.07–0.5 mg/kg/h	2–4 h	Hepatic/renal	Histamine release Accumulates in renal insufficiency
Fentanyl citrate	25–100 μg	0.7–10 μg/kg/h	2–4 h	Hepatic	May accumulate with large doses
Hydromorphone	0.2–0.6 mg	0.5–1 mg/h or 7–15 μg/kg/h	2–3 h	Hepatic	

TABLE 49.4

COMMONLY USED SEDATIVES IN THE ICU

DRUG	BOLUS DOSE	ONSET OF ACTION	INFUSION RATE	HALF-LIFE	ELIMINATION	COMMENTS
Diazepam	0.03–0.1 mg/kg	2–5 min	N/A	20–50 h	Hepatic/renal	Metabolic acidosis Active metabolites
Lorazepam	0.02–0.06 mg/kg	5–20 min	0.01–0.1 mg/kg/h	10–16 h	Hepatic/renal	Metabolic acidosis Prolonged sedation
Midazolam	2–5 mg	1–5 min	0.04–0.2 mg/kg/h	1–4 h	Hepatic/renal	Increased levels with obesity Shorter half-life
Propofol	5 μg/kg	1–2 min	5–80 μg/kg/min	3–12 h	Hepatic	Increased triglycerides, accumulates in tissues
Dexmedetomidine	1.0 μg/kg over 10 min	5–10 min	0.2–0.7 μg/kg/h	1 h	Hepatic	Alpha2 agonist Minimal respiratory depression
Haloperidol	2–10 mg	30–60 min	3–25 mg/h	18 h	Hepatic	QT prolongation Torsades de pointes Extrapyramidal side effects

illness of critical care, which would be precluded with the routine use of neuromuscular blockade. Paralytics are divided into two classes, depolarizing and nondepolarizing agents (Table 49.5). Succinylcholine, the only depolarizing paralytic agent used today, is similar to acetylcholine and binds to and activates (depolarizes) nicotinic acetylcholine receptors as manifested by muscle fasciculation. It is often used for intubation due to its rapid onset and offset. However, when hyperkalemia is present, such as in burn patients and in patients with neuromuscular disease, another agent should be considered. The nondepolarizing agents bind but do not activate acetylcholine receptors; they include the aminosteroids and benzylisoquinolinium agents. The benzylisoquinolinium drugs atracurium and cisatracurium are inactivated by ester hydrolysis and Hoffman's elimination and thus not directly dependent on renal or hepatic function.

The neuromuscular blocking agents (NMBAs) should be monitored both subjectively for skeletal and respiratory movement, and objectively with a peripheral nerve stimulator using train of four electrical impulses. Acute myopathy of critical

TABLE 49.5

COMMONLY USED PARALYTICS IN THE ICU

DRUG	BOLUS DOSE	ONSET OF ACTION	DURATION	ELIMINATION	COMMENTS
Depolarizing agent Succinylcholine	0.3–1.1 mg/kg	<1 min	4–6 min	Plasma Pseudocholinesterase	
Nondepolarizing agent (A) Aminosteroids (B) Benzylisoquinolinium					
Pancuronium (A)	0.04–0.1 mg /kg	2–3 min	60–100 min	Hepatic	Tachycardia
Vecuronium (A)	0.08–0.1 mg/kg	3–5 min	45–65 min	Biliary/renal	Prolonged effects with hepatic failure
Rocuronium (A)	0.6–1.0 mg/kg	2–4 min	30 min	Hepatic	Rapid onset
Atracurium (B)	0.4–0.5 mg/kg	2–3 min	60–70 min	Hoffman degradation	Histamine release leads to hypotension
Cisatracurium (B)	0.15–0.2 mg/kg	2–3 min	30–60 min	Hoffman degradation	
Mivacurium (B)	0.2 mg/kg	1.5–2.5 min	15–20 min	Cholinesterase	Short half-life

illness is seen with prolonged use of NMBAs and may be manifested by inability to wean from the ventilator or with symmetrical and distal muscle group weakness after discontinuing the NMBA.

ADDITIONAL THERAPY TO IMPROVE OXYGENATION

Prone Ventilation

ARDS is a life-threatening pulmonary condition that produces severe hypoxemia. ARDS leads to an accumulation of fluid in the alveoli, which hinders oxygen transport across the alveoli membrane into the bloodstream, thus creating a state of hypoxemia. First described in 1976, prone ventilation is a modality used to improve oxygenation in severe hypoxemia.[18–22] Primarily used as a rescue maneuver, prone ventilation is employed in those patients who have required a sustained elevation of the FiO_2 and/or elevation of plateau pressures despite multiple changes to conventional ventilation. It is a known fact that elevation of these specific indices can be deleterious to a patient's respiratory recovery.

While patients lie in a supine position on a flat surface, ventilation generally occurs preferentially in the anterior and nondependent areas of the lung. Hence, the posterior and dependent portion of the lung, although theoretically better perfused, experiences somewhat ineffective ventilation, leading to a shunt. By placing a patient in the prone position using a specialized bed, the pulmonary mechanics of the patient can potentially be reversed resulting in a decrease in both the shunt and dead space. This results in an increase in recruitment of the posterior alveoli, and an increase in the end-expiratory lung volume. Prone positioning has also been shown to assist with the drainage of secretions from the tracheobronchial tree. With improvement in arterial oxygenation leading to lower inspired oxygen concentrations and PEEP levels, weaning the patient from the ventilator can be facilitated.

Using computerized tomography to evaluate and measure regional lung inflation, Gattinoni and Pelosi suggested that positional changes in FRC are related to regional lung inflation gradients. This reemphasizes work published in the 1960s by West and colleagues in describing the three zone model of pulmonary perfusion. In the apical zone, Zone 1, alveolar pressure exceeds arterial pressure, which exceeds venous pressure. In zone 2 or the middle lung fields, arterial pressure exceeds alveolar pressure, which exceeds venous pressure and in zone 3 arterial pressure exceeds venous pressure, which exceeds alveolar pressure.

In 2001, Gattinoni et al. [23] published a randomized control trial detailing the use of prone ventilation in the ICU setting. In this study, prone ventilation was applied for an average of 6 hours/day for approximately 10 days. The primary endpoint was mortality at 10 days, at time of discharge from the ICU, and at 6 months. At the conclusion of the study, there was no difference observed between both the supine and prone groups at 10 days (21% vs. 25%), and at the time of discharge from the ICU (51% vs. 48%). However a secondary endpoint, improvement in respiratory failure, was seen in nearly 70% of the prone group. Although no survival benefit was proven, this study became an outline for future studies. Mancebo et al. investigated prone ventilation applied over a longer duration. Patients were placed in the prone position for an average of 17 hours/day within 48 hours of oral–tracheal intubation. Although the results were not statistically significant, there was a 15% absolute and 25% relative reduction in ICU mortality compared with those who were ventilated supine. Upon further analysis, supine position was found to be an independent risk factor for mortality. In 2009, Taccone published a study designed to correct the issues that were viewed as possible reasons for the negative findings of previous trials. The results were similar to previous trials as there was no statistically significant survival benefit in patients with ARDS regardless of severity of hypoxemia.

Prone positioning should be employed in those whose oxygenation is severely impaired. Even though previous clinical experience has been derived from its use with ventilator dependent patients with ARDS, improvement in oxygenation has been seen in other respiratory disease processes.[24–30] Prone ventilation can be used in chronic obstructive lung disease and acute cardiogenic pulmonary edema. In 2004, studies by Guerin et al.[31] found a reduction of the prevalence of nosocomial pneumonia and incidence of VAP, respectively. This may be related to improved mobilization of secretions. Once the patient's condition improves and is able to tolerate more conventional methods, prone ventilation should be discontinued.[32]

The number, and in general, types of complications associated with prone ventilation are similar to that of supine positioning. Patients requiring prone ventilation are critically ill and commonly have arterial and venous access catheters and an endotracheal or tracheostomy tube. Care should be taken to ensure there are no displacements of these tubes and catheters to prevent an adverse event from occurring since prone positioning presents a definite challenge for cardiopulmonary resuscitation. Other complication that may occur with prone ventilation includes arrhythmias, facial and periorbital edema, and pressure ulcers.

Heliox

Heliox is an 80% helium and 20% oxygen mixture with a density much lower than pure oxygen and thus able to diffuse at a rate 1.8 times greater than oxygen alone. It assists in reducing resistance seen with partial upper airway obstruction such as with post extubation stridor. Evidence based studies for its use in the surgical critical care setting are lacking at this time.

Nitric Oxide

Inhaled nitric oxide is a highly reactive gaseous radical that is a potent vasodilator, especially for the pulmonary vasculature.[33] There have been mixed results with its use in ARDS refractive to traditional forms of ventilation. Treatment is initiated at 10 parts per million (ppm), and increased to a maximum of 20 ppm if no clinical response is detected. This is an expensive mode of therapy and Box 49.1 is the policy currently used at Stony Brook University Medical Center.

EXTRACORPOREAL MEMBRANE OXYGENATION

Extracorporeal membrane oxygenation (ECMO) or extracorporeal life support is available in certain centers to provide cardiocirculatory assist in patients with severe reversible cardiac and/or pulmonary failure.[34–36] As a salvage therapy, it is used when other more conventional modalities have failed. By providing gas exchange extracorporeally the lungs

BOX 49.1

POLICY

Inhaled nitric oxide (iNO) is a selective pulmonary vasodilator approved by the FDA for use in term or near term (>34 weeks) neonates with hypoxic respiratory failure associated with clinical or echocardiographic evidence of pulmonary hypertension where it improves oxygenation and reduces the need for ECMO. Nonneonatal use of nitric oxide will be governed by this policy to ensure appropriate *and safe administration of iNO.*

SCOPE

All pediatric and adult patients treated with iNO. Administration of iNO in the Cardiac Catheterization lab for vasoreactivity determination has been addressed in a separate policy.

KEYWORDS

Inhaled nitric oxide, critical care, mechanical ventilation

DEFINITIONS

Inhaled nitric oxide (iNO): a medical gas with selective pulmonary vasodilator properties.
Vasoreactivity: evidence of acute vasodilation to a pharmacologic agent.

PROCEDURES

A. iNO delivery and safety

1. Nitric oxide administration will be performed in the intensive care unit (ICU) or Cardiac Cath lab only.
2. Nitric oxide will be administered via a device (Inovent) that precisely regulates iNO delivery and monitors concentrations of nitric oxide, nitrogen dioxide, and oxygen.
3. Nitrogen dioxide (NO_2) is a toxic byproduct of nitric oxide and oxygen. If NO_2 levels exceed five (5) ppm, lower concentrations of nitric oxide should be administered.
4. If methemoglobin levels (MetHb) increase above 5%, iNO should be weaned to a lower dose. Assure that the patient is not receiving other medications that can cause methemoglobinemia, such as dapsone, metoclopramide, sulfonamides, lidocaine, or nitroglycerin. If MetHb levels remain elevated despite iNO reduction, iNO should be discontinued and treatment with methylene blue should be considered.

B. Approved Indications

1. Vasoreactivity testing in the Cardiac Cath lab is outlined in a separate policy.
2. Refractory hypoxemia in acute respiratory distress syndrome (ARDS). Early in the course of ARDS atelectatic portions of the lungs are often recruitable. Adjunct therapies including optimum positive end expiratory pressure (PEEP), prone positioning and an open-lung ventilatory strategy may allow reduction of the inspired oxygen concentration to a nontoxic level (≤60%). If the patient remains hypoxemic (PaO_2/FiO_2) <150 despite optimizing ventilatory parameters, iNO administration may be considered.
3. Pulmonary artery hypertension (PAH).

C. Procedure

1. An open-lung ventilatory strategy should be utilized, including optimizing PEEP, airway pressure release ventilation (APRV), or high frequency oscillatory ventilation (HFOV), if appropriate.
2. ABG should be obtained prior to the initiation of iNO. Baseline calculation of PaO_2/FiO_2 will be made and may include hemodynamic measurements, pulmonary artery pressure (PAP) and pulmonary vascular resistance (PVR).
3. iNO will be started at 10 ppm.
4. ABG and MetHb analysis will be performed 1 hour after initiation of iNO to determine oxygenation response.
5. If an ICU patient is being ruled out for pulmonary hypertension and is unable to have a pulmonary artery catheter inserted, response can be assessed by improvement in PaO_2/FiO_2 ratio and/or echocardiography. Echocardiographic or hemodynamic assessment can be made within 10–20 minutes of iNO administration.
6. iNO response is considered positive if the PaO_2/FiO_2 ratio increases by 20% or if the mean PAP or PVR decreases by 20%.
7. If there is no response at 10 ppm, a trial of 20 ppm may be conducted. There has been no efficacy demonstrated in this patient population at doses > 20 ppm. Nonresponders will not be continued on iNO.
8. Responders will be continued on iNO with the goal of reducing the $FiO_2 \leq 60\%$ with an oxygen saturation ≥90%.
9. Once the FiO2 is lowered to a nontoxic range, iNO should be weaned aggressively as patients responsive to iNO become tolerant over a 96-hour period.
10. All patients managed with iNO will be evaluated on a daily basis to determine weaning readiness.

D. Weaning

1. iNO dose should be reduced by half, every 4 hours, keeping the $FiO_2 \leq 60\%$ and $SpO_2 \geq 90\%$ until the dose is 5 ppm. If the MetHb level remains low, SpO_2 monitoring may be used to guide the weaning process.
2. At 5 ppm wean by 1 ppm, every 2 hours.
3. If $SpO_2 < 90\%$ during weaning process, return to previous nitric oxide level, consider alternative lung recruitment measures, and attempt to wean again in 4 hours
4. ABG will be obtained 1 hour post wean.

TABLE 49.6

BROCHODILATORS—BETA ADERNERGIC

DRUG	METHOD	STRENGTH	DOSAGE
Albuterol	Nebulizer/MDI (metered dose inhaler)	0.5% (5 mg/mL)/90 μg/puff	2.5 mg q4–8 h/2 puffs q4–6 h
Epinephrine	Nebulizer	0.5 mL	1–3 inhalations q3 h
Isoproterenol	Nebulizer	0.5% solution	5–15 inhalations up to 5 times daily
Metaproterenol	Nebulizer/MDI	5.0% (0.3 mL/2.5 mL)/0.65 mg/puff	0.3 mL q4–6 h 2–3 puffs q4 h
Pirbuterol	MDI	200 μg/puff	2 puffs q4–6 h
Racemic epinephrine	Nebulizer	2.25% inhalation solution	**Handheld**-add 0.5 mL to nebulizer, 1–3 inhalations; not more q3 h **Jet**-add 0.5 mL to nebulizer and dilute with 3 mL of NS; administer over 15 min q3–4 h prn
Salmeterol	MDI	50 μg/puff	1 puff q12 h
Terbutaline	MDI	500 μg/puff	1 puff prn, may repeat after 5 min; avoid more than 6 inhalations in a 24 h period.

can be bypassed or its reliance on mechanical ventilation diminished, allowing the heart and the lungs to recover. These circuits usually involve an external roller pump, and either a venous–venous circuit such as femoral–jugular or arterial–venous circuit such as between the femoral artery and either femoral or internal jugular vein. Either circuit is used to retrieve the blood, oxygenate it in an extracorporeal fashion and return the blood back into the systemic circulation. Since this process requires systemic anticoagulation to prevent clot formation, bleeding is a major concern. Its use in adult patients remains controversial, especially with ALI and ARDS.

SURFACTANT THERAPY AND LIQUID VENTILATION

Surfactant therapy uses a recombinant agent to supplement the surfactant, which normally is at the air–liquid interface of the alveoli serving to reduce surface tension.[37–41] It is 90% lipid and 10% protein. Liquid ventilation uses perfluorocarbons rather than gas for respiratory support.[42–48] The use of either of these modalities remains controversial as study results have been mixed when used in patients with ARDS and ALI.

INHALATIONAL THERAPY

Inhaled aerosols delivered directly into the respiratory tract, whether through the ventilator circuit or as a metered dose inhalant by a spontaneously breathing patient, can be effective to deliver medication. The beta-adrenergic bronchodilators are used to treat reversible airflow obstruction conditions such as asthma, bronchitis, or bronchospasm. They relax bronchial smooth muscle, stimulate mucociliary activity, and provide some inhibition on inflammatory mediator release (Table 49.6). Side effects include tachycardia, palpitations, dizziness, nausea, tachyphylaxis, and bronchospasm related to the propellant.

Anticholinergic bronchodilators block cholinergic-induced bronchoconstriction and are used to maintain treatment for bronchoconstriction in such conditions as COPD (Table 49.7). They act as an antimuscarinic agent and a competitive antagonist for acetylcholine. Side effects include dry mouth, pupillary dilation, increased intraocular pressure, tachycardia, urinary retention, and altered mental status.

Aerosolized glucocorticosteroids exert an anti-inflammatory effect and are used in mild to moderate persistent asthma. As the systemic effects are less than those of systemic steroid administration, adrenal suppression is usually not seen. Local side effects include oral candidiasis (Table 49.8).

VENTILATOR-ASSOCIATED PNEUMONIA

Pneumonia has been reported in 10%–48% of patients on mechanical ventilation. VAP is the most common nosocomial infection in the ICU with an incidence of 1–20/1,000 ventilator days, with neurosurgical, surgical, and burn ICUs having the highest rates according to NNIS. VAPs increase ICU length of stay from 4 to 26 days, hospital stay from 13 to 38 days and hospital costs from \$21,620 to \$70,568. In

TABLE 49.7

BRONCHODILATORS—ANTICHOLINERGIC

DRUG	METHOD	STRENGTH	DOSAGE
Ipratropium albuterol	Nebulizer/ MDI	3.0 mL/18: 90 μg/puff	3.0 mL q4 h/2 puffs q4 h
Ipratropium bromide	Nebulizer/ MDI	500 μg/17 μg/ puff	500 μg tid-qid/2 puffs qid

TABLE 49.8

BRONCHODILATORS—AEROSOLIZED STEROIDS

DRUG	METHOD	STRENGTH	DOSAGE
Beclomethasone	MDI	40 μg/actuation 80 μg/actuation	40–80 μg bid
Budesonide	Nebulizer	90 μg/actuation 180 μg/actuation	360 μg bid
Fluticasone	MDI	44 μg/actuation 110 μg/actuation 220 μg/actuation	88 μg bid
Flunisolide	MDI	250 μg/actuation	500 μg bid

general, early onset VAP has a better prognosis and the etiology is less likely due to multidrug resistant pathogens than a VAP that develops many days after intubation. There are a number of factors that may contribute to VAP (Table 49.9). In addition, colonization of ventilator tubing, heat and moisture exchangers, in line medication nebulizers, and suction catheters are possible sources of VAP.

INITIATING MECHANICAL VENTILATION

Once the patient has been intubated and assessed, the mode of ventilation should be selected. Many will begin with an SIMV mode in the acute setting with the FiO_2 set at 100%, a volume set at 6–8 mL/kg of ideal body weight, a rate of 12–16 breaths per minute, and a PEEP of 5 cm H_2O. For ARDS patients, 6 mL/kg is initially chosen. If the patient is not exhaling the volume delivered, the circuit, ET cuff, and ET position all need to be reassessed as does the chest itself with auscultation. If a chest tube is in place and there is evidence of a pleural leak, the mechanical ventilator volume may need to be decreased with the rate increased to maintain the same MVV to decrease the peak, mean, and plateau airway pressures and thus decrease the air-leak. The rate may have to be increased for hypoxemia and hypercarbia and a slower rate given to provide for permissive hypercapnia, increased IT, or to lower the MVV. A setting of PEEP of 5 cm H_2O is considered physiologic, due the fact that we all breathe against a certain amount of water vapor and this helps avoid absorptive atelectasis. With volume modes of ventilation the inspiratory flow rate is usually set at 40–90 L/minute with rates up to 120 L/minute to improve comfort and decrease inspiratory work.

For pressure ventilator modes where the pressure is set, peak and plateau airway pressures must be followed and if the ventilator pressures for a nonneuromuscular blocked patient reach over 40 cm H_2O, an investigation should be initiated to look for the reason, such as pneumothorax, increased resistance with decreased compliance, air trapping, or another reason that would dictate a decrease in pressure without greatly compromising TV.

WEANING FROM MECHANICAL VENTILATION

There are multiple methods to wean patients from mechanical ventilation. Table 49.10 lists a number of criteria that can be used. If a patient can comprehend instructions and lift his/her head off the bed, it is a crude sign of muscular tone. In addition to clinical exam, a chest radiograph when applicable, acceptable ventilator settings with an acceptable FiO_2, acceptable

TABLE 49.9

INCREASED MORTALITY FACTORS RELATED TO VAP

Antacid or H_2 receptor antagonist use	Duration of mechanical ventilation	Multiple central lines
APACHE II > 18	Higher organ system failure	Nasogastric tube use or enteral feeding
ARDS	Inappropriate antibiotic therapy	Nonsurgical diagnosis
Blood transfusion	Infection with high risk Pathogens	Premorbid lifestyle
Bronchoscopy	*Acinetobacter*	Reintubation
Cardiothoracic surgery	*Methicillin-resistant S. aureus*	Supine head position
Chronic pulmonary disorders	*Stenotrophomonas maltophilia*	Trauma
CNS disorder	*Pseudomonas aeruginosa*	Tracheostomy
Corticosteroid use	Male > 59 years old	

TABLE 49.10

EXTUBATION PARAMETERS

Minute ventilation volume (MVV)	<10 L/min
Negative inspiratory force (NIF)	<–25 cm H_2O
Tidal volume	>5 mL/kg
Rapid shallow breath index (RSBI)	<105
Oxygen saturation (SaO_2)	≥ 92%
Arterial blood gas	If applicable
Chest x-ray	If applicable
Lack of dyspnea	
Lack of accessory muscle use	
Control of agitation	
Control of anxiety	
Control of tachycardia	

arterial blood gases (ABGs) when applicable, pulse oximetry, capnography when present, frequency, TV, and rapid shallow breathing index can all help discern if the patient is ready to be weaned and extubated. Algorithm 49.1 is the protocol currently used at Stony Brook University Medical Center.

References

1. Esmond G, Mikelsons C, eds. *Non-Invasive Respiratory Support Techniques*. UK: Wiley Blackwell; 2009.
2. MacIntyre NR, Branson RD, eds. *Mechanical Ventilation*. 2nd ed. Philadelphia, PA. Saunders; 2009.
3. Scanlan CL, Wilkins RL, Stoller JK, eds. *Egan's Fundamentals of Respiratory Care*. 7th ed. St. Louis, MO. Mosby; 1999.
4. Papadakos PJ, Lachmann B, eds. *Mechanical Ventilation: Clinical Applications and Pathophysiology*. Philadelphia, PA. Saunders; 2008.
5. Sassoon CSH, Mahutte CK, Light RW. Ventilator modes old and new. *Crit Care Clin*. 1991;100:1421-1429.
6. Lucangelo U, Pelosi P, Zin WA, Aliverti A, eds. *Respiratory System and artificial Ventilation*. Italy: Springer; 2008.
7. Lain DC, DiBenedetto R, Morris SL, et al. Pressure control inverse ratio ventilation as a method to reduce peak inspiratory pressure and provide adequate ventilation and oxygenation. *Chest*. 1989;95:1081-1088.
8. Heenan TJ, Downs JB, Douglas ME, et al. Intermittent mandatory ventilation: Is synchronization important? *Chest*. 1980;77:598-602.
9. MacIntyre NR. Weaning from mechanical ventilatory support: Volume assisting intermittent breaths versus pressure-assisting every breath. *Respir Care*. 1988;33:121-125.
10. Downs JB, Stock MC. Airway pressure release ventilation: a new concept in ventilatory support. *Crit Care Med*. 1987;15:459-461.
11. Garner W, Downs JB, Stock MC, et al. Airway pressure release ventilation (APRV): a human trial. *Chest*. 1988;94:779-781.
12. Derdak S, Mehta S, Stewart TE, et al. Multicenter oscillatory ventilation for acute respiratory distress syndrome trial (MOAT) study investigators. High frequency oscillatory ventilation for acute respiratory distress syndrome in adults: a randomized, controlled trial. *Am J Respir Crit Care Med*. 2002;166:801-808.
13. Grasso S, Puntillo F, Mascia L, et al. Compensation for increase in respiratory workload during mechanical ventilation. Pressure-support versus proportional-assist ventilation. *Am J Respir Crit Care Med*. 2000;161: 819-826.
14. Bernard GR, Artigas A, Brigham KL, et al. American-European consensus conference on ARDS. *Am J Resp Crit Care Med*. 1994;149:818-824.
15. NIH ARDS Network. Ventilation with lower tidal volumes as compared with traditional tidal volumes for acute lung injury and the acute respiratory distress syndrome. *N Engl J Med*. 2000;342:1301-1308.
16. Sevransky JE, Levy MM, Marini JJ. Mechanical ventilation in sepsis induced ALI/ARDS-an evidence based review. *Crit Care Med*. 2004;32: S548-S553.
17. Malhotra A. Low-tidal-volume ventilation in the acute respiratory distress syndrome: clinical therapeutics. *N Engl J Med*. 2007;357:1113-1120.
18. Douglas WW, Rehder K, Beynen FM, et al. Improved oxygenation in patients with acute respiratory failure: the prone position. *Am Rev Respir Dis*. 1977;115:559-566.
19. Albert RK, Leasa D, Sanderson M, et al. The prone position improves arterial oxygenation and reduces shunt in oleic-acid-induced acute lung injury. *Am Rev Respir Dis*. 1987;135:628-633.
20. Pappert D, Rossaint R, Slama K, et al. Influence of positioning on ventilation-perfusion relationships in severe adult respiratory distress syndrome. *Chest*. 1994;106:1511-1516.
21. Pelosi P, Tubiolo D, Mascheroni D, et al. Effects of the prone position on respiratory mechanics and gas exchange during acute lung injury. *Am J Resp Crit Care Med*. 1998;157:387-393.
22. Broccard A, Shapiro RS, Schmitz LL, et al. Prone position attenuates and redistributes ventilator- induced lung injury in dogs. *Crit Care Med*. 2000;28:295-303.
23. Gattinoni L, Tognoni G. Pesenti A, et al. Effect of prone positioning on the survivial of patients with acute respiratory failure. *N Engl J Med*. 2001;345:568-573.
24. Taccone P, Pesenti A, Latini R, et al. Prone positioning in patients with moderate and severe acute respiratory distress syndrome: a randomized controlled trial. *JAMA*. 2009;302(18):1977-1984.
25. Davis JW, Lemaster DM, Moore EC, et al. Prone ventilation in trauma or surgical patients with acute lung injury and respiratory distress syndrome: is it beneficial? *J Trauma*. 2007;62:1201-1206.
26. Mancebo J, Fernandez R, Blanch L, et al. A multicenter trial of prolonged prone ventilation in severe acute respiratory distress syndrome. *Am J Respir Crit Care Med*. 2006;173:1233-1239.
27. Messerole E, Peine P, Wittkopp, et al. The pragmatics of prone positioning: clinical commentary. *Am J Respir Crit Care Med*. 2002;165: 1359-1363.
28. Tiruvoipati R, Bangash M, Manktelow B, et al. Efficacy of prone ventilation in adult patients with acute respiratory failure: a meta-analysis. *J Crit Care*. 2008;23:101-110.
29. Kopterides P, Siempos I, Armaganidis A. Prone positioning in hypoxemic respiratory failure: meta-analysis of randomized controlled trials. *J Crit Care*. 2009;24:89-100.
30. Viellard-Baron A, Charron C, Caille V, et al. Prone positioning unloads the right ventricle in severe ARDS. *Chest*. 2007;132:1440-1446.
31. Guerin C, Gaillard S, Lemasson, et al. Effects of systematic prone positioning in hypoxemic acute respiratory failure: a randomized controlled trial. *JAMA*. 2004;292(19):2379-2387.
32. McAuley DF, Giles S, Fichter et al. What is the optimal duration of ventilation in the prone position in acute lung injury and acute respiratory distress syndrome? *Intensive Care Med*. 2002;28:414-418.
33. Dellinger RP, Zimmerman JL, Taylor RW, et al. Effects of inhaled nitric oxide in patients with acute respiratory distress syndrome: results of a randomized phase II trial. Inhaled Nitric Oxide in ARDS Study Group. *Crit Care Med*. 1998;26:15-23.
34. Zapol WM, Snider MT, Hill JD, et al. Extracorporeal membrane oxygenation in severe acute respiratory failure: a randomized prospective study. *JAMA*. 1979;242:2193-2196.
35. Morris AH, Wallace CJ, Menlove RL, et al. Randomized clinical trial of pressure-controlled inverse ratio ventilation and extracorporeal CO_2 removal for adult respiratory distress syndrome. *Am J Respir Crit Care Med*. 1994;149:295-305.
36. Lewandowski K. Extracorporeal membrane oxygenation for severe acute respiratory failure. *Crit Care*. 2000;4:156-168.
37. Spragg RG, Lewis JF. Surfactant therapy in the acute respiratory distress syndrome. In: Matthay MA, ed: *Acute Respiratory Distress Syndrome*. New York: Marcel Dekker; 2003:533-562.
38. Anzueto A, Baughman RP, Guntupalli KK, et al. Aerosolized surfactant in adults with sepsis-induced acute respiratory distress syndrome: Exosurf Acute Respiratory Distress Syndrome Sepsis Study Group. *N Engl J Med*. 1996;334:1417-1421.
39. Gregory TJ, Steinberg KP, Spragg R, et al. Bovine surfactant therapy for patients with acute respiratory distress syndrome. *Am J Respir Crit Care Med*. 1997;155:1309-1315.
40. Spragg RG, Lewis JF, Wurst W, et al. Treatment of acute respiratory distress syndrome with recombinant surfactant protein C surfactant. *Am J Respir Crit Care Med*. 2003;167:1562-1566.
41. Spragg RG, Lewis JF, Rathgeb F. et al. Intratracheal instillation of rSP-C surfactant improves oxygenation in patients with ARDS. *Am J Respir Crit Care Med*. 2002;165:A22.
42. Shaffer TH. A brief review: liquid ventilation. *Undersea Biomed Res*. 1987;14:169-179.
43. Shaffer TH, Douglas PR, Lowe CA, et al. The effects of liquid ventilation on cardiopulmonary function in preterm lambs. *Pediatr Res*. 1983; 17:303-306.
44. Wolfson MR, Greenspan JS, Deoras KS, et al. Comparison of gas and liquid ventilation: Clinical, physiological and histological correlates. *J Appl Physiol*. 1992;72:1024-1031.
45. Hirschl RB, Parent A, Tooley R, et al. Liquid ventilation improves pulmonary function, gas exchange, and lung injury in a model of respiratory failure. *Ann Surg*. 1995;221:79-88.

46. Hirschl RB, Tooley R, Parent AC, et al. Improvement of gas exchange, pulmonary function, and lung injury with partial liquid ventilation: a study model in a setting of severe respiratory failure. *Chest.* 1995;108:500-508.
47. Dani C, Costantino ML, Martelli E, et al. Perflurocarbons attenuate oxidative lung damage. *Pediatr Pulmonol.* 2003:322-329.
48. Hirschl RB, Croce M, Gore D, et al. Prospective, randomized controlled pilot study of partial liquid ventilation in adult acute respiratory distress syndrome. *Am J Respir Crit Care Med.* 2002;165:781-787.

CHAPTER 50 ■ CARDIOVASCULAR FAILURE AND CIRCULATORY SUPPORT—MONITORING AND ESSENTIAL ADJUNCTS

JOHN A. MORRIS, MICKEY OTT, FITZGERALD J. CASIMIR, WALTER K. CLAIR, AND MARK GLAZER

The acute care surgery patient is at increased risk of cardiovascular compromise. Whether the trauma patient with severe hemorrhage, or the emergency general surgery patient with peritonitis, these patients encounter fluid "shifts" and a systemic inflammatory response unseen in other areas of surgery or medicine. To optimize patient care, the acute care surgeon must have a firm grasp of the physiology, diagnosis, and management of cardiovascular failure.

Cardiovascular compromise leads to shock, the inadequate delivery of oxygen to supply cellular metabolic needs. In the acute care setting, the patient in cardiovascular failure will present with unique, but identifiable causes of shock that follow a predictable pattern of illness.

- *Hypovolemic shock* related to direct intravascular volume loss from hemorrhage or intravascular volume depletion from sequestration of fluid into the "third space".
- *Septic shock* related to organ dysfunction or hypoperfusion as a result of infection (Discussed in Chapter 12).
- *Cardiogenic shock related to intrinsic cardiac disease* or as a component of multiple organ dysfunction syndrome (MDS), resulting in decreased myocardial contractility that impairs oxygen delivery.
- *Cardiogenic shock related to extrinsic causes* that inhibit the heart from delivering oxygen by affecting preload, afterload, contractility, or a combination of the three.

Treatment of cardiovascular failure is focused on identification of the etiology of shock, and restoration of adequate oxygen delivery. This chapter discusses the determinants of cardiac output and oxygen delivery, techniques to diagnose and monitor the patient in shock, the clinical situations most frequently observed in the acute care setting, and the treatment and support of the patient in cardiovascular failure.

CARDIOVASCULAR PHYSIOLOGY

Oxygen must be uploaded to the blood at the pulmonary capillary level, adequately transported by the heart, and offloaded at the tissue level. Whereas factors such as pH, temperature, and alveolar and capillary membrane permeability will influence these processes, this chapter focuses specifically on the heart's ability to transport oxygen to the tissue (see Box 50.1).

Evaluation of Cardiovascular Performance

Hypotension is the harbinger of cardiovascular collapse. Although vasopressors may be appropriate in certain circumstances, the shock state should be diagnosed and categorized as a problem of preload, afterload, or contractility. Basic monitoring of oxygen saturation, continuous electrocardiography (ECG), and blood pressure measurements are vital, but other adjuncts help address this clinical scenario.

Determination of Preload

Controversy exists over the best method to determine preload.[1-8] In general, each of the devices measures a pressure in an attempt to estimate or correlate with intravascular volume.

Central Venous Pressure. Central venous catheters have the dual benefit of access to large veins for (IV) fluid resuscitation and drug delivery, but also allow the surgeon to estimate intravascular volume. The central venous pressure (CVP) is a measure of the right atrial pressure that is proportional to the right ventricular end-diastolic volume (EDV). This measurement, however, is influenced by a multitude of variables in the critically ill patient. Patients on mechanical ventilation with positive end-expiratory pressure (PEEP) demonstrate decreased venous return from increased intrathoracic pressure. These patients require higher filling pressures to maintain preload. Changes in venous capacitance, intra-abdominal pressure, or heart failure can also affect the accuracy of the CVP. Although CVP is not an exact measurement of intravascular volume, it provides a trend of the intravascular filling pressures, which is a useful guide to resuscitation[6,7,9,10]

Pulmonary Artery Catheter. Despite controversy, the use of the pulmonary artery catheter (PAC) remains widespread in intensive care units[2-6,11-17] One area where the use of the PAC has been demonstrated to improve outcomes is in the trauma population.[18] In a retrospective database analysis examining over 50,000 patients, the use of PAC was shown to improve mortality in three specific groups: (1) patients with Injury Severity Score > 25, (2) patients with initial base deficit >11, and (3) patients older than 61 years of age.[18] Given the similarities between the trauma population and the emergency general surgery population (huge volume shifts over a short period of time, the presence of a systemic inflammatory response, frequent comorbidities, and large number of elderly patients), the use of a PAC to determine adequate perfusion warrants consideration. Moreover, the PAC also provides other hemodynamic data that can potentially assist patient care, and are discussed below.

PULMONARY ARTERY OCCLUSION PRESSURE

Also known as the pulmonary artery "wedge" pressure, the pulmonary artery occlusion pressure (PAOP) approximates the left ventricular EDV. However, in the setting of increased intrathoracic pressure from positive-pressure ventilation,

BOX 50.1

The determinants of oxygen delivery are the amount of oxygen in the blood and how much blood is being pumped to the tissue:

$$DO_2 = CO\,[(Hb \times 1.34)\,SaO_2 + 0.003\,PaO_2]$$

where...

CO = Cardiac output, Hb = Hemoglobin, SaO_2 = Arterial oxygen saturation, PaO_2 = Partial pressure of oxygen in arterial blood, and DO_2 = oxygen delivery

and...

Cardiac output = Amount of blood pumped by the heart in 1 minute
= Stroke volume × heart rate

Stroke volume is determined by:

- Preload
  - The initial length of myocardial muscle fibers is proportional to the left ventricular end-diastolic volume.
  - As these fibers stretch, the energy of contraction increases proportionally until an optimal tension develops (i.e., ideal preload = ideal cardiac contraction)
- Afterload
  - Resistance to ventricular ejection
  - Measured clinically by blood pressure or SVR.
- Contractility
  - Ability of the heart to alter its contractile strength independent of fiber length (preload)
  - Decreased in intrinsic cardiac disease, contractility initially increased in sepsis but decreases in the later stages of sepsis, myocardial ischemia

structural heart defects, or certain tachyarrhythmias the PAOP becomes less reliable.[19-22]

END-DIASTOLIC VOLUME INDEX

End-diastolic volume index (EDVI) can be calculated based on the right ventricular ejection fraction and cardiac output, and provides an accurate assessment of preload.[23] Cheatham et al.[24] showed in a series of 64 critically ill patients that EDVI correlates more closely to cardiac index than PAOP, when variable levels of PEEP were applied to patients on mechanical ventilation.[24]

TRANSTHORACIC AND TRANSESOPHAGEAL ECHOCARDIOGRAPHY

The use of echocardiography has been investigated as a tool to guide resuscitation in the critically ill patient.[22,25-29] Doppler data on blood velocity and measurements of the vessel diameter of the vena cava can be used to estimate preload. Echocardiography has the added benefit of examination of the heart chambers and cardiac wall motion to estimate cardiac index. It has also becomes a useful tool for the initial evaluation of the trauma patient as part of the Focused Assessment by Sonography in Trauma (FAST) exam to demonstrate cardiac tamponade[30-35] Handheld ultrasound devices allow measurements of vessel diameter and may help guide resuscitation in critical illness.[28,36,37] Transesophageal echocardiogram has shown promise in initial studies and may replace transthoracic echo as a guide for adequate resuscitation. However, widespread use of echocardiography has been limited by availability, cost, and the skill required for interpretation.

DETERMINATION OF AFTERLOAD

Afterload can be approximated by calculating the systemic vascular resistance (SVR). SVR = (80) (MAP – CVP)/CO (where MAP is mean arterial pressure and CO is cardiac output). This can be directly calculated with the use of a PAC. High afterload leads to increased work on the heart and decreased cardiac output. In contrast, cardiovascular failure secondary to a profound decrease in afterload is the classic clinical scenario of distributive shock (e.g., septic shock).

DETERMINING CONTRACTILITY

Exact measurements of contractility are difficult to ascertain. However, the acute care surgeon can use the other above-described tools such as echocardiography or a PAC to estimate contractility. In the hypotensive patient, if values determined for preload and afterload are within normal range, it is assumed that contractility is impaired.

Oxygen Delivery. Perhaps the most important question to answer is, "is enough oxygen being provided to the tissues?" Oxygen delivery can be determined indirectly by measuring products of metabolism and monitoring acid base status, or directly by measuring the oxygen content in the blood returning to the heart. Thus, oxygen delivery is the product of cardiac output and arterial oxygen content.

MIXED VENOUS OXYGEN SATURATION

In the nonstressed setting, only 25%–30% of oxygen delivered to the tissues is actually extracted from the blood. Therefore, the blood returning to the heart from both the upper and lower parts of the body, or the mixed venous oxygen saturation (SVO_2), is normally 70%.[38] In the setting of shock, a low SVO_2 reflects inadequate delivery or increased extraction of oxygen by the tissue. The SVO_2 is most accurately measured at the coronary sinus where there is mixing of blood from the IVC and SVC, but for practical purposes it can be measured from an upper extremity central line or a PAC. SVO_2 can now be monitored in a continuous fashion with the help of continuous cardiac output PACs. Measuring SVO_2 and normalizing SVO_2 during resuscitation has been shown to improve survival.[10]

Lactate and Base Deficit

In the setting of insufficient oxygen delivery, lactate is generated as a result of altered metabolism in the pyruvate kinase pathway. Serum lactate concentration is an indirect measurement of oxygen debt. The admission lactate, highest lactate concentration, and time required to normalize lactate have all been shown to predict survival.[10,39-43] Base deficit is a measurement calculated, usually from an arterial blood gas, of the amount of alkali required to correct a pH to 7.4 with a $PaCO_2$ of 40. Base deficit has also been shown to correlate with survival in the trauma patient, and both lactate and base deficit can be used as guides to resuscitation.[10,39-43]

Several modalities have also shown promise as alternative measurements to assess cardiac performance:

- *Oxygen extraction index*—A potential variable to measure oxygen delivery[44]
- *Heart rate variability*—A biomarker that potentially can be followed to predict and monitor physiologic reserve in the critically ill patient[45-49]

In summary, the first step in treatment of the acute care surgery patient in cardiovascular failure is to determine why the patient is in failure. Elucidation of the etiology of heart failure as a problem of preload, afterload, or contractility, using the tools above, provides the necessary information to support the patient.

SUPPORT FOR CARDIOVASCULAR DYSFUNCTION

The key to treatment of the patient in cardiovascular failure is restoration of adequate oxygen delivery; think of this as "source control" first. In the case of hypovolemic shock in the trauma patient, the source is bleeding. In the case of infection, the source may be an abscess. In the case of intrinsic cardiogenic shock, the source may be the heart itself. In extrinsic cardiogenic shock, the source may be due to failure of another organ system; an adverse side effect of a medication; or a disease process that negatively affects preload, afterload, or contractility. The earlier the treatment to restore cardiovascular function is begun, the better the patient outcome.

Fluid Resuscitation

After 30 years of active investigation, controversy still exists over the use of crystalloid versus colloid for fluid replacement. Not only does the acute care surgeon need to choose what type of fluid to give, but how much. The danger of too much fluid compartment syndrome, acute respiratory distress syndrome [ARDS], versus the danger of too little fluid, (acute kidney injury tissue ischemia) must be balanced. In general, in the face of hypovolemia and shock, fluid resuscitation should be performed aggressively in the acute setting. On the other hand, resuscitation should be to specific endpoints, rather than undirected fluid infusion. Some data exist that permissive hypotension and minimal fluid resuscitation in the prehospital setting may improve outcomes in trauma patients,[50,51] the theory being that if bleeding has not been controlled, fluid resuscitation and relative hypertension will lead to more bleeding, hemodilution, and coagulopathy. Permissive hypotension assumes rapid transfer from the scene to definitive treatment, and is most applicable to the penetrating trauma population. Further study is necessary before this method can be applied outside of this every specific penetrating trauma population.

In some instances, the choice of fluid must also include the use of blood products. Blood product transfusion is potentially deleterious[52-61] As a simplified rule, when bleeding is the cause of hypotension, blood should be used as the resuscitative fluid. When bleeding is not the cause, it should not be used. Recently, the Eastern Association for the Surgery of Trauma and the Society of Critical Care Medicine published practice management guidelines for red blood cell transfusion in the critically ill[62] (Box 50.2). Another topic, which has

BOX 50.2

CLINICAL PRACTICE GUIDELINES: RED BLOOD CELL (RBC) TRANSFUSION IN ADULT TRAUMA AND CRITICAL CARE

LEVEL 1	LEVEL 2
1. RBC transfusion is indicated for patients with evidence of hemorrhagic shock	4. The use of only Hb concentration as a "trigger" for transfusion should be avoided. Decision for RBC transfusion should be based on individual patient's intravascular volume status, evidence of shock, duration and extent of anemia, and cardiopulmonary physiologic parameters.
2. RBC transfusion may be indicated for patients with evidence of acute hemorrhage and hemodynamic instability or inadequate oxygen delivery.	5. In the absence of acute hemorrhage, RBC transfusion should be given as single units, one at a time.
3. A "restrictive" strategy of RBC transfusion (transfuse when Hb <7 g/dL) is as effective as a "liberal" transfusion strategy (transfusion when Hb <10 g/dL) in critically ill patients with hemodynamically stable anemia, except possibly in patients with acute myocardial ischemia.	6. Consider transfusion if Hb <7 g/dL in critically ill patients requiring mechanical ventilation. There is no benefit of a "liberal" transfusion strategy (transfusion when Hb <10 g/dL) in critically ill patients requiring mechanical ventilation.
	7. Consider transfusion if Hb <7 g/dL in resuscitated critically ill trauma patients. There is no benefit of a "liberal" transfusion strategy (transfusion when Hb <10 g/dL) in resuscitated critically ill trauma patients.
	8. Consider transfusion if Hb <7 g/dL in critically ill patients with stable cardiac disease. There is no benefit of a "liberal" transfusion strategy (transfusion when Hb <10 g/dL) in critically ill patients with stable cardiac disease.
	9. RBC transfusion should not be considered as an absolute method to improve tissue oxygen consumption in critically ill patients.

received attention, is the ratio of blood products being transfused. Experience from the military suggests that red blood cell concentrates (packed red blood cells, PRBCs) FFP, and platelets should be given in a 1:1:1 ratio in the traumatically injured, exsanguinating patient.[63-68] This research has been confirmed in the civilian population as well by the improved survival demonstrated by the initiation of institutional massive transfusion protocols.[69,70] The ideal ratio among packed red blood cells, fresh frozen plasma, and platelets is still to be determined, but it seems clear that the transfusion of PRBCs alone in the face of bleeding is not as effective as adding the additional clotting factor products; that is, replace what the patient has lost.

Pharmacologic Support

Multiple medications are available to assist the patient in cardiovascular failure, depending on the specific cause (Table 50.1). It is important to remember that these medications have multiple effects on the cardiovascular system. Catecholamine agents (dopamine, dobutamine, epinephrine, norepinephrine) exert their effects through binding to alpha and beta receptors. Activation of alpha-1 receptors increases SVR. Activation of beta-1 receptors leads to inotropy. Activation of beta-2 receptors leads to peripheral vasodilation. Phosphodiesterase inhibitors such as milrinone cause an increase in intracellular cyclic adenosine monophosphate (cAMP), and subsequent inotropy. In general, when the cause of failure is reduced afterload, a vasopressor should be chosen. When the etiology is related to contractility, an inotrope should be used. An algorithm for the management of the patient in cardiovascular failure is presented in Algorithm 50.1. Make sure "the tank is full" (the patient is volumerepleted), and that mean arterial blood pressure, oxygen delivery, and cardiac output are adequate.

In summary:

- A thorough understanding of cardiovascular physiology is a necessity for the acute care surgeon.
- When treating the patient in cardiovascular failure, first determine whether the problem is one of preload, afterload, or contractility, and their effect on oxygen delivery.
- By using adjuncts such as a PAC, measuring pressures such as CVP or PAOP and measuring markers of oxygen delivery such as SVO_2, lactate, and base deficit, the acute care surgeon can guide the resuscitation of the patient in cardiovascular failure.
- Once the cause of the cardiovascular failure is recognized, "source control" is the key to treatment. Through the use of fluid resuscitation, vasopressor, and inotropic support, the acute care surgeon may return the critically ill patient to his/her normal physiologic state.

CLASSIFICATION OF CARDIOVASCULAR FAILURE

The acutely ill surgical patient may develop cardiovascular failure from a variety of pathologic causes. These disease processes can be simply classified into either *intrinsic* or *extrinsic* causes of heart failure. Intrinsic causes of cardiovascular failure stem from a disease of the myocardium, the heart valves, or the conducting system of the heart. Extrinsic causes of cardiovascular failure occur in the presence of a structurally normal heart; however, an external source impedes contractility or negatively affects afterload or preload. Although their etiologies differ, both extrinsic and intrinsic causes prevent adequate oxygen delivery in light of increased metabolic demand.

Intrinsic Cause of Cardiovascular Failure

There are four basic causes of intrinsic cardiovascular failure in the postoperative patient. These include myocardial ischemia, congestive heart failure (CHF), valvular heart defects, and cardiac arrhythmias. Patients with intrinsic cardiovascular failure suffer from a substantial increase in perioperative morbidity and mortality in the setting of acute surgical illness (see Table 50.2).

Myocardial Ischemia and Infarction. Myocardial infarction (MI) occurs in 5%–7% of postoperative elective general surgery patients, but is associated with a mortality

TABLE 50.1

EFFECTS OF COMMONLY USED VASOACTIVE MEDICATIONS

MEDICATION	HR	MAP	CO	SVR	ALPHA-1	BETA-1	BETA-2	DA
Primary Vasopressors								
Dopamine (low dose)	+	+	++			++		+
Dopamine (high dose)	++	++	+	+++	++	+		+
Norepinephrine	+	++	+	+++	+++	+		
Vasopressin		++		++				
Primary Inotropes								
Dobutamine	+	±	++	–		++	+	
Epinephrine	++	++	+	±	++	++	+	
Milrinone*			+++	–				

Number of plus signs reflects strength of attribute.
CO, cardiac output; HR, heart rate; MAP, mean arterial blood pressure; SVR, systemic vascular resistance; ALPHA-1, alpha-1 adrenoceptor agonist; BETA-1, beta-1 adrenoceptor agonist; DA, dopaminergic receptor agonist
*Milrinone exerts inotropic effects, but is a direct arteriolar smooth muscle relaxant and thus a direct vasodilator

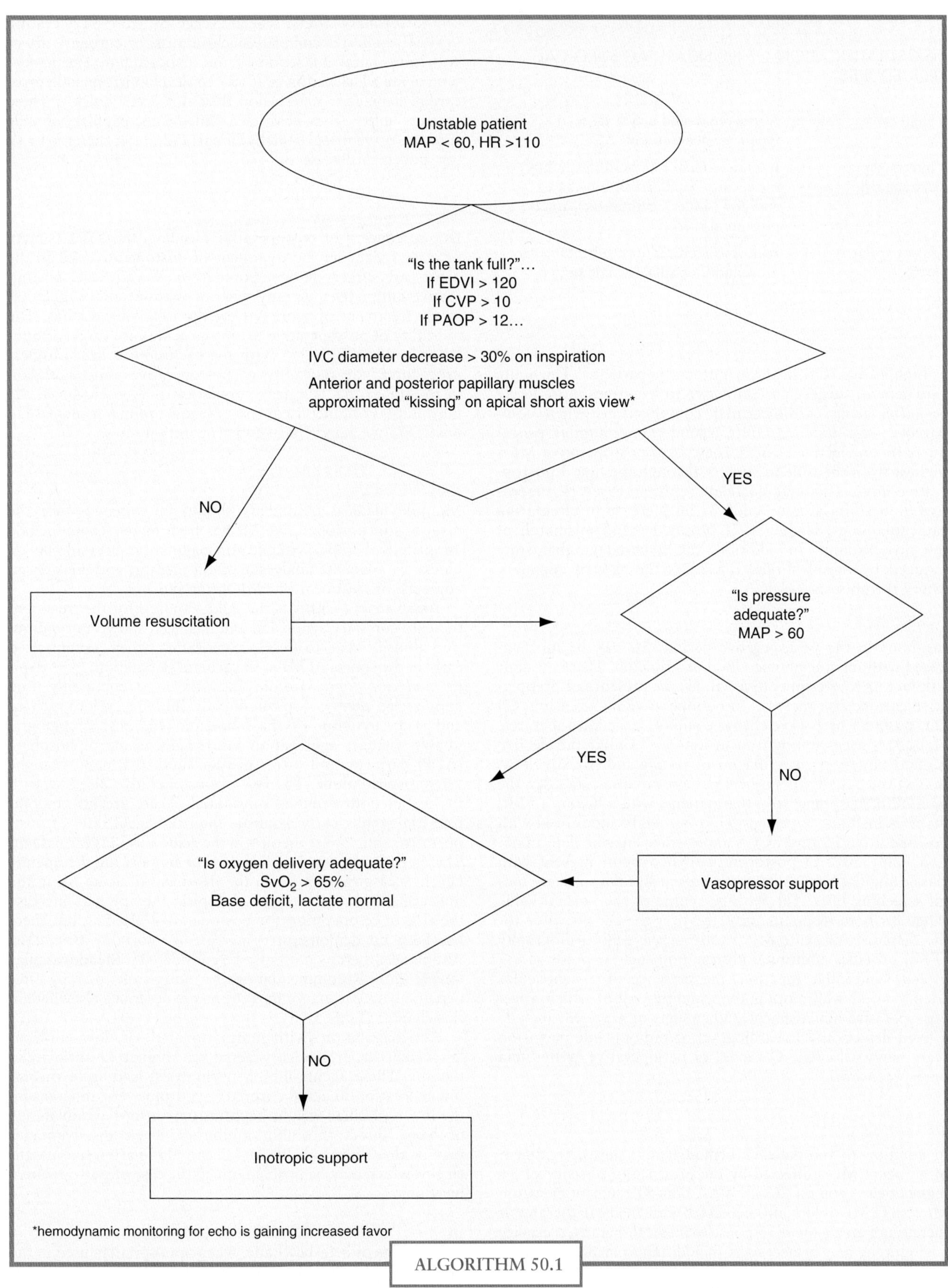

ALGORITHM 50.1 Unstable patient algorithm.
CVP, central venous pressure; EDVI, end-diastolic volume index; HR, heart rate; MAP, mean arterial blood pressure; PAOP, pulmonary artery occlusion pressure; SVO2, mixed venous oxygen saturation

TABLE 50.2

RISK STRATIFICATION OF NONCARDIAC SURGICAL PROCEDURES

High cardiac risk > 5%	Aortic repair and major vascular repair, esophagectomy
Intermediate cardiac risk 1%–5%	Intraabdominal Intraperitoneal, thoracic, carotid endarterectomy, head and neck surgery, orthopedic surgery, prostate surgery
Low cardiac risk <1%	Endoscopic procedures, subcutaneous procedures, ophthalmologic surgery

as high as 40–70% in the symptomatic patient.[71] The acute care general surgery patient is two to five times more likely to suffer from cardiovascular complications when compared to age-matched controls undergoing similar procedures on an elective basis.[71] The risk of postoperative MI is highest from the time of surgery through the first 3 postoperative days. This may correlate with increased perioperative fluid shifts accompanied by an increase in circulating catecholamines, leading to a supply/demand mismatch of the myocardium. In addition, the hypercoagulable state induced by recent surgery increases the risk of coronary artery thrombosis.[71-73]

DIAGNOSIS OF POSTOPERATIVE MI

Insidious in the postoperative period, MI can be misdiagnosed without a heightened level of suspicion. There are four risk factors for perioperative MI: (1) the presence of preoperative cardiac risk factors, (2) perioperative hypotension, (3) new onset ST or T wave changes, and (4) large intraoperative blood loss necessitating transfusion.[71,72,74] Unlike the elective general surgery patient, diagnostic testing and risk stratification in the acutely ill surgical patient often occurs *after* the operation. It is imperative that patients with a history of MI, diabetes mellitus, hypertension, or stroke be monitored with postoperative 12-lead ECG's and cardiac enzyme determination. Only 50% of postoperative MI patients present with classic anginal symptoms. ECG and cardiac enzymes are useful screening tests. The 99th percentile of the normal value range for both troponin and CK-MB is the cut off value for the diagnosis of acute MI. Transthoracic echocardiography (TTE) provides additional information such as preservation of left ventricular function, the presence of a ventricular aneurysm, or wall motion abnormalities, all of which affect postoperative management. Other signs of acute MI include a fixed defect on echocardiogram or radionuclide perfusion scan, new pathologic Q waves, or perioperative arrhythmia or hypotension.

CLASSIFICATION OF ST SEGMENT ELEVATION VERSUS NON–ST SEGMENT ELEVATION MI

In addition to the patient's hemodynamic status, treatment of an acute MI is directed by the presence or absence of ST segment elevation on ECG.[72,74-76] A non–ST segment elevation MI (NSTEMI) is initially managed with medical therapy. If there is not an adequate response to medical therapy, coronary angiography may be necessary. In addition to medical therapy, an ST segment elevation MI (STEMI) will require emergent coronary angiography to determine need for coronary revascularization. The absence of ST elevation (NSTEMI) indicates reversible subendocardial ischemia from partial occlusion of the coronary artery. The presence of acute ST elevation (STEMI) indicates complete occlusion of the coronary artery with transmural infarction of the myocardium. The patient with acute ST elevation is at risk to develop irreversible myocardial damage if reperfusion does not occur quickly. These patients suffer from ventricular aneurysm, papillary muscle rupture, or ventricular arrhythmias and are at increased risk for sudden cardiac death.

THE DILEMMA OF POSTOPERATIVE BLEEDING IN ACUTE TREATMENT OF MI

Due to concern of postoperative bleeding, there is a paucity of class 1 data on the treatment of postoperative MI in the acute care surgery patient population. We advocate postoperative antiplatelet therapy with or without anticoagulation in the treatment of acute MI for the following reasons. The mortality of postoperative MI in the acute care surgery population is 40%–70%.[72-76] With the exclusion of neurosurgical procedures, the mortality of postoperative anticoagulation in the noncardiac surgical population is low. However, the morbidity is not inconsequential, leading to major increase in postoperative hemorrhage and reoperation rates.

MEDICAL MANAGEMENT OF ACUTE MYOCARDIAL INFARCTION

Multiple medical treatments should be initiated once the diagnosis of postoperative MI has been made. These include antiplatelet therapy, systemic anticoagulation, beta-adrenergic blockade, adequate analgesia, statin therapy, and mechanical adjuncts for treatment of cardiogenic shock.[72-74,76]

Antiplatelet therapy is the gold standard for the treatment of acute coronary syndrome and has been shown in randomized clinical trials to decrease mortality when administered early in the course of MI in the general population.[74,77,78] *Aspirin and clopidogrel* are currently the most commonly used antiplatelet agents. Aspirin directly inhibits cyclooxygenase and is an inhibitor of thromboxane synthesis. Clopidogrel inhibits platelet aggregation via the adenosine diphosphate (ADP) pathway and offers greater survival benefit than the use of aspirin alone. The risk of postoperative bleeding with the use of both drugs is substantial. There are no randomized trials that clearly delineate the risk:benefit ratio of postoperative antiplatelet therapy in the acute care surgery patient. There are, however, class II data that support the therapeutic benefit of aspirin therapy in the treatment of acute MI in the noncardiac surgery patient.[72-74] Aspirin therapy may increase the risk of re-operation for postoperative bleeding but there has been no demonstrated increase in mortality from this. Antiplatelet therapy must also be considered postendovascular intervention. Recommendations for antiplatelet therapy after percutaneous coronary intervention are described elsewhere in this chapter (Table 50.3).

Anticoagulation with unfractionated or low molecular weight heparin is considered an adjunct to antiplatelet therapy. These agents inhibit fibrinolysis, leading to thrombin generation in acute coronary syndrome. For this reason, the low molecular weight heparins may afford an advantage of being direct thrombin inhibitors. Their disadvantages may be their long half-life and accumulation in renal insufficiency, which may be problematic in the case of postoperative bleeding.

BETA-BLOCKER THERAPY

The benefits of beta-blockade, when appropriately used in the treatment of acute MI, have been detailed in the literature.[71] Beta-blockers decrease tachycardia, ventricular arrhythmias, increase preload and have been proved to decrease the perioperative mortality by 28% in the first week, with the

TABLE 50.3

AMERICAN HEART ASSOCIATION/AMERICAN COLLEGE OF CARDIOLOGY RECOMMENDATIONS FOR ANTIPLATELET THERAPY AFTER PERCUTANEOUS CORONARY INTERVENTION (STENT PLACEMENT) IN THE PERIOPERATIVE PERIOD

PERCUTANEOUS INTERVENTION	ANTI-PLATELET THERAPY	TIME OF DELAY OF OPERATION
Angioplasty	Monotherapy[b]	2–4 wk elective surgery, immediately for urgent or emergent surgery
Bare metal stent	Dual therapy for 4 wk followed by monotherapy Monotherapy in surgical emergency	4–6 wk ideally, 2 wk for urgent surgery, immediate or emergent surgery however increases risk of stent occlusion 0.1% in retrospective data
DES (sirolimus)	Dual therapy[a] for 3 mo if no bleeding risk	3 mo elective surgery 3 mo nonelective surgery rethrombosis rates of 0.35%–2.60% (retrospective data)
DES (paclitaxel)	Dual therapy[a] for 6 and 12 mo if no risk of rebleeding	6 mo

Recommendations for antiplatelet therapy poststent placement.
[a]Dual therapy, aspirin plus thienopyridine (ticlopidine or clopidogrel).
[b]Monotherapy, aspirin.

most benefit achieved in the first 48 hours. All patients previously placed on a beta blocker should continue beta blockade in the peri-operative period. Premature discontinuation of beta blockade in the perioperative period is associated with an increased risk of MI.

Morphine provides analgesia and has a cardioprotective effect in patients with NSTEMI.[72,74] It decreases sympathetic tone, reduces heart rate, and lowers blood pressure. Morphine may also offer some benefit in treatment of acute pulmonary edema. Its vasodilator effects decrease afterload and left end-diastolic pressure, thus increasing cardiac output. Its vasodilatory effects, however, may induce hypotension. In addition, excessive use of narcotics in the postoperative setting has been associated with prolonged mechanical ventilation and increased length of ICU stay.[72,73]

Prophylactic use of nitroglycerin may provide symptomatic relief of anginal symptoms but does not provide a meaningful increase in survival benefit.[72-74] Indiscriminate use of nitroglycerin in the postoperative period has been associated with increased risk of hypotension.

HMG-CoA reductase inhibitors or statins have been shown to decrease mortality at 6 months to a year in patients who are considered to be at high coronary risk.[72-74] In addition, they have been shown to decrease the incidence of sudden cardiac death. Patients who have been on statin therapy previously should continue with it in the perioperative period. For patients undergoing vascular surgery with at least one coronary risk factor, the addition of statin therapy may afford meaningful survival benefit.[72-74]

Angiotensin concerting enzyme (ACE) inhibitors have also been shown to reduce morbidity in acute MI.[72-74] The greatest therapeutic benefit is in patients with a decreased left ventricular ejection fraction (<45%) and symptoms of heart failure. In addition patients who have suffered an acute MI with preexisting hypertension or documented mitral regurgitation have an elevated risk of developing ischemic cardiomyopathy, and should be started on an ACE inhibitor within 48 hours of the acute ischemic event.

There are currently no randomized clinical trials that clearly define the therapeutic benefit of cardiac catheterization in the postoperative acute general surgery patient. Indications for catheterization are listed in Table 50.4 and a decision tree regarding catheterization of the postoperative patient is presented in Algorithm 50.2.[72,74,76-78]

MECHANICAL ADJUNCTS IN THE TREATMENT OF ACUTE MYOCARDIAL INFARCTION

Intraaortic balloon pump (IABP) therapy may be necessary in the event of refractory cardiogenic shock. It decreases afterload and increases coronary perfusion. It can be used as an adjunct to reperfusion therapy because it preserves left ventricular function. IABP is contraindicated in patients with previous documented aortoiliac occlusive disease or previous

TABLE 50.4

CLASS I DATA-INDICATIONS FOR CARDIAC CATHETERIZATION

Stable angina with known left main coronary artery stenosis
Stable angina with known three vessel disease and LVEF <50%
Stable onset angina with known two vessel disease with substantial LAD stenosis
Unstable angina, dynamic ST segment changes (> 0.1 mV), hemodynamic instability, and ventricular arrhythmia.
Unstable angina in a non–ST elevation MI at high risk for coronary artery disease

LAD, left anterior descending coronary artery
LVEF, left ventricular ejection fraction
MI, myocardial infarction

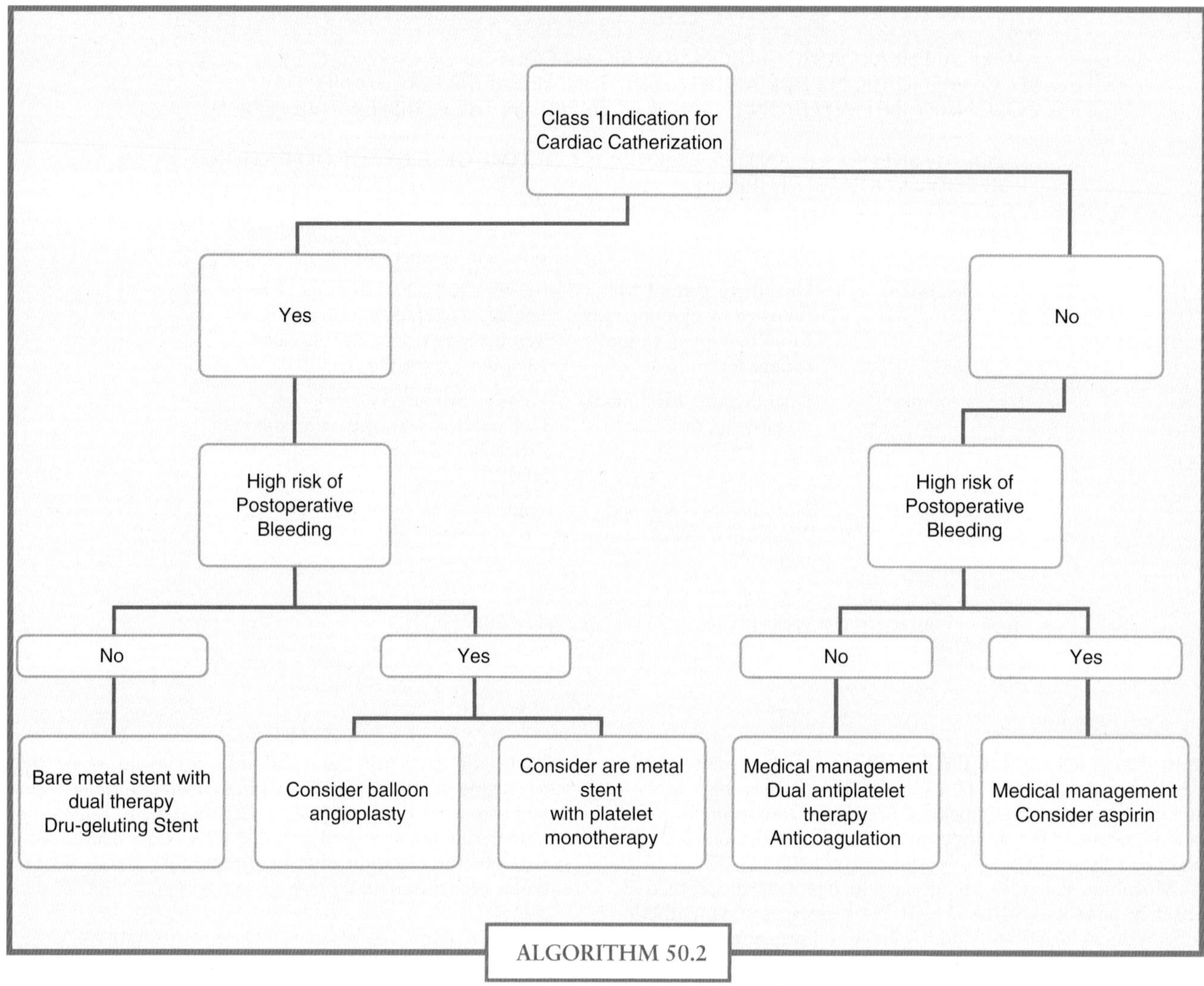

ALGORITHM 50.2 Percutaneous revascularization strategy postoperative acute care surgery

lower extremity bypass. Upon placement of an IABP, frequent peripheral vascular monitoring is mandatory.[79-81]

As a last resort, emergent venoarterial extracorporeal membrane oxygenation (ECMO) may be used as rescue therapy in the treatment of cardiogenic shock or cardiac arrest secondary to myocardial ischemia.[40,81-83] This may be required in the rare patient population with refractory cardiogenic shock despite maximal inotropic and intraaortic balloon pump support. ECMO may function as a bridge to revascularization therapy or as treatment for myocardial stunning secondary to reperfusion injury. This therapy requires anticoagulation and cannulation of the femoral artery, and may comprise lower extremity circulation. In addition, ECMO does not offload the left ventricle and is contraindicated in aortic regurgitation.

Finally, of growing interest in the acute care surgery patient is the phenomenon of "troponin leak" in the physiologically stressed and injured patient.[84-86] A poor choice of terminology once believed to be related to actual cardiac trauma, it is now being recognized that elevated troponin I concentrations can be found in patients with no previous history of ischemic heart disease and no evidence of mechanical trauma to the heart. The phenomenon likely correlates with the physiologic burden of the disease state, but scientific evidence is lacking in regards to effect on outcome. A thorough work up for acute MI is warranted in the patient with elevated troponin until the phenomenon is more clearly defined.

In summary:

- Acute myocardial ischemia is a major cause of morbidity and mortality in the acute care surgery patient.
- Acute surgical illness leads to an inflammatory cascade causing a oxygen/perfusion supply/demand mismatch of the myocardium.
- Rapid surgical correction of underlying disease and prompt treatment of myocardial ischemia according to American Heart Association (AHA)/American College of Cardiology (ACC)/AC guidelines is imperative.
- Initial medical management should include beta blockade, antiplatelet therapy with or without anticoagulation, adequate analgesia, and a high-dose statin.
- The presence of acute ST elevation, worsening anginal symptoms, or hemodynamic compromise with increasing cardiac enzymes concentrations warrants coronary angiography to determine the need for angioplasty/stent placement.
- With the exception of the neurosurgical population, postoperative anticoagulation for acute MI is problematic but

seldom fatal, whereas the mortality of untreated postoperative MI is high, generally favoring anticoagulation in the risk:benegit analysis.

- In refractory cases of cardiogenic shock, mechanical adjuncts such as placement of a IABP or ECMO may be necessary.

CONGESTIVE HEART FAILURE

Nearly 5 million people have been diagnosed with CHF and it is estimated that 500,000 new cases of CHF will be diagnosed in the United States annually. It is a common diagnosis in elderly patients, and as the population continues to age, these patients will comprise a major portion of the acute care surgery practice.

CHF is defined as a clinical syndrome that impedes the filling or emptying of the left or right ventricle and can be categorized as either right- or left-sided CHF.[72,73,87] Abnormalities of ventricular emptying are termed as systolic dysfunction whereas abnormalities of ventricular filling are referred to as diastolic dysfunction. Left-sided systolic dysfunction is the most common cause of heart failure, and is caused by impaired contractility or increased afterload. Example of systolic dysfunction from increased afterload, include hypertension and aortic stenosis. Inability of the ventricles to fill at normal pressures represents diastolic dysfunction. An example of diastolic dysfunction include left ventricular hypertrophy cardiomyopathy. Both systolic and diastolic dysfunction lead to a clinical syndrome of dyspnea, exercise intolerance, fluid retention, and pulmonary edema. Right-sided heart failure is uncommon, but it carries substantive mortality, particularly in the postoperative patient. Acute right-sided heart failure is caused by a sudden increase in afterload due to a decrease in compliance of the pulmonary artery, or intrinsic lung disease. However, the most common cause of right-sided heart failure is chronic pulmonary venous congestion from left-sided heart failure.

Uncontrolled hypertension is the most common cause of left sided CHF. Aortic stenosis is the second most common cause of left-sided heart failure. Diastolic dysfunction, impairment of left ventricular filling in diastole, is characterized by a decrease in left ventricular stroke volume, thus leading to decreased cardiac output. These patients are extremely preload dependent. Because they cannot increase stroke volume, their only compensatory mechanism to increase oxygen delivery tachycardia. This maladaptive mechanism leads to increased myocardial ischemia. Hypertrophic obstructive cardiomyopathy, left ventricular hypertrophy, ischemic cardiomyopathy of the left ventricle, mitral stenosis, or pericardial tamponade cause diastolic dysfunction.

Right-sided heart failure is less common than left-sided heart failure because the right ventricle is thinwalled and highly compliant. It is able to accept a wide range of filling volumes without an increase in the end-diastolic pressure. The right ventricle is susceptible to failure when there is a sudden increase in afterload. The three major causes of right-sided heart failure are: parenchymal pulmonary disease, primary pulmonary hypertension and pulmonary embolism. Treatment of right-sided heart failure entails successfully treating the underlying cause. Acute onset of pulmonary edema secondary to right ventricular overload should be cautiously treated with diuretic therapy. Hypoxia worsens pulmonary vasoconstriction and can worsen the effects of pulmonary hypertension. Close attention should be given to maintenance of arterial oxygen saturation. In patients with chronic obstructive pulmonary disease and pulmonary hypertension, it is important not to suppress the respiratory drive with too much oxygen therapy. In addition, this patient population will benefit from treatment of bronchospasm with beta agonist therapy, and occasionally parenteral steroids. Several medications may afford some benefit in primary pulmonary hypertension; these include calcium channel blockers and pulmonary vasodilators.

The medical treatments of heart failure includes diuretics, vasodilators, beta blockers, and drugs that inhibit the renin–angiotensin–aldosterone pathway. Fluid status and adequate perfusion should be optimized prior to administration of drugs, as the majority of heart failure regimens may exacerbate the hypotension of cardiogenic shock. If the patient is symptomatic from hypertensive heart failure with pulmonary venous congestion from volume overload, diuretics are the initial treatment. In the euvolemic hypertensive heart failure patient, peripheral vasodilators are useful. In the patient with ischemic cardiomyopathy, a beta blocker may be beneficial. Once the patient is stabilized on a beta blocker or loop diuretic, long-term therapy with an ACE inhibitor or angiotensin receptor blocker (ARB) should be initiated. Aldosterone inhibitors can be used in conjunction with the standard regimen of a beta blocker, ACE/ARB inhibitor, and loop diuretic in patients with refractory hypertensive heart failure. Digoxin was the mainstay of treatment of CHF historically and may be considered in the treatment of chronic CHF with associated atrial fibrillation. This provides a general treatment algorithm, but in the case of refractory CHF, early cardiology consultation is warranted.

Takotsubo cardiomyopathy, also known as stress-induced cardiomyopathy or "broken heart" syndrome, is a non-ischemic cardiomyopathy that causes transient weakening of the myocardium.[88,89] The usual presentation of chest pain, ST-segment changes, and cardiac enzyme abnormalities can be observed in this type of cardiomyopathy. The characteristic "apical ballooning" can often be observed by echocardiography. The etiology is unclear, but is likely multifactorial and related to the myocardial response to circulating catecholamines. It is most common in women, especially those who have undergone extreme emotional distress, or an accumulation of multiple physiologic stresses. We make special note of this rare disease process that is being diagnosed with increasing frequency in our acute care surgery patient population. Treatment is supportive and includes the diagnostic and therapeutic modalities discussed above.

In summary:

- CHF is a major cause of morbidity and mortality in the acute care surgery patient.
- There are four categories of CHF based on the location and function of the ventricles. It is either left-sided or right-sided, or an abnormality of filling (diastolic dysfunction) or emptying (systolic dysfunction).
- Cardiovascular medications used in the treatment of heart failure decrease preload (diuretics); decrease afterload (vasodilators, ACE/ARB inhibitors), or increase contractility ACE/ARB inhibitors, digoxin.

VALVULAR HEART DISEASE

Valvular heart disease is common and responsible for nearly 10% of heart failure in the United States.[90] Its prevalence continues to increase as average life expectancy increases. The severity of a patient's valvular disease may determine the patient's ability to survive an operation. When the severity of the patient's valvular disease outweighs the benefits of a high-risk operation, the acute care surgeon should reconsider the risk:benefit of surgical options. For example, placement of a cholecystomy tube, percutaneous drainage of an intra-abdominal abscess, or fecal diversion with a transverse loop colostomy are temporizing procedures, but may provide adequate source control in a moribund patient. If the operative procedure cannot be delayed, hemodynamic assessment tools such as transesophageal echocardiography (TEE) or the PAC may be essential in perioperative management (Refer to previous section on "Evaluation of Cardiac Performance"). Staffing the operative case with an anesthesiologist comfortable with TEE or emergent consultation of the interventional cardiologist may be necessary to optimize patient outcome.

Aortic stenosis is the most common valvular lesion and is most often caused by degenerative calcific disease.[90,91] The diagnostic criteria for critical aortic stenosis include an aortic valve area <0.8 cm^2 or trans-valvular gradient >50 mm Hg. Risk factors include male gender, age >65 years, hypertension, and cigarette smoking. In the asymptomatic patient, the acute care surgeon should proceed if the procedure is considered to be of low or moderate risk (Table 50.1) without further testing. If the surgery is considered highrisk, or if the patient is symptomatic, intraoperative TEE and placement of a PAC may be advisable. Particular attention should be given to the gradient across the aortic valve and evidence of left ventricular hypertrophy. Untreated severe aortic stenosis carries an intraoperative mortality of 10% and a relative risk for 1.55 of perioperative MI for an elective noncardiac surgical procedure.[90,91] An interventional cardiologist should be consulted to discuss percutaneous valvuloplasty as a therapeutic option if the patient's left ventricular failure worsens despite maximal medical therapy. Data on percutaneous valvuloplasty in the adult population shows only temporary improvement of symptoms.[90,91] It also carries a complication rate of 10% with no increase in long-term survival. Its primary function is to serve as a bridge to aortic valve replacement.

Aortic regurgitation can be caused by various etiologies such as a bicuspid aortic valve, rheumatic fever, or infective endocarditis.[90,91] An asymptomatic patient with preserved left ventricular function is considered to be lowrisk. These patients most likely have chronic aortic regurgitation, where left ventricular dilation adequately compensates for increased LVEDV. If a patient is symptomatic or has decreapressed left ventricular function, they are at elevated risk of perioperative complications such as acute onset of CHF.

Mitral stenosis is most commonly caused by rheumatic heart disease. Symptoms include orthopnea, paroxysmal nocturnal dyspnea, and hoarseness caused by compression of the recurrent laryngeal nerve by the left atrium. Mitral valve fusion leads to an increase in the left atrial pressure and increase in the pulmonary vascular pressure. A mitral valve area of <1 cm^2 is considered critical.[72,73,90,91] This leads to an inability of the left atrium to effectively empty, causing pulmonary venous congestion. Impedance of pulmonary venous flow leads to elevated pulmonary artery pressures. This mechanical cause of pulmonary hypertension may lead to right-sided heart failure. These patients are very sensitive to preload and benefit from perioperative beta blockade with adequate but not excessive volume resuscitation. Measurement of pulmonary wedge pressure, EDVI, and CVP are essential for perioperative management of mitral stenosis. Bedside TTE to determine left atrial dilation, LVEF, or respiratory variation of inferior vena cava diameter on echocardiogram also provides clinically useful information. Patients with a mitral valve area <1.5 cm^2 and a gradient of >5 mm Hg without evidence of a mural thrombus may be considered for balloon valvuloplasty.

Mitral regurgitation is the second most common valvular heart defect and is primarily caused by myxomatous degeneration.[90,91] Myocardial ischemia causing left ventricular remodeling or papillary muscle rupture is the second most common cause of mitral regurgitation. This is a high-risk population. Without surgical valve repair these patients have a 5-year survival of 19%–36%. Patients present with dyspnea on exertion with a holosystolic murmur that radiates to the axilla. Increased left atrial pressure leads to left atrial distension causing atrial fibrillation. These patients should be anticoagulated owing to increased risk of thromboembolic disease. It is important to differentiate chronic mitral regurgitation from acute-onset mitral regurgitation. In chronic mitral regurgitation, the left ventricle is distended and unable to accommodate the increased volume of the enlarged left atrium. In acute mitral regurgitation, there is discordance between the left ventricle and left atrium leading to left-sided heart failure and acute pulmonary edema. These patients are sensitive to fluid overload and may benefit from diuretics and afterload reduction.

Pathologic tricuspid regurgitation secondary to right ventricular failure is more common than primary valvular disease. Right ventricular overload, atrial septal defects, idiopathic pulmonary hypertension, or massive pulmonary embolism are causes of tricuspid regurgitation.[90,91] Treatment of tricuspid regurgitation often involves treatment of the underlying pathology leading to right-sided heart failure.

In summary:

- The elderly patient with pre-existing valvular heart disease is becoming more common in the acute care surgery practice.
- To limit perioperative morbidity and mortality the acute care surgeon must choose the operation based on the patient's physiologic reserve.
- In addition, success in this often-moribund population depends not only on the skill of the surgeon, but also on the foresight necessary to generate a treatment plan which includes capable operative staff, comprehensive critical care, and timely consultation.

Arrhythmias in the Postoperative Patient. Postoperative arrhythmias may be the continuance of preoperative (known or unknown) electrical abnormalities of the patient's cardiac electrical system. Alternatively, they may be related to or a consequence of the patient's surgery. Preoperative symptomatic arrhythmias are considered major predictors of perioperative risk; arrhythmias after cardiothoracic surgery are particularly common. The causes of postoperative arrhythmias are often multifactorial, but may be related to increased sympathetic tone, ischemia, postoperative fluid shifts, and electrolyte abnormalities that destabilize the myocardium membrane. Acute care surgeons must recognize that arrhythmias in the immediate postoperative period may indicate an undiagnosed intraoperative complication. If so, these patients may continue to deteriorate in spite of medical management without prompt surgical re-intervention.

One approach to managing postoperative arrhythmias in the acute care surgery patient is to classify them into one of three categories: benign; potentially troublesome; or dangerous. Using this classification we will discuss specific arrhythmias with their treatments.

BENIGN

Sinus tachycardia, atrial premature beats, and premature ventricular beats are typically benign. Increased sympathetic tone, missed doses of preoperative antiarrhythmic medications, postoperative fluid shifts, electrolyte abnormalities, sepsis, anemia, and postoperative pain are possible causes of these arrhythmias in surgical patients. The treatment is to identify the underlying cause and rectify it. Although listed as benign, sinus tachycardia is the most consistent sign of an enteric leak in the early postoperative period and may be an indicat or of a need for reexploration. Asymptomatic bradycardia, first-degree (AV) block or type 1 second-degree atrioventricular (AV) block (Wenckebach block) may also be observed in the postoperative patient, especially in the setting of preexisting sinus node disease, enhanced vagal tone related to nausea, pain, or narcotic medication. These arrhythmias are only specifically treated (see Dangerous below) when they result in hemodynamic compromise.

POTENTIALLY TROUBLESOME

Supraventricular arrhythmias (atrial fibrillation, atrial flutter, paroxysmal supraventricular tachycardia [PSVT] or multifocal atrial tachycardia [MAT]) and nonsustained ventricular tachycardia may have as their cause many of the same factors as the usually "benign" arrhythmias. Nonetheless, they require a more urgent assessment and imply that the patient's cardiac status may be more compromised than expected. Additionally, these arrhythmias are more likely to stress the patient's heart or lead to hemodynamic problems.

Atrial fibrillation is the most common postoperative supraventricular arrhythmia and is an insidious cause of postoperative morbidity. Tachycardia from atrial fibrillation leads to increased myocardial demand and stagnant blood flow in the fibrillating atria promotes mural thrombus formation with the potential for thromboembolic complications. In a hemodynamically unstable patient (chest pain, hypotension, altered mental status, shock) with atrial fibrillation the treatment of choice is direct-current synchronous cardioversion. In the more stable patient, the initial management is rate control with a calcium channel blocker (e.g., verapamil) or beta blocker (e.g., metoprolol), followed by pharmacologic conversion to sinus rhythm (e.g., amiodarone); digoxin is used rarely but may control both rate and thythm. Consideration of anticoagulation while precipitating causes are sought and addressed if sinus rhythm cannot be restored within 24-48 hours. Immediate cardioversion is also the appropriate approach to poorly tolerated PSVT or atrial flutter. However, MAT must be distinguished from atrial fibrillation, as MAT is likely to recur immediately if the underlying cause is not corrected. At times, an unmonitored patient is found to be in atrial fibrillation of unknown duration. This may happen when an ECG is done because of an irregular pulse or a change in the patient's clinical status. If the atrial fibrillation is not definitively confirmed to have been present for <48 hours and the patient has not been fully anticoagulated, it is safest to cardiovert with drugs or direct electrical current only after a transesophageal echocardiogram excludes a thrombus. If a thrombus is present, cardioversion should be deferred and the patient should be anticoagulated and simply rate-controlled with a beta blocker or calcium channel blocker. The cumulative risk of thromboembolism from atrial fibrillation is 1% per year or more depending on other risk factors such as CHF, hypertension, age >75 years, diabetes, or prior stroke. The acute care surgeon must weigh this against the risk of bleeding with anticoagulation.

Atrial flutter is treated in the same manner as atrial fibrillation, except that there may be a greater role for digoxin. On the other hand PSVT, which is a narrow-complex QRS tachycardia, may be initially diagnosed medically with the administration of adenosine; AV nodal reentry the tachycardia will break. In the case of an atrial tachycardia or atrial fibrillation or flutter, the transitory blockade of the AV node induced by adenosine will allow atrial activity to be parsed more clearly. Then with metabolism of adenosine, AV conduction and the tachycardia will resume within seconds. At this point, oral or intravenous calcium channel blockers or beta blockers can be used to slow the tachycardia.

Nonsustained ventricular tachycardia (VT lasting <30 seconds) in the early postoperative period must be treated as stress on the heart that may be related to a surgical complication until proven otherwise. While a surgical complication is being sought, the acute care surgeon should initiate a prompt work up for ischemia, hypoxia, and electrolyte abnormalities. In addition, central venous catheters that are advanced too far can irritate the ventricle and precipitate ventricular arrhythmias.

DANGEROUS

Sustained wide-complex QRS tachycardias are likely to compromise the postoperative patient and need to be managed emergently because of the difficulty of distinguishing between sustained VT and PSVT with aberrant conduction. If the patient is stable, a 12-lead ECG should be obtained while consultation is being requested from a cardiologist or cardiac electrophysiologist. Amiodarone-IV may be initiated and is unlikely to compromise the patient's evaluation and management. If the patient becomes hypotensive or pulseless with a wide-QRS tachycardia, immediate initiation of advanced cardiac life support protocols is mandatory.

Bradycardia with evidence of poor perfusion such as hypotension, shock, chest pain, or altered mental status is another situation in which one must be able to immediately initiate the advanced cardiac life support protocol. This would include the use of atropine, epinephrine, or dopamine. It may also require the use of transcutaneous or temporary transvenous pacing.

Ventricular fibrillation and pulseless electrical activity are the most catastrophic postoperative arrhythmias and clearly call for initiation of the appropriate resuscitation protocols. If the precipitant is in doubt and the patient continues to decline despite medical intervention, surgical exploration should be considered.

In summary:

- Acute surgical illness incites an inflammatory cascade that leads to multiple physiologic derangements, which destabilize the myocardium, leading to postoperative arrhythmias.
- A useful approach is to classify these arrhythmias as benign (sinus tachycardia, sinus bradycardia, premature atrial or ventricular beats); potentially dangerous (atrial fibrillation, atrial flutter, PSVT, and MAT), or dangerous (ventricular tachycardia and ventricular fibrillation)
- In addition to initiation of resuscitation protocols, the acute care surgeon must rectify the initiating pathologic condition.

Extrinsic Causes of Cardiovascular Failure. Pulmonary embolism is diagnosed in 650,000 new cases every year and is a major cause of morbidity and mortality in the postoperative patient.[72,73] Patients with a previous history of pulmonary embolism, recent surgery, or diagnosed hypercoagulable state are at increased risk. Physical examination is often unreliable but patients may present with tachycardia, tachypnea, or acuteonset of lower extremity swelling. The most common ECG abnormality is sinus tachycardia. In the case of a massive pulmonary embolism, the classic pattern of S1-Q3-T3 pattern of right heart strain may be present. Spiral computed tomography (CT) is the gold standard for diagnosis. In the unstable patient, an echocardiogram may be useful to exclude the presence of a massive pulmonary embolus. Treatment of acute pulmonary embolism requires prompt administration of anticoagulation with unfractionated or low-molecular-weight heparin. Massive pulmonary embolism with associated right heart failure may require operative or endovascular embolectomy. Thrombolytic therapy, although described, is not practical in the early postoperative patient because of a very high risk of bleeding.

FAT OR AIR EMBOLISM

Patients with long bone fractures are at increased risk of fat embolization to the pulmonary arterial system. Moreover, those patients undergoing orthopedic surgery are at an increased risk of fat embolism in the postoperative period. This disease process presents with the triad of hypoxemia, neurologic abnormalities, and a characteristic petechial rash. Chest CT scan may show focal areas of ground glass opacification and lobar thickening. On fundoscopic exam patients may have "cotton wool" spots as a result of fat deposition in the retinal vessels; treatment is supportive.

Air embolism is a rare, but life-threatening emergency in the perioperative period. Increasingly, the acute care surgery patient is being treated with laparoscopy for their disease process. Other potential causes include major hepatic surgery or major head and neck surgery. With insufflation and the establishment of pneumoperitoneum, air may enter the venous system and embolize to the heart. Clinically the patient will present with hypotension and tachycardia. On physical examination, the patient may demonstrate the classic "mill wheel" murmur embolus. Treatment is placement of the patient in Trendelenburg position with the right side up to avoid further embolization and to avoid obstruction of the pulmonary outflow tract. Evacuation of the air by aspiration from a PAC or central venous catheter can then be attempted.

TENSION PNEUMO-OR HEMOTHORAX

Trauma patients frequently present with hemo- or pneumothoraces; as the amount of blood or air increases in the pleural space, the patient is at an increased risk to develop tension pneumothorax. This results from a decrease in venous return to the heart. Iatrogenic pneumothorax is associated with central venous catheter placement; sudden decompensation in this patient population should trigger an immediate needle decompression followed by tube thoracostomy. Because of the clinical urgency, remember that tension pneumothorax should be a clinical diagnosis, not one made by imaging.

THYROID DYSFUNCTION

Patients with abnormalities of thyroid function often have myocardial dysfunction and are at risk for development of a dilated cardiomyopathy.[73] Hyperthyroidism has been associated with new-onset atrial fibrillation and ventricular arrhythmias. Hypothyroidism can lead to decreased contractility and left-sided heart failure if left untreated. Treatment is aimed at restoration of the patient to the euthyroid state.

ADRENAL INSUFFICIENCY

Elevated circulating concentrations of corticosteroids are part of the normal response to critical illness. However, those patients unable to mount this physiologic response can develop profound cardiovascular failure. Relative adrenal insufficiency is an important cause of cardiovascular failure in the acute care surgery population.[73,92-94] These patients fail to increase their cardiac output due to inappropriately low concentrations of cortisol in the face of acute surgical illness. They may exhibit profound hypotension due to vasodilatory shock despite maximal vasopressor therapy. The diagnosis of adrenal insufficiency can be made by measurement of serum cortisol, or by performing a cosyntropin (corticotropin [ACTH] analogue) stimulation test. Treatment of relative adrenal insufficiency with intravenous corticosteroids, (hydrocortisone 50 mg IV q6-8h) with or without mineralocorticoids, (fludrocortisone 50 mcg qd), has been shown to decrease mortality and vasopressors requirements when compared to placebo in randomized clinical trials.[95-100] However, several other studies have failed to confirm this effect. In addition, prolonged steroid use in the postoperative patient may lead to impaired wound healing and immunosuppression. At our institution we recommend treatment with a short course of intravenous steroids in patients who meet the following criteria: (1) Patients who have profound vasodilatory shock despite adequate fluid resuscitation and a maximal dose of vasopressor therapy; and (2) patients who are hypotensive and have relatively low random serum cortisol levels, or fail to stimulate appropriately on the ACTH stimulation test.

DRUG REACTIONS

Propofol infusion syndrome is rare but fatal if left untreated in the acute care surgery patient.[101] It occurs with prolonged use of propofol in the setting of a systemic immune inflammatory response. Critical illness, sepsis, and use of corticosteroids often precipitate this syndrome. The exact mechanism is unknown. It is believed that there is an interaction between the metabolites of propofol and endogenous catecholamines that leads to a massive cytokine release. These patients present with profound bradycardia, rhabdomyolysis, metabolic acidosis, hyperkalemia, and renal and hepatic failure. Treatment involves symptomatic support. However the presence of organ dysfunction with this syndrome is generally fatal.

Etomidate is a frequently used induction medication for endotracheal intubation. However, evidence exists that even one-time dosing of this medication causes adrenal suppression that can lead to adrenal insufficiency in the critically ill patient.[88,89,102,103] Many recreational drugs have been associated with cardiovascular failure. Stimulants such as cocaine or methamphetamines can lead to acute decompensated heart failure. The cardiotoxic effects of cocaine are not completely understood. However, cocaine may increase myocardial ischemia by causing coronary artery vasospasm, tachyarrhythmias, and coronary artery thrombosis. Acute treatment of cocaine toxicity with a beta-blocker is ill-advised, as it may lead to unopposed alpha adrenergic activity that may precipitate severe hypertension or may exacerbate preexisting heart failure.[73] Chronic stimulant use is associated with dilated cardiomyopathy. Chronic ethanol intoxication has been associated with a dilated cardiomyopathy.

In summary:

- Causes of intrinsic cardiovascular failure in the acute care surgery patient include myocardial ischemia, CHF, arrhythmias, and valvular heart disease, and present a unique challenge in the perioperative period (Algorithm 50.3).
- Extrinsic causes of cardiovascular failure occur in the face of a structurally normal heart, but external impedance results in decreased cardiac output. Treatment is aimed at removal of the external cause and support of the patient (Algorithm 50.4).

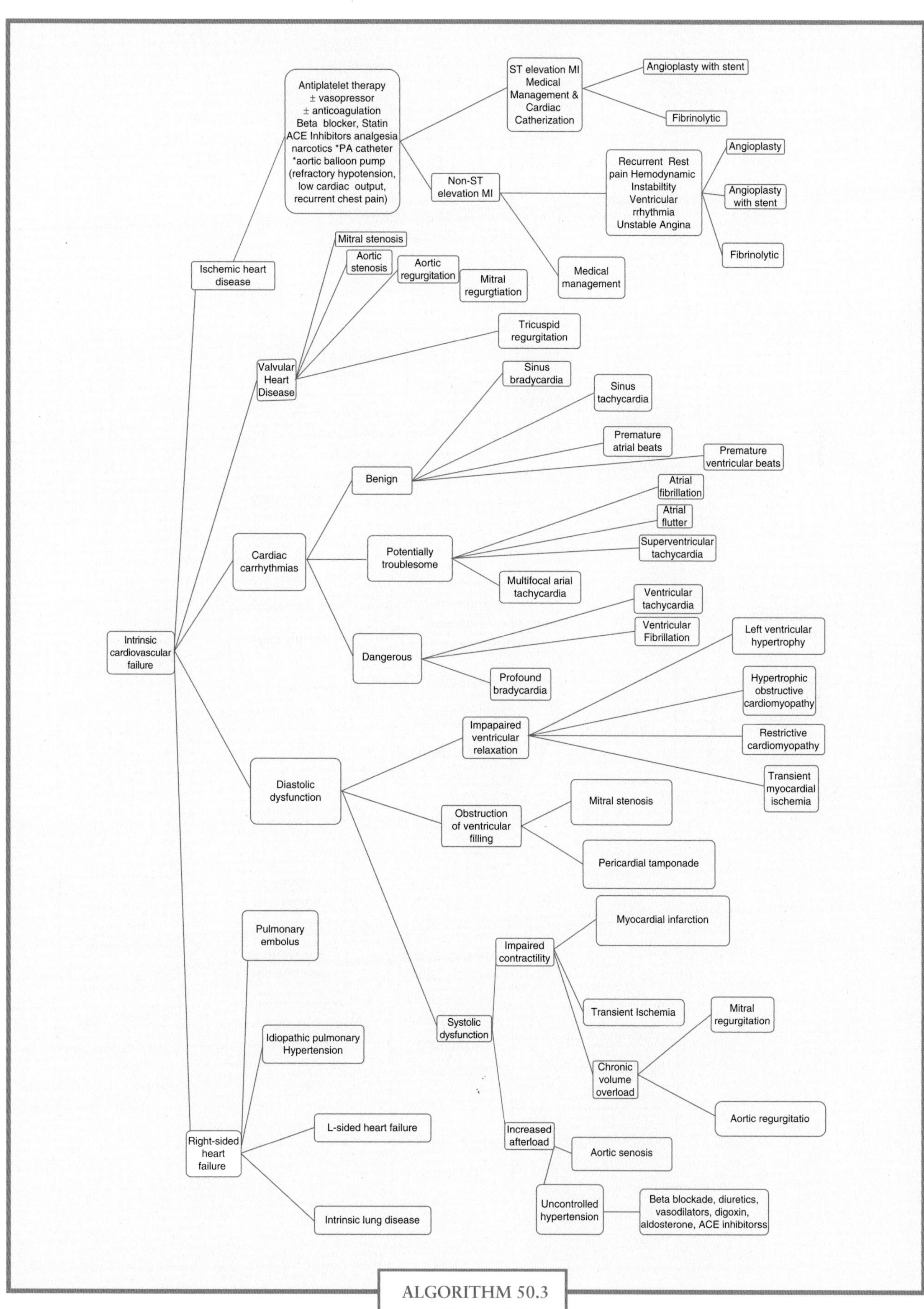

ALGORITHM 50.3 Intrinsic cardiovascular failure algorithm.
ACS, angiotensin converting enzyme; MI, myocardial infarction; PA, pulmonary artery

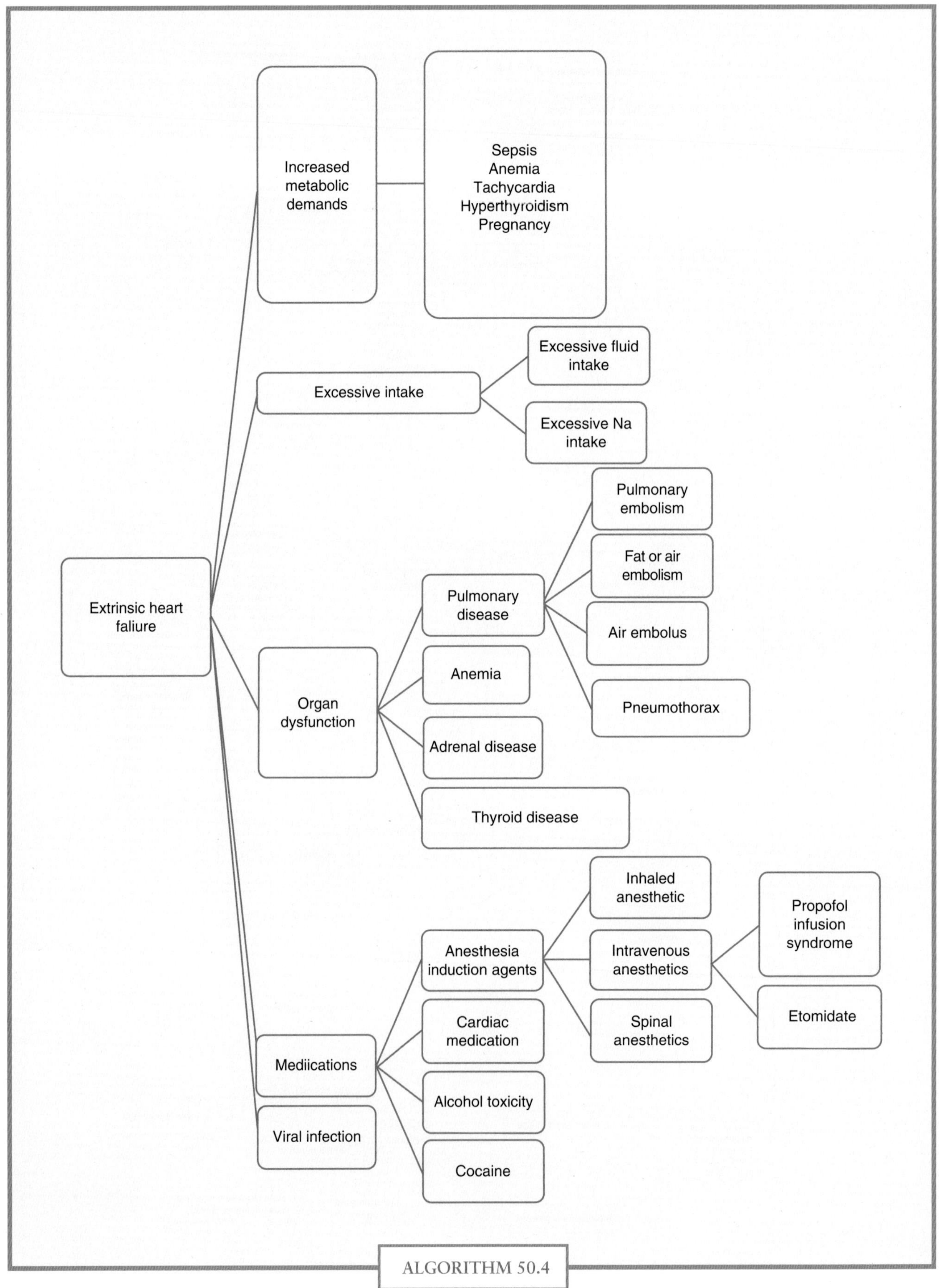

ALGORITHM 50.4 Extrinsic heart failure algorithm.

References

1. Cheatham ML. Resuscitation end points in severe sepsis: central venous pressure, mean arterial pressure, mixed venous oxygen saturation, and... intra-abdominal pressure. *Crit Care Med.* 2008;36:1012-1014.
2. Cholley BP, Payen D. Pulmonary-artery catheters in high-risk surgical patients. *N Engl J Med.* 2003;348:2035-2037.
3. Finfer S, Delaney A. Pulmonary artery catheters. *BMJ.* 2006;333:930-931.
4. Gattinoni L, Brazzi L, Pelosi P, et al. A trial of goal-oriented hemodynamic therapy in critically ill patients. SvO2 Collaborative Group. *N Engl J Med.* 1995;333:1025-1032.
5. Harvey S, Harrison DA, Singer M, et al. Assessment of the clinical effectiveness of pulmonary artery catheters in management of patients in intensive care (PAC-Man): a randomised controlled trial. *Lancet.* 2005;366:472-477.
6. McKinley BA, Sucher JF, Todd SR, et al. Central venous pressure versus pulmonary artery catheter-directed shock resuscitation. *Shock.* 2009;32:463-470.
7. Singh NK, Sangwan G, White P. Central venous pressure as popular resuscitation surrogate: not totally unjustified. *Chest.* 2008;134:1352-1353.
8. Ward KR, Tiba MH, Barbee RW, et al. A new noninvasive method to determine central venous pressure. *Resuscitation.* 2006;70:238-246.
9. Puskarich MA, Marchick MR, Kline JA, et al. One year mortality of patients treated with an emergency department based early goal directed therapy protocol for severe sepsis and septic shock: a before and after study. *Crit Care.* 2009;13:R167.
10. Tisherman SA, Barie P, Bokhari F, et al. Clinical practice guideline: endpoints of resuscitation. *J Trauma.* 2004;57:898-912.
11. Cariou A, Monchi M, Dhainaut JF. Continuous cardiac output and mixed venous oxygen saturation monitoring. *J Crit Care.* 1998;13:198-213.
12. Karkouti K, Wijeysundera DN, Beattie SW. Pulmonary-artery catheters in high-risk surgical patients. *N Engl J Med.* 2003;348:2035-2037.
13. Kaufman JL. Do critically ill patients benefit from use of pulmonary artery catheters? *JAMA.* 2000;284:1242.
14. Sandham JD, Hull RD, Brant RF, et al. A randomized, controlled trial of the use of pulmonary-artery catheters in high-risk surgical patients. *N Engl J Med.* 2003;348:5-14.
15. Shure D. Pulmonary-artery catheters—peace at last? *N Engl J Med.* 2006;354:2273-2274.
16. Simini B. Pulmonary artery catheters in intensive care. *Lancet.* 2005;366:435-436.
17. Vincent JL. A reappraisal for the use of pulmonary artery catheters. *Crit Care.* 2006;10 Suppl 3:S1.
18. Friese RS, Shafi S, Gentilello LM. Pulmonary artery catheter use is associated with reduced mortality in severely injured patients: a National Trauma Data Bank analysis of 53,312 patients. *Crit Care Med.* 2006;34:1597-1601.
19. Bellemare P, Goldberg P, Magder SA. Variations in pulmonary artery occlusion pressure to estimate changes in pleural pressure. *Intensive Care Med.* 2007;33:2004-2008.
20. Kumar A, Anel R, Bunnell E, et al. Pulmonary artery occlusion pressure and central venous pressure fail to predict ventricular filling volume, cardiac performance, or the response to volume infusion in normal subjects. *Crit Care Med.* 2004;32:691-699.
21. Pinsky MR. Clinical significance of pulmonary artery occlusion pressure. *Intensive Care Med.* 2003;29:175-178.
22. Vignon P, AitHssain A, Francois B, et al. Echocardiographic assessment of pulmonary artery occlusion pressure in ventilated patients: a transoesophageal study. *Crit Care.* 2008;12:R18.
23. Siniscalchi A, Pavesi M, Piraccini E, et al. Right ventricular end-diastolic volume index as a predictor of preload status in patients with low right ventricular ejection fraction during orthotopic liver transplantation. *Transplant Proc.* 2005;37:2541-2543.
24. Cheatham ML, Nelson LD, Chang MC, et al. Right ventricular end-diastolic volume index as a predictor of preload status in patients on positive end-expiratory pressure. *Crit Care Med.* 1998;26:1801-1806.
25. Mahjoub Y, Pila C, Friggeri A, et al. Assessing fluid responsiveness in critically ill patients: False-positive pulse pressure variation is detected by Doppler echocardiographic evaluation of the right ventricle. *Crit Care Med.* 2009;37:2570-2575.
26. Mark DG, Hayden GE, Ky B, et al. Hand-carried echocardiography for assessment of left ventricular filling and ejection fraction in the surgical intensive care unit. *J Crit Care.* 2009;24:470-477.
27. Melamed R, Sprenkle MD, Ulstad VK, et al. Assessment of left ventricular function by intensivists using hand-held echocardiography. *Chest.* 2009;135:1416-1420.
28. Poelaert J. Use of ultrasound in the ICU. *Best Pract Res Clin Anaesthesiol.* 2009;23:249-261.
29. Salem R, Vallee F, Rusca M, et al. Hemodynamic monitoring by echocardiography in the ICU: the role of the new echo techniques. *Curr Opin Crit Care.* 2008;14:561-568.
30. Chelly MR, Margulies DR, Mandavia D, et al. The evolving role of FAST scan for the diagnosis of pericardial fluid. *J Trauma.* 2004;56:915-917.
31. Kirkpatrick AW, Simons RK, Brown R, et al. The hand-held FAST: experience with hand-held trauma sonography in a level-I urban trauma center. *Injury.* 2002;33:303-308.
32. Myers J. Focused assessment with sonography for trauma (FAST): the truth about ultrasound in blunt trauma. *J Trauma.* 2007;62:S28.
33. Ollerton JE, Sugrue M, Balogh Z, et al. Prospective study to evaluate the influence of FAST on trauma patient management. *J Trauma.* 2006;60:785-791.
34. Scalea TM, Rodriguez A, Chiu WC, et al. Focused Assessment with Sonography for Trauma (FAST): results from an international consensus conference. *J Trauma.* 1999;46:466-472.
35. Speight J, Sanders M. Pericardial tamponade with a positive abdominal FAST scan in blunt chest trauma. *J Trauma.* 2006;61:743-745.
36. Hernandez C, Shuler K, Hannan H, et al. C.A.U.S.E.: Cardiac arrest ultrasound exam—a better approach to managing patients in primary non-arrhythmogenic cardiac arrest. *Resuscitation.* 2008;76:198-206.
37. Thalhammer C, Siegemund M, Aschwanden M, et al. Non-invasive central venous pressure measurement by compression ultrasound—a step into real life. *Resuscitation.* 2009;80:1130-1136.
38. Gattinoni L, Brazzi L, Pelosi P, et al. A trial of goal-oriented hemodynamic therapy in critically ill patients. SVO_2 Collaborative Group. *N Engl J Med.* 1995;333:1025-1032.
39. Andel D, Kamolz LP, Roka J, et al. Base deficit and lactate: early predictors of morbidity and mortality in patients with burns. *Burns.* 2007;33:973-978.
40. Callaway DW, Shapiro NI, Donnino MW, et al. Serum lactate and base deficit as predictors of mortality in normotensive elderly blunt trauma patients. *J Trauma.* 2009;66:1040-1044.
41. Chang MC, Rutherford EJ, Morris JA Jr. Base deficit as a guide to injury severity and volume resuscitation. *J Tenn Med Assoc.* 1993;86:59-61.
42. Kaplan LJ, Kellum JA. Initial pH, base deficit, lactate, anion gap, strong ion difference, and strong ion gap predict outcome from major vascular injury. *Crit Care Med.* 2004;32:1120-1124.
43. Paladino L, Sinert R, Wallace D, et al. The utility of base deficit and arterial lactate in differentiating major from minor injury in trauma patients with normal vital signs. *Resuscitation.* 2008;77:363-368.
44. Baenziger O, Keel M, Bucher HU, et al. Oxygen extraction index measured by near infrared spectroscopy—a parameter for monitoring tissue oxygenation? *Adv Exp Med Biol.* 2009;645:161-166.
45. King DR, Ogilvie MP, Pereira BM, et al. Heart rate variability as a triage tool in patients with trauma during prehospital helicopter transport. *J Trauma.* 2009;67:436-440.
46. Morris JA Jr, Norris PR, Moore JH, et al. Genetic variation in the autonomic nervous system affects mortality: a study of 1,095 trauma patients. *J Am Coll Surg.* 2009;208:663-668.
47. Morris JA Jr, Norris PR, Ozdas A, et al. Reduced heart rate variability: an indicator of cardiac uncoupling and diminished physiologic reserve in 1,425 trauma patients. *J Trauma.* 2006;60:1165-1173.
48. Mowery NT, Norris PR, Riordan W, et al. Cardiac uncoupling and heart rate variability are associated with intracranial hypertension and mortality: a study of 145 trauma patients with continuous monitoring. *J Trauma.* 2008;65:621-627.
49. Proctor KG, Atapattu SA, Duncan RC. Heart rate variability index in trauma patients. *J Trauma.* 2007;63:33-43.
50. Bickell WH, Wall MJ Jr, Pepe PE, et al. Immediate versus delayed fluid resuscitation for hypotensive patients with penetrating torso injuries. *N Engl J Med.* 1994;331:1105-1109.
51. Bourguignon PR, Shackford SR, Shiffer C, et al. Delayed fluid resuscitation of head injury and uncontrolled hemorrhagic shock. *Arch Surg.* 1998;133:390-398.
52. Benson AB, Moss M, Silliman CC. Transfusion-related acute lung injury (TRALI): a clinical review with emphasis on the critically ill. *Br J Haematol.* 2009;147:431-443.
53. Chant C, Wilson G, Friedrich JO. Anemia, transfusion, and phlebotomy practices in critically ill patients with prolonged ICU length of stay: a cohort study. *Crit Care.* 2006;10:R140.
54. Hebert PC, Tinmouth A, Corwin HL. Controversies in RBC transfusion in the critically ill. *Chest.* 2007;131:1583-1590.
55. Lauzier F, Cook D, Griffith L, et al. Fresh frozen plasma transfusion in critically ill patients. *Crit Care Med.* 2007;35:1655-1659.
56. Li G, Kojicic M, Reriani MK, et al. Long-term survival and quality of life after transfusion-associated pulmonary edema in critically ill medical patients. *Chest.* 2010;137:783-789.
57. Napolitano LM, Corwin HL. Efficacy of red blood cell transfusion in the critically ill. *Crit Care Clin.* 2004;20:255-268.
58. Rana R, Afessa B, Keegan MT, et al. Evidence-based red cell transfusion in the critically ill: quality improvement using computerized physician order entry. *Crit Care Med.* 2006;34:1892-1897.
59. Sarani B, Dunkman WJ, Dean L, et al. Transfusion of fresh frozen plasma in critically ill surgical patients is associated with an increased risk of infection. *Crit Care Med.* 2008;36:1114-1118.
60. Shorr AF, Jackson WL, Kelly KM, et al. Transfusion practice and blood stream infections in critically ill patients. *Chest.* 2005;127:1722-1728.
61. Vlaar AP, Binnekade JM, Prins D, et al. Risk factors and outcome of transfusion-related acute lung injury in the critically ill: a nested case-control study. *Crit Care Med.* 2009.
62. Napolitano LM, Kurek S, Luchette FA, et al. Clinical practice guideline: red blood cell transfusion in adult trauma and critical care. *J Trauma.* 2009;67:1439-1442.

63. Borgman MA, Spinella PC, Perkins JG, et al. The ratio of blood products transfused affects mortality in patients receiving massive transfusions at a combat support hospital. *J Trauma*. 2007;63:805-813.
64. Riskin DJ, Tsai TC, Riskin L, et al. Massive transfusion protocols: the role of aggressive resuscitation versus product ratio in mortality reduction. *J Am Coll Surg*. 2009;209:198-205.
65. Snyder CW, Weinberg JA, McGwin G Jr, et al. The relationship of blood product ratio to mortality: survival benefit or survival bias? *J Trauma*. 2009;66:358-362.
66. Sperry JL, Ochoa JB, Gunn SR, et al. An FFP:PRBC transfusion ratio ≥1:1.5 is associated with a lower risk of mortality after massive transfusion. *J Trauma*. 2008;65:986-993.
67. Stinger HK, Spinella PC, Perkins JG, et al. The ratio of fibrinogen to red cells transfused affects survival in casualties receiving massive transfusions at an army combat support hospital. *J Trauma*. 2008;64:S79-S85.
68. Zink KA, Sambasivan CN, Holcomb JB, et al. A high ratio of plasma and platelets to packed red blood cells in the first 6 hours of massive transfusion improves outcomes in a large multicenter study. *Am J Surg*. 2009;197:565-570.
69. Cotton BA, Au BK, Nunez TC, et al. Predefined massive transfusion protocols are associated with a reduction in organ failure and postinjury complications. *J Trauma*. 2009;66:41-48.
70. Gunter OL Jr, Au BK, Isbell JM, et al. Optimizing outcomes in damage control resuscitation: identifying blood product ratios associated with improved survival. *J Trauma*. 2008;65:527-534.
71. Fleisher LA, Beckman JA, Brown KA, et al. 2009 ACCF/AHA focused update on perioperative beta blockade incorporated into the ACC/AHA 2007 guidelines on perioperative cardiovascular evaluation and care for noncardiac surgery. *J Am Coll Cardiol*. 2009;54:e13-e118.
72. Merli GJ. Noncardiac surgery in the patient with cardiovascular disease: preoperative evaluation and perioperative care. In: Merli GJ, Weitz H, ed. *Medical Management of the Surgical Patient*. Philadelphia. Saunders Elsevier; 2008;157-258.
73. Weitz H. Cardiovascular Disease. In Smith III RB, Dotson TF, Spell NO, Walker HK, eds. Medical management of the surgical patient. A textbook of perioperative medicine. Cambridge, United Kingdom. Cambridge University Press 2010;62-101. *Medical Management of the Surgical Patient*. 2010.
74. Adesanya AO, de Lemos JA, Greilich NB, et al. Management of perioperative myocardial infarction in noncardiac surgical patients. *Chest*. 2006;130:584-596.
75. Berger PB, Bellot V, Bell MR, et al. An immediate invasive strategy for the treatment of acute myocardial infarction early after noncardiac surgery. *Am J Cardiol*. 2001;87:1100-1102, A6, A9.
76. Kushner FG, Hand M, Smith SC Jr, et al. 2009 Focused Updates: ACC/AHA Guidelines for the Management of Patients With ST-Elevation Myocardial Infarction (updating the 2004 Guideline and 2007 Focused Update) and ACC/AHA/SCAI Guidelines on Percutaneous Coronary Intervention (updating the 2005 Guideline and 2007 Focused Update): a report of the American College of Cardiology Foundation/American Heart Association Task Force on Practice Guidelines. *Circulation*. 2009;120:2271-2306.
77. Berger PB, Bell MR, Rihal CS, et al. Clopidogrel versus ticlopidine after intracoronary stent placement. *J Am Coll Cardiol*. 1999;34:1891-1894.
78. Newsome LT, Weller RS, Gerancher JC, et al. Coronary artery stents: II. Perioperative considerations and management. *Anesth Analg*. 2008;107:570-590.
79. Dhar G, Jolly N. Mechanical versus pharmacologic support for cardiogenic shock. *Catheter Cardiovasc Interv*. 2009.
80. Perera D, Stables R, Booth J, et al. The balloon pump-assisted coronary intervention study (BCIS-1): rationale and design. *Am Heart J*. 2009;158:910-916.
81. Wang SL, Liu MX, Wang XZ, et al. Efficacy and safety of intra-aortic balloon pump-assisted interventional therapy in different age groups of patients with acute coronary syndrome. *Chin Med J (Engl)*. 2009;122:2724-2727.
82. Sidebotham D, McGeorge A, McGuinness S, et al. Extracorporeal membrane oxygenation for treating severe cardiac and respiratory disease in adults: Part 1–overview of extracorporeal membrane oxygenation. *J Cardiothorac Vasc Anesth*. 2009;23:886-892.
83. Sidebotham D, McGeorge A, McGuinness S, et al. Extracorporeal Membrane Oxygenation for Treating Severe Cardiac and Respiratory Failure in Adults: Part 2-Technical Considerations. *J Cardiothorac Vasc Anesth*. 2009;23(6):886-892.
84. Edouard AR, Felten ML, Hebert JL, et al. Incidence and significance of cardiac troponin I release in severe trauma patients. *Anesthesiology*. 2004;101:1262-1268.
85. Khavandi A, Jenkins NP, Lee HS, et al. Misdiagnosis of myocardial infarction by troponin I following minor blunt chest trauma. *Emerg Med J*. 2005;22:603-604.
86. Martin M, Mullenix P, Rhee P, et al. Troponin increases in the critically injured patient: mechanical trauma or physiologic stress? *J Trauma*. 2005;59:1086-1091.
87. Hunt SA, Abraham WT, Chin MH, et al. 2009 focused update incorporated into the ACC/AHA 2005 Guidelines for the Diagnosis and Management of Heart Failure in Adults: a report of the American College of Cardiology Foundation/American Heart Association Task Force on Practice Guidelines: developed in collaboration with the International Society for Heart and Lung Transplantation. *Circulation*. 2009;119: e391-e479.
88. Bielecka-Dabrowa A, Mikhailidis DP, Hannam S, et al. Takotsubo cardiomyopathy—the current state of knowledge. *Int J Cardiol*. 2010; 142:120-125.
89. Griffin S, Logue B. Takotsubo cardiomyopathy: a nurse's guide. *Crit Care Nurse*. 2009;29:32-42.
90. Bonow RO, Carabello BA, Chatterjee K, et al. 2008 focused update incorporated into the ACC/AHA 2006 guidelines for the management of patients with valvular heart disease: a report of the American College of Cardiology/American Heart Association Task Force on Practice Guidelines (Writing Committee to revise the 1998 guidelines for the management of patients with valvular heart disease). Endorsed by the Society of Cardiovascular Anesthesiologists, Society for Cardiovascular Angiography and Interventions, and Society of Thoracic Surgeons. *J Am Coll Cardiol*. 2008;52:e1-e142.
91. Vahanian A, Baumgartner H, Bax J, et al. Guidelines on the management of valvular heart disease: The Task Force on the Management of Valvular Heart Disease of the European Society of Cardiology. *Eur Heart J*. 2007;28:230-268.
92. Guillamondegui OD, Gunter OL, Patel S, et al. Acute adrenal insufficiency may affect outcome in the trauma patient. *Am Surg*. 2009;75:287-290.
93. Morris JA Jr, Norris PR, Waitman LR, et al. Adrenal insufficiency, heart rate variability, and complex biologic systems: a study of 1,871 critically ill trauma patients. *J Am Coll Surg*. 2007;204:885-892.
94. Wu JY, Hsu SC, Ku SC, et al. Adrenal insufficiency in prolonged critical illness. *Crit Care*. 2008;12:R65.
95. Abraham E, Evans T. Corticosteroids and septic shock. *JAMA*. 2002;288:886-887.
96. Annane D, Sebille V, Charpentier C, et al. Effect of treatment with low doses of hydrocortisone and fludrocortisone on mortality in patients with septic shock. *JAMA*. 2002;288:862-871.
97. Brown JM. Corticosteroids for patients with septic shock. *JAMA*. 2003;289:41-44.
98. Coursin DB, Wood KE. Corticosteroid supplementation for adrenal insufficiency. *JAMA*. 2002;287:236-240.
99. Salvatori R. Adrenal insufficiency. *JAMA*. 2005;294:2481-2488.
100. Sprung CL, Annane D, Keh D, et al. Hydrocortisone therapy for patients with septic shock. *N Engl J Med*. 2008;358:111-124.
101. Rajda C, Dereczyk D, Kunkel P. Propofol infusion syndrome. *J Trauma Nurs*. 2008;15:118-122.
102. Kamp R, Kress JP. Etomidate, sepsis, and adrenal function: not as bad as we thought? *Crit Care*. 2007;11:145.
103. Vinclair M, Broux C, Faure P, et al. Duration of adrenal inhibition following a single dose of etomidate in critically ill patients. *Intensive Care Med*. 2008;34:714-719.

CHAPTER 51 ■ ACUTE LIVER FAILURE AND PORTAL HYPERTENSION

DEANNA BLISARD AND MICHAEL E. DE VERA

ACUTE LIVER FAILURE

Fulminant hepatic failure is synonymous with acute liver failure (ALF), a rare disorder that often leads to devastating consequences. ALF is rapid deterioration of liver function resulting in altered mutation and coagulopathy in previously normal individuals. The loss of hepatic function quickly leads to multiorgan failure and frequently death. Approximately 2,000 cases of ALF occur in the United States per year.[1] The clinical syndrome was originally described as "sudden severe impairment of hepatic function resulting in jaundice and followed by hepatic encephalopathy (HE) within 8 weeks of the onset, in the absence of prior liver disease."[2] The most widely accepted definition of ALF is the presence of coagulation abnormality and any degree of encephalopathy in a patient without preexisting cirrhosis and with an illness of <26 weeks duration.[3] ALF can be classified according to the length of illness such as hyperacute (<7 days), acute (7–21 days), or subacute (>21 days and <26 weeks), but these terms are not helpful since there is no prognostic significance distinct from the cause of the illness.

The etiology of ALF provides one of the best indicators of prognosis[4] and also dictates specific management options. ALF can be induced by viral (hepatitis A, hepatitis B, herpes, cytomegalovirus, Epstein-Barr virus), vascular (Budd-Chiari syndrome, right heart failure, shock liver), metabolic (Wilson's disease, hemolysis–elevated liver enzymes–low platelet count syndrome, acute fatty liver of pregnancy, tyrosinemia), drugs and toxins (acetaminophen, *Amanita phalloides*, *Bacillus cereus* toxin, herbal remedies), or miscellaneous/indeterminate (malignant infiltration, autoimmune hepatitis, sepsis) causes. Acetaminophen toxicity is the leading cause of ALF in the United States, accounting for 40% of cases.[1] Acetaminophen-induced ALF is suspected with evidence of excessive ingestion, usually because of a suicide attempt or supratherapeutic quantities of pain medication. Acetaminophen is a dose-related toxin with most ingestions which lead to ALF exceeding 10 g/day. Acetaminophen levels should be drawn on all patients presenting with ALF, and the agent *N*-acetylcysteine (NAC) started. Acetaminophen overdose leads to the accumulation of *N*-acetyl-*p*-benzoquinone imine, a metabolite normally conjugated by glutathione that is toxic to hepatocytes.[5] Excessive ingestion of acetaminophen leads to depletion of glutathione stores, and NAC augments glutathione levels. NAC should be started as early as possible but may still be useful even 48 hours or more after ingestion. The oral dose of NAC is 140 mg/kg diluted to 5% solution, followed by 70 mg/kg by mouth q4h × 17 doses. NAC can also be administered intravenously in patients with worsening mental status or gastrointestinal (GI) bleeding. The loading dose is 150 mg/kg in 5% dextrose over 15 minutes; maintenance dose is 50 mg/kg given over 4 hours followed by 100 mg/kg administered over 16 hours.[3] Numerous clinical trials have established the efficacy of NAC for the treatment of acetaminophen-induced ALF. ALF patients are heterogeneous but share the common disease process of acute hepatocyte necrosis and its sequelae. Presenting symptoms are often nonspecific, including fatigue, malaise, anorexia, nausea, abdominal pain, fever, and jaundice.[1] Often these symptoms progress to severe coagulopathy and encephalopathy and/or coma. The patient's clinical condition should be monitored regularly including frequent vital signs, blood glucose, and neurologic status. Initial laboratory testing should include a complete blood count, biochemical, hematologic, immunologic, hepatitis panel, and toxic drug screens. An arterial blood gas and lactate levels should be checked to assess metabolic disturbances. Radiographic tests include an abdominal ultrasound to evaluate hepatic and portal venous flow patterns, and triphasic CT to evaluate the hepatic parenchyma (unless renal insufficiency or failure is present in which case intravenous contrast use is precluded). Clinical deterioration is *often rapid and any worsening in the patient's condition should warrant urgent referral* to a transplant center. Patients who present in full-blown ALF often have severe metabolic acidosis, hypoglycemia, coagulopathy, and encephalopathy or coma.[6] Stabilization of these patients includes volume resuscitation, mechanical ventilation, and hemodynamic support. Appropriate candidates should be urgently listed for liver transplantation as quickly as possible. Next, we will discuss the systemic effects of ALF by going through each organ system in detail.

Encephalopathy and Intracranial Hypertension (IH)

The neurologic effects of ALF range from minimal to striking. Encephalopathy, the hallmark feature of ALF, may vary from subtle changes in affect, insomnia, and difficulties with concentration (stage I), to deep coma (stage IV).[1] The prognosis of ALF is inversely correlated with the degree of encephalopathy. Table 51.1 illustrates the grades of encephalopathy. The most serious complication of ALF is cerebral edema and intracranial hypertension (ICH) which affects approximately 50%-80% of patients with severe ALF (grade III or IV coma).[7] Uncal herniation can result and is uniformly fatal. Patients with grade I-II encephalopathy seldom show signs of cerebral edema. The risk of edema increases to 25%-35% with progression to grade III, and 65%-75% or more in patients reaching grade IV coma.[3] Patients with grade I-II encephalopathy should be managed in a quiet environment to minimize agitation, and sedation should be avoided. Frequent mental status checks should be performed and head imaging with CT obtained to exclude other causes of encephalopathy. Lactulose can reduce elevated ammonia levels which may play a pathogenic role in the development of cerebral edema/ICH. As patients progress to grade III or IV encephalopathy, intubation for airway protection must be undertaken. The patients should be positioned with the head elevated at 30 degrees and efforts made to avoid patient stimulation. Propofol is often used as the choice of sedation because it may reduce cerebral blood flow (CBF)[3]; however, its effectiveness has not been shown in controlled studies.

Two theories have been proposed to account for intracranial hypertension in ALF: (1) brain edema due to osmotic astrocyte

TABLE 51.1

STAGES OF ENCEPHALOPATHY IN ALF

STAGE	MENTAL STATUS	TREMOR	EEG
I	Euphoria, occasional depression, fluctuant mild confusion, slowness of mentation and affect, untidy, slurred speech	Slight	Usually normal
II	Accentuation of stage I, drowsiness, inappropriate behavior, able to maintain sphincter control	Present (easily elicited)	Abnormal, generalized slowing
III	Sleeps most of the time but is arousable, incoherent speech, marked confusion	Usually present if patient cooperative	Always abnormal
IV	Not arousable, may or may not respond to painful stimuli	Usually absent	Always abnormal

swelling secondary to ammonia-induced accumulation of glutamine, and (2) alteration of CBF regulation with increased intracranial blood volume.[8] The typical course of grade III or IV HE includes a reduction in CBF coupled with a reduction in cerebral metabolic rate early on, followed by gradual cerebral vasodilatation due to the loss of cerebral autoregulation. This results in increased cerebral blood volume and edema. The preterminal phase shows a marked reduction in CBF resulting from cerebral edema, with cerebral herniation as the end result.[7]

Clinical signs of IH include systemic hypertension, bradycardia, abnormal pupillary signs, aggravation of HE, epileptiform activity, and decerebrate posturing. However, most of these clinical signs are nonspecific. The most accurate method to diagnose IH is intracranial pressure (ICP) monitoring. Although the advantages of ICP monitoring in ALF patients have not been demonstrated by a randomized study, ICP monitoring may be helpful to establish the presence of IH and guide specific therapy.[8] ICP transducers can be placed in the brain parenchyma, epidural, or subdural spaces. Epidural devices have lower complication rates (3.8%) than subdural bolts (20%) or parenchymal monitors (22%).[9,10] In ALF, epidural transducers may be the safest choice to monitor ICP even though they are less precise than the other devices.[10] Although placement of these invasive monitors is associated with the risk of hemorrhage, the use of recombinant factor VIIa (rFVIIa) before the procedure appears to minimize this risk[11]; a single dose of 40 μg/kg of rFVIIa is recommended prior to placement.

Transcranial Doppler is a noninvasive measurement of the systolic flow velocity of the middle cerebral artery. Attenuation of the diastolic flow signal may be a sign of IH and decreased cerebral perfusion. A pulsatility index (systolic velocity–diastolic velocity/systolic velocity) >1.6 is a poor prognostic sign.[7] Jugular venous oximetry measures venous oxygenation in the superior jugular bulb of the internal jugular vein, which is representative of cerebral oxygen consumption and delivery. If one assumes that the cerebral metabolic rate remains constant, the arteriojugular venous oxygen difference (AVjDO2) will change in response to changes in CBF; this will essentially be a reflection of the ratio of the flow to metabolism. A normal AVjDO2 is 5–6 mL/100 mL; a narrow AVjDO2 difference is suggestive of cerebral hyperemia and a widened AVjDO2 difference is suggestive of cerebral ischemia. AVjDO2 measurements can be obtained at two different levels of pCO_2 to see the variability in CBF in response to CO_2 reactivity. If the AVjDO2 difference normalizes from a low value, hyperventilation may be effective to decrease cerebral hyperemia. Alternatively, an AVjDO2 difference >6 when the pCO_2 is low suggests cerebral ischemia, and elevating the pCO_2 is needed to maintain adequate CBF.

The treatment of elevated ICP involves decreasing the brain volume or decreasing the CBF and intracranial blood volume (or both). Mannitol and hypertonic saline increase blood osmolarity, thereby inducing fluid movement from the brain to the vascular space. Mannitol (0.5–1 g/kg IV) repeated once or twice as needed, provided serum osmolality does not exceed 320 mOsm/L, is recommended to treat ICH.[3] The efficacy of mannitol is affected by acute renal failure, and hemodialysis may also be needed to remove fluid. A recent controlled trial of 30% hypertonic saline to maintain serum sodium levels of 145–155 mEq/L suggests that induction and maintenance of hypernatremia may be used to prevent the rise in ICP.[12] Survival benefits could not be demonstrated in this trial however, and the role of hypertonic saline as a prophylactic measure requires larger studies.

Hyperventilation, indomethacin, thiopental, and induced hypothermia reduce ICP through vasoconstriction of cerebral blood vessels, thereby decreasing CBF. The American Association for the Study of Liver Diseases (AASLD) position paper on the management of ALF does not support prophylactic hyperventilation in patients with ALF.[3] If ICH cannot be controlled with mannitol and other general management guidelines; hyperventilation may be instituted temporarily in an attempt to acutely lower ICP and prevent impending herniation. Indomethacin induces cerebral vasoconstriction through inhibition of the endothelial cyclooxygenase pathway, alterations in extracellular pH, and reduction in cerebral temperature.[13] Studies using indomethacin are of small scale, and its use should be evaluated in a randomized, controlled study before wider use. Thiopental induces cerebral vasoconstriction possibly by inhibition of nitric oxide synthase, which is thought to be important in the pathogenesis of increased ICP in ALF. A continuous infusion is started and titrated based upon the EEG (5–10 second EEG burst suppression), ICP, and hemodynamics. Most systemic hypotension limits its use and may necessitate additional pressors or inotropes to maintain adequate mean arterial pressures. Patients who develop worsening encephalopathy and those with signs of IH must be urgently listed for liver transplantation if they are appropriate candidates; needless to say, the workup should be expeditious.

Cardiovascular

Nausea, vomiting, and loss of appetite are part of the prodrome of ALF, and patients may present with profound dehydration. Most patients will require fluid resuscitation initially with colloids primarily and complemented with crystalloid solutions.[6] Systemic vasodilation, low systemic vascular resistance, hypotension, and a compensatory increase in cardiac output are the notable clinical cardiovascular sequelae of ALF. Abnormal oxygen transport and utilization is also present; delivery of oxygen to the tissues is adequate but there is a decrease in tissue oxygen uptake,[1] resulting in tissue hypoxia and lactic acidosis.[14] Low systemic vascular resistance results in hypotension even in the volume-resuscitated patient, and a pulmonary artery catheter is often useful to assess volume status and guide further management. Inotropic or pressor support may be required to maintain an adequate mean arterial pressure. Norepinephrine and dopamine are generally used if needed to maintain vital organ perfusion.[1,3,6] Vasoconstrictive agents such as vasopressin (VP) are generally avoided unless major systemic hypotension is present.[3]

Respiratory

Patients often hyperventilate and develop a respiratory alkalosis before a metabolic acidosis as liver failure progresses.[2] Mortality in ALF escalates with the presence of pulmonary edema and acute respiratory distress syndrome (ARDS).[1,2] ARDS is present in as many as one-third of patients.[15] Ventilation–perfusion mismatch may develop acutely and worsen as the liver function deteriorates, and resulting hypoxia can contribute to neurologic injury. Positive end-expiratory pressure may compromise cardiac output and oxygen delivery, and result in increased ICP and hepatic congestion.[1,2] Treatment with increased FiO_2 is the most appropriate intervention. Patients who develop ARDS in the setting of ALF can successfully undergo liver transplantation, but the risk of death is high.[16]

Gastrointestinal/Metabolic

Upper GI bleeding is a recognized complication and often stress related. Histamine-2 receptors blocking agents and proton pump inhibitors have been shown to be efficacious in several trials. Numerous metabolic derangements are common in ALF including alkalosis, acidosis, hypoglycemia, hypophosphatemia, and hypokalemia. Hypoglycemia, seen in up to 45% of ALF patients,[1] is an indicator of major hepatic necrosis which leads to defective glycogenolysis, gluconeogenesis, and insulin metabolism. Treatment is with continuous glucose infusion. Electrolytes should be supplemented and followed closely. Enteral nutrition should be started early when feasible.

Renal Failure

Renal failure is common, with the reported incidence varying from 40% to 85%.[6] It is often multifactorial, with prerenal azotemia, renal ischemia, acute tubular necrosis, and hepatorenal syndrome (HRS) as common causes. Although few patients die of renal failure alone, it often contributes to mortality and suggests a poorer prognosis.[3] Avoidance of nephrotoxins and maintenance of adequate intravascular volume are important to maintain renal function. When hemodialysis is needed, continuous venovenous hemodialysis (CVVHD) is the preferred mode.[2,3,6,17] CVVHD tends to be better tolerated and may have more beneficial effects on ICP.[17,18] Intermittent hemodialysis has been associated with increases in ICP and decreases in CPP, whereas the opposite has been shown in patients receiving CVVHD.[18,19]

Hematologic

The normal liver is responsible for the synthesis of several clotting factors involved in the clotting cascade. The primary hematologic derangements seen in ALF include platelet dysfunction and thrombocytopenia, reduced fibrinogen, and a prolonged prothrombin time (PT).[1,3,6,18] However, spontaneous, clinically meaningful bleeding is uncommon in ALF patients (<10%).[18] The PT is used as a prognostic indicator as well as a tool to follow the progress of the liver injury; thus, correction of the PT is not necessary unless there is clinical bleeding or an invasive procedure is planned. Complete correction of the coagulopathy and thrombocytopenia is generally not achievable and can lead to volume overload and oxygenation issues, as well as exacerbation of ICH. The use of rFVIIa has been examined in treatment of the coagulopathy in ALF and may be useful in facilitating performance of invasive procedures (such as intracranial monitoring devices) in these patients, especially in the setting of renal failure and volume overload.[20] Further studies and analysis of cost–benefit ratio are needed prior to becoming standard therapy.

Infection

The liver is the site of complement synthesis, with low levels of complement reported in ALF.[6] Reduced complement has been associated with impaired opsonization[1,6] leading to sepsis. The most common pathogens are Staphylococcal species, streptococcal species, and gram-negative rods.[1,6,18] Fungal infections (particularly Candida albicans) occur in up to one-third of ALF patients with risk factors including renal failure and prolonged antibiotic therapy for existing bacterial infections. Common sites of infection include pneumonia (50%), bacteremia (20%), and urinary tract infection (25%).[17] Prophylactic antimicrobial therapy reduces the incidence of infection in certain groups of patients with ALF, but no actual survival benefit has been shown. If prophylactic antibiotics are not given, surveillance for infection including chest x-rays and periodic cultures of sputum, blood, and urine should be done.

Transplantation and Prognosis

Orthotopic liver transplantation (OLT) remains the only definitive therapy for patients who have sustained massive hepatic necrosis without regeneration of enough hepatocytes to sustain life. Overall survival rates in ALF have improved from 15% in the pretransplant era to >60% with transplantation.[3] Advances in critical care and trends toward etiologies such as acetaminophen have helped improve survival. A delay in a patient getting on the transplant list can lead to the probability of a complication precluding transplant. Contraindications to transplant include an extrahepatic malignancy, uncontrolled sepsis, irreversible brain damage, or unresponsive cerebral edema with a sustained elevation of ICP (>50 mm Hg) and a decrease in CPP (<40 mm Hg).[17]

Accurate prognosis for survival in ALF is important, given the limited organ supply and lack of good alternative therapies. The most commonly utilized and most frequently tested of the many prognostic criteria for ALF are from the King's College (Table 51.2).[21] More published data exist to support the use of acetaminophen than the nonacetaminophen criteria.

TABLE 51.2

KING'S COLLEGE CRITERIA

KING'S COLLEGE CRITERIA
• Tylenol • pH <7.3 irrespective of grade of encephalopathy or • Lactate >3.5 mmol/L following early fluid resuscitation or • Lactate >3.0 mmol/L following 12 h fluid resuscitation or • Phosphate >1.2 mmol/L at 48–96 h after ingestion or • Encephalopathy III/IV and • INR >6.5 and • Creatinine >3.4 mg/dL within 24 h
• Other etiologies • INR >6.5 or at least three of the following: • Age <10 or >40 y • Hepatitis non A-E, halothane hepatitis, idiosyncratic drug reaction • Jaundice to encephalopathy time >7 d • INR >3.5 • Serum bilirubin >17.4 mg/dL

From O'Grady J, Alexander G, Hayllar K, Williams R. Early indicators of prognosis in fulminant hepatic failure. *Gastroenterology*, (1989);97(2):439–455 with permission

Other criteria including the patient's MELD score on admission and APACHE II scores have been looked at in several studies. Currently, available prognostic scoring systems do not adequately predict outcome and determine candidacy for liver transplantation, therefore, decisions on whether to transplant a patient or not should look at the whole picture and not rely on these guidelines entirely.

PORTAL HYPERTENSION

In this section, we will discuss the critical care management of patients with complications of portal hypertension (PH), decompensated cirrhosis, and end-stage liver disease (ESLD). PH is most commonly an accompanying consequence of cirrhosis and is defined as a portal pressure gradient between the portal vein and hepatic veins (hepatic venous pressure gradient [HVPG]) of >5 mm Hg.[22] PH can be classified as prehepatic (e.g., portal or splenic vein thrombosis), intrahepatic (e.g., cirrhosis, parenchymal disease), or posthepatic (e.g., hepatic vein stenosis, Budd-Chiari syndrome, cardiac disease). The common clinical manifestations of cirrhosis and PH include GI bleeding, ascites, and encephalopathy. The ICU management of these patients can be challenging, as these patients also often have thrombocytopenia, leukopenia, or pancytopenia because of accompanying splenomegaly. Furthermore, other complications of ESLD such as HRS, coagulopathy, or malnourishment/deconditioning may also be present. Sepsis and infections are also common in these patients, further increasing the complexity of care.

The emergence of OLT as a successful and definitive therapy for ESLD has changed the approach to the care of these patients. Over 6,000 liver transplants are performed in the United States annually with excellent outcomes, with average 1-, 5-, and 10-year patient and graft survival rates of 88.4%/73.8%/60% and 84.3%/68.4%/54.1%, respectively.[23] The most common disease indications in adults for OLT in the United States are alcoholic liver disease and hepatitis C, accounting for 30%-40% of all cases. Other disease states include hepatocellular carcinoma, cholestatic liver diseases (Primary Biliary Cirrhosis, Primary Sclerosing Cholangitis), and metabolic diseases (hemochromatosis, alpha-1-antitrypsin deficiency). Nonalcoholic fatty liver disease (NAFLD) is being diagnosed with increasing frequency, and nonalcoholic steatohepatitis which is the advanced and pathologic form of NAFLD, may surpass hepatitis C in the next several years as the leading indication for OLT in the United States.[24] In patients with hepatic decompensation who are active on the liver transplant list, management is directed toward stabilizing, supporting, and ensuring that these patients continue to be viable candidates for transplantation. For patients who have not yet been evaluated for transplantation, early referral for OLT is important. The care of these patients must be multidisciplinary in nature, with the critical care team, transplant surgeons, hepatologists, nephrologists, infectious disease specialists, and ancillary support services such as social workers, involved and interacting with one another.

Upper GI (UGI) Bleeding in the Portal Hypertensive Patient

The portal-mesenteric venous system drains the entire GI tract, from the esophagus to the rectum. Because these are low-pressure venous beds that are separate from, and in normal states have no connection to the systemic venous system, PH results in the formation of either varices or shunts (collaterals). Varices occur most commonly in the distal esophagus, the umbilicus ("caput medusae"), around the spleen, and in the rectum. The GI mucosal tract can also be congested leading to portal hypertensive gastropathy (PHG) or colopathy. Natural shunts occur most frequently between the splenic and left renal veins, forming spontaneous splenorenal shunts. The presence of these shunts does not necessarily alleviate GI bleeding secondary to PH.

The prevalence of esophageal varices in patients with chronic liver disease has been reported to range from 24% to 81%,[25] and upper GI bleeding from varices account for 60%-90% of bleeding in patients with cirrhosis.[26,27] The pathophysiology of variceal hemorrhage is not completely understood. Bleeding is not wholly dependent on elevated portal pressures; on the one hand, varices are usually not encountered in patients who have a portal pressure gradient of <11–12 mm Hg.[28] However, many patients with pressures above this threshold also do not bleed from their varices. There is a correlation between the size of the varices and the risk of bleeding; the larger the varices, the greater the risk of hemorrhage. Other factors that most likely play an important role on whether varices will bleed include the patient's fluid status, respiratory cycle, meal ingestion, presence of esophagitis, and Valsalva's maneuvers.[28] The presence of red color signs (red streaks of longitudinal dilated veins) in the distal esophagus seen in endoscopy has also been shown to be an independent risk factor for variceal bleeding.[29] The mortality rate associated with esophageal variceal hemorrhage in most series ranges from 30% to 50%; mortality is greatest within the first 6 weeks of the bleed and in subjects with more advanced liver disease.[29] The Child's status is a good indicator of the severity of the liver disease (Table 51.3). In a recent study, the mortality associated with an UGI bleed in Child's B and C cirrhosis was 15% and 36%, respectively, with no deaths occurring in Child's A patients.[30]

Gastric varices (GV) are estimated to be present in 20% of patients with cirrhosis[29] and are frequently found in conjunction with esophageal varices. GV can be found in the fundus of the stomach or along the lesser curvature, with the former accounting for the majority of bleeding.[31] GV tend to bleed

TABLE 51.3

CHILD'S CLASSIFICATION

	1 POINT	2 POINTS	3 POINTS
Serum albumin (g/dL)	>3.5	2.8–3.5	<2.8
Total bilirubin (mg/dL)	<2	2–3	>3
INR	<1.7	1.7–2.2	>2.2
Ascites	None	Medically managed	Poorly controlled
Encephalopathy	None	Medically managed	Poorly controlled

Child's A: <7 points, B: 7–9 points, C: ≥10 points

less frequently but more severely than esophageal varices. PHG is a condition characterized endoscopically by gastric mucosal changes (typically a mosaic pattern) found in the setting of PH. Histologically, there is dilation of capillaries and venules in the gastric mucosa.[32] Bleeding from PHG is usually less severe compared to esophageal varices.

Management. The initial management of the portal hypertensive patient with UGI bleeding is the same as that for a trauma victim, focusing primarily on the "ABC's." Patients with acute UGI bleeding may present with hematemesis or hematochezia. The subject's airway and breathing must be protected and maintained, and circulation must be preserved. There must be a low threshold to intubate the patient, especially one with hematemesis. Along with securing the airway, mechanical ventilation reduces the risk of aspiration pneumonia and facilitates the performance of upper endoscopy. The placement of multiple large bore intravenous lines is critical, and hemodynamic monitoring with an arterial line and central venous catheterization as well as bladder catheterization to monitor urine output are recommended. Patients must be typed and crossed with blood and fresh frozen plasma, and resuscitation with blood and correction of coagulopathy and thrombocytopenia is of prime importance. Serum lactate levels are good indicators of the effectiveness of resuscitation, as well as the degree of blood loss. Placement of a nasogastric tube is important to confirm that the upper GI tract is the source of bleeding and also to decompress the stomach. The first level of treatment consists of pharmacologic therapy with vasoactive drugs. The most commonly used agent in the United States is Octreotide, a somatostatin analog. Somatostatin is a naturally occurring 14 amino acid peptide that has been shown to decrease portal pressure.[33] Its half-life in the circulation is only 1–3 minutes, thus longer acting analogs with greater potency such as octreotide have been synthesized. Octreotide (Sandostatin) is administered intravenously as a 50-μg bolus, followed by 50 μg/hour IV for 5 days. VP is a potent vasoconstricting agent with an added effect of causing splanchnic vasoconstriction. VP use, however, may be associated with a reduction in cardiac output as well as systemic vasoconstriction, so proper monitoring is essential. Concomitant nitroglycerin use has been advocated by some to decrease the systemic effects of VP but we do not routinely utilize this agent at our unit. Terlipressin, a semisynthetic VP analog, is widely used in Europe but has not yet obtained approval by the Food and Drug Administration for use in the United States. Patients are also routinely placed on proton pump inhibitors (intravenous drip) and prophylactic broad spectrum antibiotics for 5 days. A Doppler ultrasound of the liver is performed at the bedside to assess vessel patency, particularly to assess portal vein flow.

Once the patient has been stabilized, identification of the source of bleeding is the next goal of management. Esophagogastroduodenoscopy (EGD) complements vasoactive therapy and must be performed as soon as possible to determine the source of the bleed. Other causes of bleeding such as gastritis, ulcer disease, or Mallory-Weiss tears can also occur in patients with cirrhosis and PH. EGD serves as both the most important diagnostic tool and the primary therapeutic modality for variceal hemorrhage. Endoscopic strategies to stop variceal bleeding include sclerotherapy injection or rubber band ligation of bleeding varices. Sclerotherapy involves the injection of agents (e.g., ethanolamine oleate, sodium tetradecyl sulfate, absolute alcohol) either around or into a varix. This technique has largely been supplanted by band ligation which involves endoscopic placement of a rubber band around a varix, eventually causing its thrombosis. Endoscopic or pharmacologic treatments control variceal bleeding in over 90% of cases. GV are best treated with gastric variceal obliteration using endoscopic injection with cyanoacrylate rather than band ligation.[29]

In patients who continue to hemorrhage profusely despite the management and endoscopic therapies outlined above, the next option is to control bleeding with balloon tamponade using a Sengstaken-Blakemore (SB) or a Minnesota tube. These are multiluminal nasogastric tubes that have esophageal and gastric balloons that when inflated serve to tamponade varices (Fig. 51.1A). There are also esophageal and gastric ports that can be utilized for aspiration of contents or administration of medications. Once an SB tube is passed into the esophagus and stomach, its placement must be confirmed radiographically with plain films prior to inflation of the balloons (Fig. 51.1B,C). We rarely inflate the esophageal balloon; our experience has been that inflation of the gastric balloon and placement of the SB tube in traction with 1–2 lb of weight provides excellent control of bleeding esophageal varices. Balloon tamponade can typically be used for 24 hours and has been shown to be effective in controlling variceal bleeding in 80%-100% of cases, allowing the patient to be stabilized for more definitive therapy, as rebleeding occurs in up to 50% of patients once the balloon is deflated.[33]

Persistent bleeding refractory to medical management or massive GI bleeding necessitating SB tube placement requires further treatment involving either interventional radiology or surgical intervention. It is critical to involve the liver transplant team in the treatment strategy for these patients, especially for those on the transplant list. The management and treatment of these subjects depends on the severity of their liver disease (Child's Class status), whether they are transplant candidates, and their portomesenteric venous anatomy. It is also important to determine by angiography whether there is portomesenteric venous thrombosis and if so, define the location and extent. Although portal vein thrombosis is no longer a contraindication to OLT, subjects with extensive thrombosis in their portal and mesenteric venous systems may require liver/intestine or multivisceral transplantation (liver, stomach, duodenum, pancreas, and intestine). The development of the transjugular intrahepatic portosystemic shunt (TIPS) has revolutionized the care of patients with variceal bleeding and is preferred over surgical intervention as the next line of treatment, particularly in patients who are critically ill, unstable, or have massive bleeding. A TIPS is placed by interventional radiology under local anesthesia and involves a transjugular approach in which one of the hepatic veins (usually the right) is cannulated followed by the accession of a branch of the portal vein using a Rosch's needle[34] (Fig. 51.2). The tract between the veins is then widened after which a covered metal stent is placed, providing immediate reduction in portal pressures and relief of bleeding

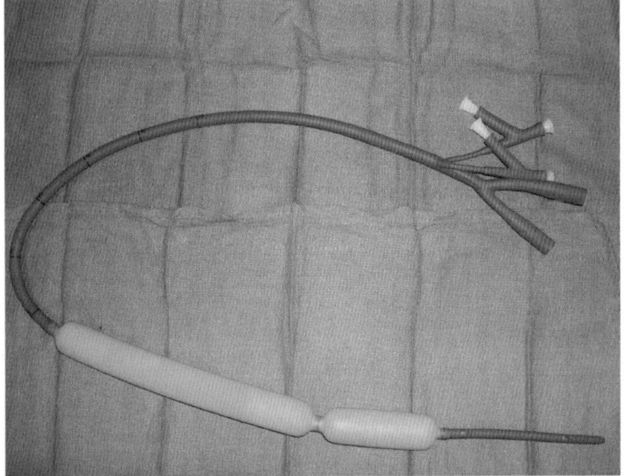
A

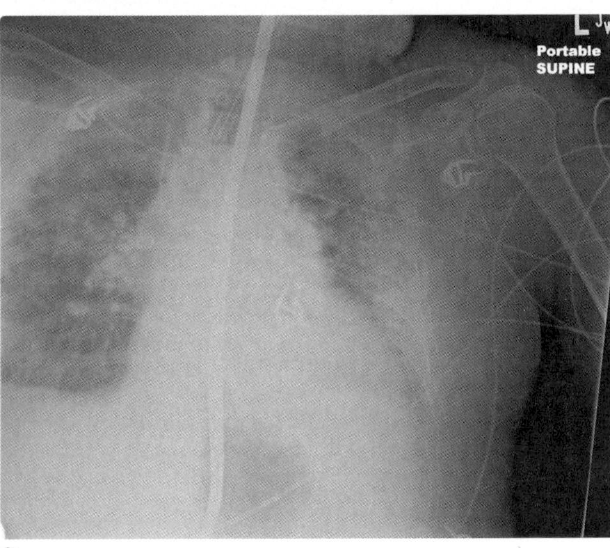

C

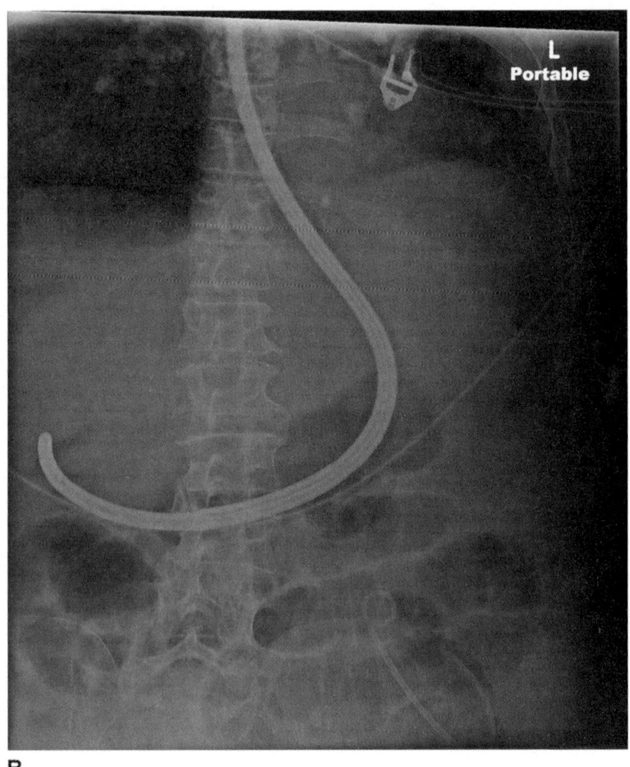

B

FIGURE 51.1. **A:** Minnesota tube. **B:** Confirmatory radiograph showing good placement. **C:** The gastric balloon is inflated.

in over 90% of cases.[33] Complications associated with TIPS placement include procedural-related bleeding (e.g., perforation of the portal vein), worsening of encephalopathy, renal failure, congestive heart failure, infection, and liver failure. Relative contraindications to placing a TIPS include portal vein thrombosis and a history of severe encephalopathy. Coil embolization of varices is another option available to interventional radiologists and can be effective in appropriate patients.

Surgical options for the treatment of portal hypertensive bleeding include shunt surgery and procedures such as gastric devascularization or esophageal transection. Although esophageal transection is effective in control of bleeding, it is rarely used currently. Emergency surgery for acute variceal bleeding has markedly declined due to the success of TIPS. Surgical shunts are effective, however, and still play a role in the treatment of variceal hemorrhage, most commonly in an elective setting and targeted toward prophylaxis from recurrent bleeding. Selective shunts, that is, the distal splenorenal shunt (DSRS), are preferred over nonselective shunts (e.g., portacaval or mesocaval shunts) because hepatic flow is preserved and no dissection is carried out at the hepatic hilum, an advantage for patients who may eventually undergo OLT. Visceral angiography is critical and helps dictate the type of shunt utilized by detailing the portomesenteric venous system and diagnosing portomesenteric venous thrombosis. Gastric devascularization is indicated for patients with portomesenteric thrombosis.[35] A TIPS functions similarly to a side-to-side portosystemic shunt but without the risk, morbidity, and mortality involved with shunt surgery. In addition, abdominal adhesions and possible dissection at the hepatic hilum are obviated, making TIPS an excellent bridge to OLT. A randomized, multicenter trial showed that TIPS was just as effective as DSRS in prevention of variceal bleeding.[36] The risk of variceal rebleeding may be up to 70% within 1 year and is greatest during the first several weeks after the index bleed.[28,33] Prophylaxis against bleeding using nonselective β-blockers or endoscopic banding is effective.[29] A recent study from Barcelona demonstrated that in a select group of patients, early placement of TIPS (within 3–4 days of acute variceal bleeding) results in substantial reduction in rebleeding rates and mortality compared to a control group treated without early TIPS.[37] Measurement of hepatic vein free and wedge pressures to calculate the HVPG has been advocated by some to help guide the management of portal hypertensive patients. In particular, reduction of HVPG by ≥20% or to <12 mm Hg in response to clinical intervention decreases the risk of rebleeding.[38]

Ascites

Another common complication of PH and cirrhosis is ascites. There are numerous physiologic alterations that eventually account for the accumulation of ascitic fluid in the cirrhotic

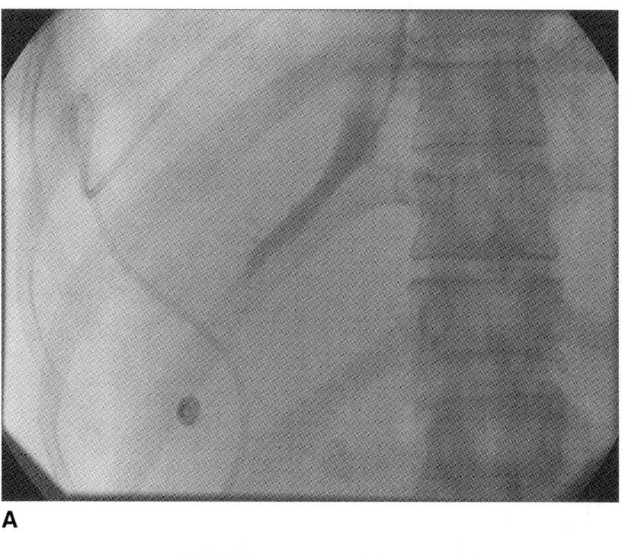

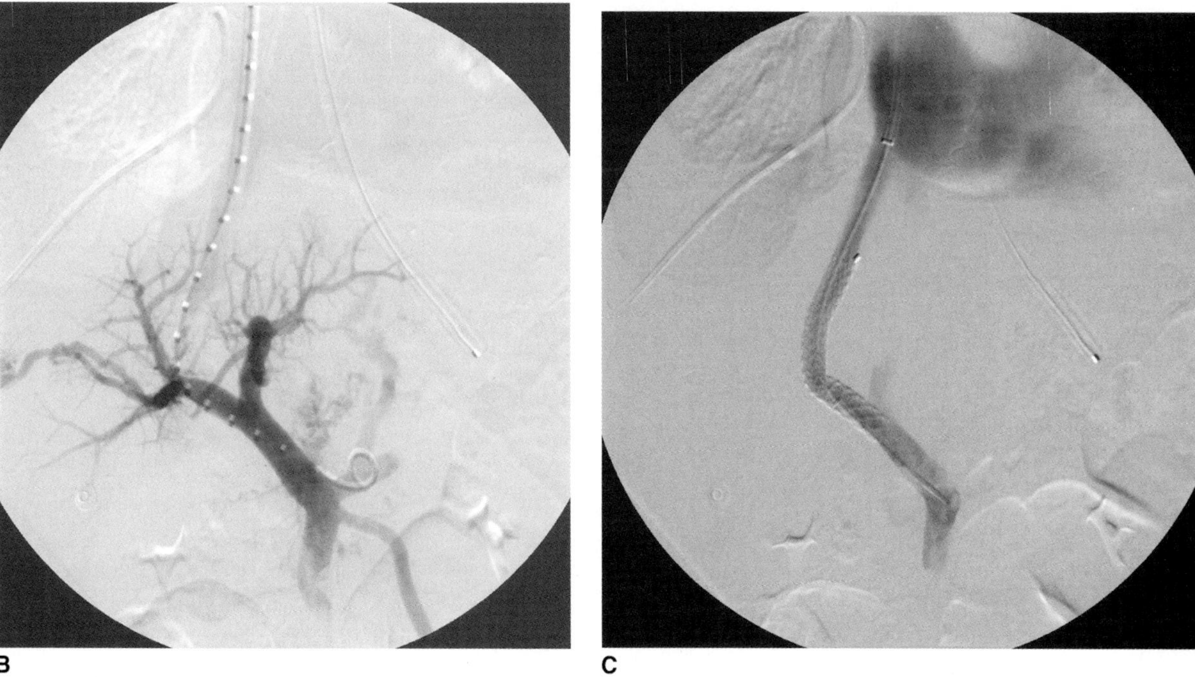

FIGURE 51.2. Placement of TIPS. **A:** Cannulation of the right hepatic vein. **B:** The portal vein has been accessed. **C:** Deployment of the stent.

patient. PH, the development of systemic vasodilation, and activation of the renin–angiotensin–aldosterone pathway are contributing factors.[39] Patients who develop refractory ascites have 1-year survival <50%.[39] Hyponatremia often accompanies ascites and is a poor prognostic indicator in patients awaiting OLT.[40] Medical management is primarily with diuretics (furosemide and aldactone). Therapeutic large volume paracentesis is indicated mainly for symptomatic relief; patients who may have respiratory compromise from tense ascites should be drained. We typically send ascites fluid for cell count and cultures. Our preference is to insert pigtail catheters and "gently" drain ascites over several days, thereby minimizing rapid shifts in volume and avoiding hypotension and dehydration/renal insufficiency. We routinely replace ascitic drainage with intravenous albumin, although some have questioned this practice. TIPS may be considered in patients who are refractory to diuretics and requiring frequent drainage. Spontaneous bacterial peritonitis (SBP) is diagnosed with either positive ascitic cultures or with ascitic neutrophil count >250/mm^3 or total WBC >500/mm^3. Broad spectrum antibiotics should be administered. Gram-positive infections are the most common followed by gram-negative infections; anaerobic infections are rare. The development of SBP does not appear to lead to increased mortality in OLT patients but is associated with higher rates of sepsis posttransplantation.[41]

Encephalopathy

HE is a common indication for admission to the ICU. The pathogenesis of HE has not been precisely elucidated but is thought to be secondary to accumulation of ammonia or excessive gamma amino butyric acid neurotransmission,[42] with the former hypothesis currently being the most popular. Standard medical therapy is with oral lactulose with or without Neomycin (500 mg po tid). Xifaxan (550 mg) is an alternative to Neomycin and has been shown to effectively reduce the occurrence of HE and the risk of hospitalization from HE.[43] The main concern with severe encephalopathy is the inability of a patient to protect the airway, in which case intubation should be performed. We administer lactulose every hour via a nasogastric tube until patient starts to have bowel movements; we also sometimes utilize lactulose enemas. HE often has a precipitating factor such as a GI bleed, new onset or worsening portal vein thrombosis, or an infection. These patients must, therefore, have blood work including a complete blood count, serum chemistries, and ammonia levels. An infectious workup is important and patients are pancultured. Ultrasound of the liver should be performed to check the patency of the portal vein.

Hepatorenal Syndrome

HRS is characterized by the development of renal insufficiency or renal failure in cirrhotic patients with advanced liver disease in the absence of intrinsic kidney disease. Clinical criteria for the diagnosis of HRS include the absence of pre- and postrenal azotemia and other causes of renal impairment (e.g., acute tubular necrosis, nephrotoxicity), the lack of improvement in renal function after withdrawal of diuretics and administration of volume, oliguria, urine sodium <10 mEq/L, urine osmolality greater than plasma osmolality, and hyponatremia (<130 mEq/L).[44] Type I HRS is a rapid and progressive form, with doubling of the serum creatinine to >2.5 mg/dL in <2 weeks, while type II HRS is slower in progression.[42] HRS is associated with high mortality; type I has a survival of <50% after 1 month while type II has a median survival of 6 months. The management of these patients involves adequate hydration, withdrawal of diuretics, and avoidance of nephrotoxic substances (e.g., drugs, IV dye). The administration of midodrine, octreotide, and albumin has been shown to improve survival and renal function in HRS patients.[45] Renal replacement therapy (RRT) should be instituted when clinically indicated. Liver transplantation is the definitive treatment for HRS. Because renal failure substantially increases the mortality risk after transplantation,[46] an increasing number of patients are undergoing combined liver and kidney transplantation. At our center, we do not consider a kidney transplant for HRS patients who have been on RRT for <8 weeks.

References

1. Sass D, Shakil O. Fulminant hepatic failure. *Liver Transplant.* 2005;11(6):594–605.
2. Shakil O, Mazariegos G, Kramer D. Fulminant hepatic failure. *Surg Clin North Am.* 1999;79(1):77–108.
3. Polson J, Lee WM. AASLD Position Paper: the Management of Acute Liver Failure. *Hepatology.* 2005;41:1179–1197.
4. Ostapowicz G, Fontana R, Schiodt F, et al. Results of a prospective study of acute liver failure at 17 tertiary care centers in the United States. *Ann Intern Med.* 2002;137:947–954.
5. Saito C, Zwingmann C, Jaeschke H. Novel mechanisms of protection against acetaminophen hepatotoxicity in mice by glutathione and *N*-acetylcysteine. *Hepatology.* 2010;51:246–254.
6. Rahman T, Hodgson H. Clinical management of acute hepatic failure. *Intensive Care Med.* 2001;27:467–476.
7. Raghavan M, Marik PE. Therapy of intracranial hypertension in patients with fulminant hepatic failure. *Neurocrit Care.* 2006;4:179–189.
8. Detry O, Roover AD, Honore P, et al. Brain edema and intracranial hypertension in fulminant heptic failure: Pathophysiology and management. *World J Gastroenterol.* 2006;12(46):7405–7412.
9. Cordoba J, Blei AT. Cerebral edema and intracranial pressure monitoring. *Liver Transplant.* 1995;1(3):187–194.
10. Blei A, Olafsson S, Webster S, et al. Complications of intracranial pressure monitoring in fulminant hepatic failure. *Lancet.* 1993;341:157–158.
11. Shami V, Caldwell S, Hespenheide E, et al. Recombinant activated factor VII for coagulopathy in fulminant hepatic failure compared with conventional therapy. *Liver Transplant.* 2003;9:138–143.
12. Murphy N, Auzinger G, Banal W, et al. The effect of hypertonic sodium chloride on intracranial pressure in patients with acute liver failure. *Hepatology.* 2002;39:464–470.
13. Jain, R. Acute liver failure: current management and future prospects. *J Hepatol.* 2005;42:S115–S123.
14. Bihari D, Gimson A, Waterson M, et al. Tissue hypoxia during fulminant hepatic failure. *Crit Care Med.* 1985;13(12): 1034–1039.
15. Baudouin S, Howdle P, O'Grady J, et al. Acute lung injury in fluminant hepatic failure following paracetamol poisoning. *Thorax.* 1995;50:399–402.
16. Doyle H, Marino I, Miro A, et al. Adult respiratory distress syndrome secondary to end-stage liver disease-successful outcome following liver transplantation. *Transplantation.* 1993;55(2):292–296.
17. Rinella M, Sanyal A. Intensive management of hepatic failure. *Semin Respir Crit Care Med.* 2006;27(3):241–261.
18. Stravitz RT, Kramer A, Davern T, et al. Intensive care of patients with acute liver failure: recommendations of the U.S. Acute Liver Failure Study Group. *Crit Care Med.* 2007;35(11):2498–2508.
19. Sass D, Shakil O. Fulminant hepatic failure. *Gastroenterol Clin North Am.* 2003;32:1195–1211.
20. Shami VM, Caldwell SH, Hespenheide EE, et al. Recombinant activated factor VII for coagulopathy in fulminant hepatic failure compared with conventional therapy. *Liver Transplant.* 2003;9:138–143.
21. O'Grady J, Alexander G, Hayllar K, et al. Early indicators of prognosis in fulminant hepatic failure. *Gastroenterology.* 1989;97(2): 439–455.
22. Mehta G, Abraldes JG, Bosch J. Developments and controversies in the management of oesophageal and gastric varices. *Gut.* 2010;59:701–705.
23. Thuluvath PJ, Guidinger MK, Fung JJ, et al. Liver transplantation in the United States, 1999–2008. *Liver Transplant.* 2010;10(pt 2):1003–1019.
24. Charlton M. Nonalcoholic fatty liver disease: a review of current understanding and future impact. *Clin Gastroenterol Hepatol.* 2004;2:1048–1058.
25. Pascal J, Cales P, Desmorat H. Natural history of esophageal varices. In: Bosch J, Rodes J, eds. Recent advances in the pathophysiology and treatment of portal hypertension. *Serono Symp Rev.* 1989;22:127–142.
26. Gatta A, Merkel C, Amodio P, et al. Evaluation of a new prognostic index predicting death after upper gastrointestinal bleeding in patients with liver cirrhosis. *Am J Gastroenterol.* 1994;89:1528–1536.
27. de Franchis R, Primignani M. Why do varices bleed? In: Groszmann R, Grace N, eds. Complications of cirrhosis. *Gastroenterol Clin North Am.* 1992;21:85–101.
28. Groszmann RJ, de Franchis R. Portal hypertension. In: Schiff ER, Sorrell MF, Madrey WC, eds. *Diseases of the Liver.* 8th ed. Philadelphia, PA: Lippincott-Raven; 1999:387–442.
29. Garcia-Tsao G, Bosch J. Management of varices and variceal hemorrhage in cirrhosis. *N Engl J Med.* 2010;362:823–832.
30. Afessa B, Kubilis PS. Upper gastrointestinal bleeding in patients with hepatic cirrhosis: clinical course and mortality prediction. *Am J Gastroenterol.* 2000;95:484–489.
31. Ryan BM, Stockbrugger RW, Ryan JM. A pathophysiologic, gastroenterologic, and radiologic approach to the management of gastric varices. *Gastroenterology.* 2004;126:1175–1189.
32. Ripoll C, Garcia-Tsao G. Management of gastropathy and gastric vascular ectasia in portal hypertension. *Clin Liver Dis.* 2010;14:281–295.
33. Sass DA, Chopra KB. Portal hypertension and variceal hemorrhage. *Med Clin North Am.* 2009;93:837–853.
34. Kalva SP, Salazar GM, Walker TG. Transjugular intrahepatic portosystemic shunt for acute variceal hemorrhage. *Tech Vasc Interv Radiol.* 2009;12:92–101.
35. Costa G, Cruz RJ, Abu-Elmagd KM. Surgical shunt versus TIPS for treatment of variceal hemorrhage in the current era of liver and multivisceral transplantation. *Surg Clin North Am.* 2010;90:891–905.
36. Henderson JM, Boyer TD, Kutner MH, et al. Distal splenorenal shunt versus transjugular intrahepatic portal systemic shunt for variceal bleeding: A randomized trial. *Gastroenterology.* 2006;130:1643–1651.
37. Garcia-Pagan JC, Caca K, Bureau C, et al. Early use of TIPS in patients with cirrhosis and variceal bleeding. *N Engl J Med.* 2010;362:2370–2379.
38. Bosch J, Abraldes JG, Berzigotti A, et al. The clinical use of HVPG measurements in chronic liver disease. *Nat Rev Gastroenterol Hepatol.* 2009;6:573–582.
39. Runyon B. Ascites and spontaneous bacterial peritonitis. In: Feldman M, Friedman LS, Brandt LJ, eds. *Sleisenger & Fordtran's Gastrointestinal and Liver Disease.* 8th ed. Philadelphia, PA: Saunders Elsevier; 2006:1935–1964.
40. Kim WR, Biggins SW, Kremers WK, et al. Hyponatremia and mortality among patients on the liver-transplant waiting list. *N Engl J Med.* 2008;359:1018–1026.
41. Mounzer R, Malik SM, Nasr J, et al. Spontaneous bacterial peritonitis prior to liver transplantation does not affect patient survival. *Clin Gastroenterol Hepatol.* 2010;8:623–628.

42. Fitz JG. Hepatic encephalopathy, hepatopulmonary syndromes, hepatorenal syndrome, and other complications of liver disease. In: Feldman M, Friedman LS, Brandt LJ, eds. *Sleisenger & Fordtran's Gastrointestinal and Liver Disease*. 8th ed. Philadelphia, PA: Saunders Elsevier; 2006:1965–1991.
43. Bass NM, Mullen KD, Sanyal A, et al. Rifaximin treatment in hepatic encephalopathy. *N Engl J Med*. 2010;362:1071–1081.
44. Arroyo V, Gines P, Gerbes AL, et al. Definition and diagnostic criteria of refractory ascites and hepatorenal syndrome in cirrhosis. *Hepatology*. 1996;23:164–176.
45. Skagen C, Einstein M, Lucey MR, et al. Combination treatment with octreotide, midodrine, and albumin improves survival in patients with type 1 and type 2 hepatorenal syndrome. *J Clin Gastroenterol*. 2009;43:680–685.
46. Papafragkakis H, Martin P, Akalin E. Combined liver and kidney transplantation. *Curr Opin Organ Transplant*. 2010;15:263–268.

CHAPTER 52 ■ ACUTE KIDNEY INJURY

SOUMITRA R. EACHEMPATI, FRANK LIU, AND PHILIP S. BARIE

The functions of the kidney can be divided into secretion of hormones and maintaining the extracellular homeostasis of pH, water, and electrolytes. The kidneys weigh approximately 300 g each but receive blood flow disproportionately, approximately 20%–25% of cardiac output. The kidneys consume more oxygen per gram of mass than any other visceral organ. The kidneys secrete renin, erythropoietin, the active form of vitamin D, and certain prostaglandins. Most importantly, the kidneys regulate fluid balance, acid–base status, and solute homeostasis.

After passing through the interlobar, arcuate, and intralobar arteries, more than 85% of renal blood flow perfuses the outer cortical glomeruli, leaving the remainder to supply the juxtamedullary glomeruli.[1]

The kidney's ability to perform many of its functions depends on three fundamental functions: filtration, reabsorption, and secretion at the level of the nephron. The nephron, the smallest functional unit of the kidney, includes a renal corpuscle, which is composed of a glomerular capillary tuft enclosed in Bowman's capsule. The glomerulus is distinct from other capillary beds in that it is situated between two muscular arterioles instead of between an arteriole and a venule. The afferent arteriole feeds into the glomerular tuft; its tone is modulated principally by a myogenic reflex, which adjusts arteriolar tone in response to perfusion pressure, and by certain prostaglandins. The efferent arteriole drains the tuft; its tone is largely determined by activity of the renin–angiotensin system. By dynamic adjustment of the tone of these two arterioles, renal blood flow and glomerular filtration pressure are autoregulated over a wide range of systemic blood pressures. Cells, proteins, and other large molecules entering the glomerulus are excluded from filtration subsequently by a fenestrated endothelium and a size- and charge-specific glomerular basement membrane. However, smaller molecules, electrolytes, and plasma fluid can pass into the Bowman space by ultrafiltration, which is driven by the capillary hydrostatic forces described above. This remaining effluent, or ultrafiltrate, then passes through the proximal tubule, the loop of Henle, the distal convoluted tubule, and finally the collecting ducts.[2] During this process, fluid is modified for water and solute regulation; the resultant fluid is urine.

The proximal tubule can be divided into an initial convoluted portion and a more distal descending portion, and functions primarily to reabsorb filtered plasma components. Fluid in the filtrate entering the proximal convoluted tubule is reabsorbed into the peritubular capillaries with approximately two-thirds of the total filtered salt and water and all the filtered organic solutes, which include primarily glucose and amino acids.[3] A substantial portion of bicarbonate reclamation also occurs here, largely due to the function of carbonic anhydrase.

The loop of Henle is a U-shaped conduit that extends from the proximal tubule and consists of descending and ascending limbs. It begins in the cortex, receiving filtrate from the straight portion of the proximal tubule, and extends into the medulla as the descending limb, before it returns to the cortex as the ascending limb to empty into the distal convoluted tubule. Its primary roles are to reabsorb 25%–35% of the filtered NaCl load via the $Na^+K^+2Cl^-$ loop diuretic–sensitive transporter, and to create gradients that allow for elaboration of either dilute or concentrated urine, depending on the immediate physiologic need.[4] The descending limb is permeable to water but impermeable to salt, whereas the ascending limb is impermeable to water. In the descending limb, the hypertonic interstitium of the renal medulla (established via active transport of sodium into the interstitium in the ascending limb) causes water to flow freely out of the descending limb by osmosis until the tonicity of the filtrate and interstitium equilibrate. The ascending limb pumps sodium continuously out of the filtrate, perpetuating a hypertonic interstitium and hypotonic tubular fluid. This process is called *countercurrent multiplication*, and results in an increasingly concentrated tubular fluid and interstitium at the bottom of the loop of Henle and a progressively more dilute filtrate by the start of the distal convoluted tubule.[4] The hypertonic interstitium eventually provides the osmotic gradients to allow water reabsorption later in the nephron, whereas the newly hypotonic filtrate (~70 mOsm/L) can be diluted further in the distal convoluted tubule if free water excretion is desired.

The distal convoluted tubule reabsorbs more salt via the NaCl thiazide-sensitive channel and, in the absence of vasopressin (antidiuretic hormone, ADH), can dilute the urine to approximately 40 mOsm/L in normal kidneys. The distal convoluted tubule is also involved in calcium reabsorption and phosphate excretion under the influence of parathyroid hormone. The filtrate then passes to the collecting tubules, where final fine-tuning of acid–base, sodium, and potassium balance occur, largely under the influence of aldosterone. The cortical and medullary collecting tubules are also the main site of ADH-directed water reabsorption. Here, the highly concentrated interstitium derived from active salt transport in the loop of Henle is used to drive passive water reabsorption. Thus, from normal kidneys, urine as dilute as 40 mOsm/L and as concentrated as 1,200 mOsm/L can be elaborated based on bodily needs.[4]

OVERVIEW OF ACUTE KIDNEY INJURY

Acute kidney injury (AKI), or acute renal failure as the entity was called previously, remains a common and lethal complication of critical illness. The literature is replete with definitions of AKI, but the occurrence of AKI in a patient is most often defined as an elevation of serum creatinine concentration (s[Cr]) of 0.5 mg/dL from baseline, or as an acute need for renal replacement therapy (RRT), for example, hemodialysis.[5] The lack of consensus on the definition of AKI has affected the ability of clinicians to compare published protocols regarding diagnosis and treatment of this prevalent disorder. As such, a workgroup called the Acute Dialysis Quality Initiative developed a consensus definition of AKI (Table 52.1) incorporating risk, injury, failure, loss, and end-stage renal failure criteria ("RIFLE") for the individual patient.[6] These criteria account for either elevation of s[Cr] or decrements of glomerular filtration rate (GFR) or urine output in the determination of the different stages of AKI. These criteria also yield prognostic information regarding the status of the critically ill patient. However, although these criteria are well accepted in the

TABLE 52.1

RIFLE CRITERIA

CATEGORY	DEFINITION	MANIFESTATION
Risk	s[Cr] > 1.5 × baseline Urine <0.5 mL/kg for 6 h	GFR decrease 25%
Injury	s[Cr] > 2.0 × baseline Urine <0.5 mL/kg for 12 h	GFR decrease 50%
Failure	s[Cr] > 3.0 × baseline *or* s[Cr] > 4.0 mg/dL Urine <0.3 mL/kg for 24 h *or* Anuria for 12 h	GFR decrease 75%
Loss	Failure > 4 wk (either GFR or urine output criterion)	
ESRD	*Failure > 3 mo (either GFR or urine output criterion)*	

s[Cr], serum creatinine concentration; ESRD, end-stage renal disease; GFR, Glomerular filtration rate; RIFLE, risk, injury, failure, loss, and end-stage renal disease criteria

research community with virtually all AKI publications using the RIFLE criteria by 2006,[7] adoption in routine clinical use remains uncommon.

The occurrence of AKI may influence profoundly the outcome of critically ill patients.[8] In a study of postoperative cardiac patients, patients with even the slightest augmentations of s[Cr] that qualified them for RIFLE R criteria of AKI had a 2.2-fold greater mortality, a 1.6-fold increase in ICU length of stay, and 1.6-fold increase in total postoperative costs compared to controls.[9] Similarly, a meta-analysis encompassing 78,855 patients found that even just a 10%–24% increase in s[Cr] was associated with an 80% increase in mortality compared with matched patients and that a s[Cr] increase >50% was associated with an eightfold increase in mortality.[10] Therefore, even small changes in s[Cr] should be of concern, and should prompt careful evaluation of potential causes and treatments.

Clinical Syndromes of AKI

The etiology of AKI is multifactorial in most patients and may represent only a portion of a patient's organ dysfunction. Whereas several etiologies may lead to AKI, each individual contributor to AKI is generally classified as being prerenal, "intrinsic" renal, or postrenal (Table 52.2).

Prerenal Azotemia. "Prerenal" AKI is believed not to be due to an actual change in the kidneys' ability to clear Cr and other solutes, but rather to a perfusion-limited decrease in solute presentation to the kidneys. Most commonly, this is due to intravascular volume depletion, such as might occur during hemorrhage, desiccation, or third spacing of intravascular fluid. However, it should be noted that "prerenal" does not necessarily mean a given patient is whole body, or even volume depleted intravascularly. Congestive heart failure, for instance, is often associated with "prerenal" increments in s[Cr], and is due to inability of the heart to generate cardiac output to perfuse the kidneys adequately. As such, prerenal azotemia is best characterized by ineffective arterial blood flow to the kidneys for any reason. AKI from prerenal causes is usually reversible, and will generally respond to correction of the underlying abnormality (i.e., fluid resuscitation for intravascular volume depletion).

Intrinsic Acute Kidney Injury. Structural injury of the kidney is the hallmark of intrinsic AKI (Table 52.2). The most common form is acute tubular necrosis (ATN), whether ischemic due to progression of prerenal azotemia or interruption of renal blood flow (e.g., trauma, thromboembolism) or cytotoxic (e.g., due to toxicity from medications or ingestion syndromes).[11] ATN may occur even absent an overt, prolonged decrease in renal blood flow or a massive exposure to nephrotoxins, usually due to a confluence of events in the acute setting. For example, doses of gentamicin insufficient to cause AKI in a normal kidney may result in substantial nephrotoxicity in the setting of hypoperfusion or concurrent exposure to other nephrotoxins.[12] However, ATN occurs most commonly when the nephrons' capacity to autoregulate blood flow is overwhelmed. As noted above, this autoregulation is dependent on modulation of the relative tones of the glomerular afferent and efferent arterioles. Moreover, oxygen tension in the renal medulla tends to be low, due to both the anatomic characteristics and energy demands of the loop of Henle. The medullary microcirculation is dependent on endothelial elaboration of vasodilators such as nitric oxide and prostaglandins, which may be impaired in acute illness, existing microvascular disease, or by medications such as radiocontrast medium or nonsteroidal anti-inflammatory drugs (NSAIDs).[13] Thus, the stressed renal microvasculature loses its autoregulatory capacity and becomes more sensitive to vasoconstrictor drugs and periods of systemic hypotension, which thus may provoke additional damage that can delay recovery from ATN.[14] Although the cellular injury is observed in proximal tubules predominantly (by contrast to apoptotic cell death, which occurs primarily in the distal nephron), necrosis of the distal nephron may also occur. The distal nephron may also become obstructed by desquamated cells and cellular debris due to sloughing of more proximal tubular cells. Endogenous growth factors regulate tissue repair and recovery; administration of growth factors exogenously has been shown experimentally to ameliorate and hasten recovery from AKI, although there have been no studies suggesting benefit in clinical trials. Depletion of neutrophils and blockade of neutrophil adhesion reduce AKI following experimental ischemia, indicating that inflammation is at least partly responsible for some features of ATN, especially in postischemic injury after transplantation.[14]

TABLE 52.2

ETIOLOGIES OF AKI

Prerenal causes (decreased renal blood flow)
Hypovolemia
Renal losses (diuretics, osmotic agents, polyuria)
Gastrointestinal losses (vomiting, diarrhea)
Cutaneous losses (burns, exfoliative syndromes)
Hemorrhage
Pancreatitis
Capillary-leak syndrome with "third spacing" of intravascular volume
Decreased cardiac output
Congestive heart failure
Pulmonary embolism
Acute myocardial infarction
Severe valvular heart disease
ACS
Renal artery obstruction (stenosis, embolism, thrombosis, dissection)
Systemic vasodilation
Sepsis
Anaphylaxis
Anesthetics
Drug overdose
Afferent arteriolar vasoconstriction
Hypercalcemia
Drugs (NSAIDs, amphotericin B, calcineurin inhibitors, norepinephrine, iodinated radiocontrast agents, aminoglycosides, vancomycin [high doses])
Hepatorenal syndrome
Efferent arteriolar vasodilation (ACE-I, aldosterone receptor blockers)
Intrinsic renal causes
Vascular (large and small vessel)
Trauma
Renal vein obstruction (thrombosis, ventilation with high-level positive end-expiratory pressure [PEEP], ACS)
Microangiopathy (thrombotic thrombocytopenic purpura [TTP], hemolytic uremic syndrome [HUS], disseminated intravascular coagulation [DIC], preeclampsia)
Malignant hypertension
Scleroderma renal crisis
Transplant rejection
Atheroembolic disease
Sickle cell disease (microinfarcts)
Glomerular
Antiglomerular basement membrane (GBM) disease (Goodpasture's syndrome)
Antineutrophil cytoplasmic antibody–associated glomerulonephritis (e.g., Wegener granulomatosis)
Immune complex glomerulonephritis (GN) (systemic lupus erythematosus [SLE], postinfectious, cryoglobulinemia, primary membranoproliferative GN, bacterial endocarditis)
Tubular
Ischemic
Cytotoxic
Heme pigment (rhabdomyolysis, intravascular hemolysis)
Crystals (tumor lysis syndrome, seizures, ethylene glycol poisoning, megadose vitamin C, acyclovir, indinavir, methotrexate)
Drugs (aminoglycosides, lithium, amphotericin B, pentamidine, cisplatin, ifosfamide, iodinated radiocontrast agents)
Interstitial
Drugs (penicillins, cephalosporins, NSAIDs, proton pump inhibitors, allopurinol, rifampin, indinavir, mesalamine, sulfonamides)
Infection (pyelonephritis, viral infection)
Systemic disease
Sjögren's syndrome, sarcoidosis, SLE, lymphoma, leukemia, tubulonephritis, uveitis
Postrenal
Ureteral obstruction (calculus, tumor [intrinsic or extrinsic], fibrosis, ligation during pelvic surgery)
Bladder neck obstruction (benign prostatic hypertrophy, prostate cancer, neurogenic bladder, tricyclic antidepressants, ganglionic blockers, bladder tumor, calculus, hemorrhage/clot)
Urethral obstruction (stricture, tumor, phimosis)
Renal calcinosis
Obstructed or malpositioned urinary catheter, ureteral stent, or ileal conduit
Trauma-pelvic retroperitoneal hematoma

Hypoperfusion-related decreases in glomerular blood flow and intrarenal vasoconstriction appear to be the dominant mechanisms for reduced GFR in ATN. The mechanisms of this vasoconstriction are not entirely clear, but tubuloglomerular (TG) feedback mechanisms appear to play a role. In the normal setting, TG feedback can modulate glomerular blood flow by causing arteriolar vasoconstriction when large amounts of chloride are presented to the macula densa, a group of cells at the end of the loop of Henle that physically abut its associated glomerulus.[4] This response is favorable from an evolutionary perspective; when there is tubular dysfunction, defects in salt and chloride reabsorption lead to activation of TG feedback and a resultant decrease in blood flow to the affected glomerulus. Salt and water losses are thereby mitigated, at the cost of some degree of GFR. Tubular obstruction from sloughed cells and interstitial edema also result in loss of the hydrostatic gradients favoring glomerular filtration.

Whereas ATN comprises the large majority of "intrinsic" causes of AKI, two other less common causes are due to host immune responses: postinfectious glomerulonephritis (PIGN) and acute interstitial nephritis (AIN). The incidence of PIGN in the acute surgical setting has not been studied but is believed to be rare, although that impression may be due to a paucity of biopsy data in this population. Although the pathophysiology of PIGN has not been elucidated, it is conceptualized as an immune complex–associated glomerulonephritis, in which antigen–antibody complexes containing bacterial (usually streptococcal) antigen deposit in the glomerulus and cause immune activation and inflammation.[15] This can result in varying degrees of renal dysfunction, from mild loss of GFR to a permanent need for RRT. Common features of PIGN include signs of acute kidney inflammation, including salt retention and edema, hypertension, hematuria, hemolysis, and proteinuria.

Interstitial nephritis is also an important contributor to intrinsic AKI. Predominantly due to allergic responses to medications, AIN was implicated as the cause in 7% of cases of AKI in a recent biopsy review.[16] Although any medication can theoretically cause AIN, the most common culprits include penicillins (especially nafcillin or methicillin [the latter now used rarely]), cephalosporins, NSAIDs, sulfa-containing medications, rifampin, fluoroquinolones, and proton pump inhibitors.[17] Time of onset of AKI is unpredictable, and can occur from 1 day to months after the second exposure to the agent. As such, awareness of and suspicion of AIN is important, especially in the setting of known potential medications, peripheral or urine eosinophilia, and rash.

Postrenal Acute Kidney Injury. "Postrenal" AKI is due to mechanical obstruction of urine flow, which results not only in failure to excrete urine, but also the eventual loss of the hydrostatic gradient favoring filtration across Bowman's capsule if the obstruction is not relieved (Table 52.2). Obstruction can occur anywhere along the urinary tract, including the ureters, bladder, and urethra. Bladder outlet obstruction due to prostate hyperplasia is the most common cause of postrenal AKI. Unilateral causes of hydronephrosis, such as a ureteral calculus or extrinsic compression of one ureter, generally do not lead to oliguria, as the contralateral kidney will continue to produce urine. As such, whereas placement of a Foley catheter does essentially rule out bladder outlet obstruction (or overcome it if present), bladder catheterization does not rule out obstructive nephropathy more proximally. In addition, although not truly "obstructive" in nature, postoperative urine leaks can also present as "postrenal" AKI. Urine leaks occur most commonly after surgical manipulation of the bladder or ureters (e.g., cystectomy, kidney transplant surgery), and can present as decreased urine output and persistently elevated or increasing s[Cr] without obvious cause. The diagnosis is usually confirmed by radionuclide imaging that detects renal excretion of tracer into a perinephric or intraperitoneal fluid collection. Alternatively, [Cr] can be measured in a sample of the fluid; if it is higher than s[Cr], the fluid collection is at least partially urine.

DETECTION OF ACUTE KIDNEY INJURY

As noted above, the RIFLE criteria have become the standard for definition of AKI, and have provided consistency to AKI diagnoses (Table 52.1). However, complicating further the evaluation and treatment of AKI is the lack of ideal biomarkers thereof. Currently, the blood urea nitrogen concentration [BUN] and s[Cr] are the tests used most commonly to monitor renal function, and as such, s[Cr] is the main laboratory parameter used in the RIFLE classification. Nevertheless, these measures are clearly imperfect. Urea nitrogen, for example, is an end product of protein metabolism, and does accumulate in the presence of AKI and chronic kidney disease (CKD). However, there are many conditions that can also result in an elevated [BUN] unrelated to renal function, including (1) states of protein catabolism (e.g., corticosteroid therapy, sepsis); (2) excessive protein intake; or (3) increased reabsorption (e.g., dehydration, gastrointestinal bleeding). Conversely, patients who cannot synthesize urea (e.g., liver cirrhosis) or have inadequate protein intake may have misleadingly low BUN concentrations even in the presence of substantial kidney dysfunction.

Although s[Cr] is accepted as the standard test to monitor renal function, it is imperfect. Steady-state s[Cr] is influenced by age, gender, and muscle mass. Severe decrements in renal function can be present even while the s[Cr] remains within the laboratory's specified "normal range,"[18] especially among elderly females. For example, a s[Cr] of 1.2 mg/dL in a 90-year-old female with a body mass of 50 kg may under-represent GFR, whereas the same s[Cr] in a 25-year-old black male with a body mass of 100 kg may be normal. Formulas such as the Cockcroft-Gault or Modification of Diet in Renal Disease (MDRD) calculations (Table 52.3) were developed to normalize demographic variations in muscle mass. Calculation tools are readily available online, and can be used to estimate renal function with reasonable accuracy. These imperfections are noted not to discourage use of [BUN] and s[Cr] for evaluation of renal function, but rather to highlight potential confounding factors that may have clinical import.

Emerging biomarkers may prove useful in the future for early detection of AKI. Potential biomarkers include both serum neutrophil gelatinase-associated lipocalin (NGAL) and cystatin C, and urinary NGAL, interleukin-18 (IL-18), and kidney injury molecule-1 (KIM-1).[19] Serum NGAL and cystatin C may be particularly useful in predicting AKI after cardiac surgery.[20] These biomarkers may also be important for drug development. With highly sensitive urinary biomarkers of kidney toxicity, drugs that have nonclinical signals of nephrotoxicity can be tested more safely in clinical trials.[21]

PREVENTION OF ACUTE KIDNEY INJURY

The best management strategy for AKI entails preventing its development. Certain patients have been identified clearly as being at high risk of developing AKI, including postoperative patients or those with sepsis, trauma, or hypovolemia,[22] including shock of any etiology. Patient groups also at risk include those receiving any nephrotoxic agents (e.g., iodinated radiocontrast medium, medications), those with CKD due to diabetes mellitus or hypertension, or patients with congestive heart failure, multiple myeloma, chronic infection (e.g., osteomyelitis), or a myeloproliferative disorder. Estimation of GFR using either the Cockcroft-Gault or MDRD GFR equation, or measurement of urine creatinine clearance (C_{Cr}) is especially important in such patients, as this may improve risk

TABLE 52.3

FORMULAS FOR ESTIMATION OF CREATININE CLEARANCE (eC_{Cr}) OR GLOMERULAR FILTRATION RATE (eGFR)

Cockroft-Gault Equation

$$eC_{Cr} = \frac{(140 - \text{Age}) \times \text{Mass (in kilograms)} \times [0.85 \text{ if female}]}{72 \times \text{Serum Creatinine (in mg / dL)}}$$

(when Cr is expressed in mg/dL)

$$eC_{Cr} = \frac{(140 - \text{Age}) \times \text{Mass (in kilograms)} \times \text{Constant}}{\text{Serum Creatinine (in } \mu\text{mol / L)}}$$

(When Cr is expressed in micromol/L, where constant is 1.23 for males and 1.04 for females.

Modification of Diet in Renal Disease (MDRD) Formula

For creatinine in mg/dL:

$$\text{eGFR} = 186 \times \text{Serum Creatinine}^{-1.154} \times \text{Age}^{-0.203} \times [1.212 \text{ if Black}] \times [0.742 \text{ if Female}]$$

For creatinine in μmol/L:

$$\text{eGFR} = 32788 \times \text{Serum Creatinine}^{-1.154} \times \text{Age}^{-0.203} \times [1.212 \text{ if Black}] \times [0.742 \text{ if Female}]$$

Creatinine levels in micromol/L can be converted to mg/dL by dividing them by 88.4. The 32,788 number above is equal to $186 \times 88.4^{1.154}$.

The MDRD equation has been validated in patients with CKD, but underestimates the GFR in healthy patients with GFRs over 60 mL/min (From Madaio M. Post-infectious glomerulonephritis. In: Schrier RW, ed. Diseases of the Kidney. Boston, MA: Little Brown; 1997:1579–1594; Prakash J, Sen D, Kumar NS, et al. Acute renal failure due to intrinsic renal diseases: review of 1122 cases. Ren Fail. 2003;25:225–233.) The equations have not been validated in AKI. These MDRD equations are to be used only if the laboratory has NOT calibrated its s[Cr] measurements to isotope dilution mass spectroscopy (IDMS). When IDMS-calibrated [sCr] is used (which is about 6% lower), the above equations should be multiplied by 175/186, or 0.94086. These formulas do not adjust for body mass, therefore, relative to the Cockcroft-Gault formula, they underestimate eGFR for heavy people and overestimate it for underweight people. See text for abbreviations.

stratification regarding administration of procedures, medications, or imaging tests. Whereas all hospitalized patients must have their intravascular volume status monitored to some degree, these at-risk patients require particularly close monitoring to ensure that hypovolemia is avoided and that exposure to nephrotoxins is minimized or avoided. Consequently, high-risk patients may need frequent measurements of vital signs, central venous pressure, serum [lactate], urine output, or short-duration (e.g., 8–12 hours) C_{Cr}.

Furthermore, medications that are not overtly "nephrotoxic" but that do affect glomerular blood flow, such as angiotensin-converting enzyme inhibitors (ACE-I) and NSAIDs, should be used with caution, especially in populations prone to AKI. For instance, in patients with cardiac or liver disease, or patients who may be volume underresuscitated, prostaglandin-mediated afferent arteriolar dilation or angiotensin II–medicated efferent arteriolar constriction may be crucial in maintaining filtration pressure. Blockade of one or both of these mechanisms with a NSAID or ACE-I can result in an abrupt decrease in GFR.

Several interventions may prevent AKI in certain patient groups. Nondiabetic cardiac patients may have a diminished risk of AKI after cardiac surgery, according to the RIFLE criteria, by maintaining tight perioperative blood glucose control. In one study, nondiabetic patients undergoing cardiac surgery had glucose concentrations controlled by insulin infusion at either a trigger of >140 mg/dL, or in a range of 80–111 mg/dL. The observed overall incidence of postoperative AKI or acute postoperative RRT was lower in the group controlled more tightly, who also demonstrated a lower mortality rate.[22] Patients with septic shock appear to be at particularly high risk for AKI. These patients may be severely hypovolemic and may also be subject to nephrotoxicity from cytokine-mediated renal vasoconstriction as part of the proinflammatory response. Notably, delays in antibiotic therapy in this cohort of patients may be particularly predictive of AKI.[23]

Certain intravenous medications have been suggested to prevent the occurrence of AKI. Historically, low-dose dopamine (1.5–3.0 mcg/kg/minute) has been used most commonly.[24] D'Orio et al. demonstrated that dopamine (3 mcg/kg/minute) caused isolated renal vasodilation, resulting in increased diuresis, natriuresis, increased renal blood flow, and enhanced GFR, without activating either alpha- or beta-adrenergic receptors.[25] The institution of low-dose dopamine in critically ill patients will augment C_{Cr} by 25% or more in individual patients,[26] but large studies have failed to demonstrate benefit to prevent development of AKI or mitigate it postonset. Marik performed a meta-analysis of 15 trials (970 patients) looking at the absolute change of s[Cr] with the use of low-dose dopamine, and found no difference.[27] Bellomo et al., through the Australian and New Zealand Intensive Care Society (ANZICS) Clinical Trials Group, performed the largest multicenter randomized trial of low-dose dopamine (by studying critically ill patients with signs of systemic inflammatory response syndrome and clinical evidence of early AKI). This trial of 328 patients in 23 ICUs found that neither the primary outcome (peak s[Cr]) nor any of the secondary outcomes (hourly urine output, requirement for RRT, duration of mechanical ventilation, duration of ICU or hospital stay, or mortality) were altered among patients treated with low-dose dopamine.[28] Currently, low-dose dopamine may be used to promote diuresis in select patients with adequate preload, as many patients do respond with increased urine output. However, low-dopamine does not alter the outcome or avert the development of AKI in critically ill patients.

Fenoldopam, a potent dopamine D_1 receptor agonist that increases blood flow to the renal cortex and outer medulla, has also been utilized to prevent AKI, but may induce hypotension. Indications for fenoldopam in critical care are not well defined, but it may be beneficial when hypertension must be treated while preserving renal perfusion. In a study using perioperative fenoldopam with *N*-acetylcysteine, investigators found the combination abrogated an early postoperative decrease of renal function in cardiac surgical patients with CKD, but did not affect other outcomes.[29] A meta-analysis of fenoldopam to prevent AKI in postoperative cardiac patients showed that fenoldopam reduced the need for RRT and perioperative mortality.[30] Another meta-analysis of randomized, controlled trials (RCTs) of fenoldopam to prevent or treat AKI in postoperative or intensive care patients demonstrated that mortality and the need for RRT were both decreased by fenoldopam.[31] However, the second meta-analysis included only small single-center studies, and doses were variable. Data are insufficient presently to support widespread use of fenoldopam for prevention or management of AKI.

SPECIAL POPULATIONS

Rhabdomyolysis

Certain patient populations are at extremely high risk of developing AKI, and warrant special consideration. Rhabdomyolysis is due most commonly to crush injury, but it can also occur with high fever or other clinical syndromes[32] (Table 52.4).

An unusual, recently described cause of rhabdomyolysis is propofol-related infusion syndrome, a complex syndrome characterized not only by rhabdomyolysis but also by metabolic acidosis, arrhythmias, myocardial failure, AKI, hepatomegaly, and death.[33] Propofol inhibits mitochondrial electron transport via the upregulation of malonyl coenzyme A, which inhibits activity of carnitine palmitoyltransferase I, thus preventing long-chain free fatty acids (FFA) from entering the mitochondria (Fig. 52.1). Beta-spiral oxidation of FFA is uncoupled and the electron transport chain is disrupted, preventing the utilization of medium- and short-chain FFAs, which leads to myocytolysis. Accumulation of FFAs may cause arrhythmias, whereas uncoupling of oxidative phosphorylation antagonizes adrenoceptor binding by β-agonists and myocardial calcium channels, thereby depressing myocardial contractility. Increased catecholamine requirements to overcome the adrenoceptor blockade (or circulating as a result of traumatic brain injury or the proinflammatory stress response) may increase propofol requirements (via increased clearance owing to the increased cardiac output), or cause direct myocyte toxicity. The negative inotropic effect of propofol, resulting in increased catecholamine requirements, could create a "vicious circle" of propofol and catecholamines driving each other to progressive myocardial depression.

TABLE 52.4

MAJOR ETIOLOGIES OF RHABDOMYOLYSIS

Crush injury
Prolonged immobilization
Muscle ischemia (prolonged hypoperfusion from hypovole mia or sepsis, extremity arterial occlusion)
Reperfusion injury
Compartment syndrome
Profound temperature elevation (high fever, heat stroke, malignant hyperthermia syndrome)
Severe exertion or muscle stimulation (marathon running, neuroleptic malignant syndrome)
Infection (*Clostridium* spp., *Streptococcus pyogenes*, Influenza A and B, Coxsackie virus)
Electrolyte disorders (hypophosphatemia, hypokalemia)
Drugs (statins or other lipid-lowering agents, daptomycin, propofol)
Toxins (alcohol, cocaine, heroin)
Genetic disorders

Another increasingly prevalent cause of rhabdomyolysis is prolonged immobilization in the bariatric setting, which may be prevented by careful padding on the operating table at all pressure points, frequent changes of patient position intraoperatively and postoperatively, or performance of certain bariatric operations in two stages.[34]

Sometimes AKI in the setting of rhabdomyolysis may be multifactorial. Factors predictive of AKI in this setting, determined by multiple logistic regression analysis, include the degree of elevation of serum creatine phosphokinase (CPK), $[K^+]$, or $[PO_4^{3-}]$, the magnitude of decrease of serum [albumin], dehydration at presentation, or sepsis as the underlying cause.[35]

The pathophysiology of rhabdomyolysis contributing to AKI has been studied extensively, and is due to renal ischemia, direct renal toxicity, and tubular obstruction. Hypotension and shock impair glomerular filtration due to reactive renal vasoconstriction, which results in decreased renal perfusion. Hypovolemia is initiated by capillary leak syndrome and extravasation of plasma into damaged muscle. As a result, oxygen delivery is reduced and renal tubular cell dysfunction impends. Likewise, tubular obstruction by cast formation (myoglobin with Tamm-Horsfall protein) can occur, resulting in oliguria.[32] Myoglobin itself is a direct tubular toxin but serum [myoglobin] peaks well before AKI is apparent, and thus is seldom measured. Myoglobin is catabolized to ferrihemate, generating reactive oxygen species (ROS) (at urine pH <5.8, both moieties are nephrotoxic) that are the likely cause of tubular toxicity.[32] The CPK may correlate with the extent of renal tubular damage, as the amount of myoglobin elaborated is also correlated.[36]

The treatment of rhabdomyolysis to prevent or minimize AKI is multifaceted. Initial therapy is focused on treating the underlying cause and resuscitating the patient. Muscle fascial compartments should be decompressed with fasciotomy and dead muscle debrided if needed, to avoid compartment syndromes. Offending toxins or drugs should be withdrawn. Intensive care unit monitoring with central venous pressure measurement and aggressive hydration optimizes intravascular volume. The next concern is to prevent AKI from myoglobinuria, especially if the serum (CPK) exceeds 5,000 U/dL, or myoglobinuria persists.[37] For these scenarios, treatment is by enforced alkaline diuresis with $NaHCO_3$ administration and an agent such as mannitol (25 g q6h being a standard dose), which is also a scavenger of ROS. Loop diuretics should be avoided as they tend to acidify the urine, which can exacerbate ROS generation and the direct toxic effects of the ferrihemate. For lesser elevations of CPK, aggressive diuresis with isotonic saline is sufficient. Many authorities recommend maintaining urine pH ≥ 6.0 by the continuous infusion of $NaHCO_3$. To maintain isotonicity, 150 mL of 8.4% $NaHCO_3$ (three standard amps of 8.4% $NaHCO_3$) is added to 850 mL D_5W to create the solution for infusion. Some authorities administer mannitol concurrently to enforce diuresis until pigmenturia disappears or [CPK] decreases, but both mannitol and $NaHCO_3$ are controversial for prevention of pigment-induced (i.e., myoglobin) nephropathy.[38]

Contrast Nephropathy

Patients at high risk of AKI also include those who have CKD and require iodinated radiocontrast medium for a diagnostic test. Patients who have baseline s[Cr] >1.5 mg/dL, or baseline C_{Cr} < 30 mg/dL, are at high risk of superimposed AKI. There is no sure-fire means of preventing contrast nephropathy. Some

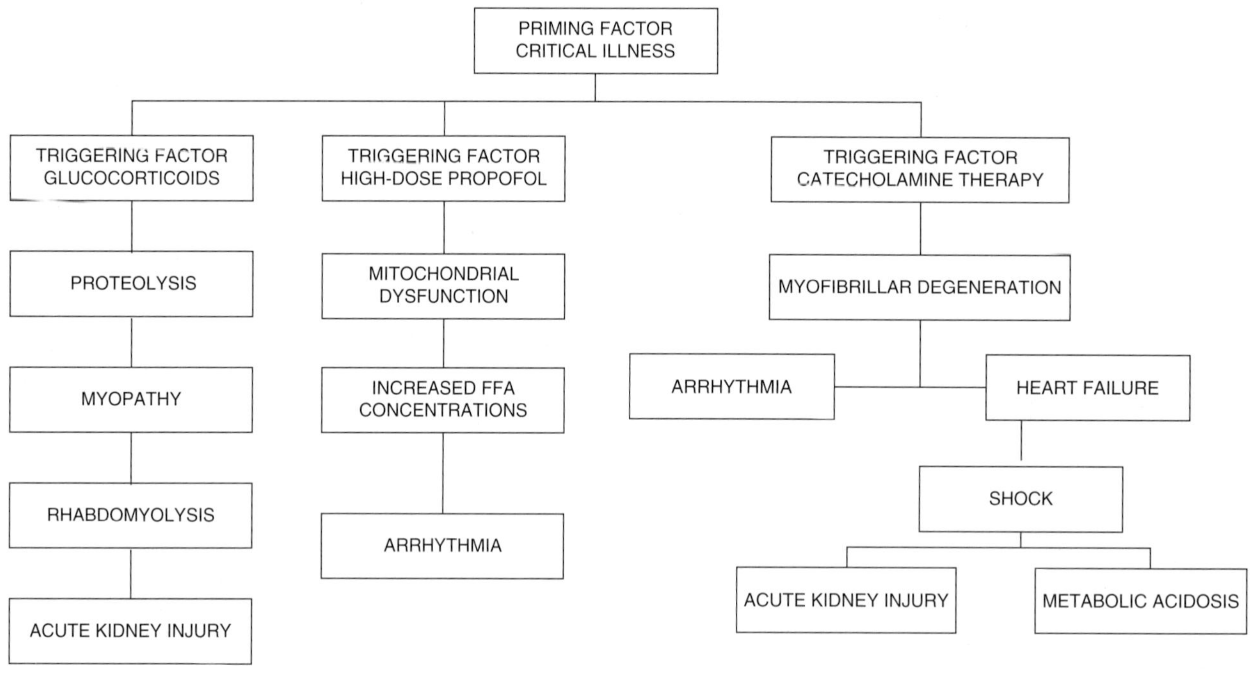

FIGURE 52.1. Pathogenesis of propofol infusion syndrome. FFA, free fatty acids.

investigators have suggested that patients at risk should receive a $NaHCO_3$ infusion (50 mL of 8.4% $NaHCO_3$ added to 950 mL D_5W) at 100 mL/hour for 1 hour prior to the contrast administration and for 6 hours thereafter. When $NaHCO_3$ is employed, patients are placed at risk of developing pulmonary edema, and consequently need careful monitoring.[39] However, whether $NaHCO_3$ infusion prevents AKI in high-risk patients is controversial. In one study, all patients who underwent cardiac catheterization with an estimated GFR < 60 mL/minute were randomized to hydration with $NaHCO_3$ versus isotonic NaCl. Neither group differed in terms of the rates of mortality, RRT, myocardial infarction, or cerebrovascular events at 30 days or 6 months.[40] This finding was corroborated in part by a meta-analysis evaluating $NaHCO_3$ infusion compared to NaCl infusion for AKI prophylaxis in high-risk patients.[41] In that study, Brar et al. found that the benefit of $NaHCO_3$ for prevention of AKI was limited to small trials of lower methodological quality; no evidence of $NaHCO_3$ was noted among larger, better-quality trials. A recent systematic review on the same topic reached the same conclusion.[42] Nonetheless, our practice is to use $NaHCO_3$ administration for prophylaxis of contrast nephropathy owing to the smaller volume of fluid.

A variety of other agents have been employed to decrease the incidence of AKI following intravenous contrast, including *N*-acetylcysteine with either NaCl or $NaHCO_3$. In a meta-analysis of 10 studies combining *N*-acetylcysteine and $NaHCO_3$, Brown et al. found this combination to be more effective than *N*-acetylcysteine plus NaCl for patients undergoing cardiac catheterization.[43] Recently, the prostaglandin analogue iloprost was found to decrease the frequency of contrast-induced nephropathy (CIN) and maintain GFR compared to controls in patients undergoing coronary angiography.[44] Atrial natriuretic peptide (ANP) has also been studied to prevent AKI from CIN. A recent Cochrane review revealed that after major surgery there was a significant reduction in RRT requirement with ANP in prevention studies, but not in treatment studies; there was no mortality difference regardless. Other interventions aimed at improving renal blood flow, such as dopamine[45] and fenoldopam[46] infusions (see above), are also of no benefit.

Low-volume nonionic low-osmolar or iso-osmolar contrast preparations have been suggested to decrease CIN when compared to high-osmolar agents. In a recent retrospective study, gadolinium was used in high-risk patients and yielded a decreased frequency of CIN when compared to standard contrast.[47] However, an RCT of 526 subjects with impaired baseline renal function and diabetes mellitus, undergoing diagnostic or therapeutic coronary angiography, showed that the renal effects of the nonionic, iso-osmolar agent iodixanol and the nonionic, low-osmolar agent iopamidol were comparable.[48] These two agents have emerged as the contrast media of choice in patients at risk of CIN who require imaging with parenteral contrast.[49]

BASIC PRINCIPLES OF TREATMENT OF ACUTE KIDNEY INJURY

Early intervention and prevention remain the optimal strategies in managing AKI, as no treatment has been proved effective in RCTs for established AKI. Nevertheless, delayed treatment of AKI may lead to worsened organ dysfunction. Although mild AKI may develop in isolation, all patients with severe AKI invariably manifest the multiple organ dysfunction syndrome (MODS). The most common pitfalls in AKI management are delay in diagnosis, incorrect assessment of the cause(s) of AKI, and failure to recognize and treat not only its complications, but also its precipitant and the other manifestations of MODS. If uncorrected, the precipitant is more likely to cause death than the AKI itself.

The most important step in diagnosing and treating AKI involves determining whether the etiology of the AKI is prerenal, renal, or postrenal (see above).[50] However, once AKI develops, the clinician must treat the underlying cause concurrently with treatment or prevention of any related complications. For example, trauma and sepsis may contribute to the development of AKI by multiple mechanisms. In trauma, blood loss and the concomitant proinflammatory response from tissue injury can lead to hypovolemia and prerenal AKI, whereas the rhabdomyolysis of trauma or the use of iodinated contrast to detect injuries can lead to intrinsic AKI. Sepsis may be the most common cause of AKI in the ICU, where it may be present in up to 50% of cases.[51] In sepsis, hypovolemia can lead to prerenal AKI but bacterial toxins, vasoconstrictor proinflammatory cytokines, or the antibiotics used to treat sepsis may contribute to intrinsic causes of AKI.

Evaluation of Oliguria

The most common manifestation of the development of AKI is oliguria, defined as urine output insufficient to excrete the daily solute load, which in patients with normal renal concentrating ability (up to ~1,200 mOsm/L) eating a normal solute diet (~600–900 mOsm/day) equates to <0.5 mL/kg/hour based on ideal body weight or <400–500 mL urine output in a 24-hour period. This more nuanced definition is important; in patients who have a high solute load (e.g., patients receiving a high protein diet for wound healing or aggressive crystalloid resuscitation) or impaired renal concentrating ability, even a daily urine output of > 1 L may be relative oliguria.

Postoperative oliguria is most likely to be due to hypovolemia or other prerenal causes. Surgical evaluation begins with a focused history and physical examination for likely causes, but if the cause is unknown or obscure, a detailed evaluation must follow. Examination of the skin may reveal petechiae, purpura, ecchymosis, or livedo reticularis, which can provide clues to inflammatory and vascular causes of AKI. Ocular examination may find evidence of uveitis suggestive of interstitial nephritis or necrotizing vasculitis, whereas ocular palsy may indicate ethylene glycol poisoning or necrotizing vasculitis. Findings suggestive of severe hypertension, atheroembolic disease, or endocarditis may be observed by fundoscopy.

The most important part of the physical examination for surgical patients is the assessment of cardiovascular and volume status.[52] Vital signs taken both supine and standing (if possible), and careful examination of the heart, lungs, jugular venous pulse, skin turgor, mucous membranes, and extremities (for peripheral edema) are essential. Accurate daily records of fluid intake and urine output and daily measurements of patient body mass are crucial. Medications must be reviewed, and doses adjusted if necessary.

Abdominal examination findings can be useful to detect obstruction at the bladder outlet (postrenal AKI). The presence of an epigastric bruit suggests renovascular hypertension. Abdominal distention may suggest intra-abdominal hypertension and abdominal compartment syndrome (ACS). Foley catheters and other urinary conduits or stents should be inspected for patency and proper positioning, and intravesical pressure measured for suspected ACS (see below).

After this initial assessment, it must be determined whether oliguria is due to prerenal or other causes.[53] Confirmatory tests may include central venous or pulmonary artery pressure monitoring or a chest radiograph (Table 52.5). Notably, the detection of pulmonary edema in critically ill patients by standard anterior–posterior chest radiography lacks sensitivity and specificity. Thus, if available, invasive monitoring with either a central venous pressure catheter or a pulmonary artery catheter may assist in determining intravascular volume status, although outcomes may be unaffected.[54]

TABLE 52.5

DIAGNOSTIC TESTS TO DISTINGUISH PRERENAL AND RENAL AKI

INDEX	PRERENAL CAUSES	RENAL CAUSES
FeNa	<1%	≤2%
Urine [Na]	<10 mmol/L	>40 mmol/L
Urine/plasma osmolality	>1.5	1–1.5
Renal failure index	<1	>2
BUN:creatinine	>20	<10

BUN, blood urea nitrogen; FeNa, fractional excretion of sodium.
Calculation of FeNa: [urine sodium × plasma creatinine]/[plasma sodium × serum creatinine] × 100.
renal failure index: urine sodium × urine creatinine/plasma creatinine.

Urine electrolytes should be measured to determine whether tubular function is intact. In general, ATN results in disruption of tubular Na and solute reabsorption, whereas prerenal causes of AKI do not. The most commonly measured urine indices include the fractional excretion of sodium (FeNa) and the fractional excretion of urea (FeUrea). If one considers that a normal daily GFR is approximately 180 L/day and that serum [Na] is approximately 140 mEq/L, then the daily filtered load of Na = 25,200 mEq. As such, the normal response of the renal tubular system is to reabsorb more than 99% of the filtered sodium (i.e., FeNa < 1%); otherwise, a diet extraordinarily high in sodium would be required in order to avoid severe negative Na balance. Thus, in an oliguric patient, a FeNa of <1% implies that the tubular Na reclamation mechanisms remain intact, and therefore unlikely that tubular necrosis is responsible for the decrease in urine output or increase in s[CR]. Conversely, if an oliguric patient is found to have a FeNa > 2%, it is likely that tubular function has been compromised, and that prerenal factors alone are not responsible for the clinical picture. If urine [Cr] is unavailable, urine [Na] < 10–20 mg/dL is also consistent with a prerenal etiology.

Whereas the FeNa is a useful tool, it may be confounded by multiple factors, including diuretic therapy, whose purpose is to induce renal sodium wasting. In these patients, the calculation of the FeUrea may be more useful. Urea excretion, as with Na excretion, decreases in prerenal azotemia, but is not affected by the vast majority of diuretics in acute clinical use (loop and thiazide diuretics). As such, a value of FeUrea <35% also suggests that tubular concentrating ability remains intact and that oliguria may be prerenal.[55]

The measurement of serial C_{Cr} may also be useful in assessing the functional status of the kidneys. These values accrue more importance if the baseline C_{Cr} is known or the patient undergoes a change in C_{Cr}. Importantly, a full 24-hour C_{Cr} is not necessary and may even be inaccurate (and therefore misleading) in patients with dynamic changes of renal function.[56] A renal ultrasound should be ordered to evaluate for hydronephrosis, and may also be useful to estimate renal blood flow. As noted above, urology and renal transplant patients pose unique diagnostic problems; the former may be leaking urine intraperitoneally and have apparent renal failure due to reabsorption of urea and creatinine, whereas the latter may have vascular complications. These cases may require measurement of [creatinine] in drain fluid, or scintigraphy to assess perfusion. Eosinophils in urine sediment may suggest a drug reaction causing AKI, most frequently from a beta-lactam antibiotic.

In certain patients, the diagnosis of ACS must be excluded. In ACS, intra-abdominal pressure exceeds renal capillary perfusion pressure, resulting in oliguria. Patients at highest risk for ACS include those with large fluid resuscitation volumes (generally >8 L), large-volume hemorrhage (generally 2 L or more), ascites, severe bowel edema, or patients with abdominal packs in place to stanch hemorrhage. Intravesical pressure is a reasonable surrogate for intra-abdominal pressure; a simple method to measure intravesical pressure is to occlude the Foley catheter after the instillation of at least 50 (preferably no more than 100) mL of saline, and then transducing the pressure via the sampling port proximal to the clamp. Measurement does carry an increased risk of nosocomial bacterial cystitis. Any measurement in excess of 20–25 mm Hg is consistent with intra-abdominal hypertension, which in the proper setting can be diagnostic for ACS. Prompt decompression of the abdomen by laparotomy is the standard treatment for patients with high suspicion of ACS. However, bladder pressure values by this method must be interpreted cautiously in patients with CKD, neurogenic or small-volume bladders, bladder cancer, recent bladder injury, or active bacterial cystitis.

Treatment of AKI of Prerenal Etiology

The management of AKI is predicated on its cause (Table 52.3). A prerenal cause is the most common etiology of AKI after surgery, due usually to severe hypovolemia if not incipient or overt shock. Treating prerenal AKI mainly entails optimizing perfusion to the kidneys and treating the cause of the hypoperfusion or shock regardless of etiology. Whereas hypovolemia is the most common etiology of shock in surgical patients, cardiogenic shock from myocardial infarction, pulmonary embolism, tension pneumothorax, or pericardial tamponade may alternatively or also be present. Other cardiac causes are manifold, including pump failure, cardiac valvular disease, or intrinsic cardiac shunts. Neurogenic shock occurs most commonly after spinal cord injury, but can also occur from epidural local anesthesia. Other forms of distributive shock from etiologies such as medication or transfusion reaction should also be considered. Whereas most of these causes require volume replacement and treatment of the underlying cause, in left ventricular pump failure, the patient may paradoxically have decreased renal perfusion but requires diuretics with afterload reduction for successful management.

Management of AKI from Intrinsic and Postrenal Causes

Regardless of the etiology, management of AKI must avoid any further insult to renal function (particularly so for intrinsic AKI) and iatrogenic complications such as fluid overload. Many patients develop secondary pulmonary dysfunction from hypervolemia, usually due to overzealous fluid administration. One important goal in AKI is to maintain euvolemia so as to avoid an additional or superimposed prerenal insult. Fluid overload in the setting of AKI can be catastrophic, resulting in endotracheal intubation and prolonged mechanical ventilation, and convert a patient with single organ failure to MODS and a propensity for nosocomial infections and substantially increased risk of mortality. Potassium and chloride should be removed from intravenous solutions, and minimized in enteral feedings and oral diets to preempt hyperkalemia and minimize metabolic acidosis. Frequent monitoring of serum electrolyte concentrations is crucial.

Presuming the point of obstruction has been identified in postrenal AKI, a decision must be made as to how to relieve the obstruction. The approach is individualized depending on the site and nature of the obstruction, the condition of the patient, and the degree of renal impairment. For critically ill patients, urinary diversion is often preferred. Options include ureteral stents, suprapubic cystostomy, or percutaneous nephrostomy, depending on the level of obstruction.

If the patient has AKI, is deemed to have adequate preload, and is making some urine, the patient may be a candidate for diuretic therapy. Diuretics are more useful if the patient has decreased ventricular function, a history of prior use, or signs of hypervolemia such as hypoxemia, rales, tachypnea absent marked metabolic acidosis, or dyspnea. Loop diuretics (e.g., furosemide, bumetanide) are generally the diuretics of first choice. Lower doses of furosemide (i.e., 10–40 mg) may be ineffective in patients with more severe AKI (s[Cr] > 4.0 mg/dL), but patients may respond to higher doses (i.e., 80–200 mg) of furosemide or bumetanide (2–5 mg; approximate furosemide:bumetanide dosage 40:1). If an oliguric patient does not respond to an initial high dose, there is little benefit to another dose. High doses of loop diuretics are ototoxic, and should not be used repeatedly if the patient is anuric and unresponsive to diuretic therapy. Importantly, diuretics do nothing to alter the natural history of the AKI, but may facilitate the management of volume and nutrition, avoid the need for RRT, or obviate the need for prolonged mechanical ventilation if some urine output is restored. Loop diuretics can cause hypokalemia, hypomagnesemia, and metabolic alkalosis, especially after large-volume diuresis, so electrolytes should be monitored closely. When a patient has oliguria and hypervolemia in the presence of metabolic alkalosis or a mixed picture of alkalosis and acidosis, loop diuretics should be used with caution, as they can exacerbate alkalosis. For patients with a serum [$NaHCO_3$] > 28 mmol/dL, acetazolamide (250–500 mg once or twice daily) is effective, provided serum [K] and [Mg] are normal and the patient still has some renal function (C_{Cr} > 25–30 mg/dL). For patients with severe metabolic alkalosis refractory to acetazolamide, intravenous HCl 1% is the next agent of choice prior to RRT. Infusion of HCl must be administered by central venous catheter because of a high risk of chemical phlebitis (or tissue necrosis should the solution extravasate), and may cause or worsen hyperkalemia.

Complications of Acute Kidney Injury

Deranged renal function impairs the maintenance of electrolyte homeostasis and the excretion of water-soluble toxins, thus complications of AKI are generally associated with these perturbations (Table 52.4). Anemia may ensue as production of erythropoietin ceases during moderate-to-severe AKI. Consequently, AKI can potentially result in fluid overload, electrolyte abnormalities, and impaired clearance of toxins such as urea. Anemia may manifest cardiovascular complications in patients with coronary artery disease, or impair oxygen delivery in patients with cardiac or pulmonary disease. Chest pain, myocardial ischemia, hypoxemia, hyperkalemia, acidosis, or uremia (avoidable if RRT is instituted timely and appropriately) is possible. Unchecked, any of these entities may be life threatening, as they may lead to arrhythmias, myocardial infarction, pericarditis, or coma. Due to the potential lethality of these complications, timely RRT is especially important for critically ill patients.

Renal Replacement Therapy. The decision to institute RRT is generally made jointly by the managing inpatient service and the consultant nephrologist. In cases of immediate life-threatening complications such as severe hyperkalemia (peaked T waves by electrocardiography, serum [K] > 6.5 mEq/dL), or pulmonary edema causing hypoxemic respiratory

TABLE 52.6

COMPLICATIONS OF AKI REQUIRING POTENTIALLY EMERGENT RRT

Fluid overload
Metabolic acidosis
Drug intoxications (dialyzable drugs)
Electrolyte abnormalities (e.g., hyperkalemia)
Uremic encephalopathy
Uremic pericarditis

failure, the decision is obvious. In other cases the timing of RRT may be subtle, depending on the clinical status of the patient.[57] Unfortunately, there are no widely accepted criteria regarding the optimal start time for RRT, as data are conflicting. Nevertheless, the strongest evidence for early initiation of dialysis (i.e., at [BUN] ~70 mg/dL, or oliguria post-CABG) is in the perioperative period[58] (Table 52.6).

The most common indications for RRT in surgical patients are hypervolemia and metabolic acidosis, two conditions that affect ventilated patients adversely in particular by increasing the risk of prolonged mechanical ventilation and consequent nosocomial pneumonia. After the indication for RRT has been determined, the modality and intensity of the RRT must be chosen (Table 52.7). Standardized methods of RRT include continuous RRT (CRRT) and intermittent hemodialysis (IHD). Peritoneal dialysis has distinct disadvantages to intravenous RRT as it is less effective in the ICU setting due to inferior clearance,[59] and it is contraindicated by recent abdominal surgery.

Both blood filtration modalities pose their own particular risks and benefits. Intermittent HD has been the traditional first-line modality for RRT in patients with AKI or end-stage renal disease (ESRD). Maintenance of outpatient IHD is often scheduled on a thrice-weekly regimen. However, in the acute setting, many patients are so catabolic that daily RRT is required, particularly at the onset. Nevertheless, because IHD only lasts 3–4 hours, it is more feasible than CRRT for critically ill patients from a nursing perspective. Furthermore, because the patient is not physically connected to the machine other than during the treatment, scheduling of imaging tests,

TABLE 52.7

INDICATIONS, ADVANTAGES, AND DISADVANTAGES OF IHD AND CRRT

MODALITY	INDICATIONS	ADVANTAGES	DISADVANTAGES
IHD	• Emergent electrolyte abnormalities (hyperkalemia and acidosis) • Emergent fluid removal (i.e., volume-related respiratory distress) • Emergent drug or intoxication treatment (i.e., ethylene glycol) • Hemodynamically stable • <3 L/d obligate fluid intake	• Superior short-term solute, acid–base, and volume control • Relatively low complexity • No extra RN requirement • Medication dosing well understood • Less risk of filter clotting and blood loss • Patent not bed-bound except during 3–4 h treatment	• Less well tolerated hemodynamically • Limited medium- and long-term solute/volume control capacity
Continuous renal replacement therapy (CRRT[a])	• Hemodynamically unstable • >3 L/d obligate fluid intake • Severe volume overload	• Superior medium- and long-term solute, acid–base, and volume control • Less hypotension during fluid removal • CVVH (continuous hemofiltration) may be associated with superior middle-molecule clearance than CVVHD	• Limited ability to rapidly correct electrolyte and acid–base abnormalities • More complex for nursing staff • Higher RN workload • Higher cost • Increased risk of filter clotting and circuit blood loss • Medication dosing less well understood • Patient continuously bed-bound • CVVH may require higher blood flows and as such may need higher access quality than CVVHD
Slow continuous ultrafiltration	• Hemodynamically unstable • Severe diuretic-resistant volume overload without renal dysfunction sufficient to require dialysis • >3 L/d obligate fluid intake • Heart failure resistant to attempts at conventional diuresis	• Superior volume control irregardless of quantity of obligate fluid intake • Less hypotension during fluid removal as compared with IHD	• Minimal solute clearance • Patient continuously bed-bound • Higher RN workload

[a]CRRT encompasses CVVH, CVVHD, and CVVHDF. There are no clearly defined outcome differences between the three modalities, and the choice of modality may be center- and program-specific
RN, registered nurse.

procedures, physical therapy, and such is relatively easy. Intermittent HD is clearly the modality of choice if rapid effect is desired. For instance, patients who have life-threatening hyperkalemia are best served with rapid reduction in serum [K]. Similarly, for marked hypervolemia and respiratory failure, IHD would be the appropriate modality to remove fluid quickly. However, these same qualities may also lead to adverse outcomes, most notably hypotension from overaggressive ultrafiltration (especially in patients with vascular leak or hypoalbuminemia).

CRRT is a basket term of continuous dialysis modalities that encompasses continuous venovenous hemofiltration (CVVH), continuous venovenous hemodialysis (CVVHD), and continuous venovenous hemodiafiltration (CVVHDF) (Table 52.7). There are no concrete differences among the various CRRT modalities in terms of outcomes, although techniques involving hemofiltration are believed to improve "middle molecule" clearance (itself, of unclear clinical importance). The main difference between CRRT techniques and "regular" dialysis is the efficiency of clearance. Because IHD was designed for stable outpatients, the goal is high-efficiency clearance in as little time as practicable to maintain reasonable clinical outcomes. On the other hand, CRRT is intended for critically ill patients with marginal or unstable hemodynamics. Many of these patients cannot tolerate rapid fluid and solute shifts, and will become hypotensive with IHD if not already, due to their underlying disease. Continuous RRT provides low efficiency clearance (15–20 mL/minute), but because it is a 24 hour/day treatment, it can accomplish much greater solute and water clearance over time. For example, even hemodynamically stable patients may have difficulty tolerating an ultrafiltration rate >1 L/hour, and so removing more than 3–4 L/3.5 hour IHD treatment may be challenging. On the other hand, most patients with adequate preload will easily tolerate an ultrafiltration rate of 200 mL/hour; if this is continued over a 24-hour CRRT treatment, 4.8 L can be removed with little hemodynamic detriment. In patients with high obligatory fluid intake (e.g., patients on total parenteral nutrition, medications such as polymyxin B that require a large-volume diluent), CRRT may be the only modality that can maintain or improve overall fluid balance. Consequently, hypotensive or vasopressor-dependent patients may be better candidates for CRRT than IHD.[60]

Despite superior filtration characteristics, CRRT does carry major disadvantages when compared with IHD[61] (Table 52.7). First, during CRRT the patient generally requires 1:1 nursing care continuously, which has implications for staffing. Second, because CRRT, by definition, entails constant connection to the dialysis machine, transport for operative procedures or diagnostic tests outside the critical care setting may be difficult. Third, the extracorporeal circuit of CRRT is more prone to clotting than IHD, likely due to prolonged contact of blood with nonbiologic dialysis membranes and tubing, even if blood pressure is maintained and anticoagulant therapy is administered. Clotting of the CRRT circuit is detrimental, as it interrupts therapy, causes the loss of approximately 200 mL blood each time, and is costly. To decrease clotting, regional or systemic anticoagulation may be employed, but clotting can still occur in the presence of therapeutic anticoagulation. Newer CRRT protocols use citrate anticoagulation rather than heparin in the extracorporeal circuit, which may be safer for the critically ill patient than systemic anticoagulation, but this method is not widely available and can lead to hypocalcemia and metabolic alkalosis.[62,63]

The intensity of the RRT has been studied.[64] Some early single-center data indicated that more intensive RRT yields better outcomes in terms of dialysis dependence and mortality,[65-67] but the issue remains controversial as larger, multicenter studies have been nonconfirmatory.[68,69] As such, there is currently no consensus on "dialysis dosing" in AKI. Although it seems plausible that higher clearances should translate to better outcomes, possible reasons for the failure of CRRT to show benefit include actual irrelevance of higher clearances to clinical outcomes in critically ill patients with MODS, or the unintended clearance of beneficial molecules such as antibiotics, anti-inflammatory cytokines, or nutrients.

Medication Dosing in Acute Kidney Injury

Consideration of the appropriate dosing of therapeutic medications is of paramount importance in patients with AKI, as both under- and overdosage may have serious consequences. Drugs that have substantial renal clearance either via glomerular filtration or tubular secretion may require either smaller doses or prolonged dosing intervals, or both. Drug clearance by both filtration or secretion can be estimated using measured or estimated C_{Cr}, although caution should be taken when dosing medications in patients whose renal function is changing dynamically, as often occurs in AKI.

Extracorporeal drug losses during RRT (both IHD or CRRT) can be substantial. Because dialysis membranes have pores that are size-exclusionary, dialytic clearance of drugs depends primarily on the molecular weight of the drug and its protein-binding characteristics. Drugs <500 kDa in size generally will require supplemental doses after dialysis, whereas extensively protein-bound drugs may require no particular adjustment.[70] A list of commonly used drugs that require supplemental dosing posthemodialysis can be found in Table 52.8.

Dosing of medications during CRRT is especially problematic due to the lack of standard CRRT protocols. For instance, the majority of published guidelines for dosing of antibiotics in CRRT patients draw on pharmacokinetic studies completed prior to the widespread adoption of high-clearance CRRT (i.e., 35 mL/kg/hour therapy fluid flow rate).[71,72] Inadvertent underdosing of antibiotics may be one factor that contributes to the lack of benefit of CRRT as compared with IHD. This may be true of nutrition as well; some studies have indicated that protein intakes in excess of 1.5–2 g/kg may be necessary to maintain positive nitrogen balance[73] Similarly, trace element replacement may be indicated, although the clinical importance is unclear.[73] Thus, in critically ill patients on CRRT, it is essential that the care team work closely with nephrology, pharmacy, and nutrition consultants to ensure proper dosing of medications and nutrients.

TABLE 52.8

COMMONLY USED DRUGS THAT REQUIRE POSTHEMODIALYSIS DOSING

Aminoglycosides
Carbapenems
Beta-lactams (penicillin derivatives, cephalosporins)
Aztreonam
Beta-blockers
Fluconazole
Chloramphenicol
ACE inhibitors
Procainamide

ACE, Angiotensin-converting enzyme.

PROGNOSIS OF ACUTE KIDNEY INJURY

The prognosis of patients with AKI is related directly to the cause of renal injury and, to some extent, to the duration of AKI prior to therapeutic intervention. Mortality rates range from 31% to 80% depending on the patient population.[74] Predictably, patients who have more severe AKI generally have a worse prognosis. For patients who require dialysis and survive hospitalization, there remains a substantive risk of dialysis dependence at discharge, especially among patients with preexisting CKD (16%–32% of patients dependent)[75] as compared with patients with previously normal function (3%).[76] Renal function may continue to improve long after the end of dialysis dependence, with optimal kidney function generally being reached between 3 and 6 months after discharge. If one also includes AKI episodes not requiring dialysis, patients without CKD generally have complete recovery assuming they survive the AKI episode, with >90% of patients enjoying "full" recovery (defined as s[Cr] below threshold for RIFLE criteria or estimated GFR >60 mL/minute). However, patients with CKD may only experience full recovery in two-thirds of cases and partial recovery in approximately30% (defined as persistent s[Cr] above threshold for RIFLE criteria).[77]

References

1. Lucas CE. The renal response to acute injury and sepsis. *Surg Clin North Am.* 1976;56:953-975.
2. Cohen AJ. Physiologic concepts in the management of renal, fluid, and electrolyte disorders in the intensive care unit. In: Rippe JM, Fink MP, Cerra FB, eds. *Intensive Care Medicine.* Boston, MA: Little, Brown; 1996:935-950.
3. Cryer HG. Acute renal failure. In: Feliciano DV, Mattox KE, Moore EE, eds. *Trauma.* 6th ed. New York, NY: McGraw-Hill Medical; 2008.
4. Rose BD, Wood TP. *Clinical Physiology of Acid-Base and Electrolyte Disorders.* 5th ed. New York, NY: McGraw-Hill; 2001.
5. Kellum JA, Bellomo R, Ronco C. Definition and classification of acute kidney injury. *Nephron Clin Pract.* 2008;109:182-187.
6. Ricci Z, Cruz D, Ronco C. The RIFLE criteria and mortality in acute kidney injury: a systematic review. *Kidney Int.* 2008;73:538-546.
7. Hoste EA, Schurgers M. Epidemiology of acute kidney injury: how big is the problem? *Crit Care Med.* 2008;36(4 suppl):S146-S151.
8. Barrantes F, Tian J, Vazquez R, et al. Acute kidney injury criteria predict outcomes of critically ill patients. *Crit Care Med.* 2008;36:1397-1403.
9. Dasta JF, Kane-Gill SL, Durtschi AJ, et al. Costs and outcomes of acute kidney injury (AKI) following cardiac surgery. *Nephrol Dial Transplant.* 2008;23:1970-1974.
10. Coca SG, Peixoto AJ, Garg AX, et al.. The prognostic importance of a small acute decrement in kidney function in hospitalized patients: a systematic review and meta-analysis. *Am J Kidney Dis.* 2007;50:712-720.
11. Rosen S, Epstein FH, Brezis M. Determinants of intrarenal oxygenation: factors in acute renal failure. *Ren Fail.* 1992;14:321-325.
12. Rosen S, Stillman IE. Acute tubular necrosis is a syndrome of physiologic and pathologic dissociation. *J Am Soc Nephrol.* 2008;19:871-875.
13. Tumlin JA. Impaired blood flow in acute kidney injury: pathophysiology and potential efficacy of intrarenal vasodilator therapy. *Curr Opin Crit Care.* 2009;15:514-519.
14. Le Dorze M, Legrand M, Payen D, et al. The role of the microcirculation in acute kidney injury. *Curr Opin Crit Care.* 2009;15:503-508.
15. Madaio M. Post-infectious glomerulonephritis. In: Schrier RW, ed. *Diseases of the Kidney.* Boston, MA: Little Brown; 1997:1579-1594.
16. Prakash J, Sen D, Kumar NS, et al. Acute renal failure due to intrinsic renal diseases: review of 1122 cases. *Ren Fail.* 2003;25:225-233.
17. Perazella MA. Drug-induced nephropathy: an update. *Expert Opin Drug Saf.* 2005;4:689-706.
18. Fliser D. Assessment of renal function in elderly patients. *Curr Opin Nephrol Hypertens.* 2008;17:604-608.
19. Venkataraman R. Can we prevent acute kidney injury? *Crit Care Med.* 2008;36(4 suppl):S166-S171.
20. Haase-Fielitz A, Bellomo R, Devarajan P, et al. Novel and conventional serum biomarkers predicting acute kidney injury in adult cardiac surgery-a prospective cohort study. *Crit Care Med.* 2009;37:553-560.
21. Goodsaid FM, Blank M, Dieterle F, et al. Novel biomarkers of acute kidney toxicity. *Clin Pharmacol Ther.* 2009;86:490-496.
22. Schrier RW, Wang W. Acute renal failure and sepsis. *N Engl J Med.* 2004;351:159-169.
23. Bagshaw SM, Lapinsky S, Dial S, et al. Acute kidney injury in septic shock: clinical outcomes and impact of duration of hypotension prior to initiation of antimicrobial therapy. *Intensive Care Med.* 2009;35:871-881.
24. Karthik S, Lisbon A. Low-dose dopamine in the intensive care unit. *Semin Dial.* 2006;19:465-471.
25. D'Orio V, el Allaf D, Juchmes J, et al. The use of low doses of dopamine in intensive care medicine. *Arch Int Physiol Biochim.* 1984;92:S11-S20.
26. Eachempati SR, Reed RL II. Use of creatinine clearances to monitor the effect of low-dose dopamine in critically ill surgical patients. *J Surg Res.* 2003;112:43-48.
27. Marik PE. Low-dose dopamine: a systematic review. *Intensive Care Med.* 2002;28:877-883.
28. Bellomo R, Chapman M, Finfer S, et al. Low-dose dopamine in patients with early renal dysfunction: a placebo-controlled randomised trial. Australian and New Zealand Intensive Care Society (ANZICS) Clinical Trials Group. *Lancet.* 2000;356(9248):2139-2143.
29. Barr LF, Kolodner K. N-acetylcysteine and fenoldopam protect the renal function of patients with chronic renal insufficiency undergoing cardiac surgery. *Crit Care Med.* 2008;36:1427-1435.
30. Landoni G, Biondi-Zoccai GG, Marino G, et al. Fenoldopam reduces the need for renal replacement therapy and in-hospital death in cardiovascular surgery: a meta-analysis. *J Cardiothorac Vasc Anesth.* 2008;22:27-33.
31. Landoni G, Biondi-Zoccai GG, Tumlin JA, et al. Beneficial impact of fenoldopam in critically ill patients with or at risk for acute renal failure: a meta-analysis of randomized clinical trials. *Am J Kidney Dis.* 2007;49:56-68.
32. Bosch X, Poch E, Grau JM. Rhabdomyolysis and acute kidney injury. *N Engl J Med.* 2009;361:62-72.
33. Vasile B, Rasulo F, Candiati A, et al. The pathophysiology of propofol infusion syndrome: a simple name for a complex syndrome. *Intensive Care Med.* 2003;29:1417-1425..
34. de Menezes Ettinger JE, dos Santos Filho PV, Azaro E, et al. Prevention of rhabdomyolysis in bariatric surgery. *Obes Surg.* 2005;15:874-879.
35. Ward MM. Factors predictive of acute renal failure in rhabdomyolysis. *Arch Intern Med.* 1988;148:1553-1557.
36. Veenstra J, Smit WM, Krediet RT, et al. Relationship between elevated creatine phosphokinase and the clinical spectrum of rhabdomyolysis. *Nephrol Dial Transplant.* 1994;9:637-641.
37. de Meijer AR, Fikkers BG, de Keijzer MH, et al. Serum creatine kinase as predictor of clinical course in rhabdomyolysis: a 5-year intensive care survey. *Intensive Care Med.* 2003;29:1121-1125.
38. Brown CV, Rhee P, Chan L, et al. Preventing renal failure in patients with rhabdomyolysis: do bicarbonate and mannitol make a difference? *J Trauma.* 2004;56:1191-1196.
39. Kelly AM, Dwamena B, Cronin P, et al. Meta-analysis: effectiveness of drugs for preventing contrast-induced nephropathy. *Ann Intern Med.* 2008;148:284-294.
40. Brar SS, Shen AY, Jorgensen MB, et al. Sodium bicarbonate vs. sodium chloride for the prevention of contrast medium-induced nephropathy in patients undergoing coronary angiography: a randomized trial. *JAMA.* 2008;300:1038-1046.
41. Brar SS, Hiremath S, Dangas G, et al. Sodium bicarbonate for the prevention of contrast induced-acute kidney injury: a systematic review and meta-analysis. *Clin J Am Soc Nephrol.* 2009;4:1584-1592.
42. Zoungas S, Ninomiya T, Huxley R, et al. Systematic review: sodium bicarbonate treatment regimens for the prevention of contrast-induced nephropathy. *Ann Intern Med.* 2009;151:631-638.
43. Brown JR, Block CA, Malenka DJ, et al. Sodium bicarbonate plus N-acetylcysteine prophylaxis: a meta-analysis. *JACC Cardiovasc Interv.* 2009;2:1116-1124.
44. Spargias K, Adreanides E, Demerouti E, et al. Iloprost prevents contrast-induced nephropathy in patients with renal dysfunction undergoing coronary angiography or intervention. *Circulation.* 2009;120:1793-1799.
45. Abizaid AS, Clark CE, Mintz GS, et al. Effects of dopamine and aminophylline on contrast-induced acute renal failure after coronary angioplasty in patients with preexisting renal insufficiency. *Am J Cardiol.* 1999;83:260-263.
46. Stone GW, McCullough PA, Tumlin JA, et al. Fenoldopam mesylate for the prevention of contrast-induced nephropathy: a randomized controlled trial. *JAMA.* 2003;290:2284-2291.
47. Yaganti V, Alani F, Yaganti S, et al. Use of gadolinium for carotid artery angiography and stenting in patients with renal insufficiency. *J Ren Care.* 2009;35:211-218.
48. Laskey W, Aspelin P, Davidson C, et al. Nephrotoxicity of iodixanol versus iopamidol in patients with chronic kidney disease and diabetes mellitus undergoing coronary angiographic procedures. *Am Heart J.* 2009;158:822-828.
49. Katholi RE. Contrast-induced nephropathy-choice of contrast agents to reduce renal risk. *Am Heart Hosp J.* 2009;7:45-49.
50. Dennen P, Douglas IS, Anderson R. Acute kidney injury in the intensive care unit: an update and primer for the intensivist. *Crit Care Med.* 2010;38:261-275.
51. Uchino S, Kellum JA, Bellomo R, et al. Acute renal failure in critically ill patients: a multinational, multicenter study. *JAMA.* 2005;294:813-818.
52. Kellum JA, Cerda J, Kaplan LJ, et al. Fluids for prevention and management of acute kidney injury. *Int J Artif Organs.* 2008;31:96-110.

53. Macedo E, Mehta RL. Prerenal failure: from old concepts to new paradigms. *Curr Opin Crit Care*. 2009;15:467-473.
54. Hadian M, Pinsky MR. Evidence-based review of the use of the pulmonary artery catheter: impact data and complications. *Crit Care*. 2006;10(suppl 3):S8-S14.
55. Carvounis CP, Nisar S, Guro-Razuman S. Significance of the fractional excretion of urea in the differential diagnosis of acute renal failure. *Kidney Int*. 2002;62:2223-2229.
56. Cherry RA, Eachempati SR, Hydo L, et al. Accuracy of short-duration creatinine clearance determinations in predicting 24-hour creatinine clearance in critically ill and injured patients. *J Trauma*. 2002;53:267-271.
57. Palevsky PM. Indications and timing of renal replacement therapy in acute kidney injury. *Crit Care Med*. 2008;36(4 suppl):S224-S228.
58. Macedo E, Mehta RL. Early vs. late start of dialysis: it's all about timing. *Crit Care*. 2010;14:112.
59. Phu NH, Hien TT, Mai NT, et al. Hemofiltration and peritoneal dialysis in infection-associated acute renal failure in Vietnam. *N Engl J Med*. 2002;347:895-902.
60. Eachempati SR, Wang JC, Hydo LJ, et al. Acute renal failure in critically ill surgical patients: persistent lethality despite new modes of renal replacement therapy. *J Trauma*. 2007;63:987-993.
61. Liu F, Mehta F.. Continuous renal replacement therapy. In: Lerma EV, Berns JS, Nissenson AR, eds. *Current Diagnosis and Treatment: Nephrology and Hypertension*. New York, NY: McGraw-Hill; 2009.
62. Kindgen-Milles D, Amman J, Kleinekofort W, et al. Treatment of metabolic alkalosis during continuous renal replacement therapy with regional citrate anticoagulation. *Int J Artif Organs*. 2008;31:363-366.
63. Burry LD, Tung DD, Hallett D, et al. Regional citrate anticoagulation for PrismaFlex continuous renal replacement therapy. *Ann Pharmacother*. 2009;43:1419-1425.
64. Palevsky PM. Clinical review: timing and dose of continuous renal replacement therapy in acute kidney injury. *Crit Care*. 2007;11:232.
65. Ronco C, Bellomo R, Homel P, et al. Effects of different doses in continuous veno-venous haemofiltration on outcomes of acute renal failure: a prospective randomised trial. *Lancet*. 2000;356(9223):26-30.
66. Saudan P, Niederberger M, De Seigneux S, et al. Adding a dialysis dose to continuous hemofiltration increases survival in patients with acute renal failure. *Kidney Int*. 2006;70:1312-1317.
67. Schiffl H, Lang SM, Fischer R. Daily hemodialysis and the outcome of acute renal failure. *N Engl J Med*. 2002;346:305-310.
68. Palevsky PM, Zhang JH, O'Connor TZ, et al. Intensity of renal support in critically ill patients with acute kidney injury. *N Engl J Med*. 2008;359:7-20.
69. Bellomo R, Cass A, Cole L, et al. Intensity of continuous renal-replacement therapy in critically ill patients. *N Engl J Med*. 2009;361:1627-1638.
70. Olyaei A dA, Bennett WM. Principles of drug dosing and prescribing in renal failure. In: Feehally RJ, ed. *Comprehensive Clinical Nephrology*. 2nd ed. London, UK: Mosby; 2003:1189-1204.
71. Choi G, Gomersall CD, Tian Q. Principles of antibacterial dosing in continuous renal replacement therapy. *Crit Care Med*. 2009;37:2268-2282.
72. Trotman RL, Williamson JC, Shoemaker DM, et al. Antibiotic dosing in critically ill adult patients receiving continuous renal replacement therapy. *Clin Infect Dis*. 2005;41:1159-166.
73. Fiaccadori E, Parenti E, Maggiore U. Nutritional support in acute kidney injury. *J Nephrol*. 2008;21:645-656
74. Macedo E, Bouchard J, Mehta RL. Renal recovery following acute kidney injury. *Curr Opin Crit Care*. 2008;14:660-665.
75. Bagshaw SM, Laupland KB, Doig CJ, et al. Prognosis for long-term survival and renal recovery in critically ill patients with severe acute renal failure: a population-based study. *Crit Care*. 2005;9:R700-R709.
76. Metcalfe W, Simpson M, Khan IH, et al. Acute renal failure requiring renal replacement therapy: incidence and outcome. *Quart J Med*. 2002;95:579-583.
77. Ali T, Khan I, Simpson W, et al. Incidence and outcomes in acute kidney injury: a comprehensive population-based study. *J Am Soc Nephrol*. 2007;18:1292-1298.

CHAPTER 53 ■ HYPOTHERMIA: TREATMENT AND THERAPEUTIC USES

MATTHEW C. BYRNES AND GREG J. BEILMAN

There is a clear distinction between hypothermia due to environmental exposure and hypothermia associated with injury. Hypothermia due to exposure can be lethal when it is extreme and persistent, such as that experienced by soldiers during the Napoleonic invasion of Russia; however, with modern medical care, patients without injury have an 80% survival when the depth of hypothermia is between 28°C and 32°C.[1] The effect of hypothermia on injured patients, however, is profound. In one large series, no patient with an initial core body temperature of <32°C survived.[2] This distinction clearly indicates that a different approach is needed for injured patients compared to medical patients suffering from hypothermia.

The triad of hypothermia, coagulopathy, and acidosis has been widely described as an important risk factor for death among injured patients.[3,4] Each component of the triad influences the other components. For instance, hypothermia can lead to worsened coagulopathy, which in turn can lead to acidosis. The presence of hypothermia worsens the physiologic condition of most patients with multisystem trauma. For decades, hypothermia has been treated aggressively in order to optimize outcomes. More recent data suggest there may be a role for induced hypothermia in certain types of injuries. This chapter reviews the physiologic aberrations that are seen with hypothermia and subsequently reviews basic science and clinical studies that guide the current clinical practice of treating injured patients with subnormal core body temperatures.

DEFINITIONS AND MEASUREMENT

There are a variety of definitions of hypothermia. The normal human core body temperature is 37°C; however, there is a normal circadian shift of ±0.5°C–1°C.[5,6] Several authors have defined hypothermia as a core body temperature of <35°C, while others have referred to hypothermia as a core body temperature of <36°C.[3,7-10] Yet another defined hypothermia as a core body temperature of <37°C.

The traditional classification of hypothermia was developed for patients with environmental exposure rather than patients with multiple injuries.[9] The traditional classification of hypothermia labels core body temperatures above 32°C as mild and core body temperatures below 28°C as severe. Profound hypothermia has been defined as core body temperature of 6°C–10°C and ultraprofound hypothermia as temperatures ≤5°C.[10] The lowest known temperature among adult survivors with environmental hypothermia is 13.7°C.

The combination of hypothermia and severe injury is associated with increased risk of death and complications. The key threshold associated with increased morbidity and mortality in injured patients appears to be 34°C.[2] The risk of mortality is further increased with temperatures below 32°C. As such, a different classification system should be utilized with injured patients. It is most appropriate to consider temperatures of 34°C–36°C as mild, 32°C–34°C as moderate, and <32°C as severe hypothermia. The existence of multiple classification systems can create confusion when interpreting descriptions of the depth of hypothermia. Whenever possible, we have described absolute temperature levels rather than qualitatively labeling the depth of hypothermia.

There are a variety of methods available to evaluate core body temperature (Fig. 53.1). The gold standard for evaluating core body temperature is the pulmonary artery catheter; however, this method is infrequently available during early evaluation and is less commonly utilized in current practice.[11] Additionally, in patients with severe hypothermia (<28°C–30°C), this catheter has the potential to induce life-threatening arrhythmias. We recommend the use of bladder or tympanic temperature probes for routine temperature evaluation in acute care surgical patients. Bladder temperatures are measured using a Foley catheter with a thermistor at its tip. Tympanic temperature is readily measurable using current technology; however, many electronic thermometers do not allow measurement of temperature below 34°C. Esophageal temperature monitoring can be used but carries no advantage over the other methods.[12] Rectal monitoring is slightly more invasive and is not as responsive to changes in core body temperature. While oral temperature probes are appropriate for healthy patients, these probes are not useful for multiply injured patients or intubated patients. Finally, axillary temperature monitoring is the most inaccurate method and has no real utility in evaluation of hypothermia in acute care surgical patients.[3]

PREVALENCE AND RISK FACTORS

Hypothermia is common in patients suffering traumatic injury. Trauma patients represent a frequent source of hypothermia.[8,9,13] The average temperature of patients in one large trauma center was 35°C.[14] Contrary to expectations, there was no seasonal variation, so hypothermia is a consideration regardless of the time of year. Previous reports have estimated that about one-half of seriously injured patients are hypothermic on presentation.[13] Patients with prolonged extrications or entrapment are at increased risk, as they often have prolonged environmental exposures. Patients at extremes of age are at increased risk, as their ability to endogenously maintain their core body temperature is reduced. Administration of anesthesia predisposes to hypothermia as these agents inhibit endogenous reflexes that increase core body temperature. Increased injury severity itself is also a risk factor for hypothermia. Submersion is a considerable risk factor, as heat losses are 32 times greater among patients submerged than patients exposed to air.[15,16]

PHYSIOLOGY

There are physiologic effects of hypothermia on nearly every organ system (Table 53.1). There is increase in metabolic activity at very mild levels of hypothermia (35°C–36°C). Beyond this level, there is a slowing of metabolic activity at the cellular level and quiescence of signs of life at the extremes of

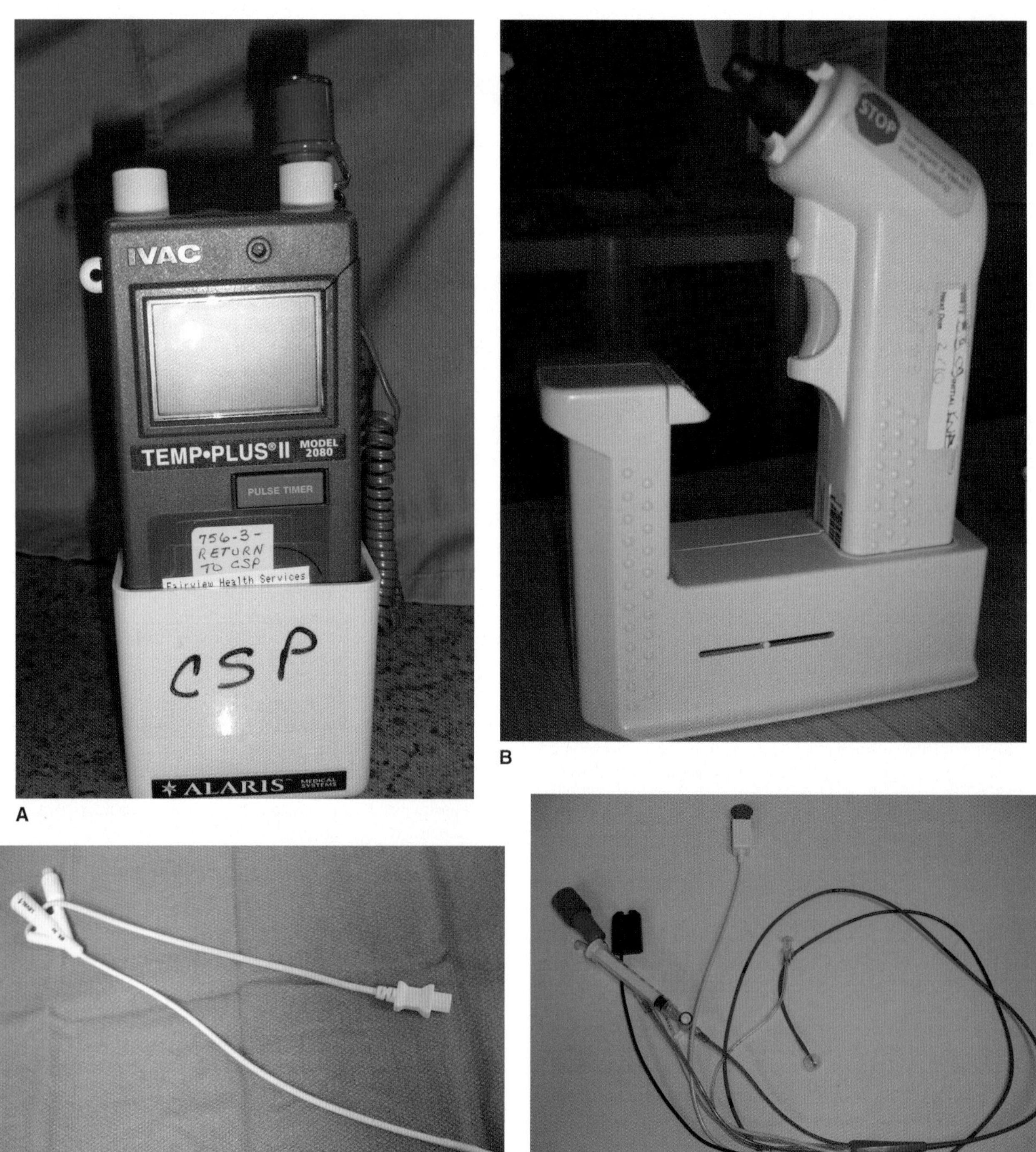

FIGURE 53.1. Current methods of measuring body temperature. A: Electronic thermometer configured for oral/rectal use. B: Electronic thermometer for tympanic measurements. C: Foley catheter with temperature-sensitive thermistor. D: Pulmonary artery catheter with temperature-sensitive thermistor.

hypothermia. In fact, the overall rate of metabolism decreases by 8% for every 1°C reduction in core body temperature.[17] Acute care surgeons must understand these physiologic changes in order to optimize treatment of patients who require either induction of hypothermia or institution of warming.

The hypothalamus is responsible for integrating signals from the body that relate to core body temperature.[18] The hypothalamus emits efferent signals that result in peripheral vasoconstriction in order to preserve heat to the body core. Shivering is induced with mild hypothermia (35°C–37°C) and can produce up to five times the normal metabolic heat production. Metabolic activity increases in order to generate heat. These mechanisms, however, are impaired as hypothermia deepens to 34°C, and they are also impaired in the multiply injured or intoxicated patient. As a result, injured patients have a reduced ability to endogenously correct hypothermia.

TABLE 53.1

PHYSIOLOGIC CHANGES ASSOCIATED WITH HYPOTHERMIA

ORGAN SYSTEM	PHYSIOLOGIC CHANGES
Neurologic	Reduction in intracranial pressure Reduction in metabolism
Respiratory	Bronchorrhea Inhibition of cilia Reduced respiratory rate
Renal	Cold diuresis
Gastrointestinal	Ileus
Cardiovascular	Arrhythmia Bradycardia Negative inotropy
Endocrine	Hyperglycemia
Coagulation	Reduced enzyme function Reduced platelet function

Respiratory system. The respiratory system is stimulated at temperatures above 34°C–35°C. This leads to tachypnea and can result in bronchospasm. As the core body temperature falls below 34°C, the respiratory drive diminishes. There is also an increase in secretions and inhibition of bronchial cilia.[8] Upon rewarming, there is often development of pulmonary edema. As core body temperature decreases below 30°C, apnea may result.

Cardiovascular system. Mild hypothermia is associated with cardiac stimulation.[8,18] The hypothalamus responds to mild hypothermia by transmitting signals that result in sympathetic activation. This results in tachycardia, peripheral vasoconstriction, and increase in cardiac output. Temperatures below a threshold level (~32°C) result in cardiac depression.[9] Negative inotropy is seen with subsequent reductions in cardiac output. Bradycardia ensues, and the myocardium becomes progressively arrhythmogenic.[17] Ventricular fibrillation (VF) may occur spontaneously at temperatures below 25°C–28°C.[19] Resuscitation from asystole or fibrillation can be difficult, if not impossible, until the patient is warmed. These arrhythmias are often resistant to chemical or electrical cardioversion until the core body temperature is raised above 28°C. Additionally, there is a reduced response to catecholamines with appreciable degrees of hypothermia.[17,20]

Neurologic. There is a temperature-dependent reduction in consciousness associated with progressive hypothermia.[21] Confusion can be expected at mild degrees of hypothermia. This will eventually give way to a comatose state at temperatures <28°C–30°C. There is a reduction in cerebral blood flow and cerebral metabolism, which leads to a reduction in intracranial pressure. Motor reflexes become diminished and ultimately become absent.[9] These cerebral effects have led to a great deal of interest in utilizing hypothermia as a therapeutic entity for conditions associated with neurologic compromise. This is described in greater detail later in the chapter.

Renal/electrolytes. "Cold diuresis" is the most obvious effect of hypothermia on the renal system.[17,22] This is seen at mild and moderate degrees of hypothermia (>32°C). This is due to increased renal blood flow and to alterations in tubular membranes. The pH measured by arterial blood gas analysis will be artificially low if the blood is warmed before the analysis is conducted. Hyperglycemia can occur as a result of reduced insulin sensitivity and decreased pancreatic secretion of insulin. Electrolytes, including potassium, phosphorus, and magnesium, can become depleted.[23]

Gastrointestinal. Bowel function in the presence of hypothermia is reduced.[17] If a nasogastric tube is inserted for an ileus in a hypothermic patient, extreme caution should be taken. Gastric intubation, along with other methods of patient manipulation, can lead to VF in patients with a core body temperature <28°C.[9]

Coagulation. Coagulation disorders represent the most important physiologic disturbance concerning hypothermic acute care surgical patients. These disorders are also the most extensively studied issues in injured patients.[24-35] Hypothermia leads to coagulopathy. Ongoing hemorrhage from coagulopathy leads to further hypothermia and acidosis. This "bloody vicious cycle" first reported by Kashuk et al.[36] has been confirmed in multiple subsequent studies. Warming hypothermic patients is a critical component to arresting this cycle.

The effect of hypothermia on standard laboratory values of prothrombin time/activated partial thromboplastin time/International Normalized Ratio (PT/PTT/INR) has been extensively reported. Cosgriff et al.[29] prospectively evaluated patients who required a massive transfusion, which was defined as transfusion of at least 10 units of blood. Coagulopathy was defined as a PT greater than two times the normal value and was present in 47% of the patients. In multivariate analysis, hypothermia was a significant risk factor for coagulopathy, with an odds ratio of 8.7. These clinical results have been confirmed by a number of laboratory studies. Reed et al.[31] submerged anesthetized rats in a water bath to achieve a core body temperature of 25°C–37°C. They observed a prolongation of the PTT and the PT when the blood was not warmed prior to analysis. When they warmed the blood *ex vivo*, the prolongation of the coagulation parameters was no longer seen. This suggests that laboratory analysis that is conducted after warming the blood *ex vivo* is likely to underestimate the degree of coagulopathy.

Rohrer and Natale[32] evaluated pooled human plasma that was known to have normal levels of clotting factors. They performed coagulation studies on the blood at temperatures ranging from 28°C–41°C. The PT in the normothermic samples was 11.8 seconds and increased to 16.6 seconds in the samples cooled to 28°C–34°C. The PTT was 36 seconds in the normothermic samples and increased to 57 seconds in the hypothermic samples. These results were confirmed clinically by Watts et al.[33] They evaluated 112 trauma patients with an injury severity score ≥9 points. They evaluated the core body temperature and performed coagulation studies. They found that 34°C was the threshold point, below which coagulation enzyme activity decreased.

Another study compared the effect of hypothermia to various clotting factor deficiencies.[30] Standard plasma was evaluated at temperatures between 25°C and 37°C, and plasma with specific clotting factor deficiencies was evaluated for comparative purposes. They found that plasma with normal factors at temperatures <33°C was functionally similar to normothermic plasma with factor deficiencies.

Hypothermia in an injured patient is often seen in combination with shock. In an animal model, hypothermia and shock were additive in their effects on coagulopathy.[28] In a human series, coagulopathy was also more common when hypothermia was paired with an increased injury severity and shock.[29]

Platelet function is also reduced in hypothermic patients. Valeri et al.[35] noted that a reduction in core body temperature in baboons was associated with a prolonged bleeding time. A similar study was conducted in healthy human volunteers. The bleeding time of hypothermic skin was significantly prolonged. This appeared to be mediated by a down regulation of P-selectin and thromboxane B_2.[34]

Whereas the most common and standard method of evaluating coagulation abnormalities involves measuring the PT/PTT/INR, Martini et al.[25] reported that thromboelastography

(TEG) is a more sensitive analysis in determining hypothermic coagulopathy. This point-of-care test evaluates the entire coagulation system in whole blood. TEG may be more accurate than are standard tests for evaluation of multiple aspects of the coagulation cascade and in directing therapy. TEG is becoming more available but has not currently been broadly adopted.

Two reports have evaluated pharmacologic manipulation of hypothermic coagulopathy.[26,27] Given that factor levels are normal, treatment with fresh frozen plasma would not be expected to reverse the coagulopathy. The administration of recombinant factor VIIa (rFVIIa), however, improved coagulation parameters of plasma that was artificially cooled. In a model of hypothermic/hemorrhagic shock, the administration of rFVIIa reduced overall blood loss. This suggests that rFVIIa can be used as an adjunct to warming when ongoing hemorrhage is severe.

In summary, there is a clear effect of hypothermia on the clotting cascade. This coagulopathy is caused by an alteration in platelet function and enzymatic activity rather than an alteration in the quantity of clotting factors. This effect is temperature-dependent, with deeper levels of hypothermia being associated with more substantial coagulopathy. Furthermore, common laboratory tests do not reflect the true degree of coagulopathy if the blood is warmed *ex vivo* prior to performing the test, as is commonly performed by most labs. The treatment of hypothermic coagulopathy is rapid warming rather than administration of blood products or supplements.

CLINICAL CONSIDERATIONS

Given the many physiologic effects of hypothermia on mammals, it is important to understand the clinical ramifications of reduced core body temperatures. There are certain responses to hypothermia that may be beneficial to acute care surgical patients, such as a reduction in metabolic rate and cerebral protection. There are other responses to hypothermia that are clearly harmful, such as coagulopathy and myocardial irritability. There is considerable of literature evaluating the effect of hypothermia on injured patients. The majority of the experimental studies have reported a beneficial effect of hypothermia on outcomes in injured patients, whereas most of the human studies have reported on a detrimental effect of hypothermia.

Numerous animal models have touted the benefit of hypothermia in injured patients.[37-43] Wu et al.[40] evaluated a model of hemorrhagic shock in pigs by creating a splenic laceration. Animals were subsequently cooled to 34°C or maintained at normothermia. Survival was greater in the hypothermic animals, and increased bleeding was not seen in the hypothermic animals. In another similar study using a model of prolonged hypotensive resuscitation, George et al.[44] demonstrated improved survival in hypothermic animals with associated decreases in resuscitation fluid requirements, organ injury, and lactate concentrations. Takasu et al.[41] reported similar findings in a rat model. Animals subjected to hemorrhagic shock that were cooled to 32°C or 34°C had a greater 72-hour survival. Another study also reported the benefits of hypothermia during hemorrhagic shock but also noted that these benefits were not realized with localized gut cooling.[38] In a rat model of hemorrhagic shock, Lee et al.[43] reported that induced hypothermia was more beneficial than spontaneous hypothermia. Another report confirmed that spontaneous hypothermia did not result in increased long-term survival.[45]

Specific organ function has also been evaluated in animal models. Severe hypothermia (28°C) in conjunction with hemorrhagic shock was associated with ventricular irritability.[46] The effect of shock on liver adenosine triphosphate (ATP) concentrations was reported by Johannigman et al.[47] In a rat model of hemorrhagic shock, ATP fell steadily with warm shock but not hypothermic shock.

The process of warming has also been evaluated in animal models. In rat and mouse models of hemorrhagic shock, there was a considerable inflammatory response associated with the warming phase.[48,49] Warming improved cardiac and hepatic function in a rat model of hemorrhage.[50] Survival was greatest among pigs that underwent a "medium" rate of warming compared with slow and fast rates of warming.[12]

In contrast to the animal data, much of the human data suggest that hypothermia in injured patients is harmful.[2,51-54] A sentinel study was reported by Jurkovich et al. in 1987. They evaluated the effect of hypothermia on a group of patients with major trauma. Mortality progressively rose with reductions in core body temperature.[2] No patients in this series survived if their core body temperature was below 32°C. Wang et al.[52] conducted a multivariate analysis of risk factors of mortality after injury and noted an odds ratio for death of 3.03 associated with hypothermia. Shafi et al. attempted to discern if hypothermia was a marker of complications or a true risk factor for death in injured patients. They evaluated nearly 40,000 patients from the National Trauma Data Bank (NTDB) and performed a multivariate regression analysis.[53] They found that hypothermia (≤35°C), independent of other factors, was associated with increased mortality. Another large review of the NTDB noted that mortality began to increase at temperatures below 36°C.[55] All of these studies were retrospective analyses. In one prospective analysis, approximately 300 seriously injured trauma patients were studied, and effects of hypothermia on outcome were evaluated.[56] Hypothermia within the first six hours of arrival was not independently associated with mortality but did predict development of multiple organ failure. In the one randomized prospective study published to date, Gentilello et al.[51] randomized patients to rapid rewarming with continuous arteriovenous rewarming (CAVR) versus standard rewarming. Patients in the CAVR group experienced faster rates of warming. Early mortality, as well as 24-hour fluid requirements, were improved in patients randomized to CAVR. However, this benefit did not result in improved survival to hospital discharge. These studies together suggest that hypothermia is harmful in injured patients.

The distinction between elective hypothermia and trauma-related hypothermia was reported by Seekamp et al. They measured plasma ATP concentrations in patients undergoing elective hypothermia during coronary artery bypass surgery and in hypothermic trauma patients.[57] They noted that there was a preservation of ATP levels in elective hypothermia but decreased level of ATP in hypothermic injured patients. This suggests that hypothermia in injured patients is due to energy exhaustion rather than being a method of energy preservation.

Several reports have noted the effect of hypothermia on injured patients who require operative intervention.[58-60] An increase in mortality was noted among hypothermic patients who required a laparotomy. Blood loss was also related to the depth of hypothermia. Notably, the degree of hypothermia was more important than the abdominal injury score in determining the amount of intraoperative blood loss.

The distinction between human and animal studies likely relates to the type of studies that have been performed. Nearly all of the human studies have been retrospective analyses. Given the uniformity of the results, surgeons have been unwilling to randomize multiply injured patients to hypothermia or normothermia in a prospective study. The animal studies have generally not involved multi-system trauma. It is unclear if single-organ models of hemorrhagic shock in animals apply to the injured patients that acute care surgeons regularly encounter. Additionally, animal models generally involve active cooling of an otherwise normothermic animal. Human studies evaluated patients who were hypothermic on presentation. Finally, animal models induce hypothermia shortly after the time of injury or before the injury. Given that there are inherent delays in transport of human trauma, it is not clear that these models are applicable to clinical settings.

Although the evidence is incomplete, we recommend warming multiply injured patients to normothermic levels. There is interesting experimental evidence suggesting that hypothermia may be beneficial during the course of injury, especially when associated with prolonged periods of hypotension,[44] but the application of this evidence is currently unclear. The bulk of the human evidence demonstrates that hypothermia is harmful to injured patients. Until the animal models are replicated in human studies, acute care surgeons should consider hypothermia to be a complicating factor in the management of their patients.

REWARMING

There are a number of methods to rewarm injured patients. These methods should be instituted early in the treatment of injured patients, as it is far easier to prevent further hypothermia than it is to treat hypothermia. An injured patient's metabolic rate may be sufficient to prevent further heat loss, but it is insufficient to produce overall warming.[61] Accordingly, the majority of severely injured patients will require adjunctive warming measures.

An average adult with a temperature of 32°C has a massive heat deficit of 300 kCal.[61] Oxygen consumption would have to increase dramatically to overcome this heat deficit, and severely injured patients generally do not have the physiologic reserve to respond to this challenge. The human body has a high specific heat (amount of energy required to raise 1 kg of material by 1°C). This, along with ongoing heat losses, makes warming injured patients challenging.

Methods of Rewarming

Methods of rewarming can be broadly categorized as passive or active (Table 53.2). Passive methods consist of blankets and a warm environment. Active methods can be characterized as either invasive or noninvasive. Noninvasive methods include forced air rewarming, circulating water blankets, radiant heat lamps, and resistive heating blankets. Invasive methods include tracheal insufflation with warmed gas, cavity lavage, cardiopulmonary bypass, and arteriovenous rewarming.

Passive Rewarming

Passive rewarming consists of provision of a warm room and blankets in order to prevent further heat loss. This modality is only appropriate for patients who are hemodynamically stable, are mildly injured, and are only minimally hypothermic. Any patient with a core body temperature <35°C and a major injury should undergo active rewarming. The effect of hypothermia on uninjured patients is much less profound. Patients without injury who become hypothermic secondary to environmental exposure can undergo passive rewarming as a long as the core body temperature is above 32°C.[62]

Active Rewarming

The majority of multiply injured patients will require some form of active rewarming. In general, the invasive methods result in more rapid warming but are also subject to more complications. The method of choice for any individual patient depends upon the degree of hypothermia as well as the urgency of the situation. A variety of warming devices are illustrated in Figure 53.2.

TABLE 53.2

METHODS OF WARMING

METHOD OF WARMING	RATE OF TEMPERATURE RISE
Passive	
Blankets, warm room	0–0.5°C/h
Active noninvasive	
Forced air rewarming	1–2.4°C/h
Resistive heating blankets	1–2.5°C/h
Radiant heating lamps	Variable
Circulating water blanket	1.5–2°C/h
Active invasive warming	
Warmed tracheal insufflation	0.5°C/h
CPB	2°C/5 min under optimal conditions; usually slower in clinical settings
CVVR	3°C/h
CAVR	8°C/h
Cavity lavage	1–4°C/h
Intravascular warming	1.5°C/h

CPB, cardiopulmonary bypass; CVVR, continuous veno-venous rewarming; CAVR, continuous arteriovenous rewarming.

The most basic method of active warming is the infusion of warmed IV fluids. The maximum amount of heat transfer, however, is limited by the volume that physicians are willing to infuse. We recommend using warmed IV fluid to 40°C as a preventive rather than a therapeutic measure. Banked blood is stored at 4°C. Accordingly, infusion of several units of banked blood can accentuate hypothermia. We recommend using an infuser with a counter-current heating mechanism, so the blood products are warmed prior to infusion. There are a number of commercial fluid warmers/infusers available. Forced air rewarming has become the modality of choice for noninvasive active rewarming in most surgical centers. One of the most commonly utilized devices is the Bair Hugger (Arizant Inc., Eden Prairie, MN). This system provides convection heating to rewarm patients.[63] It consists of a paper/plastic interface that circulates heated air over a patient. The benefits of forced air rewarming include the ease of use, the ready availability, and the noninvasive nature of the treatment.

A number of studies have demonstrated the efficacy of forced air surface rewarming. Steele et al.[63] conducted a prospective study evaluating the effect of forced air rewarming versus regular blankets. They randomized patients to forced air rewarming at 43°C or standard blankets. They noted a temperature rise of 2.4°C per hour among patients with forced air rewarming versus 1.4°C per hour among patients treated with standard blankets. This modality is generally recommended for mild to moderate forms of hypothermia, as peripheral vasoconstriction can limit the ability of surface warming to transmit heat to the body core. Nonetheless, severe hypothermia has been successfully treated with surface air rewarming. Kornberger et al.[64] evaluated 15 severely hypothermic patients with a presenting core body temperature of 24°C–30°C. All of the patients were successfully warmed with an average warming rate of 1.7°C per hour. None of the patients with a prehospital arrest survived, but the remaining patients were long-term survivors. We do not recommend this method for severely hypothermic patients with ongoing hemorrhage, as they require rapid rewarming in order to effect hemostasis.

Other methods of noninvasive warming include resistive heating blankets and circulating water mattresses. The carbon fiber resistive heating blanket has performed well in published studies. Negishi et al.[65] compared the effects of a circulating water mattress, forced air rewarming, and a resistive heating blanket on perioperative hypothermia. They found the greatest degree of heat conservation in the resistive blanket group. The touted advantage of the resistive heating blanket is the ability to cover a greater body surface area. Forced air rewarming is generally limited to the thorax while a laparotomy is being performed. Circulating water bath mattresses have the advantage of using water, which has a high specific heat and thus, the ability to transfer large amounts of heat to the patient. These mattresses, however, are generally placed posteriorly. This limits the efficacy of the mattress, as patients lose more heat anteriorly.

Another benefit of resistive heating blankets is their ease of use during transport. One study randomly allocated patients to foil blankets or resistive heating blankets during transport.[66] The patients allocated to resistive heating blankets increased their core body temperature by 0.8°C per hour, whereas the patients allocated to the foil blankets dropped their core body temperature by 0.4°C per hour.

A number of centers having access to water tanks for treatment of burn patients have described rewarming of appropriately stabilized patients (i.e., endotracheal intubation, no active surgical issues) by placing the patient in the warm water tank until warmed, but his type of warming is not widely available.

Radiant heating lamps do not serve a large role in the effort to rewarm injured patients. They can interfere with the exam of the patient or even cause a thermal burn if they are positioned too close to the patient. They are not more effective than other noninvasive methods of rewarming, and their drawbacks outweigh their benefits.

Cavity lavage was the first invasive warming technique that was widely available. This technique requires access to the peritoneal cavity or the pleural cavities. It can also be accomplished through a nasogastric tube in the stomach. The peritoneal cavity can be accessed with a peritoneal lavage catheter. The pleural cavity can be accessed with large-bore chest tubes.[67] Many liters of intravenous fluids warmed to 40°C can be instilled and withdrawn through the drainage tubes. Peritoneal warming can be more difficult to accomplish, as the rate of fluid return is often suboptimal. Pleural warming is easier to accomplish, as chest tubes are simple to place and they have a larger bore, so the rate of fluid return is much more rapid. Pleural warming also carries the benefit of directly warming the heart, which can be important in patients with clinically significant arrhythmias. Gastric lavage carries the risk of aspiration. The rate of warming with cavity lavage varies between 1°C and 4°C per hour.

Tracheal insufflation with warmed air is the least invasive method of the core rewarming modalities.[16] It is also the least effective. It is accomplished by administering warmed air through an endotracheal tube. This modality can be used as an adjunct but should not be used as the sole warming modality. The average rate of warming is 0°C-0.5°C per hour.

Extracorporeal warming is the fastest, yet most invasive, method of warming hypothermic patients.[61,68,69] Cardiopulmonary bypass can be initiated via a sternotomy or by femoral

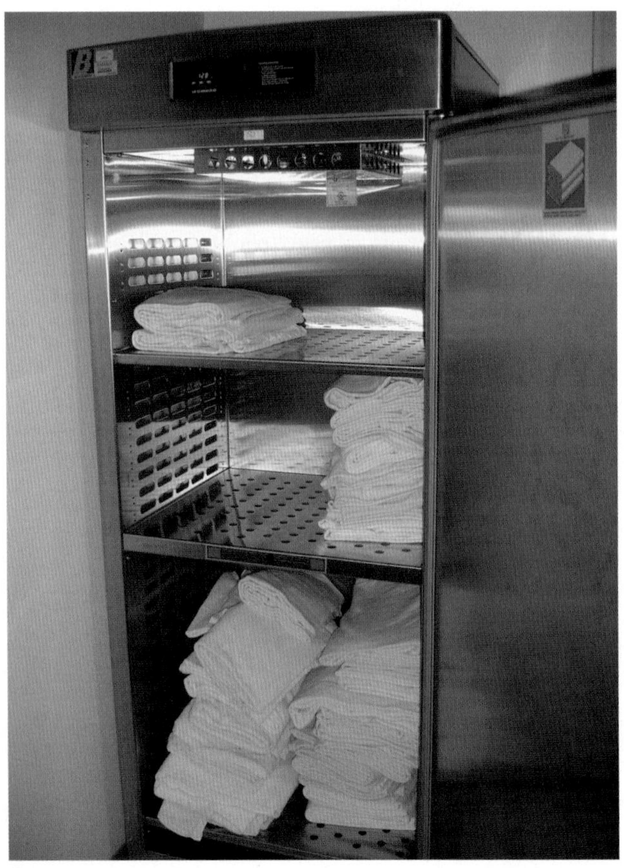

A

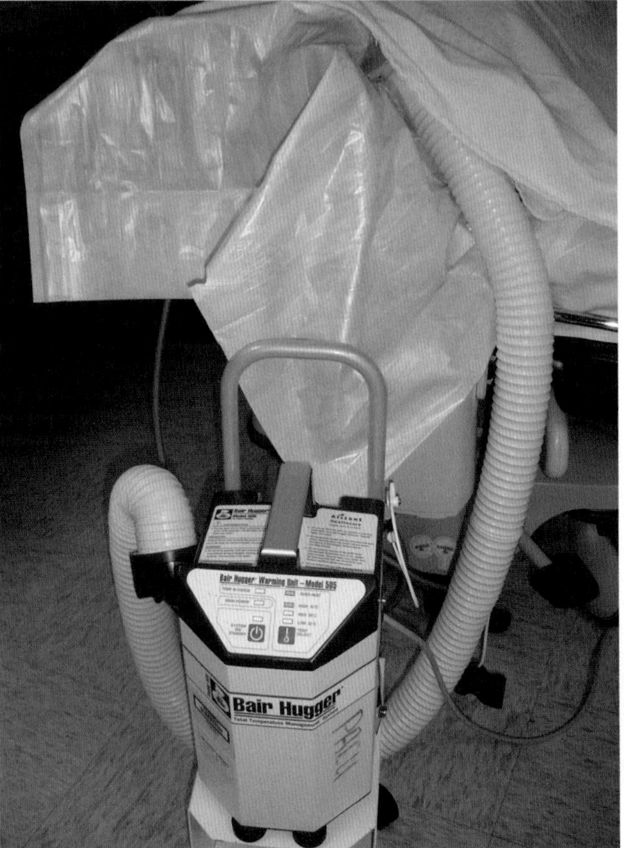

B

FIGURE 53.2. Examples of commonly used warming/cooling devices. A: Blanket/fluid warmer (set to 43°C). B: Forced-air warming device.

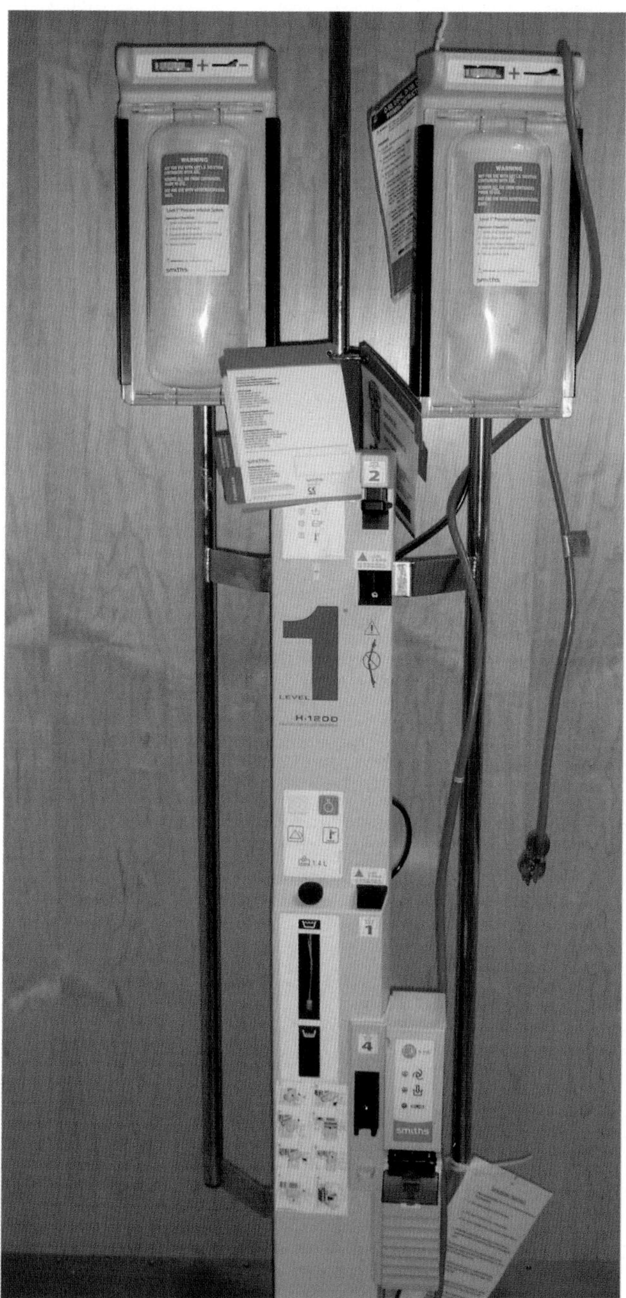

C

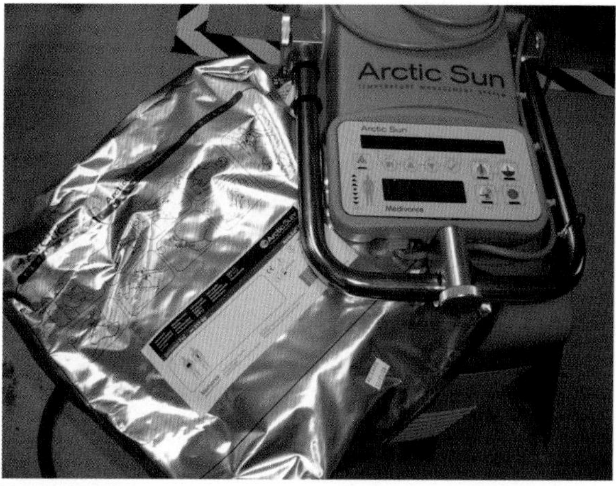

D

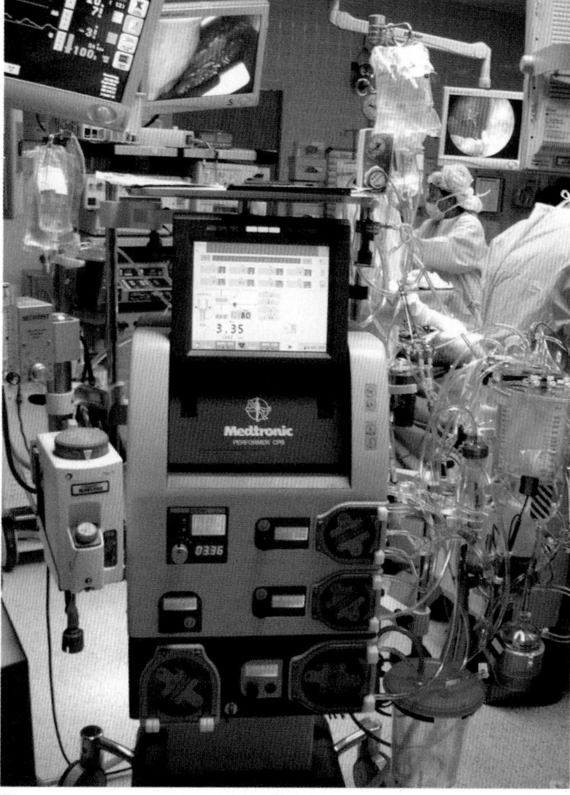

E

FIGURE 53.2. (*Continued*) C: Rapid fluid infusion device with intrinsic fluid warmer. D: Fluidized external blanket device (This device and others of similar design can be used for both warming and cooling patients). E: Cardiopulmonary bypass apparatus.

access. Blood is warmed (and can be oxygenated) extracorporeally. This will warm the majority of patients within 1–2 hours regardless of their degree of hypothermia. In fact, in optimal settings, core body temperature can be raised by 2°C every 5 minutes.[70] Cardiopulmonary bypass has the additional benefit of supporting the circulation in patients with hypothermia-induced cardiac arrest. Cardiopulmonary bypass is limited by the invasiveness of the procedure as well as the need for systemic heparinization.

To combat the limitations associated with cardiopulmonary bypass, circuits have been designed to provide either CAVR or continuous venovenous rewarming (CVVR).[70-72] This technique is accomplished by inserting large-bore catheters in the femoral vessels. CAVR utilizes the patient's blood pressure to pump blood through a warming circuit. It is then returned to the venous system. CVVR utilizes a mechanical pump to circulate venous blood through a warmer and back to the patient. This modality is similar to continuous dialysis, which can also accomplish core rewarming. The advantage of this setup compared with cardiopulmonary bypass is the lack of need for systemic heparinization and the ease of setup compared with bypass. This system can warm patients at rates of 3°C–8°C per hour.

Another technique recently developed utilizes an intravascular catheter to directly warm the blood *in vivo*. This system was developed in order to induce hypothermia as a therapeutic maneuver after cardiac arrest; however, the system also has a warming mode. A single catheter is inserted into the femoral vein, and warmed fluid is pumped through a balloon in the exterior of the catheter, directly warming the venous blood. Taylor et al.[73] reported an average warming of 1.5°C per hour with this technique.

Frostbite

Frostbite represents an additional consideration of rewarming patients. Frostbite is characterized by freezing of tissues and most often occurs in the distal extremities.[74] This can lead to tissue necrosis and potentially amputation. Whereas the adage "life over limb" always holds true, the acute care surgeon should attempt to salvage this tissue whenever possible. The most successful method of warming frostbite in the hands or feet is by submersion in warmed water (37°C–40°C). After 30–45 minutes, the temperature in the tissue will generally increase to normothermic levels, which may prevent further tissue loss. Early debridement outside of severely infected cases is not recommended, and surgery is normally delayed for a period of months.

Afterdrop

The core body temperature may initially decrease during the course of the warming process. This is referred to as the "afterdrop" phenomenon. It is likely caused by a redistribution of cooled peripheral blood to the core during the initial phases of warming. Afterdrop in patients with environmental hypothermia has been associated with cardiac arrest, as the cold, acidemic blood of the periphery is returned to the core circulation. Cardioversion is frequently not successful in this setting until the patient is warmed to a temperature above 32°C. In this setting, active core warming should take place in conjunction with cardiopulmonary support (CPR or cardiopulmonary bypass) until the patient has been warmed above 32°C, at which time cardioversion should be attempted.

THERAPEUTIC USES OF HYPOTHERMIA

The majority of this chapter has focused on the adverse effects of hypothermia and therapeutic measures to rewarm patients. There are, however, specific clinical circumstances in which hypothermia may be beneficial. These conditions are all linked by the need to minimize neurologic injury after isolated traumatic brain injury (TBI) or cerebral anoxia primarily from cardiac arrest or drowning.

Traumatic Brain Injury

The most important benefit of hypothermia revolves around cerebral protection. As such, the majority of clinical studies evaluating the efficacy of hypothermia in injured patients have focused on patients with TBIs. Unfortunately, the results of these studies have been mixed at best.

TBI evolves from the primary injury to secondary and tertiary insults.[75] The primary injury occurs at the time of the initial trauma and is unalterable. Accordingly, all interventions are aimed at preventing secondary and tertiary progression of the brain injury. These efforts focus on maintaining oxygenation and perfusion to the injured brain and to minimizing intracranial pressure. Experimental studies have revealed benefits and drawbacks to inducing hypothermia to the injured brain. An intracranial hemorrhage could theoretically expand as a result of hypothermic coagulopathy. Further, hypothermia could induce hypotension, which could worsen the injured penumbra. In contrast, however, there are a number of potential benefits. Hypothermia reliably reduces metabolic rate and cerebral oxygen demand. It also reduces excitatory neurotransmitters, which could reduce excitotoxicity to the injured brain. Other potential benefits of hypothermia include a reduction in edema formation, a reduction in intracranial pressure, and calcium antagonism. Given these experimental findings, clinicians theorized that hypothermia would improve functional outcomes after TBI.

Initial trials in the 1990s reported a benefit to inducing hypothermia in patients with TBI. On the basis of these results, a large phase 3 trial was conducted by Clifton et al.[76] in 2001. Patients were randomized to normothermia or hypothermia at 33°C for 48 hours. A poor outcome was seen in 57% of patients in both groups. Accordingly, the authors recommended against the routine use of hypothermia for TBI. Of note, however, intracranial pressure was more effectively lowered in the hypothermic patients. Hypotension and bradycardia were more common in the hypothermic patients, which may have mitigated any benefit that hypothermia may have attained. Subset analysis showed an improved outcome among patients treated with hypothermia who were already hypothermic on presentation. It is unclear if this was a result of random statistical analysis or evidence that hypothermic patients with a TBI should not be actively warmed.

Shiozaki et al.[77] evaluated the use of hypothermia for the treatment of TBI without elevated intracranial pressure. Patients were eligible for inclusion if their intracranial pressure was <25 mm Hg with standard therapeutics. Patients were randomized to receive either normothermia or hypothermia at 34°C for 48 hours. The clinical outcomes at 3 months were similar between the groups. The authors noted that infectious complications were more common among the hypothermic patients. This suggests that hypothermia is not an effective modality when intracranial pressure can be controlled with other interventions.

A phase 3 trial was conducted to evaluate hypothermia for treatment of TBI in children. The target temperature was 32.5°C and was maintained for 24 hours.[78] No benefit to neurologic function was noted in this trial.

The data on the utility of hypothermia for TBI has been summarized by six different meta-analyses.[79-84] The first four meta-analyses were conducted between 2002 and 2004, and all concluded that there was no compelling evidence to recommend the use of hypothermia. The Brain Trauma Foundation and the American Association of Neurological Surgeons have created guidelines for the management of TBI. The guideline on hypothermia was based on a subsequent meta-analysis conducted in 2008.[80] This report evaluated two additional randomized trials. They noted a reduction in mortality and an improvement in functional outcomes among patients treated with hypothermia. As a result, the guidelines include a level 3 recommendation to cautiously consider hypothermia for TBI. The most recent meta-analysis was conducted by the Cochrane group in 2009.[81] These authors found no benefit to hypothermia.

These studies have raised more questions than they have answered. The bulk of the clinical evidence argues against the routine use of hypothermia for treatment of TBI. Even if hypothermia as a general principle is beneficial, the optimal degree of hypothermia as well as the duration of treatment is unclear. It is also not clear if there is a difference between inducing hypothermia in a normothermic patient versus failing to warm a hypothermic patient. Further, patients with TBI represent a heterogeneous group of patients. It is possible that hypothermia would be beneficial in certain subgroups, such as those with diffuse axonal injury, and harmful in other groups, such as those with massive intracranial bleeding. Data to fully answer these questions are not available.

We do not routinely treat patients with TBI with hypothermia. The results of the clinical trials are mixed at best. We consider utilizing hypothermia in patients with refractory intracranial hypertension, although this is the group of patients with the most guarded prognoses. The optimal duration of hypothermia is probably at least 48 hours, and the optimal depth of hypothermia is probably around 34°C. We avoid hyperthermia as a general rule, as hyperthermia is a clear factor in increasing intracranial pressure. In most settings, our temperature goal is normothermia. We aggressively warm patients with abdominal or thoracic hemorrhagic foci. We are currently less aggressive about rapidly warming patients with isolated TBI who present with a core body temperature of <37°C.

Post–Cardiac Arrest Conditions

The rate-limiting step in the resuscitation of patients after a cardiac arrest is the eventual neurologic outcome. Whereas Advanced Cardiac Life Support (ACLS) measures are effective in resuscitating cardiac rhythms, patients are often left in a state of neurologic devastation. Permanent neurologic injury can be seen as soon as 5 minutes after cardiac arrest.

There were two landmark trials published in 2002 that demonstrated the benefit of therapeutic hypothermia.[85,86] Bernard et al. randomized 77 patients to normothermia or hypothermia at 33°C. Patients who had an out-of-hospital arrest associated with VF were eligible for enrollment. Hypothermia was achieved within 2 hours of resuscitation and was maintained for 12 hours. Good neurologic outcome was more common among patients treated with hypothermia (49% vs. 26%, $p = 0.046$). Another study evaluated 273 patients randomized to normothermia or hypothermia at 32°C–34°C for 24 hours. This study also limited the scope of patients to out-of-hospital VF arrest and also demonstrated a benefit to hypothermia.

As a result of this study, American and international guidelines have recommended therapeutic hypothermia for out-of-hospital VF arrests.[87] Unfortunately, a number of issues remain undefined. Patients with pulseless electrical activity (PEA) or asystole have a much worse prognosis, and it is not clear if hypothermia is beneficial in these patients. Since the time of the landmark trials, a variety of smaller studies and case series have emerged. One review has suggested that hypothermia should be induced after all cardiac arrest events regardless of initial rhythm (assuming exclusion criteria are not met).[88] Unfortunately, the warrant for this claim is based on much weaker evidence than what is described above, and additional randomized trials evaluating other rhythms or clinical scenarios are unlikely to be conducted.

The vast majority of patients included in trials of postarrest hypothermia were medical patients. There is sparse data to guide clinicians on the management of patients with acute care surgical conditions who develop a cardiac arrest. In our opinion, there are four main conditions associated with acute care surgical anoxia that can be considered for therapeutic hypothermia: hanging, traumatic asphyxia, drowning, and post-operative arrest.

Hanging carries a grim prognosis when the presenting neurologic condition is coma. The data on the use of hypothermia for the treatment of hanging victims is limited to case reports and a single case series. The largest case series consists of eight patients, so no conclusions can be drawn.[89] We believe that it is reasonable to consider therapeutic hypothermia in hanging patients who are comatose, are hemodynamically stable, and have no evidence of hemorrhage or a vascular injury on CT scan.

Cardiac arrest in the perioperative period is a challenging complication. This event can be caused by a multitude of factors, such as sepsis, pulmonary embolism, hemorrhage, and respiratory failure. As such, the data on out-of-hospital VF arrest have little to no application to postsurgical patients. These patients are also at a higher risk of hemorrhage from coagulopathy if hypothermia is induced. As such, we cannot make any firm recommendations on the use of hypothermia in this setting. Given the dismal prognosis of prolonged cardiac arrest, it is certainly a tempting modality to consider.

Traumatic asphyxia occasionally occurs without major additional injuries. We consider using hypothermia in this setting after all sources of hemorrhage have been ruled out with computed tomography (CT) scanning. This consideration, however, is based on animal studies of asphyxia rather than good clinical data.[90]

Drowning

Drowning victims represent a unique consideration. Again, there are no data to derive any firm recommendation on their treatment. These patients are nearly always hypothermic on presentation. They have also almost always aspirated, which is important given the effect of hypothermia on immune function. In the absence of concurrent hemorrhage and arrhythmias (and in the absence of any strong supporting data), it seems reasonable to allow these patients to passively warm slowly over 12–24 hours.

Institution of therapeutic hypothermia requires the ability to induce and maintain hypothermia and subsequently rewarm the patient. Simple measures for inducing hypothermia include ice packs and cooling blankets.[88] Infusion of 30 mL/kg of 4°C saline will drop the core body temperature by 2°C–4°C. A number of commercial devices are available that include an integral autoregulatory circuit. This provides for more precise temperature control with less nursing effort. External cooling devices include the Arctic Sun (Medivance, Louisville, CO) and others. These devices have cooling pads that are connected to the skin and have a feedback loop connected with a thermometer that maintains the temperature within a set range. Also available for internal cooling are intravascular cooling catheters (Alsius, Zoll Medical Corporation, Chelmsford, MA). This catheter is inserted in the femoral vein. Chilled water is circulated around the exterior of the catheter to directly cool venous blood. The device is connected to a temperature probe, which is able to autoregulate the core body temperature within a very narrow range. Internal devices have been demonstrated to result in more rapid cooling of patients. Current recommendations are to cool patients to 32°C–33°C for 24–48 hours. The rewarming phase must be conducted slowly—no faster than over an 8-hour period. If shivering occurs, it can be minimized by meperidine, benzodiazepines, or neuromuscular blockage. Given the propensity of these patients to develop seizures, EEG monitoring should be considered if prolonged neuromuscular blockade is instituted.

Spinal Cord Injury

Given the similarity in tissue types between the spinal cord and the brain, there has been considerable interest in treating spinal cord injuries with hypothermia. The initial neurologic damage with a spinal cord injury is irreversible; however, there is often progressive cellular injury that occurs after the initial insult. Proponents of hypothermia have suggested that reducing the core body temperature can limit the progression of neurologic deficits after the initial injury.

Initial studies in this area were conducted in the 1960s with mixed results. Many of the initial studies evaluated local hypothermia induced directly on the spinal cord during surgical procedures. More recent experimental studies have demonstrated positive outcomes. In fact, a recent review noted that 16 out of 17 experimental studies reported positive results.[91] Recent studies have utilized systemic hypothermia rather than local hypothermia. In particular, Lo et al. reported their results with a rat model. They induced systemic hypothermia at 33°C 5 minutes after inducing a spinal cord injury. Both clinical and histologic outcomes were improved in animals treated with hypothermia.[92]

Unfortunately, there are minimal clinical data to support the use of hypothermia in human beings. There are no phase 3 trials. In fact, almost all the human clinical reports were published in the 1970s. National guidelines have indicated there is not enough evidence to support the use of hypothermia for spinal cord injuries. Experimental models that induce hypothermia within 5 minutes of injury are not applicable to clinical settings, as hypothermia can almost never be induced that rapidly. This treatment received national attention after an American professional football player with a cervical spinal cord injury was treated with hypothermia and subsequently regained the ability to walk.[93] Nonetheless, we do not believe the evidence is compelling enough to recommend routine use of hypothermia.

Emergency Preservation and Resuscitation

Physicians have known for many years that neurologic recovery is possible even after an hour or more of asystole if profound hypothermia is present. This is generally seen in cases of submersion injury. Cold-water exposure induces a "diver's reflex" and is responsible for preservation of brain function during periods of prolonged circulatory arrest. Whereas postarrest studies have employed hypothermia after resuscitation, it is clearly more efficacious to achieve hypothermia before arrest. Hemorrhagic shock can lead to multiple organ dysfunction and cardiac arrest. There are certain injuries that may be reparable but not within the time frame necessary to avoid cardiac arrest. As such, the concept of the diver's reflex was introduced to injured patients. This concept involves inducing profound hypothermia, inducing circulatory arrest, repairing the injury, and resuscitating the patient.

This concept was initially referred to as "suspended animation" and subsequently became known as "emergency preservation and resuscitation," or EPR. EPR has been used in a variety of animal models.[10] It consists of inducing a core body temperature of 5°C–10°C followed by a period of circulatory arrest and resuscitation. Overall survival and cognitive function have been directly linked to the depth of hypothermia. It is possible that pharmacologic agents could induce a state of hibernation that could serve as an adjunct to hypothermia or completely replicate the benefits of hypothermia without requiring temperature modification.[94,95]

Although there is mounting evidence of the efficacy of EPR in animals, there are sparse human data. The use of EPR in humans has been limited to case reports of injuries to the inferior vena cava that were otherwise irreparable.[56] The authors of these manuscripts noted that EPR allowed them to repair retrohepatic vena cava injuries in a bloodless field. Deep hypothermia has been used in elective cardiac and neurosurgical operations, but these settings are clearly different than the patient population the acute care surgeon encounters. Accordingly, it is not clear that these results can be transferred to human settings.

In summary, EPR is a method of resuscitation that could be used at some future time period. It is not designed for most injured patients; rather, its use would be limited to injuries causing a severe state of hemorrhagic shock that are otherwise irreparable.

References

1. Danzl DF, Pozos RS, Auerbach PS, et al. Multicenter hypothermia survey. *Ann Emerg Med.* 1987;16(9):1042-1055.
2. Jurkovich GJ, Greiser WB, Luterman A, et al. Hypothermia in trauma victims: an ominous predictor of survival. *J Trauma.* 1987;27(9):1019-1024.
3. Eddy VA, Morris JA Jr, Cullinane DC. Hypothermia, coagulopathy, and acidosis. *Surg Clin North Am.* 2000;80(3):845-854.
4. Jansen JO, Thomas R, Loudon MA, et al. Damage control resuscitation for patients with major trauma. *BMJ.* 2009;338:b1778.
5. Dimopoulos G, Falagas ME. Approach to the febrile patient in the ICU. *Infect Dis Clin North Am.* 2009;23(3):471-484.
6. Laupland KB. Fever in the critically ill medical patient. *Crit Care Med.* 2009;37(7 suppl):S273-S278.
7. Segers MJ, Diephuis JC, van Kesteren RG, et al. Hypothermia in trauma patients. *Unfallchirurg.* 1998;101(10):742-749.
8. Hildebrand F, Giannoudis PV, van Griensven M, et al. Pathophysiologic changes and effects of hypothermia on outcome in elective surgery and trauma patients. *Am J Surg.* 2004;187(3):363-371.
9. Kirkpatrick AW, Chun R, Brown R, et al. Hypothermia and the trauma patient. *Can J Surg.* 1999;42(5):333-343.
10. Tisherman SA. Hypothermia and injury. *Curr Opin Crit Care.* 2004;10(6):512-519.
11. Marik PE. Fever in the ICU. *Chest.* 2000;117(3):855-869.
12. Webb GE. Comparison of esophageal and tympanic temperature monitoring during cardiopulmonary bypass. *Anesth Analg.* 1973;52(5):729-733.
13. Beilman GJ, Blondet JJ, Nelson TR, et al. Early hypothermia in severely injured trauma patients is a significant risk factor for multiple organ dysfunction syndrome but not mortality. *Ann Surg.* 2009;249(5):845-850.
14. Luna GK, Maier RV, Pavlin EG, et al. Incidence and effect of hypothermia in seriously injured patients. *J Trauma.* 1987;27(9):1014-1018.
15. Helm M, Hauke J, Lampl L, et al. Accidental hypothermia in trauma patients. *Acta Anaesthesiol Scand Suppl.* 1997;111:44-46.
16. Peng RY, Bongard FS. Hypothermia in trauma patients. *J Am Coll Surg.* 1999;188(6):685-696.
17. Polderman KH. Mechanisms of action, physiological effects, and complications of hypothermia. *Crit Care Med.* 2009;37(7 suppl):S186-S202.
18. Schmidt KD, Chan CW. Thermoregulation and fever in normal persons and in those with spinal cord injuries. *Mayo Clin Proc.* 1992;67(5):469-475.
19. Zell SC, Kurtz KJ. Severe exposure hypothermia: a resuscitation protocol. *Ann Emerg Med.* 1985;14(4):339-345.
20. Oung CM, English M, Chiu RC, et al. Effects of hypothermia on hemodynamic responses to dopamine and dobutamine. *J Trauma.* 1992;33(5):671-678.
21. Reuler JB. Hypothermia: pathophysiology, clinical settings, and management. *Ann Intern Med.* 1978;89(4):519-527.
22. Curley FJ. Hypothermia: a critical problem in the intensive care unit. *J Intensive Care Med.* 1995;10(1):1-2.
23. Polderman KH, Peerdeman SM, Girbes AR. Hypophosphatemia and hypomagnesemia induced by cooling in patients with severe head injury. *J Neurosurg.* 2001;94(5):697-705.
24. Martini WZ. Coagulopathy by hypothermia and acidosis: mechanisms of thrombin generation and fibrinogen availability. *J Trauma.* 2009;67(1):202-208; discussion 8-9.
25. Martini WZ, Cortez DS, Dubick MA, et al. Thrombelastography is better than PT, aPTT, and activated clotting time in detecting clinically relevant clotting abnormalities after hypothermia, hemorrhagic shock and resuscitation in pigs. *J Trauma.* 2008;65(3):535-543.
26. Schreiber MA, Holcomb JB, Hedner U, et al. The effect of recombinant factor VIIa on coagulopathic pigs with grade V liver injuries. *J Trauma.* 2002;53(2):252-257; discussion 7-9.
27. Kheirabadi BS, Delgado AV, Dubick MA, et al. In vitro effect of activated recombinant factor VII (rFVIIa) on coagulation properties of human blood at hypothermic temperatures. *J Trauma.* 2007;63(5):1079-1086.
28. Krause KR, Howells GA, Buhs CL, et al. Hypothermia-induced coagulopathy during hemorrhagic shock. *Am Surg.* 2000;66(4):348-354.
29. Cosgriff N, Moore EE, Sauaia A, et al. Predicting life-threatening coagulopathy in the massively transfused trauma patient: hypothermia and acidoses revisited. *J Trauma.* 1997;42(5):857-861; discussion 61-62.
30. Johnston TD, Chen Y, Reed RL II. Functional equivalence of hypothermia to specific clotting factor deficiencies. *J Trauma.* 1994;37(3):413-417.
31. Reed RL II, Johnson TD, Hudson JD, et al. The disparity between hypothermic coagulopathy and clotting studies. *J Trauma.* 1992;33(3):465-470.
32. Rohrer MJ, Natale AM. Effect of hypothermia on the coagulation cascade. *Crit Care Med.* 1992;20(10):1402-1405.
33. Watts DD, Trask A, Soeken K, et al. Hypothermic coagulopathy in trauma: effect of varying levels of hypothermia on enzyme speed, platelet function, and fibrinolytic activity. *J Trauma.* 1998;44(5):846-854.
34. Michelson AD, Barnard MR, Khuri SF, et al. The effects of aspirin and hypothermia on platelet function in vivo. *Br J Haematol.* 1999;104(1):64-68.

35. Valeri CR, Feingold H, Cassidy G, et al. Hypothermia-induced reversible platelet dysfunction. *Ann Surg*. 1987;205(2):175-181.
36. Kashuk JL, Moore EE, Millikan JS, et al. Major abdominal vascular trauma—a unified approach. *J Trauma*. 1982;22:672-678.
37. Kim SH, Stezoski SW, Safar P, et al. Hypothermia and minimal fluid resuscitation increase survival after uncontrolled hemorrhagic shock in rats. *J Trauma*. 1997;42(2):213-222.
38. Wu X, Stezoski J, Safar P, et al. Systemic hypothermia, but not regional gut hypothermia, improves survival from prolonged hemorrhagic shock in rats. *J Trauma*. 2002;53(4):654-662.
39. Prueckner S, Safar P, Kentner R, et al. Mild hypothermia increases survival from severe pressure-controlled hemorrhagic shock in rats. *J Trauma*. 2001;50(2):253-262.
40. Wu X, Kochanek PM, Cochran K, Nozari A, et al. Mild hypothermia improves survival after prolonged, traumatic hemorrhagic shock in pigs. *J Trauma*. 2005;59(2):291-299; discussion 299-301.
41. Takasu A, Stezoski SW, Stezoski J, et al. Mild or moderate hypothermia, but not increased oxygen breathing, increases long-term survival after uncontrolled hemorrhagic shock in rats. *Crit Care Med*. 2000;28(7):2465-2474.
42. Alam HB, Rhee P, Honma K, et al. Does the rate of rewarming from profound hypothermic arrest influence the outcome in a swine model of lethal hemorrhage? *J Trauma*. 2006;60(1):134-146.
43. Lee KR, Chung SP, Park IC, et al. Effect of induced and spontaneous hypothermia on survival time of uncontrolled hemorrhagic shock rat model. *Yonsei Med J*. 2002;43(4):511-517.
44. George ME, Mulier Ke, Beilman GJ. Hypothermia is associated with improved outcomes in a porcine model of hemorrhagic shock, *J Trauma*. 2010;68:1-7.
45. Wu X, Stezoski J, Safar P, et al. After spontaneous hypothermia during hemorrhagic shock, continuing mild hypothermia (34 degrees C) improves early but not late survival in rats. *J Trauma*. 2003;55(2):308-316.
46. Meyer DM, Horton JW. Effect of different degrees of hypothermia on myocardium in treatment of hemorrhagic shock. *J Surg Res*. 1990;48(1):61-67.
47. Johannigman JA, Johnson DJ, Roettger R. The effect of hypothermia on liver adenosine triphosphate (ATP) recovery following combined shock and ischemia. *J Trauma*. 1992;32(2):190-195.
48. Hildebrand F, van Griensven M, Giannoudis P, et al. Effects of hypothermia and re-warming on the inflammatory response in a murine multiple hit model of trauma. *Cytokine*. 2005;31(5):382-393.
49. Vaagenes P, Gundersen Y, Opstad PK. Rapid rewarming after mild hypothermia accentuates the inflammatory response after acute volume controlled haemorrhage in spontaneously breathing rats. *Resuscitation*. 2003;58(1):103-112.
50. Mizushima Y, Wang P, Cioffi WG, et al. Restoration of body temperature to normothermia during resuscitation following trauma-hemorrhage improves the depressed cardiovascular and hepatocellular functions. *Arch Surg*. 2000;135(2):175-181.
51. Gentilello LM, Jurkovich GJ, Stark MS, et al. Is hypothermia in the victim of major trauma protective or harmful? A randomized, prospective study. *Ann Surg*. 1997;226(4):439-447; discussion 47-49.
52. Wang HE, Callaway CW, Peitzman AB, et al. Admission hypothermia and outcome after major trauma. *Crit Care Med*. 2005;33(6):1296-1301.
53. Shafi S, Elliott AC, Gentilello L. Is hypothermia simply a marker of shock and injury severity or an independent risk factor for mortality in trauma patients? Analysis of a large national trauma registry. *J Trauma*. 2005;59(5):1081-1085.
54. Steinemann S, Shackford SR, Davis JW. Implications of admission hypothermia in trauma patients. *J Trauma*. 1990;30(2):200-202.
55. Martin RS, Kilgo PD, Miller PR, et al. Injury-associated hypothermia: an analysis of the 2004 National Trauma Data Bank. *Shock*. 2005;24(2):114-118.
56. Hartman AR, Yunis J, Frei LW, et al. Profound hypothermic circulatory arrest for the management of a penetrating retrohepatic venous injury: case report. *J Trauma*. 1991;31(9):1310-1311.
57. Seekamp A, van Griensven M, Hildebrandt F, et al. Adenosine-triphosphate in trauma-related and elective hypothermia. *J Trauma*. 1999;47(4):673-683.
58. Bernabei AF, Levison MA, Bender JS. The effects of hypothermia and injury severity on blood loss during trauma laparotomy. *J Trauma*. 1992;33(6):835-839.
59. Inaba K, Teixeira PG, Rhee P, et al. Mortality impact of hypothermia after cavitary explorations in trauma. *World J Surg*. 2009;33(4):864-869.
60. Gregory JS, Flancbaum L, Townsend MC, et al. Incidence and timing of hypothermia in trauma patients undergoing operations. *J Trauma*. 1991;31(6):795-798; discussion 8-800.
61. Gentilello LM, Moujaes S. Treatment of hypothermia in trauma victims: thermodynamic considerations. *J Intensive Care Med*. 1995;10(1):5-14.
62. Danzl DF, Pozos RS. Accidental hypothermia. *N Engl J Med*. 1994;331(26):1756-1760.
63. Steele MT, Nelson MJ, Sessler DI, et al. Forced air speeds rewarming in accidental hypothermia. *Ann Emerg Med*. 1996;27(4):479-484.
64. Kornberger E, Schwarz B, Lindner KH, et al. Forced air surface rewarming in patients with severe accidental hypothermia. *Resuscitation*. 1999;41(2):105-111.
65. Negishi C, Hasegawa K, Mukai S, et al. Resistive-heating and forced-air warming are comparably effective. *Anesth Analg*. 2003;96(6):1683-1687, table of contents.
66. Kober A, Scheck T, Fulesdi B, et al. Effectiveness of resistive heating compared with passive warming in treating hypothermia associated with minor trauma: a randomized trial. *Mayo Clin Proc*. 2001;76(4):369-375.
67. Otto RJ, Metzler MH. Rewarming from experimental hypothermia: comparison of heated aerosol inhalation, peritoneal lavage, and pleural lavage. *Crit Care Med*. 1988;16(9):869-875.
68. Gregory JS, Bergstein JM, Aprahamian C, et al. Comparison of three methods of rewarming from hypothermia: advantages of extracorporeal blood warming. *J Trauma*. 1991;31(9):1247-1251; discussion 51-2.
69. Perchinsky MJ, Long WB, Hill JG, et al. Extracorporeal cardiopulmonary life support with heparin-bonded circuitry in the resuscitation of massively injured trauma patients. *Am J Surg*. 1995;169(5):488-491.
70. Knight DA, Manifold CA, Blue J, et al. A randomized, controlled trial comparing arteriovenous to venovenous rewarming of severe hypothermia in a porcine model. *J Trauma*. 2003;55(4):741-746.
71. Gentilello LM, Cobean RA, Offner PJ, et al. Continuous arteriovenous rewarming: rapid reversal of hypothermia in critically ill patients. *J Trauma*. 1992;32(3):316-325; discussion 25-27.
72. Kirkpatrick AW, Garraway N, Brown DR, et al. Use of a centrifugal vortex blood pump and heparin-bonded circuit for extracorporeal rewarming of severe hypothermia in acutely injured and coagulopathic patients. *J Trauma*. 2003;55(3):407-412.
73. Taylor EE, Carroll JP, Lovitt MA, et al. Active intravascular rewarming for hypothermia associated with traumatic injury: early experience with a new technique. *Proc (Bayl Univ Med Cent)*. 2008;21(2):120-126.
74. Patel NN, Patel DN. Frostbite. *Am J Med*. 2008;121(9):765-766.
75. Sahuquillo J, Vilalta A. Cooling the injured brain: how does moderate hypothermia influence the pathophysiology of traumatic brain injury. *Curr Pharm Des*. 2007;13(22):2310-2322.
76. Clifton GL, Miller ER, Choi SC, et al. Lack of effect of induction of hypothermia after acute brain injury. *N Engl J Med*. 2001;344(8):556-563.
77. Shiozaki T, Hayakata T, Taneda M, et al. A multicenter prospective randomized controlled trial of the efficacy of mild hypothermia for severely head injured patients with low intracranial pressure. Mild Hypothermia Study Group in Japan. *J Neurosurg*. 2001;94(1):50-54.
78. Hutchison JS, Ward RE, Lacroix J, et al. Hypothermia therapy after traumatic brain injury in children. *N Engl J Med*. 2008;358(23):2447-2456.
79. Harris OA, Colford JM Jr, Good MC, et al. The role of hypothermia in the management of severe brain injury: a meta-analysis. *Arch Neurol*. 2002;59(7):1077-1083.
80. Peterson K, Carson S, Carney N. Hypothermia treatment for traumatic brain injury: a systematic review and meta-analysis. *J Neurotrauma*. 2008;25(1):62-71.
81. Sydenham E, Roberts I, Alderson P. Hypothermia for traumatic head injury. *Cochrane Database Syst Rev*. 2009(2):CD001048.
82. Gadkary CS, Alderson P, Signorini DF. Therapeutic hypothermia for head injury. *Cochrane Database Syst Rev*. 2002(1):CD001048.
83. Henderson WR, Dhingra VK, Chittock DR, et al. Hypothermia in the management of traumatic brain injury. A systematic review and meta-analysis. *Intensive Care Med*. 2003;29(10):1637-1644.
84. McIntyre LA, Fergusson DA, Hebert PC, et al. Prolonged therapeutic hypothermia after traumatic brain injury in adults: a systematic review. *JAMA*. 2003;289(22):2992-2999.
85. Bernard SA, Gray TW, Buist MD, et al. Treatment of comatose survivors of out-of-hospital cardiac arrest with induced hypothermia. *N Engl J Med*. 2002;346(8):557-563.
86. Mild therapeutic hypothermia to improve the neurologic outcome after cardiac arrest. *N Engl J Med*. 2002;346(8):549-556.
87. Bernard S. Hypothermia after cardiac arrest: expanding the therapeutic scope. *Crit Care Med*. 2009;37(7 suppl):S227-S233.
88. Seder DB, Van der Kloot TE. Methods of cooling: practical aspects of therapeutic temperature management. *Crit Care Med*. 2009;37(7 suppl):S211-S222.
89. Borgquist O, Friberg H. Therapeutic hypothermia for comatose survivors after near-hanging-a retrospective analysis. *Resuscitation*. 2009;80(2):210-212.
90. Katz LM, Young A, Frank JE, et al. Neurotensin-induced hypothermia improves neurologic outcome after hypoxic-ischemia. *Crit Care Med*. 2004;32(3):806-810.
91. Dietrich WD III. Therapeutic hypothermia for spinal cord injury. *Crit Care Med*. 2009;37(7 suppl):S238-S242.
92. Lo TP Jr, Cho KS, Garg MS, et al. Systemic hypothermia improves histological and functional outcome after cervical spinal cord contusion in rats. *J Comp Neurol*. 2009;514(5):433-448.
93. Cappuccino A. Moderate hypothermia as treatment for spinal cord injury. *Orthopedics*. 2008;31(3):243-246.
94. Behringer W, Safar P, Kentner R, et al. Antioxidant Tempol enhances hypothermic cerebral preservation during prolonged cardiac arrest in dogs. *J Cereb Blood Flow Metab*. 2002;22(1):105-117.
95. Aslami H, Schultz MJ, Juffermans NP. Potential applications of hydrogen sulfide-induced suspended animation. *Curr Med Chem*. 2009;16(10):1295-1303.

CHAPTER 54 ■ NOSOCOMIAL INFECTIONS

PAMELA A. LIPSETT

In order to help the clinician make decisions about empiric antibiotic selection, the classification of infections has typically been divided into the site of infection (i.e., lung, skin and soft tissue, urinary tract, and intraabdominal) and the location of the patient at the time the infection occurs.[1-3] Historically, location has been divided into community- and hospital-onset, with hospital-acquired infections (HAIs) occurring after 72 hours of hospitalization, but patient demographics, risk factors, and pathogens have changed substantially over the last two decades, making this classification schema no longer informative. Bacterial resistance to antibiotics after exposure to the health care setting, and the potential for infection due to cross-contamination from the environment or from transmission from other patients, must now be considered in the initial choice of antibiotics. Because of these changes in epidemiology, infections are now classified as health care-associated, hospital-acquired, or community-acquired.[1]

HAIs remain a leading cause of morbidity and mortality, occurring in as many as 10% of hospitalized patients. Hospitals vary substantially in rates and types of HAIs, which may relate to coding, referrals, patient demographics, use of devices and procedures, as well as actual quality of patient care.[1,4] From January 2006 to October 2007, 28,502 HAIs were reported to the National Hospital Surveillance Network (NHSN): 10,064 (35.3%) were cases of central line-associated blood stream infection (CLABSI), 8,579 (30.1%) were cases of catheter-associated urinary tract infection (CAUTI), 4,524 (15.9%) were cases of ventilator-associated pneumonia (VAP), 5,291 (18.6%) were cases of surgical site infection (SSI), and 44 (0.2%) were cases of postprocedure pneumonia.[1]

Patients in intensive care units (ICUs) suffer a disproportionally high percentage of HAI when compared with patients in non–critical care areas.[1,5-9] For example, ICU beds account for 5%–10% of all hospital beds, yet 45% of CLABSIs occur in ICUs. Thus, the clinician must consider not only the individual patient risk factors but also the location of the patient in determining the probability and source of infection.[5]

This chapter discusses some of the common HAIs encountered in surgical patients, including pneumonia, CLABSIs, and UTIs, and to a lesser extent intraabdominal infections (IAIs), emphasizing epidemiology, pathogenesis, prevention, and treatment. SSIs are discussed in detail elsewhere (see Chapter__).

PNEUMONIA

Pneumonia is one of the most common nosocomial infections of hospitalized patients.[1,6] Health care-associated pneumonia (HCAP) occurs among patients hospitalized for 90 days; who live in nursing facilities; who have received antibiotics, chemotherapy, or wound care recently; or who undergo hemodialysis.[3] These patients are at risk for the same pathogens as patients who have hospital-acquired pneumonia (HAP), which by definition occurs after 48 hours of inpatient care in previously healthy patients. Distinguishing HAP from community-acquired pneumonia (CAP) is important, as patients with HAP are susceptible to pneumonia from different, potentially more virulent pathogens. VAP is a subset of HAP that occurs among patients after more than 48–72 hours of mechanical ventilation. Each day the patient remains on mechanical ventilation, the risk for development of VAP increases.

Because the cost (increased length of stay) of VAP and HAP is substantial, prevention has become an important focus for quality improvement and pay-for-performance reporting activities.[10,11] Clear recognition of the risk factors and understanding of the probable factors in disease development can lead to rational preventive strategies. Moreover, knowledge of varying diagnostic and treatment regimens may lead to improvements in patient care and outcomes.

Epidemiology

HAP is one of the most common nosocomial infections. At a rate of 3–10 cases per 1,000 hospital admissions, HAP may increase a patient's hospital stay by more than 1 week, resulting in up to $40,000 in additional cost.[1,9-12] A large and important subset of HAP, the risk of VAP is estimated at 3% per day for the first 5 days of mechanical ventilation, 2% per day for days 6–10, and 1% per day thereafter, with each day of mechanical ventilation adding incremental risk.[12]

Pathophysiology

The pathogenesis of HAP is multifactorial; several patient and treatment risk factors have been identified (Table 54.1). Most cases of HAP are secondary to microaspiration of infected material into the normally sterile lung parenchyma.[14] Thus, patient risk factors, the amount of pathogens delivered into the respiratory tree, and the virulence of infecting pathogens influence the probability of developing HAP and potentially the severity of the disease.

Classifying pneumonia into CAP and HAP recognizes that the causative pathogens differ and even change during hospitalization.[12] Because expected pathogens differ and successful outcome depends on appropriate initial treatment, general recommendations for empiric treatment depend on whether the patient has CAP or HAP (or HCAP), and the duration of the current hospitalization.[1,14-16] Distinguishing HCAP and CAP, broad-spectrum initial treatment of HCAP followed by de-escalation, has not led to measurable changes in mortality in prospective studies. Early HAP (<5 days into the hospital course) is associated with a better prognosis than late-onset HAP (arising ≥5 days into a hospital course).[1] These two categories can then be subdivided further into patients with and without prior antibiotic exposure.

Early-onset HAP in patients with no prior antibiotic exposure tends to mirror CAP, and patients generally have susceptible pathogens. The most common pathogens include Enterobacteriaceae, *Haemophilus influenzae*, *Streptococcus pneumoniae*, and methicillin-sensitive *Staphylococcus aureus* (MSSA).[14,15] Patients with no prior antibiotic exposure who develop late-onset HAP are infected by similar bacteria; however, occasionally these patients present with gram-negative bacilli (GNB) resistant to first-generation cephalosporins. Late-onset HAP in patients with prior antibiotic exposure

TABLE 54.1

RISK FACTORS FOR THE DEVELOPMENT OF VENTILATOR-ASSOCIATED PNEUMONIA

HOST DEFENSES	INCREASED BACTERIAL LOAD	VIRULENT PATHOGENS
Nasogastric tube	Bacterial colonization, recent viral infection	Prolonged antibiotics
Endotracheal tube	Gastric colonization	Length of stay
Supine position	Re-intubation	Chronic obstructive pulmonary disease
Head injury	Sinusitis	Poor infection control techniques
Sedation	Contaminated equipment	
Malnutrition		
Steroids		
Tobacco smoking		

presents a greater problem in both the prediction and empiric treatment of likely pathogens. As many as 40% of such patients present with potentially multi–drug-resistant (MDR) pathogens, including *Pseudomonas aeruginosa, Acinetobacter baumannii*, and methicillin-resistant *Staphylococcus aureus* (MRSA).[15]

Gram-positive Bacteria. The common gram-positive cocci causing pneumonia in hospitalized patients are *S. pneumoniae* and *S. aureus*.[14-16] Patients with traumatic brain injury and early HAP may be infected with *S. aureus*. Whereas these pathogens are often seen in early-onset pneumonia, *S. aureus* can cause pneumonia at any point of the hospitalization, and MRSA is typically observed later in the hospital course. Risk factors for MRSA pneumonia include chronic obstructive pulmonary disease (COPD), longer duration of mechanical ventilation, prior antibiotic exposure, prior use of corticosteroids, prior bronchoscopy, colonization with MRSA, and adjacency to a patient identified to harbor MRSA.[16]

Gram-negative Bacteria. Gram-negative bacteria associated with early-onset HAP include *H. influenzae* and lactose-fermenting GNB such as Enterobacteriaceae, including *Escherichia coli, Klebsiella* species, and *Enterobacter* species.[14-16] Overgrowth of these organisms can be associated with prior antibiotic therapy, and their virulence may increase in critical illness. Enterobacteriaceae are increasingly demonstrating extended-spectrum beta-lactamase (ESBL) activity.[17,18] Whereas these organisms were treated frequently with broad-spectrum beta-lactam antimicrobials, plasmid-mediated resistance to these agents is increasing, and major outbreaks of VAP secondary to ESBL-producing pathogens have been identified.[17,18] Stains that produce ESBL are resistant to all beta-lactam agents and exhibit high-level resistance to fluoroquinolones, making carbapenems the recommended first-line agents for ESBL-producing strains.[17,18]

P. aeruginosa is the most common MDR GNB causing HAP/VAP,[1,16] and the most frequent VAP isolate in patients on mechanical ventilation for more than 4 days.[19] Resistance to one or more antibiotics is common and patients with MDR *P. aeruginosa* are at increased risk of severe sepsis and death.[20] *A. baumannii*, an aerobic, non–lactose-fermenting GNB that has intrinsic resistance to many antibiotics, can cause nosocomial infections that may spread rapidly among hospitalized patients[16,21-23] Due to its ability to acquire resistance rapidly to many drugs, prior antibiotic exposure is a major risk factor for resistance.[24]

Prevention

Patients scheduled for elective surgery may be identified to be at increased risk for postoperative pneumonia, and may be candidates for risk modification.[25,26] The respiratory risk index is a scoring system that categorizes patients as low-, medium-, or high risk for postoperative respiratory failure, based on factors such as emergency and complex operations, as per American Society of Anesthesiologists (ASA) score (see Chapter 10), and patient comorbidities (e.g., COPD, ascites, chronic kidney disease).[26] Potentially modifiable risk factors are indicated in Table 54.2.[27-73] The use of "ventilator bundles," such as those promulgated by the Institute for Healthcare Improvement (IHI), and similar quality improvement efforts have decreased the incidence of VAP by more than 50%.[27,28] However, the IHI paradigm contains two measures not likely to decrease the incidence of VAP (prophylaxis of stress-related gastric mucosal hemorrhage and venous thromboembolic disease, whereas other measures such as the effect of topical chlorhexidine used for oral hygiene, and recommendations about specific endotracheal tubes (e.g., silver-coated tubes) are not included in current bundles.

Diagnosis

Clinical Evaluation. The method of establishing the diagnosis of HAP remains controversial, undoubtedly due to difficulty establishing the differences among colonization, tracheobronchitis, and HAP. Neither radiological nor microbiological features in isolation can establish the diagnosis of HAP. The U.S. Centers for Disease Control and Prevention (CDC) and the NHSN have developed criteria for the diagnosis of nosocomial pneumonia, taking into account clinical factors, such as fever and leukocytosis, as well as radiological criteria, including persistent new findings on chest radiography[2,74] (Table 54.3). The controversy about whether to use clinical, noninvasive, or invasive measures to establish a diagnosis continues today.[75-91] An invasive diagnostic strategy does not alter mortality, but if antibiotic use is protocolized, the total duration of antibiotics may be lowered.[77,87,89,90]

TABLE 54.2

RISK FACTOR REDUCTION AND PREVENTION FOR VENTILATOR-ASSOCIATED PNEUMONIA

RISK FACTOR	MODIFICATION
Smoking	Stop 8 wk prior to surgery when possible[29-33]
Asthma/chronic obstructive pulmonary disease	Optimize peak flow with bronchodilators and/or steroids[29]
Congestive heart failure	Optimize fluid status and blood pressure[29]
Postoperative pain control	Neuraxial anesthesia may reduce risk by 20%[34]
Aspiration risk	Head of bed elevation >30 degree[1,10,39,40]; remove nasogastric tubes[10,13,35-40]
Oral contamination	Selective decontamination[41]; mouth care, tooth-brushing, "stress ulcer" prophylaxis[39,42-49]
Intubation route and type	Nasotracheal intubation higher risk than endotracheal; type and presence of endotracheal tube; subglottic suction ("hi-lo") endotracheal tube; silver-coated endotracheal tube[50-55]
Ventilator circuit and suctioning	Endotracheal tube suctioning.[56-60] Circuit changes only when tubing is visibly soiled and (of course) between patients[36,51,61-67]
Duration of mechanical ventilation	Shorter time on ventilator lowers risk; maximal benefit to spontaneous breathing trials linked to sedation "holidays." Protocols effective[1,68-71]
Ineffective depth of respiratory effort	Incentive spirometry, cough and deep breathing exercises[72,73]

TABLE 54.3

U.S. CENTERS FOR DISEASE CONTROL AND PREVENTION. SURVEILLANCE DEFINITION OF PNEUMONIA FOR A NON–IMMUNO-COMPROMISED ADULT PATIENT[a]

Radiology:

Two or more serial chest radiographs with at least ONE of the following:

- New or progressive AND persistent infiltrate
- Consolidation
- Cavitation

(In patients with no underlying pulmonary or cardiac disease, ONE DEFINITIVE radiograph is acceptable)

Signs/symptoms/laboratory:

At least ONE of the following:

- Fever (>38°C or >100.4°F) with no other recognized cause
- Leukopenia (<4,000 WBC/mm^3) OR leukocytosis (>12,000 WBC/mm^3)
- For adults ≥70 years old, mental status changes with no other recognized cause

AND

At least TWO of the following:

- New onset of purulent sputum, or change in character of sputum, or increased respiratory secretions, or increased suctioning requirements
- New onset or worsening cough, or dyspnea, or tachycardia
- Rales or bronchial breath sounds
- Worsening gas exchange (PaO_2:F_IO_2 ≤ 240), increased oxygen requirements, or increased ventilation demand

WBC; white blood cell count.
From http://www.cdc.gov/nhsn/PDFs/pscManual/17pscNosInfDef_current.pdf. Accessed December 29, 2010.

The Clinical Pulmonary Infection Score (CPIS)[78] includes both clinical and radiological factors that indicate an increased likelihood of the presence of pneumonia. Point values are assigned to each criterion and the total is summed. Traditionally, a threshold score of >6 points has been considered diagnostic of pneumonia[79] (Table 54.4). The clinical utility of the CPIS has been evaluated extensively, with both proponents and detractors.[78-81] In the original dataset, when the CPIS was ≤6 points, no patient satisfied microbiologic criteria for pneumonia.[79] Other investigators suggest that the CPIS, while sensitive, lacks specificity and leads to unnecessary antimicrobial treatment. Among 201 patients who underwent an invasive diagnosis of pneumonia, there was no difference in the CPIS score of patients with and without VAP. Importantly, therapy based on resolution of the CPIS would have led to 840 days of empiric antibiotics as compared to 424 days based on invasive specimen collection.[79]

Whereas most studies indicate that clinical evaluation is sensitive in identifying VAP, the specificity is low. Clinical diagnosis combined with short-course antibiotic therapy may be reasonable especially if a low [≤6 points] CPIS score is achieved after day three of treatment.[81] In a 2000 study, Singh et al.[81] examined short-course empiric therapy for patients in the ICU with suspected VAP. The rate of antimicrobial resistance or superinfection was significantly higher in patients receiving standard therapy. The duration of therapy was significantly lower in the experimental group, with no difference in mortality.

Bacteriologic Evaluation. The diagnosis of pneumonia can be established by a number of methods, including noninvasive and invasive means for sputum specimen collection and qualitative or quantitative microbiology.[82-91] Blind tracheobronchial aspiration (TBAS) is a noninvasive technique accomplished by inserting a flexible suction catheter into the distal trachea via the endotracheal tube to obtain sputum for quantitative culture.[86] The typical threshold for diagnosis of pneumonia is growth of >10^5 cfu/mL. This technique is simple

TABLE 54.4

MODIFIED CLINICAL PULMONARY INFECTION SCORE

	0 POINTS	1 POINT	2 POINTS
Temperature (°C)	36.5–38.4	38.5–38.9	≤36.4 or ≥39
Peripheral WBC	4,000–11,000	<4,000 or >11,000 > 50% bands: add one extra point	
Tracheal secretions	None	Non-purulent	Purulent
Chest x-ray	No infiltrate	Diffuse or patchy infiltrate	Localized infiltrate
Progression of infiltrate from prior radiographs	None		Progression (ARDS or CHF believed unlikely)
Culture of endotracheal tube aspirate	No growth/light growth	Heavy growth Some bacteria on gram stain: Add one extra point	
Oxygenation (PaO_2:F_IO_2)	>240 or ARDS		≤240 and no ARDS

ARDS, acute respiratory distress syndrome; CHF, congestive heart failure; WBC, white blood cell count.
Adapted from Swoboda et al. Can the clinical pulmonary infection score impact ICU antibiotic days? *Surg Infect.* 2006;7:331–339.

but does not allow specific lung segments to be sampled, and the catheter is contaminated easily.

Bronchoalveolar lavage (BAL) allows sampling of specific lung segments suspected to be involved with pneumonia, and supports quantitative microbiology. Bacterial growth of $>10^4$ cfu/mL is typically accepted as being most accurate for diagnosis of VAP, although some authors[1,89] argue that the use of 10^5 cfu/mL provides fewer false-positives and a lower likelihood of inappropriate antibiotic therapy.[90]

Specimen collection with a protected specimen brush (PSB) involves a telescoping catheter brush that is advanced blindly or through a bronchoscope, into the suspected distal airway. A diagnostic cutoff of $>10^3$ cfu/mL is typically accepted as being consistent with HAP.[1,91] Complications such as bleeding or pneumothorax may be more frequent with PSB.

Proponents of invasive diagnostic means for pneumonia suggest that fewer and more selective antibiotics be used when BAL or PSB is used to collect quantitative cultures.[89,90] Direct examination of BAL fluid for intracellular organisms (>5 cells) has overall sensitivity and specificity of 93.6% and 91.5%, respectively, for the diagnosis of VAP, with only 12% of patients receiving incorrect empiric therapy.[85] With early appropriate antibiotic therapy being an important predictor of mortality, a technique that facilitates early guidance of therapy may be useful clinically. In a randomized trial comparing PSB versus TBAS and thus quantitative versus qualitative techniques, Ruiz et al.[86] were unable to demonstrate any differences in ICU length of stay, length of mechanical ventilation, 30-day mortality, or attributable mortality between groups. However, the cost difference between groups was $368 versus $29.[86] Similarly, the Canadian Critical Care Trials Group randomized 740 patients with a clinical suspicion of pneumonia to BAL on mechanical ventilation for >4 days to quantitative culture versus TBAS, with qualitative culture controlling for the timing of empiric antibiotics.[87] The authors reported no difference in 28-day mortality. Additionally, there were no differences in the secondary outcomes of hospital and ICU length of stay, duration of mechanical ventilation, and ICU and hospital mortality.

On the other hand, Fagon et al.[88] randomized 413 patients to invasive versus noninvasive diagnosis of VAP, and found decreased 14-day mortality, improved organ function scores, and fewer days of antibiotic therapy among patients undergoing the invasive diagnosis. Interestingly, they also identified alternative infectious diseases that required intervention when pneumonia was not verified. The greatest support for the use of invasive techniques may be reflected by reducing antibiotic utilization or by more accurate use.[89,91] Shorr et al.[91] evaluated four randomized trials of diagnostic techniques, and found that invasive strategies do not affect the mortality of VAP, likely because empiric antibiotic choices must be made before results of quantitative cultures become available.

Treatment

Empiric Therapy and De-escalation of Treatment. The most important factor influencing the mortality of HAP is prompt and adequate empiric antibiotic therapy.[1,93,94] Treatment should be instituted immediately after specimen collection and should be directed against likely pathogens. The choice of antimicrobial agent(s) should account for risk factors such as current length of hospital stay, prior exposure to antibiotics, duration of mechanical ventilation, previous culture results, known antibiotic resistance locally among patient, contacts, and unit-specific microbiota, and host immunosuppression.[94,95] Several guidelines have been published suggesting agents that could be utilized for empiric antibiotics for CAP, HAP, VAP, and HCAP.[1,26,92,96,97-102] If the patient is considered low-risk by all criteria, single-agent therapy is a reasonable choice (Table 54.5).[1,26] On the other hand, patients who have risk factors as noted above should be considered for double- or triple-drug initial empiric therapy for VAP (Table 54.6).[1,26,99,100]

Whereas vancomycin is the agent used most commonly to treat MRSA in hospitalized patients, considerable debate has emerged about whether vancomycin should be used empirically as agent for suspected MRSA infection. The minimum

TABLE 54.5

EMPIRIC ANTIBIOTIC CHOICES FOR LOW-RISK PATIENTS WITH VENTILATOR-ASSOCIATED PNEUMONIA

Third-generation cephalosporin (e.g., ceftriaxone)
Extended-spectrum fluoroquinolone (e.g., moxifloxacin, levofloxacin)
Aminopenicillin (e.g., ampicillin/sulbactam)
Narrow-spectrum carbapenem (e.g., ertapenem)

SURGICAL CRITICAL CARE

TABLE 54.6

EMPIRIC ANTIBIOTIC SELECTION IN HIGH-RISK PATIENTS WITH SUSPECTED VAP

TRIPLE THERAPY FOR EMPIRIC INITIAL THERAPY IN HIGH-RISK PATIENTS WITH SUSPECTED VAP	
Antipseudomonal coverage by beta-lactam	Cefepime or ceftazadime, imipenem or meropenem or doripenem, piperacillin-tazobactam
Antipseudomonal fluoro-quinolone OR aminoglycoside	Ciprofloxacin or levofloxacin OR gentamicin, tobramycin, or amikacin
MRSA coverage	Linezolid or vancomycin
Therapy should be modified based on culture results as soon as possible, stopping unnecessary or overly-broad agents. De-escalation of therapy should occur within 72 h.	

MRSA, methicillin-resistant *S. aureus*.

inhibitory concentration (MIC) for vancomycin has been increasing among clinical isolates, and in a recent study, 73% of MRSA isolates had a MIC > 1.5 μg/mL.[103] Use of vancomycin as the primary agent for empiric use to treat high-risk patients with suspected VAP is also problematic because vancomycin has poor penetration of lung tissue.[104,105] Based on these trends, it is unclear whether vancomycin should remain the drug of choice for treating MRSA pneumonia, or whether linezolid should be considered as a first-line agent.[106-108] When compared to pneumonia caused by MSSA, MRSA is associated with prolonged ICU length of stay and increased hospital cost despite appropriate initial therapy.[108]

The decision to treat high-risk adult patients with suspected HAP/VAP with three agents (one against MRSA; two against MDR GNB) is based on the concern that MDR pathogens may be etiologic and that longer time to initial appropriate antimicrobial therapy has been linked to mortality. However, extended, overly broad antimicrobial therapy will lead to the development of additional resistance.[109,110] Some pathogens may be particularly difficult to treat; for example, as many as 50% of *Acinetobacter* isolates may be resistant to all antimicrobial agents except the polymyxins.[111,112] There is some evidence that treatment with intravenous or inhaled polymyxin E (colistin) may be safe and effective for patients with MDR *Acinetobacter* pneumonia.[111,113]

In many institutions, *P. aeruginosa* is the most common isolated pathogen responsible for VAP or HAP. In addition, the percentage of isolates sensitive to single-agent antipseudomonal therapy can be <50%.[114] This fact, along with the *in vitro* synergy observed with two-agent therapy (traditionally a beta-lactam and an aminoglycoside) has led to the suggestion that using two agents to cover possible MDR *Pseudomonas* is prudent,[108] albeit with considerable debate on the point.[115-121] Among trauma patients, Croce et al.[118] found that patients treated with a combination of a third-generation cephalosporin and gentamicin actually had increased rates of treatment failure and superinfection compared to those treated with the cephalosporin alone. However, recent investigations suggest that patients treated with initial combination therapy are more likely to receive appropriate empiric therapy, with associated improved mortality.[116,119-121] Heyland et al.[120] randomized patients with suspected VAP to empiric monotherapy versus combination therapy, and found no reduction of mortality from combination therapy. However, the percentage of patients treated effectively by combination therapy was significantly higher. Moreover, patients with one or more MDR organisms were treated adequately 84% of the time by combination therapy, versus only 19% of the time by empiric monotherapy. For these reasons, current treatment guidelines recommend initial empiric double coverage for MDR GNB for critically ill patients with suspected HAP/VAP.[1,99,100,121-123]

De-escalation of therapy should be considered within 72 hours of initiating empiric therapy and is accomplished by: (1) changing to antibiotics with a narrower spectrum; (2) eliminating unnecessary antibiotics from the treatment regimen; or (3) changing to oral therapy.[124,125] Importantly, de-escalation has not been associated with decreased response rates, higher mortality, or longer hospital or ICU lengths of stay.[124,125]

Duration of Therapy. Recommendations for duration of antimicrobial therapy for nosocomial pneumonia have evolved in recent years, with an overall trend to decrease duration of therapy. In the seminal paper by Chastre et al.,[126] patients with VAP were randomized to 8 versus 15 days of antimicrobial therapy. All-cause mortality was similar between groups (18.8% for 8 days vs. 17.2% for 15 days, risk difference 1.6, 95% confidence interval [CI], –3.7 to 6.9). Additionally, there was no difference in recurrence rate (28.9% vs. 26.0%, risk difference 2.9 [CI –3.2 to 0.1]) of VAP. In a retrospective evaluation of the same population, pneumonia secondary to non–lactose-fermenting GNB and MRSA were both independently associated with recurrence.[127] Whereas concern for recurrence exists when treating MDR infections, these results[126,127] indicate that many patients may be treated safely and effectively with shortened courses of antibiotics.

The question remains: What is the shortest course of antimicrobial therapy appropriate for nosocomial pneumonia?[131] Serial BAL has been used as a method of assessing response to therapy and allowing for a shorter duration of therapy.[82] Discontinuation of appropriate therapy after 4 days in patients with decreased bacterial growth on repeat BAL decreases antibiotic duration and total antibiotic days, with no effect on mortality, length of stay, ventilator-free days, relapse rate, or rate of superinfection,[82] indicating that shortening of antibiotic courses may be accomplished safely in appropriate patients.

Outcomes

HAP has a substantial impact, both medically and economically, with incremental cost attributed to a single episode of HAP of up to $50,000.[2,5,10] Specifically, ICU patients with VAP experience longer ICU and hospital lengths of stay, which is a major driver of cost.[2,5,10] Prevention of HAP is therefore the focus of quality improvement efforts, and is, in part, why use of ventilator "bundles" for both prevention and therapy has blossomed.[106,128-130] However, the effect of VAP on mortality is unclear. In trauma and in patients with acute respiratory distress syndrome (ARDS), VAP does not appear to increase mortality, thus mortality is not a valid endpoint in studies of prevention of VAP.[132]

CATHETER-RELATED (-ASSOCIATED) BLOOD STREAM INFECTION

Definitions, Epidemiology, and Risk Factors

Central venous catheters are used commonly in patients for hemodynamic monitoring and administration of fluids and drugs, total parenteral nutrition, and blood products, and renal replacement therapy. The main complication of catheter use is infection, which can occur at the site of insertion, within the blood stream, or result in metastatic infection.[133] Central line-associated BSI is defined from a surveillance perspective if a catheter is present within 48 hours of the culture and bacteremia occurs, irrespective of whether the catheter itself has been identified as a causative vector.[134] A laboratory-confirmed BSI (LCBSI) is defined when a patient has one of two possible conditions: (1) a recognized pathogen cultured from one or more blood cultures that is not related to infection at another site; and (2) signs and symptoms of infection and positive laboratory results not related to infection at another site; common skin contaminants must be cultured in blood from two or more sites, cultured on separate occasions.[134] These surveillance definitions overestimate the true incidence of infection because they do not account for a bacteremia from an undocumented source, such as an IAI. On the other hand, a catheter-related BSI (CRBSI) is confirmed when the catheter (cultured by the semi-quantitative "roll-plate" technique; >15 cfu—see below) and blood have identical pathogens. In the United States it is estimated that 250,000 BSIs occur annually, with rates ranging between 1.3 and 5.5 infections per 1,000 catheter-days.[135]

Catheters can become colonized or infected by two primary routes: (1) endogenous contamination from the skin alongside the catheter, causing catheter colonization and blood stream infection; or (2) endoluminal contamination from biofilm, a contaminated hub, or injection of infected fluid.[136] Catheter design and logistics must be understood to assess the associated risk.[136] For example, the catheter can be designated by the type of vessel it occupies (e.g., peripheral venous, central venous, or arterial); its intended life span (e.g., temporary or short-term vs. permanent or long-term); the insertion site (e.g., subclavian, femoral, internal jugular, or peripheral vein, peripherally inserted central catheter [PICC]); the pathway from skin to vessel (e.g., tunneled vs. nontunneled); its length; or some special characteristic of the catheter (e.g., cuffed or uncuffed, impregnation with heparin, antibiotics, or antiseptics, and the number of lumens).

Traditionally, the diagnosis of a CRBSI is established when both the catheter and blood stream yield the same pathogen.[136] A catheter may be cultured using the semi-quantitative "roll-plate" technique, whereby a 5-cm segment of catheter is rolled onto an agar plate; growth of >15 cfu is considered meaningful.[137] Pooled data suggest a sensitivity and specificity of 85% and 82%, respectively.[138] A more labor-intensive method intended to account for endoluminal pathogens subjects the catheter segment to sonication before plating. Growth of $>10^3$ cfu/mL is then considered diagnostic, with sensitivity and specificity of 83% and 87%, respectively.[138] However, both methods require catheter removal, thus alternatives have been considered. Simultaneous quantitative blood cultures can be drawn peripherally and through the catheter. A diagnosis of catheter-related infection is considered if the growth from the catheter is fivefold greater than the periphery. This method has sensitivity and specificity of 93% and 97% for long-term catheters.[138] Furthermore, if blood drawn from catheter turns positive more than 2 hours before blood drawn simultaneously from a peripheral site, CLASBI is confirmed with sensitivity and specificity of 90% and 72%.[138]

Data from the NHSN indicate that the most common pathogens isolated from CLABSIs were coagulase-negative staphylococci (34.1%), *Enterococcus* spp. (15.0%), *Candida* spp. (11.8%) and *S. aureus* (9.9%). Depending on local patterns, the frequency of resistant pathogens can vary widely, with more than one-half of *S. aureus* isolates being MRSA, 79% of *E. faecium* isolates being vancomycin-resistant (VRE), and up to 30% of *Pseudomonas* spp. resistant to more than one antimicrobial agent. More recently, *K. pneumoniae* and *Enterobacter* spp. may be resistant to cephalosporins via production of an ESBL.[139] Moreover, *A. baumannii* and *Klebsiella* spp. may be carbapenem-resistant, which can be transmitted rapidly to other GNB.

Prevention

Substantial progress has been made in preventing BSIs by implementing care bundles, including simple measures such as education, improved hand hygiene, use of full barrier precautions for catheter insertion, chlorhexidine skin antisepsis, avoidance of femoral sites, and prompt removal of unnecessary catheters.[28,140-144] After these measures proved to reduce infection substantially at Johns Hopkins, deployment in State of Michigan ICUs decreased rates of CLABSI and CRBSI from 7.7 to 1.4/1,000 catheter-days at 16–18 months.[144]

In addition to processes of care and bundles designed to reduce infection, technological advances such as catheter coatings with antiseptics or antimicrobials reduce infections when the catheter is in place for an average of 5–12 days [0.40, 95% CI, 0.27–0.58], but not 13–20 days [0.69, 0.42–1.14].[145] Ethanol lock solutions have been investigated for both prevention and treatment because resistance is unlikely and cost is modest. However, the concentration of ethanol, the dwell time, and the effect on the catheter all require elucidation.[146,147]

Antimicrobial locks have also been used in both clinical trials and in selected clinical conditions, such as in patients with tunneled hemodialysis catheters,[148-151] where CLABSI and hospitalization were reduced by 52% and 69%, respectively, albeit with concern for possible increased resistance to gentamicin in coagulase-negative *Staphylococcus* isolates.[148] Antimicrobial lock solutions are not recommended currently for routine use.[136]

The role of catheter dressings in reducing infections lacks clear recommendations as to the preferability of gauze or transparent dressings despite more than 20 years of study.[152-156] More recently, chlorhexidine gluconate-impregnated sponges have been shown consistently to reduce catheter and skin colonization, albeit with an increase in local skin reactions, especially notably in low-birth-weight infants (<1,000 g).[157-163]

URINARY TRACT INFECTION

Definitions, Epidemiology, and Risk Factors

Urinary tract infection (UTI) is the single most common HAI, representing more than 30% of all HAIs reported by acute-care hospitals.[1,2] The gold standard for diagnosis is the detection of a pathogen in the urine of a symptomatic patient. Traditionally, the microbiological quantification of a UTI has been the isolation of $>10^5$ cfu/mL from a mid-stream urine collection. However, this definition was proposed from healthy female outpatients, not from catheterized inpatients.

Several guidelines may assist clinicians in the prevention, identification, and management of UTIs.[164-169] However, sufficient evidence is lacking to support a clear definition of CAUTI versus the far more common (and often inappropriately treated) asymptomatic catheter-associated bacteriuria. In the recent guidelines of the Infectious Diseases Society of America (IDSA),[170] the term *catheter-associated asymptomatic bacteriuria* (CA-ASB) is retained, but it is omitted from the NSHN definitions (Table 54.7), and is considered by NHSN as a disease only when bacteremia ensues.[164] According to the IDSA guidelines[170]:

> *"Signs and symptoms compatible with CAUTI include new onset or worsening of fever, rigors, altered mental status, malaise, or lethargy with no other identified cause; flank pain; costovertebral angle tenderness; acute hematuria; pelvic discomfort; and in those whose catheters have been removed, dysuria, urgent or frequent urination, or suprapubic pain or tenderness."*

Furthermore, patients with spinal cord injury may present with a compendium of complaints that include spasticity,

TABLE 54.7

NHSN DEFINITION OF CAUTI

TYPE OF INFECTION	DEFINITION
Catheter associated urinary tract infection	A CAUTI occurs in a patient who had an indwelling urethral catheter in place within the 48-h period before the onset of the UTI.
Symptomatic urinary tract infection	**Criterion 1a:** Patient had an indwelling urinary catheter in place at the time of specimen collection or a catheter removed within 48 h *and* at least one of the following signs or symptoms with no other recognized cause: fever (>38°C), suprapubic tenderness, or costovertebral angle pain or tenderness *and* a positive urine culture of $\geq 10^5$ colony-forming units (cfu)/mL with no more than two species of microorganisms **Criterion 1b:** Patient did not have an indwelling urinary catheter in place at the time of specimen collection nor within 48 h prior to specimen collection *and* has at least one of the following signs or symptoms with no other recognized cause: fever (>38°C) in a patient that is ≤65 years of age, urgency, frequency, dysuria, suprapubic tenderness, or costovertebral angle pain or tenderness *and* a positive urine culture of $\geq 10^3$ cfu/mL with no more than two species of microorganisms **Criterion 2:** Patient had an indwelling urinary catheter in place at the time of specimen collection or removed within the previous 48 h *and* at least one of the following signs or symptoms with no other recognized cause: fever (>38°C), suprapubic tenderness, or costovertebral angle pain or tenderness *and* a positive urinalysis demonstrated by at least one of the following findings: (a) positive dipstick for leukocyte esterase and/or nitrite; (b) pyuria (urine specimen with ≥10 white blood cells [WBC]/mm³ or ≥3 WBC/high power field of unspun urine); (c) microorganisms seen on gram stain of unspun urine *and* a positive urine culture of $\geq 10^3$ and $<10^5$ cfu/mLwith no more than two species of microorganisms Criterion 2b Patient did not have an indwelling urinary catheter in place at the time of specimen collection nor within 48 h prior to specimen collection *and* has at least one of the following signs or symptoms with no other recognized cause: fever (>38°C) in a patient that is ≤65 y of age, urgency, frequency, dysuria, suprapubic tenderness, or costovertebral angle pain or tenderness, *and* a positive urinalysis demonstrated by at least one of the following findings: (a) positive dipstick for leukocyte esterase and/or nitrite; (b) pyuria (urine specimen with ≥10 WBC/mm³ or ≥3 WBC/high power field of unspun urine); (c) microorganisms seen on gram stain of unspun urine *and* a positive urine culture of $\geq 10^3$ and $<10^5$ cfu/mL with no more than two species of microorganisms
Asymptomatic bacteremic urinary tract infection (ABUTI)	Patient with or without an indwelling urinary catheter has no signs or symptoms (i.e., no fever (>38°C) for patients ≤65 y of age[a]; and for any age patient no urgency, frequency, dysuria, suprapubic tenderness, or costovertebral angle pain or tenderness, OR for a patient ≤1 y of age, no fever (>38°C core), hypothermia (<36°C core), apnea, bradycardia, dysuria, lethargy, or vomiting) *and* a positive urine culture of $>10^5$ cfu/mL with no more than two species of uropathogen microorganisms[b] *and* a positive blood culture with at least one matching uropathogen microorganism to the urine culture.

[a]Fever is not diagnostic for UTI in the elderly (>65 y of age) and therefore fever in this age group does not disqualify from meeting the criteria of an ABUTI.

[b]Uropathogen microorganisms are: GNB, *Staphylococcus* spp., yeasts, beta-hemolytic *Streptococcus* spp., *Enterococcus* spp., *G. vaginalis*, *Aerococcus urinae*, and *Corynebacterium* spp. (urease positive).

autonomic dysreflexia, or a "sense of unease".[170] The symptoms typical of a CAUTI are those identified also in noncatheterized patients; aside from fever, symptoms in a catheterized patient may be difficult to elicit, especially if critically ill.

Asymptomatic bacteriuria (ASB) is present when $>10^5$ cfu/mL is identified in two consecutive cultures from an asymptomatic patient. In outpatient females, ASB increases with increasing age, reaching a prevalence of 20% in those women older than 80 years.[171] In contradistinction, ASB is unusual in males before the age of 60 and is present among only 5%–10% of men older than 80 years.[172] In institutionalized older adults, as many as 50% will have ASB, which may persist for years without consequences. ASB is benign and not associated with negative outcomes.[169,173] Furthermore, the presence of pyuria is not sufficient to distinguish between asymptomatic or symptomatic UTI and does not indicate symptomatic infection.[171,173] However, absence of pyuria in a symptomatic UTI is unusual. Neither does the appearance or odor of the urine suggest presence of UTI.[174] To reiterate, ASB is not important clinically, and treatment is unlikely to confer benefit.[169,173] Moreover, inappropriate treatment leads to potential resistance, drug side effects, and increased cost. Among 510 trauma patients, fever, leukocytosis, or both were not associated with a UTI, which occurred in 42 patients (16 episodes/1,000 catheter-days).[174]

The prevalence of CAUTI is highest in ICUs, where urinary catheters are used routinely to assess urine output. According to NHSN data from 2006 to 2008, rates range from a median of 3.4 infections per 1,000 catheter-days in surgical ICUs to 6.2 infections per 1,000 catheter-days in burn ICUs.[1] Rates on general care wards tend to be higher, ranging from 6.1 infections per 1,000 catheter-days in solid-organ transplant units to 14.5 infections per 1,000 catheter-days in rehabilitation units.[1]

Perioperative use of urinary catheters is common, but this practice is being scrutinized given that a urinary catheter is the single most important risk factor for the development of a UTI, related to usage itself and duration of use.[170] The National Surgical Infection Prevention Project revealed that 86% of patients undergoing major operations had indwelling urinary catheters in the perioperative period, with one-half of the patients remaining catheterized for more than 2 days.[174] As expected, catheterization for more than 2 days was a significant risk factor for UTI (9.4% vs. 4.5%; $p < 0.004$).[175]

Additional risk factors for the development of a UTI include female gender, advanced age, diabetes mellitus, anatomic abnormalities, ureteral stents, and having had a solid-organ transplant,[165-180] In addition, conditions under which the catheter was inserted and maintained contribute to risk if not in conformance with standard infection control practices.

Pathogenesis and Microbiology

The pathogenesis of UTI can be classified according to whether infections are caused by endogenous or exogenous contamination.[170] Endogenous contamination occurs typically from contamination from the perineum and rectum by pathogens such as *E. coli*, *Klebsiella*, *Enterobacter*, and other Enterobacteriaceae. Exogenous contamination occurs via breaks in technique during insertion or aftercare. The pathogens can be typical nosocomial flora transferred to patients via contamination of the internal lumen of the catheter.

Biofilm may develop both on the internal and external surfaces of urinary catheters, and serves as a protective environment for pathogens, because antimicrobial agents penetrate poorly.[176] Biofilm can be an important factor in both forms of contamination, and is the reason why a catheter should be removed as soon as possible when a UTI is suspected, or changed if still necessary when a CAUTI is diagnosed or suspected.[171] Common nosocomial UTI pathogens are shown in Table 54.8,[139] but many may be colonists rather than pathogens. Staphylococcal UTIs may be associated with bacteremia. In a study of 102 patients with a urinary catheter and *S. aureus* bacteriuria, 33% had a CAUTI, and 13% were bacteremic. *S. aureus* bacteriuria can persist for months before causing bacteremia; bacteriuria may also reflect hematogenous pyelonephritis and urinary shedding. Therefore, all patients with *S. aureus* UTIs should be evaluated for bacteremia and possibly endocarditis (especially if blood cultures are positive.[177]

Treatment

Treatment of symptomatic CAUTI should include replacement or removal of the catheter if it has been in place for at least 1 week. Initial empiric antimicrobial therapy should be based on local epidemiologic data regarding pathogens and antimicrobial resistance patterns.[170,171] Once culture results are available, antibiotics should be adjusted accordingly, typically de-escalated and favoring an agent that is concentrated in urine. Whereas good clinical evidence is lacking regarding duration of therapy, guidelines recommend 7 days of therapy for patients who respond promptly to treatment and 10–14 days of therapy otherwise.[169] One study demonstrated that 5 days of levofloxacin treatment was sufficient if a patient was not seriously ill. Moreover, a 3-day course is recommended for females <65 years old without upper tract symptoms if the catheter has been removed.[170]

TABLE 54.8

COMMON PATHOGENS OF THE URINARY TRACT

PATHOGEN	PERCENT OF INFECTIONS
Escherichia coli	15%–25%
Enterococci	14%–18%
Candida spp.	14%–25%
Pseudomonas aeruginosa	10%–17%
Klebiella pneumoniae	5%–10%
Enterobacter spp.	4%–8%
Coagulase-negative staphylococci	1%–5%
Staphylococcus aureus	1%–4%
Acinetobacter baumannii	0.5%–2%

Prevention

The most important tactics in decreasing UTI is limiting exposure to urinary catheters and duration of their use.[165-171] Non-invasive means to measure bladder volume may reduce the "elective" use of urinary catheters during routine surgery. Specialized anti-infective catheters are not effective when catheter duration *in situ* is more than 1 week.

Because many patients become colonized with bacteria with an indwelling catheter, antibiotic prophylaxis at the time of discontinuation of a urinary catheter has been studied prospectively. A randomized trial of 239 patients given trimethoprim-sulfamethoxazole (three doses) versus placebo at the time of catheter removal demonstrated fewer infections (5/103, 4.9% vs. 22/102, 21.6%, $p < 0.001$), with only six patients requiring treatment.[178] Nevertheless, antibiotic prophylaxis of catheter removal is not recommended in the current IDSA guidelines.[170]

INTRA-ABDOMINAL INFECTION

Peritonitis

Peritonitis is a common diagnosis in surgical ICUs, often leading to severe sepsis.[179] Peritonitis is classified into three groups — primary, secondary, and tertiary, with secondary peritonitis subclassified into community- and HAIs. Primary peritonitis, previously called spontaneous bacterial peritonitis, arises without any anatomic cause, is typically mono-microbial, and is associated with ascites or peritoneal dialysis. Secondary peritonitis is most common and occurs when the peritoneal cavity is infected following perforation of a hollow gastrointestinal viscus, development of an intestinal fistula, anastomotic dehiscence, ischemic necrosis, or other injuries to the gastrointestinal tract.[179,180] Source control of the infectious focus and reduction of the bacterial inoculum are primary goals of surgical therapy, thereby allowing intraperitoneal host defenses to recover. More detailed discussion is presented elsewhere in this volume (see Chapter__).

The definition of tertiary peritonitis is controversial, but is generally considered as IAI that persists following multiple (at least two) interventions to control peritonitis. Patients with tertiary peritonitis are typically critically ill.[180-183] When compared with secondary peritonitis patients, patients with tertiary peritonitis have a higher APACHE II score (12.4 vs. 20.7 points), a greater number of organ failures (3.5 vs. 6.3 organs), and severe sepsis/septic shock (65.5% vs. 100%).[179] The mortality rate of tertiary peritonitis is quite high (30%-64%). Unlike secondary peritonitis, the microbial flora is not typically from enteric sources (e.g., *E. coli*, *Klebsiella* spp., other Enterobacteriaceae, *Bacteroides fragilis* group), but rather the common opportunistic and nosocomial facultative pathogenic bacteria and fungi (e.g., coagulase-negative staphylococci, enterococci, *P. aeruginosa*, *Candida* spp.)[179,181]; many are MDR organisms. Debate continues as to whether the presence of these microbes represents colonization of the peritoneal cavity, invasive infection, or a marker of failure of host defenses. Factors that contribute to the development of tertiary peritonitis are listed in Table 54.9.[184]

Because tertiary peritonitis is considered as a continuum of disease from secondary peritonitis, the diagnosis can be difficult to establish.[181,183] Evans et al.[183] utilized a broad definition of tertiary peritonitis that included both localized (abscess) and generalized peritonitis following inadequate surgical source control (persistent infection resulting from lack of initial source control for secondary peritonitis does not define tertiary peritonitis). Thus, it is important to determine whether the surgical team believes that adequate source control has been achieved, which is typically possible in 80%–90% of cases.

Whereas a planned "second-look" re-laparotomy has been popular in the past, it is no longer recommended to diagnose tertiary peritonitis. Computed tomography (CT) is utilized when a postoperative patient with peritonitis fails to improve (especially when fever and leukocytosis are present), or manifests continued or worsening organ dysfunction.[182,185,186] If a localized fluid collection suspicious for an abscess is identified, percutaneous drainage is preferred. Some patients with focal signs of peritonitis may need to undergo re-laparotomy, but imaging usually demonstrates the feasibility of nonoperative management as a primary tactic. Supportive care with ongoing organ support and directed antimicrobial therapy is essential.

NOSOCOMIAL DIARRHEA

Nosocomial diarrhea is defined as developing after 3 days of hospitalization. The incidence of nosocomial diarrhea varies between 6% and 30% of hospitalized patients and is most common in ICUs and geriatric wards.[187] Diarrhea can be caused by medications that affect gut mucosa such as chemotherapy, anti-inflammatory agents, and agents that increase gastrointestinal motility. Nosocomial diarrhea related to noroviruses, rotaviruses, and adenoviruses has been reported.[188] Whereas antibiotic use and infectious causes explain some cases of nosocomial diarrhea, the most common cause of nosocomial diarrhea is the enterotoxin-producing *Clostridium difficile*, which may be responsible for up to 10%–20% of all cases. Other bacteria suspected to cause antibiotic-associated diarrhea include *S. aureus*, *C. perfringens*, and *K. oxytoca*,[189] but because these bacteria are part of normal fecal flora of healthy adults, a causative role in antibiotic-associated diarrhea has not been established firmly.

Clostridium difficile

The clinical spectrum of *C. difficile*-associated disease (CDAD) varies widely, ranging from an asymptomatic carrier state to life-threatening full-thickness pan-colitis.[190,191] There has been a recent dramatic increase in the incidence of *C. difficile* infections in US hospitals, from 30 to 40 cases per100,000 admissions in 2001, to 84 per 100,000 in 2005.[192] Furthermore, CDAD has been occurring with increased severity and virulence, due to the recent emergence of a epidemic strain characterized as restriction enzyme analysis type BI, North American Pulsed-Field Type 1 (NAP1), and PCR ribotype 027, or NAP1/BI/027.[193]

Antibiotic use alters gut microbiota and proliferation of *C. difficile*. However, for colitis to develop, the bacteria must attach to colonic mucosal cells to which nonpathogenic bacteria are normally adherent. Even though binding sites may be freed by antibiotic use that inhibits growth of normal fecal flora, *C. difficile* bacteria must also move through a dense mucus layer before attachment can occur.[194] Once attachment occurs, then toxins A and B (TcdA and TcdB) are produced, potent enzymes that damage mucosa by causing cytoskeletal disorganization. In addition to TcdA and TcdB, the hypervirulent strain NAP1/BI/027 produces the binary toxin *C. difficile* transferase (CDT), and lacks a regulatory protein (tcdC) that suppresses toxin production, allowing elaboration of 10-fold more toxin than wild-type strains.[194] The NAP1/B1/027 strain also is resistant to most fluoroquinolones, a pattern not seen before 2001. Moreover, subinhibitory concentrations of clindamycin, ampicillin, metronidazole, and vancomycin can enhance *C. diffiicle* colonization, spore germination, vegetative cell growth, and toxin production.[195-198]

The diagnosis of CDAD must be suspected in any patient who has recently (<2 months) been exposed to antibiotics. The clinical syndrome of CDAD is so varied that the presence or absence of any one clinical sign or symptom is unreliable to establish the diagnosis, including the presence of diarrhea (ileus may be present in severe cases).[191,199,200] The best test for diagnosis, a cell culture cytotoxin assay that has reported sensitivity of 94% and specificity of 99%, has a turnaround time of 24–48 hours, and is expensive.[191] Stool culture, although more sensitive, allows the recovery of bacteria for typing but does not allow identification of toxin production *in vivo*, and also takes 24–48 hours for results, and therefore is used seldom. Enzyme immunoassays have been used routinely for diagnosis because they screen for the presence of toxin, most notably TcdA, and are available quickly (within 4 hours). However, sensitivity is low (40%–75%). One method used increasingly is to screen a fresh stool sample using the common-antigen (glutamate dehydrogenase [GDH]) test. Because *C. difficile* produces GDH constitutively, the test is sensitive, can be completed rapidly (<1 hour), and is inexpensive.[201] Samples that screen positive can then undergo testing by a toxin assay, because the GDH assay only identifies the likely presence of *C. difficile*, and not whether toxin is produced. False-negative tests are thus rare.

In some cases, alternative diagnostic methods may be used.[191,201] Colonoscopy may identify mucosal changes, especially the formation of pseudomembranes, which are nonspecific and present in about one-half of cases. Sigmoidoscopy may miss disease confined to the ascending colon (up to 20% of cases). Moreover, endoscopy should be used cautiously with suspected toxic megacolon, as perforation may occur.

CT may identify suggestive findings, and may be used when other etiologies of abdominal infection must be ruled out. Characteristic CT features after oral and intravenous contrast include colon wall thickening, pericolic stranding, the "accordion sign," the "double-halo sign" (also known as the "target sign"), and ascites.[202] Wall thickening may be severe; "thumb-printing" and near-total occlusion of the lumen may be identified. The accordion sign shows oral contrast with high attenuation in the colonic lumen alternating with inflamed mucosa with low attenuation. The double-halo

TABLE 54.9

PATHOGENESIS OF TERTIARY PERITONITIS

Degree of bacterial contamination-bacterial inoculum
Virulence and synergy of involved species
Presence of adjuvants supporting microbial growth:
Intestinal contents, foreign material (barium), fibrin, blood
Adequacy of host response to infection
Appropriateness of medical interventions, especially surgical source control

sign shows varying degrees of attenuation attributable to mucosal hyperemia and submucosal inflammation after intravenous contrast. There should be no small bowel involvement; *C. difficile* is typically restricted to the colon.

Treatment. Treatment of *C. difficile* should be confined to symptomatic disease and distinguished between mild and severe manifestations.[202-205] Whereas oral metronidazole and oral vancomycin have generally similar efficacy, metronidazole has been preferred for initial therapy owing to lower cost and decreased likelihood of emergence of vancomycin-resistant enterococci.[203] However vancomycin was more effective for severe disease (97% vs. 76% for metronidazole) in a randomized trial, while in mild disease the antibiotics had similar outcomes.[206] The crucial element in therapy is delivery of drug to the lumen of the colon, where it can eradicate *C. difficile*.[206] Oral vancomycin is not absorbed and reaches colon intraluminal concentrations more than 100-fold higher than the MIC for *C. difficile*. Normally, oral metronidazole is absorbed completely by the proximal gut and does not appear in feces. However, in the presence of decreased transit time associated with diarrhea, metronidazole does appear in the stool.[201] Vancomycin enemas have been recommended in cases where ileus is present, but drug may still be delivered inadequately to the proximal colon. Repopulation of fecal flora with stool enemas is marginally effective and decidedly unattractive. The use of probiotic therapy is unproved, and there is concern that systemic illness may ensue in the setting of damaged mucosal barriers seen with CDAD.

In patients with severe CDAD, a total abdominal colectomy may be indicated.[203-207] Absolute indications for surgical intervention have not been determined, and advanced surgical judgment is required to balance appropriateness and timing of colectomy. Development of organ dysfunction, signs of hypoperfusion, and the need for vasoactive agents to support blood pressure are signs associated with mortality, therefore as predictors of the need for surgery, they manifest too late.[204,207] Neither any specific degree of leukocytosis, serum [lactate], nor any combination of clinical signs and symptoms has been validated prospectively to inform surgical decision-making. Retrospective data suggest that a white blood cell count $>50 \times 10^9/L$, [lactate] >5 mmol/L, and vasopressor use are associated with a high mortality rate when compared with WBC $< 20 \times 10^9/L$, [lactate] <2.1, and no use of vasopressors.[208] If surgery is performed, total abdominal colectomy is the procedure of choice, because segmental resection has been associated with increased mortality.[204-208] One author has suggested laparoscopic creation of an ileostomy as an alternative to colectomy,[209] allowing instillation of medication directly into the bowel and ameliorating the problem of impaired colonic transit due to ileus and profound mucosal edema, but this approach is unvalidated.

References

1. Edwards JR, Peterson KD, Mu Y, et al. National Healthcare Safety Network (NHSN) report, data summary for 2006 through 200, issued December 2009. *Am J Infect Control*. 2009;37:783-805.
2. Centers for Disease Control and Prevention. Outline for healthcare associated infection surveillance. Available from: http://www.cdc.gov/nhsn/PDFS/OutlineForHAISurveillance.pdf ht. Accessed December 29, 2010.
3. Horan TC, Andrus M, Dudeck MA. CDC/NHSN surveillance definition of health care-associated infection and criteria for specific types of infections in the acute care setting. *Am J Infect Control*. 2008;35:309-332.
4. Fry DE, Pine M, Jones BL, et al. Patient characteristics and the occurrence of never events. *Arch Surg*. 2010;145:148-151.
5. Angus DC, Linde-Zwirble WT, Lidicker J, et al. Epidemiology of severe sepsis in the United States: analysis of incidence, outcome, and associated costs of care. *Crit Care Med*. 2001;29:1303-1310.
6. Martin GS, Mannino DM, Eaton S, et al. The epidemiology of sepsis in the United States from 1979 through 2000. *N Engl J Med*. 2003;348:1546-1554.
7. Vincent JL, Sakr Y, Sprung CL, et al. Sepsis in European intensive care units: results of the SOAP study. *Crit Care Med*. 2006;34:344-353.
8. Alberti C, Brun-Buisson C, Burchardi H, et al. Epidemiology of sepsis and infection in ICU patients from an international multicentre cohort study. *Intensive Care Med*. 2002;28:108-121.
9. Sopena N, Sabrià M, et al. Multicenter study of hospital-acquired pneumonia in non-ICU patients. *Chest*. 2005;127:213-219.
10. Warren DK, Shukla SJ, Oslen MA, et al. Outcome and attributable cost of ventilator-associated pneumonia among intensive care unit patients in a suburban medical center. *Crit Care Med*. 2003;31:1312-1317.
11. Safdar N, Cameron D, Collard HR, et al. Clinical and economic consequences of ventilator-associated pneumonia: a systematic review. *Crit Care Med*. 2005;33:2184-2193.
12. American Thoracic Society. Guidelines for the management of adult with hospital-acquired, ventilator-associated and healthcare-associated pneumonia. *Am J Respir Crit Care Med*. 2005;171:388-416.
13. Metheny NA, Clouse RE, Chang Y, et al. Tracheobronchial aspiration in critically ill tube-fed patients: frequency, outcomes and risk factors. *Crit Care Med*. 2006;34:1007-1015.
14. Howard LSGE, Sillis M, Pasteur MC, et al. Microbiological profile of community-acquired pneumonia in adults over the last 20 years. *J Infect*. 2005;50:107-113.
15. Chastre J. Antimicrobial treatment of hospital-acquired pneumonia. *Infect Dis Clin North Am*. 2003;17:727-737.
16. Park DR. The microbiology of ventilator-associated pneumonia. *Respir Care*. 2005;50:742-765.
17. Rupp ME, Fey PD. Extended-spectrum beta-lactamase (ESBL)-producing *Enterobacteraceae*: considerations for diagnosis, prevention and drug treatment. *Drugs*. 2003;63:353-365.
18. Colodner R. Extended-spectrum beta-lactamases: a challenge for clinical microbiologists and infection control specialists. *Am J Infect Control*. 2005;33:104-107.
19. Rello J, Ollendorf DA, Oster G, et al. Epidemiology and outcomes of ventilator-associated pneumonia in a large US database. *Chest*. 2002;122:2115-2121.
20. Zavaski AP, Barth AL, Fernandes AF, et al. Reappraisal of *Pseudomonas aeruginosa* hospital-acquired pneumonia in the era of metallo-β-lactamase-mediated multidrug resistance: a prospective, observational study. *Crit Care*. 2006;10:R114-R120.
21. Scott P, Deye G, Srinivasan A, et al. An outbreak of multidrug-resistant *Acinetobacter baumannii-caloaceticus* complex infection in the US military health care system associated with military operations in Iraq. *Clin Infect Dis*. 2007;44:1577-1584.
22. Maragakis LL, Perl TM. *Acinetobacter baumannii*: epidemiology, antimicrobial resistance and treatment options. *Clin Infect Dis*. 2008;46:1254-1263.
23. Garnacho-Montero J, Ortiz-Leyba C, Fernandez-Hinojosa E, et al. *Acinetobacter baumannii* ventilator-associated pneumonia: epidemiological and clinical findings. *Intensive Care Med*. 2005;31:649-655.
24. Bonomo RA, Szabo D. Mechanisms of multidrug resistance in *Acinetobacter* species and *Pseudomonas aeruginosa*. *Clin Infect Dis*. 2006;43(suppl 2):49-56.
25. Arozullah AM, Daley J, Henderson WG, et al. Multifactorial risk index for predicting postoperative respiratory failure in men after major noncardiac surgery: The National Veterans Administration Surgical Quality Improvement Program. *Ann Surg*. 2000;232:242-253.
26. Johnson RM, Arozullah AM, Neumayer L, et al. Multivariable predictors of postoperative respiratory failure after general and vascular surgery: results from the patient safety in surgery study. *J Am Coll Surg*. 2007;204:1188-1198.
27. Bird D, Zambuto A, O'Donnell C, et al. Adherence to ventilator-associated pneumonia bundle and incidence of ventilator-associated pneumonia in the surgical intensive care unit. *Arch Surg*. 2010;145:465-470.
28. Jain M, Miller L, Belt D, et al. Decline in ICU adverse events, nosocomial infections and cost through a quality improvement initiative focusing on teamwork and culture change. *Qual Saf Health Care*. 2006;15:235-239.
29. Qaseem A, Snow V, Fitteman N, et al. Risk assessment for and strategies to reduce perioperative pulmonary complications for patients undergoing noncardiothoracic surgery: a guideline from the American College of Physicians. *Ann Intern Med*. 2006;144:575-580.
30. Bluman LG, Masca L, Newman N, et al. Preoperative smoking habits and postoperative pulmonary complications. *Chest*. 1998;113:883-889.
31. Moller AM, Maaloe R, Pedersen T. Postoperative intensive care admittance: the role of tobacco smoking. *Acta Anaesthesiol Scand*. 2001;45:345-348.
32. Nakagawa M, Tanaka H, Tsukuma H, et al. Relationship between the duration of the preoperative smoke-free period and the incidence of postoperative pulmonary complications after pulmonary surgery. *Chest*. 2001;120:705-710.
33. Warner MA, Offord KP, Warner ME, et al. Role of preoperative cessation of smoking and other factors in postoperative pulmonary complications: a blinded prospective study of coronary artery bypass patients. *Mayo Clin Proc*. 1989;64:609-616.
34. Rodgers A, Walker N, Schug S, et al. Reduction of postoperative mortality and morbidity with epidural or spinal anaesthesia: results from an overview of randomized trials. *BMJ*. 2000;321:1493-1504.
35. Drakulovic MB, Torres A, Bauer TT, et al. Supine body position as a risk factor for nosocomial pneumonia in mechanically ventilated patients: a randomized trial. *Lancet*. 1999;354:1851-1858.

36. Ferrer M, Torsten TB, Torres A, et al. Effect of nasogastric tube size on gastroesophageal reflux and microaspiration in intubated patients. *Ann Intern Med.* 1999;130:991-994.
37. Holzapfel L, Chevert S, Madinier G, et al. Influence of long-term oro- or nasotracheal intubation on nosocomial maxillary sinusitis and pneumonia: results of a prospective, randomized clinical trial. *Crit Care Med.* 1993;8:1132-1138.
38. Magne N, Marcy PY, Foa C, et al. Comparison between nasogastric tube feeding and percutaneous fluoroscopic gastrostomy tube feeding in advanced head and neck cancer patients. *Eur Arch Otorhinolaryngol.* 2001;258:89-92.
39. Dodek P, Keenan S, Cook D, et al. Evidence-based clinical practice guideline for the prevention of ventilator-associated pneumonia. *Ann Intern Med.* 2004;141:305-313.
40. van Nieuwenhoven CA, Vandenbroucke-Graul SC, van Tiel FH, et al. Feasibility and effects of the semirecumbent position to prevent ventilator-associated pneumonia: a randomized study. *Crit Care Med.* 2006;34:396-402.
41. Kollef MH. Role of selective digestive tract decontamination on mortality and respiratory tract infections: a meta-analysis. *Chest.* 1994;105:1101-1108.
42. Cook D, Heyland D, Griffith D, et al. Risk factors for clinically important upper gastrointestinal bleeding in patients requiring mechanical ventilation; Canadian Critical Care Trials Group. *Crit Care Med.* 1999;27:2812-2817.
43. Cook D, Griffith LE, Walter SD, et al. The attributable mortality and length of intensive care unit stay of clinically important gastrointestinal bleeding in critically ill patients. *Crit Care.* 2001;5:368-375.
44. Cook D, Guyhatt G, Marshall J, et al. A comparison of sucralfate and ranitidine for the prevention of upper gastrointestinal bleeding in patients requiring mechanical ventilation. *N Engl J Med.* 1998;338:791-797.
45. de Jonge E, Schultz MJ, Spanjaard L, et al. Effects of selective decontamination of digestive tract on mortality and acquisition of resistant bacteria in intensive care: a randomized controlled trial. *Lancet.* 2003;362:1011-1016.
46. Ross A, Crumpler J. The impact of an evidence-based practice education program on the role of oral care in the prevention of ventilator-associated pneumonia. *ICCN.* 2007;23:132-136.
47. Segers P, Speekenbrink RGH, Ubbink DT, et al. Prevention of nosocomial infection in cardiac surgery by decontamination of the nasopharynx and oropharynx with chlorhexidine gluconate: a randomized controlled trial. *JAMA.* 2006;296:2460-2466.
48. Chlebicki MP, Safdar N. Topical chlorhexidine for prevention of ventilator-associated pneumonia: a meta-analysis. *Crit Care Med.* 2007;35:595-602.
49. Cook D, Guyhatt G, Marshall J, et al. A comparison of sucralfate and ranitidine for the prevention of upper gastrointestinal bleeding in patients requiring mechanical ventilation. *N Engl J Med.* 1998;338:791-797.
50. Ramirez P, Ferrer M, Torres A. Prevention measures for ventilator-associated pneumonia: a new focus on the endotracheal tube. *Curr Opin Infect Dis.* 2007;20:190-197.
51. Holzapfel L, Chastang C, Demingeon G, et al. A randomized study assessing the systematic search for maxillary sinusitis in nasotracheally mechanically ventilated patients. Influence of nosocomial maxillary sinusitis on the occurrence of ventilator-associated pneumonia. *Am J Respir Crit Care Med.* 1999;159;695-701.
52. Holzapfel L, Chevret S, Madinier G, et al. Influence of long-term oro- or nasotracheal intubation on nosocomial maxillary sinusitis and pneumonia: results of a prospective, randomized, clinical trial. *Crit Care Med.* 1993;21:1132-1138.
53. Salord F, Gaussorgues P, Marti-Flich J, et al. Nosocomial maxillary sinusitis during mechanical ventilation: a prospective comparison of orotracheal versus the nasotracheal route for intubation. *Intensive Care Med.* 1990;16:390-393.
54. Kollef MH, Skubas NJ, Sundt TM. A randomized clinical trial of continuous aspiration of subglottic secretions in cardiac surgery patients. *Chest.* 1999;116:1339-1346.
55. Lorente L, Lecuona M, Jiménez A, et al. Influence of an endotracheal tube with polyurethane cuff and subglottic secretion drainage on pneumonia. *Am J Respir Crit Care Med.* 2007;176:1079-1083.
56. Niël-Weise BS, Snoeren RIMM, van den Broed DJ. Policies for endotracheal suctioning of patients receiving mechanical ventilation: a systematic review of randomized controlled trials. *Infect Control Hosp Epidemiol.* 2007;28:178-184.
57. Combes P, Fauvage B, Oleyer C. Nosocomial pneumonia in mechanically ventilated patients, a prospective randomized evaluation of the Stericath closed suctioning system. *Crit Care Med.* 2000;26:878-882.
58. Lorente M, Lecuona M, Martin MM, et al. Ventilator-associated pneumonia using a closed versus open tracheal suction system. *Crit Care Med.* 2005;33:115-119.
59. Topeli A, Harmanci A, Cetinkaya Y, et al. Comparison of the effect of closed versus open endotracheal suction systems on the development of ventilator-associated pneumonia. *J Hosp Infect.* 2004;58:14-19.
60. Gastmeier P, Geffers C. Prevention of ventilator-associated pneumonia: analysis of studies published since 2004. *J Hosp Infect.* 2007;67:1-8.
61. Kollef MH, Shapiro SD, Fraser VJ, et al. Mechanical ventilation with and without 7-day circuit changes, a randomized controlled trial. *Ann Intern Med.* 1995;123:168-174.
62. Dreyfuss D, Djedaini K, Weber P, et al. Prospective study of nosocomial pneumonia and of patient and circuit colonization during mechanical ventilation with circuit changes every 48 hours versus no change. *Am Rev Respir Dis.* 1991;143:738-743.
63. Long MN, Wickstrom G, Grimes A, et al. Prospective, randomized study of ventilator-associated pneumonia in patients with one versus three ventilator circuit changes per week. *Infect Control Hosp Epidemiol.* 1996;17:14-19.
64. Safdar N, Crnich CJ, Redlich U. The pathogenesis of ventilator-associated pneumonia: its relevance to developing effective strategies for prevention. *Respir Care.* 2005;50:725-739.
65. Dreyfuss D, Djedaini K, Gros I, et al. Mechanical ventilation with heated humidifiers or heat and moisture exchangers: effects on patient colonization and incidence of nosocomial pneumonia. *Am J Respir Crit Care Med.* 1995;151:986-992.
66. Lacherade JC, Auburtin M, Cerf C, et al. Impact of humidification systems of ventilator-associated pneumonia. *Am J Respir Crit Care Med.* 2005;172:1276-1282.
67. Boots R, George N, Faoagali J, et al. Double-heater-wire circuits and head- and moisture exchanger and the risk of ventilator-associated pneumonia. *Crit Care Med.* 2006;34:687-693.
68. Kress JP, Pohlman AS, O'Connor MF, et al. Daily interruption of sedative infusions in critically ill patients undergoing mechanical ventilation. *N Engl J Med.* 2000;342:1461-1477.
69. Schweickert WD, Gehlbach BK, Pohlman AS, et al. Daily interruption of sedative infusions and complications of critical illness in mechanically ventilated patients. *Crit Care Med.* 2004;32:1272-1276.
70. Marelich GP, Murin S, Battistella F, et al. Protocol weaning of mechanical ventilation in medical and surgical patients by respiratory care practitioners and nurses: effect on weaning time and incidence of ventilator-associated pneumonia. *Chest.* 2000;118:459-467.
71. Girard TD, Kress JP, Fuchs BD, et al. Efficacy and safety of a paired sedation and ventilator weaning protocol for mechanically ventilated patients in intensive care (awakening and breathing controlled trial): a randomized controlled trial. *Lancet.* 2008;371:126-134.
72. Smetana GW, Lawrence VA, Cornell JE. Preoperative pulmonary risk stratification for noncardiothoracic surgery: a systematic review for the American College of Physicians. *Ann Intern Med.* 2006;144:581-595.
73. Freitas ERFS, Soares BGO, Cardoso JR, et al. Incentive spirometry for preventing pulmonary complications after coronary artery bypass graft. *Cochrane Collab.* 2007 Jul 18;(3):CD004466;1-18.
74. National Healthcare Safety Network. Criteria for defining nosocomial pneumonia. http://www.cdc.gov/nhsn/PDFs/pscManual/17pscNosInfDef_current.pdf. Accessed December 31,2010, Could replace footnote in table 54-3.
75. Andrews CP, Coalson JJ, Smith JD, et al. Diagnosis of nosocomial bacterial pneumonia in acute, diffuse lung injury. *Chest.* 1981;80:254-248.
76. Bell RC, Coalson JJ, Smith JD, et al. Multiple organ system failure and infection in adult respiratory distress syndrome. *Ann Intern Med.* 1983;99:293-298.
77. Niederman MS. The clinical diagnosis of ventilator-associated pneumonia. *Respir Care.* 2005;50:788-796.
78. Pugin J, Auckenthaler R, Mill N, et al. Diagnosis of ventilator-associated pneumonia by batcteriologic analysis of bronchoscopic and non-bronchoscopic "blind" bronchoalveolar lavage. *Am Rev Respir Dis.* 1991;143:1121-1129.
79. Luyt CE, Chastre J, Fagon JY, et al. Value of the clinical pulmonary infection score for the identification and management of ventilator-associated pneumonia. *Intensive Care Med.* 2004;30:844-852.
80. Fagon, J. Hospital acquired pneumonia: diagnostic strategies: lessons from clinical trials. *Infect Dis Clin North Am.* 2003;17:717-726.
81. Singh N, Rogers P, Atwood C, et al. Short-course empiric antibiotic therapy for patients with pulmonary infiltrates in the intensive-care unit: a proposed solution for indiscriminate antibiotic use. *Am J Respir Crit Care Med.* 2000;162:505-511.
82. Mueller EW, Croce MA, Boucher BA, et al. Repeat bronchoalveolar lavage to guide antibiotic duration for ventilator-associated pneumonia. *J Trauma.* 2007;63:1329-1337.
83. Lode H, Raffenberg M, Erbes R, et al. Nosocomial pneumonia: epidemiology, pathogenesis, diagnosis, treatment and prevention. *Curr Opin Infect Dis.* 2000;13:377-384.
84. Heyland DK, Cook DJ, Marshall J, et al. The clinical utility of invasive diagnostic techniques in the setting of ventilator-associated pneumonia. *Chest.* 1999;115:1076-1084.
85. Timsit JF, Cheval C, Gachot B, et al. Usefulness of a strategy based on bronchoscopy with direct examination of bronchoalveolar lavage fluid in the initial antibiotic therapy of suspected ventilator-associated pneumonia. *Intensive Care Med.* 2001;27:640-647.
86. Ruiz M, Torres A, Ewig S, et al. Noninvasive versus invasive microbial investigation in ventilator-associated pneumonia: evaluation of outcome. *Am J Respir Crit Care Med.* 2000;162:119-125.
87. The Canadian Critical Care Trials Group. A randomized trial of diagnostic techniques for ventilator-associated pneumonia. *N Engl J Med.* 2006;355:2619-2630.
88. Fagon JY, Chastre J, Wolff M, et al. Invasive and non-invasive strategies for management of suspected ventilator-associated pneumonia: a randomized controlled trial. *Ann Intern Med.* 2000;132:621-630.

89. Croce MA, Fabian TC, Schurr MJ, et al. Using bronchoalveolar lavage to distinguish nosocomial pneumonia from systemic inflammatory response syndrome: a prospective analysis. *J Trauma*. 1995;39:1134-1139.
90. Croce MA, Fabian TC, Waddle-Smith L, et al. Utility of Gram's Stain and efficacy of quantitative culture for posttraumatic pneumonia: a prospective study. *Ann Surg*. 1998;227:743-751.
91. Shorr AF, Sherner JH, Jackson WL, et al. Invasive approaches to the diagnosis of ventilator-associated pneumonia: a meta-analysis. *Crit Care Med*. 2005;33:46-53.
92. Ioanas M, Ferrer M, Cavalcanti M, et al. Causes and predictors of nonresponse to treatment of intensive care unit-acquired pneumonia. *Crit Care Med*. 2004;32:938-945.
93. Mueller EW, Hanes SD, Croce MA, et al. Effect from multiple episodes of inadequate empiric antibiotic therapy for ventilator-associated pneumonia on morbidity and mortality among critically ill trauma patients. *J Trauma*. 2005;58:94-101.
94. Garcia JCP, Filho OFF, Grion CMC, et al. Impact of the implementation of a therapeutic guideline on the treatment of nosocomial pneumonia acquired in the intensive care unit of a university hospital. *J Bras Pneumol*. 2007;33:175-184.
95. Kashuba ADM, Nafziger AN, Drusano GL, et al. Optimizing aminoglycoside therapy for nosocomial pneumonia caused by gram-negative bacteria. *Antimicrob Agents Chemother*. 1999;43:623-629.
96. Wall RJ, Ely EW, Talbot TR, et al. Evidence-based algorithms for diagnosing and treating ventilator-associated pneumonia. *J Hosp Med*. 2008;3:409-422.
97. Mosier MJ, Pham TN. American Burn Association Practice guidelines for prevention, diagnosis, and treatment of ventilator-associated pneumonia (VAP) in burn patients. *J Burn Care Res*. 2009;30:910-928.
98. Morrow BM, Argent AC, Jeena PM, et al. Guideline for the diagnosis, prevention and treatment of paediatric ventilator-associated pneumonia. *S Afr Med J*. 2009;99(4 pt 2):255-267.
99. Song JH; Asian Hospital Acquired Pneumonia Working Group. Treatment recommendations of hospital-acquired pneumonia in Asian countries: first consensus report by the Asian HAP Working Group. *Am J Infect Control*. 2008;36(4 suppl):S83-S92.
100. Muscedere J, Dodek P, Keenan S, et al.; VAP Guidelines Committee and the Canadian Critical Care Trials Group. Comprehensive evidence-based clinical practice guidelines for ventilator-associated pneumonia: diagnosis and treatment. *J Crit Care*. 2008;23:138-147.
101. Muscedere J, Dodek P, Keenan S, et al. VAP Guidelines Committee and the Canadian Critical Care Trials Group. Comprehensive evidence-based clinical practice guidelines for ventilator-associated pneumonia: prevention. *J Crit Care*. 2008;23:126-317.
102. Minei JP, Nathens AB, West M, et al. Inflammation and the host response to injury large scale collaborative research program investigators. Inflammation and the host response to injury, a large-scale collaborative project: patient-oriented research core—standard operating procedures for clinical care. II. Guidelines for prevention, diagnosis and treatment of ventilator-associated pneumonia (VAP) in the trauma patient. *J Trauma*. 2006;60:1106-1113.
103. Haque NZ, Cahuayme Zuniga L, Peyrani P, et al. Relationship of vancomycin MIC to mortality in patients with methicillin-resistant *Staphylococcus aureus* hospital-acquired, ventilator-associated and healthcare-associated pneumonia. *Chest*. 2010. [Epub ahead of print].
104. Steinkraus G, White R, Friedrich L. Vancomycin MIC creep in non-vancomycin-intermediate *Staphylococcus aureus* (VISA), vancomycin-susceptible clinical methicillin-resistant *S. aureus* (MRSA) blood isolates from 2001-05. *J Antimicrob Chemother*. 2007;60:788-794.
105. Wang G, Hindler JF, Ward KW, et al. Increased vancomycin MICs for *Staphylococcus aureus* clinical isolates from a university hospital during a 5-year period. *J Clin Microbiol*. 2006;44:3883-3886.
106. Adler J. The use of daptomycin for *Staphylococcus aureus* infections in critical care medicine. *Crit Care Clin*. 2008;24:349-363.
107. French GL. Bactericidal agents in the treatment of MRSA infections—the potential role of daptomycin. *J Antimicrob Chemother*. 2006;58:1107-1117.
108. Shorr AF, Combes A, Kollef MH, et al. Methicillin-resistant *Staphylococcus aureus* prolongs intensive care unit stay in ventilator-associated pneumonia, despite initially appropriate antibiotic therapy. *Crit Care Med*. 2006;34:700-706.
109. Trouillet JL, Chastre J, Vuagnat A, et al. Ventilator-associated pneumonia caused by potentially drug-resistant bacteria. *Am J Respir Crit Care Med*. 1998;157:531-539.
110. Harris AD, McGregor JC, Johnson JA, et al. Risk factors for colonization with extended spectrum beta-lactamase-producing bacteria and intensive care unit admission. *Emerg Infect Dis*. 2007;13:1144-1149.
111. Michalopoulos A, Fotakis D, Virtzili S, et al. Aerosolized colistin as adjunctive treatment of ventilator-associated pneumonia due to multidrug-resistant gram-negative bacteria: a prospective study. *Respir Med*. 2008;102:407-412.
112. Rios FG, Luna CM, Maskin B, et al. Ventilator-associated pneumonia due to colistin susceptible-only microorganisms. *Eur Respir J*. 2007;30:307-313.
113. Linden PK, Paterson DL. Parenteral and inhaled colistin for treatment of ventilator-associated pneumonia. *Clin Infect Dis*. 2006;43(suppl 2):89-94.
114. Alvarez-Lerma F, Alvarez B, Luque P, et al. Empiric broad-spectrum antibiotic therapy of nosocomial pneumonia in the intensive care unit: a prospective, observational study. *Crit Care*. 2006;10:R78-R88.
115. Pieracci FM, Barie PS. Strategies in the prevention and management of ventilator-associated pneumonia. *Am Surg*. 2007;73:419-432.
116. Lynch JP. Combination antibiotic therapy is appropriate for nosocomial pneumonia in the intensive care unit. *Semin Respir Infect*. 1993;8:268-284.
117. Arbo MD, Snydman DR. Monotherapy is appropriate for nosocomial pneumonia in the intensive care unit. *Semin Respir Infect*. 1993;8:259-267.
118. Croce MA, Fabian TC, Stewart RM, et al. Empiric monotherapy versus combination therapy of nosocomial pneumonia in trauma patients. *J Trauma*. 1993;35:303-309.
119. Ibrahim EH, Ward S, Sherman G, et al. Experience with a clinical guideline for the treatment of ventilator-associated pneumonia. *Crit Care Med*. 2001;29:1109-1115.
120. Heyland DK, Dodek P, Muscedere J, et al. Randomized trial of combination versus monotherapy for the empiric treatment of suspected ventilator-associated pneumonia. *Crit Care Med*. 2008;36:737-744.
121. Garnacho-Montero J, Sa-Borges M, Sole-Violan J, et al. Optimal management therapy for *Pseudomonas aeruginosa* ventilator-associated pneumonia: an observational, multicenter study comparing monotherapy with combination antibiotic therapy. *Crit Care Med*. 2007;35:1888-1895.
122. Trouillet JL, Chastre J, Vuagnat A, et al. Ventilator-associated pneumonia caused by potentially drug-resistant bacteria. *Am J Respir Crit Care Med*. 1998;157:531-539.
123. Harris AD, McGregor JC, Johnson JA, et al. Risk factors for colonization with extended spectrum beta-lactamase-producing bacteria and intensive care unit admission. *Emerg Infect Dis*. 2007;13:1144-1149.
124. Rello J, Vidaur L, Sandiumenge A, et al. De-escalation therapy in ventilator-associated pneumonia. *Crit Care Med*. 2004;32:2183-2190.
125. Giantsou E, Liratzopoulos N, Efraimidou E, et al. De-escalation therapy rates are significantly higher by bronchoalveolar lavage than by tracheal aspiration. *Intensive Care Med*. 2007;33:1533-1540.
126. Chastre J, Wolff M, Fagon J, et al. Comparison of 8 vs. 15 days of antibiotic therapy for ventilator-associated pneumonia in adults. *JAMA*. 2003;290:2588-2598.
127. Combes A, Luyt C, Fagon J, et al. Early predictors for infection recurrence and death in patients with ventilator-associated pneumonia. *Crit Care Med*. 2007;35:146-154.
128. Tolentino-DelosReyes AF, Ruppert SD, Shiao SPK. Evidence-based practice: use of the ventilator bundle to prevent ventilator-associated pneumonia. *Am J Crit Care*. 2007;16:20-27.
129. Cocanour CS, Peninger M, Domonoske BD, et al. Decreasing ventilator-associated pneumonia in a trauma ICU. *J Trauma*. 2006;61:122-130.
130. Salahuddin N, Zafar A, Sukhyani L, et al. Reducing ventilator-associated pneumonia rates through a staff education programme. *J Hosp Infect*. 2004;57:223-227.
131. The Johns Hopkins Hospital Antibiotic Management Program, Treatment Recommendations for Adult Inpatients. Baltimore; 2007.
132. Melsen WG, Rovers MM, Bontan. Ventilator-associated pneumonia and mortality: A systematic review of observational studies. *Crit Care Med*. 2009;37:2709-2718.
133. Raad I, Hanna H, Maki DG. Intravascular catheter-related infections: advances in diagnosis, prevention, and management. *Lancet Infect Dis*. 2007;7:645-657.
134. Anonymous. Central Line-Associated Bloodstream Infection CLABSI event. http://www.cdc.gov/nhsn/PDFs/pscManual/4PSC_CLABScurrent.pdf. Accessed December 29, 2010.
135. Klevens RM, Edward JR, et al. Estimating health care-associated infections and deaths in U.S. hospitals, 2002. *Publ Heal Rep*. 2007;122:160-166.
136. O'Grady NP, Alexander M, Dellinger EP, et al. Guidelines for the prevention of intravascular catheter-related infections. *MMWR Morbid Mortal Wkly Rep*. 2002;51:1-29.
137. Maki DG, Weise CE, Sarafin HW. A semiquantitative culture method for identifying intravenous-catheter-related infection. *N Engl J Med*. 1977;296:1305-1309.
138. Safdar N, Fine JP, Maki DG. Meta-analysis: methods for diagnosing intravascular device-related bloodstream infection. *Ann Intern Med*. 2005;142:451-466.
139. Hidron AI, Edwards JR, Patel J, et al.; National Healthcare Safety Network Team; Participating National Healthcare Safety Network Facilities. *Infect Control Hosp Epidemiol*. 2008;29:996-1011.
140. O'Grady NP, Alexander M, Burns, MA, et al.; the Healthcare Infection Control Practices Advisory Committee (HICPAC). *Guidelines for the Prevention of Intravascular Catheter-Related Infections*; 2011. www.cdc.gov/hicpac/pdf/guidelines/bsi-guidelines-2011.pdf. Accessed April 14, 2011.
141. Coopersmith CM, Rebmann TL, Zack JE, et al. Effect of an education program on decreasing catheter-related bloodstream infections in the surgical intensive care unit. *Crit Care Med*. 2002;30:59-64.
142. Berenholtz SM, Pronovost PJ, Lipsett PA, et al. Eliminating catheter-related bloodstream infections in the intensive care unit. *Crit Care Med*. 2004;32:2014-2020.
143. Pronovost P, Needham D, Berenholtz S, et al. An intervention to decrease catheter-related bloodstream infections in the ICU. *N Engl J Med*. 2006;355:2725-2732. Erratum in *N Engl J Med*. 2007;356:2660.

144. Pronovost PJ, Goeschel CA, Colantuoni E, et al. Sustaining reductions in catheter related bloodstream infections in Michigan intensive care units: observational study. *BMJ*. 2010;340:309.
145. Walder J, Pittet D, Tramer MR. Prevention of bloodstream infections with central venous catheters treated with anti-infective agents depends on catheter type and insertion time: evidence from a meta-analysis. *Infect Control Hosp Epidemiol*. 2002;23:748-756.
146. Slobbe L, Doorduijn JK, Lugtenburg PJ, et al. Prevention of catheter-related bacteremia with a daily ethanol lock in patients with tunnelled catheters: a randomized, placebo-controlled trial. *PLoS One*. 2010;5:e10840.
147. Maiefski M, Rupp ME, Hermsen ED. Ethanol lock technique: review of the literature. *Infect Control Hosp Epidemiol*. 2009;30:1096-1108.
148. Abbas SA, Haloob IA, Taylor SL, et al. Effect of antimicrobial locks for tunneled hemodialysis catheters on bloodstream infection and bacterial resistance: a quality improvement report. *Am J Kidney Dis*. 2009;53:492-502.
149. Safdar N, Maki DG. Use of vancomycin containing lock or flush solutions for prevention of bloodstream infection associated with central venous access devices: a meta-analysis of prospective, randomized trials. *Clin Infect Dis*. 2006;43:474-484.
150. Carratala J, Niubo J, Fernandez-Sevilla A, et al. Randomized, double-blind trial of an antibiotic-lock technique for prevention of Gram-positive central venous catheter-related infection in neutropenic patients with cancer. *Antimicrob Agents Chemother*. 1999;43:2200-2204.
151. Garland JS, Alex CP, Henrickson KJ, et al. A vancomycin-heparin lock solution for prevention of nosocomial bloodstream infection in critically ill neonates with peripherally inserted central venous catheters: a prospective, randomized trial. *Pediatrics*. 2005;116:e198-e205.
152. Maki DG, Ringer M. Evaluation of dressing regimens for prevention of infection with peripheral intravenous catheters: gauze, a transparent polyurethane dressing, and an iodophor-transparent dressing. *JAMA*. 1987;258:2396-2403.
153. Maki DG, Stolz SS, Wheeler S, et al. A prospective, randomized trial of gauze and two polyurethane dressings for site care of pulmonary artery catheters: implications for catheter management. *Crit Care Med*. 1994;22:1729-1737.
154. Maki DG, Stolz SS, Wheeler S, et al. A prospective, randomized trial of gauze and two polyurethane dressings for site care of pulmonary artery catheters: Implications for catheter management. *Crit Care Med*. 1994;22:1729-1737.
155. Dickerson N, Horton P, Smith S, et al. Clinically significant central venous catheter infections in a community hospital. Association with type of dressing. *J Infect Dis*. 1989;160:720-721.
156. Conly JM, Grieves K, Peters B. A prospective, randomized study comparing transparent and dry gauze dressing for central venous catheters. *J Infect Dis*. 1989;159:310-319.
157. Hoffman KK, Weber DJ, Samsa GP, et al. Transparent polyurethane film as an intravenous catheter dressing: a meta-analysis of the infection risks. *JAMA*. 1992;267:2072-2076.
158. Maki DG, Mermel LA, Kluger D, et al. The Efficacy of a chlorhexidine-Impregnated sponge (Biopatch) for the prevention of intravascular catheter-related infection—a prospective, randomized, controlled, multicenter study [Abstract]. In: *Abstracts and Proceedings of the 40th Interscience Conference on Antimicrobial Agents and Chemotherapy, Toronto, ON, Canada*. September 17-20; 2000.
159. Garland JS, Alex CP, Mueller CD, et al. A randomized trial comparing povidone -odine to a chlorhexidine gluconate-impregnated dressing for prevention of central venous catheter infections in neonates. *Pediatrics*. 2001;107:1431-1436.
160. Levy I, Katz J, Solter E, et al. Chlorhexidine-impregnated dressing for prevention of colonization of central venous catheters in infants and children. *Pediatr Infect Dis J*. 2005;24:676-679.
161. Ho KM, Litton E. Use of chlorhexidine-impregnated dressing to prevent vascular and epidural catheter colonization and infection: a meta-analysis. *J Antimicrob Chemother*. 2006;58:281-287.
162. Timsit JF, Schwebel C, Bouadma L, et al. Chlorhexidine-impregnated sponges and less frequent dressing changes for prevention of catheter-related infections in critically ill adults. *JAMA*. 2009;301:1231-1241.
163. Rasero L, Degl'Innocenti M, Mocali M, et al. Comparison of two different time interval protocols for central venous catheter dressing in bone marrow transplant patients: results of a randomized, multicenter study. *Haematologica*. 2000;85:275-279.
164. Anonymous. Catheter-Associated Urinary Tract Infections. (CAUTI) event. http://www.cdc.gov/nhsn/pdfs/pscManual/7pscCAUTIcurrent.pdf. Accessed December 29, 2010.
165. Lo E, Nicolle L, Classen D, et al. Strategies to prevent catheter-associated urinary tract infections in acute care hospitals. *Infect Control Hosp Epidemiol*. 2008;29(suppl 1):S41-S50.
166. Smith PW, Bennett G, Bradley S, et al. SHEA/APIC guideline: infection prevention and control in the long-term care facility. *Am J Infect Control*. 2008;36:504-535.
167. Tenke P, Kovacs B, Bjerklund Johansen TE, et al. European and Asian guidelines on management and prevention of catheter-associated urinary tract infections. *Int J Antimicrob Agents*. 2008;31(suppl 1):S68-S78.
168. Yokoe DS, Mermel LA, Anderson DJ, et al. A compendium of strategies to prevent healthcare-associated infections in acute care hospitals. *Infect Control Hosp Epidemiol*. 2008; 29(suppl 1):S12-S21.
169. Lin K, Fajardo K. Screening for asymptomatic bacteriuria in adults: evidence for the U.S. Preventive Services Task Force reaffirmation recommendation statement. *Ann Intern Med*. 2008;149:W20-W24.
170. Hooton TM, Bradley SF, Cardenas DD, et al.; Infectious Diseases Society of America. Diagnosis, prevention, and treatment of catheter-associated urinary tract infection in adults: 2009 International Clinical Practice Guidelines from the Infectious Diseases Society of America. *Clin Infect Dis*. 2010;50:625-663.
171. Gould CV, Umscheid CA, Agarwal RK, et al. Healthcare Infection Control Practices Advisory Committee. Guideline for prevention of catheter-associated urinary tract infections 2009. *Infect Control Hosp Epidemiol*. 2010;31:319-326.
172. Nicolle LE. Urinary tract infections in the elderly. *Clin Geriatr Med*. 2009;25:423-436.
173. Trautner BW. Management of catheter-associated urinary tract infection. *Curr Opin Infect Dis*. 2010;23:76-82.
174. Golob JF Jr, Claridge JA, Sando MJ. Fever and leukocytosis in critically ill trauma patients: it's not the urine. *Surg Infect*. 2008;9:49-56.
175. Wald HL, Ma A, Bratzler DW, et al. Indwelling urinary catheter use in the postoperative period: analysis of the national surgical infection prevention project data. *Arch Surg*. 2008;143:551-557.
176. Salo J, Sevander JJ, Tapiainen T, et al. Biofilm formation by *Escherichia coli* isolated from patients with urinary tract infections. *Clin Nephrol*. 2009;71:501-507.
177. Baraboutis IG, Tsagalou EP, Lepinski JL, et al. Primary *Staphylococcus aureus* urinary tract infection: the role of undetected hematogenous seeding of the urinary tract. *Eur J Clin Microbiol Infect Dis*. 2010;29:1095-1101.
178. Pfefferkorn U, Lea S, Moldenhauer J, et al. Antibiotic prophylaxis at urinary catheter removal prevents urinary tract infections: a prospective randomized trial. *Ann Surg*. 2009;249:573-575.
179. Weiss G, Meyer F, Lippert H. Infectiological diagnostic problems in tertiary peritonitis. *Langenbecks Arch Surg*. 2006;391:473-482.
180. Menichetti F, Sganga G. Definition and classification of intra-abdominal infections. *J Chemother*. 2009;21(suppl 1):3-4.
181. de Ruiter J, Weel J, Manusama E, et al. The epidemiology of intra-abdominal flora in critically ill patients with secondary and tertiary abdominal sepsis. *Infection*. 2009;37:522-527.
182. Chromik AM, Meiser A, Hölling J. Identification of patients at risk for development of tertiary peritonitis on a surgical intensive care unit. *J Gastrointest Surg*. 2009;13:1358-1367.
183. Evans HL, Raymond DP, Pelletier SJ, et al. Tertiary peritonitis (recurrent diffuse or localized disease) is not an independent predictor of mortality in surgical patients with intraabdominal infection. *Surg Infect*. 2001;2:255-263.
184. Malangoni MA. Evaluation and management of tertiary peritonitis. *Am Surg*. 2000;66:157-161.
185. Buijk SE, Bruining HA. Future directions in the management of tertiary peritonitis. *Intensive Care Med*. 2002;28:1024-1029.
186. Barie PS, Hydo LJ, Eachempati SR. Longitudinal outcomes of intra-abdominal infections complicated by critical illness. *Surg Infect*. 2004;5:365-373.
187. Bauer TM, Kist M, Daschner F, et al. Nosocomial diarrhoea. *Dtsch Med Wochenschr*. 2001;126:1431-1434.
188. Musher DM, Musher BL. Clinical practice: contagious acute gastrointestinal infections. *N Engl J Med*. 2004;351:2417-2427.
189. Gorkiewicz G. Nosocomial and antibiotic-associated diarrhoea caused by organisms other than *Clostridium difficile*. *Int J Antimicrob Agents*. 2009;33(suppl 1):S37-S541.
190. Bartlett JG. Historical perspectives on studies of *C difficile* and *C. difficile* infection. *Clin Infect Dis*. 2008;46:S4-S11.
191. Bartlett JG, Gerding DN. Clinical recognition and diagnosis of *Clostridium difficile* infection. *Clin Infect Dis*. 2008;46(suppl 1):S12-S518.
192. Ricciardi R, Rothenberger DA, Madoff RD, et al. Increasing prevalence and severity of *Clostridium difficile* colitis in hospitalized patients in the United States, *Arch Surg*. 2007;142:624-631.
193. McDonald LC, Killgore GE, Thompson A, et al. An epidemic, toxic gene-variant strain of *Clostridium difficile*. *N Engl J Med*. 2005;353:2433-2441.
194. Gould CV, McDonald LC. Bench-to-bedside review: *Clostridium difficile* colitis. *Crit Care*. 2008;12:203.
195. Saxton K, Baines SD, Freeman J, et al. Effects of exposure of *Clostridium difficile* PCR ribotype 027 and 001 to fluoroquinolones in a human gut model. *Antimicrob Agents Chemother*. 2009;53(2):412-420. Epub 2008 Aug 18.
196. Denève C, Delom'enie C, Barc MC, et al. Antibiotics involved in *Clostridium difficile*-associated disease increase colonization factor gene expression. *J Med Microbiol*. 2008;57:732-738.
197. Denève C, Bouttier S, Dupuy B, et al. Effects of subinhibitory concentrations of antibiotics on colonization factor expression by moxifloxacin-susceptible and moxifloxacin-resistant *Clostridium difficile* strains. *Antimicrob Agents Chemother*. 2009;53:5155-5162.
198. Denève C, Janoir C, Poilane I, et al. New trends in *Clostridium difficile* virulence and pathogenesis. *Int J Antimicrob Agents*. 2009;33(suppl 1):S24-S528.
199. Hookman P, Barkin JS. *Clostridium difficile* associated infection, diarrhea and colitis. *World J Gastroenterol*. 2009;15:1554-1580.
200. Khanna S, Pardi DS. The growing incidence and severity of *Clostridium difficile* infection in inpatient and outpatient settings. *Expert Rev Gastroenterol Hepatol*. 2010;4:409-416.

201. Gerding DN. *Clostridium difficile* 30 years on: what has, or has not, changed and why? *Int J Antimicrob Agents*. 2009;33(suppl 1):S2-S58.
202. Kawamoto S, Horton KM, Fishman EK. Pseudomembranous colitis: spectrum of imaging findings with clinical and pathologic correlation. *Radiographics*. 1999;19:887-897.
203. Halsey J. Current and future treatment modalities for *Clostridium difficile*-associated disease. *Am J Health Syst Pharm*. 2008;65:705-175. Erratum in *Am J Health Syst Pharm*. 2008;65:998.
204. Faris B, Blackmore A, Haboubi N. Review of medical and surgical management of *Clostridium difficile* infection. *Tech Coloproctol*. 2010;14:97-105.
205. Butala P, Divino CM. Surgical aspects of fulminant *Clostridium difficile* colitis. *Am J Surg*. 2010;200:131-135.
206. Zar F, Bakkanagari S, Moorthi K, et al. A comparison of vancomycin and metronidazole for the treatment of *Clostridium difficile*-associated diarrhea, stratified by disease severity. *Clin Infect Dis*. 2007;45:302-307.
207. Lipsett P, Samantaray DK, Tam ML, et al. Pseudomembranous colitis: a surgical disease? *Surgery*. 1994;116:491-496.
208. Pepin J, Vo T, Boutros M, et al. Risk factors for mortality following emergency colectomy for fulminant *Clostridium difficile* infection. *Dis Colon Rectum*. 2009;52:400-405.
209. Olivas AD, Umanskiy K, Zuckerbraun B, et al. Avoiding colectomy during surgical management of fulminant *Clostridium difficile* colitis. *Surg Infect*. 2010;11:299-305.

CHAPTER 55 ■ THROMBOEMBOLIC DISEASE

ELLIOTT R. HAUT AND EDWARD E. CORNWELL

Venous thromboembolism (VTE) disease, the composite term for deep vein thrombosis (DVT) and pulmonary embolism (PE), is a complication that deserves a prominent place in the mind of any surgeon caring for acutely ill or injured patients. As concepts of rapid triage and resuscitation accomplish their goals of optimizing the numbers of surgical patients surviving their initial physiologic insult, an ensuing challenge is represented by the attendant risk of these potentially lethal complications disproportionally seen in those who are immobilized and recuperating. The specter of the problem has reached sufficient magnitude to prompt the U. S. Congress to designate March as DVT Awareness Month[1] and the Surgeon General in 2008 to issue "A Call to Action to Prevent Deep Venous Thrombosis and Pulmonary Embolism."[2]

This chapter discusses VTE from the standpoint of incidence, risk factors, and screening philosophy and impact on "quality."

Virchow's triad composed of venous stasis, endothelial injury, and hypercoagulabilty, is the well-known classic explanation for the basic underlying pathway toward DVT. Once DVT occurs, there are many different natural outcomes that may follow. At one end of the spectrum, the body's normal fibrinolytic system can prevent propagation and lyse the clot, potentially even before the patient becomes symptomatic. At the other end of the spectrum would be the case of a large DVT traveling through the vascular system and causing sudden death from a large saddle pulmonary embolus. Other frequent scenarios include DVT that are clinically apparent with significantly swollen extremity and the potential for long-term sequelae of postthrombotic syndrome and/or PE that become symptomatic with pleuritic chest pain, shortness of breath or hypoxia requiring immediate treatment.[3]

Multiple patient populations treated by acute care surgeons are at exceedingly high risk of VTE. ICU admission is often suggested as an independent risk factor for VTE, although those patients quite likely also have multiple other well-accepted risk factors. In a study of 110 mechanically ventilated ICU patients, nearly 25% were diagnosed with DVT when the group was liberally screened with duplex ultrasound, in spite of appropriate VTE prophylaxis. In addition, 11.5% of patients with DVT in this study were diagnosed with PE as well.[4] In trauma patients, VTE remains an important clinical problem,[5] with the DVT rate as high as 58% if only high risk patients are considered in the risk pool and aggressive diagnostic surveillance is applied.[6] However, the reported rates are often lower than 1%, especially when registry data are used.[7-9] Within the field of general surgery, historical data, from the years before VTE prophylaxis was used, sheds some light on the underlying risk of VTE in certain populations. Within the group of untreated general surgery patients, the risk of DVT and PE were 19.1% and 1.6%, respectively. The rate for fatal PE was a remarkable 0.87%.[10] Even in the current era in which we frequently use prophylaxis, VTE rates of over 2.5%–3.5% are reported after some major general surgery and surgical oncology cases.[11]

Many different factors can increase a patients' risk of developing VTE.[12] Once a patient has VTE diagnosed, he/she is always at elevated risk for recurrent VTE, especially if provoked by an acute event or new diagnosis. These varied risk factors can be categorized by the patient's primary diagnosis category (i.e., trauma, cancer), other medical conditions (i.e., congestive heart failure), treatments performed (i.e., central line placement), hypercoagulable state (hereditary or acquired), or other predisposing conditions (i.e., obesity, advanced age). Some of the commonly accepted risks are listed in Table 55.1. In addition, these risk factors seem to be additive such that the more risk factors an individual patient has, the higher their risk of VTE.[12,13] Many procedures commonly performed on acute care surgery patients are also associated with elevated VTE occurrence rates including central line placement (femoral is highest risk location), major surgical procedures, chemotherapy administration, and fracture immobilization. Nearly every diagnosis that increases the odds of VTE by >10-fold is commonly treated by the acute care surgeon: fracture (hip or leg), major general surgery, major trauma, and spinal cord injury[12,13] (see Table 55.2). Additional factors specific to VTE risk in trauma patients are included in Table 55.3.

In addition to clinical impact on individual patients affected by VTE, there are significant financial implications of VTE occurring both during and following hospitalization. In one study of orthopedic surgery patients, mean hospital length of stay was more than doubled for patients with VTE compared to those without VTE. The study also reported the mean total costs of inpatient care nearly twofold higher for the VTE patients.[14] A study of cardiovascular surgery patients had similar findings; VTE patients had 14% higher inpatient costs and 68% longer length of stay as compared with those patients not having a VTE.[15] The economic burden of having DVT or PE as a secondary diagnosis during hospitalization is estimated to be \$7,594 and \$13,018, respectively.[16] In addition, this same study showed a high rate of readmission (14%) for patients with a secondary diagnosis of DVT or PE.[16]

VTE PROPHYLAXIS

According to the Agency for Healthcare Research and Quality, VTE prophylaxis in the appropriate patient populations is a top safety priority for hospitalized patients. Evidence-based guidelines published by specific specialty groups (e.g., The Eastern Association for the Surgery of Trauma [EAST])[17] and The American College of Chest Physicians [ACCP])[18] utilize risk stratification to suggest which patients are at what level of risk and allow for appropriate suggested protocols for VTE prophylaxis.

The attached risk stratification tool (Algorithm 55.1) and algorithm-based prophylaxis regimen is one example for trauma patients that takes into account several concepts from the surgical literature: (1) enoxaparin, a low molecular weight heparin (LMWH), demonstrates an efficacy advantage over unfractionated heparin in a prospective randomized trial with trauma patients with ISS ≥ 9. (2) Normal ambulation (when appropriate) is an excellent adjunct in prophylaxis. (3) No regimen is 100% effective to prevent all VTEs,[19] suggesting some role for diagnostic surveillance in some high risk patients.[20]

Prophylaxis, in general, is divided into two main categories. The first is chemical or pharmacologic prophylaxis, including unfractionated subcutaneous heparin or LWMH given prophylactically to patients. In surgical patients, there

TABLE 55.1

RISK FACTORS OBSERVED IN 1,231 CONSECUTIVE PATIENTS TREATED FOR ACUTE DVT AND/OR PE

PATIENT RISK FACTOR	(%)
Age over 40 y	88.5
Obesity	37.8
History of venous thromboembolism	26.0
Cancer	22.3
Bed rest over 5 d	12.0
Major surgery	11.2
Congestive heart failure	8.2
Varicose veins	5.8
Fracture (hip or leg)	3.7
Estrogen treatment	2.0
Stroke	1.8
Multiple trauma	1.1
Childbirth	1.1
Myocardial infarction	0.7
1 or more risks	96.3
2 or more risks	76.0
3 or more risks	39.0

Modified from Anderson FA Jr, Spencer FA. Risk factors for venous thromboembolism. *Circulation*. 2003;107(23 suppl 1):I9–I16.

TABLE 55.2

RISK FACTORS FOR VTE

STRONG RISK FACTORS (ODDS RATIO > 10)
Fracture (hip or leg)
Hip or knee replacement
Major general surgery
Major trauma
Spinal cord injury
MODERATE RISK FACTORS (ODDS RATIO 2–9)
Arthroscopic knee surgery
Central venous lines
Chemotherapy
Congestive heart or respiratory failure
Hormone replacement therapy
Malignancy
Oral contraceptive therapy
Paralytic stroke
Pregnancy/, postpartum
Previous venous thromboembolism
Thrombophilia
WEAK RISK FACTORS (ODDS RATIO < 2)
Bed rest 3 d
Immobility due to sitting (e.g., prolonged car or air travel)
Increasing age
Laparoscopic surgery (e.g., cholecystectomy)
Obesity
Pregnancy/, antepartum
Varicose veins

Modified from Anderson FA Jr, Spencer FA. Risk factors for venous thromboembolism. *Circulation*. 2003;107(23 suppl 1):I9–I16.

is also some proven benefit that the preoperative dose, given 1–2 hours before surgery, is important to help with the prevention of clots. Although there maybe some associated elevated risk of bleeding with the prophylaxis, this small elevated risk is far outweighed by the substantial drop in symptomatic VTE events and PE-related death. In the current era, nearly all admitted surgical patients will have at least some risk factors warranting pharmacologic prophylaxis. Extended prophylaxis (beyond hospitalization) is also recommended for some surgical populations treated by acute care surgeons—specifically those undergoing cancer surgery[21-24] and major abdominal and pelvic surgery.[25,26]

Mechanical prophylaxis includes sequential compression devices, intermittent pneumatic compression devices, and graduated compression stockings. These mechanical devices also have a benefit in reducing the risk VTE and are especially helpful in patients who have a specific contraindication to chemical prophylaxis and cannot get either unfractionated or LMWH. Even with the accepted improvement in VTE rates with mechanical devices, studies have shown they cannot be used in some trauma patients due to wounds, casts, immobilizers, or external fixators[27] and that compliance with these devices on surgical patients is poor even without any specific contraindications.[28]

In orthopedic surgery specifically, there are multiple other types of prophylaxis that has been recommended. There are very good data that long-term prophylaxis for up to 6 weeks with warfarin in patients after hip replacement surgery has been shown to decrease event rates for both symptomatic DVT as well as PE.[18] It is suggested that aspirin may be used for prophylaxis in certain orthopedic patient populations, although there is still much ongoing debate, and many hematologists and thrombosis experts believe that this is likely inappropriate.

The prophylactic use of IVC filters for prevention of PE in patients without proven DVT remains controversial. The use of these filters in trauma patients who are deemed to be of very high risk for PE has increased in recent years in the hopes that these prophylactic inferior vena cava filters can prevent massive PE and sudden cardiac death.[29] There is no consensus on exactly what patient population such filters should be used in, although in clinical practice they are placed for this specific indication in many trauma patients every year. There are temporary IVC filters that can be safely deployed by vascular and/or trauma surgeons in addition to interventional radiologists with a plan to remove them after the period of highest risk has ended. However, there is still ongoing concern that even with the planned removal of the devices, many filters remain *in situ* as trauma patients often lack appropriate follow up to have the filters taken out.[30]

Even with the large amount of strong evidence suggesting prophylaxis against VTE, the routine use of acceptable prophylaxis is surprisingly low both in the United States and around the world.[31-34] In surgical patients, rates of guideline-compliant prophylaxis often hover around 50%. In an attempt to increase this low compliance with best practice prophylaxis, many approaches have been taken[35] including computerized decision support[36] and electronic alerts.[37]

TABLE 55.3

RISK FACTORS INDEPENDENTLY ASSOCIATED WITH DVT IDENTIFICATION IN INDIVIDUAL TRAUMA PATIENTS BASED ON A MULTIVARIABLE LOGISTIC REGRESSION MODEL

	ODDS RATIO (OR)	95% CONFIDENCE INTERVAL
Treatment at "Screening" vs. "NonScreening" Trauma Center	2.16	1.07–4.34
Age ≥ 40 y	2.00	1.74–2.30
Extremity injury (AIS ≥ 3)	1.96	1.68–2.30
Head injury (AIS ≥ 3)	1.53	1.22–1.92
Ventilator days ≥ 3	5.14	3.66–7.22
Venous injury	2.85	1.97–4.13
Major surgery	4.79	4.08–5.62

Adapted from Haut ER, Chang DC, Pierce CA, et al. Predictors of post-traumatic deep vein thrombosis (DVT)—hospital practice vs. patient factors: an analysis of the National Trauma Data Bank (NTDB). *J Trauma*. 2009;66(4):994–999.

Diagnosis

Even as recently as 20 years ago, DVT was a difficult diagnosis to make because the test, contrast venography, was difficult to perform, invasive, painful, and likely caused more DVTs at a later date. However, presently, the duplex ultrasound is now the well-accepted standard of care for diagnosis of DVT.[17] This relatively inexpensive, noninvasive test has also likely increased the overall numbers of DVTs identified since it can be looked for more easily, even in the patient with a relatively low index of suspicion.

The Diagnosis of Pulmonary Embolism

Historically, before the modern era of diagnostic imaging, many pulmonary emboli were identified only at autopsy and were not suspected premortem. The earliest test for diagnosing a PE was pulmonary arteriogram, which was an invasive technique performed by interventional radiologists or cardiologists, whereby, contrast was injected directly into the pulmonary artery via right heart catheterization. Invasive pulmonary arteriogram gave way to the V/Q or ventilation/perfusion mismatched scan, upon which many of the major early studies regarding diagnosis of PE (i.e., PIOPED study) were based.[38]

Currently, computed tomography (CT) pulmonary angiogram is clearly the most commonly performed test to identify PE, and this test has proved appropriate for the majority of patients except for patients who cannot get IV contrast due to renal dysfunction or allergy to the contrast material for whom ventilation-perfusion scanning remains an option.[39] In addition, patients need to travel to the CT scanner for this diagnostic test, which can also be a problem for the hemodynamically unstable patient in the ICU. In this patient population, echocardiogram has been suggested to be the ideal test of choice. Echocardiogram findings of a dilated right heart and pulmonary hypertension are relatively specific for PE in the hemodynamically unstable patient. Serum testing of D-dimer levels serves as an excellent adjunct role in the diagnosis (specifically to help rule out DVT/PE) in the outpatient and emergency department settings.[39] However, in the acute inpatient

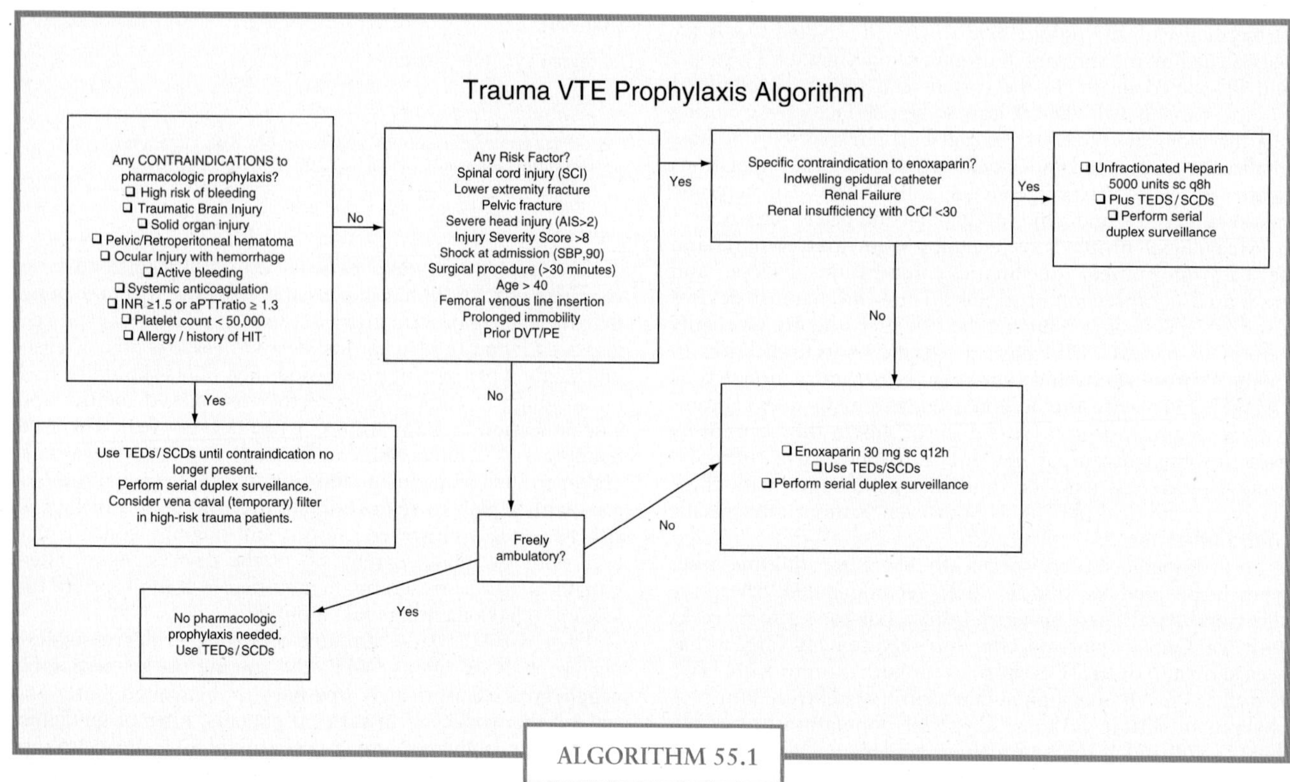

ALGORITHM 55.1 Algorithm.

setting, D-dimer levels are frequently elevated in postsurgical patients as well as in those who are systemically ill, making this test less useful.

Treatment

The mainstay of treatment for patients with all VTE is medical in the form of anticoagulation. Even as recently as just a few years ago, treatment was always in a hospital setting. Patients would receive days of intravenous heparin drip with a bridge period until they were therapeutic on their warfarin, the major vitamin-K antagonist oral anticoagulation. However, there has been a major paradigm shift in that patients with VTE are now routinely treated with either once or twice a day dosing of LMWH, and then bridging that to warfarin, which can be safely performed on an outpatient in many patient populations. It is important to remember that when a patient is started on warfarin, there must always be an overlap period with some heparin (either unfractionated or LMWH) since there may be a short period of hypercoagulability immediately after vitamin K antagonists, that is warfarin, are given. Other anticoagulants can be used specifically in patients with a history of or active heparin-induced thrombocytopenia. In this case, direct thrombin inhibitors are utilized for treatment of DVT and/or PE. Many suggest that in these complex cases, consultations with specialists such as a hematologist who are well versed in the wide range of anticoagulants are to be implemented.

Duration of Treatment for Patients with VTE or PE

Although there has been recent debate on the needed length of therapy for DVT/PE, new evidence-based guidelines from the American Heart Association have attempted to streamline expert opinions. Length of therapy should be short (3 months) for those with a first DVT episode provoked by a major risk factor. Longer treatment (at least 6 months) is suggested for patients with recurrent or unprovoked DVT. It remains unclear exactly which patients should be screened for inherited hypercoagulable states (i.e., Factor V Leiden, antithrombin deficiency, protein C or S deficiency). However, if one is identified, this may change the suggested length of therapy. There are suggestions that repeat duplex ultrasound to confirm resolution of the clot is beneficial before stopping the anticoagulation.

Some hospitalized patients with DVT/PE cannot receive first line treatment with anticoagulation due to specific contraindications. These will include recent neurologic or ophthalmologic surgery, trauma patients with solid organ injury and/or retroperitoneal hematoma), preexisting coagulopathy or thrombocytopenia, or those at significant risk for recurrent falls. In these patients, IVC filter placement is the classically accepted treatment to prevent PE, although it will not help treat the underlying DVT.

Patients with PE and hemodynamic instability present a difficult treatment decision. Fibrinolysis, or thrombolytic therapy (i.e., Alteplase), is suggested for the treatment of massive PE in patients without contraindications. This treatment may break the PE into smaller pieces and allow better blood flow to potentially resuscitate the patient, such that they can move on to the next step of therapy. If thrombolytic is going to be given, it should be done immediately as soon as possible once the diagnosis of PE is either identified definitively or in a patient with cardiac arrest and significant risk factors. In patients with submassive PE, the evidence is less clear and clinical judgment is warranted to balance the risk/benefit ratio.[40]

In patients with submassive PE, there may be a role for either catheter-directed therapies such as embolectomy/fragmentation (usually performed by vascular interventional radiologists) or potentially an open surgical pulmonary artery thrombectomy (Trendelenberg procedure). The performance of this procedure is beyond the scope of this book, as it will routinely be performed by a cardiothoracic surgeon, through either a median sternotomy or anteriolateral thoracotomy. The decision to proceed down one or the other paths should be made in team consultation and will depend on local expertise with these procedures.[40]

SCREENING PHILOSOPHY AND QUALITY

Since injured patients are at elevated risk for DVT, many authors suggest that high-risk asymptomatic patients be screened for lower extremity DVT using duplex ultrasound. However, other authors have suggested that this process may not be cost effective as it has not been proven to improve patient outcomes. Recently published data show wide variability in trauma surgeons' opinions and trauma center practices regarding the use of screening duplex ultrasound in asymptomatic trauma patients.[20] Our policy of aggressive screening is driven by a desire to identify VTE as a DVT rather than a PE; however, recent federal government health policy decisions prompts reconsideration of this approach. In this section, we offer constructive criticism of the Center for Medicare and Medicaid Services' (CMS) decision to treat DVT as a "never event"[41] and the attendant thrust to use hospital DVT incidence rates as a marker for quality of care.[19]

We have previously reported evidence for surveillance bias in DVT reporting on a national level using the National Trauma Data Bank (NTDB), as well as at a single institution.

Our first exploratory analysis of the hypothesis that DVT rates reported may be related to rates of screening asymptomatic patients for DVT with duplex ultrasound was a retrospective review of trauma registry and hospital discharge data from a single academic level 1 trauma center.[42,43] Patients admitted to the Adult Trauma Service were divided into two groups, those admitted before versus after implementation of a written guideline for DVT prophylaxis and duplex ultrasound screening of asymptomatic high-risk patients. Data were compared between these two groups. Significantly more duplex ultrasound exams were performed in the later period (20.9 vs. 81.5 per 1,000 trauma admissions, $p < 0.0001$). This outcome was expected based on the implementation of our new guideline. The proportion of patients with DVT diagnosed increased 10-fold from 0.7 to 7.0 per 1,000 admissions ($p = 0.0024$). The incidence of PE or mortality did not change significantly, but proportionately more VTEs were identified as DVTs rather than PEs.

Our next study was a hospital-level analysis of duplex ultrasound and DVT rates in the largest trauma database available, the NTDB.[44] We divided hospitals into quartiles based on their rates of duplex ultrasounds per trauma patient admission and compared the DVT rates reported from hospitals in each quartile. Hospitals in the highest quartile by duplex rate reported a DVT rate sevenfold higher than the average DVT rate in the first three quartiles (1.52% vs. 0.22%, $p < 0.001$) (see Fig. 55.1). One plausible explanation for the large disparity in DVT and ultrasound rates between quartiles was practice variation between hospitals in screening asymptomatic trauma patients. The DVT rate increased significantly and correlated with duplex ultrasound rate at hospitals that had a 2% or greater ultrasound rate.

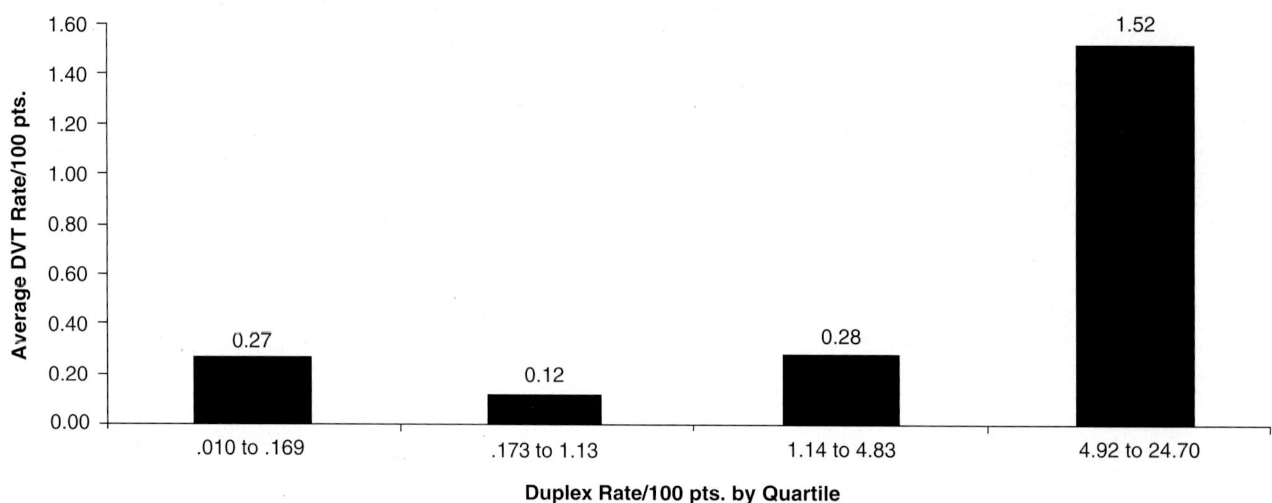

FIGURE 55.1. Hospital DVT rates in each quartile of hospitals. Raw data of the average hospital DVT rate per 100 admitted patients by duplex rate quartile. From Pierce CA, Haut ER, Kardooni S, et al. Deep vein thrombosis surveillance patterns in the National Trauma Data Bank: the more we look, the more we find. *J Trauma*. 2008;64:932–937.

We then used a multilevel analytical approach combining patient- and hospital-level characteristics within the NTDB to examine the outcome of reported DVT while controlling for differences in patient populations and individual patient characteristics that may influence rates of DVT after trauma.[8] As NTDB contains no data on hospital duplex surveillance practice, we defined "screening" trauma centers as those performing ultrasound on over 2% of patients. Multiple logistic regression was performed, using patient-level risk factor covariates (such as age, gender, injury severity score, injury mechanism, procedures, and comorbidities) as well as hospital duplex rate to compare odds of DVT diagnosis for patients at "screening" versus "nonscreening" centers. Unadjusted DVT rate was threefold higher for patients treated at "screening" trauma centers (1.18% vs. 0.35%, $p < 0.001$). Admission to a "screening " trauma center was independently associated with a twofold increased risk of having DVT reported, even after controlling for patient risk factors (odds ratio 2.16, 95% CI 1.07–4.34, $p = 0.03$) (Table 55.3).

This sequence of research suggests that DVT rates reported by trauma centers are inherently biased due to variations in local screening patterns and likely mislead rather than truly identify the quality of trauma care and should not be used for benchmarking purposes. A Journal of the American Medical Association (JAMA) editorial suggested that "aggressive screening strategies can markedly increase case-finding rates without an effect on quality of care. The absence of a standardized surveillance system could lead to a spurious association between more preventable harm and lower-quality care."[45]

We take this opinion a step further and suggest that if we ignore the issue of surveillance bias and decide to report and compare biased complication rates, there is a potential for unintended consequences to cause individual patient harm.[46] Patients may be put at elevated risk from providers who do not perform appropriate diagnostic testing in an attempt to avoid reporting complications. In the case of DVT, if the diagnosis is not considered, an ultrasound is not performed, and the DVT is not identified, the hospital may have few events to report. However, patients could be directly harmed since these DVTs may not be identified early on and intervened upon with anticoagulation to prevent propagation or PE.[19] This potential for unintended consequences was most eloquently described by Alam and Velmahos; "So if your intubated polytrauma patient develops asymptomatic DVT and you are diligent enough to screen and detect it, you are at a risk of punishment and of not being reimbursed. On the other hand, if you do not bother investing in expensive technology, developing screening protocols, or battling with the radiology department for better patient care, you are gold. No screening, no DVT, no punishment."[44]

Our ability to clearly prove harm from the CMS policy is clouded by inaccuracies in estimating which duplex exams were truly "screening," and by relatively small numbers of patients with fatal PE's in any single registry. Nonetheless, it is clear that many, if not most, patients who develop DVTs do so despite appropriate prophylaxis, and other patients escape developing a DVT despite receiving no prophylaxis. Therefore, we strongly believe that the quality marker that should be used in federal health care reimbursement policy should consider compliance with DVT prophylaxis guidelines, not merely the incidence of DVT alone.[46,47] We are hard pressed to identify a rebuttal to this premise—other than inconvenience.

SUMMARY

The experience with risk stratification, prophylaxis, diagnosis, and treatment of VTE has allowed consensus management guidelines to be generated. More work is needed, however, to achieve consensus on the utility of an aggressive screening regimen, and to resolve the controversy over the use of DVT occurrences as a marker for quality of care.

References

1. US Senate, Office of Legislative Policy and Awareness. S. Con Res. 56—Deep-Vein Thrombosis Awareness Month. http://olpa.od.nih.gov/ tracking/109/senate_res/session1/s_con_res-56.asp. Accessed July 18, 2011.
2. US Department of Health and Human Services. The Surgeon General's Call to Action to Prevent Deep Vein Thrombosis and Pulmonary Embolism; 2008. (Accessed at http://www.surgeongeneral.gov/topics/deepvein (accessed December 22, 2010).

3. Lowe GDO, Greer IA, Cooke TG, et al. Thromboembolic Risk Factors (THRIFT) Consensus Group. Risk of and prophylaxis for venous thromboembolism in hospital patients. *BMJ*. 1992;305:567-574.
4. Ibrahim EH, Iregui M, Prentice D, et al. Deep vein thrombosis during prolonged mechanical ventilation despite prophylaxis. *Crit Care Med*. 2002;30(4):771-774.
5. Rogers FB. Venous thromboembolism in trauma patients: a review. *Surgery*. 2001;130:1-12.
6. Geerts WH, Code KI, Jay RM, et al. A prospective study of venous thromboembolism after major trauma. *N Engl J Med*. 1994;331:1601-1606.
7. Knudson MM, Ikossi DG, Khaw L, et al. Thromboembolism after trauma, an analysis of 1602 episodes from the American College of Surgeons National Trauma Data Bank. *Ann Surg*. 2004;240:490-498.
8. Haut ER, Chang DC, Pierce CA, et al. Predictors of post-traumatic deep vein thrombosis (DVT)—hospital practice vs. patient factors: an analysis of the National Trauma Data Bank (NTDB). *J Trauma*. 2009;66(4):994-999.
9. Kardooni S, Haut ER, Pierce CA, et al. Hazards of benchmarking complication rates with The National Trauma Data Bank: numerators in search of denominators. *J Trauma*. 2008;64(2):273-279.
10. Clagett GP, Reisch JS. Prevention of venous thromboembolism in general surgical patients. Results of meta-analysis. *Ann Surg*. 1988;208(2):227-240.
11. Mukherjee D, Lidor AO, Chu KM, et al. Postoperative venous thromboembolism rates vary significantly after different types of major abdominal operations. *J Gastrointest Surg*. 2008;12(11):2015-2022.
12. Anderson FA Jr, Spencer FA. Risk factors for venous thromboembolism. *Circulation*. 2003;107(23 suppl 1):I9-I16.
13. Anderson FA Jr, Wheeler HB. Physician practices in the management of venous thromboembolism: a community-wide survey. *J Vasc Surg*. 1992;16:707-714.
14. Ollendorf DA, Vera-Llonch M, Oster G. Cost of venous thromboembolism following major orthopedic surgery in hospitalized patients. *Am J Health-Syst Pharm*. 2002;59:1750-1754.
15. Henke P, Froehlich J, Upchurch G Jr, et al. The significant negative impact of in-hospital venous thromboembolism after cardiovascular procedures. *Ann Vasc Surg*. 2007;21(5):545-550.
16. Spyropoulos AC, Lin J. Direct medical costs of venous thromboembolism and subsequent hospital readmission rates: an administrative claims analysis from 30 managed care organizations. *J Manag Care Pharm*. 2007;13(6);475-486.
17. Rogers FB, Cipolle MD, Velmahos G, et al. Practice management guidelines for the prevention of venous thromboembolism in trauma patients: the EAST practice management guidelines work group. *J Trauma*. 2006;53:142-164.
18. Geerts WH, Bergqvist D, Pineo GF, et al. Prevention of venous thromboembolism: American College of Chest Physicians Evidence-Based Clinical Practice Guidelines (8th Edition). *Chest*. 2008;133(6 suppl):381S-453S.
19. Streiff MB, Haut ER. The CMS ruling on venous thromboembolism after total knee or hip arthroplasty: weighing risks and benefits. *JAMA*. 2009;301(10):1063-1065.
20. Haut ER, Schenider EB, Patel A, et al. Duplex ultrasound screening for deep vein thrombosis in asymptomatic trauma patients: a survey of individual trauma surgeon opinions and current trauma center practices. *J Trauma*. 2011;70(1):27-34.
21. Muntz J. Duration of deep vein thrombosis prophylaxis in the surgical patient and its relation to quality issues. *Am J Surg*. 2010;200(3):413-421.
22. Bergqvist D, Agnelli G, Cohen AT, et al. Duration of prophylaxis against venous thromboembolism with enoxaparin after surgery for cancer. *N Engl J Med*. 2002;346:975-980.
23. Khorana AA, Streiff MB, Farge D, et al. Venous thromboembolism prophylaxis and treatment in cancer: a consensus statement of major guidelines panels and call to action. *J Clin Oncol*. 2009;27(29):4919-4926.
24. Lyman GH, Khorana AA, Falanga A, et al. American Society of Clinical Oncology guideline: recommendations for venous thromboembolism prophylaxis and treatment in patients with cancer. *J Clin Oncol*. 2007;25:5490-5505.
25. Rasmussen MS, Jorgensen LN, Wille-Jørgensen P, et al.; FAME Investigators. Prolonged prophylaxis with dalteparin to prevent late thromboembolic complications in patients undergoing major abdominal surgery: a multicenter randomized open-label study. *J Thromb Haemost*. 2006;4:2384-2390.
26. Rasmussen MS, Jørgensen LN, Wille-Jørgensen P. Prolonged thromboprophylaxis with low molecular weight heparin for abdominal or pelvic surgery. *Cochrane Database Syst Rev*. 2009;1:CD004318.
27. Shackford SR, Davis JW, Hollingsworth-Fridlund P, et al. Venous thromboembolism in patients with major trauma. *Am J Surg*. 1990;159:365-369.
28. Cornwell EE 3rd, Chang D, Velmahos G, et al. Compliance with sequential compression device prophylaxis in at-risk trauma patients: a prospective analysis. *Am Surg*. 2002;68(5):470.
29. Dossett LA, Adams RC, Cotton BA. Unwarranted national variation in the use of prophylactic inferior vena cava filters after trauma: an analysis of the national trauma databank. *J Trauma*. 2011;70(5):1066-1071.
30. Karmy-Jones R, Jurkovich GJ, Velmahos GC, et al. Practice patterns and outcomes of retrievable vena cava filters in trauma patients: an AAST multicenter study. *J Trauma*. 2007;62(1):17-25.
31. Cohen AT, Tapson VF, Bergmann JF, et al.; ENDORSE Investigators. Venous thromboembolism risk and prophylaxis in the acute hospital care setting (ENDORSE study): a multinational cross-sectional study. *Lancet*. 2008;371(9610):387-394.
32. Tapson VF, Decousus H, Pini M, et al.; IMPROVE Investigators. Venous thromboembolism prophylaxis in acutely ill hospitalized medical patients: findings from the International Medical Prevention Registry on Venous Thromboembolism. *Chest*. 2007;132(3):936-945.
33. Goldhaber SZ, Tapson VF; DVT FREE Steering Committee. A prospective registry of 5,451 patients with ultrasound-confirmed deep vein thrombosis. *Am J Cardiol*. 2004;93(2):259.
34. Yu HT, Dylan ML, Lin J, Dubois RW. Hospitals' compliance with prophylaxis guidelines for venous thromboembolism. *Am J Health Syst Pharm*. 2007;64(1):69-76.
35. Tooher R, Middleton P, Pham C, et al. A systematic review of strategies to improve prophylaxis for venous thromboembolism in hospitals. *Ann Surg*. 2005;241(3):397.
36. Durieux P, Nizard R, Ravaud P, et al. A clinical decision support system for prevention of venous thromboembolism: effect on physician behavior. *JAMA*. 2000;283:2816-2821.
37. Kucher N, Koo S, Quiroz R, et al. Electronic alerts to prevent venous thromboembolism among hospital patients. *N Engl J Med*. 2005;352(10):969-977.
38. The PIOPED Investigators. Value of the ventilation/perfusion scan in acute pulmonary embolism. Results of the prospective investigation of pulmonary embolism diagnosis (PIOPED). *JAMA*. 1990;263(20):2753-2759.
39. Agnelli G, Becattini C. Acute pulmonary embolism. *N Engl J Med*. 2010;363:266-274.
40. Jaff MR, McMurtry MS, Archer SL, et al. on behalf of the American Heart Association Council on Cardiopulmonary, Critical Care, Perioperative and Resuscitation, Council on Peripheral Vascular Disease, and Council on Arteriosclerosis, Thrombosis and Vascular Biology. Management of massive and submassive pulmonary embolism, iliofemoral deep vein thrombosis, and chronic thromboembolic pulmonary hypertension: a scientific statement from the American Heart Association. Circulation e-published ahead of print online Mar 21, 2011.
41. Haut ER. Venous thromboembolism: are regulatory requirements reasonable? *Crit Connect*. (SCCM newsmagazine), April 2008. http://www.sccm.org/Publications/Critical_Connections/Archives/April_2008/Pages/VenousThromboembolism.aspx (accessed March 23, 2011).
42. Haut ER, Noll K, Efron DT, et al. Can increased incidence of deep vein thrombosis after major trauma be used as a marker of quality of care in the absence of standardized surveillance? *J Trauma*. 2007;63(5):1132-1137.
43. Pronovost PJ, Miller MR, Wachter RM. Tracking progress in patient safety, an elusive target. *JAMA* 2006;296:696-699.
44. Pierce CA, Haut ER, Kardooni S, et al. Deep vein thrombosis surveillance patterns in the National Trauma Data Bank: the more we look, the more we find. *J Trauma*. 2008;64:932-937.
45. Pronovost PJ, Goeschel CA, Wachter RM. The wisdom and justice of not paying for "Preventable Complications". *JAMA*. 2008;299(18):2197-2199.
46. Haut ER, Pronovost PJ. Surveillance bias in outcomes reporting. *JAMA*. 2011;305(23):2462-2463.
47. Pronovost PJ, Colantuoni E. Measuring preventable harm: helping science keep pace with policy. *JAMA*. 2009;301(12):1273-1275.

CHAPTER 56 ■ THE IMMUNOCOMPROMISED PATIENT

UROGHUPATEI P. IYEGHA AND GREGORY J. BEILMAN

Immunocompromised patients present a special challenge to the acute care surgeon. Although transplant recipients, human immunodeficiency virus (HIV)-infected individuals, and chemotherapy patients are the most poignant examples, much more common are the immunocompromised states imposed by advanced age, malnutrition, chronic disease, and critical illness. As modern medicine continues to improve outcomes for such patients, they will continue to be an increasingly important part of the population that may eventually require emergency surgery. Therefore, knowledge of the various immunocompromised states and their management is of considerable importance to the acute care surgeon.

THE IMMUNE SYSTEM

As our knowledge of the immune system has grown, it has become clear that it is an extremely complex system with multiple dimensions that we are only beginning to understand. A detailed description of the immune system and our current state of knowledge is beyond the scope of this chapter. However, some basic premises remain true even if the full knowledge of the mechanisms behind them is still forthcoming. The immune system can be divided into two broad categories: innate and adaptive immunity. The innate response is the initial inflammatory response to infection or injury and is designed to proceed in a nonspecific manner. The adaptive immune system is tailored to the inciting pathogen and results in immunologic memory. While it is useful to categorize the immune system in this way, it should be pointed out that the two systems are closely integrated and each enhances the efficacy of the other. For example, the complement system as well as the host of inflammatory cytokines (tumor necrosis factor-alpha (TNFα), interferon-gamma (INFγ), interleukin (IL)-1, IL-2, etc.) play roles in both systems and illustrate their interdependence. The cells important for innate immunity are neutrophils, macrophages, natural killer (NK) cells, and dendritic cells. Mast cells, basophils, and eosinophils play a role in innate immunity as well, although their actions are classically demonstrated by type I hypersensitivity reactions. Neutrophils and macrophages phagocytose pathogens and/or cells infected with pathogens, while NK cells attack host cells that have been infected. TNFα and IL-1, primarily produced by macrophages, are the major inflammatory cytokines, and are implicated in many of the manifestations of the systemic inflammatory response syndrome.

Dendritic cells, positioned in tissues that are exposed to the external environment, link the innate immune response to the adaptive immune response by participating as antigen presenting cells (APCs). Via the major histocompatibility complex (MHC) class II, APCs present exogenous antigens to CD4+ (helper) T lymphocytes, which subsequently secrete cytokines such as INFγ, IL-2, and IL-4, which increases the activity of macrophages, CD8+ (cytotoxic) T lymphocytes and B lymphocytes, respectively. Cytotoxic T lymphocytes recognize and target cells presenting endogenous antigen (such as viral proteins) via MHC class I present on all nucleated cells. B lymphocytes recognize antigens bound to cell surface antibodies and subsequently differentiate into plasma cells that secrete antigen-specific antibodies. Perhaps the most important distinction to be made between the innate and adaptive immune response is that the adaptive immune response results in immunologic memory. Circulating memory B lymphocytes that secrete antigen-specific antibodies as well as circulating antigen-specific helper and cytotoxic T lymphocytes manifest this memory. The presence of antigen-specific immune cells allows for a much more rapid and robust response to an antigen if it is encountered again.

PROFOUND IMMUNOCOMPROMISE VERSUS RELATIVE IMMUNOCOMPROMISE

Immunocompromised patients can generally be separated into two broad categories: those with profound and those with relative immunocompromise. The most prominent example of profound immunocompromise is post solid-organ transplant immunosuppression. However, bone marrow transplantation, immunosuppressive therapy for autoimmune disorders, cancer chemotherapy resulting in neutropenia, and HIV infection/acquired immunodeficiency syndrome (AIDS) are also common etiologies of profound immunocompromise. Furthermore, an increasing number of genetic disorders, referred to as primary immunodeficiency disorders have been and continue to be elucidated (Table 56.1). While the individual conditions in this category may be rare, the aggregate should not be considered so.[1] Profoundly immunocompromised patients have a markedly increased susceptibility to infection as well as a considerable inability to combat infection once it is established. On the other hand, relative immunocompromise has many etiologies and is more difficult to quantify. Chronic illness such as diabetes mellitus, cancer, alcoholism, and drug abuse are associated with impaired innate and adaptive immunity. Advanced age and malnutrition, often synchronous with chronic disease, are also associated with impaired immune function and make up a growing portion of the general population. Additionally, intensive care units across the nation are filled with critically ill patients with immune dysfunction related to their acute illness. Similar to those with profound immunocompromise, these patients exhibit increased susceptibility to infection and demonstrate increased postoperative morbidity and mortality.

ORGAN TRANSPLANTATION

Over 20,000 organ transplants are performed annually in the United States (http://optn.transplant.hrsa.gov). The kidney is by far the most commonly transplanted organ followed by liver, heart, and lungs. A large part of the modern success of

TABLE 56.1

WELL-CHARACTERIZED PRIMARY IMMUNODEFICIENCY DISORDERS

X-linked agammaglobulinemia (Brutton's disease)
Autosomal recessive agammaglobulinemia
Common variable immunodeficiency
Selective IgA deficiency
IgG subclass deficiency
Severe combined immunodeficiency (X-linked)
Omenn's syndrome (autosomal recessive variant of SCID)
Chronic granulomatous disease
Severe congenital neutropenia
Cyclic neutropenia
Wiskott-Aldrich syndrome
DiGeorge's syndrome
Hyper IgE syndrome
Ataxia–telangiectasia

Adapted from Turvey SE, Bonilla FA, Junker AK. Primary immunodeficiency diseases: a practical guide for clinicians. *Postgrad Med J*. 2009;85:660–666.

organ transplantation has come from the development of more effective immunosuppressive agents. As organ transplantation continues to improve and becomes an increasingly viable option for a myriad of disease processes, the population of transplant recipients is likely to increase. It is well established that the rate-limiting factor in transplantation is donor availability. This observation underscores the reality that the acute care surgeon should expect to encounter transplant recipients in his or her practice and be prepared to manage them appropriately. A basic working knowledge of immunosuppressive regimens is crucial to providing proper management of transplant patients. The field of immunosuppression has undergone many changes over recent decades driven by a much better understanding of the immune system. This knowledge has allowed for the development of targeted therapies with increased efficacy. Today, most patients will receive a combination of agents to prevent rejection. While traditional corticosteroid therapy remains an integral part of immunosuppression, modern therapy includes a multiplicity of agents including antimetabolites, calcineurin inhibitors, and lymphocyte-activation inhibitors. Other agents frequently used for induction and to combat rejection include antilymphocyte antibodies and IL-2 receptor antagonists. A summary of these agents with mechanisms of action and side effects is provided in Tables 56.2 and 56.3. Corticosteroids are the most commonly encountered class of immunosuppressive agents, although arguably they are more frequently used outside of transplantation. Corticosteroids inhibit cytokine release and impair neutrophil chemotaxis, rendering patients susceptible to infection. In addition, fibroblast function, collagen production, and angiogenesis are impaired, which negatively impact wound healing. Animal data clearly demonstrate impaired wound healing with corticosteroid therapy and limited human studies have correlated increasing doses of corticosteroids with impaired wound healing and increased postoperative infectious complications.[2,3] Unfortunately, patients receiving chronic corticosteroid therapy do not have the luxury of halting therapy as this places them at risk for adrenal insufficiency due to a depressed hypothalamic–pituitary–adrenocortical (HPA) axis. For this reason, supplemental corticosteroid therapy is commonly administered during periods of acute stress.

In effect, all immunosuppressive therapy places patients at risk for infectious complications. Up to 63% of solid-organ transplant recipients experience an infectious complication within the first year of transplant.[4] The risk of infection is highest during the first 6–12 months, corresponding to the period of most intensive immunosuppression. The risk of infection also increases with treatment of rejection. The most frequent infections seen early and late after transplantation are presented in Table 56.4. Infectious complications in the first month after transplantation are frequently caused by the

TABLE 56.2

IMMUNOSUPPRESSIVE AGENTS AND MECHANISM OF ACTION

AGENT	USES	MECHANISM OF ACTION
Corticosteroids (prednisone, methylprednisolone)	Induction Maintenance Rejection	Redistribution of lymphocytes, block T-cell proliferation, IL-2 synthesis
Antilymphocyte antibodies (antithymocyte globulin, OKT-3)	Induction Rejection	Lymphocyte depletion
Humanized antibodies (Basiliximab, daclizumab)	Induction Rejection	Specific targets: IL-2 receptor
Calcineurin inhibitors (cyclosporine, tacrolimus)	Maintenance Rejection	Inhibit IL-2 production, inhibits expansion and differentiation of T cells
Proliferation signal inhibitors (sirolimus/rapamycin, everolimus)	Maintenance	Block cytokine-driven cell cycle progression
Antimetabolites (azathioprine, mycophenolate mofetil)	Maintenance	Inhibit RNA/DNA synthesis

TABLE 56.3

SIDE EFFECTS OF COMMON IMMUNOSUPPRESSIVE AGENTS

Antithymocyte globulin	Fever, leukopenia, thrombocytopenia, serum sickness
Azathioprine, mycophenolate mofetil	Leukopenia, thrombocytopenia, anemia, diarrhea, abdominal pain, hepatotoxicity, pancreatitis
Basiliximab, daclizumab	Hypersensitivity (anaphylaxis), fever
Corticosteroids	Hyperglycemia, osteoporosis, impaired wound healing, hypertension, Cushingoid facies, Addisonian crisis (from rapid withdrawal)
Cyclosporine	Nephrotoxicity, neurotoxicity, drug interactions, hypertension, hyperkalemia, hirsutism, gingival hyperplasia
Sirolimus Everolimus	Hyperlipidemia, myelosuppression, impaired wound healing, diarrhea, arthralgia, pneumonitis
Tacrolimus	Nephrotoxicity, neurotoxicity, drug interactions, hypertension, hyperkalemia, diarrhea, diabetes, tremor
OKT-3	Pulmonary edema, fevers, rigors, diarrhea, headache, bronchospasm, increased CMV infection, risk of PTLD

same organisms common to immunocompetent hosts. Thereafter, opportunistic infections predominate, correlating with the highest degree of immunosuppression. Included among the most common problems are viral infections such as cytomegalovirus (CMV) and opportunistic fungal infections such as *Candida* and *Aspergillus* species.[5] A key component to treatment of infection in transplant patients is decreasing and/or ceasing immunosuppression, allowing the host immune system a chance to respond and increasing the prospects of clearing the infection. In the balance, of course, remains the risk of developing rejection in the transplanted organ. Consequently, close collaboration with the transplant team is required to appropriately manage immunosuppressive therapy and to prevent and/or detect signs of rejection.

TABLE 56.4

RISK OF INFECTION AFTER TRANSPLANT WITH RESPECT TO TIME AFTER TRANSPLANT

WITHIN 6 wk	6 wk TO 6 mo	≥6 mo
Viral Herpes simplex Hepatitis B, C	 CMV (pneumonia) Hepatitis B, C EBV Varicella zoster Influenza Respiratory syncytial virus Adenovirus Polyoma (BK) virus	 CMV (retinitis, colitis) Hepatitis B, C Papillomavirus Posttransplant lymphoproliferative disorder
Bacterial Nosocomial infection (e.g., line, pneumonia, wound, urinary tract infection)	 Nocardiosis Listeriosis from Listeria monocytogenes Tuberculosis	 Listeriosis Tuberculosis
Fungal Candidiasis	 Candidiasis Aspergillosis Cryptococcosis Coccidioidomycosis Histoplasmosis	 Cryptococcosis Coccidioidomycosis Histoplasmosis
Parasitic	 *P. jiroveci* infection Strongyloidosis Toxoplasmosis Leishmaniasis *Trypanosoma cruzi* infection	 *P. jiroveci* infection Strongyloidosis

Modified from Snydman DR. Epidemiology of infections after solid-organ transplantation. *Clin Infect Dis.* 2001;33 (suppl 1):S5–S8.

AUTOIMMUNE DISORDERS

A multitude of chronic inflammatory and autoimmune disorders require anti-inflammatory, immunomodulating, and occasionally, immunosuppressive therapy for adequate symptom and disease control. Well-known examples include rheumatoid arthritis, systemic lupus erythematosus, and inflammatory bowel disease. Pharmacologic treatment ranges from nonsteroidal anti-inflammatory drugs (NSAIDs) and cyclooxygenase-2 (COX-2) inhibitors to corticosteroids, disease modifying anti-rheumatic drugs (DMARDs), and biologic response modifiers such as TNFα inhibitors (see Table 56.5).[58,59] By nature of their varying mechanisms of action, these drugs contribute to problems with surgical wound healing and increase rates of postoperative infectious complications. However, cessation of therapy for surgical procedures often leads to disease flares and worsening symptoms, which can decrease functional status and retard postoperative recovery. This conundrum poses a challenge to physicians and patients alike when it comes to surgical decision making.

Unfortunately, surgical outcome data in patients with chronic inflammatory and autoimmune disorders receiving various pharmacotherapies is limited. Animal studies have clearly demonstrated that NSAIDs negatively impact wound healing. However, selective COX-2 inhibitors have not been shown to negatively impact wound healing in animal models.[3] There is a paucity of human data for either class of drugs and current recommendations are based on extrapolations from the animal data. Although concerns exist regarding applicability of this data, it is generally recommended that NSAIDs be withheld for 3–4 days prior to surgery involving soft tissue and tendons. This recommendation has little applicability to the acute care surgeon, however.

There is also modest data regarding surgical outcomes and some of the more potent agents such as methotrexate, azathioprine, and other DMARDs as well as TNFα receptor inhibitors such as infliximab. Two small studies in the orthopedic literature, one retrospective review, and one prospective study, demonstrated that continuing methotrexate in rheumatoid arthritis patients in the perioperative setting is associated with increased infectious and wound healing complications. However, several other small studies, both retrospective and prospective, failed to demonstrate the same results, finding no significant difference in complication rates in patients who stopped methotrexate prior to surgery compared to those who continued methotrexate treatment perioperatively.[3] Similarly, there is conflicting data regarding outcomes in patients with inflammatory bowel disease being treated with biologic agents who are undergoing surgery. Several small studies have demonstrated equivalent postoperative complication rates in patients being treated with infliximab and other immunosuppressive agents such as azathioprine and 6-mercaptopurine for Crohn's disease and chronic ulcerative colitis compared to those who either had their medications discontinued before surgery or were not being treated with these agents.[6–9] However, multiple additional studies have noted an increased postoperative infectious complication rate in patients receiving infliximab preoperatively for

TABLE 56.5

DMARDS AND BIOLOGIC RESPONSE MODIFIERS USED IN TREATMENT OF AUTOIMMUNE AND OTHER INFLAMMATORY DISORDERS

AGENT	MECHANISM OF ACTION
Acetylsalicylic acid (ASA)	Irreversibly inhibits cyclooxygenase
NSAIDS (ibuprofen, naproxen, ketorolac, etc.)	Nonselective inhibition of cyclooxygenase
COX-2 inhibitors (celocoxib, rofecoxib, etc.)	Selective inhibition of COX-2
Corticosteroids	Specific mechanism of action unknown
Methotrexate	Folic acid analog, inhibits dihydrofolate reductase, inhibits de novo purine synthesis
D-penicillamine	Chelating agent, promotes urinary excretion of copper, mercury, zinc and lead
Gold sodium thiomalate	
Sulfasalazine	Specific mechanism of action unknown
Hydroxychloroquine	Impairs handling of heme
Azathioprine	Inhibits de novo purine synthesis
TNFα inhibitors (Infliximab, Etanercept, Adalimumab)	Prevent binding of TNFα to its receptor Infliximab—anti-TNFα monoclonal antibody Etanercept—Fused ligand binding portion of human TNFα receptor and Fc portion of human IgG_1 Adalimumab—anti-TNFα recombinant human IgG_1 monoclonal antibody
Rituximab	Chimeric monoclonal antibody against CD20 B-cell antigen
Anakinra	Recombinant IL-1 receptor antagonist
Abatacept	T-cell costimulation modulator—binds CD80 and CD86 on APCs preventing CD28 binding to T cells

Data from Brunton LL, Lazo JS, Parker KL, eds. *Goodman & Gilman's The Pharmacological Basis of Therapeutics*. 11th ed. New York: McGraw Hill; 2006; Katzung BG, Masters SB, AJ Trevor, eds. *Basic and Clinical Pharmacology*. 11th ed. New York: McGraw Hill; 2009.

SURGICAL CRITICAL CARE

treatment of Crohn's disease and ulcerative colitis.[10–13] One particular study noted that the risk of postoperative infectious complications, most notably sepsis, was mitigated by the presence of a diverting stoma in patients undergoing ileocolonic resection for Crohn's disease.[10] As a whole, these studies are small, underpowered, and possess confounding variables such as concomitant use of corticosteroids and other immunosuppressive medications. Though the authors generally attempt to compensate with multivariate analyses, the small study sizes of current reports do raise concerns about adequately detecting differences.

Despite its deficiencies, it is this data that is extrapolated to provide recommendations for other clinical scenarios. Obviously, the luxury of discontinuing immunomodulating therapy preoperatively is not typically available to acute care surgeons. The problem that most surgeons will face will revolve around the potential increased risk of postoperative infectious and wound healing complications as well as perioperative management of the primary disease state for which anti-inflammatory and immunomodulating therapy was intended. Clear guidelines are lacking given the current state of knowledge. In elective surgery, the recommended approach is to thoroughly assess risk factors and individually weigh risk versus benefit.[3,14] In some semielective instances that are encountered in acute care surgery, this approach is reasonable. In those patients in whom therapy is continued during the perioperative period, caution and vigilance is advised to detect postoperative complications early and initiate appropriate treatment in a timely fashion. When the risks clearly outweigh the benefits (e.g., intra-abdominal catastrophe), immunomodulatory therapy should be withheld until infectious concerns have subsided.

NEUTROPENIA

The most significant problem that acute care surgeons encounter in patients receiving chemotherapy is neutropenia. Defined as an absolute neutrophil count (ANC) of <1,500 cells per mL, neutropenia significantly inhibits the ability to combat bacterial infection. Moderate (ANC 500–1,000 cells per mL) and severe (ANC < 500 cells per mL) neutropenia impart the greatest risk compared to milder degrees of neutropenia. While chemotherapy is a common etiology, radiotherapy, leukemias, myelodysplastic disorders, and severe viral infections can also cause neutropenia. Neutropenic patients may experience fever and can develop life-threatening sepsis from transient bacteremia that would otherwise be clinically silent in an immunocompetent host. Common sources include the skin and oral cavity. The vast majority of infectious problems can be resolved with antimicrobial agents and cessation of the inciting agent until neutrophil counts increase. Often, granulocyte colony stimulating factor (G-CSF) has been administered to help stimulate a rise in neutrophil counts. Recently, the American Society of Clinical Oncology Update committee expanded recommendations for the use of colony stimulating factors (CSFs) to include prevention of febrile neutropenia in high-risk patients and to allow a modest to moderate increase in dose density and/or intensity of chemotherapy regimens.[15] While this decision-making process will likely fall to oncologists and hematologists, surgeons should be aware of the potential for use of CSFs in the perioperative management of neutropenic patients. Typically, surgeons become involved in the management of these patients when a gastrointestinal source is suspected for neutropenic fever or when patients complain of abdominal pain. The differential diagnosis can range from common entities such as calculous cholecystitis, peptic ulcer disease, appendicitis, diverticulitis, and bowel obstruction to less common conditions such as neutropenic enterocolitis, spontaneous intestinal perforation, and acalculous cholecystitis.

HUMAN IMMUNODEFICIENCY VIRUS/ACQUIRED IMMUNODEFICIENCY SYNDROME

HIV is a blood borne retrovirus that targets the CD4 lymphocytes of the host. It uses reverse transcriptase to translate its viral RNA into DNA in the host cell, which thereafter enables the cell to manufacture millions of viral particles. These particles are released systemically after lysis of the host cell and are free to target other CD4 lymphocytes. The end result is massive depletion of CD4 lymphocytes and subsequent host immunosuppression, referred to as AIDS. Modern antiretroviral drug therapy has improved outcomes and prolonged survival in patients with HIV infection; however, a significant portion will go on to develop AIDS, the most advanced stage of HIV infection.[16] Clinically, this corresponds with a state of profound immunosuppression and is defined by the development of an AIDS-defining illness or when CD4 counts drop to <200 cells per mm^3 (Tables 56.6 and 56.7).[16]

According to Center for Disease Control estimates, more than 1 million people in the United States are infected with HIV, one-fifth of which are unaware of their infection. Each year in the United States, an estimated 56,300 new HIV infections occur and approximately 36,000 people are newly diagnosed with AIDS. In 2007, an estimated 455,636 people were living with AIDS in the United States (http://www.cdc.gov). While the numbers are striking, they pale in comparison to the global crisis affecting millions of people.

A recent review highlighted the current state of surgical care in HIV/AIDS patients.[17] The advent of antiretroviral drug therapy has improved the overall outcomes for these patients and has concomitantly decreased the number of operations for AIDS-related surgical illnesses. However, these patients will continue to require surgical intervention for a number of intra-abdominal problems. The authors highlight that although AIDS-related conditions (CMV gastroenteritis, typhlitis, GI lymphoma and Kaposi sarcoma, mycobacterial infection, etc.) should remain in the differential diagnosis in HIV patients undergoing evaluation for abdominal pain, illnesses common in non-HIV patients and unrelated to the immunocompromised state (appendicitis, diverticulitis, peptic ulcer disease, etc.) should also be considered and are often the most likely etiology of the patient's complaints. As with any immunocompromised patient, the physical and laboratory findings may be blunted in AIDS patients. Typical findings such as peritonitis and leukocytosis may be diminished or absent. Occasionally, CD4 counts are absent or outdated and may not be available in the acute situation to impact clinical decision making. In this instance, total lymphocyte count (TLC) has been shown to be a reasonable predictor of absolute CD4+ count (specificity 97% for CD4+ count < 200 per μL when TLC $<1.0 \times 10^9$ per L) and may be useful in the acute setting to gauge the degree of immunosuppression.[18] This is typically used as prognostic information as low CD4+ counts have been correlated with increased postoperative morbidity and mortality.[19,20] However, recent reviews have not found a correlation with low CD4+ counts and adverse postoperative outcomes although an increase in postoperative pneumonia and overall 12-month mortality was noted in a cohort of HIV+ patients, irrespective of CD4+ count.[21,22] In the trauma literature, it has been recently demonstrated that no major difference in mortality exists for patients with HIV, although this

TABLE 56.6

AIDS-DEFINING CONDITIONS

- Candidiasis of bronchi, trachea, or lungs
- Candidiasis, esophageal
- Cervical cancer, invasive[a]
- Coccidioidomycosis, disseminated or extrapulmonary
- Cryptococcosis, extrapulmonary
- Cryptosporidiosis, chronic intestinal (>1 mo duration)
- CMV disease (other than liver, spleen, or nodes)
- CMV retinitis (with loss of vision)
- Encephalopathy, HIV related
- Herpes simplex: chronic ulcer(s) (>1 mo duration); or bronchitis, pneumonitis, or esophagitis
- Histoplasmosis, disseminated or extrapulmonary
- Isosporiasis, chronic intestinal (>1 mo duration)
- Kaposi's sarcoma
- Lymphoma, Burkitt's (or equivalent term)
- Lymphoma, immunoblastic (or equivalent term)
- Lymphoma, primary, of brain
- *Mycobacterium avium* complex or *Mycobacterium kansasii*, disseminated or extrapulmonary
- *Mycobacterium tuberculosis*, any site (pulmonary[a] or extrapulmonary)
- *Mycobacterium*, other species or unidentified species, disseminated or extrapulmonary
- *P. carinii* pneumonia
- Pneumonia, recurrent[a]
- Progressive multifocal leukoencephalopathy
- *Salmonella septicemia*, recurrent
- Toxoplasmosis of brain
- Wasting syndrome due to HIV

[a]From Centers for Disease Control. 1993 Revised classification system for HIV infection and expanded surveillance case definition for AIDS among adolescents and adults. *MMWR Morb Mortal Wkly Rep.* 1992;41:1–19.

patient population had a higher risk of infectious complications and a longer hospital length of stay.[23]

HEMATOPOIETIC CELL TRANSPLANTATION

Hematopoietic cell transplantation, commonly referred to as bone marrow transplantation, is achieved by ablation of a recipient's hematopoietic and immune systems with cytotoxic chemotherapy with or without radiation (known as conditioning) prior to intravenous delivery of hematopoietic stem cells obtained from bone marrow, peripheral blood, or umbilical cord blood. It is used for treatment of bone marrow failure, malignancies such as leukemia, lymphoma, and multiple myeloma, immunodeficiency syndromes and inborn errors of metabolism. The treatment produces a profound state of immunocompromise in the recipient and a markedly elevated risk of infection. The timeline of immunocompromise can be divided into three risk periods: the preengraftment period (defined from the onset of conditioning to recovery of neutrophil counts), the early postengraftment period (defined by neutrophil recovery extending until day 100, which approximates the onset of B- and T-lymphocyte functional recovery), and the late postengraftment period (which is defined by day 100 until normal immunity is achieved). Each of the periods is associated with increased risk for specific infections and necessitates appropriate prophylaxis. Bacterial infections predominate during the early time points while viral and fungal infections become more prominent as time elapses in the postengraftment period.[24] In the unfortunate circumstance of a surgical emergency prior to achievement of normal immunity, a high morbidity and mortality is anticipated.

TABLE 56.7

CD4+ T-LYMPHOCYTE STAGES

Stage 1	≥500 cells/μL[a]
Stage 2	200–499 cells/μL[a]
Stage 3 (AIDS)	<200 cells/μL[b]

[a]Without AIDS defining condition (see Table 56.6).
[b]With or without AIDS defining condition.

AGING AND MALNUTRITION

Aging is associated with a phenomenon referred to as immunosenescence—age related changes in immune function initially conceptualized as a global immune hyporesponsiveness. Although the mechanisms of these changes are extremely complex and are still being elucidated, multiple *in vitro* and *in vivo* studies in mice and humans have demonstrated impairment of both innate and adaptive immunity. Defects in multiple effectors of the immune response have been demonstrated, including neutrophil and macrophage phagocytic activity, antibody production, B and T lymphocyte proliferation, and IL-2 production.[25–27] However, aging is also associated with an increase in proinflammatory mediators resulting in a state of chronic low-grade inflammation. Several studies have demonstrated increased proinflammatory cytokines such as TNFα and IL-6 as well as an overall decrease in B and T lymphocyte receptor repertoire diversity.[28,29] As a result, immunosenescence is now thought to reflect overall dysregulation of the immune system rather than simply impaired function. The end result is an increased risk of infections, autoimmune disorders, and malignancy in elderly patients.[30–32] Complicating the issue is the synchronous issue of malnutrition in the elderly. Poor nutritional status is also recognized as a cause of immune dysfunction and a risk factor for increased mortality in elderly hospitalized patients.[33] The specific mechanisms have yet to be defined; however, studies have suggested that malnutrition impacts neutrophil chemotaxis and lymphocyte counts although this may not be reversed by improving nutrition in elderly patients.[34–36] The data is difficult to interpret in light of the complex environmental influences such as comorbid conditions, functional status, etc. Consequently, the interaction between malnutrition and the aging process that results in the immune phenotype we see clinically is still poorly understood. Despite the evidence for immune dysfunction, the impact on surgical outcomes is difficult to quantify specifically. A practical approach is to recognize age as an additional risk factor, along with the patient's nutritional state and comorbid conditions, for an impaired inflammatory response and subsequently, increased postoperative infectious complications and poorer outcomes.

BURNS/CRITICAL ILLNESS

Thermal injury is associated with an increased risk of infection that goes beyond the loss of normal barrier function of the skin. Numerous alterations in innate and adaptive immunity occur leaving the patient susceptible to infection, sepsis, and multiorgan dysfunction. Indeed, after the early postburn period, infectious complications are the leading cause of mortality. The observed immune dysfunction is postulated to be a result of alterations in the cytokine expression. Recent work has implicated macrophage hyperactivity and leads to a shift in Th-1/Th-2 balance.[37] The exact mechanisms are complex and have yet to be fully elucidated. Even in the absence of thermal injury, critical illness such as sepsis and multiorgan failure is associated with immune dysfunction. One proposed mechanism is the immunomodulating effects exerted by the sympathetic nervous system via catecholamines, which include increased IL-6 and TNFα production, depressed neutrophil function, and decreased cellular adhesion to the endothelium. Furthermore, catecholamines have been shown to increase growth of several bacteria including *Escherichia coli* and *Staphylococcus epidermidis in vivo*, purportedly because of their ability to supply iron to bacteria via interactions with iron-laden transferrin and lactoferrin.[38] Clearly, critically ill patients as a result of burns or sepsis represent an extremely complex environment with multiple concomitant factors that precludes simple description. Fortunately, heightened awareness for infectious complications is well integrated into the practices of those that care for this patient population.

SUBSTANCE ABUSE

Substance abuse has been shown to be associated with increased infection risk. While intuitively this may be attributed to the risk-taking behavior associated with substance abuse, emerging data demonstrate that the agents of abuse themselves have immunomodulatory effects. Opiates have been shown, in both animal models and human studies, to have immunosuppressive effects, likely mediated by direct action on immune cells via opioid receptors. Cannabinoids are also thought to have a receptor-mediated immunosuppressive effect, with animal and human studies implicating HPA axis and autonomic nervous system pathways. Increased susceptibility to bacterial and viral pathogens has been demonstrated in animal models. Similarly, nicotine is thought to impact the HPA axis, although via nicotinic acetylcholine receptors rather than cannabinoid receptors. Very little is known regarding the immunomodulating effect of cocaine but a receptor-mediated mechanism is also suspected. Alcohol's effect on the immune system, in contrast, is not thought to be receptor mediated, although it is associated with global depletion of circulating lymphocytes and decreased cytokine production. Animal models have demonstrated increased susceptibility to bacterial infection, and observational data suggest an increased risk of viral infection in humans who abuse alcohol.[39] Taken as a whole, substance abuse should be considered an additional risk factor for impaired immunity and increased susceptibility to infection.

DIABETES

Diabetes mellitus is associated with an increased susceptibility to infection. Diabetic patients develop infections at a higher rate and are at increased risk for severe infections such as necrotizing soft tissue infections.[40] Poor glucose control indicated by persistent fasting hyperglycemia has been linked to abnormalities in innate immunity. Specific alterations included increased basal cytokine secretion, impaired neutrophil chemotaxis, phagocytosis, and bactericidal activity, and impaired monocyte/macrophage function. In addition, the hyperglycemic environment has been shown to enhance the virulence of certain organisms including *Candida albicans* and *E. coli*.[41] Conflicting data exist on whether cell-mediated adaptive immunity is significantly affected. Even so, diabetes mellitus should not be discounted as a risk factor for severe, complicated infections and postoperative infectious complications. The data also underscores the importance of maintaining normoglycemia in the perioperative setting, especially in critically ill patients.

GENERAL CONSIDERATIONS

Diagnosis

Surgeons must possess a high degree of suspicion when evaluating for surgical pathology in the immunocompromised patient as many of the local and systemic signs of inflammation are blunted. Notoriously, immunocompromised patients may fail to demonstrate peritonitis despite significant intra-abdominal pathology. In the case of soft tissue pathology, local findings such as erythema, induration, or purulence may not correlate with the severity of infection. Patients may or may not demonstrate fever and may simply present with changes in vital signs (e.g., tachycardia and hypotension) and metabolic acidosis. White blood cell counts may be elevated, but are often normal or low. In fact, a normal white blood cell count may actually represent a relative leukocytosis in a patient who is normally leukopenic. While the physical exam is often unreliable, positive findings should be taken seriously and should prompt a vigorous workup. Radiographic imaging plays a significant role in the evaluation of abdominal complaints in these patients (Fig. 56.1). The mainstay is computed tomography (CT) scanning. As mentioned above, significant intra-abdominal pathology such as abscess or intestinal necrosis or perforation may be present without the diffuse generalized peritonitis observed in immunocompetent patients. For invasive soft tissue infection, pursuit of radiographic imaging to assist with diagnosis may cause unnecessary and dangerous delays in appropriate surgical management. If severe infection necessitating surgical debridement is suspected, prompt operative exploration is warranted and serves as a diagnostic maneuver as well as potentially life-saving intervention.

Preoperative Management

Once the decision to intervene surgically has been made, the priorities in preoperative management remain unchanged from that of immunocompetent patients. The patient should receive prompt, appropriate fluid resuscitation, invasive hemodynamic monitoring if necessary, and broad-spectrum antibiotics where applicable. Antimicrobial therapy should be directed toward the most likely etiologic organisms based on the pathophysiology of the disease process; however, the hospital-specific antibiogram and patterns of microbial resistance should play a role in antimicrobial selection. In addition, empiric antifungal therapy should be considered given the propensity of immunocompromised patients to fungal infection. Perhaps the most important consideration specific to immunosuppressed patients is for those who are receiving chronic corticosteroid therapy. These patients should receive stress dose steroids perioperatively to prevent the sequelae of adrenal insufficiency. As with immunocompetent patients, immunocompromised patients should receive appropriate surgical intervention for acute surgical conditions as rapidly as possible. Unnecessary delays in proceeding to the operating room should be avoided.

Operative Considerations

For the majority of disease processes requiring surgical intervention, the operative procedure itself changes very little in immunocompromised patients compared to immunocompetent patients. Invasive soft tissue infection should be debrided back to healthy tissue, abdominal explorations should be complete and thorough, and ischemic or infarcted bowel should be resected. If a large amount of bowel remains in question and not obviously necrotic, temporary abdominal closure with return to the operating room for a "second look" in 24–36 hours is appropriate. When bowel resection is required, the surgeon faces the decision of whether to perform a primary anastomosis or divert the fecal stream. If the patient falls into the category of profoundly immunocompromised, the patient is at increased risk of anastomotic leak and dehiscence due to impaired wound healing. The immunocompromised state further exposes the patient to increased morbidity and mortality from intra-abdominal abscess and sepsis. In these cases, fecal diversion is recommended. Similarly, cases in which significant peritoneal contamination is present, such as colonic perforation with fecal peritonitis, typically require formation of a diverting stoma. In select patients, there remains the possibility of electively reestablishing intestinal continuity after the patient has recovered from the acute process. Primary anastomosis may be considered in cases in which there is minimal peritoneal contamination or the patient only has risk factors for relative immunocompromise. In this instance the surgeon's clinical judgment is paramount. Factors such as the patient's overall presentation, comorbid conditions, operative course, and hemodynamic state play a role in the decision-making process. While frequently fecal diversion is justified based on the above factors, primary anastomosis with or without proximal diversion of the fecal stream is a viable option as well in select patients with minimal risk factors.

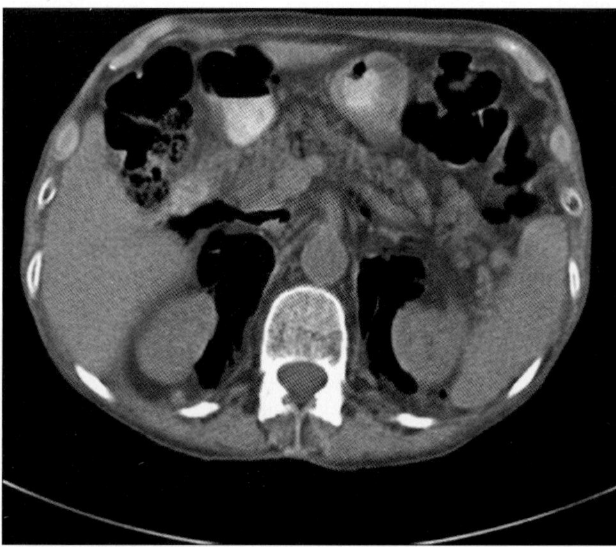

FIGURE 56.1. Massive retroperitoneal air extending medial to the bilateral kidneys secondary to descending colon perforation in a lung transplant recipient.

Abdominal closure presents another challenge in the operative management of the immunocompromised patient. These patients are at increased risk for postoperative wound infection and fascial dehiscence secondary to impaired wound healing. While closing the abdominal wall, particular attention must be paid to the strength and integrity of the fascia. Immunocompromised patients often demonstrate a thin, attenuated fascia with decreased tensile strength. Conversely, patients may have normal-appearing fascia that is still at risk for dehiscence due to an impaired inflammatory response that is essential for normal wound healing. Patients at greatest risk are those who are profoundly immunosuppressed, such as transplant recipients and cancer patients receiving chemotherapy. Likewise, elderly and/or malnourished patients and those receiving chronic corticosteroid therapy are at increased risk for poor fascial healing. If such risk factors are present or considerable concern exists over the integrity of the fascia, retention sutures may be used to prevent the catastrophic event of evisceration, should a large fascial dehiscence occur during the patient's convalescence. Postoperative incisional hernia is a predictable complication in this setting and likely represents partial fascial dehiscence during the recovery process. If the surgical wound is contaminated, standard skin closure should be avoided. In this instance, leaving an open wound to heal by secondary intention, either with daily dressings or vacuum-assisted closure is the conservative approach. Unfortunately, impaired wound healing consigns the patient to a chronic wound that may take months to heal. Alternatively, partial skin closure and delayed primary closure are both wound management strategies geared toward minimizing the postoperative wound infection risk while simultaneously attempting to decrease the size of the wound. Obviously, signs of a wound infection in a wound that is closed or partially closed should prompt immediate opening of the wound and initiation of antimicrobial therapy if considerable cellulitis is present.

Postoperative Management

Management for immunocompromised patients in the immediate postoperative period differs little from that of immunocompetent patients. Resuscitation should proceed with typical endpoints of restoring end-organ perfusion as indicated by blood pressure and urine output. Ventilatory management, invasive hemodynamic support, and pharmacologic support should proceed according to established guidelines, similar to that of immunocompetent patients. For patients who receive chronic corticosteroid therapy, stress dose steroids (typically hydrocortisone 50–100 mg intravenously every 8 hours) should be continued in the postoperative setting and gradually tapered over several days down to their preoperative dosing regimen.

Immunocompromised patients are at increased risk for postoperative infectious complications. While wound infections and intra-abdominal abscess are vivid examples, these patients are also at increased risk for pneumonia, catheter-related infection and sepsis, urinary tract infection, and antibiotic-associated diarrhea and colitis. Consequently, immunocompromised patients must be closely monitored and any indication of infectious complications should prompt a thorough workup to determine the source. Empiric antimicrobial therapy should be tailored to specific organisms based on preoperative or intraoperative culture results as soon as these are available. An abrupt decline in clinical status in which infection is suspected usually warrants broadening of the antimicrobial spectrum until the specific etiology is found.

Fungal Infections

The immunosuppression associated with solid-organ transplantation increases the risk of fungal infection. The incidence of these infections may also be increased because of the use of broad-spectrum antimicrobial agents. Agents that are useful for treating fungal pathogens include amphotericin B, azoles, and echinocandins. Amphotericin B acts to prevent fungal growth by binding to fungal cell wall sterols and causing cell death via lysis. Azoles inhibit the cytochrome P450 enzyme responsible for ergosterol synthesis. Echinocandins inhibit glucan synthesis, disrupting cell wall structure. Often the different mechanisms of action of the echinocandins and azoles are utilized simultaneously by administering dual therapy. A recent report of transplant recipients with invasive aspergillosis receiving combination therapy of voriconazole and caspofungin showed improved survival in patients with either renal failure or *Aspergillus fumigatus* infection compared to those receiving a lipid formulation of amphotericin B.[42]

The most common fungal pathogens seen in immunocompromised patients are *Candida* species. The widespread use of fluconazole has likely contributed to the increased incidence of species resistant to this agent. Suspected fungal infection should be treated initially with a broad-spectrum antifungal agent such as caspofungin or voriconazole. Unfortunately, approximately 1% of transplant patients develop infection with *Aspergillus* species and this possibility should be considered in patients who fail to respond to initial therapy. If suspected, empiric therapy is warranted rather than waiting for a definitive diagnosis as invasive aspergillosis is associated with mortality as high as 60%.[43]

Other Infectious Concerns

Viral infections are important causes of morbidity and mortality in solid-organ transplant recipients. Endemic viruses of little concern to the immunocompetent population may be life threatening in the immunosuppressed host. CMV is a common pathogen in the transplant population affecting nearly 50% of kidney transplant recipients.[44] Donor seropositivity (in seronegative recipient), high dose immunosuppression, and repeated treatment for rejection are all risk factors for CMV infection.[45] The range and severity of infection with CMV is large and the lungs, gastrointestinal tract, liver, retina, and pancreas can all be affected. CMV antigen in blood or body fluid confirms diagnosis and treatment typically consists of intravenous ganciclovir followed by oral valganciclovir (Table 56.8).

Polyoma (BK) virus has a worldwide prevalence of about 98% in the general population with near universal exposure during childhood. In kidney transplant recipients, reactivation of the virus, which typically resides in latent form in the kidney, can result in inflammatory interstitial nephritis progressing to renal failure known as BK or polyoma-associated nephropathy. Thus far, this development has only been observed in kidney transplant patients. Risk factors for reactivation include tacrolimus use and recent treatment for rejection. In patients with unexplained renal failure after renal transplant, the presence of BK virus should be evaluated using polymerase chain reaction on urine and blood samples. Patients with a viremia should undergo reduction of immunosuppression.

Pneumocystis jiroveci, previously known as *Pneumocystis carinii*, is a common cause of pneumonia in immunosuppressed patients and should be considered in any patient presenting with respiratory symptoms who is not receiving prophylactic therapy. Empirical therapy with intravenous trimethoprim/sulfamethoxazole or pentamidine is necessary before established diagnosis due to an associated high mortality with delays in treatment.

TABLE 56.8

EMPIRICAL AGENTS FOR EARLY TREATMENT OF INFECTION IN TRANSPLANT PATIENTS

CLASS OF AGENT	AGENT	DOSE[a]
Broad-spectrum antibiotic agents[b]	Piperacillin/Tazobactam Meropenem Imipenem/cilastatin	3.375 g IV q6h 0.5–1 g IV q8h 0.5–1 g IV q6–8h
Gram-positive agents[c]	Vancomycin Daptomycin[d] Quinupristin/dalfopristin Linezolid Tigecycline[e]	1–1.5 g IV q12–24h 4–6 mg/kg IV daily 7.5 mg/kg IV q8h 600 mg IV q12h 100 mg IV load, 50 mg IV q12h
Antifungal agents	Voriconazole Posaconazole Caspofungin Anidulafungin Liposomal amphotericin B	6 mg/kg IV q12h × 2, then 4 mg/kg IV q12h Oral only: 200 mg 3–4 times daily 70 mg load, 50 mg IV daily 200 mg load, 100 mg IV daily 3–10 mg/kg IV daily
Antiviral agents[f]	Ganciclovir Foscarnet	2.5–5 mg/kg IV q12h 90 mg/kg IV q12h

[a]Please note that doses given do not account for renal or hepatic insufficiency common in critically ill patients. Prior to choosing an empirical antibiotic regimen, the clinician should carefully consider the patient scenario and medication side effects related to the specific patient.
[b]Rather than a single agent, combination agents covering both gram-negative organisms and anaerobes may be chosen (e.g., fluoroquinolone plus clindamycin or metronidazole). For cases with a strong suspicion for *Pseudomonas aeruginosa* infection, additional *Pseudomonas* coverage should be added (e.g., fluoroquinolone or aminoglycoside).
[c]When vancomycin-resistant *Enterococcus faecium* infection is suspected, one of the latter four choices should be employed.
[d]Daptomycin is not indicated for treatment of pneumonia (package insert).
[e]Tigecycline is not indicated for treatment of hospital-acquired pneumonia (package insert)
[f]Antiviral agents directed toward herpesvirus family (most commonly CMV). Adjust for other viruses.

Rejection

Rejection remains a constant concern in the management of the transplant patient in whom immunosuppression has been held or decreased in order to manage infection. Indeed, this is often the case given the spectrum of pathology the acute care surgeon encounters. Particular attention must be paid to the transplanted organ in order to detect early signs of rejection. Renal allografts are monitored with serum creatinine and blood urea nitrogen determinations although these may be elevated as a result of acute renal failure secondary to the acute illness. Likewise, cardiac dysfunction, respiratory failure, liver dysfunction, and hyperglycemia all represent issues that accompany critical illness but may also be attributed to developing rejection of that particular transplanted organ. Consequently, it is imperative that the patient's transplant team be involved in the care of the patient to help with decision making in this regard. Rejection is definitively diagnosed by biopsy and histopathologic examination although empiric therapy to combat rejection may be initiated if the patient's overall condition allows and the diagnosis is strongly suspected. High-dose corticosteroids and antibody therapy are commonly used to treat rejection.

Human Immunodeficiency Virus/Acquired Immunodeficiency Syndrome

In general, surgical care in patients with HIV/AIDS should proceed similar to the patient without HIV. While CD4+ counts may offer prognostic information, this data may not always be available although TLC may be a useful predictor. Regardless, a high index of suspicion must be corroborated with adjunctive studies and vigilance must be exercised if delays in appropriate surgical care are to be avoided. Both disease processes common to HIV/AIDS patients and those unrelated to HIV/AIDS must be considered in the differential diagnosis. Postoperatively, infectious complications should be sought and treated aggressively. Collaboration with infectious disease/HIV specialists is crucial to ensure appropriate management of antiretroviral therapy postoperatively. Antiretroviral therapy should not be interrupted for any period longer than necessary since viral replication begins shortly after interruption of therapy.[46] Finally, while surgical care of this patient population does expose caretakers to the possibility of HIV transmission, the average risk is very low. The average risk of transmission after exposure to HIV-infected blood has been estimated to be 0.3% for the percutaneous route and 0.09% for mucous membrane exposure.[47,48] Care must be taken to minimize exposure; however, excessive measures are likely to be unnecessary. Exposures should be reported immediately so that post exposure prophylaxis can be initiated in a timely fashion.

SURGICAL DISEASE PROCESSES RELATED TO THE IMMUNOCOMPROMISED STATE

Posttransplant Lymphoproliferative Disorder

Posttransplant lymphoproliferative disorder (PTLD) refers to a spectrum of uncontrolled B-cell proliferation linked to Ebstein-Barr virus (EBV) infection that ranges from simple benign hyperplasia to lymphoma. This disorder is associated with increased morbidity and mortality to immunocompromised hosts, typically solid-organ and bone marrow transplant recipients. PTLD typically occurs during times of most intensive immunosuppression. The incidence of PTLD is low in renal and pancreas transplantation compared with other solid-organ transplants (2.6% at 10 years). (http://optn.transplant.hrsa.gov). The clinical presentation of this disorder can vary widely. Many patients present with nonspecific symptoms such as malaise, fever, and weight loss. Others present acutely with hemodynamic instability and markedly elevated serum lactate level that is refractory to aggressive fluid resuscitation. Patients may even present emergently with perforation, obstruction or hemorrhage requiring surgical intervention, although this represents a minority of patients.

Evaluation for suspected PTLD should include imaging of the brain, chest, and abdomen, with targeted biopsies to obtain a tissue diagnosis. Treatment of patients with PTLD has not been well standardized but includes reduction of immunosuppression, surgical resection, or radiotherapy for localized disease, or treatment with chemotherapy and/or anti–B-cell antibody (rituximab) for more extensive or refractory disease. Other treatment options include administration of antiviral therapy and interferon-α, although these modalities are under investigation.[49–51] Patients receiving chemotherapy or rituximab for gastrointestinal PTLD may suffer perforation during treatment secondary to tumor lysis and require emergent laparotomy.[52]

Neutropenic Enterocolitis

The most common gastrointestinal source of infection related to neutropenia is neutropenic enterocolitis, also known as typhlitis. The exact etiology is unknown but is postulated to be multifactorial, involving intestinal mucosal injury, neutropenia, and impaired mucosal defense against gastrointestinal microorganisms. The mucosal injury may be a direct cytotoxic effect of chemotherapy or radiotherapy or may be related to neutropenia itself in the absence of cytotoxic therapy. The mucosal injury leads to loss of gut barrier function and allows translocation of bacteria and unchecked invasion of the intestinal wall. This leads to inflammation, edema, and ultimately perforation. Treatment with antibiotics is typically sufficient but early diagnosis is imperative. CT is the mainstay of diagnosis and demonstrates sensitivity as high as 92%. Diagnostic imaging is crucial since physical exam findings are typically minimal due to the inability of neutropenic patients to mount a substantial inflammatory response and thus demonstrate peritonitis (Fig. 56.2). When present, findings may be diffuse or localized to the right lower quadrant, as the terminal ileum is the most common site of pathology. In the absence of hemodynamic instability, generalized peritonitis or imaging findings suggestive of perforation, antimicrobial therapy targeted toward gram-negative and anaerobic organisms is the standard treatment. G-CSF should be administered to normalize neutrophil counts. Surgical intervention is mandated for imaging findings suggestive of intestinal perforation, in unstable patients demonstrating shock, and in patients who fail medical management. Diverting stoma formation is obligatory in most cases if intestinal resection is required.[53]

Gastrointestinal Cytomegalovirus Infection

Profoundly immunosuppressed patients are at risk for development of upper and lower gastrointestinal tract involvement with CMV, leading to abdominal pain, bleeding, and rarely, perforation. While historically seen in patients suffering from AIDS and those receiving immunosuppressive therapy for inflammatory disorders, the rise of solid-organ transplantation has provided a growing population of susceptible patients.

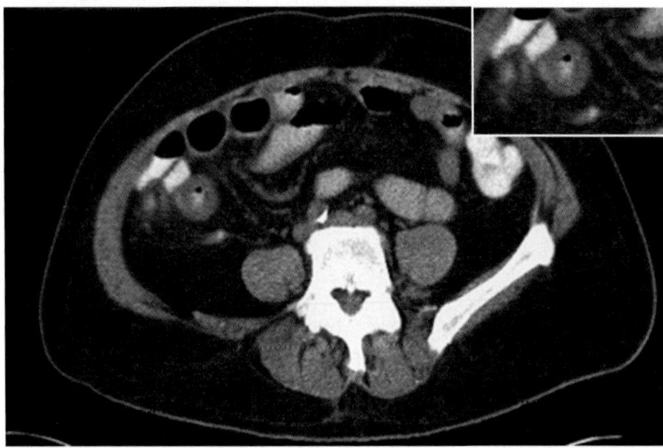

FIGURE 56.2. CT scan showing inflammation of the terminal ileum consistent with typhlitis in a neutropenic patient. Inset highlights the inflamed terminal ileum.

Initial CMV infection most commonly occurs within about 6 months of transplantation, correlating with the highest immunosuppressive load. CMV infections are more common in serologically negative patients who received organs from a CMV positive donor. CMV-related problems are also more common among patients with known CMV infection and those treated with relatively high doses of immunosuppression.[45] As a result, routine prophylaxis against CMV infection has been included in the first few months of post-organ transplantation protocols in many centers nationwide, while others perform routine surveillance for CMV for weeks to months following transplantation. While these strategies have decreased early development of CMV infection, late infection can still occur.[45] Diagnostic endoscopy should be performed early in patients with suspected gastrointestinal involvement with CMV, tissue biopsies of the stomach and/or colon should be obtained to evaluate for the presence of CMV. Initial treatment consists of intravenous ganciclovir or foscarnet, with a switch to maintenance therapy by oral agents as tolerated for a period of weeks to months. Refractory bleeding and perforation are obvious indications for surgical intervention, although intervention in the patient population susceptible to this disease process is associated with high morbidity and mortality.

Necrotizing Soft Tissue Infection and Invasive Fungal Infection

Necrotizing soft tissue infection is an entity well known to the acute care surgeon and is described in detail elsewhere in this text. Necrotizing soft tissue infection as a complication of immunosuppression such as in transplantation is a rare event, but has been reported.[54] It is associated with significant morbidity and mortality and, as in immunocompetent patients, should be treated with emergent surgical debridement and systemic antimicrobial therapy. Fungal etiologies must be considered and appropriately covered in the antimicrobial regimen if suspected. Necrotizing fasciitis caused by *Candida* species has been reported and a series of primary deep cutaneous opportunistic mycoses secondary to multiple organisms including *Alternaria*, *Aspergillus*, *Histoplasma,* and *Blastomyces* species has been published.[55–57] If not treated promptly, systemic dissemination may occur, a frequently fatal development. Timely intervention relies on early diagnosis and intervention, which is predicated on including fungal etiologies in the differential diagnosis.

Conclusion

The immunocompromised patient certainly presents a challenge that acute care surgeons must be prepared to confront in clinical practice. Patients may present with profound immunocompromise secondary to immunosuppressive medication, chemotherapy, or AIDS. It is more probable, however, that surgeons will encounter those who are relatively immunocompromised such as the diabetic, elderly, malnourished, or critically ill. Often, multiple risk factors for relative immunocompromise may be present simultaneously. While distinguishing between profound and relative immunocompromise is useful for generally assessing the risk of complications related to a compromised immune response, it also has clinical utility in formulating the differential diagnosis in patients in which the diagnosis is unclear. A high index of suspicion is necessary to treat these patients in a timely and appropriate manner. Broad-spectrum antibiotics should be instituted without delay, appropriately tailored based on culture results, and discontinued when clinically indicated. Agents active against viral and fungal pathogens should be included in the selection of antimicrobial therapy if significant risk for these pathogens exists. Likewise, surgical intervention should proceed promptly to achieve source control as rapidly as possible. Intraoperatively, special consideration must be given to the wound healing capability of the patient. Fecal diversion is indicated for those who are profoundly immunocompromised and should be considered in the relatively immunocompromised patient if additional risk factors are present. Retention sutures may also be used if fascial dehiscence is of particular concern. The postoperative care of the immunocompromised patient requires vigilance in monitoring for the development of infectious and/or wound healing complications as presenting signs may be minimal. Stress dose steroids should be administered to those patients who receive chronic corticosteroid therapy or demonstrate adrenal insufficiency. Close collaboration with specialists in transplant and HIV/AIDS patients is mandatory, as these patients will need to resume immunosuppressive or antiretroviral therapy postoperatively and the decision regarding timing may be difficult. Ultimately, as the specialty of acute care surgery expands and our ability to care for critically ill patients continues to improve, the capacity to provide safe acute care surgery services to the immunocompromised patient population should also continue to improve.

References

1. Turvey SE, Bonilla FA, Junker AK. Primary immunodeficiency diseases: a practical guide for clinicians. *Postgrad Med J*. 2009;85:660-666.
2. Aberra FN, Lewis JD, Hass D, et al. Corticosteroids and immunomodulators: postoperative infectious complication risk in inflammatory bowel disease patients. *Gastroenterology*. 2003;125:320-327.
3. Busti AJ, Hooper JS, Amaya CJ, et al. Effects of perioperative anti-inflammatory and immunomodulating therapy on surgical wound healing. *Pharmacotherapy*. 2005;25:1566-1591.
4. Rostambeigi N, Kudva YC, John S, et al. Epidemiology of infections requiring hospitalization during long-term follow-up of pancreas transplantation. *Transplantation*. 2010;89(9):1126-1133.
5. Snydman DR. Epidemiology of infections after solid-organ transplantation. *Clin Infect Dis*. 2001;33(suppl 1):S5-S8.
6. Columbel JF, Loftus EV, Tremaine WJ, et al. Early postoperative complications are not increased in patients with Crohn's disease treated perioperatively with infliximab or immunosuppressive therapy. *Am J Gastroenterol*. 2004;99:878-883.
7. Kunitake H, Hodin R, Richard S, et al. Perioperative treatment with infliximab in patients with Crohn's disease and ulcerative colitis is not associated with an increased rate of postoperative complications. *J Gastrointest Surg*. 2008;12:1730-1736.
8. Mahadevan U, Loftus EV, Tremaine, WJ, et al. Azathioprine or 6-mercaptopurine before colectomy for ulcerative colitis is not associated with increased postoperative complications. *Inflamm Bowel Dis*. 2002;8:311-316.

9. Marchal L, D'Haens G, Van Assche G, et al. The risk of post-operative complications associated with infliximab therapy for Crohn's disease: a controlled cohort study. *Aliment Pharmacol Ther*. 2004;19:749-754.
10. Appau KA, Fazio FW, Shen B, et al. Use of infliximab within 3 months of ileocolonic resection is associated with adverse perioperative outcomes in Crohn's disease patients. *J Gastrointest Surg*. 2008;12:1738-1744.
11. Mor IJ, Vogel JD, da Luz Moreira A, et al. Infliximab in ulcerative colitis is associated with an increased risk of postoperative complications after restorative proctocolectomy. *Dis Colon Rectum*. 2008;51:1202-1207.
12. Schluender SJ, Ippoliti A, Dubinski M, et al. Does infliximab influence surgical morbidity of ileal pouch-anal anastomosis in patients with ulcerative colitis? *Dis Colon Rectum*. 2007;50:1747-1753.
13. Selvasekar CR, Cima RR, Larson DW, et al. Effect of infliximab on short-term complications in patients undergoing operation for chronic ulcerative colitis. *J Am Coll Surg*. 2007;204:956-962.
14. Mushtaq S, Goodman, SM, Scanzello CR. Perioperative management of biologic agents used in treatment of rheumatoid arthritis. *Am J Ther*. 2011;18(5):426-434.
15. Smith TJ, Khatcheressian J, Lyman GH, et al. 2006 Update of recommendations for the use of white blood cell growth factors: an evidence-based clinical practice guideline. *J Clin Oncol*. 2006;4:3187-3205.
16. Centers for Disease Control. 2008 Revised surveillance case definitions for HIV infection among adults, adolescents, and children aged <18 months and for HIV infection and AIDS among children aged 18 months to <13 years—United States, 2008. *MMWR Morb Mortal Wkly Rep*. 2008;57:1-8.
17. Saltzman DJ, Williams RA, Gelfand DV, et al. The surgeon and AIDS: twenty years later. *Arch Surg*. 2005;140:961-967.
18. Blatt SP, Lucey CR, Butzin CA, et al. Total lymphocyte count as predictor of absolute CD4+ count and CD4+ percentage in HIV-infected persons. *J Am Med Assoc*. 1993;269:622-626.
19. Albaran RG, Webber J, Steffes CP. CD4 cell counts as a prognostic factor of major abdominal surgery in patients infected with the human immunodeficiency virus. *Arch Surg*. 1998;133:626-631.
20. Savioz D, Chilcott M, Ludwig C, et al. Preoperative counts of CD4 T-lymphocytes and early postoperative infective complications in HIV-positive patients. *Eur J Surg*. 1998;164:483-487.
21. Cacala SR, Mafana E, Thomson SR, et al. Prevalence of HIV status and CD4 counts in a surgical cohort: their relationship to clinical outcome. *Ann R Coll Surg Engl*. 2006;88:46-51.
22. Horberg MA, Hurley LB, Klein DB, et al. Surgical outcomes in human immunodeficiency virus-infected patients in the era of highly active antiretroviral therapy. *Arch Surg*. 2006;141:1238-1245.
23. Morrison CA, Wyatt, MM, Carrick MM. Effects of human immunodeficiency virus status on trauma outcomes: a review of the national trauma database. *Surg Infect*. 2010;11:41-47.
24. Mandell GL, Bennett JE, Dolin R, eds. *Mandell, Douglas, and Bennett's Principles and Practice of Infectious Disease*. 7th ed. Philadelphia, PA: Elsevier Incorporated; 2010.
25. Agarwal S, Busse PJ. Innate and adaptive immunosenescence. *Ann Allergy Asthma Immunol*. 2010;104:183-190.
26. Gomez CR, Nomellini V, Faunce DE, et al. Innate immunity and aging. *Exp Gerontol*. 2008;43:718-728.
27. Miller RA. The aging immune system: primer and prospectus. *Science*. 1996;273:70-74.
28. Aspinall R, Goronzy JJ. Immune senescence: editorial review. *Curr Opin Immunol*. 2010;22:497-499.
29. Shaw AC, Josi S, Greenwood H, et al. Aging of the innate immune system. *Curr Opin Immunol*. 2010;22:507-513.
30. Ahmad A, Banerjee S, Wang Z, et al. Aging and inflammation: etiological culprits of cancer. *Curr Aging Sci*. 2009;2:174-186.
31. Caruso C, Lio D, Cavallone L, et al. Aging, longevity, inflammation and cancer. *Ann N Y Acad Sci*. 2004;1028:1-13.
32. Gardner ID. The Effect of aging on susceptibility to infection. *Rev Infect Dis*. 1980;2:801-810.
33. Incalzi RA, Capparella O, Gemma A, et al. Inadequate caloric intake: a risk factor for mortality of geriatric patients in the acute-care hospital. *Age Ageing*. 1998;27:303-310.
34. Chandra RK. Nutrition and immunololgy: from the clinic to cellular biology and back again. *Proc Nutr Soc*. 1999;58:681-683.
35. Lesourd B, Mazari L. Nutrition and immunity in the elderly. *Proc Nutr Soc*. 1999;58:685-695.
36. Walrand S, Moreau K, Caldefie F, et al. Specific and nonspecific immune responses to fasting and refeeding differ in healthy young adult and elderly persons. *Am J Clin Nutr*. 2001;74:670-678.
37. Schwacha MG. Macrophages and post-burn immune dysfunction. *Burns*. 2003;29(1):1-14.
38. Dunser MW, Hasibeder WR. Sympathetic overstimulation during critical illness: adverse effects of adrenergic stress. *J Intensive Care Med*. 2009;24(5):293-316.
39. Friedman H, Newton C, Klein TW. Microbial infections, immunomodulation, and drugs of abuse. *Clin Microbiol Rev*. 2003;16(2):209-219.
40. Endorf FW, Supple KG, Gamelli RL. The evolving characteristics and care of necrotizing soft-tissue infections. *Burns*. 2005;31(3):269-273.
41. Geerlings SE, Hoepelman AI. Immune dysfunction in patients with diabetes mellitus. *FEMS Immunol Med Microbiol*. 1999;26(3-4):259-265.
42. Singh N, Limaye AP, Forrest G, et al. Combination of voriconazole and caspofungin as primary therapy for invasive aspergillosis in solid organ transplant recipients: a prospective, multicenter, observational study. *Transplantation*. 2006;81(3):320-326.
43. Singh N, Avery RK, Munoz P, et al. Trends in risk profiles for and mortality associated with invasive aspergillosis among liver transplant recipients. *Clin Infect Dis*. 2003;36:46-52.
44. Geddes CC, Church CC, Collidge T, et al. Management of cytomegalovirus infection by weekly surveillance after renal transplant: analysis of cost, rejection and renal function. *Nephrol Dial Transpl*. 2003;1(9):1891-1898.
45. Browne BJ, Young JA, Dunn TB, et al. The impact of cytomegalovirus infection ≥1 year after primary renal transplantation. *Clin Transpl*. 2010;24:572-577.
46. Paton NI. Treatment interruption strategies: How great are the risks? *Curr Opin Infect Dis*. 2008;21(1):25-30.
47. Bell DM. Occupational risk of human immunodeficiency virus infection in healthcare workers: an overview. *Am J Med*. 1997;102:9-15.
48. Ippolito G, Puro V, De Carli G, et al. The risk of occupational human immunodeficiency virus infection in healthcare workers. *Arch Intern Med*. 1993;153:1451-1458.
49. Evens AM, David KA, Helenowski I, et al. Multicenter analysis of 80 solid organ transplantation recipients with post-transplantation lymphoproliferative disease: outcomes and prognostic factors in the modern era. *J Clin Oncol*. 2010;28:1038-1046.
50. Ganne V, Siddiqi N, Kamaplath B, et al. Humanized anti-CD20 monoclonal antibody (Rituximab) treatment for post-transplant lymphoproliferative disorder. *Clin Transpl*. 2003;17:417-422.
51. Parker A, Bowles K, Bradley JA, et al. Management of post-transplant lymphoproliferative disorder in adult solid organ transplant recipients—BCSH and BTS guidelines. *Br J Haematol*. 2010;149(5):693-705.
52. Kollmar O, Becker S, Schilling MK, et al. Intestinal lymphoma perforations as a consequence of highly effective anti-CD20 antibody therapy. *Transplantation*. 2002;73(4):669-670.
53. Ullery BW, Pieracci FM, Rodney JRM, et al. Neutropenic enterocolitis. *Surg Infect*. 2009;10:307-314.
54. Audard V, Pardon A, Claude O, et al. Necrotizing fasciitis during de novo minimal change nephritic syndrome in a kidney transplant recipient. *Transpl Infect Dis*. 2005;7(2):89-92.
55. Benedict LM, Kusne S, Torre-Cisneros J, et al. Primary cutaneous fungal infection after solid-organ transplantation: report of five cases and review. *Clin Infect Dis*. 1992;15(1):17-21.
56. Tessari G, Naldi L, Piaserico S, et al. Incidence and clinical predictors of primary opportunistic deep cutaneous mycoses in solid organ transplant recipients: a multicenter cohort study. *Clin Transpl*. 2010;24:328-333.
57. Wai PH, Ewing CA, Johnson LB, et al. *Candida fasciitis* following renal transplantation. *Transplantation*. 2001;72(3):477-479.
58. Brunton LL, Lazo JS, Parker KL, eds. *Goodman & Gilman's The Pharmacological Basis of Therapeutics*. 11th ed. New York: McGraw Hill; 2006.
59. Katzung BG, Masters SB, AJ Trevor, eds. *Basic and Clinical Pharmacology*. 11th ed. New York: McGraw Hill; 2009.

CHAPTER 57 ■ SUPPORT OF THE ORGAN DONOR

DAVID M. KASHMER, SUZANNE A. FIDLER, AND MICHAEL D. PASQUALE

The gap between the availability of organs and the demand for transplantation is large. The number of potential organ donors in the United States has been estimated to be more than 10,500 per year,[1] and, clearly, not all potential donors progress to organ procurement. As of July 22, 2006, the United Network for Organ Sharing (UNOS) stated that the number of patients awaiting transplantation in the United States was 92,450. Looking at data for the period 1997 through 1999, only 50% of health care agents who were proxies approached regarding donation agreed to proceed,[1] yielding a donor conversion rate of 42%. Factors affecting procurement include the number of families approached regarding organ donation, families' perception of the donor process, religious or spiritual beliefs, cosmetic appearances, and the difficulty regarding change in provider focus from the health of their patient to the health of an unseen patient at a different location. Steps being taken to decrease the gap between demand and availability include the use of living donors, expanded criteria donors (ECDs), and donation after cardiac death (DCD, or non–heart-beating donor). As critical care surgeons, it is vitally important to understand this demand as well as our potential role in maximizing opportunities for organ procurement. At the same time, we must remain focused on the care of our patients and their families, as well as being respectful of their wishes.

In this chapter we explore the roles that the acute care surgeon plays in support of the potential organ donor. We will also examine issues surrounding the declaration of brain death, non–heart-beating donors, and medical–legal implications surrounding organ donation.

ROLES OF THE ACUTE CARE SURGEON IN CARING FOR POTENTIAL ORGAN DONORS

Determination of Death

Due to the nature of acute care surgery, surgeons practicing in this field will often be required to assist in the determination of death. This is often difficult as the focus now changes from preservation of the patient's life to declaration of death and possible salvage of a patient unknown to the surgeon. With regard to patient death and donation, one source of uncertainty that is important to manage is the application of brain death criteria or criteria for DCD.

One of the important guiding principles of organ transplantation is the "dead donor rule." This rule, a general ethical principle in organ transplantation, declares that organ procurement should occur only when the patient is dead. The Uniform Determination of Death Act (UDDA) defines death based on either the irreversible cessation of: (1) circulatory and respiratory functions, or (2) all brain functions, including the brain stem.

In 1968, an Ad Hoc Committee of Harvard Medical School defined brain death as "the irreversible cessation of all brain functions," thereby permitting transplant surgeons to harvest organs from a donor whose heart and lungs were still functioning.[2] The following are the guidelines for the determination of brain death in adults:

1. The patient must be in a deep unresponsive coma, there must be no movement or responses to stimulation, and there must be a clear understanding as to the etiology of the coma.
2. The patient must have a core temperature that is at least 32°C (90°F)
3. Drug intoxication and poisoning must be excluded.
4. There are no medical conditions that may confound the clinical assessment of brain death (e.g., no severe electrolyte, acid-base, or endocrine disturbances)
5. The patient must be apneic and must not recover spontaneous respiratory function during an apnea test.

Apnea Test:

  a. Core temperature 36.5°C (97°F)
  b. Systolic blood pressure 90 mm Hg
  c. Corrected diabetes insipidus or positive fluid balance in past 6 hours
  d. Patient on 100% oxygen at appropriate intermittent mandatory ventilation (IMV) for pCO_2 36–45 mm Hg, pH 7.35–7.44 for 30 minutes; blood gas just prior to apnea test to confirm pCO_2 36–45 mm Hg
  e. Place on continuous positive airway pressure (CPAP) at FiO_2 100% or place on T-piece 100% FiO_2 at >6 L/min
  f. Note the presence or absence of spontaneous respiration during or at the conclusion of 10-minute period of observation
  g. Check arterial blood gases (ABG) after the 10 minutes to confirm $pCO_2 \geq 60$ mm Hg (Note: if the pCO_2 is 60 mm Hg or 20 mm Hg above baseline, the apnea test supports the clinical diagnosis of brain death.

6. Two physicians must record the declarations of Brain Death in the progress notes and must sign, date, and time both declarations and document that the patient is brain dead. The clinical examinations may be up to 6 hours apart. The second clinical declaration is considered the legal time of death. The two physicians who independently determine brain death are not permitted to participate in the procedures for procuring or transplanting an organ or other body part from the patient.
7. Cranial nerve reflexes and responses:

  a. Pupils midposition (4 mm) to dilated (9 mm), fixed, and unresponsive to light.
  b. Absence of corneal reflexes.
  c. No oculocephalic reflex
  d. No deviation of the eyes to irrigation in each ear with 50 mL of ice water
  e. No swallowing or yawning
  f. No gag reflex
  g. No cough response or bradyarrhythmia to bronchial suctioning

Donation after Cardiac Death

In light of the aforementioned shortage of available organs for transplantation, DCD has emerged. Determining irreversibility depends on the circumstances; irreversible cessation of circulatory and respiratory functions may mean that the heart cannot be restarted spontaneously or that the heart cannot be restarted because of the decision to forego resuscitative measures.[2]

A "do-not-resuscitate" (DNR) order prevents the physician from engaging in resuscitation so that the patient's state of death is legally irreversible.

DCD practices pose additional legal considerations because the timing for declaring irreversible cessation of circulatory and respiratory function varies across transplant programs. Therefore, DCD protocols should clearly indicate which time period the hospitals and organ procurement organizations (OPOs) will follow, such as waiting between 2 and 5 minutes after the cessation of cardiopulmonary function before organ procurement.[2]

UNOS, which operates the Organ Procurement and Transplantation Network (OPTN), has developed rules regarding DCD, which were finalized in March 2007 and became effective on July 1, 2007, requiring that all OPOs and transplant centers must incorporate "model elements" in their DCD protocols.[2] These model elements address the withdrawal of life-sustaining measures and pronouncement of death as described below[3]:

Withdrawal of Life-sustaining Measures/ Patient Management

1. A time-out is recommended prior to the initiation of the withdrawal of life-sustaining measures. The intent of the time-out is to verify patient identification and the respective roles and responsibilities of the patient care team, OPO staff, and organ recovery team personnel.
2. No member of the transplant team shall be present for the withdrawal of life-sustaining measures.
3. No member of the organ recovery team or OPO staff may participate in the guidance or administration of palliative care, or the declaration of death.
4. There must be a determination of the location and process for withdrawal of life-sustaining measures (e.g., endotracheal tube removal, termination of blood pressure support medications) as a component of the patient management.

In pronouncing death for DCD, the physician who is authorized to declare death must not be a member of the OPO or organ recovery team, and the method of declaring cardiac death must comply in all respects with the legal definition of death by an irreversible cessation of circulatory and respiratory functions before the actual pronouncement of death.

PATHOPHYSIOLOGY OF BRAIN DEATH

Donor management begins with the neurologic determination of death (NDD, or "brain death") and consent to organ donation, and culminates in surgical organ procurement. Understanding the pathophysiology of brain death provides an important opportunity to enhance multiorgan function during this period of time and thereby improve organ utilization. It is important to realize that the resuscitation of the cardiopulmonary system benefits function of all organs and it is important to take time in the intensive care unit (ICU) to optimize organ function to improve transplant outcomes. Hence, reversible organ dysfunction can be addressed with aggressive resuscitation; once organ function is optimized, surgical procurement should be arranged emergently. The temporal changes in organ function after NDD demand flexibility in identifying the optimal time for procurement.[4]

The earliest manifestation of increased intracranial pressure (ICP) is characterized by hypertension, bradycardia, and altered breathing. When the brainstem becomes compressed as it is pushed against the foramen magnum, ischemia will result. This results in increased local neuronal activity that produces an increase in sympathetic outflow and an elevation in blood pressure in order to maintain cerebral blood flow. The hypertension will additionally produce reflex bradycardia. Herniation, however, is associated with a massive increase in catecholamines that produces hypertension and tachycardia. The catecholamine surge, which can lead to coronary vasoconstriction, subendocardial ischemia, and focal myocardial necrosis, is believed to be one of the contributing factors to cardiac dysfunction in potential organ donors. Additionally, the catecholamine surge may lead to increased filling pressures, increased afterload, and an elevated pulmonary wedge pressure (PWP), which then leads to "neurogenic pulmonary edema." The sympathetic storm lasts for only a brief period of time and is then followed by a prolonged phase of severe hypotension secondary to decreased sympathetic outflow. The hypotension may be further compounded by ventricular dysfunction requiring use of inotropes and vasopressors to maintain organ blood flow. The deterioration of cardiovascular function associated with intracranial hypertension varies with the rapidity of increase in ICP, time after herniation, and etiology of brain injury.[5] There is also evidence that brain death induces an inflammatory response and subsequent endothelial injury, which can lead to impaired graft function and graft vasculopathy.

On a cellular level, there is global mitochondrial dysfunction and a change from aerobic to anaerobic metabolism with reduced energy stores in the myocardium. This, combined with the ischemic time and ischemia–reperfusion injury, contributes to graft dysfunction. From an endocrine standpoint, there is a reduction in antidiuretic hormone (ADH, vasopressin) secretion and thyroid dysfunction. The decrease in ADH leads to the development of diabetes insipidus (DI) whereas the thyroid dysfunction generally manifests as hypothyroidism. There is data to suggest that proinflammatory cytokines may inhibit the conversion of thyroxine (T4) to the active form of thyroid hormone, tri-iodothyronine (T3). T3 via binding to specific receptors, increases oxygen utilization, the uptake of glucose and amino acids, mitochondrial size/number, and promotes a conversion to aerobic metabolism. Additionally, T3 will increase cardiac output and decrease systemic vascular resistance.

From a hematologic standpoint, release of thromboplastin from the ischemic brain can cause disseminated intravascular coagulation while the systemic inflammatory response syndrome response activates humoral and cellular components that add to the coagulopathy. As mentioned earlier, a sympathetic storm occurs during herniation which is rapidly followed by a depletion of catecholamines that can lead to significant hypothermia due to loss of central temperature control and vasodilation. Hypothermia can further exacerbate myocardial depression and further compromise oxygen delivery.

OPTIMIZATION OF THE POTENTIAL ORGAN DONOR

Subsequent to the pronouncement of death, the donor management period begins. During the donor management period, the acute care surgeon and organ procurement coordinator should focus on optimizing the patient for donation. Appropriate organ donor management then should address the pathophysiologic changes mentioned previously to optimize the number of organs transplanted per donor (OTPD). The main goals are to maintain cardiac function, minimize the deleterious effects that occur with brain death, and maintain adequate oxygen delivery to the vital organs. These goals can be met by optimizing hemodynamics with the judicious use of fluids, inotropes, and vasopressors, preserving lung function by paying close attention to mechanical ventilation and pulmonary toilet, preventing infection, and by utilizing specific measures shown to maintain and improve cardiac function. Detailed standing orders released by the Canadian Council for Donation and Transplantation are shown in Table 57.1. Note

TABLE 57.1

DATA COLLECTED FROM UNOS REGION 5 DONOR MANAGEMENT GOALS (DMG)

ADULT DONORS

Standard monitoring
- Urine catheter to straight drainage, strict intake and output
- Nasogastric tube to straight drainage
- Vital signs every hour
- Pulse oximetry, 3-lead ECG
- CVP
- Arterial line pressure
- Optional PAC

Laboratory investigations
- ABGs, electrolytes and glucose q4h and as needed
- Complete blood count q8h
- Blood urea nitrogen and creatinine q6h
- Urine analysis
- Aspartate aminotransferase (AST), alanine aminotransferase (ALT), bilirubin (total and direct), INR (or PT) and PTT q6h

Hemodynamic monitoring and therapy

General targets: heart rate 60–120 bpm, systolic blood pressure >100 mm Hg, mean arterial pressure ≥70 mm Hg
- Fluid resuscitation to maintain normovolemia, CVP 6–10 mm Hg
- If arterial blood pressure ≥ 160/90 mm Hg, then: Wean inotropes and vasopressors and, if necessary, start
  - Nitroprusside: 0.5–5.0 mcg/kg/min or
  - Esmolol: 100–500 mcg/kg bolus followed by 100–300 mcg/kg/min
- Serum lactate concentration q2–4h
- Mixed venous oximetry q2–4h; titrate therapy to MVO_2 ≥60%

Agents for hemodynamic support
- Dopamine: ≤10 mcg/kg/min
- Vasopressin: ≤2.4 U/h (0.04 U/min)
- Norepinephrine, epinephrine, phenylephrine (caution with doses >0.2 mcg/kg/min)

Indications for PAC
- 2-Dimensional echo ejection fraction ≤ 40% and/or

- Dopamine >10 mcg/kg/min (or equivalent), or
- Vasopressor support (not including vasopressin if part of hormone therapy), or
- Escalation of support

Glycemia and nutrition
- Routine intravenous dextrose infusions
- Initiate or continue enteral feeding as tolerated
- Continue parenteral nutrition if already initiated
- Initiate and titrate insulin infusion to maintain serum glucose level at 4–8 mmol/L

Fluid and electrolyte targets
- Urine output 0.5–3 mL/kg/h
- Serum Na 130–150 mmol/L
- Normal ranges for potassium, calcium, magnesium, phosphate

Diabetes insipidus

Defined as:
- Urine output >4 mL/kg/h associated with
- Increasing serum sodium ≥145 mmol/L and/or
- Increasing serum osmolarity ≥300 mosm or
- Decreasing urine osmolarity ≤200 mosm

Therapy (to be titrated to urine output ≤3 mL/kg/h):
- Intravenous vasopressin infusion at ≤2.4 U/h, or
- Intermittent D DAVP, 1–4 mcg IV then 1–2 mcg IV q6h (there is no true upper limit for dose; should be titrated to desired urine output rate, usually < 100 mL/h)

TABLE 57.1

DATA COLLECTED FROM UNOS REGION 5 DONOR MANAGEMENT GOALS (*Continued*)

Combined hormonal therapy

Defined as:

- Thyroxine (T4): 20 mcg IV bolus followed by 10 mcg/h IV infusion (or 100 mcg IV bolus followed by 50 mcg IV q12h)
- Vasopressin: 1 U IV bolus followed by 2.4 U/h IV infusion
- Methylprednisolone: 15 mg/kg (≤1 g) IV q24h

Indications:

- 2-Dimensional echocardiographic ejection fraction ≤40% or
- Hemodynamic instability (includes shock, unresponsive to restoration of normovolemia and requiring vasoactive support [dopamine > 10 mcg/min or any vasopressor agent])
- Consideration should be given to its use in all donors

Hematology

- Optimum hemoglobin: 90–100 g/L; for unstable donors, lowest acceptable level is 70 g/L
- For platelets, INR, PTT, there are no predefined targets; transfuse in cases of clinically relevant bleeding
- No other specific transfusion requirements

Microbiology

(baseline, daily and as needed)

- Daily blood cultures
- Daily urine cultures
- Daily sputum cultures
- Administer antibiotics for presumed or proven infection

Heart-specific orders

- 12-lead ECG
- Troponin I or T, q12h
- 2-Dimensional echocardiography
  - Should only be performed after fluid and hemodynamic resuscitation
  - If ejection fraction ≤40% then, insert PAC and titrate therapy to the following targets:
- PCWP: 6–10 mm Hg
- Cardiac index: >2.4 L/min/m^2
- SVR: 800–1,200 dyn/sec/cm^5
- LVSWI: >15 ml/kg/min
  - PAC data are relevant for hemodynamic therapy and evaluation for suitability of heart transplantation independent of echo findings
  - Consider repeat echocardiography at 6–12 h intervals.
- Coronary angiography

Indications:

  - History of cocaine use
  - Male > 55 years or female > 60 years
  - Male > 40 years or female > 45 years in the presence of two or more risk factors
  - Greater than or equal to three risk factors at any age.

Risk factors:

  - Smoking
  - Hypertension
  - Diabetes
  - Hyperlipidemia
  - Body mass index > 32
  - Family history of the disease
  - History of coronary artery disease
  - Ischemia on electrocardiogram
  - Anterolateral regional wall motion abnormalities on electrocardiogram
  - 2-dimensional echocardiographic assessment of ejection fraction ≤40%

Precautions:

- Ensure normovolemia
- Administer prophylactic *N*-acetylcysteine, 600–1,000 mg enterally twice daily (first dose as soon as angiography indicated) or IV 150 mg/kg in 500 mL normal saline over 30 min immediately before contrast agent followed by 50 mg/kg in 500 mL normal saline over 4 h
- Use low-risk radiocontrast agent (nonionic, iso-osmolar), using minimum radiocontrast volume, no ventriculogram

(*Continued*)

TABLE 57.1

DATA COLLECTED FROM UNOS REGION 5 DONOR MANAGEMENT GOALS (*Continued*)

Lung-specific orders

- Chest radiograph q24h and as needed
- Bronchoscopy and gram staining and culture of bronchial wash
- Routine endotracheal tube suctioning, rotation to lateral position q2h
- Mechanical ventilation targets:
  - Tidal volume: 8–10 mL/kg, PEEP: 5 cm H_2O, PIP: ≤30 cm H_2O
  - pH: 7.35–7.45, $PaCO_2$: 35–45 mm Hg, PaO_2: ≥80 mm Hg, O_2 saturation: ≥95%
- Recruitment maneuvers for oxygenation impairment may include:
  - Periodic increases in PEEP up to 15 cm H_2O
  - Sustained inflations (PIP at 30 cm H_2O times 30–60 s)
  - Diuresis to normovolemia

It is important to take the necessary time in the ICU to optimize organ function to improve transplant outcomes. Resuscitation and reevaluation can improve reversible organ dysfunction (myocardial and cardiovascular dysfunction, oxygenation impairment related to potentially reversible lung injury, invasive bacterial infections, hypernatremia) and evaluate temporal trends in hepatic AST, ALT, and creatinine or any other potentially treatable situation. This treatment period can range from 12 to 24 h and should be accompanied by frequent reevaluation to demonstrate improvement in organ function toward defined targets. Once organ function is optimized, surgical procurement procedures should be arranged emergently. There are no demographic factors or organ dysfunction thresholds that preclude giving consent for donation and offering organs for transplantation.

Reprinted with permission from CMAJ. 2006;174(6):S27.

ABGs, arterial blood gases; CVP, central venous pressure; DDAVP, 1-desamino 8-D arginine vasopressin (desmopressin); ECG, electrocardiogram; INR, International Normalized Ratio; LVSWI, left ventricular stroke work index; MVO_2, mixed venous oxygen saturation; PAC, pulmonary artery catheter; PEEP, positive end-expiratory pressure; PIP, peak inspiratory pressure; PT, prothrombin time; PTT, activated partial thromboplastin time; PWP, pulmonary wedge pressure; SVR, systemic vascular resistance; SWI, stroke work index; IV, intravenous

that the placement of invasive monitoring (central venous pressure [CVP], arterial catheter, Foley's catheter) is typically required.

The most frequent hemodynamic problem is hypotension due to either hypovolemia, neurogenic shock due to decreased sympathetic outflow, or myocardial dysfunction. Treatment begins with optimizing preload (CVP 6–10 mm Hg) with the most appropriate fluid (crystalloid, colloid, or blood product). If hypotension persists despite adequate filling pressures, an inotrope should be considered. If inotropes are initiated, consideration should be given to the placement of a pulmonary artery catheter (PAC) to assess preload, afterload, and cardiac performance. Simply stated, an escalation of support should be accompanied by escalation in monitoring. Subsequently, if inotrope dosing has to be increased due to persistent hypotension, an investigation into the exact cause must be undertaken. Echocardiography can be used to evaluate cardiac function and if this demonstrates adequate ventricular function and volume status, then severe vasodilation is the most likely cause. In such cases, a vasoconstrictor would be considered as the agent of choice. Vasopressin has been shown to be very useful in this setting because it acts synergistically with catecholamines and may allow a reduction or even discontinuation of them. Vasopressin is a special agent because it can be used in a variety of applications, i.e., hemodynamic vasopressor support, DI therapy, and hormone therapy. Second-line agents for hemodynamic support include norepinephrine, epinephrine, and phenylephrine. Escalation of doses of catecholamines should be guided by PAC data realizing that a reduction in inotropes is desired as it will reduce myocardial oxygen consumption and thereby help maintain myocardial energy stores. Optimization of these parameters, along with attention to acid-base and electrolyte balance, hematocrit, oxygenation and ventilation, and hormone supplementation has been shown to improve potential organ donor salvage.[6]

Hypoxemia can result in cardiovascular instability and may be due to pneumonia, aspiration pneumonitis, pulmonary contusions, pulmonary edema, ventilator-associated lung injury, and oxygen toxicity. The lowest inspired oxygen concentration, peak inspiratory pressure (PIP) and positive end expiratory pressure (PEEP) compatible with acceptable oxygenation should be used. The quality of donor lungs can be improved with endotracheal suctioning, bronchodilators, steroids, chest physiotherapy (PT), bronchoscopy and lavage, and judicious small-volume colloid resuscitation.

From an endocrine standpoint, central DI occurs in 50%–80% of brain dead patients. Central DI is characterized by decreased secretion of ADH, which gives rise to polyuria and polydipsia by diminishing the patient's ability to concentrate urine. This results in a loss of intravascular volume and electrolyte abnormalities. Treatment with desmopressin (1-desamino-8-D-arginine vasopressin [DDAVP]) loading followed by an infusion can reduce the volume losses and help correct the electrolyte issues. Due to the multiple endocrine abnormalities, it is now recommended that a hormonal "cocktail" consisting of T3, vasopressin, and methylprednisolone be administered to potential organ donors.[7] The weight of currently available evidence in a large retrospective cohort study by the United Network for Organ Sharing in the United States suggests a substantial benefit of triple hormone therapy with minimal risk. This study showed substantial increases in kidney, liver, and heart utilization from donors receiving triple hormonal therapy as well as improvements in 1-year kidney and heart graft survival.[8] Glycemic control should be achieved, if necessary by insulin infusion. Additionally, routine enteral feeding should be initiated or continued as tolerated, and discontinued on call to the operating room for harvesting, whereas parenteral nutrition should not be initiated, but may be continued if it had already been started.

IMPLEMENTATION OF THE ORGAN DONOR MANAGEMENT PROTOCOL

Multiple studies suggest that the use of guidelines and protocols to identify and care for the potential organ donor are effective in improving both organ donation rates and the number of OTPD.[9–15] These guidelines and protocols must provide clinical management guidance incorporating the principles mentioned previously, as well as the social support necessary to accomplish the task of obtaining consent and supporting the family and friends of the potential donor.

The clinical component of the management protocol should include early identification with admission to a monitored setting and resuscitation in accordance with the principles mentioned earlier. The combination of a clinical management protocol like the one shown in Algorithm 57.1, with standing orders as shown in Table 57.1, will facilitate the implementation of a program for aggressive organ donor management. Multiple studies have shown that adherence to these aggressive management protocols will decrease the incidence of cardiopulmonary failure and increase the number of organs recovered per donor as well as the function of the transplanted organs.[9,16–18] DuBose and Salim[19] demonstrated that adherence to their aggressive management protocol (Fig. 57.1) was associated with an 82% increase in the number of donors, a 71% increase in the number of organs recovered, and an 87% decrease in the number of donors lost due to cardiopulmonary instability. In a separate report published by the Midwest Transplant Network in 2009,[20] the number of OTPD was notably higher (p = 0.06) and the percentage of lungs transplanted was significantly higher ($p <$ 0.01) among donors who underwent optimization by critical care providers. Finally, in an unpublished report from University of Pittsburgh Medical Center (UPMC), it was noted that use of critical care providers to support potential DCD donors in the prerecovery phase of the procurement process allowed these donors to progress to donation more comfortably and more quickly.

In addition, the social aspects of the organ donation process must be addressed. Historically, consent to donation has been the largest impediment during the transplantation process, and it has been suggested that the strongest predictor of donation decisions may be the family's initial response to the request for donation.[21] Further, it has been shown that a substantial number of families deciding against organ donation cite an inadequate explanation of the process of brain death, leading to a lack of understanding of the process.[22] This stresses the involvement of critical care physicians who have a good relationship with the patient's family, are seen as advocates for the patient and family, and have a good understanding of brain death, cardiac death, and the process of organ procurement. Additionally, utilization of transplant coordinators has been shown to be useful in coordinating the efforts to facilitate both consent and refocusing of care to organ preservation and harvest. Alternatively, fully trained staff members from the regional OPOs may be used to facilitate this process. The goal is to provide consistent family support and act as liaisons between the family and the health care providers. Implementation of such programs (In-House Coordinator or IHC) has led to significant improvements in conversion and consent rates in a full range of hospital settings.[23–25]

PATHOPHYSIOLOGY OF ORGAN PRESERVATION

At least two key concepts are required to understand current thoughts regarding organ preservation: (1) warm ischemia and (2) cold ischemia. Warm ischemia is that time period when oxygen delivery (DO_2) to an organ is substantially decreased and yet that organ remains at or near a state of normothermia. An important example of warm ischemia occurs during the DCD donation process, where a patient may be extubated as part of comfort measures and becomes hypoxic, but yet is near or actually normothermic. This warm ischemia time is an important issue regarding eventual graft function and should be minimized without diminishing the important, careful respect addressed to patient comfort. In short, no matter how much warm ischemic time may be detrimental to eventual graft function, care must be taken to clearly respect patient and proxy wishes as the disease process progresses and the patient is kept comfortable prior to any declaration of death.

Tolerance for warm ischemia differs greatly across tissue types. Cornea and skin may tolerate several hours of warm ischemia, whereas the brain suffers an irreversible loss of function within a few minutes of onset.[26] Modern organ preservation methods, followed from the necessity of extending ischemic times over which organs maintained viability. Modern techniques have, prolonged the viability of grafts for transport, by utilizing cold ischemia.

Cold ischemia, describes the period of time where the temperature of an eventual graft is lowered to diminish metabolic activity, oxygen demand, and the sequelae of hypoxia that lead to irreversible cell death. The key, is cooling the eventual graft via a temperature-controlled bath and a hypothermic preservative flush solution. Cooling serves the aforementioned purposes of restraining oxygen demand as well as decreasing oxygen free radical creation, where by the preservative solution used has many important effects including pH maintenance, metabolic supply, prevention of cellular edema, and modification of intracellular calcium.[26] Cold ischemia is not simply slowing of all metabolic functions, but rather consists of both slowing those systems and preventing their discordance. Interestingly, metabolism does occur during cold storage.[27]

In order to obtain a sense of scale with regard to cold preservation techniques, consider that simple surface cooling of the kidney allows ischemia to be tolerated for 12 hours[28] whereas cooling via flush with a preservative solution allows preservation for 12–120 hours depending upon the solution used.[29] In short, cooling alone functions in an important capacity, but cooling in conjunction with flushing allows significant preservation times. Multiple different solutions are available to be used as agent for performing a cold flush of allografts.

Table 57.2 demonstrates some important solutions utilized in the cold preservation of organs: Euro-Collins solution, histidine–tryptophan–alphaketoglutarate (HTK) solution, and University of Wisconsin (UW) or ViaSpan ([DuPont Merck Pharmaceutical, Wilmington, DE]) solution are three of the most widely used agents. Each has important characteristics that may influence eventual graft outcome. For example, the potassium content of UW is substantial, and in larger solid-organ allografts, UW may yield a substantial cardioplegic effect owing to the elevated potassium content. Therefore, before reperfusion (if not earlier), it is important that the surgical and anesthesia team have some plan to offset that important, potentially deleterious effect. In the case of pancreas allografts, some centers have become concerned regarding the viscosity of HTK solution with respect to any potential influence on allograft thrombosis. These are just a few of the many important considerations regarding which flush type is used during retrieval and preservation of the allografts.

Another important consideration exists with respect to allograft storage: static versus perfusion storage. With static storage, the organ is cold-flushed as previously described and is submerged in the cold preservative solution for transport, etc. In perfusion storage, more frequently performed with renal allografts, kidneys are continuously perfused with a volume of preservative solution. Cold preservation, in the case of renal allografts, also allows potentially implanting surgeons to learn important characteristics of the organ's flow dynamics. Data from the perfusate pump, such as resistive index, are an

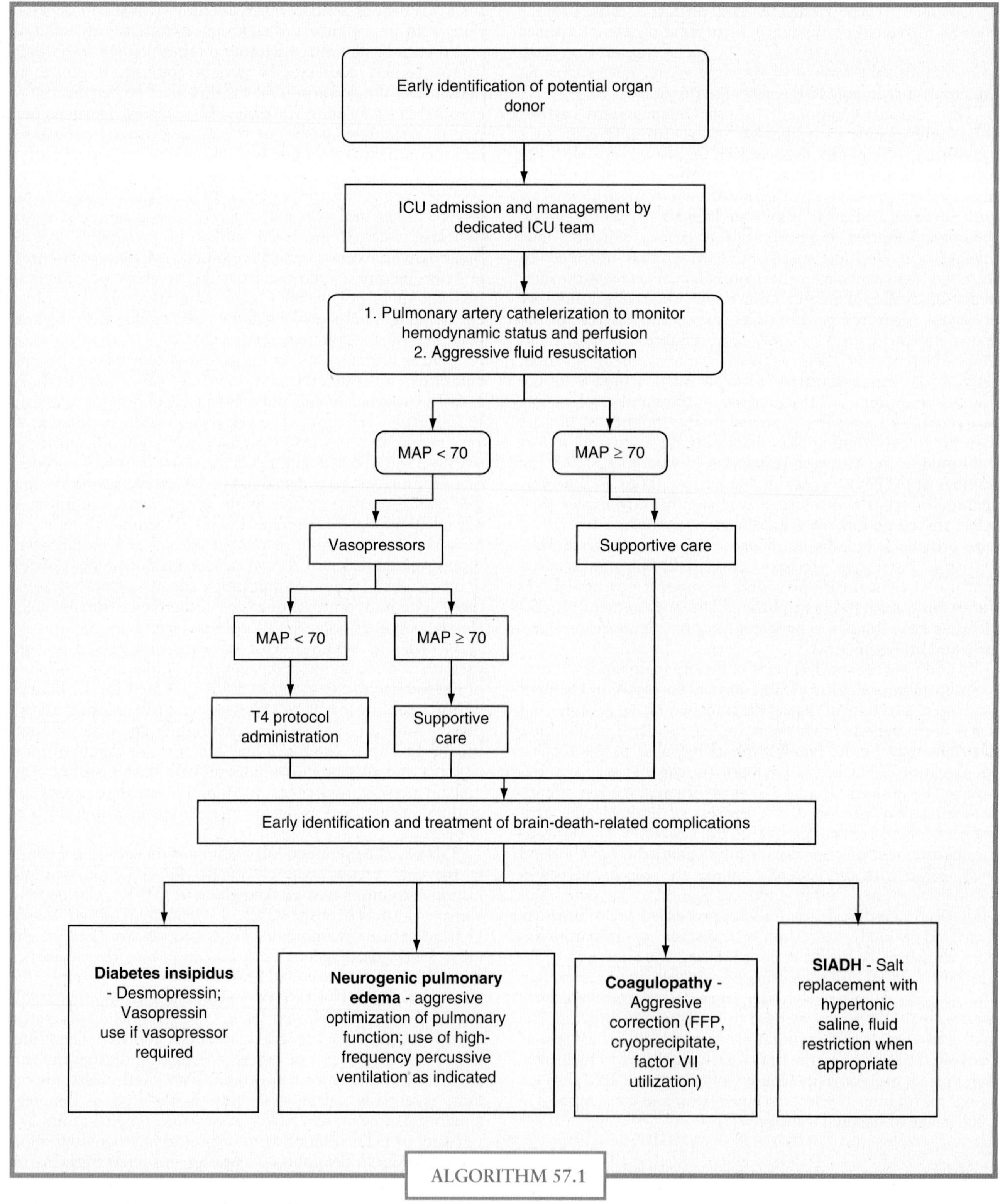

ALGORITHM 57.1 Standing orders for management of organ donors. Reprinted with permission from Shemie et al. Organ donor management in Canada: recommendations of the forum on Medical Management to Optimize Donor Organ Potential. CMAJ. 2006;174;S13–20, Appendix 3.

FFP, fresh-frozen plasma
ICU, intensive care unit
MAP, mean arterial blood pressure
SIADH, syndrome of inappropriate secretion of anti-diuretic hormone
T4, thyroxine

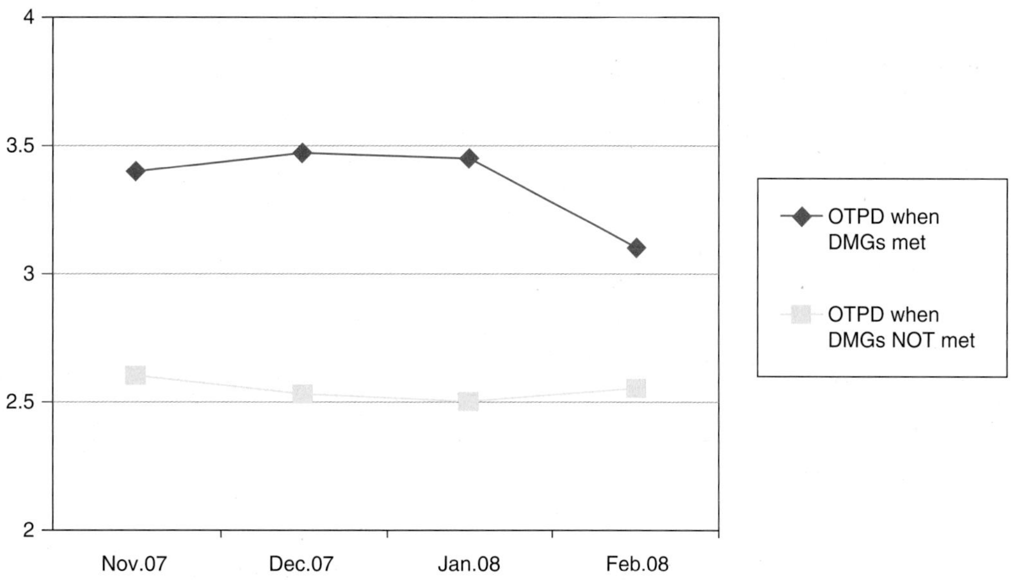

FIGURE 57.1. Organ donor clinical management protocol. Reprinted with permission from DuBose J, Salim A. Aggressive Organ Donor Management Protocol. J Intensive Care Med. 2008;23:367.
DMGs, donor management goals; OTPD,)organs transplanted per donor.

TABLE 57.2

SOLUTE COMPOSITION OF SELECTED IMPORTANT PRESERVATION SOLUTIONS

SOLUTE	EURO-COLLINS	HTK	UW
Sodium	10	15	30
Potassium	108	9	125
Magnesium	—	4	5
Bicarbonate	10	26	—
Chloride	15	26	—
Phosphate	60	—	25
Sulfate	—	—	5
Glucose	180	—	—
Osmolality	340	310	320
pH (at 0°C)	7.0	7.3	7.4
Histidine	—	198	—
Tryptophan	—	2	—
alpha-Ketoglutarate	—	1	—
Mannitol	—	30	—
Lactobionate	—	—	100
Raffinose	—	—	30
Adenosine	—	—	5
Raffinose	—	—	30
Glutathione	—	—	3
Allopurinol	—	—	1
Insulin (U L^{-1})	—	—	100
Dexamethasone	—	—	8
Bactrim (mL)	—	—	0.5
Hydroxyethyl starch (g L^{-1})	—	—	50

All units are mmol L^{-1} unless otherwise noted.
HTK, histidine–tryptophan–alphaketoglutarate solution,
UW, University of Wisconsin solution

important factor that may be used to determine the likelihood that an organ will exhibit delayed graft function post-implant. It seems, however, that preservation by perfusion is effective for approximately 3–5 days, as substantial injury to the vascular endothelium may occur with longer intervals.[30]

Those, then, are many of the practical points regarding modern organ preservation. Clearly, important messages for anyone delivering care to the potential donor exist: warm ischemia time must be minimized where possible, and cold flush via a static or perfusate system should be used. Several important consequences may act as headlines regarding the pathophysiology of organ preservation for the acute care surgeon: (1) kidney damage, for example, is predictably reversible only if renal warm ischemia time is <30 minutes,[31] and (2) recovery is rapid after 10 minutes of warm ischemia, but recovery can take ≥1 week if >30 minutes of warm ischemic time is incurred. On balance, warm ischemia is tolerated much worse than cold ischemia time.

NECESSARY INTERVENTIONS IN THE POTENTIAL ORGAN DONOR

In terms of scope of practice, surgeons are trained to recover the groin lymph nodes necessary for human leukocyte antigen (HLA) typing to begin prerecovery. Other technical interventions such as bronchoscopy, central venous catheter placement, endotracheal tube repositioning, and major vessel cannulation are reimbursed by the OPO. Some state laws mandate that a driver's license that relates a person's wishes to be an organ donor allows for the postmortem procurement of that person's organs. Therefore, as briefly described previously, it is possible that a patient who presents to the trauma bay as a "trauma code," is deemed to have a nonsurvivable injury and is declared dead may be treated as a donor owing to that patient's expressed wishes. An acute care surgeon could be contacted to heparinize that patient, cannulate the infrarenal abdominal aorta, clamp the aorta at the level of the right crus of the diaphragm, cold-flush the viscera with preservative solution, incise the inferior vena cava (IVC) in the chest to allow efflux of blood, and pack the abdomen in ice. Just as with the DCD situation, the inferior mesenteric vein need not be cannulated; a portal flush could be performed on the back table if deemed necessary at all. The process could take <10 minutes and may be performed in the trauma bay. The process could be adapted to recover more than abdominal viscera where appropriate. The potential grafts would then be preserved according to the donor's wishes as expressed via the driver's license.

In practice, this avenue is often not explored (as mentioned previously) despite frequent conjecture on the part of the procurement teams. Some OPOs across the country express concern that, despite the license's clear expression of the patient's wishes, the patient's family may potentially believe that everything was not done for the patient so the physicians could "take their organs." Whereas most physicians would bristle at the suggestion that they would withhold any care in order to enhance organ harvesting, the importance of maintaining and encouraging public perception regarding the positive nature of organ donation is commonly valued over the increased number of grafts available by procuring in this manner.

This mind-set may be changing. One OPO determined that positive public perception regarding the benefits of organ donation may be maintained (or improved) and at the same time the opportunity for increased recovery could be taken. A new dynamic has been introduced by one bellwether OPO, called Condition T. This breakthrough system honors the patient's wishes as expressed on the driver's license, such that any patient presenting as traumatically injured, or otherwise, is a candidate for cannulation and organ preservation after that patient's premanagement physician has pronounced death. Care is taken to keep separate the physician who declares death from the donation process. It is only after the patient's physicians have done all that they reasonably can for a patient that death is declared per routine. It is only after the patient has died that any consideration of Condition T is instituted.

Currently, an emergency room physician is trained to cannulate the femoral artery and begin cold flush in a specially prepared room. Other technical details regarding venting blood and effluent (via cannula or some other method) were not available at the time of publication. The donor is cooled via external techniques in addition to the flush procedure. The procurement team is called and the process is technically similar to standard retrieval in the DCD example, with one of the exceptions being that the flush has occurred.

This situation is an obvious opportunity for acute care surgeons. Cannulation and venting may be achieved via the femoral vessels or, should there be some issue, the abdomen may be opened for the more traditional aortic cannulation. The clear message is that surgeons, should they choose to participate in the process, are well equipped to manage the acute, technical nature of Condition T should the program spread across the country.

MEDICOLEGAL AND ETHICAL CONSIDERATIONS

Surgeons in the acute care setting involved in managing potential donors may encounter medicolegal issues pertaining to organ procurement. These issues include obtaining the appropriate consent to donate from the potential donor, or more often the surrogate decision maker, ensuring that the potential donor's advance directives are respected and at the same time permitting the necessary interventions for determining medical suitability to donate and preserving organs, and balancing end-of-life care with managing the prospective organ donor to maximize organ procurement.

The possibility of legal problems may create some trepidation for providers who might engage in organ transplantation opportunities. Providing some legislative support for the donation process, the National Conference of Commissioners on Uniform State Laws in 1968 drafted the Uniform Anatomical Gift Act (UAGA), which was amended in 1987 and revised in 2006. Although not all states have adopted the most recent version of the UAGA, the Act supports the organ transplantation process and creates immunity for participants.[32] Presently, the limited legal cases involving organ transplantation demonstrate that courts generally follow the legislative intent of the UAGA to promote organ donation and expand the donor pool.

The UAGA addresses who may consent to providing an anatomical gift, the interpretation of donor cards and documents for permitting an anatomical gift, the necessity for interventions to a potential donor to determine medical suitability of organs, the recognition of individuals agreeing to make an anatomical gift regardless of the jurisdiction in which the gift was initiated, and the authorization for procurement organizations to access donor registries and medical records for the purpose of coordinating organ procurement.[32] State legislation modeling the UAGA defines a framework to follow in the organ transplantation process.

Consent for organ donation is satisfied when an individual has previously signed a designation on a legal document such as a driver's license or in a donor registry. The revised UAGA in 2006 reinforced the legallybinding nature of the donor card by indicating that the donor consent for organ donation becomes irrevocable and does not require consent from anyone after the donor's death.[32] Thus, OPOs may procure organs even when families refuse donation. However, the application of the UAGA also requires a transparent process for the voluntary consent of the organ donor. Moreover, the Consolidated Omnibus Reconciliation Act of 1986 requires hospitals accepting Medicare and Medicaid to "discuss organ donation with families of deceased patients who were potential donors."[33] Requiring familial consent for donation undermines the authority of donor cards and patient autonomy and poses a conflict in those instances where the surrogate contradicts the donor's previously signed donor document. Part of the practice for obtaining consent from the family arises from the unwillingness to create tension with the family and fear of litigation from discontented family members.

A current OPO practice is to accept a presigned organ donor card or registry as legally binding regardless of family consent. Condition T, described previously, is a rapid-response protocol designed for those individuals designated as organ donors who fail resuscitative efforts. Family consent is not required, but the donor designation status must be unambiguous.[34]

Under Condition T, in the presence of a valid document for an anatomical gift, this organ procurement practice is legal and consistent with the general requirement of abiding by legally binding documented authorization.

The revised UAGA requires law enforcement officers and emergency rescue personnel to make a reasonable search for organ donation authorization and requires hospitals to cooperate in the transplantation process.[34] In the event that there is no donor card or donor registry, the UAGA specifically designates who may make an anatomical gift on behalf of the deceased based on priority: spouse, adult son or daughter, parent, adult sibling, guardian, or medical examiner.[34] Although not all in a class must be queried to exclude an objection, consent may be negated if a next of kin of the same class objects.[35] When consent from a surrogate is required, the UAGA has defined "reasonably available" as "able to be contacted by a procurement agency without undue effort and willing and able to act in a timely manner consistent with existing medical criteria necessary for making anatomical gifts," allowing hospitals to expeditiously locate a surrogate for consent.[2] The immunity protections of UAGA apply so that "persons who fail to discharge their duties to search for a donor document or discuss the option of donation with the family are not subject to criminal or civil liability."[36] But administrative actions may apply and if the behavior is truly egregious such as lying to obtain the organs, the court will not uphold the immunity protections.[37] And, because the UAGA takes effect only after death has been declared, it does not provide protection to the pronouncement of death; failure to properly declare brain death may demonstrate bad faith.

Nonetheless, the UAGA provides immunity from civil and criminal liability to those professionals involved in organ transplantation to encourage health care professionals' participation in the organ donation process.

It is generally accepted that acting in "good faith" will shield from liability those who act in accordance with the law when obtaining consent for organ recovery. Courts broadly interpret "good faith" as in *Nicoletta v. Mayo Clinic* (1987) where the court defined "good faith" as "honest belief, the absence of malice, and the absence of design to defraud or seek an unconscionable advantage."[2]

The recently revived procurement process implementing DCD, which the Institute of Medicine endorsed in 2006 to expand the donor pool, poses questions as to whether the donor card reflects a sufficiently informed consent to this type of procurement. For individuals relying on procurement organization websites, they may not have received sufficient information specifically addressing DCD, involving a more complicated process and requiring additional intervention to the prospective donor than in a procurement following brain death. Thus, institutional policies and procedures addressing DCD ensure that the potential participants understand the process and that patient autonomy and surrogate decision making are respected.[2]

The revised UAGA overrides decisions about withholding or withdrawing life support outlined in an advance directive. To address the apparent conflict in situations where a patient wishes to forgo life-sustaining treatment but is a prospective donor, the revised UAGA of 2006 included sections 14(c) and 21(b) to permit the continuation of life support and necessary measures to preserve the opportunity to donor until OPOs complete their evaluation of the suitability of the prospective donor.[38] In accordance with section 14(c), the procurement organization may conduct any reasonable examination necessary to ensure the medical suitability of a potential donor and the "measures necessary to ensure the medical suitability of the part may not be withdrawn unless the hospital or procurement organization knows that the individual expressed a contrary intent."[38] Section 21(b) specifically addresses the conflict where a prospective donor has a declaration or advance health care directive that indicates the desire to decline life-sustaining measures and yet is a potential donor.[38] In this situation, the potential donor's attending physician and prospective donor or agent shall confer to resolve the conflict as expeditiously as possible. In the meantime, "measures necessary to ensure the medical suitability of the part may not be withheld or withdrawn from the prospective donor if withholding or withdrawing the measures is not contraindicated by appropriate end-of-life care."[38]

It is recommended that facilities devise advance care planning and a team that discusses with the potential donor where possible, or family, the use of life support once the clinical triggers are met to assist in the evaluation of the medical suitability of the donor. The local OPOs are authorized by the Health Care Financing Administration and UNOS to manage the procurement of organs in their region and are responsible for organizing and overseeing the identification of donors, evaluation of potential donors, confirmation of the diagnosis of brain death, arranging consent from family, clinical management of potential donors, obtaining permission for visiting transplant surgeons to procure organs at the donor's location, preservation and packaging of organs for transplant. The OPO assists with management of the donor by preparing guidelines.[39]

Implementing a collaborative process and integrating the attending surgeon's management of the prospective donor and the OPO's role in organ procurement will aid in navigating through issues that may evolve. Collaborative practices include contacting and timely coordinating with the OPO to assist in the organ transplantation process, avoiding conflicts of interest by requiring that the health care professional involved with the donor not participate with the transplant team, assigning appropriate staff and ancillary support roles and responsibilities in the organ donation process, facilitating communication with the family, utilizing trained personnel such as an OPO representative or third party to discuss possible donation in cases where no donor card is present, designating a physician who will declare death and following donor management guidelines.[2]

NEW TRENDS IN ORGAN RECOVERY

One important new trend in organ recovery involves the utilization of the acute care surgeon in the postmortem, predonation state. Currently, select OPOs are utilizing acute care physicians to resuscitate donors and optimize organs prior to donation. Frequently, this is a physician who did not participate in the care of the patient while he or she was alive. This emerging paradigm for utilizing critical care providers is beginning to yield some important data.

Consider the number of OTPD. In a recent report by the Midwest Transplant Network, OTPD was notably higher among those donors who underwent optimization by a critical care provider ($p = 0.06$).[21] Physician involvement in the postmortem state was associated with a larger number of available organs as adjusted for the number of donors. This is not the only evidence indicating that an important opportunity exists that may benefit multiple patients. A statistically significant difference ($p < 0.01$) was noted in the percentage of lungs transplanted when optimization was guided by an acute care provider.[21] Also, note the OTPD in the standard criteria donor (SCD) and ECD conditions (Table 57.3).

TABLE 57.3

FINDINGS OF 2007 REPORT FROM MIDWEST TRANSPLANT ALLIANCE TO AMERICAN SOCIETY OF TRANSPLANT SURGEONS

	INTENSIVIST	NO INTENSIVIST
OTPD	4.05	3.30
DMGs met (PTPD 4.31 vs. 3.23)	25 (58%)	10 (23%)
Hearts transplanted	20 (47%)	21 (49%)
Lungs transplanted	37 (43%)	12 (14%)
OTPD (SCD)	4.36	3.71
OTPD (ECD)	2.43	1.50
ATN rate	12%	24%

OTPD, organs transplanted per donor; DMGs, donor management goals; SCD, standard criteria donor; ECD, expanded criteria donors; ATN, acute tubular necrosis.

Another important point regarding the current state of organ recovery involves the fact that DCD donors do not always progress to donation after extubation or withdrawal of other futile life-prolonging measures. This leaves an Operating Room Recovery team that waits for a requisite amount of time (which varies by OPO), only to be unable to recover any viable organs or able to recover only a few of the potential grafts. Equally difficult is prolongation, in the DCD situation, of what is often called the phase 2 time (time when the donor is hypoxic postextubation but still near-normothermic) which may lead to poor graft quality. In either case, failure to progress or slow donor progression yields suboptimal results.

The UPMC currently has critical care physicians manage the prerecovery phase of the procurement process. Participating physicians report (unpublished data) that they have had no DCD donors fail to progress to donation. Again, by this report, DCD donors progress both more comfortably and more quickly.

This is only a small portion of the mounting evidence that indicates how acute care providers are already influencing the process of organ recovery to the benefit of potential recipients. Also by anecdotal report, prerecovery inflammatory levels as indicated by interleukin (IL)-6 concentrations may be decreased in situations where physicians lead donor optimization; this holds a possibility for improving graft quality. A final, important anecdotal report from the UPMC program indicates that many common factors including ventilator weaning, the use of vasopressors after adequate fluid resuscitation, the weaning of vasopressors when appropriate, and resuscitation to common endpoints are greatly improved in the area of physician-led prerecovery optimization.

In short, acute care surgeons are presented with the opportunity to widen their scope of practice so as to considerably impact the current recovery process. Data are already accumulating regarding the benefits of such involvement.

FUTURE OPPORTUNITIES

Final notes regarding the potential of this important situation include reimbursement issues and scope of practice. Physicians who currently optimize donors for an OPO are reimbursed by that OPO. Because recovery is improved, it is believed there is a reasonable break-even point on the expenditure by the OPO. More viable grafts are produced and thus the situation is more easily justified. Involved parties report little discernable pushback from the OPO donor coordinators, who have been described as pleased to have physician input and guidance in the process so as to reduce uncertainty regarding resuscitation and maximization.

CONCLUSIONS

The field of acute care surgery is presented with an opportunity to expand and participate in an important emerging discipline: donor optimization and recovery. Data exist that demonstrate how, when critical care-trained physicians are involved, an increased number of allografts are available to narrow the large gap between available organs and patient demand. Further, evidence exists that describes how intervention to defined, easy to understand donor management goals (DMGs) improves the number of OTPD (Table 57.4).

Critical care-trained surgeons are uniquely poised to assist in the important work of organ recovery, as they possess the requisite cognitive and technical skills necessary to intervene so as to improve physiologic endpoints while performing necessary interventions including bronchoscopy, lymph node procurement and, perhaps in the future, cannulation. The drive to provide patients with what they need in terms of transplantable organs, while respecting donors' rights, is a guiding principle that will likely continue to bring acute care surgery toward the forefront of donor management.

TABLE 57.4

REGION 5 DATA REGARDING OTDP WHEN DMGS MET

DMG DATA (SCDS ONLY, $n = 255$)	<4 OTDP ($n = 132$)	≥4 OTPD ($n = 123$)	P VALUE
DMGs at consent (1)	4.5	5	0.001
DMGs at 12–18 h (2)	5.1	6.1	<0.001
DMGs prior to OR (3)	5.5	6.3	<0.001
Delta DMG 1–2	0.71	1.1	0.050
Delta DMG 2–3	0.3	0.19	0.522
Delta DMG 1–3	1	1.3	0.210

DMGs, donor management goals; OTPD, organs transplanted per donor.

References

1. Sheehy E, Conrad C, Brigham L, et al. Estimating the Number of Potential Organ Donors in the United States. *N Engl J Med*. 2003;349.
2. http://www.ascensionhealth.org/index.php?option=com_content&view=article&id=226&Itemid=172.
3. Fidler SA. Implementing donation after cardiac death protocols. *J Health Law Sci Law*. 2008;2(1):137. Footnote 43, quoting Alexandra K. Glazier & Glenn Krinsky, *Hot Topics in Organ Donation and Transplant,* AHLA Conference: Legal Issues Affecting Academic Medical Centers and Other Teaching Institutions (Jan. 24–25, 2008).
4. UNOS bylaws. www.unos.org.
5. Berenguer CM, Davis FE, Howington JV. Brain death confirmation: comparison of CT angiography with nuclear medicine perfusion scan. *J Trauma*. 2010;68:553–559.
6. Rosendale JD, Kauffman HM, McBride MA, et al. Aggressive pharmacologic donor management results in more transplanted organs. *Transplantation*. 2003;75:482–487.
7. Novitzky D, Cooper DK, Reichart B. Value of triiodothyronine (T3) therapy to brain-dead potential organ donors. *J Heart Transplant*. 1986;5:486–487.
8. Novitzky D, Cooper DK, Reichart B. Hemodynamic and metabolic responses to hormonal therapy in brain-dead potential organ donors. *Transplantation*. 1987;43:852–854.
9. Navarro AP, Sohrabi S, Wyrley-Birch H, et al. Dual renal transplantation for kidneys from marginal nonheart-beating donors. *Transplant Proc*. 2006;38:2633–2634.
10. Jenkins DH, Reilly PM, Schwab CW. Improving the approach to organ donation: a review. *World J Surg*. 1999;23:644–649.
11. Ullah S, Zabala L, Watkins B, Schmitz ML. Cardiac organ donor management. *Perfusion*. 2006;21:93–98.
12. Powner DJ, Darby JM, Kellum JA. Proposed treatment guidelines for donor care. *Prog Transplant*. 2004;14:16–26; quiz 27–28.
13. Salim A, Velmahos GC, Brown C, et al. Aggressive organ donor management significantly increases the number of organs available for transplantation. *J Trauma*. 2005;58:991–994.
14. Salim A, Martin M, Brown C, et al. The effect of a protocol of aggressive donor management: implications for the national organ donor shortage. *J Trauma*. 2006;61:429–433; discussion 433–435.
15. Salim A, Brown C, Inaba K, et al. Improving consent rates for organ donation: the effect of an inhouse coordinator program. *J Trauma*. 2007;62:1411–1414; discussion 1414–1415.
16. Dodd-McCue D, Tartaglia A, Veazey KW, et al. The impact of protocol on nurses' role stress: a longitudinal perspective. *J Nurs Adm*. 2005;35:205–216.
17. Wheeldon DR, Potter CD, Dunning J, et al. Haemodynamic correction in multiorgan donation. *Lancet*. 1992;339:1175.
18. Straznicka M, Follette DM, Eisner MD, et al. Aggressive management of lung donors classified as unacceptable: excellent recipient survival one year after transplantation. *J Thorac Cardiovasc Surg*. 2002;124:250–258.

19. Rosendale JD, Chabalewski FL, McBride MA, et al. Increased transplanted organs from the use of a standardized donor management protocol. *Am J Transplant.* 2002;2:761–768.
20. DuBose J, Salim A. Aggressive organ donor management protocol. *J Intensive Care Med.* 2008;23:367–375.
21. Midwest Transplant Network, Call to Action: Time for a New Partnership (presentation) at Chicago Donor Management Forum August 19–20, 2009.
22. Siminoff LA, Mercer MB. Public policy, public opinion, and consent for organ donation. *Camb Q Healthc Ethics.* 2001;10:377–386.
23. Franz HG, DeJong W, Wolfe SM, et al. Explaining brain death: a critical feature of the donation process. *J Transpl Coord.* 1997;7:14–21.
24. Shafer T, Wood RP, Van Buren CT, et al. A success story in minority donation: the LifeGift/Ben taub general hospital in-house coordinator program. *Transplant Proc.* 1997;29:3753–3755.
25. Shafer T, Wood RP, Van Buren C, et al. An in-house coordinator program to increase organ donation in public trauma hospitals. *J Transpl Coord.* 1998;8:82–87.
26. Sullivan H, Blakely D, Davis K. An in-house coordinator program to increase organ donation in public teaching hospitals. *J Transpl Coord.* 1998;8:40–42.
27. Morris Peter, ed. *Kidney Transplantation: Principles and Practice.* 5th ed. Philadelphia, PA: WB Saunders, 2001.
28. Burg, MB, Orloff, MJ. Active cation transport by kidney tubules at 0 degrees C. *Am J Physiol.* 1964;207:983.
29. Collins GM, Bravo-Shugarman M, Terasaki PI. Kidney preservation for transportation: initial perfusion and 30 hours' ice storage. *Lancet.* 1969; 2:1219.
30. Marshall VC, Howden BO, Thomas AC, et al. Extended preservation of dog kidneys with modified UW solution. *Transplant Proc.* 1991;23:2366.
31. Ueda Y, Todo S, Imventarza O, et al. The UW solution for canine kidney preservation: its specific effect on renal hemodynamics and microvasculature. *Transplantation.* 1989;48:913.
32. Florack G, Sutherland DE, Ascherl R, et al. Definition of normothermic ischemia limits for kidney and pancreas grafts. *J Surg Res.* 1986;40: 550–563.
33. Revised Uniform Anatomical Gift Act (2006), National Conference of Commissioners.
34. Omnibus Reconcillation Act Pub L. No 99–509 (1986).
35. University of Pittsburgh. http://stiresearch.health.pitt.edu/default.asp
36. Leno v. St. Joseph Hospital, 302 N.E. 2d 58 (1973).
37. Mayes Gwen. *Transplant News.* May 12, 2001.
38. Perry v. Saint Francis Hospital & Medical Center, Inc., 886 F. Supp. 1551 (1995).
39. Nicoletta v. Rochester eye and Human Parts Bank, Inc., 519 NYS 2d 928 (1987).
40. Finger, Eric- www.emedicine.com/ med TOPIC3200.htm.
41. Uniform Anatomical Gift Act, 2006. http://www.nccusl.org/Act.aspx?title=Anatomical%20Gift%20Act%20%282006%29.

CHAPTER 58 ■ PALLIATIVE CARE

RONALD M. STEWART

In the face of critical surgical illness, palliative care focuses on a set of individualized goals aimed at reducing the suffering of the patient and family members.[1,2] Ideally, this process begins prior to the patient's illness with a personal expression of the person's end-of-life choices, and extends into the bereavement period following the patient's death. Realistically, patients rarely begin palliative care planning prior to becoming ill, and most often the process is initiated only after critical illness supervenes or the patient is considered terminal. Rather, palliative care should be integrated as a routine part of the continuum of care in the surgical intensive care unit.[3,4] Stated another way, relief of suffering and pain are essential to clinical cure, so the shift from curative to primarily palliative care is largely a change in the goals of therapy.

High-quality palliative care is usually interdisciplinary in nature, and is now a recognized medical specialty. Hospice and Palliative Care Medicine was recognized in 2008 by the American Board of Medical Specialties, with certification in hospice and palliative medicine issued by 10 cosponsoring boards, including the American Boards of Anesthesiology, Emergency Medicine, Family Medicine, Internal Medicine, Obstetrics and Gynecology, Pediatrics, Physical Medicine and Rehabilitation, Psychiatry and Neurology, Radiology, and Surgery.

Considering that palliative care involves crucially important decisions that can be difficult or emotionally wrenching to make, assisting critically ill surgical patients in the transition to palliative care can be challenging for the surgeon. The proposition is no easier for the patient. Thomas Finucane pointed out two fundamental issues that ensure that this transition will continue to be difficult for the patient and his or her family.[5] There is a near-universal and fervently held desire to remain alive. Second, in spite of concerted effort, caregivers cannot predict the future sufficiently to provide a meaningful, precise estimate of when death will occur.[5] The author would make two additional points: (1) most patients have strong and unique personal beliefs about the nature of death; and (2) from a purely surgical perspective, the surgeon has a strong clinical emotional investment in the patient's care, most often manifesting as a powerful motivation for the patient to survive the operation. This chapter provides an overview of palliative care as it relates to acute care surgery, trauma, and surgical intensive care.

HISTORY

An urologic oncologist, Balfour Mount, originally coined the term *palliative care* in the establishment of a clinical service at Montreal's Royal Victoria Hospital.[6] Doctor Mount took inspiration from Elisabeth Kubler-Ross and Cicely Saunders in London.[7] The focus of the newly created palliative care unit was to provide comprehensive care of the terminally ill patient.[8] This care was aimed at understanding, anticipating, preventing, and alleviating the suffering of the dying patient, which remain the goals of palliative care today.[9]

PRINCIPLES

The American College of Surgeons (ACS) Committee on Ethics developed a statement on the principles guiding care at the end of life, which was approved by the Board of Regents and published in the Bulletin of the ACS in 1998 (Table 58.1).[10] This statement is a solid resource to the global approach to palliative care. When one reads this statement of principles and reflects on its meaning, it is clear that several crucial points were emphasized: (1) The patient has the right to determine his or her own care, and the surgeon shall respect the patient's authority to make this choice (including the right to refuse care the surgeon may recommend). (2) The provision of care based on the patient's choices should address comprehensively pain, psychosocial, family, and spiritual issues. (3) The surgeon should forego treatments that are futile.

ETHICAL CONSIDERATIONS

Although this chapter is not a primer on medical ethics, it would be incomplete without a discussion of the general philosophical framework of the principles of both palliative and curative care. The principles may not be held universally by all cultures, but are viewed widely as being applicable universally to decision making relating to the ethical practice of medicine in Western, traditional medicine. The following principles underlie the ethical structure of medical practice and palliative care: 1) honesty; 2) autonomy; 3) beneficence/nonmaleficence; 4) dignity (Table 58.2).[11] In addition, several key ethical concepts are relevant to the discussion surrounding palliative care. These include the concepts of futility, informed consent, medical uncertainty, and the principle of double effect (Table 58.3).

Palliative care is often thought of as distinct from traditional curative or supportive care; however, because most modern intensive care is supportive, meaning care that supports organ function until the patient heals, there is a natural continuum whereby palliative care can be integrated into modern intensive care.[3,4] For individual patients there may be a clear point of transition from curative to palliative care; however, in some cases the continuum may lead to indistinction, rather than a clear demarcation. For the purposes of discussion, clear transition points serve to illustrate common dilemmas or questions in the intensive care unit (ICU).

When Should Care Be Shifted from Curative/Supportive to Palliation?

In patients who are critically ill or who have major, life-threatening, or debilitating surgical and medical problems, the surgical team is often faced with the question of how much curative or supportive care to provide, or alternatively should the goals of care initiate or change to exclusively palliative care?[12] In the clinical experience of the author, these questions most often revolve around the principles of autonomy, futility, and beneficence. When the patient has outlined clearly his or her wishes and opinions related to clinical care, the treatment plan should be consistent and respectful of the patient's wishes, unless care is deemed to be futile. In the case of futility, there is no obligation on the part of the physician to provide futile care. The concept of futility is well described; however, there is considerable disagreement among experts (and applicable laws

TABLE 58.1

ACS' STATEMENT ON PRINCIPLES GUIDING CARE AT THE END OF LIFE

- Respect the dignity of both patient and caregivers.
- Be sensitive to and respectful of the patient's and family's wishes.
- Use the most appropriate measures that are consistent with the choices of the patient or the patient's legal surrogate.
- Ensure alleviation of pain and management of other physical symptoms.
- Recognize, assess, and address psychological, social, and spiritual problems.
- Ensure appropriate continuity of care by the patient's primary or specialist physician.
- Provide access to therapies that may realistically be expected to improve the patient's quality of life.
- Provide access to appropriate palliative care and hospice care.
- Respect the patient's right to refuse treatment.
- Recognize the physician's responsibility to forego treatments that are futile.

among the states) as to what constitutes futile care, except in extreme situations (e.g., brain death, anencephaly), so there is commonly disagreement over what constitutes futile care (Table 58.3).

What to Do When the Patient Wishes for Treatment, but Care Is Deemed Futile by the Physician?

This is an inherent conflict between the principle of autonomy and the concept of medical futility. The first course of action should be reassessment of the determination of futility. In most instances, futile care is assessed based on medical probability, for which there is inherent uncertainty. Oftentimes, what seems to be a disagreement over futile care is really a disagreement over the goals of care, so the next course of action should be a respectful, thoughtful, and empathetic discussion between the physician and patient/surrogate(s) concerning the goals of care and a discussion of why the care is not beneficial to the patient. This discussion should include a self-reflective reassessment of the determination of futility, including an objective internal review of biases and potential conflicts (see below).

TABLE 58.2

DEFINITIONS PRINCIPLES OF RELEVANCE TO PALLIATIVE CARE

Autonomy: The precept that the patient has the right to determine his or her care, or lack thereof.

Beneficence: The physician shall act uniformly in the best interest of the patient.

Dignity: A less well-defined term signifying that the patient has a right to respectful, ethical, and empathetic treatment.

Honesty: The precept that the patient has the right to know the truth about their condition and their planned treatment, including its likely outcome and risk.

Nonmaleficence: "First, do no harm." This is related to beneficence, but emphasizes the point that the most important principle is to not harm the patient.

TABLE 58.3

CONCEPTUAL FRAMEWORK FOR THE ETHICAL PRACTICE OF PALLIATIVE CARE MEDICINE

Double Effect: The concept that a treatment may have two effects (e.g., for opioids, that medication relieves pain, but may depress respiratory drive). In practical use, it is the intent of the treatment that is most important. Effective treatment of pain may lead to impaired respiratory drive; however, if the intent is to treat pain effectively, the treatment is ethical and warranted.

Futility: Futile care is care that provides no benefit to the patient. Practically, developing a working definition of what constitutes futile care is challenging, except at the extremes.

Informed Consent: The patient gives permission, usually in writing, to a given treatment following a thorough discussion of the risks, benefits, and alternatives.

Medical Uncertainty: Diagnoses, prognoses, and treatment decisions are based on probability, thus there is inherent uncertainty in many end-of-life situations.

Surrogate Decision Maker: The family member or significant other who is recognized to have authority to make decisions for the patient who lacks capacity for medical decision making, or there is ambiguity with respect to what the patient would have intended. Ideally, the health care agent is designated in advance by the execution of a durable power of attorney for health care, or "health care proxy." If no agent is designated, a hierarchy is defined, with the patient's spouse at the apex and children subordinate.

What to Do When the Patient Wishes No Further Treatment, but the Physician Believes the Care Is Beneficial?

In this situation, the conflict is between patient autonomy and practitioner beneficence—the patient is refusing a treatment that the surgeon considers indicated and beneficial. Again, the best first course of action is a careful self-reassessment. Provided the patient has the capacity to make medical decisions, there should follow an empathetic and respectful discussion between caregiver(s), to understand the patient's point of view, and patient/surrogate to understand the medical issues involved. For terminally ill patients, once this discussion has been held to the satisfaction of all parties, the patient's wishes should be followed, regardless of the point of view of the health care team. The patient has the right to make what the clinician may perceive to be an incorrect decision.[13]

In the author's experience, this situation is uncommon. Most often the surgical team and the patient/surrogate are in agreement as to when to transition from curative to palliative care. Even when there is disagreement initially, the parties can usually negotiate a mutually agreeable decision. Achieving this harmonious agreement should be a primary goal of the surgical team.

IDENTIFYING POTENTIAL BIAS AND CONFLICTS OF INTEREST

When there is disagreement, it is essential to perform an internal reassessment concerning one's own beliefs, potential biases, and potential conflict of interests. Even in the absence of any disagreement, it is beneficial to reexamine periodically one's own potential biases and conflicts of interest. Developing this habit assists with developing a "mindful practice".[14] One would suppose that compared to the patient and his or her family, this process would be easier for the educated, experienced surgeon or intensive care physician; however, sometimes this exercise can be more challenging than one might suppose. The most dangerous bias is one that is unrecognized by oneself. Outlined below are some of the more common potential biases of those working with critically ill patients.

Overconfidence in Predicting Outcome

> "Medicine is a science of uncertainty and an art of probability."[15]
>
> —Sir William Osler

The longer a doctor has practiced medicine, the less confident he is in his ability to predict the outcome of critical illness; any prognosticator would be well-advised to proceed with caution. Several pieces of data support this conclusion. A prospective, 1-year study of 206 critically ill French oncology patients who were considered for ICU admission found that 101 patients were not admitted: 54 because they were deemed "too sick," and 47 because they were deemed "too well."[16] Worrisome was that 17% of the "too sick" patients were still alive at 180 days, implying that this group was not terminally ill. Of the group of patients "too well" for admission, 22% were dead in 30 days. Thus the evaluators were not particularly adept at predicting either who would survive or who would not. That the data came from a group of cancer patients, for whom the end of life might seem to be easier to predict as compared to a general surgical or medical population, underscores the difficulty.

In a follow-up to the Study to Understand Prognoses and Preferences for Outcomes and Risks of Treatments (SUPPORT), a group of 2,954 critically ill, nononcology patients with chronic obstructive pulmonary disease, congestive heart failure, or end-stage liver disease were followed after hospital discharge.[17] The goal of SUPPORT was to include terminal patients who had an aggregate 6-month mortality rate of 50%. Of these patients, 347 died during the index hospitalization, leaving 2,607 patients who were followed as outpatients. Of these patients, 1,948 (66%) were alive at 6 months. None of the predictive models were accurate for the prediction of who would not survive for 6 months. Using a model predicting a <10% survival rate at 6 months, the actual survival was 41%.

The panoply of critically ill scoring and mortality prediction models (MPMs), including the Acute Physiology and Chronic Health Evaluation (APACHE), APACHE II, APACHE III, and APACHE IV scores; the Simplified Acute Physiology Score (SAPS) and SAPS II; the Sequential Organ failure Assessment (SOFA) score; and MPM and MPM II, should raise skepticism. Three points can be made about these mortality prediction tools: (1) Each of these models predicts mortality well for a population of patients. (2) From a temporal standpoint, each is more predictive the closer one comes to death. (3) Most (except APACHE III and SOFA) are not particularly useful to predict the outcome for an individual patient. Therefore, these predictive tools are not particularly helpful when trying to prognosticate for the individual patient.

Among those who care for critically ill patients, bias of overconfidence in predicting outcome can lead to an unjustified, overly pessimistic view or a similarly unjustified, overly optimistic assessment of prognosis. Based on the author's experience, a personal prognostication is offered: When physicians predict the future, one can usually predict accurately that they will be incorrect. Regardless of the author's opinion, scientific data clearly support a healthy skepticism concerning one's ability to predict the outcome of critically or terminally ill patients.

Covenant of Care

Surgeons perform operations upon patients. These operations have a permanent and immediate effect upon the patient's life. Surgeons and patients partner together to address the problem the operation is designed to remedy. As such, surgeons as a group are invested emotionally in the care of their own patients. Cassel and Buchman described this relationship as covenantal, as a simple promise: "I will care for you."[18–20] This covenantal relationship is obviously positive, and at least in the author's opinion, often makes the surgeon the most influential advocate for the patient's wishes. However, at the end of life, this relationship may lead the surgeon to push for curative care, even when it is against the patient's wishes. In a hypothetical case discussion regarding informed consent, a group of well-trained, respected, competent surgeons were asked what they would do in the following scenario[21]: A patient has a soft tissue infection of the foot that is limb-threatening. The consulting surgeon is informed by the patient that death is preferable to amputation, and operation is deferred. The surgeon is consulted again several days later after the patient has become comatose from sepsis and encephalopathy due to a necrotizing soft tissue infection, and lacks capacity to express his or her wishes or make medical decisions. The surgical panelists were unanimous in their agreement that they would amputate the lower extremity in order to save the patient's life. This was a theoretic panel discussion, but this desire to do the right thing for the patient may lead the surgeon to push curative care in contradistinction to the patient's expressed wishes. Even the language that is commonly used belies this authority—patients' "wishes," and doctors' "orders." When one is invested emotionally in the care of a patient, one should take time to reflect personally as to what the patient would choose, and then one should do what one can to honor those wishes. This may or may not be different from the surgeon's wishes or their perception of what is in the patient's best interest; clarifying any discrepancy beforehand is decidedly in the patient's best interest.

Caring for All—Distributive Justice

"Critical care resources are not only expensive, but also scarce."[18] Whereas the patient's surgeon may have an intensely personal bond with the patient, the acute care surgeon or intensive care physician caring for all patients in the ICU is often placed in the situation of determining the appropriate resource utilization for the case. Even at times of peak ICU utilization, when decision making can be particularly challenging, this responsibility must be recognized and accepted, and should not bias any decisions regarding palliative and curative care, except perhaps in mass-casualty situations. Intensive care is costly and not beneficial for every patient, but recognition of same should not bias care that is in the patient's best interest. The finite nature of resources is primarily a societal issue that must be addressed at the societal level.

Compassion Fatigue

Compassion fatigue, or "burnout," probably affects all providers of trauma and emergency care at one time or another.[22] It is common among those who provide care for terminally ill patients, particularly caregivers who are isolated and overworked. The condition tends to lead to cynicism, anger, and fatigue—a situational depression. If one is mindful of the problem, compassion fatigue can be prevented,[22] but when present it may lead to a bias in either direction. Palliative care is best provided by those fully engaged and committed to the comprehensive relief of patient suffering, which is almost impossible under conditions of burnout. A portion of the ACS Manual for the Resident on Palliative Care emphasizes self-care as a component of palliative care.[23]

The Unbiased Surgeon or Intensivist

The most dangerous bias is the unrecognized bias. Each of us has our own unique biases concerning curative and palliative care based on our own beliefs, values, previous experiences, and fund of knowledge. It is a grave mistake to consider oneself unbiased. This is well told by the late William F. Buckley, describing the story of a man without a country[24]:

> *"... It told of a man at a bar who boasted of his rootlessness, derisively dismissing the jingoistic patrons to his left and to his right. But later in the evening, one man speaks an animadversion on a little principality in the Balkans and is met with the clenched fist of the man without a country, who would not endure this insult to the place where he was born."*

So it must be with the unbiased surgeon or unbiased intensive care physician: Being mindful of our own predispositions is crucial to provide reliable guidance and advice for patients and their families when they need it most.

PROVIDING PALLIATIVE CARE IN PRACTICE

Cicely Saunders[25] and Balfour Mount[26] emphasized the concepts of the care of the whole patient and relieving all pain as essential elements of palliative care. This approach involves the more traditional domains of relief of symptoms, prevention and treatment of pain, and psychosocial support; however, the palliative approach extends beyond these domains into less traditional areas of spiritualism and existentialism. Eric Cassell broadened this view, emphasizing further that individual patient suffering is unique and is affected by a large number of holistic and subjective domains that extend beyond the typical medical assessment.[27]

As a tool to assist in addressing these domains in palliative and end-of-life care, several authors have developed tools to assist the clinician. One tool with documented effectiveness to improve care at the end of life is the PEACE Tool (Table 58.4).[28]

P reminds the practitioner to address pain and the wide range of physical ailments that afflict patients with serious medical and surgical illnesses. The acute care surgeon is well prepared to deal with this constellation of physical problems, but the important first step is a logical and systematic approach to identifying the complaints that are most distressing to the patient. Most pain management issues can be addressed by the surgeon, but consultation with a palliative care specialist or pain management practitioner is indicated when the patient's pain is not relieved completely.

TABLE 58.4
PEACE TOOL

Physical symptoms: Pain; gastrointestinal, urologic, or respiratory symptoms; skin breakdown/irritation; fatigue and energy level.
Emotive (and cognitive) symptoms: Depression, delirium, or anxiety.
Autonomy-related issues: Does the patient perceive that he/she is in control of their own care?
Communication, Contribution to others, and Closure of life affairs: Addresses relations with loved ones, one's legacy, and closure of one's personal affairs.
Economic burden and other practical issues: Addresses economic burden, care providers outside the inpatient hospital setting, insurance matters and paperwork.
Transcendent and existential issues: Is the patient at peace? Addresses issues of faith, spirituality, purpose, and what happens after death.

E is a reminder to address emotional and cognitive issues. Of these problems, the most common are depression, anxiety, and delirium. Preventing or addressing these issues requires a multifaceted approach. In particular, the identification of delirium can be challenging because as many as 70% of critically ill surgical or trauma patients may experience delirium during their hospitalization (which may persist for several days), but up to 60% of affected patients manifest a "hypoactive" delirium with no overt signs.[29,30] Validated assessment tools are available to assist the clinician, notably the Confusion Assessment Method for the Intensive Care Unit (CAM-ICU)[31,32] (Table 58.5). The CAM-ICU tool was designed for bedside use by ICU clinicians who have no psychiatric training. The assessment can be completed in as little as 2 minutes, with sensitivity, specificity, and interrater reliability all approaching 95%.[29–32]

If emotional or cognitive issues are identified, they are addressed by maintaining a relationship between patient and care providers that promotes a positive, encouraging environment, celebrating victories (past, present, and future) and allowing the patient their self-expression. The American poet Ted Rosenthal said, "Life is grim, but not necessarily serious." in his book *How Could I Not Be Among You?*, written while dying.[33] The goal is to help the patient "still smell the rose above the mould," as Osler, on his deathbed, reportedly quoted Thomas Hood repeatedly.[34] The same goals exist for the patient's family in the ICU, even when the patient is incommunicado

A is for autonomy and is a reminder to involve the patient and family in end-of-life care. It is important for the patient and family to be given voice, and to feel in control. This may be a point of friction with surgeons, who also usually have the same goals. The patient's and family's goals may not always be consistent with those of care providers, wishing (perhaps) that more aggressive care be provided than is logical or consistent with the patient's physical condition according to the medical team. As Finucane states lucidly: "The desire not to be dead coupled with an inevitable imprecision in estimates of survival for individuals makes it difficult for many severely ill patients to shift goals."[5] The author would also emphasize that the patient or their family may be correct and the medical team may be incorrect with respect to this conflict, and that it is important that the medical practitioner acknowledges with humility the uncertainty of his or her predictive powers.

TABLE 58.5

THE CONFUSION ASSESSMENT METHOD FOR THE INTENSIVE CARE UNIT

Domain 1: Acute onset of mental status changes, or fluctuating course

- Is there evidence of an acute change in mental status, from baseline?
- Has abnormal behavior fluctuated in the prior 24 h?

Sources of data: Serial Glasgow Coma Scale scores or sedation scores; input for the patient's critical care nurse, or family

Domain 2: Inattention

- Does the patient have difficulty focusing attention?
- Is there reduced ability to maintain/shift attention?

Sources of data: Attention screening examinations by picture recognition or random letter test (neither requires an oral response and can thus be used to assess patients ventilated mechanically)

Domain 3: Disorganized thinking

- Is conversation rambling or incoherent? Is there unclear or illogical flow of ideas, or unpredictable switching among subjects?
- Is the patient able to follow questions and commands?

Source of data: Clinical assessment

Domain 4: Altered level of consciousness

- Is the level of consciousness anything other than "alert?" Examples include vigilant (hyperalert), lethargic (drowsy but arousable), stuporous (difficult to arouse), or comatose.

Source of data: Clinical assessment

The CAM-ICU tool was designed and validated for use by nonpsychiatrist clinicians at the bedside. Delirium is present when both Domains 1 and 2 are positive, plus either Domain 3 or 4. Modified from Ely EW, Margolin R, Francis J, et al. Evaluation of delirium in critically ill patients: Validation of the Confusion Assessment Method for the Intensive Care Unit (CAM-ICU). *Crit Care Med.* 2001;29:1370–1379.

Alternatively, a patient may wish for less aggressive care than the medical or surgical team wishes to provide. This choice may not be linear or logical—as an example, a patient may refuse definitive care, but wish for supportive care following this decision. A patient–physician–family relationship based on respect, communication, and cooperation is beneficial to all parties. The patient's wishes for autonomy should be granted insofar as possible, and when impossible, an empathetic and thorough discussion of the rationale behind the medical decision is mandatory.

Autonomy does not mean that the physician abrogates to the patient the responsibility for the transition to palliative care. Burdening the family solely with the decision to withdraw curative or supportive care as part of the transition to palliation is at once unwise and unfair. The decision to shift from curative to palliative care is made jointly by the physician, the patient, and his or her surrogate (if applicable). As a professional who is educated, trained, and experienced in these situations, the physician is central in guiding patient and family through this situation without making them feel unheard, guilty, or abandoned. Although the task is difficult, the reward is the patient and family are often grateful for the assistance.

C is for closure for the patient and their loved ones. As much as possible, it is important for patient and family to believe that there is no unfinished business and that death will occur with no regrets. Asking about unfinished business or unfinished communication with loved ones may be therapeutic for the patient. Circumstances may not permit for critically injured patients or patients who suffer a devastating acute illness; however, it is imperative that an opportunity for closure be found insofar as possible. This may mean forgoing a declaration of brain death for a brief period of time for the family to achieve closure, or to allow a loved one to arrive after a long journey. There may be substantial guilt surrounding a violent or sudden event. To the extent possible, the skilled acute care surgeon should minimize these feelings and help the patient and family to achieve closure, which may mean the family forgives the patient or themselves, or vice versa. Forgiveness is an important part of healing, and it should start at the bedside in the ICU. Similarly, organ donation may be a part of this tactic. Many loved ones who choose to donate organs find meaning in the gift and have something positive emerge from a tragic, unexpected death, as compared to those who either choose not to donate, or were not given the opportunity.

E is for economic and other practical issues. Dying in modern Western society is a complicated, expensive, and bureaucratic event. The expense of being seriously ill may be a primary stressor to the patient. To the extent possible, the medical team can address some of these concerns. Assistance with insurance forms, social services, and simply discussing these matters with the patient and his or her family can make a positive difference.

T is for transcendental and existential issues. Religion and spirituality are extremely important to most patients and their families during their illness and surrounding the patient's death. Most terminal cancer patients in a recent survey endorsed religion as important to their care and expressed concerns about the lack of spiritual support from medicine and their community.[34] Providing faith-based support and counseling is a crucial part of palliative care.[35, 36] This should be tailored to the patient's beliefs, not those of the medical team or any physician. This spiritual care is central to addressing each of the preceding first four domains: physical complaints, emotive symptoms, autonomy, and closure. Sensitivity to these concerns is an important role for the physician.

The PEACE Tool was designed for palliative/hospice care outside of the ICU; however, it is useful to remind the practitioner of the need for total and comprehensive care across domains that are not a typical part of a surgical treatment plan. The tool also is modified easily for use in the ICU, although many of the questions may be directed toward the patient's family and loved ones, rather than the patient him- or herself. Regardless of which tools are employed, the implementation of palliative care should address the domains of physical, psychosocial, economic, and spiritual/religious issues.

SELECTED LEGAL ASPECTS OF PALLIATIVE CARE

Alleviating Pain and Hastening Death?

In many instances it is possible to treat pain without undue risk of respiratory compromise or hastening death.[37] For the patient with severe pain, respiratory depression is a small risk due to a number of factors, including opioid tolerance with chronic use.[38] In situations where pain or distress cannot be treated without risk of respiratory compromise, palliative sedation is an option. This situation arises most commonly with respiratory distress when mechanical ventilation has been withdrawn or is not indicated due to a terminal condition. Higher doses of opioids, alone or in combination with an anxiolytic, are indicated in these situations, and may be used if the intent of their use is to prevent suffering.[37]

The United States Supreme Court has differentiated palliative sedation from euthanasia and physician-assisted suicide. Euthanasia is the administration of medication by a care provider with the intent of causing death, and is illegal everywhere in the United States. Physician-assisted suicide is illegal in all US jurisdictions except the State of Oregon, and is defined as prescribing or educating the patient in the use of medication, knowing that the patient intends to use these medications to commit suicide. Palliative sedation is the administration of medication with the intent of preventing pain or suffering, even if death may be hastened. The palliation should be indicated clinically and the intent of relieving pain and suffering for the benefit of the patient should be documented. Under the principles of beneficence and double effect, the Supreme Court has ruled that palliative sedation is both legal and ethical.[39,40] Justice O'Connor wrote in Vacco v. Quill:

> *"The parties and the amici agree that in the States a patient who is suffering from a terminal illness and who is experiencing great pain has no legal barriers to obtaining medication, from qualified physicians, to alleviate suffering, even to the point of causing unconsciousness and hastening death."*[39]

Some states go further still. Both California and Florida have statutory rules mandating effective pain management. In addition, there is potential civil liability for failure to provide effective palliation and treatment of pain. Civil courts have ruled in favor of plaintiffs on the grounds of malpractice, abandonment, and elder abuse when physicians have failed to provide adequate pain relief.[37]

In summary, comfort care should be provided for the purposes of preventing and treating suffering and pain. Palliative pain relief or sedation is both ethical and legal. The palliative care plan should be documented sufficiently that an external reviewer can determine the indication and intent, describing adequately the indication for palliation and that the physician's primary intent is to relieve pain and prevent suffering.

SUMMARY

In the context of critical surgical illness, palliative care focuses on a set of individualized patient goals aimed at reducing the suffering of the patient and his or her family. The ACS' Statement on Principles Guiding Care at the End of Life provides an ethical framework for the provision of palliative care to surgical patients (Table 58.1). A mindful self-assessment of personal beliefs, potential conflicts of interest, and potential biases is a good starting point for advising and assisting patients in the transition from curative to palliative care. High-quality palliative care is interdisciplinary and deals with the total patient. The palliative care plan addresses the holistic domains of physical afflictions, psychosocial concerns, economic burdens, and spiritual/religious issues. Even with a great care plan, effective medical leadership, and superb technical implementation of treatment measures, the transition from curative to palliative care will still be challenging, because patients almost without exception have a strong desire to be among the living; and physicians are imperfect in their ability to provide meaningfully precise prognostic information as to when death will occur. These challenges should not deter us from our responsibility of providing effective guidance throughout this transition in a manner that results in comfort, dignity, and respect for the patient and their loved ones.

References

1. Dunn GP, Milch, RA. Introduction and historical background of palliative care: Where does the surgeon fit in? *J Am Coll Surg*. 2001;193:325–328.
2. Okon TR, Gomez CF. Overview of patient evaluation in palliative care. UpToDate 2011;18.3. http://www.uptodate.com/contents/overview-of-patient-evaluation-in-palliative-care?source=search_result&selectedTitle=1~150. Accessed February 23, 2011.
3. Mosenthal AC, Murphy PA. Trauma care and palliative care: time to integrate the two? *J Am Coll Surg*. 2003;197:509–516.
4. Mosenthal AC, Lee KF, Huffman J. Palliative care in the surgical intensive care unit. *J Am Coll Surg*. 2002;194:75–83.
5. Finucane TE. How gravely ill becomes dying: a key to end-of-life care. *JAMA*. 1999;282:1670–1672.
6. Duffy A. *A Moral Force: The story of Dr. Balfour Mount*. The Ottawa Citizen. Ottawa, Canada: Postmedia Network Inc.; 2005.
7. Saunders C. The evolution of palliative care. *Patient Educ Couns*. 2000;41:7–13.
8. Ajemanian I, Balfour M. *The R.V.H. Manual on Palliative/Hospice Care*. Montreal, Canada. The Palliative Care Service at Royal Victoria Hospital; 1980.
9. Dunn GP, Milch RA, Mosenthal AC, et al. Palliative care by the surgeon: How to do it. *J Am Coll Surg*. 2002;194:509–537.
10. American College of Surgeons. Principles guiding care at the end of life. *Bull Am Coll Sur*. 1998;83(4).
11. Kellum JA, Dacey MJ. Ethics in the intensive care unit: informed consent; withholding and withdrawal of life support; and requests for futile therapies. *UpToDate*, 2011;18.3. http://www.uptodate.com/contents/ethics-in-the-intensive-care-unit-informed-consent-withholding-and-withdrawal-of-life-support-and-requests-for-futile-therapies?source=search_result&selectedTitle=1~150. Accessed February 23, 2011.
12. Gunn GP. Patient assessment in palliative care: How to see the "big picture" and what to do when "there is no more we can do". *J Am Coll Surg*. 2001;193:565–573.
13. Weir RF, Gostin L. Decisions to abate life-sustaining treatment for nonautonomous patients. Ethical standards and legal liability for physicians after Cruzan. *JAMA*. 1990;264:1846–1853.
14. Epstein RM. Mindful Practice. *JAMA*. 1999;282:833–839.
15. Osler W. In: Dean WB, ed. *Aphorisms from His Bedside Teachings and Writings*. New York: H. Schuman; 1950:125.
16. Thiery G, Azoulay E, Darmon M, et al. Quality of life of long-term survivors of breast cancer and lymphoma treated with standard-dose chemotherapy or local therapy. *J Clin Oncol*. 2005;23:4406–4413.
17. Fox E, Landrum-McNiff K, Zhenshao Z, et al. Evaluation of prognostic criteria for determining hospice eligibility in patients with advanced lung, heart, or liver disease. *JAMA*. 1999;282:1638–1645.
18. Buchman TG. Invited Commentary—surgical intensivist and end-of-life issues. *J Am Coll Surg*. 2003;197:853–854.
19. Cassell J, Buchman TG, Streat S, et al. Surgeons, intensivists, and the covenant of care: administrative models and values affecting care at the end of life. *Crit Care Med*. 2003;31:1551–1557.
20. Buchman TG, Cassell J, Ray SE, et al. Who should manage the dying patient? Rescue, shame, and the surgical ICU dilemma. *J Am Coll Surg*. 2002;194:665–673.
21. GcGrath MH, Angelos P, Gewertz BL, et al. Ethical issues in surgical practice: Exploring informed consent. *Contemp Surg*. 2003;59:213–223.
22. Brandt ML. The Claude Organ Memorial Lecture: the practice of surgery: surgery as practice. *Am J Surg*. 2009;198:742–747.
23. Dunn GP, Martensen R, Weissman D, eds. *Surgical Palliative Care: A Resident's Guide*. 4th ed. Chicago, IL: American College of Surgeons and the Cunniff-Dixon Foundation; 2009.
24. Buckley WF Jr. How is it possible to believe in God? National Public Radio, May 23, 2005. Accessed February 23, 2011.
25. Clark D. 'Total pain', disciplinary power, and the body in the work of Cicely Saunders, 1958–1967. *Soc Sci Med*. 1999;49:727–736.
26. Mount BM. The problem of caring for the dying in a general hospital; the palliative care unit as a possible solution. *Can Med Assoc J*. 1976;115:119–121.
27. Cassel E. Diagnosing suffering: a perspective. *Ann Intern Med*. 1999;131:531–534.
28. Okon TR, Evans JM, Gomez CF, et al. Palliative educational outcome with implementation of PEACE tool integrated clinical pathway. *J Palliat Med*. 2004;7:279–295.
29. Pandharipande P, Cotton BA, Shintani A, et al. Prevalence and risk factors for development of delirium in surgical and trauma intensive care unit patients. *J Trauma*. 2008;65:34–41.
30. Pandharipande P, Cotton BA, Shintani A, et al. Motoric types of delirium in mechanically ventilated surgical and trauma intensive care unit patients. *Intensive Care Med*. 2007;33:1726–1731.
31. Ely EW, Margolin R, Francis J, et al. Evaluation of delirium in critically ill patients: Validation of the Confusion Assessment Method for the Intensive Care Unit (CAM-ICU). *Crit Care Med*. 2001;29:1370–1379.

32. Soja SL, Pandharipande PP, Fleming SB, et al. Implementation, reliability testing, and compliance monitoring of the Confusion Assessment Method for the Intensive Care Unit in trauma patients. *Intensive Care Med.* 2008;34:1263–1268.
33. Rosenthal T. *How Could I Not Be Among You?* New York. Persea Books; 1987.
34. Hood T. *The Poetical Works Of Thomas Hood.* Boston, MA: Crosby, Nichols, Lee and Company; 1861.
35. Balboni TA, Vanderwerker LC, Block SD, et al. Religiousness and spiritual support among advanced cancer patients and associations with end-of-life treatment preferences and quality of life. *J Clin Oncol.* 2007;25:555–560.
36. Hinshaw DB. The spiritual needs of the dying patient. *J Am Coll Surg.* 2002;195:565–568.
37. Baluss ME, Lee KF. Legal considerations for palliative care in surgical practice. *J Am Coll Surg.* 2003;197:323–330.
38. Thompson AR, Ray JB. The importance of opioid tolerance: a therapeutic paradox. *J Am Coll Surg.* 2003;196:321–324.
39. Vacco v. Quill, 521 U. S. 793 (1997).
40. Washington v. Glucksberg, 521 U. S. 702 (1997).

CHAPTER 59 ■ EMTALA AND OTHER PRINCIPLES AFFECTING THE ACUTE CARE SURGEON

KENNETH L. MATTOX

The physician engaged in trauma management, emergency surgery, acute care surgery, or surgical critical care is intricately involved with patients with immediate life-threatening emergency conditions. Issues and decisions regarding receiving such patients, evaluation, management, consultation, and even transfer are all governed by the patient's clinical condition. These issues and decision nodes have been the subject of the many chapters of this book and will not be repeated here, although some of the regulations will be reviewed in this chapter to formulate rules, misperceptions, and policies regarding patients with critical conditions.

No profession in the world is more regulated than that of physicians in the United States. Surgeons are more regulated than other medical specialists, and an "acute care surgeon" who may or may not participate in trauma and surgical critical care is subject to more regulations than any other surgeon. The Emergency Medical Treatment and Active Labor Act (EMTALA) is both the epitome and a surrogate for a long list of regulations, rules, practice guidelines, policies, and outside manipulation as to how an acute care surgeon must function. The regulations were initially designed to protect persons interacting in health care, beginning with the patient in need. Others who need regulatory protection include surgeons, hospitals, custodians of medical records, hospital administrators, nurses, and many others.

The initial EMTALA was signed into law in 1986. Minor amendments were made almost every year, with a major revision in 2003, clarifying the roles of hospitals and physicians. Unfortunately, with revisions come new areas of confusion and new areas to allow manipulations at both the sending and receiving facilities. For all EMTALA regulations, it is the hospital that bears the responsibility for complying with the law, with the physicians as representatives of the hospital care. Surgeons voluntarily accept their responsibility as "agents of the hospital" when they accept call or referred patients, as well as when they transfer patients out or refuse transfer or referral for care.

EMTALA rules were developed to ensure that a patient with an immediate life-threatening emergency in an original location, which did not have the physical and personal resources to manage that emergency condition, would be transferred to a region that possessed a facility with the capacity of diagnosing and managing that emergency. The EMTALA never *intended* these rules to be used as an economic screen. Nor was there any intent that a patient without financial resources for medical payment would automatically be sent to a facility with a higher level of care, especially when patients with payment resources with that same immediate life-threatening emergency were often kept at the original sending institution. Likewise EMTALA was never intended to be a required referral source for specialized hospitals nor a mechanism for a hospital to refuse to receive a patient in referral for an emergency merely because that patient did not have financial resources or was outside the usual payment system or program of the hospital.

DEFINITIONS WITH EMTALA RAMIFICATIONS

A number of terms or phrases have direct bearing on EMTALA and the responsibilities and interpretations by hospitals, patients, doctors, families, and governmental agencies.
"Emergency" is a word with multiple meanings; its interpretation depends on the person using the word, the situation, the venue, and combinations of these and many other variables. An emergency may be modified by ethereal politics, ethics, economics, regulations, interpretations, past experience, gender, age, culture, and ethnicity. The same person may not meet an emergency with the same response however identical the situations might be. Two persons may anticipate or define the same situation as being either an urgent emergency or a nonemergency to be handled entirely at a discretionary time.

The motivation to seek assistance during an emergency is likewise variable. Such motivations may be time limited, economic limited, culturally limited, or influenced by a previous condition, either in ones memory of another, by previous education, or by past direct experience.

Modern Western culture has imprinted on society that everything is urgent, immediate, and therefore an emergency, which must be investigated and "taken care of" that very second. Very few conditions either in personal life, politics, religion, business, or even in health care are truly "emergencies" that require an immediate response.

Most misinformation regarding the emergency nature of a medical condition is secondary to funding and payment for services issues. With regard to a medical emergency, a patient or even a payer of medical services might attempt to make a case that a condition is an emergency, either to achieve an immediate evaluation and treatment or to alter the payment source or amount. Thus the attempt to define the emergency condition might be in the mind of the patient or personnel working for a funding agency, not the physician who is evaluating and treating the patient.

"Immediate life-threatening emergency" is a condition recognized to result in the death of a patient within a reasonably short period of time, usually perceived as being within 24 hours, or in some instances 1–3 days. Such conditions have recognizable staging and classification schemes that allow a reviewer to place such a patient in an immediate life-threatening emergency. Many "highest level of code" trauma conditions, and many acute care surgery conditions, such as a perforated viscus, necrotizing infection, acute occlusion of a major blood vessel, and similar conditions are indeed universally recognized as immediately life threatening. Many acute, subacute, and chronic medical, surgical, and mental health conditions will eventually result in the disability and death of a patient, but their mere presence is not an immediate life-threatening condition. Many conditions such as neoplasia, degenerative diseases, many infections, and most vascular conditions do not require an immediate hospitalization, or even a visit to an emergency center, unless that disease process has an immediate life-threatening complication that makes it such an emergency. The immediate life-threatening emergency should be defined by the medical community as being a condition that would be readily agreed upon to be such, not just a perception on the part of a patient.

"Hospital emergency department" is a location or locations, on or off the hospital main campus, which is licensed to provide emergency services; and up to one-third of the outpatient visits to that location are seen on an urgent basis. In such instances, the hospital advertises or appears to the public as a location providing emergency medical services.

"Acute surgical emergency" is a subset of immediate life-threatening emergencies that will require a surgical or procedural approach to reversing that emergency. Such an acute surgical emergency might require surgical, nonprocedural interventions, such as might be achieved by a surgical intensivist in a surgical intensive care unit.

"Trauma" is a subset of an acute surgical emergency, requiring a specialized trauma center immediately and available 24 hours a day. Trauma conditions can be categorized by both anatomic and physiologic derangement, and sometimes by the mechanism of injury. For each body area injured classification mechanisms have been developed by the American Association for the Surgery of Trauma and are readily available on the Eastern Association for the Surgery of Trauma (EAST) website (http://www.east.org/portal/) for immediate review. The mere presence of an injury does not require the presence of a trauma center. More than 90% of injuries are of a sufficiently minor nature that it has been recommended by the Advanced Trauma Life Support course of the American College of Surgeons that only <10% of patients with major trauma be taken to a designated trauma center.

"Dumping" is a term often used to designate a transfer to a regional health facility (with or without the prior knowledge and agreement of the receiving facility) for the purpose of moving an "undesirable" patient from a sending health facility. The reason for the undesirability may be financial, complexity of conditions, unfavorable diagnosis, or a long list of other excuses.

"Reversed Dumping" is a term referring to a receiving hospital using maneuvers to prevent a sending hospital from transferring an appropriate patient with an immediate life-threatening emergency to the appropriate regional facility, when that facility clearly has a duty to accept that patient in transfer. A patient without financial means of payment for an emergency service that can be rendered at the local hospital is *not* a reason in itself to send the patient to a higher level of care.

"Innovative Dumping" is a tactic to achieve a transfer of a patient to a regional emergency facility when under some usual circumstances, the sending hospital has the resources and personnel to manage the emergency. Apparently the most recent revisions to the EMTALA law have made provisions that have encouraged many local and nonreferral hospitals to develop means of transferring patients for a variety of conditions that are only managed electively at the sending hospital. For hospitals with a single or limited specialist on the medical staff roster, a hospital may elect to develop a limited call roster with important restrictions placed on the specialist on the call roster. Even though there are specialty services and an emergency room in a facility, a hospital is not under obligation to place such specialist on a daily call roster to respond to an emergency if placing him or her on such a recurring and frequent list would cause an unreasonable work schedule for that physician, and potentially produce an unsafe call condition.

"Warranty Work" is continuity of care concept that requires a physician who started a course of treatment for a patient with an emergency to complete that course of treatment. Many surgical conditions can undergo a variety of different acceptable approaches to procedural intervention. Once begun, a surgeon who initiates such a course should complete that course, including removing sutures, external fixation devices, and secondary staged surgery. Alternatively, such a surgeon may make mutually acceptable arrangements with a professional partner, associate, or even a surgeon at another facility to participate in follow-up care of a patient. For a surgeon to unknowingly be sent a patient whose course of treatment is not completed is not considered professional. Like many other aspects of society, a tradesman has a duty to satisfactorily complete a course of work, and to redo and repair faulty work under the concept of a warranty or assurance. For a patient who received a partial completion of an emergency surgical intervention to be sent to a regional facility to a different physician or physicians, without his or her knowledge and acceptance, is a form of dumping and is considered in some states as a violation of EMTALA.

OBLIGATIONS AND ASSUMPTIONS UNDER EMTALA

A physician working in an institution or location that receives a patient with an alleged emergency medical condition has a responsibility to participate in the evaluation of that patient to determine if indeed the symptoms, complaints, and findings in that patient are immediately life threatening. A chronic condition might be life threatening sometime in the distant future, such as controlled diabetes, controlled hypertension, atherosclerosis, or cancer. With most diseases or pathologic conditions, at some point in time, the disease itself or a complication of the disease might become immediately life threatening, with an ethical requirement to make a judgment between the patient and the physician about whether or not the condition or the disease will be treated. Conversely, all medical conditions that can result in a fatal or devastating complication at some point in time, if they are *not* immediately life or limb threatening as such, are not subject to the EMTALA regulations. As an example, atherosclerosis, which can occlude a coronary artery, might have been present as a fatty streak or a small athroma for several decades, but it is the acute coronary artery syndrome with its pain, electrocardiogram and cardiac enzyme abnormalities that announce the immediate presence of an impending fatal heart attack or cardiac arrhythmia. The duty of the physician is to evaluate the patient for such immediate life-threatening conditions and take a decision with the patient about the extent and location of immediate treatment.

Under EMTALA, a hospital has an obligation to clearly state the scope of their services and capabilities, particularly the level of emergency care and capabilities. Should a patient arrive with a presumed immediate life-threatening condition, by concern, symptom, or diagnosis, the hospital has an obligation to provide the extent of the evaluation and services within its advertised limits, or to arrange for transport to a facility that can provide these services. This transport can be by prearranged transfer agreements or by communications via protocol through the hospital's transfer centers.

Hospitals, especially small hospitals with limited number of specialists on the staff who are capable of providing the emergency aspects of their specialty, are not required to have a "specialist on call" every night, weekend, and holiday. To demonstrate the extremes of such a circumstance, a single neurosurgeon, a single orthopedic surgeon, or a single general surgeon in a community with only one small hospital, but that does advertise that they take emergency patients, cannot expect the single surgeon to be available, much less operating 24 hours a day, 7 days a week. But a hospital is expected to have a published "call roster" indicating the days and hours that the specialist of that hospital who does respond to emergency calls, will indeed be on the call roster. When a hospital does not have a specialist on call, when there is such specialist on the staff of the hospital, that hospital should have prearranged methodologies for transfer of such emergency patients to another hospital.

When the need for an emergency treatment exists, a hospital might state that a transfer is required for a "higher level of care." The use of this phrase is often over used, or poorly understood. There are specific reasons that a hospital and its medical staff might not be able to provide the level of emergency care for the patient who exhibits immediate life-threatening condition, but the reasons and the details of the nonavailability should be clearly stated in the hospital's published "schedule of benefits" and/or the particular equipment, services, or personnel at a particular time. As an example, there should not be a quality difference in the general, urologic, orthopedic, or pediatric surgery available between a level 3 and level 1 trauma center. Differences between these two types of trauma centers are more in the fields of neurosurgery and thoracic surgery procedures requiring cardiopulmonary bypass. One that is often cited as needing a higher level of care is in hand and finger replantation. The skill and equipment required for replantation involves detailed microvascular surgery. However, a minor hand laceration or abrasion does *not* require the higher skills of a "hand surgeon" to evaluate such injuries, nor is a hand surgeon required to examine and treat a simple fracture of the fingers or metacarpal bones.

The status of the patient's immediate life-threatening condition and the availability of hospital and personnel resources to treat that condition should be the major driving force to prompt discussions regarding transfer to another facility. When immediate life threatening conditions exist, the availability of funding sources or methods of payment for hospital and physician services should never be the motivating factor for either keeping or transferring a patient. Over time, the economic profile of the patients transferred for emergency conditions to a facility that provides a higher level of care should be virtually identical to the overall economic profile of *all* the patients cared for in that facility.

A "DUTY" TO EVALUATE AND "DUTY" TO TREAT

A hospital whose facilities are licensed to provide emergency medical evaluation and treatment has a duty to a patient who either arrives or is transferred to this facility to evaluate that patient for the presence of that emergency condition. The operational term "EVAULATE" is key, and the extent of that evaluation must be commensurate with the ability for the physical examination, laboratory, and imaging to make a determination as to the complexity of the emergency condition and to be able to communicate to the patient and/or to secondary physicians or facilities the details of the patient's condition. A decision as to whether an emergency facility and its staff, including the physicians, are able to render the requisite interventions is a function of many factors. These factors include: available resources, adequate numbers of personnel, capability and skills of the emergency personnel, infrastructure presence, and many others. Even in the absence of optimal resources, should there be no adverse outcome, the decisions made by the emergency caregivers are rarely questioned. Should the outcomes be adverse, the hospital, outside agencies, the family and the patient, and others often have questions regarding duty, judgment, technique, timing, and process, even if the skills and treatment exceeded a local and regional standard of care and all benchmarks were higher than the normal. Thus the duty and the decisions made often have ethical, economic, moral, medical, legal, and emotional overlay, impacting judgment. Regardless of the many decision nodes involved in an acute evaluation, decision, and treatment in a patient with an immediate life-threatening condition, the physician has a duty to adequately document all actions and the reasons behind the decisions.

Can a "Treatment" Be Less Than Complete Prior to Transfer?

The various regulations relating to patient evaluation and transfer, including those of EMTALA, focus on evaluation and making plans for therapy, with appropriate disclosure and communication. It is altogether appropriate for an integrated collaborative network of care to involve a number of levels of care with a network of communications and follow-up for quality assurance and performance improvement. The epitome of such an integrated collaborative network is the sequential care given to the current wounded warrior in a military conflict in Afghanistan or Iraq, who is treated at two to three levels of care in those countries, transferred to Landsthul Army Regional Hospital in Germany, and then later to a hospital in the Continental United States for continuing care. The Joint Trauma Treatment System with its Trauma Data Base, communicates to all members of the team at all levels ensuring that the care is informed and integrated. A "damage control" or "incomplete" treatment that is then continued in an agreed-upon plan of care is appropriate for any patient with any immediate life-threatening medical condition. This integrated collaborative network is totally outside the intent and specific details of the focus of the EMTALA and other regulatory documents.

Methods of Keeping out of EMTALA Trouble with Regulatory Agencies

Hospitals and physicians evaluating and caring for patients with emergent immediate life-threatening conditions have a strong motivation to stay within existing safety regulations, including EMTALA. A few simple principles will assure that concerns from outside regulatory agencies will be kept to a minimum and when they do occur, there will be ample information available to address the intent, policy, process, and outcome of the institution and its personnel that might come into question.

- Communicate—At all levels and in all hand offs, communicate honestly with all appropriate members of the treating team, especially the physicians caring for the patient at both sending and receiving hospitals

- Document—Record in the appropriate records, both the status of the patient, the evaluation and findings, the treatment rendered, and the communications among appropriate treating personnel. Document telephone and e-mail conversations.
- Transfer centers—Utilize at your facility a transfer center that assists in both communications and permanent recording of the exact nature of the care given, the higher level of care desired, and the specifics of the information known to those involved in any patient "hand-off."
- Do not overly advertise—For both hospitals and physicians, avoid hyperbole in describing the extent and focus of the emergency care that can be provided.
- Do your warranty work—Recognize that care rendered during emergency life-threatening conditions requires the same patient–physician–hospital relationship as during elective care, if not more stringent. Care that is given is subject to the same understanding for completing the work begun by a physician, unless there are understandings from a secondary facility and physician for continuing that care. Should a complication or an untoward event occur, full disclosure of such an event is the responsibility of those who were involved in the patients' care and arrangements are made, with the full understanding of the patient as to how and who will manage the continuing care. Such continuing care, with acceptance of such continuing responsibility, should be fully understood and agreed upon by all parties.
- EMTALA during disaster situations—The principles of EMTALA equally apply during times of disaster. During such times, it is important that rescue and EMS personnel, *not* over burden a major facility that routinely receives critically ill and injured patients, with persons only needing a shelter, but to preserve such facilities for that small percentage of surviving patients with immediate life-threatening conditions that can maximally benefit from the specially focused evaluation and care.
- Regional Review Process—Many hospital systems, as well as geographic areas, including multicounty emergency, trauma, acute care organizations (both governmental and volunteer) have successfully addressed a confidential regional peer review and performance improvement emergency medical process. Such regional reviews should markedly reduce a need for continually revising national regulatory processes.

Suggested Readings

Archdeacon MT, Simon PM, Wyrick JD. The influence of insurance status on the transfer of femoral fracture patients to a level-I trauma center. *J Bone Joint Surg Am.* 2007;89(12):2625-2631.

Biffl WL, Harrington DT, Majercik SD, et al. The evolution of trauma care at a level I trauma center. *J Am Coll Surg.* 2005;200(6):922-929.

Bitterman R. *Overview of Hospital and Physician Responsibilities Mandated by EMTALS. Forste. Providing Emergency Care under Federal Law: EMTALA.* Dallas, TX: The American College of Emergency Physicians; 2000:21.

Byrne RW, Bagan BT, Slavin KV, et al. Neurosurgical emergency transfers to academic centers in Cook County: a prospective multicenter study. *Neurosurgery.* 2008;62(3):709-716.

Dozier KC, Miranda MA Jr, Kwan RO, et al. Insurance coverage is associated with mortality after gunshot trauma. *J Am Coll Surg.* 2010;210(3):280-285.

Duchesne JC, Kyle A, Simmons J, et al. Impact of telemedicine upon rural trauma care. *J Trauma.* 2008;64(1):92-97.

Esposito TJ, Crandall M, Reed RL, et al. Socioeconomic factors, medicolegal issues, and trauma patient transfer trends: is there a connection? *J Trauma.* 2006;61(6):1380-1386.

Federal Register, Vol 68, No. 174, Part II. Medicare Program; Clarifying Policies Related to the Responsibilities of Medicare-Participating Hospitals in Treating Emergency Medical Conditions: Final Rule DHHS, CMS, September 9, 2003, 53263.

Goldfarb CA, Borrelli J Jr, Lu M, et al. A prospective evaluation of patients with isolated orthopedic injuries transferred to a level I trauma center. *J Orthop Trauma.* 2006;20(9):613-617.

Green A, Showstack J, Rennie D, et al. The relationship of insurance status, hospital ownership, and teaching status with interhospital transfers in California in 2000. *Acad Med.* 2005;80(8):774-779.

Harrington DT, Connolly M, Biffl WL, et al. Transfer times to definitive care facilities are too long: a consequence of an immature trauma system. *Ann Surg.* 2005;241(6):961-966.

Hedges JR, Newgard CD, Mullins RJ. Emergency Medical Treatment and Active Labor Act and trauma triage. *Prehosp Emerg Care.* 2006;10(3):332-339.

Koval KJ, Tingey CW, Spratt KF. Are patients being transferred to level-I trauma centers for reasons other than medical necessity? *J Bone Joint Surg Am.* 2006;88(10):2124-2132.

McConnell KJ, Newgard CD, Mullins RJ, et al. Mortality benefit of transfer to level I versus level II trauma centers for head-injured patients. *Health Serv Res.* 2005;40(2):435-457.

Melkun ET, Ford C, Brundage SI, et al. Demographic and financial analysis of EMTALA hand patient transfers. *Hand (N Y).* 20109;5:72-76.

Menchine MD, Baraff LJ. On-call specialists and higher level of care transfers in California emergency departments. *Acad Emerg Med.* 2008;15(4):329-336.

Nathens AB, Maier RV, Copass MK, et al. Payer status: the unspoken triage criterion. *J Trauma.* 2001;50(5):776-783.

O'Keeffe T, Shafi S, Sperry JL, et al. The implications of alcohol intoxication and the Uniform Policy Provision Law on trauma centers; a national trauma data bank analysis of minimally injured patients. *J Trauma.* 2009;66(2):495-498.

Parks J, Gentilello LM, Shafi S. Financial triage in transfer of trauma patients: a myth or a reality? *Am J Surg.* 2009;198(3):e35-e38.

Rhee PM, Grossman D, Rivara F, et al. The effect of payer status on utilization of hospital resources in trauma care. *Arch Surg.* 1997;132(4):399-404.

Richardson JD, Cross T, Lee D, et al. Impact of level III verification on trauma admissions and transfer: comparisons of two rural hospitals. *J Trauma.* 1997;42(3):498-502

Rosen H, Saleh F, Lipsitz SR, et al. Lack of insurance negatively affects trauma mortality in US children. *J Pediatr Surg.* 2009;44(10):1952-1957.

Roszak AR, Jensen FR, Wild RE, et al. Implications of the Emergency Medical Treatment and Labor Act (EMTALA) during public health emergencies and on alternate sites of care. *Disaster Med Public Health Prep.* 2009;3(suppl 2): S172-S175.

Southard P. 2003 "clarification" of controversial EMTALA requirement for 24/7 coverage of emergency departments by on-call specialists, significant impact on trauma centers. *J Emerg Nurs.* 2004;30(6):582-583.

Southard PA, Hedges JR, Hunter JG, et al. Impact of a transfer center on interhospital referrals and transfers to a tertiary care center. *Acad Emerg Med.* 2005;12(7):653-657.

Spain DA, Bellino M, Kopelman A, et al. Requests for 692 transfers to an academic level I trauma center: implications of the emergency medical treatment and active labor act. *J Trauma.* 2007;62(1):63-67.

Taheri PA, Butz DA, Greenfield LJ. Paying a premium: how patient complexity affects costs and profit margins. *Ann Surg.* 1999;229(6):807-811.

Testa PA, Gang M. Triage, EMTALA, consultations, and prehospital medical control. *Emerg Med Clin North Am.* 2009;27(4):627-640.

Young JS, Cephas GA, Blow O. Outcome and cost of trauma among the elderly: a real-life model of a single-payer reimbursement system. *J Trauma.* 1998;45(4):800-804.

CHAPTER 60 ■ INFORMED SURGICAL CONSENT

DAVID G. JACOBS

"Patients should understand the indications for the operation, the risk involved, and the result that it is hoped to attain"

—ACS Statements on Principles of the College[1]

A chapter devoted to the topic of informed consent may, at first glance, seem to be out of place in a textbook of acute care surgery. The deliberate, sometimes painstaking, process of informing and getting the consent of patients for surgical procedures hardly seems compatible with the fast-paced decision making required of both the surgeon and the patient when acute conditions arise. Yet, given the higher likelihood of adverse outcomes (death, complications, poor quality of life, etc.) in patients undergoing acute surgical procedures, the importance of the physician and the patient being "on the same page" with respect to the anticipated risks, benefits, and outcome of the planned operative procedure cannot be overestimated. Thus, it behooves all acute care surgeons to have some familiarity with the informed consent process under both elective and nonelective situations. Furthermore, since informed consent regulations may vary from hospital to hospital, and from state to state, some familiarity with these local requirements is desirable as well.

There are perhaps several reasons why the informed consent process might be undervalued by the acute care surgeon:

- Surgeon too busy with multiple simultaneous responsibilities (acute care surgery, trauma, surgical critical care)
- Surgeon's desire to get the patient to the operating room quickly
- Surgeon's inability to adequately inform the patient regarding operative procedure since actual operative findings would be unknown to the surgeon at the time of consent
- Urgent/emergent situation precludes development of strong surgeon–patient relationship
- Surgeon under the mistaken belief that informed consent is unnecessary for acute surgical procedures
- Surgeon unsure about validity of consent for acute surgical procedures due to patient factors such as pain, sedation from medications, and anxiety
- Difficulties establishing relationship with acute surgical patients due to language or cultural barriers

This chapter will briefly review the foundation, the principles, and the practice of informed consent as it applies to the *elective* surgery arena, and will then highlight some important aspects of the consent process that are unique to the *nonelective* surgical environment. In so doing, some of the above-listed obstacles to achieving true informed consent in acute care surgical patients will be addressed, and some recommendations for perhaps improving the currently existing consent process will be offered.

INFORMED CONSENT IN ELECTIVE SURGICAL PRACTICE

Foundation of Informed Consent

A comprehensive review of the informed consent process is beyond the scope of this chapter, but the interested reader is referred to several excellent recent reviews on the topic.[2-7] However, some basic understanding of the history, as well as the components of the process, is necessary in order to place "emergent" informed consent into proper perspective. To begin with, it must be emphasized that informed consent is much more than obtaining a patient's signature on a consent form. True informed consent is a process wherein the patient is first *informed* by the surgeon of the risks, benefits, and intended outcomes of the proposed surgical procedure, followed by the patient's *consent* to undergo the procedure. Note here that it is the responsibility of the surgeon performing the procedure to both (1) inform the patient and (2) obtain the patient's consent, and that these responsibilities should not be abdicated to other members of the surgical team. Constraints of time and place occasionally preclude the surgeon from witnessing the patient's (or patient's surrogate) written signature on the consent form, especially when the procedure is being done on an emergent or urgent basis. Under these unique circumstances, it is permissible for a resident physician or nurse to obtain the patient's signature on the consent form, as the form itself is simply a legal document that attests to the fact that the informed consent process has been carried out by the surgeon. Indeed, signing, or even use of, the consent document is not a mandatory feature of the informed consent process from an ethical standpoint, although it may well be a legal requirement of a particular institution or state. All surgeons should therefore familiarize themselves with the requirements of the institutions and states within which they work. The content and structure of consent forms is discussed further elsewhere in this chapter.

Informed consent therefore really represents two separate processes and two separate tasks for the surgeon—inform and consent. In the United States, these two processes, though now inextricably linked, actually developed sequentially, separated by more than 40 years. The concept of *simple consent* was established first in 1914 in the case of *Schloendorff v. The Society of New York Hospital.*[8] In this case, consent had been obtained from the patient for an examination under ether anesthesia. However, while the patient was under anesthesia, the surgeon, without the patient's explicit consent, removed an abdominal tumor. Postoperatively the patient developed gangrene of the hand, which she claimed directly resulted from resection of the abdominal mass. The court ruled in favor of the patient, stating "*every human being of adult years and sound mind has a right to determine what shall be done with his body; and a surgeon who performs an operation without his patient's consent, commits an assault for which he is liable in damages.*"[7] Thus the concept of patient autonomy, a fundamental ethical principle and a fundamental underpinning of informed consent, was upheld by the court. No longer could surgeons unilaterally decide (and carry out) what they felt was in their patient's best interest—the patient's consent was first required. However, no further stipulations were made as to the quality of that consent until 1957, when, in *Salgo v. Leland Stanford Jr. University Board of Trustees*, the courts imposed a further duty on the surgeon to provide the patient with the information necessary to make an "intelligent" consent decision.[9] The patient in this case became paraplegic following performance, by his surgeon, of a translumbar aortogram, which involved injection of sodium urokon. This particular complication was a known, but quite rare, risk associated with this agent, one that Mr. Salgo's surgeon had not discussed with him prior to performing the aortogram. Although the case was ultimately decided in favor of the physician, the court's opinion made it quite clear that the physician had a responsibility to inform the patient as part of the consent process—"*a physician violates his duty to his patient...if he withholds any facts which are necessary to form the basis of an intelligent consent by the patient to the proposed treatment.*" Although this new requirement of the physician to provide *any* necessary facts may seem vague or overly onerous, the same opinion also provided the physician with some room for judgment in informed consent discussions—"*In discussing the element of risk a certain amount of discretion must be employed consistent with the full disclosure of facts necessary to an informed consent.*"[4] The opinion in the *Salgo* case appears to represent the first documented use of the phrase "informed consent" and clearly ushered in a new era of physician responsibility in obtaining consent for medical treatments. Decades following *Salgo*, there is still not universal agreement as to how much actual discretion a physician must employ in informed consent discussions. This aspect of the informed consent discussion will be discussed in greater detail below.

Principles of Informed Consent

The process of informed consent requires several fundamental assumptions ([10]):

- The physician has provided adequate information with which to make a decision (adequate physician disclosure)
- The patient is competent to make a decision (patient competence)
- The patient indicates full understanding of the situation and the information imparted to him by the physician (patient understanding)
- The patient voluntarily consents to the proposed intervention (absence of undue influence)

Adequate Physician Disclosure. What constitutes adequate disclosure by the consenting physician? As discussed above, the *Salgo* ruling, which established the concept of informed consent more than 50 years ago, required physicians to provide "*any facts... necessary* <for an> *intelligent consent,*" but also allowed for some physician discretion in these discussions. In response to the ambiguity of the *Salgo* decision, three ethical standards have evolved over the years [2,11]

- *The Professional Standard* (also called the "Reasonable Physician Standard" or the "Professional Community Standard")—Requires the physician to disclose what a reasonably prudent physician with the same background, training, and experience, and practicing in the same community, would disclose to a patient in the same or similar situation
- The Materiality Standard (also called the "Reasonable Patient Standard" or the "Prudent Patient Standard"—Requires the physician to disclose what a reasonable patient in the same or similar situation would need to know in order to make an appropriate decision.
- The Subjective Patient Standard—Requires the physician to disclose what a particular patient, in his or her own unique set of circumstances and conditions, would need to know in order to make an appropriate decision.

From an *ethical* perspective, none of these standards is ideal. The Professional Standard has been criticized as being too physician-centered, in that it preferentially values what the physician, not the patient, thinks is important. The Materiality Standard fails to define what a "reasonable" patient is, and the Subjective Standard perhaps makes unreasonable demands of the physician to discern the particular values, interests, and life circumstances of every patient who needs informed consent. From a *legal* perspective, most states have included language in their informed consent statutes that define which of the three standards described above is recognized in that particular state. The Encyclopedia of Everyday Law, available online, nicely summarizes these requirements for many of the 50 states, and the reader is advised to familiarize himself or herself with the standard currently being used in the particular state in which he or she practices.[11]

Although states may vary in the type of informed consent standard to which they hold physicians who practice within their borders, there does seem to be general consensus as to the basic elements of a proper informed consent discussion. In fact, several professional health care organizations have adopted formal informed consent standards for their respective organizations. The American College of Surgeons for example, in its Statement on Principles, outlines four specific items that should be included in informed consent discussions. These are

- The nature of the illness and the natural consequences of no treatment
- The nature of the proposed operation, including the estimated risks of mortality and morbidity
- The more common known complications, which should be described and discussed
- Alternative forms of treatment, including nonoperative techniques

The Joint Commission on Accreditation of Healthcare Organizations and the American Medical Association have established similar guidelines (Table 60.1). Finally, it is important to note that the health care provider is not obliged to disclose risks that are commonly understood, obvious, or already known to the patient.[12]

Patient Competence. In actuality, incompetence is a legal condition that can only be determined by the courts. Persons judged by the courts to be incompetent, by definition, are precluded from providing informed consent for themselves or for others. Similarly, minors, with very few exceptions, are legally prohibited from providing informed consent, although ethically, they should be included in informed consent discussions when they possess the maturity to do so.[10] Beyond legal considerations, and adult (nonminor) status, patients must possess adequate *capacity* for medical decision making. Capacity refers to the ability of the patient to process the information received and communicate a meaningful response, and is decision specific, so that a given patient may demonstrate capacity for medical decision making for one aspect of his or her care, yet lack decision-making capacity in other medically related areas.[6] Although there is no legal requirement for such, psychiatric consultation is frequently recommended when the loss of decision-making capacity in a given patient is suspected. However, the treating physician may actually be in the best position to assess capacity under these circumstances, since this physician likely has a better understanding of the patient's medical condition, as well as the risks, benefits, and alternatives to the proposed intervention, and is also in the best position to judge whether the patient's response to the circumstances is appropriate. Psychiatrists, however, may be helpful in working with the patient to restore capacity for medical decision making, although the time course of this restoration process may not be conducive to decision making in situations of acute surgical illness. In situations where the patient's decision-making capacity is confirmed to be lacking, or when patients have been deemed incompetent (including minors), and informed consent for a medical intervention is required, consent must be sought from the patient's surrogate. Most states have legislation that establishes the hierarchy of persons acting as a patient surrogate. Typically, a court-appointed guardian

TABLE 60.1

ELEMENTS OF INFORMED CONSENT

The Joint Commission
1. The nature of the proposed care, treatment, services, medications, interventions, or procedures
2. Potential benefits, risks, or side effects, including potential problems related to recuperation
3. The likelihood of achieving care, treatment, and service goals
4. Reasonable alternatives to the proposed case, treatment, and service goals
5. The relevant risks, benefits, and side effects related to alternatives, including the possible results of not receiving care, treatment, and services
6. When indicated, any limitations on the confidentiality of information learned from or about the patient
American College of Surgeons
1. The nature of the illness and the natural consequences of no treatment
2. The nature of the proposed operation, including the estimated risks of mortality and morbidity
3. The more common known complications, which should be described and discussed: the patient should understand the risks, as well as the benefits of the proposed operation; the discussion should include a description of what to expect during the hospitalization and posthospital convalescence
4. Alternative forms of treatment, including nonoperative techniques
American Medical Association
1. The patient's diagnosis, if known
2. The nature and purpose of a proposed treatment or procedure
3. The risks and benefits of a proposed treatment or procedure
4. Alternatives (regardless of their cost or the extent to which the treatment options are covered by health insurance)
5. The risks and benefits of the alternative treatment or procedure
6. The risks and benefits of not receiving or undergoing a treatment or procedure

From Raper SE, Sarwer DB. Informed consent issues in the conduct of bariatric surgery. *Surg Obes Relat Dis.* 2008;4(1):60–68.

heads the list, followed by a health care power of attorney. In the absence of either of these two individuals, consent would then need to be sought from spouses, adult children, parents, siblings, etc., although the precise order of these individuals in the hierarchy does vary from state to state. Once again, it is a good idea to become familiar with the regulations in force in the state in which one practices. This information can be accessed at http://new.abanet.org/aging/PublicDocuments/famcon_2009.pdf.[13]

As mentioned above, some exceptions to the "incompetent minor rule" do exist that allow for informed consent to be obtained from minors. Specifically, emancipated minors are legally permitted to provide informed consent for themselves. An emancipated minor is one who has assumed the responsibilities of adulthood, usually by willingly living apart from one's parents and by managing one's own financial affairs. Also included within this emancipated minor category are married minors and minors who are members of the armed services of the United States. These individuals are permitted to participate in the informed consent process as well. Also, minors who are parents are permitted to provide informed signature for their children. A final exception, the "mature minor doctrine" can be invoked, enabling a physician to act on the signature of a minor when parental signature cannot be obtained. Under these circumstances, the minor must be at least 15 years old, must appear capable of fully understanding the medical situation, must have received full disclosure of risks, and must grant consent to treatment.[6,14]

Patient Understanding. Even in situations where the patient's decision-making capacity is not in question, the patient may still not fully comprehend the nature of the procedure or treatment for which his/her consent is being sought. In addition to providing full disclosure, the surgeon also must ascertain whether the patient has an adequate understanding of the intervention to which he or she is being asked to consent. Several distinct thought processes have been identified in patients consenting to surgery that may interfere with their complete understanding of what their surgeons are telling them.[3] Some examples of these include

- A profound belief that surgery will result in cure
- Unrealistic expectations of the surgeon (or the institution) brought about via reputation, or by virtue of being a superspecialist (or a superspecialty hospital)
- Enhancement of physician trust as a result of being referred by family, friends, or other physicians
- Belief in medical expertise as opposed to medical information
- Resignation on the part of the patient to the risks of medical treatment
- Desire on the part of the patient to abrogate decision making to the surgeon ("do whatever you think is best, doc...")

Each of these attitudes that patients may bring with them to informed consent discussions may prevent the patient from fully engaging in, and thus fully understanding, even the most well-intentioned discussion of risks, benefits, and alternatives. Physicians need to be aware of these potential pitfalls and take the steps necessary to ensure their patient understands the information they have just imparted to them. This can be done by analyzing the types of questions being asked them by the patient, but also by asking probative questions of the patient as a means of identifying areas of incomplete comprehension. It is often helpful for the surgeon to ask patients to reiterate in their own words their understanding of the rationale, risks, and benefits of the procedure.

Absence of Undue Influence. Finally, it is also the responsibility of the surgeon to ensure that the consent obtained from the patient is voluntary and represents what the patient believes is in his or her best interest. Many external influences may exert themselves in the setting of surgical illness, particularly so under the conditions of acute surgical illness. Pain, fear, and anxiety can be powerful motivators of behavior and may propel patients to make decisions that they might not make under less stressful conditions. Steps should be taken to remove as many of these emotional and physiologic barriers to true informed consent as possible, recognizing that the pharmacologic treatment of pain and anxiety may also potentially impair the patient's capacity for decision making.[6] In addition to these external influences, family and friends may occasionally, and possibly quite unintentionally, exert unwanted influence over the consent process. Obvious examples of this can be seen in patients contemplating cosmetic or even bariatric surgery, where perhaps the patient may be considering surgery not for his or her own benefit, but rather to please others.[7] Should the surgeon suspect that the patient is experiencing unwanted external influences such as these, a private discussion with the patient (and perhaps a separate private discussion with the "unwanted influences") provides the best opportunity to understand and implement the plan of action that maximizes the best interests of the patient.[2] Recognize, too, that the surgeon may, intentionally or otherwise, act as a coercive force when it comes to informed consent. Many patients are intimidated by the stereotypical strong-willed surgeon, or by the reputation that precedes even the first encounter with a surgeon. Some surgeons may actually express displeasure or dismay when a patient questions or declines the operative plan, thereby unwittingly contributing to the coercive atmosphere, and a less than informed consent situation. A more subtle form of surgeon coercion occurs when the surgeon, uninvited, offers an opinion as to the course of action the patient should choose, and in so doing, makes it more difficult for the patient to choose an alternate path. In general, such offerings should be avoided by the surgeon unless expressly invited by the patient, and even then, the surgeon must be sure to emphasize that a different course of action chosen by the patient will be respected and honored. Another well-recognized form of surgeon coercion is "framing," a process wherein the surgeon's word choices can exert unintended influences on the patient's decision making.[2,3] These word choices, intentionally or otherwise, either overemphasize the benefits (e.g., "you'll feel like a new man") or minimize the risks (e.g., "bleeding is *never* a problem with this type of surgery") of the proposed intervention, and may lead to unrealistic expectations on the part of the patient. Exaggerating the gravity of the patient's situation, referred to as "crepe hanging," is a particularly common and unethical form of framing that preoperatively sets falsely low expectations for the postoperative outcome in order to protect the reputation of the surgeon. If the postoperative outcome turns out to be good, the patient's appreciation of, and gratitude toward, the surgeon is intensified, whereas, in the unlikely event of a bad postoperative outcome, the surgeon escapes "blame," since a poor outcome has already been predicted. These subtle and not-so-subtle forms of framing are incompatible with the ethical principles of autonomy and beneficence that underlie informed consent, and they should be scrupulously avoided. One additional common practice that may unintentionally interfere with the goal of obtaining the patient's *voluntary* consent is that of waiting until the day of surgery to obtain consent. A consent discussion that occurs in the preoperative holding area, without adequate time for a detailed explanation of the risks, benefits, and alternatives, without adequate time for questions, without adequate time to read the informed consent document, and all perhaps performed after the patient has been administered a preoperative sedative can hardly be considered "informed." In addition, the patient's awareness that the operating room has been reserved, that the surgeon has blocked out the time on his or her operating schedule, and that family or friends have taken time off from work to accompany the patient, are all potentially coercive forces that may, perhaps subconsciously, influence a patient to sign a consent document for a procedure to which he is not entirely committed to undergoing. Whenever possible, the informed consent process should be initiated well in advance of the intended procedure, with the patient being given ample time to consider, or even change, their decision. Unfortunately, this luxury of time, which works well for the informed consent process in elective surgery, is not feasible for patients needing to undergo urgent or emergent surgical procedures.

Exceptions to Informed Consent

"If a surgeon is confronted with an emergency which endangers the life and health of the patient, it is his duty to do that which the occasion demands within the usual and customary practice among physicians and surgeons in the same or similar localities, without the consent of the patient."[15]

Under some conditions, informed consent may be neither possible nor necessary, and some of these conditions are particularly germane to patients with acute surgical conditions. Occasionally, treatment of a patient without his or her consent can be mandated by law if there is a perceived risk to public health and safety. However, most exceptions to informed consent benefit the patient directly by ensuring timely access to needed medical care for that individual patient. Informed consent can legitimately be waived under the following circumstances[11,12,16]:

- Medical emergencies
- Unanticipated conditions during surgery
- Patient waiver of consent
- The therapeutic privilege

Medical Emergencies. Medical emergencies constitute the largest category of exceptions to the informed consent requirement, but this well-recognized exception should not be invoked indiscriminately simply because the patient requires "acute" surgical intervention.[16] The guiding principle here is whether delay in treatment required to obtain consent would result in harm to the patient. Harm in this context is not necessarily limited to loss of life or limb, but refers to any major adverse outcome that may occur as a result of a delay in treatment. In general, the fact that the patient has presented to the health care facility is taken as evidence of presumed consent to emergency treatment. Frequently, these patients display impaired decision-making capacity due to alterations in mental status brought on by hemodynamic instability, sepsis, or direct Central Nervous System (CNS) insult or injury. Resuscitation, including intubation and mechanical ventilation, can, and should, be undertaken immediately in this patient population without concern for obtaining informed consent based upon the fact that these patients are inherently incompetent, and based upon the assumption that most reasonable individuals under the same circumstances would desire treatment. Of course, when an appropriate patient surrogate is identified, informed consent should be obtained for all subsequent procedures. This approach can also be extended to the perhaps less straightforward situation of the emergency surgery patient with impaired decision-making capacity due to intoxication, but documentation of the patient's lack of capacity is critical if suspension of the patient's informed consent rights is to be upheld. This principle is illustrated in *Miller v Rhode Island Hospital*, where an intoxicated trauma patient was subjected to a diagnostic peritoneal lavage procedure against his will, and sued the hospital for battery. In siding with the defendants, the court held that the determination of whether a patient's intoxication would render the patient incapable of giving informed consent would depend upon the circumstances, and that medical competency (whether the patient was able to reasonably understand the medical condition, and the risks and benefits of, and alternatives to, the proposed procedure) was the relevant standard for physicians to judge conscious patients in these circumstances.[17] Thus, in order for a physician to deny a patient his or her informed consent rights on the basis of intoxication, the physician must first be absolutely convinced that intoxication has rendered the patient medically incompetent, since this is the standard required by the courts to successfully defend a charge of battery. One additional facet of the emergency exemption to informed consent that deserves mention is the issue of consent for blood transfusion. Here again, the issue of medical competency comes into play, since transfusing a medically competent patient against his or her will would clearly constitute battery. Patients deemed medically incompetent, whether due to injury, illness, or intoxication, can be transfused without their consent, even against the objections of the patient or patient's family under the compelling state interest standard.[18] The emergency exemption to informed consent also extends to the "incompetent" minor, such that the informed consent requirement can be waived when an emergency exists and immediate injury or death could result from the delay associated with attempting to obtain parental consent.[16] Emergent blood transfusion, without consent, for a minor patient has generally been upheld by the courts, even when the transfusion has been adamantly refused by the parents and the patient, again based upon the compelling state interest in preserving the life of a child. As stated in *Novak v Cobb County-Kennestone Hospital Authority*, "not even a parent has unbridled discretion to exercise their religious beliefs when the state's interest in preserving the health of the children within its borders weighs in the balance."[19] In all circumstances where the emergency exception is invoked, it is prudent to document in the patient record the nature of the emergency, and the rationale for proceeding without informed consent. If possible, a corroborating statement in the patient record from a second health care provider is also desirable.[14]

Unanticipated Conditions During Surgery. The courts have generally looked favorably on surgeons who have performed, on patients under general anesthesia, procedures for which they did not have explicit informed consent as long as (1) the procedure appeared to be in the patient's best interests and (2) there was not adequate opportunity for the surgeon to obtain consent. This is referred to as the "extension doctrine," and it assumes that the surgeon is using reasonable judgment. In order to meet the criteria for the extension doctrine, the condition must be one that was unforeseen, and the patient must not have expressly refused such an intervention.[12] These circumstances present themselves relatively frequently to the acute care surgeon when undertaking laparotomy for "peritonitis" of unknown origin. In *Barnett v Bacharach*, a patient who was thought to have an ectopic pregnancy consented only for the removal of the ectopic pregnancy itself. At laparotomy, however, the patient was found to have acute appendicitis and an appendectomy was performed. Following an uneventful recovery, the patient refused to pay for the surgical services provided because informed consent was not first obtained and thus the procedure was unauthorized. At trial, the court found that the surgeon acted properly because of the seriousness of the patient's condition.[20] However, in *Tabor v Scobee*, the court found that the surgeon had acted improperly when he removed the infected fallopian tubes from a patient who had given informed consent only for an appendectomy. Here the surgeon argued that serious harm or death could have resulted had the procedure been delayed for weeks or months, but this time frame did not fulfill the court's definition of a condition severe enough to warrant denial of the patient's informed consent rights.[21] Perhaps the patient's resulting sterility also played a role in the court's decision.

Patient Waiver of Consent. Occasionally, a patient will relinquish his or her right to informed consent by expressly waiving this right and specifically directing the physician to do what the physician thinks is in the patient's best interest. This is a relatively unusual occurrence in this day and age, and this acquiescence on the part of the patient should be clearly documented by the surgeon in the patient record.

The Therapeutic Privilege. By law, a physician has no obligation to provide informed consent if he or she believes that the patients' emotional and physical condition could be adversely affected by full disclosure of the treatment risks.[22] This is referred to as the therapeutic privilege and, although a legitimate exception, must be invoked with great caution, and with abundant physician documentation in the patient record.

Problems with Informed Consent

Even in elective surgery situations, and even with the most well-intentioned physician, the informed consent process is far from perfect. Patients seem to comprehend little about what has been explained to them, and what little they understand, they fail to retain for any substantial period of time. Falgas recently conducted a review of 23 articles that assessed the quality of the informed consent process across a variety of surgical specialties. Several different consent discussion formats were represented in these 23 articles, including verbal explanations alone, written materials alone, use of audiovisual media, and various combinations of these formats. Patient understanding was judged as either adequate (more than 80% of the participants in the study had a level of understanding graded in the highest classification category), moderate (50%–80% of the participants in the study had a level of understanding graded in the highest classification category) or inadequate (<50% of the participants in the study had a level of understanding graded in the highest classification category). Based upon these definitions, "adequate" overall understanding of the information provided was demonstrated in only 29% of the patients examined, while only 36% of the patients demonstrated "adequate" understanding of the risks associated with surgery (Table 60.2). Although one may quibble with the definitions used in this review, it is nevertheless quite clear that, regardless of how the informed consent discussion is carried out (verbal, written, with or without audiovisuals), a substantial gap exists between the information that surgeons think they transmit to their patients, and the information that patients actually understand and retain.[23]

The retention of informed consent information over time is undoubtedly less important than the information comprehension issue discussed above, but considering that many patients will go through the informed consent process in the outpatient setting days to weeks before the surgery is actually undertaken, patients may well require reeducation when they re-present for their surgical procedure. Furthermore, the retention issue can become quite problematic should accusations of inadequate disclosure be brought against the physician and the patient be required to recall specifically what he or she was or was not told in advance about the surgical procedure in question. Those items that the patient believes were not properly disclosed by the surgeon may simply have been forgotten by the patient, emphasizing the need for the physician to maintain an accurate accounting of all of the information that was exchanged as part of the consent process. Hutson and Blaha described 38 orthopedic patients who were not allowed to sign their operative consent forms until they could correctly recall all items on a questionnaire. However, 6 months after the operation, only 16% of the risks could be recalled.[24] Similar results were noted by Lavelle-Jones in general surgery patients.[25] Some have advocated the provision of written materials as a way of improving information retention, but Lavelle-Jones found that giving the patient an operation information card at the time of consent did nothing to improve long-term recall.

TABLE 60.2

SYNTHESIS OF DATA FROM DIFFERENT STUDIES REGARDING THE EVALUATION OF THE VARIOUS COMPONENTS OF THE INFORMED CONSENT PROCESS FOR SURGERY OR PARTICIPATION IN CLINICAL TRIALS

COMPONENTS OF THE INFORMED CONSENT PROCESS	STUDIES SHOWING DIFFERENT LEVELS OF UNDERSTANDING OR SATISFACTION FOR THE COMPONENTS OF INFORMED CONSENT		
	ADEQUATE (%)	MODERATE (%)	INADEQUATE (%)
Evaluation of the amount of provided information	7/12 (58)	3/12 (25)	2/12 (17)
Understanding of given information	6/21 (29)	9/21 (43)	6/21 (29)
Understanding the risks of operation	5/14 (36)	5/14 (36)	4/14 (29)
Understanding the benefits of operation	2/6 (33)	3/6 (50)	1/6 (17)

From Falagas ME, Korbila IP, Giannopoulou KP, Kondilis BK, Peppas G. Informed consent: how much and what do patients understand? *Am J Surg*. 2009;198(3):420–435.

In hopes of improving the informed consent process in their neurosurgical practice, Konndziolka developed a procedure-based consent form to facilitate patient discussion. The consent form listed specific diagnoses, procedures, alternatives, and risk, and each point discussed was checked off by the surgeon. Immediate recall of information regarding the diagnosis and planned procedure was 100%, and was 98.1% for information regarding alternative treatments, and 97.4% for information regarding risks. More impressively, recall at a mean interval of 4.5 months was still 100% for the diagnosis and procedure and was 92.4% and 91.7% for alternatives and risks, respectively.[26] In addition to improved patient recall, the new consent form provided much better documentation of the consent process and hence, better legal protection for the physicians against future claims by patients of inadequate disclosure. Since this study did not include a control group, it is not possible to attribute the authors' success to the new consent form itself, since there are likely many factors that influence patient comprehension in the context of informed consent. Fink, in a multi-institutional study of patients undergoing total hip arthroplasty, carotid endarterectomy, laparoscopic cholecystectomy, or radical prostatectomy, examined 14 variables in an attempt to define independent factors associated with improved patient understanding during the informed consent process. Patients in this study were randomized to one of two consent formats—a standard informed consent discussion or standard discussion supplemented by the "repeat back" technique, wherein the patient, after being appropriately informed about the intended procedure, is asked to describe, in his or her own words, the diagnosis, procedure, anatomic location, the risks, the benefits, and the alternatives to the proposed procedure. Factors independently associated with comprehension in this study included race, ethnicity, education, age, operation type, use of the repeat back technique, and total consent time. Total consent time was the strongest predictor of patient comprehension, with maximal comprehension being achieved when informed consent took between 15 and 30 minutes.[27] Perhaps taking more time for our informed consent discussions is the key to achieving better comprehension in surgical patients, at least in the elective surgery setting. Patients requiring more urgent surgical procedures may not be able to afford this luxury of time, and perhaps other approaches are required in this patient population. This is discussed further below.

Another problematic area in surgical informed consent is determining just how much information a given patient *wants* to know. Earlier in this chapter, we alluded to those elements that a physician should (ethically), and must (legally) disclose to the patient as part of the informed consent process, but do these requirements in any way reflect what patients really want to get out of informed consent discussions? Although very little research has been done in this area, it appears, not surprisingly, that patients are quite heterogeneous when it comes to how much information they want their physicians to divulge in informed consent discussions. Losanoff conducted a study of 98 nonhernia patients from their outpatient clinic, asking them to imagine themselves as patients requiring inguinal hernia repair. They were asked to indicate their level of interest in being informed about several different aspects of hernia surgery, including hernia natural history, pathology, management, complications, and postoperative recovery (Table 60.3) (Although the overall level of interest in this group of patients was fairly high (interest score of 5.5 out of possible 7), there

TABLE 60.3

HERNIA INFORMATION SHEET ("WOULD YOU LIKE TO KNOW ABOUT...")

Information About the Risks for Hernia Formation

- Personal risk factors
- Asymptomatic hernias
- Long-term risk of hernia
- Predisposition to hernias
- Characteristics of hernia

Types of hernias

- Demographics of hernia distribution
- Annual number of hernias repaired in the United States
- Acquired causes of hernia
- Congenital hernias
- Weakness of the abdominal muscles in patients with hernia
- Possible hernia sites

TABLE 60.3

HERNIA INFORMATION SHEET ("WOULD YOU LIKE TO KNOW ABOUT...") (*Continued*)

Management of Hernia
- Not having the surgery (watchful waiting)
- Possibility of having a "difficult" operation
- Possibility of not undergoing the surgery for medical reasons
- Growth of the hernia in case of watchful waiting
- Possibility of having a strangulation
- Signs and symptoms of strangulation
- Chance for recurrence of the hernia

Hernia Operations
- Hernia surgery in general
- Hospital trajectory during the day of surgery
- Being disrobed and with clipped hairs for the surgery
- Preoperative scrubbing
- Possible urinary catheterization
- Number of incisions
- Types of surgical repair
- Technical details of accessing the site of the hernia
- Prior experience of the surgeon

Anesthesia For Hernia Surgery
- Prior experience of the anesthesiologist
- Type of anesthesia
- Aftermath of anesthesia

Who's Who?
- Who will be around you during the day of surgery?
- Who is going to operate on you?
- Who is going to give you the anesthesia?
- Who are the nurses in the operating room?
- Who are the surgical technicians in the operating room?
- Whether an anesthesiologist or a nurse anesthetist will be providing the anesthesia

Possible Complications
- Specific complications depending on the type of procedure
- Rate of your doctor's intra- or postoperative complications
- Nonsurgical complications related to your procedure
- Complications of anesthesia
- Possible delayed effect of anesthesia
- Postoperative bleeding
- Postoperative infection
- Postoperative retention of urine
- Postoperative intestinal obstruction

Postoperative Management
- Intravenous line for medication
- Asking the nurses for pain medication
- Scarring or tissue loss after surgery
- Ipsilateral postoperative numbness
- Chronic inguinal neuralgia
- Decreased sexual function
- Hernia recurrence

Long-Term Outcome of Laparoscopic *Vs. Open Repair*

From Losanoff JE, Litwinczuk KM, Ranella MJ, et al. Elective inguinal hernia repair: a unified informed consent, or who wants to know what? *Am Surg.* 2009;75(4):29–300.

was substantial variability within the group (range 1.5–7). Patients seemed most interested in details about the operation itself, and about the postoperative period, and least interested in details about hernias in general, and in the identities of the members of the operating team.[28] This latter finding is interesting in light of a recent government recommendation that patients be specifically informed if surgical trainees (residents, students) will be involved in their operations (see following paragraph). The authors also analyzed patient demographics to identify any patterns that might help to predict which patient types might desire more or less preoperative information. Neither patient age or race was predictive of interest in obtaining more information, whereas an advanced level of education (beyond high school) was positively correlated with a desire for more information regarding the technical aspects of the operation, details of anesthetic management, and the number and type of staff present in the operating room. Similar findings were noted in a study by Keulers et al. who, in addition to surveying patients about the issues in which they were most interested in being educated on, also surveyed 24 surgeons to determine what information they thought their patients would be interested in receiving. Physicians not only consistently underestimated their patients' desire for receiving extensive information but also were wrong about the types of information their patients wanted. Patients were much more interested in receiving information about the preoperative period, anesthesia, the operation itself, and the postoperative period, including postdischarge care, than they were about the disease process itself, its cause, and its prognosis. Complexity of the procedure had no impact on the amount or types of information the patients were interested in receiving.[29] These findings underscore the need for surgeons to ensure that the consent process is a true dialogue, where the patient's desire for information is heard and met.

A final problem with the informed consent process is the consent form itself. As discussed above, there is no legal requirement for a patient to sign a consent document prior to undergoing a surgical procedure. The purpose of the form is to simply provide documentation that the informed consent process has been carried out appropriately, although even a perfectly executed consent document may not necessarily provide legal protection to the physician should the patient bring suit on the grounds of inadequate disclosure. Consent forms, however, have become synonymous with the consent process itself, and paradoxically, neither physician nor patient may actually know what is contained within the form that both parties must ultimately sign. Until recently, there was considerable latitude in the content of informed consent forms for surgery, resulting in widely disparate amounts of information being transmitted, captured, and documented. Issa reviewed 204 consent forms for 2 urologic procedures (transurethral resection of the prostate, radical prostatectomy) carried out over a 6-year period of time at the Atlanta VA Medical Center. Information on the purpose and benefits of treatment was missing in 4.4% of forms, and deficient in 22.6%. Operative risks were poorly documented as well; risk of death was documented only 62% of the time, while bleeding, infection, and deep venous thrombosis were documented in only 31%, 31%, and 1% of forms, respectively. No documentation was present on any of the forms regarding the risk of pulmonary embolus. Alternative treatment options were missing in 49% of forms and significantly deficient in the remaining 51%.[30] This study exposes some very serious flaws in the documentation phase of the informed consent process, but does not identify the source of the problem. Are the physicians simply failing to fill in completely a perfectly adequate consent form, or is the consent form itself inadequate? The answer is probably both. Bottrell graded 540 different consent forms from 157 hospitals nationwide to determine whether the forms incorporated the four basic elements of informed consent (nature of the procedure, risks, benefits, and alternatives). Only 26% of forms included all four basic elements, 35% contained three elements, 23% included two elements, 14% contained only one element, and 2% of forms included none of the four elements. Most documents, it appeared, existed to authorize treatment or to protect hospitals and caregivers from liability, as opposed to providing the patient with information that might be useful in decision making.[31] It is clear that a sizeable gap exists between the content of a good informed consent discussion and the content of most informed consent documents currently in use. Perhaps due to this fact, CMS (Centers for Medicare and Medicaid Services), in 2007, issued revised guidelines for informed consent documents.[32] Some of the more notable directives contained within these revisions include the following:

- A properly executed informed consent form should reflect the patient consent process.
- Except as specified for emergency situations in the hospital's informed consent policies, all inpatient and outpatient medical records must contain a properly executed informed consent form prior to conducting any procedure or other type of treatment that requires informed consent.
- A properly executed informed consent form contains ... [a] statement that the procedure or treatment, including the anticipated benefits, material risks, and alternative therapies, was explained to the patient or the patient's legal representative; hospitals are free to delegate to the responsible practitioner the determination of which material risks, benefits, and alternatives will be discussed with the patient.
- A well-designed informed consent form might also include the following additional information:
  - Name of the practitioner who conducted the informed consent discussion with the patient or the patient's representative
  - Indication or listing of the material risks of the procedure or treatment that were discussed with the patient or the patient's representative
  - Statement, if applicable, that physicians other than the operating practitioner, including but not limited to residents, will be performing important tasks related to the surgery, in accordance with the hospital's policies and, in the case of residents, based on their skill set and under the supervision of the responsible practitioner
  - Statement, if applicable, that qualified medical practitioners who are not physicians who will perform important parts of the surgery or administration of anesthesia will be performing only tasks that are within their scope of practice, as determined under State law and regulation, and for which they have been granted privileges by the hospital

Including all of this information on the informed consent document will not achieve the purpose intended by CMS regulations—to educate the patient—if the form is not understandable to the patient or, worse yet, if the patient doesn't actually read the form. These forms should be written on a 12-year-old (seventh grade) reading level[7], but very few actually are.[33,34] And the study by Lavelle-Jones et al.[25] cited above found that 69% of their general surgery patients admitted to not reading the consent form before signing it. Electronic consent forms that allow patients to move through and digest the educational material at their own pace have been shown to improve patient comprehension, and the interactive nature of these programs can serve to document the requisite level of comprehension, thereby providing a greater degree of medical–legal protection to the physician.[5] Unfortunately, these are not in widespread use in the United States currently. Procedure-specific or practice-specific consent forms, as discussed above, have also been suggested as better methods of transmitting the information necessary to the patient for decision making, and better methods of documenting the informed consent process, but still may suffer from the "readability" issue and provide no proof that the patient has actually read the form or understands what he or she has read.[26,30]

INFORMED CONSENT IN ACUTE SURGICAL PRACTICE

Similar Principles: Different Process

Acute care surgeons must not fall into the trap of thinking that the informed consent process can be waived for *all* acute surgical procedures. As emphasized previously, this exemption can only be invoked under those circumstances where the delay required to obtain consent would pose an unacceptable risk to the patient's life or well-being. Surgeons should not rely upon this exemption to defend against a failure-to-disclose legal action, since the courts have tended to use a rather narrow definition of "life-threatening." In *Jackovach v Yocom*, a 17-year-old boy suffered a crushed elbow joint and a profusely bleeding scalp laceration when he jumped from a moving train. The boy was subsequently taken to the operating room to stop the bleeding from the scalp wound and, while under anesthesia, the physicians determined that the boy's arm needed to be amputated because of the immediate danger it posed to his life. After the arm was amputated, the boy and his parents brought a suit against the physicians, claiming that the procedure was performed without their informed consent. In holding for the defendant physicians, the court noted that terminating the operation in order to obtain informed consent from the boy's parents would have subjected the patient to greater risk of shock because of a necessary second anesthetic induction.[15] In contrast, in *Rogers v Sells*, the court found that a defendant physician was liable for not obtaining parental informed consent before amputating a 14-year-old boy's foot following a car accident. The physician had described the extremity as "crushed and mangled...the muscles, blood vessels, and nerves were torn and some of the nerves severed, and...the foot had no circulation." However, testimony indicated that neither life-threatening ischemia nor bleeding were present at surgery. Therefore, the court held that the situation was not an emergency with the danger of immediate harm and that the physician had an obligation to obtain informed consent.[35] Recent advances in trauma, specifically the damage control philosophy, might obviate the need for such difficult intraoperative decision making for today's practicing trauma surgeon. However, the vastly different court decisions arrived at in these two very similar clinical circumstances should serve as a strong reminder to all surgeons to consider very carefully whether a true emergent situation exists before invoking the emergency exemption to informed consent.

The intensive care unit (ICU) is another venue where a patient's informed consent rights might be inappropriately or inadvertently overlooked in the name of providing "life-saving" care. As inconvenient or inefficient as it may be, informed consent must be sought from the patient or, more likely in the ICU, the patient's surrogate unless a true-life-threatening emergency exists. Unfortunately, there are no universally accepted definitions of "medical emergency," and therefore, what constitutes an emergency is left to physician judgment. That judgment, however, is reviewable by the courts, and the physician's decision may be overruled,[14] as nearly occurred in *Liguori v. Elmann, Hunter*, et al.[36] In this case, the patient, in the course of recuperating from coronary bypass surgery, developed a large pneumothorax. A chest tube was placed approximately

30 minutes later by a surgical resident without first obtaining informed consent from the patient's family. Shortly thereafter, it was discovered that the chest tube had lacerated the patient's heart, a complication that ultimately led to the patient's demise. A wrongful death suit was brought by the patient's family, claiming, among other things, that the patient had been denied her rights to informed consent and that they would have not authorized the procedure had they known it was being performed by a surgical resident. The physician defendants prevailed, based upon the "emergency exemption" to informed consent, but the case was appealed several times, ultimately to the level of the state's Supreme Court, arguing that that since the chest tube had not been placed until 30 minutes after the diagnosis of pneumothorax was established, that the circumstances did not meet the criteria of a true life-threatening emergency, and that the courts "should instead adopt a rule of law that would require physicians to secure consent, even in the context of a medical emergency, unless it is truly impossible." Ultimately, the Supreme Court found for the physicians, writing, "Although some emergencies might well present physicians with sufficient time to seek consent, we decline to adopt plaintiffs' rigid formulation of the circumstances in which their failure to do so would be permissible."[37] Some have proposed a "blanket consent" approach for ICU procedures, wherein a single consent form would be sought from the patient or the patient's surrogate for several common ICU procedures (central venous lines, arterial catheters, chest tube placement, blood transfusion, etc.).[38] Such an approach would obviate the need to enter into a separate informed consent discussion each time one of these common ICU procedures was required. Others, however, have criticized this approach as being ethically unsound, since it denies the patient (or surrogate) the detailed risk/benefit/alternative information he or she is entitled to and needs in order to make a truly informed decision about the proposed procedure.[39] Since the vast majority of acute care surgical procedures do not qualify for the informed consent emergency exemption, the acute care surgeon must be knowledgeable about the informed consent process in general, and how the process may need to be modified for patients with acute surgical conditions.

The core informed consent principles outlined above for elective surgical patients apply equally to patients with acute surgical conditions, but the process may need to be altered for acute care surgical patients to accommodate the unique needs of this patient population. Decision making in acute care surgery, by the patient and by the physician, must be, by definition, much more rapid, and less deliberate, a major difference from elective surgery patients. The ideal 15–30 minute informed consent discussion alluded to above, carried out in the outpatient setting, with the opportunity for the patient to go home, consult with friends and family, search the Internet, deliberate further, and then change his or her mind about having the operation, is a scenario that is simply not available to the patient in need of an urgent operation. In addition, the presence of severe acute pain, and the sedative and judgment-altering effects of analgesics may impair the acute care surgical patient's ability to participate fully in an informed consent discussion. The surgeon may not be able to devote the amount of time needed by the patient or family for the consent process due to other pressing demands on the surgeon's time, or due to the patient's physiologic instability, and need for urgent surgery. And even if adequate time does exist, complete disclosure by the surgeon may not be possible since the full extent of the patient's pathology (and hence the intervention required) may not be known to the surgeon until the operative procedure is under way. For all of these reasons, both patients and physicians undertaking informed consent discussions for acute surgical procedures are at a distinct disadvantage compared to their counterparts in elective surgical scenarios. Several studies, across a number of surgical disciplines, including trauma, illustrate the difficulties encountered in adapting the informed consent process to patients with acute surgical conditions. Oburo conducted postoperative interviews with 28 elective orthopedic surgery patients and 21 orthopedic trauma patients to determine any qualitative difference in the consent process.[40] All elective orthopedic surgery patients understood the nature of their operation compared to only 71% of the orthopedic trauma patients. 86% of the elective patients were knowledgeable about the possible complications of the operation, whereas only 48% of the trauma patients were familiar with this information. Only 57% of elective patients and 29% of the trauma patients had actually read the consent before signing it. All elective surgery patients had received a pamphlet preoperatively, outlining the proposed operation and its risks, whereas none of the trauma patients had access to this information. In addition, trauma patients had less contact preoperatively with senior surgeons than did elective patients and so, may not have been as completely informed about their impending surgery as were the elective patients. Finally, some trauma patients felt as if they had no choice but to sign the consent form given the circumstances of their injury. This may explain why so few of these patients actually read the consent form, since they had already resigned themselves to signing the form regardless of its content

Bhangu interviewed 41 consecutive elective orthopedic surgery patients (primarily total hip and total knee replacement) and 40 consecutive orthopedic trauma patients (primarily femur fracture) on their first postoperative day to assess the quality of the consent process[41]. Statistically significant differences were noted between the elective and the trauma patients in several different categories: knowledge of the operation performed (100% vs. 90%), recall of complications (62% vs. 22%), percentage of patients desiring more detailed information about their operation (12% vs. 30%), and the percentage of patients who wanted written information included in the preoperative consent discussion in addition to the verbal explanation (85% vs. 35%). Overall, 100% of the elective patients were happy with the consent process compared to only 90% of the trauma patients

Vessey and Siriwardena[42] carried out postoperative interviews on 49 patients who had undergone recent "urgent" abdominal surgery to determine the impact of pain and preoperative analgesia on informed consent comprehension. "Urgent" surgery was defined as "a procedure performed for a suspected acute abdominal condition where operation could not be deferred and was generally (but not exclusively) performed within 48 hours of admission." Even though all 49 patients had signed the consent document, one-third felt that preoperative pain had impaired their judgment to the point where they could not truly give informed consent, and 13% felt that preoperative analgesics had interfered with their ability to participate fully in an informed consent discussion. Sixteen percent of patients stated that inadequate exposure to, and disclosure by, the surgeon preoperatively impaired their ability to provide informed consent. Fifteen percent of patients claimed that they had not understood preoperatively why an operation was being performed, citing pain and insufficient time with the surgeon as the causative factors. Fifty-seven percent of patients stated that they had not been informed about any of the risks of, or potential complications from, the surgery, not because of pain or insufficient time with the surgeon preoperatively, but rather because the surgeon simply did not offer this information. A follow-up study performed at the same institution yielded very similar results.[43]

The largest emergency informed consent analysis to date was performed by Akkad and coworkers, who compiled 734 questionnaires received from patients undergoing either elective or emergency gynecologic surgery.[44] As in other studies, emergency surgery patients were more likely to have *not* read the consent form (49% vs. 17%) and if they had read the form, not to have understood it (51% vs. 29%). In both groups, the two most common reasons for not reading the consent form were having had "a verbal explanation," and "trust in the doctor," but patients in the emergency group were significantly more likely to report "feeling too ill" or "not being given a chance" to read the form (Table 60.4). There were also major differences in the physical and emotional conditions of the two patient groups at the time of signing the form, with 69% of emergency patients experiencing pain, or feeling "unwell, drugged, tired, or exhausted," compared to only 19% of the elective patients (Table 60.5). Emergency patients were more likely to feel as though they had no option but to sign the consent form (40% vs. 24%), and 37% of emergency patients stated they would have signed the form no matter what was on it, compared to only 15% of elective patients. Having an opportunity to ask questions of the surgeon appeared to be important to all patients, but emergency patients were much less likely than elective patients to have been given this opportunity (29% vs. 11%). Overall, elective surgical patients were more satisfied with the consent process (80%) than were emergency patients (63%). The authors also gathered information regarding those factors associated with a positive informed consent experience. Compared to the elective surgery patients, the emergency surgery patients were less interested in detailed operative information but preferred to have the consent form read to them (as opposed to reading it themselves).

What can be learned from these studies in acute care surgical patients, and what can be done to improve the consent process for these patients? Overall, acute care surgical patients

- Are less content with the overall consent process
- Have less access to materials that might aid comprehension
- Have poorer comprehension of the intended surgical procedure and its risks
- Are less likely to have been offered information about risks
- Are less likely to have read the consent form
- Are more likely to want more detailed information
- Are more likely to want consent information *read to* them
- Are less likely to have been given the opportunity to ask questions of the surgeon
- Are more likely to have IC process impaired by pain, analgesia, or by insufficient time with the surgeon

Recognizing these fundamental differences in the acute care surgery patient population is the key to crafting an informed consent process that successfully addresses these shortcomings. While the constraints of time imposed by the nature of acute surgical illness may not allow as full a disclosure as elective surgical patients receive, acute care surgical patients can, and should, be made to feel comfortable about consenting to surgery. Tailoring the informed consent discussion to the information the patient thinks is important, rather than relying on a consent form (that the patient will likely not read) to educate the patient should be the focus of the informed consent discussion. This requires first discerning from the patient what he or she understands about the nature of the illness, and what needs to be done to remedy the situation. This will help the surgeon to identify gaps in the patient's knowledge base that will need to be filled in before the patient can fully participate in the consent process. In addressing these knowledge gaps, it may not be possible, nor advisable, to provide as detailed and comprehensive an accounting of all of the risks, benefits, and alternatives as might be provided to an elective surgical patient undergoing the same procedure, but certainly any information that the surgeon thinks might possibly impact the patient's decision making must be disclosed. Some have proposed providing the patient with just the minimal amount of information necessary at this stage, and then supplementing that information with more detailed discussions in the postoperative period.[2,4,14,45] Asking then the patient to repeat back to the surgeon, in his or her own words, the purpose of the proposed operation, its major risks, and complications should provide the surgeon with additional insight into the patient's level of understanding of the situation and point out the need for further clarifications if warranted. The use of audiovisual and computer-based educational strategies may provide for increased patient comprehension and retention of important information, but their role in emergent surgical situations has

TABLE 60.4

READING AND UNDERSTANDING CONSENT FORM: ODDS RATIO WITH EMERGENCY STATUS AND REASONS FOR NOT READING CONSENT FORM

	ELECTIVE ($n = 499$)	EMERGENCY ($n = 233$)	OR (95% CI)	*P*
Patients' Recall of Consent Form				
Remember at least something about signing consent form	475 (96)	207 (90)	0.34 (0.18, 0.65)	0.001
Read at least some of consent form—handwritten part	402 (83)	114 (51)	0.22 (0.16, 0.31)	<0.0001
Found handwritten part of consent form easy to understand	342 (74)	97 (52)	0.38 (0.27, 0.54)	<0.0001
Read at least some of consent form—printed part	344 (75)	96 (44)	0.26 (0.18, 0.36)	<0.0001
Found printed part of consent form easy to understand	305 (71)	89 (49)	0.39 (0.28, 0.60)	<0.0001
Not Read Consent Form (Fully) Because...				
I was feeling too ill	5 (1)	51 (22)	27.67 (10.88, 70.46)	<0.0001
I wasn't given a chance	56 (11)	42 (18)	1.74 (1.13, 2.69)	0.011
I trusted the doctor	158 (32)	72 (31)	0.97 (0.69, 1.35)	NS
I had a verbal explanation	219 (44)	117 (50)	1.29 (0.94, 1.76)	NS
Form was too long	64 (13)	28 (12)	0.93 (0.58, 1.49)	NS
Form was standard	28 (6)	12 (5)	0.91 (0.46, 1.83)	NS

Responses are Given in N (%)
From Akkad A, Jackson C, Kenyon S, Dixon-Woods M, Taub N, Habiba M. Informed consent for elective and emergency surgery: questionnaire study. *BJOG*. 2004;111(10):1133–1138.

TABLE 60.5

PATIENTS' PHYSICAL AND EMOTIONAL STATE AT THE TIME OF SIGNING CONSENT FORM: ODDS RATIO WITH EMERGENCY STATUS

REPORTED PHYSICAL/EMOTIONAL STATE	ELECTIVE (n = 499)	EMERGENCY (n = 233)	OR (95% CI)	P
Feeling in pain, unwell, drugged, tired, or exhausted at the time of signing consent form	93 (19)	160 (69)	9.57 (6.69, 13.67)	<0.0001
Feeling scared or frightened by signing consent form	160 (33)	121 (55)	2.52 (1.82, 3.49)	<0.0001
Feeling under pressure by signing consent form	79 (17)	64 (29)	2.09 (1.43, 3.05)	<0.0001
Feeling in control by signing consent form	214 (45)	52 (23)	0.37 (0.26, 0.53)	<0.0001
Feeling reassured by signing consent form	218 (46)	67 (31)	0.53 (0.37, 0.74)	<0.0001
Feeling relieved by signing consent form	152 (32)	68 (31)	0.95 (0.68, 1.35)	NS

Responses are given in n (%).
From Akkad A, Jackson C, Kenyon S, Dixon-Woods M, Taub N, Habiba M. Informed consent for elective and emergency surgery: questionnaire study. *BJOG*. 2004;111(10):1133–1138.

yet to be elucidated.[10,46] Finally, the patient must be given an opportunity to ask any questions he or she might have, providing yet another opportunity to the surgeon to discern the patient's level of understanding of the situation, and the capacity of the patient to provide true informed consent. Once all questions have been answered to the patient's satisfaction, the consent form, if required by the medical facility, can then be offered for the patient's (or surrogate's) signature, as well as for the signature of a witness, who ideally has been present for the entire informed consent discussion. All major risks and complications that have been discussed with the patient should be listed on the consent form, and a copy of the form given to the patient after all parties have signed it. This provides an opportunity for the patient to review the form after surgery if desired, particularly if the patient chooses not to read the form preoperatively. Additional questions that occur to the patient in the postoperative period after reading the consent form can be addressed with the surgeon at that time in a less pressured environment.

CONCLUSION

Informed consent refers to a *process* wherein a physician provides to a competent patient sufficient information about the nature of the proposed intervention, its risks, benefits, and alternatives, to enable the patient to a make an informed decision about whether that intervention is in his or her best interest. As such, it is much more than obtaining a patient's signature on the consent form, and therefore, this important task should not be undervalued, or relegated to individuals (nurses, residents) who may not be as knowledgeable as is the physician concerning the details of the proposed intervention. Furthermore, since the ethical and legal underpinnings of informed consent vary across state lines and between institutions and continue to evolve over time, it would behoove all physicians to become familiar with those guidelines and regulations that could well have a direct impact on their practices. For the acute care surgeon, the informed consent process need not necessarily be altered or truncated in any way for patients requiring urgent or emergent surgical procedures unless the delay incurred in obtaining informed consent poses an immediate threat to the patient's life or well-being. The acute care surgeon should, however, recognize that pain, anxiety, sedatives and analgesics may impair the ability of the acute care surgical patient to participate fully in informed consent discussions, and therefore, the consent process may need to be tailored to fit these unique circumstances. This may entail a more limited, but also more focused, discussion of the major risks and benefits, less reliance on written materials, or even turning to a patient surrogate to obtain consent. Most importantly, providing sufficient opportunity and time for all of the patient's questions and concerns to be addressed not only leads to greater patient satisfaction, but also allows the surgeon an additional opportunity to assess whether the patient actually comprehends the circumstances and the intervention to which he or she is about to consent.

References

1. American College of Surgeons. Statement on Principles. *American College of Surgeons*. March 2004. Available at: http://www.facs.org/fellows_info/statemtns/stonprin.html. Accessed October 28, 2010.
2. Childers R, Lipsett PA, Pawlik TM. Informed consent and the surgeon. *J Am Coll Surg*. 2009;208(4):627-634.
3. Jones JW, McCullough LB, Richman BW. A comprehensive primer of surgical informed consent. *Surg Clin North Am*. 2007;87(4):903-918, viii.
4. Katz J. Reflections on informed consent: 40 years after its birth. *J Am Coll Surg*. 1998;186(4):466-474.
5. Leclercq WK, Keulers BJ, Scheltinga MR, et al. A review of surgical informed consent: past, present, and future. A quest to help patients make better decisions. *World J Surg*.34(7):1406-1415.
6. Paterick TJ, Carson GV, Allen MC, et al. Medical informed consent: general considerations for physicians. *Mayo Clin Proc*. 2008;83(3):313-319.
7. Raper SE, Sarwer DB. Informed consent issues in the conduct of bariatric surgery. *Surg Obes Relat Dis*. 2008;4(1):60-68.
8. Schleondorff v. The Society of New York Hospital: Court of Appeals of New York; 1914:92.
9. Salgo v. Leland Stanford Jr. University Board of Trustees. *P.2d vol 317: Couts of Appeals of California, First Appellate District, Division One*; 1957:170.
10. Nwomeh BC, Waller AL, Caniano DA, et al. Informed consent for emergency surgery in infants and children. *J Pediatr Surg*. 2005;40(8):1320-1325.
11. Author Unknown. Informed Consent. *enotes.com, Inc*. 2010. Available at: http://www.enotes.com/everyday-law-encyclopedia/informed-consent. Accessed October 28, 2010.
12. Tan SY. Informed Consent: Exceptions to Disclosure. May 15, 2010. Available at: http://www.internalmedicinenews.com/views/law-medicine-by-dr-s-y-tan/blog/informed-consent-exceptions-to-disclosure/32c97f872e.html. Accessed October 17, 2010.
13. Author Unknown. Default Surrogate Consent Statutes. *American Bar Association*. 2009. Available at: http://new.abanet.org/aging/PublicDocuments/famcon_2009.pdf Accessed November 24, 2010.
14. Borak J, Veilleux S. Informed consent in emergency settings. *Ann Emerg Med*. 1984;13(9 pt 1):731-735.
15. Jackovach v. Yocum: 237 N.W. 444; 1931.

16. Hartman KL, Liang BA. Exceptions to informed consent in emergency medicine. *Hosp Physician*. 1999;1999:53-59.
17. Miller v. Rhode Island Hospital: 625 A.2d 778; 1993.
18. John F. Kennedy Memorial Hospital v. Heston: 58 N.J. 576, 279 A.2d 670; 1971.
19. Novak v. Cobb County-Kennestone Hospital Authority: 849 F. Supp. 1559 (1994), aff'd, 74 F.3d 1173; 1996.
20. Barnett v. Bachrach: 34 A.2d 626; 1943.
21. Tabor v. Scobee: 254 S.W.2d 474; 1951.
22. Canterbury v. Spence 464 F.2d 772, 150 U.S. App. D.C., cert. denied, 409 U.S. 1064, 93 S. Ct 560; 1972.
23. Falagas ME, Korbila IP, Giannopoulou KP, et al. Informed consent: how much and what do patients understand? *Am J Surg*. 2009;198(3):420-435.
24. Hutson MM, Blaha JD. Patients' recall of preoperative instruction for informed consent for an operation. *J Bone Joint Surg Am*. 1991;73(2):160-162.
25. Lavelle-Jones C, Byrne DJ, Rice P, et al. Factors affecting quality of informed consent. *BMJ*. 1993;306(6882):885-890.
26. Kondziolka DS, Pirris SM, Lunsford LD. Improving the informed consent process for surgery. *Neurosurgery*. 2006;58(6):1184-1189; discussion 1184-1189.
27. Fink AS, Prochazka AV, Henderson WG, et al. Predictors of comprehension during surgical informed consent. *J Am Coll Surg*. 210(6):919-926.
28. Losanoff JE, Litwinczuk KM, Ranella MJ, et al. Elective inguinal hernia repair: a unified informed consent, or who wants to know what? *Am Surg*. 2009;75(4):296-300.
29. Keulers BJ, Scheltinga MR, Houterman S, et al. Surgeons underestimate their patients' desire for preoperative information. *World J Surg*. 2008;32(6):964-970.
30. Issa MM, Setzer E, Charaf C, et al. Informed versus uninformed consent for prostate surgery: the value of electronic consents. *J Urol*. 2006;176(2):694-699; discussion 699.
31. Bottrell MM, Alpert H, Fischbach RL, et al. Hospital informed consent for procedure forms: facilitating quality patient-physician interaction. *Arch Surg*. 2000;135(1):26-33.
32. Author Unknown. CMS New CoP's On Informed Consent—Full Text. *MedLaw.com*. July 19, 2007. Available at: http://www.medlaw.com/healthlaw/OSHA/9_4/cms-new-cops-on-informed-.shtml. Accessed October 28, 2010.
33. Hopper KD, TenHave TR, Tully DA, et al. The readability of currently used surgical/procedure consent forms in the United States. *Surgery*. 1998;123(5):496-503.
34. Paasche-Orlow MK, Taylor HA, Brancati FL. Readability standards for informed-consent forms as compared with actual readability. *N Engl J Med*. 2003;348(8):721-726.
35. Rogers v. Sells: 178 Okla. 103; 1936.
36. Sorrel A. Court Looks at Consent in Emergencies. *American Medical News*; 2006.
37. Liguori v. Elmann Supreme Court of New Jersey; 2007.
38. Davis N, Pohlman A, Gehlbach B, et al. Improving the process of informed consent in the critically ill. *JAMA*. 2003;289(15):1963-1968.
39. Boisaubin EV, Dresser R. Informed consent in emergency care: illusion and reform. *Ann Emerg Med*. 1987;16(1):62-67.
40. Oburu EO, P. An audit comparing consent taking in elective and trauma patients in the orthopaedics department. *Intern J Law Healthcare Ethics*. 2007;4(2):1-6.
41. Bhangu A, Hood E, Datta A, et al. Is informed consent effective in trauma patients? *J Med Ethics*. 2008;34(11):780-782.
42. Vessey W, Siriwardena A. Informed consent in patients with acute abdominal pain. *Br J Surg*. 1998;85(9):1278-1280.
43. Kay R, Siriwardena AK. The process of informed consent for urgent abdominal surgery. *J Med Ethics*. 2001;27(3):157-161.
44. Akkad A, Jackson C, Kenyon S, et al. Informed consent for elective and emergency surgery: questionnaire study. *Bjog*. 2004;111(10):1133-1138.
45. Agard A, Hermeren G, Herlitz J. Patients' experiences of intervention trials on the treatment of myocardial infarction: is it time to adjust the informed consent procedure to the patient's capacity? *Heart*. 2001;86(6):632-637.
46. Keulers BJ, Welters CF, Spauwen PH, et al. Can face-to-face patient education be replaced by computer-based patient education? A randomised trial. *Patient Educ Couns*. 2007;67(1-2):176-182.

CHAPTER 61 ■ ADVANCE MEDICAL DIRECTIVES

GRACE S. ROZYCKI AND WILLIAM R. SEXSON

Advances in medical care have led to life-saving interventions, but extending a patient's life in a severely compromised state may be associated with unnecessary suffering and burdensome financial consequences for the patient, family, and society. Additionally, depending upon the patient's clinical condition, prognosis, and social circumstances, the patient may not desire certain interventions, especially those that will prolong the dying process. Providing the best, yet appropriate care for a patient near the end of life requires planning and the input of multidisciplinary caregivers within the context of medical ethics principles.

Advance care planning is the process by which a patient, along with his or her physician, family members, or other close personal relations, plans for future medical care.[1] Engaging in this process eventually leads to a document called an "advance care directive" or "advance medical directive." This document provides vital information to help the patient, family, and health care provider converge on a plan to enhance the quality of end-of-life care for the patient. Although advance medical directives are not an end in themselves, they delineate the patient's preferences for medical care within a spectrum of reasonable clinical options.[1] This chapter discusses the basic terminology and evolution of advance care planning and highlights the relevant issues that the patient, physician, and family encounter when developing an advance medical directive. Also, this work discusses how the unique environment of the intensive care unit (ICU) and the unexpected medical crisis add a level of complexity to the implementation of an advance medical directive.

TERMINOLOGY

The principles of medical ethics that are most related to advance care planning include those of autonomy, informed consent, and beneficence. An understanding of these terms is important so that a quality advance medical directive can be produced that will empower the patient at the end of life (Table 61.1).

Autonomy

The principle of autonomy recognizes the rights of individuals to self-determination, that is, their ability to make informed decisions about personal matters. Over the past several decades, there has been a shift from the paternalistic physician–patient model to a more autonomous role of the patient.[3] In the paternalistic model, the physician presents selected information about an intervention or plan and encourages consent based on what the physician considers best for the patient.[3] This model is most appropriate during medical emergencies when the risk of delaying treatment to obtain informed consent outweighs the benefit to the patient. But, in nonemergent circumstances, the paternalistic model may not produce the most beneficial outcome for the patient as the physician and patient may have different values and hence, dissimilar goals of care. In contrast, the autonomous physician–patient model emphasizes the concept of the patient's control over medical decision making. When the patient uses this model to express his or her desires about medical care, the best outcomes are expected if the patient has the capacity to understand the relevant medical facts and takes responsibility for his or her actions.[4] In either model, mutual trust between the physician and the patient is the cornerstone of the relationship and the patient's autonomy is best respected when decision making takes place with open communication and informed consent.[5]

Informed Consent or Informed Decision Making

This principle refers to the patient having an understanding of the medical care or intervention and its risks and benefits. Essentially, informed consent includes the information given and the consent of the patient.[6] But, for informed consent to be effective, the patient must be competent and able to make a decision without coercion.[7] Adults are presumed to be competent, and the term implies that the decision maker is capable of understanding and retaining relevant information and then formulating and communicating a choice. Only when sufficient understanding is present can the patient assess the options and make a decision that reflects his or her values and desires. The elements of informed consent are listed in Table 61.2. Although the physician is obligated to provide information about the risks and benefits of the procedure and those of the alternative options, patients should be encouraged to ask questions, to think carefully about their choices, and to be forthright with their physicians about their goals, values, concerns, and reservations.[8]

Beneficence

As a fundamental principle of medical ethics, beneficence deals with actions that best serve the interest of patients. In general, these actions involve the restoration of health and the relief from suffering. Restoring health may not be a reasonable goal in all cases, especially for the patient who is near the end of life but, the relief from suffering usually is attainable. Beneficence should be an integral part of a physician's practice and actions taken should be in concert with the patient's values and desires.

Communication. Clear communication lies at the heart of good decision making. In one recent review, communication problems were found in 25 of 31 cases referred for ethics consultation.[9]

For example, the comment by a physician that a condition is "treatable" may be heard by the patient or family as the condition is "curable." Similarly, a surgeon may tell a patient's family that a cardiac anomaly is "fixable" but fail to mention that the patient's congenital heart disease is due to a chromosomal anomaly. Another frequently used and misunderstood term is that a patient has a "poor prognosis." Physicians use

TABLE 61.1

TERMINOLOGY RELATIVE TO ADVANCE CARE PLANNING

TERM	DEFINITION
1. Advance health care directive or advance medical directive	A written instructional health care directive and/or appointment of an agent, or a written refusal to appoint an agent or execute a directive.
2. Agent	An individual designated in a legal document known as a power of attorney for health care. Makes health care decisions for the individual who granted the power. The agent is also referred to as durable power of attorney for health care or health care representative.
3. Instructional health care directive	A "living will." A written directive describing preferences or goals for health care, or treatment preferences or willingness to tolerate health states. Its purpose is to provide information to guide future health care.
4. Advance care planning	The process of discussing, determining and/or executing treatment directives and appointing a proxy decision maker.
5. Surrogate	Proxy by default; a person who, by default, becomes the proxy decision maker for an individual who has no appointed agent.
6. Capacity	An individual's ability to understand the significant benefits, risks, and alternatives to proposed health care and to make and communicate a health care decision. The term is frequently used interchangeably with competency, but is not the same. Competency is a legal status imposed by the court.
7. Minimally conscious state	A neurologic state characterized by inconsistent but clearly discernible behavioral evidence of consciousness and distinguishable from coma and a vegetative state by documenting the presence of specific behavioral features not found in either of these conditions.
8. Palliative care	Also called "comfort care," a comprehensive approach to treating serious illness that focuses on the physical, psychological, and spiritual needs of the patient. Its goal is to achieve the best quality of life available to the patient by relieving suffering, controlling pain and symptoms, and enabling the patient to achieve maximum functional capacity. Respect for the patient's culture, beliefs, and values is an essential component.
9. Permanent vegetative state	A vegetative state is a clinical condition of complete unawareness of the self and the environment accompanied by sleep–wake cycles with either complete or partial preservation of hypothalamic and brainstem autonomic functions. The persistent vegetative state is a vegetative state present at 1 month after acute traumatic or nontraumatic brain injury, and present for at least 1 month in degenerative/metabolic disorders or developmental malfunctions. A permanent vegetative state can be diagnosed on clinical grounds with a high degree of medical certainty in most adult and pediatric patients after careful, repeated neurologic examinations by a physician competent in neurologic function assessment and diagnosis. A patient becomes permanently vegetative when the diagnosis of irreversibility can be established with a high degree of clinical certainty, that is, when the chance of regaining consciousness is exceedingly rare.
10. Patient Self-Determination Act	An amendment to the Omnibus Budget Reconciliation Act of 1990, the law became effective December 1991 requiring most United States hospitals, nursing homes, hospice programs, home health agencies, and health maintenance organizations to provide to adult individuals, at the time of inpatient admission or enrollment, information about their rights under state laws governing advance medical directives, including: (1) the right to participate in and direct their own health care decisions; (2) the right to accept or refuse medical or surgical treatment; (3) the right to prepare an advance medical directive; and (4) information on the provider's policies that govern the utilization of these rights. The act prohibits institutions from discriminating against a patient who does not have an advance medical directive. The Act further requires institutions to document patient information and provide ongoing community education on advance medical directives.

Wilkinson A, Shugarman LR. Literature Review on Advance Directives. Prepared for Office of Disability, Aging and Long-Term Care Policy. US Dept of Health and Human Services. June 2007 and Federal Patient Self Determination Act 1990 42 U. S. C. 1395 cc (a). Available at: http://www.fha.org/acrobat/Patient%20Self%20Determination%20Act%201990.pdf. Accessed April 19, 2010.

this term when death is inevitable, but the subjectivity of the term makes it almost meaningless to the patient and the family. Difficulty with communication can also be rooted in the reading or comprehension level of the patient. The average reading level of adults in the United States is approximately at the eighth-grade level.[10] Mueller et al. reviewed advanced directive forms from all 50 states. Using the Flesch-Kincaid scoring system to assess the average readability of these forms, they found them to be at the eleventh-grade level and only five states had forms with readability at the eighth-grade level or lower. Hence, many patients may not be able to comprehend the information being presented in the form and this may explain, in part, why advanced directives are commonly not completed.

TABLE 61.2

ELEMENTS OF INFORMED CONSENT

- Assessment of decision-making capacity
- Understanding of the diagnosis
- Understanding of the proposed procedure or intervention
- Understanding of the alternatives to the proposed procedure or intervention
- Understanding of the risks and benefits of each of these
- Ability to form a reasoned opinion based on this understanding
- Ability to express the desire for or against the proposed procedure or intervention

Ernst E. Informed consent in complementary and alternative medicine. *Arch Intern Med.* 2001;161:2288–2292 and Snyder L, Leffler C. Ethics manual, fifth edition. *Ann Intern Med.* 2005;142:560–582.

THE EVOLUTION OF ADVANCE CARE PLANNING

History

Based on the nationally recognized inherent right of self-determination, the law requires the physician to obtain the patient's consent for invasive medical procedures. But, as medical technology advanced, it became clear that these tools had the potential to sustain life regardless of its quality. Patients' rights advocates became concerned about this issue and by the 1960s, the "living will" was developed in an attempt to address the negative impact of futile life-sustaining treatments.[11] As the earliest form of an advance medical directive, the living will was designed to empower individuals to make medical decisions at the end of their lives. Subsequently, on November 5, 1990, Congress passed the Patient Self-Determination Act.[2] This law was in response to the United States Supreme Court case Cruzan v Director, Missouri Department of Health and Human Services.[12] Ms. Cruzan sustained a severe traumatic brain injury in 1983 following a motor vehicle crash and remained in a persistent vegetative state for years. Her parents asked that their daughter's enteral nutrition be discontinued and after several years in litigation, the case went to the United States Supreme Court. They ruled that individual states had the right to determine the requirements for surrogate decision making regarding life-sustaining therapy. In response to this ruling, Senator Danforth of Missouri sponsored the Patient Self-Determination Act, which became law on December 1, 1991. The purpose of the Patient Self-Determination Act was to give patients the right to make decisions regarding their medical care, including the right to accept or refuse treatment, and to make an advance medical directive. The law requires all Medicare-certified hospitals to ask a patient whether he or she has an advance medical directive and to make the forms available to those who do not have one. The Patient Self-Determination Act acknowledged that the patient had the right to accept or refuse treatment but also protected the physician from litigation in the end-of-life decision making for the patient.[2] Currently, advance care planning is recognized throughout the United States as a way to identify preferences for life-sustaining care when patients no longer have decision-making capacity.

Advance Medical Directives

Advance care planning constitutes the activities that lead to the development of an advance care directive. This planning process includes deciding about future health care decisions, the exploration of treatment goals, and reflection on a patient's personal values and beliefs. The process as a whole was developed to ensure patient autonomy at the end of life through the production of a document known as the "advance medical directive."[11,13] Hence, through the planning process and the generation of the advance medical directive, the patient's autonomy can be translated into treatment decisions made by physicians and families on behalf of the incapable patient.

The methods by which an individual can indicate how treatment decisions will be made in the event of loss of decision-making capacity are the development of a living will, the appointment of a proxy, or through both of these mechanisms.[14] Hence, the living will and the proxy are two distinct methods to safeguard autonomous choice. Most states have living will statutes that provide that a person's directives regarding the use of artificial life support will be honored.[15] Patients may write their own living wills or use a template that is available at their state's living will statute web site.[16] Through the living will, the patient dictates the types of medical interventions and the conditions under which they should be used. In general, the living will becomes effective when the patient becomes incompetent yet the question remains as to whether it should guide almost all medical practice. Hence, there are some valid concerns about the generation, revision, and use of a living will.[17,18] For example, patients may be concerned that the decisions they make when the living will is created will be binding even if their values and interests change. This concern is understandable as patients in a stage of advanced illness may lack decision-making capacity and are no longer able to communicate these changes. If the living will is crafted with a narrow focus or with language that is too specific, it lacks the flexibility to address unanticipated medical or social circumstances that may arise in the future. Alternatively, if it is fashioned in a very general language, it may be too ambiguous and therefore not be useful to the patient or to the physician. For example, some documents have language such as, "terminal condition," or "seriously incapacitated" leaving the interpretation of such phrases to the physician's judgment. If the patient has had a discussion with the physician, then this ambiguity may be useful. If this discussion has not occurred, then the ambiguity may lead to uncertainty as to what course to follow. Another drawback of the living will is that as patients formulate this directive, even if done with the aid of a medical professional, most will have a limited understanding about the risks and benefits of current and future medical treatments and how they may apply to the patient's condition. Therefore, the patient, family, and caregivers need to recognize that the living will has practical limits on its use and cannot encompass all circumstances. Nonetheless, physicians should encourage patients to write a living will and to ensure that it is available to their families. Patients should also be encouraged to review the document annually or whenever a significant change occurs in their health status or family relationships.[19] For further clarification on some of the legal issues surrounding this topic, the American Bar Association's Commission on Law and Aging offers information for the lay person about the myths and facts regarding advance medical directives (Table 61.3).

Another alternative to the living will or a directive that works hand-in-hand with it is the designation by the patient of a proxy decision maker. The proxy may be a family member, friend, or other person who has the authority to make medical

TABLE 61.3

MYTHS AND FACTS ABOUT HEALTH CARE ADVANCE DIRECTIVES

MYTH	FACT
1. You must have a Living Will to stop treatment near the end of life.	Treatment can be stopped without a Living Will if everyone involved agrees. However, without some kind of advance directive, decisions may be more difficult and disputes more likely. The Durable Power of Attorney for Health Care is the more useful and versatile advance directive, because it applies to all health care decisions and empowers the person you name to make decisions for you in the way you want them made.
2. You must use your state's statutory form for your advance directive to be valid.	Most states do not require a particular form, but do require witnessing or other specific signing formalities. Even if your state requires a specific form, doctors still have a legal obligation to respect your treatment wishes, regardless of the form you use.
3. Advance directives are legally binding, so doctors must follow them.	Advance directive laws merely give doctors and others immunity if they follow your valid advance directive. Doctors can always refuse to comply with your wishes if they have an objection of conscience or consider your wishes medically inappropriate. However, they may have an obligation to transfer you to another health care provider who will comply.
4. An advance directive means "Do not treat."	An advance directive can express both what you want and don't want. Never assume it simply means "Do not treat." Even if you do not want treatment to cure you, you should always be kept reasonably pain free and comfortable.
5. If I name a health care proxy, I give up the right to make my own decisions.	Naming a health care proxy or agent does not take away any of your authority. You always have the right, while you are still competent, to override the decision of your proxy or revoke the directive. If you do not name a proxy or agent, the likelihood of needing a court appointed guardian grows greater, especially if there is disagreement regarding your treatment among your family and doctors.
6. I should wait until I am sure about what I want before signing an advance directive.	No. Most of us have some ambivalence about what we would want, and that's acceptable, because treatment near the end of life can be complicated. We can't predict all the facts and circumstances that may face us in the future, and treatment wishes may change. You can, at least, appoint your proxy if you have someone whom you trust.
7. Just talking to my doctor and family about what I want is not legally effective.	Meaningful discussion with your doctor and family is actually the most important step. The question of what is "legally effective" is misleading, because even a legally effective document does not automatically carry out your wishes. The best strategy is to use a good health decisions workbook to help you clarify your wishes; talk with your physician, health care agent, and family about your wishes; put those wishes in writing in an advance directive; and make sure everyone has a copy.
8. Once I give my doctor a signed copy of my directive, my task is done!	No, you have just started. First, make sure your doctor understands and supports your wishes. Second, there is no guarantee that your directive will follow you in your medical record, especially if you are transferred from one facility to another. You or your proxy should always double-check to be sure your providers are aware of your directive and have a copy. Advance planning is an ongoing PROCESS. Review your wishes yearly or anytime your health or family status changes, make appropriate changes, and communicate those changes as needed.
9. If I am living at home and do not want to be resuscitated by an EMS team if my heart or breathing stops, my advance directive must say so.	Your advance directive will usually not help in this situation. If someone dials 9–1–1, EMS must attempt to resuscitate you and transport you to a hospital, UNLESS you have a special out-of-hospital DNR form or bracelet used in your state. This is not the same as your health care advance directive. In most states, both the patient and doctor must sign the special form and the patient then wears a special identification bracelet or necklace.
10. Advance directives are only for old people.	It is true that more older, rather than younger, people use advance directives, but every adult should have one. Younger adults actually have more at stake, because, if stricken by serious disease or accident, medical technology may keep them alive but insentient for decades

Myths and Facts About Health Care Advance Directives. Available at: http://www.abanet.org/aging/pdfs/myths_and_fact_about_HC_AD.pdf. Accessed April 19, 2010.

decisions for the patient. By understanding the patient's values, the proxy approaches medical decision making in accordance with the patient's desires and intents.[21,22] This process is commonly referred to as decision making by "substituted judgment." By appointing a proxy, there is less concern about the specificity or generality of the living will as the proxy will make medical decisions for the patient based on the patient's desires. A proxy may be appointed under a living will statute or through the creation of a durable power of attorney. In some states, the living will statute may restrict a proxy's authority to making health care decisions only in the setting of select clinical conditions such as terminal illness.[23] But, a proxy appointed as a durable power of attorney for health care has more authority and can take legally binding action on the patient's behalf. In this case, the proxy, also known as the "agent," can be a lawyer, family member, friend, or any competent adult. The durable power of attorney for health care has more authority than the living will or the proxy. For example, the durable power of attorney can be used to delegate authority for health care decisions in all cases of patient incompetence.[23] Also, the physician is able to rely on the agent's decision even when the patient's desires were not clearly expressed or did not take into account unforeseen circumstances. Although these advance medical directives are not without their drawbacks, they do provide some guidelines for the physician who needs to make difficult decisions about the care of critically ill patients with little or no chance of recovery.

To that end, the physician should plan to have an early dialog with patients about artificial life support and their treatment preferences. Despite the broad-based support for advance medical directives, few patients have them. Only about 25% of Americans have completed advance medical directives, yet studies indicate that most patients want a formal document regarding future health care and that they prefer to obtain that information from their physician.[24,25] Although this is time-consuming for physicians, studies show that one-on-one intervention with patients and brief episodic discussions seem to be the most effective strategies to increase the completion rates of advance medical directives.[26–28]

Table 61.4 lists the most common barriers to advance care planning. Discussions about advance medical directives should be rooted in the patient's values and goals for medical care, as well as the appropriateness of specific interventions. Effective measures to initiate these discussions include community education efforts and the provision of resources for the patient.[30,31] The physician can be directly instrumental in providing information such as, sample drafts of living wills, clarification of terminology, and web links where the patient can seek more information on the topic[32,33] (Table 61.5). Patients may desire more information on the ethical and legal aspects of withholding and withdrawing of life-sustaining treatments as this has been cited to be a point of confusion for patients as they develop an advance medical directive.[34] An example of a useful workbook is "Your Life, Your Choices, Planning for Future Medical Decisions: How to Prepare a Personalized Living Will."[35] This manual is a step-by-step guide that walks the patient through the process of advance care planning. Using some thought-provoking exercises and poignant questions, the authors provide useful information about the process of developing an advance medical directive including a section on how patients should articulate their desires and values to their physicians.

During an office visit, the topic of advance medical directives can be introduced in a nonthreatening way by simply asking the patient if he or she has a living will or has formally appointed a health care proxy.[24] The patient should know that advance medical directives can be revised or revoked while the patient is still competent, and that they will be implemented only when the patient is incapacitated and unable to participate in medical decision making. Understanding a patient's values is an important part of the dialog as this information will strongly influence the overall content of the document and the approach that the physician uses during a medical crisis. The importance of addressing the patient's values was highlighted in a prospective study conducted in five outpatient primary care practices in North Carolina and Pennsylvania.[36] The authors' audiotaped discussions between patients and their physicians about advance medical directives. During the discussions with their patients, all of whom were ≥65 years of age, the 56 physicians covered topics such as potential medical scenarios and their treatments, patient values, and surrogate decision makers. The authors found that the physicians covered the key areas of uncertainty and proxy well but, only 34% of them explicitly elicited information about the patient's personal values, goals for care, and reasons for

TABLE 61.4

BARRIERS TO ADVANCE CARE PLANNING

1. **Reluctance to discuss the issue.** Physicians may be reluctant to tell a patient that he or she is approaching the end of life. The patient may be in denial about their medical condition and therefore not receptive to hearing the information.
2. **Procrastination.** Patients in good health may find the discussion irrelevant.
3. **Time constraints.** End-of-life discussions with patients and families are time-consuming as they tend to be open-ended and ill-defined.
4. **Misunderstanding regarding resuscitation preferences.** Patients may not understand medical terminology and medical technology. Further, future medical technology and its applications are unknown.
5. **Unrealistic expectations.** Public awareness of CPR is promoted, but a parallel education about futile applications is not emphasized.

Butterworth AM. Reality check: 10 barriers to advance planning. *Nurse Pract.* 2003;28(5):42–43.

TABLE 61.5

HELPFUL WEB SITES FOR PATIENTS

1. "Put it in writing" is a patient-friendly document presented in a Q & A format that can help patients identify and differentiate between advance directives and their importance. Available at: http://www.putitinwriting.org.
2. Partnership for Caring. On this site, patients can learn about their end-of-life options and how to document them. Available at http://www.partnershipforcaring.org.
3. Talking about your choices. Last Acts Coalition and Partnership for Caring from the Robert Wood Johnson Foundation includes many helpful links for patients. Available at: http://www.lastacts.org.
4. The American Association of Retired Persons provides links for estate planning, hospice care, and ADs. Available at: http://www.aarp.org/families/end_life/.

Later EB, King D. Advance directives: results of a community education symposium. *Crit Care Nurse.* 2007;27:31–35.

treatment preferences. The importance of this study was that it underscored the need for physicians to adhere to standard recommendations when discussing advance medical directives with patients so that the information obtained will be useful in future decision making. To ensure that the crucial components of advance medical directives are addressed, some authors recommend the patient and the physician go through a check list that can be included in the patient's annual history and physical examination update.[24] Finally, after the advance medical directive has been completed, the document should be reviewed annually or sooner if there has been a change in the patient's health status, family relationships (that affect the appointment of the proxy), or other pertinent social circumstances.

SPECIAL CIRCUMSTANCES

Decision Making During a Medical Crisis

Making end-of-life medical decisions long before a terminal condition ensues helps to ensure that the physician and family will act in the patient's best interest and in a timely manner especially at a time when the emotional component of the decision-making process intensifies. In preparation for this time, the patient should be aware that the terminal disease may create an immediate life-threatening emergency that may not be remedied. But, even if the patient can be treated for this medical emergency, the risks are greater and the benefits usually fewer due to the patient's weakened clinical condition. Equally challenging for the physician is when a terminally ill patient's period of clinical stability is interrupted by a worsening in his or her clinical condition.[37] For example, new metastases may be detected on a follow-up computed tomography scan indicating a poor prognosis. With recognition that death is approaching soon, the decision involves pursuing treatment aimed at prolonging life or adopting an approach focused on specific end-of-life goals and comfort. Patients should understand that "doing nothing" or withholding further treatment does not equate to abandonment and that efforts will continue to ensure comfort and support for the patient during the remaining time before death.

Important issues that factor into this decision matrix during this time include the following: (1) the patient's values, (2) end-of-life goals, (3) the emotional and financial burden for the family, (4) prognosis, (5) risk-benefit analysis of the proposed intervention, (6) current symptom burden, and (7) the patient's age and life stage.[38] Further, before any decision is made, the physician should assess the patient's physical, psychological, and spiritual needs, their support system, and their end-of-life goals.[38] For example, patients who are at peace with dying and those who have accomplished their goals in life will usually decline further interventions that would prolong life.[38] In contrast, patients who have yet to fulfill an important goal or who are in denial about their terminal condition are more likely to want additional life-prolonging treatments. Patients are expected to undergo a grieving process associated with the end-of-life condition and, potentially, even feel depressed. But, physicians can best help patients and their families or surrogates prepare and navigate through this difficult time by ensuring that they understand the risks and benefits of interventions at this stage of their medical condition, their prognosis, and the principles and processes of palliative care. After having physician–patient–family discussions to address the scenarios of future medical crises, the physician can more easily affirm the patient's choices and make appropriate recommendations.[38]

End-of-Life Care in the Intensive Care Unit

Making end-of-life medical decisions for the critically ill patient in the ICU presents several challenges for the caregivers and the family. The noisy environment, visitor restrictions, and multiple monitoring instruments augment the anxiety that families and patients are feeling. The diversity of diagnoses, the presence of family and surrogates, and the urgency and complexity of the decision-making processes contribute to the challenges, rewards, and risks associated with the practice of critical care medicine. In the ICU, death is a routine occurrence to caregivers but not to the patient and the family. Given the emotional impact of decisions surrounding death and dying, conflicts are expected and are disturbing to all parties.

In this setting, end-of-life medical decisions frequently involve withholding or withdrawing support that involves transferring the patient from the ICU to a step down or ward unit. This can be difficult if the patient and the staff have developed a mutually supportive attachment. Equally difficult is transferring the patient from the ICU to a palliative care facility. When aggressive physiologic support is no longer beneficial, then equally aggressive humane supportive (palliative) care must include emotional and behavioral components as well. Also, if the patient is no longer mentally competent, the physician must rely on advance medical directives and input from the family to guide treatment decisions. If the physician has already established a good rapport and trust with the patient's family and understands the patient's values, then conflict with the family is less likely and the decision making can be both expeditious and supportive.[39] But, such a case is unlikely as the patient's primary care physician is usually not the critical care intensivist and hence conflict may arise, especially over life-sustaining treatments. Without the preestablished trust between the physician and the patient or family, the intensivist's decisions may be challenged and legal or ethical consultants may be needed to mediate these issues. It is essential to emphasize to families that their input is valued and that the health care team is committed to the patient's well being.[40] The family–physician conflicts are particularly important in the ICU because the patient is often mentally incapacitated and thus, decision making ethically and legally rests with the patient's surrogate.

As disagreements arise, some authors have suggested using a "differential diagnosis" approach so that physicians will consider all the possible explanations for the disagreements rather than dealing emotionally with the problems.[41] As this approach unfolds, the contributing factors of these family–physician conflicts fall into three categories: family features, physician features, and organizational/social features.

Families may disagree with physicians because they do not understand the medical situation or because they have been given different information in the past or conflicting information by other clinicians. In such situations, it becomes especially important to have either a single person designated to talk to the family, or better, have routine multidisciplinary conferences where all the health care team members can discuss the patient's status and can arrive at a consistent way of expressing this to the family. The physician should ask the family members to put into their own words the patient's history, what they have been told by other health care providers, and their understanding of the patient's current clinical situation. Also, the family members or proxy should be given time to explain the choices that they desire for the patients. This approach can help identify incorrect information and allows the physician to assess the family's reasoning skills. Further, through open-ended questions, the physician can elucidate information about what the family believes to be the causes, consequences, and prognosis of their loved one's illness.

In this process, the physician may discover that the family or proxy is psychologically unprepared to hear the patient's diagnosis or prognosis or may need to hear the information stated more explicitly. In addition to open-ended questions, the physician should make an effort to listen intently, have nondefensive neutral responses, and encourage the family members to write down questions as they think of them. Even if the family is not in denial about the patient's medical condition, "bad news" is often poorly processed and imperfectly remembered.[41] Suggestions to improve communication and understanding between the family and the physician include the following: (1) repeating critical information; (2) providing the information in written and verbal forms; and (3) encouraging questions to improve the information transfer and retention.[42] Finally, it is common to have numerous physicians involved in the care of the patient, and so it is helpful to choose one health care professional to serve as the primary communicator or have regular scheduled meetings with the designated family member or proxy. Another issue for the family that factors into the complexity of making decisions while the patient is in the ICU is that of guilt. The basis of this guilt may be long-standing interpersonal family disagreements or the helplessness of dealing with a critically ill or injured child, just to name a few. Hence, the family may be unwilling to make particular kinds of decisions. In general, the physician, not the family, should take responsibility for the medical decisions. Open-ended questions such as, "What do you think your sister would want us to do?" helps the family to meaningfully participate in the decision process without the burden and guilt of owning responsibility for the medical decision making. Another way that the family can comfortably participate in the medical decision making is to help set some goals for the patient, such as, to maximize comfort and minimize pain. Through this common purpose, the bond among the family members and between the family and caregivers strengthens.

Throughout the time the patient is in the ICU, the physician may also struggle on multiple levels with making end-of-life decisions. These issues include concern about prognostic uncertainty, failure, and legal repercussions. For example, medical–legal risk may be increased for the physician because of the misuse of, or complications associated with, the sophisticated diagnostic and life-support technology. To compound that risk is the urgency, complexity, and invasive nature of the procedures. Further, the physician also feels the economic pressures associated with caring for critically ill patients as ICU beds are almost always in demand and in treating patients who are nearing death, expectations for cure are low. Throughout this process, good communication remains the cornerstone of successful interactions between the physician and the family.

SUMMARY

Notwithstanding the limitations, advance care planning is an important tool that should encourage communication among the patient, physician, and family with the goal of empowering the patient at the end-of-life. The process of advance care planning and the development of a living will and choosing a surrogate should be part of an ongoing discussion intrinsic to the doctor–patient relationship. Physicians should be proactive in education and encourage patients to pursue the process of advance care planning and provide information on advance medical directives. An important part of this process is for the patient to reveal his or her values, preferences, and goals to safeguard autonomous choices and ensure that desires are honored as death ensues. As the Terry Schiavo case demonstrated, even relatively young and healthy patients should be encouraged to think about these issues that surround treatment decisions in the event of terminal illness or permanent unconsciousness.[43]

References

1. Wilkinson A, Shugarman LR. Literature Review on Advance Directives. Prepared for Office of Disability, Aging and Long-Term Care Policy. US Dept of Health and Human Services. June 2007.
2. Federal Patient Self Determination Act 1990 42 U. S. C. 1395 cc (a). Available at: http://www.fha.org/acrobat/Patient%20Self%20Determination%20Act%201990.pdf. Accessed April 19, 2010.
3. Siegler M. The Progression of medicine from physician paternalism to patient autonomy to bureaucratic parsimony. *Arch Intern Med.* 1985;145:713-715.
4. Stirrat GM, Gill R. Autonomy in medical ethics after O'Neill. *J Med Ethics.* 20005;31:127-130.
5. Prendergast T. Advance care planning: pitfalls, progress, promise. *Crit Care Med.* 2001;29:N34-N39.
6. O'Neill O. Some limits of informed consent. *J Med Ethics.*2003;29:4-7.
7. Ernst E. Informed consent in complementary and alternative medicine. *Arch Intern Med.* 2001;161:2288-2292.
8. Snyder L, Leffler C. Ethics manual, fifth edition. *Ann Intern Med.* 2005;142:560-582.
9. Førde R, Vandvik IH. Committee review of 31 cases from a clinical ethics. *J Med Ethics.*2005;31:73-77.
10. Mueller, LA, Reid KI, Puller PS. Readability of state-sponsored advance directive forms in the United States: a cross sectional study. *BMC Med Ethics.* 2010;11:6.
11. Brown BA. The history of advance directives. A literature review. *J Gerontol Nurs.* 2003;29:4-14.
12. Gaeta S, Price KJ. End-of-life issues in critically ill cancer patients. *Crit Care Clin.* 2010;26:219-227.
13. Emanuel LL, Emanuel EJ. The medical directive: a new comprehensive advance care document. *JAMA.* 1989;261:3288-3293.
14. Emanuel L. Advance directives. *Ann Rev Med.* 2008;59:187-198.
15. Surrogate Consent in the Absence of an advance directive. Available at: http://www.abanet.org/aging/legislativeupdates/docs/FamconChart-Final4–22–08.pdf. Accessed April 19, 2010.
16. State Living Will and Advance Directives Laws. Available at: http://www.livingwills-freelegal.org/state-living-will-and-advance-directives-laws.html. Accessed April 19, 2010.
17. Danis M, Southerland LI, Garrett JM, et al. A prospective study of advanced directives for life-sustaining care. *N Engl J Med.* 1991;324:882-888.
18. Ditto PH, Jacobson JA, Smucker WD, et al. Context changes choices: a prospective study of the effects of hospitalization on life-sustaining treatment preferences. *Med Decis Making.* 2006;26:313-322.
19. Tonelli MR. Pulling the plug on living wills. *Chest.* 1996;110:816-822.
20. Myths and Facts About Health Care Advance Directives. Available at: http://www.abanet.org/aging/pdfs/myths_and_fact_about_HC_AD.pdf. Accessed April 19, 2010.
21. Ditto PH, Danks JH, Smucker WD, et al. Advance directives as acts of communication. A randomized controlled trial. *Arch Intern Med.* 2001;161:421-430.
22. Shalowitz DI, Garrett-Mayer E, David W. The accuracy of surrogate decision makers. *Arch Intern Med.* 2006;166:493-497.
23. Orentlicher D. Advance medical directives. *JAMA.* 1990;263:2365-2367.
24. Maxfield CL, Pohl JM, Colling K. Advance directives: a guide for patient discussion. *Nurse Pract.* 2003;28:38-47.
25. Johnston SC. The discussion about advance directives: patient and physician opinions regarding when and how it should be conducted *Arch Intern Med.* 1995;155:1025-1030.
26. Messinger-Rapport BJ, Baum EE, Smith ML. Advance care planning: Beyond the living will. *Cleve Clin J Med.* 2009;76:276-285.
27. Jezewski MA, Meeker MA, Sessanna L, et al. The effectiveness of interventions to increase advance directives completion rates. *J Aging Health.* 2007;19:519-536.
28. Ramsaroop SD, Reid MC, Adelman RD. Completing an advance directive the primary care setting: what do we need for success? *J Am Geriatr Soc.* 2007;55:277-283.
29. Butterworth AM. Reality check: 10 barriers to advance planning. *Nurse Pract.* 2003;28(5):42-43.
30. Bravo G, Bubois MF, Wagneur B. Assessing the effectiveness of interventions to promote advance directives among older adults: a systematic review and multi-level analysis. *Soc Sci Med.* 2008;67:1122-1132.
31. Later EB, King D. Advance directives: results of a community education symposium. *Crit Care Nurse.* 2007;27:31-35.
32. Georgia Advance Directive for Health Care. Available at: http://www.aging.dhr.georgia.gov/DHR-DAS/GEORGIA%20ADVANCE%20DIRECTIVE%20FOR%20HEALTH%20CARE-07.pdf. Accessed April 20, 2010.
33. Roessel LL. Protect your patients' rights with advance directives. *Nurse Pract.* 2007;32:38-43.

34. Mueller PS. The Terri Schiavo saga. Ethical and legal aspects and implications for clinicians. *Polskie Archiwum Medycyny Wewnetrznej.* 2009;119:574-581.
35. Your Life, Your Choices. Planning for Future Medical Decisions: How to Prepare a Personalized Living Will. Available at: http://stevebuyer.house.gov/UploadedFiles/your_life_your_choices.pdf. Accessed April 20, 2010.
36. Tulksy JA, Fischer GS, Rose MA, et al. Opening the black box: How do physicians communicate about advance directives? *Ann Intern Med.* 1998;129:441-449.
37. Lunney R, Lynn J, Foley DJ, et al. Patterns of functional decline at the end of life. *JAMA.* 2003;289:2387-2392.
38. Weissman DE. Decision making at a time of crisis near the end of life. *JAMA.* 2004;292:1738-1743.
39. Tillyard ARJ. Ethics review: 'Living wills' and intensive care—an overview of the American experience. *Crit Care.* 2007;11:219-223.
40. Szalados JE. Legal issues in the practice of critical care medicine: a practical approach. *Crit Care Med.* 2007;35:S44-S58.
41. Goold SD, Williams B, Arnold RM. Conflicts regarding decisions to limit treatment. A differential diagnosis. *JAMA.* 2000;283:909-914.
42. Teno JM, Clarridge BR, Casey V, et al. Family perspective on end-of-life care at the last place of care. *JAMA.* 2004;291:88-93.
43. Gostin LO. Ethics, the Constitution and the dying process. The case of Theresa Marie Schiavo. *JAMA.* 2005;293:2403-2407.

CHAPTER 62 ■ ACUTE CARE SURGERY, ETHICS, AND THE LAW

CHARLES E. LUCAS AND ANNA M. LEDGERWOOD

The words *moral*, *ethical*, *virtuous*, and *righteous* are often used interchangeably to imply actions that are carried out "in accordance with principles or rules of right or good conduct."[1] Morality refers to personal behavior, especially in the sexual domain. Ethical behavior implies conformity with idealized standards of right and wrong, especially within medicine and the law. Virtuous behavior implies moral excellence or, more narrowly, chastity. Righteous behavior indicates freedom from guilt, such that outrage might be the justifiable response to an accusation of bad behavior. A more refined definition of ethical behavior was provided by Mark Twain:

> "*The fact that man knows right from wrong proves his intellectual superiority to other creatures; but the fact that that he can do wrong proves his moral inferiority to any creature that cannot.*"[1]

Ethical behavior is not absolute but depends upon one's rearing, education, religion, and socialization. Each culture develops its own ethic. Sanctioned behavior in an insular, parochial environment may be unacceptable in an open, cosmopolitan setting, and vice versa. This reflects the intricate balance between societal and individual rights. The United States has an open society that emphasizes individual rights, but the balance between social and individual rights permeates the legal and medical professions. In clinical medicine, an acute care encounter may challenge the caregiver's interpretation of established ethical premises; advanced technology may complicate ethical decision making even further (e.g., end-of-life care planning) as implied by General of the Army Omar Bradley: "The world has achieved brilliance without conscience. Ours is a world of nuclear giants and ethical infants."[1] The combination of advanced technology, the interrelationship of medicine and social activism, and increased medical knowledge and awareness of the civil rights of patients has stimulated interest in medical ethics, and particularly surgical ethics, where physical actions that may constitute battery outside of clinical medicine are part of every discussion between surgeon and patient.[2]

ETHICS AND THE LAW

The legal system defines how disparate members of society can interact and function in a mutually beneficial manner.[3] Acts prohibited by law are clearly unethical medically, but legal doctrine is not immutable, nor is it enforced consistently. An example of such inconsistency is the historical debate regarding assisted suicide. A prominent proponent, Doctor Jack Kevorkian, believed that sane patients have a right to die when the pain of a permanent physical illness outweighed the pleasures of living.[4] He promulgated his views within the State of Michigan in an unsuccessful attempt to change the state law against assisted suicide, but the several suicides he facilitated created discomfiture for officials reluctant to stake their political reputations on a criminal prosecution that would be deeply unpopular with the electorate, most of whom believed Kevorkian was providing ethical treatment to his patients (opponents opined that only God can terminate a human life). Only after Kevorkian defied the law openly by filming an assisted suicide and making the film public was he charged criminally. A sympathetic jury nonetheless found him guilty. After imprisonment for several years, he was paroled after promising not to be involved further in any assisted suicides. Subsequently, the State of Oregon legalized assisted suicide under specific conditions; this process has been upheld by the United States Supreme Court.[5]

The Kevorkian saga is but one of many examples of how conflict between personal medical ethics and legal doctrine can eventually lead to changes in the law. Another example of such conflict is the ongoing debate regarding abortion. Ethical and moral beliefs are widely divergent; should abortions be prohibited under any circumstance, or can they be performed in the first trimester when the mother's life is threatened or when the pregnancy resulted from rape, or is abortion permitted at any time including so-called "partial birth" abortions, whereby the fetus is destroyed prior to delivery and ligation of the umbilical cord?[6] Legal definitions regarding the propriety of abortion at different stages of pregnancy are still being tested in the courts. Individual physicians likely will act according to his or her beliefs, but certainly within the law. Although the law may not prohibit actions that many physicians would consider unethical, illegal activity should be deemed unethical regardless. Recognizing the great diversity of views present in society when human individual rights and expectations tend to outweigh societal constraints, this treatise highlights ethical surgical practice, especially as it relates to acute surgical care.

THE SURGEON AND MEDICAL ETHICS

The foundation for ethical surgical practice begins with familial encounters with parents, siblings, and neighbors. Personal relationships are formed with individuals from different backgrounds during early education, and the individual is introduced to the concept of the *golden rule*, that one should "do unto others as they would do unto you." Ethical development continues during high school and college, and especially during medical school, when exposure to physicians and patients identifies potential conflicts between personal ethics and the needs of patients. Formal teaching of surgical ethics is now incorporated into postgraduate medical education (i.e., residency training).

SURGICAL CURRICULUM IN ETHICS

Miles Little classified ethical issues as they relate to (1) rescue; (2) proximity; (3) ordeal; (4) aftermath; and (5) presence.[7] Little points out that the patient recognizes and is subject to the surgeon's power during the first encounter, especially so under emergency conditions. However, the recognition of surgical power is contingent on a perception of trust that the surgeon will act in the best interest of the patient, including obtaining appropriate help, to correct the problem (i.e., to *rescue* the patient). The surgeon's obligation is inviolate, requiring all that is legally and ethically possible to do be done. The principle of *proximity* acknowledges that the surgeon will be within the patient's body, thus the patient must trust that his or her body and mind will be treated with respect. This is particularly relevant when the physical problem cannot be corrected and the surgeon distances him- or herself from the patient as part of instinctual self-preservation. The principle of proximity dictates that the surgeon must share in this failure to heal while continuing to support the patient emotionally. The principle of *ordeal* recognizes that surgical remediation is associated with pain, discomfort, and inconvenience; however, the patient trusts that suffering will be minimized by the surgeon's concern for the overall well-being of the patient. The surgeon must strive for optimal patient care by balancing the alleviation of pain and suffering and the avoidance of treatment-related morbidity, especially when the patient requires ongoing treatment. An even greater ethical commitment is required of the surgeon when the emergency is caused by a neoplasm to which the patient will succumb eventually. The fourth principle, *aftermath*, refers to the need for the surgeon to maximize the patient's enjoyment of life to the fullest extent subsequent to the acute encounter. The surgeon must recognize the importance of frequent, regular visits as part of the treatment program. The fifth principle emphasized by Little is *presence*, which refers to the knowledge that the surgeon will always be available to answer questions, alleviate pain, and provide counsel well after the encounter has been completed.[7]

THE UNPLANNED ENCOUNTER

Occasionally, the surgeon will be in close proximity to an emergency event because of happenstance. For example, the surgeon's private life might be disrupted by a nearby restaurant patron who suddenly develops tracheal occlusion, the airplane passenger who develops acute respiratory distress, or a driver on the highway who loses control and crashes. It is easy to be passive and conceal one's surgical skills, but although the surgeon who intervenes on behalf of the endangered citizen enjoys legal protection from "Good Samaritan" laws in all 50 states, there is little statutory requirement for the surgeon to surrender anonymity while acknowledging his or her skills and providing care.[8–10] The only exception to this lack of a statutory mandate comes from the State of Vermont, which identifies that the physician in this setting has a "duty to rescue."[11] The Vermont statute states that

> *"a person who knows that another is exposed to grave physical harm shall, to the extent that the same cannot be rendered without danger or peril to himself or without interference with important duties owed to others, give reasonable assistance to the exposed person unless that assistance or care is being provided by others."*[3,11]

Although the decision to come to a patient's rescue in an unplanned encounter is not mandated in most states, it would certainly be considered proper ethical behavior. This code of ethics should stimulate the surgeon to offer assistance at the scene of a motor vehicle collision, to a pedestrian "found down," and intraoperatively to a fellow surgeon in time of need.

The American College of Surgeons (ACS) has developed a program for teaching ethics to surgical residents.[12,13] This program covers: (1) conflict of interest; (2) problems of litigation; (3) substituted decision making; (4) truth in communication; (5) end-of-life decisions; and (6) confidentiality. The practicing surgeon has to adhere to the tenets of each of the above in practicing in an ethical manner.

ADVANCE DIRECTIVES

The federal Self Determination Act of 1991 allows a citizen to define a preferred level of care that is to be provided at a future time when the said individual is unable to provide consent at the time of the encounter.[2] This act promotes advance directives as a means of controlling one's destiny even when incapacitated. Despite this option, the vast majority of people do not avail themselves of the benefit.[14] Advance directives may be part of a "living will" or may be delegated to an agent who holds the patient's Durable Power of Attorney for Health Care, also called a health care proxy. Technically, a living will addresses the implementation of care to the terminally ill patient. A decision to not provide care even though death would be imminent without care is best made in consultation by two physicians. The health care proxy transfers legal decision-making authority to an agent empowered to act when an individual lacks capacity to make health care decisions. When such documents have not been executed, decision making accrues to the relative of highest standing, usually the spouse. In cases of dispute, an opinion may be sought from the facility's legal counsel. Decisions made by surrogates are more easily supported when informed by the patient's known wishes, but sometimes only a best guess can be made as to what the surrogate believes the patient would want. Sulmasy and Terry[15] reported that judgments made by surrogates often do not represent the patient's best interests, particularly when dealing with terminal illness (i.e., there can be a powerful inclination to do "everything" to the point of futility). This dilemma is compounded when no surrogate decision maker can be identified.[16] The surgeon has the ethical responsibility to act in the best interest of the patient, based upon education and experience.[16] The golden rule that applies is that the surgeon will probably make a proper decision if the decision is to do what would be preferred for his or her own care in the same circumstance.[17] Many such decisions in acute care surgery involve endotracheal intubation and mechanical ventilation, use of catecholamines to support blood pressure, and pain management. When addressing limits to care stipulated by an advance directive or the patient's agent, the delivery of care must be modified (Table 62.1).[17] This is an example of a preventable death and unethical care in the view of the writers, but the case record provided is incomplete with respect to determination of the patient's capacity to make decisions and the involvement of a surrogate, therefore many medical ethicists might disagree. In the authors' view, decisions regarding pain management with opioids must be made in the context of the do not resuscitate (DNR) and do not intubate (DNI) orders. The surgeon is obligated to balance sedation and analgesia in the context of the DNI directive. Ideally, the discussion regarding the limits of care under the DNR order should occur as soon as practicable after admission, and the results made known to all caregivers. For example, it may be decided to adhere strictly to the advance directive (in which case care in the intensive care unit (ICU) may be unjustifiable). Alternatively, some or all aspects of care may be deemed permissible by mutual agreement, or the DNR/DNI orders may be rescinded for a period of time certain (e.g., the periprocedural period or the length of stay in the ICU. Such a discussion is decidedly less than ideal after (or during) a destabilization complication. Absent the discussion, should the patient be intubated until the opioid effects have worn off or been reversed? The authors would opine in the affirmative, after which further discussion with patient and family would determine subsequent care, because most advance directives are designed to prevent futile care or prolonged terminal care, not the short-term management of a reversible complication, but not all medical ethicists would agree.[17,18]

TABLE 62.1

EXAMPLE CASE OF HEALTH CARE LIMITED BY ADVANCE DIRECTIVE

- A 64-year-old male was thrown from an all-terrain vehicle at 15 mph.
- Unconscious for 3 min, helmet dented.
- Upon arrival at the Emergency Department, the patient had slurred speech, was amnestic to events, and complained of left leg pain. Vital signs were normal.
- Imaging studies suggested an old right hemisphere stroke.
- An advance directive specified "Do Not Resuscitate" (DNR), and "Do Not Intubate" (DNI). Morphine sulfate was administered for discomfort.
- Day 2: Increased oral secretions.
- Day 4: Increasing somnolence.
- Day 5: Gastrojejunal tube placed by interventional radiology for enteral feeding. Postprocedure restlessness treated by patient-controlled analgesia infusion of morphine sulfate at a basal rate of 2 mg/h. Respirations became labored but the patient was not intubated owing to the DNI order. The patient died that day.
- Postmortem examination showed a small subarachnoid hemorrhage at the base of the brain and a small tear of the dura mater.
- The peer review committee concluded that the death was nonpreventable due to the DNI restriction in the advance directive.

Providing optimal care in an ethical manner is more complicated when dealing with the incapacitated patient.[18] Legally, one must obtain *informed consent*.[17] The State of New York defines "lack of informed consent" to mean:

"*the failure of a person providing the professional treatment or diagnosis to disclose to the patient such alternatives thereto and the reasonably foreseeable risk and benefits involved as a reasonable medical, dental, or podiatric practitioner under similar conditions would have disclosed, in a manner permitting the patient to make a knowledgeable evaluation.*"[10,19,20]

New York further goes on to mandate that the plaintiff (in litigation regarding lack of infirmed consent):

"*establish that a reasonably prudent person in the patient's position would not have undergone the treatment or diagnosis if (s)he had been fully informed and that the lack of informed consent or diagnosis is a proximate cause of the injury or condition for which recovery is sought.*"

Obtaining informed consent prior to a major elective operation involves a thorough explanation of the anatomy, physiology, pathology, and complications of the operation. Thus, this level of informed consent is a paradigm that is never achieved unless, perhaps, the patient is another surgeon.[3] Therefore, consent is based typically upon less-complete information, because even an experienced nonsurgical physician may not really comprehend all of the potential risks of a complex operation or underlying condition.[3] Thus, the legal requirements focus on important or material risks and benefits of having surgery versus nonoperative management. The patient who is not acutely ill must be engaged seriously in the discussion, and even then may not comprehend fully. Such comprehension becomes impossible for a patient with hypotension or sepsis and impaired judgment from altered cerebral blood flow and metabolism. For example, consider a middle-aged patient who presents to the emergency department with a perforated duodenal ulcer and peritonitis. Refusal of operative intervention, in this setting, most likely will result in the death of the patient. In the setting of refusal, the surgeon is obligated to assess the patient's capacity for medical decision making by consulting a disinterested medical professional. If the individual is determined to lack capacity, then authority can be transferred to a surrogate or external legal entity,[3,16] but using the court system to appoint a guardian takes time that the situation may not afford. Often the surgeon must document in writing the life-saving nature of the intervention and the inability of the patient to consent, and then proceed with the emergency operation with the knowledge of the facility's legal representative.[3]

The ethics of surrogate consent are less defined if the incapacitated patient is not in a life-or-death situation. Each surgeon has to determine, within legality, the optimal, ethical solution to a dilemma.[3,17] For example, consider the case of a patient with schizophrenia admitted for recurrent acute pancreatitis due to neuroleptic medications. Following partial improvement with nasogastric suction, intravenous fluids, and nutrition support, a pancreatic pseudocyst associated with ductal ectasia was identified, and a lateral pancreaticojejunostomy was recommended. The patient declined operation but his legal guardian gave permission. Should the surgeon operate against the patient's wishes, or demur and instead offer to refer the patient to another surgeon?[13] In this case, the patient was discharged on a liquid diet, but recurrent dietary intolerance necessitated rehospitalization. Operation was recommended again, accepted by the patient, and carried out without complication and with a good result. Had the operation been performed initially against the patient's wishes but with the consent of the guardian, readmission and substantial additional cost would have been saved.

Refusal of consent may be influenced by temporary incapacity due to the emotional state, or alcohol, or other intoxicants. For example, consider the case of a muscular, young adult male, hypotensive and uncommunicative after a stab wound to the groin, bleeding from a presumed femoral artery injury. He responded to resuscitation and control with direct pressure. Now awake, operation was refused; angry and under the influence of cocaine, the patient was eager to exact revenge upon his assailant. The patient was observed until somnolence supervened, at which time the patient was taken to the operating room under emergency administrative consent for uneventful femoral arteriography. Postoperatively, the patient was apologetic and grateful as a result of the surgeon acting in the best interest of the patient.

A more common dilemma occurs when a patient who has capacity refuses care, such as the receipt of blood or blood products.[10] Case law is unequivocal that a patient with capacity has the legal right to refuse care.[20,21] Consequently, the surgeon who acts contrary to the patient's wish has committed battery.[2,3,13] Even more complex is the circumstance where a patient is willing to have surgery that is likely going to be associated with a need for blood transfusion but, the patient refuses to receive blood or blood products for religious reasons.[22,23] In this setting, the surgeon must determine whether the risk:benefit of the operation justifies performance without availability of blood. Surgery under that parameter increases the risk to the patient, which may be mitigated if the surgeon is experienced and believes that the operation can be performed successfully without blood bank support. Candid discussion among surgeon, patient, and family must occur and must be documented in the medical record.[24] When the surgeon is unable to accept these restrictions, referral to another surgeon must be facilitated.[24] These proscriptions do not apply when the patient is not known and cannot communicate owing to incapacity.[2,25,26] However, discovery of a wallet card prohibiting blood products constitutes valid refusal,[27] and physicians have been found liable for failure to follow such indicia of the patient's wishes (but not for adherence thereto).[27]

Restrictions to treatment do not extend to children whose consents are provided by parents. The surgeon caring for an injured child who needs blood or blood products that have been prohibited by the parents should follow his or her ethical instincts and treat the patient regardless.[21,26] Blood transfusion in this circumstance is correct ethically and protected legally in most states.[21,28] When uncertainty exists in a life-threatening situation, the surgeon is well-advised to administer blood products.[3,17,26]

An advance directive no longer applies when a patient presents after an attempted suicide.[2,3] Emergency surgical intervention is correct legally and fully compliant with ethical standards, and protects the interests of the patient, the caregivers, and the hospital.

THE UNEXPECTED FINDING

A major ethical and legal challenge related to acute care surgery is the unexpected intraoperative finding. Consider the example of an adenocarcinoma of the cecum identified rather than acute appendicitis during appendectomy through a standard low transverse incision. Should the surgeon close, or proceed with a right hemicolectomy? Again, the ethical dilemma in this situation may be resolved according to the Golden Rule.[16,17] If the colon is empty of stool, the patient has normal and stable vital signs, and the hepatic flexure can be mobilized with a modest extension of the incision, proceeding with a definitive right hemicolectomy and primary anastomosis is reasonable. Alternatively, some surgeons will believe that, because colectomy was not consented to they would therefore close, thereby subjecting the patient to subsequent reoperation. This latter approach is also legally correct, but increases the potential for morbidity and mortality. The situation can be mitigated by foresight and common sense. Presuming that a computed tomography scan was performed, identification of a large phlegmon with indistinct features may prompt a request for the patient to consent to "possible bowel resection." Put simply, the best ethical decision is to perform the procedure that provides the best (lowest) risk:benefit for the patient.[17,28]

A different situation arises when a patient is operated upon for an abdominal gunshot wound that is believed to have penetrated the peritoneal cavity near the descending colon. During exploration, the missile tract is found to be retroperitoneal, but the patient has a left-sided colon mass, probably malignant by palpation, with bulk feces within the colon. Should the surgeon close or perform a left hemicolectomy? If resection and primary anastomosis results in a leak causing fatal peritonitis, the assailant might be charged with murder even though the patient died from iatrogenesis. If resection and a colostomy is performed, the patient may be displeased. Even though it is ethically correct for the surgeon to perform the hemicolectomy, the potential for a bad result and the far-reaching consequences for a third party may favor abdominal closure followed by a second operation for cancer.

Definitive care for an unexpected finding is easy to rationalize when the preoperative symptoms are related directly to the unexpected finding, so that lack of definitive care would be detrimental to the patient. For example, a decision may be made to operate on a patient with sudden, severe upper abdominal pain and marked tenderness, even absent any evidence of pneumoperitoneum on imaging studies. At operation, a finding of a ruptured hepatic adenoma with active bleeding mandates definitive therapy. If the surgeon is not experienced with hepatic resection, a colleague should be called in.

THE DILEMMA OF PAIN MANAGEMENT

The baptism of pain as the "fifth vital sign" has created a new ethical dilemma for the acute care surgeon.[29] Physicians and other caregivers, desirous of providing optimal patient care, have promulgated a detailed system for rating the extent of pain and the caregiver response thereto.[30] The Visual Acuity Scale (VAS) has been adopted most frequently to categorize the severity of pain, rating pain from 1 to 10 and permitting both documentation in electronic medical records[29] and monitoring by "authorities" of physician performance/compliance. However, nowhere in the electronic medical record are there easily retrievable data to identify signs and symptoms of overmedication.

The Joint Commission has mandated that whenever a VAS is five or greater, the patient must be reassessed. Nurses working in a busy hospital area routinely give more narcotic because there is insufficient time to do a full reassessment.[30] This knee-jerk response to a VAS of five or greater is commonplace and possibly detrimental, but may go unchallenged for fear of personal recrimination or threatening the hospital's external credentialing.[29] All surgeons, especially acute care surgeons, recognize that pain management is a high priority, but also that preventable death from overmedication is anathema. The authors assessed the effects of this new pain management paradigm, using before-after methodology, on the incidence of preventable deaths following injury among patients treated in hospitals reviewed by the American College of Surgeons Verification Review Committee.[29] The determination of a preventable death was made locally by existing trauma center peer review performance improvement methodology; individual records were reviewed randomly. Preventable deaths due to overmedication increased by 250% following the identification of pain as the "fifth vital sign." Overmedication occurs by multiple routes of administration, including epidural catheter, patient-controlled analgesia, standing orders for medications regardless of patient status, and supplemental medication based on VAS. Taylor et al. reported that oversedation was most likely to occur within 4 hours of a patient arriving on the surgical floor after transfer from a monitored setting,[31] and identified further that a patient was at greatest risk for oversedation (usually, respiratory depression) during the first postoperative day.[32] The risk of preventable death correlated directly with age and with the use of hydromorphone. The pendulum may have swung too far in the management of perioperative pain; it is time for a scientific reassessment of current policies[31,33] and for acute care surgeons to accept personal responsibility.

THE MEDICAL-INDUSTRIAL COMPLEX

When President Dwight D. Eisenhower addressed the 1960 Republican National Convention, he alerted the citizens about the "Military-Industrial Complex." "Ike" warned that contributions to elected officials, in one form or another, could influence military contracts. His prescient predictions have been realized. The same potential conflict of interest exists in 21st century health care and might be referred to as the "Medical-Industrial Complex." Conflict of interest in the development of clinical practice guidelines has been alleged in two recent mass-market books entitled *The Truth About the*

Drug Companies and *On the Take*.[34,35] Many aspects of health care related to acute care surgery are addressed. Examples that relate to acute care surgery include medications and treatment for venous thromboembolic disease, prophylaxis of "stress gastritis," and hemopoietic agents in patients without chronic kidney disease. Commercially-sponsored symposia, designed ostensibly to educate physicians about a specific disease entity or complication, often have commercial bias.[34,35] The pharmaceutical industry is also involved in continuing medical education (CME). Rohrich et al.[36] estimated that 90% of the $1 billion spent annually on CME is supported by industry, and estimated further that the true cost of industrial promotion of pharmaceuticals may exceed $10 billion annually.[36] Acute care surgeons are presented opportunities to participate as faculty and audience members, and must consider their participation carefully.

The ethical dilemma created by industry-sponsored symposia and product self-promotion is complex.[34,35] A good working relationship between the pharmaceutical industry and physicians is necessary in order to promote excellence in health care; indeed, important, valid clinical trials can sometimes only be funded with industry support.[36] However, certain marketing tactics deserve restriction. Rohrich et al.[36] pointed out that many academic health centers no longer allow pharmaceutical companies to sponsor "journal clubs" or other on-premises meal functions. Notably, when the American Medical Association (AMA) membership proposed severance from the strong pharmaceutical support received by the AMA for their annual meetings and postgraduate courses, the leadership was resistant.[34–36] Interestingly, leadership in this arena of conflict of interest has come from younger physicians. The American Medical Student Association (AMSA) developed guidelines in 2003, updated in 2009, which define how the close relationship between medical schools and the pharmaceutical industry should evolve.[37] The AMSA guidelines address gifts (including meals), consulting relationships, industry-funded speaking relationships, disclosure of all industrial support, free pharmaceutical samples, payment to physicians involved with hospital formularies, and exposure to sales representatives, and funded educational activities including on-site support, travel, and scholarships for trainees. The AMSA encourages university oversight of these activities and willingness to implement sanctions for unethical behavior.

THE TRAINING YEARS

Jones and McCullough warned that the ethical challenge begins in the formative years during surgical residency by saying "one can not go back on their upbringing."[18] Numerous opportunities exist for the resident surgeon to be "led astray" as they relate to the ethical future practice of surgery. Residents often witness informed consent discussions.[16] Should a resident identify that certain surgeons perform procedures that are clearly outside of the permission granted by the patient as a matter of routine, the observation must be brought to the attention of the appropriate departmental officials. Hopefully, when presented such evidence, they will summon the courage to forward the information to appropriate hospital committees to sanction the surgeon as appropriate.[33] For difficult cases with a major intraoperative complication, the operative note must reflect the operation accurately, whether dictated by the attending surgeon or the resident. If not, and the dictation was made by the attending surgeon, the resident is obligated to point out to the surgeon that the dictation is inaccurate or incomplete, and offer to do the re-dictation.[24] If the offer is declined and the surgeon does not amend the dictation himself or herself, the resident again has an ethical responsibility to report this to the chief of surgery.[17] Many senior surgeons recall circumstances, during residency training, when a surgeon who no longer (or never) had the requisite technical skills to operate independently, was protected by a chief of surgery who expected the surgical residents to keep the incompetent surgeon "out of trouble."[38] Hopefully, this form of ghost surgery is no longer practiced. If faced with this practice, the resident needs to inform the program director that he or she can no longer assist that surgeon at surgery.[38]

The operating surgeon must behave ethically when obtaining consent for a complicated procedure (and serve as a role model for trainees),[3,17] explaining to the patient the surgical and nonsurgical options and the risks of a specific operation, not only on the basis of published data but also on the best estimate of his or her personal results for the operation. Adherence to the practice of having the attending surgeon obtain consent will influence the resident to be forthright and honest with his or her patients when out in practice and obtaining operative consent.[17,39]

CONFIDENTIALITY

Confidentiality is both an ethical and a legal issue. Increasing emphasis has been placed on protection of the rights of individual patients to confidentiality of their health information. State laws now define the extent to which a patient's medical records may be disclosed as part of therapy, while avoiding a breach of patient confidentiality. Illinois law cautions that "no member of a hospital's medical staff and no agent or employee of a hospital shall disclose the nature or details of services provided to patients,"[40] but makes numerous exceptions, such as for the patient's information or that of their representative regarding treatment, and for those parties providing treatment to the patient, processing payment for that treatment, instituting peer review or risk management, or defending a claim against the hospital regarding that treatment.[40] The prudent physician would be wise to review his or her own state's confidentiality statute, and should not assume that the Illinois statute is representative of that of other states. In Illinois, there are also mandated disclosures under the Abused and Neglected Child Reporting Act, the Illinois Sexually Transmitted Disease Control Act, or "where otherwise authorized or required by law."[29] At the federal level, the Emergency Medical Treatment and Active Labor Act (EMTALA) mandates, among other things, that when a critically ill or -injured patient is transferred to another center for a higher level of care, the patient's records must also be transferred.[10] Records that are not specifically transferred with the patient, but sent at a later time, should not be transmitted by e-mail, which is not secure. Such information needs to be sent by facsimile or secure package delivery after appropriate permission is obtained from the patient or the designated representative.

Safeguards are enhanced when dealing with public figures, who stimulate interest in the news media, who are often more intent on pursuing the story than protecting the individual's right to privacy.[41] Similar safeguards will likely be extended to other valid review activities. This extends to trauma conference rounds and the trauma peer review performance improvement committee meetings whereby the trauma director and other key members of the team review patient outcomes. Patients will, in the near future, likely be identified only by an identifying number rather than by name. This restriction may possibly interfere in the short term with patient care because identifying patients by name is a longstanding tradition, but confidentiality must be perserved.[3,41] While protecting confidentiality, the acute care surgery team must also respect laws of mandatory reporting, particularly those related to communicable diseases and possible abuse.

Included within the framework is the need to secure all physical evidence, such as might be present following a physical assault or rape, to preserve the "chain of evidence." Likewise, one has to protect the evidence chain as it relates to foreign bodies removed from the injured patient, particularly bullets that are needed for forensic analysis.[41] During this process, the trauma surgeon should be continually reminded that, when in doubt, do what is best for the patient.

PALLIATIVE CARE

The acute care surgeon is often faced with medical challenges that cannot be overcome. Severely injured patients with multiple organ dysfunction syndrome after hemorrhagic shock, patients with severe isolated traumatic brain injury, and patients with overwhelming sepsis are examples where even care of the highest quality may fail ultimately.[42,43] Such patients should be managed by the guidelines on palliative care established by the Institute of Medicine.[44] Many of these guidelines were developed for patients with terminal cancer, but apply equally to the acute care surgical patient. The ethical dilemma may actually begin at the time of the initial encounter. Whereas an 85-year-old patient with localized, perforated appendicitis can usually be restored to health by an appendectomy, the same patient with infarcted small bowel from congestive heart failure and mesenteric ischemia due to a low-flow state may not survive an operation. Likewise, the patient with stage IV ovarian cancer who presents with small bowel obstruction from carcinomatosis is unlikely to benefit from operative intervention. Comfort care was described many years ago by Dame Saunders; it involves four principal elements, namely, the physical dimension, the emotional or psychological component, the social and economic ramifications, and finally the spiritual aspect of pain.[45] The acute care surgeon should be comfortable providing support in all four domains.

The goal of palliative care is the physical and psychological comfort of the patient, rather than prolongation of life, and should not be restricted by typical guidelines regarding pin medication. For example, the administration of opioids to the point of respiratory depression is acceptable if other measures fail. Krizek[46] emphasized the importance of teaching these principles in medical school, during residency, and throughout one's practice, particularly, when dealing with acute emergencies. Dunn pointed out that spiritual barriers to surgeons providing palliative care may be an impediment to providing optimal care in this setting.[47] When such barriers are present, the acute care surgeon should seek consultation with a colleague who is more inclined to do whatever is necessary to make the patient comfortable.

Palliative care does not necessarily mean that operative intervention is proscribed. A gastrostomy to palliate uncorrectable bowel obstruction allows the patient to ingest liquids for pleasure, which are thence to drain freely via the gastrostomy tube, thereby avoiding the discomfort of a nasogastric tube or intractable nausea and vomiting.[48]

Often, family members are in conflict with divergent views about ongoing patient care even though the surgical ICU team recognizes that further care is futile.[45] Usually, the patient lacks the capacity to take a decision at this point on the continuum of care. The ICU team can arrange for consultants in different specialties to speak with family members (i.e., the "family meeting"). If these efforts fail to communicate that ongoing support is not in the best interest of the patient, the ethics committee, pastoral care service, and palliative care team should become involved to achieve reconciliation.

ETHICS CURRICULUM

High ethical standards are promulgated when ethical principles are emphasized throughout one's training, beginning ideally in medical school.[49] The huge debts that accrue from tuition and fees do not justify recommending surgery when nonoperative management yields comparable results.[50] Understanding the ethical dilemmas that the surgeon encounters will help the student determine whether or not surgery is a desirable career. As the surgical resident advances through training, formal conferences should emphasize ethical principles in particular. The ACS categorizes the ethics curriculum into six areas of special interest: conflict of interest; professional obligations; substitute decision making; truth-telling in communications; end-of-life issues; and confidentiality. The Royal College of Physicians and Surgeons of Canada adds: Surgical competence, resource allocation, consent taking, and research. Frequent emphasis of these principles is advantageous throughout one's surgical career. One of the last important ethical decisions that the aging surgeon must make is deciding when to retire, or at least stop operating. Part of this decision relates to what is best for one's patients.[2,49]

MEDICAL PROCEDURES ON THE NEWLY DEAD

Ethical dilemmas may extend after death. Smith, in 1824, proposed that medical procedures and dissection could be performed on unclaimed bodies to enhance knowledge of the living.[51] This concept has expanded over the years so that many program directors report that medical procedures are performed upon the newly dead for teaching purposes, without informing the family.[52] Most common is tracheal intubation, but others include central venous catheter placement, venous cutdown, pericardiocentesis, and thoracotomy.[53] Moore has reviewed this phenomenon in detail.[54] Iserson, a strong proponent of this practice without the need for consent, stated that the need to have experience in the performance of these potentially life-saving (and life-threatening) procedures overrides and supersedes any potential objections from the next of kin.[55] Iserson reasoned that this policy is not disrespectful, but rather conveys respect to the newly dead by attaching a societal value to teaching skills that may save a life in the future. Furthermore, Iserson maintained that there is neither a legal nor a moral need to obtain consent.[55] By contrast, Goldblatt concluded that a proxy consent from the next of kin is necessary both legally and ethically.[56] Goldblatt added that the cadaver is protected according to the dictates of the deceased's Last Will and Testament. That a patient dies intestate must not abrogate the rights of family members to authorize or prohibit educational medical procedures.[57] Considering this controversy, the acute care surgeon would be well advised to obtain valid consent before supervising educational procedures on the newly deceased. Although it is uncomfortable to obtain consent at a time when emotions may be running high, it may be possible to obtain consent for endotracheal intubation, tube thoracostomy, cricothyroidotomy, and central line placement.[58] The legal precedents regarding this practice are not settled. All courts would agree that the newly deceased has lost the right of self-determination. The Georgia Supreme Court ruled that harvesting corneas for transplantation did not violate the rights of the deceased or the family.[59] By contrast, the State of Ohio ruled that protection of the cadaver was a constitutionally protected right, and that the next of kin had some rights regarding the cadaver.[60] A violation of this right could lead to litigation of an allegation of "negligent infliction of emotional distress."

Although it is indisputable that the practice of medical interventions on the newly dead provides valuable training that may save lives in the future, there is also no question that many relatives would be distraught if such procedures were performed without permission. Respect for the remains of the newly dead is strongly built into the social structure from the societies of our Native Americans until the current age.[61,62,63] The acute care surgeon who would be in close proximity to many deaths would be advised to obtain consent from the next of kin before becoming involved in the teaching of technical procedures to the surgical residents.

References

1. *The American Heritage* Dictionary © 1992 by Houghton Mifflin Company.
2. Kodner IJ, Freeman DM, Whinney RR, et al. Ethical dilemmas and the law. In: Britt LD, Trunkey DD, Feliciano DV eds. *Acute Care Surgery*. 1st ed. New York: Springer; 2007:715–739.
3. Ledgerwood A, Lucas KA, Lucas CE. The convergence of trauma, medicine, and the law. In: Moore EE, Feliciano DV, Mattox KL, eds. *Trauma*. 6th ed. McGraw-Hill; 2008:1169–1180.
4. Editorial: Dr. Kevorkian's wrong way. *The New York Times*. June 5, 2007.
5. Liptak, A. Ruling upholds Oregon Law authorizing assisted suicide. *The New York Times*. May 27, 2004.
6. Martindale, M. Movie gives Kevorkian's story new life. *The Detroit News*. April 21, 2010.
7. Blow CM. Abortion's new battle lines. *The New York Times*. May 1, 2010.
8. Little M. Invited commentary: is there a distinctively surgical ethics? *Surgery*. 2001;129:668–671.
9. Sorelle R. States said to pass laws limiting liability for lay users of automated external defibrillators. *Circulation*. 1999;99:2606–2607.
10. Takata TS, Page RL, Joglar JA. Automated external defibrillators: Technical considerations and clinical promise. *Ann Intern Med*. 1002;135:990–998.
11. 42 USC SEC. 1395 dd(c)(1)(A)(ii)(2005).
12. VT. Stats. Ann. Sec. 519(a); 2005.
13. Hanlon CR. Ethics in surgery. *J Am Coll Surg*. 1998;196:41–49.
14. Hanlon CR. Surgical ethics. *Am J Surg*. 2004;187:1–2
15. Sanders AB. Advance directives. *Emerg Med Clin N Am*. 1999;17:519–526.
16. Sulmasy DP, Terry PB. More talk, less paper: predicting the accuracy of substituted judgments. *Am J Med*. 1994;96:432–438.
17. Jones JW, McCullough L. The shifting sands in senility: cancelled consent. *J Vasc Surg*. 2008;47:237–238.
18. Vanderpool HV. Surgeons as mirrors of common life: a novel inquiry into the ethics of surgery. *Texas Heart Institute J*. 2009;36:449–450.
19. Jones JW, McCullough LB. How do we guarantee trainee professional purity? *J Vasc Surg*. 2009;49:790–791.
20. Bitterman RA. Legal requirements for transferring trauma patient, in trauma management: An emergency medicine approach. St. Louis, MO, Inc.; 2001:644–649.
21. Nevarez vs. New York City Health and Hospitals Corp. 670 YS2d486 (N.Y.App.Div.1stDept.1998).
22. Goldstein J. Medical care for the child at risk: state supervision of parental authority. *Yale Law J*. 1977;86:645–670.
23. Miller vs. Rhode Island Hospital, 625A.2nd778 (R.I. 1993).
24. Siegel DM. Consent and refusal of treatment. *Emer Med Clin N Am*. 1993;11:833–840.
25. Liang NL, Herring ME, Bush RL. Dealing honestly with an honest mistake. *J Vasc Surg*. 2010;51:494–495.
26. University of Cincinnati Hospital vs. Edmond, 506N.E.2nd299 (Ohio 1986).
27. Werth vs. Taylor, 475N.W.2nd426 (MichApp.1991).
28. Rodriguez vs. Pinol. Suing healthcare providers for saving lives: Liability for providing unwanted life-saving treatment. *J Leg Med*. 1999;20:1–66.
29. Thal ER. Out of apathy. *Bulletin Am Coll Surg*. 1983;78(5):6–14.
30. Lucas CE, Vlahos AL, Ledgerwood A. Kindness kills: the negative impact of "pain" as the fifth vital sign. *J Am Coll Surg*. 2007;205(1):101–107.
31. Pain Management Standards: Joint Commission on Accreditation of Healthcare Organizations (homepage on the internet) ©2005. http://www.jcaho.org/accredited+organizations/hospitals/standards/revisions/index.htm.
32. Taylor S, Voytovich AE, Kozol RA. Has the pendulum swung too far in postoperative pain control? *Am J Surg*. 2003;186(5):472–775.
33. Taylor S, Kirton OC, Staff I, et al. Postoperative day one: a high risk period for respiratory events. *Am J Surg*. 2005;190(5):752–756.
34. *Medication Safety Alert Pain Scales Don't Weigh Every Risk*. Huntington Valley, PA. Institute for Safe Medication Practices; 2002.
35. Angell, M. *The Truth About Drug Companies: How They Deceive Us and What to do About It*. New York: Random House, Inc.; 2004.
36. Kassirer, JP. *On The Take: How Medicine's Complicity with Big Business Can Endanger Your Health*. New York: Oxford University Press, Inc.; 2005.
37. Rohrich RJ, McGrath MH, Lawrence WT, et al. Assessing the plastic surgery workforce: a template for the future of plastic surgery. *Plast Reconstr Surg*. 2010;125(2):736–746.
38. Best Practice Policies. pharmfree.org/amsascorecard.org. © 2003 AMSA PharmFree.
39. Lo B. Serving two masters—conflicts of interest in academic medicine. *N Engl J Med*. 2010;362(8):669–671.
40. Sullivan DJ. Patient discharge against medical advice. *Emerg Dept L L*. 1996;7:91–100.
41. Fields WW, Asplin BR, Larkin GL, et al. The Emergency Medical Treatment and Active Labor Act as a federal healthcare safety net program. *Acad Emerg Med*. 2001;8:1064–1069.
42. Gmoremurgy AS, Norris PA, Olson SM, et al. Pre-hospital traumatic arrest: the cost of futility. *J Trauma*. 1993;35:468–473.
43. Shimazu S, Shatney CH. Outcomes of trauma patients with no vital signs on hospital admission. *J Trauma*. 1983;23:213–216.
44. Consensus Report. Improving palliative care for cancer. Summary and recommendations. Institute of Medicine. April 2003.
45. McCahill LE, Dunn GP, Mosenthal AC, et al. Palliation as a core surgical principle: part 1. *J Am Coll Surg*. 2004;199:149–159.
46. Krizek TJ. Ethics and philosophy lecture: surgery—is it an impairing profession? *J Am Coll Surg*. 2002;194:352–366.
47. Dunn GP. Reclaiming palliative care as a surgical tradition. Palliative Care Symposium. *J Am Coll Surg*. 2004;199(1):150–156.
48. Mosenthal AC. Evidence-based outcomes in surgical palliative care. Palliative Care Symposium. *J Am Coll Surg*. 2004;199(1):156–160.
49. Kodner IJ. Ethics curricula in surgery: needs and approaches. *World J Surg*. 2003;27:952–956.
50. Jones JW, McCullough LB. Intentional over-treatment: The unmentionable conflict-of-interest. *J Vasc Surg*. 2007;46:605–607.
51. Smith TS. Use of the dead to the living. *Westminster Rev*. 1824;2:59–97.
52. Crawford T. Intubation training seems mysterious. *Physician Exec*. 1987;13:25–26.
53. Burns JP, Reardon FE, Truog RD. Sounding board: Using newly deceased patients to teach resuscitation procedures. *N Engl J Med*. 1994;331:1652–1655.
54. Moore GP. Ethics seminars: the practice of medical procedures on newly dead patients—is consent warranted? *Acad Emerg Med*. 2001;8:389–392.
55. Iserson KB. Post-mortem procedures in the emergency department: using the recently dead to practice and teach. *J Med Ethics*. 1993;19:92–98.
56. Goldblatt AD. Don't ask, don't tell: Practicing minimally invasive resuscitation techniques on the newly dead. *Ann Emerg Med*. 1995;25:86–90.
57. Alden AW, Ward KL, Moore GP. Should post-mortem procedures be practiced on recently deceased patients? A survey of relative's attitudes. *Acad Emerg Med*. 1999;6:749–751.
58. Olsen J, Spilger S, Windisch T. Feasibility of obtaining family consent for teaching cricothyroidotomy on the newly dead in the emergency department. *Ann Emerg Med*. 1995;25:660–665.
59. Georgia Lions I Bank, INC vs Lavant, 255 Ga. 60,335 S.E. 2d 127
60. Brotherton vs Cleveland, 923 F. 2d 477 (6th) Cir. 1991.
61. Perkins HS, Gordon AM. Should hospital policy require consent for practicing invasive procedures on cadavers? The arguments, conclusions, and lessons learned from one ethics committee's deliberations. *J Clin Ethics*. 1994;5:204–210.
62. Cruzan vs. Director, Missouri Department of Health, 497 UP261,279(1990).
63. Weaver WD, Hill D, Fahrenbruch D, et al. Use of automated external defibrillator in the management of out-of-hospital cardiac arrest. *N Engl J Med*. 1988;319:666–667.

CHAPTER 63 ■ SCORING SYSTEMS FOR INJURY AND EMERGENCY GENERAL SURGERY

SHAWN NESSEN AND JOHN FILDES

SCORING SYSTEMS FOR INJURY

Introduction

Modern injury severity scoring is an important aspect of managing injured patients because it allows the quantification of an injury and the probability of survival based on the injury scale score. In the field injury, scoring has been used to create field triage systems, and in smaller hospitals, it can be used to aid in the determination of which patients should be transferred to higher levels of care. An important purpose of any scoring system is to allow comparison between similarly injured patients treated at different hospitals and in different trauma systems. Injury scoring controls bias in research by allowing comparison between similarly injured patient populations. The ideal scoring system allows the correlation of increasing injury with mortality, and considers anatomic injury, physiologic derangement, and the comorbid conditions of the patient. The score should be easily calculated and reproducible. Injury scoring systems attempt to predict expected outcomes based on the severity of a given patient's injury. The ability to quantify injury in this way makes accurate scoring systems excellent quality assurance tools.

For the acute care surgeon, extending organ injury severity grading into the realm of nontrauma emergency surgery is appealing and in some cases has been attempted. An example of this is the Hinchey classification of diverticular pericolonic abscesses. Similar to injury scoring, classifying the extent of the pathologic process allows quantification that facilitates quality improvement and research, and guides treatment.

Field Triage Scoring Systems

Triage can be broadly defined as identifying those patients who, if given immediate appropriate medical treatment, will likely survive their wounds. It endeavors to separate those who are minimally or fatally injured from those who will most benefit from timely care.[1] Emergency medical system personnel usually make the first and often most critical triage decisions. For this reason, injury severity scoring systems that accurately and consistently quantify injury for triage purposes are extremely valuable. Field triage systems must categorize patients in such a way as to insure the most severely injured patients are taken to the most capable trauma facilities while ideally preventing such facilities from being overburdened with patients who have inconsequential injuries. The key components of field triage systems include injuries to the central nervous, cardiovascular, and respiratory systems.[2]

The Glasgow Coma Scale

Among the first and most successful of the trauma grading systems was the Glasgow Coma Score (GCS). Developed by Teasdale and Jennett in 1974,[3] this commonly used scale assesses the degree of head injury, and it has predictive value as to outcome. GCS includes three clinical evaluations of eye opening, verbal expression, and motor response. Each component is then assigned a numerical score (Table 63.1). The scale is graded with the best eye opening response receiving a maximum score of 4 points, the best verbal response receiving a maximum score of 5 points and the best motor response receiving a maximum score of 6 points. A lower score indicates worsening neurologic injury, and this allows for quantification of injury to mild, moderate, and severe. This has clinical implications that include indications for intubation, intracranial monitoring, and surgical decompression.[4] The GSC was revised a single time in 1977 increasing the maximum score for motor response from 5 to 6, emphasizing the relative importance of the motor response in the overall evaluation in the patient's neurologic exam.[5] The relative ease of use and reproducibility of the GCS in the context of the overall contribution of neurologic injury to subsequent morbidity and mortality of trauma patients make it an important component of field triage systems.

The Revised Trauma Score

The Revised Trauma Score (RTS) is a revision of the earlier Triage Index[6] and subsequent Trauma score. The Trauma Score was developed by Howard Champion, William Sacco, Wayne Copes and others as both a quantitative injury scale with predictive value and as a simple and reproducible triage tool for EMS personnel for which it gained wide acceptance.[7] The Trauma score assigned point values for respiratory rate (RR), respiratory effort, systolic blood pressure (SBP), capillary refill, and GCS. In revising the trauma score, the authors acknowledge respiratory effort and capillary refill were difficult to assess and some head injury patients were undertriaged. The RTS eliminated capillary refill and respiratory effort components, adopted commonly accepted intervals for GCS, adjusted values for SBP and RR, and validated the score with empirical data (see Table 63.2).

Two configurations of the score were created, one for triage (Triage RTS) and one to predict outcome (RTS).[8] The field component (T-RTS) is strictly additive and can be quickly calculated in the field. The Triage-RTS is used in the prehospital setting and assigns a maximum of 4 points to the respiratory rate, systolic blood pressure, and the GCS. The maximum point value is 12. A T-RTS of ≤ 11 is a strong indicator that a patient should be transferred to a trauma center (Table 63.2).

The second iteration of the RTS is used for predicting outcome and comparing patient data sets. The RTS is defined as

$$\text{RTS} = 0.9368\ \text{GCS} + 0.7326\ \text{SBP} + 0.2908\ \text{RR}$$

The RTS has a range from 0 to 7.841, is heavily weighted toward neurologic injury, and correlates well with the

TABLE 63.1

THE GCS IS A WEIGHTED SCORING SYSTEM FOR NEUROLOGIC INJURY WITH MOTOR RESPONSE THE MOST HEAVILY WEIGHTED COMPONENT

GLASGOW COMA SCALE	
Best motor response	**Score**
Follows commands	6
Localizes pain	5
Withdraws from pain	4
Decorticate posturing (flexion)	3
Decerebrate posturing (extension)	2
No response	1
Best verbal response	
Normal conversation	5
Disoriented comprehensible conversation	4
Inappropriate comprehensible words	3
Incomprehensible words	2
No verbalization	1
Best eye-opening response	
Spontaneous	4
To command	3
To painful stimulus	2
No eye opening	1

TABLE 63.2

THE TRIAGE-RTS IS AN ADDITIVE SCORE

TRIAGE RTS	
Respiratory rate (per minute)	**Score**
10–29	4
>29	3
6–9	2
1–5	1
0	0
Systolic blood pressure (mmHg)	
>89	4
76–89	3
50–75	2
1–49	1
0	0
GCS	
13–15	4
9–12	3
6–8	2
4–5	1
<4	0

Any score ≤11 suggests the patient should be taken to a trauma center.

probability of survival. It is an important component of the trauma injury score methodology, to be discussed later in the text.[8]

Pediatric Trauma Score

The Pediatric Trauma score is similar to the RTS but designed for children. It has six components: weight, airway, systolic blood pressure, central nervous system, open wound, and skeletal injury. Each component is given a score of –1 to 2, and patients with a score <8 should be transferred to a pediatric trauma center.[9]

Center for Disease Control National Guidelines for Field Triage of Injured Patients

In 2009, the Center for Disease Control (CDC) issued Guidelines for the field triage of injured patients. The expert panel based the criteria on physiologic criteria, anatomical criteria, mechanism-of-injury criteria and special considerations to include age <5 or >55, pregnancy, burns, and comorbidities such as diabetes mellitus and coronary artery disease. Patients with a GCS < 14, systolic blood pressure <90 mmHg, or respiratory rate <10 or >29 or <20/min in an infant under 1 year of age are triaged to a trauma center. Similarly, patients with penetrating injuries to the head, neck, torso, and extremities proximal to the knee; flail chest; two or more proximal long bone fractures; crushed, degloved, or mangled extremity; amputation proximal to the wrist or ankle; pelvic fractures; open or depressed skull fractures; or paralysis should be taken to a trauma center. Finally, it is recommended that in patients older than 55, consideration for transport to a trauma center should be undertaken. The CDC's recommendations include all of the elements of an effective injury scoring system to include physiologic, anatomical, and comorbid conditions.[10]

Anatomic Injury Scoring Systems

Abbreviated Injury Scale In 1969, a Joint Committee of the American Medical Association called the Society of Automotive Engineers and the Association for the Advancement of Automotive Medicine began to develop a scale to classify injuries and their severity. The first scale was published in the *Journal of the American Medical Association* in 1971.[11] The AIS has been revised several times by the Association for Advancement of Automotive Medicine, including the most recent 2008 update.

The AIS is not a scoring system. It is rather an anatomically based scale that classifies injuries on a 6-point scale with a score of 1 representing a mild injury and 6 representing an almost always nonsurvivable injury (Table 63.3). The scale is based on consensus opinion and simply describes the organ injury. The AIS does not attempt to predict survivability of injuries, and there is not a linear correlation to the injuries classified and patient outcome. AIS has been revised to have comparability with the Organ Injury Scales of the American Association for the Surgery of Trauma.

The use of the AIS scale can often be confusing. For example, for a given body region, a scale of 4 represents severe injury and a scale of 5 represents critical injury. To know the difference between a severe and critical injury for a given organ requires referencing the AIS manual. As an example, a grade 4 liver injury involves "parenchymal disruption of ≤75% hepatic lobe; or multiple lacerations >3 cm deep; or a 'burst' injury." A grade 5 liver injury involves "parenchymal disruption of >75% of hepatic lobe or >3 *Couinard's* segments within a single lobe or involving retrohepatic vena cava, or central hepatic veins."[12] The documentation of injury grade is sufficiently complicated to require training for coders who document scores.

The Injury Severity Score The injury severity score (ISS) was introduced in 1974 by Susan P. Baker and others. In their landmark paper, the authors pointed out the difficulty of comparing large numbers of patients with very similar injuries and

TABLE 63.3

GENERAL CATEGORIES OF THE ABBREVIATED INJURY SCALE

ABBREVIATED INJURY SCALE	
INJURY	SCORE
Minor	1
Moderate	2
Serious	3
Severe	4
Critical	5
Unsurvivable	6

instead proposed comparing patients who did not necessarily have similar injuries but instead had similar injury severity. In evaluating the AIS as a scoring system, they found that the AIS was nonlinear as mortality increased disproportionately with increasing severity. Further, the death rates for persons with two injuries of grade 4 and 3 (mortality 24%) did not have comparable mortality to patients with injuries of grade 5 and 2 (mortality 54%). They also recognized that the AIS pertained to individual injuries and state in their paper that most automotive crashes involve multiple injuries.[13]

Deducing that the simplest nonlinear equation is quadratic, the authors then determined to square the AIS grades for the most severe injury in each body region and then add the scores together. When adding the sums of the two highest squared AIS grades, death rates were found to be similar for comparable totals. The sum of the three highest squared AIS grades improved the correlation between the ISS and mortality. Adding the fourth squared AIS did not improve accuracy. The ISS was therefore defined as the "sum of the squares of the highest AIS grade in each of the three most severely injured areas."[13]

The ISS divides the body into six anatomical regions including the head or neck, face, chest, abdomen/pelvis, extremities, and external and then assigns a score to each region based on the AIS scale. The three highest scores are then squared and added together resulting in the ISS. If a patient receives an ISS of 6 in any anatomical region, a score of 75 is assigned, and the patient is presumed to have nonsurvivable injury.

The ISS has been found to correlate well with mortality and revolutionized trauma research. The immediate impact of the ISS was to allow retrospective analysis of treatment quality and effectiveness as well as comparison between similarly injured patients treated at different hospitals and in different trauma systems.[14,15] However, the ISS does have notable limitations.

The ISS only considers one injury in a body region when multiple serious injuries may exist which may result in the ISS underestimating injury in these cases. For example, a patient with a severe liver injury given an ISS score of 25 and a patient with the same liver injury and an inferior vena cava injury with an injury severity score of 16 would be given the same ISS of 25. The ISS is derived from the AIS scale, which was designed to categorize victims of motor vehicle crashes and therefore is primarily a measure of blunt trauma. Recent revisions have added penetrating injury, but the ISS may underestimate penetrating injury severity. The ISS places equal emphasis on injuries in all body regions. Because the score is not weighted, an injury to the head with an ISS score of 25 may have a different mortality compared to an extremity injury with a score of 25. The ISS is only an anatomic score as it does not consider physiologic derangement or patient comorbidities. The ISS is thought to be ordinal (well ordered) and monotonic (always increasing); however, this is not true. Kilgo and colleagues using 171,149 patients from the National Trauma Data Base demonstrated that the ISS is nonmonotonic, an example being that an ISS of 25 had a mortality of 43% while an ISS of 27 had a mortality of 14%. Further the ISS scale is from 1 to 75, but only 44 values exist, and several different combinations of injury result in the same score with disparate mortalities for the same value.[16]

Despite substantial limitations, the ISS remains the most popular injury scoring system. The ISS is simple to understand and easy to calculate. Scores from 1 to 8 have a mortality of approximately 1% (minor injury), scores from 9 to 14 have a mortality of approximately 2% (moderate injury), scores from 16 to 24 have a mortality of approximately 7% (severe injury), and scores ≥25 have a mortality of >30% (very severe injury) (Fig. 63.1).

New Injury Severity Score Turner Osler, Susan Baker, and William Long introduced the New Injury Severity Score (NISS) in 1997. This score attempted to improve on the original ISS by using the three most severe injuries regardless of anatomical region. This modification eliminated one of the primary criticisms of the ISS, and ability of the NISS to predict mortality was found by the authors to be superior to that of the ISS. In their original paper, the authors reported that approximately 60% of patients had different NISS scores compared to ISS scores with the NISS being higher than the ISS in all cases. The authors reported data from two separate hospitals and using receiver operating characteristics found the ISS to have a 0.869 predictive value in one institution compared to 0.896 using NISS. In the second institution, ISS was found to have 0.896 predictive value compared to 0.907 using NISS. In both cases the improvement was found to be statistically significant.[17] The NISS, however, like ISS is nonmonotonic, nonlinear, and not ordinal, and it has failed to replace ISS as the standard anatomical ISS.[16]

Anatomic Profile Score Wayne S. Copes, Howard R. Champion, and others identified three fundamental problems with the ISS. They felt the ISS underestimates in many cases the severity of injury because it is limited to the single worst injury in three body regions. Second, the ISS has multiple diverse injury combinations that result in similar ISS, but have clearly distinct survival differences, and third and importantly, the ISS gives the same importance or weight to the same AIS score in different body regions. Their example is that a laceration to the brain and stomach give an AIS score of 4, and an ISS of 16 would predict the same outcome.[18]

Their solution was to develop the anatomic profile (AP). The AP adjusts for severity in body regions by creating the modified components mA, mB, and mC. Each modified component includes all injuries in the given body region, and the regions are weighted differently based on the expected outcome in the body region. The mA component includes the head/brain and spinal cord, the mB component includes the thorax and neck injuries, and the mC component consists of all other injuries. AIS scores of 1 and 2 are not included. The score itself is derived by adding the squares of each AIS injury ≥3, adding the scores and then determining the square root of the total. A coefficient is then assigned to each component.

$$\text{APS} = 0.3199(\text{mA}) + 0.4381(\text{mB}) + 0.1406(\text{mC}) + 0.7961(\text{maxAIS})$$

Although the authors showed that AP better discriminated survivors from nonsurvivors compared to ISS and was more sensitive than ISS, it has failed to replace the venerable ISS.

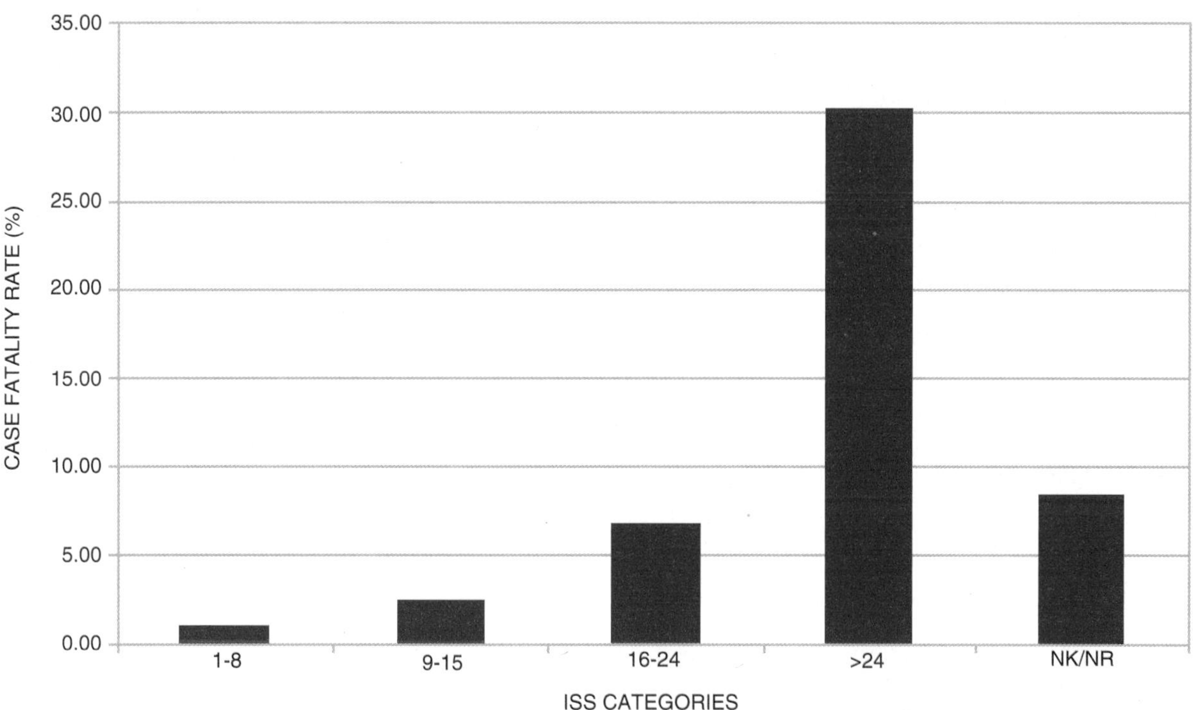

FIGURE 63.1. Case fatality rates by ISS from the 2010 National Trauma Data Base.

Scores Used to Predict Outcome

The TRISS Methodology The TRISS method combines the components of the RTS with the ISS to generate a probability of survival for individual trauma patients. Additionally, TRISS adds a calculation for age and separate coefficients for blunt and penetrating mechanisms. The TRISS method is used to quantify the severity of injury of a patient population, calculates the probability of survival of patients for identification of cases for peer review, and compares the death or survival rates of different populations.[19]

The TRISS methodology is most commonly used to generate a probability of survival for a patient using the following equation:

$$\text{Ps} = 1/(1+e^{-j})$$

$$\text{Where } j = j_0 + j_1(\text{TS}) + j_2(\text{ISS}) + j_3(A)$$

The *b* coefficients in the equation were derived using Walker-Duncan regression analysis of thousands of patients from the Major Trauma Outcome Study.[20] *A* represents age with $A = 1$ for patients age 55 and older and $A = 0$ for patients 54 and younger. Given a 55-year-old male with a GCS of 10, a systolic blood pressure of 88 mmHg, and a respiratory rate of 22/min, the RTS is 6.171. Assuming a blunt head injury with an ISS of 25:

$$j = -1.2470 + 0.9544(6.171) + -0.0768(25) + -1.9052(1)$$

$$j = 0.8174$$

$$\text{Ps} = 1/(1+2.718282^{-(0.8174)})$$

$$\text{Ps} = 1/(1 + 0.4416)$$

$$\text{PS} = 0.69$$

This patient, aged 55, with a blunt head injury has a probability of survival of 69%. The same patient with a penetrating injury would have a probability of survival of 70%. A 44-year-old with the same injury scores would have a probability of survival of 92% for a blunt injury and 88% for penetrating injury.

Once survival probabilities of a group of patients have been determined, they can be plotted against an S 50 isobar using the RTS on the vertical axis and ISS on the horizontal axis. Patients are thought to be unexpected deaths if they have a probability of survival of 50% or higher and die. Patients with a survival probability of <50% who survive are unexpected survivors. It has been suggested that patients who are unexpected deaths should undergo peer review. Using statistical analysis, survival probabilities can be used to compare subsets of patients to determine if survivors and deaths fall within expected parameters.[21]

Criticisms of the TRISS methodology are several. The MTOS database from which the coefficients were derived may be quite different than the population being evaluated. Care must be taken to assure a sufficient match among populations. The sensitivity of the S 50 isobar is also questioned. While a patient with a 52% survival probability who dies is categorized as an unexpected death, the patient had a 48% probability of dying. Therefore, care must be exercised when using the TRISS methodology for evaluating isolated patients.

A Severity Characterization of Trauma The AP score is an attempt to replace the ISS with a weighted anatomical scoring system. Champion and colleagues with a severity characterization of trauma (ASCOT) upgrade TRISS using the AP score in place of the ISS. The equation for the ASCOT methodology is similar to TRISS.

$$\text{Ps} = 1/(1+e^{-k})$$

$$\text{Where } k = k_1 + k_2\,\text{G} + k_3\,\text{S} + k_4\,\text{R} + k_5\,\text{A} + k_6\,\text{B} + k_7\,\text{C} + k_8\,\text{Age}$$

The k coefficients for ASCOT like TRISS are derived from regression analysis of patients from the Major Trauma

Outcome Study. The constants G, S, and R represent the GCS, systolic blood pressure, and respiratory rate from the RTS, and the constants A, B, and C are obtained from the first three components of the APS score. The age component of ASCOT has five categories with a numeric scale of 0–4 with the assigned value increasing as age increases.[22] ASCOT has not replaced TRISS. It is substantially more complex than TRISS, and the improvements it offers are not dramatic. A subsequent comparison of TRISS versus ASCOT found the two to be essentially equal in their predictive power.[23]

International Classification of Disease Injury Severity Score The International Classification of Disease Injury Severity Score (ICISS) instead of using AIS grades uses survival risk ratios derived from ICD-9 codes. Survival risk ratios (SRR) are derived for each ICD-9 code by determining the number of patients who survive the coded injury and dividing that number by the total number of patients with the injury. Once SRRs have been developed for a group of patients from a database, the ICISS score is determined by the formula

$$\text{ICISS} = \left(\text{SRR}_{\text{inj }1}\right)\left(\text{SRR}_{\text{inj}2}\right)\left(\text{SRR}_{\text{inj}3}\right)\left(\text{SRR}_{\text{inj}\ldots\text{last}}\right)$$

The ICISS is the product of all available SRRs for a given patient and is bounded by 0 and 1. An ICISS of 0.5 corresponds to a predicted survival of 50%.

Osler and colleagues introduced ICISS in 1996. In their original description, they developed SRRs for ICD-9 codes using 314,402 patients from the North Carolina database. Once the ratios were obtained, they compared ICISS to ISS using 3,142 trauma patients from the University of New Mexico. ICISS was found in their study to outperform ISS for both penetrating and blunt trauma.[24] They also combined RTS and age to ICISS to create a survival probability model, which they then compared to the TRISS methodology. They found the ICISS model outperformed TRISS in determining probability of survival for both penetrating and blunt injury.[22]

The appeal of a scoring system that used ICD-9–based codes is that smaller trauma centers that do not have the resources to calculate AIS and ISS scores can use the universal ICD-9 codes to predict mortality and develop probability of survival models. ICISS is derived empirically and is not determined by consensus. When large databases are used to derive SRRs, the predictive value of a specific injury is powerful. Because all injuries to a particular patient are used to calculate ICISS, the significance of lesser injuries is overestimated. This is mitigated to some degree. Indeed, Osler and his coauthors identified approximately 100 injuries that were associated with most fatalities. Chief among these were head, burn, and thoracic and abdominal vascular injuries.[22] This finding lends credibility to scoring systems that use only the worst injury like MAXAIS which in one study outperformed multi-injury scoring systems.[25]

Trauma scoring systems are useful as they allow the quantification of injury and the probability of survival based on injury scale score. They have been used to create field triage systems and allow comparison of similarly injured patients treated in different hospital and trauma systems. They are also valuable as a screening tool for quality assurance programs. They are not, however, effective for screening individual patients. A patient with a predicted survival of 55% also has 45% mortality. The variables that determine such a patient's outcome are complex and include the patient's age, comorbidities, prehospital care, and the capabilities of the hospital staff and surgeons, to name a few. The closer the probability of survival to the Survival 50 Isobar, the less able any scoring method is to discriminate outcome. For the purpose of quality improvement, scoring systems are best used to evaluate trauma populations and system outcomes.

SCORING SYSTEMS FOR EMERGENCY GENERAL SURGERY

Introduction and Background

Scoring systems for emergency general surgery must describe the severity of each surgical disease in a way that relates to treatment, complications, and outcomes. The accuracy of a scoring system can be evaluated using statistical measures such as sensitivity, specificity, positive predictive value, and the negative predictive value. The scoring systems in trauma describe the anatomic and physiologic parameters present in the patient. Cancer scoring systems describe the primary tumor, the nodal status, and metastasis. These allow for standardization of patients and comparison of treatment and outcomes. The scoring systems for emergency general surgery are not as well developed, making it difficult to construct research studies and reach firm conclusions about many of these conditions.

Emergency general surgical conditions can be broadly classified as obstruction, perforation, ischemia, infection, or bleeding affecting an organ system or specific anatomical site. Examples are found in the respiratory, cardiovascular, gastrointestinal, and genitourinary systems. These conditions include airway obstruction, pneumothorax, vascular thrombus and embolus, small bowel obstruction, cholecystitis, diverticulitis, duodenal ulcer disease, pancreatitis, and urinary retention, to name a few. There is an opportunity to develop scoring systems for many of these conditions (Table 63.4).

Scoring systems focus on three broad areas: the grade of the anatomic lesion, the physiologic response of the patient, and the patient-specific factors. Some anatomic scoring systems have been developed using the radiographic appearance, operative findings, or pathologic examination to grade the lesion. Other scoring systems describe the physiologic response of the patient to their disease. These responses can be clinical measurements such as temperature, white blood cell count, heart rate, respiratory rate, and blood pressure, or they can be physical findings like localized pain and peritonitis. The systemic inflammatory response syndrome (SIRS) score is an example of a physiologic scoring system.[26,27] Still other scoring systems use patient factors such as age, comorbid conditions, and preexisting diseases. The APACHE II score and Apache III score use physiologic data and patient factors together.[28,29] The American Society of Anesthesiologists (ASA) scoring system uses the patient's physical status, from healthy to moribund, followed by an E for emergency surgery. Anatomic, physiologic, and patient factors all affect surgical decision making, treatment, and the prediction of outcome. Combining these into multiple-factor scoring systems represents the best way to categorize patients, their disease processes, and response to therapy.

This chapter describes some of the best-known scoring systems used to describe common clinical problems in emergency general surgery. This section is also meant to highlight the gaps and opportunities for the research and the need to develop new scoring systems.

Acute Cholecystitis

Gallbladder disease is a common surgical condition with several etiologies. They include acute cholecystitis, chronic cholecystitis, acalculous cholecystitis, biliary colic, and biliary dyskinesia, or are associated with ascending cholangitis. It is crucial that a unified definition of acute cholecystitis exist. The diagnostic criteria and severity assessment of acute cholecystitis were discussed and finalized at an international consensus meeting in Tokyo in 2006.[30] The "Tokyo Guidelines" define acute cholecystitis as signs of local inflammation such

TABLE 63.4

CLASSIFICATION OF EMERGENCY GENERAL SURGERY CONDITIONS

	OBSTRUCTION	PERFORATION	ISCHEMIA	INFECTION	BLEEDING
Respiratory					
• Trachea and bronchus					
• Lung					
Cardiovascular					
• Heart					
• Cervical vascular					
• Thoracic vascular					
• Abdominal vascular					
• Peripheral vascular					
Gastrointestinal					
• Esophagus					
• Stomach					
• Duodenum					
• Small bowel					
• Colon					
• Rectum					
Hepatobiliary and pancreatic					
• Liver					
• Extrahepatic biliary tree					
• Pancreas					
Genitourinary					
• Kidney					
• Ureter					
• Bladder					
• Urethra					

Adapted from the AAST Organ Injury Scaling. Scoring systems for emergency general surgery conditions exist for some of the common problems that could be included in this array. There is little uniformity among them as you would find in trauma or cancer scoring systems.

as Murphy's sign, a mass, or localized pain and tenderness in the right upper quadrant combined with signs of systemic inflammation such as fever, elevated white blood cell count, or elevated C-reactive protein concentrations. In patients who are suspected of having acute cholecystitis, the diagnosis can be confirmed with imaging studies. The consensus group classified severity into three groups: mild (grade I), moderate (grade II), and severe (grade III). Grade I was described as mild acute cholecystitis in a patient with no systemic organ dysfunction and disease limited to the gallbladder. Cholecystectomy was viewed as a low-risk procedure in this group. Grade II was described as moderate acute cholecystitis in a patient with no systemic organ dysfunction but with extensive disease in the gallbladder. Cholecystectomy was viewed as a difficult procedure to safely perform in this group. The clinical features differentiating grade I from grade II include disease duration > 72 hours with increased fever, white blood cell count, pain and tenderness, palpable mass, and imaging studies showing substantial inflammatory changes. Grade III was described as severe acute cholecystitis in a patient with systemic organ dysfunction.

The Tokyo criteria provide an international consensus and evidence-based guideline for the definition and severity of acute cholecystitis. This is an important step in the development of similar scoring systems for other emergency surgical conditions of the gallbladder and biliary tree including ascending cholecystitis.

A scoring system for complications following cholecystectomy has been proposed.[31] This prospective nonrandomized study compared laparoscopic to open cholecystectomy. The Tokyo criteria were not used in this study. Complications were divided into four grades. Grade 1 was a deviation from the ideal postoperative course with spontaneous resolution and no increase in the length of stay. Grade 2 was a transient threat to the patient's life that may have required invasive procedures and management. Grade 3 was a persistent threat to the patient's life that required invasive procedures and was accompanied by permanent sequel. Grade 4 was death of the patient. This type of scoring system focuses on patient safety and outcomes. These are essential when evaluating treatment options in specific patient populations.

Pancreatitis

Pancreatitis is one of the best examples of an emergency general surgery condition that has had scoring systems developed and studied. Acute pancreatitis ranges from a mild self-limiting disease to a fatal illness. This unpredictability stimulated the development of objective scoring systems to predict the clinical course, identify patients for clinical trials, and to compare outcomes.[32] The best-known scoring system is the Ranson Score or Ranson Criteria, introduced in 1974.[33] Ranson developed a multiple-factor score that is calculated on admission and at 48 hours after admission. It assigns a value of 1 or 0 if the criteria are present or absent before calculating the total score. Ranson focused on measures that were related to patient factors and the pathophysiologic manifestations of the disease. The admission criteria include age, white blood cell count, serum glucose, serum lactate dehydrogenase, and serum aspartate transaminase. At 48 hours, the criteria include change in hematocrit, change in blood urea nitrogen, serum calcium, oxygenation, base deficit, and intravenous fluid requirements. These criteria have been widely used, critically evaluated, and modified over time.

The APACHE II score was introduced in 1985 as way to prognostically stratify acutely ill ICU patients.[28] It is a multiple-factor score that assigns a range of values to each criterion before calculating the total score. The criteria include temperature, mean arterial pressure, heart rate, respiratory rate, oxygenation, arterial pH, serum sodium, serum potassium, serum creatinine, hematocrit, white blood cell count, and GCS. While APACHE II was never developed for pancreatitis, it was found to be a more accurate scoring system for the prediction of outcome and attacks of severe pancreatitis than the Ranson Score.[34] It is common to see the two used in combination.

Computed tomography (CT) severity scoring was the next advance.[35] Initial and follow-up contrast-enhanced CT scans were compared to the patient's clinical course and Ranson score. These CT scans provided better prognostic accuracy. In addition, they improved clinical decision making by differentiating the anatomic lesion as pancreatic inflammation, phlegmon, the degree of necrosis, and the presence of abscess or pseudocyst. Enhanced MRI is now considered comparable to enhanced CT scan.

Further refinement of the definition and severity scoring system for severe acute pancreatitis revealed a 29% decrease in early in hospital deaths.[36] The most recent guideline for acute pancreatitis states that "severity assessment is essential for the selection of the proper initial treatment."[37] These show the relationship between scoring systems with high prognostic accuracy as a driver for clinical care and improved outcomes.

Small Bowel Obstruction

The efforts to create a scoring system for small bowel obstruction were led by radiologists. The diagnosis of intestinal obstruction is usually suspected by history and physical exam. Patients with shock, peritonitis, free air, or other compelling findings require emergency surgery. In the ambiguous case, however, diagnostic studies are helpful. The CT scan can identify the level of obstruction in the gastrointestinal tract, if high- or low-grade obstruction is present, and if strangulation or closed loop obstruction is present.[38] The use of intravenous contrast and 1-mm cuts improves the accuracy and can usually distinguish extrinsic lesions, intrinsic lesions, intussusceptions, and intraluminal foreign bodies.[39] Further experience has led to CT scoring systems that predict the need for surgery by correlating specific anatomic CT findings to the need for emergency surgery and the intraoperative findings.[40] Newer predictive models have incorporated physiologic responses and patient factors to this approach.[41]

Diverticulitis

Diverticulitis is easily diagnosed using the patient's history, physical exam, and diagnostic studies. New treatment paradigms have emerged because the anatomic, physiologic, and patient factors can be accurately described.[42] CT scans were prospectively correlated with patient's clinical course to propose a system for classifying the severity of diverticulitis and to guide clinical management.[43] CT findings consistent with mild diverticulitis included localized wall thickening (>5 mm) and inflammation of the pericolic fat. CT findings consistent with severe diverticulitis included wall thickening (>5 mm) and inflammation of the pericolic fat plus the presence of an abscess, extraluminal air, or extraluminal contrast. Patients with findings consistent with severe diverticulitis underwent operative management more frequently. These findings were also associated with recurrences in patients treated without surgery.

The timing of surgery is determined by the anatomic and physiologic severity of the disease and the patient factors.[44] These are described using the findings in the physical exam, CT scans, as well as the data associated with the ASA, APACHE II/III, or SIRS scoring systems.

Peritonitis-based scoring systems have been used to study the decision making and choice of operations for diverticulitis. Some of the best-known examples are the Hinchey classification,[45] the Mannheim peritonitis Index (MPI),[46] and the colorectal physiologic and operative severity score for the enumeration of mortality and morbidity (Cr-POSSUM).[47] The Hinchey classification system defines stage 1 as pericolic or mesenteric abscess, stage 2 as pelvic or retroperitoneal abscess, stage 3 as purulent peritonitis, and stage 4 as feculent peritonitis (Table 63.5). The Hinchey classification is widely used for research and operative decision making.[48] The MPI includes only clinical risk factors that are commonly documented for perioperative patients. The parameters include age, gender, organ failure(s), presence of malignancy, preoperative peritonitis more than 24 hours, presence of diffuse generalized peritonitis, site of primary focus, and the nature of peritoneal exudative fluid. The Cr-POSSUM appeared to be a promising tool for colorectal cancer surgery and must be evaluated for complicated diverticulitis.

Appendicitis

Acute appendicitis is a long-studied emergency general surgery condition in search of a unified scoring system. The Alvarado Score is based on eight predictive factors found to be useful in making the diagnosis of appendicitis.[49] They include localized tenderness in the right lower quadrant, increased white blood cell count, migration of pain from the umbilicus, increased polymorphonuclear neutrophils, increased temperature, nausea and vomiting, anorexia and positive acetone, and direct rebound pain. The Pediatric Appendicitis Score is a similar system that identified eight predictive findings in children.[50] They include cough-induced tenderness in the right lower quadrant, anorexia, increased temperature, nausea and vomiting, tenderness over the right lower quadrant, increased white blood cell count, increased polymorphonuclear neutrophils, and migration of pain from the umbilicus. These scoring systems have been modified by many investigators and used to direct the selection of diagnostic studies, predict the need for surgery, and correlate with the occurrence of complications. These systems focus on the patient's physiologic response to the disease. What

TABLE 63.5

THE HINCHEY CLASSIFICATION FOR INTRAPERITONEAL CONTAMINATION IN DIVERTICULITIS

HINCHEY DIVERTICULITIS CLASSIFICATION		
INTRAPERITONEAL CONTAMINATION	**SCORE**	**INITIAL TREATMENT OPTION**
Paracolonic abscess	1	Antibiotics with observation
Pelvic abscess	2	CT-guided drainage/ antibiotics
Diffuse peritonitis	3	Surgery with/without diversion
Feculent peritonitis	4	Surgery with diversion

these systems achieve in diagnostic accuracy and specificity they lack in ease of use and a simplified stage or grade approach.

Scoring systems that describe the anatomic and pathologic lesion found in the appendix have been proposed by radiologists, surgeons, and pathologists. The most common surgical and pathologic construct is to describe grade 1 as acute appendicitis, grade 2 as gangrenous appendicitis, grade 3 as perforated appendicitis, and grade 4 as a periappendicular abscess.[51] Studies have cautioned about the poor interobserver variation in the grading of appendiceal perforation by surgeons.[52] Improved accuracy has led to an increased use of CT scanning for diagnosing appendicitis. The effort to correlate CT findings with the surgical and pathologic grading has led to as many as six grades where grade 0 is normal, grade 1 is probable appendicitis and progressing to grade 5 which is complicated appendicitis with abscess or inflammatory mass.[53]

What is clear from the preceding discussion is that a unified scoring system is needed. Some large clinical studies have been difficult to interpret because of the absence of such data.[54]

SUMMARY

Scoring systems must accurately describe the anatomic lesion, physiologic responses, and the patient factors that guide treatment and surgical decision making. In addition, they must prognostically stratify outcomes.

References

1. Nesssen SC, Cronk DR, Edens J, et al. US Army split forward surgical team management of mass casualty events in Afghanistan: surgeon performed triage results in excellent outcomes. *Am J Disaster Med.* 2009;4(6):321-329.
2. Wisner DH. History and current status of trauma scoring systems. *Arch Surg.* 1992;127 (3):352-356.
3. Teasdale G, Jennett B. Assessment of coma and impaired consciousness: a practical scale. *Lancet.* 1974;2(7872):81-84
4. Bullock RM, Chestnut R, Ghajar J, et al. Surgical management of acute subdural hematomas. *Neurosurgery.* 2006;58(3 Suppl):S16-S24.
5. Jennett B, Teasdale G, Galbraith S, et al. Severe head injuries in three countries. *J Neurol Neurosurg Psychiatry.* 1977;40(3):291-298.
6. Champion HR, Sacco WJ, Hannan SD, et al. Assessment of injury severity: the triage index. *Crit Care Med.* 1980;8(4):201-208
7. Champion HR, Sacco WJ, Carnazzo AJ, et al. Trauma score. *Crit Care Med.* 1981;9(9):672-676.
8. Champion HR, Sacco WJ, Copes WS, et al. A revision of the trauma score. *J Trauma.* 1989;29(5):623-629.
9. Dierking BH, Ramenofsky ML. The pediatric trauma score: an effective method of field triage. *JEMS.* 1988;13(5):70-72.
10. Sasser SM, Hunt RC, Sullivent EE, et al. Guidelines for field triage of injured patients: recommendations of the National Expert Panelon Field Triage. *MMWR Recomm Rep.* 2009;58(RR-1):1-35.
11. Committee on Medical Aspects of Automotive Safety: rating the severity of tissue damage. *JAMA.* 1971;215:277.
12. Association for the Advancement of Automotive Medicine. *Abbreviated Injury Scale 2005.* Barrington, IL: Association for the Advancement of Automotive Medicine; 2005.
13. Baker SP, O'Neill B, Haddon W, et al. The injury severity score: a method for describing patients with multiple injuries and evaluating emergency care. *J Trauma.* 1974;14(3):18196.
14. Linn S. The injury severity score—importance and uses. *Ann Epidemiol.* 1995;5(6):440-446.
15. Senkowski CK, McKenny MG. Trauma scoring systems: a review. *J Am Coll Surg.* 1999;189(5):491-503.
16. Kilgo PD, Meredith JW, Hensberry R, et al. A note on the disjointed nature of the injury severity score. *J Trauma.* 2004;57(3):479-485.
17. Osler T, Baker SP, Long W. A modification of the injury severity score that both improves accuracy and simplifies scoring. *J Trauma.* 1997;43(6);922-926.
18. Copes WS, Champion HS, Sacco WJ, et al. Progress in characterizing anatomic injuries. *J Trauma.* 1990;30 (10):1200-1207.
19. Gabbe GJ, Cameron PA, Wolfe R. TRISS: does it get better than this? *Acad Emerg Med.* 2004;11(2):181-186.
20. Champion HS, Copes WS, Sacco WJ, et al. The major trauma outcome study: establishing national norms for trauma care. *J Trauma.* 1990;30 (11):1356-1365.
21. Boyd CR, Tolson MA, and Copes WS. Evaluating trauma care: the TRISS method. Trauma Score and the Injury Severity Score. J Trauma. 1987 Apr;27:37022. Champion HR, Copes WS, Sacco WJ, et al. A new characterization of injury severity. *J Trauma.* 1990;30(5):539-545; discussion 545-546.
23. Champion HR, Copes WS, Sacco WJ, et al. Improved predictions from a severity characterization of trauma (ASCOT) over trauma and injury severity score (TRISS): results of an independent evaluation. *J Trauma.* 1996;40 (1):42-48;discussion 48-49.
24. Osler T, Rutledge R, Deis J, et al. ICISS: an international classification of disease-9 based injury severity score. *J Trauma.* 1996; 41(3):380-386; discussion 286-288.
25. Kilgo PD, Osler TM, Meredith W. The worst injury predicts mortality outcome the best: rethinking the role of multiple injuries in trauma outcome scoring. *J Trauma.* 2003;55(4):599-606; discussion 606-607.
26. Bone RC, Balk RA, et al. Definitions for sepsis and organ failure, and guidelines for the use of innovative therapies in sepsis. The ACCP/SCCM Consensus Conference Committee. American College of Chest Physicians/ Society of Critical Care Medicine. *Chest.* 1992;136(5 Suppl):e28.
27. Talmor M, et al. Relationship of systemic inflammatory response syndrome to organ dysfunction, length of stay, and mortality in critical surgical illness: effect of intensive care unit resuscitation. *Arch Surg.* 1999;134(1):81-87.
28. Knaus WA, et al. Apache II: A severity of disease classification system. *Crit Care Med.* 1985;13(10):818-829.
29. Knaus WA, Wagner DP, Draper EA, et al. The APACHE III prognostic system. Risk prediction of hospital mortality for critically ill hospitalized adults. *Chest.* 1991;100(6):1619-1636.
30. Hirota M, et al. Diagnostic criteria and severity assessment of acute cholecystitis: Tokyo Guidelines. *J Hepatobiliary Pancreat Surg.* 2007;14(1):78-82.
31. Lujan JA, et al. Laparoscopic cholecystectomy vs open cholecystectomy in the treatment of acute cholecystitis: a prospective study. *Arch Surg.* 1998;133(2):173-175.
32. McKay CJ, et al. Staging of acute pancreatitis. Is it important? *Surg Clin North Am.* 1999;79(4):733-743.
33. Ranson JH, et al. Prognostic signs and the role of operative management in acute pancreatitis. *Surg Gynecol Obstet.* 1974;139(1):69-81.
34. Larvin M, McMahon MJ. APACHE-II score for assessment and monitoring of acute pancreatitis. *Lancet.* 1989;2(8656):201-205.
35. Balthazar EJ, et al. Acute pancreatitis: prognostic value of CT. *Radiology.* 1985;156(3):767-772.
36. Ogawa M, et al. Development and use of a new staging system for severe acute pancreatitis based on a nationwide survey in Japan. *Pancreas.* 2002;25(4)325-330.
37. Pezzilli R, Zerbi A, et al. Practical guidelines for acute pancreatitis. *Pancreatology.* 2010;10(5):523-535.
38. Balthazar EJ, George W. Holmes lecture. CT of small-bowel obstruction. *Am J Roentgenol.* 1994;162(2):255-261.
39. Furukawa A, et al. Helical CT in the diagnosis of small bowel obstruction. *Radiographics.* 2001;21(2):341-355.
40. Jones K, Mangram AJ, et al. Can a computed tomography scoring system predict the need for surgery in small-bowel obstruction? *Am J Surg.* 2007;194(6):780-783; discussion 783-784.
41. Komatsu I, et al. Development of a simple model for predicting need for surgery in patients who initially undergo conservative management for adhesive small bowel obstruction. *Am J Surg.* 2010;200(2):215-223. Epub Jul 1, 2010.
42. Hall J, Hammerich K, et al. New paradigms in the management of diverticular disease. *Curr Probl Surg.* 2010;47(9):680-735.
43. Ambrosetti P, Robert JH, et al. Acute left colonic diverticulitis: a prospective analysis of 226 consecutive cases. *Surgery.* 1994;115(5):546-550.
44. Aydin HN, Remzi FH. Diverticulitis: when and how to operate? *Digest Liver Dis.* 2004;36:435-445.
45. Hinchey EJ, Schaal PG, et al. Treatment of perforated diverticular disease of the colon. *Adv Surg.* 1978;12:85-109.
46. Linder MM, Wacha H, et al. The Mannheim peritonitis index. An instrument for the intraoperative prognosis of peritonitis. *Chirurg.* 1987;58(2):84-92.
47. Senagore AJ, Warmuth AJ, et al. P-POSSUM, and Cr-POSSUM: implementation issues in a United States health care system for prediction of outcome for colon cancer resections. *Dis Colon Rectum.* 2004;47(9):1435-1441. Epub Jul 15, 2004.
48. Constantinides VA. Operative strategies for diverticular peritonitis. A decision analysis between primary resection and anastomosis versus Hartmann's procedures. *Ann Surg.* 2007;245(1):94-103.
49. Alvarado A. A practical score for the early diagnosis of acute appendicitis. *Ann Emerg Med.* 1986;15(5):557-564.
50. Samuel M. Pediatric appendicitis score. *J Pediatr Surg.* 2002;37(6):877-881.
51. Ditillo MF, et al. Is it safe to delay appendectomy in adults with acute appendicitis? *Ann Surg.* 2006;244(5):656-660.
52. Ponsky TA, Hafi M, et al. Interobserver variation in the assessment of appendiceal perforation. *J Laparoendosc Adv Surg Tech A.* 2009;19(Suppl 1):S15-S18.
53. Raptopoulos V, Katsou G, et al. Acute appendicitis: effect of increased use of CT on selecting patient earlier. *Radiology.* 2003;226(2):521-526.
54. Ingraham AM, Cohen ME, et al. Comparison of outcomes after laparoscopic versus open appendectomy for acute appendicitis at 222 ACS NSQIP hospitals. *Surgery.* 2010;148(4):625-635; discussion 635-637. Epub Aug 24, 2004.

CHAPTER 64 ■ PROCEDURES

AMY J. GOLDBERG AND ABHIJIT S. PATHAK

OPEN TRACHEOSTOMY

Indications

1. Obstruction at or above the larynx secondary to
   a. tumor
   b. edema
   c. trauma/fracture
   d. foreign body
   e. burns
   f. severe pharyngeal or neck infection
2. Chronic/long-term respiratory issues
   a. Coma after head injury, neurosurgery
   b. Paralysis such as spinal cord injury
   c. Patients requiring prolonged ventilatory support
3. Anticipated edema/swelling in patients undergoing major operative procedures of the
   a. oropharynx
   b. mandible
   c. larynx

Preoperative Preparation

Chest x-ray and physical examination of the neck to ensure adequate external landmarks and plan for choice of tracheostomy tube size are paramount, in particular tracheostomy tube length and whether a distal extension or proximal extension tracheostomy tube may be needed. Patients with previous tracheostomy may prove to be challenging. Often, trauma patients may have a concomitant cervical spine injury or a cervical collar in place. This is important to know since the patient's neck cannot be extended and the procedure must be performed in the neutral position.

Anesthesia

Many of the patients an acute care surgeon operates on will have an existing endotracheal tube and general anesthesia. In the emergent setting, local anesthesia can be used if the clinical situation allows.

Positioning

The patient is placed in the supine position with both arms tucked to the sides. A roll (we use a tightly rolled blanket) is placed under the shoulders to allow extension of the neck if there is no contraindication (Fig. 64.1). Patients with a cervical collar (cervical spine injury or in whom the cervical spine has not been cleared) require maintenance of the neutral position, and this can be accomplished with immobilization of the patient's head and neck with sandbags on either side of the head with the anterior portion of the collar removed to gain access to the neck.

Operative Preparation

Sterile field is prepared in the usual manner and includes the anterior neck, chin, and upper chest.

Procedure

A vertical incision from just above the cricoid cartilage or transverse incision a fingerbreadth cephalad to the sternal notch is made in the skin and extended 3 cm. The skin and subcutaneous tissues are incised down to expose the strap muscles, and the median raphe of the strap muscles is identified and incised vertically (Fig. 64.2). The strap muscles are then retracted laterally to expose the isthmus of the thyroid gland. We generally divide the isthmus with electrocautery followed by suture ligation. This exposes the underlying airway. The cricoid cartilage is identified and a tracheotomy is performed through the second or third tracheal ring. This is accomplished utilizing a no. 11 or 15 scalpel to excise the anterior portion of the tracheal cartilage. Care must be taken to not extend the incision too deeply to avoid injury to the posterior wall of the trachea and esophagus. Communication between the surgeon and the anesthesiologist or person managing the airway is critical during the actual tracheotomy, withdrawal of the endotracheal tube, and insertion of the tracheostomy tube. Once the anterior portion of the tracheal cartilage is incised, the endotracheal tube is withdrawn under direct vision so the distal tip is just visible through the tracheotomy. The tracheotomy may then be dilated utilizing a tracheal dilator. The tracheostomy tube is then inserted into the trachea, the obturator removed, the balloon inflated, and the inner cannula placed and connected to the anesthesia machine to ensure end-tidal CO_2 and ventilation (Fig. 64.3). The tracheostomy tube is then secured to the skin with 2–0 nylon sutures, and a dressing may be placed under the flange of the tube. The incision usually does not need to be reapproximated.

Postoperative Care

A chest x-ray is obtained postoperatively to ensure adequate placement and to ensure that the pleura had not been violated with development of a subsequent pneumothorax. A duplicate tube should be at the patient's bedside at all times. The inner cannula should be removed and cleaned frequently to prevent buildup of secretions.

BEDSIDE TRACHEOSTOMY

A tracheostomy can be performed at the patient's bedside in the intensive care unit (ICU) via an open technique as stated above or via a semiopen or percutaneous method. The surgeon must ensure that the same equipment, lighting, monitoring, and personnel are present as in the OR. Lighting must be adequate, and electrocautery is necessary. Within the past 10–20 years,

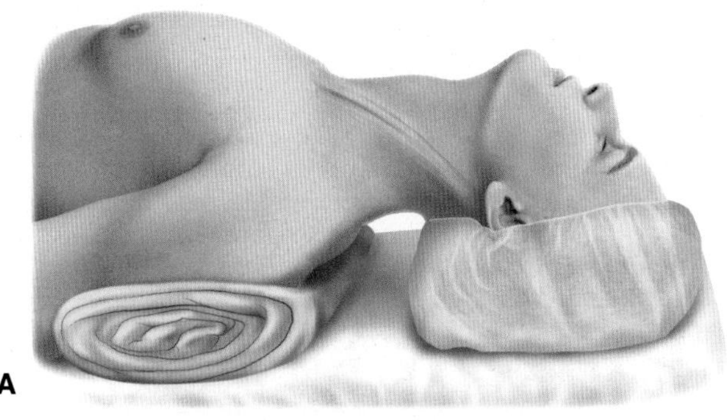

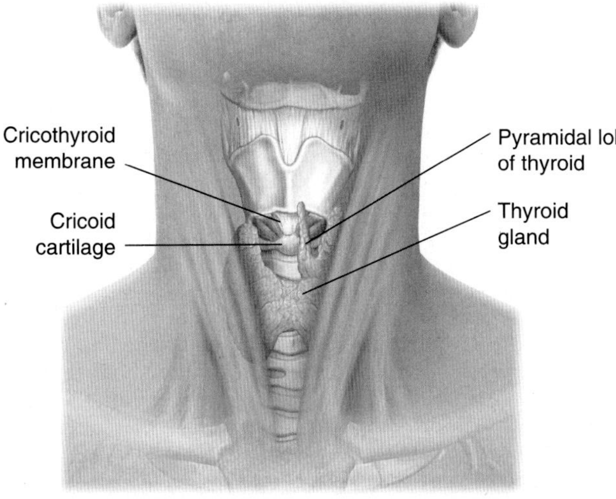

FIGURE 64.1. Patient positioning.

bedside percutaneous tracheostomy has gained popularity. We utilize the Seldinger-based blunt dilation approach (Blue Rhino Percutaneous Tracheostomy Introducer Kit, Cook Critical Care). A number of these kits are available on the market. When initiating a percutaneous tracheostomy program in your institution, patient selection is critical. Exclude patients with coagulopathy, high oxygen requirements, previous tracheostomy, morbid obesity, and unstable cervical spine injuries or an inability to hyperextend the neck.

The proper equipment must be available to ensure a successful procedure and prevent devastating complications. When beginning to utilize the percutaneous method, both percutaneous tracheostomy kit and surgical instruments should be present at the bedside. Again, adequate light is critical, and electrocautery may be beneficial. The appropriate personnel should also be present. The surgeon and his/her assistant perform the procedure; the anesthesiologist or second surgical assistant monitors the airway and performs the bronchoscopy. We recommend routine use of the bronchoscope for percutaneous tracheostomy. A nurse is necessary to assist in any parts of the procedure from monitoring vital signs to the administration of sedation (propofol and narcotic).

The patient is positioned, prepped, and draped as discussed above. The bronchoscope is passed into the endotracheal tube and positioned to adequately visualize the trachea. Local anesthetic may be infiltrated in the subcutaneous tissues prior to making a 1-cm incision over the second and third tracheal ring. Using a hemostat, the tissues are bluntly dissected to adequately palpate the second tracheal ring. Under bronchoscopic guidance, the trachea is entered percutaneously between the second and third rings. Upon entry into the airway, air bubbles are seen in the fluid-filled syringe, and the bronchoscope easily visualizes the needle. Then, in a Seldinger fashion, a wire is passed into the needle, and the needle is withdrawn (Fig. 64.4A). The track is then dilated over the wire, all under bronchoscopic visualization

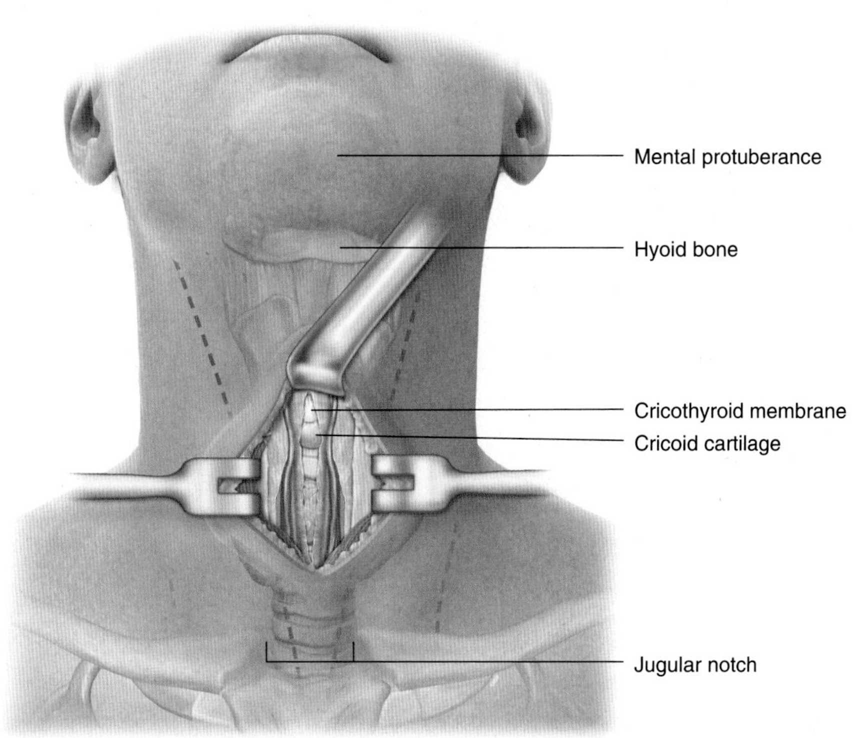

FIGURE 64.2. Dissection to the trachea.

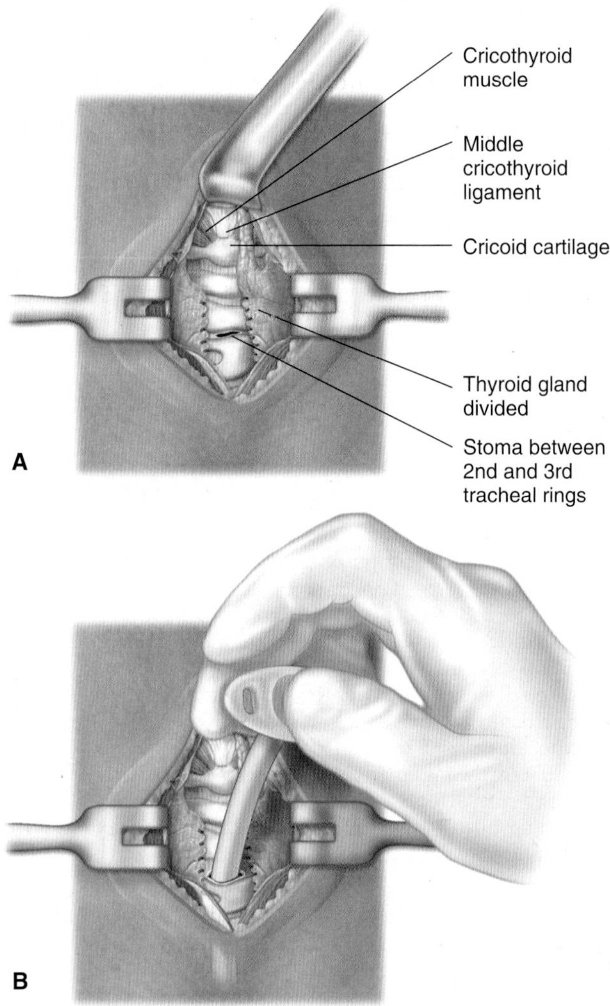

FIGURE 64.3. Exposure of the trachea and insertion of tracheostomy tube.

(Fig. 64.4B,C). The endotracheal tube is then slowly withdrawn to just above the tracheotomy, and the tracheostomy tube is placed in appropriate position (Fig. 64.4D). An end-tidal CO_2 monitor should be used to reconfirm placement.

CRICOTHYROIDOTOMY

Indications

A cricothyroidotomy is performed when an emergent airway is needed with no time to prepare for routine tracheostomy.

Preoperative Preparation

A sterile field should be attempted; however, the emergent nature of the procedure may not allow this.

Anesthesia

Local anesthesia is preferred if possible.

Positioning

Same as for tracheostomy; however, the usual emergent nature of the procedure precludes any elaborate methods for positioning. Remember that a cricothyroidotomy is performed by palpation, not visualization. If you are right-handed, you should be standing on the patient's right. The thyroid cartilage should be held between the thumb and third finger of your right hand and your index finger essentially in the cricothyroid membrane until you have incised the membrane. This technique ensures that landmarks are not lost resulting in an ill-placed incision.

Procedure

A vertical incision similar for tracheostomy is made; however, the incision is extended cranially to the mid-thyroid cartilage. It is important to avoid the anterior jugular veins that are just off the midline. Since the procedure is often performed emergently with minimal instruments and lighting, palpation of landmarks is key. The skin and subcutaneous tissue over the cricothyroid membrane is incised in a vertical fashion. A transverse incision in the cricothyroid membrane is created with a scalpel and the cricothyroidotomy may be dilated with the end of the scalpel blade or a curved hemostat (Fig. 64.5). Dilate transversely, not longitudinally. Longitudinal incision or dilatation may fracture the cricoid cartilage. Either a no. 7 endotracheal tube or no. 7 tracheostomy tube can be used in an adult male; at times a no. 6 may be necessary. A no. 6 or even a no. 5 tube may be required in a small female. Do not attempt to force too large a tube through the cricothyroid membrane as this may also fracture the cricoid cartilage. We prefer placement of an endotracheal tube, which makes subsequent conversion to formal tracheostomy easier. When utilizing an endotracheal tube, care must be taken not to insert the tube too deeply. Usually, insertion to just after disappearance of the balloon is adequate. The endotracheal tube should be properly secured the skin. If a tracheostomy tube is used, it is secured as noted above.

Postoperative Care

If an endotracheal tube is utilized, care must be taken to prevent dislodgement of the airway as well as malpositioning (usually down the right mainstem bronchus). A cricothyroidotomy is usually converted to formal tracheostomy.

DIAGNOSTIC PERITONEAL LAVAGE

Indications

In 1965, Root described the use of diagnostic peritoneal lavage (DPL) for the evaluation of the blunt trauma patient. Much has changed in the past 45 years in the care of trauma patients. Computed tomography (CT) and focused abdominal sonography for trauma (FAST) have dominated the workup of both the blunt and penetrating trauma patient. DPL remains a useful diagnostic tool. Its major disadvantages are that it is invasive and nonspecific. A positive DPL means the patient has hemoperitoneum (generally) with no information about organ injury. Thus, many laparotomies based on positive DPL in the past were nontherapeutic. In the trauma population, DPL is currently reserved for the unstable blunt trauma patient with an equivocal FAST exam. DPL is 98%

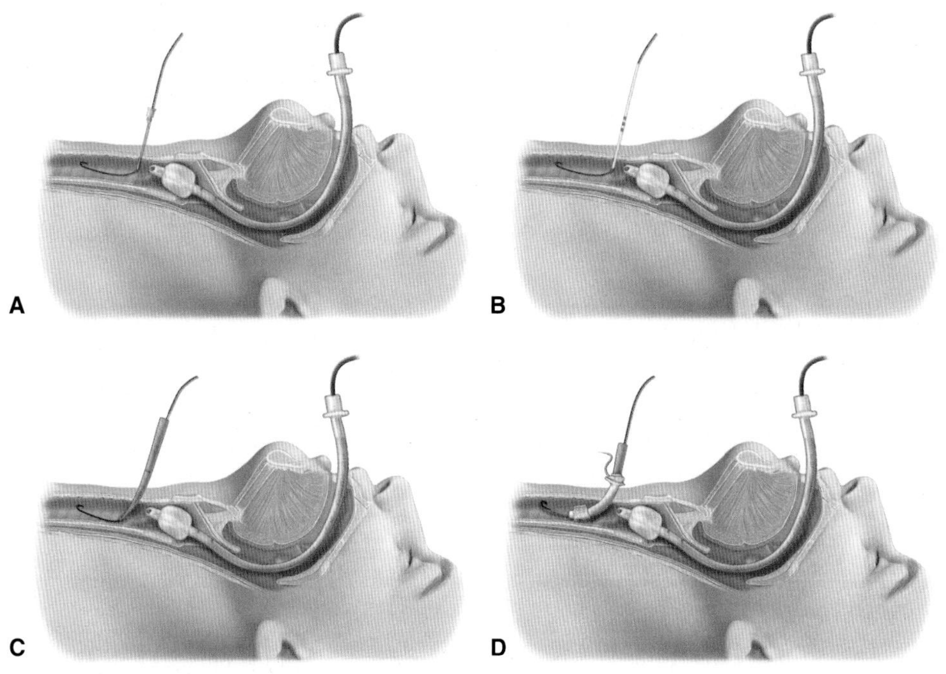

FIGURE 64.4. Percutaneous dilatational tracheostomy.

sensitive for intraperitoneal bleeding. This becomes useful when deciding where to proceed from the trauma bay, CT scan/angiography, or the operating room. DPL is also helpful in diagnosis of hollow viscus injury. Many also use DPL in the penetrating trauma patient with a positive local wound exploration.

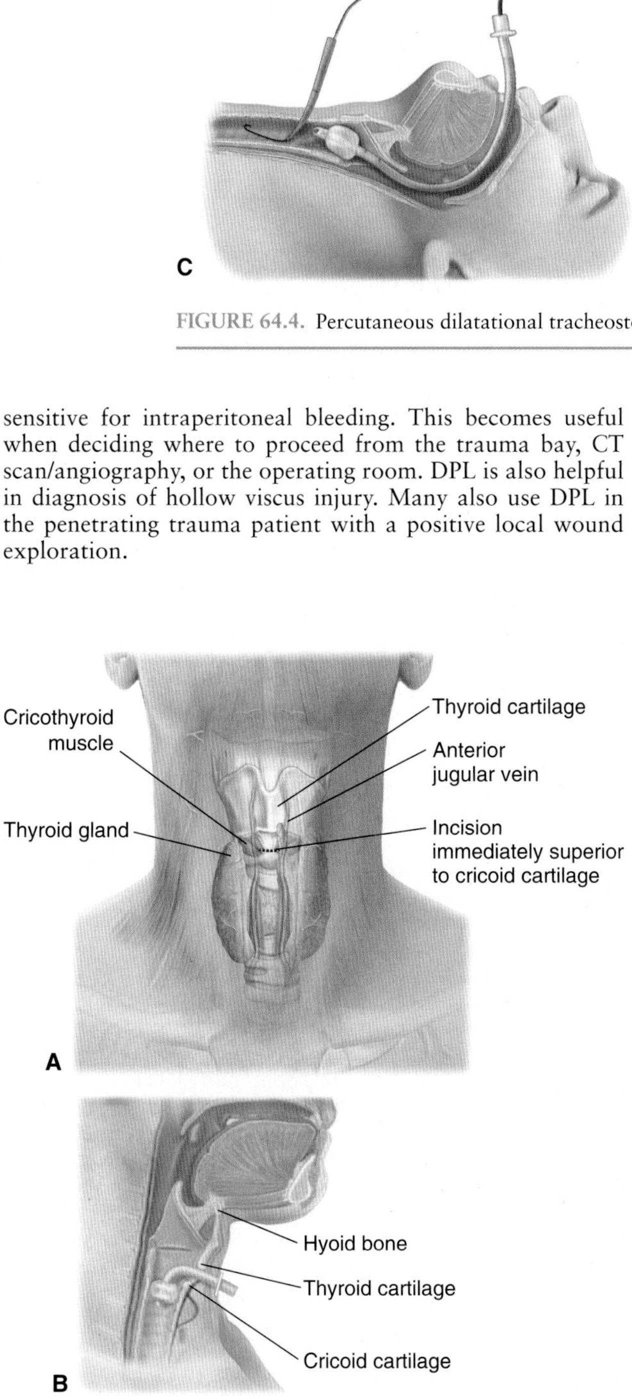

Cricothyroid muscle
Thyroid gland
Thyroid cartilage
Anterior jugular vein
Incision immediately superior to cricoid cartilage
A
Hyoid bone
Thyroid cartilage
Cricoid cartilage
B

FIGURE 64.5. Cricothyroidotomy.

DPL can also be useful in the ICU. Should the trauma patient become hemodynamically unstable several hours after admission, DPL can be performed to assess bleeding in the peritoneal cavity. Although not commonly considered, DPL can be utilized to evaluate the acute care surgery patient who may be too unstable to be transported to CT scan. A patient with dead bowel will often have a serosanguineous fluid or a positive WBC count.

Preoperative Preparation and Positioning

Prior to starting a DPL, the patient must have a Foley catheter and nasogastric tube placed. This will decrease the likelihood of puncturing these structures while performing the procedure. The patient is placed flat and supine on the trauma bay stretcher and his pulse, blood pressure, and ECG are monitored.

Anesthesia

If the patient's blood pressure permits, a small dose of intravenous narcotic can be administered. Otherwise, the procedure can be performed with local anesthesia, 1% lidocaine with epinephrine.

Operative Preparation

DPL can be performed percutaneously or utilizing the open technique. Whichever is preferred, prior to beginning the procedure, it is critical to have all the appropriate equipment necessary.

Procedure

Unless the patient is pregnant or has a pelvic fracture, the DPL should be performed in the infraumbilical location.

Figure 64.6 describes the insertion site choices. Prepackaged percutaneous DPL kits are available and should be used for the percutaneous approach. The periumbilical region is prepped and draped. After local anesthesia is infiltrated a very small incision is made in the skin inferior to the umbilicus. The abdominal wall is grasped and the blunt needle is passed through the fascia and peritoneum. This usually feels like two "pops." Saline can be placed in the hub of the needle. If it easily drains, the needle is in the peritoneal cavity. Using the Seldinger technique, the wire then is passed through the needle into the peritoneal cavity. The needle is withdrawn, as the wire remains in place. A dilator is passed over the wire and removed, and lastly, the catheter is passed over the wire, and the wire is removed.

Aspiration of 10 mL of blood or food or bowel contents is positive. If neither is returned, 1 L of warm saline is instilled into the peritoneal cavity. The saline is allowed to mix with the contents of the peritoneal cavity and then drained. Be sure that some fluid remains in the IV bag to allow for adequate drainage from the peritoneum. The fluid is then sent for RBC, WBC, and Gram stain.

A positive DPL is >100,000 red cells per cubic millimeter, 500 white cells per cubic millimeter, or the presence of bacteria on Gram stain.

After the fluid has been removed, the catheter is withdrawn. A small Steri-Strip can be placed over the incision. In a hemodynamically marginal patient, the catheter may be sewn in place and the DPL repeated.

Postoperative Care

Postoperatively, the incision should be inspected daily for the presence of infection.

TUBE THORACOSTOMY

Indications

1. Pneumothorax
2. Hemothorax
3. Hemopneumothorax
4. Pleural effusion
5. Hydrothorax
6. Empyema
7. Penetrating chest wall injury requiring positive pressure ventilation
8. Air transport of patients who are at risk for pneumothorax

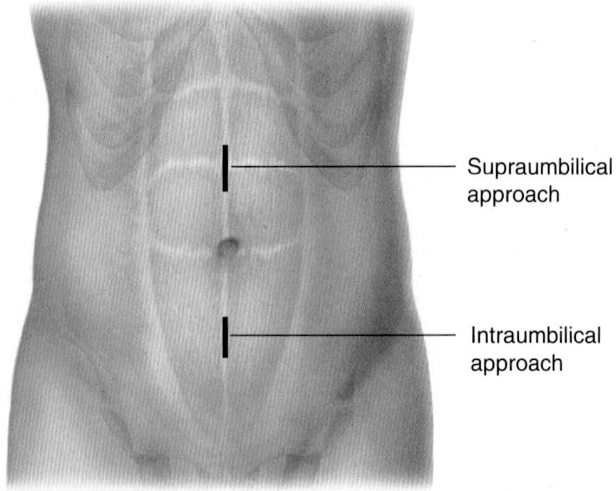

FIGURE 64.6. DPL insertion choices.

Anesthesia

Systemic analgesia such as intravenous narcotic is used in conscious patients, and sedation can be considered as well. Local anesthesia is utilized at the insertion site.

Positioning

The patient is placed in the supine position, and the ipsilateral upper extremity is abducted, and externally rotated so it is positioned above the patient's head.

Operative Preparation

For adult trauma patients undergoing chest tube placement, we usually utilize a 32–36 French chest tube, which is large enough to adequately drain a hemothorax. Consideration for a smaller caliber tube should be given for drainage of a pneumothorax or pleural effusion. Empyemas will usually require a larger caliber tube for effective drainage. The drainage system for the chest tube should be connected to suction, and the appearance of bubbles in the water chamber indicates that the device is functioning properly. A sterile field is prepared in the usual manner centered on the chest tube insertion site located in the anterior axillary line at nipple level in males and inframammary crease in females. This should correspond to the fourth or fifth intercostal space. After the sterile field is prepped, the distance between the clavicle and the incision site is measured with the chest tube. This estimates how far the tube should be inserted. This is accomplished by noting the marking on the chest tube (i.e., 12 cm from proximal end). The last hole on the chest tube must be placed sufficiently deeply in the patient's thoracic cavity. Remember that you can pull back a chest tube if placed too deeply. You cannot advance a chest tube that is too shallow on CXR as this is now contaminated externally.

Procedure

We perform insertion of a chest tube over the rib at the fifth intercostal space without creation of a subcutaneous tunnel. This is the simplest, most direct method for rapid insertion and decompression of the chest. Local anesthesia is injected in the skin and subcutaneous tissues initially. Next, a no. 10 scalpel is used to create transverse incision directly over the rib measuring approximately 2 cm. This is carried down through the subcutaneous tissues. At this point more local anesthesia is injected into the deeper tissues including the intercostal muscles, periosteum of the rib, and the parietal pleura. Next, a Kelly clamp is used to bluntly dissect the subcutaneous tissue down to the intercostal muscle. Figure 64.7 outlines placement of a chest tube. The tract is palpated with a finger to ensure that the tract extends over the top of the rib. Further blunt dissection by repeated opening and closing of the Kelly clamp along with gentle pressure is continued. Once the intercostal space is palpated, more local anesthetic can be injected into the muscle and parietal pleura. The closed Kelly clamp is then used to puncture the intercostal muscles and parietal pleura, being careful to stay along the superior margin of the rib. This maneuver requires some force and should be controlled so the Kelly clamp does not enter too far into the pleural space and injure the underlying viscera. The Kelly clamp is then opened while only the tip is in the pleural space, thereby enlarging the dissected tract. A finger is then inserted into the pleural space and rotated to ensure there are no adhesions, and if present, they can be gently broken. If adhesions are present and cannot be broken, then placement under imaging or placement at a different site should be considered if the clinical situation allows. Next the proximal end of the chest tube is grasped with a Kelly clamp such that the clamp is parallel to the tube. This allows the Kelly clamp to introduce the chest tube into the pleural cavity. Another Kelly clamp is used to clamp the distal end of the chest tube if the patient is spontaneously breathing. The Kelly clamp grasped to the proximal end of the chest tube is inserted into the tract and into the pleural cavity and directed posteriorly and superiorly, making sure that all the side holes on the chest tube are within the thoracic cavity. This is accomplished by knowing the predetermined length as noted above. The Kelly clamp is removed while the chest tube is held stationary. Rotating the chest tube 360 degrees ensures that the tube is in proper position and not within the lung parenchyma or fissure or caught in adhesions. The chest tube is then connected to the drainage system and the distal Kelly clamp removed. The chest tube is then secured to the drainage system tubing with tape and to the skin with 0-silk suture. Either a purse string or simple suture can be used, making sure to wrap the suture around the chest tube several times. The insertion site and sutures are sealed with a petrolatum gauze and an occlusive dressing placed. We utilize a mesentery fold of tape securing the chest tube to the lower thoracic wall.

Postoperative Care

A chest x-ray is obtained to ensure adequate positioning of the tube and to ensure resolution of chest pathology.

PERCUTANEOUS GASTROSTOMY TUBE

Indications

1. Enteral access for feeding
   a. Dysphagia
   b. Inability to take PO secondary to
      i. Trauma, cancer, or recent surgery of the gastrointestinal (GI) tract or respiratory tract
      ii. Prolonged ventilation
2. GI tract decompression—usually for patients with abdominal malignancies causing gastric outlet obstruction, small bowel obstruction, or ileus.

Contraindications

1. Absolute
   a. Coagulopathy or thrombocytopenia
   b. Ascites
   c. Intra-abdominal sepsis
   d. Severe gastroparesis
   e. Abdominal wall infection at site of insertion
2. Relative
   a. Oropharyngeal/esophageal malignancy
   b. Hepatomegaly
   c. Splenomegaly
   d. Gastric varices
   e. Previous abdominal surgery
   f. Ventral hernia
   g. Peritoneal dialysis
   h. History of partial gastrectomy

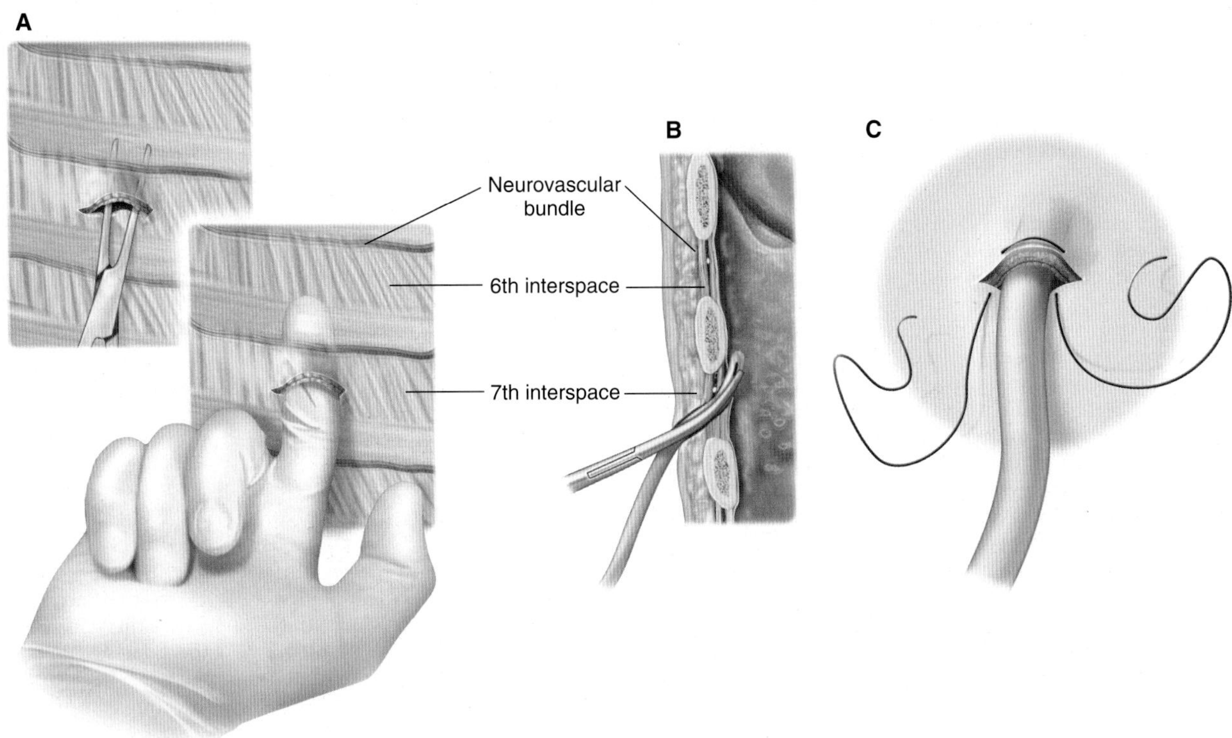

FIGURE 64.7. Tube thoracostomy insertion.

Anesthesia

The procedure can be performed with moderate to deep sedation with local anesthesia at the site of placement. It can also be performed under general anesthesia, and this is the usual technique in patients undergoing concomitant tracheostomy.

Positioning

The patient is placed in the supine position with the head of the bed elevated to about 30 degrees to prevent aspiration especially if performed with sedation and local anesthesia.

Operative Preparation

The patient should be NPO for at least 8 hours prior to the procedure. Preoperative antibiotics such as a first-generation cephalosporin should be infused prior to skin incision to prevent infection at the insertion site. An alternate antibiotic such as clindamycin to cover gram-positive organisms in penicillin-allergic patients is given. The sterile field should be prepared in the usual manner and should include the upper abdomen/lower chest.

Procedure

The procedure is performed utilizing a two-surgeon team with one surgeon performing the endoscopy and the other surgeon managing the abdominal wall portion of the procedure. An esophagogastroduodenoscopy is performed using the standard technique. When performing a percutaneous endoscopic gastrostomy (PEG) tube in conjunction with a tracheostomy, we find that PEG tube placement performed prior to the tracheostomy is technically easier since the existing endotracheal tube assists in passage of the endoscope. During the endoscopy, the stomach is inspected and any gastric contents suctioned. Any gastric outlet or duodenal obstruction is excluded (if using tube for feeding) as is any evidence of gastritis or ulcer. Next, the stomach is insufflated using the air channel of the endoscope. The OR lights are dimmed, and the abdominal wall is transilluminated using the endoscope light set at maximum intensity (many light sources have a transilluminate setting). The ideal location for placement of the PEG tube is two fingerbreadths below the left costal margin and two fingerbreadths to the left of the midline. Finger pressure is applied at this location over the previously transilluminated region, and the anterior stomach is visualized endoscopically. If transillumination is not achieved but finger pressure is visualized, one pass at insertion of the catheter may be attempted. If both are not achieved, then a decision to aborting the procedure should be taken. As finger pressure is applied and visualized endoscopically, location within the stomach is important since the tube should not be placed too close to the pylorus. The site on the abdominal wall is then anesthetized using lidocaine. Next, the catheter-over-the needle is then passed through the abdominal wall using a rapid insertion technique to avoid having the stomach fall away form the abdominal wall. The endoscopist visualizes the placement of the needle while continuously insufflating air to ensure gastric distension and apposition of the stomach to the abdominal wall. The endoscope snare is inserted through the endoscope at this time, and the needle is removed, leaving the catheter within the stomach. A looped guidewire is then inserted through the catheter and into the stomach. The endoscopist then snares the guidewire and pulls the entire endoscope with the snare/guidewire out of the mouth. The catheter is then removed by threading it back over the guidewire. At this time, a scalpel is used to make a horizontal incision measuring 0.5–1 cm in width at the guidewire insertion site on the abdominal wall, being careful not to cut the guidewire. The PEG tube is then secured to the looped end of the guidewire exiting the mouth. This is performed by passing the looped end of the guidewire through the loop of the PEG tube and then passing the PEG tube disk through the guidewire loop and pulling the entire tube through it. The PEG tube is then lubricated, and the person at the abdominal wall then pulls the guidewire so the entire PEG tube goes through the mouth, esophagus, and stomach and exits at the incision site. Meanwhile, the endoscopist reinserts the endoscope and follows the PEG tube as it is placed. The internal disk should be snug against the gastric mucosa without undue tension, and the site is inspected for bleeding. The guidewire is then cut at the tapered end of the PEG tube, and the external flange or bumper is then passed over the external portion of the PEG tube so that it sits on the abdominal wall without tension. The level of the PEG tube at the skin should be noted and recorded in the operative note. The endoscope is then withdrawn after desufflation of the stomach. The external portion of the PEG tube is then cut, and the supplied adapter is secured and the tube placed to gravity drainage or capped. The flange is secured to the skin using 2–0 nylon suture.

Postoperative Care

A drain sponge or split gauze is used as a dressing over the flange. We typically begin tube feeds on POD no. 1. The PEG tube insertion site should be cleaned daily.

FASCIOTOMY

Indications

1. Definitive compartment syndrome
2. High-risk lower extremity vascular injury
   a. Combined arterial and venous injury
   b. Associated bone fracture or massive soft tissue destruction
   c. Prolonged ischemia (>4–6 hours) prior to revascularization
   d. Treatment of major artery or vein injury by ligation

Positioning

The patient is in the supine position with both lower extremities exposed.

Operative Preparation

Circumferential sterile field preparation of the affected lower extremity.

Procedure

The double-incision technique is a safer, more effective, and preferred approach since the overlying skin can prevent decompression despite release of the underlying fascia.

There are four compartments in the lower leg (distal to knee); when performing a fasciotomy, all four compartments must be decompressed.

The anterior and lateral compartments are decompressed through one incision on the lateral aspect of the leg. A 15- to 20-cm incision that is centered over the fibula is created and taken down through the subcutaneous tissues. A flap needs to be created anteriorly (transversely) to expose the intermuscular septum. A nick in the anterior compartment fascia is performed midway between the septum and the tibia. Metzenbaum scissors are used to perform a longitudinal fasciotomy proximally and distally staying parallel to the septum. The lateral compartment is then released in the same manner by staying posterior to the intermuscular septum, and the longitudinal fasciotomy is carried out proximally, being careful not to extend it beyond the fibular head since the peroneal nerve courses around it. Likewise, the fasciotomy is carried out distally aiming for the lateral malleolus to avoid injury to the peroneal nerve that will run more anteriorly.

The medial incision is made two fingerbreadths posterior to the posterior medial margin of the tibia and is extended 15–20 cm. The subcutaneous tissue is incised and care taken to avoid the saphenous vein. This will expose the superficial posterior compartment fascia, a nick is made, and a longitudinal fasciotomy is carried out proximally and distally with Metzenbaum scissors. To expose the deep posterior compartment, the superficial posterior compartment muscles need to be dissected free of the tibia. This will expose the deep posterior compartment, which can then be released in the same manner. Bleeding is controlled with electrocautery or sutures. The two wounds are then dressed with Xeroform gauze. Alternatively, some surgeons "shoelace" the incision with vessel loops secured to the wound edges with staples and apply gentle progressive traction over several days to facilitate closure.

Postoperative Care

The fasciotomy sites are inspected daily; once the swelling has subsided, primary closure can be undertaken. If swelling continues, a vacuum assist closure device can be used to facilitate closure and promote granulation tissue if skin grafting seems necessary.

INFERIOR VENA CAVA FILTER

Indications

Inferior vena cava (IVC) filters are placed to decrease the risk of pulmonary embolism from a deep vein thrombus originating in the pelvic or lower extremity veins. IVC filters should be placed in patients who have a contraindication to anticoagulation, prophylactically in high-risk patients, and in patients who develop recurrent pulmonary emboli on therapeutic anticoagulation.

Contraindications to anticoagulation can include patients with recent trauma or surgery, recent history of a GI bleed or development of a GI bleed while on anticoagulation, or patients with intracranial bleed. Prophylactic filters may be placed in patients who are at high risk for development of a deep vein thrombosis or pulmonary embolus. In the trauma patient population, this includes patients with severe head injury, spinal cord injuries with neurologic deficits, and significant long bone and pelvic fractures.

Procedure

IVC filters can be placed at the bedside, decreasing any risks from the transport of critically ill patients from the ICUs to the operating room or interventional suite. Patients should have a venous duplex of both common femoral veins to assess patency. Only on rare occasions is an IVC filter placed from the right internal jugular vein. Bedside fluoroscopy or ultrasonography is necessary to ensure patency of the IVC, measure its diameter, and evaluate for a duplicated IVC. The right common femoral vein is accessed via a percutaneous approach, and utilizing the Seldinger approach, the guidewire is passed into the IVC, the sheath is passed over the wire, and the appropriately sized filter is deployed. The filter should be placed below the level of the right renal vein.

Retrievable

Within the last several years, retrievable filters have gained popularity. These filters are ideal for patients who are temporarily at high risk for pulmonary embolism and deep vein thrombosis or those who later become candidates for anticoagulation. The benefit of the retrievable filter is to decrease the complications from filter placement, such as migration and filter or caval thrombosis.

Note: Page numbers in *italics* indicate figures; those followed by t indicate tables.

K

L

M

T

U

V

W

Z